T0290631

CANINE and FELINE INFECTIOUS DISEASES

JANE E. SYKES, BVSc, PhD, DACVIM
Professor
Department of Medicine and Epidemiology
University of California
Davis, California

ELSEVIER

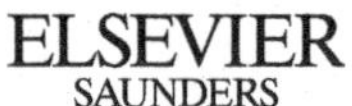

3251 Riverport Lane
St. Louis, Missouri 63043

CANINE AND FELINE INFECTIOUS DISEASES ISBN: 978-1-4377-0795-3

Library of Congress Cataloging-in-Publication Data
Sykes, Jane E.
Canine and feline infectious diseases / Jane E. Sykes.
p. ; cm.
Includes bibliographical references and index.
ISBN 978-1-4377-0795-3 (hard back)
I. Title.
[DNLM: 1. Communicable Diseases--veterinary. 2. Cat Diseases. 3. Dog Diseases. SF 781]
SF781
636.089'69--dc23 2013010391

Vice President and Publisher: Linda Duncan
Content Strategy Director: Penny Rudolph
Content Development Specialist: Brandi Graham
Publishing Services Manager: Catherine Jackson
Senior Project Manager: Mary Pohlman
Designer: Paula Catalano

Printed in the United States of America

Last digit is the print number: 9 8 7

Contributors

Gad Baneth, DVM, PhD, DECVCP
Professor of Veterinary Medicine
The Robert H. Smith Faculty of Agriculture, Food and Environment
Koret School of Veterinary Medicine
The Hebrew University of Jerusalem
Rehovot, Israel
Leishmaniosis

Stephen C. Barr, BVSc, MVS, PhD, DACVIM
Professor of Medicine
Chief, Section of Small Animal Medicine
College of Veterinary Medicine
Cornell University
Ithaca, New York
Trypanosomiasis

Malcolm Bennett, BVSc, PhD, MRCVS, FRCPath
Professor of Veterinary Pathology, Infection, and Global Health
Department of Veterinary Pathology
University of Liverpool
Liverpool, United Kingdom
Feline Poxvirus Infections

Adam J. Birkenheuer, DVM, DACVIM, PhD
Associate Professor
Department of Clinical Sciences
College of Veterinary Medicine
North Carolina University
Raleigh, North Carolina
Babesiosis

Edward B. Breitschwerdt, DVM, DACVIM
Professor of Medicine and Infectious Diseases
Department of Clinical Sciences
College of Veterinary Medicine
North Carolina State University
Raleigh, North Carolina
Rocky Mountain Spotted Fever

Bruno B. Chomel, DVM, PhD
Professor
Population Health & Reproduction
University of California
Davis, California
Rabies
Bartonellosis
Yersinia pestis (Plague) and Other Yersinioses
Tularemia

Leah A. Cohn, DVM, PhD, DACVIM
Professor, Small Animal Internal Medicine
Department of Veterinary Medicine and Surgery
College of Veterinary Medicine
University of Missouri
Columbia, Missouri
Cytauxzoonosis

Sarah D. Cramer, DVM, DACVP
Cancer Research Training Fellow
Comparative Biomedical Scientist Training Program
National Cancer Institute
National Institutes of Health
Bethesda, Maryland
Pseudorabies

Autumn P. Davidson, DVM, MS, DACVIM
Clinical Professor
Department of Medicine and Epidemiology
School of Veterinary Medicine
University of California
Davis, California;
Staff Internist
Internal Medicine/Reproduction
PetCare Veterinary Hospital
Santa Rosa, California
Canine Herpesvirus Infection
Canine Brucellosis

Steven Epstein, DVM, DACVECC
Assistant Professor of Clinical Small Animal Emergency and Critical Care
Department of Veterinary Surgical and Radiological Sciences
School of Veterinary Medicine
University of California
Davis, California
Infections of the Cardiovascular System

Janet E. Foley, DVM, PhD
Professor
Department of Veterinary Medicine and Epidemiology
School of Veterinary Medicine
University of California
Davis, California
Anaplasmosis

Craig E. Greene, DVM, MS, DACVIM
Professor Emeritus and Josiah Meigs Distinguished Teaching Professor
Departments of Infectious Diseases and Small Animal Medicine
College of Veterinary Medicine
The University of Georgia
Athens, Georgia
Bacterial Meningitis

Amy M. Grooters, DVM, DACVIM
Professor, Companion Animal Medicine
Department of Veterinary Clinical Sciences
School of Veterinary Medicine
Louisiana State University
Baton Rouge, Louisiana
Miscellaneous Fungal Diseases
Pythiosis, Lagenidiosis, and Zygomycosis

Danièlle A. Gunn-Moore, BSc, BVM&S, PhD, MACVSc, MRCVS, RCVS
Professor of Feline Medicine
Head of Companion Animal Sciences
Royal (Dick) School of Veterinary Studies
The University of Edinburgh
Easter Bush, Midlothian, United Kingdom
Mycobacterial Infections

Katrin Hartmann, Dr.med.vet, DMVH, DECVIM-CA
Professor
Center of Clinical Veterinary Sciences
Clinic of Small Animal Medicine
Ludwig-Maximilians-Universität, München
Munich, Germany
Feline Leukemia Virus Infection

Amy S. Kapatkin, DVM, MS
Associate Professor of Orthopedic Surgery
Department of Surgical and Radiological Sciences
School of Veterinary Medicine
University of California
Davis, California
Osteomyelitis, Discospondylitis, and Infectious Arthritis

Linda Kidd, DVM, PhD, DACVIM
Assistant Professor
Department of Small Animal Internal Medicine
College of Veterinary Medicine
Western University of Health Sciences
Pomona, California
Rocky Mountain Spotted Fever

Michael R. Lappin, DVM, PhD, DACVIM
Professor of Infectious Disease
Department of Clinical Sciences
College of Veterinary Medicine and Biomedical Sciences
Colorado State University
Fort Collins, Colorado
Toxoplasmosis
Giardiasis
Trichomoniasis
Cryptosporidiosis
Isosporiasis

Remo Lobetti, BVSc, MMedVet (Med), PhD, DECVIM (Internal Medicine)
Internist
Bryanston Veterinary Hospital
Bryanston, South Africa
Pneumocystosis

Jennifer A. Luff, VMD, DACVP
Veterinary Medicine
Department of Pathology, Microbiology, and Immunology
School of Veterinary Medicine
University of California
Davis, California
Viral Papillomatosis

Richard Malik, DVSc, DipVetAn, MVetClinStud, PhD, FACVSc, FASM
Valentine Charlton Veterinary Specialist
Centre for Veterinary Education
University of Sydney
Sydney, Australia
Cryptococcosis

Stanley L. Marks, BVSc, PhD, DACVIM (Internal Medicine, Oncology), DACVN
Professor
Department of Medicine and Epidemiology School of Veterinary Medicine
University of California
Davis, California
Salmonellosis
Enteric Escherichia coli Infections
Campylobacteriosis
Enteric Clostridial Infections
Gastric Helicobacter-like Infections

Lindsay K. Merkel, DVM, DACVIM
Internal Medicine Specialist
Veterinary Medical Center
College of Veterinary Medicine
University of Minnesota
St. Paul, Minnesota
Blastomycosis

Terry M. Nagle, BVSc, MACVSc, DACVD
Northern California Veterinary Specialist
Emergency & Referral Center
Sacramento, California
Malassezia Infections
Pyoderma, Otitis Externa, and Otitis Media

Jacqueline M. Norris, BVSc, MVS, PhD
Associate Professor of Veterinary Microbiology
Faculty of Veterinary Science
University of Sydney
Sydney, Australia
Coxiellosis and Q Fever

Catherine A. Outerbridge, MVSc, DVM
Associate Professor of Dermatology
Department of Medicine and Epidemiology
School of Veterinary Medicine
University of California
Davis, California
Dermatophytosis

Mark G. Papich, DVM, MS, DACVCP
Professor
Department of Molecular Biomedical Sciences
College of Veterinary Medicine
North Carolina State University
Raleigh, North Carolina
Principles of Antiinfective Therapy
Antiviral and Immunomodulatory Drugs
Antibacterial Drugs
Antifungal Drugs
Antiprotozoal Drugs

Christine A. Petersen, DVM, PhD
Associate Professor in Veterinary Pathology
Petersen and Jones Laboratory
College of Veterinary Medicine
Iowa State University
Ames, Iowa
Leishmaniosis

Shelley C. Rankin, BSc (Hons), PhD
Associate Professor (CE) of Microbiology
New Bolton Center
School of Veterinary Medicine
University of Pennsylvania
Philadelphia, Pennsylvania
Isolation in Cell Culture
Immunoassays
Isolation and Identification of Aerobic and Anaerobic Bacteria
Isolation and Identification of Fungi

Ashley B. Saunders, DVM, DACVIM (Cardiology)
Assistant Professor
Department of Small Animal Clinical Sciences
College of Veterinary Medicine and Biomedical Sciences
Texas A&M University
College Station, Texas
Trypanosomiasis

Joseph Taboada, DVM, DACVIM (Internal Medicine)
Professor and Associate Dean
Department of Veterinary Clinical Sciences School of Veterinary Medicine
Louisiana State University
Baton Rouge, Lousiana
Histoplasmosis

Séverine Tasker, BSc, BVSc, PhD, PGCert (HE), DSAM, DECVIM-CA, MRCVS
Senior Lecturer in Small Animal Medicine
School of Veterinary Sciences
University of Bristol
Bristol, Avon, United Kingdom
Hemoplasma Infections

Nancy Vincent-Johnson, DVM, MS, DACVIM (SAIM), DACVPM
Veterinary Medical Officer
Chief Clinical Services
Fort Belvoir Veterinary Treatment Facility
United States Army Veterinary Corps
Fort Belvoir, Virginia
Canine and Feline Hepatozoonosis

J. Scott Weese, DVM, DVSc, DACVIM
Professor
Department of Clinical Studies (Pathobiology)
University of Guelph
Guelph, Ontario
Infection Control Programs for Dogs and Cats

Jodi L. Westropp, DVM, PhD, DACVIM
Associate Professor
Department of Medicine and Epidemiology
School of Veterinary Medicine
University of California
Davis, California
Bacterial Infections of the Genitourinary Tract

Stephen D. White, DVM, DACVD
Professor
Department of Medicine and Epidemiology
School of Veterinary Medicine
University of California
Davis, California
Malassezia Infections
Pyoderma, Otitis Externa, and Otitis Media

To Terry Nagle, who did countless loads of laundry and cooked children's meals while I worked on this book. And to my children, Henry, Bridget, and Gillian, who through looking over my shoulder have learned a little about infectious diseases.

Perhaps readers might enjoy seeing some of what they have learned:

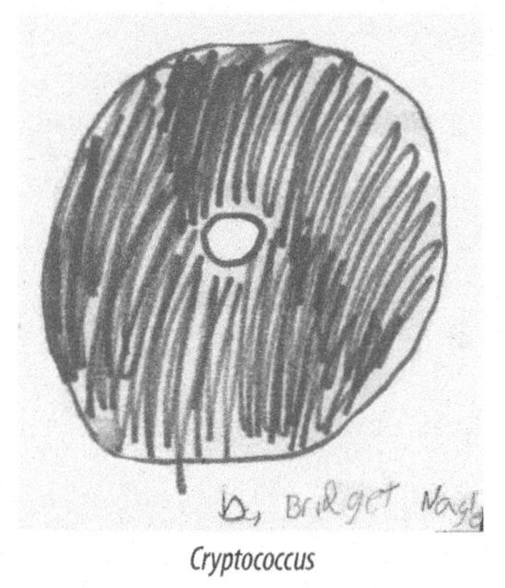

Cryptococcus

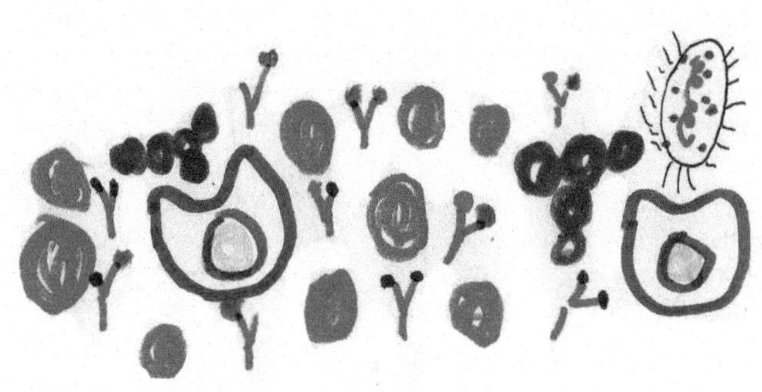

Antibodies, Phagocytes and Microbes

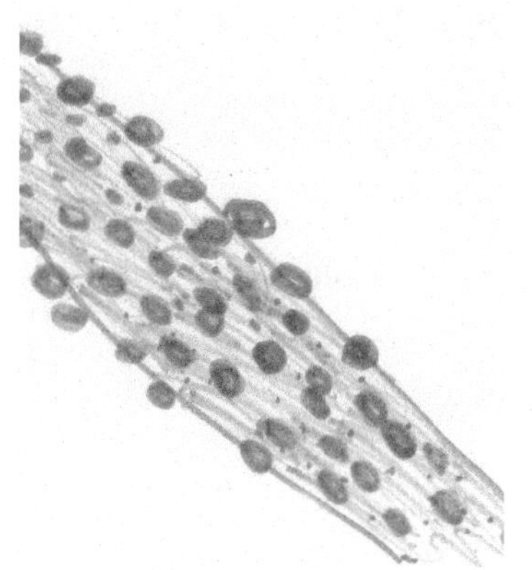

Dermatophytes

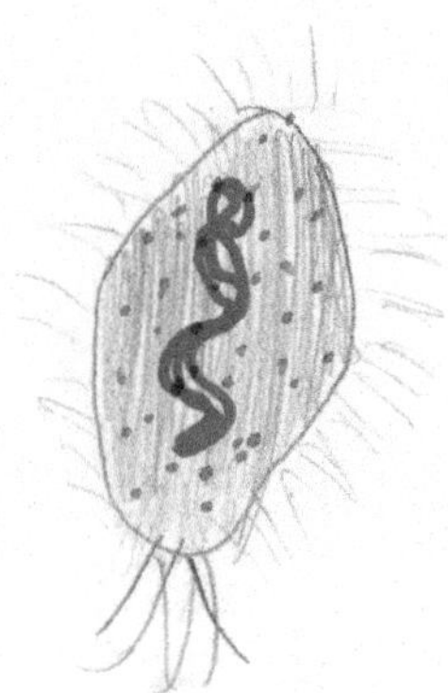

Flagellae

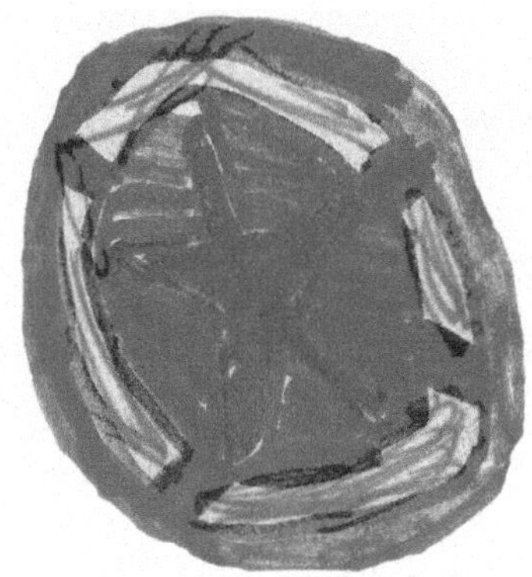

Virus

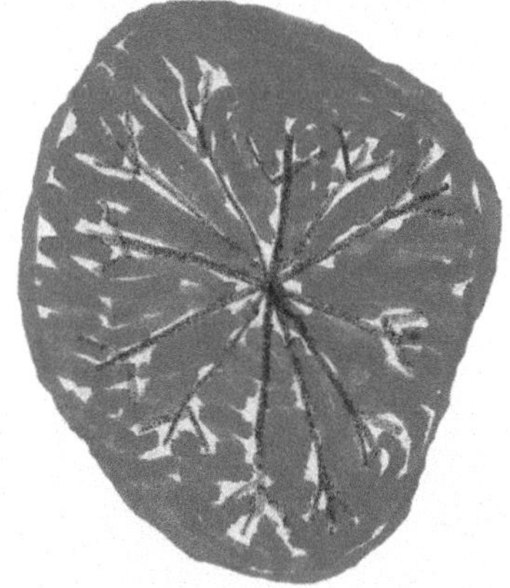

Virus

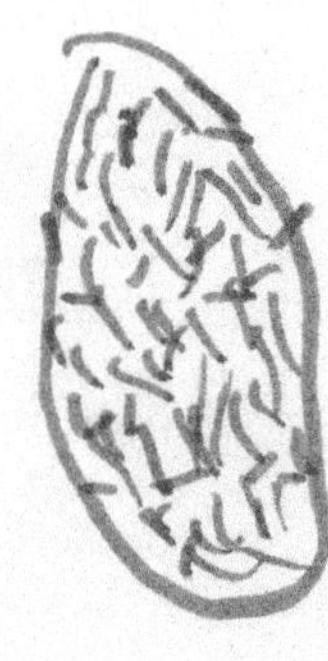

Poxvirus

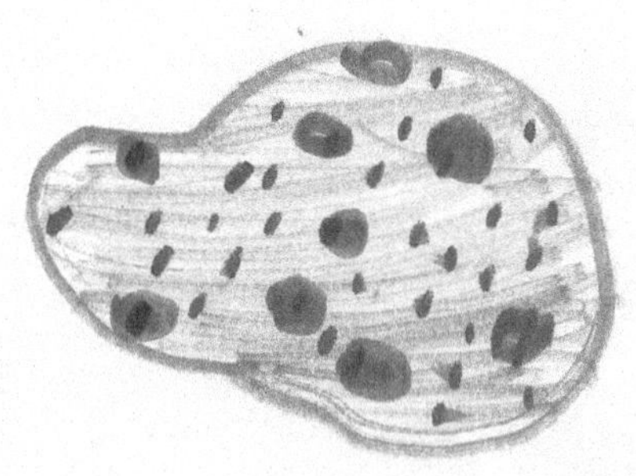

Amoeba

Preface

The goal of this first edition of *Canine and Feline Infectious Diseases* was to provide a text for veterinary students and clinicians with a strong clinical emphasis. Authorship has been limited to veterinarians who have had direct and considerable clinical experience with diagnosis and treatment of the diseases described. The chapters have been presented in a consistent and logical format with extensive use of tables, photographs, and line drawings, so that veterinarians and students can quickly find answers to questions they have that relate to infectious diseases in dogs and cats.

Organization

This book contains two parts and eight sections. The first part, *Basic Principles in the Diagnosis and Management of Small Animal Infection*, contains three sections: Laboratory Diagnosis of Infectious Diseases, Antiinfective Therapy, and Basic Principles of Infection Control. The second part, *Major Infectious Diseases and their Etiologic Agents*, systematically discusses specific infectious diseases of dogs and cats in a way that is practical and relevant to the veterinary clinician.

The first section, *Laboratory Diagnosis of Canine and Feline Infectious Diseases*, is co-authored by a small animal clinician and a clinical microbiologist. It aims to help practicing veterinarians select the best type of test for detection of an infectious disease, collect the most appropriate specimens for testing, optimally transport specimens to the laboratory, and most importantly, to interpret test results properly. The second section, *Antiinfective Therapy*, is co-authored by a clinician and a veterinary pharmacologist. The goal of this section is to help veterinarians use first principles to select the most appropriate drug for treatment of a suspected or confirmed infectious disease, understand the mechanisms of action and adverse effects of various antimicrobial drugs used in practice, and utilize treatment regimes that minimize development of antimicrobial resistance. The third section, *Basic Principles for Infection Control*, is co-authored by veterinary clinicians who have extensive practical experience with infectious disease control in veterinary hospitals. Practical protocols for the management of canine and feline patients suspected to have infectious diseases are provided, including handling, disinfection, isolation, and vaccination protocols.

The second half of this book addresses specific infectious diseases of dogs and cats, which are grouped into viral, bacterial, fungal, and protozoal diseases (Sections 1 through 4) as well as clinical syndromes (Section 5). A summary box at the beginning of the chapter provides an overview of the disease or diseases covered. Each chapter contains information on etiology and epidemiology, clinical signs and their pathogenesis; physical examination abnormalities, diagnosis, treatment and prognosis, immunity and vaccination, prevention, and public health implications. Some information on the equivalent disease in humans is provided whenever pertinent. Where relevant, maps and life cycle drawings are included, and chapters are illustrated with photographs of case material. All chapters contain a table that summarizes the performance, advantages and disadvantages of the major diagnostic assays available for each disease, and many chapters also contain a table that provides antimicrobial drug treatment recommendations and dosing. Key statements in the text are referenced in case the reader desires additional background information, although provision of an exhaustive list of references is not in the scope of this book. A few suggested readings are provided.

One (and occasionally two) case example(s) can be found in a standard format at the end of almost all of the chapters in the second half of the book. These cases are designed to emphasize key epidemiological and clinical aspects of the disease, the application of diagnostic assays, treatment, and prognosis. The cases were seen at the authors' institutions, and many include the results of full laboratory assessments, radiology, cytology, and histopathology reports. Unless otherwise specified, all urinalyses and urine cultures were performed on specimens collected by cystocentesis, and all thoracic radiographic studies consisted of left and right lateral and ventrodorsal views. Abdominal ultrasound examinations consisted of complete studies of intraabdominal structures. Because these are "real-world" examples, diagnosis, management, and outcomes are not always perfect or ideal. Nevertheless, this can provide insight into real-life problems that may confound accurate diagnosis and management of the disease, such as misdiagnosis when an infectious disease resembles other infectious or non-infectious diseases on the differential diagnosis list. Other problems illustrated include limitations of the sensitivity or specificity of diagnostic tests used, or hurdles imposed by the availability of client financial resources. A comment section at the end of the case provides the author(s') perspective on the case. It should be recognized that infectious diseases can vary widely in their clinical presentation and response to treatment, so each case just provides one "view" of the infectious disease described in the chapter.

Jane E. Sykes

Acknowledgments

I am incredibly grateful to the huge number of veterinarians, residents, and veterinary students worldwide who have encouraged me to write and edit this book. I would particularly like to acknowledge all of my colleagues at the University of California, Davis, who over the years provided a large number of the carefully collected and valuable images in this book. Special mentions go to Barbara Byrne, Patricia Pesavento, and Eileen Samitz who spent much additional time to prepare or provide material for photography for this book.

I would like to acknowledge the illustrator for the book, Ted Huff, who has performed the amazing task of converting a large number of complicated maps and life cycle drawings into crisp, clean diagrams that are easy to understand and remember. I have also been fortunate to work with a phenomenal team at Elsevier who were consistently encouraging, efficient, and made every effort to be accommodating. I would like to thank my internal medicine and infectious disease colleagues worldwide, many of whom contributed to chapters for this book, for inspiring me to have a passion for the study of small animal internal medicine and infectious diseases. Last but not least I would like to acknowledge my family, who cheered me on the whole way.

Jane E. Sykes

Contents

PART I BASIC PRINCIPLES IN THE DIAGNOSIS AND MANAGEMENT OF SMALL ANIMAL INFECTION

PART II MAJOR INFECTIOUS DISEASES AND THEIR ETIOLOGIC AGENTS

Section 2
Bacterial Diseases

Section 3
Fungal and Algal Diseases

Section 4
Protozoal Diseases

Section 5
Infections of Selected Organ Systems

PART I

Basic Principles in the Diagnosis and Management of Small Animal Infection

SECTION 1
Laboratory Diagnosis of Canine and Feline Infectious Diseases

SECTION 2
Antiinfective Therapy

SECTION 3
Basic Principles for Infection Control

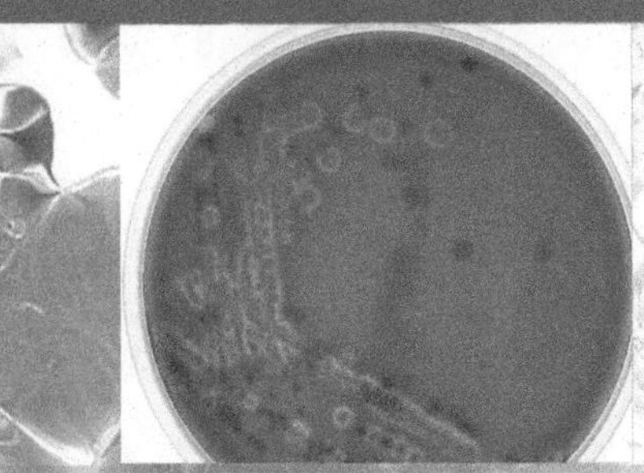

SECTION 1
Laboratory Diagnosis of Canine and Feline Infectious Diseases

Jane E. Sykes and Shelley C. Rankin

CHAPTER 1

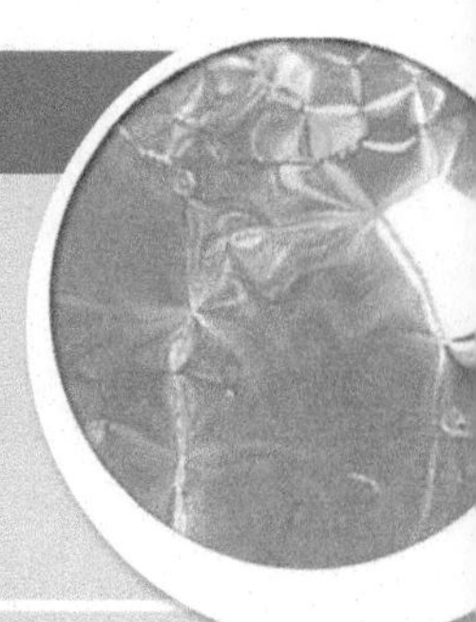

Isolation in Cell Culture

Jane E. Sykes and Shelley C. Rankin

KEY POINTS

- With the increasing availability of nucleic acid–based testing, cell culture is decreasingly used for diagnosis of infections caused by obligate intracellular pathogens in dogs and cats.
- Cell culture remains an important technique for (a) confirmation of a diagnosis when the results of molecular testing or serology are unavailable or equivocal; (b) pathogen discovery; and (c) vaccine manufacture. For some pathogens, cell culture is the most sensitive and specific method for organism detection.
- Before collection of specimens, veterinary clinicians should communicate with the laboratory that is to perform the culture to discuss the patient signalment, history, immune status, travel history, nature of the suspected infection, and number of animals affected.
- Specimens are inoculated onto monolayers, and the infecting organism is identified based on the presence of characteristic cytopathic effect after a predictable incubation period, with or without confirmatory antigen staining, electron microscopy, or nucleic acid testing.
- False-negative results may occur as a result of inadequate specimen collection, deterioration of organisms during transport, or culture contamination with bacteria or fungi.
- Positive results do not imply that the organism detected is the cause of an animal's signs, because some organisms can be present without causing disease. This is especially the case for animals with respiratory or gastrointestinal disease.

INTRODUCTION

Cell culture refers to the culture of nucleated (eukaryotic) cells under controlled conditions within the laboratory. Infectious agents that require living host cells for replication can only be isolated in cell culture. With the advent of molecular diagnostic assays based on nucleic acid detection, cell culture is being used less often for routine clinical diagnostic purposes, because of the long turnaround times (days to weeks), cost, and requirement for significant technical expertise to perform cell culture and interpret results (Table 1-1). Nevertheless, isolation of viral and intracellular bacterial and protozoal pathogens in cell culture remains an important technique for the discovery of new pathogens, identification of organisms involved in disease when the results of molecular testing or serology are unavailable or equivocal, the propagation of isolates for research purposes, the generation of organisms for vaccination purposes, and the establishment of the efficacy of novel antimicrobial drugs. Vaccines for dogs and cats that are propagated in cell culture include those for canine distemper, canine adenovirus infections, parvovirus infections, rabies, and feline viral and chlamydial respiratory tract disease. Veterinary clinicians should remain aware of situations where cell culture may be the best technique to identify the presence of an infectious agent and the optimum methods for collection and submission of specimens. Knowledge of cell culture methods can help veterinary clinicians to submit the optimum specimens and to understand laboratory turnaround times, potential complications, and how to interpret results.

Specimen Collection and Transport

Although cell culture can be used to propagate intracellular bacteria and protozoa, it is most often used by clinicians for the diagnosis of viral infections. Active communication between the clinician and the laboratory that performs viral isolation is recommended. Successful detection of viruses is highly dependent on (a) collecting the appropriate specimens, (b) the timing of specimen collection, and (c) rapid and proper specimen

TABLE 1-1

Alternatives to Cell Culture for Diagnosis of Obligate Intracellular Pathogens That Infect Dogs and Cats

System Affected and Most Common Agents	Other Diagnostic Tests Available
Respiratory Tract	
Canine respiratory coronavirus	RT-PCR
Canine adenovirus-2	PCR
Influenza viruses	RT-PCR, antibody detection
Canine parainfluenza virus	RT-PCR
Canine distemper virus	RT-PCR, antigen detection using IFA
Canine herpesvirus	PCR
Feline herpesvirus-1	PCR, IHC
Feline calicivirus	RT-PCR, IHC
Eye	
Chlamydia felis	PCR
Central Nervous System	
Canine distemper virus	RT-PCR, direct IFA, CSF antibody detection
West Nile virus	RT-PCR
Encephalitis viruses	RT-PCR
Gastrointestinal Tract	
Coronaviruses	PCR
Canine distemper virus	PCR, direct IFA/IHC
Canine and feline parvovirus	PCR, IHC
Genital	
Canine herpesvirus	PCR
Congenital and Perinatal	
Canine herpesvirus	PCR
Feline herpesvirus-1	PCR
Blood	
Feline leukemia virus	PCR, antigen detection
Feline immunodeficiency virus	PCR, antibody detection
Anaplasma phagocytophilum	PCR, antibody detection
Rickettsia rickettsii	PCR, direct IFA on skin biopsies, antibody detection
Ehrlichia canis	PCR, antibody detection

CSF, Cerebrospinal fluid; IFA, fluorescent antibody; IHC, immunohistochemistry; PCR, polymerase chain reaction; RT, reverse transcriptase.

transport and processing. Thus the actions of the veterinary clinician play a critical role in ensuring positive test results when a virus is present.

The clinician should discuss with the laboratory what types of viruses are suspected in light of the animal's clinical presentation. The patient signalment, history, clinical signs, immune status, travel history, and number of animals affected should be discussed to generate conclusions regarding the nature of the suspected infection (Box 1-1). Some viruses, such as feline coronavirus (FCoV), are difficult to isolate in cell culture or grow slowly, whereas others, such as feline calicivirus (FCV), replicate readily and rapidly in cell culture, and the sensitivity of cell culture is high. Viruses differ in respect to the cell type they prefer to replicate within. As a result, specimens should be sent to the laboratory with information on the specific viruses that are suspected.

The timing of specimen collection is particularly important for viral infections. Specimens should be collected as early as possible following the onset of clinical signs, optimally within the first week, because viral shedding may commence before the onset of signs and continue for only a few days. The duration of viral shedding depends on the type of virus and the anatomic site sampled. When multiple animals are affected, collection of specimens from more than one animal may increase the chance that an isolate will be obtained. If possible, antibody testing using acute and convalescent phase serology should be performed concurrently to help confirm the diagnosis (see Chapter 2).

Selection of the best specimen and collection site for culture is optimized based on knowledge of the pathogenesis of the infectious agent involved, because the optimum specimen collection site may not be the site where clinical signs are most severe. Attempts should be made during specimen collection to prevent contamination of the specimen with normal flora, although this is not always possible. Specimen size should also be maximized (for example, at least 5 mL of blood, body fluids, or lavage specimens, and ideally 8 to 10 mL of blood) to increase the chance of a positive isolation. In general, nasal or nasopharyngeal washes have been preferred over nasal swabs in human patients for isolation of respiratory viruses, but one study showed that nasal swab specimens were just as sensitive as nasopharyngeal washes for isolation of most respiratory viruses.[1] Nasal or oropharyngeal swab specimens are collected by placing a long-shafted swab in the area to be sampled, rotating the swab against the mucosa, and allowing the secretions to be absorbed for approximately 5 to 10 seconds.

Swabs and small tissue specimens for virus isolation should be placed in buffered virus transport medium, which contains antibiotics and protein. This can be obtained from the laboratory or purchased from other commercial sources. It is important that the medium used has not reached its expiry date.

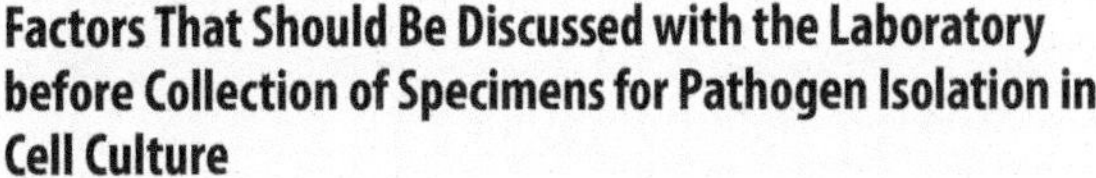

BOX 1-1

Factors That Should Be Discussed with the Laboratory before Collection of Specimens for Pathogen Isolation in Cell Culture

Patient species, breed, age, and environment
Number of animals affected
History and clinical signs
Immune status of the patient
Geographic location and travel history
Suspected infectious agents
Timing of specimen collection
Type and amount of specimen to be collected
Transport conditions, including timing and method of transportation

TABLE 1-2

Specimen Collection Guide for Diagnosis of Viral and Intracellular Bacterial Infections of Companion Animals

System Affected	Possible Agents	Specimen Type
Respiratory tract	Dogs: coronaviruses, canine adenovirus, influenza viruses, parainfluenza virus, CDV, canine herpesvirus Cats: FHV-1, FCV, influenza viruses, FCoV	Oropharyngeal swabs Nasal flushes, transtracheal wash or bronchoalveolar lavage specimens: ideally 5 to 10 mL of fluid Lung tissue obtained at biopsy or necropsy, including an area adjacent to affected tissue
Eye	Dogs: canine herpesvirus, canine adenovirus Cats: FHV-1, FCV, *Chlamydia felis*	Conjunctival swab, scraping or biopsy
Central nervous system	Dogs: CDV, West Nile virus, arboviruses	Cerebrospinal fluid: ideally at least 0.5 to 1 mL Blood: 8 to 10 mL Brain at necropsy
Gastrointestinal tract	Dogs: CDV, CPV, rotaviruses, canine coronavirus Cats: FCoV, FCV, FeLV, rotaviruses, toroviruses	Feces: ideally an olive-sized portion of formed feces or 10 mL of liquid stool Intestinal biopsies obtained using endoscopy or surgery, or intestinal tissue obtained at necropsy
Genital	Dogs: canine herpesvirus Cats: *Chlamydia felis*	Vesicle scrapings, vaginal swabs
Congenital and perinatal	Dogs: canine herpesvirus Cats: FHV-1, FeLV	Blood, tissues obtained at necropsy
Blood	Dogs: *Anaplasma phagocytophilum*, *Rickettsia rickettsii*, *Ehrlichia canis* Cats: FeLV, FIV, FCoV	Blood: ideally 8 to 10 mL

CDV, Canine distemper virus; CPV, canine parvovirus; FCoV, feline coronavirus; FCV, feline calicivirus; FeLV, feline leukemia virus; FHV-1, feline herpesvirus-1; FIV, feline immunodeficiency virus.

Liquid specimens such as blood, cerebrospinal fluid, and bronchoalveolar lavage fluid do not need to be placed in transport media. Blood samples should be collected using sterile technique, with antiseptic preparation of the site of venipuncture, and can be submitted in EDTA anticoagulant tubes.

All specimens should be refrigerated on collection and transported as quickly as possible (preferably within 24 hours) to the laboratory, because delayed transport can lead to loss of organism viability. If delays in excess of 2 to 3 days are anticipated, the specimen can be frozen. Freezing should be avoided whenever possible, as it may lead to dramatic loss of virus viability. If freezing is unavoidable, freezing at −70° C is preferable to freezing at −20° C, and shipping on dry ice is preferable, if possible. The laboratory's submission guide should be checked for specimen handling recommendations.

Table 1-2 provides a guide to the recommended specimen types for isolation of viruses or obligate intracellular bacteria from companion animals. Specimens should be labeled with the patient data, the site(s) from which the specimen(s) was collected, specific organisms suspected, and the time and date of specimen collection. Contained specimens should be placed inside leakproof triple packaging and transported on wet ice or cold packs to the laboratory, especially if transport is expected to take longer than 1 hour. Absorbent materials should be placed within the secondary container in order to absorb any spills. If specimens are to be shipped, the specimen must be labeled and handled according to governmental and International Air Transport Association (IATA) regulations for shipping materials known to contain infectious substances, which are categorized as Category A or Category B. Category A infectious substances are those capable of causing permanent disability or life-threatening or fatal disease in otherwise healthy animals and humans.[2] Most specimens submitted by veterinarians fall under Category B, which are those that do not fall under the criteria for inclusion in Category A. Updated documents providing guidance on regulations for the transport of infectious substances are provided online by the World Health Organization (WHO).[2] Import permits may be required for interstate and international transportation.

Diagnostic Methods

Maintenance of Cell Cultures in the Laboratory

In general, cells are grown as a monolayer on a plastic plate. The cells in the monolayer can be derived directly from an animal *(primary cell culture)*, which tend to have a limited life span, or they may be immortalized *(continuous cell lines)*. Primary cell cultures are needed for the isolation of some viruses, because the cells more closely resemble those present in vivo, and the replication of these viruses occurs more efficiently in primary cell lines than in continuous cell lines. Further subculture of primary cell lines often reduces their sensitivity to viral infection. Primary cell cultures are generated by placing tissues in cell culture media, often after treatment of the tissue with an enzyme such as trypsin or collagenase. Primary white blood cell cultures (such as peripheral blood mononuclear cell cultures) are generated by separation of the white cells from the other cellular elements using density gradient centrifugation, and adding them to a culture medium. Ficoll, a highly branched polysaccharide,

TABLE 1-3

Examples of Continuous Cell Lines Used for Isolation of Viruses and Intracellular Bacteria That Infect Dogs and Cats

Cell Line	Cell Origin	Pathogen(s)
Vero cells; recombinant Vero-SLAM cells	African Green monkey renal epithelial cells	CDV[11,12] *Rickettsia rickettsii*[13] *Toxoplasma gondii*[14]
Madin-Darby canine kidney cells (MDCK)	Kidney	CDV[8,15] Canine adenovirus[8,15] Canine herpesvirus-1[8,15] Parvoviruses[8,16] Canine parainfluenza virus[8] Canine calicivirus[4] Rotaviruses[17] Influenza viruses[18] FeLV[19] *Neospora caninum*[20]
Crandell-Reese feline kidney cells	Fetal kidney	FHV-1[21] FCV[21,22] FCoV[23] Parvoviruses[24] FIV[25]
HL-60	Human leukemia	*Anaplasma phagocytophilum*[26]
A-72	Canine fibroma	Canine adenovirus[27] Canine coronavirus[27] Canine parainfluenza virus[27] Canine herpesvirus[27]
McCoy	Mouse fibroblast	*Chlamydia felis*[28]
FCWF	*Felis catus* whole fetus, has characteristics of macrophages	FCoV[29] FHV-1[30]
DH-82	Monocyte/macrophage	*Ehrlichia canis*[31]

CDV, Canine distemper virus; FCoV, feline coronavirus; FCV, feline calicivirus; FeLV, feline leukemia virus; FHV-1, feline herpesvirus-1; FIV, feline immunodeficiency virus.

is an example of a medium used commonly for density gradient centrifugation. Primary cell cultures have been used widely for the isolation of intracellular pathogens of dogs and cats.[3-6]

Low-passage cell lines remain viable and sensitive to viral infections for 20 to 50 passages. *Continuous cell lines* are the type of cell line used most commonly for diagnostic, research, and commercial purposes. These are derived from cancer cells (such as the widely used HeLa cell line, derived from human cervical cancer cells of a patient named Henrietta Lacks),[7] or they result from experimental induction of cellular mutations (for example, using a carcinogen). Continuous cell lines representing a wide variety of cell types are available from commercial suppliers (Table 1-3). Laboratories that perform virus isolation for disease diagnosis may need to simultaneously inoculate multiple cell lines, because different viruses prefer to replicate in differing cell types. Mixed cell cultures are also now available commercially to simultaneously facilitate isolation of multiple different viral pathogens.

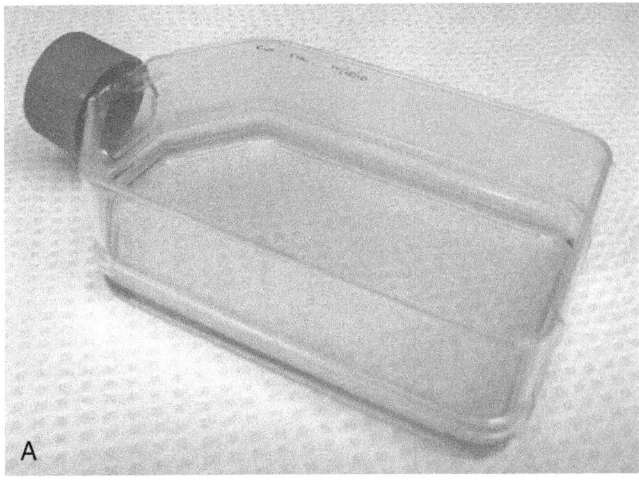

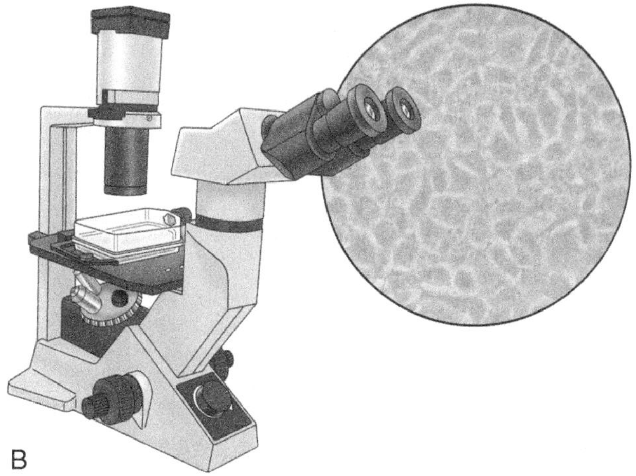

FIGURE 1-1 **A,** Plastic flask that contains cell culture medium. **B,** A confluent cell monolayer is present on the bottom of the flask and can be visualized through the top of the flask using a binocular inverted microscope.

Cells for cell culture are stored in the laboratory in liquid nitrogen tanks. The cells are thawed, dispersed in cell culture medium, and allowed to settle on the bottom of a plastic flask (Figure 1-1). The cell culture medium keeps the cells moist and provides the cells with nutrients. *Minimum essential medium* (MEM), also known as *Eagle's minimum essential medium*, and *Dulbecco's medium* are examples of widely used synthetic cell culture media. The cell culture medium contains a balanced salt solution, essential amino acids, glucose, vitamins, and a bicarbonate buffering system. Variations of MEM are available, some of which contain nonessential amino acids, the pH indicator phenol red, and the pH buffering agent HEPES (4-(2-hydroxyethyl)-1-piperazineethanesulfonic acid), which helps to maintain a physiologic pH despite an increasing concentration of CO_2 that is produced as a result of cellular respiration. The medium often requires supplementation with animal serum, most commonly fetal calf serum, which helps the cells to attach to and spread on the plate, although serum-free medium has also been used successfully for culture of canine and feline viruses.[8] Media for cell culture growth differ from media for maintenance of cells in culture, the former generally containing a higher concentration of animal serum (10% versus 2% for maintenance medium).

To prevent bacterial or fungal contamination when viral pathogens are cultured, careful attention to sterile technique is required. Manipulation of cells in the flask is performed in a laminar flow hood, and the culture medium is sometimes supplemented with antibiotics (generally ampicillin or an aminoglycoside), with or without an antifungal agent (amphotericin B or nystatin). Cell culture flasks are placed in a humidified incubator that maintains temperature usually at 37°C, and a gas mixture that typically contains 5% CO_2.

The cell culture flasks are removed from the incubator and examined daily using an inverted binocular tissue culture microscope (see Figure 1-1), which allows examination of unstained cells through the bottom of the flask. The medium is replaced with fresh medium if the pH indicator suggests it is becoming too acidic. Once the cells have multiplied sufficiently to form a semiconfluent monolayer, the cells can either be passaged or be allowed to reach confluence before inoculation with specimen. In order to passage the cells, the medium is removed, and a small volume of trypsin or EDTA solution is added to the monolayer. The monolayer is incubated with the solution for several minutes, after which the cells detach from the flask and can be resuspended in medium, which is then added to new flasks.

Occasionally, cell lines become cross-contaminated with other cell lines. The HeLa cell line is an example of a prolific and hardy cell line that commonly contaminates other cultures. Major cell line repositories such as the American Type Culture Collection (ATCC) use genetic typing methods to verify the identity of the cells in their collection. Cell lines can also become easily contaminated with *Mycoplasma* spp., which pass through filters used to exclude other bacteria. The presence of contaminating *Mycoplasma* spp. can interfere with replication of other pathogens and cause alterations of cellular morphology. *Mycoplasma* contamination is detected using stains such as Hoechst stain, culture for *Mycoplasma*, and commercially available PCR assays that specifically detect *Mycoplasma* DNA for the purpose of cell culture quality assurance.[9]

Inoculation of Cell Cultures

Infection of a cell monolayer is accomplished by removal of overlying medium and inoculation of the monolayer with a suspension of viral or bacterial organisms. If tissue specimens are provided for culture, the specimens are homogenized in culture medium before they are inoculated onto the monolayer. Specimens may first be centrifuged to remove cell debris and bacteria. Passage through a filter can also be used before inoculation to remove bacteria. The inoculum is added to the monolayer. Organisms within the inoculum are then allowed to settle on the monolayer for approximately 1 hour before the residual inoculum is removed and fresh maintenance medium is added.

For isolation of virus, the monolayer is then examined daily for evidence of cytopathic effect (CPE). Medium is replaced weekly or biweekly. CPE refers to the cellular changes induced by viral replication in the cell culture monolayer and includes cell lysis or cell fusion (syncytium formation). The presence of a particular viral pathogen is indicated by the appearance of characteristic CPE for that pathogen after a predicted incubation period (Figure 1-2). For example, CPE induced by FCV is characterized by cell rounding and detachment that can occur within 24 hours, and within 16 hours for highly virulent strains.[10] The presence of CPE is confirmed through the comparison of inoculated cultures to uninoculated (control) cultures. Examination of the cell monolayer using light microscopy after fixation and staining can reveal additional diagnostic features, such as the presence of inclusion bodies and syncytium formation. Some viruses are relatively noncytopathogenic. In some cases, the presence of these viruses can be demonstrated by adding washed erythrocytes to the monolayer and examination of the monolayer for evidence of hemadsorption (see Figure 1-2, B). Hemadsorption results from incorporation of viral surface hemagglutinin molecules into the plasma membranes of the cell culture monolayer. Examples of hemadsorbing viruses that produce minimal CPE include influenza and parainfluenza viruses. Other, more sensitive and specific methods for identification of

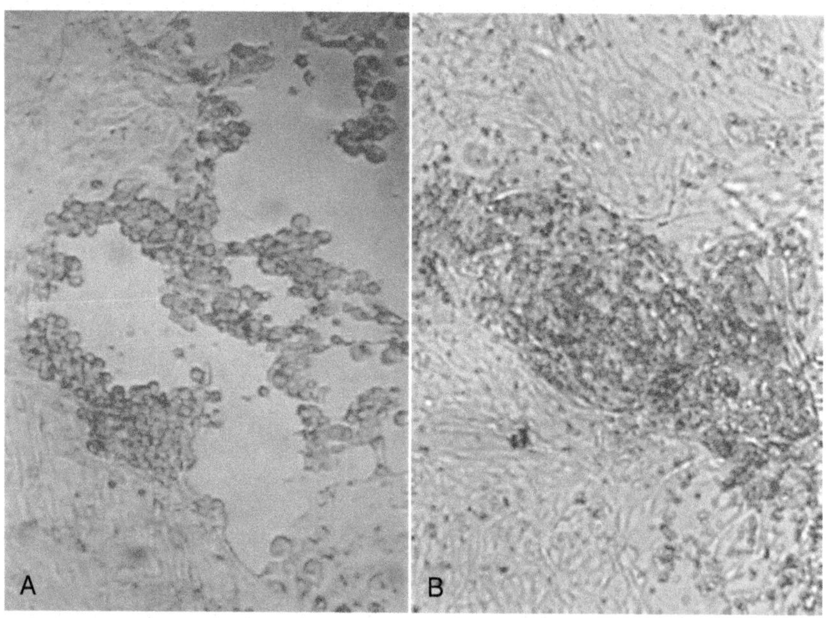

FIGURE 1-2 **A,** Cytopathic effects produced by a herpesvirus as viewed in the laboratory. Note the focal areas of rounded and detached cells. **B,** Hemadsorption: erythrocytes adsorb to infected cells that have incorporated hemagglutinin into the plasma membrane. Magnification ×60. (Courtesy of Jack I; from MacLachlan NJ, Dubovi EJ eds. Fenner's veterinary virology, 4 ed. New York: Academic Press, 2011.)

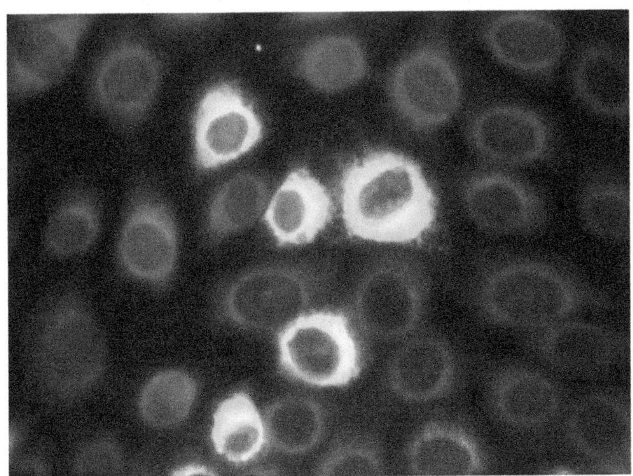

FIGURE 1-3 Indirect fluorescent antibody detection of noncytopathic virus infected cells. A cell monolayer exposed to virus for 72 hours was fixed with cold acetone. Fixed cells were stained with a mouse monoclonal antibody specific for bovine viral diarrhea virus (BVDV) followed by a goat anti-mouse serum tagged with fluorescein isothiocyanate. (From Maclachlan NJ, Dubovi EJ. Fenner's Veterinary Virology, 4 ed. New York: Academic Press, 2011.)

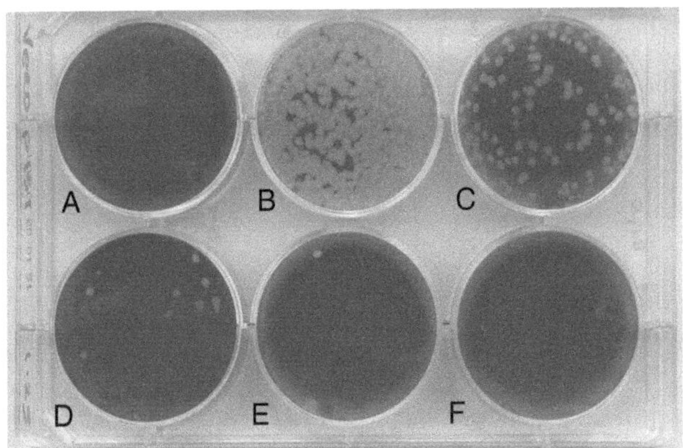

FIGURE 1-5 Determination of the concentration of infectious virus using a plaque assay. Vero cell monolayers were inoculated with serial 10-fold dilutions of vesicular stomatitis virus. After a 1-hour adsorption period, cultures were overlayed with 0.75% agarose in cell culture medium containing 5% fetal bovine serum. Cultures were incubated for 3 days at 37°C in a 5% humidified CO_2 atmosphere. The agarose overlay was removed and cultures fixed and stained with 0.75% crystal violet in 10% buffered formalin. **A,** Control culture. **B-F,** serial 10-fold dilution of virus: **B,** 10^{-3}; **C,** 10^{-4}; **D,** 10^{-5}; **E,** 10^{-6}; **F,** 10^{-7}. (From Maclachlan NJ, Dubovi EJ. Fenner's Veterinary Virology, 4 ed. New York: Academic Press, 2011.)

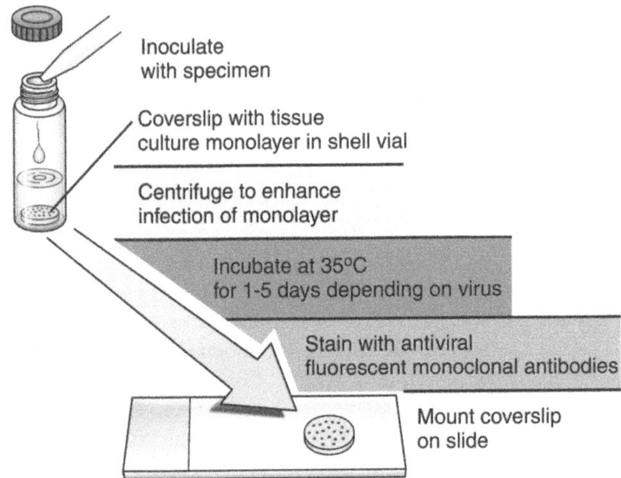

FIGURE 1-4 Schematic of the shell vial virus isolation technique. (Modified from Shelhamer JH, Gill VJ, Quinn TC, et al. The laboratory evaluation of opportunistic pulmonary infections. Ann Intern Med 1996;124(6):585-599.)

an organism that has infected a cell culture monolayer include fixation and staining of the monolayer with fluorescent antibodies that are specific for certain viruses (Figure 1-3), use of nucleic acid detection techniques such as PCR, or use of electron microscopy.

For *spin-amplified cell culture,* the monolayer is centrifuged at low speed after inoculation. This can enhance recovery of certain viruses and intracellular bacterial pathogens such as chlamydiae. Either an entire plate of cell culture wells can be spun in a plate centrifuge, or *shell vials* can be used (also known as the *shell vial technique*). Shell vials are small, flat-bottomed bottles (Figure 1-4). A monolayer is grown on a glass coverslip at the bottom of the vial, and after inoculation, the vials are centrifuged at low speed. Using this method, fluorescent antibody staining for viral or chlamydial antigen is used to detect the pathogen before CPE occurs. After 48 to 72 hours, the coverslips are fixed, stained with virus-specific fluorescent-labeled antibodies, removed from the vials, and examined with a fluorescence microscope.

Plaque Assays

Overlay of the monolayer with agar or methylcellulose after inoculation with virus minimizes subsequent viral movement through the monolayer and restricts damage by each replicating viral particle to a small area. This results in the formation of "holes" in the monolayer, or *plaques* (Figure 1-5). The monolayer can then be stained and the number of plaques can be counted in order to obtain information regarding the amount of virus in the inoculum. Plaque assays are commonly used by researchers to assess the efficacy of antiviral treatments, through reduction of plaque formation.

Laboratory Safety Concerns That Relate to Cell Culture

The processing of specimens in a biological safety cabinet not only serves to protect cultures from contamination but also acts to protect the laboratory worker from laboratory-acquired infections. Most viruses grown in veterinary diagnostic laboratories are classified as biosafety level 2 (BSL 2) agents. Biosafety levels range from 1 through 4 (Table 1-4). In the United States, the Centers for Disease Control and Prevention (CDC) assigns these levels. It is important that veterinary clinicians be aware that isolation of hazardous pathogens can only be conducted in specially designed and accredited laboratories.

Interpretation of Results

Negative Results

Reasons for negative test results using virus isolation are numerous, so the clinician should not assume that a virus is not present when a negative test result is obtained (Box 1-2). Negative test results can occur as a result of inadequate specimen size, lack of viral shedding by the animal at the time of specimen collection, the binding of antibodies to viruses within the specimen,

TABLE 1-4

Biosafety Levels Set for Diagnosis of Laboratory Practices

Level	Risk	Examples	Example Precautions
BSL 1	Minimal potential hazard to human health and the environment	Canine adenovirus-1 Nonpathogenic *Escherichia coli*	Gloves, facial protection. Standard microbiologic practices using bench-top techniques. Routine decontamination practices (hand washing, routine bench disinfection, autoclaving of infectious waste).
BSL 2	Moderate potential hazard to human health and the environment. Organisms cause mild disease or are difficult to contract as laboratory aerosols.	Most veterinary viruses, including influenza viruses	Access to the laboratory restricted when work is taking place; extreme precautions with sharp contaminated materials; use of appropriate biosafety cabinets when generation of aerosols possible. No requirement for directional airflow into the laboratory.
BSL 3	Dangerous agents that can be transmitted by aerosol within the laboratory but for which effective vaccines or treatments exist.	West Nile virus Equine encephalitis viruses *Rickettsia rickettsii* *Coxiella burnetii* *Mycobacterium tuberculosis*	Laboratory is located away from high-traffic areas. Restricted laboratory access when work in progress; double door entry, ventilation providing airflow into the room, exhaust air not recirculated; special practices and protective clothing for BSL 3, including biosafety cabinet use; special floor and ceiling materials specified.
BSL 4	Dangerous and exotic agents that pose a high risk of aerosol-transmitted laboratory infections, or which produce severe or fatal disease in humans	Ebola virus Marburg virus Smallpox	Hazmat suit and self-contained oxygen system, entrance containing multiple showers, a vacuum room, an ultraviolet light room, and multiple airlocked doors. Strict control of laboratory access to authorized personnel.

BOX 1-2

Reasons for Negative Test Results following Isolation of Viruses in Cell Culture

Virus not causing the disease
Virus causing the disease, but:
- Specimen size inadequate
- No viral shedding at the time of sampling
- No viral shedding at the site of sampling
- Antibody interference with viral infectivity for cell culture
- Inadequate organism numbers at the anatomic site of specimen collection
- Loss of organism viability during transportation to the laboratory
- Overgrowth of one viral pathogen by another
- Overgrowth by bacterial or fungal agents
- Lack of cell sensitivity for the virus (wrong cell type inoculated)
- Laboratory inexperience with techniques required for virus isolation and identification

inadequate organism numbers at the anatomic site of specimen collection, or loss of organism viability during transportation to the laboratory. Loss of viral viability is more likely to occur with enveloped viruses such as canine distemper virus than with non-enveloped, hardy viruses such as canine parvovirus or FCV. Negative test results can also occur when the cell line inoculated is not sensitive to the virus present in the specimen. Low-passage cells may also lose their infectivity for viral infection if they have undergone multiple serial passages.

False negatives can also occur if the plates are overgrown by bacteria or fungi. Although treatment of the viral transport and culture media with antimicrobials can help prevent this, resistant bacteria or fungi may still be present. Sometimes, multiple viruses are present within a specimen, and one virus overgrows another. For example, this can occur with mixed infections with FCV and feline herpesvirus-1 (FHV-1) in cats with upper respiratory tract disease. FCV rapidly infects Crandell-Reese feline kidney cells and produces CPE, which obscures the concurrent presence of FHV-1.

Positive Results

It is imperative that veterinary clinicians be aware that the detection of a virus in a specimen does not always imply that the organism is the cause of the animal's clinical signs. This is especially true for specimens collected from the respiratory or gastrointestinal tracts, where multiple infectious agents may be present concurrently, and in many cases, viruses can replicate in these locations without causing clinical signs of illness. In some animals, the development of severe clinical signs is more likely when there is simultaneous presence of multiple infectious agents. As noted previously for specimens that test negative, the presence of one agent may also obscure the presence of another, more significant organism (such as with FCV and FHV-1 co-infections), which could result in the incorrect assumption that only one organism is the cause of an animal's disease.

REFERENCES

1. Heikkinen T, Marttila J, Salmi AA, et al. Nasal swab versus nasopharyngeal aspirate for isolation of respiratory viruses. J Clin Microbiol. 2002;40(11):4337-4339.
2. World Health Organization guidance on regulations for the Transport of Infectious Substances 2009-2010. http://www.who.int/csr/resources/publications/biosafety/WHO_HSE_EPR_2008_10/en/index.html. Last accessed January 25, 2013.
3. Schobesberger M, Zurbriggen A, Summerfield A, et al. Oligodendroglial degeneration in distemper: apoptosis or necrosis? Acta Neuropathol. 1999;97(3):279-287.
4. Maeda Y, Tohya Y, Matsuura Y, et al. Early interaction of canine calicivirus with cells is the major determinant for its cell tropism in vitro. Vet Microbiol. 2002;87(4):291-300.
5. Le LP, Rivera AA, Glasgow JN, et al. Infectivity enhancement for adenoviral transduction of canine osteosarcoma cells. Gene Ther. 2006;13(5):389-399.
6. Hemphill A, Vonlaufen N, Golaz JL, et al. Infection of primary canine duodenal epithelial cell cultures with *Neospora caninum*. J Parasitol. 2009;95(2):372-380.
7. Skloot R. The Immortal Life of Henrietta Lacks. New York: Crown Publishers; 2010.
8. Mochizuki M. Growth characteristics of canine pathogenic viruses in MDCK cells cultured in RPMI 1640 medium without animal protein. Vaccine. 2006;24(11):1744-1748.
9. Young L, Sung J, Stacey G, et al. Detection of *Mycoplasma* in cell cultures. Nat Protoc. 2010;5(5):929-934.
10. Ossiboff RJ, Sheh A, Shotton J, et al. Feline caliciviruses (FCVs) isolated from cats with virulent systemic disease possess in vitro phenotypes distinct from those of other FCV isolates. J Gen Virol. 2007;88(Pt 2):506-517.
11. Narang HK. Ultrastructural study of long-term canine distemper virus infection in tissue culture cells. Infect Immun. 1982;36(1):310-319.
12. Lan NT, Yamaguchi R, Uchida K, et al. Growth profiles of recent canine distemper isolates on Vero cells expressing canine signaling lymphocyte activation molecule (SLAM). J Comp Pathol. 2005;133(1):77-81.
13. Cory J, Yunker CE, Ormsbee RA, et al. Plaque assay of rickettsiae in a mammalian cell line. Appl Microbiol. 1974;27(6):1157-1161.
14. Buckley SM. Survival of *Toxoplasma gondii* in mosquito cell lines and establishment of continuous infection in Vero cell cultures. Exp Parasitol. 1973;33(1):23-26.
15. Cornwell HJ, Weir AR, Wright NG, et al. The susceptibility of a dog kidney cell-line (MDCK) to canine distemper, infectious canine hepatitis and canine herpesvirus. Res Vet Sci. 1970;11(6):580-582.
16. Basak S, Compans RW. Polarized entry of canine parvovirus into an epithelial cell line. J Virol. 1989;63(7):3164-3167.
17. England JJ, Poston RP. Electron microscopic identification and subsequent isolation of a rotavirus from a dog with fatal neonatal diarrhea. Am J Vet Res. 1980;41(5):782-783.
18. Bao L, Xu L, Zhan L, et al. Challenge and polymorphism analysis of the novel (H1N1) influenza virus to normal animals. Virus Res. 2010;151(1):60-65.
19. Essex M, Kawakami TG, Kurata K. Continuous long-term replication of feline leukemia virus (FeLV) in an established canine cell culture (MDCK). Proc Soc Exp Biol Med. 1972;139(1):295-299.
20. Nishikawa Y, Iwata A, Nagasawa H, et al. Comparison of the growth inhibitory effects of canine IFN-alpha, -beta, and -gamma on canine cells infected with *Neospora caninum* tachyzoites. J Vet Med Sci. 2001;63(4):445-458.
21. Crandell RA, Fabricant CG, Nelson-Rees WA. Development, characterization, and viral susceptibility of a feline (*Felis catus*) renal cell line (CRFK). In Vitro. 1973;9(3):176-185.
22. Kreutz LC, Seal BS, Mengeling WL. Early interaction of feline calicivirus with cells in culture. Arch Virol. 1994;136(1-2):19-34.
23. Van Hamme E, Dewerchin HL, Cornelissen E, et al. Attachment and internalization of feline infectious peritonitis virus in feline blood monocytes and Crandell feline kidney cells. J Gen Virol. 2007;88(Pt 9):2527-2532.
24. Hirasawa T, Tsujimura N, Konishi S. Multiplication of canine parvovirus in CRFK cells. Nippon Juigaku Zasshi. 1985;47(1):89-99.
25. Talbott RL, Sparger EE, Lovelace KM, et al. Nucleotide sequence and genomic organization of feline immunodeficiency virus. Proc Natl Acad Sci USA. 1989;86(15):5743-5747.
26. Goodman JL, Nelson C, Vitale B, et al. Direct cultivation of the causative agent of human granulocytic ehrlichiosis. N Engl J Med. 1996;334(4):209-215.
27. Binn LN, Marchwicki RH, Stephenson EH. Establishment of a canine cell line: derivation, characterization, and viral spectrum. Am J Vet Res. 1980;41(6):855-860.
28. Wills PJ, Johnson L, Thompson RG. Isolation of *Chlamydia* using McCoy cells and Buffalo green monkey cells. J Clin Pathol. 1984;37(2):120-121.
29. Mochizuki M, Mitsutake Y, Miyanohara Y, et al. Antigenic and plaque variations of serotype II feline infectious peritonitis coronaviruses. J Vet Med Sci. 1997;59(4):253-258.
30. Horimoto T, Kasaoka T, Tuchiya K, et al. An improved method for hemagglutinin extraction from feline herpesvirus type 1-infected cell line. Nippon Juigaku Zasshi. 1989;51(1):177-183.
31. Iqbal Z, Chaichanasiriwithaya W, Rikihisa Y. Comparison of PCR with other tests for early diagnosis of canine ehrlichiosis. J Clin Microbiol. 1994;32(7):1658-1662.

CHAPTER 2

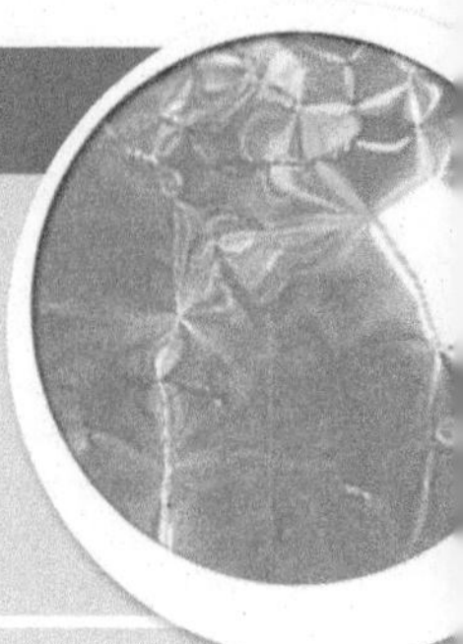

Immunoassays

Jane E. Sykes and Shelley C. Rankin

KEY POINTS

- Immunoassays are commonly used in practice to detect antigen or antibody in body fluids.
- The term *serology* is most often used to refer to assays that detect antibody in serum.
- Immunoassays that detect antigen or antibody in dogs and cats suspected to have infectious diseases include direct and indirect immunofluorescent antibody (IFA), immunohistochemistry (IHC), ELISA, Western immunoblotting, agglutination tests, gel immunodiffusion assays, and serum neutralization.
- Positive immunoassay results do not always imply infection, and negative results do not rule out infection.
- When interpreting the results of immunoassays, veterinarians should consider what is being measured (antigen or antibody), the likelihood of antigen or antibody being present in relation to the onset of illness, whether the positive test result is consistent with the animal's clinical signs, and the animal's vaccination history and immune status. The possibility of false positives due to immunologic cross-reactivity, as well as the analytical sensitivity and specificity of the test used (i.e., the test's performance), must also be considered.
- Additional assays may be required to support immunoassay test results.

INTRODUCTION

Serology refers to the measurement of antigen-antibody interactions for diagnostic purposes, but is most often used to refer to the detection of antibodies in serum. In general, a blood sample is *seroreactive* (or *seropositive*) if it contains antibodies to a particular pathogen. Assays have been designed that detect different classes of antibodies in serum, most commonly IgG or IgM. Methods used to detect antibodies can also be applied to detect antigen. They can also be used on body fluids other than serum, such as urine, cerebrospinal fluid, and aqueous humor. Assays that measure antigen-antibody interactions for diagnostic purposes are most broadly referred to as *immunoassays*. Types of immunoassays include immunofluorescent antibody (IFA) tests, ELISAs, agglutination tests, gel immunodiffusion tests (AGID or gel ID tests), and Western blotting. Many of these assays involve the use of *polyclonal antibodies*, or, more commonly, *monoclonal antibodies*, which are commercially available. Polyclonal antibodies are produced in animals (e.g., rabbits or horses) as a normal antibody response to antigen exposure. Monoclonal antibodies are produced in almost unlimited amounts in tissue culture, and have a higher degree of antigenic specificity.

Some immunoassays, such as ELISA and IFA, provide quantitative results, expressed as optical density units (ODs) or titers (e.g., 1:800, or *reciprocal titer* = 800). Exposure to an infectious agent results in a rise in antibody titer over time (Figure 2-1). Usually, the first antibody class to be produced by plasma cells is IgM, after which IgG synthesis by plasma cells occurs. When exposure to a pathogen occurs for the first time, there is a lag phase of 5 to 7 days before IgM antibodies can be detected in the blood *(primary antibody response)*. The antibody titer increases, and if the infectious agent is cleared, there is a progressive decline in the titer over weeks to months. The speed and magnitude by which the antibody titer rises depends on host factors and the infectious agent involved. For some diseases, such as leptospirosis, a significant rise occurs within 3 to 4 days of the onset of clinical signs. In secondary, or anamnestic, immune responses, the lag phase is shorter, the antibody titer increases more rapidly and to a greater magnitude, and antibodies may persist for longer periods of time (months to years).

Serologic diagnosis of infectious diseases relies on an understanding of the timing of the antibody response in relation to development of clinical signs for different infectious diseases. The results of serologic testing are interpreted differently for acute infections than they are for chronic or persistent infections. *For infections with a short incubation period,* such as leptospirosis or Rocky Mountain spotted fever, antibody titers are often negative in the first week of illness. In general, an increase in antibody titers over a 2- to 4-week period then occurs. *Seroconversion* is consistent with recent infection, and at least a fourfold increase in titer is required for the change to be considered significant. Because serologic test results can differ between laboratories that perform the same assay, the same laboratory should be used to determine the acute and the convalescent titer. Ideally, to minimize interassay variation, an aliquot of the acute specimen should be stored, frozen, and assayed at the same time as the convalescent specimen, although in reality this is often not done. A fourfold decline in antibody titer may also be consistent with recent infection, depending on the stage of illness at which serologic testing is performed. *For chronic, persistent infections,* such as FIV infection or canine leishmaniosis, a single, positive antibody titer can indicate active infection. Titer increases do not occur when infection persists beyond 1 to 2 months, and so acute- and convalescent-phase serology is not useful for diagnosis of chronic infections.

Specimen Collection and Transport

Blood collected for antibody testing should be allowed to clot, and the serum separated immediately and then refrigerated or

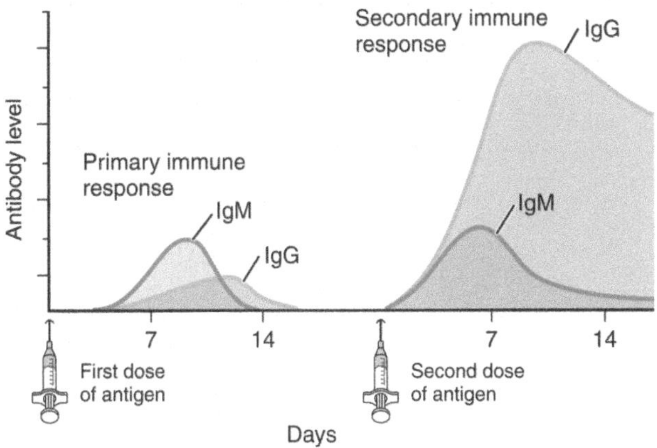

FIGURE 2-1 Time course of primary and secondary immune responses, showing relative amounts of IgM and IgG produced at different times after antigen exposure. (Modified from Tizard IR. Veterinary Immunology, 8 ed. St Louis: Saunders; 2008)

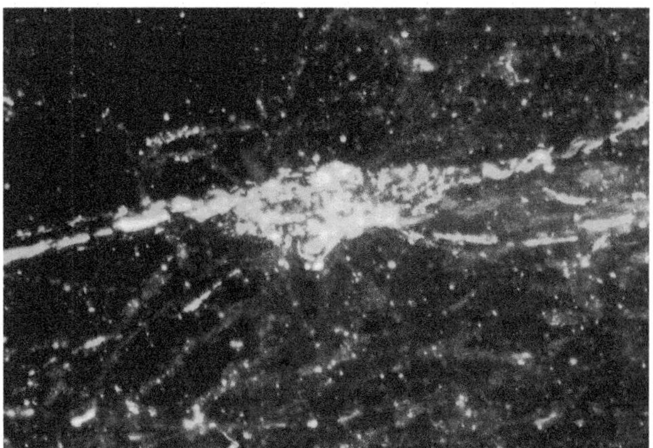

FIGURE 2-2 Direct fluorescent antibody stain of brain tissue for rabies virus. Frozen tissue sections were stained with a commercial reagent that contains three monoclonal antibodies specific for the rabies virus nucleocapsid. Antibodies were labeled with fluorescein. Positive staining is present in a Purkinje cell. (Courtesy of Galligan J. New York State Department of Health. In Maclachlan NJ, Dubovi EJ. Fenner's Veterinary Virology, 4 ed. New York: Elsevier; 2011.)

frozen. Specimens can be refrigerated for up to a week before they are shipped to the laboratory. If testing is to be delayed for longer than a week, specimens should be frozen at –20°C or –80°C. Specimens can be stored frozen for years without loss of antibody titer. For specimens collected for antigen testing, assay results may be more susceptible to variation with specimen storage. The laboratory should be contacted in order to determine specimen storage and handling requirements.

Diagnostic Methods

Immunofluorescent and Immunoperoxidase Antibody Assays

Direct IFA (also known as direct FA) detects *antigen* in clinical specimens. IFA involves the use of an antibody that has been tagged (*conjugated*) with a fluorescent label (such as fluorescein isothiocyanate) to detect the presence a specific antigen. IFA is performed directly on a glass slide, and fluorescence is detected by microscopy. The sensitivity of direct IFA is too low to detect individual virus particles or soluble antigen, so usually IFA detects antigen present in association with eukaryotic or bacterial cells. If the antigen is intracellular, pretreatment of the slide to permeabilize the cells may be necessary. The glass slide is then incubated with a solution that contains the fluorescent antibody, then washed to remove unbound antibody, and the cells are examined using a fluorescence microscope (Figure 2-2). Examples of the use of direct IFA in veterinary medicine include detection of *Giardia* oocysts, FeLV within monocytes in peripheral blood or bone marrow, or canine distemper virus within epithelial cells from a conjunctival scraping. Nonspecific fluorescence can result in false positives using these methods, but this can be overcome with the inclusion of proper controls and technical expertise. An alternative to the use of a fluorescein-conjugated antibody is the use of an antibody that has been conjugated to an enzyme such as horseradish peroxidase (immunoperoxidase). A substrate, most commonly 3,3′-diaminobenzidine (DAB), is then added to the slides. In the presence of hydrogen peroxide, DAB is converted to an insoluble brown precipitate, which can be visualized using conventional light microscopy. This technique is known as *immunocytochemistry*. The same method, when applied to tissue sections, is known as *immunohistochemistry* (IHC) (Figure 2-3).

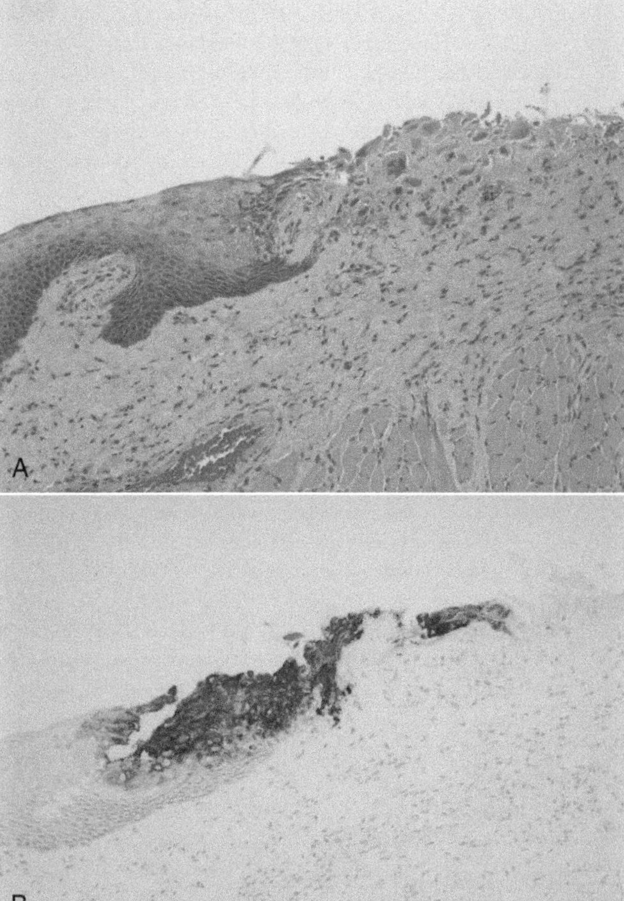

FIGURE 2-3 Immunohistochemistry. **A,** Hematoxylin and eosin stained section of a lingual ulcer from a cat infected with feline herpesvirus-1. **B,** The brown stained cells lining the ulcer are positive using an immunohistochemical stain for feline herpesvirus-1. (Courtesy of Dr. Patricia Pesavento, School of Veterinary Medicine, University of California, Davis.)

Indirect IFA (also known as IFA testing, or IFAT) is generally used to establish a serum *antibody* titer to an infectious agent, but it can also be used to detect antigen. When used to detect antigen, it is more sensitive than direct IFA. For measurement of antibody titers, patient serum is serially diluted in the laboratory

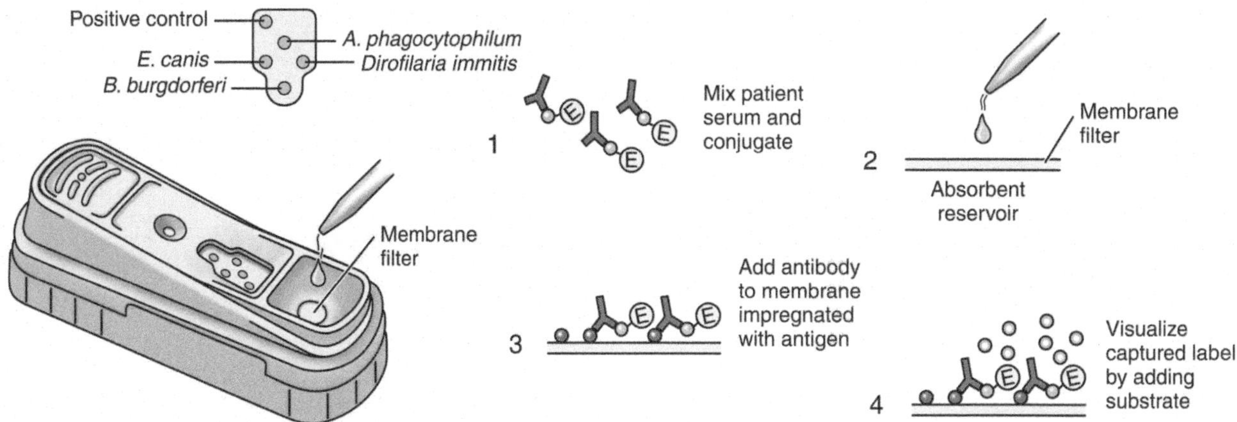

FIGURE 2-4 Flow-through immunoassay device (IDEXX Laboratories, Inc.). Specific antigen (for example, a recombinant protein) or antibody is immobilized on a membrane in the device in a spot or line. 1, Patient serum that may or may not contain target antigen or antibody is mixed with a solution that contains conjugated antibody or antigen. 2-3, The solution is allowed to flow through the device, where it becomes captured on the membrane. 4, The device is activated (snapped), which releases wash and substrate reagents within the device. A positive reaction appears as a colored bar, or in this case, a dot. Color development in designated spots on the membrane can indicate the presence of antibody to *Anaplasma* spp., *Ehrlichia canis*, and *Borrelia burgdorferi*, or the antigen of *Dirofilaria immitis*.

and reacted with a known antigen that has been fixed to glass slides. IFA slides are commercially manufactured for this purpose. Slides are then washed to remove unbound antibody. A *secondary antibody,* which is designed to react with the bound patient antibodies (e.g., dog IgG or dog IgM), is applied to the slides, which are then washed again. This secondary antibody has been conjugated to a fluorescent label. The slides are then examined using a fluorescence microscope. The highest dilution of serum that results in specific fluorescence is reported to the clinician as the antibody titer to the infectious agent of interest. Examples of the use of indirect IFA for serologic testing in dogs and cats include quantitative serology for some tick-borne infectious diseases (e.g., *Ehrlichia canis*, *Anaplasma* spp.).

More recently, veterinary immunofluorescence assays have been marketed that allow multiple antigen (or antibody) targets to be mounted on novel platforms, such as fluorescent beads or wells on the surface of a spinning silicon disc that resembles a compact disc. Automated silicon disc–based assays allow rapid and simultaneous analysis of hundreds of specimens, with dramatic reduction in labor associated with traditional IFA or ELISA assays, and reduced chance of false-positive or -negative assay results due to human error. A bead-based assay is currently available in the United States for detection of antibody to *Borrelia burgdorferi* (see Chapter 51). A silicon disc–based assay is available in the United States for detection of antibodies to *B. burgdorferi, E. canis,* and *Anaplasma phagocytophilum* and antigen to *Dirofilaria immitis* (Accuplex 4, Antech Diagnostics, Irvine, Calif). The performance of these assays in the field is under investigation.

Enzyme Linked Immunosorbent Assays

ELISA (also known as *enzyme immunoassay*) can be used to detect either antigen or antibody. In the laboratory, it is usually performed in a polystyrene microtiter plate. However, in-clinic modifications of the test, such as flow-through or lateral-flow ELISAs (e.g., SNAP, IDEXX Laboratories, Inc.), whereby antigen or capture antibody is immobilized on a membrane filter, are widely used in veterinary practices (e.g., for diagnosis of feline retroviral, heartworm, *Giardia*, *Leishmania*, and tick-borne infections) (Figure 2-4). For *antigen* detection, an unknown quantity of antigen in a clinical specimen is immobilized in the wells of the plate. The antigen is either bound directly to the surface of the plate or is bound through the use of a *capture antibody*, which is an antibody that is bound to the plate surface that specifically binds to the antigen of interest *(sandwich ELISA)*. The antigen is then detected with an antibody that is conjugated to an enzyme such as immunoperoxidase, and the substrate is added. This results in a color change, which can be read visually or using an ELISA plate reader (Figure 2-5). The plate reader records optical density of the wells in comparison to that of control wells, allowing assessment of the quantity of antigen present. The plates are washed with a detergent solution between steps, and this can be automated using an ELISA plate washer. Sandwich ELISAs have been used widely for detection of FeLV antigen in cat blood. In *competitive ELISA,* the test specimen (e.g., dog serum), which contains an unknown amount of antigen, is mixed with a known amount of labeled antigen. The mixture is added to wells that contain known amounts of a capture antibody, and the labeled and unlabeled antigens compete for antibody binding. The more labeled antigen that binds, the less antigen is present in the test specimen. Other variations of competitive ELISAs also exist.

For *antibody* detection, serial dilutions of patient serum can be added to a known amount of antigen fixed on a plate and detected using a secondary antibody.

Western Immunoblotting

Western immunoblotting, also known as *Western blotting,* is also used to detect antibodies to an infectious agent in patient serum. After physical and/or chemical disruption of an organism, the proteins are then separated on the basis of molecular mass using vertical sodium dodecyl sulfate–polyacrylamide gel electrophoresis (SDS-PAGE). The protein bands are then transferred *(blotted)* to a nitrocellulose membrane using an electric current. The membrane is cut into vertical strips, and each strip is probed with serial dilutions of patient serum. If there are antibodies in the serum to antigens from the organism of interest, the antibodies bind to the antigens on the strip. The antigen-antibody complexes can then be visualized as discrete bands using immunoperoxidase detection methods. The pattern of band reactivity is specific for an immune response to that organism (Figure 2-6). Western blotting is offered commercially

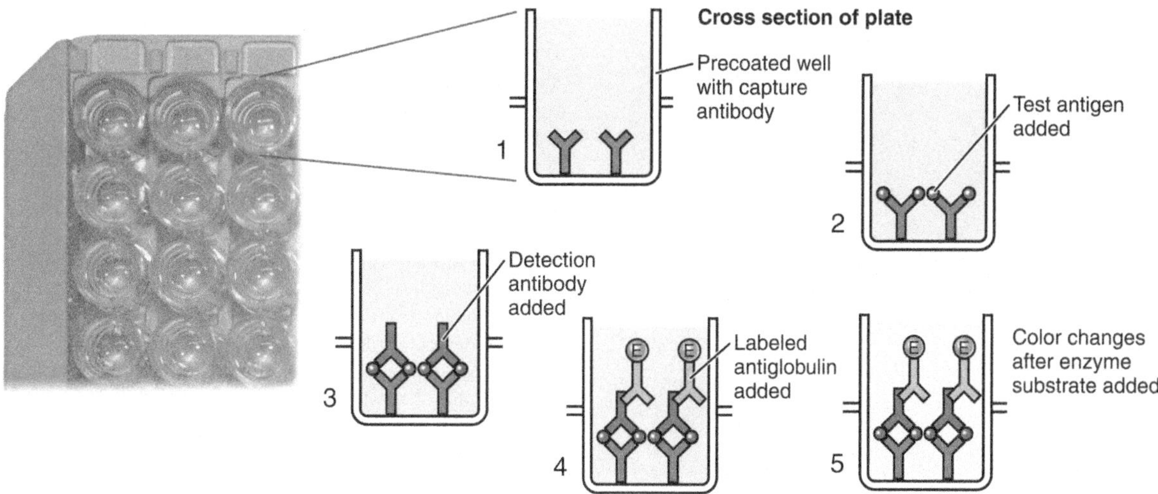

FIGURE 2-5 Sandwich ELISA. An antibody is immobilized in the plate, which binds antigen in a test specimen. The antigen is then detected using an antibody that is conjugated to an enzyme such as immunoperoxidase, and the substrate is added, which results in a color change. (Modified from Tizard IR. Veterinary Immunology, 8 ed. St Louis: Saunders; 2008.)

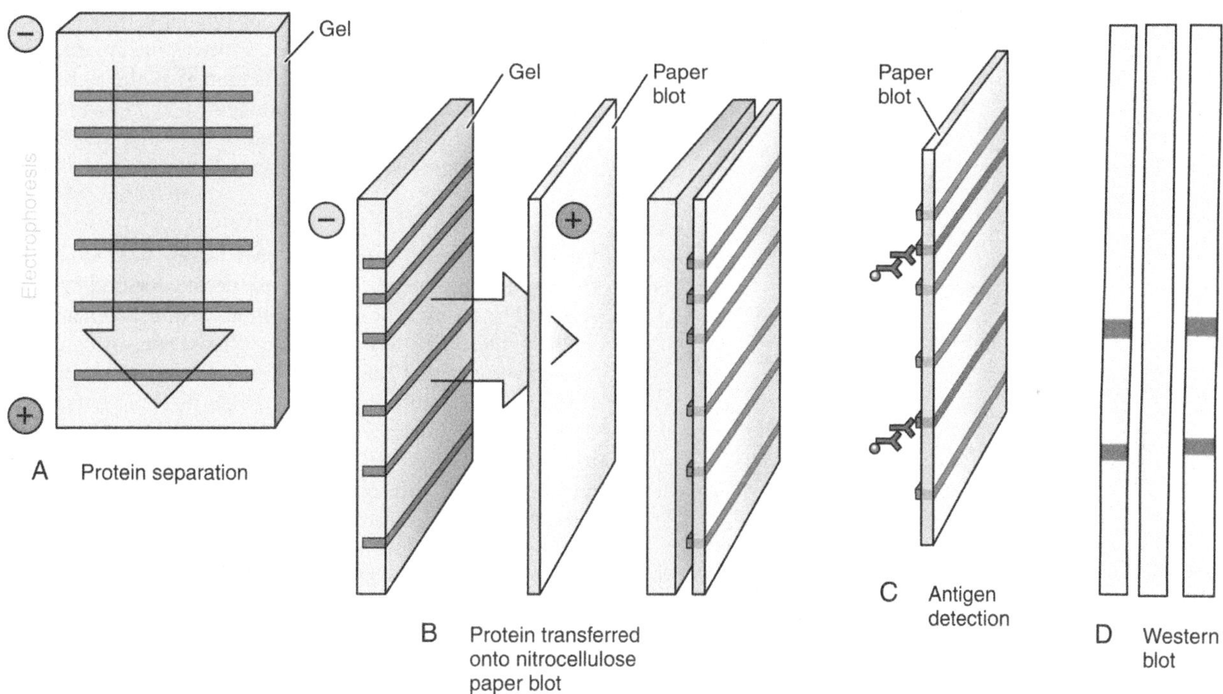

FIGURE 2-6 Western blotting (immunoblotting). Purified viruses or bacteria are disrupted and subjected to electrophoresis along the length of a polyacrylamide gel, so that the proteins are separated according to their molecular weight (**A**). The bands are then transferred to a nitrocellulose paper membrane (**B**) and probed with patient serum (**C**). The strip shown on the right is a Western blot that shows antibody reactivity to the antigens of FIV (**D**). (Original blot courtesy of IDEXX Laboratories, Inc.)

for the diagnosis of FIV and *B. burgdorferi* infection and has been used in research laboratories as the gold standard for the detection of antibody responses to vector-borne pathogens such as *E. canis*. In the case of FIV infection, Western blotting has been used to confirm positive ELISA test results.[1] In the case of *B. burgdorferi* infection, Western blotting has been evaluated for its ability to differentiate between the response to vaccination and natural exposure.[2]

Agglutination Testing

Agglutination tests detect antibody or antigen and involve agglutination of bacteria, red cells, or antigen- or antibody-coated latex particles. They rely on the bivalent nature of antibodies, which can cross-link particulate antigens. Serial dilutions of serum are tested for their ability to cause or inhibit agglutination, and the highest dilution that causes or inhibits agglutination is reported as the antibody or antigen titer. IgM causes agglutination more effectively than IgG. If excess antibody is present, particles may become so coated with antibody that agglutination is actually inhibited. This is called the *prozone effect* and can result in false-negative test results if serum is not adequately diluted. Examples of agglutination tests that are used to diagnose infectious diseases of dogs and cats include the microscopic agglutination test (MAT) for serologic diagnosis of leptospirosis

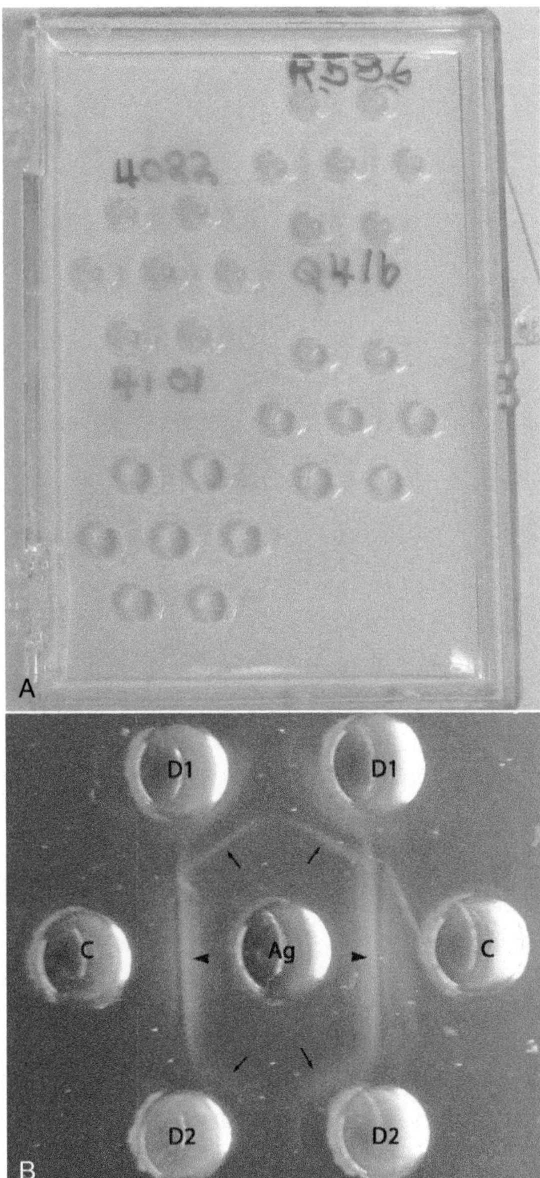

FIGURE 2-7 **A,** Gel immunodiffusion (or double diffusion) system used for detection of antibodies to *Aspergillus fumigatus, Histoplasma capsulatum, Blastomyces dermatitidis,* and *Coccidioides immitis* (Meridian Bioscience, Inc.). The kit consists of an agar diffusion medium in a small plastic tray that contains four arrays of six wells arranged around a central well. An antigen preparation for each of the fungal species is placed in the central well of each array. **B,** Positive gel immunodiffusion for *Aspergillus fumigatus*. The central well *(Ag)* contains a purified carbohydrate preparation from mycelial phase cultures of *Aspergillus fumigatus, Aspergillus niger,* and *Aspergillus flavus*. The top two wells *(D1)* and the bottom two wells *(D2)* contain serum from 2 dogs (dog 1 and dog 2) with nasal aspergillosis (performed in duplicate for each dog). After the wells are loaded, the plate is incubated at room temperature for 24 hours. Precipitin lines form when the antigen and antibody diffuse out of each well and form immune complexes. A light box is used to illuminate the plate so the precipitin bands are visible. Both dogs are positive for antibody to the *Aspergillus* species tested *(small arrows),* although the reaction is strongest for dog 1. The *arrowheads* are the precipitin lines generated by the positive control antibodies (in wells labeled *C*).

(agglutination of live leptospires) and the cryptococcal antigen latex agglutination test (agglutination of antibody-coated latex beads). Hemagglutination inhibition (HI) is used to determine antibody titers to canine parvovirus and canine influenza virus, and it evaluates the ability of serum to inhibit erythrocyte agglutination by these viruses.

Agar Gel Immunodiffusion

For *agar gel immunodiffusion* (AGID, gel ID or double diffusion) tests, round wells are cut in a layer of agar on a plastic plate using a punch. One well, usually the central well, is filled with a soluble antigen, and the other wells are filled with patient serum. A positive antibody control specimen is included in each assay. The reagents are allowed to diffuse into the agar, and when antibodies and antigen meet in optimal proportions (the *point of equivalence*), immune complexes form. This results in a visible line of precipitate between the antigen well and wells that contain positive serum (Figure 2-7). Immunodiffusion testing is most often used to detect antibodies to fungal pathogens in dogs, such as *Aspergillus fumigatus,*[3] *Coccidioides immitis,*[4] and *Blastomyces dermatitidis.*[5] It is also used to detect antibodies to *Brucella canis.*

Serum Neutralization

Serum neutralization is a technique used to determine the antibody titer to viruses. Serial dilutions of patient serum are mixed with a known quantity of virus particles. The mixture is incubated to allow the antibodies in the patient serum to bind to the virus particles, and the mixture is then added to a confluent cell monolayer. The highest dilution of patient serum that inhibits viral replication in the monolayer (as determined by examination for cytopathic effect or immunostaining) is the antibody titer reported by the laboratory. Serum neutralization can be used to detect antibodies to canine distemper virus and several respiratory viruses that infect dogs and cats.

Complement Fixation Testing

Complement fixation (CF) tests have largely been superseded by the use of ELISA tests. The CF test detects antibodies in patient serum. The serum is heat-treated to inactivate complement in the test specimen. The test uses sheep RBCs, anti–sheep RBC antibody, and unheated guinea pig serum as a source of complement. Under normal circumstances, when these three reagents are mixed, the result is hemolysis. Hemolysis occurs when complement binds to antibody-coated RBC and triggers formation of the membrane attack complex, with resultant pore formation. In the CF test, a known antigen is added to the heat-treated patient serum. When antibodies are present in the serum, the addition of this antigen leads to the formation of antigen-antibody complexes. Guinea pig complement is then added to the mixture and is consumed by the complexes. The resultant mixture is thus unable to lyse sensitized sheep RBCs. A lack of hemolysis indicates a positive CF test.

Interpretation of Results

To interpret the results of serology or immunoassay tests, the clinician first needs to consider whether the test was designed to detect antibody or antigen (Tables 2-1 and 2-2), and, if designed to detect antibody, whether it was IgM-specific (detects early antibody responses). The results also have to be interpreted in light of the pathogenesis of the infectious disease, specifically the timing of antigen and antibody appearance in the body fluid being tested. Finally, the sensitivity and specificity of the test itself need to be considered (i.e., the *analytical sensitivity and specificity*), which are determined during test validation (Table 2-3). For example, some immunoassays that detect antigen will not generate a positive result unless a large amount of antigen is present in the specimen provided (low analytical sensitivity). Test analytical sensitivity and specificity should be available from the laboratory that performs the test. False-positive test

TABLE 2-1

Guidelines for Interpretation of Test Results Using Immunoassays That Detect Antigen

Antigen Test Result	Possible Explanation	Troubleshooting Suggestions
Negative	Pathogen of interest not present	Confirm with additional diagnostic test if necessary, (e.g., alternative antigen assay, antibody or PCR assay)
	Antigen present, but quantity below limit of detection	Consider an antibody or PCR assay
	Antigen present but complexed by antibody and not available for detection	Consider an antibody or PCR assay
	Technical error or reagent failure	Identified with inclusion of appropriate laboratory controls
Positive	Pathogen of interest present	Confirm with additional diagnostic test if necessary, especially in regions with a low prevalence of infection. Antigen presence may not imply that the pathogen is the cause of disease
	Antigen present but viable microbe absent	Confirm with additional diagnostic test
	Vaccine antigen present	Obtain vaccination history and consider a test that discriminates between vaccine and wild-type organisms, if available
	Cross-reactive antigen present from another substance or pathogen	Obtain history and consider the likelihood of infection with related agents
	Technical error	Identified with inclusion of appropriate controls by the laboratory
	Poor assay analytical specificity (prone to generate false-positives)	Use alternative assay

TABLE 2-2

Guidelines for Interpretation of Test Results Using Immunoassays That Detect Antibody

Antibody Test Result	Possible Explanation	Troubleshooting Suggestions
Negative	Exposure to pathogen of interest did not occur	Confirm with additional diagnostic test if necessary
	Too early in course of infection/illness	Obtain convalescent titer; consider an antigen or PCR test for early diagnosis
	Severe immunosuppression	Consider an antigen or PCR test
	Technical error	Identified with inclusion of appropriate controls by the laboratory
	Poor assay analytical sensitivity (prone to false-negatives)	Use alternative assay
Positive	Previous natural exposure to the pathogen of interest	If infection is chronic and persistent, positive test results may equal active infection.
	Previous immunization against the pathogen of interest	Obtain vaccination history; consider use of assays that discriminate between natural exposure and vaccine antibody, if available
	Immunologic cross-reactivity	Obtain history and consider the likelihood of previous exposure to related agents
	Technical error	Identified with inclusion of appropriate controls by the laboratory
	Poor assay specificity (prone to false-positives)	Use alternative assay. Consider the use of a confirmatory test, especially in regions with low disease prevalence

TABLE 2-3

Sensitivity, Specificity, Positive and Negative Predictive Value

Test Attribute	Definition
Sensitivity	Number of truly positive animals that are identified as positive by the test, divided by the total number of animals that are truly positive (as determined by the gold standard assay) (%). A test with low sensitivity fails to detect many positive animals (many false-negative results).
Specificity	Number of truly negative animals that are identified as negative by the test, divided by the total number of animals that are truly negative (as determined by the gold standard assay) (%). A test with low specificity generates many false-positive test results.
Positive predictive value	The number of animals that are truly positive divided by the total number of animals that test positive (true positives plus false positives).
Negative predictive value	The number of animals that are truly negative divided by the total number of animals that test negative (true negatives plus false negatives).
Etiologic predictive value*	The proportion of animals with positive test results that truly have the disease of interest, as opposed to carriage of an organism in the absence of disease.

*Gunnarson, RK, Lanke J. The predictive value of microbiologic diagnostic tests if asymptomatic carriers are present. Statist Med 2002; 21:1773–1785.

results due to low analytical specificity are more likely when testing animals from populations where the prevalence of true positive test results is low. In this situation, a test has a *low positive predictive value,* and confirmatory testing may be required. A quality assurance program should be in effect within the laboratory to ensure that specimens submitted are of adequate quality, that sufficient technical expertise is present to perform the tests, and that appropriate control assays are included with each run to ensure proper assay performance.

Negative Results for Antigen Detection

Negative results for antigen will occur if the antigen is not present in the specimen being tested. They may also occur if the amount of antigen is below the limit of detection of the assay (e.g., low worm burden in heartworm disease). For some infectious agents, such as FIV, antigen testing is not performed because antigen levels during infection are typically extremely low. The amount of antigen present can also vary over the course of a particular infection. Finally, false-negative results may occur when antibody present in the specimen complexes antigen and makes it unavailable for detection by the immunoassay.

Positive Results for Antigen Detection

Positive results for antigen can indicate the presence of the suspected pathogen in the specimen. They do not necessarily imply that the pathogen is the cause of an animal's clinical signs. Antigen can also be present in the absence of intact, viable organisms. Positive results can follow recent vaccination with the pathogen of interest. For example, positive fecal parvovirus antigen tests can occasionally occur in fecal specimens obtained several days after attenuated live virus vaccination of kittens for feline panleukopenia virus.[6] False positives can occur as a result of antigenic cross-reactivity with some other substance or organism in the specimen. An example is positive serum and urine antigen assays for *Aspergillus* spp. in dogs treated with Plasmalyte infusions or those infected with other molds such as *Paecilomyces* spp.[7]

Negative Results for Antibody Detection

Negative results for antibody will occur if the patient has not been exposed to the infectious agent of interest. They may also occur if the patient has not yet had time to develop antibodies. For example, negative antibody tests early in the course of illness are common with leptospirosis and canine granulocytic anaplasmosis. In this situation, a convalescent titer is required for diagnosis using serology. Negative antibody test results can occur in severely immunosuppressed animals, such as in cats with advanced FIV infection that no longer can mount an immune response, or cats with advanced feline infectious peritonitis. Negative results may also occur because the test lacks sensitivity (i.e., low analytical sensitivity).

Positive Results for Antibody Detection

Positive results for IgG antibody suggest *previous exposure* to a pathogen and do not necessarily indicate active infection. Paired IgG titers are required to document recent infection. Single positive results for IgM-specific assays may indicate a recent infection or a chronic infection that continues to stimulate the immune system. Previous immunization may also result in positive results. If the infection is chronic and persistent, such as with FIV infection, positive results indicate active infection, provided there has been no history of previous FIV vaccination. False-positive results for antibody may also occur when antigenic cross-reactivity occurs. For example, dogs recovering from *Leptospira* infection have been shown to test positive on IFA for the related spirochete *B. burgdorferi.*

REFERENCES

1. Levy J, Crawford C, Hartmann K, et al. 2008 American Association of Feline Practitioners' feline retrovirus management guidelines. J Feline Med Surg. 2008;10(3):300-316.
2. Leschnik MW, Kirtz G, Khanakah G, et al. Humoral immune response in dogs naturally infected with *Borrelia burgdorferi* sensu lato and in dogs after immunization with a *Borrelia* vaccine. Clin Vaccine Immunol. 2010;17(5):828-835.
3. Pomrantz JS, Johnson LR, Nelson RW, et al. Comparison of serologic evaluation via agar gel immunodiffusion and fungal culture of tissue for diagnosis of nasal aspergillosis in dogs. J Am Vet Med Assoc. 2007;230(9):1319-1323.
4. Pappagianis D, Zimmer BL. Serology of coccidioidomycosis. Clin Microbiol Rev. 1990;3(3):247-268.
5. Spector D, Legendre AM, Wheat J, et al. Antigen and antibody testing for the diagnosis of blastomycosis in dogs. J Vet Intern Med. 2008;22(4):839-843.
6. Patterson EV, Reese MJ, Tucker SJ, et al. Effect of vaccination on parvovirus antigen testing in kittens. J Am Vet Med Assoc. 2007;230(3):359-363.
7. Garcia RS, Wheat LJ, Cook AK, et al. Sensitivity and specificity of a blood and urine galactomannan antigen assay for diagnosis of systemic aspergillosis in dogs. J Vet Intern Med. 2012;26:911-919.

CHAPTER 3

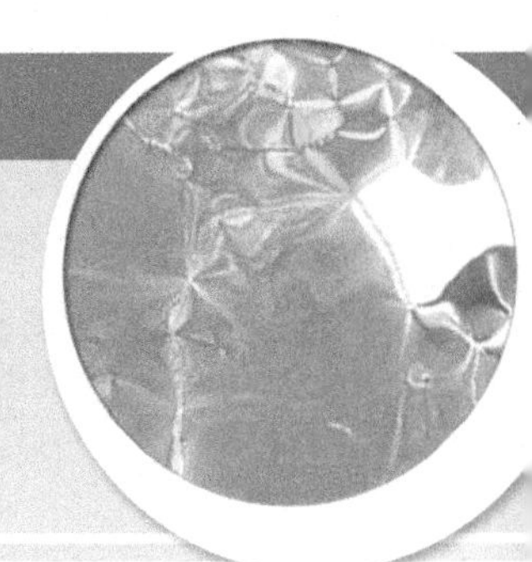

Isolation and Identification of Aerobic and Anaerobic Bacteria

Jane E. Sykes and Shelley C. Rankin

KEY POINTS

- Because of the increasing prevalence of antimicrobial drug resistance among bacteria isolated from dogs and cats, culture and susceptibility is always recommended when a bacterial infection is suspected at a normally sterile anatomic site.
- Successful isolation of aerobic and anaerobic bacteria from a clinical specimen relies on collection of a sufficient quantity of material, from the correct location, and appropriate storage and transport of the specimen to the laboratory. Care should be taken to prevent specimen contamination during collection.
- The laboratory should be provided with an appropriate history if fastidious, anaerobic, or slow-growing bacterial organisms are suspected.
- Concurrent examination of a Gram-stained smear by the laboratory assists in assessment of specimen quality and interpretation of culture results.
- Antimicrobial susceptibility testing is most commonly performed using broth microdilution or agar diffusion testing and aims to determine the minimum concentration of an antimicrobial drug that inhibits growth of the organism in vitro (minimum inhibitory concentration, or MIC). The laboratory uses MIC breakpoints, which are established and revised regularly by national standards agencies, to assess the susceptibility of an organism to a particular antimicrobial drug.

INTRODUCTION

Factors that influence the detection of clinically relevant organisms in specimens collected from dogs and cats are:

1. An appropriate level of suspicion for the presence of a bacterial infection;
2. Development of a list of differential diagnoses that reflects the types of bacterial pathogens that might be the cause of clinical signs, because of the requirement of some bacteria for special transport conditions, culture conditions, or prolonged incubation;
3. Collection of a sufficient *amount* of specimen;
4. Collection of the *correct type* of specimen;
5. Specimen collection from the *correct anatomic location;* and
6. Proper handling, storage and transport of the specimen, which should be sent with a request for culture to the laboratory within acceptable time limits.

These factors cannot be overemphasized. Without them, time and money invested in collection of specimens and culture is wasted.

Given the increasing prevalence of multidrug resistance among bacteria that infect dogs and cats, veterinarians should make attempts to confirm a bacterial infection at a normally sterile site by requesting microscopic evaluation of direct smears and culture by a laboratory whenever possible before the choice is made to administer an antimicrobial drug.

The purpose of this chapter is to provide information in regard to the correct way to collect and handle specimens for culture before they are sent to the laboratory, and to outline bacteriologic procedures performed in the microbiology laboratory that are of relevance to the small animal clinician.

Specimen Collection and Transport

Veterinary clinicians should collect specimens for culture using an *appropriate method* from the *correct anatomic site.* Collection of a sufficient *amount* of specimen is very important. Table 3-1 suggests optimal specimen types for detection of bacteria from specific anatomic sites. Attempts should always be made to prevent contamination with commensal bacteria during specimen collection. When anaerobes are suspected, aspirates or biopsies should be obtained rather than swabs, and the specimen should be stored at room temperature and not refrigerated. This is because oxygen diffuses into cold specimens more rapidly than specimens held at room temperature.

Specimens should be transported to the laboratory immediately. As a general rule for aerobic culture, if transport requires longer than 2 hours, appropriate transport medium should be used or specimens should be refrigerated without transport medium. Although specimens can be held for up to 72 hours, culture of specimens older than 24 hours should be avoided, even if they have been refrigerated or placed in transport media, because of increased likelihood of false positive and false negative results with longer storage times. Transport medium for bacterial culture is usually supplied in a plastic tube with one or two swabs attached to the tube's cap (Figure 3-1). The medium is designed to maintain bacterial viability without causing significant growth. It usually consists of a small amount of agar, reagents that maintain pH, a colorimetric pH indicator that indicates whether oxidation has occurred, and specific factors that maintain the viability of certain pathogens. Some organisms, such as chlamydiae and leptospires, have specific transport medium requirements. Specimens that are placed in transport media should not be refrigerated.

Specimens should be labeled with the patient's name, patient number, source of specimen, and the date and time of collection, and should be labeled, packaged, and transported according to regional and national regulations (see Chapter 1). Specimens for anaerobic culture should preferably be transported in an oxygen-free container.

TABLE 3-1

Suggested Specimen Types for Bacterial Culture from Selected Anatomic Sites and Likely Pathogens Present

Specimen Type	Suggested Volume for Culture	Likely Pathogens Present
Blood	≥10 mL for patients weighing >10 kg, or 1% of patient blood volume	Gram-positive and gram-negative aerobes. Common contaminants are coagulase-negative staphylococci, *Corynebacterium*, *Bacillus* spp., and propionibacteria (see Chapter 86)
CSF	≥0.5 mL	Gram-positive and gram-negative aerobes, anaerobes, *Brucella* spp. (dogs), *Nocardia*, *Actinomyces*,[1] *Mycoplasma* spp. (cats)[2] (see Chapter 90)
Middle ear	Aspirate of fluid or pus through tympanic membrane	Gram-positive and gram-negative aerobes, anaerobes, *Mycoplasma* spp., *Actinomyces* spp.[2,3] (see Chapter 84)
Skin	Swab from epidermal collarette or ruptured pustule (superficial pyoderma); biopsy from which dermis has been removed (deep pyoderma)	Gram-positive aerobes (especially staphylococci), rarely *Pseudomonas aeruginosa* (see Chapter 84)
External ear	Swab ear canal after removing debris and crusts from the canal	Gram-positive aerobes, *Pseudomonas aeruginosa* (see Chapter 84)
Cornea	Scrape or swab exposed corneal stroma and inoculate directly onto media. Referral to veterinary ophthalmologist recommended	Gram-positive aerobes, *Mycoplasma* spp., *Pseudomonas aeruginosa*[4]
Abdominal fluid	1-5 mL	Gram-negative and gram-positive aerobes, anaerobes, *Actinomyces* spp. (see Chapter 88)
Pleural fluid	1-5 mL	Gram-negative and gram-positive aerobes, anaerobes, *Actinomyces* spp., *Nocardia* spp., *Mycoplasma* spp. (see Chapter 87)
Feces	Fresh whole stools preferred. Avoid swabs or fecal loops containing fecal matter due to low specimen size. Submit in clean, dry leak-proof container.	*Escherichia coli*, *Salmonella*, *Clostridium perfringens*, *Clostridium difficile*, *Campylobacter* spp., *Anaerobiospirillum* (Chapters 45-49 and 88)
Urine	1-5 mL urine collected using cystocentesis	Gram-negative and gram-positive aerobes, *Corynebacterium urealyticum* (see Chapter 89)
Bronchoalveolar lavage specimens	1-5 mL	Gram-positive and gram-negative aerobes, anaerobes (aspiration pneumonia), *Mycoplasma* spp., rarely *Mycobacterium* spp. (see Chapter 87)

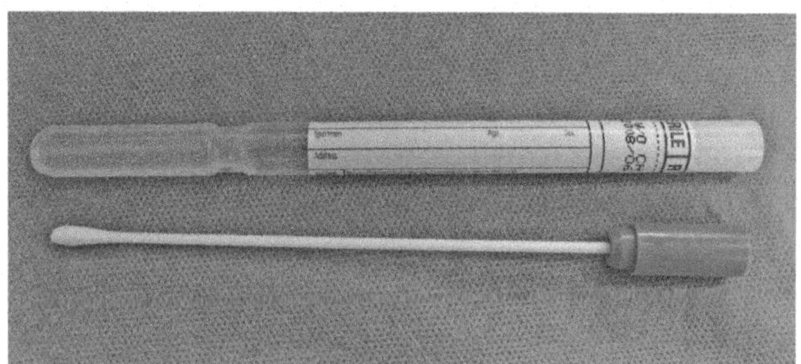

FIGURE 3-1 Swab system containing transport media for aerobic bacterial culture.

Diagnostic Methods

Microscopic Examination of Direct Smears

A Gram stain prepared from the specimen can permit the rapid preliminary diagnosis of infection and determine whether the organism(s) present are gram-positive or gram-negative (Box 3-1; Figure 3-2). This helps guide the clinician to select an appropriate empiric therapy, if necessary, while awaiting the results of culture and susceptibility testing. If sufficient material is available, examination of a direct smear also helps to determine whether a specimen is adequate for culture and aids interpretation of culture results. For swab or aspirate specimens, clinicians should consider providing a separate specimen for a direct smear in addition to a specimen for culture.

Acid-fast stains can be used on smears to assist in the identification of *Nocardia* and *Mycobacterium* spp., as well as on fecal smears to detect some parasitic oocysts, such as those of *Cryptosporidium*. These organisms stain magenta as a result of their high cell wall mycolic acid content, which in turn results in their resistance to decolorization after staining (which is often performed using an acid-alcohol solvent, hence the term *acid-fast*). Examples of acid-fast staining methods are the *Ziehl-Neelsen*, *Fite's*, and *Kinyoun* stains.

Other microscopic techniques used for bacterial identification in specialized laboratories include *darkfield microscopy*, *phase-contrast microscopy*, and *fluorescence microscopy* (see Chapter 2). Darkfield and phase contrast microscopy allow visualization of organisms without fixation and staining, so motility as well as structure can be assessed. In darkfield microscopy, the

BOX 3-1

Procedure for Gram Staining

Heat-fix specimen on the slide over a gentle flame or fix in 95% methanol for 2 min, and then air dry
Flood with crystal violet solution for 15 to 60 s (10 g of 90% dye in 500 mL absolute methanol)
Wash with water
Flood with iodine for 15 to 60 s (6 g of I_2 and 12 g of KI in 1800 mL of water)
Decolorize with acetone-alcohol (400 mL of acetone in 1200 mL of 95% ethanol)
Wash immediately
Counterstain with safranin for 15 to 60 s (10 g of dye in 1L of water)
Wash, blot dry, and examine using light microscopy

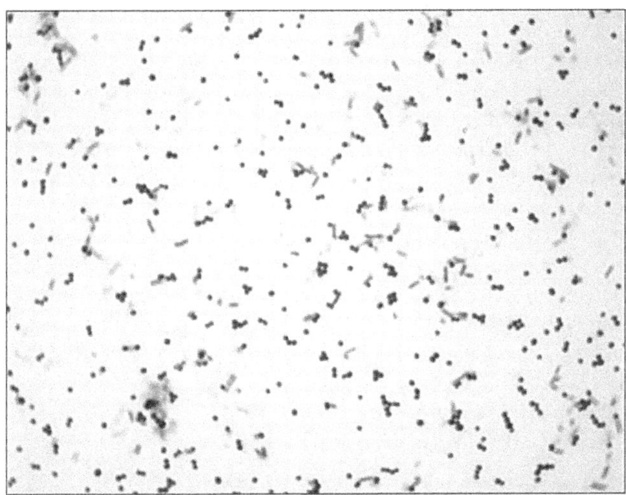

FIGURE 3-2 Gram-stained smear of gram-positive cocci *(dark blue)* and gram-negative rods *(red)* (1600× oil magnification).

condenser only permits light that bounces off an object to pass from below up into the objective, so the object appears bright against a dark background. Darkfield microscopy is used primarily for identification of fine spirochetes such as leptospires, which cannot be visualized using conventional microscopy (see Chapter 50). In phase-contrast microscopy, slowing and deflection of beams of light occur as they pass through an object.

Bacterial Culture

The performance of bacterial culture for diagnostic purposes requires appropriate laboratory facilities, proper biosafety level-2 containment, properly trained individuals, reference strains for quality control testing, and the use of standard protocols.[5] Media used for bacterial culture may be categorized as general-purpose, enriched, selective, differential, and specialized media (Table 3-2). Some media belong to more than one of these categories. For example, MacConkey agar is both a selective and a differential medium (Figure 3-3). Media for culture contains a nutrient source, most commonly peptones (hydrolyzed animal or vegetable substances), and is adjusted to a specific pH. Solid medium contains agar, which is derived from seaweed. Other nutrients may be added based on specific organism requirements. More than 100 different types of bacteriology media exist, most of which can be purchased as preprepared plates or broth.

Blood culture media contain the anticoagulant sodium polyanethol sulfonate (SPS), which is less inhibitory to bacterial growth than other anticoagulants. Some blood culture media (e.g., BD BACTEC Plus) contain resin beads that bind antimicrobial drugs in the patient's blood specimen, so they do not inhibit bacterial growth (Figure 3-4). The detection of bacterial growth in blood culture systems can be automated using instrumentation that measures emission of fluorescence or a colorimetric change in a sensor. The change occurs as CO_2 concentrations within the bottle increase, which indicates the presence of bacterial growth. Some instruments detect pressure changes in the head of the bottle. The culture is monitored at regular intervals by the instrument, to optimize early detection of bacterial growth. Positive blood culture bottles are then evaluated by performing a Gram stain of the broth, and subculture to appropriate media.

TABLE 3-2

Types of Media Used in Bacteriology

Medium Type	Attributes	Example
Transport	Nonnutritive liquid or semisolid medium. Promotes organism viability without allowing significant growth.	Amies transport medium
General-purpose	Allows growth of most aerobic and facultatively anaerobic organisms	Sheep blood agar
Enriched	Promotes growth of fastidious organisms that require specific nutrients, for example *Francisella*	Chocolate agar, which is enriched with heat-treated blood, which gives it a brown color
Selective	Selects for growth of certain organisms while inhibiting others	MacConkey agar, which selects for gram-negative bacteria
Differential	Aids in preliminary identification of organisms based on colony appearance	MacConkey agar, which promotes pink colony formation by organisms that ferment lactose
Specialized	Selects for a specific pathogen through the addition of specific nutrients	Anaerobic medium, which contains hemin, vitamin K, and reducing agents

Another blood culture system is the Isolator lysis centrifugation system (DuPont, Wilmington, DE) (See Figure 3-4, *B*). In this system, blood is added to a tube that contains anticoagulant and a reagent that induces RBC lysis. The tube is centrifuged, and the pellet is plated onto agar media and incubated. This method allows colony counts to be obtained. The tubes allow isolation not only of aerobes, but also some anaerobic bacteria.

In the laboratory, media for bacterial culture should be warmed to room temperature before inoculation, and damaged media, such as dehydrated medium or medium that has changed color, should not be used. Medium is stored in the dark at 2°C to 8°C and discarded when it reaches its expiration date. After plating, incubation is most commonly performed at 35°C to 37°C in air for a minimum of 2 days. Conditions vary for specific bacteria, and growth in 3% to 5% CO_2 is preferred by some fastidious organisms. The laboratory should be informed, by providing an adequate clinical history, when pathogens with special culture requirements are suspected, such as *Campylobacter, Mycoplasma, Actinomyces, Nocardia,* and *Mycobacterium* spp. These organisms require special media or prolonged incubation times (e.g., weeks). Specimens for anaerobic culture should be plated onto appropriate media immediately and incubated in an anaerobic environment. Anaerobic containers, which create an anaerobic environment through the use of gas-generating reagents, can be used for incubation (Figure 3-5). Because anaerobes grow more slowly than aerobes, anaerobic cultures should be held for 7 days before being reported as negative.

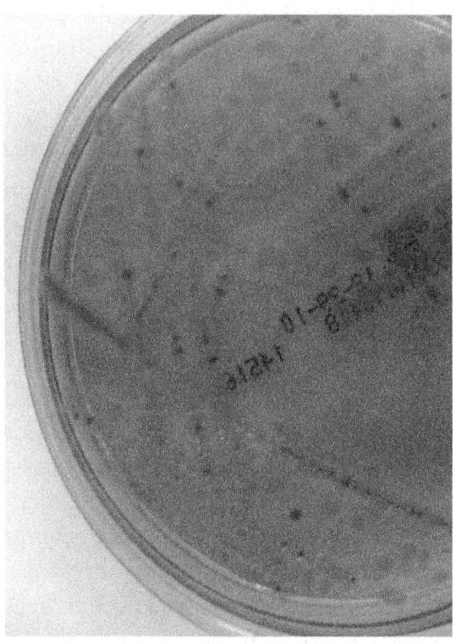

FIGURE 3-3 Growth of bacteria on MacConkey medium that shows the selective and differential qualities of the medium. The medium contains substances that inhibit the growth of gram-positive bacteria. By using the lactose available in the medium, bacteria such as *Escherichia coli*, *Enterobacter* spp., and *Klebsiella* spp. produce acid when they grow on the medium, which lowers the pH of the agar and results in the formation of red to pink colonies.

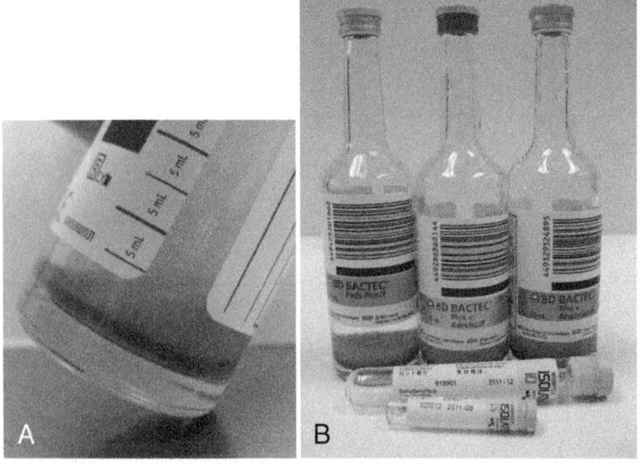

FIGURE 3-4 Blood culture systems. **A,** BACTEC system showing resin beads that bind antimicrobial drugs. **B,** Pediatric, aerobic, and anaerobic BACTEC systems for blood culture together with adult and pediatric WAMPOLE Isolator tubes (front) for lysis-centrifugation culture of blood.

Blood and Intravascular Catheters

Bacteremic animals may be continuously or intermittently bacteremic. Because of intermittent bacteremia, multiple, separate specimens, each containing greater than or equal to 10 mL of blood, are recommended. Pediatric bottles are available that can be inoculated with as little as 1.5 mL of blood, although the chance of a positive isolation increases as the blood volume drawn increases. Therefore, as much blood should be drawn as possible, provided that collection of a large volume of blood does not jeopardize the patient. Bottles should be held at room temperature and submitted immediately to the laboratory. Two, and ideally three, blood samples should be collected using meticulous sterile technique, and the timing of blood draws should depend on the severity of the animal's illness (Box 3-2). Inoculated bottles are incubated in aerobic conditions for 7 days before being reported as negative. Additional blood samples are not recommended, because they add cost without a significant increase in sensitivity.[6] The choice to inoculate anaerobic blood culture bottles is controversial. Studies in humans have shown that the prevalence of anaerobic bloodstream infections has decreased, and routine inoculation of anaerobic blood culture bottles may not be necessary. In one veterinary study, anaerobes were not identified in any of 33 dogs with endocarditis using

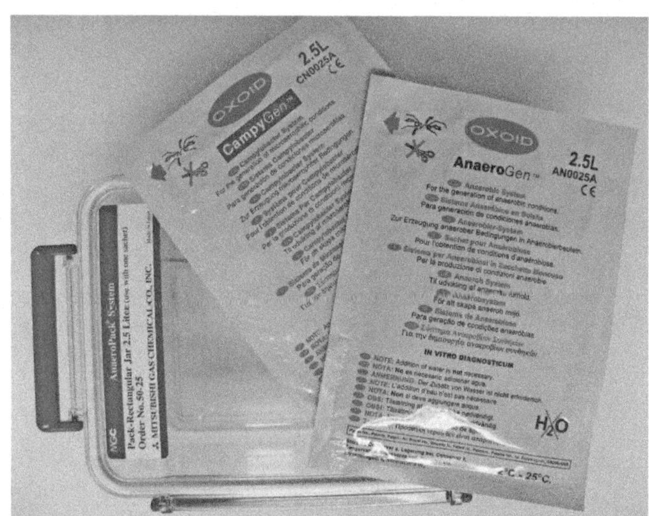

FIGURE 3-5 System for isolation of anaerobic and microaerophilic bacteria. The packets are opened, and the sachets inside are placed into the container with the inoculated plates. The container is sealed immediately. The sachets contain ascorbic acid. Atmospheric oxygen in the container is rapidly absorbed and replaced with carbon dioxide in an exothermic reaction process. After an appropriate incubation period, the container is opened and the plates inspected for growth. An anaerobic indicator can be placed within the box to ensure that the proper conditions are maintained.

anaerobic culture of blood, but anaerobic bacteremia may be occur with other underlying causes of bloodstream infections.[6] Common blood culture contaminants include coagulase-negative staphylococci, *Bacillus* spp., corynebacteria, and propionibacteria. When only one blood culture is positive for one of these organisms, contamination is likely, but the presence of multiple positive blood cultures from separate sites suggests true bacteremia.

Culture of intravascular catheter tips is performed to determine whether a catheter is a source of bacteremia and should only be performed simultaneously with blood culture. The catheter is removed after cleaning the skin around the catheter site with alcohol, and the distal 5 cm is aseptically removed into a sterile tube and submitted immediately.[7] In the laboratory, the catheter tip is rolled onto an agar plate. The result of catheter culture alone should not change treatment. Therefore, in most situations, blood culture may be all that is required.

Skin

For dogs with superficial pyoderma, specimens for culture should ideally be collected from a pustule. No surface disinfection should be performed. The hair should be clipped using sterile scissors; clippers should be avoided. A pustule is lanced with a sterile narrow-gauge needle, and pus on the needle or exuding from the pustule is applied to a sterile swab, which can then be placed in transport medium for transport to the laboratory. If a pustule cannot be found, cultures can also be obtained by lifting crusts and swabbing beneath the crust, or rolling the swab across an epidermal collarette two to three times. Papules can be cultured by biopsy after surface disinfection with 70% alcohol, allowing the surface to dry, and use of a 3- to 4-mm punch and sterile surgical instruments to collect the biopsy, which is then submitted in transport medium or a small amount of sterile saline. The biopsy site can then be sutured closed.

For deep pyoderma, a biopsy of the lesion should also be obtained after surface disinfection with 70% alcohol. The dermis should be excised with a sterile blade and the biopsy submitted as just described.

For dogs and cats with wounds, aspirates and deep tissue biopsies after surgical dissection are always preferable to swab specimens. Swab specimens are often contaminated by surface microorganisms, contain only a small amount of material, and are not amenable to optimal anaerobic transport. For this reason, collection of pus from fistulous tracts using a swab should also be avoided. If an abscess is present, an aspirate of the abscess fluid should be collected and submitted for aerobic and anaerobic culture. For dogs and cats with cellulitis, an aspirate can be attempted by injecting a small volume of sterile saline into the lesion and aspirating back into a syringe, although bacterial yields may be low and biopsy may be required in some cases.

BOX 3-2

Suggested Procedure for Obtaining Blood Cultures

Shave site.

Clean skin with 10% povidone iodine or 1-2% tincture of iodine, swabbing concentrically from the center; allow to dry (wait 1 min).

If a catheter must be used for specimen collection, clean access port with 70% alcohol and allow to dry. Avoid collection from a catheter if possible.

Clean stopper on top of the culture tube or bottle with 70% alcohol; allow to dry (wait 1 min).

Perform venipuncture using sterile gloves to palpate the vein.

Inoculate blood culture bottle without changing the needle.

Space cultures based on severity of illness, before starting antimicrobial therapy.

- Acute febrile illness: antimicrobials need to be changed or started immediately: two sets from separate sites, all within 10 minutes. Consideration could be given to drawing a third set using a resin bottle just before administering the second dose of antimicrobials (i.e., when trough drug concentrations are present)
- Acute endocarditis: 3 sets from 3 separate sites, within 1-2 hours
- Nonacute disease: 3 sets from separate sites within 24 hours, spaced at intervals of at least 3 hours

Body Fluids

Usually, 1 to 5 mL of body fluid is required for culture. Fluid can be inoculated into blood culture bottles in the laboratory or alongside the patient. Body fluids that have the potential to clot should be submitted to the laboratory in a tube that contains an appropriate ratio of anticoagulant. In the laboratory, body fluids with volumes that exceed 1 mL are generally concentrated using centrifugation and resuspension of the pellet in a smaller volume (e.g., 0.5 mL) of supernatant before they are inoculated onto agar.

For cerebrospinal fluid, the chance of organism isolation also increases when the volume submitted is maximized. If possible, at least 0.5 mL should be submitted for culture. Cerebrospinal fluid specimens should be immediately transported to the laboratory, preferably at room temperature.

Tissue Specimens

Attempts should be made to obtain as large a tissue specimen as possible for culture. The use of swabs to collect specimens for culture during surgical procedures is discouraged because of insufficient specimen size. Small pieces of tissue can be submitted in a small amount of sterile, nonbacteriostatic saline. In the laboratory, the tissue is minced using sterile procedures to release organisms before smears are prepared and media inoculated. Because an anaerobic environment can be maintained within pieces of tissue greater than or equal to 1 cm^3 in volume, these are suitable for anaerobic culture without oxygen-free transport. Such tissue specimens may be stored at room temperature for up to 24 hours.

Airway Specimens

Specimens from the upper respiratory tract are generally contaminated with commensal bacteria. Aerobic bacterial culture of a nasal wash specimen may be indicated in cats with chronic rhinosinusitis in which an antimicrobial resistant organism is suspected, in particular *Pseudomonas aeruginosa*. Isolation of *Bordetella bronchiseptica* may also have clinical significance in dogs and cats with nasal discharge. Growth of *Mycoplasma* spp. from the nasal cavity has uncertain clinical significance, because *Mycoplasma* spp. can be isolated from the nasal cavities of both healthy cats and cats with rhinosinusitis.[8-11]

Specimens from the lower respiratory tract may be collected using transtracheal, endotracheal, or bronchoalveolar lavage. Bronchial brush specimens may also be submitted for culture, after placing them in 1 mL of sterile nonbacteriostatic saline. The presence of intracellular bacteria on cytologic examination is consistent with a bacterial infection, rather than contamination. Anaerobic culture could be considered for animals with aspiration pneumonia or migrating plant awn foreign body pneumonia.

Feces

Whole stools or swabs that contain fecal matter should be processed within 1 to 2 hours or refrigerated as soon as possible after specimen collection and submitted within 24 hours. The specimens should not be contaminated with barium or urine. Rectal swabs that contain fecal material can be immersed in transport medium until processing. Testing of more than one sequential specimen may improve detection of fecal pathogens due to the low sensitivity of fecal culture methods. Selective media are required for isolation of *Salmonella* spp. Because *Clostridium perfringens* and *C. difficile* are commonly detected in normal stool specimens, toxin antigen testing may be more appropriate than culture to determine the role these organisms may be playing in diarrhea (see Chapter 48). Special medium is also required for isolation of *Campylobacter* (see Chapter 47).

Urine

Urine should be collected using cystocentesis whenever possible. Collection of urine via sterile catheterization in male dogs is acceptable when cystocentesis is not possible. Quantitative cultures should always be performed. For specimens obtained by cystocentesis, any level of bacterial growth is significant, although most urinary tract infections contain greater than or equal to 10^3 colony-forming units (CFU)/mL of bacteria. For urine specimens obtained via catheter from male dogs, bacterial growth of greater than or equal to 10^5 CFU/mL has been considered significant.[12] Only aerobic bacterial culture is routinely indicated. Anaerobic urine culture may be indicated when there is radiologic evidence of emphysematous cystitis. Urine specimens should be refrigerated and submitted to the laboratory as soon as possible. Special urine transportation tubes can be used to preserve bacteria within the specimen provided they are appropriate for the volume of urine collected (e.g., BD Vacutainer urine culture and sensitivity tube). Urine "paddles" are also available for in-house veterinary use. These allow inexpensive screening for the presence of absence of infection (Figure 3-6). The paddles have media impregnated on them, are designed to be incubated in the clinic, and can provide some information on the infecting bacterial species present and the number of CFU/mL. Positive paddles can then be submitted to the laboratory for culture and susceptibility testing, although this does not always permit accurate identification of all bacteria present in mixed infections (see also Chapter 89).

For animals with a urinary catheter in place and a suspected urinary tract infection, culture of the catheter tip is not recommended, because it is generally contaminated with commensal organisms from the urethra. Instead, a urine specimen should be obtained by aspiration from a new urinary catheter, or, if feasible, using cystocentesis. If a catheter is used to collect the specimen, several milliliters of urine should be removed and discarded first to clear the catheter. Urine culture should never be performed on collection bag specimens.

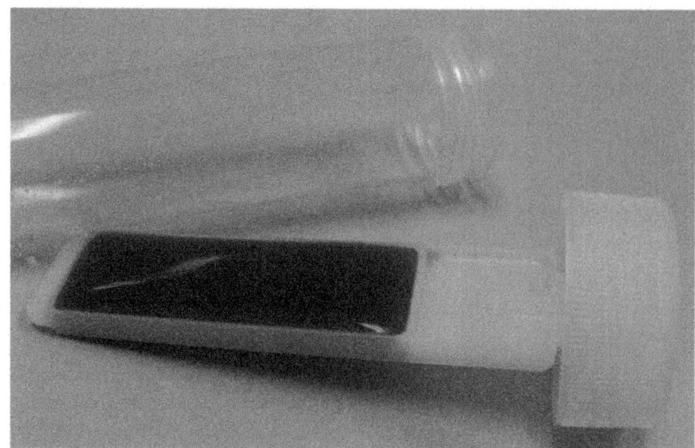

FIGURE 3-6 Media paddle available for screening urine for the presence of an aerobic bacterial infection. The paddle is impregnated on each side with selective and nonselective media (in this case eosin methylene blue medium, shown, and cysteine lactulose electrolyte-deficient media, on underside, respectively). The paddle is flooded with urine, incubated, and inspected for growth. Eosin methylene blue medium is red and selects for growth of gram-negative enteric organisms. Cysteine lactose electrolyte-deficient medium is initially green but turns yellow in the presence of lactose-fermenting organisms.

Fastidious and Unculturable Organisms

Some bacteria, such as *Bartonella* spp., *Borrelia burgdorferi*, and *Leptospira* spp., require special culture conditions (see Chapters 50 to 52). Others, such as hemotropic *Mycoplasma* species, are unculturable, and DNA amplification methods such as PCR are required for detection of these organisms. Cell culture is required to propagate certain bacteria. Examples include *Chlamydia felis* and tick-borne pathogens such as *Anaplasma phagocytophilum*.

Bacterial Identification

Following aerobic or anaerobic culture, presumptive bacterial identification can be made on the basis of colony morphology and microscopic morphology (e.g., Gram stain characteristics, rods or cocci). Further differentiation is generally based on a series of additional phenotypic tests, which are selected based on microscopic morphology and whether the organism is gram-negative, gram-positive, aerobic, or anaerobic. Microbiology laboratories use published methods to identify bacteria.[13] Preliminary tests used to identify gram-positive aerobes include the presence or absence of hemolysis on a blood agar plate (Figure 3-7), a positive or negative catalase test, and the production of coagulase. Identification of gram-negative aerobes relies on whether or not the organism ferments lactose, indole production, oxidase production, and the production of a variety of other enzymes. Assessment of motility and the ability to ferment carbohydrates are also used to differentiate bacteria. Biochemical test strips are available that allow multiple tests to be performed simultaneously (e.g., API Strips, bioMérieux) (Figure 3-8), so that identification can be made within 24 to 48 hours. Automated identification systems that consist of a 96-well microtiter tray that contains a variety of biochemical reagents (e.g., Sensititre, TREK Diagnostics, Cleveland) are also in use in some veterinary diagnostic laboratories.

Molecular methods such as 16S rRNA gene PCR and sequencing are now being used to identify organisms to the species level (see Chapter 5). Speciation of some mycobacteria requires analysis

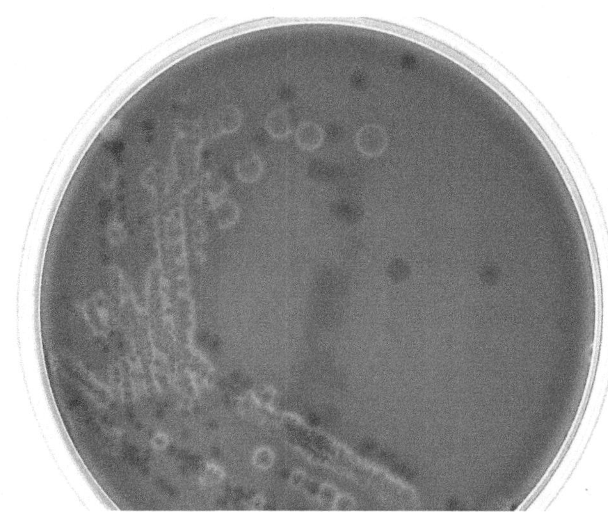

FIGURE 3-7 Mixture of beta-hemolytic and nonhemolytic enteric bacteria growing on blood agar. Beta-hemolysis is characterized by complete clearing of the agar around each colony.

of mycolic acid content using high-performance liquid chromatography. Recently, the availability of matrix-assisted laser desorption ionization time-of-flight mass spectrometry instrumentation (i.e. the Bruker Biotyper and VITEK MS systems) has revolutionized bacterial identification in the clinical microbiology laboratory. These systems use mass spectrometry to rapidly (on average in 6 minutes) and accurately (often >95%) identify organisms to the species level based on their chemical composition, provided a reference spectrum for the organism is available in the database used for comparison. Although the instrumentation is expensive, the ultimate cost is lower than with conventional biochemical methods, because of reduction in labor and reagent costs.[14]

Interpretation of Bacterial Culture Results

Specimens That Test Negative

Negative results (or lack of growth) using bacterial culture do not imply the absence of bacteria. Negative test results can occur as a result of inadequate specimen size (such as when swabs or aspirates are submitted), when there are inadequate organism numbers at the site of specimen collection, when overgrowth with commensal organisms occurs, or when there is loss of organism viability during transportation to the laboratory. The last is particularly problematic for anaerobic bacteria. In some situations, multiple bacterial species are present within a specimen, and one species (such as *Proteus* spp.) swarms the plate and obscures the presence of another. The identification of multiple bacterial types on a Gram-stained smear allows the laboratory to plan culture methods that maximize detection of all species present.

Negative test results can also occur when the organism is not inoculated onto the correct media or sufficient time is not allowed for growth. Clinicians must consider whether fastidious or slow-growing organisms might be present and inform the laboratory if they are suspected. Poor laboratory quality control procedures may also lead to false-negative test results. Use of an accredited laboratory can help minimize such problems.

Specimens That Test Positive

The detection of bacterial organisms within a specimen using culture does not imply that the organism is the cause of an animal's clinical signs. Contamination is the most common cause of false positive cultures. Isolation of only one or two colonies of coagulase-negative staphylococci, *Bacillus* spp., *Corynebacterium* spp., or propionibacteria suggests contamination. Isolation of large numbers of a single type of bacteria from a normally sterile site is usually clinically significant, especially when supported by cytologic evidence of bacteria within phagocytes.

Antimicrobial Susceptibility Testing

Importance of Antimicrobial Susceptibility Testing

Given the increasing recognition of antimicrobial resistance among bacteria that are isolated from small animal patients, determination of antimicrobial susceptibility can be as or more important to the clinician than the identity of the infecting agent. The result of antimicrobial susceptibility testing is generally available 2 to 3 days after submission of a specimen for culture. In animals that are critically ill, empiric antimicrobial therapy may already have been initiated by the time this result is available. The susceptibility results may show that the organism is resistant to a drug being used, in which case the drug should be changed to one to which the organism is susceptible. The susceptibility pattern can help to identify an alternate drug when the patient does not tolerate the initial drug prescribed. Susceptibility testing may indicate that the organism is susceptible to a more narrow-spectrum (and generally less expensive) antimicrobial drug than the drug initially prescribed, in which case the spectrum should be narrowed to minimize the development of antimicrobial resistance.

Methods of Susceptibility Testing

Susceptibility testing can be performed using dilution methods or diffusion methods. The *minimum inhibitory concentration* (MIC) is the lowest concentration of antimicrobial drug that inhibits visible growth of an organism over a defined incubation period, most commonly 18 to 24 hours. The MIC is determined using dilution methods, which involve exposing the organism to twofold dilutions of an antimicrobial drug. The concentration range used varies with the drug and the organism being tested. In vitro factors that influence MIC include the composition of the medium, the size of the inoculum, incubation conditions, and the presence of resistant bacterial subpopulations within the inoculum. Standard protocols are published by the Clinical and Laboratory Standards Institute (CLSI) that specify medium composition and pH, inoculum size, inoculation procedures, agar depth, and incubation conditions, as well as quality control requirements.[13] Failure to comply with these protocols can lead to erroneous results, so laboratories that adhere to CLSI standards should be used whenever possible. MIC testing does not take into account in vivo factors such as postantibiotic effect and the effects of protein binding on antimicrobial drug activity (see Chapter 6).

Dilution Methods

Dilution methods include *broth macrodilution, broth microdilution,* and *agar dilution.* The most widely used method in North America is broth microdilution, whereby twofold dilutions of antimicrobials are made in a broth medium in a microtiter plate (Figure 3-9). Pre-prepared frozen or freeze-dried microtiter plates for inoculation are available

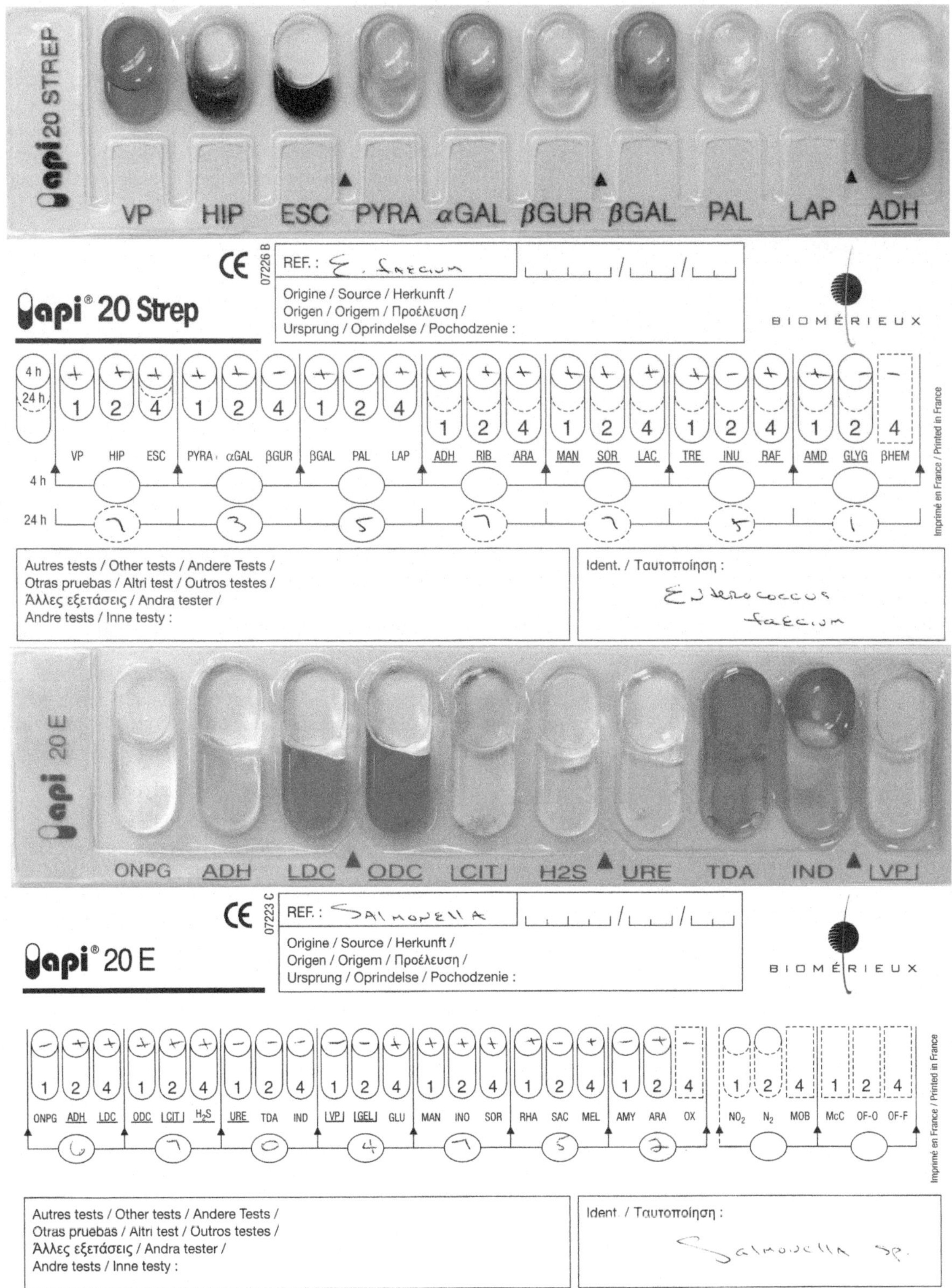

FIGURE 3-8 API bacterial identification strips. Only the left half of the reaction strip is shown. *Top (api20STREP): Enterococcus faecium. Bottom (api20E): Escherichia coli.* Positive reactions are assigned a numerical code on the handwritten strip. The codes in each three-well group are added to generate a new (seven-number) code that can be used to identify the organism.

commercially (e.g., Sensititre plates, TREK Diagnostic Systems, Cleveland). The results can be determined using visual examination of the plates for the inhibition of bacterial growth, or by the use of semiautomated or automated instrumentation. Dilutions can also be performed in agar, each dilution being poured onto a plate in a standardized fashion and allowed to set before inoculating it with the organism(s) of interest. Agar dilution can be used to perform susceptibility testing of fastidious bacteria with special medium requirements, such as *Campylobacter* spp.

The MIC for each antimicrobial drug tested against the organism is reported to the clinician on the susceptibility panel. It is the lowest concentration of antibiotic (usually in μg/mL) that inhibits growth of the organism in vitro. The lower the

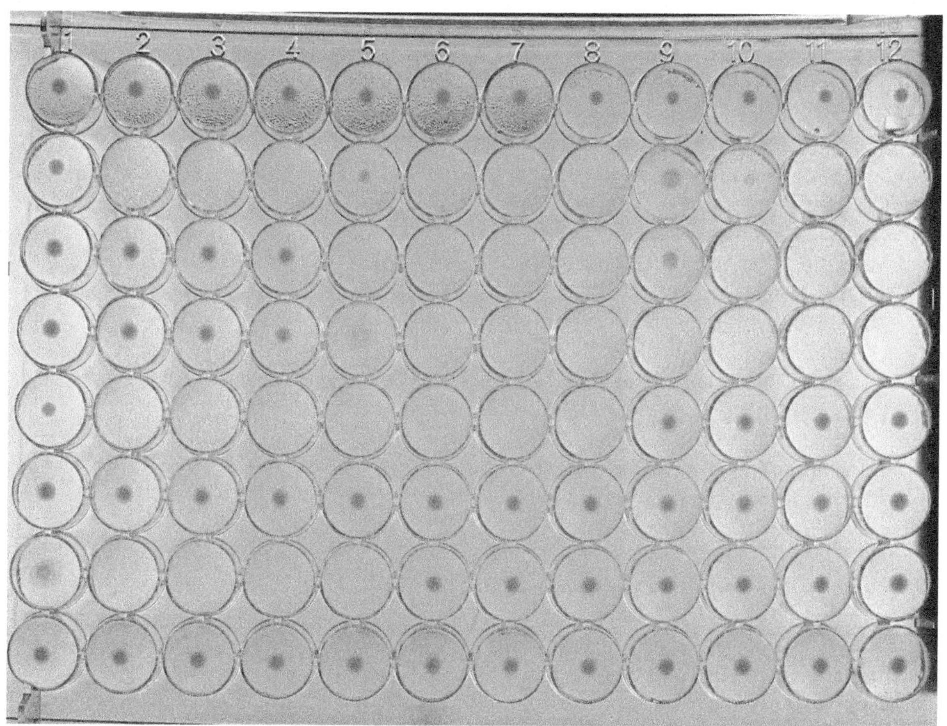

	1	2	3	4	5	6	7	8	9	10	11	12
A	AMP 0.25	AMP 0.5	AMP 1	AMP 2	AMP 4	AMP 8	AMP 16	OXA+ 0.25	OXA+ 0.5	OXA+ 1	OXA+ 2	OXA+ 4
B	AUG2 4/2	AUG2 8/4	AUG2 16/8	AUG2 32/16	AMI 4	AMI 8	AMI 16	AMI 32	FOX 2	FOX 4	FOX 8	FOX 16
C	TIC 8	TIC 16	TIC 32	TIC 64	POD 2	POD 4	POD 8	POD 16	TIM2 8/2	TIM2 16/2	TIM2 32/2	TIM2 64/2
D	SXT 0.5/9.5	SXT 1/19	SXT 2/38	FOV 0.25	FOV 0.5	FOV 1	FOV 2	FOV 4	FOV 8	FAZ 4	FAZ 8	FAZ 16
E	GEN 1	GEN 2	GEN 4	GEN 8	IMI 1	IMI 2	IMI 4	IMI 8	CLI 0.5	CLI 1	CLI 2	CLI 4
F	PEN 0.06	PEN 0.12	PEN 0.25	PEN 0.5	PEN 1	PEN 2	PEN 4	PEN 8	DOX 2	DOX 4	DOX 8	POS
G	XNL 0.25	XNL 0.5	XNL 1	XNL 2	XNL 4	MAR 0.25	MAR 0.5	MAR 1	MAR 2	RIF 1	RIF 2	POS
H	ENRO 0.25	ENRO 0.5	ENRO 1	ENRO 2	ERY 0.5	ERY 1	ERY 2	ERY 4	CHL 4	CHL 8	CHL 16	POS

AMP, ampicillin; AUG2, amoxicillin/clavulanic acid (2:1 ratio); TIC, ticarcillin; SXT, trimethoprim/sulfamethoxazole; GEN, gentamicin; PEN, penicillin; XNL, ceftiofur; ENRO, enrofloxacin; FOV, cefovecin; AMI, amikacin; POD, cefpodoxime; IMI, imipenem; ERY, erythromycin; MAR, marbofloxacin; OXA+, oxacillin + 2% NaCl; FOX, cefoxitin; TIM2, ticarcillin/clavulanic acid (constant 2); CLI, clindamycin; DOX, doxycycline; CHL, chloramphenicol; FAZ, cefazolin; RIF, rifampin; POS, positive control.

FIGURE 3-9 Broth microdilution for determination of MICs. A series of wells contain an antimicrobial drug at twofold dilutions in a standard format. One custom plate format is shown (TREK Diagnostic Systems Sensititre Companion Animal MIC plate). A pellet of bacteria (in this case, *Escherichia coli* from an infected feline esophagostomy tube site) settles on the bottom of each well when growth fails to be inhibited by the antimicrobial drug concentration tested in that well. The cutoff MICs that define susceptibility versus resistance are published by the Clinical and Laboratory Standards Institute (CLSI) in the United States. This isolate was reported as resistant to ampicillin (>16 mg/mL), susceptible to amoxicillin-clavulanic acid (8 mg/mL), susceptible to amikacin (8 mg/mL), susceptible to cefoxitin (8 mg/mL), resistant to ticarcillin (>64 mg/mL), susceptible to cefpodoxime (≤2 mg/mL), susceptible to ticarcillin-clavulanic acid (16 mg/mL), resistant to trimethoprim-sulfamethoxazole (>2 mg/mL), susceptible to cefovecin (1 mg/mL), susceptible to cefazolin (≤4 mg/mL), susceptible to gentamicin (2 mg/mL), susceptible to imipenem (≤1 mg/mL), resistant to doxycycline (>8 mg/mL), resistant to enrofloxacin and marbofloxacin (both >2 mg/mL), and resistant to chloramphenicol (>16 mg/mL). The MIC for ceftiofur was ≤0.25 mg/mL, but because a breakpoint for this drug has not been published, only the MIC was reported, and not whether the isolate was susceptible or resistant. Results for some drugs tested, such as oxacillin, are not reported for gram-negative bacteria because these drugs are used to treat gram-positive bacterial infections.

MIC, the more potent is the antimicrobial at inhibiting bacterial growth.

Diffusion Methods

Diffusion methods include gradient diffusion (also known as Etest) and disk diffusion. The *Etest* involves use of a plastic strip coated with an antimicrobial gradient on one side and an MIC interpretive scale on the other side (Figure 3-10, *A*). An agar plate is inoculated with the organism of interest so that subsequent growth of the organism forms a "lawn," rather than individual colonies (i.e., *inoculation to confluence*). At the time of inoculation, the strips are applied to the surface of the plate. The antimicrobial drug diffuses into the medium, resulting in an elliptical zone of growth inhibition around the strip. The MIC is read at the point of intersection of the ellipse with the MIC scale on the strip. Although the strips are expensive, Etests have the advantage of being adaptable to use with fastidious organisms and anaerobes.

Disk diffusion, also known as Kirby-Bauer antibiotic testing, involves application of commercially available drug-impregnated filter paper disks to the surface of an agar plate that has been inoculated to confluence with the organism of interest. Commercially available, mechanical disk-dispensing devices can be used to apply several disks simultaneously to the surface of the agar. The drug diffuses radially through the agar, the concentration of the drug decreasing logarithmically as the distance from the disk increases. This results in a circular zone of growth inhibition around the disk, the diameter of which is inversely proportional to the MIC (see Figure 3-10, *B*). The zone diameters are interpreted on the basis of guidelines published by CLSI (see Definition of Breakpoints, next), and the organisms are reported as susceptible, intermediate, or resistant. Disk diffusion can only be used to test rapidly growing organisms that have consistent growth rates, for which criteria for interpretation of zone sizes are available.

Definition of Breakpoints

Once susceptibility testing has been performed, organisms are classified on the susceptibility panel report as "susceptible" (S), "resistant" (R), and, in some cases, of "intermediate" (I) susceptibility. *This refers to a predicted in vivo situation, rather than in vitro susceptibility.* The growth of "susceptible" isolates is predicted to be inhibited by antimicrobial drug concentrations that are usually achievable in blood and tissues using normal dosage regimens. "Intermediate" isolates have MICs that approach usually attainable blood and tissue levels and for which response rates may be lower than those of susceptible isolates. This category implies clinical efficacy in body sites where the drugs are normally concentrated (e.g., enrofloxacin and amoxicillin in urine) or when a higher-than-normal dose of a drug can be used. "Resistant" isolates are predicted to grow in the face of the usually achievable concentrations of the drug in blood and tissues.[15]

So why can the laboratory predict in vivo susceptibility on the basis of MIC determination, which is an in vitro test? In order to do this, the laboratory refers to *breakpoints*, or clinical cutoff MICs (or, for disk diffusion testing, cutoff zone diameters), which are established, published, and revised regularly by committees that are affiliated with standards agencies such as the CLSI. If the MIC determined in the microbiology laboratory is lower than a published breakpoint for that organism-drug combination, the organism is defined as susceptible. *The breakpoint is not reported to the clinician.* Breakpoints are established on the basis of multiple factors (Box 3-3), which include (1) a knowledge of MIC distributions and resistance mechanisms for each organism-drug combination (Figure 3-11),[16] (2) clinical response rates in humans and animal models, (3) how the drug is distributed and metabolized in the body (pharmacokinetics), and (4) whether the drug is concentration dependent or time dependent as it relates to antibacterial effect (pharmacodynamics) (see Box 3-3).[15] Zone diameter breakpoints for disk diffusion testing are determined by correlation with MIC values. For simplicity, breakpoints are established for antimicrobial drug

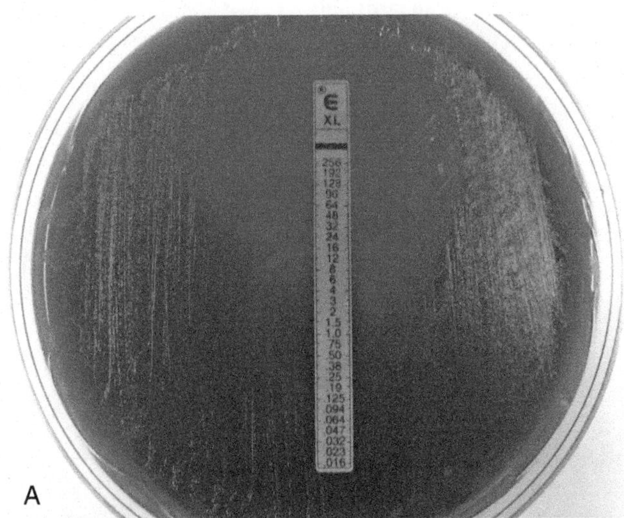

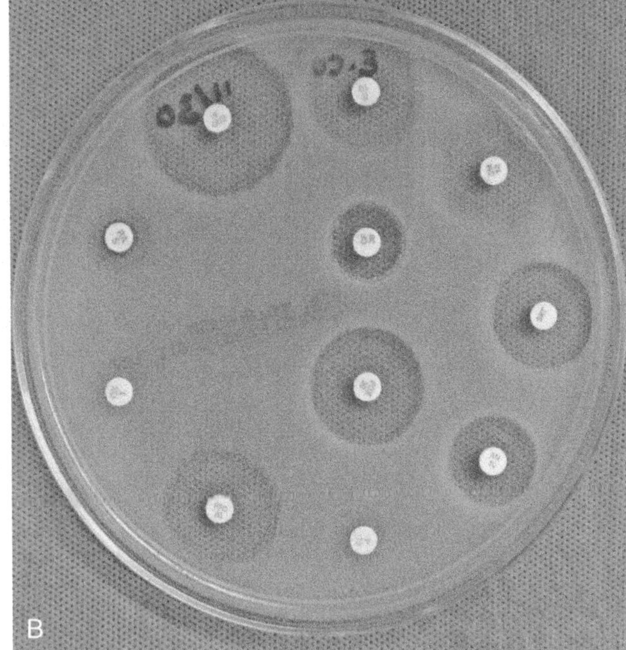

FIGURE 3-10 Alternatives to broth microdilution for antimicrobial susceptibility testing. **A,** Etest that shows susceptibility of a *Bacteroides fragilis* isolate to amoxicillin-clavulanic acid. The strip in the center is impregnated with a gradient of antimicrobial drug (in this case, amoxicill-clavulanic acid), with the highest concentration at the top of the strip. The MIC is read at the point where bacterial growth is no longer inhibited by the strip (0.19 mg/mL in this case). **B,** Disk diffusion (also known as Kirby-Bauer testing) for *Escherichia coli* showing varying degrees of resistance to different antimicrobial drugs, reflected by zones of growth inhibition around disks containing each antimicrobial drug.

concentrations in the bloodstream, and are based on a specific dosage regime for the antimicrobial drug tested. This dosage regime is selected by the standards agency involved. Because some antimicrobials are concentrated extensively in urine, some veterinary laboratories may offer urine MIC panels, which provide breakpoints for lower urinary tract infections. These breakpoints are higher than corresponding serum MIC breakpoints, so a greater proportion of organisms tested are classified as "susceptible." Urine MIC panels have been controversial because the possibility of concurrent pyelonephritis (tissue drug concentrations rather than urine concentrations) cannot always be ruled out. Breakpoints may be reevaluated when new mechanisms of resistance appear in bacteria or when new data are generated that improve understanding of the pharmacokinetics and pharmacodynamics of an antimicrobial drug.

BOX 3-3

Factors Used by Standards Agencies to Establish Breakpoints for Antimicrobial Susceptibility Testing

Bacterial Factors

- Evaluation of MIC distributions for each bacterial species. These tend to be normally distributed (see Figure 3-10; available for different antimicrobial drugs at www.eucast.org).[15]
- Knowledge of bacterial resistance mechanisms, as determined using phenotypic or genetic testing (e.g., testing for altered penicillin binding proteins in staphylococci)

Pharmacokinetics of the antimicrobial drug when used at a specific dosage regime in the animal species of interest, including protein binding, taking into account variation among individuals

Pharmacodynamic indices (e.g., whether killing is concentration or time dependent) for the antimicrobial drug as they relate to organism killing (see Chapter 6)

Clinical response rates in humans and animal models, which are based on prospective, randomized controlled clinical studies with well-defined dosage regimes

For infections in sites such as the central nervous system, the clinician needs to consider whether or not (1) an antimicrobial will penetrate that site, (2) the drug is appropriate and safe, and (3) a higher dose is necessary to achieve adequate concentrations. The clinician must also consider factors such as immunosuppression and other concurrent illness or drug therapy when treating infections on the basis of antimicrobial susceptibility test results.

The bacterial species isolated determines which antimicrobials the laboratory selects for inclusion in susceptibility panels. For example, susceptibility to cephalosporins may not be reported for enterococci because of intrinsic resistance. Some antimicrobial drugs (e.g., vancomycin, linezolid, imipenem) should be reserved for treatment of multiple-drug resistant organisms that cause life-threatening infections. Consultation with a health professional with expertise in infectious diseases or antimicrobial pharmacology is recommended before these drugs are selected.

Minimum and Serum Bactericidal Concentration

The *minimum bactericidal concentration* (MBC) is the minimum concentration of an antimicrobial drug that is bactericidal. It is determined by re-culturing *(subculturing)* broth dilutions that inhibit growth of a bacterial organism (i.e., those at or above the MIC). The broth dilutions are streaked onto agar and incubated for 24 to 48 hours. The MBC is the lowest broth dilution of antimicrobial that prevents growth of the organism on the agar plate. Failure of the organism to grow on the plate implies that only nonviable organisms are present. The use of MBCs has been advocated by some for treatment

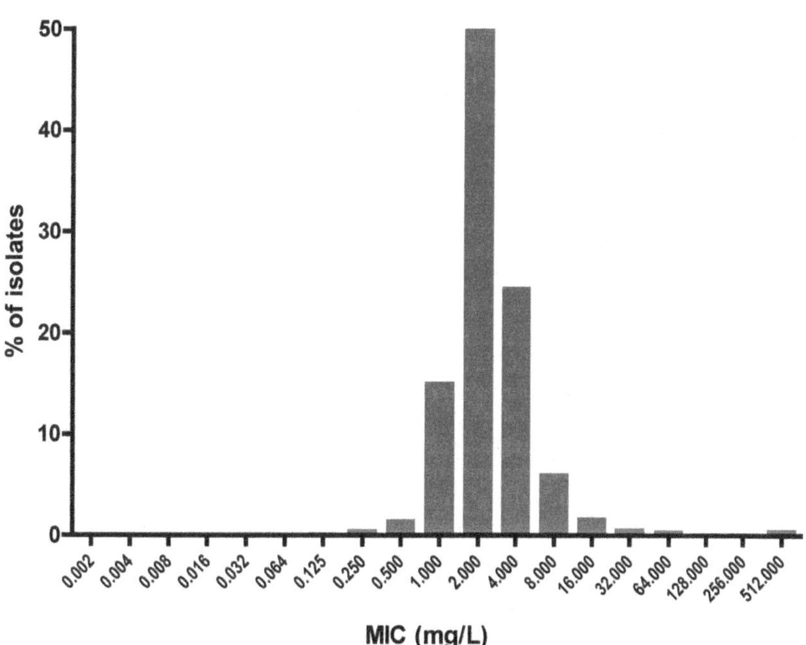

FIGURE 3-11 Histogram that shows the distribution of amikacin minimum inhibitory concentrations (MICs) for isolates of *Escherichia coli*. The MICs are normally distributed. (From www.eucast.org. Accessed May 11, 2012.)

of serious infections (such as endocarditis) or for treatment of immunosuppressed patients. Their value has been controversial, and they are not widely performed in human or veterinary medicine.

Serum bactericidal testing (SBT) is performed in the same manner as the MBC test, but uses the serum of a patient that has been treated with an antimicrobial. Serum is usually collected at expected peak and trough serum concentrations. SBC can be used to determine whether a patient has been adequately dosed, and to ensure that the antimicrobial is having the desired effect on the organism. Some data are available to support specific peak and trough SBT results required for the optimal treatment of human endocarditis, osteomyelitis, and cancer chemotherapy patients.[17-20] The SBT has not been widely used or evaluated for infections in dogs and cats and remains controversial in human medicine.

Mutant Prevention Concentration

The *mutant prevention concentration* (MPC) is the lowest antimicrobial drug concentration required to block the growth of the least susceptible bacterial cell in high density bacterial populations.[21] It is the MIC of the most resistant bacterial strain in a mixed bacterial population. Concentrations of antimicrobial between the MIC and the MPC allow selective amplification of resistant mutants (also known as the *mutant selection window*).[22] This range is considered to be a "danger zone" for therapeutic drug concentrations. Minimizing the length of time that the antimicrobial drug concentration remains in the mutant selection window in vivo may reduce the likelihood for resistance selection during treatment.[22] The MPC cannot be extrapolated from the MIC. It is estimated using the standard agar dilution method used to estimate MIC, but with a larger inoculum ($\geq 10^9$ instead of 10^5 organisms), so as to include resistant subpopulations of bacteria. Administration of higher doses of antimicrobial drugs that exceed the MPC increases the chance of toxicity to the patient, but offsets the chance of selection for resistant organisms, even though infection may be cured with lower doses.[22,23] Although first evaluated for the fluoroquinolones, data is accumulating regarding the usefulness of the MPC for other drug classes. MPC estimations are currently not routinely performed in veterinary diagnostic laboratories.

SUGGESTED READINGS

Drlica K, Zhao X. Mutant selection window hypothesis updated. Clin Infect Dis. 2007;44(5):681-688.

Turnidge JL, Paterson DL. Setting and revising antimicrobial susceptibility breakpoints. Clin Microbiol Rev. 2007;20(3):391-408.

REFERENCES

1. Radaelli ST, Platt SR. Bacterial meningoencephalomyelitis in dogs: a retrospective study of 23 cases (1990-1999). J Vet Intern Med. 2002;16(2):159-163.
2. Sturges BK, Dickinson PJ, Kortz GD, et al. Clinical signs, magnetic resonance imaging features, and outcome after surgical and medical treatment of otogenic intracranial infection in 11 cats and 4 dogs. J Vet Intern Med. 2006;20(3):648-656.
3. Cole LK, Kwochka KW, Kowalski JJ, et al. Microbial flora and antimicrobial susceptibility patterns of isolated pathogens from the horizontal ear canal and middle ear in dogs with otitis media. J Am Vet Med Assoc. 1998;212(4):534-538.
4. Tolar EL, Hendrix DV, Rohrback BW, et al. Evaluation of clinical characteristics and bacterial isolates in dogs with bacterial keratitis: 97 cases (1993-2003). J Am Vet Med Assoc. 2006;228(1):80-85.
5. Clinical and Laboratory Standards Institute. http://www.clsi.org: Last accessed May 15, 2012.
6. Sykes JE, Kittleson MD, Pesavento PA, et al. Evaluation of the relationship between causative organisms and clinical characteristics of infective endocarditis in dogs: 71 cases (1992-2005). J Am Vet Med Assoc. 2006;228(11):1723-1734.
7. Thomson RB. Specimen collection, transport, and processing: bacteriology. In: Murray PR, Barron EJ, Jorgensen JP, et al. eds. Manual of Clinical Microbiology. 9th ed. Washington, DC: ASM Press; 2007:291-333.
8. Veir JK, Ruch-Gallie R, Spindel ME, et al. Prevalence of selected infectious organisms and comparison of two anatomic sampling sites in shelter cats with upper respiratory tract disease. J Feline Med Surg. 2008;10(6):551-557.
9. Johnson LR, Drazenovich NL, Foley JE. A comparison of routine culture with polymerase chain reaction technology for the detection of *Mycoplasma* species in feline nasal samples. J Vet Diagn Invest. 2004;16(4):347-351.
10. Randolph JF, Moise NS, Scarlett JM, et al. Prevalence of mycoplasmal and ureaplasmal recovery from tracheobronchial lavages and of mycoplasmal recovery from pharyngeal specimens in cats with or without pulmonary disease. Am J Vet Res. 1993;54:897-900.
11. Tan RJS, Lim EW, Ishak B. Ecology of mycoplasmas in clinically healthy cats. Aust Vet J. 1977;53:515-518.
12. Ling GV. Lower Urinary Tract Diseases of Dogs and Cats. St Louis: Mosby; 1995:116.
13. Murray PR, Barron EJ, Jorgensen J, et al. eds. Manual of Clinical Microbiology. 9th ed. Washington, DC: ASM Press; 2007.
14. Bizzini A, Greub G. Matrix-assisted laser desorption ionization time-of-flight mass spectrometry, a revolution in clinical microbial identification. Clin Microbiol Infect. 2010;16(11):1614-1619.
15. Turnidge JL, Paterson DL. Setting and revising antimicrobial susceptibility breakpoints. Clin Microbiol Rev. 2007;20(3):391-408.
16. The European Committee on Antimicrobial Susceptibility Testing—EUCAST. http://www.eucast.org. Last accessed May 14, 2012.
17. Klastersky J, Daneau D, Swings G, et al. Antibacterial activity in serum and urine as a therapeutic guide in bacterial infections. J Infect Dis. 1974;129(2):187-193.
18. Reller LB. The serum bactericidal test. Rev Infect Dis. 1986; 8(5):803-808.
19. Weinstein MP, Stratton CW, Ackley A, et al. Multicenter collaborative evaluation of a standardized serum bactericidal test as a prognostic indicator in infective endocarditis. Am J Med. 1985;78(2):262-269.
20. Weinstein MP, Stratton CE, Hawley HB, et al. Multicenter collaborative evaluation of a standardized serum bactericidal test as a predictor of therapeutic efficacy in acute and chronic osteomyelitis. Am J Med. 1987;83(2):218-222.
21. Blondeau JM, Hansen G, Metzler K, et al. The role of PK/PD parameters to avoid selection and increase of resistance: mutant prevention concentration. J Chemother. 2004;16(suppl 3):1-19.
22. Drlica K, Zhao X. Mutant selection window hypothesis updated. Clin Infect Dis. 2007;44(5):681-688.
23. Zhao X, Drlica K. A unified anti-mutant dosing strategy. J Antimicrob Chemother. 2008;62(3):434-436.

CHAPTER 4

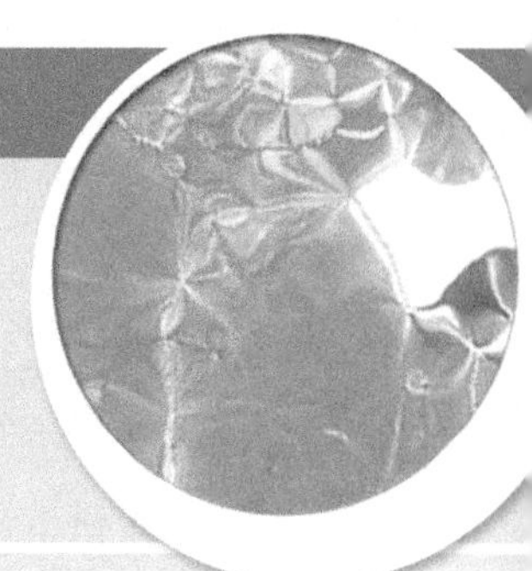

Isolation and Identification of Fungi

Jane E. Sykes and Shelley C. Rankin

KEY POINTS

- Fungi often grow more slowly than bacteria and can have specific culture media requirements. Some fungi are dangerous to culture because they produce airborne spores that may lead to laboratory-acquired infections.
- The clinician should tell microbiology laboratory personnel if a fungal infection is suspected. Providing a list of suspected pathogens facilitates safe and successful culture of pathogenic fungi. The animal's clinical abnormalities, travel history, history of immunosuppressive drug therapy, and the results of cytology or histopathology should be taken into account.
- Specimens should be collected and transported as for bacterial culture. Refrigeration inhibits growth of some fungi.
- Because of increasing drug resistance among pathogenic fungi, the demand for antifungal susceptibility testing has increased, and for some fungal pathogens, culture and susceptibility testing before beginning antifungal drug therapy may be advantageous.

INTRODUCTION AND DEFINITIONS

Fungi are eukaryotic microorganisms that secrete enzymes in order to digest organic material in the environment. The resultant nutrients are absorbed through a specialized fungal cell wall (known as *chemotrophic nutrition*). A basic understanding of fungal terminology facilitates communications between clinicians, microbiologists, and pathologists. Fungal organisms have two basic morphologic forms:

1. Molds—molds exist as filaments known as *hyphae,* which may be divided into cellular compartments *(septate hyphae).* A mass of filaments is known as a *mycelium.* A granule formed by a compacted mat of fungal filaments is a *eumycetoma* (as opposed to an *actinomycotic mycetoma;* see Chapter 42).
2. Yeasts—these are single-celled organisms that reproduce by budding. In some cases, buds do not detach from the parent cell, but instead form a chain. Elongated chains of buds may resemble hyphae. These are termed *pseudohyphae* (Figure 4-1).

Many pathogenic fungi exist as a mold in the environment, but in tissues convert to a yeast form. These fungi are called *dimorphic fungi.* An example of a dimorphic fungus is *Blastomyces dermatitidis.*

Fungi reproduce by producing *spores.* Spores can be produced following asexual or sexual reproduction. Asexual reproduction (through mitosis) generates spores that are identical to the parent cell. Sexual reproduction involves the fusion of haploid nuclei from two hyphal structures, which is followed by meiosis. The asexual stage of a fungus is known as an *anamorph*, whereas the sexual stage is known as a *teleomorph*. Many fungi have two different species names to reflect these stages. For example, the teleomorph of *Cryptococcus neoformans* is known as *Filobasidiella neoformans.* Formally, the teleomorph name is supposed to take precedence and can be used to describe both stages.[1] However, asexual reproduction predominates in most fungi, including during growth in culture. Thus, certain fungi, such as *C. neoformans*, are more widely known by their anamorph name. In addition, teleomorphs of some fungal organisms have not yet been described. Some organisms can exist in more than one asexual form, and therefore have more than two names. For example, *Pseudallescheria boydii* (teleomorph) has two asexual forms, *Graphium fruticola* and *Scedosporium apiospermum*. Currently, there is a move by mycologists to identify only a single name for a fungal organism ('one fungus = one name'). Throughout this book, the name most commonly used in the literature is used to refer to different fungal pathogens.

Specimen Collection and Transport

Isolation of fungal organisms from clinical specimens can be facilitated by the use of special media. For many fungal species, this may be hazardous to laboratory personnel. Submission of specimens for culture of dangerous organisms such as *Blastomyces dermatitidis*, *Coccidioides immitis*, and *Histoplasma*

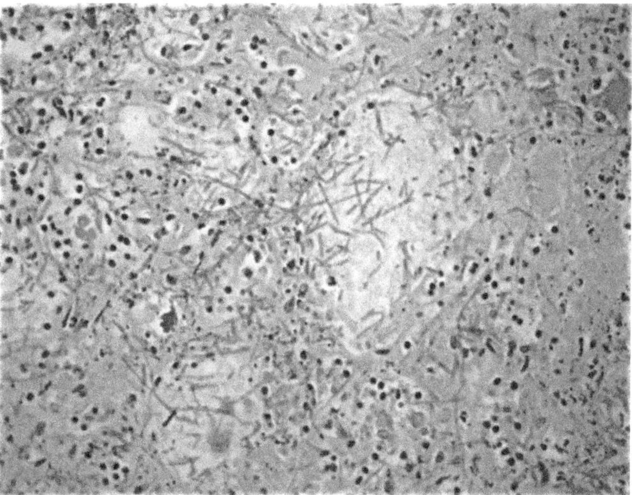

FIGURE 4-1 Histopathology of the thyroid gland from a 13-year old female spayed poodle mix with disseminated *Candida albicans* infection. The dog had been treated with prednisone, cyclosporin, and azathioprine for refractory immune-mediated hematologic disease. Note intralesional pseudohyphae. H&E stain, 400× magnification.

capsulatum is discouraged if the diagnosis can be obtained using other methods such as cytology, histopathology, and serologic testing. These organisms exist as yeasts in tissues (at 37°C) that are minimally hazardous to clinicians and laboratory personnel, but grow as hyphae at lower temperatures and on culture medium, which generate spores that can be inhaled and cause disease.

Specimens that are commonly submitted for fungal culture include lower respiratory tract wash specimens, cerebrospinal fluid, urine, other body fluids, skin, eye, hair, or biopsy specimens from the nasal cavity, bone, or skin. Guidelines for specimen collection are the same as for bacterial culture (refer to Chapter 3). The clinician should inform the laboratory what fungal species are suspected, because different fungi have different media preferences and growth conditions. As large a specimen as possible should be collected. Care should be taken to avoid collection of contaminated specimens. Blood cultures may be useful for dogs and cats with disseminated fungal disease when lesions cannot be easily accessed. Detection of fungemia can sometimes be achieved using blood culture systems for bacterial isolation. Lysis-centrifugation methods (Isolator tubes, Wampole Laboratories) may be more sensitive for detection of dimorphic and filamentous fungi in blood. Mycobacterial blood culture media (such as MB/BacT, BioMérieux) may also offer increased sensitivity for detection of fungemia.[2]

For dermatophyte culture, 10 to 12 hairs should be plucked from the edge of the lesion using sterile forceps and submitted without refrigeration in a clean dry paper envelope or sterile glass or plastic tube. Paper envelopes are preferred to tubes because tubes retain moisture that can promote overgrowth of contaminants. Scrapings of crusts at the edges of the lesion can also be submitted. Claw clippings can be collected after cleaning them with 70% alcohol to remove contaminating bacteria and fungi. Crumbling material from under the claw may be the best specimen, or the entire claw can be submitted.

If transport requires longer than 2 hours, appropriate transport media should be used or specimens should be refrigerated. When rapid transport to the laboratory is possible, storage and transport at room temperature is preferred. Fungal culture of specimens that are more than 24 hours old is not recommended because of increased likelihood of false-positive and false-negative results. The laboratory should be informed if the patient is receiving antifungal drug treatment, which may interfere with the ability to culture fungus from the specimen.

Specimens should be labeled with the patient's name, patient number, and source of specimen, as well as the date and time of collection, and labeled, packaged, and transported according to regional and global regulations for shipping of infectious substances (see Chapter 1).[3] Careful packaging and transport is particularly important for specimens suspected to contain fungal pathogens. If dangerous organisms might be present, the laboratory should be warned in advance and the specimens marked appropriately.

Diagnostic Methods

Microscopic Examination of Direct Smears

Examination of a direct smear before culture allows rapid partial or complete identification of many fungi by the laboratory (Table 4-1, Figure 4-2). This can help the clinician make initial treatment decisions and guides media selection by the laboratory. Using Gram stain, yeasts generally stain gram positive and molds tend to be gram negative.[4] A potassium hydroxide (KOH) preparation may be performed to examine a specimen for dermatophyte hyphae and arthroconidia. The KOH clears keratinaceous and cellular debris, but fungal elements are left intact. If tissue granules are present, the laboratory will crush them, examine them for hyphae, and the granules can also be cultured. Fungal morphology may be altered in specimens from dogs and cats receiving antifungal drug treatment (Figure 4-4).

Special stains used in the laboratory for fungal identification include India ink, which is used to identify cryptococcal yeasts in cerebrospinal fluid (see Figure 62-8), and calcofluor white, which binds polysaccharides in the fungal cell wall and fluoresces when examined using fluorescence microscopy (Figure 4-5, *A*). Other stains, such as lactophenol cotton blue (see Figure 4-5, *B*), are also used to identify fungi after they have been grown in culture.

In some situations, fungi are observed in tissues with histopathology but a culture of the causative organism is not available, either because it has not been performed or because the organism has failed to grow. The morphology and staining characteristics of the organism on histopathology may also be useful for preliminary identification or allow full identification of the pathogen. Special stains used include Mayer's mucicarmine stain, which stains the cryptococcal polysaccharide capsule red; Gomori's methenamine silver stain, which stains fungal organisms black; and periodic acid–Schiff, which stains fungal elements dark pink (Figure 4-6). If the identity of the fungus remains in doubt, an additional specimen should be collected for culture if possible, and the microbiology laboratory should be made aware of the morphology of the organism and the differential diagnoses. Complete identification of the organism using culture is useful for proper treatment and prognostication.

Fungal Culture

Before culture, clinical specimens must be prepared for inoculation. For example, body fluids are usually first centrifuged by the laboratory to concentrate fungal organisms. The sediment is then resuspended in a smaller volume of supernatant and inoculated onto selective media. If biopsy specimens are submitted, the tissues are finely sliced, ground, or minced, which releases the organisms before they are inoculated onto the media.

Many types of media are available for isolation of fungi, and no single medium is optimal for all organisms. Many fungi grow on blood agar plates used for primary isolation of bacteria. Special media used for initial (primary) isolation of fungal organisms from tissues and body fluids are shown in Table 4-2. Other media are available for differentiation of fungal species (see Fungal Identification, later). Media that contain antibacterial agents (usually chloramphenicol or gentamicin) are used to culture specimens that might contain bacteria. Cycloheximide is added to dermatophyte test medium to inhibit the growth of contaminant saprophytic mold species. This allows selective isolation of dermatophytes such as *Microsporum canis*.

Plates for fungal culture are sealed with an air-permeable tape in order to prevent exposure of laboratory personnel to potentially dangerous spores and to minimize plate contamination with airborne fungal organisms. Plates that grow filamentous fungi are opened only in a biological safety cabinet. Laboratories prefer to use media in tubes or bottles to reduce occupational exposure to aerosolized fungal elements. Fungal cultures are incubated at room temperature (22°C to 25°C)

TABLE 4-1

Microscopic Descriptions of Some Common Fungal Pathogens of Dogs and Cats

Organism	Yeast or Hyphae	Diameter (μm)	Description	Geographic Distribution
Blastomyces dermatitidis	Yeast	8-15	Round with thick, often refractile cell wall and broad-based budding (see Figure 60-8).	Southeastern and south central United States, upper Midwest region
Histoplasma capsulatum	Yeast	2-5	Oval to round, often found in clusters within macrophages (see Figure 61-7).	Ohio and Mississippi river valleys, especially in southern United States. Also Central America
Cryptococcus spp.	Yeast	2-15	Round to oval, narrow-based budding, sometimes forming chains of organisms. Large capsule (see Figures 4-4 and 62-8). Poorly encapsulated variants are rarely encountered.	Worldwide, common in Australia and western North America
Coccidioides spp.	Spherule	10-200	Spherules vary in size and may contain endospores ("pomegranate-like"). Using cytology, they appear as empty and collapsed, deeply basophilic structures (see Figure 63-8).	Central California, Arizona, Nevada, Central and South America
Sporothrix schenckii	Yeast	2-6	Oval, round, or cigar-shaped, occasionally budding (see Figure 64-4). May be found intracellularly and extracellularly. Difficult to find in dogs but may be abundant in cats.	Temperate and tropical zones worldwide. Most common in South and Central America
Malassezia spp.	Yeasts and pseudohyphae	3-8 (yeast), 5-10 (pseudohyphae)	Round to oval; when budding, have the appearance of "footprints" (see Figure 59-2).	Worldwide
Candida spp.	Yeast and pseudohyphae	3-4 (yeast), 5-10 (pseudohyphae)	Usually yeasts with a single bud or pseudohyphae with multiple constrictions (see Figure 67-3).	Worldwide
Dermatophytes	Hyphae	3-15	Septate hyaline hyphae, arthroconidia may be visible along hair shafts (see Figure 58-8)	Worldwide
Aspergillus spp.	Hyphae	4-6	Septate hyaline hyphae with uniform diameter that branch at 45° angles (see Figure 4-2).	Worldwide
Scedosporium spp., *Paecilomyces* spp.	Hyphae	3-12	Septate hyaline hyphae that tend to branch at wider angles than *Aspergillus* spp. (45° to 90°) (see Figure 4-6).	Worldwide
Basidiobolus and *Conidiobolus* (zygomycosis)	Hyphae	10-30	Wide, non- or poorly septate irregular hyaline hyphae, branching at right angles, may be twisted or folded. Poorly stained using hematoxylin and eosin stain (see Figure 4-3).	Tropical and subtropical regions of the Americas, Africa, southeast Asia, and Australia
Phialophora, *Exophiala*, *Cladophialophora*, *Bipolaris* (phaeohyphomycosis or dematiaceous molds)	Hyphae	1.5-6	Pigmented hyphae, budding cells with single septa and chains of swollen round cells (see Figure 68-5). May form granules.	Worldwide
Pythium insidiosum	Hyphae	4-9	Sparsely septate, hyaline hyphae with 90° branches, detectable using hematoxylin and eosin stain	Tropical, subtropical, and some temperate regions of the world.

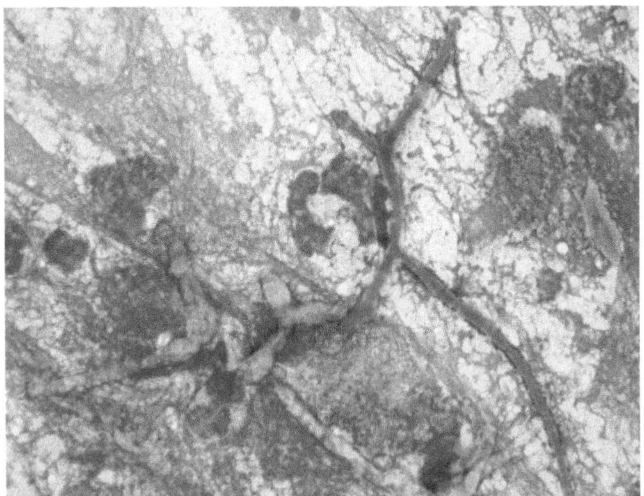

FIGURE 4-2 Direct smear of an aspirate from a mediastinal mass of a 6-year-old female spayed labrador retriever with disseminated *Aspergillus deflectus* infection. Note hyphae with parallel walls that branch at 45° angles. Stain uptake by some hyphae is poor. Wright's stain, 1000× oil magnification. (Image courtesy Dr. William Vernau, University of California, Davis.)

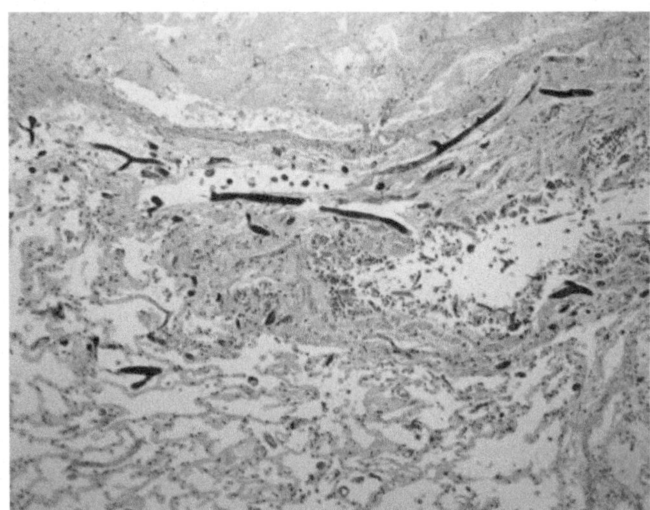

FIGURE 4-3 Histopathology showing severe pulmonary zygomycosis at necropsy in an 11-year-old mixed-breed dog that had been diagnosed with diabetic ketoacidosis before euthanasia. H&E stain, 100× magnification.

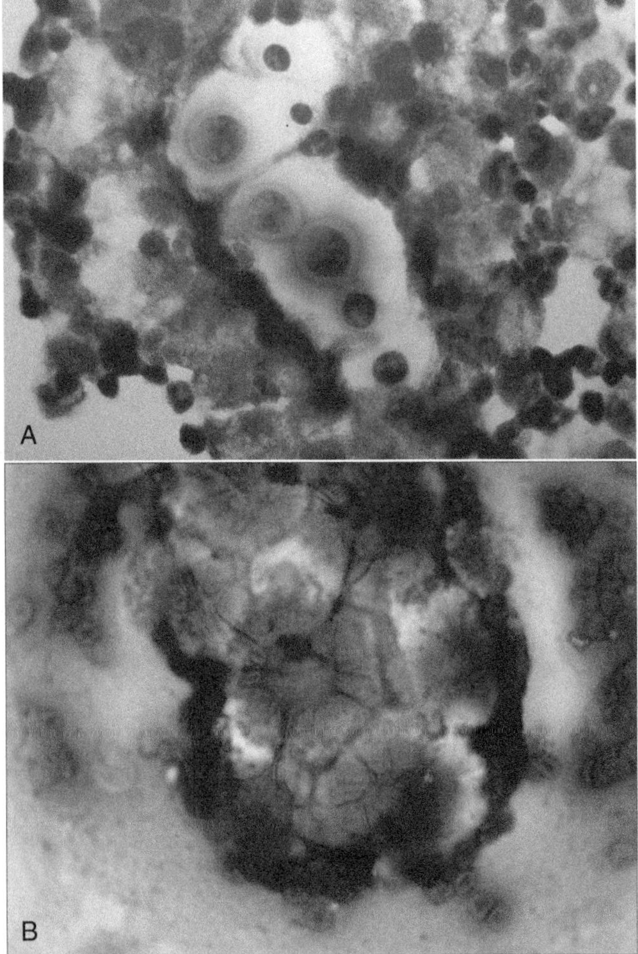

FIGURE 4-4 **A,** Cerebrospinal fluid cytology (Cytospin preparation) from a dog with newly diagnosed cryptococcosis. Note the thick capsule, which appears as a halo around the organism, and narrow-based budding. Wright-Giemsa stain, 1000× oil magnification. **B,** Cytology of a lymph node aspirate from a cat that had been treated for cryptococcosis with antifungal drugs. The architecture of the organisms is distorted. Diff Quik stain, 1000 × oil magnification.

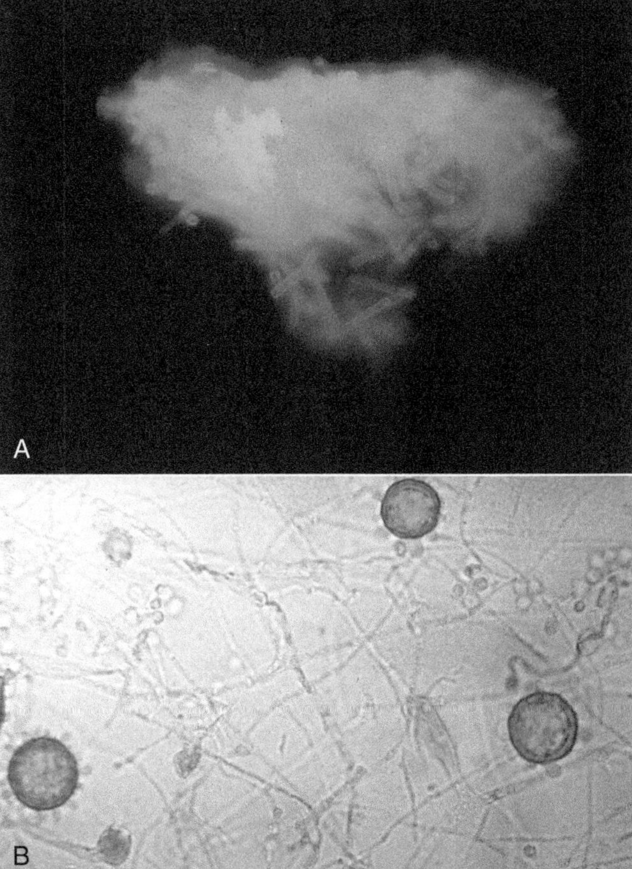

FIGURE 4-5 Special stains used for identification of fungal isolates following direct smear preparation. **A,** Calcofluor white stain of a mass of *Aspergillus fumigatus* hyphae. 1000× oil magnification. **B,** Lactophenol cotton blue preparation of the mold phase of *Histoplasma capsulatum*. 1000 × oil magnification.

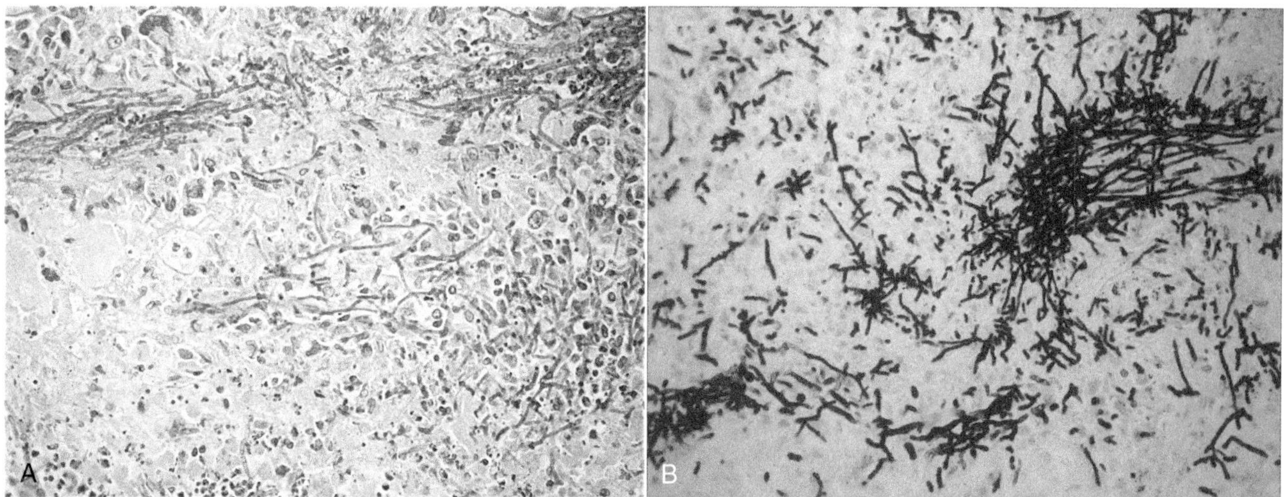

FIGURE 4-6 Histopathology of the kidney from a 2-year-old female spayed German shepherd with disseminated paecilomycosis. **A,** Periodic acid Schiff stain. The fungal hyphae stain bright pink. **B,** Gomori's methenamine silver stain, which stains the fungal hyphae black. 400× magnification.

TABLE 4-2

Special Medium Types Used to Culture Fungi That Infect Dogs and Cats

Type of Medium	Additives	Indications
Sabouraud dextrose agar	None	Cultivation of all fungi.
Brain-heart infusion agar	None	Cultivation of all fungi.
Potato dextrose agar or potato flake agar	None	Cultivation of all fungi. Especially useful for opportunistic molds. Induces sporulation.
Inhibitory mold agar	Chloramphenicol, sometimes gentamicin	Cultivation of all fungi when bacterial contamination is suspected or possible.
Dermatophyte test medium	Chloramphenicol, gentamicin, cycloheximide	Dermatophyte isolation. Shows a color change when dermatophytes grow on the medium.

or 30°C, a lower temperature than that used for routine culture of bacteria. In general, cultures should be examined daily for 2 weeks and twice weekly for an additional 2 to 4 weeks, because the growth of some organisms may be very slow. In general, rapidly growing fungi grow in 1 to 3 days, those with intermediate growth in 5 to 9 days, and slow growers take up to 4 weeks. Yeast colonies are smooth and resemble bacterial colonies, and molds grow in colonies that are dry, wrinkled, or heaped (Figure 4-7).

Fungal Identification

After growth in culture, fungi are identified based on visual characteristics such as colony morphology and color. Light microscopy is useful to evaluate the microscopic morphology of yeasts and to determine the presence of septate or nonseptate hyphae and fruiting structures for molds (Table 4-3). Increasingly, DNA sequence information has been used to identify fungi (such as after PCR of D2 or ITS regions of the 23S rRNA gene). Matrix-assisted laser desorption ionization time-of-flight (MALDI-TOF) mass spectrometry holds considerable promise for identification of fungi in the future (see Chapter 3).[5] Molds that produce pigment are known as *dematiaceous* fungi (see Figure 4-7, *B*), and those that do not are known as *hyaline* fungi. A variety of broth or solid media are also used for fungal identification. For example, *Candida* species can be differentiated using *Candida* bromcresol green (BCG) agar, because each species has a specific colonial morphology and color on this medium. Test strips are commercially available that allow multiple biochemical identification tests for yeasts to be performed simultaneously (e.g., API 20C AUX Yeast Identification Kit, bioMérieux) (see Figure 3-8), so identification can be made within 1 to 2 days.

Interpretation of Fungal Culture Results

False-negative and false-positive results are very common with fungal culture, and results must be interpreted in light of the organism grown, the animal's clinical condition, and the results of cytology and histopathology.

Specimens That Test Negative

Negative test results can occur as a result of inadequate specimen size (such as when swabs or aspirates are submitted), when there are inadequate organism numbers at the site of specimen collection, when overgrowth with contaminating bacteria or saprophytic fungi occurs, or when there is loss of organism

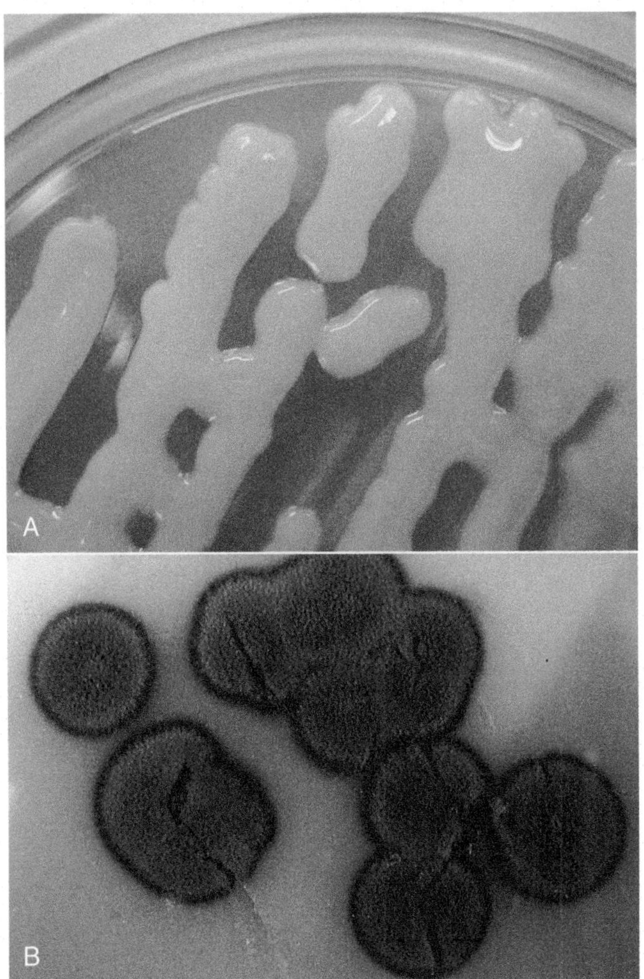

FIGURE 4-7 **A,** Growth of *Cryptococcus gattii* yeasts on potato flake agar. **B,** *Cladophialophora bantiana*, a pigmented (dematiaceous) mold, isolated from canine brain tissue on potato flake agar.

viability during specimen transportation. If the patient is receiving antifungal drugs but has not completely cleared the infection, culture may be negative.

False-negative test results also occur when the organism is not inoculated onto the correct media or sufficient time is not allowed for growth. It is critical that clinicians inform the laboratory if a fungal infection is suspected, and what organism might be involved. Poor laboratory quality control procedures may also lead to false-negative test results. Use of an accredited laboratory can help minimize such problems.

Specimens That Test Positive

The detection of fungal organisms within a specimen does not always imply that the organism is causing the animal's clinical signs. Contamination by saprophytic fungi, especially *Aspergillus*, is the most common cause of false-positive fungal cultures. Organisms are more likely to be clinically significant when cytologic examination of a stained smear also demonstrates the presence of fungal organisms.

Antifungal Susceptibility Testing

Increasing resistance to antifungal agents has been documented for a variety of fungal pathogens. This has led to an increased demand for antifungal susceptibility testing by clinicians. Fortunately, the reproducibility of antifungal susceptibility testing has improved greatly in recent years, and breakpoints (see Chapter 3) have been established for treatment of many fungal infections in human patients. Although breakpoints are still lacking for veterinary patients, antifungal susceptibility testing allows comparison of the activity of two or more antifungal drugs, and serial testing of isolates from a single patient allows the development of resistance to be monitored over time. Methods of susceptibility testing that have been adapted for yeast and mold infections include broth microdilution, the Etest, and disk diffusion (see Chapter 3).

TABLE 4-3

Classification of Fungi That Are Known to Infect Dogs and Cats

Phylum	Class	Example	Characteristics
Zygomycota	Zygomycetes	*Absidia, Rhizopus, Conidiobolus, Basidiobolus*	Aseptate hyphae. In asexual reproduction, spores are abundantly produced in a closed sac called a sporangium. Sexual reproduction results in a single, large thick-walled zygospore.
Basidiomycota	Basidiomycetes	*Cryptococcus, Malassezia*	Sexual reproduction leads to haploid production of basidiospores on a basidium.
Ascomycota	Archiascomycetes Hemiascomycetes Euascomycetes	*Pneumocystis* *Candida* spp. *Histoplasma, Blastomyces, Microsporum, Trichophyton* *Aspergillus* spp. *Fusarium* spp. *Pseudallescheria* spp. (teleomorph of *Scedosporium* spp.)	Sexual reproduction leads to haploid production of ascospores in a sac-like structure (ascus). Organisms are more commonly identified based on characteristics of asexual reproduction.

Common antifungal agents tested include amphotericin B, itraconazole, fluconazole, voriconazole, posaconazole, caspofungin, griseofulvin, and flucytosine (Figure 4-8). Limitations of antifungal susceptibility testing include the slow growth of fungal pathogens when compared to bacteria, and the fact that fungi may grow as yeasts or molds depending on media and incubation conditions. Partial inhibition of growth over a wide range of antifungal drug dilutions may also occur (a phenomenon known as *trailing*). Criteria have been set for interpretation of MICs in the presence of trailing for different antifungal drugs.[6] MALDI-TOF mass spectrometry can be used to determine antifungal drug susceptibility among fungal pathogens and in future may overcome some of the difficulties that currently exist.[7]

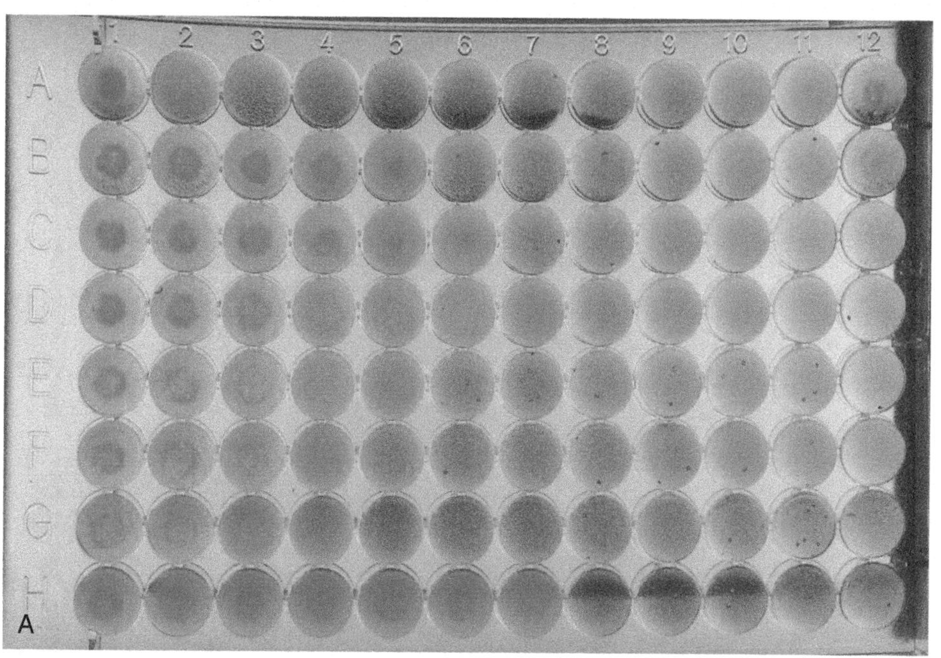

	1	2	3	4	5	6	7	8	9	10	11	12
A	POS	AND 0.015	AND 0.03	AND 0.06	AND 0.12	AND 0.25	AND 0.5	AND 1	AND 2	AND 4	AND 8	AB 0.12
B	MF 0.008	MF 0.015	MF 0.03	MF 0.06	MF 0.12	MF 0.25	MF 0.5	MF 1	MF 2	MF 4	MF 8	AB 0.25
C	CAS 0.008	CAS 0.015	CAS 0.03	CAS 0.06	CAS 0.12	CAS 0.25	CAS 0.5	CAS 1	CAS 2	CAS 4	CAS 8	AB 0.5
D	FC 0.06	FC 0.12	FC 0.25	FC 0.5	FC 1	FC 2	FC 4	FC 8	FC 16	FC 32	FC 64	AB 1
E	PZ 0.008	PZ 0.015	PZ 0.03	PZ 0.06	PZ 0.12	PZ 0.25	PZ 0.5	PZ 1	PZ 2	PZ 4	PZ 8	AB 2
F	VOR 0.008	VOR 0.015	VOR 0.03	VOR 0.06	VOR 0.12	VOR 0.25	VOR 0.5	VOR 1	VOR 2	VOR 4	VOR 8	AB 4
G	IZ 0.015	IZ 0.03	IZ 0.06	IZ 0.12	IZ 0.25	IZ 0.5	IZ 1	IZ 2	IZ 4	IZ 8	IZ 16	AB 8
H	FZ 0.12	FZ 0.25	FZ 0.5	FZ 1	FZ 2	FZ 4	FZ 8	FZ 16	FZ 32	FZ 64	FZ 128	FZ 256

POS, positive control; AND, anidulafungin; MF, micafungin; CAS, caspofungin; FC, 5-flucytosine; PZ, posaconazole; VOR, voriconazole; IZ, itraconazole; FZ, fluconazole; AB, amphotericin B.

B

FIGURE 4-8 **A,** Minimum inhibitory concentration (MIC) assay for a *Candida krusei* isolate. Growth in the presence of the antifungal drug is characterized by formation of a pellet on the bottom of the well and a change in the color of the medium from purple to pink. **B,** Schematic of the same microtiter plate showing antifungal drug dilutions. Organisms are defined as susceptible, intermediate, or resistant based on MIC cutoffs (breakpoints or interpretive criteria) set by regulatory bodies such as the Clinical and Laboratory Standards Institute in the United States. The report to the clinician would read susceptible to anidulafungin (0.12 µg/mL), susceptible to micafungin (0.25 µg/mL), susceptible to caspofungin (1 µg/mL), intermediate susceptibility to flucytosine (8 µg/mL), susceptible to voriconazole (0.12 µg/mL), susceptible to itraconazole (0.25 µg/mL), and resistant to fluconazole (128 µg/mL). The MICs for posaconazole and amphotericin B were reported as 0.25 µg/mL and ≤0.12 µg/mL, but the organism was not classified as susceptible or resistant because interpretive criteria for this organism-drug combination were not available.

REFERENCES

1. Pitt JI, Samson RA. Nomenclatural considerations in naming species of *Aspergillus* and its teleomorphs. Stud Mycol. 2007;59:67-70.
2. Taniguchi T, Ogawa Y, Kasai D, et al. Three cases of fungemia in HIV-infected patients diagnosed through the use of mycobacterial blood culture bottles. Intern Med. 2010;49:2179-2183.
3. World Health Organization. A guide for shipping infectious substances. 2009. http://www.who.int/ihr/infectious_substances/en/index. Last accessed May 11, 2012.
4. Shea YR. General approaches for direct detection of fungi. In: Versalovic J, Carroll KC, Funke G, et al. eds. Manual of Clinical Microbiology. 10th ed. Washington, DC: ASM Press; 2011:1776-1792.
5. Iriart X, Lavergne RA, Fillaux J, et al. Routine identification of medical fungi by MALDI-TOF: performance of the new VITEK MS using a new time-effective strategy. J Clin Microbiol. 2012;50(6):2107-2110.
6. Johnson EM, Espinel-Ingroff AV, Pfaller MA. Susceptibility test methods: yeasts and filamentous fungi. In: Versalovic J, Carroll KC, Funke G, et al. eds. Manual of Clinical Microbiology. 10th ed. Washington, DC: ASM Press; 2011:2020-2037.
7. Marinach C, Alanio A, Palous M, et al. MALDI-TOF MS-based drug susceptibility testing of pathogens: the example of *Candida albicans* and fluconazole. Proteomics. 2009;9:4627-4631.

CHAPTER 5

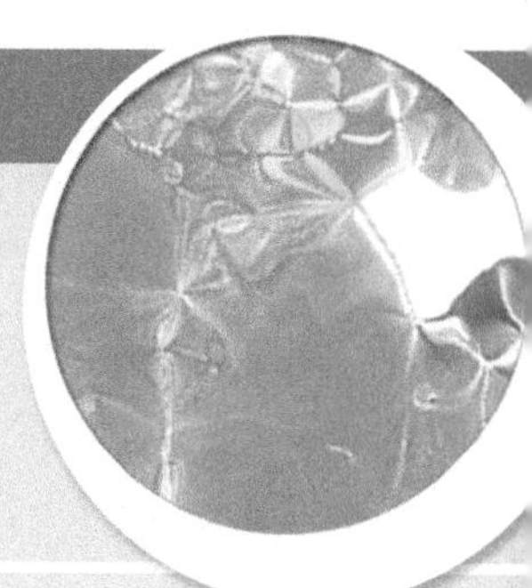

Nucleic Acid Detection Assays

Jane E. Sykes and Shelley C. Rankin

KEY POINTS

- Assays for detection of nucleic acid such as polymerase chain reaction assays are increasingly available commercially for diagnosis of companion animal infectious diseases.
- Molecular diagnostic assays include those that involve amplification (the copying of nucleic acid so that it can be more readily detected) or probe-based assays that do not involve nucleic acid amplification.
- Specimens for these assays should be collected using sterile technique in order to minimize contamination.
- Interpretation of the results of molecular diagnostic tests requires knowledge of the problems and pitfalls of each type of assay. The results of testing at one laboratory may differ from that at another because of variations in assay design.
- With increased automation, laboratory proficiency testing, improved quality assurance, and standardization of reporting, the availability and utility of molecular diagnostic tests for companion animal infectious diseases will increase.

INTRODUCTION

Assays that detect nucleic acid, also known as molecular diagnostic assays, include probe-based assays such as in situ hybridization, and methods that amplify DNA, such as the polymerase chain reaction (PCR).

DNA or RNA probes are short, single-stranded nucleic acids (usually <50 base pairs) that have a sequence that hybridizes to (i.e., is complementary to) a specific segment of DNA from the target microorganism (Figure 5-1). For in situ hybridization, the probe is labeled with a fluorescent or chemical tag so that the bound probe can be detected. The probe is reacted with a tissue specimen on a microscope slide in order to determine if the organism is present in the specimen. For PCR, two specific short (approximately 20 bases) DNA sequences called *primers*, which are complementary to the target microorganism's DNA, are used in conjunction with a machine called a *thermocycler* to amplify a specific segment of DNA from just one copy to millions of copies that can be more easily detected. In situ PCR is a combination of these two techniques.[1]

Nucleic acid detection methods are ideally suited to detection of organisms that are not easily found using cytology or histopathology, are slow-growing, or are difficult to culture, as well as when a rapid (<12 hours) diagnosis is required. Other applications are shown in Box 5-1.

The use of nucleic acid–based assays for diagnosis has increased dramatically in veterinary medicine over the past 10 years. Because of the exquisite sensitivity of some assays, especially those that involve DNA amplification, positive results may reflect contamination that occurs in the laboratory. Contamination problems have decreased with increased automation and the use of real-time PCR assays (see later). In human medicine, proficiency testing programs have helped to overcome quality assurance problems in laboratories that perform molecular diagnostic assays.[2] Not all PCR assays for a specific pathogen are equal, because the nucleic acid primers and probes and the equipment used to run each assay may be different. So a PCR assay for *Leptospira* performed in one laboratory may perform differently than an assay used in another laboratory.

A plethora of nucleic acid detection methods have been developed since the advent of PCR, many of which are commercially available for diagnosis of human infectious diseases but are not yet being widely used in veterinary medicine. These are described in detail elsewhere.[1,3,4] The purpose of this chapter is to outline (1) the indications for nucleic acid detection methods, (2) the best ways to collect and transport specimens for these assays, (3) the most commonly used methods in veterinary medicine, and (4) guidelines for their interpretation.

Specimen Collection and Transport

The recommendations for specimen collection and transport presented here are based on the guidelines published by the Clinical and Laboratory Standards Institute (CLSI).[5] These guidelines are updated on a regular basis and ensure that detection of nucleic acids within clinical specimens is optimal. In some instances, nucleic acid may be present and detectable in a specimen even when the specimen has not been handled in a manner that is consistent with the guidelines. Many laboratories publish their own specific guidelines for specimen collection and transport. Specimens should be properly packaged and labeled (see Chapter 3).

Nucleic Acid Probe Assays

In situ hybridization is generally performed on formalin-fixed, paraffin-embedded tissue specimens. Specimens that have been archived for several years may still be adequate, even for detection of RNA, which is more labile than DNA.[6,7] The optimum specimen for fluorescence in situ hybridization (see later for discussion) is tissue that has been snap frozen in liquid nitrogen after being embedded in optimal cutting temperature (OCT) medium.[5]

Polymerase Chain Reaction

When collecting specimens for PCR, the timing of collection relative to the course of disease and the best specimen type must be considered. For acute diseases, PCR is often most useful early in the course of disease. For chronic diseases, timing is less critical.

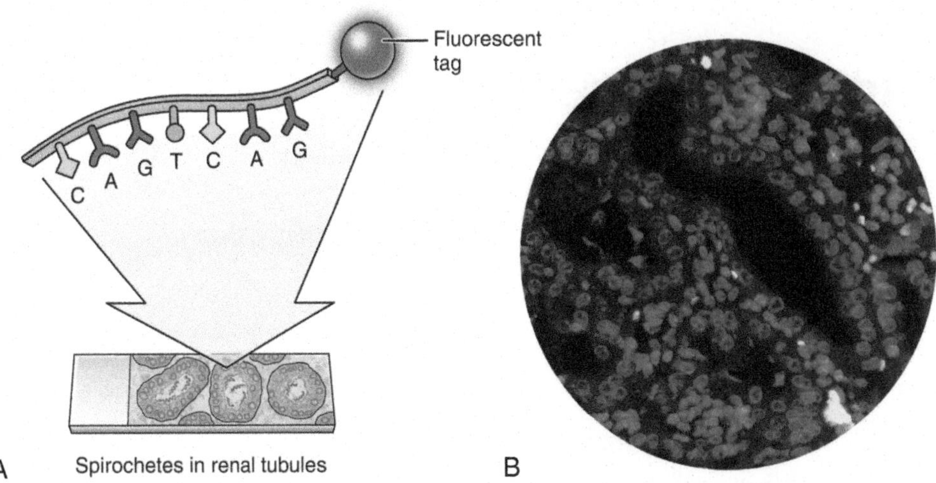

FIGURE 5-1 Fluorescence in situ hybridization (FISH). **A,** A nucleic acid probe that is complementary to a segment of leptospiral DNA is tagged with a fluorescent label and incubated with a tissue section on a slide. **B,** Unbound probe is washed away, and the section is examined using fluorescence microscopy. (*Leptospira* FISH image courtesy Dr. Richard Goldstein.)

BOX 5-1

Applications of Nucleic Acid Based Assays

Application	Examples
Detection of microbes that are not easily detected using light microscopic examination of tissues or smears	*Bartonella* spp., viral pathogens
Detection of microbes that are difficult or impossible to culture	Hemotropic mycoplasmas, *Bartonella* spp., *Mycobacterium* spp., *Brucella* spp.
Rapid detection of microbes to allow early institution of infection control measures	Influenza virus, hypervirulent FCV, rabies virus, *Mycobacterium tuberculosis*
Detection of microbes that are hazardous to culture in the laboratory	H1N1 influenza virus, *Francisella tularensis*
Detection of microbes in the face of inactivating substances such as antimicrobials or formalin	Retrospective identification of an infecting microorganism in formalin-fixed, paraffin-embedded tissues after histopathology
Detection of antimicrobial resistance genes	Possession of *mecA*, the gene for methicillin resistance, by staphylococci
Detection of novel pathogens using broad-spectrum PCR and sequencing	*Bartonella henselae*,* hemotropic mycoplasmas†
Monitoring organism load as a measure of disease progression or response to treatment	FIV viral load
Identification of a cultured organism to the species level	*Nocardia* and *Actinomyces* spp., many molds

FCV, Feline calicivirus.

*Anderson B, Sims K, Regnery R, et al. Detection of *Rochalimaea henselae* DNA in specimens from cat scratch disease patients by PCR. J Clin Microbiol 1994;32:942-948.

†Willi B, Boretti FS, Cattori V, et al. Identification, molecular characterization, and experimental transmission of a new hemoplasma isolate from a cat with hemolytic anemia in Switzerland. J Clin Microbiol 2005;43:2581-2585.

Knowledge of organism shedding patterns can help to determine the most appropriate timing of specimen collection. For example, *Leptospira* organisms are primarily present in blood in the first week of acute illness, after which they may be shed in the urine.[8]

Because contamination can occur outside the PCR laboratory as well as within the laboratory, collection of specimens for nucleic acid testing should be performed aseptically. Gloves should be worn, and disposable instruments should be used (e.g., disposable blades, punch biopsy instruments).

In general, for detection of pathogens that contain DNA (i.e., all bacteria, fungi, some viruses), either fresh or frozen specimens should be submitted. In general, DNA is stable in tissue for up to 24 hours at 2°C to 8°C, at least 2 weeks at −20°C, and at least 2 years at −20°C or below −70°C.[5] Specimens held at room temperature should be submitted immediately and reach the laboratory within 24 hours. Specimens can also be refrigerated and submitted on wet ice within 72 hours. Provided the target of the assay is not an erythrocyte pathogen, erythrocytes should be removed before storage if possible. Specimens should not be stored in frost-free freezers, as these undergo repeated freeze-thaw cycling, which can be associated with DNA degradation.[9] Box 5-2 outlines recommendations based on specimen type.

BOX 5-2

Guidelines for Collection and Transport of Specimens for Polymerase Chain Reaction Assays

Specimen Type	Collection and Transport Recommendations
Whole blood and bone marrow	Use only EDTA or acid citrate dextrose (ACD) anticoagulant. Heparin inhibits PCR.* The use of hemolyzed specimens and frozen blood should be avoided if possible. DNA: Submit specimens held at room temperature within 24 hours of collection. Specimens can be stored at 2°C to 8°C for 72 hours, or at −20°C or ≤−70°C for prolonged storage (removal of erythrocytes recommended). RNA: Use stabilization solution or send immediately to the laboratory on wet ice. For storage, freeze serum, plasma, or buffy coat specimens at or below −70°C.
Tissue specimens	Optimal specimen is 1 to 2 g of fresh tissue. Rinse blood from tissue using sterile saline. Wrap in saline-moistened gauze or paper. Avoid excessive dilution. Formalin-fixed, paraffin-embedded tissues can be used when no other specimen is available but are not optimal. DNA: Transport fresh tissue immediately to the laboratory on wet ice. Any storage should be at or below −70°C, preferably after snap freezing in liquid nitrogen. RNA: Use stabilizing solution, process within 1 hour of collection, or snap freeze in liquid nitrogen and store at or below −70°C
Cerebrospinal fluid	DNA: Transport at 2°C to 8°C or freeze at −20°C or at or below −70°C RNA: Chill immediately on wet ice and deliver to the laboratory within 4 hours. Otherwise freeze immediately (removal of contaminating erythrocytes recommended) and ship on dry ice.
Bronchoalveolar lavage specimens	Transport at room temperature within 24 hours of collection. If a delay is anticipated, store for up to 72 hours at 2°C to 8°C or freeze at or below −70°C.
Urine	Minimize storage at room temperature. Storage and transport should be according to the specific assay performed.
Feces	Use preserved specimen transport container, or transport under refrigeration at 2°C to 8°C.

Adapted from the CLSI guidelines MM13-A.
*Beutler E, Gelbart T, Kuhl W. Interference of heparin with the polymerase chain reaction. Biotechniques 1990;9:166.

RNA is highly susceptible to degradation during storage and transport. For detection of RNA viruses, some laboratories provide an RNA stabilizing solution into which specimens are collected to prevent RNA degradation. If stabilizing solution is not readily available at the time of specimen collection, swabs and body fluids should be immediately sent to the laboratory on wet ice. Tissue should ideally be snap frozen at −70°C within half an hour of collection and shipped on dry ice without being thawed in the interim. RNA is stable for at least 2 years at or below −70°C. Ribonucleases can continue to degrade RNA at −20°C.

For tissue specimens, the optimal amount is 1 to 2 g, although more or less may be required depending on the cellularity of the specimen.[5] Tissues stored in formalin, especially for prolonged periods, are suboptimal for PCR because the formalin cross-links the DNA in the specimen. Tissues fixed briefly in formalin and then paraffin-embedded are preferable to tissues stored in formalin, because the formalin is removed during the embedding process. Paraffin-embedded specimens should only be used when no other specimens are available.[5]

Although PCR can be performed on feces, its sensitivity may be lower than with other specimens because inhibitors of PCR are particularly abundant in fecal material.[10] The use of appropriate amplification controls by the laboratory facilitates detection of false negatives due to the presence of inhibitors.

Diagnostic Methods

Nucleic Acid Probes

A variety of nucleic acid probes are available commercially as kits for detection of microorganisms that infect humans. Some of these can also be used to detect the same pathogens in specimens from dogs or cats. Probes are available for use in the clinical microbiology laboratory to identify organisms that have grown in culture (e.g., Gen-Probe Inc., San Diego), and these probes are widely used in human clinical microbiology laboratories.

Probe hybridization can be performed on a nitrocellulose membrane *(solid-phase hybridization)*; on formalin-fixed, paraffin-embedded sections mounted on a microscope slide (*in situ hybridization*); or in solution *(liquid-phase hybridization)*. For solid-phase hybridization, the probe is reacted with microorganism DNA that has been immobilized on the membrane. Unbound probe is washed away, and the bound probe is detected using fluorescence, chemiluminescence, radioactivity, or color development (in the same way that bound antibody or antigen is detected in an ELISA or immunofluorescent antibody assay). For in situ hybridization, formalin-fixed, paraffin-embedded specimens are sectioned and mounted on a special slide. The sections are deparaffinized, dried, and incubated with a solution that contains the probe, so both the presence and the location of the target pathogen within tissues can be identified. In situ hybridization assays that include a fluorescent-labeled probe are referred to as *fluorescence in situ hybridization* (FISH) assays (see Figure 5-1).

Because liquid-phase hybridization occurs in solution, unbound probe cannot be washed away. To overcome this problem, a chemiluminescent acridinium ester label is attached to the probe. A subsequent chemical hydrolysis step selectively degrades only unbound probe. On addition of peroxides, the intact (hybridized) probe then emits light.[11]

Although not yet widely used for veterinary applications, *peptide nucleic acid (PNA) probes* are now increasingly available to detect target DNA. PNA probes are uncharged peptides that mimic DNA and bind to complementary DNA sequences just as a nucleic acid probe would.[12,13] PNA probes lack the net negative charge of nucleic acid probes; therefore, the electrostatic repulsion that normally occurs when two negatively charged DNA strands hybridize does not occur. The result is a more stable and specific binding of the probe to its target, which in turn can be associated with increased assay sensitivity and specificity.

Branched DNA assays and *hybrid capture assays* are highly sensitive hybridization methods that include steps to intensify the signal generated from probe hybridization.[3,4] They are not yet widely used in veterinary medicine.

The Polymerase Chain Reaction

PCR allows the specific amplification of DNA sequences from just one copy to millions of copies, which can be more readily detected. The DNA from a clinical specimen is extracted using a commercially available DNA extraction kit. A pair of primers, roughly 20 nucleotides long, is then used to bracket a desired DNA sequence, which is subsequently copied using a DNA polymerase enzyme (Figure 5-2).

PCR assays are broadly divided into *conventional PCR assays* and *real-time PCR assays*. Conventional PCR assay is the simplest PCR method and although still widely for research purposes, its use for diagnostic purposes is decreasing. In conventional PCR, the PCR product is detected as a band on an agarose gel after agarose gel electrophoresis. In real-time PCR, a fluorescent signal is generated *as PCR products accumulate*, allowing them to be detected in "real time." A major advantage of real-time PCR methods is that the tube in which the PCR takes place does not need to be opened for detection of the PCR product. This greatly reduces the likelihood of contamination and false positive test results. Real-time PCR assays are amenable to automation, and reactions are generally loaded onto covered 96- or 384-well plates. This can be done robotically, further reducing the possibility of contamination and manual loading errors.

Regardless of the type of PCR assay, extracted DNA is added to aliquots of a PCR *mastermix*. The mastermix is a solution

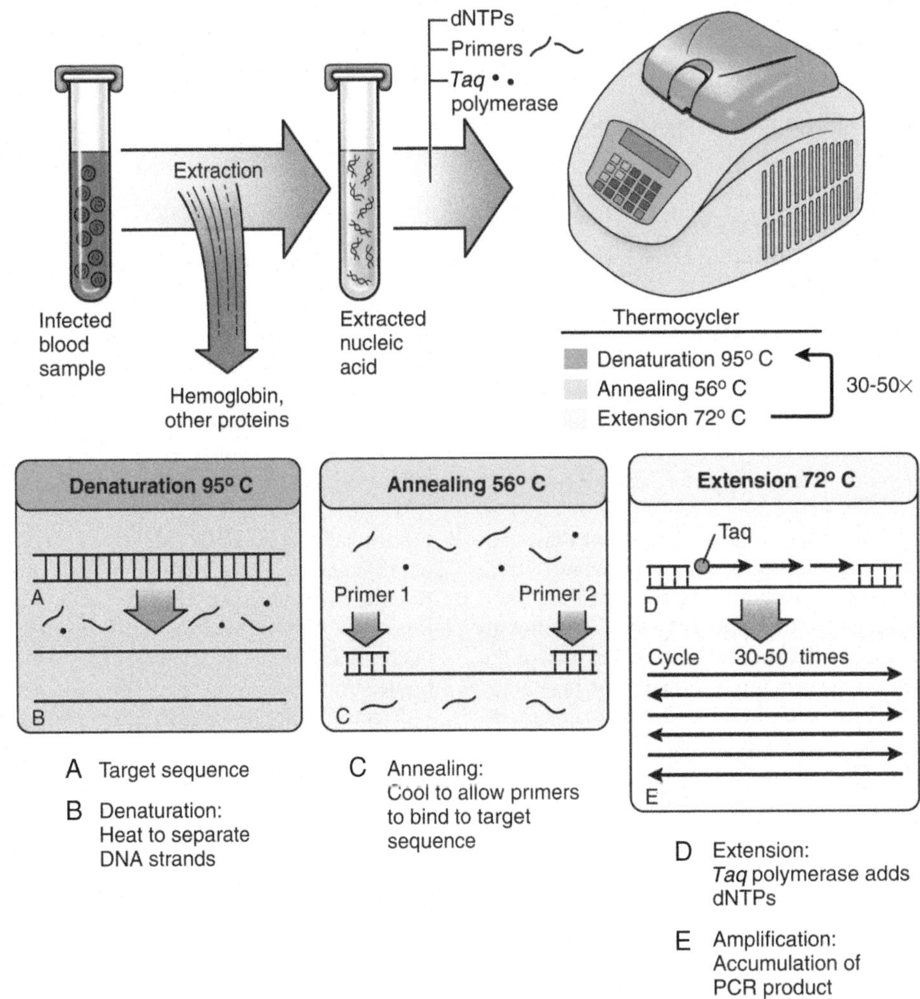

FIGURE 5-2 Basic PCR assay. Nucleic acid is extracted from a clinical specimen through removal of contaminating proteins such as hemoglobin. Two primers are added that hybridize at each end of a specific segment of a pathogen's DNA. Also present in the reaction mixture are the enzyme *Taq* polymerase (*dots*) and free nucleotides (dNTPs) for new DNA. A thermocycler is used to rapidly and repeatedly heat and cool the tubes through denaturation, annealing, and extension steps. Denaturation separates double-stranded DNA. Annealing occurs at a specific temperature that causes the primers to bind only to their target sequences. When the reaction mixture is then heated to 72°C, the *Taq* enzyme uses the primers as initiation points for DNA extension, and the target sequence is copied. The process is repeated 30 to 50 times, with logarithmic accumulation of the PCR product, so there are millions of copies of the target pathogen's DNA. These can then be detected using agarose gel electrophoresis (see Figure 5-3).

that contains the two primers, dNTPs (G, T, A, and C) for making new DNA, and a DNA polymerase. The DNA polymerase used most commonly (*Taq* DNA polymerase) is a heat-stable polymerase derived from *Thermophilus aquaticus*, a bacterium that is adapted to live in hot springs. Typical PCR assay reaction volumes are 10 to 50 µL.

The next step is performed in a thermocycler, a machine that is programmed to heat and cool the tubes repeatedly, so that the DNA can be amplified (see Figure 5-2). Initially the DNA is heated to 95°C, which causes the paired strands of DNA to *denature*. Next, the tubes are cooled to a specific *annealing temperature* (usually around 50°C to 65°C), which allows the primers bind to their respective sequences. Finally, the tubes are heated to 72°C. This is the temperature at which the DNA polymerase adds dNTPs in the mastermix to the primers, extending the primers as it copies the sequence of the template DNA. The 3-step cycle is repeated 30 to 50 times, which results in logarithmic accumulation of a PCR product that is an exact copy of the segment of DNA between the two primers. The amplified segments of DNA are called *amplicons*.

Detection of the PCR Product: Conventional versus Real-time PCR

In conventional PCR, amplified DNA is loaded into wells in an agarose gel then passed through the gel using horizontal electrophoresis, stained with a DNA stain, and visualized using ultraviolet transillumination. The longer the PCR product, the more slowly it moves through the gel during electrophoresis. When a series of molecular weight markers are run alongside the end product of PCR, the size of the PCR product can be estimated (Figure 5-3). The true identity of the product can then be confirmed using sequencing or by transferring it to a membrane and performing DNA hybridization with a specific probe. The process of loading the PCR product in agarose wells requires that the PCR tubes be opened, which can lead to aerosolization of PCR amplicons. These amplicons can then contaminate reagents, equipment, and tubes that are used for running subsequent PCR assays. Unless proper controls are included, false positives resulting from such contamination may go unidentified and lead to erroneous reporting of results.

Two major types of real-time PCR assays are in use in veterinary medicine: fluorescent probe–based assays and SYBR Green PCR assays.

Fluorescent probe real-time PCR assays incorporate one or more specific DNA probes into the PCR mastermix, in addition to the two primers used in conventional PCR. The probe(s) are tagged with a dye that emits fluorescent light. Inclusion of a probe adds specificity to the test, because it is less likely that both primers *and* the probe will bind to DNA other than that of the target organism. Three types of probes may be used:

1. *TaqMan (5′ nuclease) probes.* Many veterinary laboratories that offer probe-based PCR assays use TaqMan probes. These are tagged with a fluorescent reporter dye at one end, and a quencher dye at the other end of the probe. The close proximity of the quencher dye to the reporter dye inhibits the reporter dye from emitting fluorescence. When the *Taq* DNA polymerase copies the section of DNA between the two primers, it encounters the probe and chops it into pieces, because it has inherent exonuclease activity. This causes the reporter dye to separate from the quencher dye. The reporter dye then emits fluorescence, which can be measured using a spectrophotometer (Figure 5-4, *A*).
2. *Molecular beacons.* A molecular beacon is a probe with fluorescent reporter and quencher dyes at each end, but when not bound to the target sequence, it forms a hairpin loop that brings each dye in close proximity and stops the reporter dye from emitting fluorescence. When the probe anneals, the dyes separate, and the reporter dye emits fluorescence (see Figure 5-4, *B*).
3. *FRET probes.* FRET (fluorescent resonance energy transfer) probe assays use two probes that are expected to lie next to one another on the target sequence. One of the probes is tagged at the 3′ end with a green fluorescent dye, the other at the 5′ end with a red fluorescent dye. When the two dyes come together during annealing, the green fluorescent dye transfers its energy to the red probe, causing it to emit fluorescence, which can then be detected (see Figure 5-4, *C*). Currently there are only rare reports of the use of this technology for diagnosis in veterinary medicine.

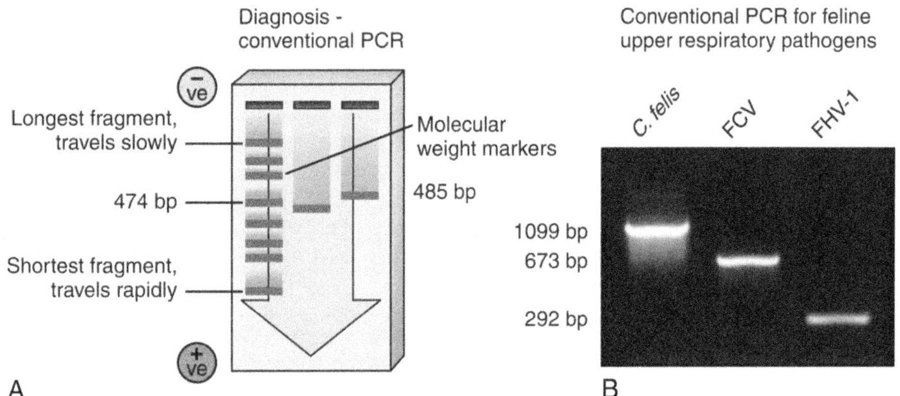

FIGURE 5-3 **A,** Detection of PCR products by agarose gel electrophoresis. At the end of the PCR process, the reaction mixture that results is loaded into wells at the top of an agarose gel. An electric current is applied across the gel, and because DNA is negatively charged, any amplified DNA in the reaction mixture migrates through the gel toward the positive terminal. The longer the DNA sequence that has been amplified, the more slowly it moves through the gel. Simultaneous electrophoresis of a molecular weight standard in an adjacent lane (*left* lane) allows estimation of the size of any PCR products amplified. The molecular weight standard contains DNA fragments of known size. After electrophoresis, the gel is stained with a DNA stain. If the target pathogen's DNA was successfully amplified, it appears as a band of an expected size (in this case, 485 base pairs [*bp*] long). Bands that are the wrong size ("aberrant PCR products") may represent nonspecific amplification of DNA from a different microorganism or host DNA (*middle* lane). **B,** Photograph of PCR products in an agarose gel after agarose gel electrophoresis and staining. DNA bands amplified from *Chlamydia felis*, feline calicivirus (*FCV*), and feline herpesvirus-1 (*FHV-1*) are shown. The primers were designed to amplify different-length products from each pathogen so that if multiple pathogens were present in a single specimen, they could be distinguished from one another.

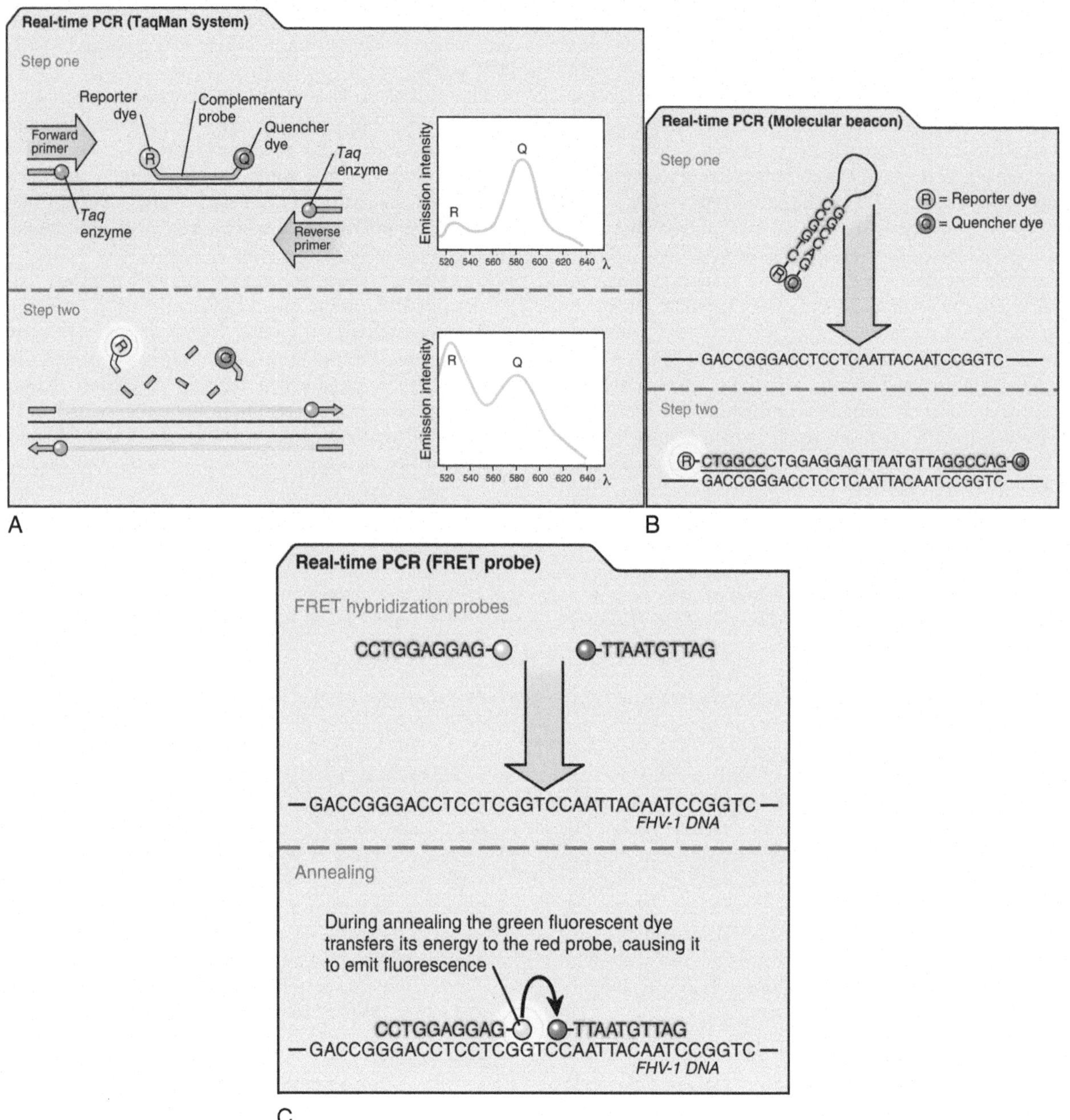

FIGURE 5-4 Probe-based real-time PCR assays. **A,** TaqMan probe PCR system. In addition to the forward and reverse primers used in conventional PCR, an additional short probe is used that binds specifically to the DNA of the pathogen of interest (step one). Emission of fluorescence by a reporter dye located at one end of the probe is quenched by another dye at the other end of the probe. When the *Taq* enzyme extends the primers, an inherent exonuclease activity of the enzyme results in the digestion of the probe. The quencher and reporter dyes separate, causing the quencher dye to emit fluorescence. Other probe-based real-time PCR assays include molecular beacon assays **(B)** and fluorescent resonance energy transfer probe assays **(C)**.

SYBR Green Real-time PCR assays use a double-stranded DNA binding dye (SYBR Green) that fluoresces when bound to double-stranded DNA as it forms during PCR amplification. Because there is no probe, carefully designed primers are required to ensure high assay specificity for the organism of interest.

The amount of fluorescence emitted during real-time PCR is proportional to the number of copies of template DNA in the specimen, so real-time PCR assays can be quantitative. A plot of PCR cycle number against fluorescence is generated by an attached computer and interpreted by the laboratory technician (Figure 5-5). The number of cycles that elapse before fluorescence is detectable above a certain threshold value is the CT (cycle threshold) value. Most laboratories run approximately 40 cycles, and so specimens that generate CT values less than 40 are considered positive. Said another way, if PCR proceeds to 40 cycles without emission of fluorescence (CT = 40), then the target DNA is not detectable in the specimen, and the result is reported as negative. The lower the CT value, the more target DNA (= organism load) is present in the sample, because fewer cycles elapse before fluorescence is detected. Because specimen size can vary, the CT value may be normalized to the number of host cells present in the sample. Knowledge of organism load may have prognostic value for some infections, can allow infection to be monitored over time with treatment, and may be useful to differentiate low-level colonization from active infection causing clinical signs (see Interpretation of Results, later). At the time of writing, organism loads are variably reported by veterinary diagnostic laboratories performing PCR assays.

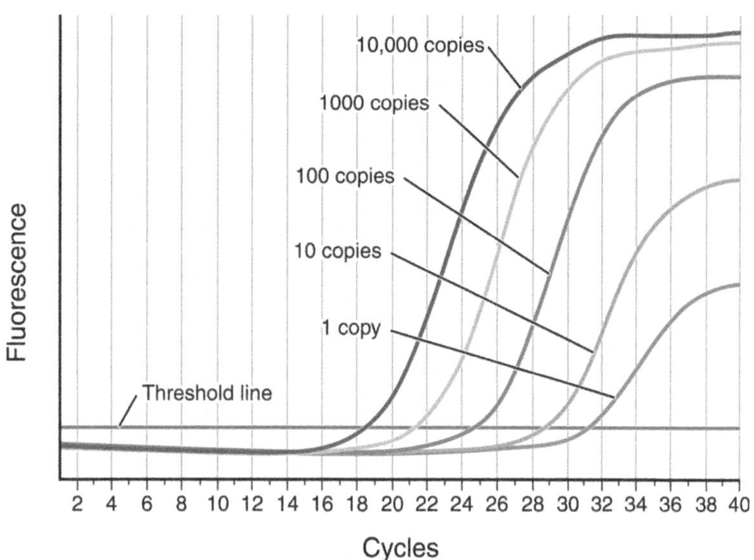

FIGURE 5-5 Plot that shows the emission of fluorescence during PCR product formation over time in real-time PCR as the number of cycles of denaturation, annealing, and extension increases from 0 to 40 (*x*-axis). The cycle threshold (CT) value is the number of PCR cycles required for the fluorescent signal (*y*-axis) to rise above a threshold value for fluorescence (threshold line). The more copies of target pathogen DNA that are present in a clinical specimen (which correlates with the number of organisms present), the earlier fluorescence is emitted and the lower the CT value. Thus, for example, if only one organism is present in a submitted specimen, the CT value for this particular PCR assay is 32, but if 10,000 organisms are present, the CT value is around 19.

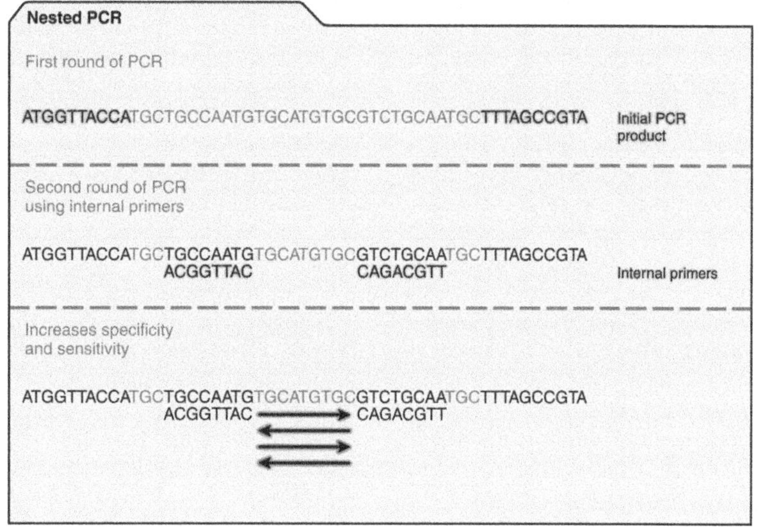

FIGURE 5-6 Nested PCR. After the first round of PCR amplification, a second set of internal primers *(green)* is used in yet another round of PCR amplification, which generates a second, shorter PCR product.

Rapid thermocyclers are available in several different formats. Special carousel thermocyclers have been developed that rapidly heat and cool the reactions, which are placed in specially designed glass capillaries. As a result, PCR assays can be completed in 45 minutes, instead of the usual 4 to 5 hours.[14]

Polymerase Chain Reaction Variations

Variations on the basic PCR assay include reverse-transcriptase PCR, nested PCR, and multiplex PCR.

Reverse-transcriptase PCR is used for RNA detection. After extraction of RNA from the clinical specimen using a commercial kit, the enzyme *reverse transcriptase* is added to the RNA, together with dNTPs that will be used to make DNA. The starting point for reverse transcription can be a single complementary DNA primer that binds to the RNA, or alternatively, *random hexamers*, which are a mixture of six-nucleotide primers that represent all possible combinations of dNTPs. The reverse transcriptase then uses the primers to make a DNA copy of the RNA (known as *cDNA*), which is subsequently subjected to PCR amplification.

For *nested PCR*, a small amount of amplified PCR product is subjected to a second round of conventional PCR using another set of internal primers (Figure 5-6). Having an additional set of primers increases the specificity of the PCR assay and also greatly increases its sensitivity.[15] Unfortunately, the increased sensitivity means that false positives due to contamination can be extremely problematic with this method, and it has lost popularity for diagnostic purposes.

Multiplex PCR assays use multiple sets of primers *in the same reaction tube* to simultaneously detect multiple organisms (or multiple genes from the same organism). Duplex PCR assays can detect two organisms, and triplex PCR assays can detect three organisms. The potential downside of multiplex reactions is that if both organisms are present, and one organism is present in relative abundance, amplification of this organism can consume reagents, which reduces the sensitivity of the assay for the other target organism.

Verification of Polymerase Chain Reaction Assay Performance

Before being used for diagnostic purposes, PCR assays must be shown to be *sensitive, specific, reproducible,* and *efficient.*

For PCR, *the limit of detection* is the lowest number of copies of the target DNA or RNA sequence that the assay can detect. Serial dilutions of known amounts of the template DNA are tested using the PCR assay of interest, until template can no longer be detected.

From a diagnostic standpoint, a PCR assay may lack sensitivity (many false negatives) if the assay fails to detect all possible strains of a target organism. This can occur if the probe or primers are strain, rather than species-specific, and many strains of the target organism exist with variable sequences (as is the case with RNA pathogens such as feline calicivirus). As part of the verification process, the assay should be shown to detect as many strains as possible.

A PCR assay has poor analytical specificity if false positives occur as a result of contamination or because of manual loading error. Specificity may also be poor if the primers bind to and initiate amplification of DNA from unrelated organisms or the host animal (i.e., cat, dog, human DNA). Specificity is tested during the verification process by showing that the PCR assay fails to amplify DNA from specimens that contain organisms that are genetically related to the target organism, as well as organisms that may be expected to be contaminating normal flora.

The results of PCR assays must also be repeatable. Repeatability is determined for real-time PCR assays by determining whether the CT value varies significantly for the same specimen when tested multiple times. Usually intraassay (within the same run) and interassay (within different runs) variations are measured.

A real-time PCR assay that has an *efficiency* of 100% doubles the number of copies of template in every PCR cycle. Efficiencies below 90% are unacceptable for quantitative assays, and ideally efficiency should be greater than 95%. The efficiency is determined by testing serial dilutions of a target DNA standard and by creating a chart of copy number versus CT value. Ideally, this is compared with a similar chart using dilutions of the standard DNA spiked into a clinical specimen, to show that inhibitors within the specimen will not affect efficiency.

Prevention of Contamination and Quality Control

Prevention of PCR contamination relies on good laboratory practices, some of which are outlined in Box 5-3. Contamination can be difficult to eradicate once it occurs, so prevention of contamination is critical. Laboratories should include negative controls with every run, and a positive control should be included to ensure that the assay is working, preferably one that is put through the nucleic acid extraction process. The positive control should contain a low concentration of DNA, as abundant DNA in a positive control sample may be a source of contamination. Many laboratories run two separate negative controls. One of the negative controls contains mastermix and nuclease-free water in place of specimen DNA. The other consists of water or a known negative specimen that is placed through the extraction process to ensure that contamination does not occur during extraction (negative extraction control). When 96- or 384-well plate formats are used, negative control wells are interspersed among the test wells to monitor for plate contamination.

In order to prevent contamination, some laboratories use deoxyuracil triphosphate (dUTP) instead of deoxythymidine triphosphate (dTTP) in the PCR mastermix. The PCR products therefore contain uracil (U) in place of thymidine (T). The enzyme uracil-*N*-glycosylase (UNG) is also added to the mix. This enzyme destroys DNA amplicons that contain deoxyuracil residues, and eliminates any contaminating DNA amplicons from previous reactions before PCR amplification begins. When the specimen is heated in the initial denaturation step, the UNG is destroyed.

The presence of substances that inhibit the PCR assay can be detected using a *housekeeping gene* control PCR assay. This is performed on a separate aliquot of the specimen at the same time as the assay for the target pathogen. Housekeeping genes are host (dog or cat) genes that are expected to be present in the specimen. Examples of commonly used housekeeping gene PCR assays are those for canine or feline glyceraldehyde-3-phosphate dehydrogenase (GAPDH), histone, or 18S DNA. A negative housekeeping gene PCR assay result (or a high CT value for the assay, which is equivalent to a weak positive result) suggests that inhibitors may be present in the specimen, or that the DNA in the submitted specimen may have degraded during storage or transport. Some PCR assays use an *internal housekeeping gene control*, in which a housekeeping gene PCR is multiplexed with the PCR assay for the target microorganism.

BOX 5-3

Methods That May Be Used to Minimize Contamination in Diagnostic Laboratories That Perform Nucleic Acid Amplification Assay

Separation of rooms for DNA extraction, PCR, and PCR product detection
Robotic DNA extraction
Automated detection of PCR products (real-time PCR)
Opening one specimen tube at a time
Use of screw-top caps rather than snap-top tubes to prevent splashing
Use of filter-plugged pipette tips
Use of negative extraction controls and negative template controls in every run
Routine monitoring for contamination using wipes
Standard cleanup protocol that inactivates nucleic acids
Use of positive control samples of low concentration
Use of dUTP and uracil-*N*-glycosylase in the PCR mastermix

Interpretation of Results

Because some PCR assays can detect as few as one or two organisms, and both viable and nonviable organisms are detected, it may be difficult to determine the significance of a positive PCR test result in light of an animal's disease. An understanding of the pathogenesis of infectious diseases and organism shedding patterns is crucial in interpreting positive PCR results. Correct interpretation of the results relies on knowledge of the methods used by a laboratory and their advantages and disadvantages.

BOX 5-4

Factors That Should Be Considered When Interpreting Nucleic Acid Amplification Assay Results

Negative Test Result

Organism not present
Too few organisms present
Insufficient specimen size
Wrong specimen type
Improper timing of specimen collection
Patient receiving antimicrobial therapy
Specimen degradation during storage or transport
Assay reagent failure
Assay inhibitors present or extraction failure
Reagents consumed in a multiplex assay
Assay does not detect all strains

Positive Test Result

Viable or nonviable organisms present and causing disease
Viable or nonviable organisms present but not causing disease
Vaccine organisms present
Contamination
Loading errors
Assay cross-reaction with other pathogens or host DNA in the sample

Specimens That Test Negative

Factors that lead to negative test results are shown in Box 5-4. An example of the use of the wrong specimen type would be submission of blood for a *Borrelia burgdorferi* PCR test, when *B. burgdorferi* is found predominantly in connective tissue.[16] Assay inhibition and specimen degradation can be identified by interpretation of housekeeping gene control assay results, which should be performed by the laboratory. Assay reagent failure is identified by the laboratory when the positive control tests negative.

Specimens That Test Positive

Factors that must be considered when interpreting positive test results are shown in Box 5-4. The most common reason for false-positive test results for assays that involve DNA amplification is contamination. Loading errors, in which specimens are inadvertently loaded into the wrong wells on a microtiter plate, may also lead to false-positive results and are reduced with the use of automated methods. Because of the exquisite sensitivity of PCR, it may be difficult to determine the significance of a true positive result. The organism may be part of the normal flora, carried subclinically (e.g., latent feline herpesvirus-1 in a nasal biopsy), or simply colonizing the anatomic site sampled. Several U.S. veterinary laboratories offer PCR "panels" for diagnostic purposes. Individual PCR assays for several different pathogens are performed on nucleic acid extracted from a single specimen. This high-throughput panel format allows assays to be offered at a substantial discount over the cost of multiple individual assays. This type of testing can result in unexpected positive test results, such as a positive result for the *Clostridium perfringens* toxin gene in a cat with diarrhea that is suspected to have trichomoniasis. As with any laboratory test, positive results need to be interpreted in light of the clinical history, clinical signs, and the pathogenesis of the disease in question.

A positive result can occur if an attenuated live vaccine for the target organism was recently administered. Because PCR detects both viable and nonviable organisms, PCR can be positive for days after antimicrobials have been administered, when culture is negative.[17-19] The duration of PCR positivity after treatment depends on the specimen type tested and the target pathogen.

REFERENCES

1. Komminoth P, Werner M. Target and signal amplification: approaches to increase the sensitivity of in situ hybridization. Histochem Cell Biol. 1997;108:325-333.
2. Quality Control for Molecular Diagnostics. 2012. http://www.qcmd.org/. Last accessed May 11, 2012.
3. Andras SC, Power JB, Cocking EC, et al. Strategies for signal amplification in nucleic acid detection. Mol Biotechnol. 2001;19:29-44.
4. Nolte FS, Caliendo AM. Molecular microbiology. In: Versalovic J, Carroll KC, Funke G, et al. eds. Manual of Clinical Microbiology. 10th ed. Washington, DC: ASM Press; 2011:27-59.
5. Clinical and Laboratory Standards Institute. Collection, transport, preparation, and storage of specimens for molecular methods; approved guideline. MM13-A. 2005;25:7-18.
6. Illig R, Fritsch H, Schwarzer C. Breaking the seals: efficient mRNA detection from human archival paraffin-embedded tissue. RNA. 2009;15:1588-1596.
7. Tan LH, Do E, Chong SM, et al. Detection of ALK gene rearrangements in formalin-fixed, paraffin-embedded tissue using a fluorescence in situ hybridization (FISH) probe: a search for optimum conditions of tissue archiving and preparation for FISH. Mol Diagn. 2003;7:27-33.
8. Greenlee JJ, Bolin CA, Alt DP, et al. Clinical and pathologic comparison of acute leptospirosis in dogs caused by two strains of *Leptospira kirschneri* serovar *grippotyphosa*. Am J Vet Res. 2004;65:1100-1107.
9. Lahiri DK, Schnabel B. DNA isolation by a rapid method from human blood samples: effects of $MgCl_2$, EDTA, storage time, and temperature on DNA yield and quality. Biochem Genet. 1993;31:321-328.
10. Oikarinen S, Tauriainen S, Viskari H, et al. PCR inhibition in stool samples in relation to age of infants. J Clin Virol. 2009;44:211-214.
11. Arnold Jr LJ, Hammond PW, Wiese WA, et al. Assay formats involving acridinium-ester-labeled DNA probes. Clin Chem. 1989;35:1588-1594.
12. Padilla E, Manterola JM, Rasmussen OF, et al. Evaluation of a fluorescence hybridisation assay using peptide nucleic acid probes for identification and differentiation of tuberculous and non-tuberculous mycobacteria in liquid cultures. Eur J Clin Microbiol Infect Dis. 2000;19:140-145.
13. Zhang N, Appella DH. Advantages of peptide nucleic acids as diagnostic platforms for detection of nucleic acids in resource-limited settings. J Infect Dis. 2010;201(suppl 1):S42-S45.
14. Cockerill 3rd FR. Application of rapid-cycle real-time polymerase chain reaction for diagnostic testing in the clinical microbiology laboratory. Arch Pathol Lab Med. 2003;127:1112-1120.
15. Lu JJ, Chen CH, Bartlett MS, et al. Comparison of six different PCR methods for detection of *Pneumocystis carinii*. J Clin Microbiol. 1995;33:2785-2788.
16. Aguero-Rosenfeld ME, Wang G, Schwartz I, et al. Diagnosis of Lyme borreliosis. Clin Microbiol Rev. 2005;18:484-509.
17. Bockenstedt LK, Mao J, Hodzic E, et al. Detection of attenuated, noninfectious spirochetes in *Borrelia burgdorferi*-infected mice after antibiotic treatment. J Infect Dis. 2002;186:1430-1437.
18. Braddock JA, Tasker S, Malik R. The use of real-time PCR in the diagnosis and monitoring of *Mycoplasma haemofelis* copy number in a naturally infected cat. J Feline Med Surg. 2004;6:161-165.
19. Sykes JE, Studdert VP, Browning GF. Comparison of the polymerase chain reaction and culture for the detection of feline *Chlamydia psittaci* in untreated and doxycycline-treated experimentally infected cats. J Vet Intern Med. 1999;13:146-152.

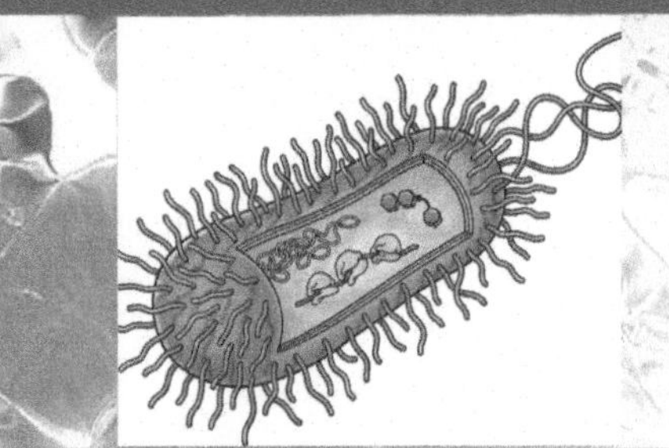

SECTION 2

Antiinfective Therapy

Jane E. Sykes and Mark G. Papich

CHAPTER 6

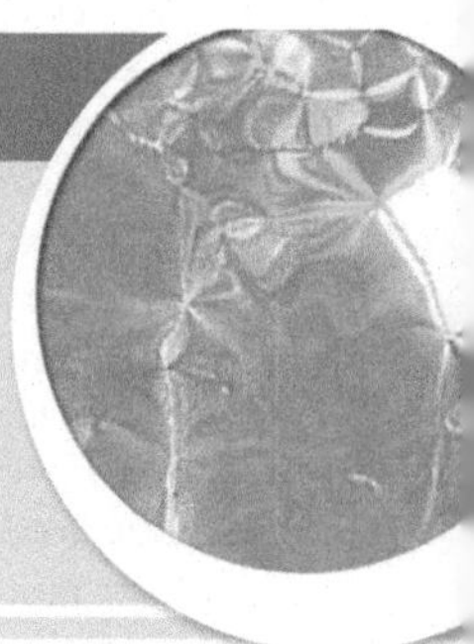

Principles of Antiinfective Therapy

Jane E. Sykes and Mark G. Papich

KEY POINTS

- The use of antimicrobial drugs (AMDs) can lead to selection of resistant bacterial populations, within the targeted bacterial population and also other commensal bacteria.
- Bacterial mechanisms of drug resistance include production of enzymes that inactivate AMDs, drug exclusion through membrane alterations and efflux pumps, and modification of the site of action of the AMD.
- Strategies that minimize selection for drug resistance include (1) confirmation of the presence of infection before AMD treatment is commenced, (2) proper identification of the infecting organism, (3) selection of agents with activity specific to the pathogen present, (4) administration of an adequate dose of AMD, and (5) administration of AMD for the proper duration of time.
- Selection of an appropriate AMD should be based on the activity of the agent against the suspected pathogen; knowledge of drug pharmacokinetics, which includes bioavailability and tissue penetration; consideration of host factors such as concurrent illness, medications, or immunosuppression; and knowledge of drug pharmacodynamics, that is, whether the drug exhibits concentration- or time-dependent antibacterial effects.

INTRODUCTION

Antibiotics have been considered one of the greatest inventions of the 20th century. The modern era of antimicrobial drug (AMD) treatment began with the discovery of sulfonamides in 1935.[1] In the 1940s, the therapeutic value of penicillin and streptomycin was discovered, and by 1950, the "golden age" of AMD therapy was underway. With the increasing use of AMDs, there has been a transition to an era of widespread antimicrobial resistance among important veterinary and human pathogens. This has been compounded by a declining rate of development of new classes of AMDs.

Antimicrobial resistance genes have existed in microbes long before antimicrobial agents were used in therapy. Microbe populations generally consist of a mixture of genetically susceptible and resistant organisms. The use of AMDs exerts pressure that favors selection of the resistant microbes ("survival of the fittest"), within both the targeted bacterial population and other commensal bacteria (which have the potential to become pathogenic when host defenses are impaired). The chance that resistant bacterial populations will emerge depends on the ability of the population to rapidly acquire mutations, the ability of host defenses to eliminate resistant bacteria, and the AMD concentrations at the site of infection.

Guidelines for prudent antimicrobial use have been published by several professional veterinary organizations in order to reduce selection for resistant bacterial pathogens.[2-6] Individual hospitals are encouraged to develop antimicrobial guidelines based on evaluation of their local prevalence of AMD resistance. Strategies that minimize selection for antimicrobial resistance include documentation of the presence of infection; proper identification of the infecting organism; and the use of agents that are as specific for the pathogen as possible, at the proper dose and for the proper duration of time. These strategies are described in more detail in this chapter.

Identification of the Infecting Organism

The detection of fever or leukocytosis does not imply bacterial infection and the need for antibiotic treatment, especially given the relatively high prevalence of sterile inflammatory and immune-mediated diseases in dogs and viral infections in cats. Selection of the most appropriate AMD relies on knowledge of (1) the presence of an infectious agent, (2) the type of infectious agent present, and (3) the susceptibility of the agent to different AMDs. In some cases, treatment with antibiotics may not be necessary even though the cause of disease is bacterial. Some infections undergo spontaneous cures without the aid of an antibiotic. For example, a cat bite abscess can often be drained and resolved without the need to administer an antibiotic (see Chapter 57).

In some situations, collection of a specimen for cytology or histopathology permits a diagnosis of infection to be established.

The identity of some infectious agents, such as rickettsial and fungal pathogens, may be presumptively identified to the genus or species level based on their morphology. If skin cytology from a dog reveals cocci (a Gram stain is not necessary to confirm the presence of gram-positive cocci), then the presence of *Staphylococcus pseudintermedius* is highly probable. If, on the other hand, cytology from an ear swab reveals rods, the possibility of *Pseudomonas aeruginosa* must be considered. In either case, this knowledge is valuable for selecting initial antibacterial therapy. The use of molecular diagnostic techniques, such as PCR assays, can also allow rapid identification of an infecting organism, which can help to guide antimicrobial drug selection. For example, identification of a vector-borne pathogen (e.g., *Rickettsia* spp., *Ehrlichia canis*) is helpful because doxycycline is usually the first drug of choice for the majority of these pathogens. Unfortunately, unless susceptibility to a particular AMD is predictable, these techniques do not typically provide information about AMD susceptibility. Given the emergence of widespread AMD resistance, especially among bacteria and some fungi, collection of specimens for culture and susceptibility before treatment with AMDs is commenced has become more and more important. Although there is an initial cost to the client for culture and susceptibility testing, long-term costs to the client may be reduced considerably because of decreased prescription of unnecessary or inappropriate AMDs, improved likelihood of rapid resolution of the underlying disorder with early diagnosis and appropriate treatment, and reduced need for more expensive, second- or third-line AMDs. Administration of AMDs without identification of the infectious agent can also decrease subsequent chances of successful culture and proper diagnosis if the disorder does not resolve.

In animals with life-threatening infections, institution of AMD treatment is necessary before the results of culture and susceptibility become available. The choice of treatment at this stage can be based on cytology and knowledge of the type of infections that most commonly occur at the anatomic site involved (also known as *bacteriologic statistics*). Because of the life-threatening nature of these infections, the practice of "de-escalation" (as opposed to "escalation") is employed. This is the practice of initially selecting a highly active agent that has a high probability of successful elimination of the pathogen; then once the infectious agent has been identified, the drug spectrum should be changed or narrowed according to culture and susceptibility results. If the infection is life threatening, highly active agents such as an aminoglycoside or fluoroquinolone with or without a β-lactam can be selected initially. Then, if culture and susceptibility show susceptibility to β-lactams, treatment should be continued with these agents alone.

Classification of Antimicrobial Drugs

Antimicrobial drugs may be classified based on their structure (e.g., β-lactams, fluoroquinolones), spectrum of activity (gram-positive versus gram-negative bacteria), mechanism of action (Table 6-1, Figure 6-1), whether they are *bacteriostatic* (inhibit or slow growth) or *bactericidal* drugs, and their pharmacodynamic properties (see Pharmacodynamics of Antimicrobial Drugs, later). Bactericidal drugs interfere with cell wall or nucleic acid synthesis, whereas bacteriostatic drugs inhibit protein synthesis or cause changes in bacterial physiology. When a bacteriostatic drug is removed, in the absence of host defense mechanisms, organism growth resumes, and any decline in bacterial numbers that occurs when the drug concentration drops below the minimum inhibitory concentration (MIC) reflects clearance by the host immune response. However, the line that separates bactericidal and bacteriostatic is not as precise as previously thought. Some bacteriostatic drugs become bactericidal when present in high concentrations at the site of infection, or if concentrations are maintained above the MIC for the entire dosing interval. Even macrolides and chloramphenicol, which are traditionally considered as bacteriostatic drugs, can be bactericidal against some organisms. A drug may be bactericidal against gram-positive cocci, but bacteriostatic against gram-negative bacilli. Therefore, from a clinical perspective, it is more useful to describe drugs as time versus concentration-dependent, rather than as bactericidal or bacteriostatic. This allows the clinician to consider the dosage regimen and dosing interval to optimize therapy. There are rare instances where a bactericidal agent is preferred over a bacteriostatic one. It may be preferable to prescribe a bactericidal drug to treat life-threatening infections (such as vegetations in endocarditis or in a systemically immunocompromised host).[7]

Antibacterial drugs have also been classified for veterinary use as first-line, second-line, or third-line drugs.[8] First-line drugs are those that could be used for empirical selection in the absence of or pending the results of culture and susceptibility testing, and include amoxicillin, cephalexin, doxycycline, and trimethoprim-sulfonamides. Second-line drugs are those to be used on the basis of culture and susceptibility testing and because of the lack of any appropriate first-line options. These include ticarcillin, piperacillin, amikacin, and third-generation cephalosporins. Fluoroquinolones were also included in this group because in human medicine, excessive fluoroquinolone use has been associated with emergence of antimicrobial resistance and treatment failures.[9] Fluoroquinolones could be considered as first-line drugs for dogs and cats suspected to have serious gram-negative bacterial infections that require treatment pending the results of culture and susceptibility testing. The use of third-line drugs, including vancomycin, linezolid, and carbapenems such as imipenem and meropenem, is usually reserved for situations when certain criteria are met[8]:

1. Infection must be documented based on clinical abnormalities and culture.
2. The infection is serious and has the potential to be life-threatening if left untreated.
3. Resistance is documented to all other reasonable first- and second-line options.
4. The infection is potentially treatable.
5. The clinician may seek advice from an infectious disease clinician or a clinical microbiologist to discuss antimicrobial susceptibility test results, and to discuss the use of these agents if there is unfamiliarity with their use. In some instances, there may be other viable options (e.g., topical therapy).

Pharmacodynamics of Antimicrobial Drugs

Pharmacokinetic and pharmacodynamic parameters (PK-PD exposure relationships) are important determinants of the efficacy of AMDs and serve as the basis for determination of clinically effective dosage regimens and susceptibility breakpoints and for the development of guidelines for AMD use for specific types of infections.[10]

The killing of microbes by AMDs may be classified as *concentration dependent* or *time dependent*. AMDs that exhibit

TABLE 6-1

Classification of Antimicrobial Drugs Based on Their Mechanism of Action

Mechanism of Action	Antimicrobial Drug	Examples
Inhibition of cell wall synthesis	β-Lactams, glycopeptides	Penicillin, cephalexin, meropenem, vancomycin
Protein synthesis inhibition	Tetracyclines, aminoglycosides, chloramphenicol, lincosamides, macrolides	Doxycycline, gentamicin, erythromycin, clindamycin, azithromycin
Inhibition of DNA replication	Fluoroquinolones	Enrofloxacin, marbofloxacin
Inhibition of folic acid metabolism	Trimethoprim-sulfonamides	Trimethoprim-sulfamethoxazole

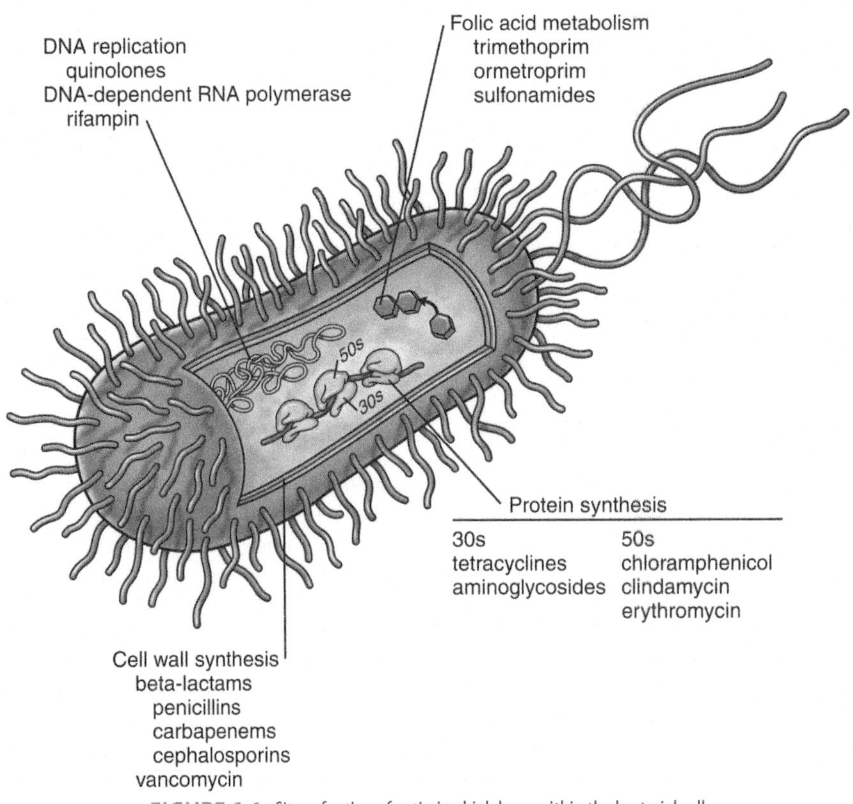

FIGURE 6-1 Sites of action of antimicrobial drugs within the bacterial cell.

concentration-dependent killing are fluoroquinolones and aminoglycosides. These drugs work optimally when the peak concentration in the plasma (C_{max}), or the area under the curve (AUC) exceeds the MIC by a defined factor (Figure 6-2). These are typically bactericidal agents and the ability to kill bacteria increases as the AMD concentrations increase. Target concentrations have been defined for laboratory animals and humans and have been extrapolated to veterinary patients. For example, the peak concentration to MIC ratio (C_{max}/MIC) should exceed 8 to 10 for optimum dosing of aminoglycosides. The AUC for a 24-hour interval to MIC ratio (AUC_{24}/MIC) should exceed 100 for fluoroquinolones. For some infections, a ratio of 125 is better, and in some patients (e.g., immunocompromised patients with life-threatening infections), a ratio of 250 may be desirable. Drugs that exhibit concentration-dependent killing also have *postantibiotic effect* (PAE). The PAE is the persistence of antimicrobial effects after drug concentrations at the site of infection fall below the MIC. The exact cause of the PAE varies with the drug, but it may result from irreversible binding of a drug to the target site. The duration of the PAE is influenced by the duration of antibiotic exposure, the drug concentration, the bacterial species present, and the class of antibiotic. For concentration-dependent antibiotics, administration of the total daily dose as a single dose every 24 hours is preferred to a smaller divided dose, in order to maximize C_{max} or AUC. For aminoglycosides, this also reduces drug toxicity.[7]

β-lactams (penicillins and cephalosporins), macrolides, and lincosamides (clindamycin) exhibit *time-dependent killing*. As concentrations of these drugs increase, bacterial killing plateaus, and outcome is correlated with the *time* that the AMD concentration spends above the MIC at the site of infection. This is usually expressed as the percent of time above the MIC during a 24-hour interval (T > MIC). For β-lactam drugs apart from carbapenems, PAEs are minimal. As a result, these drugs work best when administered multiple times a day or as continuous-rate infusions, in order to maintain drug concentrations at the site of infection. For some drugs (e.g., some

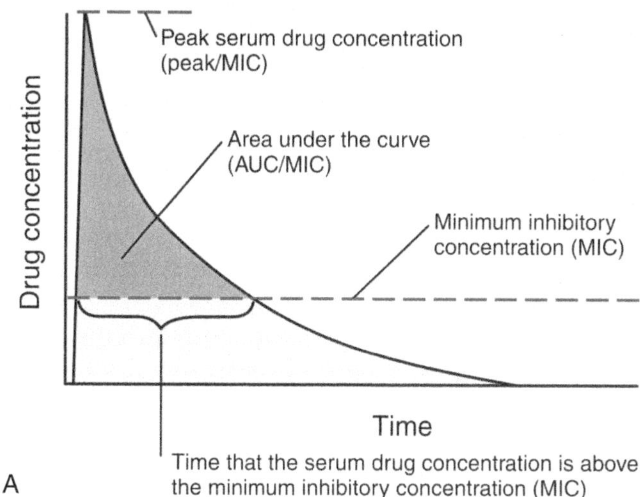

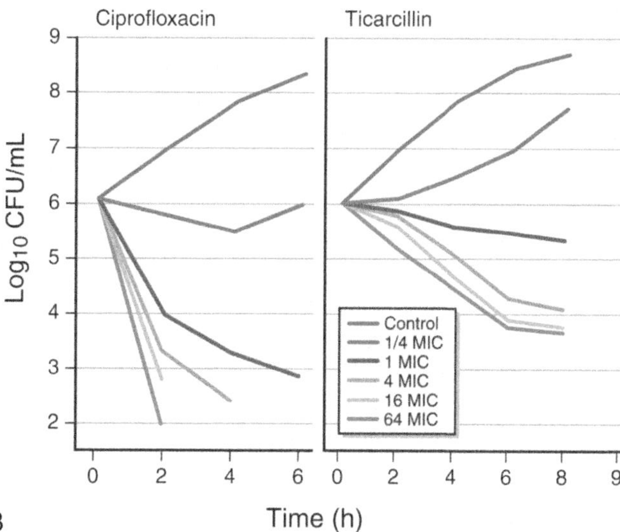

FIGURE 6-2 **A,** Antimicrobial drug (AMD) pharmacodynamics. Concentration-dependent drugs are most active when the peak concentration (C_{max}), or the area-under-the-curve (AUC) in the plasma exceeds the MIC by a defined factor. For time-dependent drugs, outcome is correlated with the time that the AMD concentration at the site of infection spends above the MIC. This is usually expressed as the percent of time above the MIC during a 24-hour interval (T > MIC). **B,** As AMD concentrations increase, the ability of concentration-dependent drugs such as fluoroquinolones (in this case, ciprofloxacin) to kill bacteria increases. As concentrations of time-dependent drugs such as β-lactam drugs (in this case, ticarcillin) increase, bacterial killing plateaus. MIC, minimum inhibitory concentration.

cephalosporins), a long T > MIC is achieved by virtue of a long half-life. The required time above the MIC for an AMD varies with the pathogen present, the drug, and the site of infection, but in general it should be 40% to 50% of the dosing interval.[7,10] Drug dosages that achieve concentrations in excess of an MIC for these periods can be calculated based on pharmacokinetic data. For time-dependent AMD with long half-lives (such as macrolides, clindamycin, and tetracyclines), efficacy is determined primarily by the extent to which the area under the curve exceeds the MIC. As the MIC of an organism increases, it becomes more difficult to achieve these PK-PD targets, and organisms are regarded as resistant.

In animals with renal failure, AMD clearance may be greatly diminished. In this case, T > MIC and AUC/MIC are achieved with a reduced dose or less frequent dosing. For β-lactam antibiotics, it is logical to increase the dose interval. For fluoroquinolones, it is better to decrease the dose.

Site of Infection

In general, the concentration of an AMD at the site of infection should at least equal the MIC for the infecting organism, but the exact concentration and the duration of the concentration at the site varies with the class of antimicrobial. For some AMDs, the serum or plasma total (bound and unbound) drug concentrations may not reflect the drug concentration in tissues. Examples are the highly lipophilic macrolide antibiotics (e.g., azithromycin) for which the tissue drug concentration greatly overestimates the plasma drug concentration. On the other hand, tissue concentrations greatly underestimate the plasma or serum drug concentration for poorly lipophilic agents such as aminoglycosides or β-lactams. Antimicrobial selection for different body sites is outlined in Box 6-1.

The concentration of an AMD at the site of infection is affected by factors such as lipid solubility, protein binding, and other factors reducing permeability, such as the presence of large amounts of pus, scar tissue, foreign material, devitalized tissue, and bone. Lipid-soluble drugs such as chloramphenicol, rifampin, fluoroquinolones, and trimethoprim are most adept at crossing membranes, including the blood-brain, alveolar, and prostatic barriers. In contrast, poorly lipophilic, polar drugs such as penicillins and aminoglycosides do not cross lipid membranes and will not achieve adequate tissue levels in tissues in which there is a barrier to penetration (e.g., prostate, brain, eye, or intracellular sites). In human patients, aminoglycosides and amphotericin B have been administered intrathecally to treat central nervous system infections.[11,12] In order to use β-lactam antibiotics to treat these infections, high doses are required because of a poorly penetrated blood-brain barrier. Even in the face of inflammation, the brain/blood concentration ratio of these drugs is low. Water-soluble AMDs that are excreted in active form by the liver and concentrated in bile, such as doxycycline and ampicillin, make excellent choices for susceptible hepatobiliary infections (see Chapter 88). Urinary tract infections are ideally treated with drugs such as amoxicillin and trimethoprim-sulfonamides, which are highly concentrated in the urine (see Chapter 89).

Other Host Factors

Other host factors that should be considered in AMD selection and route of administration include the following:

1. History of adverse drug reactions. These are most commonly gastrointestinal in dogs and cats, but may include hypersensitivity reactions.
2. Age. With the exception of doxycycline, the use of systemic tetracyclines is contraindicated in young animals because of the potential for teeth discoloration (see Figure 8-5). Fluoroquinolones have the potential to cause cartilage and joint toxicity in dogs between the ages of 7 and 28 weeks. The clinical significance of this has been questioned.[13,14]
3. Species. Dogs and cats differ in their susceptibility to adverse drug reactions. For example, dogs can develop severe cutaneous reactions to 5-flucytosine. Cats are susceptible to acute retinal degeneration following treatment with high doses of

BOX 6-1

Examples of Appropriate Initial Antimicrobial Drug Choices for Treatment of Bacterial Infections in Different Anatomic Sites*

Skin
Cephalexin
Amoxicillin-clavulanate
Clindamycin

Urinary Tract
Amoxicillin
Trimethoprim-sulfamethoxazole

Prostate
Trimethoprim-sulfamethoxazole

Respiratory tract
Doxycycline
Fluoroquinolones

Intestinal Tract (e.g., for animals with hepatic encephalopathy)
Ampicillin
Neomycin

Biliary Tree
Amoxicillin-clavulanate
Doxycycline
Fluoroquinolones

Brain
Metronidazole
Fluoroquinolones
Trimethoprim-sulfonamides

Bone
Clindamycin
Cephalosporins
Amoxicillin-clavulanate

*The identity of the pathogen present must also be used to guide antimicrobial drug selection.

enrofloxacin. Cats also are prone to esophageal ulceration from oral doxycycline hyclate or clindamycin unless the medication is administered with a bolus of water or food.

4. Breed. Doberman pinschers may be more susceptible to hypersensitivity reactions following trimethoprim-sulfonamide administration.
5. Gastric acidity. The absorption of some AMDs, such as ketoconazole and itraconazole, is impaired by medications that suppress gastric acid production.
6. Concurrent medications. Drug interactions, such as concurrent use of drugs that require metabolism using cytochrome P450 enzymes, can affect the choice or dose of AMD used. For example, chloramphenicol and ketoconazole are well-known P450 enzyme inhibitors, whereas rifampin is an enzyme inducer.
7. Pregnancy. Penicillins, cephalosporins, aminoglycosides, and macrolides are generally considered safe during pregnancy. The volume of distribution in pregnancy is greater, and so higher doses may be required to achieve equivalent serum concentrations.
8. Renal and hepatic function. The dose of AMDs that are dependent on renal elimination may require reduction in these animals with impaired renal function in order to minimize toxicity. For example, fluoroquinolones may be more likely to cause seizures or retinal toxicity in animals with renal failure. The use of nephrotoxic drugs such as amphotericin B or aminoglycosides may be relatively contraindicated in animals with renal dysfunction. Adverse effects may be more common when drugs that require hepatic metabolism, such as metronidazole or chloramphenicol, are administered to animals with impaired liver function.

Route of Administration

The most common routes of administration for AMDs in dogs and cats are topical, intravenous, intramuscular, subcutaneous, and oral. For localized infections of the skin, eye, or ear canal, topical administration has the advantage of delivering a high concentration of the AMD to the site, which may overcome bacterial resistance mechanisms, and avoid any systemic exposure to the drug. Parenteral administration, especially intravenous administration, provides maximum bioavailability and is recommended for (1) treatment of life-threatening infections, (2) systemic administration of antimicrobials with poor oral bioavailability (such as aminoglycosides), and (3) when gastrointestinal signs or malabsorption preclude effective drug administration via the oral route. Because parenteral AMDs are generally administered in hospital, compliance with this mode of administration is also likely to be greater. Absorption may be delayed after subcutaneous or intramuscular administration when perfusion of these tissues is impaired, and so these routes are not recommended for use when intravenous administration is possible. Peak plasma drug concentrations are achieved quickly after intravenous bolus administration. Therefore, bolus administration is an optimum approach for a concentration-dependent antimicrobial provided rapid injection does not produce toxicity (such as may occur with fluoroquinolones). For a time-dependent drug such as a β-lactam, a slow infusion (even a slow constant-rate infusion) optimizes the time-dependent activity.

Provided gastrointestinal function is healthy, administration of many oral AMDs results in acceptable bioavailability, even though many popular antimicrobials have oral absorption that is far less than 100%. Drugs with the highest oral bioavailability in dogs and cats are the fluoroquinolones; β-lactams have low and variable bioavailability. Nevertheless, once the animal can tolerate oral medications and its clinical condition becomes stable, a switch can be made from parenteral to oral antimicrobials. Peak plasma concentrations are always lower with oral administration than those achieved with intravenous administration, but for time-dependent drugs or for drugs that achieve efficacy on the basis of an AUC/MIC exposure relationship, this route is acceptable for a cure. Early switch from intravenous to oral therapy in human patients has gained increased favor in recent years because of reduced lengths of hospitalization, lowered costs, fewer intravascular catheter-related infections, and decreased selective pressure on nosocomial bacterial infections.[15,16] The oral bioavailability of some drugs can be maximized if they are administered with food (e.g., clavulanic acid-amoxicillin) or

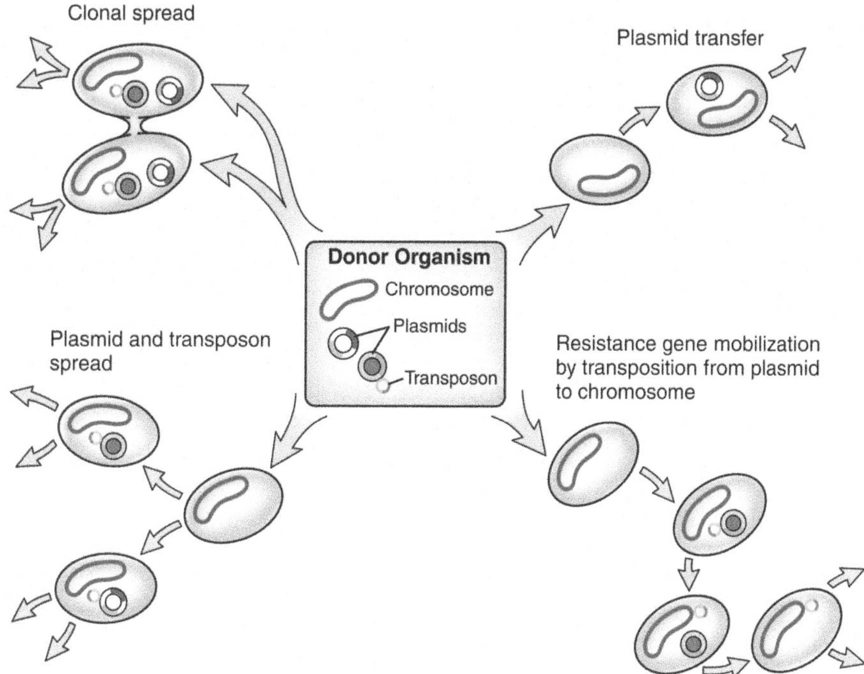

FIGURE 6-3 Genetic mechanisms of resistance in bacteria.

without food (e.g., azithromycin). Some drugs are simply not absorbed orally and must be administered parenterally or by the topical route. These drugs include penicillin G, piperacillin, ticarcillin, aminoglycosides, many cephalosporins (cefazolin, cefotaxime, cefoxitin), meropenem, imipenem, and vancomycin. Some drugs are not absorbed orally unless administered as a prodrug. An example is cefpodoxime proxetil. The proxetil portion of the molecule is cleaved off at the time of intestinal absorption to allow for adequate systemic concentrations.[17]

Antimicrobial Resistance

Infectious agents may be intrinsically resistant to an AMD, or be resistant as a result of genetic variations. *Intrinsic* or *innate resistance* refers to the innate ability of an organism to resist the effects of an AMD owing to structural or functional characteristics of that organism. For example, enterococci are intrinsically resistant to cephalosporins, because they lack the penicillin-binding proteins that bind these antibiotics.[18] Anaerobic bacteria are intrinsically resistant to aminoglycosides because oxygen is required for entry of the drug to the bacteria. The microbiology laboratory may "suppress" the results of susceptibility tests for antimicrobials to which organisms are intrinsically resistant (i.e., they are not listed in the susceptibility report to the clinician). Resistance can also be defined via pharmacokinetic-pharmacodynamic targets. For example, an organism may not express complete resistance to an antimicrobial, but the organism is effectively resistant when standard dosage regimens cannot reach a particular peak concentration or AUC.

Genetic resistance to an AMD may occur as a result of point mutations, DNA rearrangements, or acquisition of foreign DNA. Point mutations can result in alteration of the target site of an AMD, such as the susceptibility of bacterial DNA gyrase to fluoroquinolones.[19] DNA rearrangements may include inversions, deletions, duplications, insertions, or transpositions (including chromosome to plasmid) of large segments of DNA. The single most important mechanism of antibacterial resistance is acquisition of foreign DNA by horizontal transfer, especially that carried by plasmids and transposons.[20] Plasmids are circular, double-stranded DNA molecules that are capable of independent replication and can be transferred from one bacterial strain or species to another through the process of bacterial conjugation. Transposons are small, mobile segments of DNA that are flanked by inverted repeats and encode one or more resistance genes (Figure 6-3). They depend on the chromosome or plasmids for replication. Plasmid-associated genes that confer AMD resistance are frequently on transposons and can move from the plasmid to the bacterial chromosome. A single plasmid may contain resistance genes for more than five different AMDs.

Mechanisms of Antimicrobial Resistance

Antimicrobial Inactivation

Bacterial enzymes capable of inactivation of AMDs include β-lactamase enzymes, enzymes that modify aminoglycoside structure, chloramphenicol acetyltransferase, and erythromycin esterase. β-Lactamase production is the most important mechanism of resistance to β-lactam antibiotics among gram-negative bacteria.[20] A vast array of β-lactamase enzymes have been discovered, which have been extensively classified into groups.[21,22] Extended-spectrum β-lactamases (ESBLs) can hydrolyze not only penicillins and first-generation cephalosporins, but also extended-spectrum cephalosporins such as cefotaxime and ceftazidime (which contain an oximino group). To date, ESBLs have only been described in gram-negative bacilli and are most commonly produced by *Escherichia coli* and *Klebsiella pneumoniae*. ESBLs are often inhibited by β-lactamase inhibitors such as clavulanic acid. The ESBL with the most importance at the present time for small animals are the CTX-M β-lactamases, which hydrolyze cefotaxime and other third-generation cephalosporins. Other types of β-lactamase enzymes include AmpC β-lactamases, which are encoded by chromosomal genes, and metallo-β-lactamases.[20,23] These types of β-lactamase enzymes

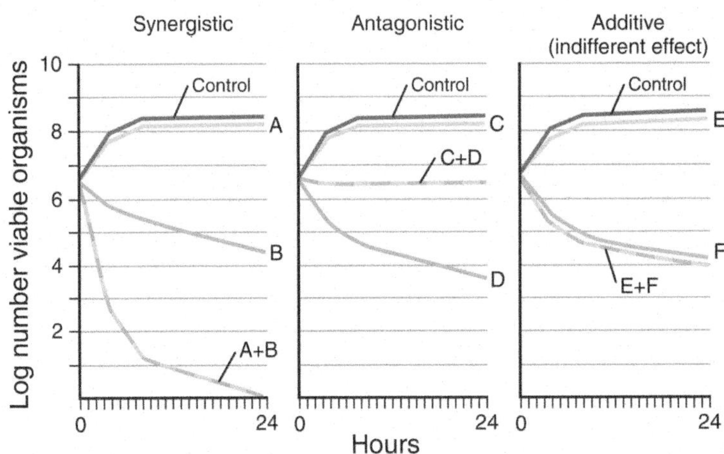

FIGURE 6-4 Synergistic, antagonistic, and additive effects of antimicrobial drug combinations. Drugs used are referred to using letters of the alphabet. Control = no drug.

are resistant to clavulanic acid. Metallo-β-lactamases can inactivate carbapenems such as meropenem and imipenem.

Membrane Alteration

Protein channels called *porins* facilitate the passage of hydrophilic AMDs into gram-negative bacteria. Acquisition of porin mutations can result in conformational changes of or reduced expression of porins. The result is exclusion of AMDs such as β-lactams and fluoroquinolones.[24]

Efflux Pump Induction

Expression of efflux pumps by bacteria allows them to exclude certain AMDs. This is a major mechanism of resistance to tetracyclines in gram-negative bacteria. A huge variety of efflux pumps have been described.[25] Efflux pumps may not be specific for one particular class of antimicrobial. Therefore, these have been termed "multidrug" efflux pumps and mediate multidrug resistance (MDR). The acquisition of MDR mechanisms greatly reduces the effective options for therapy. Multidrug-resistant organisms such as *Pseudomonas aeruginosa* and *Acinetobacter baumannii* can utilize multidrug efflux pumps in concert with a variety of other resistance mechanisms, including β-lactamase enzyme production, drug target alterations, and AMD modification enzymes.

Target Modification

Methylation of ribosomal targets by bacterial methyltransferases can lead to resistance to tetracyclines, lincosamides, aminoglycosides, and especially macrolide antibiotics. Expression of altered penicillin binding proteins (PBPs) is an important mechanism of resistance to β-lactam antimicrobials. Expression of PBP2a by staphylococci, which is encoded by the *mecA* gene, confers resistance to all β-lactam antimicrobials, including β-lactamase resistant penicillins such as methicillin and oxacillin (methicillin-resistant staphylococci). Mutations of DNA gyrase can confer resistance to fluoroquinolones.[20] Resistance to trimethoprim sulfonamides can result from altered dihydropteroate synthetase and dihydrofolate reductase enzymes.[26]

Novel Approaches to Antimicrobial Drug Resistance

With rapid spread of multidrug-resistant bacterial pathogens, alternatives to antibiotics have been investigated. One approach is bacteriophage therapy. Bacteriophages are viruses that infect bacteria, and because of their specificity for certain bacterial species, they can deliver targets to one type of organism without harming others.[27,28] Bacteriophage treatment may also be more successful than AMD treatment in the presence of biofilms, which impair antibiotic penetration. Other approaches that are under investigation include use of bacterial cell wall hydrolases, cationic antimicrobial peptides, and antisense antibiotics. Cationic antimicrobial peptides are derived from eukaryotic cells, have immunomodulatory properties, and rapidly kill a variety of bacteria.[29] Although it is difficult for bacteria to develop resistance to these peptides, multiple resistance mechanisms have been described. Antisense antibiotics are oligonucleotides that bind to the DNA of pathogenic microorganisms and inhibit gene expression.[30]

Antimicrobial Drug Combinations

When an infectious agent is suspected but has not yet been identified, the use of AMD combinations is tempting because of the added broad spectrum of coverage that they provide. However, use of AMD combinations does not necessarily reduce the chance of selection for a resistant organism, adds expense, and may predispose to drug toxicity. Theoretically, drug combinations may have additive, synergistic, or antagonistic effects (Figure 6-4). These properties are not as well established in clinical situations. For example, antagonism between a bacteriostatic antibiotic (such as tetracycline) and a bactericidal antibiotic that requires bacterial growth for efficacy (such as a β-lactam) is also theoretically possible, but there is only one clinical example of this occurrence, published in the 1950s.[31] Such antagonism has not been replicated since that time.

Several reasons have been suggested for the use of AMD combinations:

1. Some drugs must be administered in combination with other drugs because of rapid development of resistance to them when they are used as a sole agent. Examples are 5-flucytosine and rifampin.
2. If a polymicrobial infection is present, one drug may not have a sufficient spectrum of activity.
3. If the nature of an infection is not known and infection is life-threatening, it is reasonable to commence treatment with a broad-spectrum combination (such as a fluoroquinolone and a β-lactam), based on knowledge of the likely pathogen present and local prevalence of AMD resistance, pending the results of culture and susceptibility testing. Once the results

of culture and susceptibility testing are available, deescalation should be performed.

4. Certain combinations of AMD are synergistic for treatment of specific infections. For example, the combination of a β-lactam and an aminoglycoside is synergistic for treatment of enterococcal endocarditis. The relatively slow bactericidal activity of the β-lactam is greatly enhanced by the addition of the aminoglycoside, such that shorter durations of treatment or extension of the dosing interval becomes possible without affecting outcome.[7]
5. Some drugs are not effective against anaerobic bacteria (e.g., fluoroquinolones with the exception of pradofloxacin). They should be combined with an agent active against anaerobes (e.g., clindamycin or metronidazole) when a mixed infection with anaerobic and aerobic bacteria is suspected.
6. When a vector-borne pathogen is suspected, doxycycline may be administered until the results of further diagnostic tests confirm or eliminate this suspicion. In these cases, patients are frequently administered doxycycline in combination with another active agent to treat alternative bacterial infections that have not yet been ruled out.

Monitoring the Response to Treatment

The response to antimicrobial treatment is best monitored based on clinical assessment, which includes follow-up cytologic examination or cultures. Therapeutic drug monitoring can be used to ensure adequate serum drug concentrations when treating with aminoglycosides, vancomycin, and azole antifungal drugs. It should be remembered that in some cases, infections resolve because of the host immune response alone.

SUGGESTED READINGS

Hawkey PM, Jones AM. The changing epidemiology of resistance. J Antimicrob Chemother. 2009;64(suppl 1):i3-i10.

Levison ME, Levison JH. Pharmacokinetics and pharmacodynamics of antibacterial agents. Infect Dis Clin North Am. 2009;23(4):791-815.

Weese JS. Investigation of antimicrobial use and the impact of antimicrobial use guidelines in a small animal veterinary teaching hospital: 1995-2004. J Am Vet Med Assoc. 2006;228(4):553-558.

REFERENCES

1. Domagk G. Ein Beitrag zur Chemotherapie der bakteriellen Infektionen. Deut Med Wochenschr. 1935;61:250-253.
2. Weese JS, Blondeau JM, Boothe D, et al. Antimicrobial use guidelines for treatment of urinary tract disease in dogs and cats: antimicrobial guidelines working group of the international society for companion animal infectious diseases. Vet Med Int. 2011:2011:263768.
3. American Association of Feline Practitioners. Basic guidelines of judicious therapeutic use of antimicrobials in cats. 2001. http://www.catvets.com/uploads/PDF/antimicrobials.pdf. Last accessed May 12, 2012.
4. American Veterinary Medical Association. American Association of Feline Practitioners/American Animal Hospital Association basic guidelines of judicious therapeutic use of antimicrobials. 2006. (updated April 2009) http://www.avma.org/issues/policy/jtua_aafp_aaha.asp. Last accessed May 12, 2012.
5. Morley PS, Apley MD, Besser TE, et al. Antimicrobial drug use in veterinary medicine. J Vet Intern Med. 2005;19:617-629.
6. Canadian Veterinary Medical Association. Guidelines on the prudent use of antimicrobial drugs in animals. 2000. http://canadianveterinarians.net/Documents/Resources/Files/85_Resources_Prudent-Use-of-Antimicrobial-Drugs-in-Animals.pdf. Last accessed May 12, 2012.
7. Levison ME, Levison JH. Pharmacokinetics and pharmacodynamics of antibacterial agents. Infect Dis Clin North Am. 2009;23:791-815:vii.
8. Weese JS. Investigation of antimicrobial use and the impact of antimicrobial use guidelines in a small animal veterinary teaching hospital: 1995-2004. J Am Vet Med Assoc. 2006;228:553-558.
9. Bakken JS. The fluoroquinolones: how long will their utility last? Scand J Infect Dis. 2004;36:85-92.
10. Jacobs MR. Optimisation of antimicrobial therapy using pharmacokinetic and pharmacodynamic parameters. Clin Microbiol Infect. 2001;7:589-596.
11. Preston SL, Briceland LL. Intrathecal administration of amikacin for treatment of meningitis secondary to cephalosporin-resistant *Escherichia coli*. Ann Pharmacother. 1993;27:870-873.
12. Johnson RH, Einstein HE. Amphotericin B and coccidioidomycosis. Ann N Y Acad Sci. 2007;1111:434-441.
13. Rosanova MT, Lede R, Capurro H, et al. Assessing fluoroquinolones as risk factor for musculoskeletal disorders in children: a systematic review and meta-analysis. Arch Argent Pediatr. 2010;108:524-531.
14. Sansone JM, Wilsman NJ, Leiferman EM, et al. The effect of fluoroquinolone antibiotics on growing cartilage in the lamb model. J Pediatr Orthop. 2009;29:189-195.
15. Mertz D, Koller M, Haller P, et al. Outcomes of early switching from intravenous to oral antibiotics on medical wards. J Antimicrob Chemother. 2009;64:188-199.
16. Scheinfeld NS, Allan JM. Intravenous-to-oral switch therapy. 2011. http://emedicine.medscape.com/article/237521-overview. Last accessed May 12, 2012.
17. Papich MG, Davis JL, Floerchinger AM. Pharmacokinetics, protein binding, and tissue distribution of orally administered cefpodoxime proxetil and cephalexin in dogs. Am J Vet Res. 2010;71:1484-1491.
18. Williamson R, Calderwood SB, Moellering Jr RC, et al. Studies on the mechanism of intrinsic resistance to beta-lactam antibiotics in group D streptococci. J Gen Microbiol. 1983;129:813-822.
19. Arai K, Hirakata Y, Yano H, et al. Emergence of fluoroquinolone-resistant *Streptococcus pyogenes* in Japan by a point mutation leading to a new amino acid substitution. J Antimicrob Chemother. 2011;66:494-498.
20. Hawkey PM, Jones AM. The changing epidemiology of resistance. J Antimicrob Chemother. 2009;64(suppl 1):i3-i10.
21. Bush K, Jacoby GA. Updated functional classification of beta-lactamases. Antimicrob Agents Chemother. 2010;54:969-976.
22. Jacoby GA, Munoz-Price LS. The new beta-lactamases. N Engl J Med. 2005;352:380-391.
23. Jacoby GA. AmpC beta-lactamases. Clin Microbiol Rev. 2009;22:161-182.
24. Pages JM, James CE, Winterhalter M. The porin and the permeating antibiotic: a selective diffusion barrier in gram-negative bacteria. Nat Rev Microbiol. 2008;6:893-903.
25. Li XZ, Nikaido H. Efflux-mediated drug resistance in bacteria: an update. Drugs. 2009;69:1555-1623.
26. Sköld O. Resistance to trimethoprim and sulfonamides. Vet Res. 2001;32:261-273.
27. Górski A, Miedzybrodzki R, Borysowski J, et al. Bacteriophage therapy for the treatment of infections. Curr Opin Invest Drugs. 2009;10:766-774.
28. O'Flaherty S, Ross RP, Coffey A. Bacteriophage and their lysins for elimination of infectious bacteria. FEMS Microbiol Rev. 2009;33:801-819.
29. Findlay B, Zhanel GG, Schweizer F. Cationic amphiphiles, a new generation of antimicrobials inspired by the natural antimicrobial peptide scaffold. Antimicrob Agents Chemother. 2010;54:4049-4058.
30. Bai H, Xue X, Hou Z, et al. Antisense antibiotics: a brief review of novel target discovery and delivery. Curr Drug Discov Technol. 2010;7:76-85.
31. Lepper MH, Dowling HF. Treatment of pneumococcic meningitis with penicillin compared with penicillin plus Aureomycin; studies including observations on an apparent antagonism between penicillin and Aureomycin. AMA Arch Intern Med. 1951;88:489-494.

CHAPTER 7

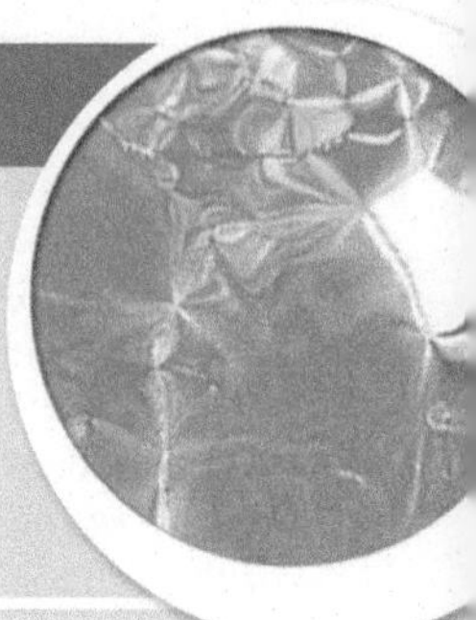

Antiviral and Immunomodulatory Drugs

Jane E. Sykes and Mark G. Papich

KEY POINTS

- Most antiviral drugs available for treatment of canine and feline viral infections are nucleoside analogues with greatest activity against herpesvirus and retrovirus infections.
- Because antiviral drugs also affect the function of host cell machinery, they have considerable potential for toxicity.
- Antiviral drugs are widely used in human medicine for treatment of herpesvirus, HIV and other viral infections. Much less is known about these medications in dogs and cats and there are few diseases of dogs and cats for which efficacy has been demonstrated.
- Because of important differences between human and animal virus infections, one should never assume that an antiviral agent used in people should be used in animals unless there is proof of safety and efficacy.
- Antiviral drugs used to treat feline herpesviral infections include famciclovir, idoxuridine, and cidofovir. Zidovudine is the only antiretroviral drug that has demonstrated efficacy for treatment of cats, primarily for FIV infections.
- Antiviral drugs can act synergistically with immunomodulators.
- Immunomodulators include microbial products, plant-derived immunomodulators, naturally occurring mammalian proteins, glucocorticoids, and synthetic compounds such as pentoxifylline and opioids. The effect of many of these drugs on outcome in dogs and cats with infectious diseases has not been fully evaluated using large, prospective, randomized, masked, controlled clinical trials.
- The parenteral use of natural or recombinant human protein immunomodulators in dogs and cats may result in the formation of neutralizing antibodies after 1 to 2 weeks of treatment, which can cross-react with endogenous proteins.

INTRODUCTION

The purpose of this chapter is to describe the mechanisms of action, spectrum of activity, and adverse effects of the major antiviral and immunomodulatory drugs that have exhibited utility or have potential for treatment of companion animal infectious diseases. An enormous number of different compounds have been considered or evaluated in vitro and in vivo with variable success. Only those currently in use for treatment of dogs and cats with naturally occurring infections, those that show considerable promise for the future, or those evaluated in controlled clinical trials are discussed in this chapter.

Antiviral Drugs

Antiviral agents interfere with virus-specific events in replication, including viral attachment, uncoating, assembly, and virus-directed macromolecular synthesis. As a result, antiviral agents typically have a restricted spectrum of activity. In contrast to most antibacterial drugs, antiviral drugs can also affect the function of host cell machinery and thus antiviral drugs have a greater risk of toxicity. In addition to acute toxicities such as marrow suppression, many antiviral agents are immunosuppressive, carcinogenic, and teratogenic. Many are given topically in order to minimize systemic toxicity. Antiviral agents are more likely to be effective when an intact host immune response is present. Combinations of antiviral drugs with different mechanisms of action and combinations of antiviral and immunomodulatory drugs are increasingly being used to treat human viral infections, especially HIV infection, with an associated decrease in toxicity and reduction in selection for drug-resistant mutants.

Although all antiviral drugs used to treat small animals were originally developed for treatment of human viral infections, the application of these drugs to treat viral infections of small animals has not proven straightforward. This relates to differences in the composition of human and companion animal viruses (which affect their susceptibility to inactivation by antiviral drugs), or problems relating to toxicity of human antiviral drugs in dogs and cats.

Antiviral drugs can be classified based on their spectrum of activity (i.e., family of viruses that are inhibited) and their mode of action. Antiviral drugs used in small animal medicine are primarily effective against herpesviruses or retroviruses, and most are *nucleoside analogues*. Nucleoside analogues resemble host nucleosides, which are nitrogenous bases with an attached sugar molecule used as a building block for the formation of DNA or RNA (Figure 7-1). Use of nucleoside analogues by viruses during replication leads to the formation of abnormal nucleic acids or termination of nucleic acid synthesis. Latent viral infections are not affected because the replication of latent virus is suspended. However, reactivation of these infections can be reduced in frequency or prevented. Examples of nucleoside analogues and their spectrum of activity are shown in Figure 7-1 and Table 7-1. Other antiviral drugs that have been used in clinical veterinary medicine include *amino acids* (L-lysine) and *neuraminidase inhibitors* (oseltamivir). The value of other treatments such as small inhibitory RNA molecules for viral infections of small animals is also under investigation.[1]

Antiherpesviral Drugs

The standard antiviral treatments for herpesviral infections in human patients are the nucleoside analogues acyclovir and penciclovir, and their prodrugs valacyclovir and famciclovir, respectively. These drugs are activated by the herpesviral enzyme thymidine kinase (TK), which phosphorylates them to a monophosphate form. Host cell enzymes then phosphorylate the drugs further to triphosphate forms, which concentrate in virus-infected cells and interfere with viral DNA replication via inhibition of the viral DNA polymerase enzyme. Because the DNA polymerases of different herpesviruses are inhibited to varying degrees by acyclovir triphosphate, not all herpesviral infections are equally susceptible. Drug resistance results from reduced viral TK activity, altered viral TK, or altered viral DNA polymerase. The antiherpesviral drugs cidofovir, idoxuridine, trifluridine, and vidarabine are not dependent on viral TK for phosphorylation and so have greater host cell toxicity. In small animal medicine, these four drugs have been used topically to treat ocular feline herpesviral infections.

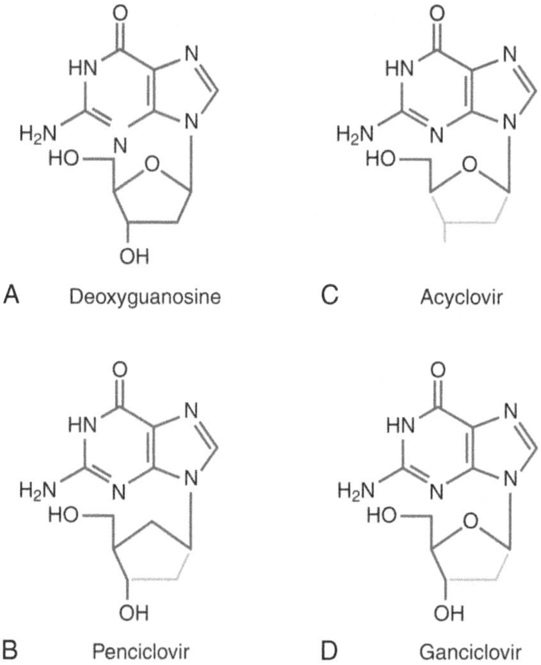

FIGURE 7-1 Chemical structures of deoxyguanosine (a nucleoside) and antiherpesviral nucleoside analogues. the grey portion is missing in the nucleoside analogues. **A,** Deoxyguanosine. **B,** Acyclovir. **C,** Penciclovir. **D,** Ganciclovir.

Acyclovir and Valacyclovir

Acyclovir is a synthetic analogue of the purine nucleoside deoxyguanosine (see Figure 7-1). In human patients, acyclovir is widely used to treat herpes simplex and varicella-zoster virus infections, both of which are α-herpesviruses. In small animal medicine, acyclovir has primarily been used to treat feline herpesvirus-1 (FHV-1) infections, although FHV-1 has a much lower susceptibility to the drug compared with the human herpesviruses.[2] Acyclovir has also been used to treat canine herpesvirus-1 (CHV-1) infections in puppies (see Chapter 16). Other nucleoside analogues (trifluridine, idoxuridine, cidofovir, ganciclovir, and penciclovir) show much greater activity than acyclovir against FHV-1 in vitro.[2-4]

Topical acyclovir has been used with limited success to treat feline herpetic dermatitis[5] and keratitis.[6] Topical treatment requires frequent (>4 times a day) application for beneficial effect.[6] The oral bioavailability of acyclovir is low in cats, and high doses are required to achieve adequate serum drug concentrations.[7] Valacyclovir, the prodrug for acyclovir, is rapidly converted to acyclovir by a first-pass effect after oral administration, and administration of the prodrug results in improved oral bioavailability of acyclovir. Unfortunately, administration of high doses of acyclovir or valacyclovir to cats has resulted in significant toxicity, including myelosuppression, renal tubular

TABLE 7-1

Antiviral Drugs in Use in Small Animals

Antiviral Drug	Mechanism of Action	Human Applications	Small Animal Applications
Acyclovir/ valacyclovir	Guanosine analogue; interferes with viral DNA polymerase and DNA synthesis. Activity requires viral TK.	Herpesviruses, especially HSV and varicella-zoster virus	Poorly effective against FHV-1
Penciclovir/ famciclovir	See acyclovir	Herpesviruses, especially HSV and varicella-zoster virus	FHV-1 infections
Cidofovir	Deoxycytidine monophosphate analogue. Activity independent of viral TK.	Systemically to treat cytomegalovirus retinitis; topically to treat papillomavirus infections	Topical treatment of FHV-1 ocular infections
Idoxuridine	Iodinated thymidine analogue. Interferes with viral DNA synthesis.	Topical treatment of HSV keratoconjunctivitis	Topical treatment of FHV-1 keratitis
Trifluridine	Fluorinated thymidine analogue. Interferes with viral DNA synthesis.	See idoxuridine	See idoxuridine
Vidarabine	Adenosine analogue. Interferes with viral DNA synthesis.	See idoxuridine	See idoxuridine
Zidovudine	Thymidine analogue. Interferes with viral DNA synthesis.	Systemic treatment of HIV infections	Systemic treatment of FIV and FeLV infections

FHV-1, feline herpesvirus-1; HSV, herpes simplex virus; TK, thymidine kinase.

necrosis, and hepatic necrosis, without effective suppression of viral replication.[8] Thus the use of systemic acyclovir and valacyclovir to treat cats with herpesvirus infections is not recommended.

Penciclovir and Famciclovir

Of all antiviral drugs used to treat small animal patients, penciclovir and famciclovir have shown the greatest promise. Penciclovir is another guanosine analogue (see Figure 7-1). It is present at much higher concentrations and for longer duration in cells than is acyclovir, which permits less frequent dosing. In humans, the prodrug famciclovir is well absorbed orally and rapidly converted to penciclovir, leading to increased oral bioavailability of penciclovir. Most of the drug is eliminated unchanged in the urine, and so dose reduction may be required for animals with decreased kidney function. In human patients, the concurrent administration of food decreases peak plasma concentrations without affecting overall bioavailability. In humans with herpes simplex virus and herpes zoster infections, famciclovir is as effective as acyclovir. In contrast, penciclovir (and thus famciclovir) have been shown to be potent inhibitors of FHV-1 replication (which is not the case for acyclovir). Penciclovir-resistant mutants of FHV-1 with altered TK enzymes have been described.[9]

Administration of famciclovir to cats at dosages comparable to those used in other species results in much lower plasma concentrations and a longer time to development of peak plasma concentrations of penciclovir when compared with other animal species, which suggests altered absorption or metabolism of famciclovir in cats.[10] High doses of famciclovir have been required to achieve adequate plasma drug concentrations. Nevertheless, famciclovir is well tolerated when administered orally to cats at doses that produce clinical responses.[5,10,11] Treatment of cats with experimentally induced FHV-1 conjunctivitis with famciclovir at 90 mg/kg PO q8h for 21 days resulted in lower clinical and pathologic disease scores and decreased viral shedding when compared with placebo-treated cats.[11] Clinical responses also occur in naturally infected cats with both acute and chronic manifestations of disease with negligible adverse effects.[5] Because of saturation of the metabolism of famciclovir to penciclovir, equivalent serum and tear penciclovir concentrations can be achieved in cats with 40 or 90 mg/kg PO q8h of famciclovir, so 40 mg/kg PO q8h is considered equally efficacious.[12,13] Clinical improvement often occurs within a week of treatment.

Ganciclovir

Ganciclovir resembles acyclovir except that it has an additional hydroxymethyl group on its acyclic side chain (see Figure 7-1). In human patients, ganciclovir is widely used specifically for the treatment of human cytomegalovirus infections, which can be life threatening in the immunocompromised. Cytomegaloviruses are β-herpesviruses. Systemic administration of ganciclovir to human patients is associated with a high prevalence of adverse drug reactions, especially cytopenias and central nervous system (CNS) signs, and so the use of ganciclovir is limited to patients with life-threatening or sight-threatening infections. A topical ophthalmic gel formulation of ganciclovir (0.15%) is now available for treatment of keratitis caused by herpes simplex virus-1. Ganciclovir is highly inhibitory to FHV-1 replication in vitro.[4,14] Pharmacokinetic, safety, and efficacy studies in cats have not yet been performed, but topical ganciclovir holds promise for treatment of feline ocular herpesviral infections.

Cidofovir

Cidofovir is a nucleotide analogue of deoxycytidine monophosphate. Because the drug already has a monophosphate group, its metabolism to the active diphosphate form by host cellular enzymes is not dependent on viral TK, and so it has been used to treat acyclovir- and penciclovir-resistant infections. In human patients, cidofovir is primarily used to treat cytomegalovirus retinitis. Cidofovir also has efficacy against other DNA virus infections, such as poxvirus and papillomavirus infections, and has been used topically as a cream to treat viral warts in people. Because the oral bioavailability of cidofovir is extremely low (<5%), it is always administered intravenously, intravitreally, or topically. Cidofovir has a prolonged intracellular half-life, which enables infrequent parenteral dosing regimens in human patients (once weekly, and then every other week for maintenance therapy).

Like ganciclovir, cidofovir is highly active in vitro against FHV-1.[4,14,15] Twice-daily administration of a 0.5% cidofovir ophthalmic solution significantly decreases viral shedding and the severity of clinical disease in cats with experimentally induced ocular FHV-1 infection (Table 7-2).[16] Local irritation and scarring of the nasolacrimal duct has been reported with topical administration of cidofovir to humans and rabbits with keratoconjunctivitis.

Idoxuridine and Trifluridine

Idoxuridine and trifluridine are halogenated thymidine analogues that interfere with the replication of FHV-1 in vitro, although they are more potent inhibitors of herpes simplex virus replication.[2,14] They have been used to treat herpesviral keratitis in humans and in cats.[17] These drugs are highly toxic when given systemically, because host cell and viral DNA synthesis are equally affected. Frequent topical application is required (five to six times daily), and prolonged use can cause corneal irritation or ulceration. Trifluridine has better corneal penetration than idoxuridine and is available as a 1% ophthalmic solution. Unfortunately, trifluridine is expensive, and ocular administration of trifluridine is often extremely irritating to cats.[18] In contrast, topical idoxuridine administration is generally well tolerated.

Vidarabine

Vidarabine is an adenosine analogue that is phosphorylated by host cellular enzymes to vidarabine triphosphate, which interferes with DNA synthesis by both the virus and host cells. It is effective against idoxuridine-resistant herpesviral strains because its mechanism of action differs from that of idoxuridine. It is reportedly well tolerated by cats when administered five to six times daily to cats as a 3% ophthalmic ointment.[18]

Lysine

Lysine is an amino acid that interferes with herpesviral replication by a poorly understood mechanism. Antagonism of arginine may somehow be involved, because a high lysine-to-arginine ratio appears to be important for efficacy. However, arginine itself was also shown to interfere with the replication of herpes simplex virus in vitro.[19]

Lysine has shown efficacy when administered as tablets to cats with FHV-1 conjunctivitis[20] and, in another study, it reduced shedding of reactivated virus by latently infected cats.[21]

TABLE 7-2

Antiviral Drugs Used for Treatment of Feline Herpesvirus Infections

Drug	Dose	Interval	Route	Comments
Famciclovir	62.5 mg/cat, 125 mg/cat, or 40-90 mg/kg	q8h	PO	Reduce dose for cats with renal insufficiency. Compound suspensions are bitter and poorly tolerated. Broken tablets are best administered in a gel cap. Safe in kittens.
Cidofovir	0.5% solution	q12h	Topical ophthalmic	Monitor for ocular irritation. Solution prepared from commercial 7.5% intravenous solution by dilution in sterile saline. Store diluted solution up to 6 months at 4°C, −20°C, and −80°C. Can also be obtained from compounding pharmacies.
Idoxuridine	0.1% solution or 0.5% ointment	5-6 times daily	Topical ophthalmic	Monitor for ocular irritation and ulceration. Compounding may be required.
Trifluridine	1% solution	5-6 times daily	Topical ophthalmic	May be poorly tolerated.
Vidarabine	3% ointment	5-6 times daily	Topical ophthalmic	Well tolerated. Compounding may be required.
Lysine	250 mg (kittens) 500 mg (cats)	q12h	PO	Questionable efficacy. Bolus administration preferred to dietary supplementation.
Zidovudine	5 to 15	q12h	PO, SC	Monitor CBC weekly during treatment for the first month, then monthly. Use low end of the dose range in renal failure. Use higher dose with caution.

When administered as tablets to cats in a shelter, there was no reduction in upper respiratory tract disease.[22] There was concern that the stress of tablet administration may have contributed to disease in these cats. However, in two other studies, dietary supplementation with lysine was not effective for management of upper respiratory tract disease in a shelter.[23,24] In fact, cats that received the lysine-supplemented diet had more severe disease and more frequent viral shedding than cats that received a nonsupplemented ration, despite having increased plasma lysine concentrations. The lysine-supplemented diet did not affect plasma arginine concentration, so altered arginine levels did not appear to contribute to the increased severity of disease.

Antiretroviral Drugs

All antiviral drugs used to treat cats with retrovirus infections have been nucleoside analogues, which inhibit the DNA polymerase function of the retroviral reverse transcriptase (RT) enzyme. Unfortunately, many drugs used for treatment of HIV infections (such as protease inhibitors) are not effective for treatment of feline retrovirus infections, because they only act on HIV enzymes. The only antiretroviral that has shown benefit in naturally infected cats is zidovudine (AZT). At the time of writing, an integrase inhibitor known as raltegravir has shown early promise for treatment of FeLV infections both in vitro and in vivo.[25,26] Many drugs that have activity against feline retroviruses in vitro, such as ribavirin and adefovir (PMEA), are toxic when given to cats, which limits their use in practice.

Zidovudine and Fozivudine

Zidovudine (azidothymidine; AZT; Retrovir) is a thymidine analogue and was one of the first drugs shown to be effective against HIV. Inside host cells, it is converted to the active triphosphate form. AZT inhibits the replication of FIV, reduces plasma viral load, improves stomatitis, and increases CD4/CD8 ratios in cats naturally infected with FIV.[27,28] Some FIV isolates are resistant as a result of mutations in the RT enzyme. Although AZT is active against FeLV in vitro, when compared with FIV-infected cats, it has not performed as well for treatment of naturally infected, sick cats with chronic FeLV infection. Nevertheless, improvement in stomatitis, reduced antigenemia, and reduction in development of lymphoma have been reported in studies of naturally and experimentally FeLV-infected cats that were treated with AZT.[28,29]

AZT is available as a10 mg/mL syrup and a 10 mg/mL injection. It has good oral bioavailability and is well distributed to tissues, including the CNS. It is metabolized to an inactive form by the liver and excreted by the kidneys. Dosage reduction has been recommended for cats with renal failure. Unfortunately, some cats treated with AZT can develop dose-related hematologic adverse effects, most commonly nonregenerative anemia and neutropenia, so the CBC must be monitored during treatment. Adverse effects may be confused with retrovirus-induced cytopenias. In human patients with HIV infection, cytopenias are more likely to occur when disease is advanced.

Fozivudine is a thioether lipid-zidovudine conjugate that undergoes intracellular cleavage to zidovudine monophosphate and subsequent phosphorylation to the active triphosphate form. Cleavage preferentially occurs in lymphocytes and monocytes compared with RBC and marrow stem cells, and so hematologic toxicity is less likely to occur. Fozivudine reduces viremia in cats experimentally infected with FIV, without significant adverse effects.[30] Further study is required to evaluate this drug for treatment of chronic FIV and FeLV infections in cats.

Lamivudine

Lamivudine (3TC), a cytidine analogue, is synergistic when combined with AZT for treatment of HIV infection, and the combination is in common use in human medicine. AZT/3TC prevented FIV infection when given to cats shortly after experimental inoculation, but did not appear to be beneficial for treatment of cats with chronic FIV infection.[31] In addition, severe hematologic adverse effects and fever occurred in some cats.

Other Antiretroviral Drugs

Raltegravir inhibits the retroviral integrase enzyme. Integrase incorporates transcribed viral DNA into the host chromosome. In human patients, raltegravir is approved for treatment of HIV infections and is used in combination with other antiretroviral drugs. Although expensive, raltegravir has shown great promise for treatment of FeLV infections in vitro and also in vivo.[25,26] Other drugs that have shown promise in vitro for treatment of FeLV infections, with no evidence of toxicity to cell cultures, are the nucleoside analogues tenofovir, decitabine, and gemcitabine.[26] Tenofovir is used as part of combination therapy to treat HIV infections. It is administered as a prodrug. Decitabine and gemcitabine are cytidine analogues used in human patients to treat myelodysplastic syndromes and carcinomas, respectively. The use of combinations of gemcitabine and carboplatin to treat carcinomas in cats has been reported, but cytopenias and gastrointestinal toxicity occurred in some of the cats.[32]

Plerixafor is a bicyclam derivative that selectively blocks the chemokine receptor, CXCR4. This receptor is used by FIV to enter cells (see Chapter 21). In a placebo-controlled, masked clinical trial, administration of plerixafor to cats with FIV infection for 6 weeks reduced proviral load but did not lead to improvement in clinical or immunologic variables.[33]

Antiinfluenza Viral Drugs

The main drugs used in human medicine to treat influenza virus infections are neuraminidase inhibitors, such as oseltamivir and zanamivir, and the tricyclic amines amantadine and rimantadine, which inhibit the M2 ion channel protein that is present in influenza A viruses (Figure 7-2). Only oseltamivir has been used to any great extent in small animals. Amantadine, which also has antagonistic effects at the NMDA (*N*-methyl-D-aspartate) receptor, has been used to treat osteoarthritis in animals in combination with other drugs.[34]

Oseltamivir

Oseltamivir (Tamiflu) is the prodrug of oseltamivir carboxylate (GS4071), a potent inhibitor of influenza virus neuraminidase. Oseltamivir was developed because of the poor oral bioavailability of zanamivir, a neuraminidase inhibitor that is structurally similar to GS4071. Neuraminidase is a surface glycoprotein of both influenza A and influenza B viruses (see Figure 7-2). The viral neuraminidase cleaves sialic acid residues on the surface of infected cells, which allows new virus particles to be released from host cells. It also prevents aggregation of virus particles after they are released and facilitates spread of the virus through the mucus of the respiratory tract by cleaving sialic acid residues in mucin.

In humans and dogs, oseltamivir has high oral bioavailability.[35] Esterase enzymes in the liver then convert oseltamivir to its active form, which is well distributed to most body fluids, including surface epithelial cells throughout the upper and lower respiratory tract. Elimination of the drug relies on renal excretion. The drug is well tolerated in humans, with gastrointestinal signs being the most frequently reported adverse effects.

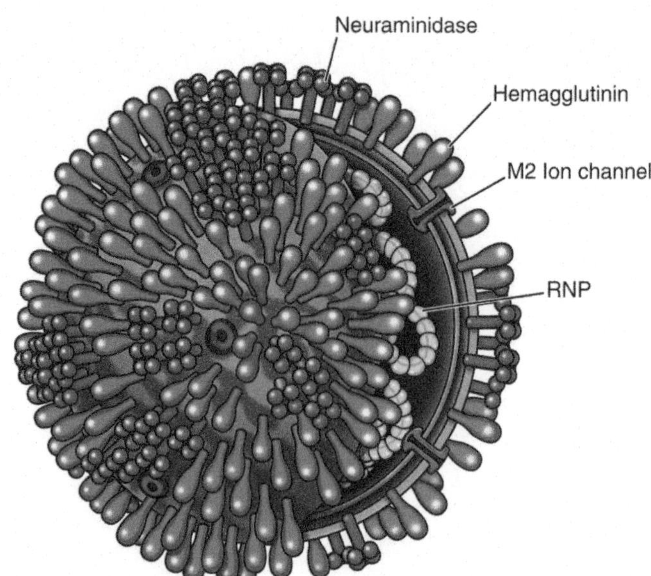

FIGURE 7-2 Structure of an influenza virus. The M2 protein, which is only present in influenza A viruses, is inhibited by tricyclic amines such as amantadine. Oseltamivir inhibits the viral neuraminidase.

The prevalence of resistance to oseltamivir among influenza virus isolates is generally low (<5%). High-level resistance results from mutations in the viral neuraminidase. Neuraminidase inhibitors could play a critical role in prevention of mortality in human influenza virus pandemics, so strategies that minimize the selection of resistant mutants are important. The Centers for Disease Control and Prevention recommends prioritizing antiviral treatment to human patients at risk of complications of influenza, such as the very young and very old.[36]

Oseltamivir has been used to treat canine parvovirus (CPV) enteritis in puppies, with anecdotal reports of improved outcome. A single prospective, randomized, masked, placebo-controlled trial of 35 dogs with CPV enteritis showed that dogs treated with oseltamivir (2 mg/kg PO q12h) had no significant drop in their white blood cell count, whereas untreated dogs had a significant drop in their white blood cell count in the first 5 days of hospitalization.[37] Treated dogs also gained weight during hospitalization, whereas untreated dogs lost weight. However, there was no difference in hospitalization time, treatments needed, clinical scores, morbidity, or mortality between the two groups, and the number of dogs in each group was small. No significant adverse drug effects were observed, but oseltamivir was administered as a 1:1 dilution with water, in order to reduce reactions to the taste of the drug and vomiting shortly after drug administration. The authors acknowledged that there were potential concerns that related to administration of an oral medication to dogs with enteritis, with variability in drug absorption.

As CPV has no neuraminidase, it was hypothesized that oseltamivir instead may act on the neuraminidases of bacteria that are normally responsible for secondary bacterial infections in CPV enteritis, which are primarily those of the gastrointestinal tract. The role of bacterial neuraminidases in the pathogenesis of enteric bacterial infections and bacterial translocation is unknown. Bacterial neuraminidase enzymes may play a role in biofilm formation and help bacteria to invade mucin layers of the respiratory tract.[38] It has been suggested that gut bacteria may use neuraminidase enzymes to cleave sialic acid residues on gastrointestinal epithelial cells, which exposes receptor sites for bacterial adherence.

A major concern that relates to treatment of CPV enteritis with oseltamivir is the possibility of selection for resistant mutants among influenza viruses if widespread use of the drug occurs in veterinary clinics. Given the restrictions on the use of this drug for treatment of human influenza virus infections, further investigation is required before the use of oseltamivir can be recommended for treatment of CPV enteritis.

Other Antiviral Drugs

Although not useful for treatment of cats because of toxicity, the nucleoside analogue ribavirin has shown promise in vitro for treatment of canine distemper virus (CDV) infections. Another drug, 5-ethynyl-1-beta-D-ribofuranosylimidazole-4-carboxamide (EICAR), has also shown activity against CDV in vitro[39] and for treatment of measles virus, which is closely related to CDV.[40] Ribavirin is primarily used to treat hepatitis C virus infections in humans. The pharmacokinetics and toxicity of ribavirin and EICAR in dogs require further study.

Nelfinavir is a protease inhibitor used to treat HIV infection. It also limits the replication of severe acute respiratory syndrome (SARS) coronavirus in vitro,[41] but its mode of action against coronaviruses is poorly understood. Nelfinavir was not effective in a mouse model of SARS.[42] Although nelfinavir alone was not completely effective, a combination of nelfinavir and *Galanthus nivalis* agglutinin (GNA) inhibited the replication of feline coronavirus in vitro and may have application for the treatment of feline infectious peritonitis (FIP).[43] GNA appears to bind the viral outer envelope glycoproteins and prevent cellular entry. The use of nelfinavir was reported in a few cats with naturally occurring coronavirus infections,[43,44] but the toxicity and pharmacokinetics of nelfinavir and GMA in cats and efficacy of these drugs for treatment of FIP remains unknown.

Immunomodulators

An immunomodulator is any drug that alters immune system function. Immunomodulators are also referred to as *biologic response modifiers*. Their use for treatment of infectious diseases may be beneficial when compromise of the immune system impairs effective antimicrobial drug treatment. Alternatively, immunomodulators can be used to dampen an excessive host inflammatory response.

A variety of immunomodulators have been used to treat feline retroviral infections, FIP, FHV-1 infections, and canine and feline parvoviral enteritis (Table 7-3). Immunomodulators used in veterinary medicine can be divided into six main groups: (1) microbial products; (2) plant-derived biologic response modifiers; (3) naturally occurring cytokines, such as colony-stimulating factors, and interferons; (4) immunoglobulins; (5) glucocorticoids; and (6) synthetic compounds with immunomodulatory activity, such as pentoxifylline.

Treatment of canine and feline viral infections with immunomodulators has frequently been associated with disappointing results, and data from large, prospective, controlled clinical trials are generally not available. Frequently, an immunomodulator shows antiviral activity in vitro but this does not correlate with treatment responses in vivo. Sometimes, mild to moderate clinical improvement is observed, but treatment does not result in cure. The use of human recombinant cytokines beyond 1 or 2 weeks of treatment has been associated with the development of antibodies against the cytokines, which have the potential to cross-react with endogenous cytokines. In the absence of data from randomized, placebo-controlled clinical trials to support their use, immunomodulators should be used with caution, because they may have the potential to accelerate disease. This may occur for viruses that are dependent on rapidly dividing cells for replication (such as parvovirus) or those that replicate only in activated lymphocytes (such as FIV). Promotion of an inflammatory response may also have detrimental effects if immune-mediated processes play an important role in the pathogenesis of disease (such as for FIP).

Microbial Products

Microbial products with immunomodulatory activity include bacillus Calmette-Guérin extract (a mycobacterial cell wall extract from *Mycobacterium bovis*), purified staphylococcal protein A, killed *Propionibacterium acnes* (ImmunoRegulin, ImmunoVet), *Staphylococcus aureus* phage lysate (Staphage Lysate, Delmont Laboratories, USA), *Serratia marcescens* abstract, and inactivated poxviruses (Baypamun, Bayer). To date, controlled clinical trials with these products have not demonstrated significant efficacy for treatment of viral infections in dogs and cats. Staphylococcal phage lysate, which contains components of *S. aureus* and a bacteriophage, and *Propionibacterium acnes* immunotherapy have shown efficacy for treatment of pyoderma in dogs and are available commercially for this purpose (see Table 7-3; also see Chapter 84).[45]

Plant-Derived Biologic Response Modifiers

Acemannan (Carrisyn, Carrington Laboratories, Irving, TX) is a mucopolysaccharide derived from aloe vera plant leaves that induces cytokine production and dendritic cell maturation. It stimulates macrophages to secrete a variety of cytokines, including IFN-γ, TNF-α, prostaglandin E2, Il-1, and Il-6. It has been used to treat FIV and FeLV infections, either by oral or parenteral administration,[46,47] and a veterinary product is available for treatment of canine and feline fibrosarcomas. Controlled trials are needed to understand the efficacy of this treatment in naturally infected cats.

Polyprenyl immunostimulant (Sass & Sass, Inc., Oakridge, TN) is a plant-derived investigational veterinary biological that is made up of phosphorylated, linear polyisoprenols. In vitro, it upregulates synthesis of Th1 cytokines and has antiviral properties. Cats with experimentally induced FHV-1 infection had a decreased severity and duration of upper respiratory tract signs when treated with polyprenyl immunostimulant, in comparison to placebo-treated cats.[47a] Long-term (>2 years) survival has been reported in a few cats with noneffusive FIP that were treated with polyprenyl immunostimulant. The response in cats with effusive FIP has been disappointing.[48]

Naturally Occurring Mammalian Proteins

Colony-Stimulating Factors

Colony-stimulating factors (CSFs) are naturally occurring glycoproteins that stimulate production, differentiation, survival, and activation of white blood cells. Examples include erythropoietin; thrombopoietin; Il-5 (which stimulates eosinophil and basophil production); Il-3; stem cell factor; and macrophage CSF, granulocyte CSF (G-CSF), and granulocyte-macrophage CSF (GM-CSF). Recombinant G-CSF has been used most

TABLE 7-3

Commercially Available Immunomodulators That May Have Benefit for Treatment of Infectious Diseases of Dogs and Cats

Drug	Dose	Interval	Species	Route	Comments
Acemannan	2 mg/kg	Weekly	C	SC	For treatment of fibrosarcomas, efficacy unclear for FIV and FeLV infections
Feline recombinant interferon omega	1 million U/kg	q24h for 5 consecutive days on days 0, 14, and 60	C, D	SC	For FeLV infections
	0.1 million U/kg	q24	C	Oromucosal	For refractory caudal stomatitis associated with FCV infection
Filgrastim	5 μg/kg	q24h	C, D	SC	Monitor CBC weekly during treatment. Long-term use (>2 weeks) can lead to development of neutralizing antibodies.
Lactoferrin	200 mg powder or 40 mg/kg solution	q24h	C	Topical	For refractory gingivitis and stomatitis. Must be purchased from chemical suppliers
Lymphocyte T-cell immunomodulator	1 mL	Weekly	C	SC	For treatment of FeLV and FIV infections
Human recombinant interferon alpha	10^4 to 10^6 U/kg	q24h	C	SC	Monitor CBC weekly during parenteral treatment. Long-term parenteral use can lead to development of neutralizing antibodies
	1 to 50 U/cat	q24h		PO	
Pentoxifylline	15 mg/kg	q8h	D	PO	Benefits for treatment of FIP unclear. Co-administration of cytochrome P450 inhibitors may increase serum drug concentrations
	¼ of a 400 mg tablet	q8h	C		
Polyprenyl immunostimulant	3 mg/kg	Three times weekly	C	PO	Possible benefit for treatment of noneffusive FIP
Prednisolone	1 to 2 mg/kg	q24h	C	PO	For FIP
Propionibacterium acnes, killed	0.1 mg dogs <7 kg 0.2 mg 7-20 kg 0.4 mg 20-34 kg 0.8 mg > 34 kg	Twice weekly. After 14 d, weekly until remission, and monthly thereafter to maintain remission	D	IV	For pyoderma. Available as a 0.4 mg/mL solution
Staphylococcus aureus phage lysate	0.5 mL	Once or twice weekly	D	SC	For pyoderma

C, Cats; *D*, dogs.

widely in veterinary medicine as an immunomodulator. The use of these drugs may be limited by their cost and immunogenicity.

Granulocyte colony-stimulating factor. Granulocyte CSF stimulates growth and differentiation of the neutrophil cell line. It also stimulates neutrophil function, including chemotaxis, phagocytosis, antibody-dependent cellular cytotoxicity, and superoxide production. Nonglycosylated, recombinant human G-CSF is available under the trade name Neupogen. Pegfilgrastim (Neulasta) is a pegylated form with a long half-life and single-dose administration. Lenograstim is a glycosylated form available outside the United States. These three forms have similar efficacy and adverse effects in humans. G-CSF is approved for use in humans for treatment of chemotherapy-induced myelosuppression, for treatment of severe chronic neutropenia, for mobilization and collection of peripheral blood stem cells for bone marrow transplantation, and to accelerate myeloid reconstitution after hematopoietic stem cell transplantation.[49] G-CSF and GM-CSF have been used to treat pneumonia and severe sepsis in humans without neutropenia, but significant benefit has not been identified.[50,51]

When G-CSF is administered as a daily subcutaneous injection to dogs and cats, the neutrophil count increases over several days. This results from an enhanced rate of granulopoiesis and a shortened neutrophil maturation time. Slight increases in monocyte and lymphocyte counts can also occur.[52] Counts return to normal 5 days after discontinuation of treatment.

In veterinary medicine, filgrastim has been used to treat chemotherapy-induced neutropenia and cyclic neutropenia in gray collies. Filgrastim was not effective for treatment of leukopenia in experimentally induced CPV infection.[53,54] Repeated administration of filgrastim to dogs and cats has been associated with development of antibodies to the protein within 2 to 3 weeks of treatment, which can cross-react with endogenous G-CSF. Thus, although it can increase neutrophil counts in some FIV-infected cats, long-term use of filgrastim is not recommended.[55] Recombinant canine G-CSF (rcG-CSF) may be safer for long-term use in dogs, and possibly also cats. One recombinant canine formulation mobilized neutrophils in dogs within 24 hours of administration.[56] Recombinant canine G-CSF reduces the severity and duration of bone marrow suppression induced by cyclophosphamide in dogs.[57] In a prospective, non-randomized clinical trial for treatment of CPV infection, neutrophil counts were higher and hospital times were shorter in dogs treated with rcG-CSF, but survival times were decreased.[58] Treatment of canine and feline parvovirus infections with G-CSF might cause harm, because the increased cell turnover induced by the drug might promote parvovirus replication. Further studies are required to evaluate the utility of rcG-CSF for treatment of neutropenias associated with canine parvoviral enteritis, feline retrovirus infections, and chronic canine monocytic ehrlichiosis.

In dogs and cats, exogenous G-CSF is well tolerated. In human patients, the main adverse effects of treatment are bone and musculoskeletal pain, headache, anemia, thrombocytopenia, and splenomegaly. Long-term use in humans can be associated with osteopenia as a result of upregulation of osteoclast activity. Rare complications in people include splenic rupture and exacerbation of autoimmune disorders.

Granulocyte-macrophage colony-stimulating factor. GM-CSF stimulates growth and function of neutrophils, monocytes, and eosinophils. Commercial GM-CSF formulations available for treatment of hematologic disorders in human patients include sargramostim, molgramostim, and regramostim, which vary slightly in amino acid sequence and degree of glycosylation. When used to treat cats with FIV, viral load increased,[59] and so the use of GM-CSF is not recommended for treatment of FIV-induced cytopenias. Interestingly, sargramostim has been used to treat some human patients with AIDS-associated opportunistic infections, which include oropharyngeal candidiasis and disseminated mycobacterial infections. Administration of recombinant human GM-CSF to dogs was associated with antibody development after 10 days.[60]

Interferons

Interferons are cytokines with antiviral properties. IFN-α, IFN-β, and IFN-ω are type I interferons, which are produced by leukocytes and fibroblasts in response to a viral infection. Type I interferons activate natural killer (NK) cells, increase expression of major histocompatibility complex (MHC) class I molecules, and have antitumor activity. IFN-γ is the only type II interferon and is produced by T lymphocytes and NK cells in response to antigenic stimulation. IFN-γ plays a critical role in the clearance of intracellular pathogens by macrophages. Recombinant human IFN-γ has been used to treat chronic granulomatous disease in humans as well as chronic infections caused by intracellular bacteria and fungi, but recombinant veterinary preparations are not available.

Interferon alpha. Naturally occurring IFN-α represents a group of more than 20 molecules that vary slightly in composition and inhibit viral nucleic acid and protein synthesis. A variety of recombinant human and natural IFN-α preparations are available, including pegylated forms that have prolonged biologic half-lives. In human patients, IFN-α is used in conjunction with antiviral drugs to treat hepatitis B and hepatitis C virus infections, papillomavirus infections, and HIV-associated Kaposi's sarcoma. It is generally administered for 24 or 48 weeks.

Recombinant human IFN-α (rhIFN-α) has been administered parenterally and orally to cats for treatment of feline retroviral infections, feline upper respiratory viral infections, and FIP. It inhibits replication of FeLV, FIV, FHV-1, and feline coronavirus in vitro. Unfortunately, mixed results have been obtained after parenteral and oral administration to cats with retrovirus infections, and parenteral IFN-α was not effective for treatment of FIP.[61] Parenteral administration can lead to the development of neutralizing antibodies and apparent loss of activity after 3 or 7 weeks.[62]

Oral administration of a low dose of rhIFN-α to treat viral infections of animals has been controversial because of proteolytic degradation of rhIFN-α by gastric acid. Nevertheless, beneficial outcomes have been reported in some cats with FHV-1, FeLV, and FIV infections, presumably because immunomodulation follows mucosal absorption of the drug. Topical application of rhIFN-α to the eye has been used to treat FHV-1 keratitis, but controlled studies using this treatment are lacking. With the availability of more effective antiviral drugs such as famciclovir, it is likely that the use of these antiviral drugs may take precedence over, or be used in combination with, treatment with IFN-α.

Feline recombinant interferon-omega. IFN-ω is a Type 1 interferon closely related to IFN-α. It is secreted by virus-infected leukocytes. Its precise mechanism of action is not known. In dogs it increases macrophage and NK cell activity, and it has antiviral activity against several feline viruses in vitro, including FeLV, FHV-1, feline calicivirus (FCV), canine and feline parvoviruses, and feline coronavirus. It also has antitumor activity.[63] A recombinant feline formulation of IFN-ω produced in silkworms is available in Europe and Canada for veterinary use (rfIFN-ω, Virbagen omega, Virbac). Because it has similar activity in canine and feline cells, it has potential for treatment of both canine and feline viral infections. The optimal dosing regimen is unknown, but the manufacturer recommends three cycles of treatment, on days 0, 14, and 60, for 5 consecutive days.

Preliminary data suggested that treatment of cats with FIP with rfIFN-ω might increase survival times,[64] but a randomized, placebo-controlled study of naturally infected cats demonstrated no improvement in quality of life or survival time.[65] When cats with naturally occurring FeLV-related disease were treated with rfIFN-ω in a placebo-controlled trial, survival time over a 2-month follow-up period increased.[66] Improvement in clinical scores and laboratory parameters was also documented in some sick cats that were naturally infected with FeLV and FIV, despite no significant changes in viral load.[67] The drug also has been used topically, orally, and parenterally to treat FHV-1 infections, and subcutaneously to treat refractory FCV-associated stomatitis.[68-71] Oromucosal administration of rfIFN-ω to cats with refractory FCV-associated stomatitis led to significant clinical improvement when compared with placebo.[68] Treatment of puppies with naturally and experimentally induced CPV enteritis with rfIFN-ω in a number of placebo-controlled trials was associated with reduced disease severity and, in some studies, significantly reduced mortality. In contrast, there was no improvement in survival in cats from a cattery with feline panleukopenia virus infection that were treated with rfIFN-ω when compared with an untreated control group.[72]

Recombinant fIFN-ω is well tolerated by dogs and cats. Transient lethargy, fever, vomiting, mild diarrhea, and anorexia have been documented in some treated cats, especially at higher doses (2.5×10^6 U/kg). Mild neutropenia, eosinophilia, and reversible increases in the activity of serum AST have also been described following treatment.[73] Additional studies of the efficacy and safety of rfIFN-ω in larger numbers of sick cats with retroviral infections and cats and dogs with other viral infections are required.

Lymphocyte T-cell Immunomodulator

Lymphocyte T-cell immunomodulator (T-cyte Therapeutics, Inc.) is a protein derived from thymus epithelial cells. According to the product brochure, LTCI upregulates Il-2 production in vitro and regulates CD4 T-cell function. It was also reported to stimulate platelet production in mice with chemotherapy-induced thrombocytopenia. LTCI has been conditionally approved by the U.S. Department of Agriculture as an aid for treatment of FIV and FeLV infections, and for the associated signs of cytopenias and opportunistic infections. Controlled independent studies of the efficacy of LTCI in cats are required.

Immunoglobulins

In human patients, human intravenous immune globulin (IVIG) has been used for treatment of immunodeficiencies, as well as autoimmune disorders (Figure 7-3). A single infusion of human IVIG has been used successfully to treat immune-mediated thrombocytopenia in dogs,[74] but repeated administration to animals may lead to transfusion reactions. Intravenous immunoglobulin preparations have been commercially available for passive immunization of cats or dogs in Europe. These contain antibodies to FPV, FHV-1, and FCV (Feliserin, IDT Biologika GmbH, Rodelben, Germany), or CDV, canine adenovirus, and CPV (Stagloban, IDT Biologika GmbH). The efficacy of these preparations has not been reported. Subcutaneous and intraperitoneal administration of adult cat serum to kittens with failure of passive transfer can provide IgG concentrations equivalent to those in kittens that suckle normally.[75] In general, when given parenterally in high doses, specific immunoglobulins are only effective for prevention, and not treatment of an infectious disease.[76] Oral administration is not effective. Passive administration of antitoxins is also used to treat tetanus (see Chapter 54) and for neutralization of snake venom components. Passive immunization may be associated with allergic reactions, which can be severe, and it has the potential to interfere with subsequent active immunization attempts. Administered antibodies are generally eliminated over a period of 2 to 3 weeks.

Lactoferrin

Bovine lactoferrin is a glycoprotein with immunomodulatory properties that is normally present in exocrine secretions and neutrophils. It reduces cytokine secretion by mononuclear cells and lymphocyte activation in cats infected with FIV. In vitro, bovine lactoferrin has antiviral activity against FCV and FHV-1.[77,78] Topical application (40 mg/kg q24h for 14 days) to the mouth of a small number of FIV-positive and FIV-negative cats with stomatitis was associated with improved appetite and reduced oral inflammation, salivation, and pain, and increased neutrophil phagocytic activity.[79] Chronic oral administration of bovine lactoferrin to a dog with β_2-integrin-related neutrophil dysfunction was associated with increased neutrophil function and recovery from opportunistic infections.[80]

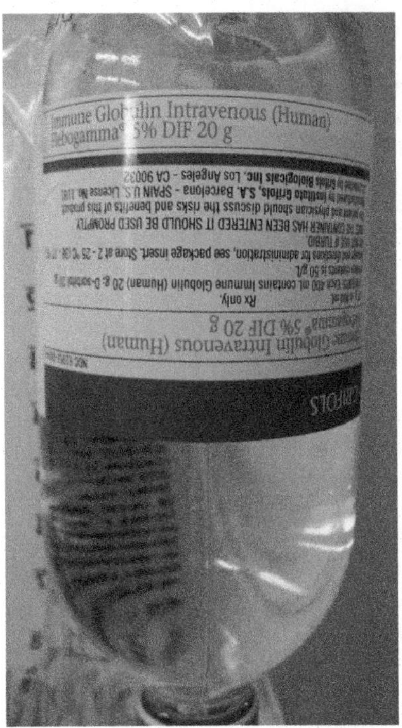

FIGURE 7-3 Human intravenous immune globulin solution (inverted for administration).

Glucocorticoids

In animals and humans with infectious diseases, treatment with glucocorticoids is sometimes used to dampen an overzealous immune response that contributes to the pathology of infection. Glucocorticoids have potent antiinflammatory and immunosuppressive properties. They suppress cytokine synthesis, decrease antibody production, cause lymphocytolysis and eosinopenia, decrease neutrophil margination, interfere with cyclooxygenase-2, and reduce the activity of phospholipase A2, and thus initiation of the arachidonic acid cascade. However, glucocorticoid administration also has the potential to worsen outcome through excessive immune suppression, so their use has been advocated only for specific infectious diseases under certain circumstances. Glucocorticoids can also contribute to development of secondary infections even when they are used to treat another disease. For example, it is not unusual in dogs or cats for a latent infection to emerge, or for a secondary infection to develop (e.g., demodicosis, staphylococcal pyoderma, dermatophytosis, systemic mycoses) when glucocorticoids are used to produce immunosuppression.

An example of the beneficial effect of glucocorticoids for treatment of an infectious disease is in FIP, where inflammation plays a major role in pathogenesis. Although controlled clinical trials comparing prednisone treatment with a placebo have not been performed, for many cats, treatment with prednisolone (1 to 2 mg/kg PO q24h) is associated with transient complete or partial remission and as a result is generally accepted as the standard of care for treatment of FIP (see Chapter 20).[65]

A short course of prednisolone using immunosuppressive doses (1 mg/kg PO q12h) has also been used to suppress secondary immune-mediated hemolysis in cats infected with *Mycoplasma haemofelis*,[81] but given that glucocorticoids can reactivate hemoplasma infections, additional studies are needed to determine whether this practice improves outcome. Similarly, glucocorticoid treatment has been used to suppress immune-mediated consequences of infection with the tick-borne pathogens *Ehrlichia canis* and *Babesia* spp, when antimicrobial treatment alone is not followed by complete resolution of clinical abnormalities. Adjunctive glucocorticoid treatment did not worsen outcome in dogs with Rocky Mountain spotted fever.[82] In contrast, glucocorticoid administration may have a negative impact in dogs with Lyme arthritis.[83] There are anecdotal reports of improved outcome for dogs with suspected Lyme glomerulonephritis that are treated with methylprednisolone sodium succinate in conjunction with other immunosuppressive drugs, such as mycophenolate mofetil or azathioprine (see Chapter 51).

Many large human studies have assessed the role of glucocorticoid treatment in septic shock (see Chapter 86). Treatment with high doses of hydrocortisone for less than 5 days is contraindicated because of secondary infection and gastrointestinal bleeding. Treatment with physiologic doses of glucocorticoids has been advocated to overcome relative adrenal insufficiency, which occurs in severe septic shock in both humans and dogs.[84] Recent consensus guidelines for human patients with septic shock recommend adjunctive hydrocortisone treatment in patients who are unresponsive to fluid resuscitation and treatment with vasopressors.[85]

Infections that generate inflammation within the eye and CNS are frequently treated with anti-inflammatory doses of topical or systemic glucocorticoids, respectively, in conjunction with antimicrobial drugs. The goal of such treatment is to minimize or prevent loss of vision or deterioration of neurologic status, especially when organism death is followed by a profound inflammatory response. For CNS infections, the effect of concurrent glucocorticoid treatment may depend on the specific pathogen present and the immune response of the infected individual. Prospective studies that evaluate outcome after adjunctive glucocorticoid treatment in CNS infections of dogs and cats are lacking. In a retrospective study, treatment of dogs and cats with CNS cryptococcosis with antiinflammatory doses of glucocorticoids increased survival in the first 15 days after starting antifungal drug treatment.[86]

Other

Pentoxifylline

Pentoxifylline is a synthetic methylxanthine derived from theobromine. It is a broad-spectrum phosphodiesterase inhibitor with a variety of immunomodulatory properties. In rodents and humans it inhibits TNF-α, Il-1, Il-6, and Il-12 production, as well as the activation of T and B cells, and increases neutrophil mobility and chemotaxis. It increases erythrocyte cAMP levels, which results in increased erythrocyte deformability, lowered blood viscosity, and improved microcirculation and tissue perfusion. Pentoxifylline also decreases platelet aggregation, and increases tissue plasminogen activator in patients with hyperaggregable platelets, so may be useful for treatment of disorders that result in hypercoagulable states. The value of pentoxifylline for treatment of endotoxemia has been primarily studied in horses. Despite significant decreases in TNF and IL-6 activity after incubation of equine monocytes with pentoxifylline in vitro, these effects did not occur in horses in vivo.[87] Beneficial effects of pentoxifylline are limited in horses when administered IV after challenge with endotoxin.[88]

In dogs, pentoxifylline has been used to treat a variety of skin diseases, including canine atopic dermatitis, dermatomyositis, and cutaneous vasculopathies.[89,90] In cats it has been used to treat FIP, but a masked, placebo-controlled study of the related drug propentofylline showed no benefit of treatment.[91] In dogs, pentoxifylline has a low and unpredictable oral bioavailability and a short half-life, and so three-times-daily administration has been recommended. Adverse effects include vomiting and decreased appetite, which are more likely to occur when the tablets are crushed. Crushed tablets are also unpalatable to cats.

Antimicrobial Drugs with Immunomodulatory Properties

Antimicrobial drugs with immunomodulatory properties include the macrolides, doxycycline, and metronidazole. The mechanisms of these activities are discussed in Chapter 8.

SUGGESTED READINGS

Maggs DJ. Antiviral therapy for feline herpesvirus infections. Vet Clin North Am Small Anim Pract. 2010;40:1055-1062.

REFERENCES

1. McDonagh P, Sheehy PA, Norris JM. In vitro inhibition of feline coronavirus replication by small interfering RNAs. Vet Microbiol. 2011;150:220-229.
2. Nasisse MP, Guy JS, Davidson MG, et al. In vitro susceptibility of feline herpesvirus-1 to vidarabine, idoxuridine, trifluridine, acyclovir, or bromovinyldeoxyuridine. Am J Vet Res. 1989;50:158-160.
3. Williams DL, Fitzmaurice T, Lay L, et al. Efficacy of antiviral agents in feline herpetic keratitis: results of an in vitro study. Curr Eye Res. 2004;29:215-218.
4. van der Meulen K, Garre B, Croubels S, et al. In vitro comparison of antiviral drugs against feline herpesvirus 1. BMC Vet Res. 2006;2:13.
5. Malik R, Lessels NS, Webb S, et al. Treatment of feline herpesvirus-1 associated disease in cats with famciclovir and related drugs. J Feline Med Surg. 2009;11:40-48.
6. Williams DL, Robinson JC, Lay E, et al. Efficacy of topical acyclovir for the treatment of feline herpetic keratitis: results of a prospective clinical trial and data from in vitro investigations. Vet Rec. 2005;157:254-257.
7. Owens JG, Nasisse MP, Tadepalli SM, et al. Pharmacokinetics of acyclovir in the cat. J Vet Pharmacol Ther. 1996;19:488-490.
8. Nasisse MP, Dorman DC, Jamison KC, et al. Effects of valacyclovir in cats infected with feline herpesvirus 1. Am J Vet Res. 1997;58:1141-1144.
9. Hussein IT, Menashy RV, Field HJ. Penciclovir is a potent inhibitor of feline herpesvirus-1 with susceptibility determined at the level of virus-encoded thymidine kinase. Antiviral Res. 2008;78:268-274.
10. Thomasy SM, Maggs DJ, Moulin NK, et al. Pharmacokinetics and safety of penciclovir following oral administration of famciclovir to cats. Am J Vet Res. 2007;68:1252-1258.
11. Thomasy SM, Lim CC, Reilly CM, et al. Evaluation of orally administered famciclovir in cats experimentally infected with feline herpesvirus type-1. Am J Vet Res. 2011;72:85-95.
12. Thomasy SM, Covert JC, Stanley SD, et al. Pharmacokinetics of famciclovir and penciclovir in tears following oral administration of famciclovir to cats: a pilot study. Vet Ophthalmol. 2012;15:299-306.
13. Thomasy SM, Whittem T, Bales J, et al. Pharmacokinetics of penciclovir following oral famciclovir and intravenous penciclovir administration in cats. Am J Vet Res. 2012;73(7):1092-1099.
14. Maggs DJ, Clarke HE. In vitro efficacy of ganciclovir, cidofovir, penciclovir, foscarnet, idoxuridine, and acyclovir against feline herpesvirus type-1. Am J Vet Res. 2004;65:399-403.
15. Sandmeyer LS, Keller CB, Bienzle D. Effects of cidofovir on cell death and replication of feline herpesvirus-1 in cultured feline corneal epithelial cells. Am J Vet Res. 2005;66:217-222.

16. Fontenelle JP, Powell CC, Veir JK, et al. Effect of topical ophthalmic application of cidofovir on experimentally induced primary ocular feline herpesvirus-1 infection in cats. Am J Vet Res. 2008;69:289-293.
17. Stiles J. Treatment of cats with ocular disease attributable to herpesvirus infection: 17 cases (1983-1993). J Am Vet Med Assoc. 1995;207:599-603.
18. Maggs DJ. Antiviral therapy for feline herpesvirus infections. Vet Clin North Am Small Anim Pract. 2010;40:1055-1062.
19. Naito T, Irie H, Tsujimoto K, et al. Antiviral effect of arginine against herpes simplex virus type 1. Int J Mol Med. 2009;23: 495-499.
20. Stiles J, Townsend WM, Rogers QR, et al. Effect of oral administration of L-lysine on conjunctivitis caused by feline herpesvirus in cats. Am J Vet Res. 2002;63:99-103.
21. Maggs DJ, Nasisse MP, Kass PH. Efficacy of oral supplementation with L-lysine in cats latently infected with feline herpesvirus. Am J Vet Res. 2003;64:37-42.
22. Rees TM, Lubinski JL. Oral supplementation with L-lysine did not prevent upper respiratory infection in a shelter population of cats. J Feline Med Surg. 2008;10:510-513.
23. Drazenovich TL, Fascetti AJ, Westermeyer HD, et al. Effects of dietary lysine supplementation on upper respiratory and ocular disease and detection of infectious organisms in cats within an animal shelter. Am J Vet Res. 2009;70:1391-1400.
24. Maggs DJ, Sykes JE, Clarke HE, et al. Effects of dietary lysine supplementation in cats with enzootic upper respiratory disease. J Feline Med Surg. 2007;9:97-108.
25. Cattori V, Weibel B, Lutz H. Inhibition of feline leukemia virus replication by the integrase inhibitor raltegravir. Vet Microbiol. 2011;152:165-168.
26. Greggs 3rd WM, Clouser CL, Patterson SE, et al. Discovery of drugs that possess activity against feline leukemia virus. J Gen Virol. 2012;93:900-905.
27. Gomez NV, Castillo VA, Gisbert MA, et al. Immune-endocrine interactions in treated and untreated cats naturally infected with FIV. Vet Immunol Immunopathol. 2011;143:332-337.
28. Hartmann K, Donath A, Beer B, et al. Use of two virustatica (AZT, PMEA) in the treatment of FIV and of FeLV seropositive cats with clinical symptoms. Vet Immunol Immunopathol. 1992;35:167-175.
29. Nelson P, Sellon R, Novotney C, et al. Therapeutic effects of diethylcarbamazine and 3'-azido-3'-deoxythymidine on feline leukemia virus lymphoma formation. Vet Immunol Immunopathol. 1995;46:181-194.
30. Fogle JE, Tompkins WA, Campbell B, et al. Fozivudine tidoxil as single-agent therapy decreases plasma and cell-associated viremia during acute feline immunodeficiency virus infection. J Vet Intern Med. 2011;25:413-418.
31. Arai M, Earl DD, Yamamoto JK. Is AZT/3TC therapy effective against FIV infection or immunopathogenesis? Vet Immunol Immunopathol. 2002;85:189-204.
32. Martinez-Ruzafa I, Dominguez PA, Dervisis NG, et al. Tolerability of gemcitabine and carboplatin doublet therapy in cats with carcinomas. J Vet Intern Med. 2009;23:570-577.
33. Hartmann K, Stengel C, Klein D, et al. Efficacy and adverse effects of the antiviral compound plerixafor in feline immunodeficiency virus-infected cats. J Vet Intern Med. 2012;26: 483-490.
34. Lascelles BD, Gaynor JS, Smith ES, et al. Amantadine in a multimodal analgesic regimen for alleviation of refractory osteoarthritis pain in dogs. J Vet Intern Med. 2008;22: 53-59.
35. Li W, Escarpe PA, Eisenberg EJ, et al. Identification of GS 4104 as an orally bioavailable prodrug of the influenza virus neuraminidase inhibitor GS 4071. Antimicrob Agents Chemother. 1998;42:647-653.
36. Centers for Disease Control and Prevention. Guidance on the use of influenza antiviral agents. 2011. http://www.cdc.gov/flu/professionals/antivirals/antiviral-use-influenza.htm: Last accessed May 13, 2012.
37. Savigny MR, Macintire DK. Use of oseltamivir in the treatment of canine parvoviral enteritis. J Vet Emerg Crit Care (San Antonio). 2010;20:132-142.
38. Soong G, Muir A, Gomez MI, et al. Bacterial neuraminidase facilitates mucosal infection by participating in biofilm production. J Clin Invest. 2006;116:2297-2305.
39. Dal Pozzo F, Galligioni V, Vaccari F, et al. Antiviral efficacy of EICAR against canine distemper virus (CDV) in vitro. Res Vet Sci. 2010;88:339-344.
40. Wyde PR, Moore-Poveda DK, De Clercq E, et al. Use of cotton rats to evaluate the efficacy of antivirals in treatment of measles virus infections. Antimicrob Agents Chemother. 2000;44:1146-1152.
41. Yamamoto N, Yang R, Yoshinaka Y, et al. HIV protease inhibitor nelfinavir inhibits replication of SARS-associated coronavirus. Biochem Biophys Res Commun. 2004;318:719-725.
42. Barnard DL, Day CW, Bailey K, et al. Evaluation of immunomodulators, interferons and known in vitro SARS-CoV inhibitors for inhibition of SARS-CoV replication in BALB/c mice. Antivir Chem Chemother. 2006;17:275-284.
43. Hsieh LE, Lin CN, Su BL, et al. Synergistic antiviral effect of *Galanthus nivalis* agglutinin and nelfinavir against feline coronavirus. Antiviral Res. 2010;88:25-30.
44. Tsai HY, Chueh LL, Lin CN, et al. Clinicopathological findings and disease staging of feline infectious peritonitis: 51 cases from 2003 to 2009 in Taiwan. J Feline Med Surg. 2011;13:74-80.
45. Becker AM, Janik TA, Smith EK, et al. *Propionibacterium acnes* immunotherapy in chronic recurrent canine pyoderma. An adjunct to antibiotic therapy. J Vet Intern Med. 1989;3:26-30.
46. Yates KM, Rosenberg LJ, Harris CK, et al. Pilot study of the effect of acemannan in cats infected with feline immunodeficiency virus. Vet Immunol Immunopathol. 1992;35:177-189.
47. Sheets MA, Unger BA, Giggleman Jr GF, et al. Studies of the effect of acemannan on retrovirus infections: clinical stabilization of feline leukemia virus-infected cats. Mol Biother. 1991;3:41-45.
47a. Legendre A. Personal communication. 2011.
48. Legendre AM, Bartges JW. Effect of polyprenyl immunostimulant on the survival times of three cats with the dry form of feline infectious peritonitis. J Feline Med Surg. 2009;11:624-626.
49. Page AV, Liles WC. Immunomodulators. In: Mandell GL, Bennett JE, Dolin R, eds. Principles and Practice of Infectious Diseases. 7th ed. Philadelphia, PA: Churchill Livingstone, Elsevier; 2010:611-623.
50. Schefold JC. Immunostimulation using granulocyte- and granulocyte-macrophage colony stimulating factor in patients with severe sepsis and septic shock. Crit Care. 2011;15:136.
51. Cheng AC, Stephens DP, Currie BJ. Granulocyte-colony stimulating factor (G-CSF) as an adjunct to antibiotics in the treatment of pneumonia in adults. Cochrane Database Syst Rev. 2007: CD004400.
52. Fulton R, Gasper PW, Ogilvie GK, et al. Effect of recombinant human granulocyte colony-stimulating factor on hematopoiesis in normal cats. Exp Hematol. 1991;19:759-767.
53. Rewerts JM, McCaw DL, Cohn LA, et al. Recombinant human granulocyte colony-stimulating factor for treatment of puppies with neutropenia secondary to canine parvovirus infection. J Am Vet Med Assoc. 1998;213:991-992.
54. Mischke R, Barth T, Wohlsein P, et al. Effect of recombinant human granulocyte colony-stimulating factor (rhG-CSF) on leukocyte count and survival rate of dogs with parvoviral enteritis. Res Vet Sci. 2001;70:221-225.

55. Phillips K, Arai M, Tanabe T, et al. FIV-infected cats respond to short-term rHuG-CSF treatment which results in anti-G-CSF neutralizing antibody production that inactivates drug activity. Vet Immunol Immunopathol. 2005;108:357-371.
56. Yamamoto A, Iwata A, Saito T, et al. Expression and purification of canine granulocyte colony-stimulating factor (cG-CSF). Vet Immunol Immunopathol. 2009;130:221-225.
57. Yamamoto A, Fujino M, Tsuchiya T, et al. Recombinant canine granulocyte colony-stimulating factor accelerates recovery from cyclophosphamide-induced neutropenia in dogs. Vet Immunol Immunopathol. 2011;142:271-275.
58. Duffy A, Dow S, Ogilvie G, et al. Hematologic improvement in dogs with parvovirus infection treated with recombinant canine granulocyte-colony stimulating factor. J Vet Pharmacol Ther. 2010;33:352-356.
59. Arai M, Darman J, Lewis A, et al. The use of human hematopoietic growth factors (rhGM-CSF and rhEPO) as a supportive therapy for FIV-infected cats. Vet Immunol Immunopathol. 2000;77:71-92.
60. Mayer P, Werner FJ, Lam C, et al. In vitro and in vivo activity of human recombinant granulocyte-macrophage colony-stimulating factor in dogs. Exp Hematol. 1990;18:1026-1033.
61. Weiss RC, Cox NR, Oostrom-Ram T. Effect of interferon or *Propionibacterium acnes* on the course of experimentally induced feline infectious peritonitis in specific-pathogen-free and random-source cats. Am J Vet Res. 1990;51:726-733.
62. Zeidner NS, Myles MH, Mathiason-DuBard CK, et al. Alpha interferon (2b) in combination with zidovudine for the treatment of presymptomatic feline leukemia virus-induced immunodeficiency syndrome. Antimicrob Agents Chemother. 1990;34:1749-1756.
63. Penzo C, Ross M, Muirhead R, et al. Effect of recombinant feline interferon-omega alone and in combination with chemotherapeutic agents on putative tumour-initiating cells and daughter cells derived from canine and feline mammary tumours. Vet Comp Oncol. 2009;7:222-229.
64. Ishida T, Shibanai A, Tanaka S, et al. Use of recombinant feline interferon and glucocorticoid in the treatment of feline infectious peritonitis. J Feline Med Surg. 2004;6:107-109.
65. Ritz S, Egberink H, Hartmann K. Effect of feline interferon-omega on the survival time and quality of life of cats with feline infectious peritonitis. J Vet Intern Med. 2007;21:1193-1197.
66. de Mari K, Maynard L, Sanquer A, et al. Therapeutic effects of recombinant feline interferon-omega on feline leukemia virus (FeLV)-infected and FeLV/feline immunodeficiency virus (FIV)-coinfected symptomatic cats. J Vet Intern Med. 2004;18:477-482.
67. Domenech A, Miro G, Collado VM, et al. Use of recombinant interferon omega in feline retrovirosis: from theory to practice. Vet Immunol Immunopathol. 2011;143:301-306.
68. Hennet PR, Camy GA, McGahie DM, et al. Comparative efficacy of a recombinant feline interferon omega in refractory cases of calicivirus-positive cats with caudal stomatitis: a randomised, multi-centre, controlled, double-blind study in 39 cats. J Feline Med Surg. 2011;13:577-587.
69. Haid C, Kaps S, Gonczi E, et al. Pretreatment with feline interferon omega and the course of subsequent infection with feline herpesvirus in cats. Vet Ophthalmol. 2007;10:278-284.
70. Southerden P, Gorrel C. Treatment of a case of refractory feline chronic gingivostomatitis with feline recombinant interferon omega. J Small Anim Pract. 2007;48:104-106.
71. Gutzwiller ME, Brachelente C, Taglinger K, et al. Feline herpes dermatitis treated with interferon omega. Vet Dermatol. 2007;18:50-54.
72. Paltrinieri S, Crippa A, Comerio T, et al. Evaluation of inflammation and immunity in cats with spontaneous parvovirus infection: consequences of recombinant feline interferon-omega administration. Vet Immunol Immunopathol. 2007;118:68-74.
73. Hampel V, Schwarz B, Kempf C, et al. Adjuvant immunotherapy of feline fibrosarcoma with recombinant feline interferon-omega. J Vet Intern Med. 2007;21:1340-1346.
74. Bianco D, Armstrong PJ, Washabau RJ. A prospective, randomized, double-blinded, placebo-controlled study of human intravenous immunoglobulin for the acute management of presumptive primary immune-mediated thrombocytopenia in dogs. J Vet Intern Med. 2009;23:1071-1078.
75. Levy JK, Crawford PC, Collante WR, et al. Use of adult cat serum to correct failure of passive transfer in kittens. J Am Vet Med Assoc. 2001;219:1401-1405.
76. Day MJ, Horzinek MC, Schultz RD. WSAVA guidelines for the vaccination of dogs and cats. J Small Anim Pract. 2010;51:1-32.
77. McCann KB, Lee A, Wan J, et al. The effect of bovine lactoferrin and lactoferricin B on the ability of feline calicivirus (a norovirus surrogate) and poliovirus to infect cell cultures. J Appl Microbiol. 2003;95:1026-1033.
78. Beaumont SL, Maggs DJ, Clarke HE. Effects of bovine lactoferrin on in vitro replication of feline herpesvirus. Vet Ophthalmol. 2003;6:245-250.
79. Sato R, Inanami O, Tanaka Y, et al. Oral administration of bovine lactoferrin for treatment of intractable stomatitis in feline immunodeficiency virus (FIV)-positive and FIV-negative cats. Am J Vet Res. 1996;57:1443-1446.
80. Kobayashi S, Abe Y, Inanami O, et al. Oral administration of bovine lactoferrin upregulates neutrophil functions in a dog with familial beta2-integrin-related neutrophil dysfunction. Vet Immunol Immunopathol. 2011;143:155-161.
81. Tasker S, Lappin MR. *Haemobartonella felis*: recent developments in diagnosis and treatment. J Feline Med Surg. 2002;4:3-11.
82. Breitschwerdt EB, Davidson MG, Hegarty BC, et al. Prednisolone at anti-inflammatory or immunosuppressive dosages in conjunction with doxycycline does not potentiate the severity of *Rickettsia rickettsii* infection in dogs. Antimicrob Agents Chemother. 1997;41:141-147.
83. Chang YF, Novosel V, Chang CF, et al. Experimental induction of chronic borreliosis in adult dogs exposed to *Borrelia burgdorferi*-infected ticks and treated with dexamethasone. Am J Vet Res. 2001;62:1104-1112.
84. Peyton JL, Burkitt JM. Critical illness-related corticosteroid insufficiency in a dog with septic shock. J Vet Emerg Crit Care (San Antonio). 2009;19:262-268.
85. Dellinger RP, Levy MM, Carlet JM, et al. Surviving Sepsis Campaign: international guidelines for management of severe sepsis and septic shock: 2008. Crit Care Med. 2008;36:296-327.
86. Sykes JE, Sturges BK, Cannon MS, et al. Clinical signs, imaging features, neuropathology, and outcome in cats and dogs with central nervous system cryptococcosis from California. J Vet Intern Med. 2010;24:1427-1438.
87. Baskett A, Barton MH, Norton N, et al. Effect of pentoxifylline, flunixin meglumine, and their combination on a model of endotoxemia in horses. Am J Vet Res. 1997;58:1291-1299.
88. Barton MH, Moore JN, Norton N. Effects of pentoxifylline infusion on response of horses to in vivo challenge exposure with endotoxin. Am J Vet Res. 1997;58:1300-1307.
89. Marsella R, Olivry T. The ACVD task force on canine atopic dermatitis (XXII): nonsteroidal anti-inflammatory pharmacotherapy. Vet Immunol Immunopathol. 2001;81:331-345.
90. Nichols PR, Morris DO, Beale KM. A retrospective study of canine and feline cutaneous vasculitis. Vet Dermatol. 2001;12:255-264.
91. Fischer Y, Ritz S, Weber K, et al. Randomized, placebo controlled study of the effect of propentofylline on survival time and quality of life of cats with feline infectious peritonitis. J Vet Intern Med. 2011;25:1270-1276.

CHAPTER 8

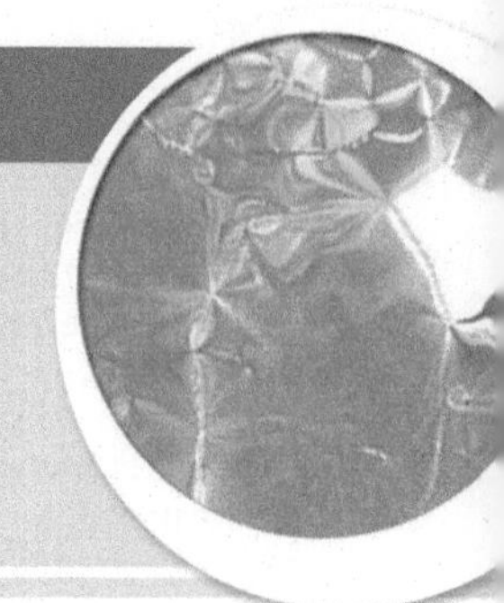

Antibacterial Drugs

Jane E. Sykes and Mark G. Papich

KEY POINTS

- An understanding of the mechanisms of action, spectrum of activity, pharmacokinetics, pharmacodynamics, and adverse effects of antibacterial drugs facilitates optimal treatment of bacterial infections while minimizing the chance for (1) selection of resistant bacteria, (2) adverse reactions, and (3) drug interactions.
- The importance of appropriate administration of antibiotics, compliance issues, and potential adverse effects of the drug chosen should be discussed with the pet owner when antibiotics are prescribed.

INTRODUCTION

This chapter reviews the classification, mechanisms of action, spectrum of activity, resistance mechanisms, tissue penetration, clinical use, and adverse effects of the major classes of antibiotics used to treat dogs and cats. Antimicrobials have been grouped together alphabetically according to their mechanism of action (cell wall synthesis, nucleic acid, and then protein synthesis inhibitors). Tables are dispersed throughout the text with drug dosages for each group of antibiotics. The reader is encouraged to review the accompanying text when using the tables. Not all antibiotics are reviewed here. Antibiotics that have specific uses, such as certain antimycobacterial drugs and nitrofurantoin, are reviewed in the relevant chapters of this book. Chapter 6 provides an overview of the basic principles of antimicrobial treatment.

Inhibitors of Cell Wall Synthesis

Beta-Lactam Antibiotics

β-Lactam antibiotics have a β-lactam ring in their molecular structure (Figure 8-1). They include penicillins, cephalosporins, monobactams, and carbapenems. They are bactericidal antibiotics (see Chapter 6) that bind covalently to and inhibit penicillin binding proteins (PBPs). These PBPs are needed to catalyze the cross-linking (or *transpeptidation*) of the peptidoglycan layer of bacterial cell walls, which is continuously remodeled by bacteria (Figure 8-2). When PBPs are inactivated by β-lactam antibiotics, bacterial enzymes that hydrolyze the peptidoglycan cross-links during cell wall remodeling continue to function, which breaks down the cell wall further. The accumulation of peptidoglycan precursors also triggers activation of cell wall hydrolases, with further digestion of intact peptidoglycan. The end result is bacterial rupture.

The peptidoglycan layer of gram-positive bacteria is 50 to 100 times thicker than that of gram-negative bacteria and is highly cross-linked, which maintains the structural integrity of gram-positive bacteria.[1] Therefore, compared to gram-negative bacteria, gram-positive bacteria are more easily inactivated by β-lactam antibiotics. Bacteria possess multiple PBPs, which are assigned numbers based on their molecular weight. PBPs vary in their affinities for different β-lactam antibiotics, which in part explains the difference in spectrum of activity and bactericidal action of β-lactam antibiotics. For example, inhibition of PBP1a and PBP1b leads to cell lysis, whereas inhibition of PBP2 results in rounded cells called spheroblasts. Drugs that produce rapid lysis (e.g., carbapenems) are the most bactericidal and have highest affinity for PBP1.

Resistance to β-lactam antibiotics is now widespread and results primarily from β-lactamase production.[2] It can also result from production of altered PBPs (such as PBP2a) and, among gram-negative bacteria, exclusion of drugs that normally diffuse through porins to their site of action. Gram-negative β-lactamases are strategically located just beneath the outer lipopolysaccharide layer, which acts as the barrier to drug penetration. Gram-positive bacteria secrete β-lactamases into their immediate surroundings. There are many different β-lactamase enzymes that vary in their specificity for β-lactam drugs.[3]

β-Lactam antibiotics have a short half-life and exhibit time-dependent pharmacodynamics (see Chapter 6). Drug concentrations should be maintained above the minimum inhibitory concentration (T > MIC) for at least 50% of the dosing interval. For penicillins and carbapenems, T > MIC can be less than 50%, but aiming for a target of 50% ensures that most patients will have adequate exposure. To maintain this target, some β-lactam antibiotics with short half-lives require frequent administration or slow infusion. For other drugs, a long half-life prolongs the

Beta-lactam ring — Penicillin (R–C(=O)–NH–, CH_3, CH_3, COOH)

Beta-lactam ring — Cephalosporin (R_1–C(=O)–NH–, S, R_2)

Beta-lactam ring — Imipenem (H_3C, OH, SCH_2CH_2NH–CH=NH, COOH)

Beta-lactam ring — Clavulanate (O, $CHCH_2OH$, COOH)

FIGURE 8-1 Structure of β-lactam antibiotics.

T > MIC to allow for infrequent administration. For example, cefpodoxime proxetil has a half-life longer than those of other oral cephalosporins, so it can be administered only once per day. Cefovecin has an extremely long half-life in dogs and cats and can be effective for some infections when administered at 14-day intervals. For other cephalosporins (e.g., injectable drugs with short half-lives such as cefotaxime), three- to four-times-daily dosing may be required for treatment of gram-negative bacterial infections.

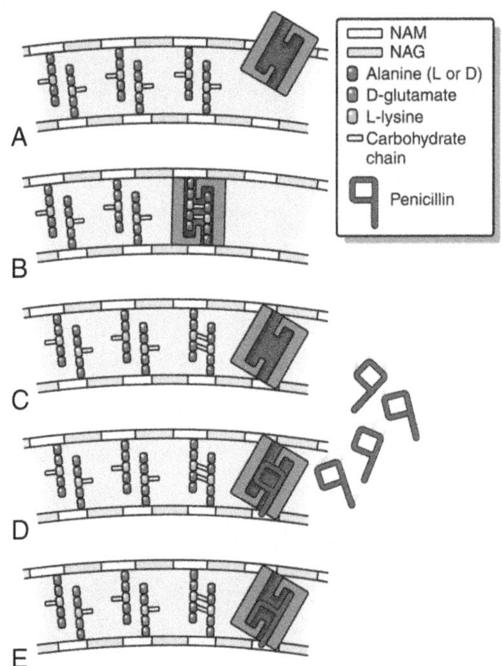

FIGURE 8-2 Interference of peptidoglycan production by β-lactam antibiotics. The bacterial cell wall consists of *N*-acetylglucosamine (NAG) and *N*-acetylmuramic acid (NAM) subunits. **A,** The penicillin binding protein (PBP, *brown squares*) binds peptide side chains and forms a cross-link **(B)**. **C,** The PBP dissociates from the wall once the cross-link has been formed. **D,** Penicillins enter the active site of the PBP. **E,** The β-lactam ring of the penicillin is irreversibly opened when it reacts with the PBP, which permanently blocks the active site.

Penicillins

Classification, Spectrum of Activity, and Resistance Mechanisms

Penicillins are derived from *Penicillium* molds. They are classified as naturally occurring penicillins such as penicillin G (benzyl penicillin), the semisynthetic aminopenicillins such as ampicillin and amoxicillin, penicillinase-resistant penicillins, and extended-spectrum penicillins. Table 8-1 shows the classification of the penicillins and their respective spectra of activity.

Penicillin G must be given parenterally because of poor oral bioavailability. Gram-positive bacteria that are susceptible to penicillin G are more susceptible to penicillin G than aminopenicillins such as ampicillin. The aminopenicillins have some activity against gram-negative bacteria, although many gram-negative bacteria are resistant because they produce β-lactamases. Ampicillin has limited absorption from the gastrointestinal tract, so it should be given parenterally for treatment of systemic infections. Amoxicillin has approximately twice the oral absorption of ampicillin and can be given orally.

Penicillinase-resistant penicillins (antistaphylococcal penicillins) such as methicillin have a structure that resists inactivation by β-lactamase enzymes. Methicillin is no longer used clinically. Drugs such as flucloxacillin and dicloxacillin have replaced the use of methicillin, because they can be administered orally and have fewer adverse effects. These drugs are highly protein-bound, which delays their elimination and maintains plasma drug concentrations, but tissue penetration is sufficient for treatment of skin and soft-tissue infections. Although dosages of penicillinase-resistant penicillins have been published for dogs and cats,[4] they are rarely used because other alternatives exist such as the combination of amoxicillin and the β-lactamase inhibitor clavulanic

TABLE 8-1

Classification and Spectrum of Activity of Penicillin Antibiotics

Penicillin Group	Examples	Antibacterial Spectrum
Natural penicillins	Penicillin G	Gram-positive aerobic bacteria (especially streptococci) and anaerobes. *Pasteurella multocida* may also be susceptible.
Aminopenicillins	Ampicillin Amoxicillin	Gram-positive aerobic bacteria (cocci and bacilli) and anaerobes; some susceptible gram-negative bacteria.
Penicillinase-resistant penicillins	Methicillin Oxacillin Cloxacillin Dicloxacillin	Susceptible β-lactamase producing gram-positive aerobic bacteria. Less active against penicillinase-susceptible organisms than penicillin G.
Extended spectrum carboxypenicillins	Ticarcillin Carbenicillin	Increased activity against susceptible gram-negative aerobes, which includes *Pseudomonas aeruginosa*, *Proteus* spp., *Klebsiella*, and anaerobes. Some reduction in gram-positive spectrum. Destroyed by β-lactamases.
Ureidopenicillins	Mezlocillin Piperacillin	Susceptible gram-positive and gram-negative aerobes, which includes *Pseudomonas aeruginosa*. Some loss of anaerobic spectrum. Destroyed by β-lactamases.
Penicillin–β-lactamase inhibitor combinations	β-Lactamase inhibitors: clavulanic acid, sulbactam, tazobactam	Susceptible β-lactamase producing gram-positive and gram negative aerobic bacteria and anaerobes.

acid. Methicillin and oxacillin are used in the laboratory for susceptibility testing. Resistance to methicillin results from bacterial production of an altered penicillin-binding protein (PBP2a), which leads to resistance to all β-lactam antibiotics.[5]

Extended-spectrum penicillins (antipseudomonal penicillins) have enhanced activity against gram-negative bacteria, but must be given parenterally. They include the carboxypenicillins, such as ticarcillin and carbenicillin, and piperacillin, an ureidopenicillin.

Clavulanic acid, sulbactam, and tazobactam are β-lactamase inhibitors that are administered in conjunction with penicillins, which increases the spectrum of activity. β-Lactamase inhibitors possess weak intrinsic antibacterial activity. Clavulanate has been combined not only with amoxicillin (oral), but also ticarcillin (parenteral). Sulbactam has been combined with ampicillin for intravenous (IV) injection. Sulbactam is not as active as clavulanic acid against some gram-negative β-lactamases. Tazobactam is combined with piperacillin.

Clinical Use

Penicillin dosages for dogs and cats are listed in Table 8-2. Penicillins are distributed to the extracellular fluid of most tissues. Because of low penetration across the blood-brain barrier and blood-ocular barrier, high doses are needed in order to attain effective levels in these tissues. Penicillins undergo rapid renal elimination, and active drug is concentrated in the urine, so they are useful for treatment of bacterial urinary tract infections (UTIs). Liver impairment has little effect on the pharmacokinetics of penicillins. Increasing the length of the dose interval is important in order to minimize toxicity in animals with renal failure.

Because of a short half-life, frequent dosing is necessary, especially when treating gram-negative bacterial infections with aminopenicillins. Penicillin MICs are generally higher for gram-negative bacteria than gram-positive bacteria; therefore, higher penicillin dosages may also be needed for gram-negative bacterial infections.

Adverse Effects

Penicillins are generally well tolerated by dogs and cats. The most common adverse effects in dogs and cats are vomiting, diarrhea, and inappetence. These are more likely to occur with amoxicillin when clavulanic acid is administered concurrently. Hypersensitivity reactions that include fever, cutaneous

TABLE 8-2

Suggested Penicillin Dosages for Small Animals

Drug	Dose (mg/kg)	Interval (hours)	Species	Route	Comments	CLSI Breakpoints (μg/mL)
Penicillin G potassium or sodium	20,000-40,000 U/kg	6-8	D, C	IV, IM		≤8 enterococci; ≤0.12 staphylococci and streptococci
Ampicillin sodium	10-20	6-8	D, C	IV, IM, SC	Administer IV over 3 minutes. When reconstituted with sterile water to 250 mg/mL, vials should be used within 1 hour. When reconstituted with 0.9% NaCl to 45 mg/mL, stability is maintained for 48 hours if refrigerated.	≤0.25 staphylococci, streptococci, and gram-negative bacilli; ≤8 canine urinary tract pathogens
Ampicillin-sulbactam	10-20	8	D, C	IV, IM	See ampicillin. Dose according to ampicillin component.	≤8/4* staphylococci and gram-negative bacteria
Amoxicillin	10-20	8-12	D, C	PO		See ampicillin.
Amoxicillin-clavulanate potassium	12.5-25	12	D, C	PO	More frequent or higher doses recommended for gram-negative infections.	≤0.25/0.12* staphylococci, streptococci, *Escherichia coli* and *Pasteurella multocida*
Ticarcillin disodium, ticarcillin-clavulanate†	33-50	4-6	D, C	IV	When reconstituted with 0.9% NaCl, stable for up to 14 days when refrigerated.	≤64/2* *Pseudomonas aeruginosa* ≤16/2 gram-negative enteric bacteria
Piperacillin sodium/piperacillin-tazobactam†	40	6	D, C	IV	Reconstituted solution should be used within 7 days if refrigerated.	See ticarcillin.

C, Cats; CLSI, Clinical and Laboratory Standards Institute; D, dogs.
*The "/" distinguishes the ticarcillin from clavulanic acid concentrations.
†It is recommended that the use of these drugs be reserved for life-threatening infections that are susceptible to these drugs but resistant to other drugs, on the basis of culture and susceptibility testing.

reactions, immune-mediated cytopenias, and anaphylaxis are possible, especially in dogs, but are less common than in human patients. The use of penicillins should be avoided in animals with a history of such reactions. Rapid intravenous infusion or administration of high doses of penicillins to animals with coexisting renal failure is rarely followed by development of neurologic signs, such as seizures. Pain or tissue reactions can occur when penicillins are administered intramuscularly or subcutaneously. High doses of extended-spectrum penicillins such as ticarcillin have been associated with platelet function abnormalities and significant bleeding in human patients.[6]

Cephalosporins

Classification and Spectrum of Activity

The cephalosporins were originally derived from *Acremonium* spp. (previously known as *Cephalosporium* spp.). They have been broadly grouped into first-, second-, third-, and fourth-generation cephalosporins based on their spectrum of activity. As the generation increases, there is an increase in gram-negative spectrum, and fourth-generation drugs have truly broad-spectrum activity (Table 8-3). An exception to this pattern is the newest addition to the group, ceftaroline. It has activity against methicillin-resistant staphylococci as a result of an affinity for PBP2a and has been considered a "fifth-generation" cephalosporin. Cephalosporins are resistant to staphylococcal β-lactamase, and the extended-spectrum cephalosporins (primarily the third-generation drugs) are resistant to many gram-negative β-lactamases. However, extended-spectrum β-lactamase (ESBL) enzymes can hydrolyze even third-generation cephalosporins and present an important therapeutic challenge.

Clinical Use

Cephalosporin dosages for cats and dogs are listed in Table 8-4. First-generation cephalosporins such as cephalexin are moderately absorbed orally and distributed into extracellular fluids. In general, they have poor penetration of blood-brain barrier, even in the face of inflammation. Most are excreted unchanged in the urine, and so are useful for treatment of UTIs. Cefazolin has greater activity against a wider range of bacterial isolates than the oral first-generation cephalosporins (e.g., cephalexin and cefadroxil).[7] Cefazolin has been a popular injectable antibiotic for perioperative use in small animals. This perioperative use of cefazolin is with the intention to prevent postsurgical infections, particularly in orthopedic surgery (see Chapter 85).

Use of second-, third-, and fourth-generation cephalosporins may be indicated when there is resistance to first-generation cephalosporins and there are no other reasonable alternatives available. Three third-generation cephalosporins are approved by the U.S. Food and Drug Administration (FDA) for use in small animals: ceftiofur, cefpodoxime proxetil, and cefovecin. These agents are approved for treatment of skin and soft-tissue infections (cefpodoxime proxetil and cefovecin) and UTIs in dogs (ceftiofur). Although their use in small animal medicine has been controversial because of concerns that relate to selection for resistant bacteria, there is no evidence at this time that the use of these agents has been associated with increased resistance among isolates from dogs and cats. The injectable third-generation cephalosporins approved for people have greater in vitro activity than cefpodoxime or cefovecin and occasionally have been used in dogs and cats (e.g., cefotaxime, ceftazidime, cefoperazone). These drugs have a high degree of activity, but are expensive and must be administered frequently by injection. Distribution and excretion into urine and bile is variable. Some third-generation cephalosporins have a longer duration of activity than first- and second-generation drugs by virtue of long half-lives. Cefpodoxime proxetil is the most commonly used oral third-generation drug in small animals, approximately 50% of which is excreted in the urine in active form. Cefovecin is approved for use in dogs and cats in Europe and North America as a subcutaneous injection. The high protein binding and slow clearance result in a very long half-life in these species (approximately 7 days in cats and 5 days in dogs). Administration of cefovecin to cats results in a duration of activity of at least 14 days, and for at least 7 to 14 days in dogs

TABLE 8-3

Classification and Spectrum of Activity of Cephalosporin Antibiotics

Cephalosporin Generation	Examples	Antibacterial Spectrum
First	Cephalexin Cefazolin Cefadroxil	Methicillin-susceptible staphylococci and streptococci and aerobes; some activity against gram-negative aerobes (especially cefazolin). Unpredictable activity against anaerobes.
Second	Cefaclor Cefotetan Cefoxitin	Improved activity against gram-negative aerobes and anaerobes compared with first-generation drugs. Cefoxitin has greater stability against anaerobic β-lactamases (such as those produced by *Bacteroides*) than other second-generation drugs.
Third	Cefixime Cefpodoxime Ceftiofur Cefotaxime Ceftriaxone Cefovecin Ceftazidime	Activity primarily against gram-negative bacteria. Some drugs in this group have less activity against gram-positive bacteria and anaerobes.
Fourth	Cefepime	Gram-positive cocci, gram-negative bacilli, many β-lactamase-producing gram-negative bacteria. Reserve for life-threatening infections where no other alternative is available.

TABLE 8-4

Suggested Cephalosporin Dosages for Small Animals

Drug	Dose (mg/kg)	Interval (hours)	Route	Species	Comments	CLSI Breakpoints (μg/mL)
Cephalexin	10-30 15-20	6-12 12	PO	D C	Use 30 mg/kg q12h for pyoderma. More frequent dosing (q6-8h) is required for gram-negative bacterial infections.	≤2 susceptible organisms. Cephalothin can be used to test susceptibility for all other 1st generation drugs.
Cefadroxil	22	12 24	PO	D C		See cephalexin.
Cefazolin sodium	20-35	8	IV, IM	D, C	22 mg/kg q2h during surgery if indicated.	See cephalexin.
Cefaclor†	15-20	8	PO	D, C		≤8 all susceptible organisms
Cefoxitin sodium†	30	6-8	IM, IV	D, C	Pain on injection IM.	See cefaclor.
Cefixime†	10	12	PO	D, C	Use 5 mg/kg q12-24h for urinary tract infections.	≤1 all susceptible organisms
Cefpodoxime proxetil†	5-10	24	PO	D*	Of all third-generation cephalosporins, most active against staphylococci. Less active against gram-negative and anaerobic infections.	≤2 all susceptible organisms
Ceftiofur sodium†	2.2-4.4	24	SC	D*	For treatment of otherwise resistant urinary tract infections.	Not established for dogs and cats
Cefotaxime sodium†	50 20-80	12 6	IV, IM	D C	Partially metabolized by the liver to desacetyl cefotaxime which contributes to antibacterial activity. Good CNS penetration. Stable for 5 days in the refrigerator after reconstitution.	See cefpodoxime.
Ceftazidime†	30	6	IV	D, C	Potent antipseudomonal activity.	≤4 *Enterobacteriaceae*, ≤8 *Pseudomonas aeruginosa* and staphylococci
Cefovecin†	8	14 days	SC	D, C	Approved for use for skin and soft tissue infections and in some countries, urinary tract infections. Efficacy for treatment of infections in other sites not established.	No approved breakpoint. ≤2 all susceptible organisms is suggested
Cefepime†	40	6	IV, IM	D*	Reduce frequency in dogs with renal failure (q12-24h).	≤ 8 all susceptible organisms

C, Cats; CLSI, Clinical and Laboratory Standards Institute; CNS, central nervous system; D, dogs.

*Dose not established for cats.

†It is recommended that the use of most second-, third-, and fourth-generation cephalosporins be reserved for serious infections that are susceptible to those drugs but resistant to other reasonable alternatives on the basis of culture and susceptibility testing.

(depending on the pathogen). Injections can be repeated in dogs at 14-day intervals if necessary.

Adverse Effects

Adverse effects of cephalosporins in dogs and cats are similar to those of penicillins, with gastrointestinal signs and hypersensitivity reactions being most frequent. Although the incidence is low, cross-sensitivity can occur between penicillins and cephalosporins, so cephalosporins should be avoided or used with caution in animals that have a history of reactions to penicillin. Injectable cephalosporins can cause phlebitis and pain on injection. Cephalosporins have the potential to cause false-positive results on test strips that use copper reduction for urine glucose detection. Certain cephalosporins, such as cefotetan and ceftriaxone, may exacerbate bleeding tendencies due to vitamin K antagonism.[8] Reversible bone marrow suppression has been reported in dogs given high doses of ceftiofur, cefonicid, and cefazedone long-term.[9]

Monobactams (Aztreonam)

Aztreonam is a synthetic β-lactam antibiotic that is resistant to some β-lactamases. It is effective against a wide range of

TABLE 8-5

Suggested Carbapenem Dosages for Small Animals

Drug	Dose (mg/kg)	Interval (hours)	Species	Route	Comments	CLSI Breakpoints (μg/mL)
Imipenem-cilastatin	5	6-8	D, C	IV, IM, SC	250 to 500 mg of reconstituted drug should be added to no less than 100 mL of fluids and administered IV over 30-60 minutes. Stable for 24 hours after reconstitution when refrigerated. For IM injections, reconstitute with 1% lidocaine.	≤1 Enterobacteriaceae, ≤2 *Pseudomonas aeruginosa*
Meropenem	8.5 24	12 12	D, C D, C	SC IV	SC injections may cause alopecia at the injection site. For *Pseudomonas aeruginosa* or infections with MIC values approaching the breakpoint, use 12 mg/kg q8h SC or 24 mg/kg q8h IV.	See imipenem.

Carbapenems should be used for serious infections resistant to other reasonable alternatives, on the basis of culture and susceptibility testing.
C, Cats; CLSI, Clinical and Laboratory Standards Institute; D, dogs; MIC, minimum inhibitory concentration.

gram-negative bacteria, including *Pseudomonas aeruginosa,* but not gram-positive or anaerobic bacteria. In human medicine, aztreonam is used to treat patients with serious gram-negative infections who are allergic to penicillins and cannot tolerate aminoglycosides.[10] Dosages have not been established for dogs.

Carbapenems

Spectrum of Activity and Clinical Use

Carbapenems are highly resistant to almost all bacterial β-lactamases and include imipenem, meropenem, ertapenem, and doripenem. They penetrate the outer membrane of gram-negative bacteria more effectively than many other β-lactam antibiotics and bind to a variety of PBPs, which leads to rapid lysis of a broad spectrum of bacteria.[11] In contrast to other β-lactam antibiotics, carbapenems have a postantibiotic effect (see Chapter 6) similar to that of aminoglycosides and fluoroquinolones. Although effective against many gram-positive, gram-negative, and anaerobic bacterial infections, the use of carbapenems is reserved for treatment of serious, multiple drug-resistant (MDR) gram-negative infections, especially *Escherichia coli, Klebsiella pneumoniae,* and *P. aeruginosa,* that are resistant to other antibiotics. Methicillin-resistant staphylococci are resistant to carbapenems. Dosages for dogs and cats are listed in Table 8-5.

The identification of carbapenemase production by some strains of gram-negative bacteria has raised great concern, because this confers resistance to a broad range of β-lactam antibiotics. Carbapenemase-producing *K. pneumoniae* (KPC) are resistant not only to all β-lactam antibiotics, but also to fluoroquinolones and aminoglycosides.[12] *K. pneumoniae* that produce a plasmid-encoded metallo-β-lactamase enzyme (NDM-1) appeared in India in 2008 and have subsequently spread worldwide.[13] The only options left for treatment of these infections are tigecycline and polymyxins, both of which have been associated with emergence of resistance during treatment.[14] The potential for spread of *K. pneumoniae* isolates that are resistant to all commercially available antibiotics now exists. Carapenemase (NDM-1) production was recently detected in an *E. coli* isolate from a cat in the United States.

Adverse Effects

Imipenem is degraded by dehydropeptidase-1, a brush border enzyme in the proximal renal tubules, which results in production of an inactive metabolite that is nephrotoxic. In order to prevent nephrotoxicity and maximize imipenem's antibacterial activity, imipenem is administered with cilastatin, which inhibits the dehydropeptidase-1 enzyme. Newer carbapenems such as meropenem are resistant to dehydropeptidase-1.

Adverse effects of carbapenems are otherwise rare and include vomiting, nausea, and pain on injection. Neurologic signs, including tremors, nystagmus, and seizures, can occur following rapid infusion of imipenem-cilastatin or in animals with renal insufficiency. Imipenem must be administered slowly in intravenous fluids (see Table 8-5). Slow administration is not required for meropenem, which is more soluble. Subcutaneous injections of meropenem have produced alopecia at the injection site,[4] but otherwise these injections have been very well tolerated and have eradicated infections associated with MDR gram-negative bacteria.

Glycopeptides

Mechanism of Action and Clinical Use

Glycopeptides are cyclic glycosylated peptide antimicrobials that inhibit the synthesis of peptidoglycan by binding to amino acids (D-alanyl-D-alanine) in the cell wall, preventing the addition of new units. Vancomycin, teicoplanin, and decaplanin are all glycopeptides, but only vancomycin has been used in small animals.

Vancomycin was discovered in the 1950s, but has not been frequently used in small animals because it is not absorbed orally, so IV infusion is required for treatment of systemic infections. When administered IV, it can be valuable for treatment of MDR gram-positive bacterial infections, such as methicillin-resistant staphylococcal infections, resistant enterococcal infections, and encrusting cystitis caused by *Corynebacterium urealyticum.* The last is an emerging infection of dogs, cats, and immunocompromised human patients, treatment of which requires surgical debridement of the bladder in conjunction with glycopeptide administration.[15,16] Vancomycin is a valuable agent for treatment of methicillin-resistant staphylococci, because resistance among these organisms is extremely rare, and the bactericidal activity can be an advantage when treating immunocompromised patients. In human patients, oral vancomycin has been used to treat gastrointestinal infections caused by resistant *Clostridium difficile*.

Vancomycin-resistant methicillin-resistant *Staphylococcus aureus* (MRSA) isolates are extremely rare in people and have only been described in specific geographic locations. Vancomycin-resistant *Staphylococcus pseudintermedius* isolates have not yet been described. Vancomycin-resistant enterococci (VRE) are well documented in human patients and can present a therapeutic challenge. Although currently rare, the existence of VRE has been reported in companion animals.[17] Resistance to vancomycin results from bacterial alteration of the terminal amino acid to which vancomycin binds. In order to reduce inappropriate use of vancomycin, some laboratories do not report results for vancomycin susceptibility unless reporting is indicated on the basis of resistance in the remainder of the susceptibility panel.

Teicoplanin has a longer half-life and is up to 100 times more lipophilic than vancomycin. It is not commercially available in the United States but is used in Europe. Vancomycin and teicoplanin appear to be equally efficacious in human patients.[18]

Adverse Effects

Vancomycin is not commonly used to treat small animals, and so adverse reactions have not been well documented. The most common reaction in human patients is the "red man syndrome" caused by histamine release after rapid infusion. This can be prevented through the use of antihistamines and slower infusion rates. Other adverse reactions are rare. Previously cited nephrotoxicity from vancomycin may be exaggerated because of its frequent co-administration with aminoglycosides. Current formulations are of better quality and purity and less likely to produce kidney injury. Vancomycin is given by IV infusion over 30 to 60 minutes through a central or peripheral catheter (Table 8-6). Trough plasma concentrations can be monitored and should be greater than 10 μg/mL for skin and soft tissue infections, and 10 to 20 μg/mL for more complicated infections. Intramuscular administration is painful and irritates tissues.

Nucleic Acid Inhibitors

Fluoroquinolones

Classification and Mechanism of Action

The fluoroquinolones bind to DNA gyrase (also known as topoisomerase II) and topoisomerase IV, enzymes that cleave DNA during DNA replication. The result is disruption of bacterial DNA and protein synthesis. For the veterinary fluoroquinolones enrofloxacin, orbifloxacin, and marbofloxacin, DNA gyrase is the primary target for gram-negative bacteria and topoisomerase IV is the primary target for gram-positive bacteria. Because topoisomerase IV has a lower affinity than DNA gyrase for this group of drugs, higher MICs are observed for gram-positive bacteria compared to the Enterobacteriaceae.

Fluoroquinolones were created by addition of a fluorine group to nalidixic acid, which improves its spectrum of activity. Examples are enrofloxacin, ciprofloxacin, difloxacin, orbifloxacin, and marbofloxacin. Newer-generation fluoroquinolones inhibit *both* DNA gyrase and topoisomerase IV in gram-positive bacteria, leading to enhanced activity for treatment of gram-positive and anaerobic bacterial infections and reduced likelihood of selection for resistant mutants. Pradofloxacin, levofloxacin, moxifloxacin, and gatifloxacin are third-generation fluoroquinolones. The only antibiotic in this group approved for use in companion animals is pradofloxacin, which is approved for use in cats in the United States, and approved for both dogs and cats in European countries.

Resistance to fluoroquinolones results from DNA gyrase mutations, decreased bacterial permeability, and increased drug efflux.[19] Susceptibility to one fluoroquinolone generally predicts susceptibility to others, with the exceptions of third-generation fluoroquinolones (such as pradofloxacin) and ciprofloxacin, which has higher in vitro activity against *P. aeruginosa* than other fluoroquinolones.[20,21] Limited use of fluoroquinolones has been recommended by some human and veterinary medical authorities in order to minimize further development of resistance, but a clear association between prescription of fluoroquinolones and increased resistance has not been established in companion animals. Nevertheless, other "first line" drugs are often available for most infections, and the valuable fluoroquinolones can be reserved for cases that cannot tolerate other drugs, or when resistance to other drugs is more likely.

TABLE 8-6

Suggested Vancomycin Dosages for Small Animals

Drug	Dose (mg/kg)	Interval (hours)	Species	Route	Comments	CLSI Breakpoints (μg/mL)
Vancomycin*	15 12-15	6-8 8	D C	IV	Reconstituted drug is added to 0.9% NaCl or 5% dextrose and administered over 30 to 60 minutes. It can also be administered in 5% dextrose as a CRI, with a loading dose of 3.5 mg/kg, and then 1.5 mg/kg/hr IV. Therapeutic drug monitoring recommended.	≤4 *Enterococcus* and *Staphylococcus*

C, Cats; CLSI, Clinical and Laboratory Standards Institute; CRI, continuous-rate infusion; D, dogs.

*The use of vancomycin should be reserved for gram-positive infections that are susceptible to vancomycin but resistant to all other reasonable alternatives, on the basis of culture and susceptibility testing.

A sufficiently high dose should be used to minimize selection of resistant isolates.

Clinical Use

Fluoroquinolones are most valuable to treat gram-negative infections, because there are often few oral medication alternatives for these infections. The fluoroquinolones are also effective for infections caused by staphylococci, but staphylococci tend to have higher MICs for fluoroquinolones than gram-negative bacteria. The activity of fluoroquinolones against anaerobes is variable. Pradofloxacin has the greatest activity, followed by marbofloxacin and enrofloxacin.[22] Fluoroquinolones are concentration-dependent antibiotics, so they are best administered as a single high daily dose. Doses for fluoroquinolones are listed in Table 8-7.

Fluoroquinolones are usually well absorbed after oral administration. Poor absorption occurs when they are complexed by divalent and trivalent cation-containing medications (e.g., antacids) and supplements (aluminum, calcium, iron, zinc). Use of these should be avoided if animals are receiving fluoroquinolones by the oral route. Oral absorption of the human drug ciprofloxacin is lower and more variable in dogs than in people, which necessitates administration of a higher dose. In one study, oral absorption of generic ciprofloxacin tablets in dogs was 58%, but the coefficient of variation was 45%.[23] In cats, only 22% to 33% of orally administered ciprofloxacin is absorbed. Most fluoroquinolones are highly concentrated in the urine, so they are useful for treatment of UTIs. Enrofloxacin is metabolized to ciprofloxacin, which is subsequently excreted in the urine. Approximately half of the administered dose of marbofloxacin and orbifloxacin is excreted as unchanged drug in the urine. In contrast, difloxacin is excreted primarily in bile, and little drug enters the urine.[24]

TABLE 8-7

Suggested Fluoroquinolone Dosages for Small Animals

Drug	Dose (mg/kg)	Interval (hours)	Species	Route	Comments	CLSI Breakpoints (μg/mL)
Enrofloxacin	5-20 5	24 24	D C*	IV, IM, PO IM, PO	Interactions can occur with certain oral medications (see text). Reduce dose or increase dosage interval with renal failure. Dilute in fluids (e.g., 1:10 dilution) and infuse IV over 30 minutes.	≤0.5 susceptible infections. Use higher dosages (10-20 mg/kg) for organisms with MICs of 1 or 2 (except in cats). A dose of 5 mg/kg may be sufficient for UTIs.
Ciprofloxacin hydrochloride	20-30 10	24 24	D, C D, C	PO IV	See enrofloxacin. Oral absorption may be limited (see text).	In humans, ≤1 susceptible infections. More active against *Pseudomonas aeruginosa* than other fluoroquinolones
Marbofloxacin	2.75-5.5	24	D, C	PO	See enrofloxacin.	≤1 susceptible infections. Use higher doses for bacteria with higher MICs.
Orbifloxacin	2.5-7.5	24	D, C	PO	See enrofloxacin. Orbifloxacin suspension provides lower and more variable plasma levels than the tablets. A dose of 7.5 mg/kg should be used.	See marbofloxacin.
Difloxacin hydrochloride	5-10	24	D	PO	Urine concentrations may not be sufficient for treating UTIs.	≤0.5 susceptible infections
Moxifloxacin	10	24	D, C	PO	Moxifloxacin has enhanced activity against gram-positive bacteria and anaerobes. In humans, urine concentrations are not sufficient for treatment of UTIs.	See marbofloxacin.
Pradofloxacin	3† 5-7.5‡	24	D, C C	PO	See moxifloxacin for spectrum of activity. Food reduces bioavailability. Appears effective for treatment of UTIs.	Not established

C, Cats; CLSI, Clinical and Laboratory Standards Institute; D, dogs; MIC, minimum inhibitory concentration; UTI, urinary tract infection.

*The use of enrofloxacin to treat cats is controversial because of the potential for irreversible retinal toxicity and blindness. Do not exceed a dose of 5 mg/kg in cats. The use of alternative fluoroquinolones such as marbofloxacin, orbifloxacin, or pradofloxacin should be considered for cats.

†Tablet formulation. The use of pradofloxacin at high doses in dogs has been associated with myelosuppression and is off-label in the United States, but it is approved for both dogs and cats outside the United States at a dose of 3 mg/kg (tablets).

‡Oral suspension for cats. The dose of the oral suspension for cats is higher (5-7.5 mg/kg) owing to reduced bioavailability.

Fluoroquinolones have variable protein binding, but this does not inhibit distribution to tissue fluids. Because of good lipophilicity, these drugs penetrate the prostate and respiratory secretions. They also penetrate the ear canal, but high doses may be required for treatment of bacteria with relatively high MIC values.[25] Fluoroquinolones can attain high intracellular concentrations and can be used to treat infections caused by intracellular pathogens such as *Mycoplasma* spp. and some *Mycobacterium* spp.

Adverse Effects

Fluoroquinolones can occasionally produce gastrointestinal signs in dogs and cats, such as decreased appetite and vomiting. Rapid IV administration can cause systemic hypotension, tachycardia, and cutaneous erythema, possibly as a result of histamine release.[26] Neurologic signs, including tremors, ataxia, and seizures, can occur in dogs and cats treated with high doses of parenteral fluoroquinolones. Although not well understood, this is thought to result from fluoroquinolone interference with the binding of γ-aminobutyric acid to its receptors in the central nervous system (CNS).[27] In general, fluoroquinolones should be used cautiously in animals prone to seizures. Enrofloxacin causes hallucinations in humans and so is not marketed or approved for treatment of humans.

Cats treated with high doses of enrofloxacin (generally >5 mg/kg/day), especially parenteral enrofloxacin, have developed blindness resulting from acute retinal degeneration, manifested as bilateral mydriasis with tapetal hyperreflectivity.[28,29] This results from a functional defect in a fluoroquinolone transport protein in the cat, with subsequent accumulation of photoreactive drug in the retina.[30] In general, the blindness is irreversible, but if it is detected early and medication is discontinued, some resolution may occur. Orbifloxacin also can produce retinal injury in cats, but the dose needed for this reaction is much higher than doses used therapeutically. Studies of marbofloxacin (reported by the manufacturer) and pradofloxacin[31] showed no evidence of retinal toxicity in cats, even with high doses, although there are reports to the FDA of blindness in cats associated with the use of marbofloxacin. Cats with renal insufficiency or those treated with medications that increase plasma fluoroquinolone concentrations may be more likely to develop this adverse effect.

Because they inhibit proteoglycan synthesis and chelate magnesium, fluoroquinolones can cause cartilage and joint toxicity in young animals, although the clinical importance of this has been questioned.[32,33] In general, prolonged (>7 days) use of fluoroquinolones during the period of rapid growth in dogs (from about 1 to 2 months of age to 28 weeks) should be avoided if possible. Cats are thought to be more resistant to development of cartilage toxicity. Pradofloxacin has been associated with myelosuppression in dogs at doses greater than 10 mg/kg.

Fluoroquinolones inhibit some cytochrome P450 enzymes, which decreases metabolism of other drugs. This occurs with theophylline in dogs; therefore, the dose of theophylline should be adjusted if administered concurrently. Like cephalosporins, fluoroquinolones can cause false-positive results on test strips for urine glucose detection. Cutaneous photosensitization occurs in human patients but is rare in animals. Other adverse effects reported in humans, but not in dogs and cats, include cardiac arrhythmias, tendinitis and tendon rupture, altered glucose metabolism, and hepatic dysfunction.[34]

Metronidazole

Mechanism of Action and Spectrum of Activity

Metronidazole is a bactericidal nitroimidazole drug that is used primarily to treat anaerobic bacterial infections (both gram-negative and gram-positive), which includes those caused by *Bacteroides fragilis* and *Clostridium* spp., and infections with certain protozoa, such as *Giardia* spp. Metronidazole diffuses into bacterial cells as a prodrug and is activated in the cytoplasm. Once within the cell, the nitro group of metronidazole preferentially accepts electrons from electron transport proteins such as ferredoxin. A short-lived nitroso free radical is thus generated that damages DNA. The intermediate compounds then decompose into non-toxic, inactive end products.

Metronidazole has antioxidant properties that are believed to result from its ability to scavenge reactive oxygen species and modulation of neutrophil activity.[35] It is often used at low doses to treat inflammatory bowel disease in dogs and cats,[36] but it is not known if the benefit is from the antibacterial activity or direct effects on inflammatory cells.

Resistance to metronidazole is rare among anaerobes.[37] Mechanisms of resistance include reduced drug uptake and decreased reduction activity. Other proposed mechanisms include increased efflux, drug inactivation, and accelerated DNA repair.

Clinical Use

In dogs and cats, metronidazole is used to treat anaerobic bacterial and protozoal infections in a variety of tissues. Suggested

TABLE 8-8

Suggested Metronidazole Dosages for Small Animals

Drug	Dose (mg/kg)	Interval (hours)	Species	Route	Comments
Metronidazole	15 10-15	12 24	D C	PO	Reduce dose by 50% in animals with hepatic dysfunction. An intravenous solution, metronidazole hydrochloride, is available but is highly acidic. It should be diluted in 100 mL of IV crystalloids and neutralized with 5 mEq sodium bicarbonate per 500 mg for a pH of 6-7. Diluted solutions are stable for 24 hours.
Metronidazole benzoate	25	12	C	PO	More palatable formulation for cats may be available from some compounding pharmacies.

C, Cats; D, dogs.

doses are listed in Table 8-8. Metronidazole is rapidly and almost completely absorbed from the gastrointestinal tract, diffuses across lipid membranes, and achieves therapeutic concentrations in tissue fluids. Metronidazole is metabolized by the liver. The metabolites, along with intact drug, are excreted in the urine.

Adverse Effects

The main adverse effect of metronidazole is neurotoxicity, which tends to occur with high doses (>30 mg/kg/day) or in animals with hepatic dysfunction. Clinical signs of neurotoxicity are reversible on discontinuation of the drug and include lethargy, truncal ataxia, hypermetria, intention tremors, head tilt, falling, vertical nystagmus, extensor rigidity, opisthotonos and seizures, and reflect damage to the vestibular system.[38,39] Although not fully understood, neurotoxicity is believed to result from antagonism of γ-aminobutyric acid in the cerebellar and vestibular systems. Neurologic signs resolve more quickly when treated with a low dose of diazepam (0.4 mg/kg PO q8h for 3 days).[38] Bilateral symmetrical cerebellar lesions, most commonly in the dentate nucleus have been reported on magnetic resonance imaging in human patients with metronidazole toxicity,[40] and multifocal necrotic foci were detected at necropsy in the brainstem of a cat.[39] Administration of metronidazole to animals with a history of metronidazole toxicosis is not recommended.[38]

Less commonly, metronidazole causes decreased appetite, vomiting, and diarrhea. Metronidazole suspension has a bitter taste that may be unpalatable to cats, which can be overcome by administration of the drug in gel capsules. Although not approved by the FDA, metronidazole benzoate is a more palatable formulation for cats and pharmacokinetic studies have demonstrated good absorption.[41] There have been concerns that relate to toxicity from the benzoic acid component of the formulation, which can cause CNS signs, blindness, and respiratory problems at high doses. However, this possibility is considered to be unlikely.[41] Because metronidazole benzoate is only 62% metronidazole, dosage adjustment is required when this formulation is used. Metronidazole inhibits hepatic microsomal enzymes and so may increase the concentration of drugs such as warfarin and cyclosporine. It also lowers serum lipid concentrations (including cholesterol concentrations) in human patients.[42]

Rifamycins

Mechanism of Action and Spectrum of Activity

Named after the French crime movie *Rififi*, rifamycins are bactericidal antimicrobials that inhibit the β-subunit of DNA-dependent RNA polymerase in bacteria. This leads to impaired RNA synthesis. Only the semisynthetic drug rifampin (also known as rifampicin) has been used to any great extent in small animal medicine. Rifampin is active against staphylococci, streptococci, and only a few gram-negative organisms. When used as a component of antimycobacterial treatment regimes, it increases the chance of treatment success. Rifabutin is effective for treatment of some mycobacterial infections that are resistant to rifampicin.[43]

It has been recommended that rifampin be used in combination with other antimicrobials to reduce the risk of emergence of rifampin resistance, which occurs quickly when rifampin is used alone. However, this applies primarily when it is used for long-term treatment, such as for mycobacterial infections. Monotherapy has been successful when rifampin has been used to treat methicillin-resistant *Staphylococcus* infections, which accounts for most of the current small animal use. If combination treatment is pursued for treatment of methicillin-resistant staphylococci, there are often few effective alternatives with which to combine rifampin, because these infections are typically multidrug resistant. Resistance to rifampin results from a single mutation that leads to an altered RNA polymerase that does not effectively bind rifampin.

Clinical Use

One of the major advantages of rifampin is its high degree of lipid solubility, which provides the degree of intracellular penetration required for treatment of infections caused by intracellular bacteria such as *Mycobacterium* spp. and *Brucella canis* infections. Rifampin has been used to treat bartonellosis in combination with doxycycline.[44,45] Because of its activity against staphylococci and the fact that it can be administered orally, it has been used for treatment of methicillin-resistant staphylococcal infections in small animals. For other infections, rifampin is less attractive because of its adverse effect profile.

Rifampin dosing is shown in Table 8-9. Rifampin is rapidly absorbed from the gastrointestinal tract and metabolized by the liver. Active metabolites are excreted in bile and to a lesser extent the urine.

Adverse Effects

Vomiting and anorexia are common in dogs treated with rifampin. The drug can impart a red-orange color to the urine and, to a lesser extent, tears, saliva, the sclera, and mucous membranes. Rifampin can also be associated with increased

TABLE 8-9

Suggested Rifampin Dose for Small Animals

Drug	Dose (mg/kg)	Interval (hours)	Species	Route	Comments	CLSI Breakpoints (μg/mL)
Rifampin	5	12	D, C	PO	Preferably use in combination with other drugs. Avoid in animals with hepatic dysfunction. Do not administer with fatty meals. Drug interactions may occur (see text). Monitor liver enzymes with prolonged treatment. May impart a red-orange color to the urine and tears.	≤1 for susceptible organisms (usually MICs of gram-positive bacteria fall below this breakpoint)

C, Cats; CLSI, Clinical and Laboratory Standards Institute; D, dogs; MIC, minimum inhibitory concentration.

serum liver enzyme activities and hepatopathy. Doses that exceed 10 mg/kg per day in dogs increase the risk of liver injury. In humans, fever, cutaneous reactions, thrombocytopenia, acute intravascular hemolytic anemia, and acute tubulointerstitial nephritis have been reported, which appear to have an immune-mediated pathogenesis.[46] Rarely, pancreatitis has been reported in human patients receiving rifampin. Adverse effects have not been reported in cats, but some of these risks may apply to cats as well as dogs. Because of poor palatability, it is a challenge to administer to cats.

Rifampin is one of *the* most potent inducers of hepatic microsomal enzymes and efflux proteins, such as P-glycoprotein. Subsequently, it can increase the clearance of several co-administered drugs (thereby decreasing their efficacy), such as glucocorticoids, cyclosporin, itraconazole, and digoxin. In human patients, recovery from the effect of rifampin on hepatic microsomal enzymes can take 4 weeks.[47]

Trimethoprim-Sulfonamides

Mechanism of Action

Trimethoprim and sulfonamides act synergistically to inhibit folic acid metabolism by bacteria. The combination interferes with purine and therefore DNA synthesis. Trimethoprim inhibits bacterial dihydrofolate reductase. Sulfonamides are chemical analogs of para-aminobenzoic acid (PABA), and competitively inhibit the incorporation of PABA into dihydropteroic acid by the enzyme dihydropteroate synthetase, which also leads to decreased folic acid synthesis. When administered separately, each drug is bacteriostatic, but the combination is bactericidal. Preparations used to treat dogs and cats include a 1:5 ratio of trimethoprim to sulfonamide. Because folic acid is of dietary origin in animals, only bacterial purine synthesis is affected.

Resistance to trimethoprim-sulfonamide (TMS) antibiotics most commonly results from plasmid-mediated production of altered dihydrofolate reductase or dihydropteroate synthetase, with reduced binding affinities. Other mechanisms include overproduction of dihydrofolate reductase or PABA by bacteria, and reduced bacterial permeability to trimethoprim and sulfonamides. Multiple mechanisms may operate simultaneously.[48]

Clinical Use

TMS antibiotics have a broad spectrum of activity and can be used to treat gram-positive and many gram-negative bacterial infections, as well as some protozoal infections. Enterococci are intrinsically resistant to TMS antibiotics. Many anaerobic bacteria are not treated successfully because despite in vitro susceptibility, the drugs are less active in tissues where anaerobes proliferate. TMS antibiotics are the treatment of choice for nocardiosis. They have also been used successfully for prevention of bacterial infections in dogs being treated with myelosuppressive chemotherapeutics such as doxorubicin.[49] Prophylactic protocols have selected for resistant bacteria in humans,[50] but this has not been reported in animals. TMS combinations are available as either trimethoprim-sulfadiazine or trimethoprim-sulfamethoxazole (the latter is a human medical preparation), which are used interchangeably. However, the veterinary formulation of trimethoprim-sulfadiazine is rarely available commercially, and most veterinarians rely on trimethoprim-sulfamethoxazole. No difference in activity between the two formulations has been documented, but this has never been evaluated. The primary difference between the formulations is that sulfadiazine is more water soluble and is excreted in the urine in an unchanged form. A similar formulation to the trimethoprim-sulfonamides for use in veterinary medicine is ormetoprim sulfadimethoxine, which has been used for the same indications as trimethoprim-sulfonamides. Doses for TMS combinations are listed in Table 8-10.

TMS is well absorbed after oral administration. As a weak base, trimethoprim is able to penetrate the blood-prostate barrier and can be used to treat prostatic infections. Both trimethoprim and sulfonamides are metabolized to some extent by the liver. Both active drug and inactive metabolites appear in the urine. Active TMS is highly concentrated in urine and is an appropriate first choice for treatment of UTIs in dogs and cats.[51]

Adverse Effects

TMS antimicrobials cause a wide range of adverse effects, which have somewhat limited their use. These reactions are primarily caused by the sulfonamide component. Some of the adverse

TABLE 8-10

Suggested Trimethoprim-Sulfonamide Dosages for Small Animals

Drug	Dose (mg/kg)	Interval (hours)	Species	Route	Comments	CLSI Breakpoints (µg/mL)
Trimethoprim-sulfamethoxazole, trimethoprim-sulfadiazine	30*	12	D, C	PO, IV	Avoid in animals with hepatic failure. Reduce dose in animals with renal insufficiency. Obtain baseline Schirmer tear test and monitor this and the CBC with prolonged treatment. Each 5-mL vial of the injectable preparation should be diluted in 75-125 mL of 5% dextrose and administered IV over 1 hour.	≤2/38 for susceptible infections
Ormetoprim-sulfadimethoxine	55 on first day, and then 27.5*	24	D	PO	See trimethoprim-sulfamethoxazole.	Use information for TMS.

C, Cats; CLSI, Clinical and Laboratory Standards Institute; D, dogs; TMS, trimethoprim-sulfonamide.
*Dose listed is for combined components, (e.g., 5 mg of trimethoprim and 25 mg of sulfonamide).

effects may be attributed to the inability of dogs to acetylate sulfonamide compounds. People who are "slow acetylators" are also more prone to adverse effects from sulfonamides.

Gastrointestinal signs such as vomiting can occur. Other common adverse effects in dogs are hypersensitivity reactions and include keratoconjunctivitis sicca, fever, polyarthritis, cutaneous drug eruptions,[52,53] immune-mediated thrombocytopenia, hemolytic anemia, hepatitis, pancreatitis, meningitis, interstitial nephritis, glomerulonephritis, and aplastic anemia (Figure 8-3).[54-57] These events are relatively uncommon, but have been documented well enough in dogs that it has discouraged their routine use among some veterinary clinicians. Reversible hypothyroidism can occur after periods of treatment as short as 10 days.[58] Hepatic necrosis can occur as an idiosyncratic reaction.[59] Ormetoprim has been associated with neurologic signs in dogs, including tremors, anxiety, and seizures. Schirmer tear tests should be performed before sulfonamides are administered to dogs, tear tests should be monitored when prolonged treatment is required (e.g., greater than 1 week), and the drug should be avoided in dogs with keratoconjunctivitis sicca. Sulfonamide cystolithiasis can occur in dogs treated with high doses of sulfonamides.[60] Doberman pinschers may be more susceptible than other breeds to adverse effects of TMS because of their inability to detoxify certain sulfonamide metabolites; in another study, Samoyeds and miniature schnauzers also appeared to be more susceptible.[55,61]

Protein Synthesis Inhibitors

Aminoglycosides

Mechanism of Action

All aminoglycosides contain an essential six-membered ring with amino-group substituents and are highly positively charged. Aminoglycosides with names that end in *-mycin* derive directly or indirectly from *Streptomyces* spp. (e.g., neomycin). Those with names ending in *-micin* are derived from *Micromonospora* (e.g., gentamicin).

Aminoglycosides have multiple mechanisms of action. They bind electrostatically to the bacterial outer membrane and displace cell wall Mg^{2+} and Ca^{2+}, which normally link adjacent lipopolysaccharide molecules. This initial binding is greater in gram-negative bacteria than gram-positive bacteria because of a greater presence of an outer membrane in gram-negative organisms. The end result is disrupted cell permeability. Subsequently, the bacterial cell takes up the aminoglycoside molecules, and they become trapped irreversibly within the cytoplasm. Because this is an oxygen-dependent process, anaerobes are intrinsically resistant to aminoglycosides. Once within the cell, aminoglycosides bind to the 30S subunit of the bacterial ribosome, which results in decreased protein synthesis.

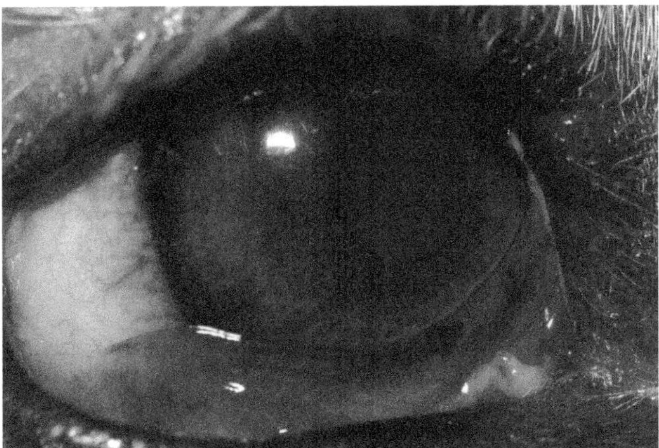

FIGURE 8-3 Right eye of a 7-year-old intact male golden retriever that developed keratoconjunctivitis sicca after administration of trimethoprim-sulfamethoxazole for 3 weeks for septic peritonitis. The owner noticed the dog pawing at his eyes. Mucoid ocular discharge is present at the medial canthus. Schirmer tear test strip results were 0 mm for both eyes. (Image courtesy University of California, Davis Veterinary Ophthalmology service.)

Aminoglycosides, particularly gentamicin, amikacin, and tobramycin, are highly active compounds for which resistance is uncommon. The most common mechanism of aminoglycoside resistance is enzymatic modification of the drug by bacteria. More than 50 modifying enzymes have been identified.[62] Reduced drug uptake by bacteria may also occur. Enterococci are intrinsically resistant to low levels (4 to 250 μg/mL) of aminoglycosides because of their anaerobic metabolism, and thus they require testing for high-level resistance using higher concentrations of aminoglycosides. Resistance to one aminoglycoside does not imply resistance to others. For example, tobramycin and amikacin are consistently more active than gentamicin, and kanamycin is one of the least active aminoglycosides. Because of these differences, a susceptibility panel should include gentamicin and either amikacin or tobramycin.

Clinical Use

Aminoglycosides are primarily used to treat gram-negative bacterial infections and MDR staphylococcal infections. They should not be used to treat anaerobes, and *Streptococcus* species are better treated with β-lactams. Aminoglycosides have usually been administered together with cell wall–active antimicrobial drugs (β-lactams and glycopeptides), but this is no longer believed to be a therapeutic advantage. They are very water soluble and poorly lipid soluble, so they penetrate tissue fluids well, but do not readily penetrate tissues that are dependent on lipid diffusion (prostate, brain, eye, or cerebrospinal fluid). Penetration of bile is also poor. Oral absorption is negligible, and they should not be administered orally unless specifically intended to treat intestinal bacteria (e.g., oral neomycin for treatment of hepatic encephalopathy). Doses are shown in Table 8-11. Aminoglycosides also may be administered topically. Because they penetrate bronchial secretions poorly, nebulization has been used in order to overcome this problem in human patients as well as dogs with resistant gram-negative bacterial bronchopneumonia (see Table 8-11).[63] Aminoglycosides are excreted unchanged by the kidney and concentrate 25- to 100-fold in urine within an hour of drug administration, so they can be used to treat resistant gram-negative bacterial UTIs. They also accumulate in renal tissue and remain active for several days after dosing is discontinued. Because they are not well distributed into fat, dose reduction may be indicated for obese animals.

Despite their primary mechanism of action being protein synthesis inhibition, aminoglycosides are rapidly bactericidal with a prolonged, concentration-dependent postantibiotic effect. Transient high peak drug concentrations result in faster killing and greater bactericidal activity than lower concentrations over a prolonged period of time (i.e., they are concentration-dependent antimicrobial drugs). Once-daily dosing of a high dose of an aminoglycoside is therefore preferred because it achieves optimal bacterial killing but minimizes toxicity. In order to further minimize toxicity, aminoglycosides are generally infused slowly. In human patients, it is recommended they

TABLE 8-11

Suggested Aminoglycoside Dosages for Small Animals

Drug	Dose (mg/kg)	Interval (hours)*	Species	Route	Comments	CLSI Breakpoints (μg/mL)
Gentamicin sulfate	9-14 5-8	24 24	D C	IV, IM, SC	Ensure adequate fluid and electrolyte balance during treatment. Avoid in animals with renal impairment. Monitor BUN and creatinine. Amikacin and tobramycin are more active against some gram-negative bacteria than gentamicin, but gentamicin is preferred for *Serratia* infections. Do not mix in vials with other drugs.	≤2 susceptible infections
Amikacin	15-30 10-14	24 24	D C	IV, IM, SC	See gentamicin.	≤16 susceptible infections
Tobramycin sulfate	9-14 5-8	24 24	D C	IV, IM	See gentamicin. For nebulization, 160 mg of nebulization solution† q12h for 28 days. Preferred aminoglycoside for *Pseudomonas* infections.	≤4 susceptible infections
Kanamycin sulfate	20	24	D, C	IV or IM	See gentamicin. Less active than gentamicin and amikacin.	≤16 susceptible infections
Neomycin	10-20	6-12	D, C	PO	Not absorbed systemically; used to treat hepatic encephalopathy. Use cautiously in animals with renal disease and avoid use for >14 days.	Not applicable

C, Cats; CLSI, Clinical and Laboratory Standards Institute; D, dogs; MIC, minimum inhibitory concentration.

*Once-daily administration is preferred except for enterococcal endocarditis, where the continuous presence of both an aminoglycoside and a penicillin is recommended (see Chapter 86).

†TOBI nebulization solution. Injectable tobramycin or gentamicin can be used but may be associated with bronchospasm. They should be diluted in 3 mL of sterile saline, and albuterol should be administered just before nebulization.

be administered over a 15- to 30-minute period. Subcutaneous and intramuscular injections of water-soluble formulations of aminoglycosides are also acceptable routes of administration, although they may cause pain in some animals.

Adverse Effects

Aminoglycosides have the potential to cause nephrotoxicity, ototoxicity, and neuromuscular blockade. Their cationic structure and the high anionic phospholipid concentrations in the kidney and inner ear play an important role in toxicity. In the presence of gastrointestinal ulceration, systemic absorption of orally administered aminoglycosides can occur, with associated nephrotoxicity or ototoxicity.[64]

Nephrotoxicity results from apoptosis and necrosis of renal tubular epithelial cells, and direct damage to the glomerulus as well. The mechanisms involved are complex.[65] Recovery can occur when the aminoglycoside is removed, but because aminoglycosides accumulate in renal tissue, the insult can persist for some time even after treatment is discontinued. Efforts to understand the mechanism of nephrotoxicity should lead to improved preventative measures and increased applications for aminoglycoside antibiotics. Aminoglycosides bind to megalin-cubulin complexes on the surface of the cell and are endocytosed into the cytoplasm, where they accumulate in lysosomes. The lysosomes break down, with resultant drug leakage into the cytoplasm, where interference with mitochondrial function occurs. Aminoglycosides also bind membrane phospholipids and alter their turnover. Damaged renal tubular epithelial cells are shed into and obstruct the tubular lumen, which leads to a build-up of pressure within the glomerulus, leading to decreased glomerular filtration rate. Disrupted proximal tubular cell function leads to delivery of excessive water and electrolytes to the distal nephron, which in turn triggers tubuloglomerular feedback, with constriction of afferent arterioles and further decreases in the glomerular filtration rate.[65] Tubuloglomerular feedback is designed to protect the body from massive loss of water and electrolytes.

Risk factors for nephrotoxicity include older age, reduced renal function, concomitant liver disease, dehydration, sodium depletion, hypokalemia, and concurrently administered nephrotoxic drugs, most commonly nonsteroidal antiinflammatory drugs but also furosemide and cyclosporin. Although gentamicin nephrotoxicity can occur in young animals,[66] young age is not a contraindication to use of aminoglycosides, which are used widely to treat human neonatal sepsis.[67] The chance of toxicity increases with more prolonged treatment periods (≥3 days). Gentamicin and amikacin are more toxic than tobramycin. Volume and salt loading do not decrease toxicity, but high levels of dietary calcium and protein have protective effects.[68] The best preventative measure is to avoid these drugs in any

TABLE 8-12

Suggested Chloramphenicol Dosages for Small Animals

Drug	Dose (mg/kg)	Interval (hours)	Species	Route	Comments	CLSI Breakpoints (μg/mL)
Chloramphenicol, chloramphenicol sodium succinate	40-50 12.5-20	6-8 12	D C	PO, IV, IM	Avoid long-term use in cats. Monitor CBC with long-term use. Warn owners that human exposure to chloramphenicol may cause bone marrow disease. Drug interactions may occur (see text). Avoid in animals with hepatic failure.	≤4 for streptococci, ≤8 for other susceptible bacteria
Florfenicol	20 22	6 8	D, C	PO, IM	Not approved for use in dogs and cats. Doses and adverse effects have not been well studied.	See chloramphenicol.

C, Cats; CLSI, Clinical and Laboratory Standards Institute; D, dogs.

patients with preexisting renal disease. If renal disease develops after initiating treatment, the drug should be substituted with a safer drug.

Ototoxicity results from damage to the cochlear or the vestibular apparatus and is more likely to occur in animals with renal impairment or that are dehydrated. Cochlear toxicity results from damage to the hair cells of the organ of Corti, whereas vestibular toxicity results from damage to hair cells at the tip of the ampullae cristae. Auditory toxicity may be more common in dogs, whereas cats tend to develop vestibular toxicity.[69] Cochlear toxicity in dogs and cats may be underrecognized, because it may be overlooked by pet owners. In human patients, signs of vestibular toxicity can disappear with time because of compensatory mechanisms. Ototoxicity is generally irreversible, but in some human patients, gradual improvement in hearing can occur.[70]

Neuromuscular blockade is a rare but potentially life-threatening complication of aminoglycoside treatment. Severe neuromuscular blockade has not been reported in cats and dogs, but experimental studies show it does occur when aminoglycosides are used in conjunction with some anesthetic agents.[71-73] Neuromuscular blockade results from decreased release of acetylcholine at neuromuscular junctions, and decreased sensitivity of the postsynaptic neuron to acetylcholine. Autonomic blockade can also occur. The use of aminoglycosides should be avoided in animals with neuromuscular disease such as myasthenia gravis, because aminoglycosides have the potential to exacerbate the clinical signs.[74]

Measurement of serum aminoglycoside concentrations can be used to ensure adequate plasma concentrations or to minimize toxicity.[75] Assays are offered by specialized veterinary pharmacology laboratories or through human hospitals. Aminoglycoside doses that result in peak plasma concentrations approximately 8 to 10 times the MIC produce the optimal bactericidal effect. The effective volume of distribution for aminoglycosides is often higher in septic patients or animals that have a "third space" problem (such as pleural effusion), which may necessitate a higher dose. To perform therapeutic drug monitoring, the optimum time points are 1 hour after injection (C_{max}), followed by two additional time points in order to estimate the slope of the elimination curve. Trough levels could also be performed to minimize the chance of toxicity, with the recommendation that if high trough levels are detected, the drug should be discontinued. In patients with normal renal function, trough levels with once-daily dosing should be in the "undetectable" range.

Chloramphenicol

Mechanism of Action and Spectrum of Activity

Chloramphenicol binds to the 50S subunit of the bacterial ribosome and inhibits bacterial protein synthesis. It is usually described as bacteriostatic, but there is some evidence that chloramphenicol may be more bactericidal than previously thought. Like other ribosomal inhibitors, chloramphenicol has a broad spectrum of activity, which includes gram-positive and gram-negative bacteria, anaerobes, and some rickettsial pathogens. Because chloramphenicol can cause aplastic anemia in humans, its use in humans has greatly diminished, and it is only used for the treatment of MDR bacterial infections where few or no other antimicrobial drugs are useful. Thiamphenicol and florfenicol are related compounds, the availability of which varies from country to country. Although thiamphenicol was initially promoted as not inducing aplastic anemia in humans, cases of aplastic anemia have now been identified.[76] Florfenicol is more active than chloramphenicol and thiamphenicol, but has a shorter half-life in dogs and thus requires more frequent dosing (e.g., more often than every 8 hours) in this species. It was developed for food animal species where use of chloramphenicol is illegal.

Resistance to chloramphenicols results from porin mutations, drug efflux, or production of chloramphenicol acetyltransferase enzymes, which inactivate the antibiotic.[77] Resistance to one chloramphenicol derivative predicts resistance to the others.

Clinical Use

Doses are shown in Table 8-12. Chloramphenicol is absorbed orally with or without food. Tablets and capsules have similar oral absorption, but the extent of oral absorption varies considerably among dogs. Chloramphenicol distributes well to extracellular fluids of most tissues. Because of its high degree of lipid solubility, it also diffuses to tissues with barriers, such as the CNS and the eye. Topical ophthalmic preparations achieve high concentration in the aqueous humor. In dogs, most absorbed chloramphenicol is metabolized by glucuronidation in the liver, with inactive metabolites excreted by the kidney. The use of chloramphenicol should therefore be avoided in animals with hepatic failure. Provided renal failure is not present, sufficient active drug is excreted in the urine to enable treatment of UTIs that are resistant to other drugs, such as methicillin-resistant staphylococci and resistant enterococci.

Adverse Effects

Exposure of humans to even small amounts of chloramphenicol has the potential to lead to irreversible aplastic anemia, an idiosyncratic reaction, weeks to months after discontinuing treatment. The reaction is rare (1 in 24,000 to 1 in 40,000 exposed humans) and most commonly occurs when human patients are treated with oral formulations.[78] Whether use of ophthalmic preparations in human patients poses a risk has been controversial.[79] Nevertheless, it is recommended that owners of pets that are being treated with chloramphenicol wear gloves when handling the drug and to avoid splitting tablets at home. Chloramphenicol commonly causes gastrointestinal adverse effects in dogs and cats, including anorexia, hypersalivation, and vomiting. High doses or prolonged treatment can result in *reversible* bone marrow suppression, which usually resolves within days after discontinuation of treatment. High doses and prolonged treatment are needed to produce this effect in dogs, but cats are more susceptible and can be at risk within 2 weeks of administration. Chloramphenicol is a potent inhibitor of P450 enzymes, and so the potential for significant drug interactions exists. Florfenicol has not been widely used in dogs and cats, and adverse effects have not yet been reported.

Macrolides and Lincosamides

Classification and Mechanism of Action

The macrolides and lincosamides (clindamycin and lincomycin) are not chemically related but possess similar mechanisms of action, resistance, and antimicrobial activity. Macrolides and lincosamides inhibit protein synthesis by binding to the 50S subunit of bacterial ribosomes. Because they are weak bases, they concentrate in the relatively acidic interior of leukocytes. The high concentrations in leukocytes may also produce immunomodulatory effects. Macrolides, particularly the newer agents such as azithromycin, can impair leukocyte function, interfere with superoxide production by mast cells, suppress proinflammatory cytokine release, and produce apoptosis.[80,81] These effects may suppress inflammatory reactions in some tissues, but the significance of these effects has not been explored in small animal infections.

The first macrolide antibiotic to be discovered was erythromycin, a derivative of *Streptomyces erythreus*. Despite the common occurrence of gastrointestinal adverse effects, poor gastrointestinal absorption, and an extremely short half-life, erythromycin continues to have application in human medicine because of its safety in pregnancy and utility in human patients who are allergic to penicillin. Because these concerns are less important in dogs and cats, erythromycin is less commonly used in small animal patients.

Since the discovery of erythromycin, several semisynthetic macrolides have become available. Azithromycin and other new macrolide antibiotics, such as clarithromycin and roxithromycin, have been referred to as "advanced-generation" macrolides. These have an extended spectrum of activity, with greater efficacy against atypical and some gram-negative bacteria, a longer duration of antimicrobial activity, ... improved gastrointestinal absorption, greater intracellular concentrations, and a marked reduction in gastrointestinal adverse effects. Clarithromycin has improved activity against streptococci and staphylococci compared with erythromycin.

Azithromycin is an *azalide*, because unlike other macrolides, it contains nitrogen. Azithromycin is extensively concentrated within cells and is retained in tissues for prolonged periods, with a half-life of 30 hours in the dog and 35 hours in the cat. In human patients, a 5-day course provides therapeutic tissue concentrations for at least 10 days. Although azithromycin has an improved spectrum against gram-negative bacteria, it has less activity against gram-positive bacteria than erythromycin.[82,83]

Susceptibility to erythromycin often predicts susceptibility to other macrolide antimicrobial drugs. Resistance to macrolides and lincosamides results from decreased bacterial permeability (for gram-negative bacteria), alteration in the target site, increased drug efflux, and enzymatic inactivation of certain macrolides by bacterial esterases. Alteration in the target site involves production of a ribosomal methylase that adds a methyl group to the 50S subunit RNA, preventing the macrolide from binding to the ribosome. Expression of the methylase enzyme confers high-level resistance to azithromycin, clarithromycin, and also clindamycin.

Clinical Use

Macrolides and lincosamides are primarily used to treat gram-positive bacterial infections. They are generally considered to be bacteriostatic. Doses are shown in Table 8-13. Erythromycin tablets have a protective coating to prevent degradation by gastric acid. After absorption, erythromycin is distributed well to most tissues and body fluids, with the exception of the CNS and urine. It is excreted in high concentrations in bile, followed by enterohepatic circulation, and ultimately eliminated in the feces. Non-absorbed drug is also present in the feces. It has activity against some anaerobes, spiral bacteria (particularly *Campylobacter*), and many intracellular bacteria. Tylosin has been used to treat chronic colitis in dogs[84] and is also active against *Campylobacter* and enteric *Clostridium* spp.

Clarithromycin and azithromycin have considerably longer half-lives than erythromycin. The intracellular concentration of clarithromycin is about two- to sixfold that in plasma. Clarithromycin is preferred over erythromycin or azithromycin for treatment of rapidly growing mycobacterial infections in dogs and cats (usually in combination with rifampin) (see Chapter 44). In humans, clarithromycin is extensively metabolized by the liver to a variety of specific active and inactive metabolites, with some excretion of active drug and its metabolites into urine. Formation and excretion of these metabolites have not been well studied in dogs and cats. Azithromycin is largely excreted unchanged in bile.

Because of its prolonged tissue retention, serum concentrations of azithromycin do not reflect tissue concentrations, and so the antibiotic can still be effective even if the serum concentration is less than the MIC. Intracellular concentrations of azithromycin are 10- to 100-fold those in serum, concentrations that are considered bactericidal. Concentrations can remain high within tissues several days after the drug has been

TABLE 8-13

Suggested Macrolide and Lincosamide Dosages for Small Animals

Drug	Dose (mg/kg)	Interval (hours)	Species	Route	Comments	CLSI Breakpoints (μg/mL)
Erythromycin	10-20	8	D, C	PO	Do not administer to rabbits or rodents, as this may cause fatal diarrhea. Drug interactions may occur (see text).	≤0.25 for streptococci and ≤0.5 for other susceptible organisms
Tylosin	7-15 8-11	12-24 12	D, C	PO IM	See erythromycin. For colitis in dogs, use 20 mg/kg q8h with food, and taper to q24h if a response occurs.*	
Clarithromycin	7.5	12	D, C	PO	Drug interactions may occur (see text). Consider dosage reduction in severe renal failure.	≤2 for staphylococci. Respiratory cures may be possible for organisms with MICs up to 8, because drug concentrates within the lung.
Azithromycin	5-10	24	D, C	PO		≤ 2 for susceptible bacteria. Serum MIC values may not predict tissue concentrations.
Lincomycin hydrochloride	15-25	12	D, C	PO	See erythromycin. A dose of 10 mg/kg PO q12h has been suggested for pyoderma.	0.25 for streptococci and ≤ 0.5 for other susceptible organisms
Clindamycin hydrochloride, clindamycin phosphate	11-33 11 10	12 24 12	D C D, C	PO PO IV, IM	See erythromycin. For IV administration, dilute 1:10 in 0.9% saline and administer over 30-60 minutes. The oral suspension may be unpalatable to cats. For toxoplasmosis, use 25 mg/kg q12h PO.	See lincomycin.

C, Cats; CLSI, Clinical and Laboratory Standards Institute; D, dogs; MIC, minimum inhibitory concentration.
*20 mg/kg is equal to 1/8th teaspoon of tylosin phosphate (Tylan) for a 20-kg dog.

discontinued. Despite the improved spectrum of activity of clarithromycin and azithromycin, with activity against some gram-negative bacteria and intracellular pathogens, many of these organisms are resistant. The primary indication for these antibiotics in small animals is in combination with other drugs such as rifampin for treatment of mycobacteriosis or bartonellosis, or atovaquone for treatment of certain systemic protozoal infections such as babesiosis and cytauxzoonosis. Azithromycin has been used to treat secondary bacterial infections in cats with upper respiratory tract disease because its long half-life permits convenient dosing on an every-48- or every-72-hour basis. Despite its popularity for treating upper respiratory infections in cats, one study showed no benefit to this protocol over use of amoxicillin,[85] and the potential for overuse of azithromycin in this setting raises concerns in regard to selection for resistance to azithromycin.

Lincomycin is active against gram-positive bacteria and has been used to treat staphylococcal pyoderma. However, the use of lincomycin has largely been replaced by clindamycin, which has similar activity, favorable pharmacokinetics, and widely available formulations (tablets, capsules, oral liquid, and injection). Clindamycin is also used to treat anaerobic bacterial infections, as well as toxoplasmosis and neosporosis (see Chapters 72 and 73).

Adverse Effects

Although otherwise very safe, erythromycin frequently causes vomiting, decreased appetite and nausea because of stimulation of receptors of the gastrointestinal hormone motilin, which increases gastrointestinal smooth muscle activity.[86] Like other poorly absorbed oral antimicrobials, it can produce diarrhea due to changes in the gastrointestinal flora. Although diarrhea and pseudomembranous colitis are serious complications of clindamycin treatment in people, these problems are uncommon in small animals. Adverse effects are rarely reported for clarithromycin and azithromycin. Erythromycin and azithromycin inhibit P450 enzymes and so can increase the concentration of other drugs that are administered concurrently.

Clindamycin and lincomycin can cause vomiting and diarrhea, especially when clindamycin is used at high doses. Oral clindamycin hydrochloride can cause esophagitis in cats.[87,88]

TABLE 8-14

Suggested Linezolid Dose for Small Animals

Drug	Dose (mg/kg)	Interval (hours)	Species	Route	Comments	CLSI Breakpoints (μg/mL)
Linezolid*	10	8	D	PO, IV	If administered with other drugs IV, the administration line should be flushed first.	≤4 for staphylococci, ≤2 for *Enterococcus* spp.

CLSI, Clinical and Laboratory Standards Institute; D, dogs.

*The use of linezolid should be reserved for gram-positive infections that are susceptible to linezolid but resistant to all other reasonable alternatives, on the basis of culture and susceptibility testing.

Oxazolidinones (Linezolid)

Mechanism of Action and Spectrum of Activity

Linezolid is a synthetic antibiotic used to treat life-threatening infections caused by gram-positive bacteria that are resistant to other antimicrobial drugs, especially methicillin-resistant and vancomycin-resistant staphylococci. Linezolid binds to the 50S ribosome and prevents formation of the initiation complex for protein synthesis.[89] This is a unique mechanism, because other protein synthesis inhibitors interfere with polypeptide extension. Resistance to other protein synthesis inhibitors does not correlate with resistance to linezolid. Rarely, resistance to linezolid is due to modification of the drug's target site, but this is extremely rare because several step mutations are necessary before resistance can occur. The high cost of oral linezolid currently limits its application in small animals. Currently, its use has been limited to dogs and cats with resistant staphylococcal or enterococcal infections for which other antibiotics are not effective or have produced adverse effects. Linezolid has favorable pharmacokinetics in dogs,[90] with nearly 100% oral absorption, which is not influenced by food (Table 8-14). The pharmacokinetics in cats has not been published. Because linezolid is bacteriostatic, plasma concentrations should be maintained above the MIC throughout the dosing interval.

In human patients, adverse effects include vomiting, diarrhea, and, rarely, thrombocytopenia or reversible pure red cell aplasia (PRCA). Linezolid is a type A monoamine oxidase inhibitor and so can interact with serotonin reuptake inhibitors.[92] Linezolid appears to be well tolerated by dogs and cats. Despite the concern about monoamine oxidase inhibition and bone marrow suppression in human patients, these effects have not yet been documented in dogs or cats, although one of the authors is aware of a cat that developed reversible PRCA after treatment with linezolid.

Tetracyclines

Mechanism of Action

Tetracyclines are bacteriostatic, time-dependent antibiotics that have a broad spectrum of activity that includes gram-positive and gram-negative bacteria, some anaerobes, and atypical and intracellular pathogens such as spirochetes, *Mycoplasma* spp., and rickettsiae. In contrast to the macrolides and clindamycin, which bind to the 50S ribosomal subunit, tetracyclines inhibit bacterial protein synthesis by binding to the 30S subunit. Thus, resistance to macrolides does not imply resistance to tetracyclines. Examples of tetracyclines used to treat dogs and cats are tetracycline, oxytetracycline, and the semisynthetic tetracycline doxycycline. Doxycycline and minocycline are longer-acting tetracyclines that are more lipophilic than the older tetracyclines. Doxycycline and minocycline also have antiinflammatory and immunomodulatory properties that result from inhibition of inducible nitric oxide synthase and proinflammatory cytokines such as TNF-α.[91] These properties have led to the use of tetracyclines for treatment of immune-mediated dermatopathies in dogs[92] and plasmacytic pododermatitis in cats.[93] Delayed-release formulations that produce subantimicrobial doses have been developed for use in human patients with the inflammatory skin disease rosacea. Although development of tetracycline resistance in bacterial flora has not been documented in association with the use of these preparations, the possibility has not been ruled out.[94]

Resistance to tetracyclines primarily results from porin mutations that exclude tetracyclines from the bacterial cell, and increased drug efflux, mediated by the *tetK* gene. Some bacteria with tetK may still be susceptible to minocycline. Resistance mediated by *tetM* confers resistance to all tetracyclines.[95] In diagnostic laboratories, tetracycline is used to assess the susceptibility of bacteria to all other tetracyclines except the glycylcycline antibiotic tigecycline, a new antibiotic derived from minocycline that is reserved for treatment of multidrug-resistant bacterial infections.[96] In addition, resistance to doxycycline does not always imply resistance to minocycline.[97]

Clinical Use

Doses are shown in Table 8-15. Doxycycline is the most commonly used tetracycline in dogs and cats and has fewer adverse effects when compared with other tetracyclines. It is the drug of choice for treatment of a variety of tick-borne infectious diseases, feline chlamydiosis, salmon poisoning disease, and leptospirosis. The long half-life of doxycycline permits once-daily dosing, although twice-daily dosing is frequently recommended. Doxycycline is well absorbed from the gastrointestinal tract and distributed to a variety of tissues, including the lung, bronchial secretions, liver, kidney, and, to some extent, the CNS. If doxycycline is not available, minocycline can be used as a substitute. Minocycline is more lipophilic than doxycycline, it is better absorbed orally, and can be administered at similar doses as doxycycline. Absorption of other tetracyclines from the gastrointestinal tract is not as efficient. All tetracyclines are concentrated in bile. Sufficient drug is excreted in the urine to permit treatment of UTIs caused by bacteria that are resistant to other drugs.

TABLE 8-15

Suggested Tetracycline Dosages for Small Animals

Drug	Dose (mg/kg)	Interval (hours)	Species	Route	Comments	CLSI Breakpoints (μg/mL)
Tetracycline	15-20 4.4-11	8	D, C	PO IV, IM	Do not mix with food containing cations such as calcium, zinc, magnesium, iron, aluminum.	≤2 for streptococci, ≤4 for other susceptible bacteria. Consider use of ≤1 for susceptible bacteria.
Oxytetracycline	20 7.5-10	12	D, C	PO IV	See tetracycline.	See doxycycline.
Doxycycline	5 10	12 24	D, C	PO, IV	For IV administration, dilute in 100 to 1000 mL of LRS or 5% dextrose and administer over 1 to 2 hours.	≤2 for streptococci, ≤0.25 for *Staphylococcus pseudintermedius,* ≤4 for other susceptible bacteria
Minocycline	5-12.5	12	D, C	PO		See doxycycline, but the pharmacokinetics of minocycline in dogs and cats require further study.

C, Cats; CLSI, Clinical and Laboratory Standards Institute; D, dogs; LRS, lactated Ringer solution.

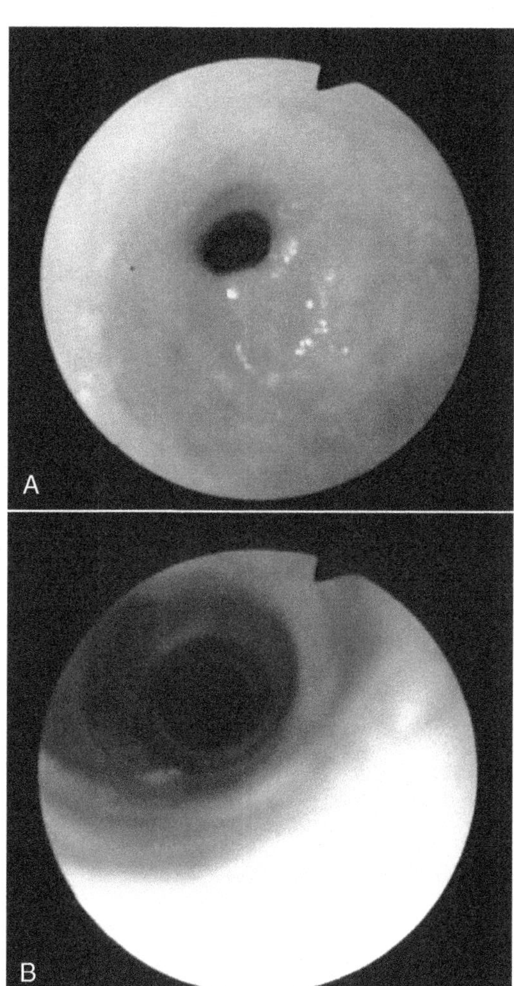

FIGURE 8-4 **A,** Esophageal stricture in a 9-year-old female spayed domestic shorthair that had been treated with doxycycline for possible hemoplasmosis. Regurgitation after eating commenced shortly after treatment was initiated. **B,** The stricture was treated via repeated balloon dilatation; the image is immediately after the ballooning procedure was performed.

Adverse Effects

The most common adverse effects of tetracyclines in dogs and cats are vomiting, decreased appetite, nausea, and diarrhea. These may be reduced when doxycycline hyclate tablets are administered intact (rather than being split or crushed) and by administering doxycycline with food. Administration of other tetracyclines with food can lead to significantly reduced drug absorption, because of extensive binding with divalent and trivalent cations in the gastrointestinal tract. The hyclate salt of doxycycline (doxycycline hydrochloride) has been associated with esophagitis and esophageal strictures in cats (Figure 8-4),[98] and life-threatening esophageal ulceration in a dog.[99] This is also a complication in people.[100] A bolus of water or food should be administered immediately after dosing in order to prevent this complication, or a suspension rather than tablets should be used. Compounded, high-concentration (e.g., 33.3 mg/mL or 167 mg/mL) suspensions in aqueous vehicles have limited stability; suspensions in some vehicles do not retain their potency beyond 7 days.[101]

In dogs and cats with renal failure, tetracyclines other than doxycycline should be avoided. Doxycycline is excreted in the intestinal tract in this situation. Tetracyclines other than doxycycline can interfere with bone growth and cause significant and permanent gray-brown or yellow discoloration of the teeth (Figure 8-5), and so their use is not recommended in puppies and kittens. Doxycycline is not likely to produce this effect because it binds calcium less avidly. As a result, the use of doxycycline in human pediatric medicine is now accepted.[102] All tetracyclines, including doxycycline, have the potential to cause hepatic failure and renal tubular necrosis. Cutaneous reactions occur rarely in animals treated with tetracycline, but have been reported in humans.

Intravenous preparations of doxycycline are available but can be considerably more expensive than the oral formulations. They must be given over 1 to 2 hours. Thrombophlebitis can occur at the site of injection, and anaphylactic shock has been reported following parenteral administration of tetracycline to a dog.[103]

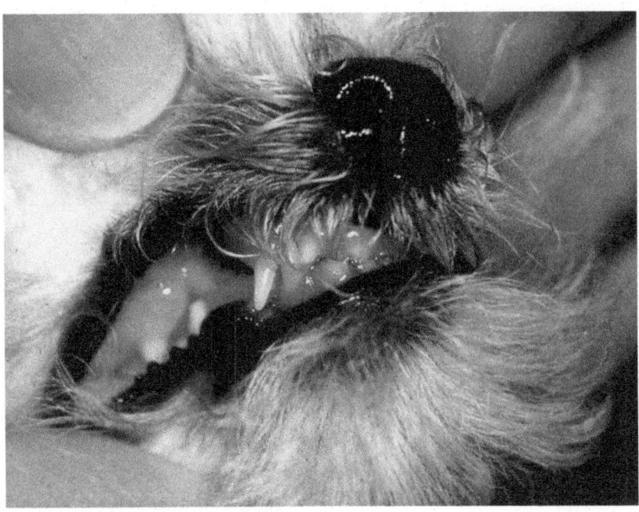

FIGURE 8-5 Yellow discoloration of the teeth in a "puppy mill" puppy that was presumably treated with tetracycline antibiotics.

REFERENCES

1. Silhavy TJ, Kahne D, Walker S. The bacterial cell envelope. Cold Spring Harb Perspect Biol. 2010;2:a000414.
2. Gold HS, Moellering Jr RC. Antimicrobial-drug resistance. N Engl J Med. 1996;335:1445-1453.
3. Bush K, Jacoby GA. Updated functional classification of beta-lactamases. Antimicrob Agents Chemother. 2010;54:969-976.
4. Papich MG. Saunders Handbook of Veterinary Drugs: Small and Large Animal. 3rd ed. St. Louis, MO: Saunders; 2011.
5. Stapleton PD, Taylor PW. Methicillin resistance in *Staphylococcus aureus*: mechanisms and modulation. Sci Prog. 2002;85:57-72.
6. Fass RJ, Copelan EA, Brandt JT, et al. Platelet-mediated bleeding caused by broad-spectrum penicillins. J Infect Dis. 1987;155:1242-1248.
7. European Committee on Antimicrobial Susceptibility Testing (EUCAST). MIC Distributions. 2011. http://www.eucast.org/mic_distributions/. Last accessed May 12, 2012.
8. Williams KJ, Bax RP, Brown H, et al. Antibiotic treatment and associated prolonged prothrombin time. J Clin Pathol. 1991;44:738-741.
9. Deldar A, Lewis H, Bloom J, et al. Cephalosporin-induced changes in the ultrastructure of canine bone marrow. Vet Pathol. 1988;25:211-218.
10. Asbel LE, Levison ME. Cephalosporins, carbapenems, and monobactams. Infect Dis Clin North Am. 2000;14:435-447, ix.
11. Zhanel GG, Wiebe R, Dilay L, et al. Comparative review of the carbapenems. Drugs. 2007;67:1027-1052.
12. Bratu S, Landman D, Alam M, et al. Detection of KPC carbapenem-hydrolyzing enzymes in *Enterobacter* spp. from Brooklyn, New York. Antimicrob Agents Chemother. 2005;49:776-778.
13. Marra A. NDM-1: a local clone emerges with worldwide aspirations. Future Microbiol. 2011;6:137-141.
14. Peleg AY, Hooper DC. Hospital-acquired infections due to gram-negative bacteria. N Engl J Med. 2010;362:1804-1813.
15. Bailiff NL, Westropp JL, Jang SS, et al. *Corynebacterium urealyticum* urinary tract infection in dogs and cats: 7 cases (1996-2003). J Am Vet Med Assoc. 2005;226:1676-1680.
16. Briscoe KA, Barrs VR, Lindsay S, et al. Encrusting cystitis in a cat secondary to *Corynebacterium urealyticum* infection. J Feline Med Surg. 2010;12:972-977.
17. Abbott Y, Kirby BM, Karczmarczyk M, et al. High-level gentamicin-resistant and vancomycin-resistant *Enterococcus faecium* isolated from a wound in a dog. J Small Anim Pract. 2009;50:194-197.
18. Svetitsky S, Leibovici L, Paul M. Comparative efficacy and safety of vancomycin versus teicoplanin: systematic review and meta-analysis. Antimicrob Agents Chemother. 2009;53:4069-4079.
19. Robicsek A, Jacoby GA, Hooper DC. The worldwide emergence of plasmid-mediated quinolone resistance. Lancet Infect Dis. 2006;6:629-640.
20. Phillips I, King A. Comparative activity of the 4-quinolones. Rev Infect Dis. 1988;10(Suppl 1):S70-S76.
21. Rubin J, Walker RD, Blickenstaff K, et al. Antimicrobial resistance and genetic characterization of fluoroquinolone resistance of *Pseudomonas aeruginosa* isolated from canine infections. Vet Microbiol. 2008;131:164-172.
22. Silley P, Stephan B, Greife HA, et al. Comparative activity of pradofloxacin against anaerobic bacteria isolated from dogs and cats. J Antimicrob Chemother. 2007;60:999-1003.
23. Papich MG. Ciprofloxacin pharmacokinetics and oral absorption of generic tablets in dogs. Am J Vet Res. 2012;73:1085-1091.
24. Frazier DL, Thompson L, Trettien A, et al. Comparison of fluoroquinolone pharmacokinetic parameters after treatment with marbofloxacin, enrofloxacin, and difloxacin in dogs. J Vet Pharmacol Ther. 2000;23:293-302.
25. Cole LK, Papich MG, Kwochka KW, et al. Plasma and ear tissue concentrations of enrofloxacin and its metabolite ciprofloxacin in dogs with chronic end-stage otitis externa after intravenous administration of enrofloxacin. Vet Dermatol. 2009;20:51-59.
26. Mori K, Maru C, Takasuna K. Characterization of histamine release induced by fluoroquinolone antibacterial agents in-vivo and in-vitro. J Pharm Pharmacol. 2000;52:577-584.
27. Christ W. Central nervous system toxicity of quinolones: human and animal findings. J Antimicrob Chemother. 1990;26(Suppl B):219-225.
28. Wiebe V, Hamilton P. Fluoroquinolone-induced retinal degeneration in cats. J Am Vet Med Assoc. 2002;221:1568-1571.
29. Ford MM, Dubielzig RR, Giuliano EA, et al. Ocular and systemic manifestations after oral administration of a high dose of enrofloxacin in cats. Am J Vet Res. 2007;68:190-202.
30. Ramirez CJ, Minch JD, Gay JM, et al. Molecular genetic basis for fluoroquinolone-induced retinal degeneration in cats. Pharmacogenet Genomics. 2011;21:66-75.
31. Messias A, Gekeler F, Wegener A, et al. Retinal safety of a new fluoroquinolone, pradofloxacin, in cats: assessment with electroretinography. Doc Ophthalmol. 2008;116:177-191.
32. Rosanova MT, Lede R, Capurro H, et al. Assessing fluoroquinolones as risk factor for musculoskeletal disorders in children: a systematic review and meta-analysis. Arch Argent Pediatr. 2010;108:524-531.
33. Sansone JM, Wilsman NJ, Leiferman EM, et al. The effect of fluoroquinolone antibiotics on growing cartilage in the lamb model. J Pediatr Orthop. 2009;29:189-195.
34. Committee on Infectious Diseases. The use of systemic fluoroquinolones. Pediatrics. 2006;118:1287-1292.
35. Narayanan S, Hunerbein A, Getie M, et al. Scavenging properties of metronidazole on free oxygen radicals in a skin lipid model system. J Pharm Pharmacol. 2007;59:1125-1130.
36. Jergens AE, Crandell J, Morrison JA, et al. Comparison of oral prednisone and prednisone combined with metronidazole for induction therapy of canine inflammatory bowel disease: a randomized-controlled trial. J Vet Intern Med. 2010;24:269-277.
37. Lofmark S, Edlund C, Nord CE. Metronidazole is still the drug of choice for treatment of anaerobic infections. Clin Infect Dis. 2010;50(Suppl 1):S16-S23.
38. Evans J, Levesque D, Knowles K, et al. Diazepam as a treatment for metronidazole toxicosis in dogs: a retrospective study of 21 cases. J Vet Intern Med. 2003;17:304-310.
39. Olson EJ, Morales SC, McVey AS, et al. Putative metronidazole neurotoxicosis in a cat. Vet Pathol. 2005;42:665-669.

40. Moosa AN, Perkins D. Neurological picture. MRI of metronidazole induced cerebellar ataxia. J Neurol Neurosurg Psychiatry. 2010;81:754-755.
41. Sekis I, Ramstead K, Rishniw M, et al. Single-dose pharmacokinetics and genotoxicity of metronidazole in cats. J Feline Med Surg. 2009;11:60-68.
42. Jenkins DJ, Kendall CW, Hamidi M, et al. Effect of antibiotics as cholesterol-lowering agents. Metabolism. 2005;54:103-112.
43. Cavusoglu C, Karaca-Derici Y, Bilgic A. In-vitro activity of rifabutin against rifampicin-resistant *Mycobacterium tuberculosis* isolates with known rpoB mutations. Clin Microbiol Infect. 2004;10:662-665.
44. Dutta A, Schwarzwald HL, Edwards MS. Disseminated bartonellosis presenting as neuroretinitis in a young adult with human immunodeficiency virus infection. Pediatr Infect Dis J. 2010;29:675-677.
45. Liston TE, Koehler JE. Granulomatous hepatitis and necrotizing splenitis due to *Bartonella henselae* in a patient with cancer: case report and review of hepatosplenic manifestations of bartonella infection. Clin Infect Dis. 1996;22:951-957.
46. De Vriese AS, Robbrecht DL, Vanholder RC, et al. Rifampicin-associated acute renal failure: pathophysiologic, immunologic, and clinical features. Am J Kidney Dis. 1998;31:108-115.
47. Reitman ML, Chu X, Cai X, et al. Rifampin's acute inhibitory and chronic inductive drug interactions: experimental and model-based approaches to drug-drug interaction trial design. Clin Pharmacol Ther. 2011;89:234-242.
48. Then RL. Mechanisms of resistance to trimethoprim, the sulfonamides, and trimethoprim-sulfamethoxazole. Rev Infect Dis. 1982;4:261-269.
49. Chretin JD, Rassnick KM, Shaw NA, et al. Prophylactic trimethoprim-sulfadiazine during chemotherapy in dogs with lymphoma and osteosarcoma: a double-blind, placebo-controlled study. J Vet Intern Med. 2007;21:141-148.
50. Jacoby GA. Perils of prophylaxis. N Engl J Med. 1982;306:43-44.
51. Weese JS, Blondeau JM, Boothe D, et al. Antimicrobial use guidelines for treatment of urinary tract disease in dogs and cats: antimicrobial guidelines working group of the international society for companion animal infectious diseases. Vet Med Int. 2011;2011:263768.
52. Nuttall TJ, Malham T. Successful intravenous human immunoglobulin treatment of drug-induced Stevens-Johnson syndrome in a dog. J Small Anim Pract. 2004;45:357-361.
53. Noli C, Koeman JP, Willemse T. A retrospective evaluation of adverse reactions to trimethoprim-sulphonamide combinations in dogs and cats. Vet Q. 1995;17:123-128.
54. Weiss DJ, Adams LG. Aplastic anemia associated with trimethoprim-sulfadiazine and fenbendazole administration in a dog. J Am Vet Med Assoc. 1987;191:1119-1120.
55. Trepanier LA, Danhof R, Toll J, et al. Clinical findings in 40 dogs with hypersensitivity associated with administration of potentiated sulfonamides. J Vet Intern Med. 2003;17:647-652.
56. Trepanier LA. Idiosyncratic toxicity associated with potentiated sulfonamides in the dog. J Vet Pharmacol Ther. 2004;27: 129-138.
57. Vasilopulos RJ, Mackin A, Lavergne SN, et al. Nephrotic syndrome associated with administration of sulfadimethoxine/ormetoprim in a dobermann. J Small Anim Pract. 2005;46: 232-236.
58. Brenner K, Harkin K, Schermerhorn T. Iatrogenic, sulfonamide-induced hypothyroid crisis in a Labrador Retriever. Aust Vet J. 2009;87:503-505.
59. Twedt DC, Diehl KJ, Lappin MR, et al. Association of hepatic necrosis with trimethoprim sulfonamide administration in 4 dogs. J Vet Intern Med. 1997;11:20-23.
60. Osborne CA, Lulich JP, Bartges JW, et al. Drug-induced urolithiasis. Vet Clin North Am Small Anim Pract. 1999;29:251-266, xiv.
61. Cribb AE, Spielberg SP. An in vitro investigation of predisposition to sulphonamide idiosyncratic toxicity in dogs. Vet Res Commun. 1990;14:241-252.
62. Ramirez MS, Tolmasky ME. Aminoglycoside modifying enzymes. Drug Resist Updat. 2010;13:151-171.
63. Sykes JE, Mapes S, Lindsay LL, et al. *Corynebacterium ulcerans* bronchopneumonia in a dog. J Vet Intern Med. 2010;24: 973-976.
64. Gookin JL, Riviere JE, Gilger BC, et al. Acute renal failure in four cats treated with paromomycin. J Am Vet Med Assoc. 1999;215:1821-1823, 1806.
65. Lopez-Novoa JM, Quiros Y, Vicente L, et al. New insights into the mechanism of aminoglycoside nephrotoxicity: an integrative point of view. Kidney Int. 2011;79:33-45.
66. Cowan RH, Jukkola AF, Arant Jr BS. Pathophysiologic evidence of gentamicin nephrotoxicity in neonatal puppies. Pediatr Res. 1980;14:1204-1211.
67. Rao SC, Ahmed M, Hagan R. One dose per day compared to multiple doses per day of gentamicin for treatment of suspected or proven sepsis in neonates. Cochrane Database Syst Rev. 2006:CD005091.
68. Grauer GF, Greco DS, Behrend EN, et al. Effects of dietary protein conditioning on gentamicin-induced nephrotoxicosis in healthy male dogs. Am J Vet Res. 1994;55:90-97.
69. Papich MG, Riviere JE. Aminoglycoside antibiotics. In: Riviere JE, Papich MG, eds. Veterinary Pharmacology and Therapeutics. 9th ed. Ames, IA: Wiley-Blackwell; 2009:915-935.
70. Gooi A, Hochman J, Wellman M, et al. Ototoxic effects of single-dose versus 19-day daily-dose gentamicin. J Otolaryngol Head Neck Surg. 2008;37:664-667.
71. Singh YN, Marshall IG, Harvey AL. Some effects of the aminoglycoside antibiotic amikacin on neuromuscular and autonomic transmission. Br J Anaesth. 1978;50:109-117.
72. Forsyth SF, Ilkiw JE, Hildebrand SV. Effect of gentamicin administration on the neuromuscular blockade induced by atracurium in cats. Am J Vet Res. 1990;51:1675-1678.
73. Martinez EA, Mealey KL, Wooldridge AA, et al. Pharmacokinetics, effects on renal function, and potentiation of atracurium-induced neuromuscular blockade after administration of a high dose of gentamicin in isoflurane-anesthetized dogs. Am J Vet Res. 1996;57:1623-1626.
74. Harnett MT, Chen W, Smith SM. Calcium-sensing receptor: a high-affinity presynaptic target for aminoglycoside-induced weakness. Neuropharmacology. 2009;57:502-505.
75. Papich MG. Therapeutic drug monitoring. In: Riviere JE, Papich MG, eds. Veterinary pharmacology and therapeutics. 9th ed. Ames, IA: Wiley-Blackwell; 2009:1328.
76. De Renzo A, Formisano S, Rotoli B. Bone marrow aplasia and thiamphenicol. Haematologica. 1981;66:98-104.
77. Schwarz S, Kehrenberg C, Doublet B, et al. Molecular basis of bacterial resistance to chloramphenicol and florfenicol. FEMS Microbiol Rev. 2004;28:519-542.
78. Wiholm BE, Kelly JP, Kaufman D, et al. Relation of aplastic anaemia to use of chloramphenicol eye drops in two international case-control studies. BMJ. 1998;316:666.
79. Rayner SA, Buckley RJ. Ocular chloramphenicol and aplastic anaemia. Is there a link? Drug Saf. 1996;14:273-276.
80. Giamarellos-Bourboulis EJ. Macrolides beyond the conventional antimicrobials: a class of potent immunomodulators. Int J Antimicrob Agents. 2008;31:12-20.
81. Schultz MJ. Macrolide activities beyond their antimicrobial effects: macrolides in diffuse panbronchiolitis and cystic fibrosis. J Antimicrob Chemother. 2004;54:21-28.
82. Sivapalasingham S, Steigbigel N. Macrolides, clindamycin and ketolides. In: Mandell GL, Bennett JE, Dolin R, eds. Mandell, Douglas, and Bennett's Principles and Practice of Infectious Diseases. 7th ed. Philadelphia, PA: Churchill Livingstone Elsevier; 2011:427-448.

83. Piscitelli SC, Danziger LH, Rodvold KA. Clarithromycin and azithromycin: new macrolide antibiotics. Clin Pharm. 1992;11:137-152.
84. Westermarck E, Skrzypczak T, Harmoinen J, et al. Tylosin-responsive chronic diarrhea in dogs. J Vet Intern Med. 2005; 19:177-186.
85. Ruch-Gallie RA, Veir JK, Spindel ME, et al. Efficacy of amoxicillin and azithromycin for the empirical treatment of shelter cats with suspected bacterial upper respiratory infections. J Feline Med Surg. 2008;10:542-550.
86. Peeters TL. Erythromycin and other macrolides as prokinetic agents. Gastroenterology. 1993;105:1886-1899.
87. Beatty JA, Swift N, Foster DJ, et al. Suspected clindamycin-associated oesophageal injury in cats: five cases. J Feline Med Surg. 2006;8:412-419.
88. Glanemann B, Hildebrandt N, Schneider MA, et al. Recurrent single oesophageal stricture treated with a self-expanding stent in a cat. J Feline Med Surg. 2008;10:505-509.
89. Livermore DM. Linezolid in vitro: mechanism and antibacterial spectrum. J Antimicrob Chemother. 2003;51(Suppl 2):ii9-i16.
90. Beekmann SE, Gilbert DN, Polgreen PM. Toxicity of extended courses of linezolid: results of an Infectious Diseases Society of America Emerging Infections Network survey. Diagn Microbiol Infect Dis. 2008;62:407-410.
91. Leite LM, Carvalho AG, Ferreira PL, et al. Anti-inflammatory properties of doxycycline and minocycline in experimental models: an in vivo and in vitro comparative study. Inflammopharmacology. 2011;19:99-110.
92. White SD, Rosychuk RA, Reinke SI, et al. Use of tetracycline and niacinamide for treatment of autoimmune skin disease in 31 dogs. J Am Vet Med Assoc. 1992;200:1497-1500.
93. Bettenay SV, Mueller RS, Dow K, et al. Prospective study of the treatment of feline plasmacytic pododermatitis with doxycycline. Vet Rec. 2003;152:564-566.
94. McKeage K, Deeks ED. Doxycycline 40 mg capsules (30 mg immediate-release/10 mg delayed-release beads): anti-inflammatory dose in rosacea. Am J Clin Dermatol. 2010;11:217-222.
95. Thaker M, Spanogiannopoulos P, Wright GD. The tetracycline resistome. Cell Mol Life Sci. 2010;67:419-431.
96. Pankey GA. Tigecycline. J Antimicrob Chemother. 2005; 56:470-480.
97. Weese JS, Sweetman K, Edson H, et al. Evaluation of minocycline susceptibility of methicillin-resistant *Staphylococcus pseudintermedius*. Vet Microbiol. 2013;162:968-971.
98. German AJ, Cannon MJ, Dye C, et al. Oesophageal strictures in cats associated with doxycycline therapy. J Feline Med Surg. 2005;7:33-41.
99. Sykes JE, Bailiff NL, Ball LM, et al. Identification of a novel hemotropic mycoplasma in a splenectomized dog with hemic neoplasia. J Am Vet Med Assoc. 2004;224:1945-1951, 1930-1931.
100. Morris TJ, Davis TP. Doxycycline-induced esophageal ulceration in the U.S. Military service. Mil Med. 2000;165:316-319.
101. Papich MG, Davidson G. Doxycycline potency after storage in a compounded formulation for animals. American College of Veterinary Internal Medicine Forum. 2011. Denver, CO, USA.
102. Volovitz B, Shkap R, Amir J, et al. Absence of tooth staining with doxycycline treatment in young children. Clin Pediatr (Phila). 2007;46:121-126.
103. Ward GS, Guiry CC, Alexander LL. Tetracycline-induced anaphylactic shock in a dog. J Am Vet Med Assoc. 1982;180:770-771.

CHAPTER 9

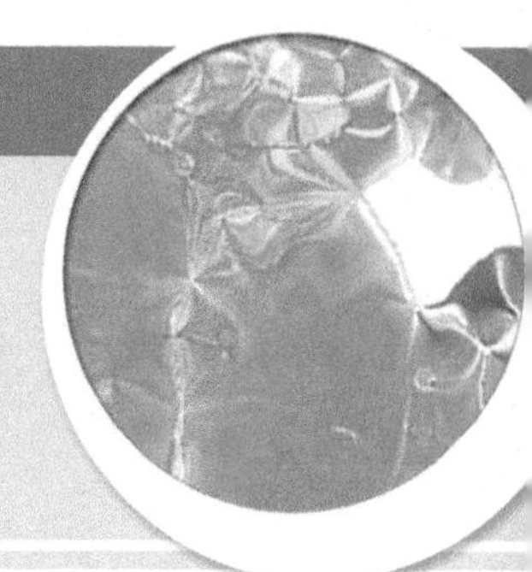

Antifungal Drugs

Jane E. Sykes and Mark G. Papich

KEY POINTS

- Compared to antibacterial drugs, the range of antifungal drug classes available is very limited, with most systemic treatment accomplished with the azole group of medications. The azoles have a similar mechanism of action and share other properties such as spectrum of activity, pharmacokinetics, tissue penetration, and adverse effect profiles. Proper understanding of these factors is most likely to result in successful treatment with minimal adverse effects.
- Drug interactions occur with many antifungal drugs.
- Although therapeutic drug monitoring would improve treatment with the azole antifungals and 5-flucytosine, this is rarely done because of variable availability of clinical assays and uncertainty in interpretation of the measured concentrations.
- Fungal infections often require prolonged treatment durations. This may be costly for some pet owners and can increase the risk of adverse effects to pets.
- Fungal organisms that are resistant to certain antifungal drugs are increasingly recognized. Although antifungal susceptibility testing can identify resistant organisms, this is often not performed because there are no standards for veterinary pathogens and drugs used in veterinary medicine, and few laboratories perform these tests.

INTRODUCTION

The use of antifungal drugs in human and veterinary medicine has increased in recent years. In humans, increased susceptibility to fungal infections has arisen because of immunosuppression secondary to HIV infection or treatment with potent immunosuppressive drugs. In animals, opportunistic fungal infections also result from immunosuppression, and the importance of fungal infections in dogs and cats is increasingly recognized. Antifungal drugs used in dogs and cats are generally not approved for use in these species. Therefore, veterinarians use human antifungal drugs off-label, with indications and dosing protocols often extrapolated from the human use. Because of differences in pharmacokinetics among species for these drugs, and differences in susceptibility to adverse effects in dogs and cats compared to people, this approach is not optimal. Fortunately, the clinical experience and pharmacokinetic data have expanded for these human drugs, which will improve antifungal treatment in animals. Efforts also have focused on the development of new, less toxic, and more efficacious antifungal drugs. This chapter reviews the classification, mechanisms of action, spectrum of activity, resistance mechanisms, tissue penetration, clinical use, and adverse effects of the major systemic antifungal drugs used to treat dogs and cats. Topical antifungal treatments are reviewed in the relevant chapters of this book. Basic principles of antimicrobial drug treatment are discussed in Chapter 6.

Antifungal drug treatment is often more prolonged than antibacterial drug treatment. One reason for this difference is that fungal organisms grow more slowly, and the drugs used (primarily azoles) are fungistatic, not fungicidal. Therefore, long-term treatment is needed to inhibit fungal growth and allow for the animal's immune system, which is often compromised, to eradicate the infection. Treatment of animals with deep mycoses with antifungal drugs must often be continued for months, and in some animals it may be weeks before clinical improvement is evident. Sometimes, disease worsens in the first week of treatment, because of the host's inflammatory response to killed organisms. This may have severe consequences for the host when there is extensive involvement of the pulmonary parenchyma or the central nervous system (CNS). Concurrent treatment with a nonsteroidal antiinflammatory drug (NSAIDs) or, when CNS involvement is present, judicious use of a short course of antiinflammatory glucocorticoids may improve outcome in these situations.[1]

The prognosis for animals with disseminated mold infections that have reversible underlying immunosuppression (such as drug-induced immunosuppression) may be better than the prognosis for animals with no apparent underlying immunosuppressive disease. This is because the latter group of animals are likely to have underlying (irreversible) genetic defects in immunity.

Azole Antifungals

Mechanism of Action, Classification, and Spectrum of Activity

Azole antifungal drugs inhibit sterol 14α-demethylase, a cytochrome P450–dependent fungal enzyme involved in synthesis of ergosterol, a key component of the fungal cell wall, from lanosterol. The result is the accumulation of 14α-methylsterols, which disrupt the fungal cell membrane (Figure 9-1). The majority of the adverse effects and drug interactions observed with these drugs relate to the cross-inhibition of mammalian P450 enzymes. All of the azole antifungals have the potential to be teratogenic, and their use should be avoided in pregnancy.

Azole antifungals are classified as imidazoles or triazoles based on whether they possess two or three nitrogen molecules

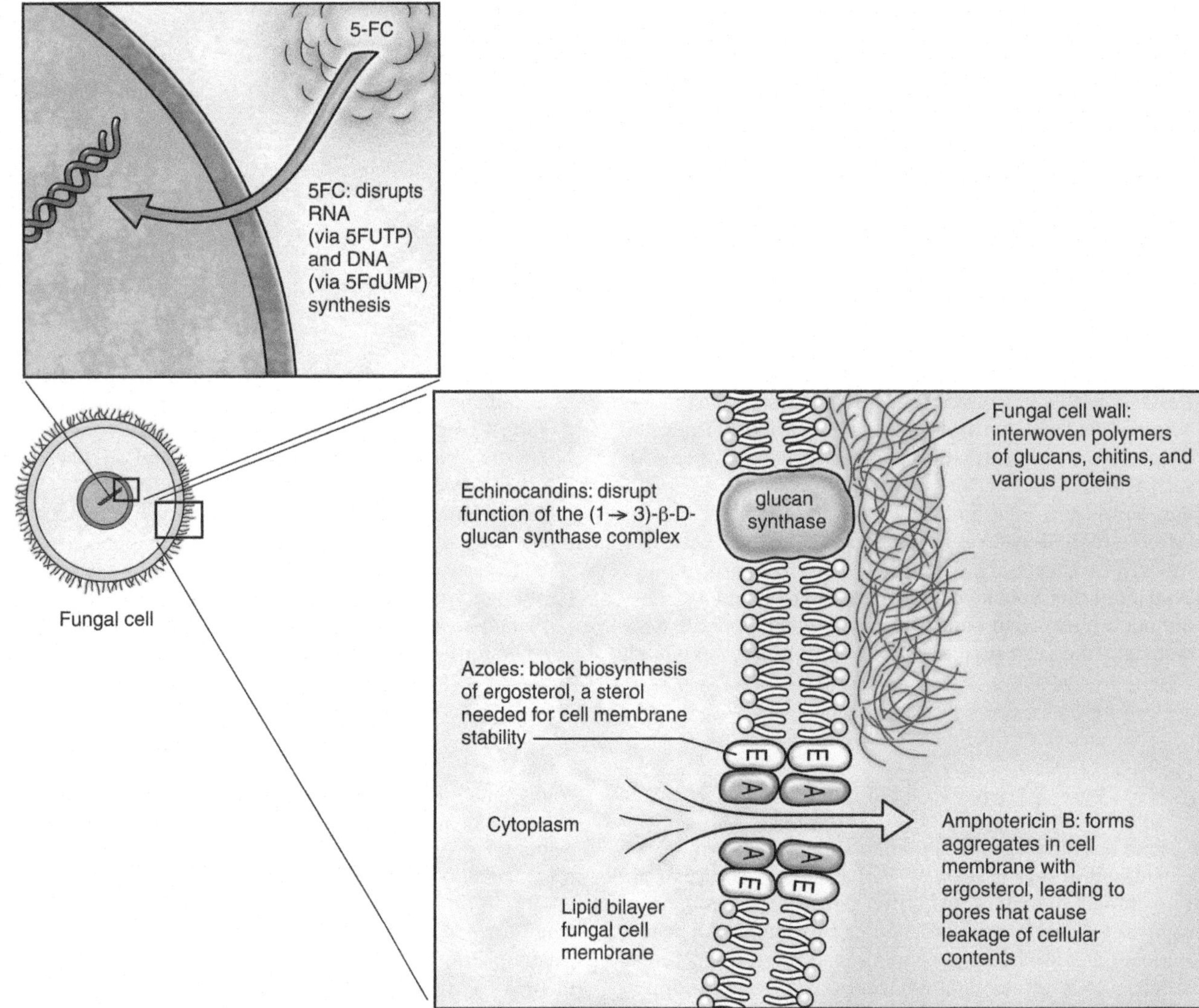

FIGURE 9-1 Mechanism of action of antifungal drugs. 5FC, 5-flucytosine; 5FUTP, 5-fluorouridine triphosphate; 5FdUMP, 5-fluorodeoxyuridine monophosphate; A, amphotericin B; E, ergosterol. Modified from Rex JH, Stevens DA. Systemic antifungal agents. In: Mandell GL, Bennett JE, Dolin R, eds. Mandell, Douglas and Bennett's Principles and Practice of Infectious Diseases, 7 ed. Philadelphia, PA: Churchill Livingstone Elsevier; 2011:549-563.

in their azole ring. Ketoconazole, enilconazole, and clotrimazole are imidazoles. The latter two drugs have poor oral bioavailability and are used topically in veterinary medicine for the treatment of superficial mycoses (see Chapters 65 and 67). Triazole antifungal drugs, such as itraconazole and fluconazole, are more slowly metabolized and have less impact on mammalian sterol synthesis than do imidazoles. Imidazoles and triazoles have been widely used to treat a variety of mycoses, which include candidiasis, cryptococcosis, blastomycosis, histoplasmosis, coccidioidomycosis, dermatophytosis, sporotrichosis, and aspergillosis (Tables 9-1 and 9-2).

Unfortunately, resistance to azole antifungal drugs has emerged among some fungi. Resistance results from mutations in the gene encoding the demethylase enzyme, increased production of C-14α demethylase, and increased azole efflux by fungal cell membrane transporters. Methods for in vitro susceptibility testing have become more standardized,[2,3] with improved correlation between the results of in vitro susceptibility testing and clinical response, but breakpoints (criteria that define susceptible versus resistant minimum inhibitory concentration values) are still needed for many drug-fungus combinations. Increasingly, it is apparent that resistance to one azole does not always imply resistance to other azole antifungal drugs.

Ketoconazole

Spectrum of Activity and Clinical Use

The use of ketoconazole has largely been replaced by itraconazole for treatment of many mycoses, because of the greater toxicity and reduced efficacy of ketoconazole when compared with triazole antifungal drugs. Because of its low cost, ketoconazole continues to be used in veterinary medicine when the cost of other antifungal drugs is prohibitive to the client, and it remains efficacious for treatment of *Malassezia* dermatitis[4] and feline nasal and cutaneous cryptococcosis. The absorption of ketoconazole is improved when it is administered with food, but it is inhibited by concurrent use of antacids. Ketoconazole is highly protein bound and is metabolized extensively by the liver. Nevertheless, moderate hepatic dysfunction does not alter blood levels of ketoconazole. Inactive products are excreted in bile and, to a lesser extent, the urine. Because of poor CNS penetration, it is ineffective for treatment of meningeal cryptococcosis and aspergillosis.[5]

TABLE 9-1

Spectrum of Activity and Tissue Distribution of Different Antifungal Drugs

Drug	Spectrum of Activity	Tissue Distribution
Ketoconazole	Dimorphic fungi, *Malassezia*. Ineffective for aspergillosis	Skin, bone, joint, lung. Poor CNS penetration
Itraconazole	Dimorphic fungi and molds, *Malassezia* spp.	Skin, bone, lung. May enter the CNS and eye with inflammation
Fluconazole	Some *Candida* spp., *Malassezia* spp., some dimorphic fungi. Poor activity against molds. *Aspergillus* spp. are intrinsically resistant	Widely distributed, including to the skin, lung, CNS, urine, and eye
Voriconazole	Dimorphic fungi, yeasts, and molds with the exception of *Sporothrix schenckii* and zygomycetes	CNS, eye, lung, bone
Posaconazole	Dimorphic fungi, yeasts, and molds including zygomycetes	Widely distributed
Amphotericin B	Broad spectrum. Also active against *Leishmania*	Limited penetration of the CNS and eye
5-Flucytosine	*Cryptococcus* and *Candida* spp.	Widely distributed, which includes the CNS, eye, and urine
Griseofulvin	Dermatophytes	Concentrates in skin
Terbinafine	Activity highest for dermatophytes. To a lesser extent may have activity against other dimorphic and filamentous fungi	Concentrates in skin and hair
Caspofungin	*Candida* and *Aspergillus* spp. Not active against *Cryptococcus* spp. or when given alone to treat *Coccidioides*	Widely distributed. Poor penetration of the CNS and eye

CNS, Central nervous system.

TABLE 9-2

Suggested Azole Antifungal Drug Doses for Dogs and Cats

Drug	Dose (mg/kg)	Interval (hours)	Species	Route	Comments
Ketoconazole	10 to 15 5 to 10	12	D C	PO	Do not administer to pregnant animals. Monitor liver enzymes monthly during treatment. Drug interactions may occur (see text). Inhibits adrenal function. Antacids impair absorption.
Itraconazole	5	12 to 24	D, C	PO	Do not administer to pregnant animals. Monitor liver enzymes monthly during treatment. Drug interactions may occur. Use of the oral suspension warrants dose reduction to 3 mg/kg. Monitor serum drug concentrations after 2 weeks if there is inadequate response to treatment (see text). Compounded formulations are unstable.
Fluconazole	5 to 10 50 mg/cat	12 12 to 24	D C	PO	Do not administer to pregnant animals. Monitor liver enzymes monthly during treatment. Drug interactions may occur.
Voriconazole	4 to 5	12	D	PO	Do not use in cats. Use cautiously in animals with liver disease. Also see fluconazole. Consider therapeutic drug monitoring (see text).
Posaconazole	5 to 10 5	12 to 24 24	D C	PO	Absorption may be improved when daily dose is split into 2 to 4 doses. Consider therapeutic drug monitoring. Also see fluconazole. Antacids impair absorption.

C, Cats; D, dogs.

Adverse Effects

The most common adverse effects of ketoconazole in dogs and cats are vomiting, anorexia, lethargy, and diarrhea.[6,7] Administration of ketoconazole with food may reduce gastrointestinal adverse effects. Mild increases in the activity of serum transaminases occur commonly during treatment, but do not warrant discontinuation of the drug. Less commonly, ketoconazole causes hepatitis, which may be accompanied by anorexia, vomiting, lethargy, increasing activities of serum ALT and ALP, and hyperbilirubinemia. The drug should be discontinued if this occurs and serum chemistry values checked 1 to 2 days later. Hepatitis can occur at any time, and the onset may be extremely rapid. Pruritis and cutaneous erythema have been reported in fewer than 1% of dogs treated with ketoconazole.[6] Lightening of the hair coat color and cataract formation occur rarely.

Ketoconazole is a potent inhibitor of mammalian cytochrome P450 enzymes and efflux transporter proteins such as P-glycoprotein. It also inhibits testosterone and cortisol synthesis. As a result, it has been used to treat pituitary-dependent hyperadrenocorticism in dogs[8] and also to deliberately inhibit the metabolism of cyclosporin, allowing a reduction in dose and, therefore, cost,[9] although there are concerns about whether use of ketoconazole in this way could contribute antifungal drug resistance and it increases the risk of adverse drug reactions. Transient infertility can occur during treatment of intact male animals. Ketoconazole can interfere with P-glycoprotein transport of ivermectin, which predisposes dogs to ivermectin toxicity.[6,10]

Itraconazole

Spectrum of Activity and Clinical Use

Itraconazole is one of the most widely used azoles in veterinary medicine. It has been used to treat blastomycosis, sporotrichosis, aspergillosis, coccidioidomycosis, dermatophytosis, histoplasmosis, phaeohyphomycosis, paecilomycosis, cryptococcosis, and *Malassezia* infections. It is available in capsules (which contain itraconazole granules) and an oral solution. The IV solution has been withdrawn.[11] Itraconazole in capsules is best absorbed when given with food because the acid secretion stimulated with feeding increases the drug solubility, which is necessary for dissolution and absorption. However, the oral solution is complexed with cyclodextrin to improve solubility, and administration of food does not influence absorption of this formulation. Absorption of the oral solution is consistently better than absorption of the capsule formulation, regardless of feeding.[12] As with ketoconazole, concurrent administration of gastric acid suppressants (H_2-blockers, proton pump inhibitors) may reduce absorption of the oral capsule. In cats, the oral solution is very well absorbed, and dose reduction is indicated to reduce the chance of toxicity (see Table 9-2). In addition to hydroxypropyl-β-cyclodextrin, this formulation contains sorbitol, propylene glycol, hydrochloric acid, cherry flavor, and saccharin, which may be unpalatable for cats. In Europe and Canada an oral solution for cats is available (Itrafungol, 10 mg/mL). Compounded formulations prepared by pharmacists have highly variable, poor, and even negligible oral absorption in animals, in addition to being unstable formulations. As a result, compounded formulations should never be used.

Like ketoconazole, itraconazole undergoes hepatic metabolism and inhibits metabolism of other P450-dependent drugs (e.g., cisapride, diazepam, cyclosporin). It is the only triazole antifungal drug that is converted to an active metabolite, hydroxylitraconazole.[11] Itraconazole is highly (99%) plasma protein bound and does not appear in urine, cerebrospinal fluid (CSF), or ocular tissues, although penetration of the CSF and eye can occur in the presence of inflammation. Itraconazole accumulates in the skin and claws and is the drug of choice for treatment of dermatophytosis in cats. Itraconazole is also a good choice for treatment of fungal osteomyelitis. Although loading doses have been recommended, these initial high doses can increase the risk of toxicity and do not appear to improve outcome.[13] Advanced liver disease increases itraconazole concentrations. Because of the variable absorption of oral itraconazole, monitoring of steady-state plasma concentrations (e.g., 3 weeks after initiating treatment) may be helpful if clinical responses are suboptimal.[14] Trough plasma itraconazole concentrations should be 0.5 to 1 μg/mL as determined using high-performance liquid chromatography.[15,16]

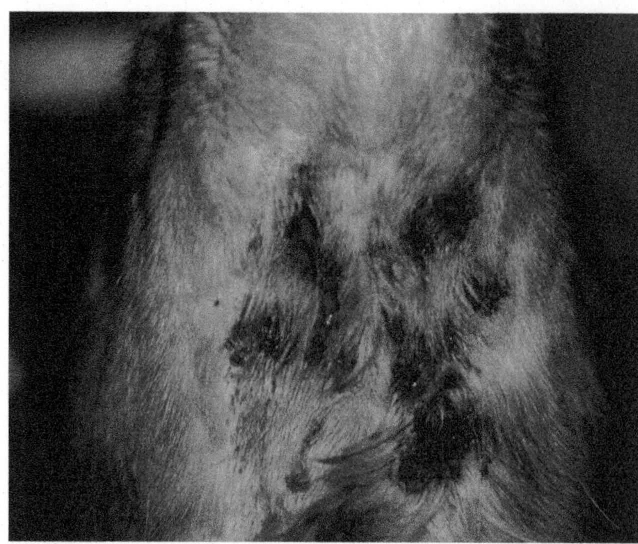

FIGURE 9-2 Submandibular ulcerative skin lesions in a golden retriever that had been treated with itraconazole for systemic blastomycosis.

Adverse Effects

The most common adverse effects of itraconazole in dogs and cats are vomiting and anorexia. Division of the total dose for twice-daily administration has been associated with decreased gastrointestinal signs and improved absorption in human patients.[5] Gastrointestinal adverse effects may be more common with the oral solution. Mild to moderate increases in serum ALT activity commonly occur during treatment. Provided these are not accompanied by inappetence, treatment need not be discontinued. Significant hepatotoxicity, accompanied by anorexia, vomiting, and hyperbilirubinemia, is less likely to occur than with ketoconazole but has been reported in humans as well as cats and dogs.[13,17-19] Hepatotoxicity more commonly occurs in dogs treated with 10 mg/kg/day.[13] Ulcerative skin lesions can occur in dogs, especially when doses of 10 mg/kg/day or higher are used (Figure 9-2). Development of hepatitis or severe cutaneous ulceration should prompt discontinuation of the drug. It may be possible to reinstitute treatment at a lower dose once the adverse effects have resolved. Occasionally mild, focal cutaneous ulcerative lesions can resolve spontaneously, without discontinuation of treatment.

Itraconazole does not suppress adrenal and testicular function like ketoconazole, but can inhibit the metabolism of other P450 enzyme-dependent drugs, including cyclosporine, digoxin, cisapride, and vinca alkaloids. It can also interfere with P-glycoprotein transport of ivermectin, which results in increased plasma ivermectin concentrations.[20]

Fluconazole

Spectrum of Activity and Clinical Use

Fluconazole is the least active azole antifungal drug and has the narrowest spectrum. The activity of fluconazole is limited to some *Candida* spp., *Cryptococcus* spp., *Malassezia* spp., and some dimorphic fungi. Fluconazole has poor activity against molds, and *Aspergillus* species are intrinsically resistant to fluconazole. Some *Cryptococcus* isolates are resistant to fluconazole, and resistance can develop during treatment. Itraconazole is preferable to fluconazole for treatment of histoplasmosis, blastomycosis, sporotrichosis, and dermatophytosis, although fluconazole has been successfully used to treat coccidioidomycosis, blastomycosis, and *Malassezia* infections in dogs.[19]

Fluconazole is available as tablets, an oral suspension, and as an IV solution. The availability of generic fluconazole has greatly reduced its cost and increased its use in veterinary medicine. Approved generic fluconazole tablets are bioequivalent to the brand name formulation in people. Similar bioequivalence is likely in animals. Fluconazole is more water-soluble and stable than itraconazole, and the compounded oral suspensions can be used in animals with a 14-day beyond-use-day (BUD). Some compounded preparations may have reduced activity. Fluconazole is almost completely absorbed after oral administration, and bioavailability is not altered by food or gastric acidity. In contrast to itraconazole and ketoconazole, fluconazole is only weakly protein bound. Because it is more water soluble than other azoles, fluconazole diffuses into body fluids such as saliva, urine, synovial fluid, and CSF. Therefore, it is the drug of choice for treatment of susceptible meningeal and urinary tract fungal infections. Renal excretion accounts for more than 90% of the elimination of fluconazole. The dosage should be decreased in animals with renal failure; this is especially important in patients receiving other P450-dependent drugs.

Adverse Effects

Adverse effects of fluconazole are uncommon to rare. When they occur, they are similar to those of itraconazole and include vomiting, anorexia, diarrhea, and increased liver enzymes. Dogs that fail to tolerate itraconazole may tolerate fluconazole without increases in liver enzymes.[19] Cutaneous rash, cytopenias, and retinal edema with impaired vision have been reported in human patients.[21,22] In contrast to itraconazole, cutaneous ulceration has not been reported in dogs.

Voriconazole

Spectrum of Activity and Clinical Use

Voriconazole is a second-generation triazole that is derived from fluconazole. In humans, it is the drug of choice for treatment of invasive aspergillosis.[23] It is also used to treat serious and refractory mold infections caused by *Scedosporium* spp., *Paecilomyces* spp., and *Fusarium* spp. Voriconazole is at least as active as itraconazole against veterinary isolates of *Cryptococcus* spp., *Candida* spp., and *Aspergillus fumigatus*.[24] It is not active against *Sporothrix* spp. or the zygomycetes.

Voriconazole is available as a tablet, an oral suspension, and an IV solution in a sulfobutylether–β-cyclodextrin base. Like fluconazole, it has excellent oral bioavailability, but its absorption is significantly reduced in the presence of food. Voriconazole is poorly water soluble and moderately protein bound. It is extensively metabolized by hepatic cytochrome P450 enzymes and eliminated into bile. The degree to which active drug enters the urinary tract in dogs is not clear. It has good CNS penetration. Voriconazole has been used with some success to treat systemic mold infections in dogs.[25] If therapeutic drug monitoring can be performed, the recommended trough concentration target is between 1 and 5 mg/L, and peak concentrations below 6 mg/L.[15,16,23]

Adverse Effects

In humans, adverse effects of voriconazole include reversible visual effects such as photophobia and blurred vision, hallucinations, peripheral neuropathies, and photosensitization, as well as the same toxicities as other triazoles. Of all the triazoles, it is the most potent inhibitor of P450 enzymes. Voriconazole can induce its own metabolism over time.[26] Because of its high cost, adverse effects have not been well documented in dogs. The author has observed inappetence, increased serum liver enzyme activities, and, uncommonly, CNS signs, including ataxia and staring. Tachypnea and marked pyrexia after IV infusion was observed in one dog. Cats are extremely sensitive to adverse effects of voriconazole and predictably develop inappetence, as well as ocular and CNS signs that have included ataxia, pelvic limb paresis, mydriasis, apparent blindness, decreased pupillary light responses, and a decreased menace response.[27] Cardiac arrhythmias and hypokalemia also occur in cats. A safe dose has not been established for cats.

Posaconazole

Posaconazole is an itraconazole analogue that has demonstrated good efficacy for treatment of several refractory deep mycoses in animals, which includes aspergillosis and mucormycosis in cats and invasive aspergillosis in dogs.[25,28-30] It has the broadest spectrum of activity of all the azoles. Its spectrum of activity is similar to that of voriconazole, but also includes the zygomycetes.[11] Posaconazole is available as an oral suspension. As with itraconazole, its absorption is *promoted* by the concurrent presence of fatty food. Gastric acid suppression can reduce the bioavailability of posaconazole.[31] Absorption is improved when the total daily dose is divided into two to four doses.[32] Therapeutic drug monitoring is recommended in human patients; target peak concentrations are greater than 1.48 mg/L.[15,16] Posaconazole is highly protein bound (>95%) and undergoes hepatic metabolism, with some inhibition of P450 enzymes. Most administered posaconazole is eliminated in the feces. Data on CSF concentrations of posaconazole are not yet available but it appears to be effective for treatment of CSF cryptococcosis. Adverse effects are less common in cats when compared with voriconazole, but information is limited at the time of writing.[28-30,33]

Other Azole Antifungals

Other azole drugs that are undergoing clinical trials in humans are ravuconazole and isavuconazole. Ravuconazole is a fluconazole derivative with good oral bioavailability. Isavuconazole is a water-soluble triazole with a spectrum similar to that of posaconazole but is available in oral and IV formulations. It is metabolized by P450 enzymes and does not achieve therapeutic concentrations in the urine. The CNS penetration of isavuconazole has not yet been evaluated.[34]

Amphotericin B

Mechanism of Action and Spectrum of Activity

Amphotericin B (AMB) is a polyene macrolide antibiotic produced by *Streptomyces nodosus*. It is closely related to nystatin. AMB irreversibly binds sterols in fungal cell membranes, forming pores or channels with subsequent leakage of ions. Although generally considered to be fungistatic, at high doses it may be fungicidal. AMB also possesses immunomodulatory effects; it activates macrophages and enhances macrophage-killing capacity. This may help explain its efficacy against pathogens such as *Pythium insidiosum*, which lack cell wall ergosterol.

Amphotericin B has antifungal activity against all of the important small animal fungal pathogens. It is also active against *Leishmania* spp.[35,36] In human medicine, AMB is the preferred drug for treatment of rapidly progressive mycoses,

BOX 9-1

Suggested Amphotericin B Infusion Protocols for Dogs and Cats

Formulation	Protocol
All formulations	Obtain baseline CBC, kidney panel, and UA and ensure adequate hydration before starting treatment. Recheck a kidney panel before each infusion. Administer three times weekly for 4 weeks or until azotemia is detected. For some patients, monthly administration of a single dose may be required to maintain remission.
Amphotericin B deoxycholate (IV route)	Reconstitute vial contents in sterile water to 5 mg/mL. Administer 0.9% NaCl IV at 1.5-2 times the calculated maintenance rate for 1 hour before and after AMB treatment. Ensure lines are flushed with D5W before infusing AMB. Dogs: Transfer 0.5 mg/kg to a 250-mL to 1000-mL bag of D5W (total fluid volume administered should be based on body weight and ability to tolerate a fluid load). Administer IV over 4-6 hours. Cats: Dilute 0.25 mg/kg in 30 mL of D5W and administer IV over 30 minutes to 1 hour.
Amphotericin B deoxycholate (SC route)	Transfer 0.5 mg/kg (cats) or 0.8 mg/kg (dogs) to bag containing 400 mL (cats) or 500 mL (dogs) of 0.45% sodium chloride in 2.5% dextrose. Administer subcutaneously. Fractious cats may need to be sedated or placed in a restraint bag. Sterile injection site abscess formation may occur with this protocol, especially with concentrations of amphotericin B > 20 mg/L.
Amphotericin B lipid complex (Abelcet)	Dilute to 1 mg/mL in D5W. Administer calculated dose IV over 1 to 2 hours. Dogs: 3 mg/kg Cats: 1 mg/kg

AMB, Amphotericin B; D5W, 5% dextrose in water; UA, urinalysis.

immunosuppressed hosts, or fungal meningitis. Resistance to AMB is rare, although high minimum inhibitory concentrations have been observed for some molds, including some isolates of *Aspergillus terreus*, *Paecilomyces* spp., and *Scedosporium* spp., as well as *Sporothrix schenckii*. The mechanism of resistance is not well understood, but it may relate to decreased cell wall ergosterol content.[37]

Clinical Use

Amphotericin B has poor aqueous solubility and is not absorbed from the gastrointestinal tract, so it is formulated for IV infusion in lyophilized form as a complex with the bile salt deoxycholate (Fungizone, AMB-D) (Box 9-1). The complex forms a colloid in water. Addition of electrolytes to the solution causes it to aggregate, so it is administered in 5% dextrose (D5W). It is not necessary to protect the infusion from light, as recommended in the past. In the bloodstream, AMB dissociates from deoxycholate and binds extensively to plasma proteins and cholesterol in membranes throughout tissues. Penetration of the vitreous humor and CSF is poor, but some animals with CNS infections still respond to treatment. In human patients, AMB-D has been given intrathecally to treat fungal meningitis and intraocularly following vitrectomy.[38]

A protocol for subcutaneous administration of AMB-D has been reported for treatment of cryptococcosis,[39] which may be less costly than IV administration. Sterile injection site abscesses occur in some animals treated using this protocol, so IV administration is preferred if possible.

Adverse Effects

The major adverse effect of AMB-D is nephrotoxicity, which is dose dependent and transient if it is detected early and the drug is discontinued. Both an acute effect caused by renal vasoconstriction and a chronic cumulative effect from repeated administration occurs. Renal tubular acidosis, nephrogenic diabetes insipidus, hypokalemia, and hypomagnesemia uncommonly occur with treatment. Rarely, aggressive IV fluid therapy and potassium supplementation to counteract these may be required. Loading with sodium before the infusion may decrease nephrotoxicity.[40] Slow administration in a large volume of fluid also decreases nephrotoxicity. Concurrent use of other nephrotoxic drugs, such as aminoglycosides, should be avoided. In humans, AMB-D can also cause fever, chills, headache, nausea, vomiting, and, rarely, cytopenias and anaphylaxis.[40] Fever, inappetence, and vomiting also appear to occur in some dogs treated with AMB-D. Phlebitis can occur at the IV infusion site. Other adverse effects noted in humans include infusion-related hypotension and hypochromic, normocytic anemia. NSAIDs can be administered to decrease pyrexia during treatment.

Lipid Formulations of Amphotericin B

Three lipid formulations of AMB are marketed in the United States. These are less nephrotoxic than AMB-D but are considerably more expensive. Decreased nephrotoxicity results from a reduced rate of transfer of AMB to mammalian cell membranes and increased drug clearance from the blood by the mononuclear phagocyte system. This allows administration of a higher dose of the drug, sometimes with improved treatment efficacy. Nevertheless, renal function should still be monitored.

Amphotericin B colloidal dispersion (ABCD, Amphotec) contains AMB and cholesterol sulfate, which form disc-shaped particles. It is more likely to cause chills, fever, and hypotension in humans than AMB-D (80% compared with 12% for AMB-D), so it is given over 3 to 4 hours and with premedication.

Liposomal amphotericin B (Ambisome) is a widely used formulation for treatment of human patients. It consists of AMB and a lipid mixture (phosphatidylcholine, cholesterol, and distearoyl phosphatidylglycerol). After reconstitution in D5W, it forms 80-nm vesicles. Nephrotoxicity and infusion-related reactions are much less common with liposomal amphotericin B than with ABCD or AMB-D, and the drug appears to reach higher concentrations in the eye.[41] In human patients, it is used as salvage therapy for aspergillosis, cryptococcosis, and candidiasis.

TABLE 9-3

Suggested 5-Flucytosine Drug Doses for Cats

Drug	Dose (mg/kg)	Interval (hours)	Species	Route	Comments
5-Flucytosine	25 to 50	6 to 8	C	PO	Monitor CBC. Use cautiously in animals with impaired renal function. Avoid use in dogs. Serum concentration monitoring is recommended in humans.

C, Cats.

Amphotericin B lipid complex (ABLC, Abelcet) is a mixture of AMB, dimyristoyl phosphatidylcholine, and dimyristoyl phosphatidylglycerol that forms ribbon-like sheets. ABLC is the most common formulation used in veterinary medicine. In humans, nephrotoxicity and infusion-related reactions are intermediate between AMB-D and liposomal amphotericin B. ABLC has been used in small animals to treat refractory cryptococcosis and cryptococcal meningitis and disseminated coccidioidomycosis, aspergillosis, blastomycosis, histoplasmosis, and pythiosis.

AMB cochleates are phosphatidylserine-calcium precipitates in the form of a continuous lipid bilayer sheet rolled up in a spiral. This formulation permits oral administration of AMB. Cochleates have been effective when used to treat mouse models of candidiasis and aspergillosis without significant toxicity. They remain under investigation on a research basis.

5-Flucytosine

Mechanism of Action and Spectrum of Activity

Flucytosine is a fluorinated pyrimidine related to fluorouracil. It has activity only against *Cryptococcus* spp. and *Candida* spp. These fungi deaminate flucytosine to 5-fluorouracil, which interferes with DNA replication and protein synthesis. Mammalian cells cannot convert flucytosine into 5-fluorouracil, so toxicity to mammalian cells is limited. Marked drug resistance arises during treatment (secondary drug resistance), and so flucytosine must always be used in combination with other drugs, most commonly AMB. Flucytosine may be synergistic with AMB. Resistance results from modifications in fungal enzymes that are required for flucytosine uptake and metabolism.[37]

Clinical Use

Flucytosine is absorbed rapidly and well from the gastrointestinal tract and is minimally bound to plasma proteins. Penetration of the CSF and aqueous humor is excellent. In cats, flucytosine may be considered to treat severe or refractory cryptococcosis in combination with other agents. Because about 80% of the dose is excreted unchanged in the urine, high urinary concentrations can be achieved. For the same reason, flucytosine toxicity is greatly increased in animals with renal failure, so the drug should be avoided in these animals or the dose lowered and plasma drug concentrations monitored carefully (Table 9-3). In human patients, toxicity is correlated with 2-hour postpill concentrations greater than 100 mg/L, and concentrations of 30 to 80 mg/L are suggested for treatment of cryptococcosis.[15] Because AMB can cause impaired renal function, careful monitoring for toxicity is indicated when flucytosine is used in conjunction with AMB. The use of flucytosine in animals has mostly been limited by its high cost.

Adverse Effects

Administration of flucytosine should be avoided in dogs, which often develop a severe (but reversible) drug eruption within 2 to 3 weeks of starting treatment. The most common adverse effects of flucytosine in cats are myelosuppression and gastrointestinal signs. The CBC should be monitored during treatment, and therapeutic drug monitoring should be considered. Myelosuppression is more likely to occur in human patients receiving other myelosuppressive drugs. Other adverse effects in humans include rash and reversible increases in liver enzyme activities. Flucytosine toxicity may result from conversion of flucytosine to 5-fluorouracil by the intestinal microflora.

Griseofulvin

Mechanism of Action and Spectrum of Activity

Griseofulvin is an oral antifungal drug derived from *Penicillium griseofulvum* that binds to fungal tubulin, leading to impaired microtubule function and mitotic arrest. It also has antiinflammatory properties.[42] After administration, griseofulvin is rapidly deposited in keratin precursor cells in the skin and hair, but disappears from the stratum corneum within 48 to 72 hours of discontinuation of treatment. Griseofulvin is fungistatic and has a limited spectrum of activity. It is used primarily to treat dermatophytosis and is not effective against yeasts such as *Candida* spp. and *Malassezia* spp. Resistance has been documented in some dermatophytes and may be due to altered tubulin.

Clinical Use

The absorption of griseofulvin is increased when it is administered with a fatty meal or whole milk. The drug is available in microsized and ultramicrosized formulations, which improve absorption from the stomach and small intestine. Most veterinary preparations are microsized. The dose of the ultramicrosized formulation can be reduced by 50%, because of improved absorption, but efficacy remains unchanged (Table 9-4). Prolonged treatment periods (months) are required for dermatophytosis (see Chapter 58).[43]

Adverse Effects

Griseofulvin is a potent inducer of cytochrome P450 enzymes and so decreases the efficacy of other drugs that are metabolized to inactive metabolites by P450 enzymes. It is teratogenic, so it should not be used to treat pregnant animals. Other adverse effects of griseofulvin include inappetence, vomiting, and diarrhea. In cats, it can cause myelosuppression, which is generally reversible on discontinuation of treatment, but irreversible pancytopenia has been reported.[44] Myelosuppression may be more likely to occur in cats with FIV infection.[45] The CBC should be monitored every 2 weeks during treatment.

TABLE 9-4

Suggested Griseofulvin and Terbinafine Doses for Dogs and Cats

Drug	Dose (mg/kg)	Interval (hours)	Species	Route	Comments
Griseofulvin (microsized)	25	12	D, C	PO	Administration with fatty food improves absorption. Dose may be increased to 50 mg/kg q12h for refractory infections. Avoid in cats with FIV infections. Do not use in pregnancy. Drug interactions possible. Monitor CBC.
Griseofulvin (ultramicrosized)	15	12	D, C	PO	Avoid in cats with FIV infections. Do not use in pregnancy. Drug interactions possible. Monitor CBC.
Terbinafine hydrochloride	30 to 40	24	D, C	PO	Administer with food.

C, Cats; D, dogs.

Terbinafine

Mechanism of Action and Spectrum of Activity

Terbinafine is a synthetic allylamine that inhibits fungal squalene epoxidase, which blocks fungal lanosterol and ergosterol synthesis and leads to accumulation of toxic squalene, with resultant fungal cell lysis. It is most effective for treatment of dermatophytosis. It has also been used to treat *Malassezia* spp. dermatitis in dogs.[46] The efficacy of terbinafine for treatment of invasive fungal infections has not been well investigated. It has been used both successfully[47] and unsuccessfully[48] in combination with other drugs to treat pythiosis in dogs, and as an alternative to itraconazole to treat human sporotrichosis.[49] It also has in vitro activity against other dimorphic fungi and molds, although its activity is highest for dermatophytes.[50,51] Terbinafine may be synergistic when administered with other antifungal drugs, which may provide enhanced efficacy for treatment of refractory mycoses.[52] However, nondermatophyte molds including *Aspergillus* spp. and *Fusarium* spp. have been detected in people with onychomycosis that failed to respond to terbinafine treatment.[53] Resistance has been reported in dermatophytes as a result of altered squalene epoxidase.[54]

Clinical Use

Terbinafine is available in tablet form (Lamasil). It is well absorbed in dogs when given with food (see Table 9-4).[55] The drug is highly lipophilic and accumulates in skin, claws, hair, and fat, where it persists for weeks after treatment is discontinued. Hepatic and renal failure increase plasma levels unpredictably, and dosage reduction may be required.

Adverse Effects

Terbinafine is generally well tolerated. Gastrointestinal signs, especially vomiting and increased liver enzyme activities, are uncommon. Facial pruritis has been reported in cats.[56]

Echinocandins

The echinocandins are lipopeptide antifungals that inhibit the formation of β-1,3-D-glucans in the fungal cell wall, a mechanism of action that is completely different from that for AMB and the azoles. The prototype drug is caspofungin acetate (Cancidas). Other drugs in this class are micafungin and anidulafungin. Caspofungin is fungicidal against *Candida* spp. and fungistatic against *Aspergillus* species. Treatment with caspofungin induced remission in a dog with disseminated aspergillosis (1 mg/kg IV in 250 mL 0.9% NaCl over 1 hour, q24h).[25] Synergism has been reported when echinocandins are used in combination with other antifungal drugs.[57] The echinocandins are ineffective against *Cryptococcus* spp., which possess little glucan synthase, and were only effective for treatment of *Coccidioides* spp. in a mouse model when used in conjunction with AMB.[58] In human patients, caspofungin is approved for treatment of refractory invasive aspergillosis, but it is also effective for mucosal candidiasis.

Caspofungin is given once daily as a slow IV infusion. In human patients, it is extensively protein bound and metabolized slowly by the liver, with some renal excretion. It has limited ability to penetrate the CNS and eye.[59,60] The cost is similar to that of lipid formulations of amphotericin B. Adverse effects noted in humans include fever, phlebitis, and increased activity of serum ALT (<20% of patients). The proper dose and extent to which adverse effects occur in dogs and cats is unknown, but administration of anidulafungin to the dog treated with caspofungin was associated with the development of a severe diffuse urticarial reaction.[25]

Other Antifungal Treatments

In human patients, hyperbaric oxygen therapy has been used to treat some fungal infections in combination with antifungal drugs. Whether this is beneficial or harmful is controversial and requires further study.[61]

SUGGESTED READINGS

Arthur RR, Drew RH, Perfect JR. Novel modes of antifungal drug administration. Expert Opin Investig Drugs. 2004;13(8):903-932.

Goodwin ML, Drew RH. Antifungal serum concentration monitoring: an update. J Antimicrob Chemother. 2008;61:17-25.

Hope WM, Billaud EM, Lestner J, et al. Therapeutic drug monitoring for triazoles. Curr Opin Infect Dis. 2008;21:580-586.

Pound MW, Townsend ML, Dimondi V, et al. Overview of treatment options for invasive fungal infections. Med Mycol. 2011;49:561-580.

REFERENCES

1. Sykes JE, Sturges BK, Cannon MS, et al. Clinical signs, imaging features, neuropathology, and outcome in cats and dogs with central nervous system cryptococcosis from California. J Vet Intern Med. 2010;24:1427-1438.
2. Clinical and Laboratory Standards Institute. M27–A3: Reference method for broth dilution antifungal susceptibility testing of yeasts. 2008. Available from www.clsi.org.
3. Clinical and Laboratory Standards Institute. M38–A2: Reference method for broth dilution antifungal susceptibility testing of filamentous fungi. 2008. Available from www.clsi.org.
4. Negre A, Bensignor E, Guillot J. Evidence-based veterinary dermatology: a systematic review of interventions for *Malassezia* dermatitis in dogs. Vet Dermatol. 2009;20:1-12.
5. Rex JH, Stevens DA. Systemic antifungal agents. In: Mandell GL, Bennett JE, Dolin R, eds. Mandell, Douglas and Bennett's Principles and Practice of Infectious Diseases. 7th ed. Philadelphia, PA: Churchill Livingstone Elsevier; 2011:549-563.
6. Mayer UK, Glos K, Schmid M, et al. Adverse effects of ketoconazole in dogs—a retrospective study. Vet Dermatol. 2008;19:199-208.
7. Medleau L, Chalmers SA. Ketoconazole for treatment of dermatophytosis in cats. J Am Vet Med Assoc. 1992;200:77-78.
8. Lien YH, Huang HP. Use of ketoconazole to treat dogs with pituitary-dependent hyperadrenocorticism: 48 cases (1994-2007). J Am Vet Med Assoc. 2008;233:1896-1901.
9. Mouatt JG. Cyclosporin and ketoconazole interaction for treatment of perianal fistulas in the dog. Aust Vet J. 2002;80:207-211.
10. Hugnet C, Lespine A, Alvinerie M. Multiple oral dosing of ketoconazole increases dog exposure to ivermectin. J Pharm Pharm Sci. 2007;10:311-318.
11. Pound MW, Townsend ML, Dimondi V, et al. Overview of treatment options for invasive fungal infections. Med Mycol. 2011;49:561-580.
12. Barone JA, Moskovitz BL, Guarnieri J, et al. Enhanced bioavailability of itraconazole in hydroxypropyl-beta-cyclodextrin solution versus capsules in healthy volunteers. Antimicrob Agents Chemother. 1998;42:1862-1865.
13. Legendre AM, Rohrbach BW, Toal RL, et al. Treatment of blastomycosis with itraconazole in 112 dogs. J Vet Intern Med. 1996;10:365-371.
14. Pasqualotto AC, Denning DW. Generic substitution of itraconazole resulting in sub-therapeutic levels and resistance. Int J Antimicrob Agents. 2007;30:93-94.
15. Goodwin ML, Drew RH. Antifungal serum concentration monitoring: an update. J Antimicrob Chemother. 2008;61:17-25.
16. Hope WW, Billaud EM, Lestner J, et al. Therapeutic drug monitoring for triazoles. Curr Opin Infect Dis. 2008;21:580-586.
17. Gupta AK, Chwetzoff E, Del Rosso J, et al. Hepatic safety of itraconazole. J Cutan Med Surg. 2002;6:210-213.
18. McKay JS, Cox CL, Foster AP. Cutaneous alternariosis in a cat. J Small Anim Pract. 2001;42:75-78.
19. Foy DS, Trepanier LA. Antifungal treatment of small animal veterinary patients. Vet Clin North Am Small Anim Pract. 2010;40:1171-1188.
20. Ballent M, Lifschitz A, Virkel G, et al. Modulation of the P-glycoprotein-mediated intestinal secretion of ivermectin: in vitro and in vivo assessments. Drug Metab Dispos. 2006;34:457-463.
21. Bradbury BD, Jick SS. Itraconazole and fluconazole and certain rare, serious adverse events. Pharmacotherapy. 2002;22:697-700.
22. Magrath GN, Pulido JS, Montero J, et al. Cystoid macular edema secondary to fluconazole toxicity. Ocul Immunol Inflamm. 2010;18:472-474.
23. Lat A, Thompson 3rd GR. Update on the optimal use of voriconazole for invasive fungal infections. Infect Drug Resist. 2011;4:43-53.
24. Okabayashi K, Imaji M, Osumi T, et al. Antifungal activity of itraconazole and voriconazole against clinical isolates obtained from animals with mycoses. Nihon Ishinkin Gakkai Zasshi. 2009;50:91-94.
25. Schultz RM, Johnson EG, Wisner ER, et al. Clinicopathologic and diagnostic imaging characteristics of systemic aspergillosis in 30 dogs. J Vet Intern Med. 2008;22:851-859.
26. Roffey SJ, Cole S, Comby P, et al. The disposition of voriconazole in mouse, rat, rabbit, guinea pig, dog, and human. Drug Metab Dispos. 2003;31:731-741.
27. Quimby JM, Hoffman SB, Duke J, et al. Adverse neurologic events associated with voriconazole use in 3 cats. J Vet Intern Med. 2010;24:647-649.
28. Evans N, Gunew M, Marshall R, et al. Focal pulmonary granuloma caused by *Cladophialophora bantiana* in a domestic short haired cat. Med Mycol. 2011;49:194-197.
29. Wray JD, Sparkes AH, Johnson EM. Infection of the subcutis of the nose in a cat caused by *Mucor* species: successful treatment using posaconazole. J Feline Med Surg. 2008;10:523-527.
30. McLellan GJ, Aquino SM, Mason DR, et al. Use of posaconazole in the management of invasive orbital aspergillosis in a cat. J Am Anim Hosp Assoc. 2006;42:302-307.
31. Krishna G, Moton A, Ma L, et al. Pharmacokinetics and absorption of posaconazole oral suspension under various gastric conditions in healthy volunteers. Antimicrob Agents Chemother. 2009;53:958-966.
32. Li Y, Theuretzbacher U, Clancy CJ, et al. Pharmacokinetic/pharmacodynamic profile of posaconazole. Clin Pharmacokinet. 2010;49:379-396.
33. Krockenberger MB, Martin P, Halliday C, et al. Localised *Microsphaeropsis arundinis* infection of the subcutis of a cat. J Feline Med Surg. 2010;12:231-236.
34. Thompson 3rd GR, Wiederhold NP. Isavuconazole: a comprehensive review of spectrum of activity of a new triazole. Mycopathologia. 2010;170:291-313.
35. Oliva G, Roura X, Crotti A, et al. Guidelines for treatment of leishmaniasis in dogs. J Am Vet Med Assoc. 2010;236:1192-1198.
36. Sundar S, Chakravarty J, Agarwal D, et al. Single-dose liposomal amphotericin B for visceral leishmaniasis in India. N Engl J Med. 2010;362:504-512.
37. Espinel-Ingroff A. Mechanisms of resistance to antifungal agents: yeasts and filamentous fungi. Rev Iberoam Micol. 2008;25:101-106.
38. Arthur RR, Drew RH, Perfect JR. Novel modes of antifungal drug administration. Expert Opin Investig Drugs. 2004;13:903-932.
39. Malik R, Craig AJ, Wigney DI, et al. Combination chemotherapy of canine and feline cryptococcosis using subcutaneously administered amphotericin B. Aust Vet J. 1996;73:124-128.
40. Laniado-Laborin R, Cabrales-Vargas MN. Amphotericin B: side effects and toxicity. Rev Iberoam Micol. 2009;26:223-227.
41. Goldblum D, Rohrer K, Frueh BE, et al. Ocular distribution of intravenously administered lipid formulations of amphotericin B in a rabbit model. Antimicrob Agents Chemother. 2002;46:3719-3723.
42. Moossavi M, Bagheri B, Scher RK. Systemic antifungal therapy. Dermatol Clin. 2001;19:35-52.
43. Moriello KA. Treatment of dermatophytosis in dogs and cats: review of published studies. Vet Dermatol. 2004;15:99-107.
44. Rottman JB, English RV, Breitschwerdt EB, et al. Bone marrow hypoplasia in a cat treated with griseofulvin. J Am Vet Med Assoc. 1991;198:429-431.
45. Shelton GH, Grant CK, Linenberger ML, et al. Severe neutropenia associated with griseofulvin therapy in cats with feline immunodeficiency virus infection. J Vet Intern Med. 1990;4:317-319.
46. Rosales MS, Marsella R, Kunkle G, et al. Comparison of the clinical efficacy of oral terbinafine and ketoconazole combined with cephalexin in the treatment of *Malassezia* dermatitis in dogs—a pilot study. Vet Dermatol. 2005;16:171-176.
47. Hummel J, Grooters A, Davidson G, et al. Successful management of gastrointestinal pythiosis in a dog using itraconazole, terbinafine, and mefenoxam. Med Mycol. 2011;49:539-542.
48. Pereira DI, Schild AL, Motta MA, et al. Cutaneous and gastrointestinal pythiosis in a dog in Brazil. Vet Res Commun. 2010;34:301-306.

49. Francesconi G, Francesconi do Valle AC, Passos SL, et al. Comparative study of 250 mg/day terbinafine and 100 mg/day itraconazole for the treatment of cutaneous sporotrichosis. Mycopathologia. 2011;171:349-354.
50. Ryder NS. Activity of terbinafine against serious fungal pathogens. Mycoses. 1999;42(Suppl 2):115-119.
51. Gupta AK, Kohli Y, Batra R. In vitro activities of posaconazole, ravuconazole, terbinafine, itraconazole and fluconazole against dermatophyte, yeast and non-dermatophyte species. Med Mycol. 2005;43:179-185.
52. Revankar SG, Nailor MD, Sobel JD. Use of terbinafine in rare and refractory mycoses. Future Microbiol. 2008;3:9-17.
53. Baudraz-Rosselet F, Ruffieux C, Lurati M, et al. Onychomycosis insensitive to systemic terbinafine and azole treatments reveals non-dermatophyte moulds as infectious agents. Dermatology. 2010;220:164-168.
54. Osborne CS, Leitner I, Hofbauer B, et al. Biological, biochemical, and molecular characterization of a new clinical *Trichophyton rubrum* isolate resistant to terbinafine. Antimicrob Agents Chemother. 2006;50:2234-2236.
55. Sakai MR, May ER, Imerman PM, et al. Terbinafine pharmacokinetics after single dose oral administration in the dog. Vet Dermatol. 2011;22:528-534.
56. Foust AL, Marsella R, Akucewich LH, et al. Evaluation of persistence of terbinafine in the hair of normal cats after 14 days of daily therapy. Vet Dermatol. 2007;18:246-251.
57. Chen SC, Slavin MA, Sorrell TC. Echinocandin antifungal drugs in fungal infections: a comparison. Drugs. 2011;71:11-41.
58. Gónzalez GM, Gónzalez G, Najvar LK, et al. Therapeutic efficacy of caspofungin alone and in combination with amphotericin B deoxycholate for coccidioidomycosis in a mouse model. J Antimicrob Chemother. 2007;60:1341-1346.
59. Goldblum D, Fausch K, Frueh BE, et al. Ocular penetration of caspofungin in a rabbit uveitis model. Graefes Arch Clin Exp Ophthalmol. 2007;245:825-833.
60. Flattery AM, Hickey E, Gill CJ, et al. Efficacy of caspofungin in a juvenile mouse model of central nervous system candidiasis. Antimicrob Agents Chemother. 2011;55:3491-3497.
61. Grahl N, Shepardson KM, Chung D, et al. Hypoxia and fungal pathogenesis: to air or not to air? Eukaryot Cell. 2012;11:560-570.

CHAPTER 10

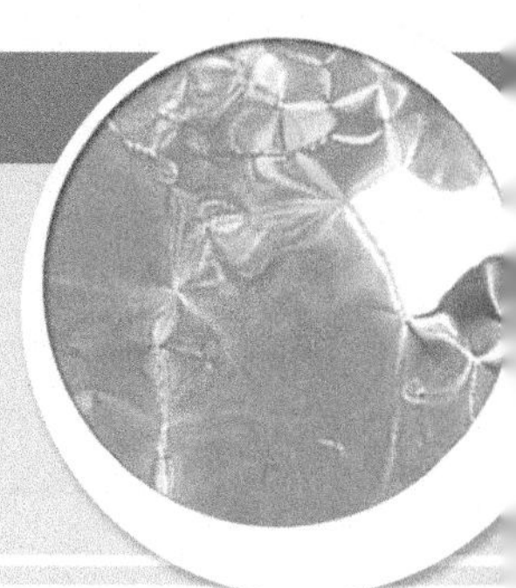

Antiprotozoal Drugs

Jane E. Sykes and Mark G. Papich

KEY POINTS

- Antiprotozoal drugs often have a restricted spectrum of activity, although some are also active against bacteria and fungi. Many interfere with enzyme pathways specific to certain protozoal species.
- Treatment with antiprotozoal drugs may not consistently clear an infection.
- Resistance to antiprotozoal drugs is a growing problem among protozoal pathogens.
- Some antiprotozoal drugs have minimal to no adverse effects, whereas for others, adverse effects severely limit use.
- The availability of antiprotozoal drugs is restricted in some countries.

INTRODUCTION

The use of antiprotozoal drugs in dogs and cats is frequently extrapolated from their use in human patients or food animal species. Almost all antiprotozoal drugs are not specifically approved for treatment of protozoal infections in dogs and cats. Some antibacterial and antifungal drugs also have antiprotozoal activity (see Chapters 8 and 9 for the use and adverse effects of these drugs). In vitro activity of antiprotozoal drugs, and monitoring of resistance, is more difficult for antiprotozoal drugs because standardized susceptibility testing is not routinely performed for these pathogens. In addition, many antiprotozoal drugs are designed to be active in the lumen of the intestine for treatment of intestinal protozoal infections and the concentration of active drug in the intestinal lumen after oral administration is difficult to measure. Therefore, the concentration of drug to which these pathogens are exposed is often not known. The activity and dosage regimens of antiprotozoal drugs are often based on the results of clinical trials, rather than concentration-exposure relationships between antiprotozoal drugs and the organism of interest.

Many antiprotozoal drugs are active only against a restricted range of protozoal species. To reflect this, drugs in this chapter are organized into antiprotozoal drugs primarily used for gastrointestinal infections; those with a broad spectrum of activity; those used to treat systemic protozoal infections (such as hepatozoonosis, toxoplasmosis, neosporosis, and sarcocystosis); antiprotozoal drugs used to treat leishmaniosis; and those used to treat Chagas' disease. For many infections, treatment does not consistently result in parasitologic cure.

Antiprotozoal Drugs Used Primarily for Gastrointestinal Infections

Amprolium

Amprolium is a thiamine analogue that is used to prevent and treat intestinal coccidiosis (Table 10-1). It is available as a feed additive for livestock and is sometimes administered in food or drinking water to puppies and kittens. Adverse effects of anorexia or diarrhea are rare and primarily occur at high doses and with prolonged use. Central nervous system (CNS) signs can result from thiamine deficiency, which is reversible on addition of thiamine to the diet. However, thiamine supplementation may interfere with the drug's efficacy.

Benzimidazoles

Fenbendazole and Albendazole

Benzimidazoles bind to β-tubulin within a variety of helminths and protozoa. This leads to inhibition of tubulin polymerization and the formation of microtubules, with impaired cell division. Glucose uptake by parasites is also impaired. Resistance can result from production of altered β-tubulin by parasites, which reduces binding of benzimidazole drugs.

Fenbendazole is widely used to treat giardiasis in dogs and cats. It is safer than metronidazole, can be administered to young animals, and has higher efficacy, although treatment failure can still occur. A second course of treatment or administration of fenbendazole in combination with metronidazole can be effective in refractory cases. Administration with food may improve absorption, but the fat content of the food does not influence absorption.[1] Adverse effects of fenbendazole are very rare but can include decreased appetite, vomiting, diarrhea, and rarely reversible pancytopenia.[2] At high doses used to treat *Mesocestoides* spp. peritonitis (100 mg/kg q12h), neurologic signs have been observed.[3] Febantel is metabolized to a benzimidazole compound and has been used in combination with praziquantel and pyrantel (Drontal Plus) to treat *Giardia* spp. infection in dogs, although efficacy at label dosages has been variable and some dogs can re-shed low numbers of cysts when treatment is discontinued.[4] Albendazole has an affinity for rapidly dividing cells, and although it is used extensively for treatment of parasitic infections in human patients, it been associated with anorexia and reversible bone marrow suppression in dogs and cats especially when high doses are administered for more than 5 days.[5] As a result, fenbendazole is used more commonly in small animals.

Nitroimidazoles

Protozoa reduce nitroimidazoles to nitro anion free radicals, which cause damage to parasite DNA. Some nitroimidazoles are mutagens and carcinogens, but carcinogenesis has not been demonstrated in dogs and cats with long-term use. Metronidazole,

TABLE 10-1

Suggested Doses of Drugs That Are Primarily Used to Treat Protozoal Infections of the Gastrointestinal Tract in Small Animals

Drug	Dose (mg/kg)	Interval (hours)	Species	Route	Duration (days)	Comments
Fenbendazole	50	24	C, D	PO	5	Giardiasis. May be administered with food. Safe in pregnancy.
Albendazole	25	12	C, D	PO	3	Giardiasis. May cause bone marrow suppression. Do not use in pregnancy.
Metronidazole	15	12	C, D	PO	8	Giardiasis. Use caution with hepatic insufficiency. Dose for metronidazole benzoate is 25 mg/kg.
Tinidazole	15	12 24	D C	PO	5	Giardiasis. Administer with food or in capsules to reduce bitterness.
Ronidazole	30	24	C	PO	14	Tritrichomoniasis. Avoid doses ≥60 mg/kg/day. Compounded from powder.
Paromomycin	10	8	D	PO	5-10	Cryptosporidiosis. Caution in animals with diarrhea due to possible systemic absorption. Avoid in cats.
Nitazoxanide	100 mg/animal	12	D, C	PO	3	Cryptosporidiosis. Efficacy and safety unclear. Vomiting common in cats.
Amprolium	1.25 g of 20% powder or 30 mL of 9.6% solution to 3.8 L of water	24	D, C	PO	7	Isosporiasis. Add to food. Do not administer for prolonged periods.
Sulfadimethoxine	55 on day 1, 27 thereafter	24	D, C	PO	3-23 or for 48 hr after signs resolve	Isosporiasis with or without a dihydrofolate reductase inhibitor.

C, Cats; D, dogs.

ronidazole, and tinidazole have primarily been used to treat enteric protozoal infections. Benznidazole is specifically used to treat infections with *Trypanosoma cruzi.*

Metronidazole

Metronidazole is used to treat giardiasis in dogs and cats, although efficacy may be as low as 50%. It also has activity against amoebic infections. The clinical use and adverse effects of metronidazole are described in Chapter 8. Doses of metronidazole used for treatment of giardiasis have the potential to be associated with neurotoxicity, so fenbendazole is preferred because of greater safety and efficacy. Metronidazole can be combined with fenbendazole for refractory giardiasis.

Tinidazole

Tinidazole is a 5-nitroimidazole that has amoebicidal, giardicidal, trichomonicidal, and anaerobic bactericidal activity. It is sometimes used as a single-dose treatment for giardiasis in human patients. The efficacy of tinidazole for treatment for giardiasis in dogs and cats has not been evaluated, and the half-life in dogs (4.4 hours) and cats (8.4 hours) is shorter than that in human patients (>12 hours).[6,7] Tinidazole is very well absorbed in dogs and cats, with a bioavailability of 100%. Adverse effects are similar to those of metronidazole. Like metronidazole, tinidazole has a bitter taste.

Ronidazole

Ronidazole is the drug of choice for treatment of *Tritrichomonas foetus* infections, which are less responsive to metronidazole and tinidazole.[8-10] Resistance to ronidazole has been identified in some isolates of *T. foetus* and is associated with treatment failure in infected cats.[11] Resistance is thought to result from increased oxygen-scavenging capacity by the parasite, whereby oxygen competes effectively with ronidazole and other nitroimidazoles for ferredoxin-bound electrons.

Ronidazole is absorbed rapidly and completely after oral administration to cats. Some compounded formulations may have decreased efficacy as a result of low ronidazole content or differences in drug release at the site of action (the large bowel). A modified-release formulation that is delivered to the colon may have improved efficacy.[12] Decreased appetite, vomiting, and neurologic signs can occur in dogs and cats, especially at doses above 30 mg/kg q12h in cats and at doses as low as 10 mg/kg/d in dogs.[13] Once daily dosing is probably sufficient because of the long half-life of the drug in cats.[12] Doses of 20 mg/kg or less may not effectively clear infection with *T. foetus*. Neurologic signs result from γ-aminobutyric acid (GABA) antagonism in the CNS and include ataxia, decreased mentation, agitation, tremors, and hyperesthesia, which occur up to 9 days after the start of treatment and resolve when the drug is discontinued.[13]

Nitozoxanide

Nitazoxanide is a nitrothiazolyl-salicylamide derivative that has activity against *Giardia* spp., *Cryptosporidium* spp., *Sarcocystis neurona,* some anaerobic bacteria, *Helicobacter* spp., and *Campylobacter jejuni.* It inhibits the pyruvate-ferredoxin/flavodoxin oxidoreductase enzyme-dependent electron transfer reaction that is essential for anaerobic metabolism in these organisms. Resistance has been documented in *Giardia* spp.[14]

Reports of nitazoxanide use in dogs and cats have been rare, and its efficacy in dogs and cats is largely unknown. An equine formulation (Navigator) that was used to treat equine protozoal meningoencephalitis caused by *Sarcocystis neurona* has been removed from the market. Doses have been extrapolated from those used for human patients. Nitazoxanide treatment of cats co-infected with *Cryptosporidium* spp. and *T. foetus* led to cessation of shedding during treatment, but infection was not eliminated.[15] Vomiting occurred frequently, especially at higher doses (75 mg/kg PO q12h). In humans, nitazoxanide is rapidly absorbed from the gastrointestinal tract and metabolized to the active metabolite tizoxanide, which is highly protein bound. After hepatic glucuronidation, it is excreted in urine and bile.

Antibacterial Drugs with Broad-Spectrum Antiprotozoal Activity

Folic Acid Antagonists

Trimethoprim, pyrimethamine, ormetoprim, and sulfadiazine inhibit parasite replication through folate antagonism. Synergistic combinations of sulfadiazine with trimethoprim or pyrimethamine are primarily used to treat toxoplasmosis, neosporosis, and intestinal coccidiosis (*Isospora* spp. infections) in dogs and cats. A combination of pyrimethamine, trimethoprim-sulfadiazine, and clindamycin has also been used to treat *Hepatozoon americanum* infections.[16] The mechanisms of action, use, and adverse effects of trimethoprim and sulfonamides are discussed in Chapter 8.

Pyrimethamine

Like trimethoprim, pyrimethamine inhibits dihydrofolate reductase, which is necessary for synthesis of thymidine. However, in contrast to trimethoprim, it has a greater affinity for the protozoal enzyme than the bacterial enzyme. Resistance to pyrimethamine can occur when parasites synthesize dihydrofolate reductase enzymes with an altered drug target site. Pyrimethamine is well absorbed after oral administration and penetrates a variety of tissues including the CNS. Hepatic metabolism and some renal excretion occur. Although clearance of pyrimethamine is not affected by renal disease, the use of caution with hepatic or renal insufficiency has been recommended in human patients.

Pyrimethamine is well tolerated. Gastrointestinal signs such as vomiting, diarrhea, and decreased appetite occur in some treated animals. Bone marrow suppression can occur with prolonged treatment at higher doses as a result of folic acid deficiency. In human patients, concurrent administration of folinic acid is recommended when high doses are used for treatment of toxoplasmosis. Folinic acid, but not folic acid supplementation also reverses marrow suppression in dogs treated with pyrimethamine.[17] The CBC should be monitored weekly during treatment, and supplementation should be provided if leukopenia develops and continued treatment is necessary. Stomatitis, ulcerative glossitis, and exfoliative dermatitis have also been described in human patients as a result of folic acid deficiency.[18] Other adverse effects of pyrimethamine-sulfadiazine combinations result from the sulfadiazine component (see Chapter 8).

Unlike trimethoprim-sulfadiazine, there are no approved formulations of pyrimethamine-sulfonamides for dogs and cats. Pyrimethamine is available as a single agent in tablets but should be administered with a sulfonamide for the best efficacy. Another alternative is the combination of pyrimethamine-sulfadiazine, which is available in an oral liquid suspension for horses (ReBalance). Although off-label, it is a convenient formulation for small animal veterinarians. This formulation can be administered at a dose of 1 mg/kg pyrimethamine + 20 mg/kg sulfadiazine PO q24h. This is equivalent to 0.33 mL of the equine formulation per 4 kg of body weight for dogs and cats.

Macrolides and Lincosamides

Clindamycin, azithromycin, and clarithromycin have antiprotozoal activity. The use of these macrolides and lincosamides in dogs and cats and their adverse effects are discussed in Chapter 8. Clindamycin is the most widely used antiprotozoal for treatment of toxoplasmosis and neosporosis in dogs and cats. Although clindamycin inhibits shedding of *Toxoplasma gondii* oocysts by cats,[19] clinical efficacy of clindamycin for treating toxoplasmosis in dogs and cats has been questioned by experts and in published studies. Trimethoprim-sulfonamides are a suitable alternative, or if clindamycin is used, pyrimethamine may be used in combination. In human patients, pyrimethamine and clindamycin are used as a substitute for pyrimethamine and sulfadiazine for treatment of toxoplasmosis in sulfadiazine-sensitive individuals. Azithromycin is used in combination with atovaquone for treatment of babesiosis and cytauxzoonosis.

Paromomycin

Paromomycin is the only aminoglycoside antibiotic that has efficacy against protozoa. It is poorly absorbed from the gastrointestinal tract and so has been used to treat enteric protozoal infections, particularly cryptosporidiosis. It is ineffective for treatment of tritrichomoniasis in cats.[10] Furthermore, when used to treat intestinal protozoal infections in cats, paromomycin has been absorbed systemically because of intestinal mucosal compromise, with resultant acute renal failure, deafness, and cataract formation.[20] As a result, its use has been limited. In human patients, paromomycin has been used topically to treat cutaneous leishmaniasis and parenterally to treat visceral leishmaniasis.[21]

Tetracyclines and Ciprofloxacin

Doxycycline has primarily been used for malaria prophylaxis in humans. Ciprofloxacin is thought to inhibit DNA gyrase within a chloroplast organelle (the apicoplast) of apicomplexan parasites (see the triazines, later). It is an alternative to sulfadiazine for treatment of isosporiasis in human patients.[18] Tetracyclines and ciprofloxacin have not been widely used for prevention or treatment of protozoal infections in dogs and cats with the possible exception of doxycycline as part of combination treatment for babesiosis (see Chapter 75).

Antiprotozoal Drugs Used for Systemic Protozoal Infections

Quinolone Derivatives

Atovaquone

Atovaquone is a hydroxynaphthoquinone that inhibits electron transport in protozoa by targeting the cytochrome bc_1 complex (Table 10-2). It has been used in combination with other antiprotozoal drugs as an alternative treatment for malaria,

TABLE 10-2

Suggested Doses of Drugs Primarily Used to Treat Systemic Protozoal Diseases Excluding Leishmaniosis and Trypanosomiasis in Small Animals

Drug	Dose (mg/kg)	Interval (hours)	Species	Route	Duration (days)	Comments
Pyrimethamine	1 0.5-1	24	D C	PO	14-28	Primarily neosporosis, toxoplasmosis, and American hepatozoonosis. Use with a sulfonamide. Use caution with hepatic and renal insufficiency. Monitor CBC. Folinic acid supplementation (5 mg/day) may be required.
Clindamycin	22	12	D, C	PO		Toxoplasmosis, neosporosis, sarcocystosis, and American hepatozoonosis.
Azithromycin	10	24	D, C	PO	10	Babesiosis and cytauxzoonosis. Used with atovaquone.
Atovaquone	13.3 15	8	D C	PO	10	Babesiosis and cytauxzoonosis with azithromycin. Administer with food.
Decoquinate	10-20	12	D	PO	≥365	American hepatozoonosis and sarcocystosis. Powder (6% decoquinate; 60 mg active ingredient per gram) is mixed with food. This equates to 0.5 to 1 tablespoon/10 kg body weight q12h.
Imidocarb dipropionate	6.6 5	Once, repeat in 14 days	D C	Deep IM	N/A	Large *Babesia* spp. infections. Caution with hepatic or renal insufficiency. Avoid use with other cholinesterase inhibitors.
Diminazene aceturate	3-5	Once	D	Deep IM	N/A	Babesiosis and African trypanosomiasis. Narrow therapeutic range.
Ponazuril	20-50	12-24	D	PO	3-28	Toxoplasmosis, neosporosis, isosporiasis. Optimal dose, duration, efficacy, and adverse effects unknown.
Toltrazuril	5-10 18	12-24	D C	PO	1-14	Hepatozoonosis, isosporiasis. One dose may be effective for isosporiasis. Optimal dose and duration for hepatozoonosis unknown.

C, Cats; D, dogs; N/A, not applicable.

toxoplasmosis, and pneumocystosis in human patients.[18] In veterinary medicine, atovaquone is used in combination with azithromycin for treatment of *Babesia gibsoni* and *Babesia conradae* infections and cytauxzoonosis (see Chapters 75 and 76), but is expensive. Resistance has been reported in *Plasmodium* spp., *T. gondii, Pneumocystis jirovecii,* and canine *B. gibsoni* strains as a result of mutations in the cytochrome bc_1 complex.

Atovaquone is highly lipophilic and extensively protein bound. Little is known about atovaquone metabolism in dogs and cats. Its oral bioavailability increases significantly when food is administered concurrently. Atovaquone is available alone or in a formulation with proguanil for treatment and prevention of malaria in human patients. The combination formulation may cause vomiting and diarrhea in dogs, but otherwise atovaquone appears well tolerated by both dogs and cats.[22-24] In human patients, adverse effects have included gastrointestinal signs, headache, fever, and increased liver enzyme activities. Coadministration with metoclopramide, tetracycline, or rifampin significantly decreases plasma drug concentrations in humans.

Decoquinate

Decoquinate is a 4-hydroxyquinolone coccidiostat that inhibits electron transport in protozoal mitochondria and interferes with sporozoite development. It likely has a similar mechanism of action to atovaquone, because resistance to atovaquone can result in cross-resistance to decoquinate.[25] Although developed as a food additive for use in production animals, decoquinate can be used successfully and without adverse effects to prevent relapses in dogs that are chronically infected with *Hepatozoon americanum*.[16] Decoquinate also appeared to be effective for treatment of *Sarcocystis* spp. myositis in a dog.[26] Its distribution and metabolism in dogs and cats have not been described.

Aromatic Diamines

The aromatic diamines include imidocarb dipropionate, diminazene aceturate, pentamidine isethionate, and phenamidine isethionate. These drugs inhibit DNA synthesis in protozoa. In dogs, imidocarb and diminazene have been used most widely, primarily for treatment of *Babesia* spp. and *Hepatozoon canis* infections. In general, the use of imidocarb has been preferred over diminazene because of diminazene's narrow therapeutic index. Pentamidine and phenamidine have also been used in dogs. Pentamidine isethionate is a second-line treatment for leishmaniasis in human patients and is used as an alternative to diminazene for treatment of African trypanosomiasis (see Chapter 78). Treatment of protozoal infections using the aromatic diamines may not result in complete parasite elimination.

Imidocarb Dipropionate

Imidocarb dipropionate is primarily used to treat large *Babesia* spp. and *Hepatozoon canis* infections in dogs. More effective agents have replaced imidocarb for treatment of canine monocytic ehrlichiosis and feline cytauxzoonosis.

Imidocarb is given by intramuscular injection, twice, 2 weeks apart. It is generally well tolerated, although it can cause transient pain at the site of injection. It appears to be eliminated in urine and feces.[27] Acute adverse effects result from its anticholinergic activity and include vomiting, shivering, hypersalivation, lacrimation, diarrhea, agitation, lethargy, pyrexia, and periorbital swelling. These generally resolve within a few hours. A possible association between imidocarb treatment and acute renal tubular necrosis has been reported in dogs.[28] Massive hepatic necrosis was described after overdosage of dogs with 10 times the recommended dose.[29]

Diminazene Aceturate

Diminazene aceturate is administered parenterally, primarily to dogs, for treatment of babesiosis, African trypanosomiasis, and, most recently, infections with *Rangelia vitalii*, a novel protozoal pathogen of dogs from Brazil.[30] Diminazene aceturate is not readily available in the United States. Resistance to diminazene has been described in *Babesia gibsoni*.[31]

Although formulations for small animals are not available, a powdered commercial drug formulation (Veriben) has been reconstituted with sterile water to a concentration of 7 mg/mL and administered intramuscularly at a dose of 3 mg/kg diminazene diaceturate for a pharmacokinetic study in cats.[32] The dose was well tolerated, and diminazene was eliminated with a half-life of only 1.7 hours and a peak concentration of only 0.5 μg/mL. Development of clinically effective doses from these data requires further studies. Diminazene was administered to seven cats experimentally infected with *Trypanosoma evansi* at a dose of 3.5 mg/kg intramuscularly on five consecutive days.[33] The treatment was 85.7% efficacious for elimination of the parasite, and no adverse effects were observed.

Effective doses of diminazene approach doses that are toxic, so it should be used with caution.[34] Adverse effects include tachycardia and CNS signs such as ataxia, nystagmus, and opisthotonos. A single treatment can be given, or the dose can be repeated 72 to 96 hours after drug administration. In some protocols for *B. gibsoni* infections, diminazene administration has been followed a day later by treatment with imidocarb.

Triazine Antiprotozoals (Toltrazuril and Ponazuril)

Toltrazuril and its major metabolite ponazuril (toltrazuril sulfone, Marquis) are triazine-based antiprotozoal drugs that have specific activity against apicomplexan coccidial infections. Toltrazuril is not available within the United States. Ponazuril and toltrazuril appear to act on a plastid-like chloroplast organelle (the *apicoplast*) in apicomplexan protozoa, which may have originally been acquired from a green alga.[35] This organelle contains a small circular genome and operates key biochemical pathways. Although their mechanism of action is unclear, triazines may inhibit metabolic enzymes or decrease pyrimidine synthesis within the apicoplast. Ponazuril and toltrazuril have been used in animals to treat isosporiasis, toxoplasmosis, neosporosis, and equine protozoal meningoencephalitis. Triazine resistance has been described in coccidia from production animals.[36]

In dogs and cats, toltrazuril has been used to treat isosporiasis and hepatozoonosis, although infection may persist in some animals.[16,37-42] In Europe it is available in combination with the anthelmintic emodepside (Procox Oral Suspension for Dogs, Bayer Animal Health) for treatment of isosporiasis and roundworm infections in puppies over 2 weeks of age. The suspension contains 18 mg/mL of toltrazuril, and a single 9-mg/kg dose is recommended. Toltrazuril appeared to be as effective as trimethoprim-sulfadiazine-clindamycin-pyrimethamine for treatment of canine American hepatozoonosis.[16] One dog with *Hepatozoon canis* infection recovered after treatment with toltrazuril and trimethoprim-sulfamethoxazole,[42] but a toltrazuril and imidocarb combination did not offer benefit over treatment of *H. canis* infection with imidocarb alone.[43] Dogs with *H. canis* infection respond clinically within 72 hours of starting treatment with toltrazuril. Anecdotal reports exist of the use of ponazuril to treat *Isospora* spp. infections in dogs and cats, but its efficacy is unclear. Doses of ponazuril used have ranged from 20 to 50 mg/kg for 2 to 5 days. In one dog, ocular toxoplasmosis that was refractory to clindamycin resolved after treatment with ponazuril for 28 days.[44]

The pharmacokinetics of the triazines in dogs has not been reported. In horses, ponazuril crosses the blood-brain barrier to some extent and achieves concentrations in the cerebrospinal fluid sufficient to inhibit protozoa. It has long half-life in horses (>4 days) and in cattle (2 to 3 days). Because of its specific activity against apicomplexan parasites, significant toxicity in mammalian species has not been reported.

Antileishmanial Antiprotozoal Drugs

Antifungal Agents

Amphotericin B

Amphotericin B is a treatment of choice for human visceral leishmaniasis.[18] It is thought to bind to ergosterol in the protozoal membrane, and blocks the ability of *Leishmania* spp. to bind to and enter macrophages.[45] Lipid amphotericin B formulations have been used to treat visceral leishmaniosis in dogs, although organism persistence and relapse have been reported in some dogs after twice-weekly treatment for up to 10 administrations (0.8 to 3.3 mg/kg intravenously).[46,47] In an effort to reduce selection for resistant parasites, the World Health Organization recommends against the use of amphotericin B for treatment of canine leishmaniosis.[48] A full discussion of amphotericin B is provided in Chapter 9.

Azole Antifungals

Azole antifungals such as fluconazole have been used to treat cutaneous leishmaniasis in human patients. More effective antiprotozoal drugs are substituted for visceral leishmaniasis. Posaconazole and ravuconazole also have activity against *Trypanosoma cruzi* (see Chapter 78), and fluconazole may have activity against *Toxoplasma* (see Chapter 72).

Antimony Compounds

Sodium stibogluconate (Pentostam) and *N*-methylglucamine antimoniate (meglumine antimoniate, Glucantime) are derived from the heavy metal antimony (Sb). They are called pentavalent antimony compounds (symbol Sb^{v}) because they contain Sb atoms that have five electrons in their outer shell. Pentavalent antimonials have been recommended as the first choice for treatment of *Leishmania* infections in humans and in dogs.[49] Their mechanism of action is still not completely clear, but it is thought that pentavalent antimony undergoes reduction to the more toxic trivalent version, possibly within macrophage phagolysosomes or within the parasite itself.[50] The trivalent compound inhibits protozoal enzymes and damages protozoal

TABLE 10-3

Suggested Doses of Drugs Primarily Used to Treat Leishmaniosis or Chagas' Disease in Dogs

Drug	Dose (mg/kg)	Interval (hours)	Route	Duration (days)	Comments
Meglumine antimoniate	75-100	24	SC	30-60	Leishmaniosis. Use with allopurinol. Available in ampules. Dose based on concentration of meglumine antimoniate. Caution in dogs with renal insufficiency.
Allopurinol	10	12	PO	At least 6-12 months	Leishmaniosis. Use with meglumine or miltefosine. Monitor CBC and serum chemistry in dogs with hepatic and renal insufficiency.
Miltefosine	2	24	PO	28	Leishmaniosis. Use with allopurinol.
Benznidazole	5-10	24	PO	60	Chagas' disease

DNA.[51] Resistance to antimonials is an emerging problem in human *Leishmania* spp. isolates. This has led to the use of higher drug dosages, with an associated rise in the rate of drug toxicity. The availability of antimonial drugs is limited in the United States.

Both sodium stibogluconate and meglumine antimoniate are administered subcutaneously (Table 10-3). The treatment of choice for canine leishmaniosis is a combination of meglumine antimoniate and allopurinol.[48,49] Complete clearance of the infection may not always occur.[52] After subcutaneous administration, more than 80% of meglumine antimoniate is eliminated by the kidneys. Pain at the site of injection is the most common adverse effect, and cutaneous abscesses or cellulitis may also occur.[53] Systemic adverse effects such as lethargy, vomiting, diarrhea, inappetence, and increased serum liver enzyme activities may be more likely to occur in the presence of renal failure, which can be a complication of leishmaniosis. Of concern, the administration of meglumine antimoniate to healthy dogs has led to renal tubular necrosis, in the absence of azotemia.[54] In human patients, other adverse effects include generalized arthralgias, abdominal pain, mild cytopenias, cardiotoxicity, and chemical pancreatitis.[21] Novel formulations of antimony compounds are being developed for treatment of leishmaniasis, including lipid formulations and preparations that could be administered orally.[50]

Allopurinol

Allopurinol is a purine analogue. In parasites, allopurinol is metabolized to derivatives that are incorporated into RNA, which leads to impaired protein synthesis. Resistance can occur and appears to result from reduced activity of purine transporters and a reduced ability to accumulate purine.[55] Although it has been used alone for treatment of canine leishmaniosis, allopurinol is most commonly used in combination with meglumine or miltefosine.

Allopurinol is rapidly absorbed from the gastrointestinal tracts of dogs. Peak drug concentrations occur 1 to 3 hours after administration.[56] Allopurinol is not bound to plasma proteins. Allopurinol rarely causes adverse effects in dogs. It inhibits mammalian xanthine oxidase, which results in decreased uric acid production from xanthine. As a result, long-term use can result in xanthine urolithiasis.[57] In human patients, allopurinol most commonly causes skin rashes. Gastrointestinal signs can also occur. Rarely administration of allopurinol to humans results in aplastic anemia or a hypersensitivity syndrome characterized by toxic epidermal necrolysis with hepatic and renal failure.[58,59] Serious adverse reactions are more likely to occur in human patients with renal insufficiency. At usual doses, allopurinol treatment leads to improvement in kidney lesions in dogs with leishmaniosis that have renal insufficiency.[60] Nevertheless, careful monitoring for adverse effects is indicated in these dogs (see Table 10-3). Serious drug interactions can occur when allopurinol is administered with azathioprine.

Miltefosine

Miltefosine is an effective alternative to pentavalent antimonials for treatment of leishmaniosis.[61] It is a phospholipid analogue that activates cellular proteases in *Leishmania* spp., which results in apoptosis. Miltefosine is the first highly active oral drug for treatment of leishmaniosis. Nevertheless, despite clinical improvement in treated dogs, elimination of the parasite may not always occur.[62,63] Resistance to miltefosine can result from increased P-glycoprotein–mediated drug efflux and decreased drug uptake. Because miltefosine has a long half-life and must be administered for 28 days, selection for resistant isolates has been a concern. The World Health Organization has recommended that veterinary use of miltefosine in dogs with leishmaniosis be avoided in order to minimize the rate of selection for resistant strains.[64]

Over 90% of miltefosine is absorbed from the gastrointestinal tract of dogs after oral administration.[54] The half-life of miltefosine in the dog is approximately 6 days, so it accumulates until a steady-state plasma concentration is reached after 3 to 4 weeks of treatment. Clearance is believed to result from slow hepatic metabolism and excretion in bile. In dogs, adverse effects of treatment are mild and transient and consist of occasional vomiting and diarrhea.[65] In contrast to meglumine antimoniate, miltefosine does not appear to contribute to renal pathology in dogs.[54,66]

Antiprotozoal Drugs for Treatment of Chagas' Disease

Benznidazole

Benznidazole is a nitroimidazole that is used to treat acute Chagas' disease (see Chapter 78). Benznidazole is activated by a parasite-specific nitroreductase to produce toxic metabolites.[67] Resistance can result from reduction in the level of activity of the nitroreductase and confers cross-resistance to nifurtimox.

Benznidazole is lipophilic, is readily absorbed from the gastrointestinal tract, and undergoes hepatic metabolism. In the United States, it is available from the Centers for Disease Control and Prevention (CDC). The main adverse effect of treatment in dogs is vomiting. In human patients, it can cause skin rashes, peripheral neuropathy, and less commonly bone marrow suppression. It also has the potential to be carcinogenic.

Nifurtimox

Nifurtimox is a nitrofuran derivative used to treat Chagas' disease in humans. It has limited efficacy, with 70% parasitologic cure for acute disease and at best 20% for chronic disease.[18] As with benznidazole, metabolic reduction of the nitro group by a trypanosome-specific nitroreductase leads to the formation of toxic metabolites. In human patients, it is well absorbed orally and undergoes hepatic metabolism. Gastrointestinal and neurologic signs are the primary adverse effects of nifurtimox, and like benznidazole, it has carcinogenic properties.[68] Severe adverse effects have precluded the use of nifurtimox in dogs.[69]

SUGGESTED READING

Rossignol JF. *Cryptosporidium* and *Giardia*: treatment options and prospects for new drugs. Exp Parasitol. 2010;124(1):45-53.

REFERENCES

1. McKellar QA, Galbraith EA, Baxter P. Oral absorption and bioavailability of fenbendazole in the dog and the effect of concurrent ingestion of food. J Vet Pharmacol Ther. 1993;16:189-198.
2. Gary AT, Kerl ME, Wiedmeyer CE, et al. Bone marrow hypoplasia associated with fenbendazole administration in a dog. J Am Anim Hosp Assoc. 2004;40:224-229.
3. Boyce W, Shender L, Schultz L, et al. Survival analysis of dogs diagnosed with canine peritoneal larval cestodiasis (*Mesocestoides* spp.). Vet Parasitol. 2011;180:256-261.
4. Bowman DD, Liotta JL, Ulrich M, et al. Treatment of naturally occurring, asymptomatic *Giardia* sp. in dogs with Drontal Plus flavour tablets. Parasitol Res. 2009;105(Suppl 1):S125-S134.
5. Stokol T, Randolph JF, Nachbar S, et al. Development of bone marrow toxicosis after albendazole administration in a dog and cat. J Am Vet Med Assoc. 1997;210:1753-1756.
6. Lamp KC, Freeman CD, Klutman NE, et al. Pharmacokinetics and pharmacodynamics of the nitroimidazole antimicrobials. Clin Pharmacokinet. 1999;36:353-373.
7. Sarkiala E, Järvinen A, Välttilä S, et al. Pharmacokinetics of tinidazole in dogs and cats. J Vet Pharmacol Ther. 1991;14:257-262.
8. Gookin JL, Copple CN, Papich MG, et al. Efficacy of ronidazole for treatment of feline *Tritrichomonas foetus* infection. J Vet Intern Med. 2006;20:536-543.
9. Gookin JL, Stauffer SH, Coccaro MR, et al. Efficacy of tinidazole for treatment of cats experimentally infected with *Tritrichomonas foetus*. Am J Vet Res. 2007;68:1085-1088.
10. Kather EJ, Marks SL, Kass PH. Determination of the in vitro susceptibility of feline *Tritrichomonas foetus* to 5 antimicrobial agents. J Vet Intern Med. 2007;21:966-970.
11. Gookin JL, Stauffer SH, Dybas D, et al. Documentation of in vivo and in vitro aerobic resistance of feline *Tritrichomonas foetus* isolates to ronidazole. J Vet Intern Med. 2010;24:1003-1007.
12. LeVine DN, Papich MG, Gookin JL, et al. Ronidazole pharmacokinetics after intravenous and oral immediate-release capsule administration in healthy cats. J Feline Med Surg. 2011;13:244-250.
13. Rosado TW, Specht A, Marks SL. Neurotoxicosis in 4 cats receiving ronidazole. J Vet Intern Med. 2007;21:328-331.
14. Müller J, Sterk M, Hemphill A, et al. Characterization of *Giardia lamblia* WB C6 clones resistant to nitazoxanide and to metronidazole. J Antimicrob Chemother. 2007;60:280-287.
15. Gookin JL, Levy MG, Law JM, et al. Experimental infection of cats with *Tritrichomonas foetus*. Am J Vet Res. 2001;62:1690-1697.
16. Macintire DK, Vincent-Johnson NA, Kane CW, et al. Treatment of dogs infected with *Hepatozoon americanum*: 53 cases (1989-1998). J Am Vet Med Assoc. 2001;218:77-82.
17. Castles TR, Kintner LD, Lee CC. The effects of folic or folinic acid on the toxicity of pyrimethamine in dogs. Toxicol Appl Pharmacol. 1971;20:447-459.
18. Moore TA. Agents active against parasites and *Pneumocystis*. In: Mandell GL, Bennett JE, Dolin R, eds. Mandell, Douglas and Bennett's Principles and Practice of Infectious Diseases. 7th ed. Philadelphia, PA: Churchill Livingstone Elsevier; 2011:631-668.
19. Malmasi A, Mosallanejad B, Mohebali M, et al. Prevention of shedding and reshedding of *Toxoplasma gondii* oocysts in experimentally infected casts treated with oral clindamycin: a preliminary study. Zoonoses Public Health. 2009;56(2):102-104.
20. Gookin JL, Riviere JE, Gilger BC, et al. Acute renal failure in four cats treated with paromomycin. J Am Vet Med Assoc. 1999;215: 1821-1823:1806.
21. Murray HW, Berman JD, Davies CR, et al. Advances in leishmaniasis. Lancet. 2005;366:1561-1577.
22. Birkenheuer AJ, Levy MG, Breitschwerdt EB. Efficacy of combined atovaquone and azithromycin for therapy of chronic *Babesia gibsoni* (Asian genotype) infections in dogs. J Vet Intern Med. 2004;18:494-498.
23. Cohn LA, Birkenheuer AJ, Brunker JD, et al. Efficacy of atovaquone and azithromycin or imidocarb dipropionate in cats with acute cytauxzoonosis. J Vet Intern Med. 2011;25:55-60.
24. Matsuu A, Koshida Y, Kawahara M, et al. Efficacy of atovaquone against *Babesia gibsoni* in vivo and in vitro. Vet Parasitol. 2004;124:9-18.
25. Pfefferkorn ER, Borotz SE, Nothnagel RF. Mutants of *Toxoplasma gondii* resistant to atovaquone (566C80) or decoquinate. J Parasitol. 1993;79:559-564.
26. Sykes JE, Dubey JP, Lindsay LL, et al. Severe myositis associated with *Sarcocystis* spp. infection in 2 dogs. J Vet Intern Med. 2011;25(6):1277-1283.
27. Vial HJ, Gorenflot A. Chemotherapy against babesiosis. Vet Parasitol. 2006;138:147-160.
28. Máthé A, Dobos-Kovács M, Vörös K. Histological and ultrastructural studies of renal lesions in *Babesia canis* infected dogs treated with imidocarb. Acta Vet Hung. 2007;55:511-523.
29. Kock N, Kelly P. Massive hepatic necrosis associated with accidental imidocarb dipropionate toxicosis in a dog. J Comp Pathol. 1991;104:113-116.
30. Da Silva AS, Franca RT, Costa MM, et al. Experimental infection with *Rangelia vitalii* in dogs: acute phase, parasitemia, biological cycle, clinical-pathological aspects and treatment. Exp Parasitol. 2011;128:347-352.
31. Hwang SJ, Yamasaki M, Nakamura K, et al. Development and characterization of a strain of *Babesia gibsoni* resistant to diminazene aceturate in vitro. J Vet Med Sci. 2010;72:765-771.
32. Lewis KM, Cohn LA, Birkenheuer AJ, et al. Pharmacokinetics of diminazene diaceturate in healthy cats. J Vet Pharmacol Ther. 2012;35:608-610.
33. Silva ASD, Zanette RA, Wolkmer P, et al. Diminazene aceturate in the control of *Trypanosoma evansi* infection in cats. Vet Parasitol. 2009;165:47-50.
34. Solano-Gallego L, Baneth G. Babesiosis in dogs and cats—expanding parasitological and clinical spectra. Vet Parasitol. 2011;181:48-60.
35. Wiesner J, Reichenberg A, Heinrich S, et al. The plastid-like organelle of apicomplexan parasites as drug target. Curr Pharm Des. 2008;14:855-871.
36. Stephen B, Rommel M, Daugschies A, et al. Studies of resistance to anticoccidials in *Eimeria* field isolates and pure *Eimeria* strains. Vet Parasitol. 1997;69:19-29.
37. Altreuther G, Gasda N, Adler K, et al. Field evaluations of the efficacy and safety of emodepside plus toltrazuril (Procox oral suspension for dogs) against naturally acquired nematode and *Isospora* spp. infections in dogs. Parasitol Res. 2011;109(Suppl 1):S21-S28.

38. Altreuther G, Gasda N, Schroeder I, et al. Efficacy of emodepside plus toltrazuril suspension (Procox oral suspension for dogs) against prepatent and patent infection with *Isospora canis* and *Isospora ohioensis*-complex in dogs. Parasitol Res. 2011;109(Suppl 1):S9-20.
39. Daugschies A, Mundt HC, Letkova V. Toltrazuril treatment of cystoisosporosis in dogs under experimental and field conditions. Parasitol Res. 2000;86:797-799.
40. Lloyd S, Smith J. Activity of toltrazuril and diclazuril against *Isospora* species in kittens and puppies. Vet Rec. 2001;148:509-511.
41. Petry G, Kruedewagen E, Bach T, et al. Efficacy of Procox oral suspension for dogs (0.1% emodepside and 2% toltrazuril) against experimental nematode (*Toxocara cati* and *Ancylostoma tubaeforme*) infections in cats. Parasitol Res. 2011;109(Suppl 1):S37-S43.
42. Voyvoda H, Pasa S, Uner A. Clinical *Hepatozoon canis* infection in a dog in Turkey. J Small Anim Pract. 2004;45:613-617.
43. Pasa S, Voyvoda H, Karagenc T, et al. Failure of combination therapy with imidocarb dipropionate and toltrazuril to clear *Hepatozoon canis* infection in dogs. Parasitol Res. 2011;109:919-926.
44. Swinger RL, Schmidt Jr KA, Dubielzig RR. Keratoconjunctivitis associated with *Toxoplasma gondii* in a dog. Vet Ophthalmol. 2009;12:56-60.
45. Paila YD, Saha B, Chattopadhyay A. Amphotericin B inhibits entry of *Leishmania donovani* into primary macrophages. Biochem Biophys Res Commun. 2010;399:429-433.
46. Oliva G, Gradoni L, Ciaramella P, et al. Activity of liposomal amphotericin B (AmBisome) in dogs naturally infected with *Leishmania infantum*. J Antimicrob Chemother. 1995;36:1013-1019.
47. Cortadellas O. Initial and long-term efficacy of a lipid emulsion of amphotericin B desoxycholate in the management of canine leishmaniasis. J Vet Intern Med. 2003;17:808-812.
48. Solano-Gallego L, Koutinas A, Miro G, et al. Directions for the diagnosis, clinical staging, treatment and prevention of canine leishmaniosis. Vet Parasitol. 2009;165:1-18.
49. Oliva G, Roura X, Crotti A, et al. Guidelines for treatment of leishmaniasis in dogs. J Am Vet Med Assoc. 2010;236:1192-1198.
50. Frézard F, Demicheli C, Ribeiro RR. Pentavalent antimonials: new perspectives for old drugs. Molecules. 2009;14:2317-2336.
51. Lima MI, Arruda VO, Alves EV, et al. Genotoxic effects of the antileishmanial drug Glucantime. Arch Toxicol. 2010;84:227-232.
52. Manna L, Reale S, Vitale F, et al. Real-time PCR assay in *Leishmania*-infected dogs treated with meglumine antimoniate and allopurinol. Vet J. 2008;177:279-282.
53. Ikeda-Garcia FA, Lopes RS, Ciarlini PC, et al. Evaluation of renal and hepatic functions in dogs naturally infected by visceral leishmaniasis submitted to treatment with meglumine antimoniate. Res Vet Sci. 2007;83:105-108.
54. Bianciardi P, Brovida C, Valente M, et al. Administration of miltefosine and meglumine antimoniate in healthy dogs: clinicopathological evaluation of the impact on the kidneys. Toxicol Pathol. 2009;37:770-775.
55. Kerby BR, Detke S. Reduced purine accumulation is encoded on an amplified DNA in *Leishmania mexicana amazonensis* resistant to toxic nucleosides. Mol Biochem Parasitol. 1993;60:171-185.
56. Ling GV, Case LC, Nelson H, et al. Pharmacokinetics of allopurinol in Dalmatian dogs. J Vet Pharmacol Ther. 1997;20:134-138.
57. Ling GV, Ruby AL, Harrold DR, et al. Xanthine-containing urinary calculi in dogs given allopurinol. J Am Vet Med Assoc. 1991;198:1935-1940.
58. Kim YW, Park BS, Ryu CH, et al. Allopurinol-induced aplastic anemia in a patient with chronic kidney disease. Clin Nephrol. 2009;71:203-206.
59. Fagugli RM, Gentile G, Ferrara G, et al. Acute renal and hepatic failure associated with allopurinol treatment. Clin Nephrol. 2008;70:523-526.
60. Plevraki K, Koutinas AF, Kaldrymidou H, et al. Effects of allopurinol treatment on the progression of chronic nephritis in canine leishmaniosis (*Leishmania infantum*). J Vet Intern Med. 2006;20:228-233.
61. Miró G, Oliva G, Cruz I, et al. Multicentric, controlled clinical study to evaluate effectiveness and safety of miltefosine and allopurinol for canine leishmaniosis. Vet Dermatol. 2009;20:397-404.
62. Manna L, Vitale F, Reale S, et al. Study of efficacy of miltefosine and allopurinol in dogs with leishmaniosis. Vet J. 2009;182:441-445.
63. Andrade HM, Toledo VP, Pinheiro MB, et al. Evaluation of miltefosine for the treatment of dogs naturally infected with *L. infantum* (=*L. chagasi*) in Brazil. Vet Parasitol. 2011;181:83-90.
64. World Health Organization. Report of a WHO informal consultation on liposomal amphotericin B in the treatment of visceral leishmaniosis. 2007. http://www.who.int/entity/neglected_diseases/resources/AmBisomeReport.pdf: Last accessed January 25, 2013.
65. Woerly V, Maynard L, Sanquer A, et al. Clinical efficacy and tolerance of miltefosine in the treatment of canine leishmaniosis. Parasitol Res. 2009;105:463-469.
66. Mateo M, Maynard L, Vischer C, et al. Comparative study on the short term efficacy and adverse effects of miltefosine and meglumine antimoniate in dogs with natural leishmaniosis. Parasitol Res. 2009;105:155-162.
67. Wilkinson SR, Taylor MC, Horn D, et al. A mechanism for cross-resistance to nifurtimox and benznidazole in trypanosomes. Proc Natl Acad Sci U S A. 2008;105:5022-5027.
68. Castro JA, de Mecca MM, Bartel LC. Toxic side effects of drugs used to treat Chagas' disease (American trypanosomiasis). Hum Exp Toxicol. 2006;25:471-479.
69. Barr SC. Canine Chagas' disease (American trypanosomiasis) in North America. Vet Clin North Am Small Anim Pract. 2009;39:1055-1064:v-vi.

SECTION 3

Basic Principles for Infection Control

Jane E. Sykes and J. Scott Weese

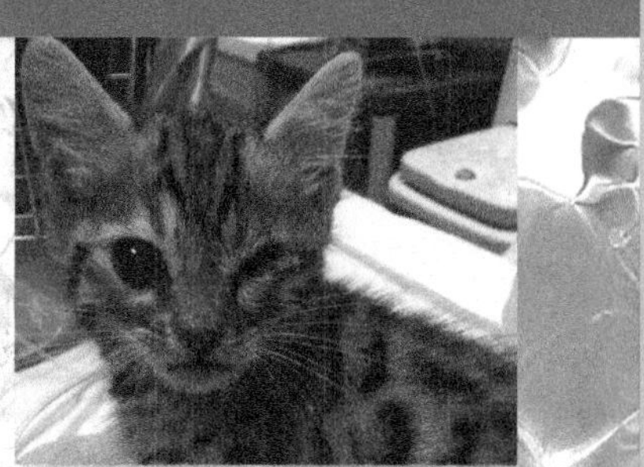

CHAPTER 11

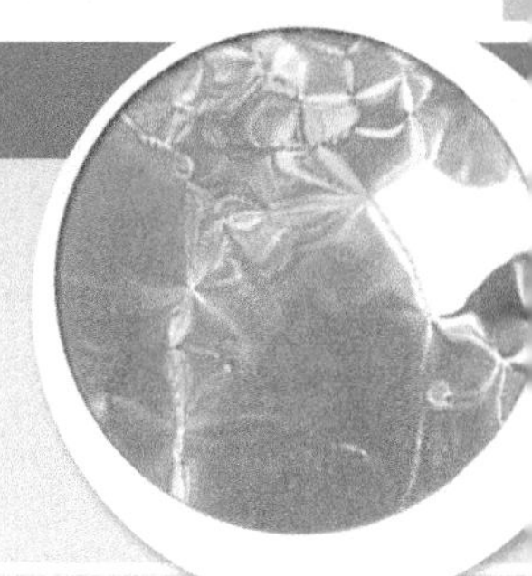

Infection Control Programs for Dogs and Cats

Jane E. Sykes and J. Scott Weese

KEY POINTS

- A hospital infection control program consists of infectious disease control personnel, a written protocol, training, and documentation. The aim of such a program is to reduce the incidence of hospital-acquired infections among patients, staff, and visitors to a small animal hospital.
- The infection control program describes the requirement for practices that optimize hygiene such as hand washing, the use of protective clothing, cleaning and disinfection, and appropriate disposal of infectious agents. The protocol can also be used to educate staff about specific transmission precautions for infectious diseases seen within a practice.
- This chapter describes the infection control program and important components of an infection control protocol, including the advantages and disadvantages of various methods of sterilization, disinfection, and antisepsis used in small animal hospitals.
- Information in this chapter also has relevance to infection control in shelters and in breeding and boarding facilities.

INTRODUCTION

The primary role of an infection control program is to reduce the incidence of hospital-acquired infections (HAIs) by patients, staff, and visitors to a small animal hospital. Infection control programs in veterinary hospitals have largely evolved from evidence and protocols from the human health care setting, together with our understanding of transmission pathways for veterinary pathogens. In recent years, several factors have led to an increased rate of adoption of infection control programs by veterinary hospitals, such as an increased prevalence of multidrug-resistant bacterial infections among small animal patients, the appearance of more studies that support the common occurrence of transmission of hospital-associated and zoonotic pathogens in the veterinary setting, the requirement for an infection control program in veterinary teaching hospitals for accreditation purposes, and increased scrutiny of hospital-associated and zoonotic infections to protect hospitals against litigation.

Infection Control Programs

Every small animal hospital should have an infection control program. At a minimum, this should consist of an infectious disease control officer, a written infection control protocol, regular training of staff, and documents that record all training and surveillance efforts. In large hospitals, formation of an infectious disease control committee may be required. In this situation, the infectious disease control committee could consist of an internist or criticalist with an interest or training in infectious diseases, a veterinary clinical microbiologist, a nursing supervisor, a safety officer, the hospital administrator, and the hospital director. There should be adequate personnel and communication so that proper coverage is maintained when one individual is absent or unavailable. All personnel who work in a veterinary hospital, as well as visitors, should be familiar with the infectious disease control personnel as well as procedures and policies listed in the infection control protocol. Documentation of training should be maintained for all hospital personnel.

The Hospital Infection Control Protocol

The objective of a hospital infection control protocol is to provide a standard procedure for the control of infectious diseases in the hospital, in order to minimize animal-to-animal, animal-to-human, and human-to-animal transmission of pathogens. Adherence to the infection control protocol can also reduce transmission of infectious agents between personnel through increased hand washing and reduction of fomite contamination. The infection control protocol is a legal document and should be regularly updated by a designated hospital infection control officer or committee. Each hospital should develop a protocol that is tailored to address specific practice requirements and the hospital design, purpose, and equipment used. Additional special precautions may need to be described for hospitals that see avian and exotic pet animal species, and in geographic locations where serious zoonotic diseases such as rabies and plague are endemic (see Chapters 13 and 55).

The infection control protocol details practices that optimize hygiene such as hand washing, the use of protective clothing, cleaning and disinfection, and appropriate disposal of infectious agents. Specific infectious disease control procedures to be followed in different areas of the hospital (radiology, surgery, the intensive care unit, isolation, wards) can be included, as well as policies on antimicrobial use. The protocol can also be used to educate staff about routes of transmission, the potential for zoonotic transmission, specific transmission precautions for infectious diseases that are seen within the practice, and immunization requirements, such as those for rabies (see Chapter 13).

Standard Precautions

All animals that enter a veterinary hospital are potential carriers of pathogens that may be spread to other animals or people. Animals may be colonized with multidrug-resistant bacteria, often without showing evidence of disease due to these organisms. Pet owners may carry these organisms on their hands and clothing. Standard precautions such as hand hygiene and the wearing of routine protective clothing can minimize the spread of these bacteria around the hospital and to immunocompromised animals.

Hand Hygiene

Frequent and proper hand and wrist washing to remove transient flora on the hands has been proven as the most important component for prevention of the spread of infectious diseases in human hospitals.[1] Signs that outline proper hand-washing technique, including the use of paper towels to turn off the faucet, posted adjacent to basins around the hospital can improve compliance among staff. Online videos that demonstrate proper hand-washing technique are available for educational purposes.[2] Guidelines for hand washing are shown in Box 11-1. Antibacterial soap should be used, and all surfaces of the hands should be rubbed together, which should include the backs of the hands, between the fingers, and under the fingernails, for a total hand-washing time of at least 20 seconds. In order to prevent chapped skin, which can harbor bacteria, water used for hand washing should not be too hot, and hand lotion should be applied regularly. Behaviors such as keeping fingernails short, avoidance of artificial and/or polished fingernails or hand jewelry, or wearing jewelry on a chain around the neck instead of on the hand can be encouraged. Meticulous hand hygiene is particularly important for personnel who work frequently with immunocompromised animals, such as emergency and critical care personnel. The use of touch-free taps and paper towel dispensers can also reduce transmission of bacteria during hand washing.

Alcohol-based hand sanitizers are a more convenient form of sanitization. These can be provided in multiple locations around a hospital, or travel-sized bottles can be carried in a coat pocket. At least one to two full pumps or a 3-cm diameter pool of the product should be dispensed onto one palm. All surfaces of the hands and wrists should be rubbed with the product until it has dried. Use of soap and water, rather than hand sanitizer, is recommended when there is gross contamination with organic matter, or when exposure to alcohol-resistant pathogens such as *Clostridium* spp. spores or parvovirus might have occurred. However, the availability of hand sanitizers improves compliance in busy hospital situations, is associated with lower rates of dermatitis than medicated soaps, and is recommended for routine hand sanitation in human health care settings by the Centers for Disease Control and Prevention (CDC) and the World Health Organization (WHO).[3,4]

The use of gloves prevents contamination of the hands with microorganisms, prevents exposure to bloodborne pathogens, and reduces the risk of transmission of microorganisms from personnel to animals. However, gloves are not a substitute for proper hand hygiene. Guidelines for wearing disposable gloves are shown in Box 11-1. Gloves should be promptly removed after use, before other surfaces are touched, and hands should then be washed. If a glove is torn or punctured, it should be removed and replaced as soon as possible.

BOX 11-1

Guidelines for Hand Washing and the Wearing of Disposable Gloves

Situations That Require Hand Washing

Immediately before handling a patient
Immediately after handling a patient
Immediately before and after procedures that involve nonintact skin
Before and after gloves are worn for procedures
After blood, body fluids, secretions, excretions, or contaminated items are touched
After cages are cleaned
Before and after eating, smoking, or leaving the hospital
After going to the restroom

Situations When Disposable Gloves Should Be Worn

Contact with broken skin and bodily fluids (blood, urine, and feces)
Handling of disinfectants
Handling of animals with suspected or known infectious diseases
Handling of all animals for immunocompromised people

Hospital Attire

Nonsurgical Areas

Staff should be encouraged to wear dedicated hospital attire that is not worn elsewhere, so that hospital pathogens are not transported to and from locations outside the hospital. At the minimum, protective clothing such as clean laboratory coats or hospital scrubs and closed-toe shoes must be worn in nonsurgical areas. Sleeves must be short enough or rolled up to expose the wrists, and laboratory coats changed whenever gross soiling occurs. In the absence of gross soiling, coats should be changed daily. If neckties are worn, they must be secured in place by an outer layer of clothing or a tie pin so that they cannot be contaminated as a result of contact with patients or environmental

TABLE 11-1

Transmission Precautions for Selected Infectious Diseases of Dogs and Cats

	Infectious agent	Specific precautions
Airborne	*Mycobacterium tuberculosis* *Yersinia pestis* *Francisella tularensis*	Isolation, preferably in negative pressure facility Properly fitted N95 respirator masks Contact precautions
Droplet	Canine and feline transmissible respiratory disease pathogens (e.g., canine distemper virus, canine respiratory coronavirus, feline herpesvirus-1, feline calicivirus)	Isolation Space animals at least 4 feet apart Contact precautions
Contact	Multidrug-resistant bacteria Dermatophytes *Leptospira* spp. *Salmonella* spp. Parvoviruses	Warning signage Gown, gloves, dedicated equipment Isolation for select pathogens (see Box 11-2) Limitation of movement Standard hand hygiene precautions Proper cleaning, disinfection, and disposal of medical waste

surfaces and act as fomites, as has been shown to occur in human hospital environments.[5] Long hair must be tied back so that it does not drape on animals and hospital surfaces. Face shields and a clean gown should be worn during procedures that are likely to generate splashes or sprays of blood and body fluids. Gowns must be made of impervious material and tied on securely and correctly. Soiled gowns must be removed as soon as they are no longer required and face shields cleaned.

Surgical Areas

Dedicated operating room attire should be worn in surgical areas and should be changed after gross soilage and when leaving the operating room for the day. Caps and masks should be worn and hands thoroughly washed on entry to the operating room. There is no evidence that dedicated footwear or foot protection should be worn for prevention of surgical site infections in human patients, and major human guidelines do not advocate that footwear be addressed.[6] Protective wear should be removed whenever staff members leave the operating room. Traffic in and out of the operating room should be limited to the minimum required for patient care.

General Animal Handling Precautions

All animals seen at a veterinary hospital should undergo a history and physical examination by a veterinarian to determine the likelihood and nature of any transmissible infections that might be present. Ideally, client beds, blankets, collars, and leashes should not be brought into the hospital, where they could become contaminated. Animals should always be placed in cages that have been cleaned and disinfected appropriately. Disposable thermometer sleeves should always be used on thermometers. Equipment should not be shared between animals unless it has been cleaned and disinfected. Diets that contain raw meat and bones should not be fed or stored in the hospital, because they commonly contain and can potentially transmit foodborne gastrointestinal pathogens.[7] The handling of sick animals should be minimized, unless required for patient care.

Because some infections can be transmitted through bites and scratches, staff should be educated on bite and scratch avoidance, such as the use of restraint devices, protective gloves, and warning signage on cages and medical records. Should bites or scratches occur, they should be vigorously flushed and immediately washed with water and chlorhexidine or a dilute iodophor solution, and the bite reported to appropriate officials as necessary. Deep wounds could be irrigated with pressure using a syringe without an attached needle. If a bite occurs, medical attention should be sought as soon as possible. All bites or scratches must be documented and consideration be given as to why the injury occurred, so that procedures or training to prevent future injuries can be implemented if necessary.

Consumption of food and drink should be limited to parts of a hospital where patient care and the handling of biologic specimens and medications do not occur. Food and beverages should not be left out open on benches for long periods. Microwaves used for animal care purposes should not be used to heat food intended for people.

Transmission-Based Precautions

Transmission-based precautions are instituted for selected patients that are confirmed to be or suspected to be infected or colonized with important transmissible pathogens. Transmission-based precautions are used in combination with standard precautions. In the human hospital setting, three types of transmission-based precautions have been developed—airborne, droplet, and contact precautions (Table 11-1).[8] *Airborne precautions* are used to prevent the transmission of diseases by droplet nuclei (particles <5 μm). Transmission by droplet nuclei occurs with diseases such as measles, varicella, and pulmonary tuberculosis. The precautions for human patients involve isolation in a single-bed, negative-pressure room and the wearing of high-density respirator (N95) masks. These resemble surgical masks but filter 1-μm particles with an efficiency of at least 95% and must be properly fitted. Airborne contact precautions are rarely necessary in hospitals that treat only dogs and cats, but could be considered when animals suspected to have pneumonic plague, tularemia, or *Mycobacterium tuberculosis* infection. *Droplet precautions* are used to prevent transmission by large-particle aerosols and do not require a negative-pressure room. Droplet precautions apply to dogs and cats with transmissible respiratory disease. *Contact precautions* are indicated for animals with infections that can be transmitted by direct contact with the patient or through fomite contact.

If it is known in advance that an animal with a suspected or known transmissible disease is to be seen at the hospital, arrangements should be made to have the pet owner take the animal from the parking area directly to an examination room, so that the animal does not contaminate the waiting area. After the animal has been examined, appropriate signage should be placed on the door of the examination room to prevent use until it has been properly cleaned and disinfected.

If hospitalization is required, animals with known or suspected transmissible disease must be admitted either to an isolation ward or to regular hospital cages with handling precautions, based on the pathogen suspected. Immediately after hospitalization, the name of the suspected or known pathogen should be posted on the cage or run, together with a handling precautions notice. Animals that require contact precautions should be placed in cages away from other animals in the ward and should not be moved from one cage to another, unless there is a medical need. Animals with transmissible respiratory disease should be placed in isolation and separated both horizontally and vertically from other patients by at least 4 feet. Gloves and a gown should be put on before the patient is handled, and then removed and disposed of immediately afterward. Hands should be washed after the gloves are removed. Additional items of personal protective equipment (masks, gowns, gloves, booties) may be required in some circumstances. Soiled linen and equipment should be handled, transported, and processed in a manner that prevents skin and mucous membrane exposures and contamination of clothing and that avoids transfer of microorganisms to other patients and environments. All equipment that contacts the patient (scales, examination tables, stethoscope heads, floor) should be cleaned and disinfected immediately after use. Medications and fluids from these patients should not be returned to the hospital pharmacy. When possible, personnel who handle these animals should not work with other immunosuppressed animals in the hospital, or they should work with the infectious disease cases last. If animals with contact precautions must be moved within the hospital, personnel should ensure that precautions are maintained throughout and that equipment and environmental surfaces that come into contact with the patient are properly disinfected and/or disposed of. The cleaning and bandaging of wounds infected with multidrug-resistant bacteria should be conducted in low-traffic areas that can be properly cleaned and disinfected.

The owners of dogs and cats that have transmissible diseases should be provided with general information regarding the risk of disease transmission to in-contact animals and people that includes the mode of transmission, duration of organism shedding, and if there are special implications for young children or other immunosuppressed individuals. If dogs and cats are diagnosed with a zoonotic disease, the owners should be notified without delay. The owners should be told to see their physicians if they become unwell or, in some circumstances, immediately, and to advise a physician of the potential exposure.

Isolation

In contrast to human hospitals where patients can be more readily isolated in single-bed rooms or cubicles, isolation of veterinary patients can be more difficult because of the close proximity of one animal to another. Floor contamination with secretions and excretions can also occur more readily. Isolation rooms are available in many veterinary hospitals, but they may be poorly visible and/or accessible and may not provide access to an oxygen source or be amenable to intensive monitoring and care. For some animals (especially puppies and kittens) suspected to have a transmissible disease, housing in a general ward or ICU area with as much physical and procedural separation as possible, and with strict infection control practices, may be acceptable (if perhaps not optimal). Once a diagnosis is confirmed, the animal should be moved immediately to isolation whenever possible. Patients chosen for strict isolation vary based on the specific situation and facilities available, but suggestions are provided in Box 11-2.

Only the individuals directly involved in the care of the patient should enter isolation. Pet owners should not be allowed into the isolation ward. No equipment used outside isolation (pens, thermometers, stethoscopes, cell phones) should be brought into isolation. Laboratory coats should be removed, and personnel must put on protective wear such as a disposable gown, gloves, and booties when entering the isolation ward. Face protection may also be required, depending on the situation. A notice that outlines the required precautions should be posted on the door of isolation. Protective clothing should be removed before leaving isolation, and hands should be washed. Once a patient has been discharged, the room should be properly disinfected.

Handling of Potentially Infectious Materials and Waste

The risk of human infection from patient blood and body fluids in small animal hospitals is clearly lower than that in human hospitals. However, a number of zoonotic pathogens have the potential to be spread from dogs or cats to humans through contact with medical waste, and a number of emerging zoonotic infectious agents are bloodborne. Examples include *Bartonella* spp., *Anaplasma phagocytophilum*, *Brucella* spp., and hemoplasmas. Proper handling of blood and body fluids also has the potential to protect staff against as-yet-unrecognized zoonotic pathogens. Improper disposal of medical waste in veterinary hospitals risks injuring others who handle the waste and has the potential to result in serious penalties or fines.

Potentially contaminated waste should be disposed of in an approved plastic bag in a container labeled on all exposed sides

BOX 11-2

Examples of Infectious Agents of Dogs and Cats for Which Strict Isolation Is Indicated

- *Salmonella* spp.
- *Francisella tularensis*
- *Yersinia pestis*
- *Mycobacterium tuberculosis* or *Mycobacterium bovis*
- *Microsporum canis*
- Rabies virus
- Enteric viruses, such as parvoviruses
- Canine transmissible respiratory disease pathogens (*Bordetella*, canine distemper virus, influenza viruses, canine respiratory coronavirus, canine adenovirus, canine parainfluenza virus)
- Feline upper respiratory tract disease pathogens (feline herpesvirus-1, feline calicivirus, influenza virus, *Chlamydia*)

with "biohazardous waste." Blood-soaked materials, infected materials, and empty fluid bags should all be placed in biohazardous waste containers. Care should be taken not to contaminate the outside of the container during disposal. The lid of the biohazardous waste container must close properly. Blood and body fluids should be inactivated with an appropriate disinfectant (e.g., bleach or accelerated hydrogen peroxide) and allowed to stand for 10 minutes before disposal. Disposal regulations may vary depending on local laws, but liquid waste should not be disposed of into storm drains.

Specimens for laboratory testing that are collected from a patient with suspected zoonotic infectious diseases should be placed in an outer plastic bag, taking care not to contaminate the outside of the plastic bag, and labeled with an appropriate warning label. Fecal material should be picked up using a tongue depressor while wearing gloves, and placed in a sealed plastic cup and clearly labeled. Urine specimens should be submitted in a sealed container.

Sharps Handling

Sharps handling practices receive considerable attention in human medicine because of the risk of transmission of various bloodborne pathogens. Although the risks are less in veterinary medicine, significant injury or illness can follow sharps injuries, such as transmission of infectious agents from the patient, allergic or inflammatory reactions from exposure to medication, and inoculation of opportunistic pathogens from the injured person's own skin microflora. Care should be taken to prevent injuries when needles, scalpels, and other sharp instruments are used, cleaned, or disposed of. Used needles should never be recapped, and they should not be removed from the barrel of a disposable syringe. Personnel should be instructed not to walk with uncapped needles and not to hold syringe or needle caps in the mouth. Used needles should not be carried in a pocket. Animals suspected of having an infectious disease that could be transmitted to humans through a needle-stick injury should be sedated before skin masses or peripheral lymph nodes are aspirated or venipuncture is performed. Contaminated sharps (slides, scalpel blades, broken glass, needles with attached syringes) must immediately be placed into an approved puncture-resistant sharps disposal biohazard container. Personnel who perform necropsy examinations should take care to use sharp knives in the proper manner and to avoid rushed situations. If a contaminated sharps injury occurs, medical attention should be sought immediately if necessary.

Hospital Cleaning, Disinfection, and Sterilization

Definitions

Sterilization refers to complete elimination of all microbes, including bacterial spores, and is accomplished in hospital settings using processes such as pressurized steam, dry heat, ethylene oxide gas, or liquid chemicals.

Disinfection is the process that eliminates many or all microbes from inanimate objects, but not bacterial spores. Factors that influence the efficacy of disinfection include the type of microorganism present, their number, the amount and type of organic matter present, the presence of biofilms, and the porosity of the surface to be disinfected. Some disinfectants kill spores at high concentrations and with prolonged exposure times. These are known as *chemical sterilants*. At low concentrations and short contact times, chemical sterilants inactivate all microbes except large numbers of bacterial spores and are known as *high-level disinfectants*. *Low-level disinfectants* inactivate most vegetative bacteria, some fungi, and enveloped viruses, but not bacterial spores. *Intermediate-level disinfectants* inactivate mycobacteria, vegetative bacteria, most viruses, and most fungi (Tables 11-2 and 11-3).

Antisepsis is the process that reduces the number of microbes from *living tissue and skin*. Disinfectants are rarely used for skin antisepsis because they can injure tissues and skin. *Sanitation* is the reduction in the number of microorganisms *on a surface* to a safe level. *Germicides* are agents that inactivate microorganisms and include disinfectants, antiseptics, and sanitizers.

TABLE 11-2

Characteristics of Selected Disinfectants

Disinfectant Category	Activity in the Presence of Organic Matter	Advantages	Disadvantages	Precautions	Comments
Alcohols: Ethyl alcohol, isopropyl alcohol	Rapidly inactivated	Fast-acting No residue Relatively nontoxic	Rapid evaporation	Flammable	Not appropriate for routine environmental disinfection Primarily used as antiseptics
Aldehydes: Formaldehyde, glutaraldehyde	Good	Broad spectrum Relatively noncorrosive	Highly toxic	Irritant Carcinogenic Requires ventilation	Used as an aqueous solution or as a gas (fumigation)
Alkalis: Ammonia			Unpleasant odor Irritating	Do not mix with bleach.	Not recommended for general use
Biguanides: Chlorhexidine	Rapidly inactivated	Nontoxic	Incompatible with anionic detergents		Not appropriate for environmental disinfection Primarily used as antiseptics

Continued

TABLE 11-2

Characteristics of Selected Disinfectants—cont'd

Disinfectant Category	Activity in the Presence of Organic Matter	Advantages	Disadvantages	Precautions	Comments
Halogens: Hypochlorites (bleach)	Rapidly inactivated	Broad spectrum, sporicidal Inexpensive Can be used on food preparation surfaces	Inactivated by cationic soaps/ detergents and sunlight. Frequent application required.	Corrosive Irritant May produce toxic gas when mixed with other chemicals	Used to disinfect clean environmental surfaces Only commonly available sporicidal disinfectant
Oxidizing agents	Good	Broad spectrum Environmentally friendly	Breakdown with time	Corrosive	Excellent choice for environmental disinfection
Phenolics	Good	Broad spectrum Noncorrosive Stable in storage	Toxic to cats Unpleasant odor Incompatible with cationic or non-ionic detergents	Irritant	Some residual activity after drying
Quaternary ammonium compounds (QUATs)	Moderate	Stable in storage Nonirritating to skin Low toxicity Can be used on food preparation surfaces Effective at high temperatures and pH	Incompatible with anionic detergents		Commonly used primary environmental disinfectant Some residual activity after drying

Source: Modified from the Canadian Committee on Antibiotic Resistance. Infection Prevention and Control Best Practices for Small Animal Veterinary Clinics, 2008; http://www.wormsandgermsblog.com/2008/04/promo/services/infection-prevention-and-control-best-practices-for-small-animal-veterinary-clinics/. Last accessed May 15, 2012.

TABLE 11-3

Antimicrobial Spectrum of Selected Disinfectants

Agent	Alcohols	Aldehydes	Alkalis: Ammonia	Biguanides: Chlorhexidine	Halogens: Hypochlorite (Bleach)	Oxidizing Agents	Phenolics	Quaternary Ammonium Compounds
Mycoplasmas	++	++	++	++	++	++	++	+
Gram-positive bacteria	++	++	+	++	++	++	++	++
Gram-negative bacteria	++	++	+	+	++	++	++	+
Pseudomonads	++	++	+	±	++	++	++	±
Enveloped viruses	+	++	+	++	++	++	++	+
Non-enveloped viruses	–	+	±	–	++	+	±*	–
Fungal spores	±	+	+	±	+	±	+	±
Mycobacteria	+	++	+	–	+	±	++	–
Bacterial spores	–	+	±	–	++	+	–	–

++, Highly effective; +, Effective; ±, Limited activity; –, No activity.

*In general, phenols are not active against non-enveloped viruses but they do have some activity against rotaviruses. Activity against parvoviruses has not been documented.

Examples of microorganisms from each category:

Mycoplasmas: *Mycoplasma cynos*, *Mycoplasma felis*; **Gram-positive bacteria:** *Staphylococcus* spp., *Streptococcus* spp.; **Gram-negative bacteria:** *Bordetella bronchiseptica*, *Salmonella* spp.; **Pseudomonads:** *Pseudomonas aeruginosa*; **Enveloped viruses:** influenza virus, herpesvirus; **Non-enveloped viruses:** feline panleukopenia virus, canine parvovirus, feline calicivirus; **Fungal spores:** *Aspergillus* spp.; **Acid-fast bacteria:** *Mycobacterium fortuitum*; **Bacterial spores:** *Clostridium difficile*, *Clostridium perfringens*.

Source: Modified from the Canadian Committee on Antibiotic Resistance. Infection Prevention and Control Best Practices for Small Animal Veterinary Clinics, 2008; http://www.wormsandgermsblog.com/2008/04/promo/services/infection-prevention-and-control-best-practices-for-small-animal-veterinary-clinics/. Last accessed May 15, 2012.

TABLE 11-4

Recommended Conditions for Heat Sterilization

	Conditions	Time
Gravity displacement steam sterilization	121°C (250°F), 106 kPa (15 lb/in^2)* 132°C (270°F), 30 lb/in^2	30 min wrapped items, 20 min unwrapped 15 min wrapped items
High-speed prevacuum steam sterilization	132°C (270°F), 30 lb/in^2	4 min
Dry heat sterilization	160°C (320°F) 170°C (340°F)	2 hours at temperature, 3 to 3.5 hours with cooling 1 hour at temperature, 2 to 2.5 hours with cooling

*Pressure settings may vary between incubators. When possible, follow manufacturer's recommendations.

Cleaning involves the removal of all visible organic and inorganic material from objects and surfaces through the use of manual or mechanical processes and detergent or enzymatic solutions.

According to the Spaulding method of classification, items to be sterilized or disinfected can be grouped into *critical, semicritical,* and *noncritical* items.[9] Critical items enter tissue or the vascular system, or devices through which blood flows. Critical items require sterilization before they can be used. Semicritical items are items that contact mucous membranes or nonintact skin and include endoscopes and balloon dilation catheters. These generally require high-level disinfection. Noncritical items are items that contact intact skin. Noncritical items generally require low-level or intermediate-level disinfection and contact times of 1 to 10 minutes.[9]

All personnel should be educated regarding the standard hospital germicides used for disinfection and antisepsis, how they should be diluted and applied, and the hazards associated with their use. Gloves and eye protection should be worn when disinfectant solutions are handled or mixed. In large hospitals, posters on hospital walls can be used to guide selection of appropriate germicides for different situations. Disinfectant solution should be readily accessible throughout the hospital. Because mops can spread infection, cotton mops should be laundered daily, or mops with detachable microfiber heads should be used. Microfiber heads absorb a large amount of water and are not returned to the mop bucket after use. They can be laundered and reused the following day.

Methods of Sterilization

Steam sterilization. Steam sterilization involves the use of saturated steam under pressure in an autoclave to achieve sterilization. This is the most effective form of sterilization, is nontoxic and inexpensive, and as a result is the most widely used as well. The use of steam under pressure allows lower temperatures to be used for shorter periods of time when compared with dry heat sterilization (Table 11-4). The most common temperatures used for steam sterilization are 121°C (250°F) and 132°C (270°F). Cycle times vary depending on the autoclave used and whether items are wrapped or unwrapped, but are generally less than 30 minutes (see Table 11-4). There are two basic types of autoclaves: gravity displacement autoclaves, and high-speed prevacuum sterilizers. Gravity displacement autoclaves admit steam at the top or sides of the autoclave, which displaces air through a drain vent at the bottom of the chamber (Figure 11-1). High-speed prevacuum sterilizers rapidly pump air out of the sterilizer before steam is admitted. This leads to rapid penetration of steam into all surfaces. As a result, cycle times can be reduced to less than 15 minutes. Drying times are also reduced with prevacuum sterilizers.

Sterilizers should be located away from potential sources of contamination, such as sinks, trash disposal, or high-traffic areas. Before steam sterilization is performed, instruments should be cleaned thoroughly to remove organic and inorganic material, and then dried. All jointed items should be opened or unlocked, and items should not be crowded in the autoclave, so that steam can circulate freely. At least 3 inches should be left between the autoclave wall and items to be sterilized. The manufacturer's instructions for autoclave operation should be followed.

The efficacy of autoclaving must be tested for every autoclaved item, with additional quality control performed on a periodic basis. Autoclave indicator tape is routinely used; although this only indicates conditions on the outside of the package. Steam indicator strips should be included in each surgical pack and evaluated by the person opening the pack. Biological indicators provide a more definitive assessment of autoclave efficacy and should be used periodically (e.g., weekly) and the results documented. These consist of a standardized population of bacterial spores, usually on a filter paper strip or contained within a vial. The strip is then sent to the microbiology laboratory for culture, or cultured in-house, to ensure that the spores have been completely inactivated by the sterilization process. Any indicator failure should result in immediate inspection of the autoclave. Sterilization indicators should never be used as a substitute for proper autoclave operation and careful preparation, packing, and loading of equipment to be sterilized.

After steam sterilization, instruments should be allowed to dry before they are removed, which typically takes an additional 30 minutes. Items should then be stored in a location and manner that prevents further contamination.

Flash sterilization. Flash sterilization refers to the rapid sterilization of unwrapped instruments and is usually performed as an emergency procedure in an operating room setting when time is insufficient to perform the preferred sterilization of wrapped items. In general it is performed for 3 minutes at 270°F and 27 to 28 lb/in^2. Each instrument must be carefully protected to ensure it does not become recontaminated during transport back to the operating room, usually in a "flash pan." Flash sterilization has occasionally been associated with intraoperative infections and should not be used for routine disinfection purposes.

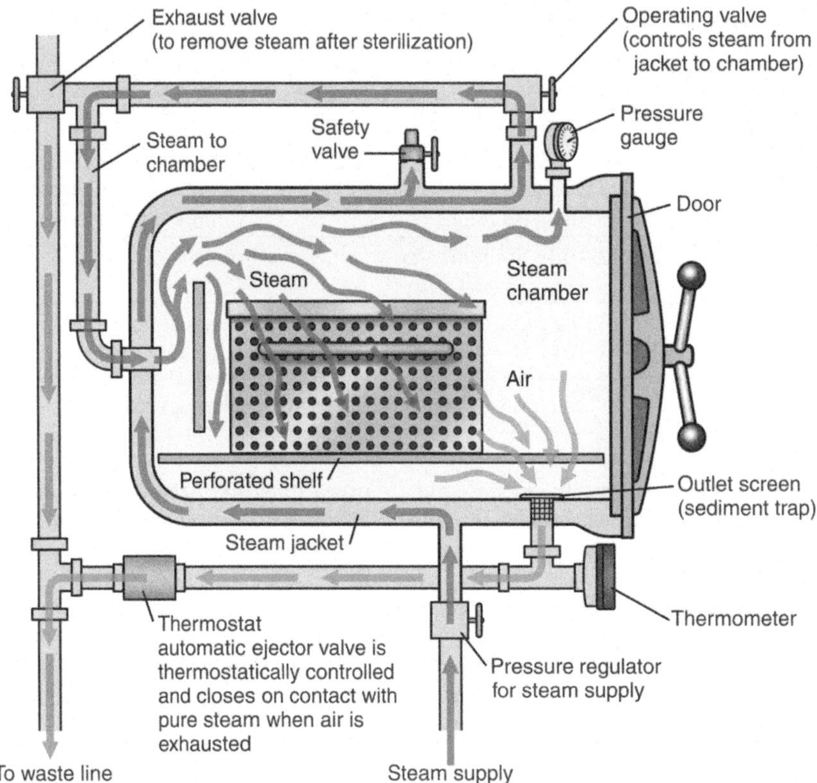

FIGURE 11-1 Gravity displacement sterilization. Steam is admitted at the top or sides of the autoclave, which displaces air through a drain vent at the bottom of the chamber.

Gas sterilization. Gas sterilization is used for sterilization of heat- and moisture-sensitive instruments but can have significant toxicity. Gases that can be used for sterilization include formaldehyde, ethylene oxide (ETO), hydrogen peroxide vapor, and ozone gases. The most commonly used gas in veterinary medicine, ETO, has strong alkylating properties and causes protein coagulation, enzyme inactivation, and damage to nucleic acid. When compared with heat sterilization, ETO sterilization takes longer (24 hours or more including the time required to allow ETO to diffuse out of packages at the end of sterilization) and is more expensive. In addition, it only achieves surface sterilization and requires sophisticated equipment and trained staff. The gas is extremely flammable, irritates the eyes and mucous membranes, is mutagenic and carcinogenic, and has a misleadingly pleasant smell.

Irradiation. Gamma irradiation uses a cobalt-60 radiation source to destroy microorganisms through generation of high-energy photons. Health care product manufacturers use gamma irradiation to sterilize disposable medical supplies, such as catheters, gloves, syringes, and pharmaceuticals.

Chemical sterilants. Chemical sterilants are used when heat or ETO gas sterilization is not available or would otherwise damage instruments, such as endoscopes or laparoscopes. Disinfectants that act as sterilants when they are used at high concentrations and for adequate contact periods include certain solutions that contain glutaraldehyde (e.g., >2.4% glutaraldehyde solutions, 0.95% glutaraldehyde with 1.64% phenol/phenate), 0.55% *ortho*-phthalaldehyde (OPA), 7.5% hydrogen peroxide, or greater than or equal to 0.2% peracetic acid (see section on Disinfectants following). Chemical sterilants must be rinsed repeatedly with sterile water and dried once sterilization is complete. Chemical sterilants must be used with the proper contact times and at the right concentration. Solutions may lose efficacy, become diluted, or become contaminated with bacteria over time. They should be replaced frequently according to the manufacturer's recommendations, and they should never be used in procedures that involve sterile body sites unless there is no other sterilizing option.

Disinfectants

Glutaraldehyde. Glutaraldehyde is a saturated dialdehyde. Glutaraldehyde solutions are relatively inexpensive, are noncorrosive, and can be used to disinfect rubber, plastics, and endoscopic equipment. Aqueous solutions require activation by alkalinization to a pH of 7.5 to 8.5 for sporicidal activity to occur. When alkalinized glutaraldehyde is used at a concentration of 2.4% for adequate periods of time, either chemical sterilization or high-level disinfection occurs, depending on the contact time (e.g., Cidex). Contact times of at least 20 minutes (at or above 20°C) are effective for high-level disinfection. Sterilization requires a 10-hour contact time and higher concentrations of glutaraldehyde (e.g., Cidex Plus, which contains 3.4% glutaraldehyde), or formulations that combine glutaraldehyde with another disinfectant.

Once activated, 2.4% glutaraldehyde solution retains activity for 14 days, provided inadvertent dilution does not occur. The solution is active in the presence of 2% organic matter. Inadvertent dilution can occur when endoscopes that contain fluid within their channels are immersed in the solution. Test strips are available from the manufacturer to monitor the activity of the solution, but should not be used to extend the solution's expiration date. They indicate inactivity when the concentration drops below 1.5%, the minimum concentration required for activity.

Glutaraldehyde irritates mucous membranes of the respiratory and gastrointestinal tracts, and so endoscopes must be rinsed properly after disinfection. It can also cause allergic contact dermatitis, but it is not mutagenic or carcinogenic. The wearing of nitrile rubber or butyl rubber gloves is recommended. Because of its relative expense and toxicity, it is not used to disinfect noncritical surfaces.

***ortho*-Phthalaldehyde.** OPA (e.g., Cidex OPA) is favored over glutaraldehyde for high-level disinfection in the United States, because it does not require activation, is stable over a wide pH range, does not cause irritation of mucous membranes, and it has a barely perceptible odor. Its activity is greater than that of glutaraldehyde, and high-level disinfection is achieved with a contact time of 12 minutes at or above 20°C.[10,11] The primary disadvantage of OPA is that it stains tissues and mucous membranes gray. Protective equipment must be worn when handling the solution, and it must be rinsed thoroughly from items after treatment. Irritation can occur with eye contact. OPA is also more expensive than glutaraldehyde.[12] Solutions can be reused for a maximum of 14 days.

Hydrogen peroxide. Hydrogen peroxide (H_2O_2) is a potent oxidizer. Hydrogen peroxide solutions are widely available, are inexpensive, and can enhance removal of organic matter. When used at concentrations of 7.5% for contact periods of at least 6 hours, hydrogen peroxide is a chemical sterilant (e.g., Sporox). High-level disinfection can be achieved with contact times of 12 to 30 minutes. Unfortunately 7.5% hydrogen peroxide causes discoloration and functional changes within endoscopes and so is not suitable for endoscope reprocessing. Although nonirritating to mucous membranes, serious ocular damage can occur with eye contact.

Accelerated hydrogen peroxide (AHP) is a patented hydrogen peroxide solution that contains surfactants, an acid, and hydrogen peroxide. Use of a 4.5% AHP gel with contact times of 10 minutes can inactivate bacterial spores.[13] Even 0.5% solutions have some sporicidal activity and can inactivate non-enveloped viruses such as canine parvovirus.[14,15] AHP has gained popularity as a disinfectant among health care institutions because it is odorless, does not generate volatile gas, is nonirritating, and is noncorrosive at dilutions used in health care settings.

Peracetic acid. Peracetic acid belongs to the peroxygen family of compounds. When used at 50°C to 56°C in a specific peracetic acid reprocessing system (Steris System 1, Steris), 0.2% solutions achieve sterilization in very short time periods (30 to 45 minutes). Peracetic acid is active in the presence of organic matter and may actually enhance its removal. Nevertheless endoscopes must still be thoroughly cleaned before sterilization to avoid fixation of blood onto the instrument. After sterilization, the processor rinses the instrument thoroughly. Peracetic acid is stable but can be corrosive and causes discoloration of endoscopes over time. It is more expensive than other chemical sterilants. Peracetic acid concentrates can cause irritation to mucous membranes and are corrosive to the eye and skin, but 0.2% solutions are generally nonirritating.

Potassium peroxymonosulfate (Trifectant, Virkon S). Like peracetic acid, potassium peroxymonosulfate is an oxidizing agent, and 1% solutions are high-level disinfectants that are capable of inactivation of non-enveloped viruses when contact times of 10 minutes are used.[16] Thus it is suitable for inactivation of canine parvovirus and feline calicivirus. Potassium peroxymonosulfate retains some activity in the presence of organic matter. Solutions are prepared from powder and remain active for 7 days. The powder is corrosive and can cause serious skin and ocular burns, but the solution is nonirritating and less corrosive than bleach. The solution stains fabric and may damage surfaces, particularly metal, over time if rinsing is not performed.

Sodium Hypochlorite (Bleach). Household bleach, which contains 5.25% to 6.15% sodium hypochlorite, is widely available, inexpensive, and active in the presence of hard water. When used at a 1:10 dilution for a 10-minute contact time, household bleach is sporicidal but is irritating and can be highly corrosive to metal surfaces. This 1:10 dilution is used to control outbreaks of clostridial diarrhea. For most hospital situations, 1:30 to 1:50 dilutions of household bleach provide more than 1000 ppm available chlorine and are effective for intermediate-level disinfection. Noncritical surfaces can be disinfected with 1:500 dilutions of household bleach (>100 ppm available chlorine), with contact times of at least 1 minute. Sodium hypochlorite is inactivated by organic matter, so cleaning is required before disinfection is performed. Solutions lose 50% of their activity over a 1-month period unless they are stored in closed brown bottles. Other disadvantages of bleach solutions are bleaching of colored fabric and the release of toxic chlorine gas when they are combined with other disinfectants such as quaternary ammonium compounds (QUATs).

Quaternary Ammonium Compounds. QUATs are often used as low-level disinfectants for noncritical surfaces in health care facilities. Although they are generally fungicidal, bactericidal, and virucidal for enveloped viruses, some bacteria resist and even grow within QUATs, and such contamination has resulted in HAIs.[17] Contact times vary by product so manufacturer recommendations should be followed; however, 10-minute contact times are often used. Advantages of QUATs include their low cost, high stability, and low toxicity. QUATs are inactivated by hard water, organic materials, soaps, and detergents.

Phenolics. Phenolics are one of the oldest known disinfectant classes. Phenol derivatives that are available for hospital disinfection include *ortho*-phenylphenol and *ortho*-benzyl-*para*-chlorophenol (e.g., Qualitrol, Vetnex). Effective contact times vary with the product. They are active against enveloped viruses and bacteria, but they are not sporicidal and have limited activity against fungi and non-enveloped viruses. Phenol derivatives are active in the presence of organic matter and hard water, are stable, and are noncorrosive. They irritate skin and mucous membranes, and have the potential to be highly toxic if ingested by cats. Because of these limitations and the availability of other effective disinfectants, phenolics are rarely used in veterinary hospitals.

Antiseptics

Alcohol. Ethyl alcohol and isopropyl alcohol are bactericidal, virucidal (for enveloped viruses), and variably fungicidal. The optimum bactericidal concentration is 60% to 90% in water (volume/volume). They do not destroy bacterial spores or penetrate proteinaceous material and so are not recommended for high-level disinfection. They can be used to disinfect noncritical items such as hospital fomites and have very low toxicity, so they are often included in waterless hand sanitizer products together with emollients to prevent drying of the skin. They are flammable and dry quickly, so it can be difficult to achieve adequate contact times (≥1 minute). As a result, alcohol should not be used for routine environmental disinfection.

Iodophors. Iodine solutions are primarily used as skin antiseptics. Formulations for disinfection are also available, which contain higher concentrations of free iodine than antiseptic preparations. An iodophor is a combination of iodine and a solubilizing agent (e.g., polyvinylpyrrolidone in povidone-iodine), which serves to provide a sustained-release form of iodine. Dilutions of iodophors are more active against microbes than concentrated povidone-iodine, so iodophores must be diluted correctly. Iodophors are bactericidal and virucidal. Their antibacterial activity does not persist for long periods on skin or in tissues, so frequent reapplication is required. Iodophors are relatively nontoxic and nonirritating. They are stable in solution but are inactivated by organic material and they can stain plastics and, to some extent, tissues.

Chlorhexidine. Chlorhexidine is a cationic bisbiguanide that disrupts microbial cell membranes and precipitates cell contents. It is used widely for skin antisepsis in veterinary medicine. Chlorhexidine has persistent activity on the skin, is nonirritating, is active in the presence of body fluids, and has rapid bactericidal activity. Like iodophors, chlorhexidine has limited activity against fungi and mycobacteria. A 2% chlorhexidine solution is preferred over 70% alcohol or povidone-iodine for skin preparation of central venous catheter sites in human patients[18] and is the skin antiseptic of choice for collection of blood for blood cultures. Chlorhexidine may have slightly lower activity against gram-negative bacteria and fungi than povidone-iodine, and both chlorhexidine and iodophors have a slower antimicrobial activity than 60% to 90% alcohol solutions.

Principles of Cleaning and Disinfection

Standard operating procedures that describe preparation and application of disinfectants for all surfaces and objects used in a veterinary hospital, as well as waste management, should be developed, and staff and visitors should receive education about the location of protocols and their use. Wards and procedure and examination rooms should remain uncluttered in order to facilitate effective cleaning. Because organic matter can inactivate disinfectants, all visible debris should be removed before disinfection. Disinfectants are only active when applied to clean, nonporous surfaces. Porous surfaces such as dirt and wood cannot be effectively disinfected using routine procedures. Hard porous surfaces should be scrubbed with disinfectant using brushes, and then rinsed with water after the contact time has elapsed.

When hospital surfaces are cleaned, attention should be paid to corners, under cabinets, chairs, the bases of examination tables, door handles, elevator buttons, shelves, sinks, faucets, and other surfaces that might otherwise be ignored. Personal items such as cell phones and stethoscope heads should be regularly disinfected with disinfectant wipes. Cell phones should be disinfected at least daily, and stethoscope heads wiped between patients. Stethoscope tubing should be cleaned regularly with soap and water. Disinfection of other fomites should be performed on a regular (at least daily) basis. These include digital thermometers, computer keyboards and mice, land-line telephones, calculators, microscopes, otoscopes, and blood pressure cuffs.

Cleaning staff should wear gloves when general hospital disinfection is performed. This may not be necessary for spot cleaning of areas such as examination room tables or fomites. Depending on the disinfectant, additional protective attire, such as a gown, boots, or face mask, may be required if there is a probability of significant splashing during the disinfection process. After disinfection is complete, protective clothing should be removed and handwashing performed. The individuals responsible for cleaning and disinfection at each time point, situation, and location in the hospital should be clearly identified. A plan for the cleaning of outdoor areas that become contaminated with excretions or other biohazardous material should be outlined.

When disinfection of cages or runs is performed, animals should be removed and placed in a clean holding cage or run, away from other patients. Solid waste and soiled laundry or paper should be removed and placed directly in waste or laundry containers, taking care to avoid dripping onto the floor. If laundry is contaminated with potentially infectious material, it must be bagged and labeled with the contents and suspected infectious agent. Proper contact times should be used after application of disinfectant solution. Runs and cages should be allowed to dry completely before a new patient is introduced.

Immunocompromised People and Children

People are considered immunocompromised if they (1) have various comorbidities such as diabetes mellitus, chronic kidney failure, leukopenia, immune-mediated disease, HIV/AIDS, congenital immunodeficiencies, hepatic cirrhosis, cancer, or splenectomy; (2) are being treated with immunosuppressive drugs or chemotherapeutics; (3) are very young (5 and under) or very old; or (4) are pregnant, although the immunosuppressive effects of pregnancy are considerably lower than those of the preceding disorders.

Immunocompromised staff members who work in small animal hospitals should discuss any necessary work restrictions and precautions in light of their specific condition with their physician or an infectious disease doctor. The risks for a diabetic, for example, may be significantly different from those for a transplant recipient. In general, immunosuppressed individuals who work in small animal hospitals should avoid handling patients with suspected or known infectious diseases. Gloves should always be worn when handling animals and animal fluids or excreta, and strict attention to general hand hygiene and any bites, scratches, or sharps injuries is critical. Children 5 years of age or younger should be kept out of patient care areas. Strict attention to hygiene and protective apparel is necessary when handling soiled cat litter or animal feces, because of the risk for transmission of enteropathogens. The reader is referred to other chapters in this book for public health implications of specific infectious diseases that may be encountered in small animal hospitals. If possible, small animal clinics should establish a relationship with a doctor who is prepared to consult on zoonotic exposures with staff members.

Transmissible Disease Surveillance and Reporting

A transmissible disease surveillance program allows collection of baseline data that establishes the prevalence of certain infectious diseases, so that possible outbreak situations can be readily identified. It can also provide background prevalence information on antimicrobial drug susceptibility patterns, which can assist in the initial selection of antibacterial drugs for individual animal patients while culture and susceptibility test results are in progress. Information is generally collected for multidrug-resistant bacterial infections, zoonotic diseases, highly contagious diseases, pathogens that are difficult to inactivate with disinfectants, or agents of regulatory concern. Although surveillance may seem like a difficult, time-consuming, and expensive measure, in reality, it can be easy and cost-effective and can provide important information.

There are two main forms of infection control surveillance applicable to veterinary hospitals: active and passive. *Active surveillance* involves collection of data specifically for infection control purposes. This can provide the highest quality and most relevant information, but it can be expensive and time consuming. Examples of this would be collection of swab specimens to screen for infection with methicillin-resistant *Staphylococcus pseudintermedius* (MRSP) from dogs before surgery as part of MRSP outbreak investigation. Active surveillance is a core component of infection control in most human hospitals, but it is only sporadically used in veterinary medicine and is rarely needed in most veterinary clinics. It is typically reserved for large facilities with increased infection control risks and personnel available to direct such testing, or as a part of outbreak control.

In contrast, *passive surveillance* is a practical, easy, and cost-effective surveillance approach that can and should be performed in every veterinary clinic. It involves the use of data that are already available, such as information about surgical site infections collected during routine follow-up or culture results from clinical testing. The quality of passive surveillance data can be limited by poor or incomplete record keeping or sporadic use of appropriate diagnostic tests, but if properly collected and if potential biases are understood, passive surveillance data can provide important insight into aspects such as endemic disease rates, common pathogens, and antimicrobial susceptibility trends. To facilitate passive surveillance, clinicians should be encouraged to use appropriate diagnostic testing to determine the etiology of nosocomial infections, even if the clinical consequences are not severe. They also should be encouraged to confirm a diagnosis in animals with suspected transmissible disease. This allows clients to protect their other animals and their families and friends who might be in contact with the pet, and it benefits the hospital.

Another form of surveillance that is easy to perform and potentially very useful is *syndromic surveillance.* This involves surveillance for readily identifiable syndromes (i.e., diarrhea, cough) instead of specific diagnoses. Although syndromes do not indicate a specific disease, they can indicate an increased risk of infectious disease. Syndromic surveillance is an initial screening tool that can be used by all personnel, including lay personnel, to flag potentially high-risk cases and allow for early implementation of enhanced infection control practices. All clinic personnel should be made aware of certain syndromes that indicate the need either for isolation or for further investigation, such as diarrhea, fever of unknown origin, acute neurologic disease, wound infections, and acute respiratory tract disease. Protocols to deal with these animals on arrival should be developed. As an example, a dog with an acute onset of cough should be considered potentially infectious, and if front office personnel note this syndrome at the time the appointment is made, the dog can be handled appropriately on arrival (e.g., admitted directly to isolation or an examination room, with personnel wearing enhanced barrier precautions from the onset). The role of lay staff (i.e., front office stall) is critical, as these people are the ones who are most able to identify such cases before they enter the clinic and ensure that they are properly handled to prevent nosocomial or zoonotic transmission.

BOX 11-3

Infectious Diseases of Dogs and Cats That Are Reportable or Potentially Reportable to Public Health Agencies

Amebiasis
Granulocytic anaplasmosis
Brucellosis
Campylobacteriosis
Coccidioidomycosis
Cryptococcus gattii infection
Cryptosporidiosis
Giardiasis
Leishmaniosis
Leptospirosis
Lyme disease
Q fever
Rabies
Salmonellosis
Tularemia
Tuberculosis
MRSA (not MRSP)
Novel H1N1 influenza virus infections
West Nile Virus infection
Yersinia infections

Environmental cultures are rarely informative and so are not considered a useful routine infection control tool. They may be used to detect a specific pathogen if an outbreak of an HAI is suspected when there is suspicion that the environment is a source of exposure. However, it is often difficult to distinguish cause from effect (i.e., environmental contamination that leads to transmission vs. environmental contamination that occurs as a result of contamination from a patient in the absence of a risk of transmission).

Although surveillance programs require time, effort, and expense, in the long term they may save morbidity and mortality and reduce costs that relate to control of large outbreak situations or the legal ramifications of HAIs.

When zoonotic diseases are identified, all in-contact individuals and, if necessary, public health authorities should be notified in the appropriate manner. The specific diseases that must be reported to authorities vary among geographic locations. Examples of diseases that may be of interest to public health authorities are listed in Box 11-3.

Surgical Preparation

Surgical site infections (SSIs) are an uncommon but important and sometimes devastating complication of surgery. Every patient undergoing a surgical procedure is at some risk of SSI. Standard practices have been developed to reduce the risk of SSIs. Although a wide range of practices are relevant, preparation of the patient and preparation of the surgeon are critical.

Patient Preparation

The patient's endogenous microflora is an important source of pathogens that cause SSIs. Careful preparation of the patient, therefore, can help reduce contamination of the surgical site during surgery. The goal of preoperative surgical site management is to eliminate potential pathogens while not creating a physical environment that is more conducive to bacterial colonization or infection postoperatively. Bathing of the patient preoperatively is reasonable if there is significant contamination of the haircoat[19] and if the patient's coat can be dried by the time of surgery. In most situations, bathing is not required. Rather, careful hair removal and skin antisepsis are the main measures.

The goals of surgical scrubbing of patients are to reduce bacterial counts, reduce debris, and facilitate later antisepsis. Scrubbing should be done as atraumatically as possible. Minimizing skin damage during clipping and scrubbing is essential, because skin damage from excessive attempts to clip all remaining pieces of hair or from forceful scrubbing of the surgical site can create an environment that is more amenable to bacterial growth. This predisposes to infection rather than reducing the risk. Clipping should be performed after anesthesia, to reduce the risk of trauma associated with a struggling patient and to minimize the time between clipping and surgery. Clipping should be done outside the operating environment. There is currently no information that relates to optimal methods of cleaning and disinfecting clippers. Repeated use of clipper blades without sterilization not surprisingly results in higher levels of bacterial contamination of blades[20]; however, the clinical relevance of this is unclear, because the surgical site is cleaned and disinfected after clipping. Regular cleaning and disinfection of clippers are probably useful, and they should be thoroughly cleaned and disinfected after use on an animal with a potentially transmissible infection (e.g., an animal with diarrhea), on an area where the skin is broken, or on any area where the skin or hair is significantly contaminated with feces, urine, blood, or other body fluids.

After hair removal, various approaches for skin antisepsis can be used. There is little outcome-based evidence of the relative efficacy of different approaches in the human literature. Typically, a three-step process is used, with initial scrubbing of the site with biocidal (i.e., chlorhexidine, povidone-iodine) soap, followed by application of alcohol for biocidal effects and to remove oils, and a final application of a biocidal solution with residual activity (e.g., chlorhexidine).

Surgeon Preparation

The surgeon's body and clothing are potential sources of SSI pathogens, and standard practices have been developed to reduce the risk of contamination of the surgical site. One aspect is the use of proper protective clothing. Every person in the operating environment should wear clean surgical scrubs. These scrubs should be dedicated for use only in the operating room or should be covered with a clean laboratory coat whenever the individual is outside of the operating room.

Surgical hand antisepsis is critical because of the close contact of the hands with the surgical site and the relatively high incidence of grossly evident breaks or micro-breaks in gloves. Surgical hand antisepsis is designed to greatly reduce bacterial burdens on the hands, particularly the abundant transient microflora that contains most of the relevant pathogens that cause SSIs. Surgical antisepsis must find a balance between effective elimination of pathogens, minimization of trauma to the skin (because skin irritation facilitates bacterial growth), and time constraints. The traditional approach to surgical hand antisepsis has involved structured scrubbing of the hands for a predetermined time. Recommended scrub times vary between products but are typically 2 to 4 minutes.

Application of alcohol-chlorhexidine combinations has been evaluated as a replacement for surgical scrubbing and has been shown to be more effective than standard surgical scrub methods.[21,22] Specific manufacturer instructions should be followed, and hands and arms must be dry before application of gloves. The use of alcohol-based surgical hand antisepsis products is encouraged as a replacement for traditional scrubbing.

BOX 11-4

Example of Criteria Specified within a Hospital for Use of Restricted Antimicrobial Drugs

- Infection must be documented based on clinical abnormalities *and* culture.
- Subclinical infections should not be treated with these antibiotics. These antibiotics should be reserved for infections that are life threatening.
- Resistance to all other reasonable options and susceptibility to the chosen antimicrobial must be documented.
- The infection must be potentially treatable.
- The clinician should contact the infectious disease control officer or a clinical microbiology faculty member by email or telephone to discuss antimicrobial susceptibility test results, determine whether there are any other viable options, and confirm that a restricted antimicrobial is necessary.

Regardless of the method used, a thorough handwash with careful cleaning under the fingernails must be performed at the beginning of each day.[23] Long (>¼-inch) and artificial nails are prohibited in many human health care facilities and some veterinary hospitals because they harbor pathogenic bacteria[24] and are associated with surgical glove tears.

A cap and mask must be worn during hand antisepsis, and sterile gown and gloves must then be donned using appropriate technique.

Antimicrobial Drug Use

The use of antimicrobial drugs contributes to the selection for antimicrobial-resistant bacteria. Inclusion of a policy on antimicrobial drug use in the infection control protocol may help to reduce the prevalence of multidrug-resistant HAIs. On their own, fever and leukocytosis are not justification for antimicrobial drug treatment. Whenever possible, when infection is suspected, attempts to obtain material for culture and susceptibility testing should be made before antimicrobial drug treatment is initiated. When secondary bacterial infection is likely, attempts to identify and treat the underlying cause should be made. In an effort to minimize the emergence of resistance in bacterial flora of animals in the hospital and decrease the risk of resistant HAIs, the use of several antimicrobials (e.g., certain parenteral third generation cephalosporins, vancomycin, linezolid, and carbapenems such as imipenem and meropenem) may be restricted unless criteria must be met (Box 11-4).

Prevention of Infectious Disease in Shelters and Breeding and Boarding Facilities

Attention to hand hygiene and proper disinfection of fomites and the environment as outlined for hospitals can also be used to reduce transmission of infectious pathogens in shelters and in breeding and boarding facilities (Box 11-5). Disinfectants with activity against parvoviruses and feline calicivirus should be used routinely, such as a 1:30 dilution of household bleach,

BOX 11-5

Factors That Should Be Considered for the Reduction of Infectious Disease Transmission in Animal Housing Facilities

Adequate ventilation and air quality
Adequate temperature
Adequate lighting conditions (including provision of darkness at night)
Population density/space per animal
Daily removal of fecal and urine contamination and disinfection
Adequate drainage
Separate housing areas for dogs and cats
Isolation for sick animals
Separate housing areas for young and adult animals
Individual housing or small groups of two to four compatible animals
Separation of elimination, feeding, and resting areas
Elevated resting areas
Elevated cages for cats
Provision of hiding areas
Sound control
Use of surfaces that can be readily disinfected
Proper use of appropriate disinfectants
Hand hygiene and protective clothing
Fomite control
Use of appropriate vaccination protocols
Order of care (young animals, healthy adults, and then sick animals)
Proper nutrition
Pain management
Free access to clean water
Rodent and pest control
Parasite control
Daily monitoring by properly trained individuals
Proper diagnosis of disease outbreaks

potassium peroxymonosulfate, or accelerated hydrogen peroxide solutions. Removal of organic matter, the use of surfaces that can be adequately disinfected, and proper contact times are essential.

Factors that increase stress should also be minimized, such as high population densities, the grouping of animals, and poor nutrition. Cats and dogs should be separated from one another. In cats, the use of methods that reduce stress, such as provision of a low-stress cage environment, can dramatically reduce the frequency of upper respiratory tract disease. Compartmentalized housing allows animals to urinate and defecate away from areas where they rest and eat, and provision of a hiding area so that animals can retreat from visual stimulation can also reduce stress. A total of 10 to 20 air changes per hour is often recommended for animal housing, but higher levels of ventilation may be needed with increased population density and concentration of airborne contaminants. Cages should be cleaned and disinfected at least daily. The use of compartmentalized housing areas also facilitates cleaning and disinfection without requiring an animal to be removed from the housing area. Isolation areas for sick animals should be present and these should have separate airflow from areas that house healthy animals. Mass treatment of dogs and cats with upper respiratory tract disease with antimicrobials without attention to the underlying causes only results in selection for antimicrobial drug resistant organisms and is not recommended. Detailed information on the control of infectious diseases in shelter environments is beyond the scope of this book but can be found elsewhere.[25] The American Association of Shelter Veterinarians and the Humane Society of the United States have published guidelines for operation of animal shelters.[26,27]

SUGGESTED READINGS

Association of Shelter Veterinarians. Guidelines for standards of care in animal shelters. 2010. oacu.od.nih.gov/disaster/ShelterGuide.pdf. Last accessed November 17, 2012.

Boyce JM, Pittet D. Guideline for hand hygiene in health-care settings. MMWR. 2002;51. http://www.cdc.gov/handhygiene/Guidelines.html. Last Accessed November 17, 2012.

Canadian Committee on Antibiotic Resistance. Infection prevention and control best practices for small animal veterinary clinics. 2008. http://www.wormsandgermsblog.com/2008/04/promo/services/infection-prevention-and-control-best-practices-for-small-animal-veterinary-clinics/. Last accessed November 17, 2012.

WHO guidelines on hand hygiene in health care. http://www.cdc.gov/handhygiene/guidelines.html. Last accessed November 17, 2012.

REFERENCES

1. Edmond EB, Wenzel RP. Isolation. In: Mandell GL, Bennett JE, Dolin R, eds. Principles and Practice of Infectious Diseases. 7th ed. Philadephia, PA: Elsevier; 2010:3673-3676.
2. Longtin Y, Sax H, Allegranzi B, et al. Hand hygiene. N Engl J Med. 2011:e24.
3. WHO guidelines on hand hygiene in health care. 2009. http://www.cdc.gov/handhygiene/Guidelines.html. Last accessed November 17, 2012.
4. Guideline for hand hygiene in health-care settings. 2002. http://www.cdc.gov/handhygiene/Guidelines.html. Last accessed November 17, 2012.
5. McGovern B, Doyle E, Fenelon LE, et al. The necktie as a potential vector of infection: are doctors happy to do without? J Hosp Infect. 2010;75:138-139.
6. Centers for Disease Control and Prevention. Guideline for the prevention of surgical site infection. 1999. http://www.cdc.gov/HAI/ssi/ssi.html. Last accessed November 17, 2012.
7. Lenz J, Joffe D, Kauffman M, et al. Perceptions, practices, and consequences associated with foodborne pathogens and the feeding of raw meat to dogs. Can Vet J. 2009;50:637-643.
8. Guideline for isolation precautions: preventing transmission of infectious agents in healthcare settings. 2008. http://www.cdc.gov/hicpac/2007ip/2007isolationprecautions.html. Last accessed November 17, 2012.
9. Rutala WA, Weber DJ. Disinfection, sterilization, and control of hospital waste. In: Mandell GL, Bennett JE, Dolin R, eds. Principles and Practice of Infectious Diseases. 7th ed. Philadephia, PA: Elsevier; 2010:3677-3695.
10. Akamatsu T, Minemoto M, Uyeda M. Evaluation of the antimicrobial activity and materials compatibility of orthophthalaldehyde as a high-level disinfectant. J Int Med Res. 2005;33:178-187.
11. Hession SM. Endoscope disinfection by ortho-phthalaldehyde in a clinical setting: an evaluation of reprocessing time and costs compared with glutaraldehyde. Gastroenterol Nurs. 2003;26:110-114.
12. Cooke RP, Goddard SV, Whymant-Morris A, et al. An evaluation of Cidex OPA (0.55% ortho-phthalaldehyde) as an alternative to 2% glutaraldehyde for high-level disinfection of endoscopes. J Hosp Infect. 2003;54:226-231.

13. Omidbakhsh N. Evaluation of sporicidal activities of selected environmental surface disinfectants: carrier tests with the spores of *Clostridium difficile* and its surrogates. Am J Infect Control. 2010;38:718-722.
14. Alfa MJ, Lo E, Wald A, et al. Improved eradication of *Clostridium difficile* spores from toilets of hospitalized patients using an accelerated hydrogen peroxide as the cleaning agent. BMC Infect Dis. 2010; 10:268.
15. Howie R, Alfa MJ, Coombs K. Survival of enveloped and non-enveloped viruses on surfaces compared with other micro-organisms and impact of suboptimal disinfectant exposure. J Hosp Infect. 2008;69:368-376.
16. Eleraky NZ, Potgieter LN, Kennedy MA. Virucidal efficacy of four new disinfectants. J Am Anim Hosp Assoc. 2002;38:231-234.
17. Weber DJ, Rutala WA, Sickbert-Bennett EE. Outbreaks associated with contaminated antiseptics and disinfectants. Antimicrob Agents Chemother. 2007;51:4217-4224.
18. Maki DG, Ringer M, Alvarado CJ. Prospective randomised trial of povidone-iodine, alcohol, and chlorhexidine for prevention of infection associated with central venous and arterial catheters. Lancet. 1991;338:339-343.
19. Stick JA. Preparation of the surgical patient, the surgery facility, and the operating team. In: Auer JA, Stick JA, eds. Equine Surgery. 3rd ed. Philadelphia, PA: Saunders Elsevier; 2006:123-140.
20. Masterson TM, Rodeheaver GT, Morgan RF, et al. Bacteriologic evaluation of electric clippers for surgical hair removal. Am J Surg. 1984;148:301-302.
21. Mulberrry G, Snyder AT, Heilman J, et al. Evaluation of a waterless, scrubless chlorhexidine gluconate/ethanol surgical scrub for antimicrobial efficacy. Am J Infect Control. 2001;29:377-382.
22. Hobson DW, Woller W, Anderson L, et al. Development and evaluation of a new alcohol-based surgical hand scrub formulation with persistent antimicrobial characteristics and brushless application. Am J Infect Control. 1998;26:507-512.
23. Larson EL. APIC guideline for handwashing and hand antisepsis in health care settings. Am J Infect Control. 1995;23:251-269.
24. Pottinger J, Burns S, Manske C. Bacterial carriage by artificial versus natural nails. Am J Infect Control. 1989;17:340-344.
25. Miller L, Hurley KF. Infectious Disease Management in Animal Shelters. Ames, IA: Wiley-Blackwell; 2009.
26. Humane Society of the United States. HSUS guidelines for standard operating procedures for animal shelters. http://dev.animalsheltering.pub30.convio.net/resource_library/policies_and_guidelines/guidelines_for_standard_operating_procedures.html. Last accessed November 17, 2012.
27. Association of Shelter Veterinarians. Guidelines for standards of care in animal shelters. 2010. oacu.od.nih.gov/disaster/ShelterGuide.pdf. Last accessed November 17, 2012.

CHAPTER 12

Immunization

Jane E. Sykes

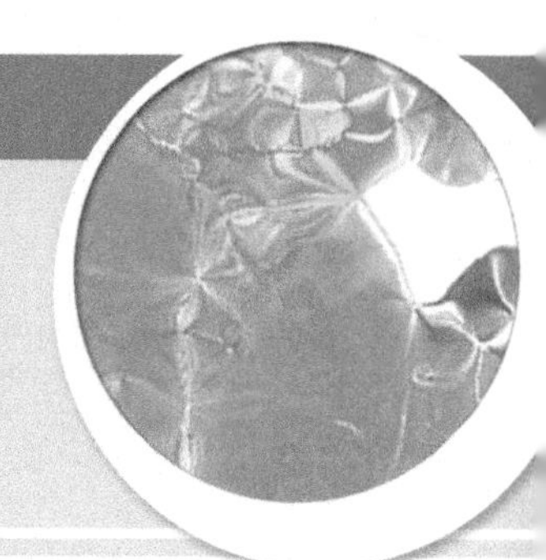

KEY POINTS

- Active immunization can partially or completely protect dogs and cats from severe consequences of infection with a variety of different pathogens, and in some cases it reduces shedding of these pathogens.
- Vaccines contain attenuated live microorganisms, inactivated microorganisms, or portions of these organisms. They also contain preservatives and adjuvants.
- Failure of immunization can occur with improper storage or administration of vaccines, a large challenge dose, host factors such as concurrent infections or disease, and interference by maternal antibody.
- Other adverse effects of vaccine administration are uncommon to rare but include hypersensitivity reactions, disease induced by live attenuated vaccine organisms, and injection-site sarcomas in cats.
- The decision to administer a vaccine should be based on discussion of risks and benefits between the veterinarian and pet owner. This should be documented in the medical record.
- Guidelines for vaccine selection and administration have been published by a number of veterinary bodies, such as the AAFP, AAHA, AVMA, and WSAVA; suggestions can also be found in Appendix I.

INTRODUCTION

Immunization refers to artificial induction of immunity or protection from infectious disease and may be *active* or *passive*. *Active immunization* involves administration of vaccines that stimulate cell-mediated or humoral immunity, or both, to a specific pathogen. *Passive immunization* refers to the administration of antibodies in order to provide temporary protection from disease and can occur through acquisition of maternally derived antibody (MDA) transplacentally, in colostrum, or milk; or treatment with preparations that contain specific or nonspecific immunoglobulins (see Immunomodulators, Chapter 7, and post-exposure prophylaxis for rabies, Chapter 13). Readers are referred to advanced immunology texts for detailed descriptions of the physiology of active and passive immunity.[1]

The goal of immunization is to generate a protective immune response of prolonged duration against a specific infectious disease, with minimal adverse effects. Because of the potential for adverse effects, vaccination should be performed only if there is a risk for significant morbidity or mortality from an infectious disease. Since the 1950s, a huge number of vaccines for dogs and cats have been developed and marketed worldwide, and more are in development. Nevertheless, it is estimated that even in developed countries such as the United States, only 30% to 50% of dogs are properly immunized, and possibly an even smaller proportion of cats.[2,3] Appropriate vaccination of a larger proportion of the pet population may assist in reduction of the prevalence of infectious diseases through the induction of herd immunity.

With the appearance of injection-site sarcomas in cats, increased emphasis has been placed on vaccine safety, and a change from annual to 3-yearly immunization protocols for some vaccines has been recommended, with administration of other vaccines based on exposure risk. Vaccines have had a profound influence in the control of infectious disease, and for many vaccines the benefits of vaccination outweigh the risks.

Vaccine Composition and Types of Vaccines

A vaccine is a suspension of attenuated live or inactivated microorganisms, or parts thereof, that is administered to induce immunity. In addition to protective antigens, vaccines may contain preservatives and stabilizers as well as specific antibiotics to preserve the antigen and inhibit bacterial and fungal growth within the vaccine. Some vaccines also contain an *adjuvant* to enhance the immune response to the antigen. Although the mechanisms are not completely clear, adjuvants can delay the release of antigen from the site of injection and induce the secretion of chemokines by leukocytes.[4] The most widely used adjuvants are particulate adjuvants, such as those that contain aluminum salt precipitates such as aluminum hydroxide.[5] Other particulate adjuvants include immunostimulators such as saponin, which is present in a canine *Leishmania* vaccine.

Attenuated live vaccines (or modified live vaccines) contain microorganisms that are artificially manipulated so as to negate or greatly reduce their virulence, or are field strains of low virulence. Repeated passage through cell culture is the most common means of attenuation. Because they replicate in the host, organisms in attenuated live vaccines usually stimulate an immune response that most closely mimics the protection that results from natural infection. Vaccination with attenuated live canine parvovirus (CPV) and canine distemper virus (CDV) vaccines in the absence of MDA can result in protective immune responses within 3 days of a single injection, which may be followed by immunity that lasts many years, if not for life.[6-8] Partial immunity after vaccination with attenuated live CDV and feline panleukopenia virus (FPV) vaccines can occur within hours.[3,9,10] In addition, vaccine organisms that are shed can serve to immunize other animals in a population. However, the potential for reversion to virulence or vaccine-induced disease exists. Vaccine-induced disease is most likely to occur in highly immunosuppressed animals. Attenuated live vaccines also have the potential to cause some immunosuppression in their

TABLE 12-1

Advantages and Disadvantages of Attenuated Live and Inactivated Vaccines

	Attenuated Live	Inactivated
Advantages	Rapid onset of immunity Sustained immunity after single dose May immunize others in populations Improved breakthrough of maternal antibody interference	Safe, even in immunocompromised and pregnant animals Do not interfere with development of immunity from other vaccines Stable in storage
Disadvantages	Potential for reversion to virulence Virulence in the immunocompromised Contraindicated in pregnancy May cause immune suppression Can interfere with development of immunity if administered within days to 2 weeks of another vaccine Less stable in storage Potential for vaccine contamination	Slow onset of immunity Multiple boosters required Often highly adjuvanted, with greater potential for adverse effects Reduced degree of protection compared with attenuated live vaccines Poor breakthrough of maternal antibody interference

own right,[11,12] or they may shift the balance from Th1 to Th2 immune responses.[13] Rarely, this can lead to clinical disease. For example, an outbreak of salmonellosis was reported in cats after use of a high-titered attenuated live FPV vaccine.[14] Very rarely, contamination of attenuated live vaccines has occurred with other pathogenic microorganisms present within cell cultures used to propagate the vaccine.

Generally speaking, *inactivated vaccines* are less effective than attenuated vaccines, because replication in the host does not occur. They produce weaker immune responses of shorter duration, and more frequent booster immunizations may be required. Two initial doses of vaccine 3 to 4 weeks apart are essential to produce an effective immune response, and if more than 6 weeks elapses between these doses, it has been recommended that the series should be repeated.[15] Beyond the initial vaccination series, it is not clear whether lapsed annual boosters require the series to be restarted. This is not considered necessary for human immunization[16] but has been suggested for dogs when more than 2 or 3 years elapses between boosters.[15] Inactivated vaccines usually contain adjuvant as well as a large infectious dose to improve immunogenicity. They are safer than live attenuated vaccines for use during pregnancy and in very young or debilitated animals. Although bacterins have traditionally been associated with a greater likelihood of allergic reactions than live attenuated vaccines, newer inactivated vaccines are safer and have reaction rates that more closely approach those of live attenuated vaccines. The maximum duration of immunity that is induced by commercially available bacterins for dogs and cats remains largely unknown, partly because challenge studies that evaluate long-term duration of immunity are prohibitively expensive. However, some inactivated viral vaccines have been shown to have durations of immunity in excess of 7 years in cats.[17] Caution is required when extrapolation is made from the duration of immunity for one product to that for a similar product from a different manufacturer, because it may not be equivalent. Although bacterins usually do not protect all animals from infection, they may prevent clinical illness. In some cases, natural infection of vaccinated animals serves to further boost the immune response, and this can influence duration of immunity in the field. The advantages and disadvantages of attenuated live and inactivated vaccines are shown in Table 12-1.

Subunit vaccines contain specific structural components of a microbe that stimulate a protective immune response, together with adjuvant. They contain reduced amounts of foreign protein, which minimizes the potential for hypersensitivity reactions.

Recombinant DNA vaccines are created through manipulation of the DNA of a pathogen in the laboratory, with the negation of pathogen virulence. Sometimes this also can allow diagnostic tests to differentiate naturally infected from vaccinated animals (DIVA), because of differences in the antibody response evoked by the vaccine. There are several different types of recombinant DNA vaccines:

1. Recombinant subunit vaccines. These are produced by cloning one or more genes for a protective antigen into an expression vector, such as in *Escherichia coli.* The protein expressed by the bacteria is then purified and used in the vaccine (Figure 12-1, *A*). An example of a recombinant subunit vaccine is the Lyme recombinant OspA vaccine.
2. Deletion mutant vaccines. These are produced by deleting virulence genes from a pathogen while protective antigens are left in place. There are currently no such vaccines for dogs and cats.
3. Vectored vaccines. These are produced by inserting genes for one or more protective antigens into the genome of a virus. The virus replicates in the host and expresses the antigens but is nonpathogenic (see Figure 12-1, *B*). Currently available vectored vaccines for dogs and cats use canarypox virus as a vector.
4. DNA vaccines. These consist of naked DNA that encodes the antigens required for protective immunity. The DNA is injected directly to the animal using an inoculation system. The DNA is then taken up by host cells and translated into antigen. Both humoral and cell-mediated immune responses are produced. DNA vaccines are not currently available commercially for use in dogs and cats.

Vaccine Storage, Handling, and Administration

Vaccines should be stored and administered according to label recommendations. Inactivation of vaccines can occur if they

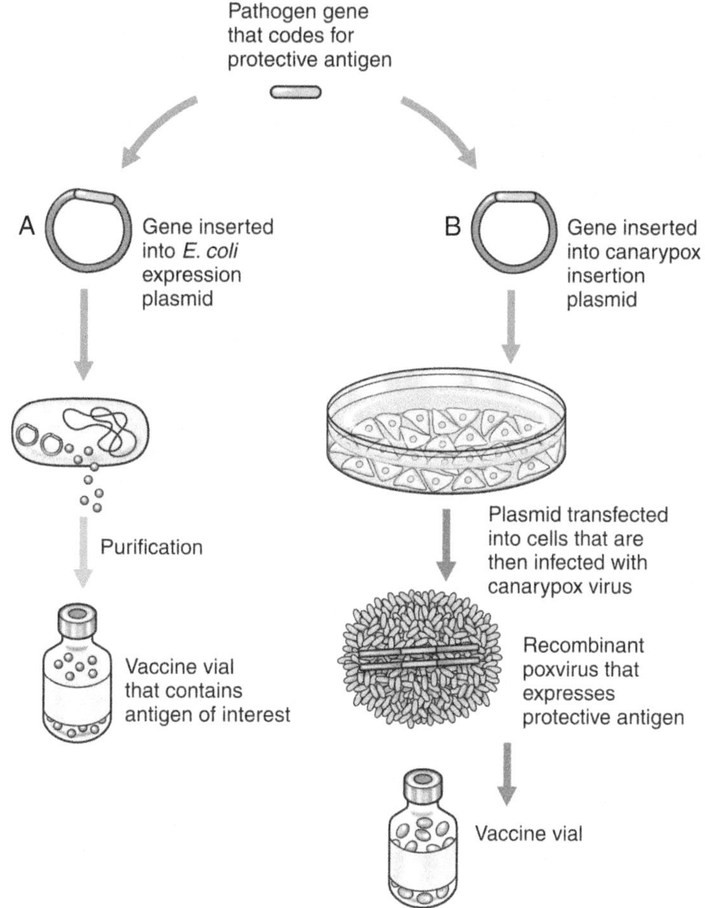

FIGURE 12-1 Examples of recombinant DNA vaccines. **A,** Recombinant subunit vaccine. The gene of interest is inserted into an expression vector such as a plasmid taken up by *Escherichia coli,* which subsequently produces large amounts of an immunogenic protein. This is purified and used in the vaccine. **B,** Vectored vaccine. The gene or genes of interest are inserted into a canarypox or vaccinia vector, which is then inoculated into an animal. Replication of the vector within the host is followed by expression of the immunogenic protein.

are inadvertently frozen or heated to excessive temperatures, exposed to excessive amounts of light, or used beyond their expiration date. Hands should be washed before preparation and administration of the vaccine. Lyophilized products should be reconstituted with the proper diluent, and different vaccines should not be mixed in the same syringe or vial. Reconstituted products should be used immediately. It has been recommended that attenuated live vaccines be discarded if more than 1 hour has lapsed since reconstitution,[15] although no published reports exist of the viability of vaccine organisms over time after reconstitution or of the ability of stored, reconstituted vaccine to elicit an immune response. Vaccines should only be used in the animal species for which they are labeled, or serious adverse effects or failure of immunization can occur.

If vaccines for multiple different pathogens are to be administered simultaneously, they should be injected at distant sites or, if possible, a combination vaccine should be used. Simultaneous vaccination for more than one pathogen does not appear to interfere with immune responses to each component of the vaccine,[18-20] and vaccine manufacturers must demonstrate that the protection that occurs for a specific pathogen after vaccination with a combination product equals the protection that occurs when a vaccine for only that pathogen is given. In contrast, successive parenteral administration of different attenuated live vaccines at 3 to 14 day intervals has the potential to interfere with immune responses. An interval of 4 weeks is preferred for human patients.[16,21] Inactivated vaccines do not produce interference in this way.[16] If possible, administration of vaccines to animals that are under anesthesia should be avoided because adverse reactions may be difficult or impossible to recognize in this situation. It is not necessary to re-administer an intranasal vaccine if the animal coughs or sneezes after administration.

The site and route of administration, product, serial number, expiry date, and individual who administered the vaccine should be recorded for each vaccine administered.[2] Vaccine vials often possess adhesive labels that can be easily removed and applied to a paper medical record.

Components of the Immune Response

The immune response is divided into innate and adaptive immune responses. The innate immune response is nonspecific and acts as an immediate line of defense against an infection. Components of the innate immune response consist of natural killer cells, which recognize host cells that are infected by viruses; complement, which is activated by bacterial cell wall components; and phagocytes, such as macrophages and dendritic cells. The adaptive immune response develops over several days and involves presentation of antigen by dendritic cells in association with the major histocompatibility complex and stimulation of B and T cell responses, together with the

BOX 12-1

Factors That Can Affect Immune Responses to Vaccines

Target pathogen (e.g., respiratory versus systemic pathogen)
Vaccine composition (e.g., inadequate adjuvant)
Route of administration
Young age
Breed/genetic factors
Nutrition
Pregnancy status
Concurrent moderate to severe illness
Fever
Immunosuppressive drugs
Presence of maternal antibody
Improper vaccine storage and administration
Vaccination with an attenuated live viral vaccine within last 3 days to 2 weeks
Inadequate time allowed for immunization before exposure to field organisms

formation of memory B cells. The nature of the innate response influences the subsequent adaptive response. Cells of the innate immune system possess pattern recognition receptors that can recognize patterns that are characteristic for various pathogens (pathogen-associated molecular patterns, or PAMPs), including Toll-like receptors and NOD-like receptors. PAMPs are under investigation for use as adjuvants in human and animal vaccines in order to create improved T cell immune responses.[4,22]

Determinants of Immunogenicity

All vaccines that are available for dogs and cats induce cell-mediated immunity (CMI) with induction of immunologic memory and a booster effect on repeat administration. Although the presence of antibody correlates with protection for some pathogens, such as CDV and CPV, a lack of antibody does not infer a lack of protection, because of the presence of CMI, which is more difficult to measure.

Vaccines rarely protect all vaccinated individuals from infection and disease. In particular, vaccines for canine and feline respiratory pathogens do not prevent disease but can reduce the prevalence and severity of disease as well as reduce the number of organisms shed. Limited immunity following vaccination is especially likely for infections for which immunity after natural infection is partial or short-lived.

The ability of a vaccine to induce an immune response depends not only on the target pathogen, vaccine composition, and route of administration, but also on host factors such as age, nutrition, pregnancy status, stress, concurrent infections, and immune status, including the presence or absence of passively acquired antibody (Box 12-1). Some of these factors may also influence vaccine safety. Some animals, particularly dogs of the Rottweiler breed, may have an impaired ability to respond to vaccination. These dogs have been termed *nonresponders*.[2,23] This situation is probably rare if efficacious vaccines are used and booster vaccines are administered. Young dogs, less than 1 year of age, have a significantly reduced response to vaccination with rabies virus vaccines when compared with adult dogs.[24] Small-breed dogs have a greater serologic response to rabies vaccines than large-breed dogs.[25] Administration of vaccines to febrile animals or animals with moderate to severe illness should be avoided if possible until recovery has occurred, because the immune response to the vaccine may be suboptimal.

Failure of immunization can result from an inadequate dose of antigen. Thus, division of a single vaccine dose for administration to a larger number of dogs and cats, or small-breed dogs as opposed to large-breed dogs, may lead to failure of immunization. Veterinarians should not split vaccine doses because this shifts the liability from the vaccine manufacturer to the veterinarian if vaccine failure occurs. Immunization can also fail in the face of an overwhelming challenge dose.

The route of administration can influence the type of immune response generated. Subcutaneous administration is associated primarily with an IgG response, and rarely induces high levels of secretory IgA antibodies. In contrast, intranasal administration results in an IgA and, to a lesser extent, an IgG response. Immunogenicity and safety may be compromised when a vaccine is administered using the incorrect route.

In young animals, MDA can neutralize vaccine antigens and interfere with effective immunization. This is one of the most common reasons for vaccine failure in dogs and cats. Any MDA titer against CPV has the potential to interfere with immunization. The amount of MDA in a puppy or kitten at any one point in time cannot be predicted because it varies depending on the titer of the dam and the amount of colostrum ingested after birth. As a result, a series of vaccinations are administered in order to increase the chance that successful immunization will occur soon after the decline of MDA titers to sufficiently low concentrations (Figure 12-2). Nevertheless, a window always exists when MDA concentrations are high enough to interfere with immunization, but not sufficient to prevent natural infection. This window is known as the *window of susceptibility* or the *window of vulnerability*. The use of recombinant vectored vaccines can overcome the interference by MDA, although the extent to which this applies in animals that have passive immunity to the vector virus (i.e., immunity transferred from a dam that was immunized with a recombinant vector vaccine) requires clarification. Because replication of the vector is aborted, the immune response to the vector itself may be reduced. As a result, passive transfer of neutralizing antibody titers to the vector may not occur. Mucosal vaccines can also provide greater protection in the face of MDA; the mucosal immune system matures shortly after birth.[26,27]

Whenever possible, animals should be isolated until sufficient time has elapsed for proper immunization. For most parenteral and mucosal vaccines, this is 1 week (and at the absolute minimum, 3 days) after inoculation. Vaccine failure can also occur in animals that are incubating the disease for which vaccination is performed at the time of vaccination.

Measurement of the Immune Response

For some vaccines, such as rabies, CDV, CPV, and FPV, the presence of circulating antibodies correlates with protection (Table 12-2). Thus, serologic assays have been used in dogs and cats to decide whether vaccination is necessary or likely to be effective. These serologic assays have also been used to clear pets for travel.

Although tests that measure antibody responses in dogs and cats have improved in recent years, different laboratories can report significantly different values for the same serum

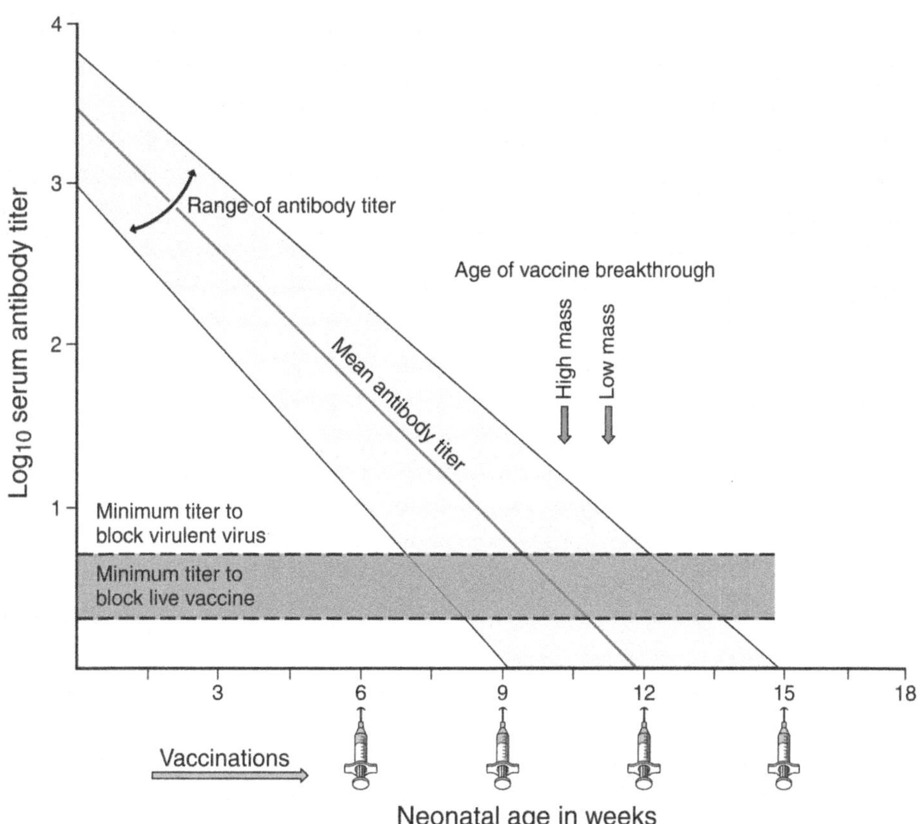

FIGURE 12-2 Influence of maternal antibody (MDA) on immunization. Puppies and kittens acquire variable amounts of MDA transplacentally and through colostrum after birth. This binds to vaccine antigens and inhibits the immune response. A series of vaccines are administered to maximize the chance of inducing an immune response as MDA concentrations decline. The *window of susceptibility* is the period of time when MDA concentrations are high enough to interfere with immunization, but not sufficient to prevent natural infection. High antigen mass vaccines provide protection earlier than low mass vaccines. (From Greene CE, Schultz RD. Immunoprophylaxis. In: Greene CE, ed. Infectious Diseases of the Dog and Cat, 3 ed. St Louis, MO: Saunders; 2006.)

TABLE 12-2

Antibody Titers That Correlate with Protection against Distemper, Parvovirus, and Rabies

Pathogen	Minimum Protective Titer	Methodology Used
Canine distemper virus	≥1:16 to 1:20	Serum neutralization (SN)
Canine parvovirus	≥1:80 to 1:100	Hemagglutination inhibition (HI)
Rabies	≥0.5 IU/mL	Fluorescent antibody virus neutralization (FAN)

specimen, and there is a lack of validated sensitivity and specificity for these assays. Sometimes use of these assays increases costs significantly and delays immunization. In-practice assays also are available for detection of antibody responses, and these have the potential to overcome problems associated with laboratory quality control and delays in immunization. In-practice assays are generally not quantitative. Although high antibody titers are generally associated with greater protection, an animal with no titer may still be resistant to challenge because of CMI, which is not measured. Conversely, an animal with a titer that is generally regarded as protective has the potential to develop disease after challenge, possibly because of overwhelming exposure or immune suppression. Measurement of antibody titers may be considered for animals that have had previous adverse responses to vaccination, particularly susceptible breeds (e.g., Rottweilers and CPV infection). The World Small Animal Veterinary Association (WSAVA) has suggested that puppies could be tested at least 2 weeks after the final puppy vaccine to decide whether further vaccination for CDV or CPV is necessary.[2] Negative titers should prompt additional vaccination for these puppies.

Rapid in-house serologic assays have also been used to make decisions regarding isolation or euthanasia in shelter situations, through identification of immune animals.[28] Unfortunately, it is not always be possible to know if positive titers represent recent infection, and animals that test positive may still shed virus and pose a risk to other animals. In young puppies and kittens, positive results may represent persistent MDA or the presence of active immunity, and MDA does not have the same ability to protect against infection. In-house serologic assays can also be used to decide whether pregnant animals are susceptible in a shelter environment and thus minimize adverse reactions to attenuated live vaccines in this group of animals (see Appendix I). A study that evaluated the performance of one ELISA assay (Synbiotics TiterCHEK CPV/CPV) found that for CPV antibodies, the sensitivity and specificity of the assay was 92% and 94%, respectively, when compared with hemagglutination inhibition; and for CDV was 76% and 92%, respectively, when compared with serum neutralization.[29]

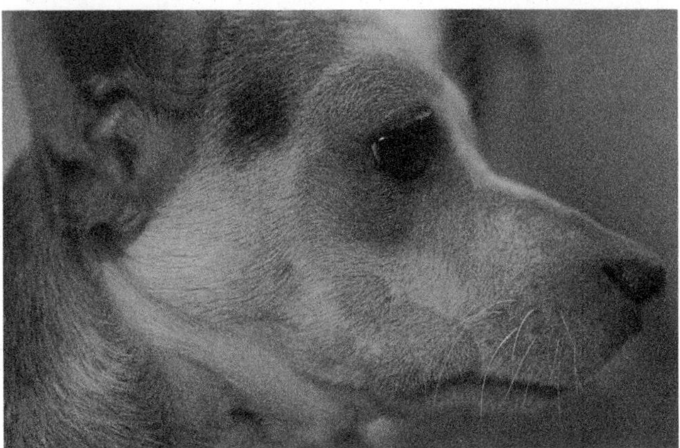

FIGURE 12-3 Facial edema and hyperemia in a 4-month old intact male Chihuahua mix after vaccination with a bacterin vaccine. (Courtesy Dr. Stephen D. White, University of California, Davis Veterinary Dermatology Service.)

Adverse Reactions to Vaccines

A vaccine is needed if an infectious disease causes significant morbidity and mortality. Vaccines should prevent more disease than they cause. In order to produce protective immunity, a vaccine *must* stimulate a reaction in an animal, both at the site of injection and systemically. This may cause clinical signs. Ideally, the signs are mild and either unnoticeable or acceptable to the pet owner. In rare situations, adverse reactions are severe enough to threaten a pet's life. Sometimes, enhanced efficacy leads to a reduction in vaccine safety. Veterinarians are encouraged to report adverse reactions to vaccines to a technical service veterinarian employed for this purpose by the vaccine manufacturer. In some countries, the drug company then reports details of the adverse reaction to drug regulatory authorities. An understanding of the true nature and incidence of adverse effects associated with vaccination has been hampered by underreporting and variable delays between vaccination and the inconsistent appearance of potential, more chronic systemic adverse effects.[30] In addition, correlation of adverse reactions to vaccine administration in young animals may be difficult because of the uniform and frequent administration of vaccines to this group. For example, it has been difficult to prove a connection between vaccination for distemper and development of hypertrophic osteopathy in Weimaraner dogs.

Immune-Mediated Vaccine Reactions

Type I Hypersensitivity Reactions

Type I hypersensitivity reactions occur when allergens cross-link IgE molecules that are bound to receptors on mast cells and basophils and trigger degranulation. Clinical signs of type I hypersensitivity responses that occur after vaccine administration include facial or periorbital edema, urticaria, cutaneous hyperemia, generalized pruritus, salivation, hypotensive shock, tachypnea, vomiting, diarrhea, collapse, and even death (Figure 12-3). Vomiting and respiratory distress are common in cats. These signs generally occur within 24 hours of vaccine administration; anaphylaxis usually begins within minutes. The estimated incidence of anaphylaxis after vaccination of dogs and cats is 1 in 5000 to 1 in 50,000 and depends on the vaccines used. One retrospective study evaluated 1.23 million dogs and nearly 0.5 million cats from more than 300 Banfield hospitals in the United States in 2002 through 2005. In this study, vaccine-associated adverse effects that were listed as vaccine reactions, allergic reactions, anaphylaxis, urticaria, and/or cardiac arrest were documented within 3 days of vaccine administration in 38.2 per 10,000 dogs and 47.4 per 10,000 cats.[20,31] Reactions coded as "allergic" or "anaphylaxis" were reported in approximately 1 in 785 dogs and 1 in 1200 cats. Reactions coded as anaphylaxis constituted only 5% of these reactions. Death occurred in 1 in 400,000 dogs and 1 in 125,000 cats that received vaccines, and all 3 dogs and 1 of the 4 cats that died received four or more doses of a vaccine (i.e., more than one vaccine product administrated simultaneously). Most reactions in dogs (73%) occurred on the day the vaccine was administered (day 0), 19% occurred on day 1, 6% on day 2, and 3% on day 3. Data from the UK Veterinary Products Committee report indicated anaphylaxis in 1 in 385,000 vaccinated dogs and 1 in 555,000 cats.[23]

Vaccines that contain large amounts of adjuvant, certain preservatives, or inactivated bacteria with proinflammatory outer surface components are more likely to cause reactions. Proteins present in fetal calf serum and stabilizers such as gelatin within the vaccine may also be responsible for allergic reactions.[32] In the Banfield study, the risk of reactions increased with the number of vaccine doses (i.e., volume of vaccine in milliliters) administered per office visit.[20] Small-breed dogs, such as miniature dachshunds, pugs, Boston terriers, miniature pinschers, and Chihuahuas, were more susceptible to development of acute vaccine reactions, and the risk of a vaccine-related adverse increased as body weight decreased. The risk of vaccine-related adverse events was 4 times greater in dogs that weighed 5 kg or less than in those that weighed more than 45 kg (Figure 12-4). Adverse events increased in frequency with age up until 2 years of age in dogs and 1 year of age in cats, after which the frequency progressively declined to rates lower than that observed in animals less than 1 year of age (see Figure 12-4). The decrease in frequency with older age may have occurred because of owners' unwillingness to have their pets vaccinated if a previous reaction occurred. Sexually intact dogs were less likely to develop adverse reactions than neutered dogs, but the opposite was true for cats.[20,31] Female cats were more likely to exhibit reactions than male cats.

The treatment of choice for anaphylaxis is epinephrine, together with other supportive treatments such as intravenous fluids and supplemental oxygen if necessary. Antihistamines and corticosteroids can be administered to dogs with less severe reactions. Vaccination should be avoided in animals with a history of severe reactions. Pretreatment with an antihistamine could be considered in animals with a history of mild reactions. These animals should also be monitored closely in the hospital for several hours after vaccine administration. It has been suggested that in the future, commercial production of low-dose vaccines for small-breed dogs might be more appropriate, given their increased risk of reactions and more marked serologic responses to vaccination.[33]

Other Hypersensitivity Reactions, including Autoimmune Disease

Type II hypersensitivity reactions occur when IgG and IgM bind to cell surface antigens and fix complement, with target cell lysis or removal of target cells by macrophages within reticuloendothelial tissues. Concerns have been raised that vaccination may predispose certain genetically susceptible individuals to immune-mediated cytopenias, although as in human medicine, studies of dogs and cats to date have failed to conclusively document vaccines as causes of these and other chronic diseases.[21,34]

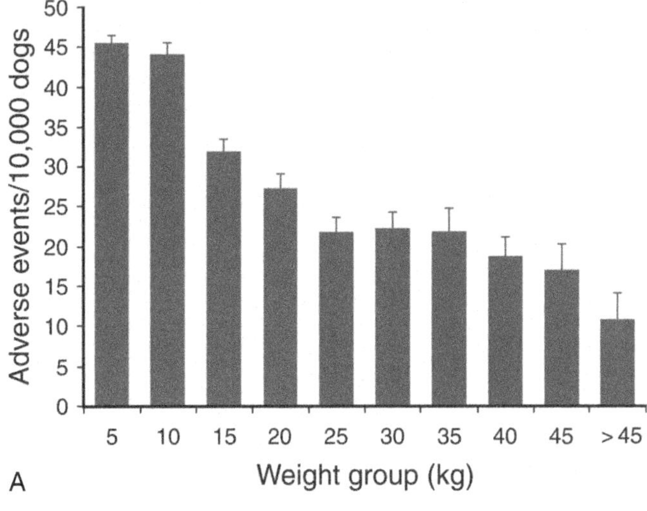

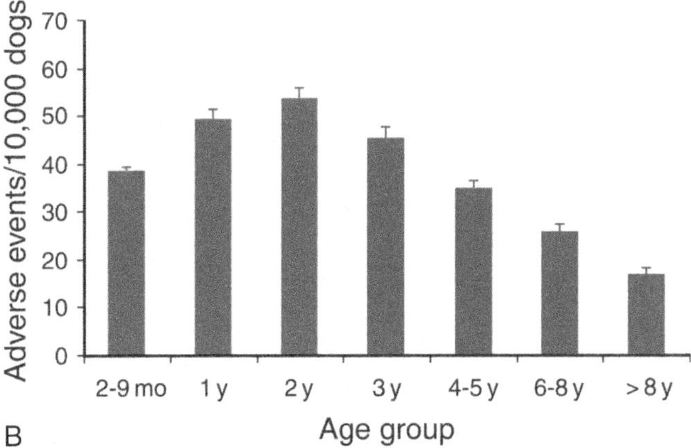

FIGURE 12-4 Correlation between **(A)** body weight and **(B)** age and the occurrence of vaccine-associated adverse effects within 3 days of vaccination in dogs. (From Moore GE, Guptill LF, Ward MP, et al. Adverse events diagnosed within three days of vaccine administration in dogs. J Am Vet Med Assoc 2005;227(7):1102-1108.)

Immune-mediated hemolytic anemia was suspected to occur following parvovirus vaccination, possibly due to the hemagglutinating properties of the virus and the high antigen mass in some of these vaccines,[35] but a later retrospective case-control study found no association.[36] Transient thrombocytopenia can occur after vaccination in some dogs.[37] In one study, dogs developed antithyroglobulin antibodies after vaccination, although this was not associated with development of hypothyroidism.[38] Cats that are vaccinated with Crandell-Rees feline kidney (CRFK) cell-derived vaccines develop antibodies against the CRFK proteins alpha-enolase and annexin A2.[39] Whether production of these antibodies has clinical significance remains to be determined.

Type III hypersensitivity reactions are characterized by immune-complex deposition in tissues and may be a consequence of immunization with certain vaccines. For example, anterior uveitis and subclinical nephritis developed in 0.4% of dogs receiving the canine adenovirus-1 (CAV-1) vaccine. This vaccine has now been replaced by CAV-2 vaccines, which rarely produce these lesions. A cutaneous vasculitis has been described after vaccination of dogs and cats with rabies virus vaccines ("rabies vaccine-induced vasculitis")[40-42] (Figure 12-5). This can occur at the site of vaccine administration, and in some animals, a multifocal ischemic dermatopathy and myopathy that affects sites such as the pinnal margins, periocular areas, tail tip, and paw pads has been reported to occur 1 to 5 months after the appearance of the initial skin lesion.[40] The multifocal dermatopathy and myopathy has been reported to resolve after treatment with pentoxifylline and vitamin E. Additional evidence is required to strengthen the association between the multifocal condition and rabies vaccination. Similarly, concerns have been raised about a possible temporal association between vaccination and immune-mediated polyarthritis in some dogs,[43] but this association remains unproven. Immune-mediated polyradiculoneuritis, a type IV hypersensitivity reaction (delayed-type hypersensitivity), occurred after vaccination of dogs with suckling-mouse brain-derived inactivated rabies vaccines, which are no longer

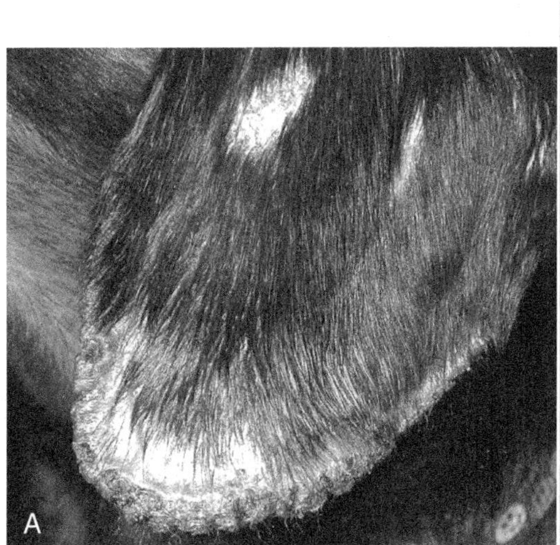

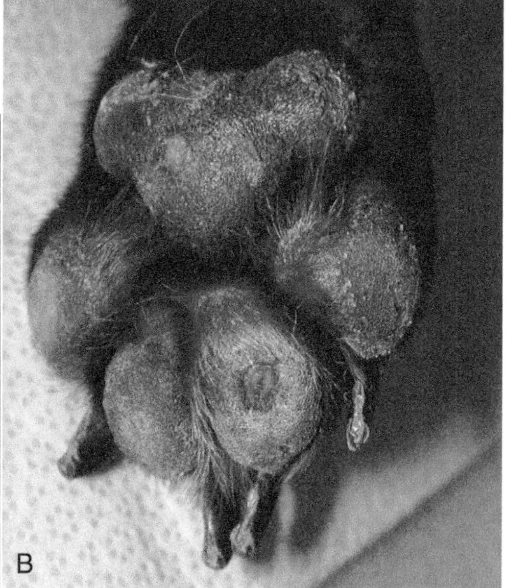

FIGURE 12-5 Ischemic dermatopathy suspected to be associated with rabies virus vaccination that involved the pinnae **(A)** and footpads **(B)** of a 1-year-old male dachshund. The rabies vaccine was administered several months before the onset of signs. (Courtesy Dr. Stephen D. White, University of California, Davis Veterinary Dermatology Service.)

available.[44] Subsequent reexposure resulted in more severe and prolonged paralysis. Granuloma formation at the site of vaccine administration also represents a type IV hypersensitivity reaction.

Despite the lack of conclusive evidence for an association between vaccination with currently available vaccines and autoimmune disease, it is possible that vaccination may be associated with dysregulation of the immune response in predisposed individuals. Therefore, vaccination is often withheld if not absolutely necessary in dogs and cats with a history of autoimmune disease. Serum titers could also be assessed to gauge the need for specific immunization in these animals.

Vaccine Organism-Induced Disease

Disease occasionally results from replication of microorganisms present in a vaccine, although severe disease is uncommon with currently available vaccines. Fever and lethargy are the most common adverse effects of vaccination and result from cytokine production in response to the vaccine. These are transient and usually resolve within 1 to 2 days.

In the past, the use of attenuated rabies virus vaccines resulted in ascending paralytic disease in a proportion of cats and dogs. This led to a change to inactivated, adjuvanted rabies vaccines. Administration of attenuated parvovirus vaccines to pregnant cats and dogs can lead to cerebellar disease in the fetus, and these vaccines have the potential to cause severe disease if shed vaccine virus infects colostrum-deprived neonates that are less than 2 weeks of age.[2] Some CDV vaccines have been associated with postvaccinal distemper in young puppies.[45] As a result, vaccination with live attenuated CDV and CPV (dogs) and feline panleukopenia virus (cats) vaccines should be avoided in pregnant animals, puppies and kittens less than 6 weeks of age, and animals receiving potent anticancer chemotherapy drugs. Some CDV vaccine strains, such as Rockborn-like strains, are more virulent than others, and these may continue to circulate and contribute to distemper in the dog population.[46] The safest attenuated live CDV vaccines contain the Onderstepoort strain. Vaccination of certain exotic pet, zoo, and wild animal species, such as ferrets, with any attenuated live CDV vaccine for dogs can also lead to postvaccinal distemper.[47,48] For animals with chronic immunocompromise, the use of inactivated vaccines has been recommended if immunization is deemed necessary. However, inactivated vaccines may have reduced efficacy in immunocompromised animals compared with healthy animals.

The use of mucosal (e.g., intranasal) vaccines for respiratory pathogens in dogs and cats can be followed by development of mild to moderate, transient upper respiratory tract signs. There have been concerns that mucosal *Bordetella bronchiseptica* vaccines may cause respiratory disease in immunosuppressed humans who inhale the vaccine directly during administration or who contact vaccine organisms that are subsequently shed by the vaccinated dog,[49,50] but definitive proof of this is still required. Inadvertent parenteral administration of the avirulent live intranasal *B. bronchiseptica* vaccine to dogs can lead to local injection-site reactions and, occasionally, fatal hepatic necrosis.[51] Inadvertent parenteral administration of mucosal *B. bronchiseptica* vaccines should be treated with subcutaneous fluids at the site of administration and treatment with an oral antibiotic likely to be effective against *B. bronchiseptica*, such as doxycycline. The ASPCA Poison Control Center also recommends injection of a gentamicin sulfate solution into the affected area (2 to 4 mg/kg gentamicin sulfate in 10 to 30 mL of saline).[4] Doxycycline treatment could be continued for 5 to 7 days. Dogs that develop hepatic necrosis may need more aggressive supportive care.

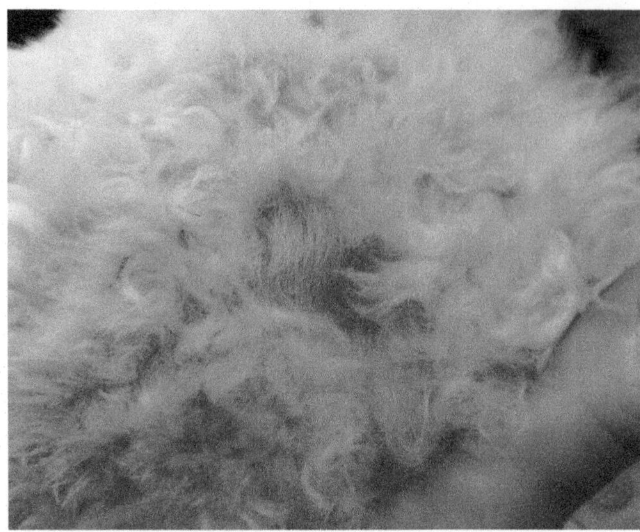

FIGURE 12-6 Two-year-old female toy poodle/maltese terrier mix that developed focal alopecia at the site of vaccination followed by regrowth of hair with an altered color and texture. (Courtesy Nicole Pierce, University of California, Davis, Class of 2013.)

Local Cutaneous Reactions and Injection-Site Sarcomas

Local cutaneous reactions are common adverse effects of vaccination, especially in cats, and include pain, swelling, irritation, and abscess formation. In dogs, focal alopecia or discoloration of the haircoat at the vaccination site can also occur (Figure 12-6). Inactivated, adjuvanted vaccines have been most commonly incriminated. Focal cutaneous granulomas and sometimes permanent focal alopecia have been most commonly reported after inactivated rabies vaccine administration to breeds such as Maltese terriers and bichon frisé.

In the late 1980s, an increase in inflammatory injection-site reactions at the site of rabies vaccine administration were noted in canine and feline biopsy specimens sent to the University of Pennsylvania. Shortly thereafter, sarcomas were observed at these sites in cats in the United States, with a 25% increase each year from 1987 to 1991 (Figure 12-7).[52] This followed (1) the change from attenuated live to inactivated rabies vaccines, (2) increased use of rabies vaccines in cats, and (3) the introduction of FeLV vaccines. The national incidence of sarcoma formation is estimated to be 0.6 to 2 sarcomas per 10,000 cats that are vaccinated.[53,54] In contrast, in the United Kingdom, it was 0.21 per 10,000 vaccine doses sold between 1995 and 1999.[22] The interval between tumor development and the last rabies vaccine typically ranges from 3 months to 3.5 years. Most tumors are fibrosarcomas, but other types of sarcomas can also occur. Although development of injection-site sarcomas is clearly linked to administration of FeLV, rabies, and other vaccines, development of sarcomas is not related to the use of specific brands or types of vaccine within an antigen class (with the possible exception of recombinant vaccines[56]), reuse of syringes, needle gauge, use and shaking of multidose vials, or concomitant viral infection.[55] There is also no evidence that aluminum-containing vaccines are associated with a higher risk of sarcoma development than aluminum-free vaccines, but there has been concern that adjuvant stimulates an inflammatory response that predisposes to sarcoma formation. A recent study showed that

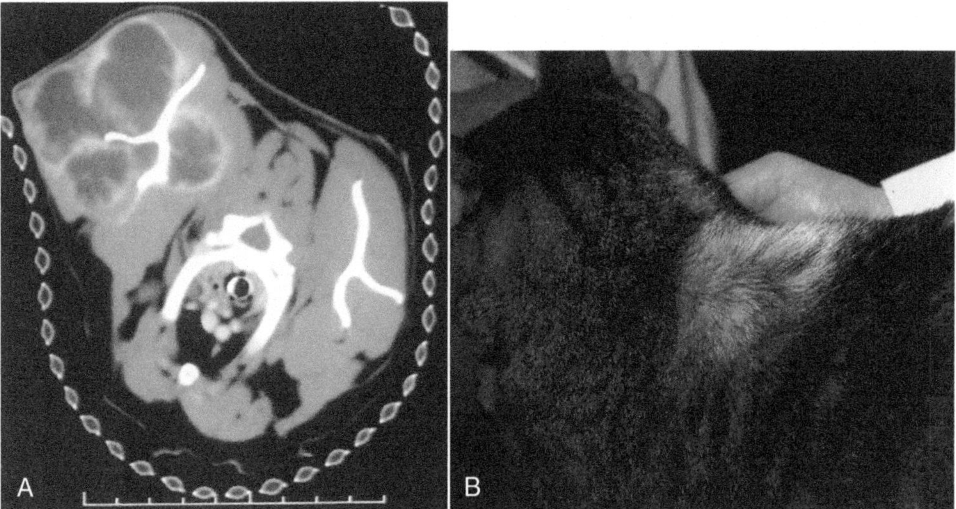

FIGURE 12-7 **A,** Computed tomographic image of an injection-site sarcoma over the scapula of a 12-year old male neutered domestic shorthair cat. **B,** Discoloration of the haircoat after radiation therapy.

inactivated vaccines were approximately 10 times more likely to be associated with injection-site sarcomas when administered at the pelvic limb site than nonadjuvanted recombinant vaccines.[56] However, neither attenuated live, recombinant, nor inactivated vaccines are risk-free, and injection of certain long-acting injectable medications (especially glucocorticoids) can also be associated with sarcoma formation in cats years later.[56,57] There is some evidence that administration of cold vaccine may also be more likely to be associated with sarcoma formation, but this requires verification.[55] It is currently hypothesized that an individual cat's genetically programmed wound healing response is responsible for the development of injection-site sarcomas.

Treatment of injection-site sarcomas involves aggressive surgical resection followed by full-course post-operative radiation therapy, because of the high incidence of recurrence. Possible adverse effects of radiation include mild to moderate cutaneous burns, hypopigmentation of the hair in the field (see Figure 12-7, *B*), and damage to the spinal cord, lungs, and kidneys within the field, although the last is rare. In one study, the median survival time for cats treated with postsurgical curative radiation therapy was 43 months.[57] Most of these cats had clean margins after surgical resection of the tumor. In contrast, the median survival times for cats treated with coarse fractionated radiation therapy was 24 months. These cats generally had macroscopic disease or dirty margins. Adjuvant chemotherapy with carboplatin or single-agent doxorubicin also has been associated with improved outcome.[57]

In order to prevent death from sarcoma formation in cats, the Vaccine-Associated Feline Sarcoma Task Force (VAFSTF) in North America recommended that rabies vaccines be administered as distally as possible on the right pelvic limb, and leukemia vaccines be administered as distally as possible on the left pelvic limb (rabies right, leukemia left). Care should be taken not to administer the vaccine too proximally or in the flank region, because tumors in these locations cannot be resected as effectively.[58] Other core vaccines should be administered over the right shoulder. These recommendations were not adopted by the WSAVA, which suggested that the skin of the lateral thorax and abdomen be used for vaccination, and vaccination sites be rotated from year to year.[2] Both groups recommended that the interscapular region be avoided, because vaccine constituents can pool in this region and contribute to a chronic inflammatory response. In addition, both groups recommended that the sites of administration and the product and batch number be documented to facilitate the reporting of adverse events. Excessive administration of vaccines to cats should be minimized, and alternative routes, such as intranasal immunization, should be considered. Owners should be advised to monitor injection sites for 3 months after vaccines are administered. If a lump forms and increases in size 1 month after vaccination, or persists beyond 3 months, the owner should have the mass evaluated by the veterinarian.

In accordance with the VAFSTF recommendations, the anatomic location, shape, and size of masses that develop at injection sites should be documented, and an incisional or tru-cut biopsy performed. Fine-needle aspiration is not recommended. If the mass is malignant, routine laboratory tests and thoracic radiography should be performed, together with computed tomography or magnetic resonance imaging of the mass if client finances allow. A veterinary oncologist should be consulted, and if possible, referral to a specialist surgeon or oncologist is recommended. Wide excision that includes at least a 2-cm margin is necessary, and the entire piece of tissue excised should be submitted for histopathology and evaluation of surgical margins. Additional treatment, such as chemotherapy and radiation therapy, is often necessary. Cats should be reevaluated at 3-month intervals for a year after surgery.

Interference with Diagnostic Test Results

Vaccination has the potential to interfere with the results of assays that detect the antibody response to infection or assays that detect components of a pathogen itself.

Interference with antibody test results can be specific or nonspecific. Nonspecific interference is rarely identified, but results from cross-reactivity between antibodies to vaccine components (such as albumin) and the reagents used in serodiagnostic tests. More commonly, specific interference with serodiagnostic tests for the infection that is targeted by the vaccine occurs. This especially problematic if (1) vaccination does not completely protect against infection, (2) the results of serologic tests are required for diagnosis, and (3) infection is chronic and persistent, and so identification of recent natural infection through seroconversion is usually not possible. For example, the inactivated FIV vaccine does not provide 100% protection, but vaccinated cats develop antibodies to the vaccine virus. These antibodies are detected by ELISA and Western blot immunoassays used for diagnosis of FIV infection. In the absence of a history of vaccination, positive antibody test results indicate active infection.[59] PCR can be used to detect FIV infection in infected cats that have a history of vaccination with FIV vaccines, but PCR can occasionally be negative in cats with active infection, so a negative PCR result does not rule out natural infection with FIV. Vaccine interference with serodiagnosis can occur after vaccination of dogs for influenza or leptospirosis, but because both of these diseases are acute, seroconversion can be used for diagnosis of recent infection in vaccinated dogs. Some serologic assays differentiate between vaccinated and naturally infected animals (DIVA). For example, serologic assays that detect the C6 antigen of *Borrelia burgdorferi* do not detect antibodies that result from immunization with Lyme vaccines. The development of recombinant vaccines that stimulate a pattern of antibody responses that differ from those that result from natural infection can help to overcome issues related to differentiation of naturally infected and vaccinated animals.

Interference with the results of assays *that detect the pathogen itself (as opposed to the antibody response)* occurs after vaccination with attenuated live vaccines that are shed by animals after vaccination. For example, cats may test positive using ELISA assays for FPV antigen after vaccination with attenuated live FPV vaccines, although for some assays, the rate at which this occurs is very low.[60] PCR tests can be positive for extended periods after vaccination with attenuated live vaccines. In some cases, sequence analysis of the PCR product can sometimes allow differentiation between vaccine and field strains, but this is currently performed only on a research basis.[61] Rapid PCR assays have also been designed that differentiate between vaccine and field strains of some pathogens, such as CDV or *B. bronchiseptica*.[62,63] Quantification of organism numbers present in a specimen through the use of real-time PCR assays (e.g., for CDV) may shed light on whether natural infection (high organism load) or vaccination (low organism load) has occurred.

Vaccine Selection

The advantages and disadvantages of vaccines and vaccine combinations that are currently available on the market are provided in the relevant sections of this book for each infection entitled "Immunity and Vaccination." Suggested vaccination schedules for individual pets and shelter animals that are based on recommendations provided by the American Animal Hospital Association (AAHA), the American Association for Feline Practitioners (AAFP), the European Society for Feline Medicine (ESFM), and WSAVA are summarized in tables in Appendix.[2,15,64-73]

To facilitate vaccine selection, vaccines for dogs and cats have been divided by various task forces into core vaccines, noncore vaccines, and those that are generally not recommended.

Core vaccines are recommended for all animals with an unknown vaccination history. The diseases involved have significant morbidity and mortality and are widely distributed, and in general, vaccination results in good protection from disease. All shelter animals should be vaccinated with core vaccines before entry to a shelter or at the time of entry if immunization ahead of time is not possible. Canine core vaccines include vaccines for CPV, CDV, CAV, and rabies for countries where rabies is endemic. The core feline vaccines are those for feline herpesvirus-1 (FHV-1), feline calicivirus (FCV), FPV, and rabies.

Noncore vaccines are optional vaccines that should be considered in light of exposure risk, that is, based on geographic distribution and the lifestyle of the pet. Vaccines considered as noncore vaccines for dogs are canine parainfluenza virus, canine influenza virus, *B. bronchiseptica, Leptospira* spp., and *Borrelia burgdorferi*. Optional or noncore vaccines for cats include FeLV, FIV, virulent FCV, *Chlamydia felis,* and *B. bronchiseptica* vaccines.

Several other vaccines are currently available on the market. For dogs, these are vaccines for canine coronavirus, CAV-1, and rattlesnake envenomation. The reports of the American Veterinary Medical Association (AVMA) and the AAHA canine vaccine task force have listed the first two vaccines as not generally recommended, because "the diseases are either of little clinical significance or respond readily to treatment," evidence for efficacy of these vaccines is minimal, and they may "produce adverse events with limited benefit." Currently, information regarding the efficacy of the canine rattlesnake vaccine is insufficient. For cats, the feline infectious peritonitis (FIP) vaccine is not generally recommended by the AAFP.

SUGGESTED READINGS

Baker C, Pickering L, Chilton L, et al. General recommendations on immunization—recommendations of the Advisory Committee on Immunization Practices (ACP). MMWR Recomm Rep. 2011;60(2):1-64.

Day MJ, Horzinek MC, Schultz RD. Guidelines for the vaccination of dogs and cats. Compiled by the Vaccination Guidelines Group of the World Small Animal Veterinary Association. J Small Anim Pract. 2007;48(9):528-541.

Larson LJ, Newbury S, Schultz RD. Canine and feline vaccinations and immunology. In: Miller L, Hurley K, eds. Infectious Disease Management in Animal Shelters. Ames, IA: Wiley-Blackwell; 2009:61-82.

Moore GE, HogenEsch H. Adverse vaccinal events in dogs and cats. Vet Clin North Am Small Anim Pract. 2010;40:393-407.

Paul MA, Appel M, Barrett R, et al. Report of the American Animal Hospital Association (AAHA) Canine Vaccine Task Force: executive summary and 2003 canine vaccine guidelines and recommendations. J Am Anim Hosp Assoc. 2003;39(2):119-131.

The 2006 American Association of Feline Practitioners Feline Vaccine Advisory Panel Report. J Am Vet Med Assoc 229:1405–1441 (also http://www.aafponline.org/resources/practice_guidelines.htm).

REFERENCES

1. Delves PJ, Martin SJ, Burton DR, et al. eds. Roitt's Essential Immunology. 12th ed. Ames, IA: Wiley-Blackwell; 2011.
2. Day MJ, Horzinek MC, Schultz RD. WSAVA guidelines for the vaccination of dogs and cats. J Small Anim Pract. 2010;51(6):1-32.
3. Larson LJ, Newbury S, Schultz RD. Canine and feline vaccinations and immunology. In: Miller L, Hurley K, eds. Infectious Disease Management in Animal Shelters. Ames, IA: Wiley-Blackwell; 2009:61-82.
4. De Gregorio E, D'Oro U, Wack A. Immunology of TLR-independent adjuvants. Curr Opin Immunol. 2009;21(3):339-345.
5. Cox JC, Coutler AR. Adjuvants—a classification and review of their modes of action. Vaccine. 1997;15(3):248-256.
6. Abdelmagid OY, Larson L, Payne L, et al. Evaluation of the efficacy and duration of immunity of a canine combination vaccine against virulent parvovirus, infectious canine hepatitis virus, and distemper virus experimental challenges. Vet Ther. 2004;5(3):173-186.
7. Schultz RD. Duration of immunity for canine and feline vaccines: a review. Vet Microbiol. 2006;117(1):75-79.

8. Schultz RD, Thiel B, Mukhtar E, et al. Age and long-term protective immunity in dogs and cats. J Comp Pathol. 2010;142(Suppl 1): S102-S108.
9. Larson LJ, Schultz RD. Effect of vaccination with recombinant canine distemper virus vaccine immediately before exposure under shelter-like conditions. Vet Ther. 2006;7(2):113-118.
10. Brun A, Chappuis G, Précausta P, et al. Immunisation against panleukopenia: early development of immunity. Comp Immunol Microbiol Infect Dis. 1979;1(4):335-339.
11. Phillips TR, Jensen JL, Rubino MJ, et al. Effects of vaccines on the canine immune system. Can J Vet Res. 1989;53(2):154-160.
12. Mastro JM, Axthelm M, Mathes LE, et al. Repeated suppression of lymphocyte blastogenesis following vaccinations of CPV-immune dogs with modified-live CPV vaccines. Vet Microbiol. 1986;12(3):201-211.
13. Strasser A, May B, Teltscher A, et al. Immune modulation following immunization with polyvalent vaccines in dogs. Vet Immunol Immunopathol. 2003;94(3-4):113-121.
14. Foley JE, Orgad U, Hirsh DC, et al. Outbreak of fatal salmonellosis in cats following use of a high-titer modified-live panleukopenia virus vaccine. J Am Vet Med Assoc. 1999;214(1):67-70:43-44.
15. Welborn LV, DeVries JG, Ford R, et al. 2011 AAHA canine vaccination guidelines. J Am Anim Hosp Assoc. 2011;47:1-42.
16. Baker C, Pickering L, Chilton L, et al. General recommendations on immunization—recommendations of the Advisory Committee on Immunization Practices (ACP). MMWR Recomm Rep. 2011;60(2):1-64.
17. Scott FW, Geissinger CM. Long-term immunity in cats vaccinated with an inactivated trivalent vaccine. Am J Vet Res. 1999;60(5):652-658.
18. King GE, Hadler SC. Simultaneous administration of childhood vaccines: an important public health policy that is safe and efficacious. Pediatr Infect Dis. 1994;13(5):394-407.
19. Offit PA, Quarles J, Gerber MA, et al. Addressing parents' concerns: do multiple vaccines overwhelm or weaken the infant's immune system? Pediatrics. 2002;109(1):124-129.
20. Moore GE, Guptill LF, Ward MP, et al. Adverse events diagnosed within three days of vaccine administration in dogs. J Am Vet Med Assoc. 2005;227(7):1102-1108.
21. Orenstein WA, Pickering LK, Mawle A, et al. Immunization. In: Mandell GL, Bennett JE, Dolin R, eds. Principles and Practice of Infectious Diseases. 7th ed. Philadephia, PA: Elsevier; 2010:3917-3949.
22. Coffey TJ, Werling D. Therapeutic targeting of the innate immune system in domestic animals. Cell Tissue Res. 2011;343(1):251-261.
23. Day MJ. Vaccine adverse effects: fact and fiction. Vet Microbiol. 2006;117:51-58.
24. Kennedy LJ, Lunt M, Barnes A, et al. Factors influencing the antibody response of dogs vaccinated against rabies. Vaccine. 2007;25(51):8500-8507.
25. Berndtsson LT, Nyman AK, Rivera E, et al. Factors associated with the success of rabies vaccination of dogs in Sweden. Acta Vet Scand. 2011;53:22.
26. Jónsdóttir I. Maturation of mucosal immune responses and influence of maternal antibodies. J Comp Pathol. 2007;137(Suppl 1): S20-S26.
27. Siegrist CA. The challenges of vaccine responses in early life: selected examples. J Comp Pathol. 2007;137(Suppl 1):S4-S9.
28. Crawford PC, Levy JK, Leutenegger C. Use of antibody titers and quantitative PCR as risk assessment tools for management of an outbreak of canine distemper and parvovirus. Denver, CO: Proceedings of the 2011 American College of Veterinary Internal Medicine; 2011.
29. Litster AL, Pressler B, Volpe A, et al. Accuracy of a point-of-care ELISA test kit for predicting the presence of protective canine parvovirus and canine distemper virus antibody concentrations in dogs. Vet J. 2012;193:363-366.
30. Moore GE, HogenEsch H. Adverse vaccinal events in dogs and cats. Vet Clin North Am Small Anim Pract. 2010;40:393-407.
31. Moore GE, DeSantis-Kerr AC, Guptill LF, et al. Adverse events after vaccine administration in cats: 2,560 cases (2002-2005). J Am Vet Med Assoc. 2007;231:94-100.
32. Ohmori K, Masuda K, Maeda S, et al. IgE reactivity to vaccine components in dogs that developed immediate-type allergic reactions after vaccination. Vet Immunol Immunopathol. 2005;104(3-4):249-256.
33. Day MJ. Vaccine safety in the neonatal period. J Comp Pathol. 2007;137:S51-S56.
34. Edwards DS, Henley WE, Ely ER, et al. Vaccination and ill-health in dogs: a lack of temporal association and evidence of equivalence. Vaccine. 2004;22(25-26):3270-3273.
35. Duval D, Giger U. Vaccine-associated immune-mediated hemolytic anemia in the dog. J Vet Intern Med. 1996;10(5):290-295.
36. Carr AP, Panciera DL, Kidd L. Prognostic factors for mortality and thromboembolism in canine immune-mediated hemolytic anemia: a retrospective study of 72 dogs. J Vet Intern Med. 2002;16(5):290-295.
37. Straw B. Decrease in platelet count after vaccination with distemper-hepatitis (DH) vaccine. Vet Med Small Anim Clin. 1978;73(6):725-726.
38. Scott-Moncrieff JC, Azcona-Olivera J, Glickman NW, et al. Evaluation of antithyroglobulin antibodies after routine vaccination in pet and research dogs. J Am Vet Med Assoc. 2002;221:515-521.
39. Whittemore JS, Hawley JR, Jensen WA, et al. Antibodies against Crandell Rees feline kidney (CRFK) cell line antigens, alpha-enolase, and annexin A2 in vaccinated and CRFK hyperinoculated cats. J Vet Intern Med. 2010;24(2):306-313.
40. Vitale CB, Gross TL, Magro CM. Vaccine-induced ischemic dermatopathy in the dog. Vet Dermatol. 1999;10:131-142.
41. Wilcock BP, Yager JA. Focal cutaneous vasculitis and alopecia at sites of rabies vaccination in dogs. J Am Vet Med Assoc. 1986;188(10):1174-1177.
42. Nichols PR, Morris DO, Beale KM. A retrospective study of canine and feline cutaneous vasculitis. Vet Dermatol. 2001;12(5): 255-264.
43. Kohn SL, Garner M, Bennett D, et al. Polyarthritis following vaccination in four dogs. Vet Comp Orthoped Traumatol. 2003;16:6-10.
44. Gehring R, Eggars B. Suspected post-vaccinal acute polyradiculoneuritis in a puppy. J S Afr Vet Assoc. 2001;72(2):96.
45. Cornwell HJ, Thompson H, McCandlish IA, et al. Encephalitis in dogs associated with a batch of canine distemper (Rockborn) vaccine. Vet Rec. 1988;122(3):54-59.
46. Martella V, Blixenkrone-Møller M, Elia G, et al. Lights and shades on an historical vaccine canine distemper virus, the Rockborn strain. Vaccine. 2011;29(6):1222-1227.
47. Carpenter JW, Appel MJ, Erickson RC, et al. Fatal vaccine-induced canine distemper virus infection in black-footed ferrets. J Am Vet Med Assoc. 1976;169(9):961-964.
48. Bush M, Montali RJ, Brownstein D, et al. Vaccine-induced canine distemper in a lesser panda. J Am Vet Med Assoc. 1976;169(9):959-960.
49. Gisel JJ, Brumble LM, Johnson MM. *Bordetella bronchiseptica* pneumonia in a kidney-transplant patient after exposure to recently vaccinated dogs. Transpl Infect Dis. 2010;21(1):73-76.
50. Berkelman RL. Human illness associated with the use of veterinary vaccines. Clin Infect Dis. 2003;37(3):407-414.
51. Toshach K, Jackson MW, Dubielzig RR. Hepatocellular necrosis associated with the subcutaneous injection of an intranasal *Bordetella bronchiseptica*–canine parainfluenza vaccine. J Am Anim Hosp Assoc. 1997;33(2):126-128.
52. Hendrick MJ, Shofer FS, Goldschmist MH, et al. Comparison of fibrosarcomas that developed at vaccination sites and nonvaccination sites in cats: 239 cases (1991-1992). J Am Vet Med Assoc. 1994;205(10):1425-1429.
53. Richards JR, Elston TH, Ford RB, et al. The 2006 American Association of Feline Practitioners Feline Vaccine Advisory Panel Report. J Am Vet Med Assoc. 2006;229(9):1405-1441.

54. Gobar GM, Kass PH. World Wide Web-based survey of vaccination practices, postvaccinal reactions, and vaccine site-associated sarcomas in cats. J Am Vet Med Assoc. 2002;220(10):1477-1482.
55. Kass PH, Spangler WL, Hendrick MJ, et al. Multicenter case-control study of risk factors associated with development of vaccine-associated sarcomas in cats. J Am Vet Med Assoc. 2003;223(9):1283-1292.
56. Srivastav A, Kass PH, McGill LD, et al. Comparative vaccine-specific and other injectable-specific risks of injection-site sarcomas in cats. J Am Vet Med Assoc. 2012;241:595-602.
57. Eckstein C, Guscetti F, Roos M, et al. A retrospective analysis of radiation therapy for the treatment of feline vaccine-associated sarcoma. Vet Comp Oncol. 2009;7(1):54-68.
58. Shaw SC, Kent MS, Gordon IK, et al. Temporal changes in characteristics of injection-site sarcomas in cats: 392 cases (1990-2006). J Am Vet Med Assoc. 2009;234(3):376-380.
59. Levy JK, Crawford PC, Slater MR. Effect of vaccination against feline immunodeficiency virus on results of serologic testing in cats. J Am Vet Med Assoc. 2004;225(10):1558-1561.
60. Patterson EV, Reese MJ, Tucker SJ, et al. Effect of vaccination on parvovirus antigen testing in kittens. J Am Vet Med Assoc. 2007;230(3):359-363.
61. Hirasawa T, Yono K, Mikazuki K. Differentiation of wild- and vaccine-type canine parvoviruses by PCR and restriction-enzyme analysis. Zentralbl Veterinarmed B. 1995;42(10):601-610.
62. Si W, Zhou S, Wang Z, et al. A multiplex reverse transcription-nested polymerase chain reaction for detection and differentiation of wild-type and vaccine strains of canine distemper virus. Virol J. 2010;7:86.
63. Iemura R, Tsukatani R, Micallef MJ, et al. Simultaneous analysis of the nasal shedding kinetics of field and vaccine strains of *Bordetella bronchiseptica*. Vet Rec. 2009;165(25):747-751.
64. American Animal Hospital Association (AAHA) Canine Vaccine Taskforce. 2006 AAHA canine vaccine guidelines. J Am Anim Hosp Assoc. 2006;42(2):80-89.
65. Klingborg DJ, Hustead DR, Curry-Galvin EA, et al. AVMA's principles of vaccination. J Am Vet Med Assoc. 2001;219:575-576: (also http://www.avma.org/policies/vaccination.htm).
66. Truyen U, Addie D, Belçk S, et al. Feline panleukopenia. ABCD guidelines on prevention and management. J Feline Med Surg. 2009;11(7):538-546.
67. Thiry E, Addie D, Belçk S, et al. Feline herpesvirus infection. ABCD guidelines on prevention and management. J Feline Med Surg. 2009;11(7):547-555.
68. Radford AD, Addie D, Belçk S, et al. Feline calicivirus infection. ABCD guidelines on prevention and management. J Feline Med Surg. 2009;11(7):556-564.
69. Lutz H, Addie D, Belçk S, et al. Feline leukemia. ABCD guidelines on prevention and management. J Feline Med Surg. 2009;11(7):565-574.
70. Frymus T, Addie D, Belçk S, et al. Feline rabies. ABCD guidelines on prevention and management. J Feline Med Surg. 2009;11(7):585-593.
71. Addie D, Belçk S, Boucraut-Baralon C, et al. Feline infectious peritonitis. ABCD guidelines on prevention and management. J Feline Med Surg. 2009;11(7):594-604.
72. Gruffydd-Jones T, Addie D, Belçk S, et al. *Chlamydophila felis* infection. ABCD guidelines on prevention and management. J Feline Med Surg. 2009;11(7):605-609.
73. Egberink H, Addie D, Belçk S, et al. *Bordetella bronchiseptica* infection in cats. ABCD guidelines on prevention and management. J Feline Med Surg. 2009;11(7):610-614.

PART II

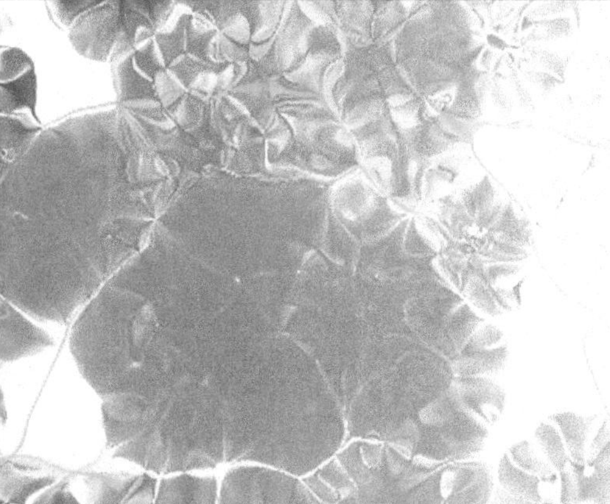

Major Infectious Diseases and Their Etiologic Agents

SECTION 1
Viral Diseases

SECTION 2
Bacterial Diseases

SECTION 3
Fungal and Algal Diseases

SECTION 4
Protozoal Diseases

SECTION 5
Infections of Selected Organ Systems

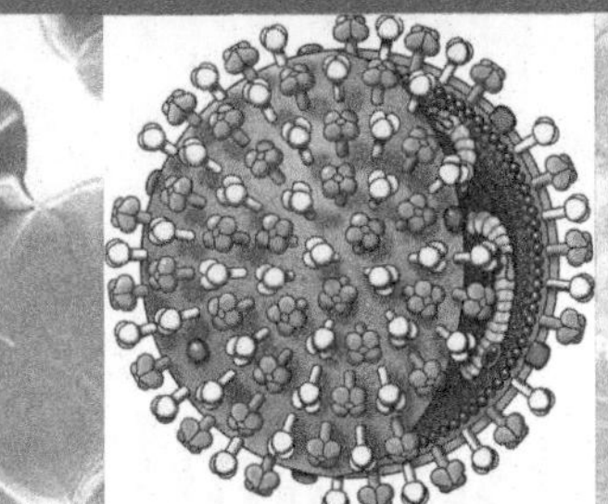

SECTION 1 Viral Diseases

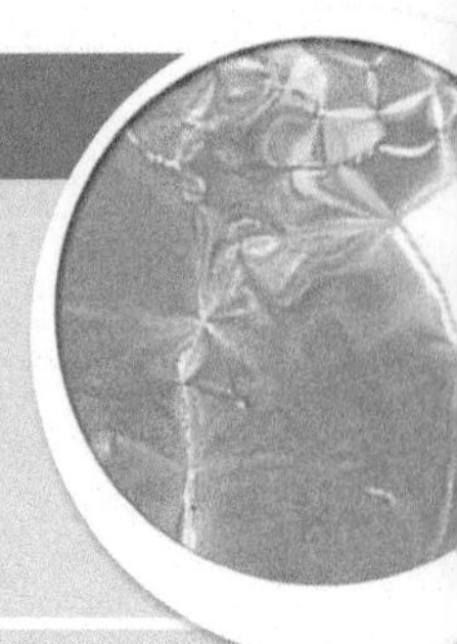

CHAPTER 13

Rabies

Jane E. Sykes and Bruno B. Chomel

Overview of Rabies

First Described: Circa the second millennium BC, Mesopotamia[1]

Cause: Rabies virus (Family Rhabdoviridae, Genus *Lyssavirus*)

Primary Mode of Transmission: biting, with inoculation of saliva containing the virus

Affected Hosts: All warm-blooded animals. Highly susceptible hosts include wolves, foxes, coyotes, jackals, dogs, cattle, raccoons, skunks, bats, and mongooses. Moderately susceptible hosts include cats, ferrets, primates, sheep, goats, and horses.

Geographic Distribution: Classic (genotype 1) rabies is found worldwide except for Australia, New Zealand, Iceland, the United Kingdom, Japan, most of western Europe, Fiji, Hawaii, and Guam.

Major Clinical Signs: Fever, lethargy, behavioral changes, pupillary dilation, ataxia, lower motor neuron paresis or paralysis (including of the muscles of mastication), vestibular signs (including a head tilt), dysphagia, dysphonia, tremors, seizures, ptyalism.

Differential Diagnoses: Distemper virus infection; West Nile virus infection; equine encephalitis virus infection; bacterial, protozoal, or fungal meningoencephalitis; toxins such as strychnine; central nervous system trauma; spinal neoplasia; granulomatous meningoencephalitis.

Public Health Significance: Rabies is a deadly zoonosis and dogs are a major natural reservoir of the virus. In the United States, most human rabies is associated with bat contact.

Etiologic Agent and Epidemiology

Rabies is a deadly, zoonotic, neurologic disease caused by a bullet-shaped, enveloped RNA virus that belongs to the genus *Lyssavirus* (from Lyssa, the Greek goddess of madness, rage, and frenzy) (Figure 13-1). The virus is fragile in the environment, and readily inactivated by a variety of disinfectants, soaps, ultraviolet light, and heat. It can survive up to 3 to 4 days in carcasses at 20°C, and longer with refrigeration.[2,3] Freezing tissues at temperatures less than −20°C may prolong survival of the virus for years.

There are seven lyssavirus genotypes (Table 13-1). Classical rabies virus belongs to genotype 1. The remaining six lyssavirus genotypes primarily infect bats and less frequently cause fatal human encephalitis, which is clinically indistinguishable from classical rabies.[4] Thus, although Australia, New Zealand, Iceland, the United Kingdom, Japan, most of western Europe, Fiji, Hawaii, and Guam are designated terrestrial rabies-free, lyssaviruses capable of causing fatal encephalitis in humans exist in some of these regions, including Australia, Western Europe, and the United Kingdom (Figure 13-2). The remaining information in this chapter pertains only to genotype 1 rabies virus infections.

Infection with rabies virus most commonly occurs as a result of inoculation of virus-containing saliva into a bite wound, in the large majority of the cases after a dog bite. Other routes of transmission reported in species other than dogs and cats

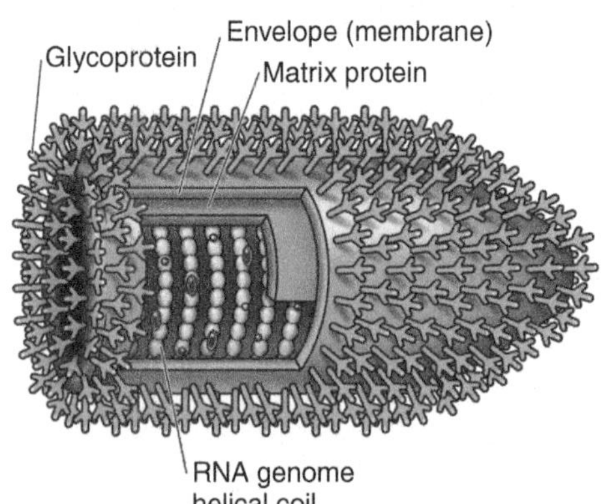

FIGURE 13-1 Structure of a rabies virus virion.

TABLE 13-1

Lyssaviruses Belonging to the Family Rhabdoviridae

Genotype	Virus	Source	Distribution
1	Rabies virus	Dog, fox, raccoon, bat, others	Widespread
2	Lagos bat virus	Bats, cats, not in human beings	Africa (rare)
3	Mokola	Shrews, cats, dog	Africa
4	Duvenhage	Insectivorous bats	Africa (rare)
5 and 6	European bat lyssavirus types 1 and 2	Insectivorous bats	Netherlands, United Kingdom, Denmark, Germany, Spain, France, Poland, Hungary, Russian Federation, Ukraine, Switzerland
7	Australian bat lyssavirus	Flying fox (fruit bats); insectivorous bats	Australia; Philippines (serologic evidence)

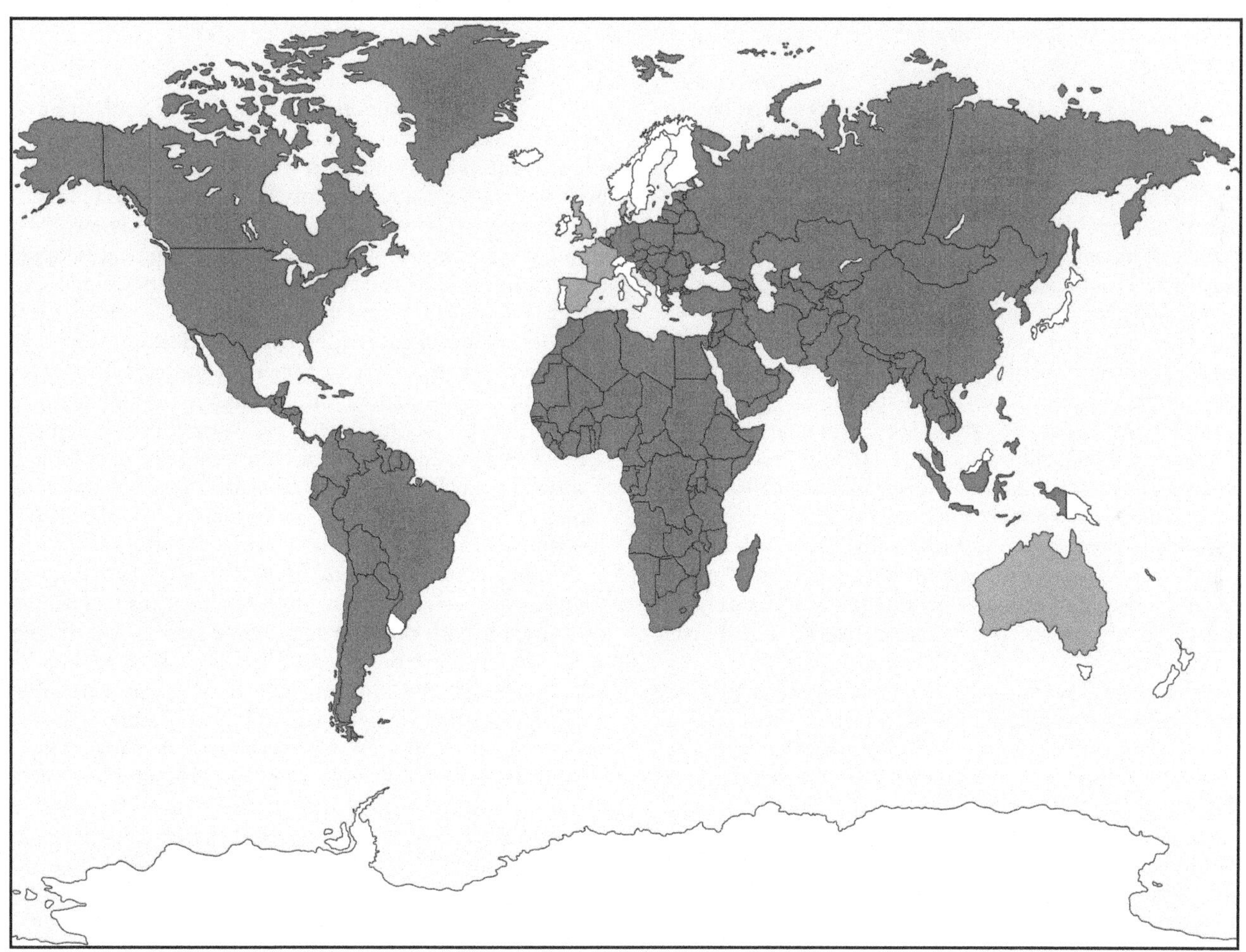

FIGURE 13-2 Global distribution of lyssaviruses. Distribution of rabies virus *(red)*. Areas where rabies-related viruses only, and not classic rabies genotype 1, are documented are classified by the WHO as "rabies free" *(dark blue)*. White areas are free of rabies and rabies-related viruses. (Redrawn from Warrell MJ, Warrell DA. Rabies and other lyssavirus diseases. Lancet 2004;363:959-969.)

are rare and include corneal or solid-organ transplantation in human patients[5]; aerosol transmission, such as that occurring within caves containing large numbers of bats[6,7]; and transmission after ingestion of infected tissues or milk.[6,8]

All warm-blooded animals are susceptible to rabies, although dogs, wild carnivores, and bats are considered the main natural reservoirs of rabies virus. In general, wolves, foxes, coyotes, jackals, dogs, cattle, raccoons, skunks, bats, and mongooses are highly susceptible to infection. Moderately susceptible hosts include cats, ferrets, primates, sheep, goats, and horses. Marsupials, including opossums, have a low degree of susceptibility. Some bird species can be experimentally infected but do not develop clinical signs and are unlikely hosts.[9]

Not every bite from a rabid animal leads to rabies virus infection, and infection may not always culminate in death, unless clinical signs develop. Factors influencing the outcome after a

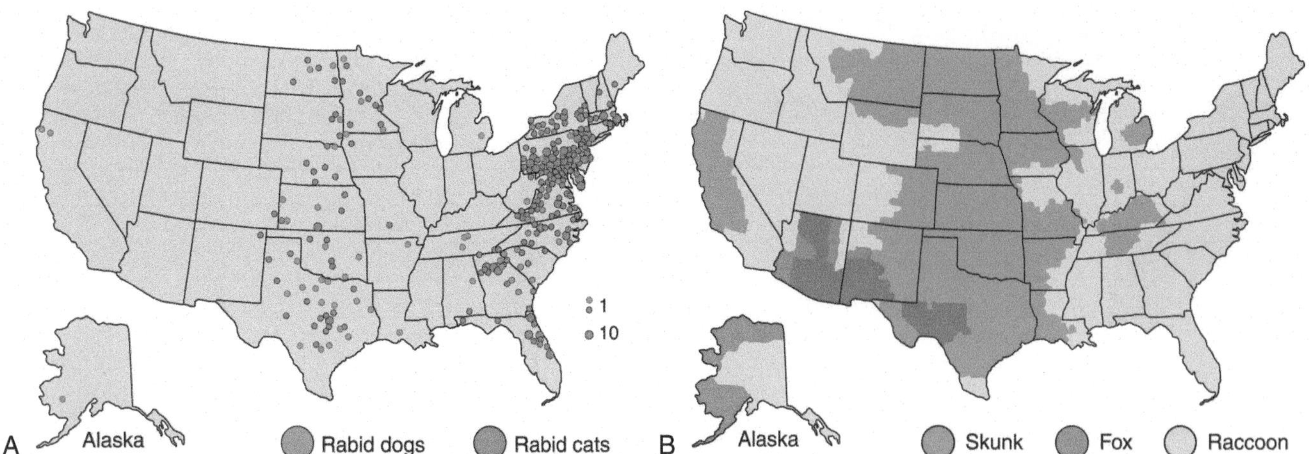

FIGURE 13-3 **A,** Reported cases of rabies that involve cats and dogs, by county, 2010. Histogram represents numbers of counties in each category for total number of cats and dogs submitted for testing. Note the overlap with the distribution of wildlife reservoir hosts in **B. B,** Distribution of major rabies virus variants among mesocarnivore reservoirs in the United States. (A and B modified from Blanton JD, Palmer D, Dyer J, et al. Rabies surveillance in the United States during 2010. J Am Vet Med Assoc 2011;239:773-783.)

bite from a rabid animal include the proximity of the bite site to the central nervous system (CNS), the degree of innervation of the bite site, the age of the host (young animals are more susceptible), the amount of virus inoculated, and the neuroinvasiveness of the rabies virus variant involved. If left untreated, up to 60% of humans bitten by a rabid dog on the head or neck develop rabies, compared with up to 40% of those bitten on the hand, and 10% of those bitten on the trunk or leg.[10]

Rabies viruses that circulate within a certain geographic region are adapted to specific dominant reservoir hosts (e.g., bat rabies virus variants or raccoon rabies virus variants). All rabies virus variants can infect and cause disease in animals other than their reservoir hosts (spillover hosts). In all host species, rabies is usually an acute fatal illness, although some animals, such as bats and skunks, have a more prolonged course of illness than others, such as foxes, coyotes, or raccoons. The possibility of a subclinical carrier state, especially in bats, has been suggested based on the detection of rabies virus antibody and, rarely, the virus itself in some reservoir host species that are not showing signs of illness.[4]

Over the past 50 years, owing to mandatory vaccination and control programs, domestic animal rabies in the United States has decreased in prevalence, whereas wildlife rabies has increased. The dog rabies virus variant was considered eradicated from the United States at the beginning of the 21st century. Currently, cats are more commonly reported with rabies in the United States (about 300 cases/year) than dogs (fewer than 100 cases/year), most likely reflecting rabies vaccination practices (Figure 13-3, *A*). No feline rabies virus variant has been described. The geographic distribution of feline and canine rabies follows that of regions where wildlife rabies is endemic. Most cats and dogs are infected with the rabies virus variant that is associated with the major wildlife reservoir host in their respective geographic location (see Figure 13-3, *B*). Rabid cats are most often reported from the northeastern United States, mid-Atlantic, and south-Atlantic states, with lesser numbers from the north and south central states. The eastern distribution of feline rabies follows the distribution of raccoon rabies.[11,12] Rarely, cats are infected from bats. Rabies in dogs and cats is most commonly reported from the north central, south central, and Atlantic states (see Figure 13-3, *A*). Dogs may be infected with rabies virus variants from skunks or raccoons. Infected dogs have also been imported into the United States from other countries where canine rabies variants are endemic.[13,14] In Europe, the major wildlife reservoir species have been foxes and raccoon dogs, and in South Africa, jackals and mongooses predominate. In western Europe, fox rabies has largely been eliminated as a result of mass vaccination campaigns. Spillover occurs from wildlife reservoir hosts to domestic animal species, which subsequently contact humans. Nevertheless, the vast majority of human cases in North America result from contact with infected bats, which are present in all states except Hawaii (see Public Health Aspects). Rabies in rodents and lagomorphs is rare, possibly because they are always killed by the bite of a rabid animal. In the United States, most reports have been from woodchucks in raccoon endemic areas.[15] A few cases of rabies in pet ferrets, rabbits, and a pet guinea pig have been described.[16]

Although rabies occurs in cats and dogs of any age, it is most frequently reported in young dogs and cats, with a median age of 1 year for both cats and dogs in one study; 75% of animals were 3 years of age or younger.[17] Rabies can occur in puppies and kittens that have not yet reached the age at which routine rabies vaccination is approved, which is an emerging issue as a result of illegal importation of pet dogs from Mexico through California and Texas. Male dogs may be slightly more predisposed, and most dogs and cats with rabies have not been neutered and live in rural environments, frequently being unrestrained at night.[11,17] In the United States, some degree of seasonality occurs for rabies in dogs and cats, which correlates with seasonal increases in rabid raccoons and skunks.[11,17] For the majority of cats and dogs with rabies, a history of known contact with wild animals or a wound is lacking.

Clinical Features

Signs and Their Pathogenesis

After inoculation into the subcutaneous tissues and muscle, rabies virus replicates locally within muscle cells and then attaches to peripheral nerve endings. Local replication around the bite site can continue for months before the virus enters peripheral sensory and motor nerve endings, with the nicotinic acetylcholine receptor being the main receptor for the virus. The virus then travels in a retrograde fashion up nerve axons at a

TABLE 13-2

Major Clinical Findings in 183 Cats and 119 Dogs with Rabies in the United States

Sign	Percent of Cats	Percent of Dogs
Aggression	55	31
Ataxia	30	49
Irritability	34	23
Anorexia	22	38
Lethargy	20	37
Hypersalivation	14	41
Dysphagia	10	30
Lameness	18	16
Limb paralysis	17	29
Jaw paralysis	3	29
Dysphonia	16	9
Hyperesthesia	10	17
Seizures	8	14
Fever	3	14

From Eng TR, Fishbein DB. Epidemiologic factors, clinical findings, and vaccination status of rabies in cats and dogs in the United States in 1988. National Study Group on Rabies. J Am Vet Med Assoc 1990;197:201-209.

rate of 3 mm/hr.[6] Once the virus is within the CNS, there is massive viral replication, with cell-to-cell transmission of the virus across synaptic junctions. The spinal cord, medulla oblongata, periaqueductal gray matter, limbic system, and cerebellum are particularly affected. The virus also moves outwards from the CNS in somatic and autonomic nerves and is deposited in a variety of tissues, including cardiac and skeletal muscle, the eye, the kidney, pancreas, nerves around hair follicles, and the salivary glands. Production of new virions through budding from the plasma membranes occurs primarily within the salivary glands, which results in the shedding of virus that can be transmitted to other hosts. Thus, the presence of virus in the saliva indicates that the CNS has been infected. In some animals, death occurs before the saliva becomes infected. Virus is shed by some dogs for up to 13 days before the onset of clinical signs.[18]

Clinical signs probably result from impaired neuronal function[6] and occur after an incubation period that ranges from just over a week to 6 months. Most dogs and cats develop disease 1 to 2 months after exposure. In general, the closer the bite site is to the CNS, the shorter the incubation period. The incubation period is also influenced by the host species, age, degree of innervation of the bite site, neuroinvasiveness of the rabies virus variant, and the amount of virus inoculated. Although 90% of humans develop disease within 6 months of exposure, incubation periods of 6 years or more have been reported.[19-21]

The clinical presentations of rabies virus infection have been divided into excitatory ("furious") and paralytic ("dumb") forms. Three phases have been described in the progression of the disease, the prodromal, furious, and paralytic phases, but the stages are variable and may overlap, and signs may be atypical (Table 13-2). Infrequently, there is a history of a wound, or wounds are still present at the time neurologic signs occur. Unfortunately, rabies is infrequently suspected as the possible diagnosis at the time rabid animals are examined by veterinarians.[11,17]

When it occurs, the *prodromal phase* lasts 2 to 3 days in dogs and 1 to 2 days in cats, and is characterized by a variable fever, licking or chewing at the bite site, and behavioral changes. Dogs and cats may become lethargic, anorexic, apprehensive, restless, or reclusive, and vomiting may occur.[11] Some animals become more docile or affectionate. Pupillary dilation, sometimes with decreased pupillary light reflexes, may occur. The *furious phase* occurs in approximately two thirds of affected cats and dogs[22] and lasts 0 to 7 days. Clinical signs result from forebrain involvement and include irritability, anxiousness or excitability, hyperesthesia, hypersalivation, vocalization, roaming, and aggression. Affected animals may try to eat foreign objects, which may become lodged within the gastrointestinal tract, or they may attack their surroundings or moving objects. Some animals develop ataxia, vestibular signs, and grand mal seizures. Tremors; staring, or a wild, spooky, or blank look in the eyes; increased vocalization; and compulsive running can occur cats, which also often develop aggressive behavior.[11,17,23] The *paralytic phase* develops 1 to 10 days after the onset of clinical signs and is characterized by flaccid paralysis, which is ascending and often initially involves the bitten extremity. Neurologic examination reveals flaccid paralysis with absent segmental reflexes. Laryngeal paralysis may lead to a change in the sound or pitch of a dog's bark or cat's meow. Hypersalivation results from paralysis of the pharyngeal muscles, and a "dropped jaw" can occur as a result of masticatory muscle paralysis, especially in dogs, which may appear to owners as if they are choking.

If euthanasia is not performed, coma and death usually occurs within a week of the onset of signs, with a few animals dying as long as 10 days after the onset of illness. Death is associated with multiorgan failure, especially cardiac and respiratory failure. Recovery from rabies is extremely rare. Experimentally, some dogs have recovered from clinical rabies days to months after being infected with certain rabies virus strains.[24,25]

Diagnosis

Rabies should be suspected in dogs and cats evaluated for sudden onset of behavioral changes and flaccid paralysis, especially in rabies-endemic regions, or in animals imported from rabies-endemic countries. Although a particularly high degree of suspicion is warranted for animals that lack a vaccination history for rabies, the disease has been reported in partially and completely vaccinated dogs and cats,[11,17,23] so a history of rabies vaccination should not be used to dismiss suspicion for rabies.

Laboratory Abnormalities

No specific or characteristic hematological or biochemical changes have been reported in dogs and cats with rabies. Mild anemia was reported in one dog.[26] Analysis of the cerebrospinal fluid (CSF) may be unremarkable or show an increase in CSF protein concentration and mild to marked CSF pleocytosis. Small lymphocytes account for most of the differential cell count.[26]

Electromyography in one dog revealed abnormalities consistent with impaired neuromuscular transmission, including moderate fibrillations, positive sharp waves, and an absent M wave.[26] Changes suggestive of denervation have also been described in humans with rabies.[27]

TABLE 13-3

Diagnostic Assays Available for Rabies in Dogs and Cats

Assay	Specimen type	Target	Performance
Direct fluorescent antibody staining or immunohistochemistry	Brain, spinal cord, skin biopsies (latter not recommended in animals), other extracranial tissues	Rabies virus N (nucleocapsid) protein	High sensitivity and specificity on brain tissue; because a single negative result does not rule out rabies, confirmatory tests such as mouse inoculation or reverse-transcription polymerase chain reaction (RT-PCR) are required for specimens testing negative. Sensitivity when used on extracranial tissues is relatively low.
Serology	Serum or cerebrospinal fluid (CSF)	Antirabies virus antibodies	Virus neutralization assays are the gold standard for serology, although ELISA assays are also available. Rarely useful for diagnosis of rabies, as the antibody response is delayed and so titers are often negative. Titers often determined before importation of animals into rabies-free countries.
Histopathology	Brain, spinal cord	Intracytoplasmic eosinophilic inclusions (Negri bodies)	Detection of Negri bodies has low sensitivity.
RT-PCR	Brain, spinal cord, saliva, CSF, extracranial tissues	Rabies virus RNA	Rapid (within hours), has the potential to be very sensitive and specific; can be used to identify rabies genotypes and strains.

Diagnostic Imaging

Magnetic Resonance Imaging Findings

Findings on MRI in dogs with rabies have included hyperintense lesions on T2-weighted images, especially in the midbrain, thalamus, and basal ganglia, that do not enhance with contrast.[28] In human patients with rabies, no significant abnormalities may be present on MRI, or it may show hyperintensities on T2-weighted images, especially in association with the gray matter. Lesions are frequently described in the medulla, pons, basal ganglia, and thalamus and reflect concentrations of rabies virus antigen.[29] Contrast enhancement can be present in comatose human patients but is usually not detected early in the course of illness. Computed tomography commonly does not reveal lesions in humans with rabies.

Microbiologic Testing

Diagnostic assays for rabies in dogs and cats are listed in Table 13-3.

Direct Fluorescent Antibody Testing and Immunohistochemistry

Rabies virus diagnosis is generally based on direct fluorescent antibody (DFA) staining for virus on impression smears of brain tissue obtained at necropsy. This is rapid, sensitive, and economical and is performed only in qualified laboratories that have been approved by local or state public health departments. In the United States, a national standardized protocol for rabies testing is published by the Centers for Disease Control and Prevention.[30] False-negative results with DFA staining are rare when compared with mouse inoculation testing,[31] and all animals with virus in their saliva test positive. A direct rapid immunohistochemistry test is also available, which has a similar sensitivity and specificity and does not require a fluorescence microscope.[32]

If rabies is suspected, the animal should be handled with extreme caution (see Prevention). Humane euthanasia should be performed, and the entire head should be submitted as soon as possible to public health authorities, so as not to delay postexposure prophylaxis measures for exposed individuals (see Public Health Aspects). Opening the skull using a saw generates aerosols and is not recommended. Although not optimal, if the head is not available, the spinal cord can be submitted. Tissues should be refrigerated and not frozen for optimal test sensitivity. Approved shipping containers should be used, which must be labeled with appropriate warnings.

Antemortem, DFA testing has been used to detect rabies virus in corneal touch impressions and frozen skin biopsy sections from the nuchal area in humans[33,34] or the region of the whiskers in dogs and cats. The sensitivity of this method is as low as 25%, and it should not be used for clinical diagnosis in dogs and cats suspected to have rabies. DFA staining has also been used for detection of rabies virus antigen in extracranial tissues at necropsy, including the tongue, salivary glands, adrenal glands, pancreas, gastrointestinal tract, and myocardium.[35,36]

Serologic Diagnosis

Serologic tests for rabies virus antibodies are often negative in affected animals, as a result of immune evasion by the virus during the incubation period and possibly also virus-induced immunosuppression after the onset of clinical signs. If seroconversion occurs, it is typically late in the course of illness. Prior vaccination for rabies may result in confusing results. Determination of acute and convalescent titers on serum and determination of CSF antibody titers can aid diagnosis of human rabies.[34] In dogs and cats, serologic testing is most commonly used to document proof of prior vaccination, which is required for importation into rabies-free countries. It is not suitable for determining the need for booster vaccinations.[37]

Serologic methods include virus neutralization assays and ELISA assays.[38] The gold standard of rabies serology is the rapid fluorescent focus inhibition test (RFFIT), a virus neutralization assay, which assesses the ability of antibodies to prevent viral replication in cell culture. The fluorescent antibody virus neutralization (FAVN) test has been accepted as an alternative for determining titers in animals before importation. A minimum titer of 0.5 U/mL is required before importation to rabies-free countries is permitted.

Virus Isolation and Mouse Inoculation

Rabies virus can be isolated in a variety of cell culture lines, although isolation may be less sensitive than nucleic acid-based detection methods.[39] Virus isolation and inoculation of mice with tissue from affected patients can be used to confirm rabies virus infection by public health authorities when direct fluorescent antibody testing of brain tissue is negative.

Molecular Diagnosis Using the Polymerase Chain Reaction

Nucleic acid detection techniques are increasingly employed to detect rabies virus in tissues and may ultimately replace techniques such as isolation and histopathology.[40] Reverse-transcriptase polymerase chain reaction (RT-PCR) assays have been used to rapidly detect rabies virus RNA in dogs and humans and, when used on brain tissue, are sensitive and specific, the results correlating with those of DFA testing.[41,42] RT-PCR can be used to detect virus in decomposing tissue, when the results of other assays might be negative.[43,44] Genetic analysis of resultant PCR products can also be used to identify lyssavirus genotypes and rabies virus variants (see Table 13-1).[45] For antemortem diagnosis in human patients, saliva is more likely to test positive than CSF. A nuchal biopsy specimen can also be tested.[46] The same appears to be true in dogs, although again, attempts to make an antemortem diagnosis of rabies are not recommended in animals.[47] The sensitivity of RT-PCR for detection of rabies virus in the saliva of rabid dogs was 87%, so a negative result does not rule out a diagnosis of rabies.

Pathologic Findings

Gross Pathologic Findings

Gross lesions are generally absent in the CNS of dogs and cats with rabies. Lesions consistent with a previous wound or traumatic event may be present elsewhere on the body.

Histopathologic Findings

Rabies virus infection results in a remarkably mild, nonsuppurative polioencephalomyelitis. Changes include mild neuronal degeneration and neuronophagia, which may be followed by neuronal necrosis.[26] Lymphoplasmacytic perivascular cuffing and focal microglial hyperplasia are frequently described. The longer the duration of illness, the more pronounced the nonsuppurative inflammatory response. Sometimes, a spongiform encephalopathy with vacuolization in the gray matter is present.[16] In some animals, eosinophilic intracytoplasmic viral inclusion bodies (Negri bodies) are identified. Negri bodies are considered a hallmark of rabies virus infection and are most commonly seen in tissues such as the pons, thalamus, hypothalamus, and hippocampus. They are generally only seen once neurologic signs have developed, and only in about 50% of animals that test positive using direct fluorescent antibody testing. Inclusions that resemble Negri bodies have been described in the brain of nonrabid cats, and so the potential for confusion and a false positive diagnosis of rabies exists.[48]

Treatment and Prognosis

Immediate euthanasia and testing of dogs and cats suspected to have rabies is recommended. Once clinical signs have developed, rabies is almost always fatal and very few humans have survived. Most have been children, and several of those individuals had been vaccinated for rabies before the onset of illness. In all individuals, moderate to severe neurologic sequelae persisted. A person in Texas appeared to survive rabies without the need for intensive care.[49] After treatment with induced coma (the "Milwaukee protocol"), an 8-year old girl survived rabies that may have been acquired after a scratch from a stray cat.[50] Rarely, dogs inoculated experimentally with certain canine rabies virus variants have recovered from rabies encephalitis, sometimes with intermittent shedding of rabies virus in saliva after recovery.[25]

Immunity and Vaccination

In most cases of human rabies, no immune response is detectable at 7 to 10 days after the onset of clinical signs. Rabies virus may evade immune recognition through inhibition of apoptosis and destruction of invading T cells, which may explain the relative lack of an inflammatory response within the CNS.[51]

Currently available vaccines contain inactivated virus or are canarypox-vectored recombinant rabies (cats) vaccines. Modified live rabies vaccines are no longer available in the United States because of their association with occasional postvaccinal rabies encephalitis in dogs and cats.[52] Vaccinia poxvirus-vectored glycoprotein recombinant vaccines are used for wildlife vaccination.

All dogs and cats should be vaccinated for rabies at 3 or 4 months of age (depending on state legislation), with a booster dose 1 year later, then every 3 years with approved inactivated vaccines, or annually with recombinant vaccines (see Chapter 12). It has been recommended that rabies vaccines be administered as distally as possible in the right pelvic limb, to allow better understanding of which vaccines are associated with sarcoma formation and to permit complete removal of sarcomas by amputation should they develop.[53,54] Canine rabies vaccination is required by law within most of the United States, and vaccines must be administered only by (or under the direct supervision of) a veterinarian.[37] Effective vaccination of at least 70% of the dog population is required to prevent rabies epizootics.[55] Owners who fail to comply with state or local requirements should be reported to the public health authorities.

Although rare, rabies has been reported in vaccinated animals, especially when vaccinations are not up to date.[23] Dogs and cats less than 1 year of age are not considered immunized until 28 days after the initial vaccination.[37] Because of a rapid anamnestic response, an animal is considered fully vaccinated immediately after booster vaccination.

The use of inactivated rabies virus vaccines in cats has been associated with formation of injection-site sarcomas.[56,57] More commonly, rabies virus vaccination is associated with pain at the injection site, lameness, transient fever, and local cutaneous reactions, such as alopecia, focal cutaneous vasculitis, and focal granulomas.[58] A more generalized ischemic skin disease characterized by variable alopecia, crusting, erosions, and ulcers on the pinnal margins, periocular areas, tail tip, and paw pads has been described that occurs several months after rabies virus vaccination of dogs and begins with a lesion at the site of vaccination (see Chapter 12).[59]

TABLE 13-4

Procedures Required by Public Health Officials for Prevention of Rabies According to the 2011 Compendium of Animal Rabies Prevention and Control[37]

Situation	Rabies Vaccination History	Procedure	Rationale
Dog or cat exposed* to a rabid wild animal or wild animal that is unavailable for testing	Unvaccinated, dog or cat	Euthanize immediately or place in strict isolation for 6 months. Administer rabies vaccine on isolation or up to 28 days before release.	The quarantine period is based on the known incubation period for rabies. Animals that develop signs consistent with rabies during quarantine should be euthanized and tested for rabies.
	Not up to date with booster vaccinations	Contact public health authorities, who decide procedures (revaccination or euthanasia) based on biting species, local prevalence of rabies, timing of previous vaccinations.	
	Vaccinated, dog or cat	Revaccinate, and keep under owner's control and observation for 45 days.	
Person bitten by a healthy dog or cat	Any	Confine animal and observe daily for 10 days; report illness that develops immediately to public health authorities. If signs of rabies develop, euthanize and test for rabies. Vaccination should not be performed until after the isolation period is complete.	Dogs and cats shedding rabies virus within the saliva will develop illness and die within the 10-day quarantine period.
Human bitten by a stray or unwanted dog or cat		Euthanize biting animal immediately and submit for rabies testing.	
Human bitten by a known rabid animal	Vaccinated, human	Vaccinate on day 0 and day 3 intramuscularly, in the upper deltoid muscle.	
	Unvaccinated, human	Postexposure prophylaxis (injection of human rabies immune globulin infiltrated at the bite site, followed by vaccination on days 0, 3, 7, 14, and 28)	

Modified from Brown CM, Conti L, Ettestad P, et al. Compendium of animal rabies prevention and control, 2011. J Am Vet Med Assoc 2011;239:609-617. Compendium updates are available online at http://www.nasphv.org/documentsCompendia.html.

*Exposure for rabies constitutes introduction of the virus into bite wounds, open cuts in skin, or onto mucous membranes from saliva or other potentially infectious material such as neural tissue.

Oral vaccinia-vectored recombinant rabies vaccines, which express the rabies virus glycoprotein, have been used in North America and Europe to control the spread of rabies in wild animals such as raccoons, coyotes, and gray foxes.[60] Canine and feline rabies vaccines are not approved for use in wild animals, which include wild animal hybrids such as wolf hybrids and Savannah cats. Wolf hybrids and Savannah cats are considered unvaccinated when decisions must be made regarding quarantine and euthanasia (Table 13-4).

Prevention

Prevention of rabies is dependent on widespread education of the public regarding the need to vaccinate dogs and cats for rabies, and the risks of wildlife contact. Control of stray dogs and cats and wild animal vaccination programs also help to prevent the disease. Ownership and importation of wild animals and hybrids is discouraged. Puppies and kittens that have not yet reached the age for rabies vaccination should be kept away from wildlife.

According to U.S. regulations, unvaccinated dogs and cats that have been exposed to a rabid animal should be euthanized immediately or vaccinated and placed in strict isolation, without direct contact with people or other animals, for 6 months.[37] If the biting animal is a wild animal that is unavailable for testing, the biting animal is presumed to be rabid. Animals that are overdue for a booster vaccination are evaluated on a case-by-case basis by public health authorities. Dogs and cats that are currently vaccinated should be revaccinated immediately (within 48 hours), kept under the owner's control, and observed for 45 days. Any illness in isolated or confined animals should be reported to local public health officials. If clinical signs suggestive of rabies develop, euthanasia and rabies testing should be performed.

Animals suspected to have rabies should be isolated from other animals and humans and handled with extreme caution, using heavy gloves, catch poles, and cages for restraint. Care should be taken not to allow people's skin to come into contact with salivary secretions. Signs that warn of the possibility of rabies should be placed on the cages of animals that are hospitalized for any period of time. If the risk of rabies is low, the animal should be confined and observed for 10 days. The clinician in charge should keep a list of all in-contact personnel during that period, and procedures should be minimized. High-risk rabies suspects should be confined in isolation using an established hospital protocol (see Chapter 11). Marked improvement in an animal's condition that occurs during a 10-day period is not consistent with a diagnosis of rabies. All specimens submitted to the laboratory should be labeled with warning labels.

Public Health Aspects

Each year, 50,000 to 55,000 people die from rabies worldwide. Approximately half those numbers occur in India alone, and it has been estimated that 3 billion people continue to be at risk of rabies virus infection in more than 100 countries.[61] A large proportion of these people are children who have been attacked by rabid dogs. In the United States, human deaths due to rabies have decreased from more than 100 per year in the early 20th century to 2 to 3 per year.[62] Most humans in the United States are infected as a result of contact with insectivorous bats, which often appear injured or are behaving abnormally (including flying during the day), and, depending on the bat species, around 5% to 40% of dead or ill bats submitted for testing have rabies.[63,64] Seemingly insignificant contact with tiny bats, particularly the eastern pipistrelle and silver-haired bats, is reported in many human rabies cases (cryptic bat rabies). Despite the high prevalence of raccoon rabies in the eastern United States, the only human death associated with a raccoon rabies variant was reported in 2003.[65]

Prodromal signs of rabies in humans include malaise, fever, and pain, itching, or paresthesia at the site of the bite. People with furious rabies become nervous and hyperexcitable, after which signs of hydrophobia, aerophobia, confusion, and aggression develop. Autonomic signs such as hypersalivation, vomiting, miosis or mydriasis, excessive sweating, and priapism may occur. Paralytic rabies can be confused with Guillain-Barré syndrome.[34]

Sick domestic and wild animals that bite humans in regions where rabies is endemic and that subsequently die should be tested for rabies without delay. Prompt and aggressive treatment of wounds including irrigation under pressure with 20% aqueous soap solution, and application of a greater than 50% ethanol solution or povidone-iodine, can dramatically reduce the risk of contracting rabies after a bite.

The chain of events that must occur after a dog or cat bites a human are listed in Table 13-4 and depend on whether the animal is owned or stray and the animal's vaccination status.[37] Public health authorities must be notified when potential exposure occurs and make the final decision as to how these animals are handled.

Postexposure prophylaxis (PEP) is administered to humans after a bite from a known or suspected rabid animal. In the United States it consists of an injection of human rabies immune globulin (H-RIG), ideally with at least half of the whole dose in the region of a bite site as soon as possible within the first 7 days of the bite, followed by vaccination by the intramuscular route on days 0, 3, 7, 14, and 28 in the upper deltoid muscle. Fewer than 5 humans develop rabies each year in the United States, but PEP is given to 20,000 to 40,000 people each year, with on average 50 humans receiving PEP for each rabies case investigated.

Depending on risk, certain individuals may receive prophylactic vaccines against rabies. These individuals include veterinarians, veterinary students and staff, dog catchers, rabies researchers, rabies diagnosticians, wildlife workers, and travelers visiting rabies-enzootic regions. After exposure to a rabid animal, administration of immunoglobulin to these individuals is not necessary. Instead, rabies vaccine boosters are given immediately and 3 days later. The major vaccine in use in the United States is the human diploid cell vaccine (HDCV), although in developing countries, access to this vaccine is limited. Among animal workers, antibody titers are generally checked every 2 years, with administration of a booster dose if necessary.

SUGGESTED READINGS

Dietzschold B, Li J, Faber M, et al. Concepts in the pathogenesis of rabies. Future Virol. 2008;3:481-490.

Lackay SN, Kuang Y, Fu ZF. Rabies in small animals. Vet Clin North Am Small Anim Pract. 2008;38:851-861:ix.

Public health response to a rabid kitten-four states, 2007. MMWR Morb Mortal Wkly Rep. 2008;56(51-52):1337-1340.

Recovery of a patient from clinical rabies–California, 2011. MMWR Morb Mortal Wkly Rep. 2012;61:61-65.

REFERENCES

1. Adamson PB. The spread of rabies into Europe and the probable origin of this disease in antiquity. J R Asiat Soc GB Irel. 1977;2:140-144.
2. Lewis VJ, Thacker WL. Limitations of deteriorated tissue for rabies diagnosis. Health Lab Sci. 1974;11:8-12.
3. Matouch O, Jaros J, Pohl P. Survival of rabies virus under external conditions. Vet Med (Praha). 1987;32:669-674.
4. Warrell MJ, Warrell DA. Rabies and other lyssavirus diseases. Lancet. 2004;363:959-969.
5. Maier T, Schwarting A, Mauer D, et al. Management and outcomes after multiple corneal and solid organ transplantations from a donor infected with rabies virus. Clin Infect Dis. 2010;50:1112-1119.
6. Dietzschold B, Li J, Faber M, et al. Concepts in the pathogenesis of rabies. Future Virol. 2008;3:481-490.
7. Davis PL, Bourhy H, Holmes EC. The evolutionary history and dynamics of bat rabies virus. Infect Genet Evol. 2006;6:464-473.
8. Fischman HR, Ward 3rd FE. Oral transmission of rabies virus in experimental animals. Am J Epidemiol. 1968;88:132-138.
9. Jorgenson RD, Gough PM, Graham DL. Experimental rabies in a great horned owl. J Wildl Dis. 1976;12:444-447.
10. Cleaveland S, Fevre EM, Kaare M, et al. Estimating human rabies mortality in the United Republic of Tanzania from dog bite injuries. Bull World Health Organ. 2002;80:304-310.
11. Fogelman V, Fischman HR, Horman JT, et al. Epidemiologic and clinical characteristics of rabies in cats. J Am Vet Med Assoc. 1993;202:1829-1833.
12. McQuiston JH, Yager PA, Smith JS, et al. Epidemiologic characteristics of rabies virus variants in dogs and cats in the United States, 1999. J Am Vet Med Assoc. 2001;218:1939-1942.
13. Blanton JD, Robertson K, Palmer D, et al. Rabies surveillance in the United States during 2008. J Am Vet Med Assoc. 2009;235:676-689.
14. Castrodale L, Walker V, Baldwin J, et al. Rabies in a puppy imported from India to the USA, March 2007. Zoonoses Public Health. 2008;55:427-430.
15. Childs JE, Colby L, Krebs JW, et al. Surveillance and spatiotemporal associations of rabies in rodents and lagomorphs in the United States, 1985-1994. J Wildl Dis. 1997;33:20-27.
16. Lackay SN, Kuang Y, Fu ZF. Rabies in small animals. Vet Clin North Am Small Anim Pract. 2008;38:851-861,ix.
17. Eng TR, Fishbein DB. Epidemiologic factors, clinical findings, and vaccination status of rabies in cats and dogs in the United States in 1988. National Study Group on Rabies. J Am Vet Med Assoc. 1990;197:201-209.
18. Fekadu M, Shaddock JH, Baer GM. Excretion of rabies virus in the saliva of dogs. J Infect Dis. 1982;145:715-719.
19. Dimaano EM, Scholand SJ, Alera MT, et al. Clinical and epidemiological features of human rabies cases in the Philippines: a review from 1987 to 2006. Int J Infect Dis. 2011;15:e495-e499.
20. Johnson N, Fooks A, McColl K. Human rabies case with long incubation, Australia. Emerg Infect Dis. 2008;14:1950-1951.

21. Shankar SK, Mahadevan A, Sapico SD, et al. Rabies viral encephalitis with probable 25 year incubation period! Ann Indian Acad Neurol. 2012;15:221-223.
22. Tepsumethanon V, Lumlertdacha B, Mitmoonpitak C, et al. Survival of naturally infected rabid dogs and cats. Clin Infect Dis. 2004;39:278-280.
23. Murray KO, Holmes KC, Hanlon CA. Rabies in vaccinated dogs and cats in the United States, 1997-2001. J Am Vet Med Assoc. 2009;235:691-695.
24. Fekadu M, Baer GM. Recovery from clinical rabies of 2 dogs inoculated with a rabies virus strain from Ethiopia. Am J Vet Res. 1980;41:1632-1634.
25. Fekadu M, Shaddock JH, Baer GM. Intermittent excretion of rabies virus in the saliva of a dog two and six months after it had recovered from experimental rabies. Am J Trop Med Hyg. 1981;30:1113-1115.
26. Barnes HL, Chrisman CL, Farina L, et al. Clinical evaluation of rabies virus meningoencephalomyelitis in a dog. J Am Anim Hosp Assoc. 2003;39:547-550.
27. Gadre G, Satishchandra P, Mahadevan A, et al. Rabies viral encephalitis: clinical determinants in diagnosis with special reference to paralytic form. J Neurol Neurosurg Psychiatry. 2010;81:812-820.
28. Laothamatas J, Wacharapluesadee S, Lumlertdacha B, et al. Furious and paralytic rabies of canine origin: neuroimaging with virological and cytokine studies. J Neurovirol. 2008;14:119-129.
29. Tirawatnpong S, Hemachudha T, Manutsathit S, et al. Regional distribution of rabies viral antigen in central nervous system of human encephalitic and paralytic rabies. J Neurol Sci. 1989;92:91-99.
30. Centers for Disease Control and Prevention. http://www.cdc.gov/rabies/specific_groups/laboratories/index.html. Last accessed November 19, 2012.
31. Beauregard M, Boulanger P, Webster WA. The use of fluorescent antibody staining in the diagnosis of rabies. Can J Comp Med Vet Sci. 1965;29:141-147.
32. Lembo T, Niezgoda M, Velasco-Villa A, et al. Evaluation of a direct, rapid immunohistochemical test for rabies diagnosis. Emerg Infect Dis. 2006;12:310-313.
33. Crepin P, Audry L, Rotivel Y, et al. Intravitam diagnosis of human rabies by PCR using saliva and cerebrospinal fluid. J Clin Microbiol. 1998;36:1117-1121.
34. Madhusudana SN, Sukumaran SM. Antemortem diagnosis and prevention of human rabies. Ann Indian Acad Neurol. 2008;11:3-12.
35. Li Z, Feng Z, Ye H. Rabies viral antigen in human tongues and salivary glands. J Trop Med Hyg. 1995;98:330-332.
36. Jogai S, Radotra BD, Banerjee AK. Rabies viral antigen in extracranial organs: a post-mortem study. Neuropathol Appl Neurobiol. 2002;28:334-338.
37. Brown CM, Conti L, Ettestad P, et al. Compendium of animal rabies prevention and control, 2011. J Am Vet Med Assoc. 2011;239:609-617.
38. Moore SM, Hanlon CA. Rabies-specific antibodies: measuring surrogates of protection against a fatal disease. PLoS Negl Trop Dis. 2010;4:e595.
39. Panning M, Baumgarte S, Pfefferle S, et al. Comparative analysis of rabies virus reverse transcription-PCR and virus isolation using samples from a patient infected with rabies virus. J Clin Microbiol. 2010;48:2960-2962.
40. Fooks AR, Johnson N, Freuling CM, et al. Emerging technologies for the detection of rabies virus: challenges and hopes in the 21st century. PLoS Negl Trop Dis. 2009;3:e530.
41. Kamolvarin N, Tirawatnpong T, Rattanasiwamoke R, et al. Diagnosis of rabies by polymerase chain reaction with nested primers. J Infect Dis. 1993;167:207-210.
42. Gupta PK, Singh RK, Sharma RN, et al. Preliminary report on a single-tube, non-interrupted reverse transcription-polymerase chain reaction for the detection of rabies virus in brain tissue. Vet Res Commun. 2001;25:239-247.
43. David D, Yakobson B, Rotenberg D, et al. Rabies virus detection by RT-PCR in decomposed naturally infected brains. Vet Microbiol. 2002;87:111-118.
44. Lopes MC, Venditti LL, Queiroz LH. Comparison between RT-PCR and the mouse inoculation test for detection of rabies virus in samples kept for long periods under different conditions. J Virol Methods. 2010;164:19-23.
45. Wacharapluesadee S, Hemachudha T. Ante- and post-mortem diagnosis of rabies using nucleic acid-amplification tests. Expert Rev Mol Diagn. 2010;10:207-218.
46. Human rabies—Virginia, 2009. MMWR Morb Mortal Wkly Rep. 2010;59:1236-1238.
47. Saengseesom W, Mitmoonpitak C, Kasempimolporn S, et al. Real-time PCR analysis of dog cerebrospinal fluid and saliva samples for ante-mortem diagnosis of rabies. Southeast Asian J Trop Med Public Health. 2007;38:53-57.
48. Szlachta HL, Habel RE. Inclusions resembling Negri bodies in the brains of nonrabid cats. Cornell Vet. 1953;43:207-212.
49. Presumptive abortive human rabies—Texas, 2009. MMWR Morb Mortal Wkly Rep. 2010;59:185-190.
50. Recovery of a patient from clinical rabies—California, 2011. MMWR Morb Mortal Wkly Rep. 2012;61:61-65.
51. Lafon M. Subversive neuroinvasive strategy of rabies virus. Arch Virol Suppl. 2004:149-159.
52. Pedersen NC, Emmons RW, Selcer R, et al. Rabies vaccine virus infection in three dogs. J Am Vet Med Assoc. 1978;172:1092-1096.
53. Morrison WB, Starr RM. Vaccine-associated feline sarcomas. J Am Vet Med Assoc. 2001;218:697-702.
54. Shaw SC, Kent MS, Gordon IK, et al. Temporal changes in characteristics of injection-site sarcomas in cats: 392 cases (1990-2006). J Am Vet Med Assoc. 2009;234:376-380.
55. World Health Organization. http://www.who.int/mediacentre/factsheets/fs099/en/. Last accessed August 26, 2012.
56. Kass PH, Spangler WL, Hendrick MJ, et al. Multicenter case-control study of risk factors associated with development of vaccine-associated sarcomas in cats. J Am Vet Med Assoc. 2003;223:1283-1292.
57. Srivastav A, Kass PH, McGill LD, et al. Comparative vaccine-specific and other injectable-specific risks of injection-site sarcomas in cats. J Am Vet Med Assoc. 2012;241:595-602.
58. Wilcock BP, Yager JA. Focal cutaneous vasculitis and alopecia at sites of rabies vaccination in dogs. J Am Vet Med Assoc. 1986;188:1174-1177.
59. Vitale CB, Gross TL, Magro CM. Vaccine-induced ischemic dermatopathy in the dog. Vet Dermatol. 1999;10:131-142.
60. Sidwa TJ, Wilson PJ, Moore GM, et al. Evaluation of oral rabies vaccination programs for control of rabies epizootics in coyotes and gray foxes: 1995-2003. J Am Vet Med Assoc. 2005;227:785-792.
61. Wunner WH, Briggs DJ. Rabies in the 21 century. PLoS Negl Trop Dis. 2010;4:e591.
62. Nigg AJ, Walker PL. Overview, prevention, and treatment of rabies. Pharmacotherapy. 2009;29:1182-1195.
63. Balsamo GA, Ratard RC. Epidemiology of animal rabies and its practical application to pre- and postexposure prophylaxis, Louisiana, 1988 to 2007. Vector Borne Zoonotic Dis. 2010;10:283-289.
64. Shankar V, Orciari LA, De Mattos C, et al. Genetic divergence of rabies viruses from bat species of Colorado. USA. Vector Borne Zoonotic Dis. 2005;5:330-341.
65. First human death associated with raccoon rabies—Virginia, 2003. MMWR Morb Mortal Wkly Rep. 2003;52:1102-1103.

CHAPTER 14

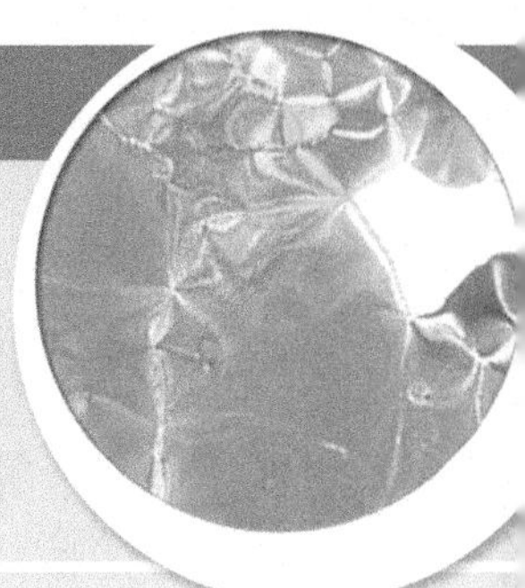

Canine Parvovirus Infections and Other Viral Enteritides

Jane E. Sykes

> **Overview of Canine Parvoviral Enteritis**
>
> First Described: 1978, worldwide, Appel and others[1]
>
> Cause: Canine parvovirus-2 variants (Family Parvoviridae, subfamily Parvovirinae, Genus *Parvovirus*)
>
> Affected Hosts: Dogs and other Canidae such as coyotes, foxes, and wolves; cats
>
> Geographic Distribution: Worldwide
>
> Route of Transmission: Direct contact with virus in feces and vomitus as well as contact with contaminated fomites
>
> Major Clinical Signs: Fever, lethargy, inappetence, vomiting, diarrhea, dehydration. Sudden death or tachypnea due to myocarditis occurs rarely.
>
> Differential Diagnoses: Canine distemper virus infection, other canine viral enteritides, dietary indiscretion, toxins, gastrointestinal foreign body, enteric parasitic infections such as giardiasis and helminth infections, enteric bacterial infections such as salmonellosis, salmon poisoning disease, pancreatitis, hypoadrenocorticism, inflammatory bowel disease
>
> Human Health Significance: CPV-2 variants do not infect humans

Etiology and Epidemiology

Canine parvovirus is the most widely recognized cause of transmissible viral diarrhea in dogs and one of the most common infectious diseases of dogs worldwide. It is caused by variants of canine parvovirus-2 (CPV-2), which are members of the genus *Parvovirus*. CPV-2 emerged in the early to mid-1970s and caused a worldwide pandemic of illness in dogs.[2] The spread of the virus worldwide occurred over a remarkable period of about 6 months. CPV-2 may have been derived from feline panleukopenia virus (FPV) or a closely related virus of wild carnivores. It has since mutated to CPV-2a in 1979, CPV-2b in 1984, and, most recently, CPV-2c, which was first detected in Italy in 2000 and has subsequently been found worldwide, with the exception of Australia. Separate lineages have been identified in different geographic locations worldwide.[3] The virus uses the transferrin receptor to enter host cells. With the mutation from CPV-2 to CPV-2a, the virus developed the ability to replicate readily in feline cells, and CPV-2a, CPV-2b, and CPV-2c are now responsible for some cases of feline viral enteritis.[4,5] Feline parvoviral enteritis is further discussed in Chapter 19. CPV-2 variants must be differentiated from CPV-1, also known as canine minute virus, which belongs to the genus *Bocavirus*. In general, CPV-1 is thought to have minimal pathogenic potential, but it has been associated with abortion in pregnant dogs; respiratory, cardiac, and gastrointestinal signs in neonatal dogs; severe gastroenteritis in adult dogs; and possibly neurologic signs in dogs.[6-8]

Parvoviruses are small, non-enveloped single-stranded DNA viruses (Figure 14-1, *A*) that can survive for long periods (over 1 year) in the environment. As a result, contact with virus that persists in the environment is an important means of transmission. Insects and rodents may also serve as mechanical vectors for the virus. Canine parvovirus requires the presence of mitotically active cells in order to replicate. Young animals (6 weeks to 6 months, and especially those less than 12 weeks of age) are more likely to develop severe illness; however, disease can also occur in unvaccinated or improperly vaccinated adult dogs. In North America, Rottweilers, American pit bull terriers, Doberman pinschers, English springer spaniels, and German shepherd dogs appear to be at increased risk for development of parvoviral enteritis,[9,10] but this has not been the case in other geographic locations. A seasonal distribution of disease has been reported in some geographic locations, which may reflect times when dogs access the outdoors and contact virus in the environment. For example, in Saskatoon, Canada, dogs were three times more likely to be admitted with parvoviral enteritis in July, August, and September, compared with the rest of the year.[9] In other locations, the seasonal pattern of disease has differed or been nonexistent.[11,12] For dogs older than 6 months of age, intact males were twice as likely as females to develop parvoviral enteritis.[9] A surveillance study from Australia found a correlation between clusters of parvoviral enteritis and regions of relative socioeconomic disadvantage.[12]

Other viral pathogens that have been associated with enteritis and diarrhea in dogs are canine distemper virus (CDV) (see Chapter 15), canine enteric coronavirus (Figure 14-1, *B*), rotaviruses, astroviruses, adenoviruses, caliciviruses, and novel viruses that include a norovirus, kobuvirus, sapovirus, and possibly also a circovirus.[13-17] Canine enteric coronavirus primarily causes mild diarrhea in puppies that are less than 6 weeks of age and may be found in co-infections with other viral causes of gastroenteritis, including CPV-2 variants. Rarely, it has been identified as a more significant cause of diarrhea in young dogs.[18] This chapter focuses on canine parvoviral enteritis, which is the most widely recognized and pathogenic viral enteritis of dogs.

Clinical Features

Signs and Their Pathogenesis

Transmission of parvovirus and other viral causes of gastroenteritis occurs by the fecal-oral route, after exposure to virus in feces or vomit, or importantly, virus that persists on fomites.

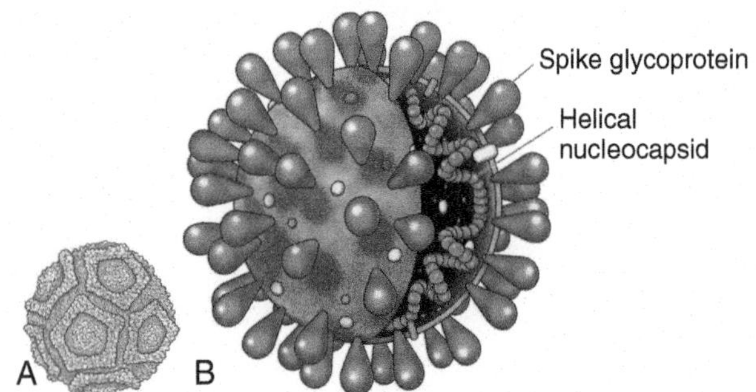

FIGURE 14-1 **A,** General structure of canine parvovirus. The virus is non-enveloped, is 25 nm in diameter, and has icosahedral symmetry. **B,** Structure of a coronavirus, which is an enveloped virus. Canine parvovirus is about one-quarter the size of a coronavirus.

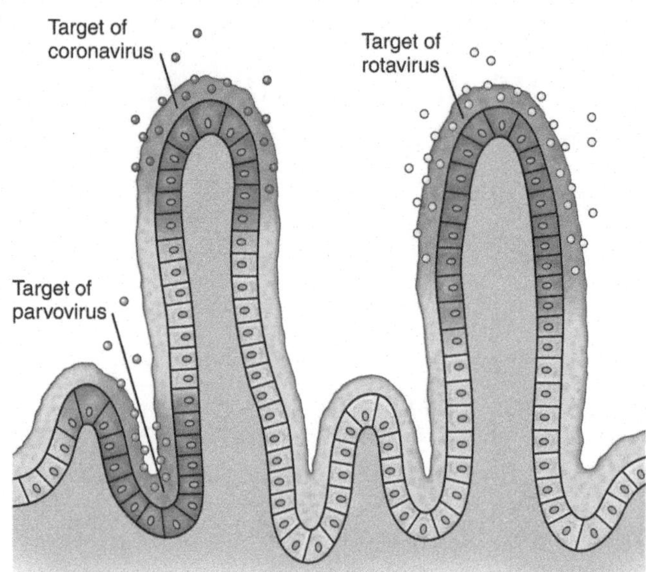

FIGURE 14-2 Target sites of replication of selected enteric viral pathogens. The most pathogenic enteric viruses, such as canine parvovirus, replicate and destroy crypt epithelial cells.

Virus is shed for a few days before the onset of clinical signs, and shedding declines considerably after 7 days.[19] The severity of clinical signs depends on factors such as virus strain and host immunity, which is affected by stressors such as weaning and overcrowding, maternal antibody, and the presence of concurrent infections such as other enteric viral and parasitic infections. Subclinical infections are probably widespread.

The incubation period for canine parvoviral enteritis is 7 to 14 days in the field, but shorter incubation periods (as short as 4 days) have been observed with experimental infections. The virus replicates in oropharyngeal lymphoid tissues, after which viremia occurs. Damage occurs to rapidly dividing cells in the gastrointestinal tract, thymus, lymph nodes, and bone marrow. Affected gastrointestinal tissues include the epithelium of the tongue, oral cavity, esophagus, and intestinal tract, and especially the germinal epithelial cells of the intestinal crypts. Neutropenia results not only from infection of the marrow but also sequestration of neutrophils in damaged gastrointestinal tissue. Malabsorption and increased intestinal permeability result. Secondary bacterial infections of the gastrointestinal tract, which may be followed by bacterial translocation, bacteremia, and endotoxemia, play a key role in the pathogenesis of the disease. Mucosal candidiasis has also been described in puppies with parvoviral enteritis (see Chapter 67). The outcome is clinical signs of fever, lethargy, inappetence, vomiting, diarrhea, rapid dehydration, and abdominal pain. Diarrhea is often liquid, foul-smelling, and may contain streaks of blood or frank blood. Ascarid nematodes may be identified in the vomitus of some dogs. Dogs with canine parvoviral enteritis have evidence of disordered coagulation, with decreased antithrombin activities, prolonged activated partial thromboplastin time, increased thromboelastography maximum amplitude, and increased fibrinogen concentrations. Catheter and organ thrombosis may occur.[20] Secondary bacteremia may be associated with multiple organ failure and death.

Infection of the dam by CPV-2 variants early in gestation can lead to infertility, resorption, or abortion. Puppies that are infected in utero or up to 2 weeks of age may develop viral myocarditis, which results in signs of sudden death or congestive heart failure.[21-23] Damage to the developing myocardium usually occurs up to the first 2 weeks of life, but clinical signs of myocardial damage may be delayed until up to 2 months of age. Cerebellar hypoplasia has been rarely reported in dogs after in utero infection[24] but is more common in kittens infected with FPV (see Chapter 19). Generalized infection has been reported in neonatal puppies, with hemorrhage and necrosis within the brain, liver, lungs, kidneys, lymphoid tissues, and gastrointestinal tract.[25] Because maternal antibody protects puppies during this period, the incidence of neonatal complications of parvovirus infection and myocarditis has declined dramatically since the virus first emerged, because of widespread vaccination and exposure of adult animals.

Neurologic signs in puppies with parvoviral enteritis may result from hypoxia secondary to myocarditis, hypoglycemia, or intracranial thrombosis or hemorrhage. The possibility of co-infection with CDV should also be considered. The DNA of CPV-2 variants has also been detected in the central nervous system,[26] and there have been rare reports of leukoencephalomalacia in association with infection.[27,28]

In contrast to canine CPV-2 variants, the replication of less pathogenic enteric viruses is restricted to the intestinal tract, and the crypt epithelial cells are generally spared (Figure 14-2). Canine enteric coronavirus, for example, infects the mature enterocytes at the tips of the villi. Crypt cell hyperplasia occurs to replace the damaged cells. The villi become shortened or distorted, which leads to malabsorption and diarrhea.

Physical Examination Findings

Physical examination of puppies with parvoviral enteritis often reveals fever (up to 41°C or 105°F), lethargy, weakness, dehydration, and abdominal tenderness and a fluid-filled intestinal tract on palpation (Figure 14-3). Vomiting or diarrhea may occur during the examination, or there may be evidence of diarrhea or frank blood on the perineum or the rectal thermometer. Occasionally abdominal palpation reveals a tubular mass as a result of intestinal intussusception. Ulcerative glossitis can occur in some puppies. Mucosal pallor, prolonged capillary refill time, or rarely hypothermia may be observed in some dogs.[29] Septic shock may be associated with tachycardia or bradycardia, mental obtundation, and poor pulse quality. Uncommonly, neurologic signs such as tremors and seizures are observed. Puppies with myocarditis may be tachypneic and have increased lung sounds as a result of congestive heart failure. Erythema multiforme has been reported in dogs with canine parvoviral enteritis; these dogs had generalized cutaneous and mucosal ulceration as well as swelling of the pinnae and paws.[30,31]

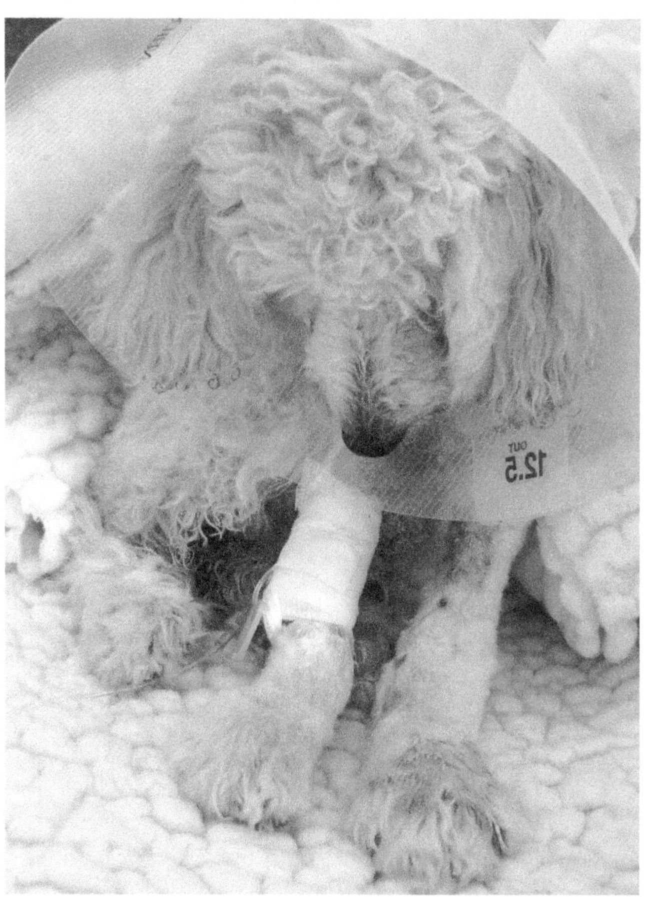

FIGURE 14-3 Obtundation in a 3-month-old intact male standard poodle puppy with canine parvovirus enteritis. The dog had been vaccinated for canine parvovirus at 8 and 10 weeks of age.

Diagnosis

Laboratory Abnormalities

Complete Blood Count

The most common abnormalities found on the CBC are leukopenia, neutropenia, and lymphopenia (Table 14-1). Toxic neutrophils and monocytopenia may also be present. Only around one third of dogs had leukopenia in one study.[29] Leukopenia can develop after the onset of gastrointestinal signs, when puppies are first brought for examination. Some dogs have leukocytosis due to a neutrophilia and monocytosis. Although the presence of leukopenia supports a diagnosis of parvoviral enteritis, other severe gastrointestinal infections such as salmonellosis can also cause leukopenia and diarrhea, so it is not specific for diagnosis of the disease. Thrombocytosis or, less commonly, thrombocytopenia may also occur.[29] Some puppies develop anemia as a result of gastrointestinal blood loss, which may be non regenerative or become regenerative.

Serum Biochemical Tests

The serum biochemistry panel in dogs with parvoviral enteritis often shows hypoproteinemia, hypoalbuminemia, and hypoglycemia. Mild hyperglycemia has also been reported. Electrolyte abnormalities such as hyponatremia, hypochloremia, and hypokalemia may occur (Table 14-2). Occasionally severe dehydration results in prerenal azotemia. Puppies with bacterial sepsis may develop increased liver enzyme activities and hyperbilirubinemia.

Coagulation Profile

Coagulation abnormalities have been reported in a small number of dogs with parvoviral enteritis. When abnormalities occur, findings include prolonged activated partial thromboplastin time, decreased antithrombin activity, increased fibrinogen

TABLE 14-1

Complete Blood Count Findings at Admission in 45 Dogs Diagnosed with Canine Parvoviral Enteritis at the UC Davis VMTH

Test	Reference Range	Percent below the Reference Range	Percent within the Reference Range	Percent above the Reference Range	Range for Dogs with CPV Enteritis	Number Tested
Hematocrit (%)	40-55	71	29	0	21-53	45
MCV (fL)	65-75	29	71	0	54-74	45
MCHC (g/dL)	33-36	24	69	7	30-37	45
Neutrophils (cells/μL)	3000-10,500	56	31	13	8-22,453	45
Band neutrophils (cells/μL)	0-rare	0	31	69	0-1582	45
Monocytes (cells/μL)	150-1200	20	60	20	11-2475	45
Lymphocytes (cells/μL)	1000-4000	49	22	0	165-3698	45
Eosinophils (cells/μL)	0-1500	0	100	0	0-1236	45
Platelets (cells/μL)	150,000-400,000	5	60	35	103,000-639,000	43

Note: Adult reference ranges were used by the laboratory.
CPV, Canine parvovirus.

TABLE 14-2

Findings on Serum Biochemistry Analysis in 27 Dogs with Canine Parvoviral Enteritis at the UC Davis VMTH

Test	Reference Range	Percent below the Reference Range	Percent within the Reference Range	Percent above the Reference Range	Range for Dogs with Parvoviral Enteritis	Number of Dogs Tested
Sodium (mmol/L)	145-154	85	15	0	132-147	26
Potassium (mmol/L)	3.6-5.3	4	92	4	3.4-5.9	26
Chloride (mmol/L)	108-118	65	31	4	94-120	26
Bicarbonate (mmol/L)	16-26	8	92	0	14-25	26
Calcium (mg/dL)	9.7-11.5	30	70	0	7.4-11.5	27
Phosphorus (mg/dL)	3.0-6.2	0	52	48	3.1-12.3	27
Creatinine (mg/dL)	0.3-1.2	37	59	4	<0.2-1.6	27
BUN (mg/dL)	5-21	0	85	15	5-48	27
Albumin (g/dL)	3.0-4.4	70	30	0	0.9-3.8	27
Globulin (g/dL)	1.8-3.9	26	67	7	1.4-4.5	27
Cholesterol (mg/dL)	135-361	4	89	8	108-460	26
Total bilirubin (mg/dL)	0-0.2	0	89	12	0-1.7	26
ALT (U/L)	19-67	15	62	23	10-165	26
ALP (U/L)	21-170	0	42	58	56-397	26

Note: Adult reference ranges were used by the laboratory.

concentrations, and increased thromboelastography maximum amplitude.[20] An increase in D-dimers or fibrin degradation products has not been reported. More research is warranted to understand the range of coagulation abnormalities that can occur in parvoviral enteritis.

Diagnostic Imaging

Plain Radiography

Plain abdominal radiography in dogs with parvoviral enteritis may show poor serosal detail (often due to lack of intra-abdominal fat in puppies) and a fluid- and gas-filled gastrointestinal tract. Abdominal radiography is usually performed to assess for the presence of a gastrointestinal foreign body.

Sonographic Findings

Findings on abdominal ultrasonography in canine parvoviral enteritis are nonspecific but can include a thickened gastrointestinal mucosa, mild peritoneal effusion, fluid distention of the gastrointestinal tract, and decreased gastrointestinal motility. Mild mesenteric lymphadenopathy may be present. Abdominal ultrasound is useful to confirm a diagnosis of secondary intestinal intussusception.

Microbiologic Tests

Diagnostic assays for canine parvoviral enteritis in dogs are listed in Table 14-3.

Fecal Parvovirus Antigen ELISA

The most widely used assay for diagnosis of canine parvoviral enteritis is an in-house fecal antigen ELISA, which is performed on a rectal swab specimen. Several assays are available, and although they detect all variants of CPV-2 including CPV-2c, their sensitivities and specificities vary.[32,33] Sensitivity is particularly problematic, because viral shedding is transient, and antibody present may bind viral antigen so that it is unavailable for reaction with the assay. The sensitivities of three commercially available fecal antigen assays (SNAP Parvo antigen, IDEXX Laboratories GmbH; FASTest Parvo Strip, Scil Animal Care Company GmbH; Witness Parvo Card, Selectavet GmbH) were 50%, 40%, and 60%, respectively, when compared to immunoelectron microscopy, and 18%, 16%, and 26%, respectively, when compared with results of a fecal PCR assay.[33] Because some dogs that lack evidence of gastrointestinal signs can be positive using PCR assay, immunoelectron microscopy may be a more appropriate gold standard for disease (although it is not widely available for routine diagnosis). In another study, the sensitivity of a fecal antigen test for detection of CPV-2a, CPV-2b, and CPV-2c, on specimens that contained high CPV DNA loads (>10^5 copies/mg of feces as determined with real-time PCR) was 80%, 78%, and 77%, respectively.[32]

When compared with PCR and immunoelectron microscopy of stool, the specificities of the three commercially available antigen assays above were 98%, 98%, and 92%, respectively,[33] so false positives were uncommon. It has been suggested that false-positive antigen tests can occur 4 to 8 days after vaccination with attenuated live CPV-2 vaccines.[34] In kittens, false-positive test results did occur after vaccination for FPV, but they were more likely to occur with some assays as opposed to others, were generally weak positives, and occurred even after vaccination with inactivated vaccines.[35] Similar studies have not been reported for CPV.

TABLE 14-3

Diagnostic Assays Available for Canine Parvoviral Enteritis in Dogs

Assay	Specimen type	Target	Performance
Fecal antigen ELISA	Feces	CPV antigen	Specificity for detection of virus nears 100%, but weak false positives have the potential to occur after immunization with attenuated live vaccines. False negatives are common (low sensitivity).
Hemagglutination assay	Feces	CPV antigen	Inexpensive and rapid. Sensitivity and specificity in naturally infected dogs has not been well established.
Histopathology	Usually necropsy specimens, especially gastrointestinal tissues	Crypt necrosis with intranuclear inclusions; parvovirus antigen with IHC or parvovirus DNA with in situ hybridization	Can be used for diagnosis at necropsy. In situ hybridization may be most sensitive for detection of virus in tissues.
Polymerase chain reaction (PCR)	Feces, tissue species	CPV DNA	Sensitivity and specificity may vary depending on assay design. Attenuated live vaccine virus may be detected in feces for days to weeks after vaccination, but some assays differentiate between vaccine and field virus. Because of the high sensitivity of some assays, the significance of a positive result may be difficult to interpret. False negative results may occur as a result of inhibition of PCR by components of feces. Degradation of nucleic acid during specimen transport is more problematic for RNA viruses such as canine coronavirus.
Fecal electron microscopy	Feces	Virus particles	Not widely available, turnaround time can be slow, and may be expensive. Requires the presence of large amounts of virus.
Virus isolation	Feces, tissues	CPV	Difficult, not widely available. Used as a research tool.

CPV, Canine parvovirus (refers to CPV-2 variants); IHC, immunohistochemistry.

Hemagglutination Testing

Canine parvovirus agglutinates erythrocytes, and so the presence of the virus in stool can be detected with a simple hemagglutination test that involves mixing a suspension of feces with porcine erythrocytes. Agglutination of erythrocytes in a microwell plate or on a slide indicates the presence of parvovirus in the feces.[36] The sensitivity and specificity of these assays in dogs with and without natural parvoviral infections in the field require further investigation.

Molecular Diagnosis Using the Polymerase Chain Reaction

Several commercial veterinary diagnostic laboratories now offer real-time PCR assays for detection of CPV-2 variants and other enteric viral pathogens (such as canine coronavirus). Assays may detect as few as 1000 copies of viral DNA per milligram of stool. Turnaround times are less than 24 hours in some laboratories. PCR assays are useful when fecal antigen tests are negative but parvoviral enteritis is still suspected as a diagnosis, or when canine enteric coronavirus infection is a potential cause of illness (because PCR panels that assay for parvovirus DNA also often include an assay for canine enteric coronavirus RNA). Unfortunately, although infrequent, positive PCR assay results for CPV can occur in dogs without signs of gastroenteritis or in dogs with chronic diarrhea, and so it may be difficult to ascertain whether a positive parvovirus PCR result indicates that CPV is the cause of a dog's illness. Attenuated live vaccine virus can also be detected in the feces with PCR assays after vaccination, although assays have been designed that can differentiate between vaccine and wild-type virus.[37] It is not yet clear for how long after vaccination false-positive PCR results might occur, and this could vary based on the design of the PCR assay used. Both vaccine and field virus have been detected simultaneously in some dogs using these assays. In the future, quantitation of virus loads in feces using real-time PCR may be helpful for interpretation of the significance of a positive PCR assay result.

Fecal Electron Microscopy

Fecal electron microscopy is still offered by some institutions for diagnosis of viral enteritis. It is generally used on a research basis when viral enteritis is suspected but a diagnosis cannot be made with antigen tests or PCR assays. Fecal electron microscopy may facilitate diagnosis of other viral infections such as rotavirus, norovirus, and coronavirus infections. Turnaround time may be slow. Generally speaking, large amounts of virus must be present for results to be positive, and technical expertise is required to accurately identify virus in the stool.

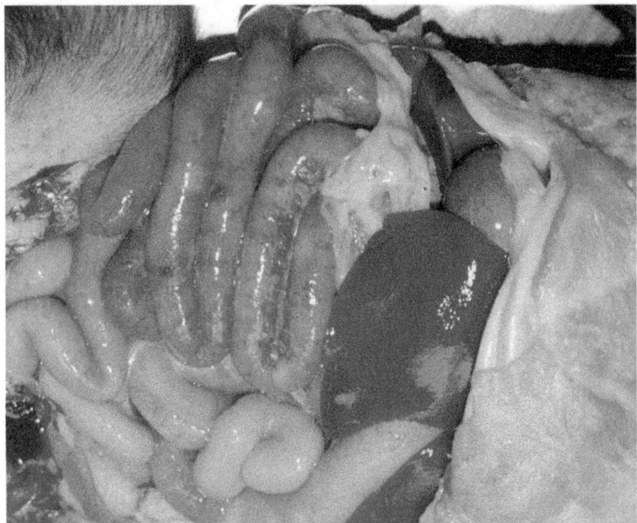

FIGURE 14-4 Discoloration of the small intestinal wall and serosal hemorrhage in a puppy that died of canine parvoviral enteritis. (Courtesy University of California, Davis Veterinary Anatomic Pathology Service.)

Virus Isolation

Canine parvovirus variants can be isolated in canine and feline cells, but isolation is difficult, and the virus shows minimal cytopathic effects. As a result, virus isolation is rarely used for diagnosis and is not widely available. It remains important as a research tool.[38]

Serology

Antibodies to CPV-2 can be measured in the laboratory using hemagglutination inhibition (see Chapter 2). In addition, an in-clinic ELISA assay is available for semiquantitative measurement of antibodies to CPV-2. These assays are generally used to assess the need for vaccination, rather than for diagnosis of CPV-2 enteritis, because affected dogs are either seronegative or previous vaccination or material antibodies confound early serodiagnosis.

Pathologic Findings

Gross Pathologic Findings

Gross pathologic findings in dogs with CPV enteritis include thickening and discoloration of the intestinal wall with serosal hemorrhage (Figure 14-4) and enlarged, edematous abdominal lymph nodes. The intestine may contain bloody liquid contents, and mucosal hemorrhage may be identified. Pale areas may be seen within the myocardium of dogs with parvoviral myocarditis.

Histopathologic Findings

The major histopathologic finding is necrosis of the crypt epithelium in the small intestine, with widespread systemic lymphoid depletion and necrosis. The crypts can be dilated and distended with cellular debris and mucus (Figure 14-5). Proliferation of crypt enterocytes may be observed as part of the recovery response. Intestinal villi are collapsed, shortened, and fused, with attenuation of the epithelial lining, and there may be mild to severe fibrinous inflammation and hemorrhage. Myeloid depletion may be found in the bone marrow. Parvoviral myocarditis is characterized by myocardial degeneration and necrosis, with a lymphocytic inflammatory infiltrate. Myocardial fibrosis can also be present. Rarely, central nervous system lesions consisting of leukoencephalomalacia have been described.[27] Viral intranuclear inclusions may be visible in some cells, especially the intestinal crypt epithelium. Immunohistochemistry can be used to detect viral antigen in the gastrointestinal tract, marrow, lymphoid tissues, and rarely in the myocardium. In situ hybridization (see Chapter 5) can also be used to detect virus in histopathology specimens and may have greater sensitivity than immunohistochemistry.[39,40]

Treatment and Prognosis

Antimicrobial Treatment and Supportive Care

Treatment of CPV enteritis involves supportive care and treatment of secondary bacterial infections with antimicrobial drugs (Table 14-4). Whenever possible, the patient should be hospitalized in isolation. Appropriate fluid therapy and maintenance of adequate blood glucose concentrations are the most critical aspect of treatment. Whenever possible, fluids should be given intravenously and supplemented as needed with potassium chloride and dextrose. Blood glucose concentrations should be monitored at least twice daily, and more frequent monitoring may be indicated if hypoglycemia is present. Although not generally recommended for puppies that are vomiting or dehydrated, administration of subcutaneous fluids and antimicrobial drugs in the home can sometimes result in recovery when client finances do not permit treatment in hospital. Fluids administered subcutaneously should never be supplemented with dextrose, because dextrose is hyperosmotic and can cause further dehydration, as well as injection-site reactions. Unfortunately, the owners of many dogs with parvoviral enteritis lack financial resources for treatment. In these situations, the inability to afford vaccination may have been a reason the puppy develops parvoviral enteritis in the first place.

An antimicrobial drug or drug combination with activity against gram-negative and anaerobic bacteria should be administered parenterally. Injectable ampicillin or cefazolin alone may be sufficient for many dogs, but puppies that have hemorrhagic diarrhea or evidence of the systemic inflammatory response syndrome (SIRS) should probably be treated with a combination of a penicillin and a fluoroquinolone, or a combination of a penicillin and an aminoglycoside. Use of fluoroquinolones in young, rapidly growing animals has been associated with cartilage damage (see Chapter 8), but when used for the short periods of time required to treat parvoviral enteritis, this may not be of significant concern. Proper hydration is critical before aminoglycosides are used because of their potential for nephrotoxicity.

Treatment with antiemetics (such as a constant rate infusion of metoclopramide or parenteral ondansetron), H2 blockers such as famotidine, whole blood or plasma transfusions, colloids such as hetastarch, or partial or total parenteral nutrition may be indicated in some dogs. Placement of a central line or multilumen catheter may be necessary in severely ill puppies, but strict sterile technique must be adhered to because of the potential for hospital-associated infection. In general, unless absolutely necessary, invasive surgical procedures and the use of parenteral nutrition solutions should be avoided in puppies with severe neutropenia. Whether plasma or hetastarch is the treatment of choice for dogs with low colloid oncotic pressure requires further study. Plasma may offer benefit over hetastarch in that it contains antibodies from immune dogs, but titers may not be sufficient to be beneficial, and most puppies

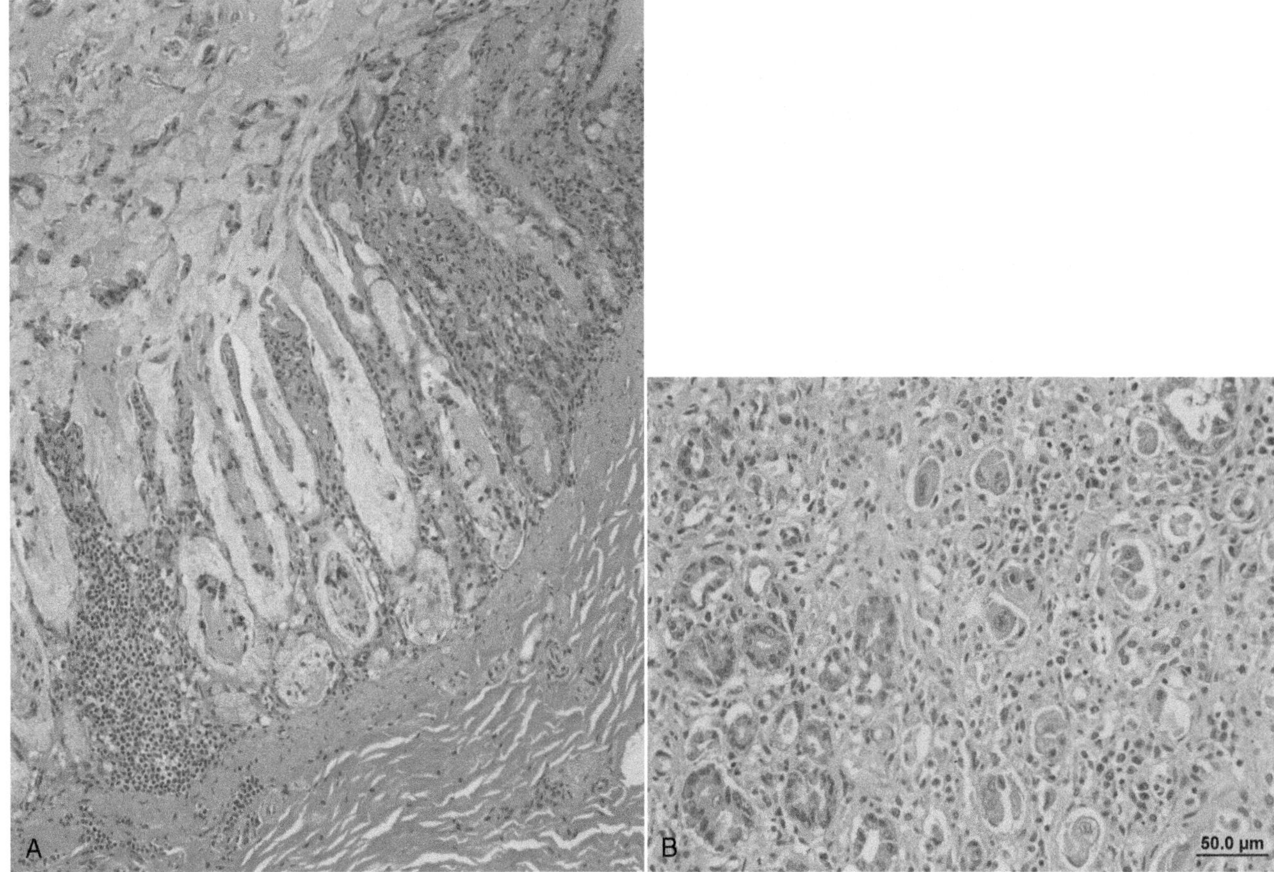

FIGURE 14-5 **A,** Segmental crypt necrosis in the ileum of a dog infected with a CPV-2 variant. There is severe loss of crypt epithelial cells. Hematoxylin and eosin (H&E) stain. **B,** Jejunum of a dog after infection by a CPV-2 variant. Regenerating epithelial cells, which here are nested in an inflamed jejunal lamina, have a large and bizarre appearance and resemble adenoma cells. As a result, the disease has been termed *adenomatosis*. Parvovirus antigen was no longer detectable by immunohistochemistry at this stage. The crypts in the bottom left corner have a more normal appearance. H&E stain. (Courtesy Dr. Patricia Pesavento, University of California, Davis Veterinary Anatomic Pathology Service.)

TABLE 14-4

Medications That May Be Used in Conjunction with Fluid Therapy to Treat Canine Parvoviral Enteritis

Drug	Dose (mg/kg)	Route	Interval (hours)
Ampicillin sodium	20	IV	6
Cefazolin sodium	20	IV	8
Enrofloxacin*	5	IV	24
Ondansetron	0.5 to 1	IV	12
Maropitant citrate	1	SC	24
Metoclopramide	1-2 mg/kg/d	IV	CRI
Famotidine	0.5	IV	12 to 24

CRI, Constant-rate infusion.
*Has been associated with cartilage injury in growing animals. Prolonged use (>7 days) is not recommended. See Chapter 8.

show evidence of an antibody response within 3 days after onset of clinical signs. Hetastarch has anticoagulant properties that could be beneficial in light of the hypercoagulable state that has been documented in canine parvoviral enteritis, but these effects also have the potential to increase mortality, and hetastarch has been associated with acute kidney injury in critically ill human patients.[41] Early enteral nutrition with a nasogastric feeding tube was associated with reduced hospitalization times in one study, as compared to withholding food until vomiting had ceased (Figure 14-6).[42] Gastric suction should be performed through the tube before food is administered.

Other treatments that have been investigated include anti-endotoxin sera, recombinant bactericidal permeability-increasing (BPI) protein, recombinant granulocyte colony-stimulating factor (G-CSF), recombinant feline interferon-omega (rfIFN-ω, Virbagen omega), and oseltamivir. Anti-endotoxin sera, recombinant BPI protein, and human recombinant G-CSF were not found to be beneficial. Although neutrophil counts were higher and hospital times were shorter in dogs treated with recombinant canine G-CSF, survival times in these dogs were decreased.[43] Treatment of parvovirus infections with G-CSF might cause harm, because the increased cell turnover induced by the drug might promote parvovirus replication. Treatment of puppies with parvoviral enteritis with rfIFN-ω in a number of placebo-controlled trials has been associated with reduced disease severity and, in some studies, significantly reduced mortality, but it has not been beneficial for treatment of FPV infections (see Chapter 19).

Oseltamivir inhibits the neuraminidase of influenza viruses and does not have specific anti-parvoviral activity, but it has been widely used for treatment of canine parvoviral enteritis. As canine parvovirus does not possess a neuraminidase, it has been

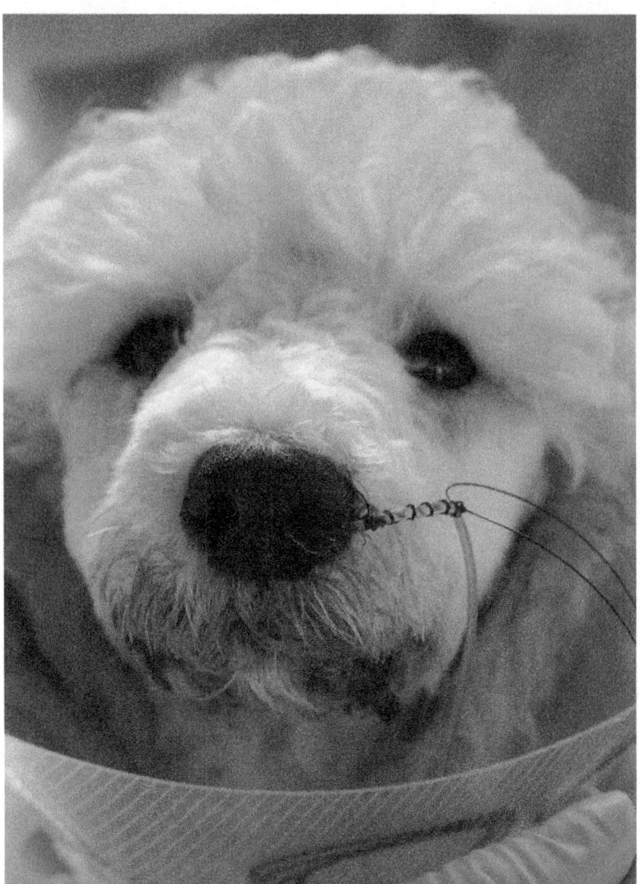

FIGURE 14-6 Puppy in Figure 14-2 after placement of a nasogastric feeding tube.

hypothesized that oseltamivir instead may act on the neuraminidases of bacteria that are normally responsible for secondary bacterial infections in parvovirus enteritis, primarily those of the gastrointestinal tract. A single prospective, randomized, masked, placebo-controlled trial of 35 dogs with parvovirus enteritis showed that dogs treated with oseltamivir (2 mg/kg PO q12h) had no significant drop in their leukocyte count, whereas untreated dogs had a significant drop in their leukocyte count in the first 5 days of hospitalization.[44] Treated dogs also gained weight during hospitalization, whereas untreated dogs lost weight. However, there was no difference in hospitalization time, clinical scores, morbidity, or mortality between the two groups, and the number of dogs in each group was small. The authors acknowledged the potential concerns that relate to administration of an oral medication to dogs with enteritis, with possible variability in drug absorption. A major concern that relates to treatment of canine parvoviral enteritis with oseltamivir is the possibility of selection for resistant mutants among influenza viruses if widespread use of the drug occurs in veterinary clinics. Given the restrictions on the use of this drug for treatment of human influenza virus infections, further investigation is required before the widespread use of oseltamivir can be recommended for treatment of CPV enteritis. More information on canine G-CSF, rfIFN-ω, and oseltamivir can be found in Chapter 7 of this book.

After recovery from viral enteritis, intestinal parasites should be treated with a broad-spectrum anthelmintic such as fenbendazole.

Prognosis

The prognosis for viral enteritis in puppies varies with the severity of illness and the owners' ability to afford appropriate treatment. Survival rates for puppies with CPV-2 enteritis have ranged from 9% in untreated puppies to greater than 90% with aggressive treatment in tertiary referral hospitals.[10,45-47] Factors that have been related to mortality include the presence of initial leukopenia or lymphopenia, monocytopenia, neutropenia, and evidence of SIRS.[29,48,49] SIRS was defined as the presence of at least three of the following four criteria: heart rate greater than 140 beats/min, temperature above 102.5°F or below 100°F, and white blood cell counts greater than 17,000 or less than 6000 cells/μL (see Chapter 86). Survival may also be lower in Rottweilers when compared to other breeds and in young puppies (less than 7 to 12 weeks of age).[50] In Australia, euthanasia was more likely to occur in summer; among pedigree dogs, in hounds, gundogs, and non-sporting breed dogs; and in puppies less than 6 months of age.[47] Vomiting and lethargy at admission as well as lymphopenia and hypoalbuminemia have been associated with prolongation of hospitalization times by approximately 2 days.[29] Positive changes in leukocyte counts (and especially lymphocyte counts) as early as 24 hours after admission have also been associated with survival.[48] In general, puppies that survive the first 3 to 4 days of treatment make complete recoveries. Complications of infection include bacteremia and septic shock, intestinal intussusception, aspiration pneumonia, and esophageal strictures.

Immunity and Vaccination

Immunity that follows natural infection by CPV-2 variants is probably lifelong. Immunization with attenuated live viral vaccines also provides sterile immunity that may even be lifelong. Both attenuated live and inactivated CPV vaccines are available. With the possible exception of shelter environments, attenuated live vaccines should never be administered to pregnant bitches because they may cause disease in the developing fetus. If possible, pregnant bitches introduced into shelter environments should be tested for antibody to CPV before vaccination with attenuated live vaccines, and these dogs should only be vaccinated if they test negative. The use of inactivated vaccines is not recommended in contaminated environments, because the window of vulnerability and the time to onset of protection is too long. The *window of vulnerability* is the period when maternal antibody interferes with the vaccine's ability to stimulate an effective immune response, but does not prevent infection with virulent field virus (see Chapter 12 for a discussion of this concept). Small quantities of attenuated live vaccine virus are shed from the intestinal tract after immunization, but this should not be relied on to immunize other in-contact animals. Protection against challenge with field virus occurs for at least 3 years and possibly for life after the initial puppy series is administered (see Chapter 12). Exposure of dogs to virus in the environment may also serve to booster immunity after vaccination.

The initial immunization series should be given every 3 to 4 weeks from 6 to 8 weeks of age, until no sooner than 14 to 16 weeks (16 to 20 weeks in breeding kennels), because of persistence of sufficient titers of maternal antibody in some puppies until this age. After that, a booster should be given at 1 year of age, and every 3 years thereafter (see Appendix). Puppies should be isolated in the home environment until 7 to 10 days after the last booster. Attendance at organized puppy classes has been advocated as a way to promote socialization in this period, and currently there is no evidence that such activities increase risk for parvoviral enteritis. Serum antibody titers of at least 1:80 as determined with hemagglutination-inhibition correlate well with protection.

Concern has been raised that currently available CPV vaccines may not provide adequate protection against CPV-2c infection, because of reports of CPV-2c enteritis in vaccinated dogs.[51] Furthermore, the serum of animals immunized against CPV-2, CPV-2a, and CPV-2b poorly recognized CPV-2c.[52] However, experimental challenge studies have demonstrated strong protection against CPV-2c challenge when dogs are immunized with vaccines that contain CPV-2.[53,54] The extent to which maternal antibody against non-CPV-2c strains protects against infection with CPV-2c requires investigation.

Both inactivated and attenuated live vaccines are available for prevention or reduction of canine enteric coronavirus infection, but because the disease is generally mild or inapparent and primarily occurs in puppies younger than 6 weeks of age, their use has not been generally recommended.[55]

Prevention

Prevention of CPV-2 enteritis requires immunization and appropriate quarantine, isolation, cleaning, and disinfection procedures. Proper immunization is the most effective method. Puppies that are incompletely vaccinated should not be introduced into environments where there has been a history of parvoviral enteritis and adequate environmental disinfection cannot be guaranteed. Although extremely resistant to disinfectants, parvoviruses can be inactivated with a 1 in 30 dilution of household bleach; potassium peroxymonosulfate (Trifectant, Virkon S); accelerated hydrogen peroxide; or high-level chemical disinfectants such as glutaraldehyde and *ortho*-phthalaldehyde, when contact times of at least 10 minutes are used (see Chapter 11 for more information on disinfection). These disinfectants will also inactivate other enteric viruses. Steam cleaning should be used on surfaces that cannot be otherwise disinfected, and dishwashers that attain temperatures of at least 75°C should be used to wash dishes. For shelters, quarantine periods of 2 weeks have been recommended before introduction of puppies that might be shedding virus, because shedding rarely continues for longer than 10 days.[56] The bathing of recovered puppies can help to remove virus that persists on the haircoat. Rodent and insect vector control can also be used to prevent spread of the virus in the environment. Outdoor grassy areas and dirt are difficult or impossible to adequately disinfect, and so only immunized animals should be allowed on these areas. The use of bleach on these areas is not recommended because of adverse environmental effects from runoff.

The prevalence and impact of enteric viral infections can also be reduced through regular removal of fecal contamination, prolonged exposure of contaminated surfaces to sunlight and drying, and elimination of stressors such as overcrowding, transport, poor nutrition, and concurrent infections such as intestinal parasites.

Public Health Aspects

Enteric viral pathogens of dogs, including CPV-2 variants, do not infect humans. However, other infectious causes of gastroenteritis in puppies have the potential to be zoonotic, and co-infections with these pathogens can occur, so caution should be maintained when handling puppies with diarrhea. Precautions used in isolation should be sufficient to prevent enteric zoonoses (see Chapter 11).

CASE EXAMPLE

Signalment: "Sam", an 8-week old intact male Hungarian vizsla puppy from northern California.

History: Sam was acquired 6 days ago from a breeder, and at that time was eating and active. The next day Sam was examined at a local veterinary clinic, and a routine fecal examination revealed infection with *Giardia* and *Isospora* spp. Treatment with sulfamethoxazole was initiated, but 1 day later the puppy developed diarrhea. The next day, lethargy and vomiting were noted. Vomiting and diarrhea occurred every few hours. The diarrhea contained fresh blood and the vomitus consisted of clear, frothy fluid. Inappetence and intermittent vomiting continued for the next 2 days.

Current Medications: None

Other Medical History: Vaccination with an attenuated live CDV, CPV-2, and canine parainfluenza vaccine was performed when Sam was 6 weeks of age. There were no other dogs in the household, only one adult cat.

Physical Examination:

Body weight: 4.2 kg

General: Quiet, alert, responsive. Estimated to be 7% to 8% dehydrated, T = 103.4°F (39.7°C), HR = 240 beats/min, RR = 36 breaths/min, mucous membranes pale pink and tacky, CRT = 2 seconds.

Integument: Full, shiny haircoat. No ectoparasites were seen.

Eyes, ears, nose, and throat: Enophthalmos and a dry nasal planum were present.

Musculoskeletal: Body condition score 2/9. The dog was ambulatory, but emaciated and weak.

Cardiovascular: Weak but synchronous femoral pulses. No murmurs or arrhythmias ausculted.

Respiratory: No clinically significant findings.

Gastrointestinal: No evidence of abdominal pain on palpation. Fluid-filled intestinal tract. Full urinary bladder noted.

Rectal examination: Bloody diarrhea was present on the thermometer. Rectal examination was not performed.

Lymph nodes: All lymph nodes were within normal limits.

Laboratory Findings:

CBC:

HCT 31.5% (40-55%)
MCV 62.6 fL (65-75 fL)
MCHC 35.6 g/dL (33-36 g/dL)
WBC 530 cells/μL (6000-13,000 cells/μL)
Neutrophils 16 cells/μL (3000-10,500 cells/μL)
Lymphocytes 504 cells/μL (1000-4000 cells/μL)
Monocytes 11 cells/μL (150-1,200 cells/μL)
Platelets clumped but appeared adequate.

Serum Chemistry Profile:

Sodium 143 mmol/L (145-154 mmol/L)
Potassium 3.8 mmol/L (3.6-5.3 mmol/L)

Continued

Chloride 106 mmol/L (108-118 mmol/L)
Bicarbonate 23 mmol/L (16-26 mmol/L)
Phosphorus 4.8 mg/dL (3.0-6.2 mg/dL)
Calcium 10.3 mg/dL (9.7-11.5 mg/dl)
BUN 6 mg/dL (5-21 mg/dL)
Creatinine <0.2 mg/dL (0.3-1.2 mg/dL), glucose 133 mg/dL (64-123 mg/dL)
Total protein 4.3 g/dL (5.4-7.6 g/dL)
Albumin 2.4 g/dL (3.0-4.4 g/dL)
Globulin 1.9 g/dL (1.8-3.9 g/dL)
ALT 22 U/L (19-67 U/L), AST 15 U/L (19-42 U/L)
ALP 179 U/L (21-170 U/L)
Creatine kinase 274 U/L (51-399 U/L)
Gamma GT <3 U/L (0-6 U/L)
Cholesterol 278 mg/dL (135-361 mg/dL)
Total bilirubin 0.1 mg/dL (0-0.2 mg/dL)
Magnesium 2.0 mg/dL (1.5-2.6 mg/dL).

Imaging Findings:

Abdominal radiographs: The stomach wall appeared thickened. Numerous round gas opacities were present in a loop of intestine in the right cranial abdomen, which were believed to represent gas in the ascending colon or duodenum. Multiple additional gas opacities were present in a loop of intestine in the mid right abdomen at the level of the fourth lumbar vertebra. There was reduced serosal detail compatible with the age of the animal. Changes were considered consistent with the presence of gastroenterocolitis.

Microbiologic Testing:

Fecal Parvovirus Antigen ELISA: Negative

Fecal Enteric Real-time PCR Panel: PCR positive for CPV in fecal specimen. PCR negative for *Clostridium difficile* toxin A and toxin B genes, *Cryptosporidium* spp., *Salmonella* spp., and *Giardia* spp. DNA.

Fecal Zinc Sulfate Centrifugal Flotation: Negative for parasite ova.

Diagnosis: Enteritis and leukopenia secondary to canine parvoviral infection.

Treatment: Sam was admitted to isolation and treated aggressively with intravenous lactated Ringer's solution that was supplemented with 20 mEq KCl/L, famotidine (0.5 mg/kg IV q12h), ondansetron (0.5 mg/kg IV q12h), ampicillin (22 mg/kg IV q6h), and enrofloxacin (5 mg/kg IV q24h). Because of persistent vomiting, maropitant citrate (1 mg/kg IV q24h) was added as a second antiemetic. Blood glucose concentration was monitored three times daily, but supplementation with dextrose was not required. Bloody diarrhea that contained sloughed intestinal mucosa occurred every few hours for the first 24 hours. The neutrophil count was 9 cells/μL the following day, but by day 4 of hospitalization was 261 cells/μL, with 241 moderately toxic bands/μL and a lymphocyte count of 1226 cells/μL. There was gradual clinical improvement during this time, and Sam began to ingest small quantities of cottage cheese and rice on day 4. He was discharged from the hospital on day 5.

Comments: Despite the negative fecal antigen ELISA assay, CPV enteritis was suspected in this dog based on the history, clinical signs, and severe leukopenia. The finding of leukopenia and diarrhea is not diagnostic for parvoviral enteritis, because it can also be caused by other severe enteritides such as salmonellosis. The positive fecal real-time PCR assay for CPV supported the diagnosis, but because positive fecal PCR results can occur in healthy dogs with some assays, and also after vaccination, the fecal PCR result alone did not confirm the diagnosis of CPV enteritis. The diagnosis was therefore made on the basis of the combination of findings. The neutropenia in this dog was profound. Infection likely occurred before the owner acquired the puppy because the diarrhea began only 2 days after the puppy was purchased.

SUGGESTED READINGS

Carmichael LE. An annotated historical account of canine parvovirus. J Vet Med Ser B. 2005;52(7-8):303-311.

Iris K, Leontides LS, Mylonakis ME, et al. Factors affecting the occurrence, duration of hospitalization and final outcome in canine parvovirus infection. Res Vet Sci. 2010;89:174-178.

REFERENCES

1. Carmichael LE. An annotated historical account of canine parvovirus. J Vet Med Ser B. 2005;52(7-8):303-311.
2. Hoelzer K, Parrish CR. The emergence of parvoviruses of carnivores. Vet Res. 2010;41:39.
3. Clegg SR, Coyne KP, Parker J, et al. Molecular epidemiology and phylogeny reveal complex spatial dynamics in areas where canine parvovirus is endemic. J Virol. 2011;85:7892-7899.
4. Ikeda Y, Nakamura K, Miyazawa T, et al. Feline host range of canine parvovirus: recent emergence of new antigenic types in cats. Emerg Infect Dis. 2002;8:341-346.
5. Battilani M, Balboni A, Ustulin M, et al. Genetic complexity and multiple infections with more *Parvovirus* species in naturally infected cats. Vet Res. 2011;42:43.
6. Pratelli A, Buonavoglia D, Tempesta M, et al. Fatal canine parvovirus type-1 infection in pups from Italy. J Vet Diagn Invest. 1999;11:365-367.
7. Ohshima T, Kawakami K, Abe T, et al. A minute virus of canines (MVC: canine bocavirus) isolated from an elderly dog with severe gastroenteritis, and phylogenetic analysis of MVC strains. Vet Microbiol. 2010;145:334-338.
8. Eminaga S, Palus V, Cherubini GB. Minute virus as a possible cause of neurological problems in dogs. Vet Rec. 2011;168:111-112.
9. Houston DM, Ribble CS, Head LL. Risk factors associated with parvovirus enteritis in dogs: 283 cases (1982-1991). J Am Vet Med Assoc. 1996:542-546.
10. Glickman LT, Domanski LM, Patronek GJ, et al. Breed-related risk factors for canine parvovirus enteritis. J Am Vet Med Assoc. 1985;187:589-594.
11. Kalli I, Leontides LS, Mylonakis ME, et al. Factors affecting the occurrence, duration of hospitalization and final outcome in canine parvovirus infection. Res Vet Sci. 2010;89:174-178.
12. Brady S, Norris JM, Kelman M, et al. Canine parvovirus in Australia: the role of socio-economic factors in disease clusters. Vet J. 2012;193:522-528.

13. Li L, Pesavento PA, Shan T, et al. Viruses in diarrheic dogs include novel kobuviruses and sapoviruses. J Gen Virol. 2011;92:2534-2541.
14. Pesavento PA, Li L, Leutenegger C, et-al. Canine circovirus is associated with vascular damage in dogs. Proceedings of the 2nd symposium of the International Society for Companion Animal Infectious Diseases. San Francisco, CA. 2012;A01.
15. Ntafis V, Xylouri E, Radogna A, et al. Outbreak of canine norovirus infection in young dogs. J Clin Microbiol. 2010;48:2605-2608.
16. Mesquita JR, Barclay L, Nascimento MS, et al. Novel norovirus in dogs with diarrhea. Emerg Infect Dis. 2010;16:980-982.
17. Martella V, Lorusso E, Decaro N, et al. Detection and molecular characterization of a canine norovirus. Emerg Infect Dis. 2008;14:1306-1308.
18. Evermann JF, Abbott JR, Han S. Canine coronavirus-associated puppy mortality without evidence of concurrent canine parvovirus infection. J Vet Diagn Invest. 2005;17:610-614.
19. Macartney L, McCandlish IA, Thompson H, et al. Canine parvovirus enteritis 2: pathogenesis. Vet Rec. 1984;115:453-460.
20. Otto CM, Rieser TM, Brooks MB, et al. Evidence of hypercoagulability in dogs with parvoviral enteritis. J Am Vet Med Assoc. 2000;217:1500-1504.
21. Hayes MA, Russell RG, Babiuk LA. Sudden death in young dogs with myocarditis caused by parvovirus. J Am Vet Med Assoc. 1979;174:1197-1203.
22. Lenghaus C, Studdert MJ, Finnie JW. Acute and chronic canine parvovirus myocarditis following intrauterine inoculation. Aust Vet J. 1980;56:465-468.
23. Bastianello SS. Canine parvovirus myocarditis: clinical signs and pathological lesions encountered in natural cases. J S Afr Vet Assoc. 1981;52:105-108.
24. Schatzberg SJ, Haley NJ, Barr SC, et al. Polymerase chain reaction (PCR) amplification of parvoviral DNA from the brains of dogs and cats with cerebellar hypoplasia. J Vet Intern Med. 2003;17:538-544.
25. Lenghaus C, Studdert MJ. Generalized parvovirus disease in neonatal pups. J Am Vet Med Assoc. 1982;181:41-45.
26. Decaro N, Martella V, Elia G, et al. Tissue distribution of the antigenic variants of canine parvovirus type 2 in dogs. Vet Microbiol. 2007;121:39-44.
27. Schaudien D, Polizopoulou Z, Koutinas A, et al. Leukoencephalopathy associated with parvovirus infection in Cretan hound puppies. J Clin Microbiol. 2010;48:3169-3175.
28. Agungpriyono DR, Uchida K, Tabaru H, et al. Subacute massive necrotizing myocarditis by canine parvovirus type 2 infection with diffuse leukoencephalomalacia in a puppy. Vet Pathol. 1999;36:77-80.
29. Iris K, Leontides LS, Mylonakis ME, et al. Factors affecting the occurrence, duration of hospitalization and final outcome in canine parvovirus infection. Res Vet Sci. 2010;89:174-178.
30. Woldemeskel M, Liggett A, Ilha M, et al. Canine parvovirus-2b-associated erythema multiforme in a litter of English Setter dogs. J Vet Diagn Invest. 2011;23:576-580.
31. Favrot C, Olivry T, Dunston SM, et al. Parvovirus infection of keratinocytes as a cause of canine erythema multiforme. Vet Pathol. 2000;37:647-649.
32. Decaro N, Desario C, Beall MJ, et al. Detection of canine parvovirus type 2c by a commercially available in-house rapid test. Vet J. 2010;184:373-375.
33. Schmitz S, Coenen C, Konig M, et al. Comparison of three rapid commercial canine parvovirus antigen detection tests with electron microscopy and polymerase chain reaction. J Vet Diagn Invest. 2009;21:344-345.
34. Greene CE, Decaro N. Canine viral enteritis. In: Greene CE, ed. Infectious Diseases of the Dog and Cat. 4th ed. St Louis, MO: Elsevier Saunders; 2012.
35. Patterson EV, Reese MJ, Tucker SJ, et al. Effect of vaccination on parvovirus antigen testing in kittens. J Am Vet Med Assoc. 2007;230:359-363.
36. Marulappa SY, Kapil S. Simple tests for rapid detection of canine parvovirus antigen and canine parvovirus-specific antibodies. Clin Vaccine Immunol. 2009;16:127-131.
37. Decaro N, Elia G, Desario C, et al. A minor groove binder probe real-time PCR assay for discrimination between type 2-based vaccines and field strains of canine parvovirus. J Virol Methods. 2006;136:65-70.
38. Mochizuki M, Ohshima T, Une Y, et al. Recombination between vaccine and field strains of canine parvovirus is revealed by isolation of virus in canine and feline cell cultures. J Vet Med Sci. 2008;70:1305-1314.
39. Nho WG, Sur JH, Doster AR, et al. Detection of canine parvovirus in naturally infected dogs with enteritis and myocarditis by in situ hybridization. J Vet Diagn Invest. 1997;9:255-260.
40. Waldvogel AS, Hassam S, Stoerckle N, et al. Specific diagnosis of parvovirus enteritis in dogs and cats by in situ hybridization. J Comp Pathol. 1992;107:141-146.
41. Groeneveld AB, Navickis RJ, Wilkes MM. Update on the comparative safety of colloids: a systematic review of clinical studies. Ann Surg. 2011;253:470-483.
42. Mohr AJ, Leisewitz AL, Jacobson LS, et al. Effect of early enteral nutrition on intestinal permeability, intestinal protein loss, and outcome in dogs with severe parvoviral enteritis. J Vet Intern Med. 2003;17:791-798.
43. Duffy A, Dow S, Ogilvie G, et al. Hematologic improvement in dogs with parvovirus infection treated with recombinant canine granulocyte-colony stimulating factor. J Vet Pharmacol Ther. 2010;33:352-356.
44. Savigny MR, Macintire DK. Use of oseltamivir in the treatment of canine parvoviral enteritis. J Vet Emerg Crit Care (San Antonio). 2010;20:132-142.
45. Otto CM, Jackson CB, Rogell EJ, et al. Recombinant bactericidal/permeability-increasing protein (rBPI21) for treatment of parvovirus enteritis: a randomized, double-blinded, placebo-controlled trial. J Vet Intern Med. 2001;15:355-360.
46. Otto CM, Drobatz KJ, Soter C. Endotoxemia and tumor necrosis factor activity in dogs with naturally occurring parvoviral enteritis. J Vet Intern Med. 1997;11:65-70.
47. Ling M, Norris JM, Kelman M, et al. Risk factors for death from canine parvoviral-related disease in Australia. Vet Microbiol. 2012;158:280-290.
48. Goddard A, Leisewitz AL, Christopher MM, et al. Prognostic usefulness of blood leukocyte changes in canine parvoviral enteritis. J Vet Intern Med. 2008;22:309-316.
49. Mason MJ, Gillett NA, Muggenburg BA. Clinical, pathological, and epidemiological aspects of canine parvoviral enteritis in an unvaccinated closed beagle colony: 1978-1985. J Am Anim Hosp Assoc. 1987;23:183-192.
50. Horner GW. Canine parvovirus in New Zealand: epidemiological features and diagnostic methods. N Z Vet J. 1983;31:164-166.
51. Decaro N, Desario C, Elia G, et al. Evidence for immunisation failure in vaccinated adult dogs infected with canine parvovirus type 2c. New Microbiol. 2008;31:125-130.
52. Cavalli A, Martella V, Desario C, et al. Evaluation of the antigenic relationships among canine parvovirus type 2 variants. Clin Vaccine Immunol. 2008;15:534-539.
53. Siedek EM, Schmidt H, Sture GH, et al. Vaccination with canine parvovirus type 2 (CPV-2) protects against challenge with virulent CPV-2b and CPV-2c. Berl Munch Tierarztl Wochenschr. 2011;124:58-64.
54. Larson LJ, Schultz RD. Do two current canine parvovirus type 2 and 2b vaccines provide protection against the new type 2c variant? Vet Ther. 2008;9:94-101.
55. Welborn LV, DeVries JG, Ford R, et al. 2011 AAHA canine vaccination guidelines. J Am Anim Hosp Assoc. 2011;47:1-42.
56. Appel LD, Barr SC. Canine parvovirus and coronavirus. In: Miller L, Hurley KF, eds. Infectious Disease Management in Animal Shelters. Ames, IA: Wiley-Blackwell; 2009:197-208.

CHAPTER 15

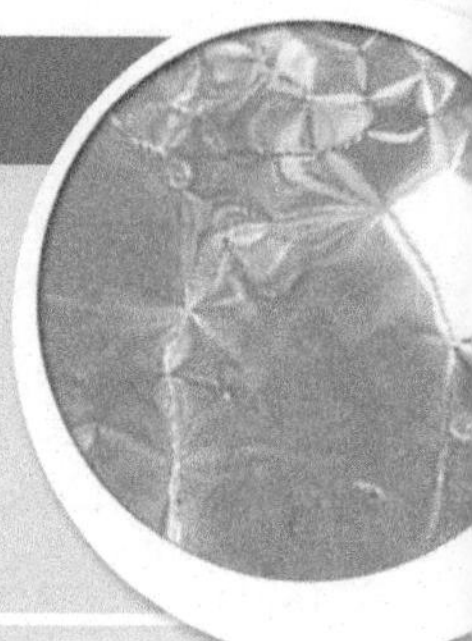

Canine Distemper Virus Infection

Jane E. Sykes

Overview of Canine Distemper

First Described: 1905, Henri Carré, France[1]

Cause: Canine distemper virus (family Paramyxoviridae, subfamily Paramyxovirinae, genus *Morbillivirus*)

Affected Hosts: Dogs and other Canidae such as coyotes, foxes, and wolves; Procyonidae (raccoons, pandas); Mustelidae (ferrets, mink, skunks, otters). Large wild Felidae can also be affected.

Geographic Distribution: Worldwide

Mode of Transmission: Oronasal contact with virus in secretions or excretions, droplet nuclei, and large particle aerosol transmission

Major Clinical Signs: Fever, lethargy, inappetence, vomiting, diarrhea, dehydration, tachypnea, cough, conjunctivitis, neurologic signs, footpad, and nasal planum hyperkeratosis

Differential Diagnoses: Canine parvovirus infection, other infectious causes of gastroenteritis, other causes of canine infectious respiratory disease, rabies, parasitic gastrointestinal and respiratory disease, toxins such as lead and ethylene glycol, gastrointestinal foreign body, dietary indiscretion, protozoal meningoencephalitis, systemic fungal infections such as cryptococcosis, portosystemic shunting with hepatic encephalopathy

Human Health Significance: CDV has been used as a model to study measles virus infection. There is some evidence that it may be involved in the pathogenesis of Paget's disease, a chronic, focal skeletal disorder of the elderly.

Etiology and Epidemiology

Canine distemper is an important disease of domestic dogs and wild animals worldwide. It is caused by canine distemper virus (CDV), an enveloped, pleomorphic RNA virus that belongs to the genus *Morbillivirus* (family Paramyxoviridae). CDV is closely related to human measles virus and rinderpest virus and has been used as a model to study the pathogenesis of measles virus infections. The outer envelope of CDV contains hemagglutinin (H) and fusion (F) proteins, which are important in cellular attachment and entry (Figure 15-1). Infection of dogs can lead to a severe, multisystemic disease that primarily affects the gastrointestinal, respiratory, and neurologic systems (Figure 15-2).

Ferrets also are highly susceptible to distemper, but domestic cats are not affected. In addition, distemper occurs in a variety of wildlife species that belong to the families Canidae, Mustelidae, Procyonidae, and Felidae (see Overview). Virus shed by wildlife species such as raccoons can infect domestic dogs, but virus that is shed by dogs may also be a significant threat to wildlife populations, with catastrophic outbreaks of disease and high mortality rates. In domestic dogs with signs of infectious upper respiratory disease ("kennel cough"), distemper is an important differential diagnosis, and distemper can also mimic canine parvovirus (CPV) enteritis. In fact, dual infections with CDV and CPV are probably underrecognized.

Worldwide, at least eight different geographic lineages (also referred to as genotypes or clades) of CDV exist based on sequence analysis of the H gene: Asia-1, Asia-2, America-1, America-2, Europe-1/South America-1, Europe-2 (European wildlife), Europe-3 (Arctic-like), and South Africa. In addition, strains recognized in Argentina, Africa, Asia, and Mexico may represent separate geographic lineages.[1,2] In the United States, vaccine strains belong to the America-1 lineage, whereas most field strains belong to the America-2 lineage. Strains that belong to the Europe-2 and Europe-3 lineages have also been detected in North American dogs.[3]

Although vaccination has reduced the incidence of the disease, distemper still remains important where large numbers of

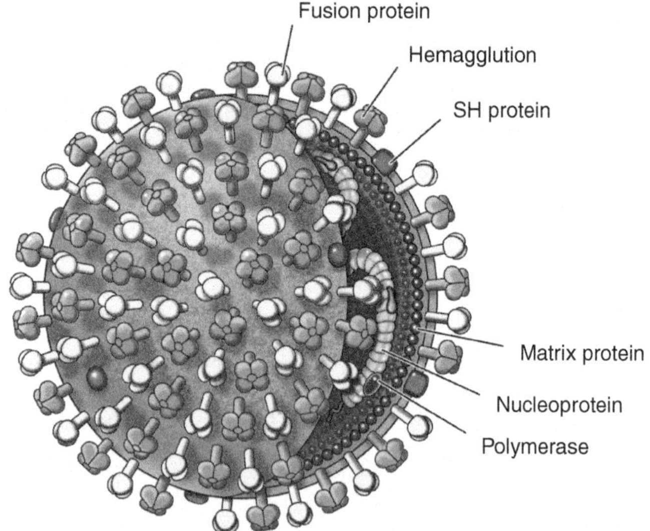

FIGURE 15-1 Structure of CDV. The outer envelope contains hemagglutinin (H) and fusion (F) proteins, which are connected to the nucleocapsid by a matrix (M) protein, which is the most abundant protein in the virion.

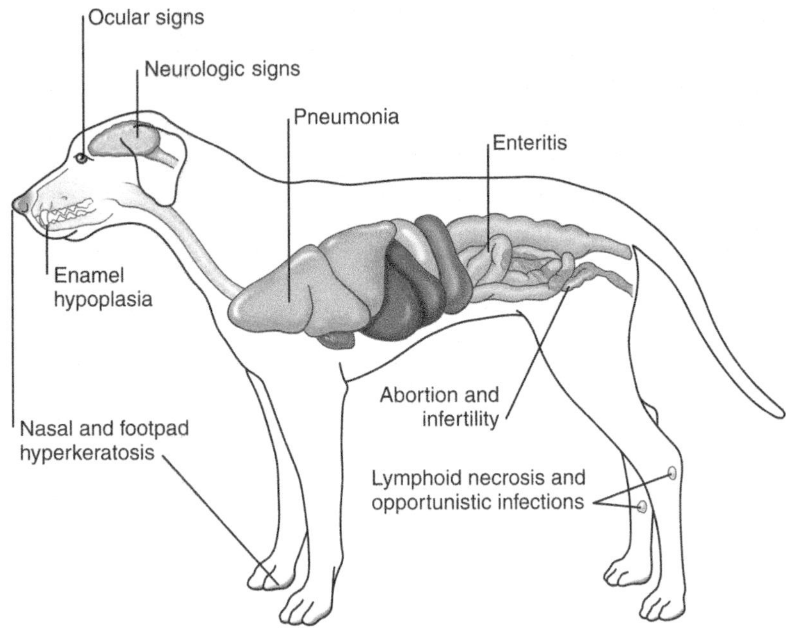

FIGURE 15-2 Anatomic sites targeted by CDV infection.

young dogs with inadequate immunity are housed together, such as in kennels, large breeding facilities, and shelter environments. Puppies that have lost their maternal antibody are predisposed in regions where vaccination is performed, but occasionally disease occurs in older, vaccinated dogs.[4-6] Distemper also occurs in regions where vaccination of dogs is not performed or is poorly timed. As an enveloped virus, CDV is susceptible in the environment (surviving less than 1 day at room temperature) and is readily inactivated by heat, drying, and disinfectants; thus, contact between infected dogs is important to maintain transmission of the virus.

Clinical Features

Signs and Their Pathogenesis

CDV is highly contagious and is spread through droplet nuclei and large-particle aerosol transmission. Dogs are generally exposed to CDV through contact with infected oronasal secretions, which may be shed by subclinically or clinically affected dogs. The virus initially infects monocytes within lymphoid tissue in the upper respiratory tract and tonsils and is subsequently disseminated via the lymphatics and blood to the entire reticuloendothelial system. The viral hemagglutinin binds to a molecule on the surface of host cells known as the signaling lymphocytic activation molecule (SLAM, also known in humans as CD150). SLAM is a membrane glycoprotein of the immunoglobulin superfamily. It is important for cell entry by CDV as well as other morbilliviruses and is a key molecule in the pathogenesis of disease.[7] SLAM is expressed by immature thymocytes, activated lymphocytes, macrophages, and dendritic cells. Direct viral destruction of a significant proportion of the lymphocyte population, and especially CD4+ T cells, occurs within the blood, tonsils, thymus, spleen, lymph nodes, bone marrow, mucosa-associated lymphoid tissue, and hepatic Kupffer cells (Figure 15-3).[8-10] Massive destruction of lymphocytes results in an initial lymphopenia and transient fever, which occurs a few days after infection. Subsequently, there is a second stage of cell-associated viremia and fever

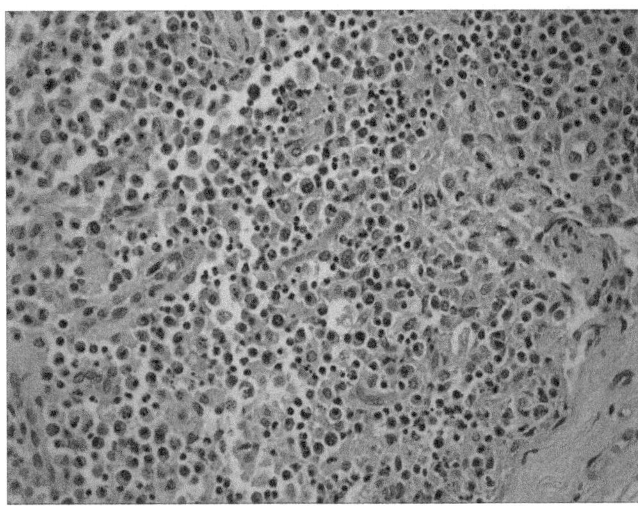

FIGURE 15-3 Lymph node histopathology of a 5-month-old German shepherd mix with distemper. The dog had been adopted from a shelter and subsequently developed neurologic signs, diarrhea, and pneumonia. There is marked lymphoid necrosis. H&E stain.

(8 to 9 days after infection), after which CDV infects cells of the respiratory, gastrointestinal tract, central nervous system (CNS), urinary tract, and skin, as well as red and white blood cells, including additional lymphoid cells. In this stage of infection, CDV infects a variety of cell lineages, including epithelial, mesenchymal, neuroendocrine, and hematopoietic cells, and forms intracytoplasmic but also intranuclear inclusions (Figure 15-4). Infection of epithelial cells by the virus is inefficient and occurs relatively late in the course of infection, through a SLAM-independent mechanism that appears to involve the nectin 4 receptor, as is true for measles virus.[11] CDV is shed in all secretions and excretions from as early as day 5 after infection, before the onset of clinical signs. Shedding of virus can continue for as long as 3 to 4 months, but usually resolves after 1 to 2 weeks.

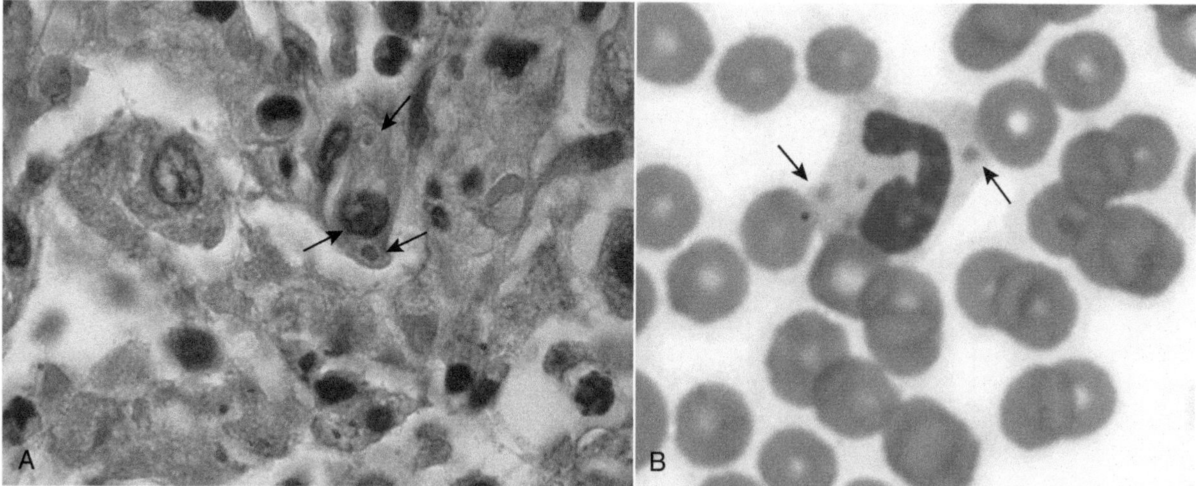

FIGURE 15-4 **A,** Eosinophilic intracytoplasmic and intranuclear viral inclusions *(arrows)* in the lung of the dog from Figure 15-3. Hematoxylin and eosin stain, 1000× oil magnification. **B,** Intracytoplasmic inclusions *(arrows)* in a circulating leukocyte of a 4-month-old Border collie mix with distemper.

The clinical signs of distemper in dogs vary dramatically and are highly dependent on virus strain and the age and immune status of the host, as well as concurrent infections with other viruses and bacteria. Many dogs experience subclinical infection, whereas others experience rapidly progressive infection followed by death. The incubation period ranges from 3 to 6 days. Respiratory or gastrointestinal tract signs may be indistinguishable from those caused by other respiratory or enteric viruses and bacteria, or signs may be so mild that they go unnoticed by the owner. Dogs with respiratory involvement may exhibit fever, bilateral serous and nasal ocular discharges, conjunctivitis, and a nonproductive cough. Secondary bacterial infection, which occurs unhindered as a result of virus-induced immunosuppression, can lead to the development of mucopurulent nasal and ocular discharges and bacterial bronchopneumonia, with tachypnea, productive cough, lethargy, and decreased appetite. Viral destruction of the gastrointestinal tract epithelium can result in inappetence, vomiting, diarrhea, electrolyte abnormalities, and dehydration. Dogs that mount an intermediate or delayed immune response may recover from acute illness but fail to eliminate the virus completely, which leads to a spectrum of more chronic disease manifestations, which often involve the uvea, lymphoid organs, footpads, and especially the CNS. Opportunistic infections can also develop in these dogs.

Up to 30% of infected dogs develop CNS signs. These usually occur 1 to 6 weeks after the onset of acute illness but can occur even when initial infection is subclinical. Neurologic signs are more likely to develop following infection with certain CDV strains, such as the Snyder Hill strain.[12] The types of brain cells that are infected differ with the strain of CDV involved,[13] but neuronal necrosis and atrophy can occur.[14] Neurologic signs are often progressive and generally do not resolve, so dogs that recover often have residual neurologic deficits. "Old dog encephalitis" is a poorly characterized, progressive immune-mediated demyelinating leukoencephalomyelitis induced by CDV that occurs weeks to years after recovery from the acute infection and is difficult to diagnose. The term "old dog encephalitis" is a misnomer, because affected dogs are not necessarily old. Both CDV and measles virus have been incriminated as possible agents of multiple sclerosis because of the resemblance of demyelinating CDV encephalitis to the pathology of this disease.[15] Virus has been detected within the brains of these dogs with immunohistochemistry and reverse-transcriptase PCR assays.[16] Persistent infection of astrocytes in the CNS by some CDV strains has been postulated as a mechanism for this chronic manifestation of infection, with transmission from cell to cell through induction of cell-cell fusion and resultant evasion of the host immune response.[17]

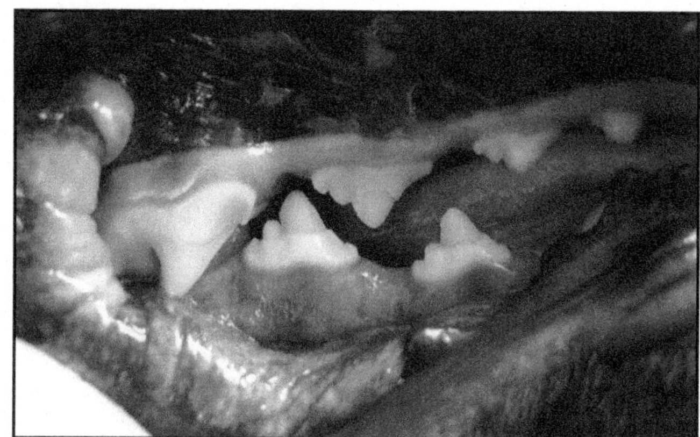

FIGURE 15-5 Enamel hypoplasia induced by CDV infection.

Ocular signs of persistent CDV infection include uveitis, chorioretinitis, keratoconjunctivitis sicca (KCS), keratitis, and optic neuritis, which may be associated with blindness. KCS is thought to result from damage to the lacrimal gland by CDV.[18] It may be transient or permanent, and can lead to keratitis and corneal ulceration. The virus itself can also infect the corneal epithelial and stromal cells. Enamel and dentin hypoplasia, manifested as irregularities of the teeth, is an incidental finding in recovered dogs due to infection of the stratum intermedium of developing teeth (Figure 15-5). Retention and partial eruption of teeth has also been reported as a sequela of CDV infection.[19,20] Infection of the skin can lead to a cutaneous measles-like rash, although this is uncommonly recognized. Persistent infection of the footpad and nasal planum epithelium leads to hyperkeratosis in these regions (Figure 15-6).

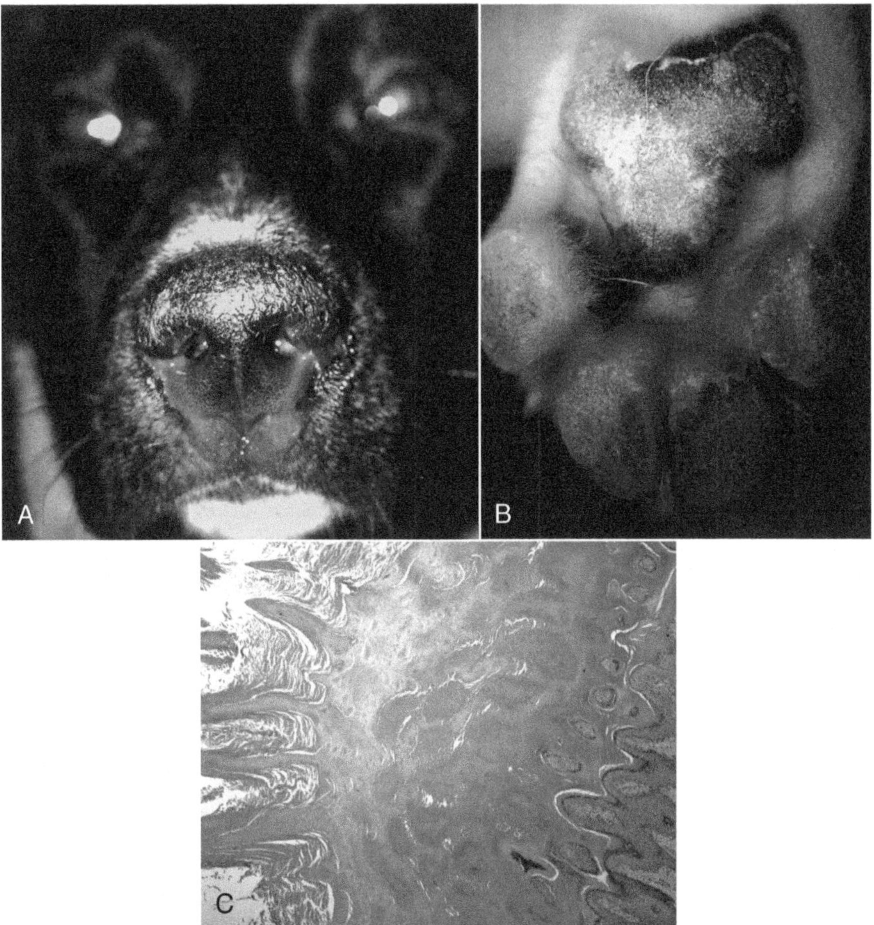

FIGURE 15-6 Nasal planum **(A)** and footpad **(B)** hyperkeratosis induced by CDV infection in a 4-month-old Border collie mix with conjunctivitis, mucopurulent nasal and ocular discharge, and myoclonus. Blepharospasm is also present. **C,** Histopathology of the footpad of a 1-year old German shepherd mix with distemper. Marked hyperkeratosis is evident. H&E stain, 40× magnification.

Immunosuppression results from lymphopenia, necrosis of hematopoietic cells in the bone marrow, and dendritic cell malfunction. Lymphocyte apoptosis also occurs independent of viral infection of lymphocytes.[21] The viral V protein allows CDV to replicate rapidly in T cells and is critical in CDV-mediated immunosuppression. This protein almost completely antagonizes IFN-α, TNF-α, Il-6, IFN-γ, and Il-2 in the acute phase of infection.[10] Finally, the nucleocapsid (N) protein of morbilliviruses binds to the CD32 (Fc-γ) receptor on B cells, which results in impaired differentiation of B cells into plasma cells.[22] When the virus binds this receptor on dendritic cells, impaired antigen presentation by dendritic cells results, which disrupts T-cell function. The most common secondary infections in distemper are secondary bacterial infections that contribute to bronchopneumonia. *Bordetella bronchiseptica* is a common copathogen. Dogs may be diagnosed with bordetellosis in the early stages of distemper, and the underlying CDV infection may be overlooked. Other opportunistic infections that have been identified in dogs with distemper include toxoplasmosis,[23] salmonellosis,[24] nocardiosis,[25,26] and generalized demodecosis. Infection with *Pneumocystis carinii* was associated with CDV infection in a mink,[27] and concurrent neosporosis and canine distemper was reported in a raccoon.[28]

Uncommonly, CDV infection has been associated with metaphyseal bone lesions in young dogs as a result of infection of osteoclasts, osteoblasts, and osteocytes.[29] Infected cells undergo degeneration and necrosis, and metaphyseal osteosclerosis occurs (Figure 15-7). This may lead to pain and lameness. CDV RNA has also been detected in bone cells of dogs with hypertrophic osteodystrophy, and CDV may play a role in this disease.[30]

Finally, transplacental infections with CDV may be associated with infertility, stillbirth, or abortion and with neurologic signs in puppies that are less than 4 to 6 weeks of age.

Physical Examination Findings

Physical examination findings in dogs with distemper depend on the severity and chronicity of the disease, but include fever (occasionally up to 106°F or 41.1°C), conjunctivitis, serous to mucopurulent ocular and nasal discharges, blepharospasm and photophobia, tonsillar enlargement and hyperemia, tachypnea, and increased lung sounds (see Figure 15-6). Cough may occur during the examination. Dehydration may also be present, especially in dogs with gastrointestinal and severe neurologic signs. Rarely, a measles-like cutaneous rash or pustular dermatitis is evident.

Dogs with chronic disease can be thin or emaciated and show hyperkeratosis of the nasal planum and footpads. Puppies with hyperkeratosis, also known as "hardpad," have thickened, crusty footpads that resemble those of adult dogs (see Figure 15-6). Myoclonus (involuntary twitching of isolated muscle groups) is common and, when mild, is most readily detected

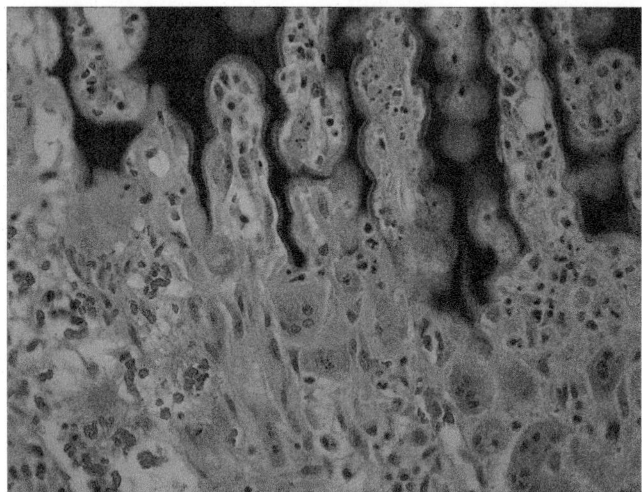

FIGURE 15-7 Severe, neutrophilic osteomyelitis with submetaphyseal osteonecrosis and extensive bony resorption in a 4-month-old intact male Labrador retriever mix with distemper. The dog was seen for lethargy, mild diarrhea, fever, and reluctance to stand; joint pain was detected on physical examination. Direct IFA on urine sediment was positive for CDV, but a conjunctival scrape tested negative with direct IFA. Necropsy also revealed pneumonia with intracytoplasmic and intranuclear viral inclusions. H&E stain.

when affected puppies are at rest. Other neurologic signs include obtundation, seizures, tremors, opisthotonos, tetraparesis, paraparesis, delayed placing reactions, ataxia, and, less commonly, behavioral abnormalities, compulsive pacing, and vestibular signs such as a head tilt, nystagmus, strabismus, and circling.[4] Focal seizures may be localized to the head and jaw, with accompanying foamy hypersalivation ("chewing gum" seizures). Vocalization and apparent blindness can also occur. In addition to conjunctivitis and ocular discharge, an ophthalmologic examination may reveal corneal edema, corneal ulceration, aqueous flare, chorioretinitis, and uveitis, or optic neuritis. Markedly decreased Schirmer tear test results and positive fluorescein tests may be present.[18] Optic neuritis appears as a large, pale, fluffy, optic disc with no physiologic depression. Rarely, lameness may be observed.

Dogs that have recovered from CDV infection may have evidence of dental abnormalities and enamel hypoplasia (see Figure 15-5); healed chorioretinitis lesions, which appear as hyperreflective circular lesions ("gold medallion lesions"); keratoconjunctivitis sicca; or residual neurologic signs, especially myoclonus.

Diagnosis

Establishment of a diagnosis of distemper is most easily accomplished in dogs that have the full spectrum of clinical abnormalities, and especially when myoclonus is present, because there are few other diseases that cause this array of clinical signs. In dogs with isolated respiratory, gastrointestinal, or neurologic signs, antemortem diagnosis is more challenging because these signs are less specific, laboratory diagnostic assays can be insensitive, and the presence of attenuated live vaccine virus can lead to false-positive results. A combination of laboratory tests may be required to establish the diagnosis, and the finding of a negative result for any assay does not rule out distemper. Sensitivity for detection of CDV using assays that detect virus may also be increased by testing of multiple specimens from different anatomic locations, such as various combinations of blood, urine, conjunctival smears, and CSF. In dogs with respiratory signs, the presence of conjunctivitis, blepharospasm, and ocular discharge should raise suspicion for distemper. Distemper should always be considered as a diagnosis in young dogs with neurologic signs, whether or not respiratory or gastrointestinal signs are present. Finally, clinicians should maintain a high suspicion for the presence of concurrent infections such as parvoviral enteritis, concurrent respiratory viral infection, or bordetellosis.

Laboratory Abnormalities

Complete Blood Count

The CBC in dogs with acute distemper most commonly reveals mild anemia and lymphopenia (Table 15-1). However, the lymphocyte count may also be normal, especially with more chronic distemper. Neutropenia, monocytopenia, and thrombocytopenia can occur, and occasionally these are severe. Neutrophilia with a left shift and toxic neutrophils may be present. Rarely, examination of Romanowsky-stained blood smears using light microscopy reveals CDV inclusions in the cytoplasm of circulating erythrocytes and leukocytes (see Figure 15-4, *B*).

Serum Biochemical Tests

Abnormalities on the serum biochemistry panel in dogs with distemper are nonspecific and include electrolyte changes that occur with vomiting and diarrhea such as hyponatremia, hypokalemia, and hypochloridemia (Table 15-2). Hypoalbuminemia and associated hypocalcemia are also common. Mild increases in liver enzyme activities occur in some dogs, which may reflect hypoxia or secondary infections that occur as a result of translocation of intestinal bacteria.

Urinalysis

No specific urinalysis findings are reported in dogs with distemper.

CSF Analysis

CSF analysis may show no clinically significant findings in dogs with distemper, especially when chronic demyelinating encephalitis is present. In some dogs with CNS involvement, a mild to moderate increase in CSF protein concentration is present (usually <100 mg/dL), and there is lymphocytic or monocytic pleocytosis, sometimes with reactivity. Nucleated cell counts are usually less than 50 cells/μL and rarely less than 100 cells/μL.[4]

Diagnostic Imaging

Plain Radiography

When present, abnormalities on thoracic radiography in dogs with distemper include pulmonary interstitial to alveolar infiltrates and consolidation compatible with bronchopneumonia, especially in the cranial and ventral lung lobes.

Magnetic Resonance Imaging

Dogs with distemper encephalomyelitis can have normal magnetic resonance imaging findings. Hyperintense lesions and loss of contrast between gray and white matter in the cerebellum and/or the brainstem have been described in T2-weighted images, which correspond to demyelination on histopathology.[31] Multifocal T2 and fluid-attenuated inversion recovery (FLAIR) hyperintensities can occur in other locations in the brain, and there may be mild meningeal contrast enhancement.

TABLE 15-1

Complete Blood Count Findings at Admission in 50 Dogs Diagnosed with Distemper at the UC Davis VMTH

Test	Reference Range	Percent below the Reference Range	Percent within the Reference Range	Percent above the Reference Range	Range for Dogs with Distemper
Hematocrit (%)	40-55	80	20	0	17-53
MCV (fL)	65-75	26	72	2	58-80
MCHC (g/dL)	33-36	10	74	16	28-37
Neutrophils (cells/μL)	3000-10,500	12	32	56	16-27,765
Band neutrophils (cells/μL)	0-rare	0	72	28	0-4442
Monocytes (cells/μL)	150-1200	4	62	34	24-5202
Lymphocytes (cells/μL)	1000-4000	54	42	4	110-5575
Eosinophils (cells/μL)	0-1500	0	100	0	0-1114
Platelets (cells/μL)	150,000-400,000	14	66	20	17,000-594,000

Note: Adult reference ranges were used.

TABLE 15-2

Findings on Serum Biochemistry Analysis in 27 Dogs with Distemper at the UC Davis VMTH

Test	Reference Range	Percent below the Reference Range	Percent within the Reference Range	Percent above the Reference Range	Range for Dogs with Distemper	Number of Dogs Tested
Sodium (mmol/L)	145-154	56	40	5	106-158	26
Potassium (mmol/L)	3.6-5.3	12	79	9	2.8-5.9	26
Chloride (mmol/L)	108-118	40	56	5	65-130	26
Bicarbonate (mmol/L)	16-26	0	86	14	16-34	26
Calcium (mg/dL)	9.7-11.5	25	68	7	5.1-12.7	27
Phosphorus (mg/dL)	3.0-6.2	7	50	43	2.6-10.0	27
Creatinine (mg/dL)	0.3-1.2	11	89	0	0-1.2	27
BUN (mg/dL)	5-21	7	91	2	0.6-25	27
Albumin (g/dL)	3.0-4.4	68	32	0	0.9-3.7	27
Globulin (g/dL)	1.8-3.9	7	82	11	1.5-5.3	27
Cholesterol (mg/dL)	135-361	9	86	5	88-385	26
Total bilirubin (mg/dL)	0-0.2	0	80	20	0-0.8	26
ALT (U/L)	19-67	7	75	18	8-389	26
ALP (U/L)	21-170	0	77	23	28-322	26

Note: Adult reference ranges were used by the laboratory.

Microbiologic Tests

Microbiological tests for CDV infection are shown in Table 15-3.

Virus Isolation

CDV can be readily isolated in SLAM transfected Vero cell lines, which show cytopathic effects within 24 hours of inoculation. Isolation is generally used as a research tool rather than for commercial diagnostic purposes. Wild-type virus must be distinguished from vaccine virus in dogs that have been recently vaccinated with attenuated live vaccines.

Cytologic Demonstration of CDV Inclusions

Intracytoplasmic viral inclusions can occasionally be seen in circulating blood cells of affected dogs, especially early in infection (see Figure 15-4, *B*). Inclusions may also be visible in the cytoplasm of conjunctival epithelial cells. Epithelial cells can be scraped from the conjunctiva using a curette after application of a topical ophthalmic local anesthetic preparation. The cells are smeared onto a glass slide, stained with a Romanowsky stain and examined with light microscopy. Unfortunately, this has low sensitivity for diagnosis of distemper.

Immunostaining for CDV Antigen

Direct immunofluorescent antibody (IFA) techniques are often used in practice to detect CDV antigen in a variety of cell types, including conjunctival epithelial cells, leukocytes in a buffy coat smear, urine sediment, or tissues obtained at necropsy. Immunoperoxidase antibody can also be used. Immunostaining is more sensitive than identification of CDV inclusions with routine stains, but false negatives still occur when low quantities of virus are present in the specimen.

Transient false positive results might occur after vaccination with attenuated live vaccines, so the results must be interpreted with caution in recently vaccinated dogs. False positives also have the potential to occur if nonspecific fluorescence is interpreted as a positive result by inexperienced laboratory technicians. Further research is required to understand the prevalence of, and influence of vaccination on false positive direct IFA results for diagnosis of distemper.

Antigen Detection ELISA Assays

ELISA assays that detect CDV antigen in serum (Table 15-3) are available commercially as in-practice kits in some countries. The sensitivity and specificity of these assays has not been well studied, and there are no published reports in the scientific literature of the performance of commercially available assays, only those in the research and development phase. One assay had a low sensitivity in dogs that were naturally infected with distemper, with positive results in only 27% of 26 dogs at initial examination and 12% when the dogs were examined 2 to 3 weeks later.[32] False-positive results occurred for up to 4 weeks after vaccination in 20% of 40 dogs immunized with attenuated live viral vaccines. Another lateral flow (immunochromatography) assay had sensitivity equivalent to that of an RT-PCR assay when applied to conjunctival swab specimens, but sensitivity was 90% and 86% when the assay was applied to blood lymphocytes and nasal swab specimens from dogs with distemper.[33]

Molecular Diagnosis Using the Polymerase Chain Reaction

Reverse transcriptase-PCR (RT-PCR) assays are offered by a number of commercial veterinary diagnostic laboratories for diagnosis of distemper, sometimes as part of a panel that includes assays for other canine respiratory pathogens (see Chapter 17). Most assays detect a portion of the N protein gene. RT-PCR can be performed on whole blood, buffy coat, skin biopsies, conjunctival scrapings, urine, CSF, transtracheal washes, nasal and oropharyngeal swabs, and a variety of other tissues collected at necropsy (e.g., lung, small intestine, stomach, kidney, brain, bladder, lymphoid tissues). In one study of a limited number of experimentally infected dogs, conjunctival swabs were superior to whole blood, nasal flushes, and urine for PCR diagnosis of CDV infection,[34] whereas another study of naturally infected dogs showed highest viral loads in blood, followed by conjunctival swabs, and then urine.[35] RT-PCR is more sensitive than direct IFA, but false positives may be more likely to occur after vaccination with attenuated live virus vaccines, because RT-PCR assays that are currently available for routine diagnostic purposes do not distinguish between vaccine and wild-type strains. Assays have been developed that differentiate between field and vaccine strains of CDV.[36] False-positive test results should not occur after use of *recombinant* CDV vaccines. More research is needed to clarify the influence of vaccination on the results of RT-PCR for distemper. Quantitation of RT-PCR results may ultimately be helpful in differentiating vaccination with attenuated virus vaccines (low viral load) and natural infection (high viral load).

False-negative RT-PCR results can occur if the virus is present in low levels at the site from which specimens are collected. Because RNA is labile, degradation of viral RNA during specimen collection and transport to the laboratory can also lead to false-negative PCR results. In outbreak situations, collection of specimens from multiple dogs (at least 5 to 10) may increase the chance of positive test results.[37] The diagnosis is strengthened when positive PCR assay results are combined with positive results of other assays such as direct IFA.

Serology

Antibodies to CDV can be measured in the laboratory using serum neutralization (SN) assays (see Chapter 2). ELISA assays that detect IgG and IgM are also available for routine diagnosis of distemper in dogs, which have improved sensitivity and specificity over SN.[38] In one study, IgM antibodies appeared 1 week before SN titers.[39] Use of serology for diagnosis of distemper is complicated by the confounding effect of vaccination. This is especially true in shelter environments where all dogs are vaccinated on intake. Nevertheless, a fourfold rise in titer over a 2- to 4-week period supports recent infection. Acute and convalescent sera should be submitted to the same laboratory, because interlaboratory variation in assay results occurs. Ideally, an aliquot of the acute serum specimen should be retested at the same time the convalescent titer is determined. Antibodies within the CSF can be quantified and compared to those in serum to determine whether local production of antibody in the CSF is likely. Dogs with delayed-onset CDV encephalomyelitis have high levels of antibody in the CSF when compared with serum.[40]

The results of serologic tests can be used to assess the need for vaccination, and also to determine which dogs are protected and therefore of low risk for development of disease and to some extent, virus shedding in outbreak situations. Serum neutralization titers of at least 1:16 to 1:20 correlate with protection after vaccination. Titers of 1:100 or more correlate with protection in puppies that have received maternal antibodies.[41] Because of the presence of cell-mediated immunity, negative serologic results do not imply lack of protection. Point-of-care ELISA assays are also available for semiquantitative measurement of antibodies to CDV. One assay (Synbiotics TiterCHEK CDV/CPV) had a sensitivity of 76% and a specificity of 92% compared with SN when performed as a point-of-care assay.[42] The low sensitivity would tend to overestimate the need for vaccination, which is preferable to an assay with low specificity, which might result in unnecessary exposure of a susceptible dog to infected dogs.

Pathologic Findings

Gross Pathologic Findings

In addition to physical examination abnormalities described earlier, gross pathologic findings in canine distemper include thymic atrophy, pulmonary congestion and consolidation, liquid intestinal contents, and lymph node congestion and enlargement. Less common findings are mild pleural, pericardial, and/or peritoneal effusion and, uncommonly, visceral congestion and ecchymotic

TABLE 15-3

Diagnostic Assays Available for Distemper in Dogs

Assay	Specimen Type	Target	Performance
Virus isolation	Conjunctival and nasal swabs, blood, urine, transtracheal wash specimens, necropsy specimens	CDV	False negatives can occur in specimens that contain low numbers of virus particles. Attenuated live vaccine virus may also be isolated. Not widely offered for routine diagnostic purposes.
Direct immunostaining (such as direct fluorescent antibody)	Smears made from conjunctival scrapings, urine sediment, respiratory lavage specimens, impression smears of tissue specimens	CDV antigen	False negatives can occur in specimens that contain low numbers of virus particles. False positives can occur if nonspecific fluorescence is incorrectly interpreted as a positive result. Possibility of false positives after recent vaccination with attenuated live CDV vaccines.
Distemper ELISA antigen assay	See Virus isolation	CDV antigen	Inexpensive and rapid. Sensitivity and specificity in naturally infected dogs have not been well established. False positives can occur for weeks after vaccination with attenuated live CDV vaccines.
RT-PCR	See Virus isolation	CDV RNA	Sensitivity and specificity can vary depending on assay design. Testing specimens from multiple anatomic sites or combining PCR assays with other diagnostic tests for CDV improves sensitivity. Attenuated live vaccine virus may be detected for days to weeks after vaccination. Because of the high sensitivity of some assays, the significance of a positive result in relation to disease may be difficult to interpret. False-negative results can occur when virus levels are low or as a result of degradation of viral nucleic acid during specimen transport.
Serology (IgG and IgM ELISA; SN)	Serum and/or CSF	Antibodies against CDV antigens	Acute and convalescent sera are required for diagnosis of acute distemper, so diagnosis is retrospective. False positives can occur with recent CDV vaccination.
Histopathology	Usually necropsy specimens, but also skin biopsies (such as footpad biopsies)	Eosinophilic intracytoplasmic and intranuclear inclusions; CDV antigen with immunostaining or CDV RNA with in situ hybridization	If available, in situ hybridization may be most sensitive for detection of virus in tissues.

CDV, Canine distemper virus; RT, reverse transcriptase; SN, serum neutralization.

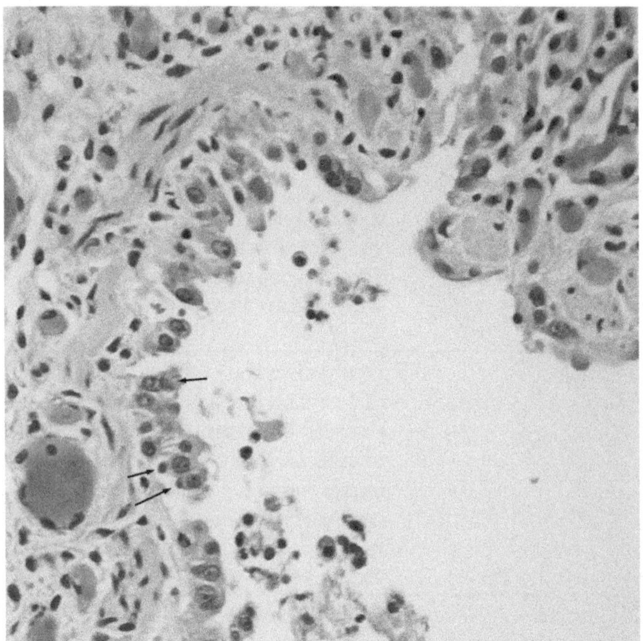

FIGURE 15-8 Bronchial epithelium from a dog infected with CDV. Intracytoplasmic inclusions are abundant *(arrows)*. H&E stain. (Image courtesy Dr. Patricia Pesavento, University of California, Davis Veterinary Anatomic Pathology service.)

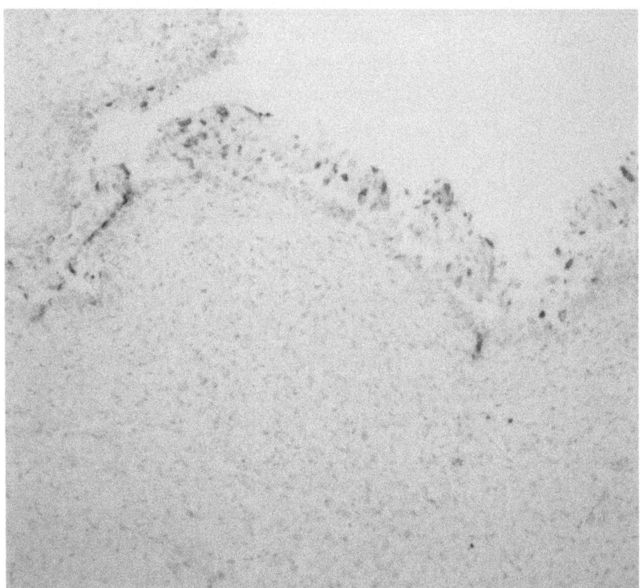

FIGURE 15-9 Immunohistochemistry that shows CDV antigen (brown staining) in bladder transitional epithelial cells from a 2-year-old male neutered Australian cattle dog infected with CDV that had been recently adopted from a shelter and developed cough, ataxia, blindness, and seizures.

hemorrhages and meningeal congestion. In some dogs, gross necropsy abnormalities are minimal. Concurrent external and intestinal parasitic infections may also be identified.

Histopathologic Findings

Histopathologic findings in the brain and spinal cord are variable and depend on the CDV strain, the immune status of the host, the presence of secondary infections, and disease chronicity. Findings in the brain and spinal cord include neuronal necrosis and degeneration, and demyelination with subacute to chronic infection. Multifocal gliosis, astrocytosis, vacuolization, and lymphoplasmacytic perivascular cuffing may be present. The virus has a predilection for white matter of the lateral cerebellar peduncles, the cerebellum, and the dorsolateral medulla adjacent to the fourth ventricle, but lesions can also occur elsewhere, such as the thalamus, midbrain, and pyriform lobes of the cerebral cortex. Less commonly, nonsuppurative meningitis is observed. Infection of the lungs leads to a lymphocytic and histiocytic interstitial pneumonia with proliferation of the alveolar epithelium; neutrophilic bronchopneumonia occurs as a result of secondary bacterial infection. There is often widespread lymphoid depletion and necrosis in all reticuloendothelial tissues (see Figure 15-3), although lymphoid hyperplasia may be observed in dogs with chronic distemper. Epithelial cell necrosis may be noted in the dental ameloblast layer, trachea, and bladder mucosa.

The diagnosis of CDV infection is supported by the identification of eosinophilic intracytoplasmic or intranuclear inclusion bodies, which are 1 to 5 μm in diameter and occur in a variety of cell types, but especially in neurons, astrocytes, microglial cells, conjunctival epithelial cells, bladder epithelium, footpad epithelium, and sometimes lymphocytes (Figure 15-8). Less commonly, syncytia may be identified, such as within the meninges, and lymph nodes. Confirmation of the presence of CDV in tissues can be established with the use of immunostaining, in situ hybridization, or RT-PCR (Figure 15-9).

Treatment and Prognosis

When required, the mainstay of treatment for CDV infection is supportive care. No specific antiviral drug is available for treatment of CDV infection, although ribavirin and 5-ethynyl-1-β-D-ribofuranosylimidazole-4-carboxamide (EICAR) have shown efficacy in vitro[43] and for treatment of measles in a rodent model.[44] The pharmacokinetics and toxicity of these drugs in dogs require further study.

Dogs with mild respiratory or gastrointestinal distemper may recover spontaneously without treatment. Dogs with severe respiratory and gastrointestinal disease may require hospitalization and treatment with IV fluids, antimicrobial drugs for secondary bacterial pneumonia, oxygen supplementation, nebulization, and coupage. Ideally, these dogs should be housed in isolation, although in many veterinary hospitals, isolation may not permit treatment with oxygen and adequate monitoring. Under these circumstances, dogs could be housed under strict barrier precautions where oxygen and critical care can be provided (see Chapter 11). When possible, collection of a transtracheal lavage specimen for culture and susceptibility is recommended for dogs with secondary bacterial pneumonia. When this is not possible, the use of antimicrobial drugs likely to be effective against *Bordetella bronchiseptica* (such as doxycycline) is recommended (see Chapter 38). Dogs with severe bronchopneumonia may require treatment with parenteral broad-spectrum antimicrobial drug combinations, such as ampicillin and a fluoroquinolone. Other supportive treatments include enteral nutrition, artificial tears for dogs with KCS, and antiemetics. Parenteral nutrition should be used only if absolutely necessary, because of the immunosuppression that occurs with CDV infection and possibility of nosocomial infections. Vitamin A supplementation before experimental infection reduced morbidity and mortality associated with CDV infection in ferrets,[45] but its usefulness as a treatment for canine distemper requires further investigation. Administration of daily oral vitamin A for 2 days to children younger than 2 years of age with measles reduces the risk of mortality and pneumonia-specific mortality.[46] Ascorbic acid has also been advocated as a treatment for distemper in dogs, but its efficacy remains unproven.[41]

Owners of dogs with respiratory and gastrointestinal illness should be warned that CNS signs have the potential to develop weeks to even months after apparent recovery. Unfortunately, the development of CNS signs is unpredictable. When neurologic signs occur, they rarely resolve and may be progressive. The prognosis for dogs with severe neurologic signs is poor, but some neurologic signs, such as mild myoclonus, may still be compatible with normal daily activities and do not interfere with quality of life. Euthanasia is recommended for dogs with neurologic signs that are progressive and not compatible with a good quality of life.

A single IV dose of dexamethasone or tapering antiinflammatory doses of glucocorticoids has been advocated to halt or reduce the severity of progressive CNS signs,[41] although controlled prospective studies are required to fully evaluate the usefulness of this treatment in dogs with distemper. Anticonvulsants such as diazepam and, for chronic management, potassium bromide or phenobarbital can be used to treat seizures and prevent the spread of a seizure focus. However, they do not prevent progressive CDV infection of the CNS and are sometimes poorly effective. Mexiletine and procainamide have also been suggested as treatments for distemper myoclonus, but their true efficacy is unreported. To date, the author has had disappointing results using these treatments in a limited number of dogs with persistent distemper myoclonus.

Immunity and Vaccination

Immunity to CDV requires antibodies as well as cell-mediated immunity. Recovery from natural infection provides lifelong immunity. Distemper can be effectively prevented through immunization with attenuated live or recombinant vaccines. Inactivated vaccines do not provide sufficient protection and are not available in the United States. In contrast, proper vaccination with attenuated live vaccines can provide long-lasting (at least 3 to 5 years), sterile immunity.[47] Attenuated live vaccines should be given every 3 to 4 weeks, commencing no earlier than 6 weeks of age. Maternal antibodies are usually absent by 12 to 14 weeks of age, and so the last vaccine should be given no sooner than 14 to 16 weeks of age (consider extension to 16 to 20 weeks in breeding kennels and shelters).[47] Ideally pups should be isolated for at least 7 to 10 days after the last vaccine is administered (see Appendix). For dogs older than 16 weeks of age that are brought to the veterinarian for their first vaccination, two doses of vaccine should be given 3 to 4 weeks apart, although a single dose may provide protection. A booster is recommended at 1 year and then no earlier than every 3 years thereafter.[47] For shelter dogs, vaccination should be performed as soon as possible before entry into the shelter. A single vaccine given even hours before entry can provide protection from severe disease.[48] Infection can still occur, but disease severity is lessened.

Although generally safe and effective when used according to label recommendations, attenuated live CDV vaccine virus can cause encephalitis when administered to immunocompromised dogs and puppies less than 6 weeks of age, and severe disease can occur in susceptible species such as ferrets and certain wildlife species. Administration of attenuated live CDV vaccines to dams immediately after whelping has been associated with the development of encephalitis in the puppies, and it was suggested that vaccine virus shed by the dam may cause disease in the pups.[49] Postvaccinal encephalitis usually occurs 3 to 20 days after vaccination and has been associated with certain batches of vaccines that contain the Rockborn strain.[50] Neurologic signs such as ataxia may be reversible in some dogs. Seizures may be progressive and irreversible. Some distemper vaccines available on the market still contain the Rockborn strain, and Rockborn-like viruses have been isolated from dogs with distemper, which may represent residual virulence of vaccine virus or circulation of vaccine-derived Rockborn-like viruses in the dog population.[51] Attenuated live CDV vaccines have been incriminated as a cause of hypertrophic osteodystrophy, especially in young Weimaraner dogs,[41,52] but there is a paucity of published evidence that supports the association (see Chapter 12).

A canarypox-vectored recombinant vaccine that expresses the H and F glycoproteins of CDV is also available for prevention of canine distemper (Merial Limited). This vaccine induces a 3-year duration of immunity, protects dogs from severe disease when administered hours before shelter admission, can protect puppies from virulent CDV infection in the face of maternal antibody, and can be used in pregnant bitches and puppies as young as 4 weeks of age in the face of an outbreak or in heavily contaminated environments.[48,53] The recombinant vaccine has replaced the use of canine measles vaccines, which were previously used to overcome maternal antibody in the face of distemper outbreaks. Whether the recombinant vaccine overcomes maternal antibody that is directed against the canarypox vector vaccine virus as effectively as it overcomes maternal antibody against the attenuated CDV vaccine virus requires further evaluation. Further study of the relative efficacy of the recombinant and attenuated live vaccines in heavily contaminated environments such as shelters is also required. The canarypox vectored recombinant vaccine is also the vaccine of choice for ferrets, and a specific ferret vaccine is available at the time of writing (Purevax Ferret Distemper, Merial Limited).

Vaccine strains of CDV, such as Onderstepoort, Snyder Hill, and Lederle, belong to the America-1 lineage, but field strains that circulate in North America belong primarily to the America-2 lineage. Concern has been raised that these vaccines may not adequately protect against infection with field strains, but cross-neutralization studies suggest that antigenic differences are not sufficient to warrant changes in the current vaccines. The development of distemper in vaccinated dogs may reflect failure of vaccine efficacy as a result of the improper administration of vaccines, improperly timed vaccination series, or the use of vaccines that have been stored and handled inappropriately. The last is especially important for CDV vaccines because attenuated live vaccine virus is so labile. Vaccines should be stored in a refrigerator that maintains an internal temperature of 0°C to 4°C and reconstituted with the proper diluent immediately (within 1 hour) before administration. It has been recommended that vaccine held for longer than 1 hour after reconstitution be discarded.[47] A second dose should be given if some of the vaccine is found on the haircoat after administration.

Prevention

Properly timed vaccination is the key to prevention of CDV infection. Puppies with declining maternal antibody titers should be kept away from other dogs until the vaccination series is complete. In shelter situations, dogs with signs of respiratory or gastrointestinal disease should be held well away from other dogs (at least 25 feet has been suggested[37]) and handled only after apparently healthy dogs have been cared for. Puppies should always be separated from adult dogs using equipment designated only for that area, and overcrowding should be prevented. Quarantine for CDV is difficult because the incubation period for development of neurologic signs may be as long as 6 weeks. Wildlife species such as raccoons can also shed CDV and were suspected as a source of infection in an outbreak that occurred in a Chicago shelter, when raccoons and dogs were co-transported in the back of a vehicle.[37] Routine cleaning and disinfection of contaminated surfaces readily eliminates virus in the environment. Proper nutrition may also help to prevent disease due to CDV. Isolated vitamin A deficiency is a major risk factor for severe measles and death in humans and distemper in ferrets. Retinoids interfere with replication of measles virus in vitro through a type I IFN-dependent mechanism.[54] The impact of nutritional status on disease due to CDV requires further investigation.

Public Health Aspects

In general, CDV is not believed to infect human cells or cause disease in people. However, both CDV and measles virus have played a controversial role in Paget's disease of bone, a common skeletal disorder characterized by focal abnormalities of increased bone turnover, which is associated with bone pain, deformity, and pathologic fractures.[55] Paget's disease most often occurs in the elderly, men are more likely to be affected than women, and the overall prevalence of the disease has decreased in many geographic locations.[56] Genetic factors clearly play a role in the disease, but in some studies, the RNA of paramyxoviruses that include CDV has been detected within lesions.[57] Other studies have failed to detect the nucleic acid of CDV in lesions, and contamination has been suggested as a reason for positive test results.[55] However, CDV has been shown to infect and replicate in human osteoclast precursors, further raising concern about the possibility of zoonotic transmission of CDV.[58]

CASE EXAMPLE

Signalment: "Molly", a 1.5-year-old female spayed golden retriever from Sacramento, CA

History: Molly was evaluated for a 1-month-long history of abnormal behavior that included stumbling, failure to catch balls, and loss of interest in activity. She also had a 1-year history of seizures, which were thought to be due to idiopathic epilepsy and which were treated with phenobarbital (4 mg/kg PO q12h) and potassium bromide (17 mg/kg PO q12h). This was associated with a decrease in seizure frequency. Two weeks after the onset of abnormal behavior, Molly was taken to a local veterinary clinic. A serum phenobarbital level at that time was 50 µg/mL (therapeutic range, 10 to 40 µg/mL). The phenobarbital dose was decreased (1.4 mg/kg PO q24h), but Molly began circling to the left, head pressing, pacing, and vocalizing. She also stopped responding to the owners when they called her name, and two episodes of vomiting were noted. In the week before evaluation, Molly refused to eat dry food, but ate canned dog food. Her thirst had decreased and she was voluntarily urinating in the house. A serum phenobarbital level was repeated 2 days before she was evaluated and was 13 µg/mL. Molly had been immunized regularly (CDV, CPV, CAV-2, and parainfluenza) and received monthly flea, tick, and heartworm prophylaxis.

Current medications: Phenobarbital (1.4 mg/kg PO q24h); potassium bromide (17 mg/kg PO q12h).

Physical Examination:

Body weight: 23.2 kg

General: Obtunded but hydrated. T = 101.7°F (38.7°C), HR = 60 beats/min, RR = 36 breaths/min, mucous membranes pink, CRT = 1 sec.

Integument, eyes, ears, nose and throat: No clinically significant abnormalities were identified. A full ophthalmologic examination was also unremarkable.

Musculoskeletal: Body condition score was 5/9. Molly was ambulatory on all four limbs.

Cardiovascular, respiratory, gastrointestinal, and urogenital systems: No clinically significant findings were identified. All peripheral lymph nodes were normal sized. Average systolic blood pressure (10 measurements) was 120 mm Hg.

Neurologic Examination:

Mentation: Obtunded and not responsive to verbal and most tactile stimuli; head pressing.

Gait/Posture: Compulsive circling and leaning to the left was present.

Cranial nerves: No clinically significant abnormalities were identified.

Postural reactions: Placing reactions were absent in the left thoracic and left and right pelvic limbs.

Segmental reflexes: Diminished biceps and withdrawal reflexes were present, left thoracic limb only.

Panniculus: No abnormalities detected.

Spinal palpation: Pain was elicited in several regions along the spine. Resisted cervical ventroflexion.

Neuroanatomic localization: Diffuse cerebral or thalamic disease; C6 to T2 myelopathy.

Laboratory Findings:

CBC:

HCT 37.9% (40-55%)
MCV 68 fL (65-75 fL)
MCHC 35.4 g/dL (33-36 g/dL)
WBC 7510 cells/µL (6000-13,000 cells/µL)
Neutrophils 4859 cells/µL (3000-10,500 cells/µL)
Lymphocytes 2155 cells/µL (1000-4000 cells/µL)
Monocytes 338 cells/µL (150-1200 cells/µL)
427,000 platelets/µL (150,000-400,000 platelets/µL).

Serum Chemistry Profile:

Sodium 141 mmol/L (145-154 mmol/L)
Potassium 4.4 mmol/L (4.1-5.3 mmol/L)
Chloride 109 mmol/L (105-116 mmol/L)
Bicarbonate 21 mmol/L (16-26 mmol/L)
Phosphorus 3.9 mg/dL (3.0-6.2 mg/dL)
Calcium 12.2 mg/dL (9.9-11.4 mg/dl)
BUN 6 mg/dL (8-31 mg/dL)

Creatinine 0.6 mg/dL (0.5-1.6 mg/dL)
Glucose 109 mg/dL (70-118 mg/dL)
Total protein 6.1 g/dL (5.4-7.4 g/dL)
Albumin 2.7 g/dL (2.9-4.2 g/dL)
Globulin 3.4 g/dL (2.3-4.4 g/dL)
ALT 132 U/L (19-67 U/L)
AST 62 U/L (21-54 U/L)
ALP 155 U/L (15-127 U/L)
Creatine kinase 399 U/L (46-320 U/L)
Gamma GT 10 U/L (0-6 U/L)
Cholesterol 291 mg/dL (135-345 mg/dL)
Total bilirubin 0.2 mg/dL (0-0.4 mg/dL).

Serum ionized calcium: 1.39 mmol/L

Urinalysis: SGr 1.014; pH 7.0, few amorphous crystals. No other abnormalities detected.

Serum bromide concentration: 1.1 mg/mL (therapeutic range, 1.0 to 2.0 mg/mL)

Serum phenobarbital concentration: 1.4 μg/mL (therapeutic range, 15 to 40 μg/mL)

Serum bile acids: Pre-meal, 14 μmol/L (reference range, 0-12 μmol/L); post-meal, 16 μmol/L (reference range, 0-16 μmol/L)

Imaging Findings:

Thoracic radiographs: No clinically significant abnormalities were present.

Spinal radiographs: Disc space narrowing was present between the sixth and seventh cervical vertebrae and to a greater extent between the seventh cervical and first thoracic vertebrae.

Abdominal ultrasound: No significant lesions were identified.

Magnetic resonance imaging: Precontrast: Multiple small regions of hyperintensity were noted on dual echo and FLAIR sequences, one of which was in the left thalamus along the third ventricle and another diffusely along the lateral aspect of the right thalamus. There was a linear region of hyperintensity along the right parietal and temporal lobes. On T1-weighted postcontrast images, a small focus of contrast enhancement was noted in the ventral aspect of the right thalamus in the region of hyperintensity on the precontrast fluid-weighted sequences. Impressions: Multifocal, relatively non–contrast-enhancing lesions in the cerebrum and thalamus suggestive of cerebral edema, encephalitis, or small infarcts.

Electroencephalography: No abnormalities were detected.

CSF Analysis:

	Lumbar	Cisternal
Protein (mg/dL)	31	21
Total RBC (cells/μL)	111	2
Total nucleated cells (cells/μL)	1	3
Neutrophils (%)	0	0
Small mononuclear cells (%)	92	80
Large mononuclear cells (%)	8	20
Microscopic evaluation	Mild to moderate lymphocytic reactivity	Marginal mononuclear (lymphocytic) pleocytosis

Treatment and Outcome: Molly was hospitalized for a week during the diagnostic work-up and treated with intravenous fluids and potassium bromide (35 mg/kg PO q12h). She became progressively more obtunded and showed additional neurologic signs of circling to the right and positional horizontal nystagmus with a fast phase to the right. The narrowed disc spaces were thought to represent intervertebral disc disease, and granulomatous meningoencephalitis was suspected. Potassium bromide was discontinued, and treatment with phenobarbital (5 mg/kg PO q12h) reinstituted. Dexamethasone was administered (0.2 mg/kg, IV q24h), but there was minimal improvement, and euthanasia was elected.

Necropsy Findings:

- Brain, cerebrum: severe, generalized, chronic neuronal loss, axonal necrosis, and myelin degeneration with abundant eosinophilic inclusion bodies and canine distemper antigen (immunohistochemistry)
- Brain and spinal cord (C1 to T7), corticospinal tracts: severe, diffuse axonal necrosis and myelin degeneration
- Brain, cerebrum, and meninges: generalized, lymphoplasmacytic, perivascular cuffing
- Tonsil, lymph nodes (mandibular, mesenteric, thoracic): mild, multifocal lympholysis with intranuclear and intracytoplasmic eosinophilic inclusion bodies and canine distemper antigen

Diagnosis: Chronic distemper encephalitis with demyelination ("old dog encephalitis")

Comments: Distemper was not suspected in this dog because of the dog's older age and history of vaccination. Initial infection may have occurred before vaccination was complete, vaccination may have been improperly performed, or the dog may have been a vaccine nonresponder, which is believed to occur rarely. The previous diagnosis of epilepsy further complicated the identification of distemper as an underlying cause. This case example highlights the importance of including distemper on the differential diagnosis list for young adult dogs with neurologic signs, because of the chronic course of disease that can occasionally occur. Additional laboratory tests that might or might not have been helpful for diagnosis of distemper in this dog include comparison of serum antibody titers to CDV in the CSF and serum, and RT-PCR for CDV on CSF. Neurologic signs were progressive in this dog and largely unresponsive to anticonvulsant drugs, and so the prognosis was extremely poor.

SUGGESTED READINGS

Beineke A, Puff C, Seehusen F, et al. Pathogenesis and immunopathology of systemic and nervous canine distemper. Vet Immunol Immunopathol. 2009;127:1-18.

Newbury S, Larson LJ, Schultz RD. Canine distemper virus. In: Miller L, Hurley K, eds. Infectious disease management in animal shelters. Ames, IA: Wiley-Blackwell; 2009:161-172.

REFERENCES

1. Gamiz C, Martella V, Ulloa R, et al. Identification of a new genotype of canine distemper virus circulating in America. Vet Res Commun. 2011;35:381-390.
2. Panzera Y, Gallo Calderón M, Sarute N, et al. Evidence of two co-circulating genetic lineages of canine distemper virus in South America. Virus Res. 2012;163:401-404.
3. Kapil S, Allison RW, Johnston 3rd L, et al. Canine distemper virus strains circulating among North American dogs. Clin Vaccine Immunol. 2008;15:707-712.
4. Amude AM, Alfieri AA, Alfieri AF. Clinicopathological findings in dogs with distemper encephalomyelitis presented without characteristic signs of the disease. Res Vet Sci. 2007;82:416-422.
5. Blixenkrone-Moller M, Svansson V, Have P, et al. Studies on manifestations of canine distemper virus infection in an urban dog population. Vet Microbiol. 1993;37:163-173.
6. Richards TR, Whelan NC, Pinard CL, et al. Optic neuritis caused by canine distemper virus in a Jack Russell terrier. Can Vet J. 2011;52:398-402.
7. Yanagi Y, Takeda M, Ohno S. Measles virus: cellular receptors, tropism and pathogenesis. J Gen Virol. 2006;87:2767-2779.
8. Beineke A, Puff C, Seehusen F, et al. Pathogenesis and immunopathology of systemic and nervous canine distemper. Vet Immunol Immunopathol. 2009;127:1-18.
9. von Messling V, Milosevic D, Cattaneo R. Tropism illuminated: lymphocyte-based pathways blazed by lethal morbillivirus through the host immune system. Proc Natl Acad Sci U S A. 2004;101:14216-14221.
10. von Messling V, Svitek N, Cattaneo R. Receptor (SLAM [CD150]) recognition and the V protein sustain swift lymphocyte-based invasion of mucosal tissue and lymphatic organs by a morbillivirus. J Virol. 2006;80:6084-6092.
11. Pratakpiriya W, Seki F, Otsuki N, et al. Nectin4 is an epithelial cell receptor for canine distemper virus involved in neurovirulence. J Virol. 2012;86:10207-10210.
12. Appel MJ. Pathogenesis of canine distemper. Am J Vet Res. 1969;30:1167-1182.
13. Pearce-Kelling S, Mitchell WJ, Summers BA, et al. Virulent and attenuated canine distemper virus infects multiple dog brain cell types in vitro. Glia. 1991;4:408-416.
14. Rudd PA, Bastien-Hamel LE, von Messling V. Acute canine distemper encephalitis is associated with rapid neuronal loss and local immune activation. J Gen Virol. 2010;91:980-989.
15. Summers BA, Appel MJ. Aspects of canine distemper virus and measles virus encephalomyelitis. Neuropathol Appl Neurobiol. 1994;20:525-534.
16. Headley SA, Amude AM, Alfieri AF, et al. Molecular detection of canine distemper virus and the immunohistochemical characterization of the neurologic lesions in naturally occurring old dog encephalitis. J Vet Diagn Invest. 2009;21:588-597.
17. Wyss-Fluehmann G, Zurbriggen A, Vandevelde M, et al. Canine distemper virus persistence in demyelinating encephalitis by swift intracellular cell-to-cell spread in astrocytes is controlled by the viral attachment protein. Acta Neuropathol. 2010;119:617-630.
18. de Almeida DE, Roveratti C, Brito FL, et al. Conjunctival effects of canine distemper virus–induced keratoconjunctivitis sicca. Vet Ophthalmol. 2009;12:211-215.
19. Bittegeko SB, Arnbjerg J, Nkya R, et al. Multiple dental developmental abnormalities following canine distemper infection. J Am Anim Hosp Assoc. 1995;31:42-45.
20. Boutoille FF, Hennet PR. Diagnostic imaging in veterinary dental practice. Enamel hypoplasia. J Am Vet Med Assoc. 2011;238:1251-1253.
21. Schobesberger M, Summerfield A, Doherr MG, et al. Canine distemper virus–induced depletion of uninfected lymphocytes is associated with apoptosis. Vet Immunol Immunopathol. 2005;104:33-44.
22. Kerdiles YM, Cherif B, Marie JC, et al. Immunomodulatory properties of morbillivirus nucleoproteins. Viral Immunol. 2006;19:324-334.
23. Ehrensperger F, Pospischil A. Spontaneous mixed infections with distemper virus and *Toxoplasma* in dogs. Dtsch Tierarztl Wochenschr. 1989;96:184-186.
24. Smith HW, Buxton A. Incidence of salmonellae in faces of dogs suffering from distemper. Nature. 1950;166:824.
25. Fawi MT. Tag el Din MH, el-Sanousi SM. Canine distemper as a predisposing factor for *Nocardia asteroides* infection in the dog. Vet Rec. 1971;88:326-328.
26. Ribeiro MG, Salerno T, Mattos-Guaraldi AL, et al. Nocardiosis: an overview and additional report of 28 cases in cattle and dogs. Rev Inst Med Trop Sao Paulo. 2008;50:177-185.
27. Dyer NW, Schamber GJ. Pneumocystosis associated with canine distemper virus infection in a mink. Can Vet J. 1999;40:577-578.
28. Lemberger KY, Gondim LF, Pessier AP, et al. *Neospora caninum* infection in a free-ranging raccoon (*Procyon lotor*) with concurrent canine distemper virus infection. J Parasitol. 2005;91:960-961.
29. Baumgartner W, Boyce RW, Alldinger S, et al. Metaphyseal bone lesions in young dogs with systemic canine distemper virus infection. Vet Microbiol. 1995;44:201-209.
30. Mee AP, Gordon MT, May C, et al. Canine distemper virus transcripts detected in the bone cells of dogs with metaphyseal osteopathy. Bone. 1993;14:59-67.
31. Bathen-Noethen A, Stein VM, Puff C, et al. Magnetic resonance imaging findings in acute canine distemper virus infection. J Small Anim Pract. 2008;49:460-467.
32. Soma T, Ishii H, Hara M, et al. Detection of canine distemper virus antigen in canine serum and its application to diagnosis. Vet Rec. 2003;153:499-501.
33. An DJ, Kim TY, Song DS, et al. An immunochromatography assay for rapid antemortem diagnosis of dogs suspected to have canine distemper. J Virol Methods. 2008;147:244-249.
34. Kim D, Jeoung SY, Ahn SJ, et al. Comparison of tissue and fluid samples for the early detection of canine distemper virus in experimentally infected dogs. J Vet Med Sci. 2006;68:877-879.
35. Elia G, Decaro N, Martella V, et al. Detection of canine distemper virus in dogs by real-time RT-PCR. J Virol Methods. 2006;136:171-176.
36. Si W, Zhou S, Wang Z, et al. A multiplex reverse transcription-nested polymerase chain reaction for detection and differentiation of wild-type and vaccine strains of canine distemper virus. Virol J. 2010;7:86.
37. Newbury S, Larson LJ, Schultz RD. Canine distemper virus. In: Miller L, Hurley K, eds. Infectious disease management in animal shelters. Ames, IA: Wiley-Blackwell; 2009:161-172.
38. von Messling V, Harder TC, Moennig V, et al. Rapid and sensitive detection of immunoglobulin M (IgM) and IgG antibodies against canine distemper virus by a new recombinant nucleocapsid protein-based enzyme-linked immunosorbent assay. J Clin Microbiol. 1999;37:1049-1056.
39. Noon KF, Rogul M, Binn LN, et al. Enzyme-linked immunosorbent assay for evaluation of antibody to canine distemper virus. Am J Vet Res. 1980;41:605-609.
40. Johnson GC, Fenner WR, Krakowka S. Production of immunoglobulin G and increased antiviral antibody in cerebrospinal fluid of dogs with delayed-onset canine distemper viral encephalitis. J Neuroimmunol. 1988;17:237-251.

41. Greene CE, Appel MJ. Canine distemper. In: Greene CE, ed. Infectious diseases of the dog and cat. 3rd ed. St. Louis, MO: Saunders Elsevier; 2006:25-41.
42. Litster AL, Pressler B, Volpe A, et al. Accuracy of a point-of-care ELISA test kit for predicting the presence of protective canine parvovirus and canine distemper virus antibody concentrations in dogs. Vet J. 2012;193:363-366.
43. Dal Pozzo F, Galligioni V, Vaccari F, et al. Antiviral efficacy of EICAR against canine distemper virus (CDV) in vitro. Res Vet Sci. 2010;88:339-344.
44. Wyde PR, Moore-Poveda DK, De Clercq E, et al. Use of cotton rats to evaluate the efficacy of antivirals in treatment of measles virus infections. Antimicrob Agents Chemother. 2000;44:1146-1152.
45. Rodeheffer C, von Messling V, Milot S, et al. Disease manifestations of canine distemper virus infection in ferrets are modulated by vitamin A status. J Nutr. 2007;137:1916-1922.
46. Huiming Y, Chaomin W, Meng M. Vitamin A for treating measles in children. Cochrane Database Syst Rev. 2005:CD001479.
47. Welborn LV, DeVries JG, Ford R, et al. 2011 AAHA canine vaccination guidelines. J Am Anim Hosp Assoc. 2011;47:1-42.
48. Larson LJ, Schultz RD. Effect of vaccination with recombinant canine distemper virus vaccine immediately before exposure under shelter-like conditions. Vet Ther. 2006;7:113-118.
49. McCandlish IA, Cornwell HJ, Thompson H, et al. Distemper encephalitis in pups after vaccination of the dam. Vet Rec. 1992;130:27-30.
50. Cornwell HJ, Thompson H, McCandlish IA, et al. Encephalitis in dogs associated with a batch of canine distemper (Rockborn) vaccine. Vet Rec. 1988;122:54-59.
51. Martella V, Blixenkrone-Moller M, Elia G, et al. Lights and shades on an historical vaccine canine distemper virus, the Rockborn strain. Vaccine. 2011;29:1222-1227.
52. Harrus S, Waner T, Aizenberg, et al. Development of hypertrophic osteodystrophy and antibody response in a litter of vaccinated Weimaraner puppies. J Small Anim Pract. 2002;43:27-31.
53. Larson LJ, Schultz RD. Three-year duration of immunity in dogs vaccinated with a canarypox-vectored recombinant canine distemper virus vaccine. Vet Ther. 2007;8:101-106.
54. Trottier C, Colombo M, Mann KK, et al. Retinoids inhibit measles virus through a type I IFN-dependent bystander effect. FASEB J. 2009;23:3203-3212.
55. Ralston SH, Afzal MA, Helfrich MH, et al. Multicenter blinded analysis of RT-PCR detection methods for paramyxoviruses in relation to Paget's disease of bone. J Bone Miner Res. 2007;22:569-577.
56. Cooper C, Harvey NC, Dennison EM, et al. Update on the epidemiology of Paget's disease of bone. J Bone Miner Res. 2006;21(suppl 2):P3-P8.
57. Mee AP, Dixon JA, Hoyland JA, et al. Detection of canine distemper virus in 100% of Paget's disease samples by in situ-reverse transcriptase-polymerase chain reaction. Bone. 1998;23:171-175.
58. Selby PL, Davies M, Mee AP. Canine distemper virus induces humanosteoclastogenesisthroughNF-kappaBandsequestosome1/P62 activation. J Bone Miner Res. 2006;21:1750-1756.

CHAPTER 16

Canine Herpesvirus Infection

Autumn P. Davidson

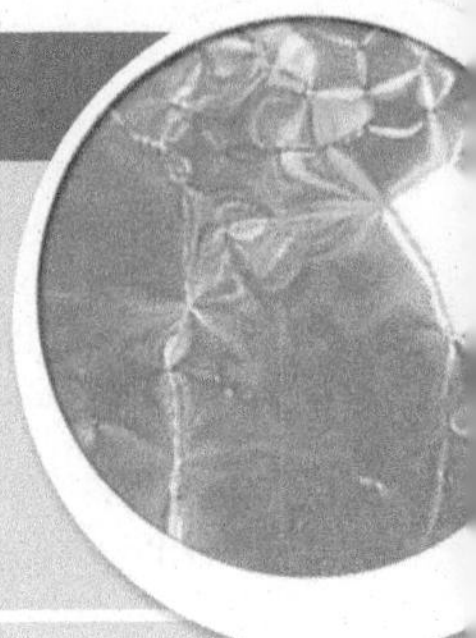

Overview of Canine Herpesvirus Infection

First Described: New York State, United States, 1965[1]

Cause: Canine herpesvirus-1 (Family Herpesviridae)

Affected Hosts: Domestic and wild Canidae

Geographic Distribution: Worldwide

Mode of Transmission: Direct oronasal contact with infected secretions, transplacental transmission

Major Clinical Signs: Abortion in bitches; upper respiratory disease and keratitis in adult dogs; in neonates, inappetence, failure to thrive, vocalization, tachypnea, diarrhea, neurologic signs, abdominal pain, nasal discharge, weight loss, mucosal petechiation, death

Differential Diagnoses: Bacterial sepsis, infections with other viruses such as canine distemper virus and canine parvovirus

Human Health Significance: Canine herpesvirus-1 does not infect humans.

Etiology and Epidemiology

Canine herpesvirus (CHV-1) is an enveloped virus that belongs to the family Herpesviridae (Figure 16-1). It has been reported from the United States, Canada, Australia, Japan, England, and Germany. CHV-1 was first recognized in the mid-1960s in association with a fatal disease in puppies.[2] The virus is commonly blamed for acute neonatal puppy death or failure to thrive, sometimes termed the "fading puppy syndrome." When confirmed as a cause of disease, untreated CHV-1 infection in neonates can cause high (up to 100%) mortality among littermates. The virus is temperature sensitive and prefers to replicate at temperatures less than 37°C. It is not stable in the environment and is readily inactivated by disinfectants. As with other herpesviral infections, recovery from disease is associated with lifelong latent infection of the neural ganglia, with periodic reactivation of shedding in association with stress or immunosuppression, such as that which results from overcrowding and pregnancy. CHV-1 infection has not been reported in cats.

Clinical Features

Signs and Their Pathogenesis

Transmission of CHV-1 can occur subsequent to close contact with infectious vaginal fluids during whelping or with vulvar or oronasal secretions in the postpartum period. Exposure of a naïve bitch to CHV-1 during the last 3 weeks of gestation results either in late-term abortion of a litter or neonatal death within the first few weeks of life, because inadequate periparturient maternal antibodies exist to allow passive immunity to be acquired by the neonates. Puppies born to a naïve bitch may also become infected as a result of contact with other dogs that shed the organism. The incubation period of CHV-1 disease is 6 to 10 days. The virus replicates in the epithelial cells of the oronasal and pharyngeal mucosa, the genital tract, and the regional lymphatics. Replication and spread of the virus is facilitated by the presence of a low body temperature (<38°C or 100°F), which is normal for canine neonates.

Older (>3 to 5 weeks of age) puppies that are exposed to CHV-1 may develop subclinical infection, or the course of disease is less severe, as a result of their ability to mount a febrile response. Latent infection also may develop. Concerns have been raised about latency and the possibility of late development of neurologic signs.[3]

Clinical signs are more likely to occur in animals that are hypothermic or immunosuppressed. Signs in the neonate are not specific and include incessant vocalization, anorexia (with poor weight gain), dyspnea, abdominal pain, incoordination, diarrhea, serous to hemorrhagic nasal discharge, and petechiation of the mucous membranes. The mortality rate in litters infected in utero or during birth can approach 100%, with deaths occurring during the first few days to a week of life. Exposed, surviving older neonates may develop a late onset of central nervous signs including blindness, ataxia, and deafness; apparent complete recovery has also been reported.

The recently infected brood bitch generally shows no clinical signs. Healthy adult dogs of either gender can develop mild upper respiratory signs (sneezing, serous oculonasal discharge, keratitis) for a few days but are otherwise usually clinically unaffected.[4-6] Additional information on respiratory and ocular disease caused by CHV-1 can be found in Chapter 17.

Diagnosis

Antemortem diagnosis of CHV-1 infection in neonates can be challenging. Necropsy of a deceased littermate is usually required.

Virus Isolation and Molecular Diagnosis Using the Polymerase Chain Reaction

Tissues obtained at necropsy can be submitted for virus isolation or molecular diagnosis using the PCR. Diagnosis by virus isolation takes days. CHV-1–specific PCR assays can also confirm infection, in a more timely fashion. Clinicians should confirm the availability and turnaround time of commercially available diagnostic tests when attempting to investigate a possible outbreak of CHV-1 infection in puppies.[7-9]

Pathologic Findings

Gross Pathologic Findings

Gross changes in the kidneys at necropsy of pups infected with CHV-1 include multifocal petechial to ecchymotic subcapsular hemorrhages (Figure 16-2). The pleural surfaces may be mottled pink and red due to coagulation necrosis (Figure 16-2, *B*). Multifocal random acute necrosis of other organs, including the liver, pancreas, intestine and adrenal glands, may also be apparent. Lesions may resemble those of bacterial sepsis.

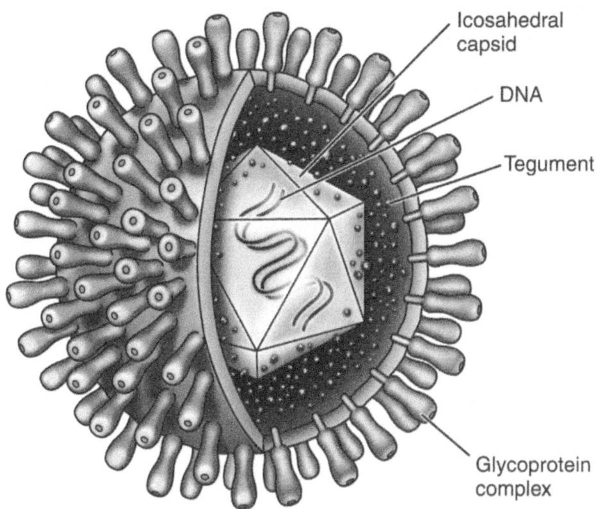

FIGURE 16-1 Structure of a herpesvirus. Herpesviruses are large, enveloped DNA viruses. The DNA is contained within an icosahedral capsid.

Histopathologic Findings

Histopathology can be used to confirm CHV-1 infection but may be unrewarding in the clinical scenario unless very timely. Characteristic viral intranuclear inclusion bodies can be difficult to find. Histopathologic evaluation commonly reveals severe nephrosis (proximal renal tubular epithelial necrosis and renal pelvic epithelial apoptosis with swollen vesicular nuclei); diffuse severe hepatic congestion and inflammation with vacuolar hepatopathy (neutrophilic, histiocytic, and lymphocytic infiltration with apoptosis); acute severe necrotizing bronchointerstitial pneumonia with pulmonary edema and hemorrhage (terminal bronchiolar hemorrhage and edema with fibrin accumulation, macrophage infiltration, necrosis, and alveolar disruption); and thymic, lymph node, and splenic lympholysis (severe diffuse cortical lympholysis with sinus congestion).

Treatment

Treatment of puppies with CHV-1 infection is unrewarding and rarely effective, and residual cardiac and neurologic damage can occur in recovered animals. Treatment with immune serum from seroconverted dams is typically ineffective in sick puppies, and warming also has little effect.

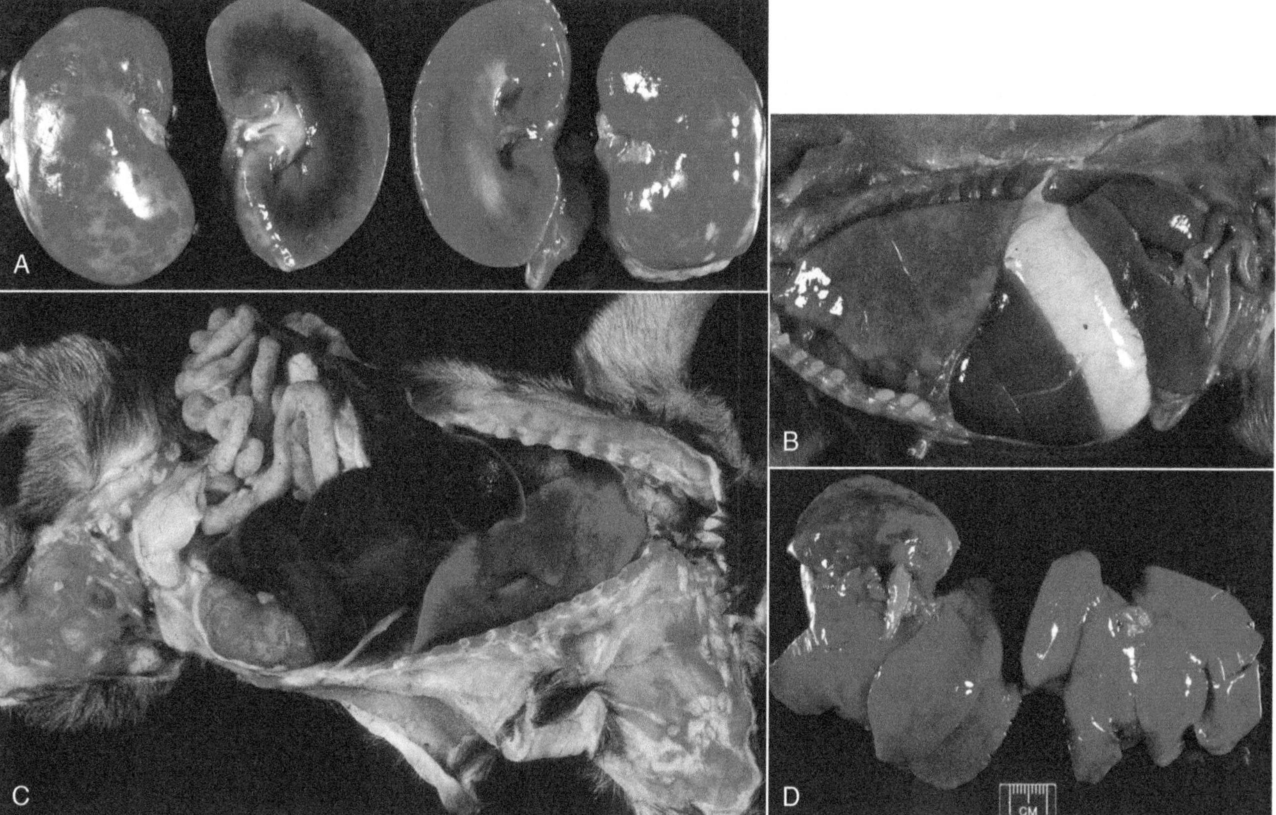

FIGURE 16-2 **A,** Kidneys from 12-day-old mastiff puppy from a litter of 17 puppies, 14 of which died. CHV-1 was isolated from the puppy. Gross changes include subcapsular hemorrhagic foci typical of (but not pathognomonic for) herpetic nephritis. On cut section, white and red cortical streaks are evident; a hemorrhagic medulla is evident. **B,** Multifocal pink and red pleural mottling in the puppy described in **A**. Serosanguineous pleural fluid was present. Histopathology identified multiple areas of pulmonary necrosis and bronchopneumonia. **C,** Small-intestinal serosal petechiation in the same puppy. Histopathology identified enterocyte necrosis consistent with CHV-1 infection. **D,** Liver of the same puppy showing uniform firmness and diffuse mottle with rounded edges. Histopathology identified scattered multiple foci of acute hepatic coagulation necrosis; eosinophilic intranuclear inclusions typical of herpes viral inclusions were seen within viable hepatocytes. (Images courtesy JR Peauroi.)

An incompletely developed immune system and inadequate thermoregulation during the first days of life means neonates are vulnerable to systemic infection (by both bacterial and viral pathogens). The umbilicus of neonates should be treated with tincture of iodine immediately after birth to reduce contamination and prevent bacterial ascent into the peritoneal cavity (omphalitis-peritonitis). Neonatal bacterial peritonitis with bacteremia can cause rapid neonatal death if not recognized and treated promptly (see Figure 34-1). Factors that predispose puppies to bacteremia and sepsis include endometritis in the bitch, a prolonged delivery/dystocia, feeding of replacement formulas, the use of ampicillin, stress, low birth weight (<350 g), and chilling with body temperatures less than 35.5°C or 95°F. Bacterial organisms most frequently associated with bacteremia are *Escherichia coli*, streptococci, staphylococci, and *Klebsiella* spp. Commonly, a decrease in weight gain, failure to suckle, hematuria, persistent diarrhea, unusual vocalization, abdominal distention and pain, and sloughing of the extremities indicate sepsis may be present. These signs are similar to those encountered with CHV-1 infection. Prompt therapy with broad-spectrum, bactericidal antibiotics; optimal nutrition via supported nursing, tube feeding, or bottle feeding; maintenance of body temperature; and appropriate fluid replacement are indicated. The third-generation cephalosporin ceftiofur sodium is an appropriate choice for treatment of neonatal sepsis, because it alters normal intestinal flora minimally and is usually active against the causative organisms.

Failure of neonatal sepsis to respond to antibacterial drug treatment should prompt consideration of CHV-1 infection. Specific antiviral therapy, if instituted in a timely manner, may reduce mortality from CHV-1. Acyclovir has activity against herpes simplex virus (see Chapter 7). Its use in veterinary medicine is not well established, and it should be used with caution and only in situations where indicated. The safety and effectiveness in humans less than 2 weeks of age is not established. The dose (20 mg/kg PO q6h for 5 days) is extrapolated from that for humans.[10] The efficacy of famciclovir for treatment of CHV-1 infection requires study, but the pharmacokinetics of famciclovir in dogs resembles that in humans,[11] so much lower doses may be required when compared with cats.

Immunity, Vaccination, and Prevention

Minimal transplacental transfer of immunity occurs in the dog. Adequate ingestion of colostrum must occur promptly postpartum for puppies to acquire passive immunity. The transmission of protective passive immunity (placental or colostral antibodies) between a bitch and her puppies depends on the prior existence of adequate serum maternal antibodies. Therefore, breeding bitches with exposure to CHV-1 earlier in life have the best opportunity to seroconvert and develop protective antibodies. This commonly occurs in kennels or at crowded canine events such as dog shows and trials. Documentation of positive CHV-1 serology generally indicates the presence of adequate maternal antibodies.

Bitches who are naïve to CHV-1 during pregnancy must be strictly isolated from potential exposure during gestation and for at least 6 weeks postpartum to prevent transmission of the virus to her fetuses or neonates. Subsequent litters of the infected pregnant or postpartum bitch are usually normal because of acquisition of maternal antibodies.

Vaccine development has been hampered by the poor immunogenicity characteristic of the herpesviral vaccines developed for other species, such as feline herpesvirus-1 vaccines. In Europe, a vaccine (Eurican Herpes 205) has been available since 2003. Administration of two doses of the vaccine is recommended, first during estrus or early pregnancy and again 1 to 2 weeks before whelping. No suggestion for an evaluation of the bitch's serologic status prior to vaccination is made by the manufacturer. Revaccination with two doses of the vaccine is recommended at each pregnancy. No independent, nonproprietary studies exist corroborating this vaccine's efficacy or benefit. The vaccine is not currently available in the United States.[12,13]

Public Health Aspects

In general, herpesviruses are very host specific, and CHV-1 is not known to infect humans.

CASE EXAMPLE

Two, 25-day-old, female Labrador retriever puppies were examined because of acute tachypnea and vocalization. The puppies belonged to a litter of eight. Whelping occurred without incident, and the pups showed normal weight gain and behavior until the last 24 hours. Four days previously, the litter was vaccinated with an intranasal *Bordetella bronchiseptica* vaccine and dewormed with pyrantel pamoate according to routine preventative health care practice. The litter nursed from birth, and the dam was normal.

Physical examination of both puppies revealed hypothermia (rectal temperature 36.3°C [97°F] and 36.0°C [97°F], respectively), tachypnea, a markedly tense abdomen, and continuous vocalization. Despite supportive care (exogenous warming, supplemental feeding with artificial bitch's milk [Esbilack Pet Ag, Inc.], subcutaneous lactated Ringer's solution, and ceftiofur sodium [2.5 mg/kg SC q12h]), the puppies died within 12 hours and then underwent necropsy examination. Tissues collected for histopathologic evaluation included kidney, liver, lung, thymus, mesenteric lymph node, and spleen.

Because of gross findings of hemorrhagic foci in the lungs and kidneys, renal tissue was submitted for a CHV-1–specific PCR assay. The PCR assay later confirmed the presence of CHV-1 DNA in the renal tissue. Gross (foci of hemorrhage in the lungs and kidneys) and histopathologic evaluations of the deceased puppies were typical of CHV-1 but were not confirmatory because of the similarity of findings to those of neonatal bacterial sepsis. Intranuclear inclusion bodies were suspected in macrophages from the lung of one puppy. Aerobic bacterial culture of the peritoneal cavity was negative for bacterial growth.

Poor weight gain and vocalization were reported in two additional puppies. The primary differentials included neonatal bacterial sepsis and CHV-1 infection. Because of the lack of response to therapy for bacterial infection in the two deceased puppies, the remaining six puppies were treated with acyclovir suspension (20 mg/kg PO q6h) for 7 days, and exogenous warming adequate to raise the rectal temperature to just above 37.7°C (100°F). Therapy was initiated the day before the PCR assay confirmed infection with CHV-1.

All six treated puppies survived and were successfully weaned between 5 and 6 weeks of age. All were placed in private homes and had uneventful subsequent health histories and normal behavior. Physical examinations including complete fundic evaluations were performed at 12 to 14 months of age and were normal in all. Two of the dogs have become active guide dogs for the blind, and one is an assistance dog for the hearing impaired. All remain physically normal at more than 26 months of age.

Comments: The epizootiology of this outbreak suggests that the puppies were born from a naïve bitch and exposed to CHV-1 from another carrier dog at days 14 to 17 after birth. Two of 8 (25%) succumbed to the disease; 2 of the remaining 6 showed early clinical signs, after which antiviral therapy was initiated for all dogs.

REFERENCES

1. Carmichael LE, Squire RA, Krook L. Clinical and pathological features of a fatal viral disease of newborn pups. Am J Vet Res. 1965;26:803-814.
2. Carmichael LE, Greene CE. Canine herpesvirus infection. In: Greene CE, ed. Clinical Microbiology and Infectious Diseases of the Dog and Cat. Philadelphia, PA: WB Saunders; 1990:252-258.
3. Carmichael LE. Herpesvirus canis: aspects of pathogenesis and immune response. J Am Vet Med Assoc. 1976;156:1714-1725.
4. Johnson SD, Root Kustritz MV, Olson PN. The neonate—from birth to weaning. Canine and Feline Theriogenology. Philadelphia, PA: WB Saunders; 2001:146-167.
5. Carmichael L. Neonatal viral infections of pups: canine herpesvirus and minute virus of canines (canine parvovirus-1). In: Carmichael L, ed. Recent Advances in Canine Infectious Diseases. Ithaca, NY: International Veterinary Information Service (www.Ivis.org); 1999.
6. Percy DH, Carmichael LE, Albert DM, et al. Lesions in puppies surviving infections with canine herpesvirus. Vet Pathol. 1971;8:37-53.
7. Evermann JF. Diagnosis of canine herpetic infections. In: Kirk RW, Bonagura JD, eds. Current Veterinary Therapy. Philadelphia, PA: WB Saunders; 1989:1313-1316.
8. Burr PD, Campbell ME, Nicolson L, et al. Detection of canine herpesvirus 1 in a wide range of tissues using the polymerase chain reaction. Vet Microbiol. 1996;53:227-237.
9. Decaro N, Amorisco F, Desario C, et al. Development and validation of a real-time PCR assay for specific and sensitive detection of canid herpesvirus 1. J Virol Methods. 2010;169:176-180.
10. Plumb DC, ed. Plumb's Veterinary Drug Handbook. Pocket Size. 6th ed. Hoboken, NJ: Wiley-Blackwell; 2008:18-19.
11. Filer CW, Ramji JV, Allen GD, et al. Metabolic and pharmacokinetic studies following oral administration of famciclovir to the cat and dog. Xenobiotica. 1995;25:477-490.
12. Malone EK, Ledbetter EC, Rassnick KM, et al. Disseminated canine herpesvirus-1 infection in an immunocompromised adult dog. J Vet Intern Med. 2010;24(4):965-968.
13. Verstegen J, Dhaliwal G, Verstegen-Onclin K. Canine and feline pregnancy loss due to viral and non-infectious causes: a review. Theriogenology. 2008;70(3):304-319.

CHAPTER 17

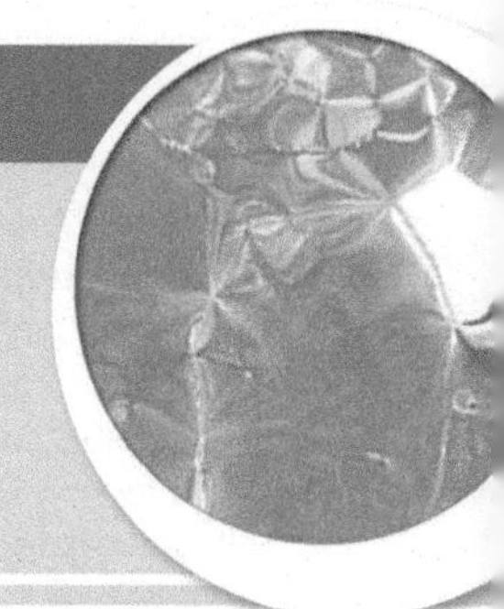

Canine Viral Respiratory Infections

Jane E. Sykes

Overview of the Canine Viral Respiratory Infections

First Described: Respiratory disease in dogs (due to canine adenovirus-2) was first described in 1961 in Canada.[1] The most newly recognized virus, canine pneumovirus, was described in the United States in 2010.[2]

Proposed Causes: Canine adenovirus, canine influenza virus, parainfluenza virus, canine respiratory coronavirus, canine herpesvirus, possibly reoviruses and canine pneumovirus

Geographic Distribution: Worldwide

Mode of Transmission: Aerosol transmission or close contact, sometimes fomites

Major Clinical Signs: Harsh or honking cough, serous nasal discharge, conjunctivitis, fever (uncomplicated disease). Fever, lethargy, inappetence, tachypnea, productive cough, mucopurulent nasal and ocular discharge, rarely death (complicated disease).

Differential Diagnoses: Upper and lower respiratory diseases such as airway collapse, bordetellosis, *Streptococcus equi* subsp. *zooepidemicus* infection, fungal or protozoal pneumonia, respiratory tract neoplasia, airway foreign bodies, chronic bronchitis, eosinophilic bronchopneumopathy or granulomatosis, parasitic infections (such as *Filaroides, Oslerus, Capillaria, Paragonimus, Dirofilaria*), aspiration bronchopneumonia, left-sided congestive heart failure

Human Health Significance: Viruses that cause canine infectious respiratory disease generally are not considered zoonotic. Canine parainfluenza and reoviruses represent potential zoonoses, but the significance of this is unknown.

Etiology and Epidemiology

Canine viral respiratory disease is a widespread problem where large numbers of dogs are housed indoors together, such as in shelters, commercial dog colonies, and breeding facilities. The longer dogs are housed in a shelter situation, the greater the risk that respiratory illness will occur.[3] In shelter environments, transmissible respiratory disease (or canine infectious respiratory disease complex [CIRDC], previously referred to as "kennel cough" or canine infectious tracheobronchitis) delays the placement of dogs in homes and can result in unmanageable costs related to treatment, quarantine, and isolation. Transmissible respiratory disease occasionally occurs in owned dogs after a period of contact with large numbers of other dogs at dog parks, dog sporting events such as fly ball, or dog behavior classes. It can also occur after dogs (or dog owners) visit veterinary hospitals, boarding facilities, or pet daycare centers.

With the widespread clinical application of molecular diagnostic assays, it is increasingly apparent that the number of viruses that can infect the canine respiratory tract is much larger than previously thought. This has led to exciting new discoveries in the field of canine infectious respiratory disease, and our knowledge of the pathogens involved continues to expand. Co-infections with multiple viruses and bacteria such as *Mycoplasma* spp., *Bordetella bronchiseptica*, and *Streptococcus equi* subspecies *zooepidemicus* are common and contribute to an increased severity of disease.[4-6] Viruses believed to play a role in canine respiratory disease include canine herpesvirus-1 (CHV-1), canine adenovirus-2 (CAV-2), canine distemper virus (CDV), canine parainfluenza virus (CPiV), canine pneumovirus, canine respiratory coronavirus (CRCoV), and canine influenza virus (CIV) (Table 17-1). CAV-1 may also play a role when vaccination is not performed or when it is performed improperly.[7] Reoviruses may also play a role.[8] CDV, CHV-1, and CAV are discussed in more detail in Chapters 15, 16, and 18, respectively. The major bacterial causes of canine transmissible respiratory disease are covered in Part II, Section 2 of this book (Chapters 34, 38, and 40). Although most of the canine respiratory viruses have a worldwide distribution, their relative prevalence varies from year to year and between geographic locations. Even within a state or city, predominant pathogens may differ from one shelter and boarding kennel to another.

CDV, CHV-1, CPiV, CRCoV, and CIV are enveloped viruses, so they survive poorly in the environment and are susceptible to a variety of disinfectants. Despite this, contact with virus that persists in the environment may be important for transmission in densely housed populations of dogs. CAV-2 is a non-enveloped virus and has the potential to survive several weeks on fomites.

Canine Adenovirus-2

Adenoviruses are icosahedral DNA viruses that infect a variety of animal species. CAV-2 is found worldwide and primarily infects the respiratory tract of dogs. Rarely, it has been implicated as a cause of enteritis in dogs, and it was found in the brains of puppies with neurologic signs.[9] The virus replicates in nonciliated bronchiolar epithelial cells; epithelial cells of the nasal mucosa, pharynx, and tonsillar crypts; mucous cells in the trachea and bronchi; and type 2 alveolar epithelial cells. CAV-2 can also be isolated from retropharyngeal and bronchial lymph nodes as well as epithelial cells of the intestinal tract. Shedding typically ceases 1 to 2 weeks after initial infection.

TABLE 17-1

Potential Causes of Transmissible Respiratory Disease in Dogs

Organism	Incubation Period (days)*	Shedding Period*	Environmental Survival
Canine adenovirus-1	4 to 9	6 to 9 months	Weeks to months
Canine adenovirus-2	3 to 6	1 to 2 weeks	Weeks to months
Canine distemper virus	3 to 6, longer for neurological signs	Weeks to months	Hours
Canine herpesvirus-1	6 to 10; may be longer with stress-induced reactivation	Unknown	Hours
Canine influenza virus	2 to 4	7 to 10 days	Hours
Canine parainfluenza virus	3 to 10	8 to 10 days	Hours
Canine respiratory coronavirus	Probably days	6 to 8 days	Hours
Bordetella bronchiseptica	2 to 6	Months	Has the potential survive and grow in environmental water for several weeks
Mycoplasma cynos	3 to 10	Months	Hours
Streptococcus equi subspecies *zooepidemicus*	Probably days	At least 2 weeks	Unknown; other streptococci can survive weeks

*Incubation and shedding periods are approximate and may differ when co-infections or immunosuppression operate.

Canine Herpesvirus-1

The extent to which CHV-1 plays a role in respiratory disease in dogs has been debated.[10] Experimental infections of dogs can result in rhinitis or signs of tracheobronchitis, and intraocular infection results in conjunctivitis and keratitis.[11-14] There is evidence of widespread exposure to CHV-1 in dogs worldwide,[10] and a substantial proportion of the dog population may be latently infected. Like other herpesviruses, CHV-1 becomes latent in neurologic tissues, with precipitation of virus shedding by stress. Consistent with the time delay required for reactivation after stress, CHV-1 was most frequently detected 3 to 4 weeks after dogs were introduced to a rehoming center, whereas CRCoV and CPiV were most frequently detected in the first and second week. Dogs infected with CHV-1 were more likely to have severe respiratory disease, although severe respiratory disease itself might predispose dogs to the shedding of CHV-1.[10] Infection with CHV-1 was reported in association with fatal hepatic necrosis in an adult dog that lacked any evidence of immunosuppression.[15] Refer to Chapter 16 for information on CHV-1 infections in neonates.

Canine Influenza Virus

Influenza viruses are enveloped viruses with segmented single-stranded RNA genomes that belong to the family Orthomyxoviridae. Influenza viruses that cause disease in domestic animals belong to the genus Influenzavirus A, whereas influenza B and influenza C viruses primarily circulate among humans. Influenza A viruses are classified based on the genetic composition of their hemagglutinin (H) and neuraminidase (N) genes. To date, 16 H types and 9 N types have been identified, each of which are antigenically distinct.[16] The names of influenza viruses are specified as follows: influenza genus (A, B, or C)/host/geographic origin/strain number/year of isolation and, in parentheses, H and N type—for example, A/canine/Florida/43/2004 (H3N8).[17] Extensive genomic rearrangements that occur within influenza A viruses allow for occasional cross-species transmission among birds and mammals. These rearrangements occur when two different viruses simultaneously infect a host, with subsequent genetic reassortment. Occasionally, cross-species transmission occurs without alteration of the viral genome.

In the United States, CIV emerged in racing greyhounds in Florida in 2003 and 2004,[17] where it caused hemorrhagic pneumonia and a high mortality. However, serologic evidence of infection in the greyhound dog population dates back to 1999.[18] Infections spread slowly and were subsequently reported in racing greyhounds and non-greyhounds in at least 38 U.S. states. Outbreaks have continued to occur in shelter situations for nearly a decade after the virus was discovered. The virus that currently circulates in the United States is an H3N8 virus that closely resembles an equine influenza virus, which suggested that an interspecies jump occurred without genetic reassortment.[17] Instead, accumulation of point mutations with minor amino acid changes occurred, with sustained transmission among dogs. The most significant outbreaks of disease due to CIV have occurred in Florida, New England, Colorado, Wyoming, and Texas. In many other states, sustained transmission of the virus from one dog to another has not occurred. The most significant risk factor for infection has been indoor housing.[19] Virtually all cases to date have involved dogs in kennels, animal shelters, or dog daycare facilities. Dogs of all ages and breeds are susceptible, but to date severe hemorrhagic pneumonia has occurred only in greyhounds.[20] The virus is shed for up to 7 to 10 days. CIV has retained the ability to infect horses, but horses develop only mild disease or no clinical signs.[20]

Avian-lineage H3N2 CIV emerged in South Korean dogs in 2007, and a similar virus was subsequently isolated from dogs in China.[21,22] Experimentally, cats are also susceptible to infection by this virus.[23] Korean isolates were associated with epidemics of respiratory disease in kennels within veterinary clinics.[22] A novel H3N1 virus was also detected in South Korean dogs that lacked signs of respiratory disease.[24] A novel H5N2 influenza virus was recently detected in a dog with respiratory disease in China.[25] Dogs are susceptible to infection with human influenza virus H1N1[26,27] and avian H5N1,[28] but sustained transmission of these viruses in the dog population has not been reported. Limited infection of dogs with equine H3N8 viruses was detected in hounds in England[29] and during an equine influenza outbreak in Australia.[30] In England, disease was so severe that several hounds had to be euthanized, and subacute bronchointerstitial pneumonia was detected at necropsy.[29] The Australian dogs developed inappetence, lethargy, nasal discharge, and a cough that persisted for several weeks, but dog-to-dog transmission was not identified. Experimental transmission of H3N8 influenza virus from horses to dogs was documented in Japan, but infected dogs did not show signs of illness.[31]

Canine Parainfluenza Viruses

CDV, CPiV, and canine pneumovirus belong to the family Paramyxoviridae, which are enveloped RNA viruses. CPiV belongs to the genus *Rubulavirus.* Although previously referred to as canine parainfluenza virus-2, it is probably the same virus as simian virus 5, which was originally isolated from monkey cell cultures. It has been proposed that it be renamed parainfluenza virus 5.[32] Unlike CDV, the outer envelope possesses not only hemagglutinin but also neuraminidase activity (HN attachment glycoprotein). The virus infects dogs worldwide, replicates in epithelial cells of the upper respiratory tract, and often causes no signs or mild respiratory illness. Respiratory disease may be more severe when co-infections with other pathogens such as *B. bronchiseptica* are present.[33] Viremia seems to be uncommon, but occasionally CPiV has been isolated from the liver, spleen, and kidneys. A strain of CPiV was also isolated from a dog with neurologic signs.[34] There is some evidence that cats may be infected with CPiV or a closely related virus.[35] Virus is shed for up to 10 days after infection.

Canine pneumovirus belongs to the genus *Pneumovirus.* It was first isolated from dogs with acute respiratory disease in shelters in the United States in 2010.[2] The virus is most closely related to a murine pneumovirus and in fact can replicate in mice and cause severe inflammatory pathology.[36]

Canine Reoviruses

Reoviruses (family Reoviridae, genus *Orthoreovirus*) are nonenveloped viruses with a segmented, double-stranded RNA genome. Mammalian reoviruses infect a variety of host species and have a worldwide distribution. The prefix *reo-* stands for *r*espiratory *e*nteric *o*rphan virus, which highlights the tropism of reoviruses for cells of the respiratory and gastrointestinal tract, and their uncommon association with disease. Despite serologic evidence of widespread exposure to reoviruses in dogs, they have been found only rarely in dogs with respiratory disease[8,37] and dogs with enteritis.[38] There are three mammalian reovirus (MRV) serotypes, and all three have been detected in dogs. The role of reoviruses in disease causation in dogs is unclear, because disease has not been reproducible experimentally. It has been speculated that reoviruses might act synergistically with other respiratory pathogens to cause disease.[10]

Canine Respiratory Coronavirus

Coronaviruses are enveloped RNA viruses that possess large, club-shaped spikes on their outer surface, also known as peplomers (see Figure 14-1, *B*). CRCoV is a relatively newly identified cause of contagious respiratory disease in dogs. The virus is a group 2a coronavirus (family Coronaviridae, genus *Coronavirus*) and is distinct from canine enteric coronavirus, a group 1a coronavirus (Box 17-1).[39] Minimal serologic cross-reactivity exists between these two viruses. Group 2a coronaviruses possess a gene that encodes hemagglutinin esterase, an outer membrane protein glycoprotein. This gene is absent in group 1 and 3 coronaviruses. CRCoV is most closely related to a bovine coronavirus but also resembles human coronavirus OC43.[40]

CRCoV was first reported in 2003, in a group of dogs with respiratory disease in a rehoming facility in England that had been vaccinated against CAV-2, CDV, and CPiV.[6,40] Some of the dogs were co-infected with CPiV and CHV-1.[6] CRCoV spread rapidly and primarily was detected in the first week that dogs were introduced to the kennel, after which time CPiV and CHV-1 were detected. Alone, CRCoV causes subclinical infections or mild respiratory disease, but like human respiratory coronaviruses, it can cause reversible damage to, or loss of, the cilia on respiratory epithelial cells (Figure 17-1). As a result, infected dogs are predisposed to secondary infections. Serologic evidence of exposure to CRCoV is widespread in dogs from North America, Great Britain and continental Europe, Japan, Korea, and New Zealand,[10,41-43] and the virus has been detected widely using PCR-based methods in dogs with respiratory disease from many of these countries. To date, there is no evidence that cats can be infected with CRCoV.

BOX 17-1

Genetic Relationships between Coronaviruses

Group 1a
Feline coronavirus
Canine enteric coronavirus
Transmissible gastroenteritis virus of swine
Porcine respiratory coronavirus
Ferret and mink coronaviruses

Group 1b
Bat coronavirus HKU8
Human coronavirus 229E
Human coronavirus NL63
Porcine epidemic diarrhea virus

Group 2a
Canine respiratory coronavirus
Bovine coronavirus
Human coronavirus OC43
Human coronavirus HKU3
Mouse hepatitis virus
Porcine hemagglutinating encephalomyelitis virus

Group 2b
SARS coronavirus (humans)
Bat SARS coronavirus HKU3

Group 3
Avian infectious bronchitis virus
Turkey coronavirus

SARS, Severe acute respiratory syndrome

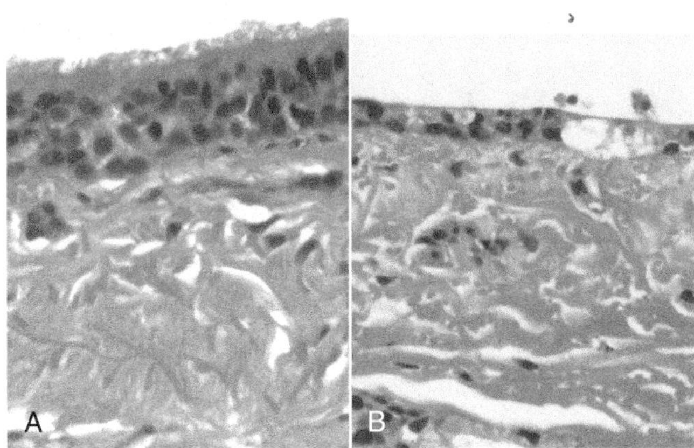

FIGURE 17-1 Effect of canine respiratory coronavirus infection on ciliated respiratory epithelial cells. **A,** Respiratory epithelium immediately before inoculation with CRCoV. **B,** The same cells 48 hours after inoculation with CRCoV. There is marked loss of cilia, thinning of the epithelium with individual cell necrosis, and sloughed necrotic cells on the surface. There are also occasional large vacuoles within the epithelium, which likely represent foci of cell loss secondary to viral replication. (Courtesy Dr. Simon Priestnall and Professor Joe Brownlie, Royal Veterinary College, UK.)

Infection with pancytotropic strains of canine enteric coronavirus has recently been associated with severe systemic disease in puppies from Europe. Affected pups have fever, mucoid to hemorrhagic enteritis, lymphopenia, neurologic signs such as seizures, and bronchopneumonia.[44,45] Co-infections with CPV-2 were present in some puppies, but the disease has been reproduced by experimental infection by canine enteric coronavirus alone. Death occurred in some puppies, but others developed transient gastrointestinal signs and recovered.[46]

Clinical Features

Signs and Their Pathogenesis

The incubation period for viral respiratory disease is generally less than 2 weeks and can be as short as 2 to 3 days. Influenza virus infections, in particular, have been associated with very short incubation periods.[20] Transmission occurs by aerosol, but direct contact between dogs and fomite transmission (hands, clothing, contaminated food and water bowls, common hallways and exercise areas) are important routes in population-dense environments. Cells of the larynx, trachea, bronchi, and sometimes the nasal mucosa, bronchioles, and alveoli are infected, and although viral shedding patterns differ between pathogens, shedding may occur before the onset of clinical signs. The duration of shedding for CIV and CPiV is very short, typically a few days, and in some dogs, shedding has ceased by the time clinical signs are most apparent. In contrast, CDV can be shed for weeks (see Chapter 15).

Infection with respiratory viruses may be associated with no signs, or complicated pneumonia and death can occur. In general, morbidity is high, but mortality is low. Moderate to severe signs may be more likely to occur in very young puppies, genetically susceptible animals, and when stress and co-infections with multiple viral and bacterial pathogens are present. Infection with CDV is especially effective at predisposing dogs to other respiratory viral infections, because of its immunosuppressive properties, but other viruses that damage ciliated epithelial cells, such as CRCoV and CPiV, also predispose to co-infections. Clinical signs of acute respiratory disease include

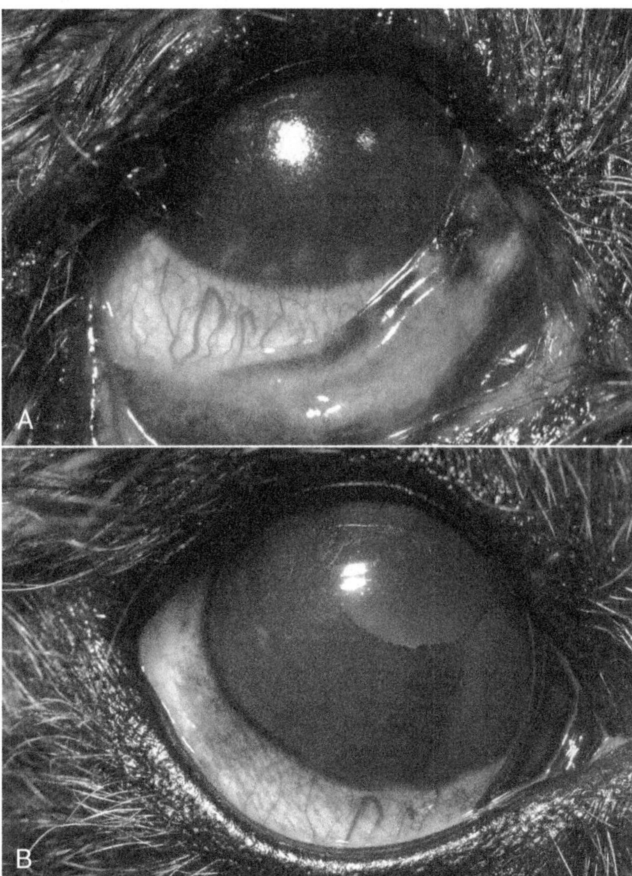

FIGURE 17-2 **A,** Right eye of a 10-year-old male neutered miniature schnauzer infected with bilateral conjunctivitis and dendritic ulceration associated with canine herpesvirus infection. Fluorescein uptake can be seen in a branching pattern at the limbus of the right eye. **B,** The same dog 1 month later. Note diffuse stain uptake over at least 25% of the corneal surface. (Courtesy University of California, Davis Veterinary Ophthalmology Service.)

mild fever, a paroxysmal harsh or "honking" cough, serous nasal discharge, and sometimes sneezing, but usually otherwise affected dogs are often alert, active, and appetent. The cough may be followed by gagging or retching, which may be followed by the production of frothy mucus. An altered bark or stridor may occur in dogs that develop laryngitis, tonsillitis, and/or pharyngitis. CAV-2 and CHV-1 may cause conjunctivitis.[47] In addition, CHV-1 has been associated with ulcerative and nonulcerative keratitis, which may be precipitated by immunosuppression (Figure 17-2).[48-50] Infections with CIV or CDV, or infections with multiple respiratory pathogens, may be more likely to produce systemic signs of fever and lethargy. Dogs that develop secondary bacterial infections may show fever, inappetence, lethargy, a mucopurulent nasal discharge, tachypnea, and a moist, productive cough.

Physical Examination Findings

On physical examination, dogs with uncomplicated transmissible respiratory disease are typically bright, alert, and active with a paroxysmal cough. The cough is often easily elicited on tracheal palpation. Conjunctivitis and serous ocular and/or nasal discharge may be present, and the tonsils may be enlarged and hyperemic. Dogs with secondary bacterial infections may be pyrexic, lethargic, and tachypneic with increased respiratory effort and

TABLE 17-2

Diagnostic Assays Available for Respiratory Viruses in Dogs

Assay	Specimen Type	Target	Performance
Virus isolation	Conjunctival, nasal, and caudal pharyngeal swabs; transtracheal and bronchoalveolar wash specimens; airway and lung specimens collected at necropsy	Virus	False negatives can occur in specimens that contain no or low numbers of virus particles. Attenuated live vaccine virus may also be isolated. May take several days and requires specialized techniques and expertise.
Influenza ELISA antigen assay	Same as virus isolation	CIV antigen	Inexpensive and rapid. Sensitivity and specificity in naturally infected dogs have not been well established, so results should be interpreted with caution.
PCR or RT-PCR	Same as virus isolation	Viral nucleic acid	Sensitivity and specificity may vary with assay design. Sensitivity may be low because of brief shedding for some viruses. Assays may not be available for all viruses or may not detect all virus strains. Testing specimens from multiple different anatomic sites or combining PCR with other diagnostic tests can increase sensitivity. Attenuated live vaccine virus may be detected after vaccination. Because of subclinical shedding, the significance of a positive result may be difficult to interpret. False-negatives may occur as a result from degradation of viral nucleic acid during specimen transport.
Serology	Serum	Antibodies against respiratory viral antigens	Interpretation complicated by previous vaccination and exposure. May be useful when the exposed population is naïve and unvaccinated for the virus of interest. Acute and convalescent sera required for diagnosis.
Histopathology	Necropsy specimens	Viral inclusions; immunostaining	Can be used for diagnosis at necropsy. Detection of inclusions has low sensitivity, and immunostaining and/or PCR is required to definitively identify the infecting virus.

CIV, Canine influenza virus; RT, reverse transcriptase.

increased lung sounds on thoracic auscultation. A mucopurulent nasal discharge may also be present. Ulcerative or nonulcerative keratitis may be present in dogs infected with CHV-1.

Diagnosis

It is not possible to identify the cause of transmissible respiratory disease in dogs based on clinical signs alone, because each pathogen produces a similar spectrum of signs. The high prevalence of co-infections further complicates diagnosis. In addition, other, noncontagious causes of respiratory disease in dogs can lead to signs that closely resemble transmissible respiratory disease. A history of exposure to other dogs can support the diagnosis.

Most dogs experience self-limiting disease. Attempts to obtain an etiologic diagnosis should be made when disease persists for longer than 7 to 10 days or is complicated by bacterial pneumonia, with lethargy and inappetence. When outbreaks occur in shelters or the pattern of endemic respiratory disease changes, attempts to make an etiologic diagnosis are also indicated and encouraged (Table 17-2). Collection of multiple specimen types from several dogs with and without clinical signs in an outbreak situation can facilitate diagnosis and allow interpretation of the significance of positive test results. Organism detection methods, such as PCR assays, are likely to be of highest yield early in the course of illness (e.g., the first 1 to 3 days) or in exposed dogs that have not yet developed clinical signs. Use of a combination of serology and organism detection methods also facilitates diagnosis. In shelter situations or outbreaks where severe disease occurs, necropsies can provide valuable information and should be performed by a veterinary pathologist as soon as possible after death or euthanasia. Tissues should be submitted for histopathology (in formalin), bacterial and virus cultures (fresh tissue), and PCR assay for respiratory viruses and bacteria (fresh or frozen tissue; see Chapter 5).

Laboratory Abnormalities

There are no specific abnormalities in the CBC, serum biochemistry profile, or urinalysis that aid in a diagnosis of canine viral respiratory disease. The CBC may be normal or show a mild to moderate neutrophilia. Band neutrophils and neutrophil toxicity may be apparent in dogs with secondary bacterial pneumonia. Severe infections may be associated with leukopenia, which may be followed by leukocytosis in dogs that recover.

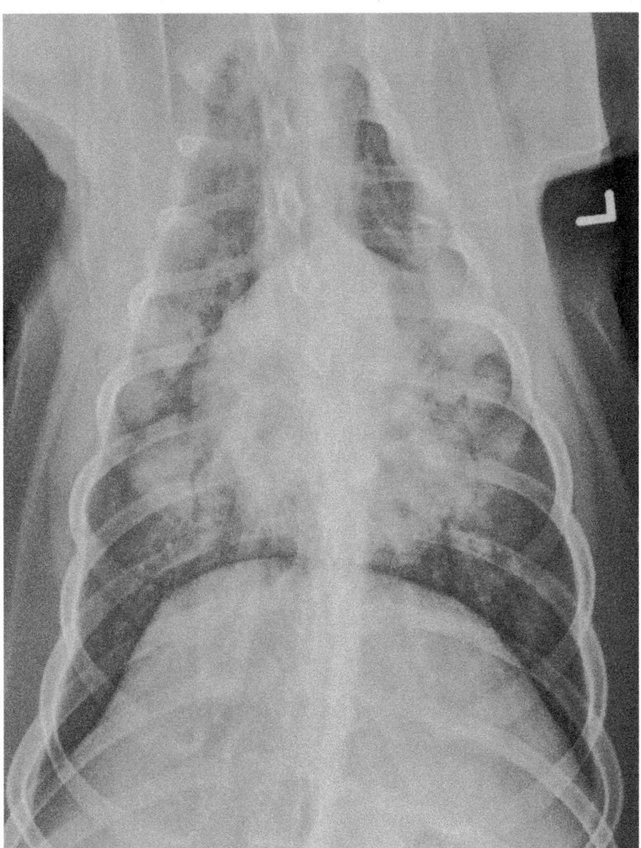

FIGURE 17-3 Dorsoventral thoracic radiograph from a 2-year-old male neutered coonhound that had left a boarding facility 6 days previously with a moist, productive cough that subsequently progressed and was complicated by the development of fever and a mucopurulent nasal discharge. A CBC showed neutrophilia (17,840 cells/μL), increased numbers of band neutrophils (223 cells/μL), and monocytosis (3,345 cells/μL). Bronchopneumonia is present that involves the right cranial, right middle, and left cranial lung lobes. Interestingly, canine herpesvirus DNA was detected in a pooled extract from nasal, conjunctival, and oral swab specimens, as well as a whole blood sample using a PCR assay.

Transtracheal wash and bronchoalveolar lavage specimens from dogs with viral pneumonia typically show a suppurative or mixed exudate, sometimes with evidence of intracellular bacteria. Culture for aerobic bacterial culture and *Mycoplasma* spp. are indicated on wash specimens, and antimicrobial susceptibilities should be obtained for any aerobic bacteria isolated. Organisms such as *Pasteurella* spp., *Staphylococcus pseudintermedius, Streptococcus canis, Escherichia coli, Klebsiella pneumoniae,* and some *Mycoplasma* spp. infect the airways as opportunists and are not considered to be primary pathogens. Bacterial culture of nasal swabs is generally not recommended because it often leads to growth of normal flora, which has no clinical relevance.

Diagnostic Imaging

Plain Radiography

In uncomplicated viral infections, plain thoracic radiography in dogs often shows no significant abnormalities, or there may be a mild diffuse interstitial or bronchointerstitial pattern. Secondary bacterial bronchopneumonia may be characterized by development of peribronchial and alveolar infiltrates or lobar consolidation (Figure 17-3).

Microbiologic Tests

Virus Isolation

Efforts to isolate viruses from dogs with acute respiratory disease have been most useful for identification of novel or reemerging pathogens.[2,38,40] Despite the increased availability of molecular diagnostic assays, virus isolation is still offered to veterinarians for routine diagnostic purposes by laboratories that specialize in virology (e.g., the Animal Health Diagnostic Laboratory at Cornell University in Ithaca, NY). Suitable specimens for respiratory virus isolation are nasal and pharyngeal swab specimens, transtracheal or bronchoalveolar lavage specimens, or upper airway or lung tissue obtained at necropsy. If swabs are used to collect specimens, polyester-tipped swabs and specific virus transport media should be used. Cotton swabs should be avoided, because influenza viruses adhere to the cotton, which can lead to reduced sensitivity.[20] Virus isolation is a specialized process that may take several days. As with PCR assays, sensitivity may be low because shedding of respiratory viruses occurs early in the course of illness and may be transient. CRCoV fails to replicate in many cell lines, but was successfully isolated in HRT-18 cells.[51] This may explain its relatively recent discovery relative to other respiratory viral pathogens.

Fluorescent Antibody Testing

Fluorescent antibody can be applied to smears made from swabs from the upper respiratory tract, or tissues collected at necropsy, such as fresh lung tissue. Assays are available for detection of CPiV, CAV, CDV (see Chapter 15), and CHV-1. Attenuated live vaccination with intranasal vaccines for CPiV and CAV has the potential to interfere with fluorescent antibody results, but this requires further study. The sensitivity of fluorescent antibody testing is likely to be lower than that of PCR assays, and inexperienced personnel may misinterpret nonspecific fluorescence as a positive result.

Enzyme-Linked Immunosorbent Assays for Influenza Virus Antigen

Point-of-care ELISAs are available for detection of nucleoprotein antigen of human influenza A viruses. The assays are easily performed and provide rapid results. Unfortunately, such assays have had limited sensitivity and specificity for diagnosis of CIV infections, and so their use is not recommended. False positives may especially be a problem in shelters where canine influenza is not endemic.

Molecular Diagnosis Using the Polymerase Chain Reaction

Panels of real-time PCR assays that detect respiratory pathogens are offered by some commercial veterinary diagnostic laboratories. These may include assays for CRCoV, parainfluenza virus, and CIV, as well as bacterial pathogens such as *B. bronchiseptica* and *Mycoplasma* spp. Swabs of the nasal cavity and/or caudal pharynx, or respiratory lavage specimens could be submitted for testing. At necropsy, CRCoV is most readily detected in upper respiratory tract specimens, such as the nasal mucosa, nasal tonsil, and trachea.[52] Lung specimens may also yield positive results. Unfortunately, false-negative PCR results are common, especially in antemortem specimens, because of transient or low-level shedding of many respiratory viruses. In addition, because many respiratory viruses are RNA viruses and RNA is very labile when compared with DNA, false negatives can occur when viral RNA degrades during specimen transport.

In outbreak situations, false-positive PCR results may occur if swab specimens become contaminated with virus from the environment or the hands of personnel. Clean examination gloves should be worn for each dog, and the swab should only touch the anatomic site to be tested. Vaccination with live attenuated vaccines (especially intranasal vaccines) may cause positive test results with real-time PCR assays, but the extent to which this occurs in dogs with respiratory viral illness requires further study. Because CIV vaccines are parenteral inactivated vaccines, they would not be expected to lead to false-positive PCR assay results. The detection of nucleic acid from a respiratory virus in a specimen may not imply disease causation.

Serologic Diagnosis

Diagnostic laboratories that specialize in veterinary virology may offer serologic assays for antibodies to canine respiratory viral pathogens on a commercial basis to practitioners. Serology has limited use for diagnosis because of vaccine titer interference for some organisms, and the high prevalence of subclinical exposure to organisms endemic in the dog population. Titers may be negative in the first 10 days of illness, and some dogs may not show a significant increase in antibody titer after infection. Despite these limitations, serologic assays have been key to identification of infection and disease caused by emerging pathogens such as CIV, when the disease is not endemic.[20] In this situation, analysis of paired serum specimens collected 2 weeks apart can be used to document recent infection. In some dogs, no other diagnostic test may be useful for antemortem diagnosis because virus shedding is so transient and difficult to detect.

Serologic assays for CIV exposure are based on serum neutralization or hemagglutination-inhibition (see Chapter 2). Assays for CIV that use equine influenza virus antigen for antibody detection have suboptimal sensitivity, whereas an assay based on H3N8 CIV antigen was sensitive and specific when compared with serum neutralization.[53] Seroconversion to CRCoV in a bovine coronavirus antigen ELISA assay helped identify the association between infection with this virus and respiratory disease in dogs in the rehoming kennel in the United Kingdom.[6] Serum neutralization assays can be performed for detection of antibodies to CAV-2, CPiV, and CHV-1. Antibodies to CAV-2 and CPiV can also be detected by hemagglutination-inhibition.

Pathologic Findings

Gross Pathologic Findings

Necropsy of dogs with viral respiratory infections may show no gross lesions, or pulmonary consolidation and hyperemia of the tracheal mucosa may be present. Purulent exudate may be present in the bronchi. Greyhounds that died of CIV infection had extensive hemorrhage within the lungs, mediastinum, and pleural space, together with mild, fibrinous pleuritis.[17]

Histopathologic Findings

Histopathology of the airways of dogs with viral respiratory infections may show loss or irregularity of normal respiratory cilia and epithelial necrosis and ulceration within the trachea, bronchi, and bronchioles. With secondary bacterial infection, a neutrophilic or mixed inflammatory infiltrate may be seen in the airway mucosa, submucosa, and alveoli.[54] Bronchial and bronchiolar lumina may contain neutrophils, macrophages, and cellular debris. Thickening of the alveolar walls with type 2 pneumocyte hyperplasia and interstitial edema has also been described. Hemorrhagic interstitial and bronchointerstitial pneumonia, vasculitis, and thrombus formation have been observed in greyhounds with CIV infection.[20] CAV-2 can produce large, basophilic intranuclear inclusion bodies within bronchial, bronchiolar, and alveolar cells. These must be differentiated from the eosinophilic inclusions of CDV (see Chapter 15).[55] Reoviruses can also produce intracytoplasmic inclusions within bronchial epithelial cells.[8] Use of immunohistochemistry can facilitate definitive identification of viral antigen within cells of the respiratory tract.[5,55]

Treatment and Prognosis

Like the common cold in humans, contagious respiratory disease in dogs resolves without treatment in the vast majority of dogs, regardless of the underlying cause. For dogs with signs of respiratory disease that have been present for less than 7 to 10 days and that remain bright and appetent, no treatment is indicated. In some dogs, cough persists for as long as 10 to 30 days. Cough suppressants such as hydrocodone could be used for dogs with a nonproductive, honking cough that occurs throughout the day and night. Cough suppressants should not be used in dogs that have productive cough, because they suppress normal clearing mechanisms. Use of a harness or gentle leader for leash walking rather than a neck collar may also reduce cough. The efficacy and optimal dosage of neuraminidase inhibitors such as oseltamivir (see Chapter 7) is unknown, and because of this and the fact that oseltamivir is a first-line treatment for pandemic influenza in humans, it should not be used to treat dogs with respiratory disease, even when CIV infection is present. For dogs with confirmed ocular CHV-1 infections that are associated with corneal ulceration, topical antiviral ophthalmic preparations such as idoxuridine or cidofovir could be considered (see Chapter 7).[50]

Antimicrobial drug treatment could be considered for dogs with signs that persist beyond 7 to 10 days, but is primarily indicated when there is evidence of secondary bacterial bronchopneumonia, such as pulmonary alveolar infiltrates and consolidation on thoracic radiography, lethargy, mucopurulent oculonasal discharges, and/or decreased appetite. Because antimicrobial drug resistance is increasingly reported among secondary bacterial pathogens and *B. bronchiseptica*, treatment of dogs with secondary bacterial bronchopneumonia is optimally based on the results of culture of a transtracheal wash specimen from each affected dog and antimicrobial susceptibility testing. For dogs with severe pneumonia, initial treatment should involve the use of broad-spectrum parenteral antimicrobial drugs such as a combination of a fluoroquinolone and a penicillin or clindamycin. When infection with *B. bronchiseptica* or *Mycoplasma* spp. is suspected, doxycycline may be the best first choice. Indiscriminate use of antimicrobial drugs leads only to widespread bacterial resistance and failure of antimicrobial drug treatment in dogs that develop severe disease.

Dogs with pneumonia may also require treatment with intravenous fluids, supplemental oxygen, nebulization, and coupage. Nutritional support in the form of feeding tubes may be required for dogs that are inappetent.

Prognosis depends on the virulence of the causative agent(s), the presence of co-infections, and other factors that contribute to host immunosuppression. Prognosis is generally excellent for dogs with uncomplicated infections with a single pathogen. For CIV infection, mortality rates have been less than 8% and could be lower with rapid diagnosis and appropriate treatment.[20]

Immunity and Vaccination

Vaccines are available for reduction of disease due to CPiV, CAV-2, CDV, and CIV. With the exception of CDV vaccines, none of the available vaccines completely prevent infection and shedding, but they can lessen the severity of disease, provided other factors such as overcrowding and appropriate disinfection and reduction of other stressors are also addressed. Parenteral and mucosal (intranasal and oral) attenuated live vaccines are available for CPiV and CAV-2. The vaccine for CIV is an inactivated vaccine. Vaccines for canine transmissible respiratory disease are considered noncore vaccines, so they should be administered to dogs at risk of exposure, such as those that enter shelters, boarding kennels, shows, sporting competitions, popular dog parks, or pet daycare facilities.

Canine Adenovirus-2

Mucosal and parenteral vaccines are available for prevention of disease due to CAV-2. Parenteral CAV-2 vaccines also protect against CAV-1 infection. Maternal antibodies persist for up to 12 to 14 weeks after birth. Mucosal vaccines may be useful to overcome maternal antibodies in young dogs that are introduced to shelter environments. However, parenteral vaccines are still required for adequate protection against CAV-1.

Canine Herpesvirus

An inactivated vaccine for CHV-1 is available in Europe for pregnant bitches to protect puppies against neonatal infections (see Chapter 16). It is not intended to reduce respiratory disease due to CHV-1 infection.

Canine Influenza Virus

Inactivated, parenteral vaccines are available for reduction of disease and shedding caused by H3N8 CIV.[56] One vaccine also reduced the severity of illness caused by co-challenge with CIV and *Streptococcus equi* subspecies *zooepidemicus*.[4] The use of these vaccines could be considered for dogs that are likely to contact other dogs in regions where CIV is endemic, especially those that enter boarding or pet daycare facilities. Vaccination against CIV is required for importation of North American dogs to Australia.[57] The initial vaccine can be given as early as 6 weeks of age. Because CIV vaccines are inactivated, two initial doses are required 3 to 4 weeks apart, and maximum immunity does not occur until 1 week after the second dose. As a result, CIV vaccines may not protect dogs that enter shelters where canine influenza is endemic, unless newly introduced dogs are separated from dogs that might be shedding CIV until immunization is complete. Annual boosters are recommended for dogs that remain at risk of infection, but the maximum duration of immunity is unknown.

Canine Parainfluenza Virus

Intranasal vaccination with CPiV significantly reduces clinical signs and virus shedding after challenge.[58-60] One study showed that intranasal CPiV vaccination reduced clinical signs even when dogs were challenged as long as 1 year after immunization.[58] Few studies have compared the efficacy of parenteral and intranasal vaccines. In a study reported in the early 1980s, the parenteral vaccine was less effective at reducing shedding than the intranasal vaccine,[59] but a study reported in the 1970s showed reduction of clinical signs and shedding after parenteral vaccination.[61] The use of one parenteral CPiV vaccine resulted in antibody titers that persisted for at least 2 years.[62] Use of intranasal CPiV vaccines, as opposed to parenteral vaccines, has been advocated, because they produce local immunity, reduce shedding, and can be used in puppies as young as 3 to 4 weeks of age.[63] However, proper administration of mucosal vaccines may be difficult in aggressive dogs or dogs that refuse to be restrained. Mucosal vaccines may also be associated with transient respiratory illness for 3 to 10 days after immunization in a small percentage of dogs. This may be problematic in shelter and boarding environments, because these signs cannot be distinguished from those that result from natural infection with wild-type viruses. More studies that evaluate the relative efficacy of mucosal and parenteral CPiV vaccines are required.

Prevention

Although vaccination can reduce the prevalence of respiratory disease in dogs,[3] current vaccines do not provide protection against all the organisms that cause respiratory disease in dogs, and immunity is not sterile, so infection and mild clinical signs can still occur. When factors such as stress, immunosuppression, co-infections, and overwhelming challenge doses are present, vaccine-induced protection may be overwhelmed. Prevention of transmissible respiratory tract disease in dogs therefore involves not only vaccination, but also control methods that include quarantine of dogs introduced into densely populated environments, early identification and isolation of dogs with signs of respiratory disease through proper training of shelter personnel, avoidance of overcrowding and mixing of dogs, use of solid walls between runs, reduction of time dogs spend in a shelter environment, optimum nutrition, fomite control, control of noise such as barking, and proper ventilation and disinfection (see Box 11-5). Distances traveled by aerosols generated by dogs are unknown. Dogs with respiratory disease should be separated from other dogs in shelter environments by at least 25 feet (or as far as possible) and ideally placed in an enclosed room with a separate ventilation system. Isolated dogs should not be moved back into the general shelter population, but adopted out of isolation or a separate recovery room. Provided proper cleaning and contact times are used, use of disinfectants with activity against parvovirus should also kill respiratory viruses, with CAV-2 being the respiratory virus that is most resistant to disinfection. The order of inspection of dogs in shelters should be healthy dogs, then quarantined dogs, and finally dogs in isolation.

When outbreaks occur, attempts should be made to identify the pathogen(s) involved. This allows potential routes of transmission of infection and shedding patterns to be identified, proper vaccination and control strategies to be implemented, and adequate disinfectants to be selected. For example, quarantine for 2 weeks and isolation or removal of any dogs that develop illness may be effective for diseases such as canine influenza, because of the short incubation and shedding periods. However, it is less likely to be successful for distemper and bordetellosis, which can have prolonged incubation and shedding periods. For some viral respiratory diseases such as canine influenza, discontinuation of intake and adoptions for 2 to 3 weeks may be necessary while the disease runs its course. Exposed dogs could also be transferred to foster care in a household with no other dogs. Because of a lack of adequate resources for treatment, diagnostic evaluation, and management, some shelters have elected to euthanize large numbers of affected dogs.

Shelters should provide written information on transmissible respiratory disease to clients who adopt shelter animals, regardless of the presence or absence of clinical signs at the time of adoption, and communicate fully about diseases that are endemic in the shelter. Whenever possible, dogs that leave shelters should be kept away from other dogs for at least 2 weeks (consider 4 weeks if bordetellosis is endemic), and informed about follow-up medical care. Other dogs in the household should be vaccinated before they are placed in contact with the shelter animal. Clients should also be instructed to ensure their local veterinary clinic is aware that their dog is newly adopted from a shelter, so that precautions can be taken to prevent contamination of the hospital environment when the dog is examined a few days after leaving the shelter.

Public Health Aspects

Viruses related to simian virus 5 (parainfluenza virus 5) have been detected in humans, but the role of CPiV as a human pathogen is controversial. Reoviruses have a broad host range, and human infection has been associated with enteritis and respiratory disease; MRV-3 infection was associated with meningitis in a child.[64] Thus they represent a potential zoonosis. Although adenoviruses, influenza viruses, coronaviruses, and paramyxoviruses cause respiratory disease in humans, there is no evidence that CAV-2, CIV, CDV, CHV-1, or CRCoV can be transmitted to humans. Human influenza viruses such as H1N1 can cause disease in dogs and may have the potential to spread from infected dogs back to humans.

CASE EXAMPLE

Signalment: "Winnie", a 10-year old male neutered miniature Schnauzer from Sacramento, CA

History: Winnie was brought to his local veterinarian because of a 1-day history of serous ocular and nasal discharge, and sneezing. Fever (103.5°F or 39.7°C) was documented on physical examination, and enrofloxacin (2 mg/kg PO q24h), bacitracin-neomycin-polymyxin ophthalmic ointment (both eyes q8h), and diphenhydramine (2.2 mg/kg PO q12h) were prescribed, without clinical improvement. A day later, he became lethargic, inappetent, and polydipsic, and the owners described continuous nasal discharge, and a moist cough. Winnie was brought to the UC Davis VMTH for a second opinion. He had been vaccinated regularly for CDV, CAV-2, CPV, rabies, *Bordetella bronchiseptica,* and CPiV. He was recently cared for in a boarding facility for a week and had been home for the past 11 days. He also regularly visited dog parks. There were two other miniature Schnauzers at home, and both were currently well.

Current Medications: Enrofloxacin, 2 mg/kg PO q24h

Other Medical History: Increased activity of serum ALP was noted at a senior care visit 2 months before the onset of respiratory signs.

Physical Examination:

Body Weight: 9.4 kg

General: Lethargic but hydrated. T = 100.8°F (38.2°C), HR = 104 beats/min, respiratory rate = 12 breaths/min, mucous membranes pink, CRT = 1 to 2 s.

Eyes, Ears, Nose, and Throat: Severe chemosis, hyperemia, and mucoid ocular discharge were present bilaterally. There was also profuse bilateral serous nasal discharge and decreased nasal airflow, hypersalivation, and right tonsillar enlargement.

Musculoskeletal: Body condition score 5/9.

Respiratory: Stertorous respiratory noises were noted. Increased respiratory effort with a normal respiratory rate was also present. Auscultation revealed referred wheezing noises in all lung fields.

Gastrointestinal: Tense abdomen, hepatomegaly was detected on abdominal palpation.

All Other Systems: No abnormalities were detected.

Ophthalmologic Examination: Pupillary light reflexes (PLRs) (direct and consensual) were brisk and complete. There was no evidence of anisocoria. Menace response, dazzle, and palpebral reflexes were all complete. Globe position and movements were normal bilaterally (OU). Periorbital palpation and globe retropulsion were also normal. The dog behaved as if sighted. The eyelids were normal. Both nictitans were hyperemic and edematous, and there was moderate conjunctival hyperemia, chemosis, and mucoid ocular discharge OU. Bilateral iris atrophy and lens nuclear sclerosis were also present. The cornea, anterior chamber, vitreous, and dilated fundic examination were normal OU. In the left eye (OS), a pinpoint incipient anterior cortical cataract was identified just ventral to the center of the lens. In the right eye (OD), a linear pigment deposition on the anterior lens capsule was present at the 5 o'clock position.

Schirmer Tear Test: 8 mm/min OU

Intraocular Pressure: 16 mm Hg OS, 17 mm Hg OD

Fluorescein Stain: Multiple dendritic ulcers were identified at the ventral peripheral cornea OD (see Figure 17-2).

Laboratory Findings:

CBC:

HCT 53.5% (40-55%)
MCV 67.7 fL (65-75 fL)
MCHC 35.3 g/dL (33-36 g/dL)
1 nucleated red cell/100 WBCs
WBC 14,600 cells/μL (6000-13,000 cells/μL)
Neutrophils 10,804 cells/μL (3000-10,500 cells/μL)
Band neutrophils 438 cells/μL
Lymphocytes 1752 cells/μL (1000-4000 cells/μL)
Monocytes 1460 cells/μL (150-1200 cells/μL)
Eosinophils 0 cells/μL (0-1500 cells/μL)
Platelets 216,000 platelets/μL (150,000-400,000 platelets/μL)
A few highly reactive lymphocytes were noted.

Serum Chemistry Profile:

Sodium 142 mmol/L (145-154 mmol/L)
Potassium 6.1 mmol/L (3.6-5.3 mmol/L)
Chloride 102 mmol/L (105-116 mmol/L)
Bicarbonate 25 mmol/L (16-26 mmol/L)
Phosphorus 6.7 mg/dL (3.0-6.2 mg/dL)
Calcium 9.5 mg/dL (9.9-11.4 mg/dl)
BUN 20 mg/dL (8-31 mg/dL)
Creatinine 0.7 mg/dL (0.5-1.6 mg/dL)

Glucose 80 mg/dL (60-104 mg/dL)
Total protein 5.7 g/dL (5.4-7.4 g/dL)
Albumin 2.2 g/dL (2.9-4.2 g/dL)
Globulin 3.5 g/dL (2.3-4.4 g/dL)
ALT 564 U/L (19-67 U/L)
AST 116 U/L (21-54 U/L)
ALP 1024 U/L (15-127 U/L)
Gamma GT 10 U/L (0-6 U/L)
Cholesterol 195 mg/dL (135-345 mg/dL)
Total bilirubin 0.4 mg/dL (0-0.4 mg/dL).

Urinalysis: SGr 1.009; pH 8.5, negative for protein, bilirubin, hemoprotein, glucose; rare WBC/HPF, 0 RBC/HPF, 0-3 hyaline casts/HPF, few amorphous crystals, moderate degenerated cells and amorphous debris in the sediment.

Imaging Findings:

Thoracic and Cervical Radiographs: A mild to moderate bronchial and interstitial pattern was identified and was most prominent in the caudal lung fields. Cervical radiographs were unremarkable. The pulmonary changes were considered nonspecific, but more significant than those expected due to age.

Abdominal Ultrasound: The cranial pole of the right adrenal was mildly to moderately enlarged. The liver appeared sonographically normal. A 3 mm stone was identified in the urinary bladder.

Microbiologic Testing: A nasal swab specimen was submitted for real-time PCR panel for canine respiratory pathogens, which included CHV-1, CIV, CDV, CPiV, CAV-2, and *B. bronchiseptica*. The results were available 3 days later, and the specimen was positive for CHV-1 DNA.

Diagnosis: Upper respiratory disease and keratitis associated with CHV-1 infection.

Treatment: Winnie was hospitalized in isolation and treated with 0.9% NaCl (30 mL/hr IV), nebulization for 15 min q8h, clavulanic acid-amoxicillin (13.5 mg/kg PO q12h), and lubricating eye ointment (1 inch OU q4h). Clinical improvement occurred a day later, electrolyte abnormalities normalized, and the dog was discharged with instructions to administer topical idoxuridine (0.1% ophthalmic solution, 2 drops OU q4-6h). Unfortunately a caretaker of the dog did not regularly administer the idoxuridine. At a recheck 5 weeks after the dog was first seen, the owner reported 80% improvement in Winnie's respiratory signs, but he continued to sneeze approximately six times a day and was pawing at his eyes. Examination revealed persistent conjunctivitis, and a fluorescein stain showed large, superficial areas of uptake over the central cornea OU (see Figure 17-2). A Schirmer tear test (STT) was 13 mm/min OS and 8 mm/min OD. A CBC was normal, and the serum biochemistry profile showed persistently increased ALP (835 U/L) and GGT activities (12 U/L) and improvement in the serum ALT activity (124 U/L). The owner was instructed to administer idoxuridine for an additional 2 weeks, as well as lubricating ointment, bacitracin-neomycin ophthalmic ointment (q8h OU), and L-lysine gel (2 mL [400 mg] q12h PO), separating the ophthalmic medications with administration of the idoxuridine first. At a recheck 2 weeks later, all signs had resolved and there was no fluorescein uptake. STT results were 14 mm/min OS and 10 mm/min OD. The idoxuridine was discontinued. Winnie had another episode of respiratory signs 4 months later, at which time the STT results were 15 mm/min OU. Treatment with lubricating eye ointment and L-lysine was continued.

Comments: This was an unusual case of ocular and respiratory herpesviral infection. The early detection of dendritic ulcers allowed a connection to be made between the clinical signs and positive PCR assay result. The negative PCR assay results for other respiratory pathogens did not rule out the possibility of co-infections, because shedding of these organisms may have ceased or been at undetectable levels. Although idoxuridine was used to treat this dog, topical cidofovir may also have been effective.[50] Approximately 2 years later, mild serous nasal discharge and depigmentation of the planum nasale developed. A biopsy of the nasal planum showed epitheliotropic lymphoma. The dog was treated with multiagent chemotherapy for over a year without relapse of herpetic keratitis.

SUGGESTED READINGS

Buonavoglia C, Martella V. Canine respiratory viruses. Vet Res. 2007;38:355-373.

Crawford PC, Dubovi EJ, Castleman WL, et al. Transmission of equine influenza virus to dogs. Science. 2005;310:482-485.

Ellis JA, Krakowka GS. A review of canine parainfluenza virus infection in dogs. J Am Vet Med Assoc. 2012;240:273-284.

Erles K, Dubovi EJ, Brooks HW, et al. Longitudinal study of viruses associated with canine infectious respiratory disease. J Clin Microbiol. 2004;42:4524-4529.

REFERENCES

1. Ditchfield J, Macpherson LW, Zbitnew A. Association of canine adenovirus (Toronto A 26/61) with an outbreak of laryngotracheitis ("kennel cough"): a preliminary report. Can Vet J. 1962;3:238-247.
2. Renshaw RW, Zylich NC, Laverack MA, et al. Pneumovirus in dogs with acute respiratory disease. Emerg Infect Dis. 2010;16:993-995.
3. Edinboro CH, Ward MP, Glickman LT. A placebo-controlled trial of two intranasal vaccines to prevent tracheobronchitis (kennel cough) in dogs entering a humane shelter. Prev Vet Med. 2004;62:89-99.
4. Larson LJ, Henningson J, Sharp P, et al. Efficacy of the canine influenza virus H3N8 vaccine to decrease severity of clinical disease after cochallenge with canine influenza virus and *Streptococcus equi* subsp. *zooepidemicus*. Clin Vaccine Immunol. 2011;18:559-564.
5. Damian M, Morales E, Salas G, et al. Immunohistochemical detection of antigens of distemper, adenovirus and parainfluenza viruses in domestic dogs with pneumonia. J Comp Pathol. 2005;133:289-293.
6. Erles K, Dubovi EJ, Brooks HW, et al. Longitudinal study of viruses associated with canine infectious respiratory disease. J Clin Microbiol. 2004;42:4524-4529.
7. Decaro N, Campolo M, Elia G, et al. Infectious canine hepatitis: an "old" disease reemerging in Italy. Res Vet Sci. 2007;83:269-273.
8. Lou TY, Wenner HA. Natural and experimental infection of dogs with reovirus type 1: pathogenicity of the strain for other animals. Am J Hygiene. 1963;77:293-304.
9. Benetka V, Weissenbock H, Kudielka I, et al. Canine adenovirus type 2 infection in four puppies with neurological signs. Vet Rec. 2006;158:91-94.
10. Buonavoglia C, Martella V. Canine respiratory viruses. Vet Res. 2007;38:355-373.

11. Appel MJ, Menegus M, Parsonson IM, et al. Pathogenesis of canine herpesvirus in specific-pathogen-free dogs: 5- to 12-week-old pups. Am J Vet Res. 1969;30:2067-2073.
12. Karpas A, Garcia FG, Calvo F, et al. Experimental production of canine tracheobronchitis (kennel cough) with canine herpesvirus isolated from naturally infected dogs. Am J Vet Res. 1968;29:1251-1257.
13. Ledbetter EC, Dubovi EJ, Kim SG, et al. Experimental primary ocular canine herpesvirus-1 infection in adult dogs. Am J Vet Res. 2009;70:513-521.
14. Ledbetter EC, Kim SG, Dubovi EJ, et al. Experimental reactivation of latent canine herpesvirus-1 and induction of recurrent ocular disease in adult dogs. Vet Microbiol. 2009;138:98-105.
15. Gadsden BJ, Maes RK, Wise AG, et al. Fatal canid herpesvirus 1 infection in an adult dog. J Vet Diagn Invest. 2012;24:604-607.
16. Webster RG, Bean WJ, Gorman OT, et al. Evolution and ecology of influenza A viruses. Microbiol Rev. 1992;56:152-179.
17. Crawford PC, Dubovi EJ, Castleman WL, et al. Transmission of equine influenza virus to dogs. Science. 2005;310:482-485.
18. Anderson TC, Bromfield CR, Crawford PC, et al. Serological evidence of H3N8 canine influenza-like virus circulation in USA dogs prior to 2004. Vet J. 2012;191:312-316.
19. Barrell EA, Pecoraro HL, Torres-Henderson C, et al. Seroprevalence and risk factors for canine H3N8 influenza virus exposure in household dogs in Colorado. J Vet Intern Med. 2010;24:1524-1527.
20. Crawford C, Spindel M. Canine influenza. In: Miller L, Hurley K, eds. Infectious Disease Management in Animal Shelters. Ames, IA: Wiley-Blackwell; 2009:173-180.
21. Lin Y, Zhao Y, Zeng X, et al. Genetic and pathobiologic characterization of H3N2 canine influenza viruses isolated in the Jiangsu Province of China in 2009-2010. Vet Microbiol. 2012;158:247-258.
22. Song D, Kang B, Lee C, et al. Transmission of avian influenza virus (H3N2) to dogs. Emerg Infect Dis. 2008;14:741-746.
23. Kim H, Song D, Moon H, et al. Inter- and intraspecies transmission of canine influenza virus (H3N2) in dogs, cats, and ferrets. Influenza and Other Respiratory Viruses. May 2012.
24. Song D, Moon HJ, An DJ, et al. A novel reassortant canine H3N1 influenza virus between pandemic H1N1 and canine H3N2 influenza viruses in Korea. J Gen Virol. 2012;93:551-554.
25. Zhan GJ, Ling ZS, Zhu YL, et al. Genetic characterization of a novel influenza A virus H5N2 isolated from a dog in China. Vet Microbiol. 2012;155:409-416.
26. Lin D, Sun S, Du L, et al. Natural and experimental infection of dogs with pandemic H1N1/2009 influenza virus. J Gen Virol. 2012;93:119-123.
27. Dundon WG, De Benedictis P, Viale E, et al. Serologic evidence of pandemic (H1N1) 2009 infection in dogs. Italy. Emerg Infect Dis. 2010;16:2019-2021.
28. Chen Y, Zhong G, Wang G, et al. Dogs are highly susceptible to H5N1 avian influenza virus. Virology. 2010;405:15-19.
29. Daly JM, Blunden AS, Macrae S, et al. Transmission of equine influenza virus to English foxhounds. Emerg Infect Dis. 2008;14:461-464.
30. Kirkland PD, Finlaison DS, Crispe E, et al. Influenza virus transmission from horses to dogs, Australia. Emerg Infect Dis. 2010;16:699-702.
31. Yamanaka T, Nemoto M, Tsujimura K, et al. Interspecies transmission of equine influenza virus (H3N8) to dogs by close contact with experimentally infected horses. Vet Microbiol. 2009;139:351-355.
32. Chatziandreou N, Stock N, Young D, et al. Relationships and host range of human, canine, simian and porcine isolates of simian virus 5 (parainfluenza virus 5). J Gen Virol. 2004;85:3007-3016.
33. Ellis JA, Krakowka GS. A review of canine parainfluenza virus infection in dogs. J Am Vet Med Assoc. 2012;240:273-284.
34. Evermann JF, Lincoln JD, McKiernan AJ. Isolation of a paramyxovirus from the cerebrospinal fluid of a dog with posterior paresis. J Am Vet Med Assoc. 1980;177:1132-1134.
35. Hsiung GD. Parainfluenza-5 virus. Infection of man and animal. Prog Med Virol. 1972;14:241-274.
36. Percopo CM, Dubovi EJ, Renshaw RW, et al. Canine pneumovirus replicates in mouse lung tissue and elicits inflammatory pathology. Virology. 2011;416:26-31.
37. Binn LN, Marchwicki RH, Keenan KP, et al. Recovery of reovirus type 2 from an immature dog with respiratory tract disease. Am J Vet Res. 1977;38:927-929.
38. Decaro N, Campolo M, Desario C, et al. Virological and molecular characterization of a mammalian orthoreovirus type 3 strain isolated from a dog in Italy. Vet Microbiol. 2005;109:19-27.
39. MacLachlan NJ, Dubovi EJ. Coronaviridae. In: Fenner's Veterinary Virology. 4th ed. Philadelphia, PA: Elsevier; 2011:393-413.
40. Erles K, Toomey C, Brooks HW, et al. Detection of a group 2 coronavirus in dogs with canine infectious respiratory disease. Virology. 2003;310:216-223.
41. Bryan HM, Darimont CT, Paquet PC, et al. Exposure to infectious agents in dogs in remote coastal British Columbia: possible sentinels of diseases in wildlife and humans. Can J Vet Res. 2011;75:11-17.
42. Knesl O, Allan FJ, Shields S. The seroprevalence of canine respiratory coronavirus and canine influenza virus in dogs in New Zealand. N Z Vet J. 2009;57:295-298.
43. An DJ, Jeong W, Yoon SH, et al. Genetic analysis of canine group 2 coronavirus in Korean dogs. Vet Microbiol. 2010;141:46-52.
44. Zicola A, Jolly S, Mathijs E, et al. Fatal outbreaks in dogs associated with pantropic canine coronavirus in France and Belgium. J Small Anim Pract. 2012;53:297-300.
45. Buonavoglia C, Decaro N, Martella V, et al. Canine coronavirus highly pathogenic for dogs. Emerg Infect Dis. 2006;12:492-494.
46. Decaro N, Campolo M, Lorusso A, et al. Experimental infection of dogs with a novel strain of canine coronavirus causing systemic disease and lymphopenia. Vet Microbiol. 2008;128:253-260.
47. Ledbetter EC, Hornbuckle WE, Dubovi EJ. Virologic survey of dogs with naturally acquired idiopathic conjunctivitis. J Am Vet Med Assoc. 2009;235:954-959.
48. Ledbetter EC, Kim SG, Dubovi EJ. Outbreak of ocular disease associated with naturally-acquired canine herpesvirus-1 infection in a closed domestic dog colony. Vet Ophthalmol. 2009;12:242-247.
49. Ledbetter EC, Riis RC, Kern TJ, et al. Corneal ulceration associated with naturally occurring canine herpesvirus-1 infection in two adult dogs. J Am Vet Med Assoc. 2006;229:376-384.
50. Gervais KJ, Pirie CG, Ledbetter EC, et al. Acute primary canine herpesvirus-1 dendritic ulcerative keratitis in an adult dog. Vet Ophthalmol. 2012;15:133-138.
51. Erles K, Shiu KB, Brownlie J. Isolation and sequence analysis of canine respiratory coronavirus. Virus Res. 2007;124:78-87.
52. Mitchell JA, Brooks H, Shiu KB, et al. Development of a quantitative real-time PCR for the detection of canine respiratory coronavirus. J Virol Methods. 2009;155:136-142.
53. Anderson TC, Crawford PC, Katz JM, et al. Diagnostic performance of the canine Influenza A Virus subtype H3N8 hemagglutination inhibition assay. J Vet Diagn Invest. 2012;24:499-508.
54. Castleman WL, Powe JR, Crawford PC, et al. Canine H3N8 influenza virus infection in dogs and mice. Vet Pathol. 2010;47:507-517.
55. Rodriguez-Tovar LE, Ramirez-Romero R, Valdez-Nava Y, et al. Combined distemper-adenoviral pneumonia in a dog. Can Vet J. 2007;48:632-634.
56. Deshpande M, Abdelmagid O, Tubbs A, et al. Experimental reproduction of canine influenza virus H3N8 infection in young puppies. Vet Ther. 2009;10:29-39.
57. Australian Government Department of Agriculture, Fisheries, and Forestry. http://www.daff.gov.au/aqis/cat-dogs/cat4?name=theUSA (not including Hawaii). Last accessed January 28, 2013.
58. Jacobs AA, Theelen RP, Jaspers R, et al. Protection of dogs for 13 months against *Bordetella bronchiseptica* and canine parainfluenza virus with a modified live vaccine. Vet Rec. 2005;157:19-23.
59. Kontor EJ, Wegrzyn RJ, Goodnow RA. Canine infectious tracheobronchitis: effects of an intranasal live canine parainfluenza–*Bordetella bronchiseptica* vaccine on viral shedding and clinical tracheobronchitis (kennel cough). Am J Vet Res. 1981;42:1694-1698.

60. Chladek DW, Williams JM, Gerber DL, et al. Canine parainfluenza–*Bordetella bronchiseptica* vaccine immunogenicity. Am J Vet Res. 1981;42:266-270.
61. Emery JB, House JA, Bittle JL, et al. A canine parainfluenza viral vaccine: immunogenicity and safety. Am J Vet Res. 1976;37:1323-1327.
62. Mouzin DE, Lorenzen MJ, Haworth JD, et al. Duration of serologic response to five viral antigens in dogs. J Am Vet Med Assoc. 2004;224:55-60.
63. Welborn LV, DeVries JG, Ford R, et al. 2011 AAHA canine vaccination guidelines. J Am Anim Hosp Assoc. 2011;47:1-42.
64. Tyler KL, Barton ES, Ibach ML, et al. Isolation and molecular characterization of a novel type 3 reovirus from a child with meningitis. J Infect Dis. 2004;189:1664-1675.

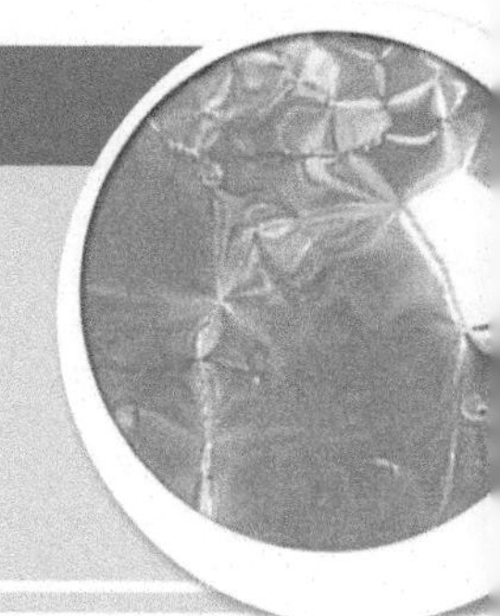

Infectious Canine Hepatitis

Jane E. Sykes

Overview of Infectious Canine Hepatitis

First Described: First described as infectious canine hepatitis (ICH) in 1947 in Sweden by Rubarth[1]; CAV-1 was first isolated in chick embryos in 1951[2]

Cause: Canine adenovirus-1 (family Adenoviridae, genus *Mastadenovirus*)

Affected Hosts: Dogs, coyotes, foxes, wolves, bears, skunks

Geographic Distribution: Worldwide

Mode of Transmission: Direct contact with infected saliva, feces and urine, and contaminated fomites

Major Clinical Signs in Dogs: Fever, lethargy, inappetence, vomiting, hemorrhagic diarrhea, abdominal pain, dehydration, conjunctivitis, petechial hemorrhages, tachypnea, cough, corneal edema ("blue eye"), rarely icterus or neurologic signs.

Differential Diagnoses: Other systemic viral diseases such as parvoviral enteritis and canine distemper, enteric viral and bacterial infections, hepatotoxicosis (e.g., mushrooms), Rocky Mountain spotted fever, gastrointestinal foreign body, dietary indiscretion, leptospirosis, portosystemic shunting with hepatic encephalopathy, disseminated fungal infections (especially systemic candidiasis), systemic protozoal infections (especially sarcocystosis, toxoplasmosis or African trypanosomiasis), hemic neoplasia (especially lymphoma).

Human Health Significance: CAV-1 does not infect humans.

Etiology and Epidemiology

Infectious canine hepatitis (ICH) is an uncommonly recognized disease of dogs that is caused by canine adenovirus type 1 (CAV-1), a non-enveloped, icosahedral double-stranded DNA virus that is antigenically related to CAV-2 (see Chapter 17) (Figure 18-1). CAV-1 also causes disease in wolves, coyotes, skunks, and bears, as well as encephalitis in foxes, but the diversity of wildlife hosts is not as great as that for CDV. Ferrets are not susceptible.[3] ICH has also been referred to as Rubarth's disease, after Carl Sven Rubarth, a veterinarian who first described the disease in the late 1940s.[1] Over the subsequent 10 years, ICH was described worldwide, including the United States, Canada, United Kingdom, Australia, Japan, Brazil, and throughout Europe. The virus can survive for months at room temperature, but should be readily inactivated by disinfectants with activity against canine parvovirus (CPV).[4] Disease most commonly occurs in dogs that are less than 1 year of age, but was reported in adult dogs before widespread vaccination for ICH was introduced.

The strong antigenic relationship between CAV-1 and CAV-2 is clinically important, because vaccines that contain CAV-2 protect against infection with CAV-1 and vice versa. After the introduction of CAV-1 vaccines, ICH largely disappeared, but over the past decade it has reemerged, with published reports of disease from Italy, Switzerland, and the United States.[5-8] Disease in Europe has been associated with puppy trading from kennels in eastern European countries and possibly spillover of virus circulating in wildlife.[9] In Italy, three outbreaks occurred in shelters in southern Italy, and the others involved purebred puppies imported from Hungary a few days before the onset of clinical signs. Several of the dogs were co-infected with other viruses, such as canine distemper virus (CDV), CPV, or canine enteric coronavirus. Encephalopathy due to CAV-1 infection was described in nine 5-week-old Labrador retriever puppies from Arkansas in the United States, all of which belonged to the same litter.[8] The litter was from an unvaccinated bitch. These case descriptions confirm that CAV-1 continues to circulate in the dog population and can result in severe disease in young dogs when vaccination does not occur, is improperly timed, and stress, co-infections, and overcrowded conditions prevail.

Clinical Features

Signs and Their Pathogenesis

CAV-1 is shed in saliva, feces, and urine, and transmission occurs through direct dog-to-dog contact or contact with contaminated fomites such as hands, utensils, and clothing. Ectoparasites such as fleas and ticks are also potential mechanical vectors.[4] Airborne transmission does not appear to be important. Initial infection occurs through the nasopharyngeal, conjunctival, or oropharyngeal route, and the virus replicates within the tonsils, after which it spreads to regional lymph nodes and the bloodstream via lymphatics. Subsequently, infection of hepatocytes and endothelial cells within a variety of tissues occurs, such as the lungs, liver, kidneys, spleen, and eye with resultant hemorrhage, necrosis, and inflammation. The virus replicates in the nucleus of host cells, where crystalline arrays of virions form. There is severe condensation and margination of nuclear chromatin, with inclusion body formation (Figure 18-2). The virions are released by cell lysis, which leads to tissue injury and disseminated intravascular coagulation (DIC). Within the liver, the virus initially infects Kupffer's cells and subsequently spreads to hepatocytes.

Clinical signs generally occur after an incubation period of 4 to 9 days, although many dogs probably show no signs of illness.[4] Three overlapping disease syndromes have been described. The first is peracute disease with circulatory collapse, coma, and death after a brief illness that lasts less than 24 to 48 hours. The second, most commonly described syndrome is acute disease, which is associated with high morbidity and reported mortality rates of around 10% to 30%.[4] Dogs with acute disease

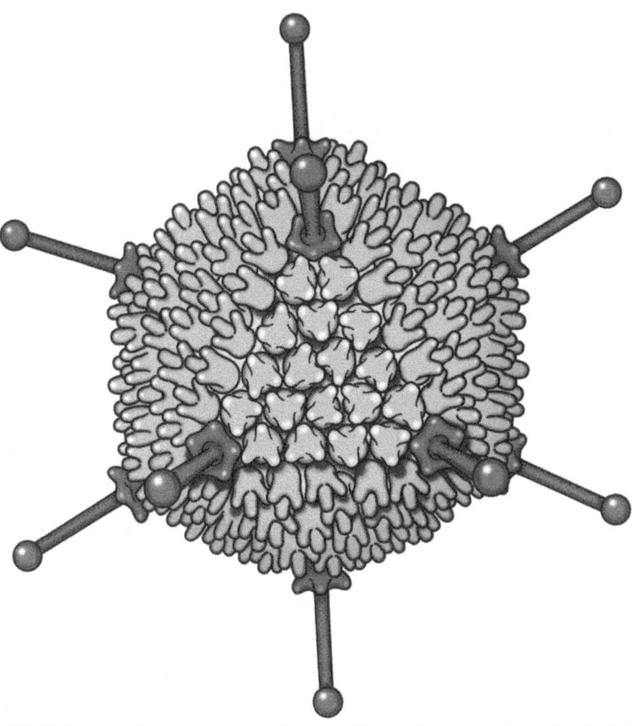

FIGURE 18-1 Structure of canine adenovirus. The virus is a non-enveloped, Icosahedral virus with fibers (purple) that radiate outwards from the virion.

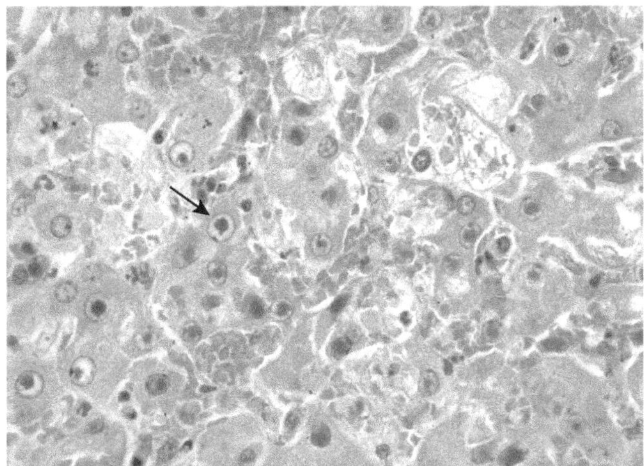

FIGURE 18-2 Infection of hepatocytes and endothelial cells with CAV-1 produces characteristic basophilic intranuclear inclusions surrounded by a clear zone that separates them from the marginated chromatin *(arrow)*. H&E stain. (Courtesy Dr. W. Crowell, College of Veterinary Medicine, The University of Georgia and Noah's Archive, College of Veterinary Medicine, The University of Georgia. In Zachary JF, McGavin M. Pathologic Basis of Veterinary Disease, 5 ed. St. Louis, MO: Mosby; 2012.)

either recover or die within a 2-week period. The third is a more chronic form that occurs in dogs with partial immunity, with death due to hepatic failure weeks (subacute disease) or months (chronic infection) after initial infection.[10]

Acute disease is variably characterized by the presence of fever, tonsillitis, conjunctivitis, inappetence, lethargy, weakness, polydipsia, vomiting, hematemesis, diarrhea, cough, tachypnea, and icterus. Diarrhea may contain frank blood or melena. Widespread petechial and ecchymotic hemorrhages and hematuria can be seen. Corneal edema ("blue eye") occurs in the first week of illness and results from replication of virus within corneal endothelial cells (Figure 18-3). Rarely, neurologic signs such

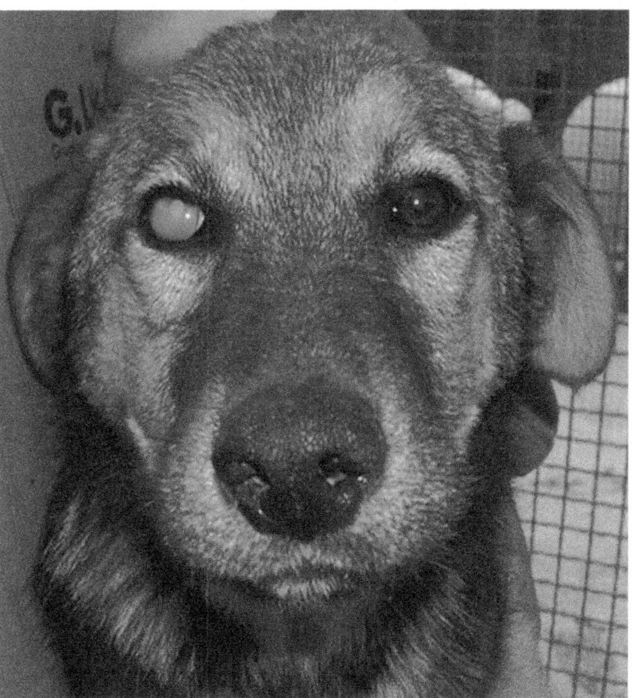

FIGURE 18-3 Young adult dog with corneal edema from an Italian shelter outbreak of CAV-1 infection. (Courtesy Dr. Nicola Decaro, Department of Veterinary Public Health, Faculty of Veterinary Medicine of Bari, Italy.)

as seizures, ataxia, circling, apparent blindness, head pressing, and nystagmus have been reported in association with CAV-1 encephalitis.[7,8] The development of neurologic signs may also represent hepatic encephalopathy, intracranial thrombosis or hemorrhage, or, as occurred in one outbreak, concurrent infection with CDV.[7]

The antibody response appears 7 days after infection and limits tissue damage. Viral persistence within the renal glomeruli, uveal structures of the eye (the iris and ciliary body), and the cornea can trigger immune complex formation in dogs that recover from acute illness. This leads to glomerulonephritis with proteinuria, severe uveitis, and persistent corneal edema in some surviving dogs. Glomerulonephritis usually occurs about 1 to 2 weeks after the acute signs resolve. Glomerular lesions contain deposits of viral antigen, IgG, IgM, and C3.[11,12] Infection of the glomerular endothelium is followed by a persistent tubular infection, development of interstitial nephritis, and viruria, but chronic renal failure has not been described. Viral shedding in the urine can occur for up to 6 to 9 months after infection. Anterior uveitis is associated with massive influx of inflammatory cells into the anterior chamber. Occasionally persistent corneal edema fails to resolve for months and may be associated with complications such as glaucoma.[13] The Afghan hound is reportedly susceptible to this complication.[14]

In experimental infections with CAV-1, chronic hepatitis with extensive fibrosis was observed in some dogs that recovered from acute illness, with survival for up to 8 months.[10] The virus could not be found in hepatic lesions from these dogs. Attempts to detect CAV-1 in the liver of other dogs with chronic active hepatitis using PCR assays have to date been unrewarding.[15-17]

Physical Examination Findings

Physical examination findings in dogs with acute ICH vary, but might include lethargy, dehydration, fever (up to 106°F or 41°C),

TABLE 18-1

Diagnostic Assays Available for Infectious Canine Hepatitis

Assay	Specimen Type	Target	Performance
Histopathology	Usually necropsy specimens, but also liver biopsy	Hepatic necrosis with intranuclear inclusions; CAV-1 antigen with immunohistochemistry	True sensitivity and specificity of inclusion visualization unknown. Liver biopsy may not be feasible because of coagulopathies.
Polymerase chain reaction (PCR)	Blood; rectal, conjunctival and nasal swabs; urine; tissues collected at necropsy	CAV-1 DNA	Sensitivity and specificity may vary depending on assay design. Specific CAV-1 assays are not widely offered by commercial veterinary diagnostic laboratories. Some assays differentiate between vaccine (CAV-2) and field virus (CAV-1). The significance of a positive result from urine may be difficult to interpret due to subclinical shedding. False-negative results may occur as a result of PCR assay inhibition by components of feces or in dogs with subacute or chronic presentations.
Virus isolation	All body secretions, tissues	CAV-1	Sensitive and specific, but generally only available as a research tool.

CAV, Canine adenovirus.

congestion and enlargement of the tonsils (which may be severe), pallor, conjunctivitis, peripheral lymphadenopathy, tachypnea, increased lung sounds, and tachycardia. In some reports, serous to mucopurulent ocular and nasal discharge have been observed, but these may have resulted from co-infections with other respiratory viruses.[4] Abdominal palpation may reveal hepatomegaly, splenomegaly, or abdominal pain. Icterus is uncommon but can occur in dogs with a more prolonged course of disease. Peripheral edema that involves the head, neck, and ventral abdomen has been described.[18] Puppies with CAV-1 encephalitis may show signs of circling, vocalization, head pressing, ataxia, and blindness.[8] Coagulopathies may be manifested as cutaneous or mucosal petechial hemorrhages; gingival hemorrhages; epistaxis; or prolonged bleeding from venipuncture sites.

Ocular complications occur in at least 20% of affected dogs. Unilateral or, less commonly, bilateral corneal edema may be observed, which initially develops at the limbus and is occasionally associated with blepharospasm, photophobia, and a serous ocular discharge.[13] Unilateral involvement may progress to bilateral involvement over several days. Using a slit lamp, the cornea is markedly thickened, and there is episcleral and ciliary injection. Uveitis may also be apparent. Corneal ulceration and increased intraocular pressure has also been described in dogs with corneal edema, the latter of which may result in blindness.[13]

Diagnosis

ICH should be suspected in any dog less than 1 year of age that has a questionable vaccination history and signs of fever, respiratory, gastrointestinal, and hepatic disease, and certainly in any young dog that develops corneal edema. Diagnosis is easily achieved at necropsy when characteristic intranuclear inclusion bodies are seen in tissues, but the sensitivity and specificity of this finding is unknown. Inclusion bodies may be seen on impression smears of liver biopsies or tissue obtained at necropsy. At the time of writing, antemortem diagnosis is challenging owing to the lack of commercially available assays that specifically detect the virus or viral DNA, and the disease may be underdiagnosed (Table 18-1). Serologic assays are available, but they provide only retrospective diagnosis, and interpretation of these assays may be a challenge when there is a history of vaccination.

Laboratory Abnormalities

Complete Blood Count

Findings reported on the CBC are variable and include leukopenia, anemia, increased nucleated red blood cells, and moderate to severe thrombocytopenia. Leukopenia occurs early in the course of infection and may be profound. Initially there is a lymphopenia, after which neutropenia occurs and worsens progressively until death.[18] Increased band neutrophils and toxic changes may also be present. Occasionally leukocytosis is observed.[19] Leukocytosis and lymphocytosis may occur as part of the recovery process.

Serum Biochemical Tests

Changes on the serum biochemistry profile include increased activity of serum ALT (sometimes >1000 U/L) and ALP, hyperbilirubinemia, hypoglycemia, and hypoalbuminemia.[20] Determination of serum ammonia concentration may facilitate diagnosis of hepatic encephalopathy in dogs with neurologic signs.

Urinalysis

The urinalysis of dogs with ICH may reveal proteinuria, hyaline and granular cylindruria, hematuria, and bilirubinuria.

Coagulation Profile

In addition to thrombocytopenia, coagulation abnormalities reported in ICH reflect the presence of DIC and hepatic failure and include prolonged prothrombin time, markedly prolonged activated partial thromboplastin time (to 6 to 7 times control values), decreased factor VIII activity, hypofibrinogenemia, and increased fibrinogen degradation products. Platelet function assays have shown reduced platelet adhesion.[18]

Diagnostic Imaging

Findings on plain radiography and abdominal sonography in dogs with ICH have not been reported. Plain radiography might reveal a normal to slightly enlarged liver, and poor detail as a result of abdominal effusion or the young age (and therefore low intra-abdominal fat content) of affected dogs.

Microbiologic Tests

Virus Isolation

CAV-1 can be readily isolated in a variety of cell types, such as Madin-Darby canine kidney cells.[7,8] In dogs with acute illness, any body fluid or tissue is likely to contain sufficient virus for isolation. Cultures are evaluated for a cytopathic effect with intranuclear inclusions, and the presence of CAV-1 is confirmed using immunostaining. Isolation is not widely offered by commercial veterinary diagnostic laboratories.

Serologic Diagnosis

Serologic tests are available commercially for detection of IgG and IgM against CAV-1, which include ELISA assays, hemagglutination-inhibition, and serum neutralization. Unfortunately, dogs with acute disease may die before they develop antibodies to the virus.[10] For dogs that recover from illness, a recent history of vaccination may complicate interpretation of acute and convalescent phase serology. In the absence of a vaccination history, a fourfold rise in titer over a 2- to 3-week period together with compatible clinical signs is supportive of the diagnosis of ICH. Titers that follow natural infection may be higher than those that follow vaccination.

Molecular Diagnosis Using the Polymerase Chain Reaction

Conventional PCR assays for detection of CAV-1 in clinical specimens such as nasal, rectal, and ocular swabs and blood, as well as tissue obtained at necropsy, have been described. These include assays that differentiate between CAV-1 and CAV-2[21] and represent one of the most rapid means of antemortem diagnosis. Because of the rarity of the disease, the clinical sensitivity and specificity of these assays are not well understood. Real-time PCR assays that specifically detect CAV-1 infection were not available at the time of writing (see Chapter 5 for a discussion of the differences between conventional and real-time PCR assays). The results of PCR assays on urine may be more difficult to interpret than those for other specimens, because of the potential for chronic shedding from this site in the absence of clinical signs. Assays that specifically detect CAV-1 differentiate between virulent CAV-1 virus and vaccine virus, because vaccines for ICH all contain only CAV-2.

Pathologic Findings

Gross Pathologic Findings

Gross pathologic findings in dogs with ICH include blood-tinged ascites or hemoabdomen; a slightly enlarged, congested or mottled liver; mild splenomegaly; enlarged, congested, and edematous lymph nodes; and fibrin deposition on the surface of abdominal viscera (Figure 18-4). The gallbladder wall is typically markedly thickened and edematous. Petechial and ecchymotic subserosal hemorrhages may be apparent in multiple viscera, and the intestinal tract may contain bloody fluid. The brain may also contain petechial hemorrhages or areas of gray discoloration.[8] Parenchymal organs may contain fibrin thrombi. Occasionally, multifocal pulmonary consolidation and/or serosanguineous pleural fluid is noted.

Histopathologic Findings

Histopathologic findings are variable and depend on the course of infection and possibly the virus strain. The most characteristic finding is hepatocellular necrosis and intranuclear viral inclusion bodies within Kupffer's cells and hepatocytes, and a mixed

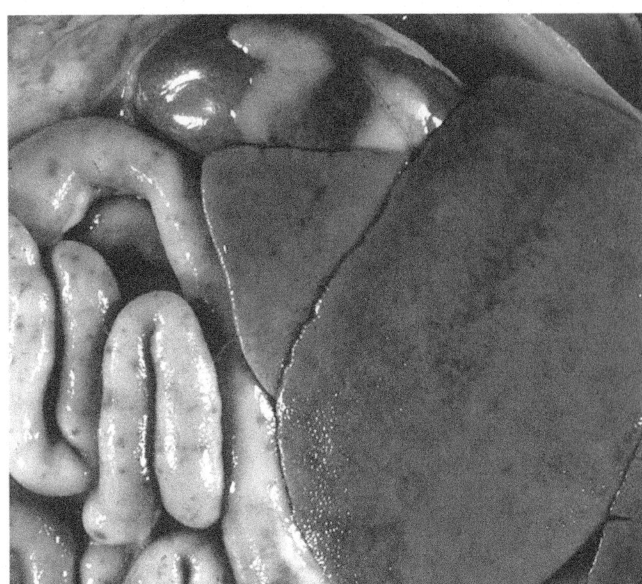

FIGURE 18-4 Infectious canine hepatitis, hepatic necrosis, liver, dog. The liver from dogs with ICH can be slightly enlarged and friable with a blotchy yellow discoloration. Sometimes fibrin is evident on the capsular surface. Note the petechiae on the serosal surface of the intestines caused by vascular damage. (Courtesy Dr. M.D. McGavin, College of Veterinary Medicine, University of Tennessee. In Zachary JF, McGavin MD. Pathologic Basis of Veterinary Disease, 5 ed. St. Louis, MO: Mosby; 2012.)

inflammatory cell infiltrate (see Figure 18-2). Fibrosis may be observed in dogs with chronic liver injury. Interstitial nephritis, with focal accumulations of neutrophils, mononuclear cells, and fibrosis, may also be present,[22] as well as evidence of widespread hemorrhage, thrombosis, and necrosis as a result of DIC. Findings in dogs with CAV-1 encephalitis have included mild spongiosis, neuronal necrosis, hemorrhage, and perivascular cuffing with mononuclear cells.[8] Viral inclusion bodies may be found in endothelial cells of meningeal vessels, the cornea, renal glomeruli, and the tonsils. Immunohistochemistry can be used to confirm the presence of the virus within tissues.

Treatment and Prognosis

Supportive Care

Treatment of dogs with acute ICH is purely supportive and consists primarily of fluid therapy, including crystalloid fluids and blood products. Fluid therapy should be aggressive with careful monitoring and avoidance of overhydration, because of increased vascular permeability and hypoalbuminemia. Fluids should be supplemented with electrolytes and dextrose as required. Other medications that may be indicated include antiemetics, antacids, sucralfate, whole blood or plasma transfusions, and colloids such as hetastarch. Partial or total parenteral nutrition may be indicated for severely affected dogs that do not tolerate enteral feeding. Dogs with DIC may require treatment with heparin in addition to plasma. Management of hepatic encephalopathy with lactulose enemas, oral lactulose (in the absence of vomiting), and poorly absorbed oral antimicrobial drugs such as ampicillin may also be indicated. The use of parenteral broad-spectrum antimicrobial drugs should be considered for dogs with hemorrhagic gastroenteritis that may develop bacteremia as a result of bacterial translocation. After fluorescein staining has shown no evidence of corneal ulceration, dogs with severe corneal edema and uveitis should be treated with topical ophthalmic preparations that contain glucocorticoids and atropine to prevent development of glaucoma.

Prognosis depends on the severity of disease, which reflects the immune status of the affected dog and possibly the virus strain. There is a possibility that recovered dogs may develop chronic hepatitis or chronic glomerulonephritis, but the extent to which this truly occurs is unknown.

Immunity and Vaccination

Immunity to natural infection with CAV-1 is probably lifelong. Effective vaccines have been available and widely used as part of core vaccine programs for dogs for many years. Immunity after immunization with attenuated live vaccines lasts at least 3 years and probably longer. Early vaccines, which contained CAV-1, were associated with the development of corneal edema and glomerulonephritis in a small percentage (<1%) of immunized dogs. Replacement of attenuated live CAV-1 with CAV-2 occurred after 1980 and eliminated this complication.[23] These vaccines have the potential to cause transient respiratory signs and tonsillitis in dogs if accidental inhalation occurs, so care should be taken not to aerosolize the vaccine during administration. Maternal antibody persists until puppies are 12 weeks of age and interferes with immunization when virus neutralization titers exceed 1:100. Vaccines should be administered every 3 to 4 weeks from 6 weeks of age, with the last vaccine given no earlier than 16 weeks of age (see Appendix). Vaccine virus may be shed from the respiratory tract by dogs after vaccination, which has the potential to immunize other dogs as well. It has been suggested that this phenomenon may have been responsible for the virtual disappearance of the disease in the dog population in regions where vaccination is widely performed.[24]

Prevention

The best means of prevention of ICH is proper vaccination. Additional control measures that could be considered in locations where outbreaks occur, such as in shelters, include proper disinfection, isolation, and prevention of overcrowding and other co-infections, which may worsen disease. Because contact with wild animal species such as coyotes, wolves, and foxes that might be shedding the virus may also be a source of infection for dogs, exclusion of these species from interactions with domestic dogs may also serve to prevent the disease.

Public Health Aspects

There is no evidence that CAV-1 infects humans.

SUGGESTED READINGS

Decaro N, Campolo M, Elia G, et al. Infectious canine hepatitis: an "old" disease reemerging in Italy. Res Vet Sci. 2007;83:269-273.

Gocke DJ, Preisig R, Morris TQ, et al. Experimental viral hepatitis in the dog: production of persistent disease in partially immune animals. J Clin Invest. 1967;46:1506-1517.

REFERENCES

1. Rubarth S. An acute virus disease with liver lesion in dogs (hepatitis contagiosa canis): a pathologico-anatomical and etiological investigation. Acta Path Microbiol Scand. 1947(Suppl):69.
2. Miles JA, Parry HB, Larin NM, et al. Cultivation of canine hepatitis virus in embryonated hen's eggs and its subsequent transmission to dogs. Nature. 1951;168(4277):699-700.
3. Hudson JR, Mansi W. Rubarth's disease (canine virus hepatitis) II. The insusceptibility of ferrets to experimental infection. J Comp Pathol. 1953;63:335-345.
4. Cabasso VJ. Infectious canine hepatitis virus. Ann N Y Acad Sci. 1962;101:498-514.
5. Pratelli A, Martella V, Elia G, et al. Severe enteric disease in an animal shelter associated with dual infections by canine adenovirus type 1 and canine coronavirus. J Vet Med B Infect Dis Vet Public Health. 2001;48:385-392.
6. Muller C, Sieber-Ruckstuhl N, Decaro N, et al. [Infectious canine hepatitis in 4 dogs in Switzerland]. Schweiz Arch Tierheilkd. 2010;152:63-68.
7. Decaro N, Campolo M, Elia G, et al. Infectious canine hepatitis: an "old" disease reemerging in Italy. Res Vet Sci. 2007;83:269-273.
8. Caudell D, Confer AW, Fulton RW, et al. Diagnosis of infectious canine hepatitis virus (CAV-1) infection in puppies with encephalopathy. J Vet Diagn Invest. 2005;17:58-61.
9. Decaro N. Infectious canine hepatitis—a re-emerging disease. Sevilla, Spain: 21st ECVIM-CA Congress; 2011:78–79.
10. Gocke DJ, Preisig R, Morris TQ, et al. Experimental viral hepatitis in the dog: production of persistent disease in partially immune animals. J Clin Invest. 1967;46:1506-1517.
11. Morrison WI, Nash AS, Wright NG. Glomerular deposition of immune complexes in dogs following natural infection with canine adenovirus. Vet Rec. 1975;96:522-524.
12. Hervas J, Gomez-Villamandos JC, Perez J, et al. Focal mesangial-sclerosing glomerulonephritis and acute-spontaneous infectious canine hepatitis: structural, immunohistochemical and subcellular studies. Vet Immunol Immunopathol. 1997;57:25-32.
13. Curtis R, Barnett KC. The ocular lesions of infectious canine hepatitis. 1. Clinical features. J Small Anim Pract. 1973;14:375-389.
14. Curtis R, Barnett KC. Canine adenovirus-induced ocular lesions in the Afghan hound. Cornell Vet. 1981;71:85-95.
15. Chouinard L, Martineau D, Forget C, et al. Use of polymerase chain reaction and immunohistochemistry for detection of canine adenovirus type 1 in formalin-fixed, paraffin-embedded liver of dogs with chronic hepatitis or cirrhosis. J Vet Diagn Invest. 1998;10:320-325.
16. Boomkens SY, Slump E, Egberink HF, et al. PCR screening for candidate etiological agents of canine hepatitis. Vet Microbiol. 2005;108:49-55.
17. Bexfield NH, Andres-Abdo C, Scase TJ, et al. Chronic hepatitis in the English springer spaniel: clinical presentation, histological description and outcome. Vet Rec. 2011;169(16):415.
18. Wigton DH, Kociba GJ, Hoover EA. Infectious canine hepatitis: animal model for viral-induced disseminated intravascular coagulation. Blood. 1976;47:287-296.
19. Kobayashi Y, Ochiai K, Itakura C. Dual infection with canine distemper virus and infectious canine hepatitis virus (canine adenovirus type 1) in a dog. J Vet Med Sci. 1993;55:699-701.
20. Beckett SD, Burns MJ, Clark CH. A study of the blood glucose, serum transaminase, and electrophoretic patterns of dogs with infectious canine hepatitis. Am J Vet Res. 1964;25:1186-1190.
21. Hu RL, Huang G, Qiu W, et al. Detection and differentiation of CAV-1 and CAV-2 by polymerase chain reaction. Vet Res Commun. 2001;25:77-84.
22. Wright NG. Interstitial nephritis in a dog associated with infectious canine hepatitis virus. Vet Rec. 1970;86:92-93.
23. Bass EP, Gill MA, Beckenhauer WH. Evaluation of a canine adenovirus type 2 strain as a replacement for infectious canine hepatitis vaccine. J Am Vet Med Assoc. 1980;177:234-242.
24. MacLachlan NJ, Dubovi EJ. Adenoviridae. Fenner's Veterinary Virology. 4th ed. Elsevier; 2011:203-212.

CHAPTER 19

Feline Panleukopenia Virus Infection and Other Viral Enteritides

Jane E. Sykes

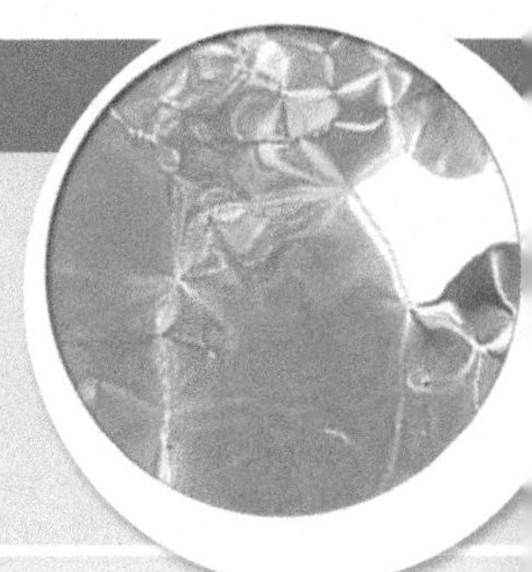

Overview of Feline Parvoviral Enteritis

First Described: 1928, Verge and Christoforoni, France[1]

Cause: Feline panleukopenia virus (FPV); also canine parvovirus (CPV)-2a, CPV-2b, and CPV-2c (Family Parvoviridae, subfamily Parvovirinae, genus *Parvovirus*)

Affected Hosts: Domestic and wild cats; foxes, mink, and raccoons

Geographic Distribution: Worldwide

Mode of Transmission: Direct contact with virus in feces and vomitus and contaminated fomites.

Major Clinical Signs: Fever, lethargy, inappetence, vomiting, diarrhea, dehydration, sudden death. Neurologic signs (primarily cerebellar signs) may also occur.

Differential Diagnoses: Other feline viral enteritides, toxins, gastrointestinal foreign body, enteric parasitic infections such as giardiasis and nematode infections, enteric bacterial infections such as salmonellosis, pancreatitis, or inflammatory bowel disease. Congenital central nervous system defects should be considered in cats with neurologic signs.

Human Health Significance: FPV is not known to infect humans, but was isolated from a monkey.

Etiology and Epidemiology

Feline panleukopenia virus (FPV) is a parvovirus that causes enteritis and panleukopenia in domestic and wild cat species worldwide.[2] It has also been associated with disease in raccoons, mink, foxes, and a monkey, and can replicate in ferrets without causing disease. Feline panleukopenia is sometimes confusingly referred to as "cat plague" and "feline distemper." FPV is a small, single-stranded non-enveloped DNA virus that is closely related to CPV-2, but in contrast to CPV-2, which emerged in the late 1970s, the existence of FPV has been known since the 1920s.[1] FPV has the same ability as CPV-2 to survive long periods in the environment and resist disinfection, and has the same preference for replication in rapidly dividing cells (see Chapter 14).

Feline panleukopenia is most likely to occur in cats younger than 1 year of age, but it can occur in unvaccinated or improperly vaccinated cats of all ages. The median age of affected cats in one study was 4 months, and when disease occurred in vaccinated cats, it occurred only in cats that had not received a booster vaccine after 12 weeks of age.[3] However, kitten deaths have been reported in households of fully vaccinated kittens, possibly because of exposure to large amounts of virus in the environment.[4] Outbreaks of panleukopenia in cats correlate seasonally with increases in susceptible newborn kitten numbers. Panleukopenia occurs most commonly in multicat households, and especially in enclosed, shelter environments. It can also occur in cats with outdoor exposure, such as barn, feral, and stray cats. In one study, the prevalence of protective antibody titers to FPV in feral cats in Florida was only 33%, which suggested a low rate of exposure to the virus.[5] In some North American shelters, devastating outbreaks of panleukopenia have led to euthanasia of large numbers of cats. Contact with other cats may not be present in the history, because fomite transmission is so effective.[3] FPV replicates to a limited extent in dogs, without disease or virus shedding. Some feline panleukopenia results from infection of cats by the related mink enteritis virus, CPV-2a, CPV-2b, or CPV-2c.[6-8] Mixed infections with FPV and CPV-2 variants have been detected in cats, and there is evidence for recombination between FPV and CPV-2 variants.[7,9] Infection of cats with CPV-2 variants is uncommon in Europe but predominated among cats with panleukopenia in Asia.[10]

Other viral pathogens that have been associated with gastroenteritis in cats include feline enteric coronavirus (see Chapter 20), FeLV, rotaviruses, caliciviruses, reoviruses, and astroviruses. A torovirus-like agent has been associated with a syndrome of diarrhea and protrusion of the nictating membranes in cats.[11] Togavirus-like and picornavirus-like particles have been identified in the feces of Australian cats, but their significance is uncertain.[12]

Clinical Features

Signs and Their Pathogenesis

The pathogenesis of FPV infection is similar to that of CPV infection (see Chapter 14). Transmission is by the fecal-oral route, and indirect transmission through contaminated fomites represents the most important means of infection. Like CPV, FPV enters cells using transferrin receptors[13] and replicates in cells that are in the S-phase of the mitotic cycle. Initially, the virus replicates in oropharyngeal lymphoid tissue, after which it disseminates in blood to all tissues. Infection of lymphoid tissues leads to lymphoid tissue necrosis. Infection of the marrow is associated with leukopenia, which is compounded by neutrophil sequestration in damaged gastrointestinal tissue. The virus replicates in the intestinal crypt epithelial cells, with shortening of villi, increased intestinal permeability, and malabsorption.

Subclinical infection is probably widespread, especially in young adult or adult, immune-competent cats. Disease severity depends on factors such as age, immune status, and concurrent infections with other bacterial or viral pathogens, which increase the turnover rate of intestinal epithelial cells and enhance viral replication and cellular destruction. Co-infections can occur with feline enteric coronavirus, *Clostridium piliforme, Salmonella* spp., FeLV, or astroviruses.[14-17] Disease generally occurs after an incubation period of 2 to 10 days. The peracute form of disease involves death without apparent premonitory signs. Infection of kittens or adult cats results in clinical signs of fever, lethargy, vocalization, weakness, and inappetence, which may progress to profound dehydration, vomiting, sometimes watery to hemorrhagic diarrhea, and rapid loss of weight. Some cats develop only anorexia and lethargy, in the absence of vomiting, diarrhea, or leukopenia.[3] Secondary bacterial infections appear to be essential for signs of disease to occur. Death usually results from complications relating to dehydration, electrolyte imbalances, hypoglycemia, hemorrhage, or bacteremia and endotoxemia.

In the developing fetus or neonate, FPV replicates in a variety of tissues. Abortion, congenital abnormalities, or infertility can result from infection early in pregnancy, although the queen is generally otherwise unaffected. Later in pregnancy or in neonates up to approximately 1 week of age, viral destruction of Purkinje cells and granule precursor cells located in the cerebellar external granular layer leads to cerebellar hypoplasia (Figure 19-1). The severity of infection can vary between kittens in a litter. Sometimes a portion of the litter fails to survive and the remainder develop neurologic signs.[18] Signs of cerebellar ataxia are nonprogressive and are most apparent when kittens begin to walk at about 2 to 3 weeks of age, although mentation and appetite are otherwise normal, and these kittens can sometimes make acceptable pets. Other developmental central nervous system (CNS) abnormalities have been reported less commonly, and include hydrocephalus, porencephaly (cystic lesions within the cerebral hemispheres), or hydranencephaly (complete replacement of the cerebral hemispheres with cystic lesions). These abnormalities may be accompanied by signs of forebrain damage, such as seizures and behavioral changes. Unlike canine parvoviruses, FPV appears to be able to infect neurons other than the cerebellar Purkinje cells, which are terminally differentiated cells.[19] Ocular lesions can also develop and include retinal folding, dysplasia and degeneration, and optic nerve hypoplasia.

The DNA of FPV has been detected in the myocardium of cats with hypertrophic, dilated, and restrictive cardiomyopathy, but was not detected in a subset of healthy control cats.[20] Additional studies to assess the role of FPV in feline myocarditis and cardiomyopathy are needed.

Fecal shedding of virus usually lasts for several days, and in some cats, it may persist for up to 6 weeks. Kittens infected in utero have been reported to develop immune tolerance to the virus, with viral persistence in the kidneys and lungs for up to 1 year in the absence of shedding.

Physical Examination Findings

The most common physical examination findings are weakness, lethargy, and dehydration. Fever (103°F to 107°F or 39.5°C to 42.5°C) may be present early in the course of illness. Pain may be noted on palpation of the abdomen, or a hunched posture may be present. The perianal region may be contaminated with feces. Oral ulceration and mucosal pallor may be present in severely affected cats, and rarely, bacteremia may be accompanied by icterus. Terminally, affected cats may be hypothermic, bradycardic, and comatose.

Kittens with cerebellar signs are generally bright and alert but exhibit intention tremors, incoordination, ataxia, hypermetria, a broad-based stance, decreased postural reactions, a truncal sway, and absence of a menace response. Cats with forebrain disease may show abnormal behavior, such as aggression or decreased mentation. Examination of the ocular fundus may reveal folding of the retina, evidence of retinal degeneration with discrete gray spots, and optic nerve hypoplasia. Retinal lesions may be an incidental finding in older, recovered cats, which includes surviving cats with cerebellar hypoplasia.

Diagnosis

Laboratory Abnormalities

Complete Blood Count

The most common abnormality on the CBC in feline panleukopenia is leukopenia, which is due to a neutropenia and lymphopenia (Box 19-1).[3] Total leukocyte counts may be as low as 50 cells/μL, and toxic band neutrophils may be present. In one study, only 65% of 187 cats with panleukopenia were leukopenic, so an absence of leukopenia does not rule out FPV infection. Recovery may be associated with lymphocytosis and

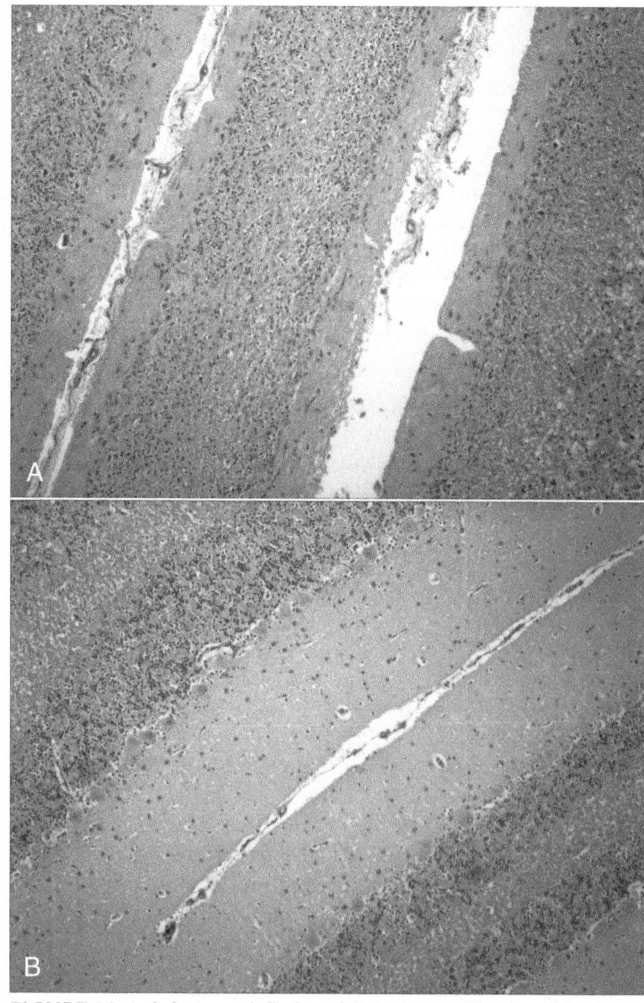

FIGURE 19-1 **A,** Severe cerebellar hypoplasia in a 1-year-old male neutered domestic shorthair that was euthanized for cerebellar signs and seizures. The neurologic signs had been present since the cat was found at approximately 4 months of age. There is a paucity of neurons and glial cells in all layers. **B,** Normal feline cerebellum. Note the dramatically increased width of the molecular layer when compared to (A).

leukocytosis. Thrombocytopenia and mild anemia are also common. Thrombocytopenia may result from damage to the marrow or, possibly, disseminated intravascular coagulation (DIC).

BOX 19-1

Prevalence of Laboratory Abnormalities in Cats with Panleukopenia

Leukopenia: 122/187 (65%)
Thrombocytopenia: 83/153 (54%)
Anemia: 91/187 (48%)
Neutropenia: 64/137 (47%)
Lymphopenia: 53/137 (39%)
Hypoalbuminemia: 45/101 (45%)
Hypochloremia: 40/112 (36%)
Hyponatremia: 41/127 (32%)
Hypoproteinemia: 46/153 (30%)
Hyperglycemia: 48/168 (29%)
Increased AST activity: 26/98 (27%)
Hyperkalemia: 30/132 (23%)
Increased BUN: 36/168 (21%)
Hyperbilirubinemia: 19/134 (14%)
Increased ALT activity: 18/135 (13%)
Increased creatinine: 12/155 (8%)
Hypokalemia: 9/132 (7%)
Hypernatremia: 8/127 (6%)
Hypoglycemia: 10/168 (6%)

Modified from Kruse BD, Unterer S, Horlacher K, et al. Prognostic factors in cats with feline panleukopenia. J Vet Intern Med 2010;24:1271-1276.

Serum Biochemical Tests

Serum biochemistry analysis may show hypoalbuminemia, hypoglobulinemia, and/or hypocholesterolemia; electrolyte abnormalities such as hyponatremia or hypernatremia, hypochloremia, hyperkalemia, or, less commonly hypokalemia; and acid-base abnormalities (see Box 19-1). In severely affected cats, azotemia, increased serum activities of AST or ALT, or hyperbilirubinemia may be present. Hyperglycemia or hypoglycemia may also be identified.

Diagnostic Imaging

Plain Radiography

As in dogs with parvoviral enteritis, abdominal radiography in cats with panleukopenia may show evidence of poor serosal detail and a fluid- and gas-filled gastrointestinal tract.

MRI Findings

MRI of cats with neurologic signs due to FPV may reveal evidence of cerebellar agenesis or hypoplasia. Rarely, hydrocephalus, porencephaly, or hydranencephaly can be detected.[18]

Microbiologic Tests

Diagnostic assays available for feline panleukopenia are listed in Table 19-1.

Serologic Diagnosis

Use of serology for diagnosis of feline panleukopenia is complicated by widespread exposure or immunization, so serologic assays that detect antibody against FPV are generally used to assess the need for vaccination rather than for diagnosis. They can also be used in outbreak situations in order to determine which cats are at risk for development of disease and virus shedding, and which cats are protected and therefore at low risk. The gold standard method for FPV serology is hemagglutination

TABLE 19-1

Diagnostic Assays Available for Feline Panleukopenia

Assay	Specimen Type	Target	Performance
Canine parvovirus fecal antigen ELISA	Feces	Parvoviral antigen	Sensitivity varies with the assay used and the timing of specimen collection. False negatives are common, but a positive result generally indicates infection.
Histopathology	Usually necropsy specimens, especially gastrointestinal tissues	Crypt necrosis with intranuclear inclusions; FPV antigen with IHC or IFA	Can be used for necropsy diagnosis.
Polymerase chain reaction (PCR)	Feces, tissue samples	FPV DNA	Sensitivity and specificity varies depending on assay design. The extent to which attenuated live vaccine virus can be detected after vaccination is not well understood. Because of the high sensitivity of some assays, the significance of a positive result may be difficult to interpret. False-negative results may occur as a result of inhibition of PCR by components of feces.
Fecal electron microscopy	Feces	Virus particles	Not widely available, turnaround time can be slow, and may be expensive. Requires the presence of large amounts of virus.
Virus isolation	Feces, tissues	FPV	Difficult, not widely available. Used primarily as a research tool.

FPV, feline panleukopenia virus; IFA, immunofluorescent antibody; IHC, immunohistochemistry.

inhibition, which measures the ability of serum to prevent agglutination of erythrocytes by the virus (see Chapter 2). Serum neutralization assays may also be used. Point-of-care assays designed to detect antibody titers to CPV have a low sensitivity (28%) for detection of antibodies to FPV in cats.[21] A point-of-care assay designed to detect feline antibodies (ImmunoComb Feline VacciCheck Test Kit, Biogal, Galed Labs, Israel) also had a low sensitivity (49%), although specificity was high.[21] The use of this test for risk analysis in shelter situations may lead to inappropriate removal or isolation of cats with false-negative results for protective antibody titers, which might waste time, space, and financial resources.[21] However, positive results should reliably indicate protection. The test can be performed quickly (30 minutes) and requires as little as 5 μL of serum or plasma, so provided it is understood that a negative result means either a protected or susceptible status, and a positive result equates to protection, the test still has the potential to provide useful information.

Antigen Detection Enzyme Linked Immunosorbent Assay

FPV can be detected in feces or rectal swabs using antigen assays designed to detect CPV.[22,23] The sensitivity and specificity of these assays varies from one assay to another and with the stage of infection, because virus shedding may be transient. In general, false-negative results are common with these assays, but false positives are uncommon, so a positive test result in a cat with consistent clinical signs suggests a diagnosis of feline panleukopenia. The specificity of one point-of-care device (SNAP Parvo, IDEXX Laboratories, Westbrook, ME) was high; 54 of 55 positive assay results were confirmed with a PCR assay. Another study of 52 cats with diarrhea and 148 healthy cats showed variability in the sensitivity and specificity of five different test kits when compared with fecal electron microscopy.[23] Sensitivity ranged from 50% to 80%, and specificity ranged from 94% to 100%. This study included only 10 cats with FPV as determined with electron microscopy. Additional studies are warranted that evaluate the sensitivity and specificity of these assays in larger numbers of cats with FPV infection when both real-time PCR and electron microscopy are used as the gold standard. False-positive fecal antigen assay results after vaccination with attenuated live viral vaccines appear to be uncommon, but again vary with the test used.[24] Of the SNAP Parvo (IDEXX Laboratories), AGEN CPV (AGEN Biomedical Ltd., Brisbane, Australia), and the Witness CPV (Synbiotics Corp, San Diego, CA), the SNAP Parvo was least likely to yield positive results after vaccination.

Fecal Electron Microscopy

Fecal electron microscopy is still offered by some institutions for diagnosis of viral enteritis. It may also facilitate diagnosis of other infections such as rotavirus, astrovirus, torovirus, and coronavirus infections. Turnaround time may be slow. Generally speaking, large amounts of virus must be present for results to be positive, and technical expertise is required to accurately identify virus in the stool.

Virus Isolation

FPV can be isolated in feline cells, but as with CPV, isolation can difficult, and the virus shows minimal cytopathic effects. As a result, isolation of FPV is a specialized procedure that is uncommonly used for diagnosis.

Molecular Diagnosis Using the Polymerase Chain Reaction

Specific real-time PCR assays have been developed for detection of FPV and differentiation of FPV from CPV-2 variants and are offered by veterinary diagnostic laboratories. Clinicians should contact their laboratory to determine the specificity of the assay offered.[25] These assays can be used on whole blood or feces. The extent to which these assays detect attenuated live vaccine virus after vaccination requires further study. Assays have also been developed that differentiate between field and vaccine strains of FPV.[26]

Pathologic Findings

Gross Pathologic Findings

Gross pathologic findings in feline panleukopenia include thymic involution; thickening, distention, and discoloration of the intestinal wall with serosal hemorrhage (Figure 19-2); and enlarged, edematous mesenteric lymph nodes. The intestine may contain bloody liquid contents, and mucosal hemorrhage may be identified. Hemorrhages may be visible on the surface of other organs as well. In some cats, mild pleural or peritoneal effusion is present. Cats infected prenatally may have cerebellar aplasia, or more commonly a small cerebellum (often half to three-quarters normal size).[27] Rarely other developmental CNS abnormalities such as hydrocephalus, hydranencephaly, or porencephaly are observed.[18]

Histopathologic Findings

Histopathologic findings in the intestinal tract are similar to those described for CPV-2 infection, with crypt dilation and necrosis of crypt epithelial cells, accumulation of cellular debris, neutrophil infiltration, loss of villi, and submucosal edema throughout the small and large intestines; the jejunum and ileum are usually most severely affected (Figure 19-3, *A*). Acutely affected cats show widespread lymphoid depletion and there may be hyperplasia of mononuclear phagocytes. Intranuclear inclusions are found in some cats (Figure 19-3, *B*). Examination of the bone marrow may reveal bone marrow hypoplasia. Examination of the cerebellum shows cellular depletion; reactive astrocytosis may be present. Immunohistochemistry or immunofluorescent

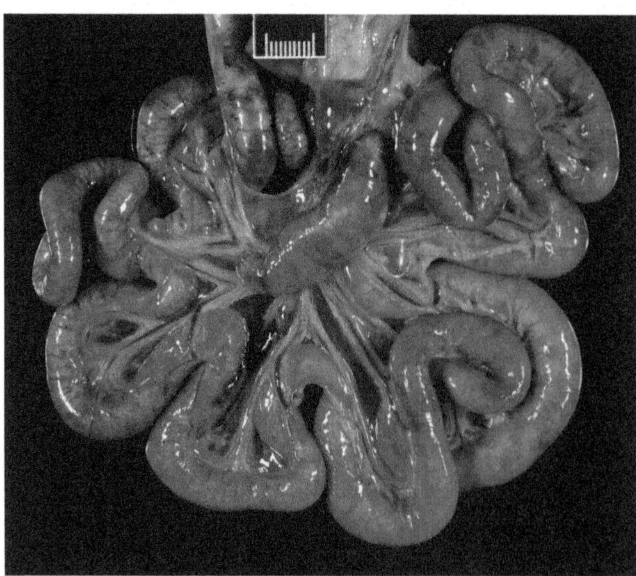

FIGURE 19-2 Intestinal tract of a 2-year-old intact female domestic longhair cat with severe feline panleukopenia. The intestinal loops are dilated and flaccid and discolored red to purple. Ruler = 1 cm.

antibody may be used to document the presence of the virus within tissues (see Figure 19-3, C).

Treatment and Prognosis

Antimicrobial Treatment and Supportive Care

Treatment of cats with feline panleukopenia is with supportive care, especially intravenous crystalloids and parenteral antimicrobial drug treatment as for CPV-2 infections (see Chapter 14). Dextrose supplementation of the fluids may be required, and blood glucose concentration should be monitored. Oral intake of food and water should be withheld until vomiting has ceased. Experience with early enteral nutrition has not been reported in cats, and extreme care is warranted to prevent aspiration pneumonia. Antiemetics such as metoclopramide or ondansetron may be effective. In contrast to canine parvoviral enteritis, treatment with rfIFN-ω has not been beneficial for treatment of feline panleukopenia, although increased antibody production and a reduced acute inflammatory response was observed.[28]

Prognosis

Cats with panleukopenia that survive the first 5 days of treatment usually recover, although recovery is often more prolonged than it is for dogs with parvoviral enteritis. In 244 cats with feline panleukopenia from Europe, the survival rate was 51.1%.[3] Nonsurvivors had lower leukocyte and platelet counts than survivors, and cats with white cell counts below 1000/μL were almost twice as likely to die than those with white cell counts above 2500/μL. Only total leukopenia, and not lymphopenia, was correlated with mortality. Hypoalbuminemia and hypokalemia were also associated with an increased risk of mortality. In contrast to dogs with parvoviral enteritis, mortality in cats does not appear to be correlated with age.

Cerebellar signs in kittens with cerebellar hypoplasia typically do not progress and may improve slightly as a result of compensatory responses from other senses such as vision.[29]

Immunity and Vaccination

Recovery from feline panleukopenia is thought to confer lifelong immunity. Effective vaccines are widely available, and include both parenteral inactivated and attenuated live viral vaccines. An intranasal FPV, FHV-1 and feline calicivirus vaccine is available; its use has been controversial, because panleukopenia is a systemic disease. An outbreak of salmonellosis and panleukopenia occurred in one cattery that used an intranasal FPV vaccine.[4] No difference was noted in seroconversion rates between five cats vaccinated with the intranasal vaccine and five cats vaccinated with a parenteral attenuated live vaccine, but the number of cats in this study was small, and a larger number of cats that were vaccinated with the parenteral vaccine had protective antibody titers on day 7.[30]

Both inactivated and attenuated live vaccine types induce protective antibody titers after vaccination in a high proportion of cats,[5] although the attenuated live vaccine may be more likely to induce protective titers than the inactivated vaccine.[24] Provided maternally-derived antibody (MDA) is absent, immunity occurs within 1 week after a single vaccination with an attenuated live viral vaccine[31] and lasts for at least 3 years, and possibly for life.[32] Nevertheless, two doses, 3 to 4 weeks apart, have been recommended for initial vaccination with attenuated live vaccines in the absence of MDA. Two injections are always required for inactivated vaccines, and maximal immunity does not occur until 1 week after the second dose. However, even with an inactivated vaccine, challenge 7.5 years after vaccination was associated with protection.[33] The use of inactivated vaccines should be reserved for immunosuppressed cats or colostrum-deprived neonates that are less than 4 weeks of age, or when there is a need to vaccinate pregnant cats. In shelter situations, the use of attenuated live vaccines is always recommended because of the slow onset of immunity with inactivated vaccines.[34] FPV vaccines protect cats against challenge with CPV-2b strains.[35,36] However, cross-reactivity of antibodies induced by FPV vaccination to CPV-2 strains was lower than that to FPV as determined using hemagglutination inhibition.[37] The extent to which FPV vaccines protect against infection with other CPV-2 variants requires further investigation.[38]

The most common reason for vaccine failure is interference by MDA. Maternal antibody persists until at least 12 weeks, and possibly longer in some cats. Virus neutralization titers above 1:10 are likely to interfere with vaccination, and kittens with titers below 1:40 are generally considered to be susceptible to infection by FPV. Kittens should be vaccinated every 3 to 4 weeks from 6 to 8 weeks of age, and it is recommended

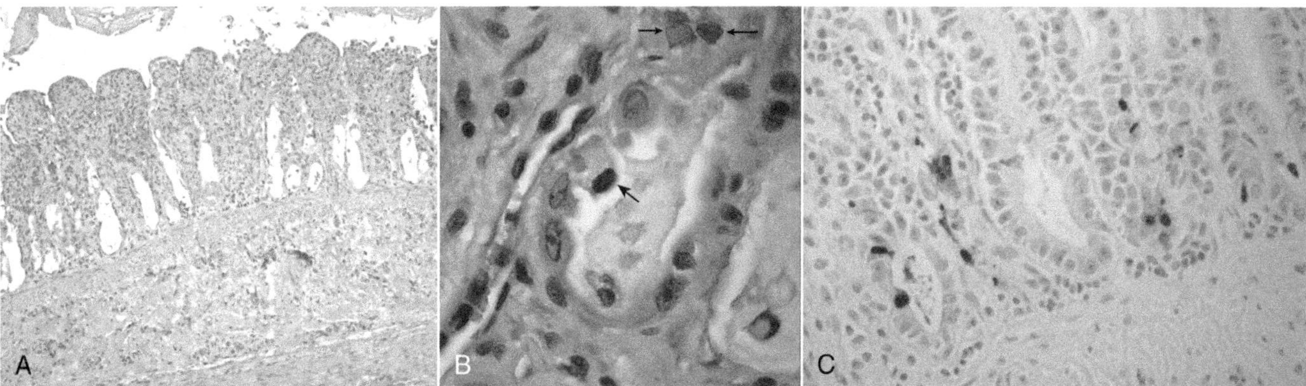

FIGURE 19-3 **A,** Histopathology of the jejunum from a kitten with panleukopenia. Villi are rounded and blunted with nearly complete epithelial loss and crypt dilation. H&E stain. **B,** Histopathology of the jejunum from a young barn cat that died after several days of profound weakness and neurologic signs. Six other cats in the barn died with the same signs. Mucosal crypts are dilated and contain debris, and intranuclear inclusions are present *(small arrows)*. Another cell *(large arrow)* is foamy and degenerate and has a hyperchromatic nucleus. H&E stain. **C,** Same cat as in **B.** The presence of FPV in the intestinal tract is confirmed with immunohistochemistry (brown stain). (Courtesy Dr. Patricia Pesavento, University of California, Davis Veterinary Anatomic Pathology Service.)

that the last vaccine in the kitten series be given no earlier than 14 to 16 weeks of age. When there is a history of an outbreak situation, the final booster could be given no earlier than 18 to 20 weeks of age.[39] In all situations, a booster should be administered at 1 year, and every 3 years thereafter.

Vaccination of pregnant queens with attenuated live viral vaccines can cause cerebellar hypoplasia or fetal losses. The frequency with which this occurs is unknown. As a result, it has been suggested that pregnant queens only be vaccinated with attenuated live FPV vaccines if they are being introduced into a shelter and quarantine while immunization with inactivated vaccines is performed is not possible. Alternatively, assessment for protective antibody titers with an in-house test kit (where available) could be performed.

Prevention

New kittens should not be introduced into households that previously contained cats infected with FPV unless they are fully vaccinated. In the face of an outbreak, exposed and susceptible kittens may be effectively protected for 2 to 4 weeks through subcutaneous or intraperitoneal administration of 2 mL of type-matched serum from cats with a high antibody titer.[39,40] However, this is only effective when administered before the onset of clinical signs, and it can interfere with subsequent vaccination. For these kittens, it has been recommended that vaccination be withheld for 3 weeks after the serum has been administered.[39] Passive immunization may be useful when cats are introduced into a shelter situation where a known problem exists. Repeated treatment with serum should be avoided because hypersensitivity reactions may occur. Prevention of feline panleukopenia should also include proper disinfection with disinfectants that are effective against parvoviruses, such as bleach, accelerated hydrogen peroxide, or potassium peroxymonosulfate (see Chapter 11) and, in shelter situations, isolation or removal of cats that develop gastrointestinal illness, and separate housing for healthy kittens.

Public Health Aspects

Although FPV is not known to infect humans, a unique strain of FPV was recently isolated from a diarrheic monkey in China.[41] This strain was shown to cause panleukopenia in inoculated cats.

CASE EXAMPLE

Signalment: "Callie", a 2 year-old, female intact domestic longhair from Woodland, CA

History: Callie was brought to an emergency clinic for acute onset of collapse and severe illness. The current owner had fostered the cat for 1 week after she was found as a stray. The cat had been nursing a litter of kittens. The kittens were 4 weeks old, being weaned and apparently healthy. Since being fostered, the cat had exhibited a progressive decrease in appetite and thirst, and her feces had become soft and pasty. The night before she was brought to the emergency clinic, she had been bathed, and afterwards she vomited bile-stained fluid twice and was placed on a heating pad. The following morning she was found laterally recumbent and minimally responsive.

Physical Examination:

Body Weight: 2.3 kg

General: Stuporous mentation, estimated to be 8% to 10% dehydrated, T < 92°F (<33°C), HR = 132 beats/min, RR = 32 breaths/min, mucous membranes pale and tacky, unable to assess CRT. Fecal and urinary stains were present around the perineum and on the caudal aspect of the pelvic limbs.

Musculoskeletal: Body condition score 2/9. Diffuse muscle wasting was present. The cat was laterally recumbent and nonambulatory.

Cardiovascular: Weak femoral pulses. No murmurs or arrhythmias were detected.

Gastrointestinal and Urogenital: The abdomen was soft and nonpainful on palpation. Fluid-filled intestinal loops were palpated, and the urinary bladder was small (<5 cm) and soft.

All Other Systems: No abnormalities were detected.

Laboratory Findings:

CBC:

HCT 46% (30-50%)
MCV 49.8 fL (42-53 fL)
MCHC 30.4 g/dL (30-33.5 g/dL)
WBC 150 cells/μL (4500-14,000 cells/μL)
Neutrophils 0 cells/μL (2000-9000 cells/μL)
Lymphocytes 141 cells/μL (1000-7000 cells/μL)
Highly reactive lymphocytes 6 cells/μL
Monocytes 3 cells/μL (50-600 cells/μL)
Platelets 32,000 platelets/μL (180,000-500,000 platelets/μL).

Serum Chemistry Profile:

Sodium 141 mmol/L (151-158 mmol/L)
Potassium 4.0 mmol/L (3.6-4.9 mmol/L)
Chloride 111 mmol/L (117-126 mmol/L)
Bicarbonate 23 mmol/L (15-21 mmol/L)
Phosphorus 6.0 mg/dL (3.2-6.3 mg/dL)
Calcium 7.4 mg/dL (9.0-10.9 mg/dl)
BUN 24 mg/dL (18-33 mg/dL)
Creatinine 0.5 mg/dL (1.1-2.2 mg/dL)
Glucose 68 mg/dL (63-118 mg/dL)
Total protein 3.2 g/dL (6.6-8.4 g/dL)
Albumin 1.6 g/dL (2.2-4.6 g/dL)
Globulin 1.6 g/dL (2.8-5.4 g/dL)
ALT 125 U/L (27-101 U/L)
AST 143 U/L (17-58 U/L)
ALP 4 U/L (14-71 U/L)
Creatine kinase 2409 U/L (73-260 U/L)
Gamma GT <3 U/L (0-4 U/L)
Cholesterol 68 mg/dL (89-258 mg/dL)
Total bilirubin 0.2 mg/dL (0-0.2 mg/dL)
Magnesium 2.5 mg/dL (1.5-2.5 mg/dL).

Imaging: An abdominal ultrasound showed marked fluid distention of the small intestines.

Microbiologic Testing: In-clinic ELISA serology for FeLV antigen and FIV antibody: negative.

Treatment and Outcome: Callie was treated with active warming, and a central venous access line was placed. Intravenous crystalloids (four warmed 60-mL boluses of lactated Ringer's solution [LRS], each given over 20 minutes) were administered, after which an venous acid-base panel showed a pH of 7.267 (7.31-7.46), bicarbonate of 17.5 mmol/L (14-22 mmol/L), base excess of −8.1 mmol/L (−4 to +2 mmol/L), pCO_2 of 39.7 mm Hg (25-37 mmHg), lactate of 4.5 mEq/L (<2 mEq/L), glucose of 52 mg/dL, potassium of 3.1 mEq/L, sodium of 141 mEq/L, and ionized calcium of 1.17 (1.1-1.4 mmol/L). A dextrose bolus and ticarcillin-clavulanic acid (22 mg/kg, q6h, IV) were administered. The cat repeatedly vomited blood-tinged fluid, and so treatment with metoclopramide (0.02 mg/kg/hr) and famotidine (0.5 mg/kg IV q12h) was initiated. Aggressive crystalloid fluid therapy was continued (LRS supplemented with 30 mEq/L KCl and 2.5% dextrose), and treatment with hetastarch was also initiated. Systolic blood pressure (Doppler) was 60 to 90 mm Hg, heart rate increased to 170 beats/min, and rectal temperature increased to 100°F. When the CBC results were available, the cat was placed in the isolation ward.

Pasty diarrhea that contained sloughed mucosa occurred every 1 to 2 hours, which transitioned to liquid red feces over 24 hours. A CBC again showed absolute neutropenia and 15,000 platelets/µL. After another 24 hours, the cat's condition deteriorated despite aggressive treatment and monitoring. Partial parenteral nutrition was initiated. That evening, pyrexia developed (104.6°F) as well as tachypnea and increased respiratory effort. The owner elected euthanasia. The cat regurgitated approximately 200 mL of dark brown fluid at the time of euthanasia.

Gross Necropsy Findings: Ten mL of semiopaque red fluid was present in the peritoneal cavity. Streaks of hemorrhage were noted throughout the skeletal muscle. Between the pylorus and the ileocecocolic junction, the serosa of the small intestinal tract was dark red to purple to black (see Figure 19-2). The entire small and large intestinal tract was dilated and flaccid. The small intestinal mucosa was dark red to purple and contained a small amount of dark red mucoid material. The mesenteric lymph nodes were prominent, and their cut surface was discolored red to dark pink. The liver was pale yellow and extended beyond the costal arches. Numerous petechial hemorrhages were present on the serosal surface of the urinary bladder.

Histopathologic Findings: Within the duodenum, jejunum, and ileum there was severe, subacute, diffuse necrotizing and fibrinohemorrhagic enteritis. The villi were necrotic, fused, and markedly blunted with a minimal inflammatory response. Necrosis extended into the crypts, and there was some evidence of a regenerative response that included enterocyte hypertrophy, karyomegaly, and rare mitotic figures. Mixed bacteria, which included small gram-negative rods and large numbers of gram-positive cocci, lined and effaced the denuded villi. There was diffuse lymphoid depletion in lymph nodes, as well as the mucosa-associated lymphoid tissue in the cecum and colon. Marked depletion of erythroid and myeloid precursors was present in the bone marrow. There were multifocal areas of hemorrhage in the skeletal and cardiac muscle, intestinal tract, and lungs, as well as fibrin thrombi in the lungs. FPV antigen was identified in intestinal epithelial cells using immunohistochemistry. Culture of the jejunum for *Salmonella* spp. was negative.

Diagnosis: Feline panleukopenia

Comments: The cat in this report was a stray with an unknown vaccination history, which demonstrates that severe disease can occur even in adult cats. Antemortem diagnostic testing for FPV with a fecal antigen ELISA assay or PCR assay was discussed with the owner, but was declined because of the high degree of suspicion for the disease and the lack of impact that a positive or negative result would have had on the treatment plan. Secondary bacterial sepsis was suspected. Additional co-infections with other viruses, such as feline coronavirus, or enteropathogenic bacteria could not be ruled out. During the cat's treatment, one of the kittens in the litter died suddenly and the other developed signs of illness.

SUGGESTED READINGS

Kruse BD, Unterer S, Horlacher K, et al. Prognostic factors in cats with feline panleukopenia. J Vet Intern Med. 2010;24:1271-1276.

Neuerer FF, Horlacher K, Truyen U, et al. Comparison of different in-house test systems to detect parvovirus in faeces of cats. J Feline Med Surg. 2008;10:247-251.

Truyen U, Addie D, Belak S, et al. Feline panleukopenia. ABCD guidelines on prevention and management. J Feline Med Surg. 2009;11:538-546.

REFERENCES

1. Verge J, Christoforoni N. La gastroenterite infectieuse des chats; est-elle due a un virus filtrable. C R Seances Soc Biol Fil. 1928;99:312.
2. Steinel A, Parrish CR, Bloom ME, et al. Parvovirus infections in wild carnivores. J Wildl Dis. 2001;37:594-607.
3. Kruse BD, Unterer S, Horlacher K, et al. Prognostic factors in cats with feline panleukopenia. J Vet Intern Med. 2010;24:1271-1276.
4. Addie DD, Toth S, Thompson H, et al. Detection of feline parvovirus in dying pedigree kittens. Vet Rec. 1998;142:353-356.
5. Fischer SM, Quest CM, Dubovi EJ, et al. Response of feral cats to vaccination at the time of neutering. J Am Vet Med Assoc. 2007;230:52-58.
6. Decaro N, Desario C, Miccolupo A, et al. Genetic analysis of feline panleukopenia viruses from cats with gastroenteritis. J Gen Virol. 2008;89:2290-2298.
7. Battilani M, Balboni A, Ustulin M, et al. Genetic complexity and multiple infections with more *Parvovirus* species in naturally infected cats. Vet Res. 2011;42:43.
8. Nakamura K, Sakamoto M, Ikeda Y, et al. Pathogenic potential of canine parvovirus types 2a and 2c in domestic cats. Clin Diagn Lab Immunol. 2001;8:663-668.
9. Ohshima T, Mochizuki M. Evidence for recombination between feline panleukopenia virus and canine parvovirus type 2. J Vet Med Sci. 2009;71:403-408.
10. Ikeda Y, Mochizuki M, Naito R, et al. Predominance of canine parvovirus (CPV) in unvaccinated cat populations and emergence of new antigenic types of CPVs in cats. Virology. 2000;278:13-19.
11. Muir P, Harbour DA, Gruffydd-Jones TJ, et al. A clinical and microbiological study of cats with protruding nictitating membranes and diarrhoea: isolation of a novel virus. Vet Rec. 1990;127:324-330.
12. Marshall JA, Kennett ML, Rodger SM, et al. Virus and virus-like particles in the faeces of cats with and without diarrhoea. Aust Vet J. 1987;64:100-105.

13. Goodman LB, Lyi SM, Johnson NC, et al. Binding site on the transferrin receptor for the parvovirus capsid and effects of altered affinity on cell uptake and infection. J Virol. 2010;84:4969-4978.
14. Moschidou P, Martella V, Lorusso E, et al. Mixed infection by feline astrovirus and feline panleukopenia virus in a domestic cat with gastroenteritis and panleukopenia. J Vet Diagn Invest. 2011;23:581-584.
15. Lutz H, Castelli I, Ehrensperger F, et al. Panleukopenia-like syndrome of FeLV caused by co-infection with FeLV and feline panleukopenia virus. Vet Immunol Immunopathol. 1995;46:21-33.
16. Ikegami T, Shirota K, Goto K, et al. Enterocolitis associated with dual infection by *Clostridium piliforme* and feline panleukopenia virus in three kittens. Vet Pathol. 1999;36:613-615.
17. Mochizuki M, Osawa N, Ishida T. Feline coronavirus participation in diarrhea of cats. J Vet Med Sci. 1999;61:1071-1073.
18. Sharp NJ, Davis BJ, Guy JS, et al. Hydranencephaly and cerebellar hypoplasia in two kittens attributed to intrauterine parvovirus infection. J Comp Pathol. 1999;121:39-53.
19. Url A, Truyen U, Rebel-Bauder B, et al. Evidence of parvovirus replication in cerebral neurons of cats. J Clin Microbiol. 2003;41:3801-3805.
20. Meurs KM, Fox PR, Magnon AL, et al. Molecular screening by polymerase chain reaction detects panleukopenia virus DNA in formalin-fixed hearts from cats with idiopathic cardiomyopathy and myocarditis. Cardiovasc Pathol. 2000;9:119-126.
21. Digangi BA, Gray LK, Levy JK, et al. Detection of protective antibody titers against feline panleukopenia virus, feline herpesvirus-1, and feline calicivirus in shelter cats using a point-of-care ELISA. J Feline Med Surg. 2011;13:912-918.
22. Abd-Eldaim M, Beall M, Kennedy M. Detection of feline panleukopenia virus using a commercial ELISA for canine parvovirus. Vet Ther. 2009;10:E1-E6.
23. Neuerer FF, Horlacher K, Truyen U, et al. Comparison of different in-house test systems to detect parvovirus in faeces of cats. J Feline Med Surg. 2008;10:247-251.
24. Patterson EV, Reese MJ, Tucker SJ, et al. Effect of vaccination on parvovirus antigen testing in kittens. J Am Vet Med Assoc. 2007;230:359-363.
25. Decaro N, Desario C, Lucente MS, et al. Specific identification of feline panleukopenia virus and its rapid differentiation from canine parvoviruses using minor groove binder probes. J Virol Methods. 2008;147:67-71.
26. Horiuchi M, Yuri K, Soma T, et al. Differentiation of vaccine virus from field isolates of feline panleukopenia virus by polymerase chain reaction and restriction fragment length polymorphism analysis. Vet Microbiol. 1996;53:283-293.
27. De Lahunta A. Comments on cerebellar ataxia and its congenital transmission in cats by feline panleukopenia virus. J Am Vet Med Assoc. 1971;158(Suppl 2):901-906.
28. Paltrinieri S, Crippa A, Comerio T, et al. Evaluation of inflammation and immunity in cats with spontaneous parvovirus infection: consequences of recombinant feline interferon-omega administration. Vet Immunol Immunopathol. 2007;118:68-74.
29. Penderis J. The wobbly cat. Diagnostic and therapeutic approach to generalised ataxia. J Feline Med Surg. 2009;11:349-359.
30. Lappin MR, Veir J, Hawley J. Feline panleukopenia virus, feline herpesvirus-1, and feline calicivirus antibody responses in seronegative specific pathogen-free cats after a single administration of two different modified live FVRCP vaccines. J Feline Med Surg. 2009;11:159-162.
31. Jas D, Aeberle C, Lacombe V, et al. Onset of immunity in kittens after vaccination with a non-adjuvanted vaccine against feline panleucopenia, feline calicivirus and feline herpesvirus. Vet J. 2009;182:86-93.
32. Gore TC, Lakshmanan N, Williams JR, et al. Three-year duration of immunity in cats following vaccination against feline rhinotracheitis virus, feline calicivirus, and feline panleukopenia virus. Vet Ther. 2006;7:213-222.
33. Scott FW, Geissinger CM. Long-term immunity in cats vaccinated with an inactivated trivalent vaccine. Am J Vet Res. 1999;60:652-658.
34. Day MJ, Horzinek MC, Schultz RD. WSAVA guidelines for the vaccination of dogs and cats. J Small Anim Pract. 2010;51:1-32.
35. Gamoh K, Senda M, Inoue Y, et al. Efficacy of an inactivated feline panleucopenia virus vaccine against a canine parvovirus isolated from a domestic cat. Vet Rec. 2005;157:285-287.
36. Chalmers WS, Truyen U, Greenwood NM, et al. Efficacy of feline panleucopenia vaccine to prevent infection with an isolate of CPV2b obtained from a cat. Vet Microbiol. 1999;69:41-45.
37. Nakamura K, Ikeda Y, Miyazawa T, et al. Characterisation of cross-reactivity of virus neutralising antibodies induced by feline panleukopenia virus and canine parvoviruses. Res Vet Sci. 2001;71:219-222.
38. Decaro N, Buonavoglia D, Desario C, et al. Characterisation of canine parvovirus strains isolated from cats with feline panleukopenia. Res Vet Sci. 2010;89:275-278.
39. Truyen U, Addie D, Belak S, et al. Feline panleukopenia. ABCD guidelines on prevention and management. J Feline Med Surg. 2009;11:538-546.
40. Levy JK, Crawford PC, Collante WR, et al. Use of adult cat serum to correct failure of passive transfer in kittens. J Am Vet Med Assoc. 2001;219:1401-1405.
41. Yang S, Wang S, Feng H, et al. Isolation and characterization of feline panleukopenia virus from a diarrheic monkey. Vet Microbiol. 2010;143:155-159.

CHAPTER 20

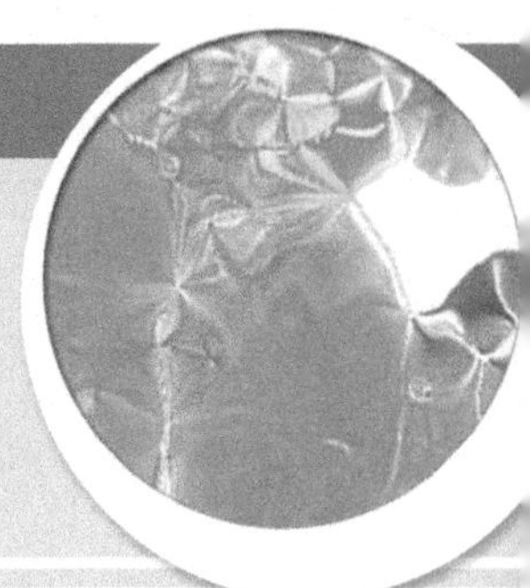

Feline Coronavirus Infection

Jane E. Sykes

> **Overview of Feline Coronavirus Infections**
>
> First Described: 1963[1]; a viral etiology was not identified until the 1970s.
>
> Cause: Feline coronavirus (Family Coronaviridae, genus *Coronavirus*)
>
> Affected Hosts: Cats and wild felids, especially cheetahs
>
> Mode of Transmission: Fecal-oral
>
> Geographic Distribution: Worldwide
>
> Major Clinical Signs: Fever, lethargy, inappetence, vomiting, diarrhea, dehydration, icterus, tachypnea, uveitis, neurologic signs, abdominal distention due to ascites.
>
> Differential Diagnoses: Toxoplasmosis, congestive heart failure, carcinomatosis, lymphoma, pancreatitis, rabies, cryptococcosis, bacterial peritonitis, pyothorax, bacterial meningitis, chronic stomatitis, multiple myeloma, infection with FeLV or FIV.
>
> Human Health Significance: Feline coronaviruses do not infect humans.

Etiology and Epidemiology

Coronaviruses are large, enveloped, single-stranded RNA viruses with club-shaped spikes on their outer surface (see Figure 14-1, *B*). They have the largest RNA genomes of all known viruses. Feline coronaviruses (FCoV), like canine enteric coronavirus, belong to the Group 1a coronaviruses (see Box 17-1). In fact, even canine enteric coronavirus has the potential to infect cats and cause diseases similar to those caused by FCoV.[2] Among FCoVs, there are two different serotypes, type I and type II, which use different receptors for cellular entry in vitro[3,4] but cause the same clinical manifestations. Type I strains predominate worldwide.[5-7] Type II strains, which are thought to have evolved from genetic recombination between canine enteric coronavirus and FCoV, are more readily grown in culture and so have been more extensively studied; they possess a spike protein that resembles that of canine enteric coronavirus.

FCoVs cause enteric disease in cats as well as feline infectious peritonitis (FIP), a serious systemic pyogranulomatous to granulomatous disease that progresses over a period of weeks to months and, once it occurs, is ultimately always fatal. FIP is a major cause of death in young and young adult cats, especially cats from multicat environments such as purebred catteries and shelters. Wild cats, especially cheetahs, are also susceptible.[8] The vast majority of domestic cats that develop FIP are 3 months to 3 years of age, with at least 50% of affected cats aged 12 months or younger (Figure 20-1). However, FIP can occur at any age, and there is a secondary peak of incidence in geriatric cats (>10 years of age), possibly as a result of suboptimal immune function. Males and sexually intact cats have been predisposed in some studies,[9-11] and a disease peak may exist in the fall and winter.[12] Although the disease occurs in all breeds, purebred cats are more susceptible; Abyssinians, Australian mist, Bengals, birmans, Burmese, British shorthairs, Himalayans, ragdolls, rexes, and possibly Scottish folds may be predisposed.[9-14] Breed predispositions may vary geographically and temporally depending on the preferences of breeders in a region, and specific lines may be more predisposed than the breeds themselves.[6] The molecular basis of genetic susceptibility to FIP is currently unclear. Siblings of cats that die of FIP may be at increased risk for FIP.[15]

In multiple-cat household situations, cats are repeatedly infected, shed virus, and recover, but some cats remain persistently infected and chronically shed FCoV in the absence of clinical signs (Figure 20-2). More than half, and as many as 100% of cats in environments with more than six cats, become infected with FCoVs.[6] The seroprevalence is lower in cats from single-cat households and among feral cats.[16] However, even though the prevalence of infection in multicat households is high, fewer than 10% of cats from large, multicat households ultimately develop FIP. Thus, although the incidence of *infection* is high, the incidence of *disease* in single- or two-cat households is only around 1 in 5000; in catteries it is around 5% to 10%.[17,18] Provided they are unrelated by birth, cats in households with a history of FIP are not more likely to develop FIP than cats in households without FIP.[19] Thus, FIP is usually a sporadic disease that does not spread from one cat to another. However, every few years, epidemics of disease can occur in catteries or shelters, with mortality rates that exceed 10%.[12] Because it is an enveloped virus, FCoV is readily inactivated by disinfectants and generally survives less than a day or two at room temperature. However, the possibility of prolonged survival (up to 7 weeks) in the environment under certain conditions has been suggested.[15,20] In this situation, fomites might play an important role in transmission.

The epidemiology and pathogenesis of FIP has both fascinated and confused veterinary virologists worldwide for decades. The most widely accepted theory (the "internal mutation hypothesis") is that cats are initially infected with a low-pathogenicity coronavirus after oronasal exposure, which results either in no signs, or mild enteric disease. This low-pathogenicity virus has been referred to as *feline enteric coronavirus* in some publications in order to distinguish it from virulent FIP virus. The use of this name has been controversial, because although the virus is primarily confined to the gastrointestinal tract (and especially colonic epithelial cells), FCoV RNA can also be found in blood

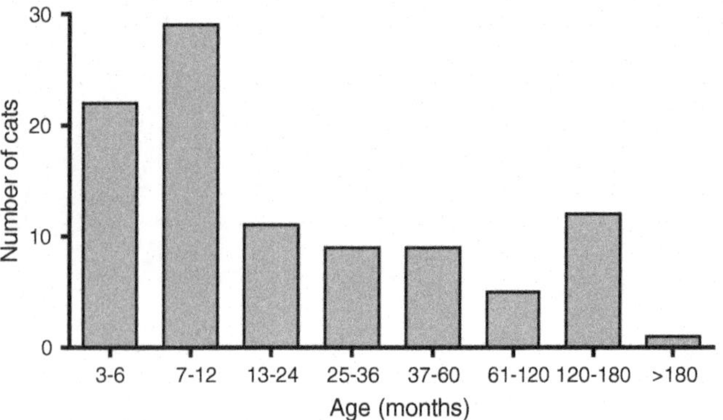

FIGURE 20-1 Age distribution of 99 cats with necropsy-confirmed FIP at the UC Davis VMTH. An additional six cats were reported to be "juvenile" or kittens. There were 38 females (17 intact) and 66 males (22 intact).

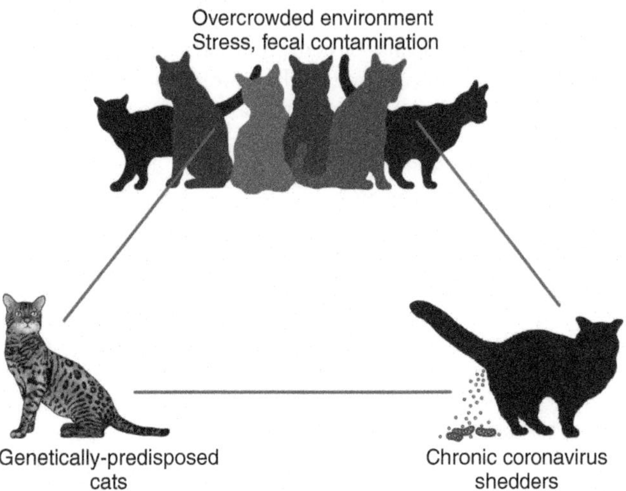

FIGURE 20-2 Interplay between genetics, virus shedding, and environment in feline coronavirus infections and FIP.

and tissue macrophages of cats that do not have FIP.[21,22] In some infected cats, the low-pathogenicity virus is believed to mutate to a virulent strain that can multiply within macrophages without hindrance by the immune system and incite a systemic pyogranulomatous vasculitis. The mutation may occur shortly after initial infection, or years later, which may explain why some indoor cats from single-cat households develop FIP several years after they are acquired. Virulent strains may not be able to replicate effectively within the gut,[23] which may be the reason why cat-to-cat transmission of FIP does not occur, yet the disease can be transmitted effectively by inoculating naïve cats with effusion from a cat with FIP. Factors that contribute to immunosuppression, such as concurrent viral infection, stress due to overcrowding, surgery, or transport, and especially genetic factors may allow viral replication and mutation to proceed unchecked. Simultaneous immune compromise of a large number of cats, such as in a shelter situation, may explain epidemics of FIP. Other risk factors for FIP include regular introduction of new cats to a cattery and the proportion of cats in a cattery that shed coronavirus chronically.[12] There is no distinct mutation that allows avirulent FCoV strains to be differentiated from virulent strains, and therefore no diagnostic test exists that distinguishes FIP from benign FCoV strains. However, mutations in the spike protein gene,[24,25] membrane protein gene,[26] and the nonstructural *3c* and *7b* genes[23,27-29] may play a role. In particular, the *3c* gene appears to be disrupted in many (but not all) virulent FCoV strains.

The other hypothesis proposed to explain the pathogenesis of FIP is that distinct circulating virulent and avirulent FCoV strains exist, and the combination of infection with a virulent FCoV and an individual cat's genetic and environmental predispositions leads to FIP.[25] It has also been suggested that both hypotheses may play a role.[30]

Clinical Features

Signs and Their Pathogenesis

Cats are usually infected with FCoV by oronasal exposure to virus in feces or fomites contaminated with fecal material. Shared litter boxes are thought to play a major role in transmission.[15] Replication of low-pathogenicity strains of FCoV in epithelial cells at the tips of intestinal villi may be associated with no signs, or acute or chronic, persistent or intermittent small-bowel diarrhea, and less commonly, vomiting and/or inappetence. Transient upper respiratory signs have been reported in some cats on initial infection with FCoV.[15] Virus is shed in the feces from 1 week after infection. Some cats then shed large quantities of virus continuously for life.[12,22,31-33]

Both serotype I and serotype II strains appear to enter macrophages via a lectin receptor known as fDC-SIGN (feline dendritic cell-specific intercellular adhesion molecule grabbing non-integrin receptor).[3,34] Replication of virulent FCoV strains within macrophages results in two forms of disease, which reflect the immune response mounted by the host. FIP is an immune complex disease. *Noneffusive* ("dry") FIP occurs in cats that mount a partial CMI response and is characterized by pyogranulomatous to granulomatous inflammation within a variety of organs, but especially the mesenteric lymph nodes, kidneys, liver, lungs, brain, and eye. Solitary or multifocal granulomas of the intestinal wall also occasionally develop, especially in the region of the ileocecal junction (Figure 20-3).[15] *Effusive* ("wet") FIP occurs in cats that are unable to mount an immune response and is characterized by accumulation of high protein exudates in the thorax and/or abdomen, which typically contain low numbers of cells. Production of vascular endothelial growth factor by infected monocytes may be lead to increased vascular permeability and contribute to cavitary effusion.[35] Many cats have a mixture of both forms of the disease, and noneffusive disease may progress to effusive disease. Infection itself results in immune dysregulation, with a profound, virus-induced depletion of CD4+ and CD8+ cells; production of TNF-α, granulocyte-macrophage colony stimulating factor (GM-CSF), and granulocyte colony-stimulating factor (G-CSF) by infected macrophages; impaired IFN-γ production; and hypergammaglobulinemia.[36-38] The mechanism of T-cell depletion is not clear, as the virus does not infect lymphocytes, only monocytes and macrophages. Infection of antigen-presenting cells, specifically dendritic cells, has been hypothesized to lead to T-cell apoptosis. Progressive immune system failure may be associated with a conversion to predominantly effusive disease manifestations. Despite the profound T-cell deficiency that accompanies FIP, opportunistic infections are rarely reported. Nevertheless, concurrent infections with retroviruses and *Toxoplasma gondii* and opportunistic bacterial infections can occur;[6] the author is aware of one cat that was co-infected with *Sporothrix schenckii*.

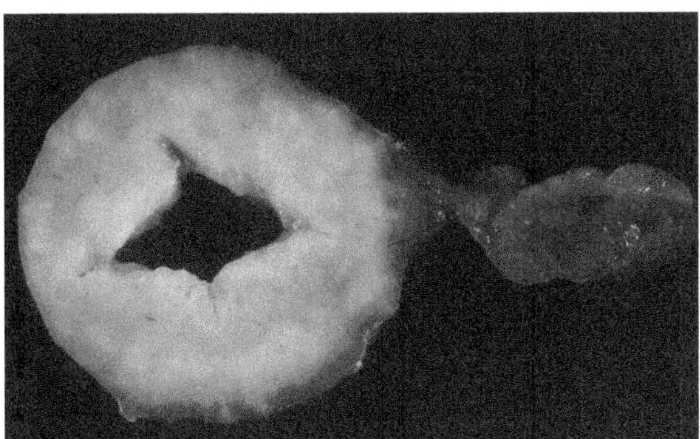

FIGURE 20-3 Colonic mass removed at surgery from a 7-month-old female spayed domestic shorthair with anorexia and hematochezia. Histopathology showed severe, multifocal coalescing pyogranulomatous colitis and lymphadenitis. (Courtesy of the University of California, Davis Veterinary Anatomic Pathology service.)

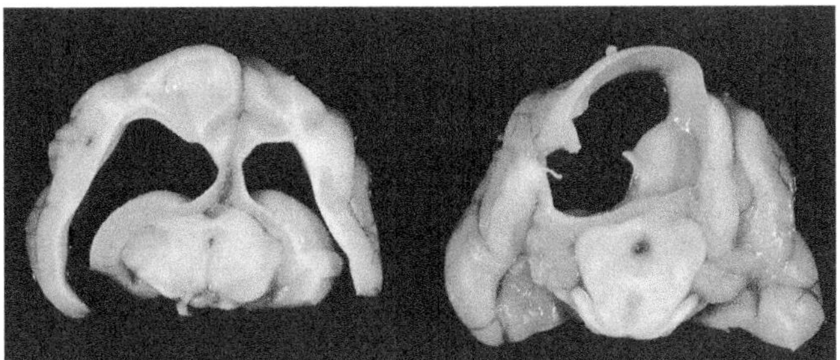

FIGURE 20-4 Obstructive hydrocephalus in an 8-month-old male neutered exotic shorthair cat that developed ataxia and head tremors. Hydrocephalus and secondary cerebellar herniation were found at necropsy. Histopathology revealed severe, multifocal pyogranulomatous meningoencephalitis, choroiditis, and ventriculitis, and pyogranulomatous inflammatory lesions were also found throughout the thoracic and abdominal viscera. (Courtesy of the University of California, Davis Veterinary Anatomic Pathology service.)

The incubation period for FIP is highly variable. Kittens usually become infected at 4 to 8 weeks of age, when maternal antibody begins to wane, but infections have been reported in kittens as young as 2 weeks of age.[20] Disease may occur a few weeks after infection or years later, but most often it occurs 6 to 18 months after initial infection.[19] Even after the onset of systemic pyogranulomatous inflammatory disease, clinical signs may not be apparent for months. In support of this, lesions consistent with FIP have been found incidentally in cats during abdominal surgery such as ovariohysterectomy.[20]

The clinical signs of FIP often change over time and depend on the organs affected and the relative predominance of inflammatory versus effusive disease manifestations. The most common signs are lethargy and inappetence, as well as a fluctuating fever that does not respond to antibacterial drug treatment. Nevertheless, many cats are bright, appetent, and in good body condition early in the course of illness. Some cats have increased thirst and urination, possibly secondary to pyrexia. Ultimately, weight loss develops, but owners of cats that develop abdominal distention may mistake the distention for weight gain or pregnancy. Stunted growth may occur in affected kittens. Pleural effusion may be associated with tachypnea and respiratory distress. Testicular enlargement may occur in cats with serositis that involves the tunica vaginalis. FIP is responsible for approximately 10% of pericardial effusions in cats, the third most common cause of pericardial effusion after cardiomyopathy and

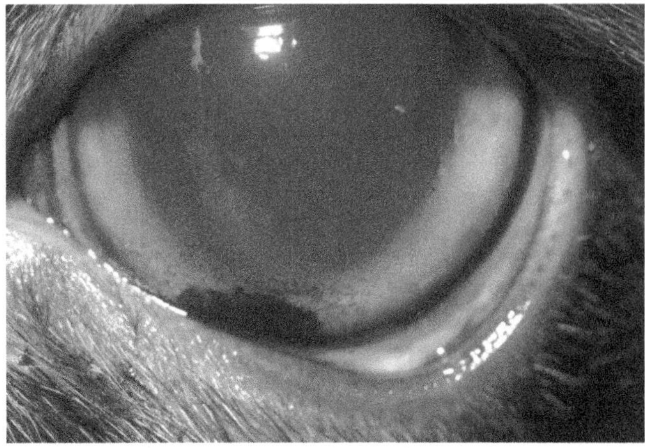

FIGURE 20-5 Keratic precipitates in a 5-year-old intact male Burmese cat with FIP. (Courtesy of the University of California, Davis Veterinary Ophthalmology service.)

neoplasia.[39] Rarely, pericardial effusion results in cardiac tamponade. Pyogranulomatous or granulomatous inflammation may lead to mesenteric lymphadenomegaly, irregular renomegaly, intestinal masses, hepatomegaly, icterus, pneumonia, uveitis, chorioretinitis, and, rarely, nodular skin lesions. Neurologic signs, which can include focal or generalized seizures, occur in at least 10% of cats with FIP and result primarily from meningoencephalitis, meningomyelitis, ependymitis, choroiditis, and obstructive hydrocephalus. Obstructive hydrocephalus occurs secondary to choroiditis and ependymitis (Figure 20-4). In one study, FIP was responsible for almost half of all neurologic disease in 97 cats due to infectious or inflammatory causes.[40] Occasionally profound anemia occurs secondary to immune-mediated hemolysis[13,14] or possibly microangiopathic damage, whereby erythrocytes are lysed as they travel through inflamed blood vessels. Immune-mediated glomerulonephritis has also been reported, and FIP should always be considered in cats with protein-losing nephropathy, which is otherwise rare in cats.[41] Uncommonly, lameness occurs as a result of synovitis.[6]

Physical Examination Findings

Physical examination findings in cats with FIP reflect the type of disease present (effusive versus noneffusive) and the location where lesions occur. Cats with respiratory tract involvement may show tachypnea, and if there is pleural effusion, a rapid, shallow breathing pattern and muffled heart and lung sounds may be present. Other signs include pyrexia, dehydration, mucosal pallor or icterus, a thin body condition, and evidence of ascites. Abdominal palpation may reveal hepatomegaly, irregular renomegaly, and/or abdominal mass lesions that result from mesenteric lymphadenomegaly or intestinal pyogranulomas. Sometimes pain is appreciated on abdominal palpation, which may reflect pancreatic involvement in some cats. Testicular enlargement may be detected in intact male cats. A wide range of neurologic signs may be present, such as obtundation, twitching, tremors, behavioral changes, nystagmus, hyperesthesia, exaggerated segmental reflexes, ataxia, urinary incontinence, or cranial nerve defects. Ocular signs include conjunctivitis, mucopurulent ocular discharge, thickening and hyperemia of the nictitans, uveitis with dyscoria or anisocoria, aqueous flare, keratic precipitates, hypopyon, hyphema, chorioretinitis, perivascular infiltrates, retinal detachment, or blindness (Figure 20-5).

TABLE 20-1

Complete Blood Count Findings at Admission in 38 Cats with Necropsy-Confirmed Feline Infectious Peritonitis at the UC Davis VMTH

Test	Reference Range	Percent below the Reference Range	Percent within the Reference Range	Percent above the Reference Range	Range for Cats with FIP	Number Tested
Hematocrit (%)	30-50	68	32	0	17-53	38
MCV (fL)	65-75	18	82	0	36-52	38
MCHC (g/dL)	33-36	5	58	37	28-36	38
RDW (%)	14-18	0	30	70	14-33	27
Neutrophils* (cells/μL)	2000-9000	3	26	71	416-49,313	38
Band neutrophils* (cells/μL)	0-rare	0	50	50	0-3251	38
Metamyelocytes (cells/μL)	0	0	95	5	0-276	38
Monocytes (cells/μL)	50-600	5	71	24	0-820	38
Lymphocytes (cells/μL)	1000-7000	58	42	0	89-6886	38
Eosinophils (cells/μL)	150-1100	71	29	0	0-770	38
Platelets (cells/μL)	180,000-500,000	37	44	19	30,000-874,000	27†

FIP, Feline infectious peritonitis; RDW, red cell distribution width.
*22 (58%) had evidence of toxic neutrophils.
†A smear was evaluated manually for 37 of the 38 cats. The presence of macroplatelets were reported for 18 (49%) of cats.

Diagnosis

Currently, definitive diagnosis of FIP is made only by immunohistochemical staining for coronavirus antigen within lesions characterized by pyogranulomatous or granulomatous vasculitis. Because it can be difficult or impossible to safely obtain biopsy specimens from cats with FIP, antemortem diagnosis is often only suspected on the basis of history, signalment, and clinical and laboratory findings, and by ruling out other causes of disease. Provided it is correctly performed and interpreted, immunocytochemistry may be helpful. Because the presence of the characteristic effusion is most helpful for antemortem diagnosis, efforts should be always made to identify and analyze any fluid that is present in body cavities. When owner funds are limited, laboratory analysis of effusion, rather than blood, may be the most economic diagnostic approach. Unfortunately, the lack of a definitive noninvasive diagnostic assay for FIP and the extremely poor prognosis sometimes leads clinicians to perform large numbers of diagnostic tests in the hope that an answer will appear. In other situations, the diagnosis of FIP is made too hastily, and euthanasia is performed without sufficient clinical and laboratory justification.

Laboratory Abnormalities

Complete Blood Count

A mild, nonregenerative anemia is often present in cats with FIP, and sometimes severe anemia occurs, which is usually poorly regenerative or nonregenerative (Table 20-1). Microcytosis may be present. Examination of erythrocyte morphology occasionally reveals schistocytosis, mild normoblastosis, or agglutination. There may be a leukocytosis due to a neutrophilia and monocytosis, or leukopenia. Lymphopenia occurs in more than 50% of affected cats, and eosinopenia is also common. In some cats, a left shift and evidence of toxic neutrophils are seen. Mild to moderate thrombocytopenia is common in cats with noneffusive disease and may reflect the presence of disseminated intravascular coagulation or immune-mediated platelet destruction. However, thrombocytosis can also occur.

Serum Biochemical Tests

Many cats with FIP have hyperproteinemia due to hyperglobulinemia, which results from a polyclonal gammopathy (Figure 20-6). Rarely, a monoclonal gammopathy can occur.[42] Total protein concentrations may be as high as 12 g/dL (Table 20-2).[20] In one study, hyperglobulinemia was present in 50% of cats with effusion and 70% of cats without effusion.[43] Globulin concentration may decrease terminally, so cats with advanced disease may have protein concentrations that are within the reference range.[14] Hypoalbuminemia is often present because of liver involvement, leakage from damaged vessels, urinary loss in cats with glomerulonephritis, or inflammation (albumin is a negative acute-phase reactant protein). Thus, the serum albumin:globulin ratio

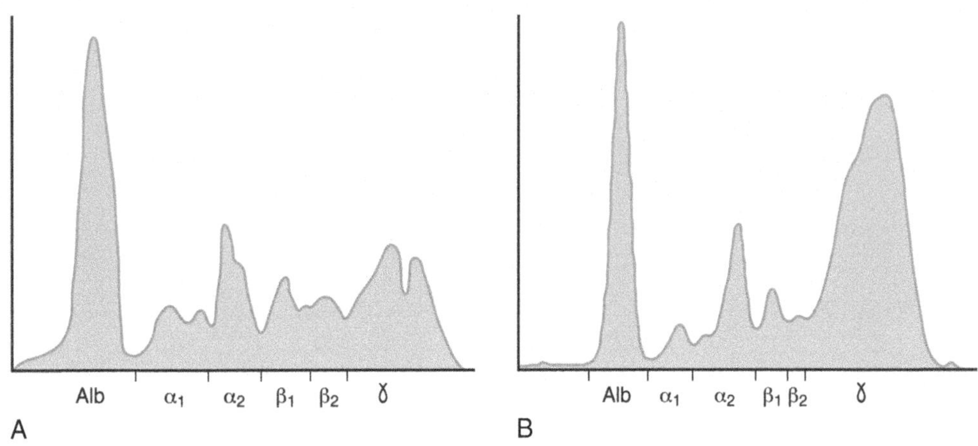

FIGURE 20-6 **A,** Densitometric scan of serum protein electrophoresis of normal feline serum. **B,** Scan from a 9-month-old male neutered domestic shorthair cat with FIP. There is a polyclonal gammopathy, represented by a broad peak in the γ-globulin region, with a mild decrease in the albumin and mild increases in the α_2 and β_1 fractions. (A redrawn from Baker RJ, Valli VE. Electrophoretic and immunoelectrophoretic analysis of feline serum proteins. Am J Vet Res 1988;52[3]:308-304.)

TABLE 20-2

Findings on Serum Biochemistry Analysis in 36 Cats with Necropsy-Confirmed Feline Infectious Peritonitis at the UC Davis VMTH

Test	Reference Range	Percent below the Reference Range	Percent within the Reference Range	Percent above the Reference Range	Range for cats with FIP	Number of Cats Tested
Sodium (mmol/L)	151-158	94	6	0	129-152	35
Potassium (mmol/L)	3.6-4.9	26	74	0	2.2-5.4	35
Chloride (mmol/L)	117-126	91	9	0	94-121	35
Bicarbonate (mmol/L)	15-21	8	75	17	12-25	36
Calcium (mg/dL)	9.0-10.9	56	44	0	6.6-10.6	36
Phosphorus (mg/dL)	3.2-6.3	8	69	22	1.9-8.4	36
Creatinine (mg/dL)	1.1-2.2	69	28	3	0.4-2.8	36
BUN (mg/dL)	18-33	56	31	14	10-58	36
Glucose (mg/dL)	63-118	0	47	53	63-381	36
Total protein (g/dL)	6.6-8.4	31	28	42	4.1-11.9	36
Albumin (g/dL)	2.2-4.6	50	50	0	0.9-3.6	36
Globulin (g/dL)	2.8-5.4	3	42	56	2.5-9.4	36
Cholesterol (mg/dL)	89-258	17	83	0	56-247	36
Total bilirubin (mg/dL)	0-0.2	0	40	60	0-5.3	36
ALT (U/L)	27-101	50	25	25	18-648	36
AST (U/L)	17-58	6	43	51	0-1554	36
ALP (U/L)	14-71	28	61	11	0-161	36
GGT (U/L)	0-4	0	96	4	0-5	23

FIP, feline infectious peritonitis.

may be more useful than the globulin alone for diagnosis; ratios less than 0.8 are uncommon (but not impossible) in cats with FIP, so they help to rule out (but not to rule in) a diagnosis of FIP.[44,45] Other variable findings include hyponatremia, hypokalemia, hypochloremia, hyperglycemia, azotemia, increased liver enzyme activities, hypocholesterolemia, and hyperbilirubinemia. The cause of hyperbilirubinemia is not clear, but it may result from hemolysis, hepatic necrosis, and/or cholestasis.

Measurement of α_1-acid glycoprotein (an acute phase protein) has been suggested for diagnosis, because serum concentrations often exceed 1500 μg/mL in cats with FIP.[20,46,47] However, α_1-acid glycoprotein concentrations also increase with other inflammatory diseases.[20]

TABLE 20-3

Composition of Body Cavity Effusions from 21 Cats with Necropsy-Confirmed Feline Infectious Peritonitis at the UC Davis VMTH

Test	Range	Mean ± SD	Number of Cats Tested
Total protein (g/dL)	2.9-8.1	5.1 ± 1.8	21
RBC (cells/μL)	<100-38,600	ND	18
TNC (cells/μL)	200-13,200	3683 ± 3474	19
Neutrophils (%)	3-97	61 ± 28	21
Lymphocytes (%)	0-22	6 ± 6	21
Monocytes (%)	1-96	33 ± 26	21

Nineteen specimens were abdominal and two were pleural effusions. ND, Not determined; SD, standard deviation; TNC, total neutrophil count.

TABLE 20-4

Composition of Cerebrospinal Fluid from 10 Cats with Necropsy-Confirmed Feline Infectious Peritonitis at the UC Davis VMTH

Test	Range	Median	Reference Range	Number of Cats Tested
Total protein (mg/dL)	44-4079	639	<25	4*
RBC (cells/μL)	3-850	340	0	9
TNC (cells/μL)	26-2637	303	0-2	10
Neutrophils (%)	4-90	73		10
Lymphocytes (%)	5-89	19		10
Monocytes (%)	0-20	7		10

TNC, total neutrophil count.
*Insufficient quantity available from some cats for determination of protein concentration.

Urinalysis

The urinalysis in cats with FIP may be unremarkable or contain protein due to glomerular or tubular damage. Hematuria and, less commonly, pyuria and cylindruria may be present. Bilirubinuria may be detected in cats with liver injury.

Coagulation Profile

In addition to thrombocytopenia, abnormalities of coagulation in cats with FIP include prolonged prothrombin time and partial thromboplastin time as a result of severe liver injury, and increased fibrin degradation product or D-dimer concentrations.[15]

Analysis of Effusion Fluid

The "classic" FIP effusion fluid is a high-protein (greater than 3.5 g/dL) exudate that contains a low number of nucleated cells (<5000 cells/μL), usually nondegenerate to mildly degenerate neutrophils and macrophages (Table 20-3). Erythrophagocytosis, leukophagia, and reactive mesothelial cells can be observed in the fluid from some cats. Grossly, the fluid has a yellow appearance and may contain fibrin clots. However, the total protein content and cell counts of abdominal and pleural effusions vary considerably, which complicates the diagnosis for some cats with effusive disease. Very rarely, chylous effusions occur.[48] An effusion albumin/globulin ratio below 0.4 is suggestive of FIP.[49]

The *Rivalta test* is a simple test that can differentiate between transudates and exudates. In this test, a drop of 98% glacial acetic acid is mixed with 7 to 8 mL of distilled water in a transparent 10-mL tube. A drop of effusion is then added to the tube, and if it dissipates in the solution, the test is negative. If it retains its shape, stays attached to the surface, or moves slowly down in the solution, then the test is positive.[20] In a study of cats with effusion, 35% of which had FIP and a conclusive Rivalta test, the positive predictive value of this test for the diagnosis of FIP was 58% (58% chance that a cat that tests positive truly has FIP), and the negative predictive value was 93% (93% chance that a cat that tests negative does not have FIP).[50] In younger cats, the positive predictive value of the test is higher, because diseases such as lymphoma and bacterial peritonitis are less common. Positive test results indicate only the presence of an exudate, so cytologic examination of the fluid must still be performed.

Cerebrospinal Fluid Analysis

The cerebrospinal fluid (CSF) of cats with neurologic FIP often has increased protein content (30 to more than 1000 mg/dL, reference range less than 25 mg/dL) and increased total nucleated cell count (20 to 10,000 cells/μL), usually consisting of a mixed but predominantly neutrophilic cellular pleocytosis (Table 20-4). In some cats, protein content and leukocyte counts are normal.[51,52]

Diagnostic Imaging

Plain Radiography

Plain thoracic radiography may reveal pleural effusion, enlargement of the cardiac silhouette in cats with pericardial effusion, and pulmonary nodular or peribronchial infiltrates in cats with pyogranulomatous pneumonia (Figure 20-7). Abdominal radiographs may show loss of peritoneal or retroperitoneal detail due to peritoneal effusion, hepatomegaly, splenomegaly, renomegaly, or mass lesions associated with the gastrointestinal tract or abdominal lymph nodes.

Sonographic Findings

Abdominal ultrasound findings in FIP include the presence of anechoic or mildly echogenic peritoneal fluid; hyperechogenicity and "clumping" of the mesentery; enlarged and hypoechoic abdominal lymph nodes (Figure 20-8, *A*); enlargement and diffuse or focal hypoechogenicity of the liver and spleen;[53] renal asymmetry with increased cortical echogenicity, hypoechoic nodules, subcapsular fluid accumulation, or loss of corticomedullary distinction (see Figure 20-8, *B*); and/or thickening of all intestinal wall layers or intestinal mass lesions. Pleural effusion or comet-tail artifacts (due to pulmonary infiltrates) may be seen through the diaphragm.

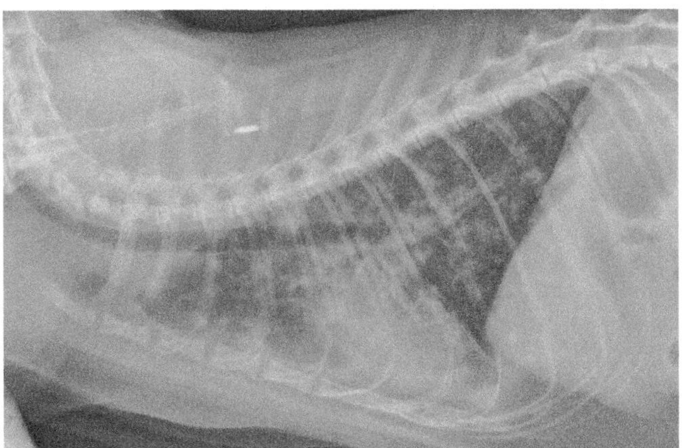

FIGURE 20-7 Lateral thoracic radiograph from a 9-month-old male neutered domestic shorthair cat with FIP and pyogranulomatous pneumonia. There is a severe, diffuse, patchy alveolar and nodular interstitial pattern with thickening of the bronchial walls and mild pleural effusion.

Magnetic Resonance Imaging of the Central Nervous System

Findings on MRI that suggest FIP consist of ventricular dilatation and variable contrast enhancement of the periventricular regions, choroid, and meninges. In some cats, MRI findings are unremarkable.

Microbiologic Tests

Serologic Diagnosis

Detection of antibodies to FCoV can be performed using immunofluorescent antibody testing, ELISA, or virus neutralization.[54] The methods used, as well as the titers themselves, vary considerably between laboratories. For example, some laboratories use related coronaviruses as a source of antigen for the test, rather than FCoV.[15] Use of a reliable laboratory that reports quantitative titers (to the endpoint dilution, as well as down to 1:100) is critical. Even when performed correctly, a positive FCoV antibody titer is not diagnostic for FIP, because cats that have been exposed to avirulent FCoV strains or even other related coronaviruses are also seropositive. Therefore, serology is a "coronavirus antibody test" and not an "FIP test." It has been suggested that more cats have been killed as a result of misinterpretation of FCoV antibody tests than by the disease itself.[20] Certainly a diagnosis of FIP should *never* be made based on the presence of nonspecific clinical or laboratory abnormalities such as fever or leukocytosis and a positive coronavirus antibody test. Occasionally (up to 10% of the time), cats with advanced disease are seronegative, because of failure of antibody production with severe immunosuppression, or the complexing of antibody by the large quantities of virus present. In one study, titers of 1:1600 or higher were highly suggestive (94% chance) of FIP in the presence of compatible clinical signs.[44] In addition, strong positive titers (e.g., ≥ 1:6400) in cats with consistent signs and laboratory abnormalities support a diagnosis of FIP if a cat resides in a household that contains only one or two cats, because cats often become seronegative within a few months once they are removed from households that contain large numbers of cats.

Other body fluids can also be analyzed for antibodies to FCoV. In one study, positive antibody titers in effusion had a positive predictive value of 90% and a negative predictive value of 79%, but the magnitude of the titer did not correlate with the diagnosis of FIP.[44] The presence of anti-FCoV

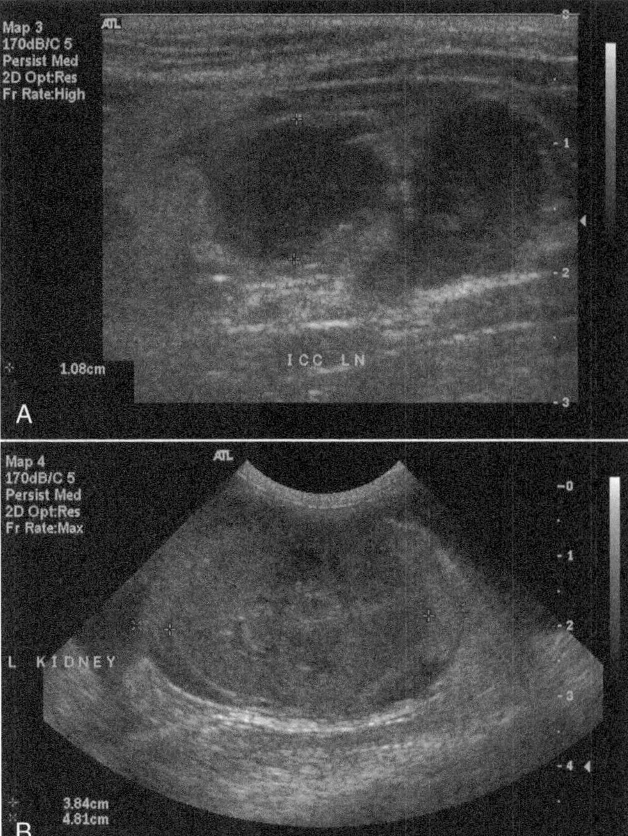

FIGURE 20-8 **A,** Abdominal ultrasound image from a 9-month-old male neutered domestic shorthair cat with FIP and ileocecocolic lymphadenopathy. The lymph nodes are enlarged and hypoechoic. **B,** Abdominal ultrasound image from a 1-year-old male intact Scottish fold with FIP. There is renal irregularity and subcapsular fluid, as well as moderate peritoneal effusion.

antibody in the CSF correlated well with a diagnosis of FIP in one study,[52] but not in another study.[51] In addition, the presence of sufficient quantities of CSF for serology are frequently not available.

Molecular Diagnosis Using the Polymerase Chain Reaction

Real-time reverse transcriptase–PCR (RT-PCR) assays have been developed for detection of FCoV, but these do not differentiate between virulent and avirulent strains. In addition, avirulent strains can be found in the blood and tissues of cats that do not have FIP,[21,22] so the finding of virus in locations other than the gastrointestinal tract is not helpful for diagnosis. False-negative test results can occur when there are low quantities of virus present or if degradation of RNA occurs during specimen transport. Some RT-PCR assays do not detect all strains of FCoV. Positive RT-PCR results in blood or effusion fluid from cats with other clinical abnormalities that suggest FIP do indicate the presence of a coronavirus and, in that respect, may help to support the diagnosis made, provided the limitations of the test are recognized.

Immunostaining of FCoV Antigen

FCoV antigen can be detected in macrophages with immunocytochemistry or immunohistochemistry (Figure 20-9). Either fluorescent antibody or immunoperoxidase methods

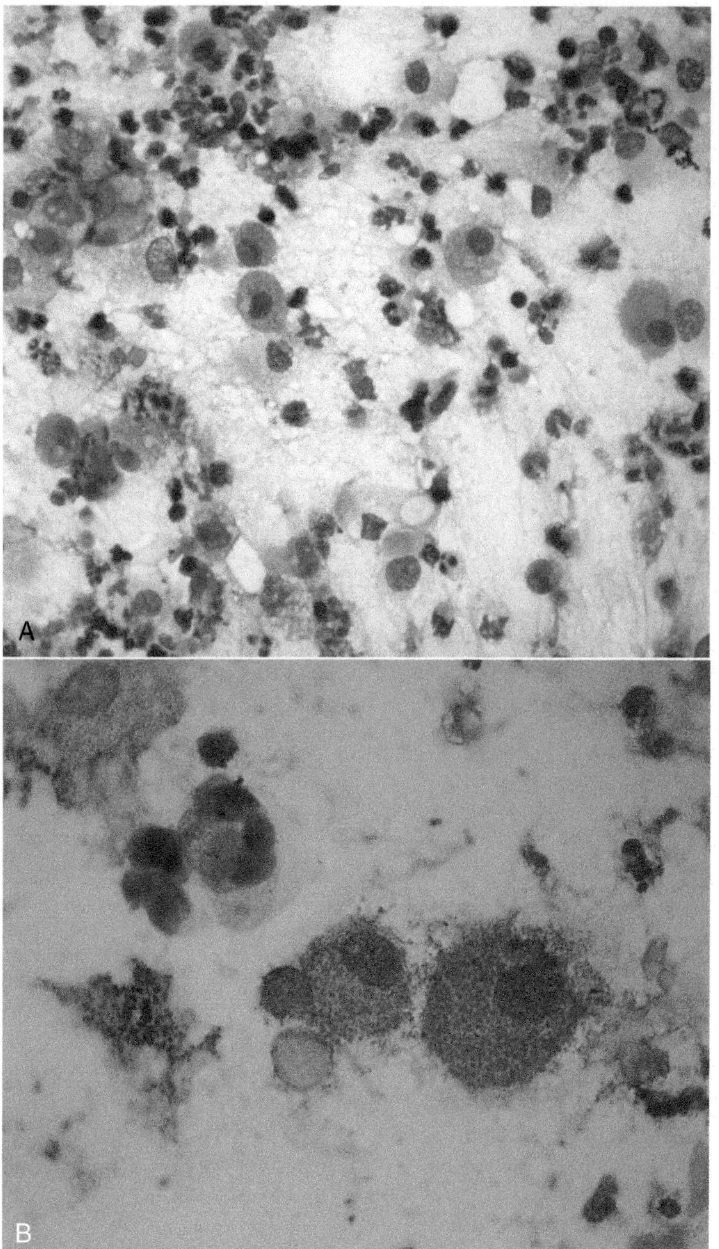

FIGURE 20-9 **A,** Cytospin preparation of a tracheobronchial lavage from the cat in Figure 20-7. The specimen was highly cellular (4400 cells/μL) and the cells consisted of 42% degenerate and nondegenerate neutrophils, 5% lymphocytes, and 53% macrophages. **B,** Immunocytochemistry stain on the same specimen for coronavirus antigen showing positive staining in association with macrophages.

may be used (Table 20-5). When antigen tests are positive, provided the test is performed and interpreted properly (with use of positive and negative control slides), studies suggest that only cats with FIP have positive test results.[44,55] False-negative results occur when there are insufficient numbers of infected cells, when low quantities of virus are present, or when antigen is unavailable for detection because of complexing by antibody.

Pathologic Findings

Gross Pathologic Findings

At necropsy, gross findings in cats with FIP include variable quantities of pleural, pericardial, and peritoneal effusion (Figure 20-10, *A*). Fibrin adhesions may be present and the mesentery may be clumped. Abdominal organs may be enlarged or irregular. Granulomas appear as variably sized multifocal white, cream, tan, or yellow nodular lesions on serosal surfaces and within the parenchyma of organs such as the lungs, spleen, kidneys, pancreas, and liver (see Figure 20-10, *B*). Lesions have also been described within the nasal cavity and sinuses. Pyogranulomas may be visible grossly as miliary lesions, or they may be several centimeters in diameter. Thoracic and/or abdominal lymphadenomegaly is a common finding. Diffuse or focal thickening of the intestinal wall or intestinal mass lesions may be present. Examination of the brain can reveal fibrinous exudate in association with the meninges, with or without ventricular dilation and hydrocephalus (see Figure 20-4). Thymic involution may also be present.

TABLE 20-5

Assays Available for Diagnosis of Feline Infectious Peritonitis

Assay	Specimen Type	Target	Performance
Fluorescent or immunoperoxidase antibody staining	Wash or effusion specimens, tissue aspirates, tissues obtained at biopsy or necropsy	FCoV	Gold standard for diagnosis. False negatives can occur in specimens that contain low numbers of macrophages or virus particles, or when virus is complexed by antibody. Immunofluorescence is more sensitive than immunoperoxidase methods. Non-specific staining may be interpreted as positive results by untrained personnel.
Serology	Blood, CSF, aqueous humor, effusion fluid	FCoV antibody	Positive antibody titers reflect only antibodies to a coronavirus and are not specific for a diagnosis of FIP. Most cats in multicat households test positive. Negative titers can occur in cats with advanced FIP. High titers in cats that do not reside in multicat households and that have signs suggestive of FIP may support the diagnosis. Interlaboratory variation in methodology and titer reporting occurs.
RT-PCR	Blood, wash or effusion specimens, tissue aspirates, tissues obtained at biopsy or necropsy	FCoV RNA	Does not differentiate between virulent and avirulent FCoV strains, and avirulent strains may be found in tissues and blood. Sensitivity and specificity can vary depending on assay design. False negative results occur when virus levels are low, when variant virus strains are present, or as a result of degradation of viral nucleic acid during specimen transport.
Histopathology	Usually necropsy specimens, but also biopsies	Inflammatory lesions induced by FCoV (pyogranulomatous vasculitis)	Biopsy is often not feasible antemortem as a result of critical illness and coagulopathies.

FCoV, feline coronavirus; FIP, feline infectious peritonitis; RT-PCR, reverse transcriptase–polymerase chain reaction.

Histopathologic Findings

The characteristic histopathologic findings of FIP are systemic perivascular, multifocal to coalescing pyogranulomatous or granulomatous inflammatory lesions (Figure 20-11). Lesions predominantly contain macrophages and neutrophils, with lesser numbers of lymphocytes and plasma cells, although occasionally the histiocytic or the lymphoplasmacytic component of the inflammatory response is more florid. Necrosis may be present within the lesions. Lesions in the central nervous system consist of pyogranulomatous meningoencephalomyelitis and choroiditis. Other findings that may be identified include lymphoid depletion, which results from apoptosis, and membranous glomerulonephritis.

Treatment and Prognosis

Currently, no cure for FIP exists; it is a progressive, invariably fatal disease. The goal of treatment is to prolong life span and improve quality of life through reduction of inflammation and supportive care. The most effective treatment known is prednisolone, administration of which results in temporary remissions in some cats (Table 20-6). Other immunosuppressive drugs, such as chlorambucil and cyclophosphamide, have been used in addition to prednisolone, but whether these drugs improve outcome is unknown, and they have the potential to be toxic. A variety of immunomodulators and antiviral drugs have been tried, such as ribavirin and oral and parenteral human recombinant IFN-α, but none have convincingly shown benefit in vivo. Prolonged remissions were reported in several cats treated with a combination of glucocorticoids and feline IFN-ω,[56] but a randomized, placebo-controlled clinical trial reported no effect of feline IFN-ω.[57] Other drugs used to treat cats with FIP include the immunomodulatory drugs pentoxifylline and Polyprenyl Immunostimulant (see Chapter 7)[58]; ozagrel hydrochloride, a thromboxane synthetase inhibitor[59]; and the antiviral drug nelfinavir.[14,60] Controlled clinical trials are required to assess the efficacy and safety of these treatments. Because FIP is an immune-mediated disease, nonspecific immune stimulation has the potential to cause harm. The use of small interfering RNA molecules, which bind viral RNA and prevent viral replication, has recently shown promising results in vitro.[61] Cyclosporin inhibits FIPV replication in vitro;[62] studies are required to determine if cyclosporin treatment benefits infected cats or whether harm results from immunosuppression.

Supportive treatments that may be required include subcutaneous fluid therapy and nutritional support. Inappetent cats can benefit from enteral nutrition through a feeding tube. The use of broad-spectrum antimicrobial drugs to treat cats with FIP is controversial; it may only promote opportunistic infections with resistant bacteria.

The prognosis for cats with FIP is generally grave. Almost all cats with effusion at the time of diagnosis die within weeks. Very rarely, more prolonged survival times (1 to 2 years) have been documented after glucocorticoid treatment (see Case Example).

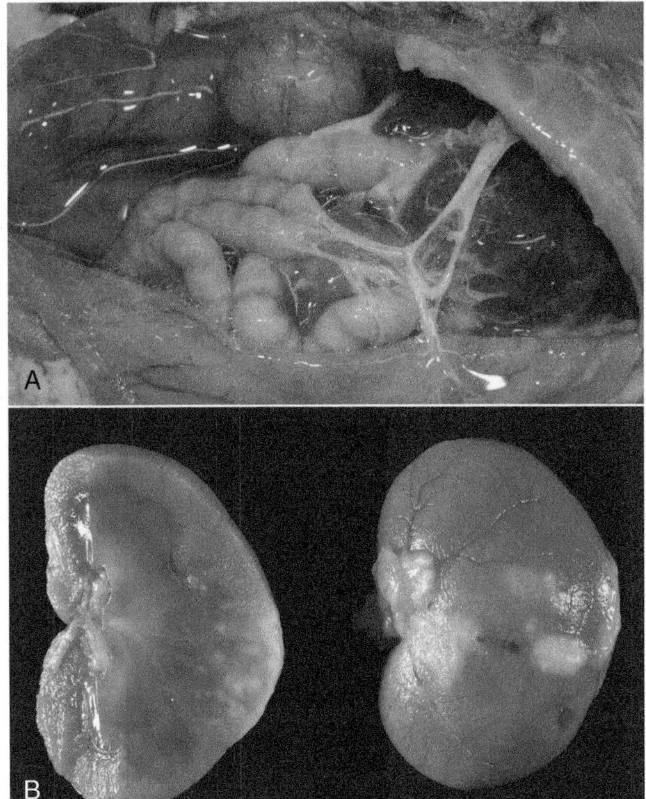

FIGURE 20-10 **A,** Gross necropsy findings in a 10-month-old male intact domestic shorthair cat with effusive FIP. Approximately 1.2 liters of yellow fluid was present in the abdomen, and there are abundant fibrin strains adherent to the visceral and parietal peritoneal surfaces. **B,** Kidneys of the cat in Figure 20-8. Multiple, pale tan firm nodules expand the renal cortices and protrude from the cortical surfaces. (Courtesy of the University of California, Davis Veterinary Anatomic Pathology service, D. Gasper and M. Jones.)

The median survival time in one study of 37 cats was 9 days (range, 3 to 200 days).[57] In another it was 21 days (range, 1 to 99 days) for 30 cats with effusive disease, 38 days (range, 1 to 171 days) for 12 cats with noneffusive disease, and 111 days (range, 7 to 477 days) for 9 cats with mixed effusive and noneffusive disease.[14] Hyperbilirubinemia, the presence of effusion, and lymphopenia are negative prognostic factors[20]; in one study, the hematocrit, lymphocyte count, and serum albumin, potassium, sodium, and globulin concentrations decreased as disease progressed, and total bilirubin concentration and serum liver enzyme activities increased.[14] Euthanasia should be considered for cats with severe illness that fail to respond to treatment within a 3-day period.[20]

Immunity and Vaccination

Although antibodies to the spike protein can neutralize virus, antibodies are required for FIP to occur, because FIP is an immune complex disease. Cell-mediated immunity is important for protection,[6] but if immunity is incomplete, granulomatous or pyogranulomatous disease results.

The development of vaccines for FIP has been complicated by the fact that stimulation of antibody production against FCoV can accelerate the disease, should FIP develop after vaccination has been performed. Antibodies may bind to Fc receptors on macrophages and accelerate virus uptake in a phenomenon known as *antibody-dependent disease enhancement* (ADDE). Currently, an intranasal, temperature-sensitive mutant serotype II FIP virus vaccine is available on the market, but its use has been controversial. The vaccine virus replicates in the lower temperatures found in the respiratory tract. It is licensed for administration from 16 weeks of age, by which time most kittens have already been exposed to FCoV. The vaccine does not appear to cause ADDE,[63-65] but its efficacy and ability to induce

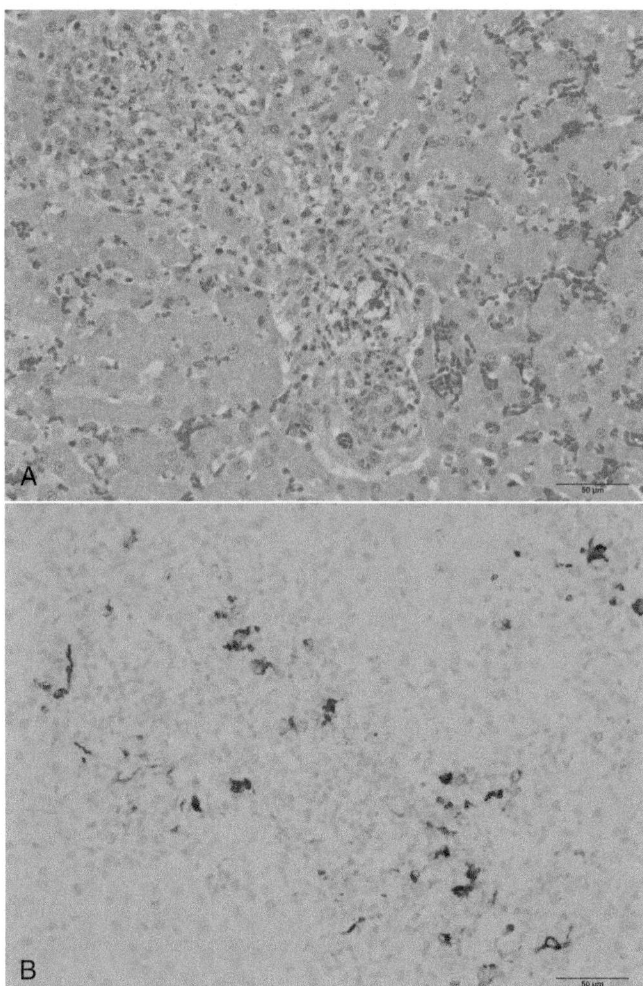

FIGURE 20-11 **A,** Histopathology of the liver of a cat with FIP. There is pyogranulomatous hepatitis. Hematoxylin and eosin stain. **B,** Macrophages stain strongly positive for feline coronavirus antigen with immunohistochemistry. (Courtesy Dr. Patricia Pesavento, University of California, Davis Veterinary Anatomic Pathology service.)

TABLE 20-6

Suggested Drug Dosages for Treatment of Feline Infectious Peritonitis

Drug	Dose (mg/kg)	Route	Interval (hours)
Prednisolone	1-2	PO	12-24
Chlorambucil*	2 mg/cat	PO	48-72

*Monitor the CBC during treatment.

immunity against heterologous strains is controversial. In a study of 138 cats that belonged to 15 different cat breeders, virtually all of which were seropositive, there was no difference in prevalence of FIP in vaccinated versus placebo-treated cats.[63] A slight reduction in the prevalence of FIP occurred when the vaccine was used in cats that had not been exposed to FCoV before vaccination, but protection was not convincing based on the small numbers of cats that developed the disease in each group.[6,65]

Prevention

In households that contain only one or a few cats, young cats that develop FIP likely become infected with FCoV before they are acquired. They may or may not have FIP at the time of acquisition. When a cat from a single-cat household dies with FIP, it is suggested that the owner wait at least 2 months before a new cat is obtained, so that any virus in the environment becomes inactivated.[20] Selection of a new cat from a different genetic background than the previous cat should be considered, and if possible, the breeder should be informed if a purebred cat develops FIP. If a low number of other cats remain in the household, they may or may not continue to shed virus. These cats often have a positive antibody titer, but this in no way predicts that they will develop FIP. Before a new cat is introduced to a household that has a history of FIP, factors that could reduce stress and overcrowding should be identified and addressed.

The risk of transmission and disease can be reduced through attention to hygiene, prevention of overcrowding, maintenance of a larger ratio of adult to juvenile cats, and ensuring that cats are in stable groups of three or fewer per room. Cats should have sufficient numbers of regularly cleaned litter trays located in a different area from where they are fed. Methods to control FIP in cattery situations, such as identification and removal of chronic shedders with serial fecal RT-PCR assays and removal of kittens from the queen followed by isolation at 5 to 6 weeks of age (before maternal antibody has declined), have limitations and are difficult to achieve properly in large catteries.[20] For example, cats that do not shed FCoV may still be infected with avirulent FCoV strains, and shedding may recommence at a later date.[22] Isolation of kittens may be useful if reexposure is prevented until after they are 16 weeks of age, when their immune system is more mature.[6] In shelter situations, FIP may be reduced when overcrowding and prolonged stays are minimized, especially during kitten season.[6] If possible, owners that adopt cats from shelter environments should be provided with a handout that provides basic information on the disease (and other major infectious diseases of shelter cats such as retrovirus infections, bartonellosis, and feline upper respiratory tract disease) and the ubiquitous nature of infection.

Further understanding of genetic factors that contribute to FIP is required, because selective breeding may reduce the risk of the disease. In the meantime, the breeding of cats that produce litters that succumb to FIP should be avoided. This is especially true for male cats, because a single male cat can have an effect on far more kittens and litters than a single queen. It is recommended that no more than six breeding animals be maintained if possible.[6]

Public Health Aspects

There is no evidence that humans can become infected with FCoV. The closest human coronavirus relative is the severe acute respiratory syndrome (SARS) coronavirus. Other coronaviruses cause FIP-like disease in nonfelids such as ferrets and mice. If a coronavirus emerged that could cause similar clinical manifestations and outcomes in humans as FIPV can in cats, it would represent a major threat to humans and would be the subject of intense research.

CASE EXAMPLE

Signalment: "Ricky", a 9-month-old male castrated domestic shorthair from Sacramento, CA

History: Ricky was brought to a local veterinary clinic because of increased thirst and urination. A serum chemistry panel showed hyperglobulinemia (7.7 mg/dL), and urinalysis showed a specific gravity (SGr) of 1.025 with an inactive sediment; aerobic bacterial urine culture was negative. Three days later, Ricky became inappetent and was returned to the local veterinary clinic. Laboratory abnormalities included mature neutrophilia (11,904 cells/μL), lymphocytosis (5104 cells/μL), eosinophilia (1536 cells/μL), hyperglobulinemia (6.9 mg/dL), and hypoalbuminemia (2.4 mg/dL). A feline coronavirus antibody titer was 1:400. Serology for *Toxoplasma gondii* was negative. Plain thoracic radiographs showed a mild interstitial pattern. Abdominal ultrasound showed mesenteric lymphadenomegaly, and an aspirate of the lymph nodes showed lymphoid reactivity. Treatment with cyproheptadine was initiated, and Ricky's appetite recovered, after which treatment was discontinued. For the 3 weeks that followed, the cat had been appetent and energetic, but occasional soft feces had been noticed in the litter box. The owners were concerned about the possibility of FIP.

Ricky was obtained at 3 months of age from a rescue group, who rescued him as an 8-week-old stray kitten. As a kitten he had multiple upper respiratory tract infections, but since adoption he had been healthy and shared a household with one other cat. He was an indoor cat that was sometimes walked briefly outdoors. He was fed commercial dry and wet cat food.

Physical Examination:

Body Weight: 4.2 kg

General: Bright, alert and responsive, hydrated. T = 103°F (39.4°C), HR = 200 beats/min, eupneic.

All Systems: No clinically significant abnormalities of any body system were detected. Body condition score was 5/9.

Laboratory Findings:

CBC:

HCT 27.3% (30%-50%)
MCV 42.1 fL (42-53 fL)

MCHC 34.1 g/dL (30-33.5 g/dL)
WBC 24,950 cells/μL (4500-14,000 cells/μL)
Neutrophils 17,141 cells/μL (2000-9000 cells/μL)
Lymphocytes 6886 cells/μL (1000-7000 cells/μL)
Monocytes 724 cells/μL (50-600 cells/μL)
Eosinophils 200 cells/μL (150-1100 cells/μL)
Basophils 25 cells/μL (0-50 cells/μL)
Platelets 518,000/μL (180,000-500,000 platelets/μL).

Serum Chemistry Profile:
Sodium 147 mmol/L (151-158 mmol/L)
Potassium 4.5 mmol/L (3.6-4.9 mmol/L)
Chloride 116 mmol/L (117-126 mmol/L)
Bicarbonate 18 mmol/L (15-21 mmol/L)
Phosphorus 6.4 mg/dL (3.2-6.3 mg/dL)
Calcium 9.5 mg/dL (9.0-10.9 mg/dl)
BUN 22 mg/dL (18-33 mg/dL)
Creatinine 1.1 mg/dL (1.1-2.2 mg/dL)
Glucose 83 mg/dL (63-118 mg/dL)
Total protein 10.7 g/dL (6.6-8.4 g/dL)
Albumin 2.6 g/dL (2.2-4.6 g/dL)
Globulin 8.1 g/dL (2.8-5.4 g/dL)
ALT 31 U/L (27-101 U/L)
AST 17 U/L (17-58 U/L)
ALP 35 U/L (14-71 U/L)
Gamma GT <3 U/L (0-4 U/L)
Cholesterol 143 mg/dL (89-258 mg/dL)
Total bilirubin < 0.1 mg/dL (0-0.2 mg/dL).

Serum Protein Electrophoresis: A polyclonal gammopathy with a mild decrease in albumin concentration and mild increases in the α_2 and β_1 fractions was present (see Figure 20-4). These changes were consistent with the acute-phase inflammatory response.

Imaging Findings: Abdominal ultrasound: The spleen was moderately enlarged. There was diffuse mesenteric lymphadenopathy (see Figure 20-8, *B*).

Mesenteric Lymph Node Aspirate Cytology: Intact nucleated cells were composed of a heterogenous population of lymphocytes, predominated by small, mature lymphocytes. Lower numbers of intermediate and large reactive lymphocytes, moderate numbers of mildly degenerate neutrophils, and scattered plasma cells and histiocytes were noted. Immunocytochemistry using two different monoclonal antibodies against FCoV was negative, but macrophages were low in number.

Microbiologic Testing: FeLV antigen and FIV antibody serology: negative

Serology (IFA) and blood culture for *Bartonella clarridgeiae* and *Bartonella henselae*: negative

Serology (IFA) for vector-borne diseases: negative for antibodies to *Ehrlichia canis, Neorickettsia risticii, Anaplasma* spp., and *Rickettsia* spp.

PCR for FCoV (whole blood): negative

PCR panel for other bloodborne pathogens *(Anaplasma phagocytophilum, Anaplasma platys, Bartonella* spp., *E. canis, N. risticii, Mycoplasma haemofelis):* negative

Aerobic and anaerobic bacterial culture of mesenteric lymph node aspirate: negative

Serology for FCoV: positive at 1:102,400

Diagnosis: A tentative diagnosis of FIP was made on the basis of Ricky's background, the marked polyclonal gammopathy, and the strongly positive coronavirus titer.

Treatment and Outcome: Biopsy of the enlarged mesenteric node was offered, but the owners declined. Ricky was treated with prednisolone (5 mg PO q12h for 7 days, followed by 5 mg PO q24h thereafter), chlorambucil (2 mg PO every 3 days), and pentoxifylline (50 mg PO q8h). Six weeks later, the cat was well and CBC variables within reference ranges. Serum total protein concentration was 8.5 g/dL, with a globulin concentration of 4.5 g/dL. Abdominal ultrasound examination showed persistent but mild mesenteric lymphadenomegaly (0.5 to 0.75 cm in diameter). A feline coronavirus titer was 1:25,600. Treatment with feline interferon-ω was commenced (4.5 million units SC once weekly). Ricky was seen again 3 months later, at which time he continued to be playful and appetent, with a stable body weight of 4.5 kg. A CBC showed mild anemia (HCT 29%), a neutrophil count of 4439 cells/μL, and lymphopenia (468 cells/μL). A chemistry panel and abdominal ultrasound showed no abnormalities. Chlorambucil and interferon-ω were discontinued. The next time the cat was reexamined was 12 months after the onset of illness, at which time he continued to be apparently healthy. CBC findings were unchanged, and the serum globulin concentration was 4.7 g/dL. The prednisolone dose was decreased to 5 mg q48h and pentoxifylline treatment was discontinued. One month later, albumin and globulin concentrations were 3.3 and 5.1 g/dL, respectively, and the prednisolone dose was reduced to 2.5 mg q48h. At the next 1-month recheck, a CBC was unremarkable but globulin was 5.7 g/dL. Abdominal ultrasound showed mildly enlarged mesenteric lymph nodes, and the serum coronavirus antibody titer was 1:409,600. The prednisolone dose was increased to 5 mg PO q24h; 1 month later, the serum globulin concentration was 4.9 g/dL. One and a half years after the onset of illness, Ricky was still apparently healthy according to the owner, but a midabdominal mass was palpated on physical examination, and the serum globulin concentration had increased again (5.6 g/dL). Abdominal ultrasound showed several moderately enlarged and hypoechoic lymph nodes in the ileocolic region, the largest of which was 0.9 cm in diameter. The surrounding mesentery was focally hyperechoic. There was also focal hyperechoic retroperitoneal tissue surrounding the right kidney with scant retroperitoneal fluid. Attempts to obtain aspirates from the lymph nodes were unsuccessful. The prednisolone dose was increased to 5mg PO q12h, and treatment with chlorambucil and pentoxifylline was reinstituted.

One week later, Ricky developed lethargy and inappetence. A CBC showed macrocytic anemia (HCT 24.3%, MCV 57.2 fL) and lymphopenia (782 cells/μL). A serum chemistry panel showed only hyperglobulinemia (5.8 g/dL). FeLV and FIV serology was repeated and was again negative, and the coronavirus antibody titer was 1:25,600. Treatment with cyproheptadine was initiated and the chlorambucil and pentoxifylline discontinued. However, inappetence continued, and persistent pyrexia (103.4° to 104°F), hematochezia, and tachypnea developed over the next few days. The hematocrit dropped to 16.5%, and hypokalemia, hyponatremia, and hypochloremia were identified. Ricky was hospitalized and treated with 1 unit of packed RBC, IV crystalloids, and parenteral antimicrobial drugs. Thoracic radiographs showed a severe, diffuse, patchy alveolar and nodular interstitial pattern with thickening of the bronchial walls and mild pleural effusion (see Figure 20-7). A tracheobronchial lavage showed marked mixed, predominantly pyogranulomatous inflammation with moderate epithelial hyperplasia and some degenerate neutrophils (see Figure 20-9). Immunocytochemistry with an anti-FCoV antibody was strongly positive in macrophages. Aerobic and anaerobic bacterial cultures of the wash specimen were negative. The cat subsequently seizured and was euthanized.

Necropsy Findings: Necropsy showed moderate to severe, multifocal to coalescing pyogranulomatous capsulitis and serositis that involved the spleen, liver, kidney, intestines, diaphragm, thoracic and abdominal walls, and pericardium. There was also multifocal pyogranulomatous splenitis, hepatitis, nephritis, meningoencephalitis, and pneumonia with necrosis. Straw-colored effusion was present in the abdominal cavity, thoracic cavity, and pleural space. Immunohistochemistry was strongly positive for FCoV antigen (see Figure 20-11).

Comments: The course of disease and survival time (587 days) in this cat was unusually prolonged for FIP, and on many occasions the diagnosis was questioned. However, the persistently increased FCoV antibody titer in a cat that lived with only one other cat raised suspicion for the disease. Chronic, smoldering FIP may be more common than recognized.[6] The initial clinical signs in this cat were mild and may have been overlooked by some owners. Although the cat appeared to respond to prednisolone treatment, it was not known whether the other medications used had any effect. Ultimately, disease progressed, and a diagnosis of FIP was confirmed with immunocytochemistry on the tracheobronchial lavage specimen. Although effusion developed, the amount was too low to permit collection of the fluid for analysis. The initial negative PCR and immunocytochemistry results may have reflected the presence of low quantities of virus.

SUGGESTED READINGS

Addie D, Belak S, Boucraut-Baralon C, et al. Feline infectious peritonitis. ABCD guidelines on prevention and management. J Feline Med Surg. 2009;11:594-604.

Brown MA. Genetic determinants of pathogenesis by feline infectious peritonitis virus. Vet Immunol Immunopathol. 2011;143:265-268.

Pedersen NC. A review of feline infectious peritonitis virus infection: 1963-2008. J Feline Med Surg. 2009;11:225-258.

REFERENCES

1. Holzworth J. Some important disorders of cats. Cornell Vet. 1963;53:157-160.
2. McArdle F, Bennett M, Gaskell RM, et al. Induction and enhancement of feline infectious peritonitis by canine coronavirus. Am J Vet Res. 1992;53:1500-1506.
3. Van Hamme E, Desmarets L, Dewerchin HL, et al. Intriguing interplay between feline infectious peritonitis virus and its receptors during entry in primary feline monocytes. Virus Res. 2011;160:32-39.
4. Tekes G, Hofmann-Lehmann R, Stallkamp I, et al. Genome organization and reverse genetic analysis of a type I feline coronavirus. J Virol. 2008;82:1851-1859.
5. Pedersen NC, Black JW, Boyle JF, et al. Pathogenic differences between various feline coronavirus isolates. Adv Exp Med Biol. 1984;173:365-380.
6. Pedersen NC. A review of feline infectious peritonitis virus infection: 1963-2008. J Feline Med Surg. 2009;11:225-258.
7. Hohdatsu T, Okada S, Ishizuka Y, et al. The prevalence of types I and II feline coronavirus infections in cats. J Vet Med Sci. 1992;54:557-562.
8. Heeney JL, Evermann JF, McKeirnan AJ, et al. Prevalence and implications of feline coronavirus infections of captive and free-ranging cheetahs (*Acinonyx jubatus*). J Virol. 1990;64:1964-1972.
9. Rohrbach BW, Legendre AM, Baldwin CA, et al. Epidemiology of feline infectious peritonitis among cats examined at veterinary medical teaching hospitals. J Am Vet Med Assoc. 2001;218:1111-1115.
10. Pesteanu-Somogyi LD, Radzai C, Pressler BM. Prevalence of feline infectious peritonitis in specific cat breeds. J Feline Med Surg. 2006;8:1-5.
11. Worthing KI, Wigney DI, Dhand NK, et al. Risk factors for feline infectious peritonitis in Australia. J Fel Med Surg. 2012;14:405-412.
12. Foley JE, Poland A, Carlson J, et al. Risk factors for feline infectious peritonitis among cats in multiple-cat environments with endemic feline enteric coronavirus. J Am Vet Med Assoc. 1997;210:1313-1318.
13. Norris JM, Bosward KL, White JD, et al. Clinicopathological findings associated with feline infectious peritonitis in Sydney, Australia: 42 cases (1990-2002). Aust Vet J. 2005;83:666-673.
14. Tsai HY, Chueh LL, Lin CN, et al. Clinicopathological findings and disease staging of feline infectious peritonitis: 51 cases from 2003 to 2009 in Taiwan. J Feline Med Surg. 2011;13:74-80.
15. Hartmann K. Feline infectious peritonitis. Vet Clin North Am Small Anim Pract. 2005;35:39-79, vi.
16. Bell ET, Toribio JA, White JD, et al. Seroprevalence study of feline coronavirus in owned and feral cats in Sydney, Australia. Aust Vet J. 2006;84:74-81.
17. Pedersen NC. Serologic studies of naturally occurring feline infectious peritonitis. Am J Vet Res. 1976;37:1449-1453.
18. Addie DD, Jarrett O. A study of naturally occurring feline coronavirus infections in kittens. Vet Rec. 1992;130:133-137.
19. Addie DD, Toth S, Murray GD, et al. Risk of feline infectious peritonitis in cats naturally infected with feline coronavirus. Am J Vet Res. 1995;56:429-434.
20. Addie D, Belak S, Boucraut-Baralon C, et al. Feline infectious peritonitis. ABCD guidelines on prevention and management. J Feline Med Surg. 2009;11:594-604.
21. Gunn-Moore DA, Gruffydd-Jones TJ, Harbour DA. Detection of feline coronaviruses by culture and reverse transcriptase-polymerase chain reaction of blood samples from healthy cats and cats with clinical feline infectious peritonitis. Vet Microbiol. 1998;62:193-205.
22. Kipar A, Meli ML, Baptiste KE, et al. Sites of feline coronavirus persistence in healthy cats. J Gen Virol. 2010;91:1698-1707.
23. Chang HW, de Groot RJ, Egberink HF, et al. Feline infectious peritonitis: insights into feline coronavirus pathobiogenesis and epidemiology based on genetic analysis of the viral *3c* gene. J Gen Virol. 2010;91:415-420.
24. Rottier PJ, Nakamura K, Schellen P, et al. Acquisition of macrophage tropism during the pathogenesis of feline infectious peritonitis is determined by mutations in the feline coronavirus spike protein. J Virol. 2005;79:14122-14130.
25. Chang HW, Egberink HF, Halpin R, et al. Spike protein fusion peptide and feline coronavirus virulence. Emerg Infect Dis. 2012;18(7):1089-1095.
26. Brown MA, Troyer JL, Pecon-Slattery J, et al. Genetics and pathogenesis of feline infectious peritonitis virus. Emerg Infect Dis. 2009;15:1445-1452.
27. Vennema H, Poland A, Foley J, et al. Feline infectious peritonitis viruses arise by mutation from endemic feline enteric coronaviruses. Virology. 1998;243:150-157.

28. Pedersen NC, Liu H, Dodd KA, et al. Significance of coronavirus mutants in feces and diseased tissues of cats suffering from feline infectious peritonitis. Viruses. 2009;1:166-184.
29. Takano T, Tomiyama Y, Katoh Y, et al. Mutation of neutralizing/antibody-dependent enhancing epitope on spike protein and *7b* gene of feline infectious peritonitis virus: influences of viral replication in monocytes/macrophages and virulence in cats. Virus Res. 2011;156:72-80.
30. Brown MA. Genetic determinants of pathogenesis by feline infectious peritonitis virus. Vet Immunol Immunopathol. 2011;143:265-268.
31. Addie DD, Schaap IA, Nicolson L, et al. Persistence and transmission of natural type I feline coronavirus infection. J Gen Virol. 2003;84:2735-2744.
32. Addie DD, Jarrett O. Use of a reverse-transcriptase polymerase chain reaction for monitoring the shedding of feline coronavirus by healthy cats. Vet Rec. 2001;148:649-653.
33. Pedersen NC, Allen CE, Lyons LA. Pathogenesis of feline enteric coronavirus infection. J Feline Med Surg. 2008;10:529-541.
34. Regan AD, Ousterout DG, Whittaker GR. Feline lectin activity is critical for the cellular entry of feline infectious peritonitis virus. J Virol. 2010;84:7917-7921.
35. Takano T, Ohyama T, Kokumoto A, et al. Vascular endothelial growth factor (VEGF), produced by feline infectious peritonitis (FIP) virus-infected monocytes and macrophages, induces vascular permeability and effusion in cats with FIP. Virus Res. 2011;158:161-168.
36. Kiss I, Poland AM, Pedersen NC. Disease outcome and cytokine responses in cats immunized with an avirulent feline infectious peritonitis virus (FIPV)-UCD1 and challenge-exposed with virulent FIPV-UCD8. J Feline Med Surg. 2004;6:89-97.
37. Takano T, Azuma N, Satoh M, et al. Neutrophil survival factors (TNF-alpha, GM-CSF, and G-CSF) produced by macrophages in cats infected with feline infectious peritonitis virus contribute to the pathogenesis of granulomatous lesions. Arch Virol. 2009;154:775-781.
38. de Groot-Mijnes JD, van Dun JM, van der Most RG, et al. Natural history of a recurrent feline coronavirus infection and the role of cellular immunity in survival and disease. J Virol. 2005;79:1036-1044.
39. Davidson BJ, Paling AC, Lahmers SL, et al. Disease association and clinical assessment of feline pericardial effusion. J Am Anim Hosp Assoc. 2008;44:5-9.
40. Bradshaw JM, Pearson GR, Gruffydd-Jones TJ. A retrospective study of 286 cases of neurological disorders of the cat. J Comp Pathol. 2004;131:112-120.
41. Hayashi T, Ishida T, Fujiwara K. Glomerulonephritis associated with feline infectious peritonitis. Nihon Juigaku Zasshi. 1982;44:909-916.
42. Taylor SS, Tappin SW, Dodkin SJ, et al. Serum protein electrophoresis in 155 cats. J Feline Med Surg. 2010;12:643-653.
43. Sparkes AH, Gruffydd-Jones TJ, Harbour DA. Feline infectious peritonitis: a review of clinicopathological changes in 65 cases, and a critical assessment of their diagnostic value. Vet Rec. 1991;129:209-212.
44. Hartmann K, Binder C, Hirschberger J, et al. Comparison of different tests to diagnose feline infectious peritonitis. J Vet Intern Med. 2003;17:781-790.
45. Jeffery U, Dietz K, Hostetter S. Positive predictive value of albumin:globulin ratio for feline infectious peritonitis in a mid-western referral hospital population. J Fel Med Surg. 2012;14:903-905.
46. Duthie S, Eckersall PD, Addie DD, et al. Value of alpha 1-acid glycoprotein in the diagnosis of feline infectious peritonitis. Vet Rec. 1997;141:299-303.
47. Giori L, Giordano A, Giudice C, et al. Performances of different diagnostic tests for feline infectious peritonitis in challenging clinical cases. J Small Anim Pract. 2011;52:152-157.
48. Savary KC, Sellon RK, Law JM. Chylous abdominal effusion in a cat with feline infectious peritonitis. J Am Anim Hosp Assoc. 2001;37:35-40.
49. Shelly SM, Scarlett-Kranz J, Blue JT. Protein electrophoresis on effusions from cats as a diagnostic test for feline infectious peritonitis. J Am Anim Hosp Assoc. 1988;24:495-500.
50. Fischer Y, Sauter-Louis C, Hartmann K. Diagnostic accuracy of the Rivalta test for feline infectious peritonitis. Vet Clin Pathol. 2012;41:558-567.
51. Boettcher IC, Steinberg T, Matiasek K, et al. Use of anti-coronavirus antibody testing of cerebrospinal fluid for diagnosis of feline infectious peritonitis involving the central nervous system in cats. J Am Vet Med Assoc. 2007;230:199-205.
52. Foley JE, Lapointe JM, Koblik P, et al. Diagnostic features of clinical neurologic feline infectious peritonitis. J Vet Intern Med. 1998;12:415-423.
53. Lewis KM, O'Brien RT. Abdominal ultrasonographic findings associated with feline infectious peritonitis: a retrospective review of 16 cases. J Am Anim Hosp Assoc. 2010;46:152-160.
54. Pratelli A. Comparison of serologic techniques for the detection of antibodies against feline coronaviruses. J Vet Diagn Invest. 2008;20:45-50.
55. Tammer R, Evensen O, Lutz H, et al. Immunohistological demonstration of feline infectious peritonitis virus antigen in paraffin-embedded tissues using feline ascites or murine monoclonal antibodies. Vet Immunol Immunopathol. 1995;49:177-182.
56. Ishida T, Shibanai A, Tanaka S, et al. Use of recombinant feline interferon and glucocorticoid in the treatment of feline infectious peritonitis. J Feline Med Surg. 2004;6:107-109.
57. Ritz S, Egberink H, Hartmann K. Effect of feline interferon-omega on the survival time and quality of life of cats with feline infectious peritonitis. J Vet Intern Med. 2007;21:1193-1197.
58. Legendre AM, Bartges JW. Effect of Polyprenyl Immunostimulant on the survival times of three cats with the dry form of feline infectious peritonitis. J Feline Med Surg. 2009;11:624-626.
59. Watari T, Kaneshima T, Tsujimoto H, et al. Effect of thromboxane synthetase inhibitor on feline infectious peritonitis in cats. J Vet Med Sci. 1998;60:657-659.
60. Hsieh LE, Lin CN, Su BL, et al. Synergistic antiviral effect of *Galanthus nivalis* agglutinin and nelfinavir against feline coronavirus. Antiviral Res. 2010;88:25-30.
61. McDonagh P, Sheehy PA, Norris JM. In vitro inhibition of feline coronavirus replication by small interfering RNAs. Vet Microbiol. 2011;150:220-229.
62. Tanaka Y, Sato Y, Osawa S, et al. Suppression of feline coronavirus replication in vitro by cyclosporin A. Vet Res. 2012;41-43.
63. Fehr D, Holznagel E, Bolla S, et al. Placebo-controlled evaluation of a modified live virus vaccine against feline infectious peritonitis: safety and efficacy under field conditions. Vaccine. 1997;15:1101-1109.
64. Postorino Reeves NC, Pollock RV, Thurber ET. Long-term follow-up study of cats vaccinated with a temperature-sensitive feline infectious peritonitis vaccine. Cornell Vet. 1992:82.
65. Postorino Reeves NC. Vaccination against naturally-occurring FIP in a single large cat shelter. Feline Pract. 1995;23:81-82.

CHAPTER 21

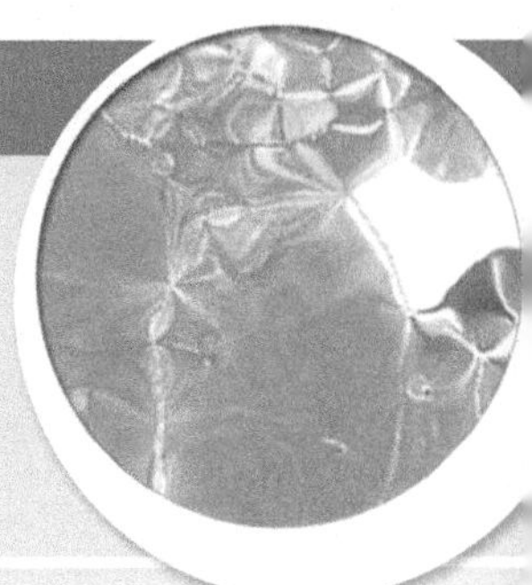

Feline Immunodeficiency Virus Infection

Jane E. Sykes

> **Overview of Feline Immunodeficiency Virus Infection**
>
> First Described: California, 1986 (Pedersen)[1]; serologic evidence of infection dates back to the 1960s[2,3]
>
> Cause: Feline immunodeficiency virus (FIV) (family Retroviridae, subfamily Orthoretrovirinae, genus *Lentivirus*)
>
> Affected Hosts: Domestic and wild cats; hyenas
>
> Geographic Distribution: Worldwide
>
> Mode of Transmission: Biting, and to a lesser extent transplacental, through milk, possibly venereal, blood transfusion
>
> Major Clinical Signs: Lethargy, fever, pallor, stomatitis, diarrhea, muscle atrophy, neurologic signs, signs of underlying neoplastic or immune-mediated disorders or opportunistic infections
>
> Differential Diagnoses: FeLV infection, bartonellosis, other causes of stomatitis such as feline calicivirus infection, immune-mediated disease, other chronic inflammatory and neoplastic diseases of cats that occur in the absence of detectable infection with FIV.
>
> Human Health Significance: FIV does not infect humans.

Etiology and Epidemiology

Feline immunodeficiency virus (FIV) is an enveloped, RNA virus that belongs to the *Lentivirus* genus of the Retroviridae. It infects domestic and wild cats worldwide, as well as hyenas.[4] Like HIV, FIV establishes a chronic, persistent infection that, in some cats, ultimately culminates in immunodeficiency. Because of its similarities to HIV, FIV infection in cats has been used as a research model for HIV infection and acquired immunodeficiency syndrome (AIDS),[5] and relative to other viral infections of companion animals, much is known about its pathogenesis.

Knowledge of retroviral structure and replication is required in order to understand diagnostic, treatment, and prevention strategies that target these viruses. Like other retroviruses, FIV has a three-layered structure that is composed of an innermost genome-nucleocapsid complex with helical symmetry, an icosahedral capsid, and an envelope with glycoprotein spikes (Figure 21-1). The FIV genome contains three major genes: *gag*, which encodes the virion core proteins (capsid [p24], nucleocapsid, and matrix); *pol*, which encodes the reverse transcriptase, protease and integrase enzymes; and *env*, which encodes surface (gp120) and transmembrane virion (gp41) envelope glycoproteins. Several other accessory and regulatory genes are also present. FIV invades cells via the primary receptor CD134, which is expressed on feline CD4+ T cells, B cells, and activated macrophages,[6,7] and the secondary receptor CXCR4, which is normally a chemokine receptor. The viral envelope fuses with the cell membrane, and the capsid enters the cytoplasm, where reverse transcription occurs and a double-stranded DNA (dsDNA) copy of the retroviral genome is made. Additional sequences, known as *long terminal repeats* (LTRs), are added to either end of the viral genome. The virus then passes into the nucleus where the dsDNA copy integrates into the host genome; at this point the integrated dsDNA becomes a *provirus*. Transcription of this DNA, which is controlled by the LTRs, leads to synthesis of new virion components, and virus assembly and budding occur at the cell surface (Figure 21-2). Depending on the cellular environment, proviral DNA may either be *latent*, whereby transcription does not occur, or be transcriptionally active. Latency is one mechanism by which retroviruses can evade the host immune system. Because the reverse transcriptase enzyme is prone to error, the mutation rate of retroviruses is high, and a diversity of viral variants continuously emerges from infected hosts. Integration of retroviral DNA into host cell DNA can disrupt genes that are responsible for cell growth and differentiation (proto-oncogenes). Alternatively, cellular oncogenes captured and carried by retroviruses develop mutations during retroviral replication, and are then re-inserted into host cell DNA. The end result is abnormal cell growth and differentiation, which results in tumor formation by some retroviruses.

Based on sequence diversity of the *env* gene, there are six different subtypes of FIV, A through F. Subtypes A and B are distributed most widely, followed by subtype C[8-10]—although a recent study from the United States showed an equal distribution of subtypes A, B, and C (Table 21-1).[11-31] In addition, a number of recombinant subtypes have been recognized, such as A/B, A/C, B/D, B/E, and A/B/C recombinants, and additional subtypes also likely exist.[9,11] The heterogeneity of the virus complicates the design of molecular diagnostic tests and vaccines for FIV. Whether differences in the clinical manifestations of disease relate to infection by different subtypes requires further study.[9,10,31]

Retroviruses survive only minutes outside the host and are very susceptible to disinfection. FIV is shed in high concentrations in saliva, and the major mode of transmission is through bites. Transplacental transmission, transmission during parturition, and through milk have been documented experimentally, but these modes appear to be uncommon in naturally infected cats, and kittens infected by this route may not sustain productive infection.[32,33] Venereal transmission has not been demonstrated, but FIV can be recovered from semen, and experimental inoculation of FIV into the vaginas of queens results in transmission.[34,35] Transmission also has the potential to occur through blood donation.

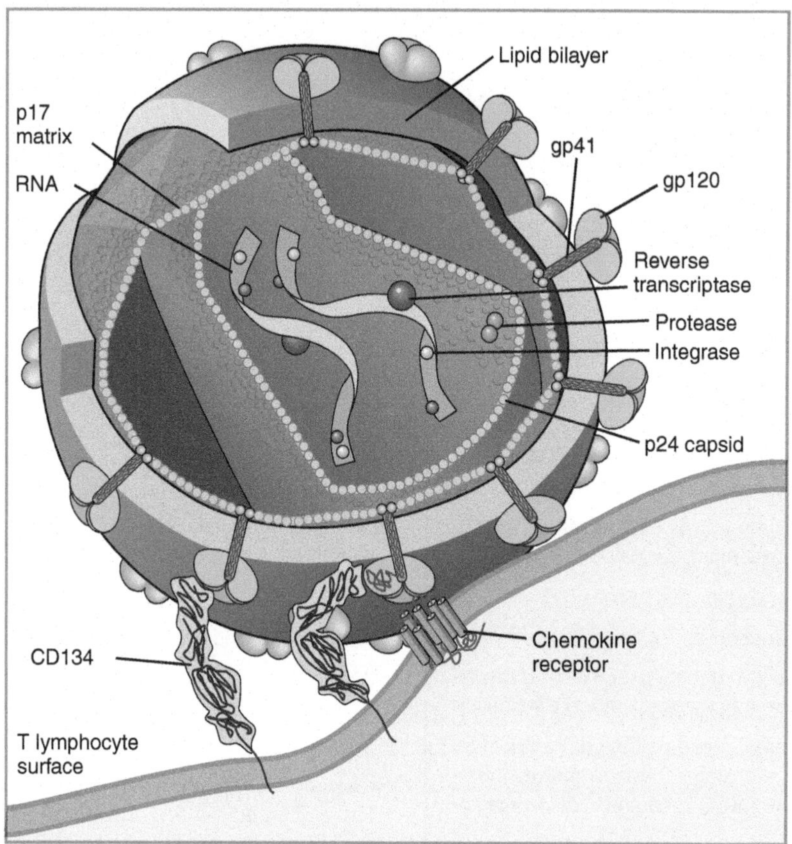

FIGURE 21-1 Structure of FIV. An FIV virion is shown adjacent to the surface of a CD4+ T cell. Lentiviruses contain two identical strands of RNA (the viral genome) and associated enzymes, which include reverse transcriptase, integrase, and protease, packaged into a core composed of the p24 capsid protein with a surrounding p17 protein matrix, all enclosed by a phospholipid membrane envelope that is derived from the host cell. Viral encoded membrane proteins (gp41 and gp120) are bound to the envelope. CD134 and CXCR4 (chemokine) receptors on the host cell surface function as the receptors for FIV.

Seropositivity to FIV (which is equivalent to infection because of viral persistence) is consistently associated with a history of bite wounds, older age, male sex, illness, and outdoor access (Table 21-2).[12,36-41] Being of mixed breed has also been a risk factor in some studies. The mean age at diagnosis is around 6 to 8 years, and 80% to 90% of cats are more than 2 years of age. Male cats are up to 4.7 times more likely to be seropositive than female cats.[40] Indoor housing decreases transmission but does not eliminate it.[42] Worldwide, the seroprevalence of FIV in domestic pet cats ranges from around 1% to 12%.[9,40,41] A study that included more than 18,000 North American cats estimated the overall prevalence of FeLV and FIV infections as around 2.3% and 2.5%, respectively.[5] Higher prevalences are found in feral and free-ranging cats and sick cats. In the North American study, the prevalence of FIV infection in sick, feral cats was 18.2%, whereas that in healthy indoor cats was only 0.7%. A study from France showed a seroprevalence of 21% in unowned cats, compared with 10% in owned cats.[43] In Japan, the overall seroprevalence is very high (23% in one study), and as many as one-third of male cats test positive.[12] Occasionally, co-infections with FeLV occur, and infection with one retrovirus is a risk factor for infection with the other.[36,37]

Clinical Features

Signs and Their Pathogenesis

The main cellular target for FIV is the CD4+ T cell. However, FIV also infects CD8+ T cells, B cells, macrophages, and dendritic cells, microglia, and astrocytes. The subsequent effects of the virus on the immune system are complex, incompletely understood, and seem to result in both immune suppression and immune activation.

Three phases of disease have been delineated, *acute (primary), subclinical,* and *terminal,* although not all phases are recognized in many naturally infected cats. After inoculation, the virus replicates in lymphoid tissues, and high concentrations of virus are present in blood 2 weeks after infection. A peak of viremia occurs 8 to 12 weeks after infection (Figure 21-3). There is a decline in CD4+ and CD8+ T cells in peripheral blood. This may be associated with transient illness, which lasts 3 to 6 months and is often unrecognized by cat owners. Some cats show lethargy, fever, anorexia, diarrhea, stomatitis, weight loss, and/or lymphadenopathy during the acute phase. Lymphadenopathy results from lymphoid hyperplasia, and can persist for weeks to months. Neutropenia can also occur,[44] possibly as a result of neutrophil apoptosis. CD4+/CD25+ T regulator (Treg) cells are infected and activated during the acute phase. These cells then inhibit the proliferation of activated CD4+ and CD8+ T cells, and cause them to undergo apoptosis. This may contribute to persistence of FIV and further immunosuppression.[45-47] Altered dendritic cell function may also occur.[48,49] In general, impaired T cell function in acute infection is thought to result from cytokine dysregulation, immunologic anergy (failure to respond to specific antigens), and increased apoptosis.[45] Nevertheless, most cats survive this phase because of a rebound in CD8+ T cell numbers and a strong humoral immune response.

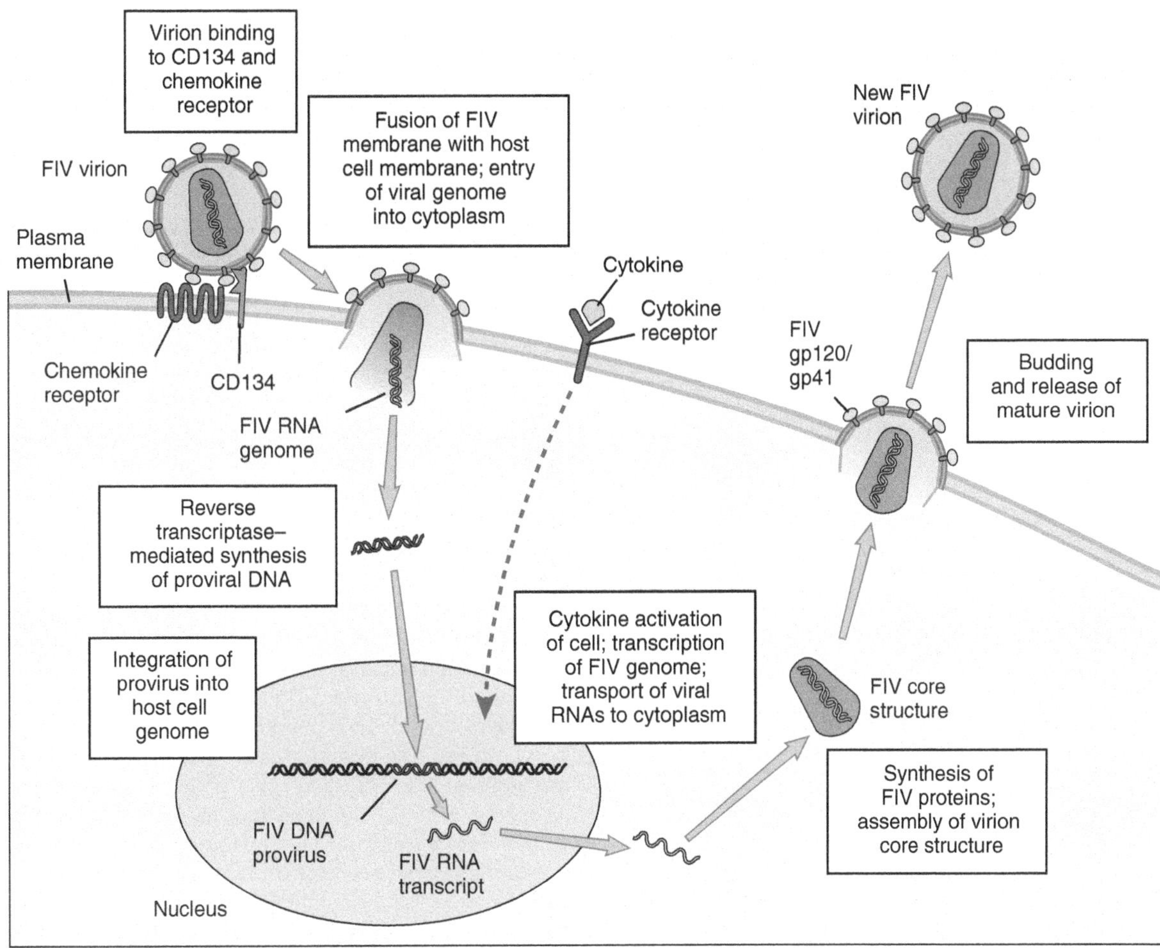

FIGURE 21-2 The life cycle of FIV. The sequential steps in FIV reproduction are shown, from initial infection of a host cell to release of a new virus particle. An infected cell produces many virions, each capable of infecting nearby cells, with subsequent spread of the infection.

TABLE 21-1

Distribution of FIV Subtypes Worldwide

A	Australia, New Zealand, United States (especially western United States), South Africa, northwestern Europe, Japan, United Kingdom[11-19]
B	Central and eastern United States, Caribbean, central and western Europe, Brazil, eastern Japan[11,14,20-25]
C	United States, Canada, New Zealand, southeast Asia[11,12,26-29]
D	Japan, Vietnam, rarely United States[21,27,31]
E	Argentina[10,30]
F	United States[10,31]

In the subclinical (or asymptomatic) phase, CD4+ T cell numbers rebound, and the plasma virus load declines to very low levels. Cats remain subclinically infected, often for years or even for life. This is not latent infection, because virus production continues at low levels; a slow, progressive decline in CD4+ T cell numbers; reduction in the CD4+:CD8+ T cell ratio; and in some cats, hyperglobulinemia, which results from B cell hyperactivation. Some studies also describe a sustained increase in CD8+ T cell numbers. Although activated, paradoxically, T cells have a reduced ability to respond to antigenic stimulation. Altered lymphocyte expression of cell surface molecules (including CD4 and cytokine receptors, and MHC II antigens), and continued alteration of dendritic cell and neutrophil function also contribute to immunosuppression. Dysregulation of cytokine production occurs. For example, cats that are chronically infected with FIV fail to produce Il-2, Il-6, and Il-12 in response to *Toxoplasma gondii* infection and instead produce elevated levels of the antiinflammatory cytokine Il-10.[45,50] There is a slow influx of immune cells into the brain, with gradual progression of central nervous system (CNS) disease.[51] The rate of progression of the subclinical phase depends on factors such as the virus strain, co-infections with other agents that activate virus transcription, and host immunity.

In some cats, these changes ultimately lead to the terminal phase, which is characterized by clinical signs of opportunistic infections, neoplastic disease, myelosuppression, and neurologic disease. This is the phase most commonly recognized in naturally infected cats (Table 21-3). However, many infected cats never develop FIV-related clinical signs, even when CD4+ T cell counts are low, and instead die from other causes. The terminal phase of FIV infection is commonly associated with moderate to severe periodontal disease, lymphoplasmacytic stomatitis (Figure 21-4), gingivitis, and feline odontoclastic resorptive

TABLE 21-2

Risk Factors for FIV Infection in Cats Seen at the UC Davis VMTH

Variable	Number of FIV+ Cats*	Number of Control Cats†	Odds Ratio	P-value‡
Sex				
Male neutered	100	117	—	
Male intact	10	5	2.729	0.08
Female/female neutered	17	88	0.24Åò	<0.001
Breed				
Mixed	116	170	—	
Purebred	11	40	0.37	0.02
Environment				
Indoor	15	57	—	
Outdoor	85	107	2.58	0.01
Stray history				
No	101	195	—	
Yes	26	15	3.73	<0.001
Cats in household				
<3	34	70	—	
≥3	39	61	1.25	0.53

Modified from Trott KA, Kass PH, Sparger EE, et al. A clinical case control study: clinical presentation of FIV-positive cats. University of California, Davis, STARS in Science Day. 2007; abstr.

*All cats were >6 months of age and none had a history of FIV vaccination.

†All control cats were negative for FIV antibody at their visit to the University of California, Davis.

‡P-values <0.05 were significant.

ÅòIn other words, female cats were four times less likely to be FIV+ than male neutered cats.

lesions,[52] which may result from opportunistic bacterial and viral infections. Other opportunistic infections include chronic bacterial skin and ear infections, persistent viral upper respiratory tract infections, dermatophytosis, mycobacterial infections, fungal infections such as cryptococcosis and sporotrichosis, hemoplasmosis, toxoplasmosis, and/or parasitic infections such as demodecosis and severe flea burdens. With the exception of stomatitis, the relationship between many of these opportunistic infections and FIV infection is somewhat unclear, because the prevalence of many of these infections in cats with FIV infection is similar to that in cats without FIV infection. However, infections are often more severe and less responsive to treatment than the same infections in immunocompetent cats.

The development of neoplasia in FIV-infected cats is thought to result primarily from immune suppression, although there is serologic evidence that cats may be infected with a gammaherpesvirus similar to Epstein-Barr virus that might be reactivated in cats infected with FIV.[53] Lymphomas are the most commonly reported FIV-associated tumor, especially B cell lymphomas, but also T cell and non-B, non-T cell lymphomas.[54] FIV-infected cats are 5 times more likely to develop lymphoma than cats not infected with FIV and are more likely to develop it an earlier age. Leukemia and squamous cell carcinomas (SCCs) are also common tumors in cats with FIV, although the association with SCC may be confounded by outdoor exposure. Other tumors include mast cell tumors, fibrosarcomas, meningiomas, and metastatic carcinomas; some infected cats develop more than one type of neoplasia. Rarely, lymphoma may develop as a result of viral integration into the genome and disruption of proto-oncogenes.[54,55]

Immune dysregulation and increased circulating immune complexes in the terminal phase can lead to immune-mediated disorders, such as immune-mediated glomerulonephritis and uveitis.[56] Myelodysplasia develops in some cats,[57,58] which may be manifested by clinical signs of lethargy, inappetence, pallor, or evidence of bleeding tendencies such as petechial hemorrhages.

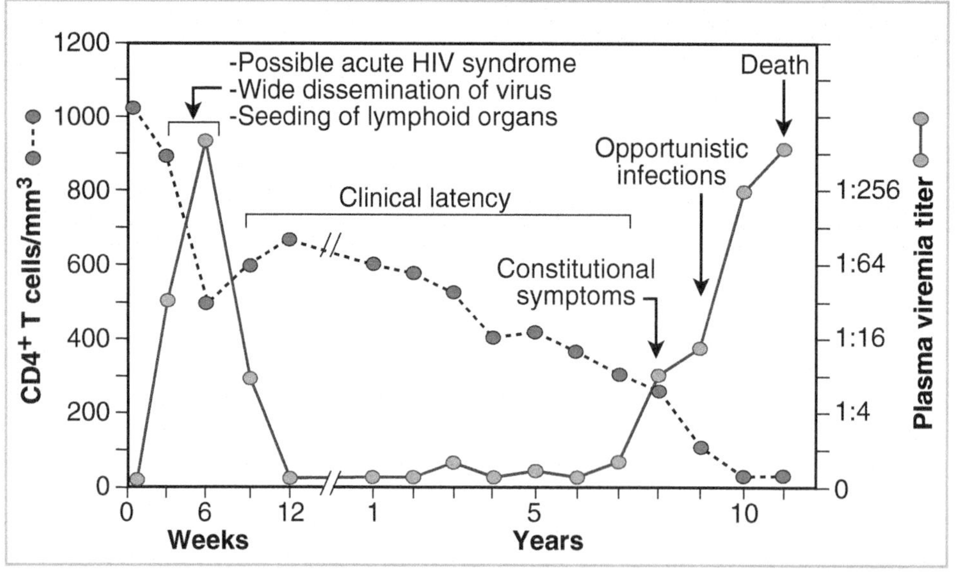

FIGURE 21-3 Changes in virus load and CD4+ T Cell numbers over the course of infection with HIV. A similar clinical course of infection occurs for FIV infection. Viremia is detected early after infection and may be accompanied by systemic signs (acute phase). Plasma viremia then falls to very low levels and remains this way for many years (subclinical phase). Although this period is referred to here as "clinical latency," the virus itself is not latent during this time, because there is ongoing production of virus and a steady decline in CD4+ T cell counts. In the terminal phase of infection, signs of immunodeficiency develop and plasma viremia increases. Some infected cats never reach this phase. Antibody production declines, and antibody tests may be negative in cats with advanced terminal-phase disease, but PCR assays are more likely to be positive.

TABLE 21-3

Disease Diagnoses in 127 Cats with FIV Infection and 210 Age-Matched Control Cats Seen over the Same Time Period at the UC Davis VMTH*

Disease	Cats Infected with FIV (n = 127)†	Controls (n = 210)‡	P-value§
Intraocular inflammation	16	17	0.18
Stomatitis	21	11	< 0.001
Cardiomyopathy	21	17	0.02
Upper respiratory tract disease	13	9	0.03
Neurologic signs	16	24	0.75
Chronic kidney disease	23	40	0.83
Diabetes mellitus	9	18	0.63
Hyperthyroidism	11	14	0.49
Lymphoma	23	20	0.02
Squamous cell carcinoma (SCC)	12	9	0.057
Fibrosarcoma	2	9	0.17
Carcinomas other than SCC	4	12	0.28

Modified from Trott KA, Kass PH, Sparger EE, et al. A clinical case control study: clinical presentation of FIV-positive cats. University of California, Davis, STARS in Science Day. 2007; abstr.

*Results should be interpreted with caution because the data were retrospectively collected. Some cats may have had undiagnosed disease, such as subclinical chronic kidney or cardiac disease. The pathogenesis of a disease process in FIV-positive cats might also differ from that found in FIV-negative cats.

†All cats were >6 months of age and none had a history of FIV vaccination.

‡All control cats were negative for FIV antibody at their visit to the University of California, Davis.

§As determined by chi-square (univariate) analysis. P-values <0.05 were significant.

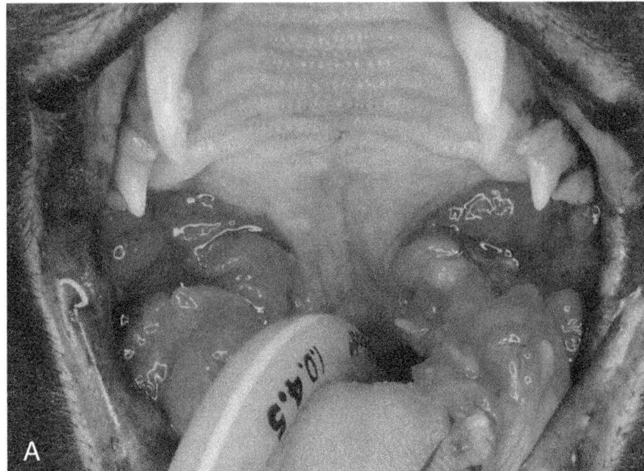

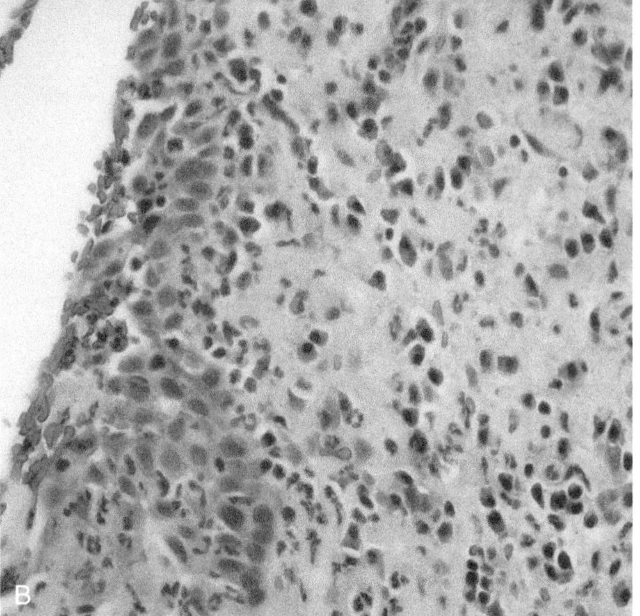

FIGURE 21-4 severe lymphoplasmacytic stomatitis in a cat infected with feline immunodeficiency virus. **A,** There is marked hyperemia, ulceration, and proliferative lesions in the palatoglossal folds. (From Bonello D, Roy CG, Verstraete FJM. Non-neoplastic proliferative oral lesions. In: Verstraete FJM, Lommer MJ, eds. Oral and Maxillofacial Surgery in Dogs and Cats. Philadelphia, PA: Saunders; 2011.) **B,** Histopathology of a biopsy from a cat with severe stomatitis associated with FIV infection.

The end result of infection by neurovirulent strains of FIV can be progressive behavioral changes such as increased aggression and cognitive disturbances, tremors, sleep disturbances, anisocoria, delayed reflexes, abnormal cranial nerve function, urinary and fecal incontinence, and seizures. Decreased nerve conduction velocities and abnormal electroencephalograms and brainstem evoked potentials have been documented.[59] The virus does not infect neurons, but neuronal cell death occurs through multiple incompletely defined mechanisms.[51]

Inflammatory lesions can develop in a variety of organs in cats infected with FIV. An inflammatory myopathy has been described,[60] and terminally, severe muscle atrophy can occur. Infection is associated with gut inflammation and intestinal epithelial cell damage (also known as AIDS enteropathy), which may result in chronic diarrhea and failure to gain weight.[61] The extent to which chronic FIV infection contributes to inflammatory or degenerative changes in other organs, such as the myocardium and the kidneys, is not well understood, because the prevalence of cardiomyopathy and interstitial nephritis in geriatric cats not infected with FIV is high (see Table 21-3).

When transplacental transmission occurs in FIV-infected queens, only some kittens in a litter may be infected. In the first year of infection, the overall rate of such transmission is around 70%.[62] Rates of mother-to-kitten transmission are highest in queens that have a CD4+ count less than 200 cells/μL, those with signs of immunodeficiency, and those infected within the past 15 months.[63] In utero transmission can lead to arrested fetal development, abortion, stillbirth, low birth weights, and the birth of T cell deficient kittens.[62,64]

Physical Examination Findings

Many cats infected with FIV have no signs of illness, or clinical signs that are unrelated to FIV infection. Cats in the acute

TABLE 21-4

Diagnostic Assays Available for Feline Immunodeficiency Virus Infection

Assay	Specimen Type	Target	Performance
Serology (ELISA, Western blotting, IFA)	Blood, serum	Antibody to FIV	Positive test results in cats >6 months of age that have not been vaccinated for FIV equal infection, but confirmation is recommended in healthy cats using a second test from a different manufacturer or Western blot. False positives occur in cats <6 months of age (maternal antibody) and cats vaccinated with the FIV vaccine. False negatives can occur in the first 2 months of infection or with advanced disease and severe immunosuppression.
PCR	Blood	FIV proviral DNA or viral RNA	Sensitivity and specificity vary between laboratories. Even well-designed assays may be insensitive because of viral variability and low-level viremia. PCR assays are the only assay that can definitively diagnose infection in cats vaccinated for FIV. Never use without performing serology.
Virus isolation	Blood	FIV	Difficult, not widely available. Used primarily as a research tool.

IFA, immunofluorescent antibody.

phase of FIV infection may be febrile or show generalized peripheral lymphadenopathy. Behavioral abnormalities such as obtundation, aggression, and cognitive impairment may be evident in cats with terminal neurologic disease; other neurologic abnormalities include ataxia, anisocoria, and abnormal segmental reflexes. Ocular abnormalities may be present as a result of the FIV infection itself, opportunistic infections, or lymphoma, and include anterior uveitis, hyphema, pars planitis, chorioretinitis, and/or glaucoma.[65] Other common physical examination findings in cats with terminal disease are periodontal disease and chronic stomatitis, signs of chronic upper respiratory tract infection, otitis externa, pyoderma, cutaneous abscesses, and a diverse and variable spectrum of disease manifestations that relate to other underlying opportunistic infections or neoplasia.

Diagnosis

For many cats, infection with FIV is diagnosed during screening efforts. Screening for infection should be performed with tests that detect antibody against FIV, because these assays have the highest overall sensitivity and are rapid and widely available (Table 21-4). It has been recommended that the retrovirus status of all cats be known regardless of the presence of absence of illness.[66] Indications for testing as recommended by the American Association of Feline Practitioners (AAFP) are shown in Box 21-1. In practice, compliance with retrovirus testing is low. In a study that evaluated 967 cats with bite wounds or cutaneous abscesses that presented to veterinary practitioners from 134 practices in 30 states, the combined FeLV-FIV status of only 96 (9.9%) of the cats was known.[38] In addition, despite the availability of a financial incentive for retesting, only 64 of 478 cat owners returned their cats for retesting after treatment.

When positive test results occur in sick cats, the role that FIV plays as a cause of the signs may be unclear, although it is reasonable to assume that FIV may be playing a role in cats with severe stomatitis, unusual infections with intracellular pathogens such as mycobacteria, and lymphoma. With refinement and improved availability of test methodologies in the future, clinical assessment of CD4+ T cell counts, the CD4+/CD8+ ratio, and plasma viral loads may facilitate interpretation of the relationship between disease manifestations and infection and provide prognostic information, as in human patients infected with HIV.[67]

BOX 21-1

Indications for Serologic Testing for FIV and FeLV

- Sick cats, even if tested negative in the past
- All newly acquired cats or kittens (2 tests, at least 60 days apart)
- After exposure to a retrovirus-infected cat or a cat with unknown status, and especially after a bite wound (2 tests, at least 60 days apart)
- Cats that live in a household with other retrovirus-infected cats (annual retesting unless isolated)
- Before initial vaccination with FeLV or FIV vaccines
- Before use as a blood donor (in conjunction with real-time PCR)
- On entry to a shelter or before adoption (2 tests, at least 60 days apart); if financial resources are not available for this, cats should be held singly and postadoption testing (2 tests, at least 60 days apart) recommended before mingling with other cats occurs. The status of the other cats in the household should be known before new cats are introduced.
- For group-housed cats, before introduction (2 tests, at least 60 days apart if possible) and on an annual basis
- Testing is considered optional for feral cat trap-neuter-return programs

Modified from Levy J, Crawford C, Hartmann K, et al. 2008 American Association of Feline Practitioners' feline retrovirus management guidelines. J Feline Med Surg 2008;10:300-316.

Laboratory Abnormalities

Complete Blood Count

Common abnormalities on the CBC in cats infected with FIV include mild anemia, lymphopenia, and neutropenia. Occasionally severe anemia, thrombocytopenia, thrombocytosis, monocytopenia, or leukocytosis occur. In one large European study, neutrophil counts of FIV-infected cats were lower than those of control cats, and lymphocyte counts were higher than those of control cats.[68] Leukopenia and neutropenia were more likely to be present in FIV-infected cats.

Serum Biochemical Tests

The most common and significant abnormality on the chemistry panel in cats infected with FIV is hyperproteinemia, which results from increased γ-globulin concentrations and is a direct result of FIV infection (rather than the result of opportunistic infection). Total protein concentrations that ranged from 4.5 to 11 g/dL were reported in one study.[68] Other findings are variable and relate to the presence of concurrent disease, neoplasia, or opportunistic infections.

Urinalysis

Urinalysis may reveal proteinuria in cats with glomerulonephritis.

Coagulation Testing

Cats infected with FIV can have mild prolongations in their APTT, thrombin time, and fibrinogen concentrations, although the PT and platelet function are generally normal.[69]

Cytologic Evaluation of Bone Marrow

Bone marrow cytologic evaluation in FIV-infected cats with cytopenias and nonregenerative anemias may show mild dysplasia (usually not as severe as in FeLV infections); erythroid hypoplasia; and/or myeloid hyperplasia despite peripheral leukopenia, sometimes with a left shift. The latter suggests ineffective hematopoiesis or maturation arrest.

Microbiologic Tests

Serologic Diagnosis

The initial assay of choice for diagnosis of, and screening for, FIV infection is an ELISA assay that detects antibody to FIV. Provided there has not been a history of vaccination for FIV and the tested cat is less than 6 months of age, positive antibody test results equate with infection, because the virus establishes a lifelong, persistent infection. Point-of-care, lateral-flow ELISA assays and diagnostic laboratory-based ELISA assays are in widespread use and have rapid turnaround times and high sensitivities and specificities.[70] These assays usually detect antibodies to the FIV p24 core protein, and sometimes to the gp40 transmembrane protein. False positive test results occur rarely as a result of operator error or nonspecific reactivity against tissue culture components after vaccination.[71] When Western immunoblotting was used as the gold standard, the sensitivities, specificities, and positive and negative predictive values of six different ELISA assays (Synbiotics Witness, Viracheck FIV, IDEXX SNAP Combo Plus, PetChek Plus Anti-FIV, MegaCor Fastest, and Bio Veto Duo Speed) in one U.S. study of 535 cats with an overall FIV seroprevalence of 10.3% ranged from 94.5% to 100%, 98.5% to 100%, 91.2% to 100%, and 99.2% to 100%, respectively.[70] The Mapic FIV test had a high (23.1%) rate of invalid test results and was not recommended for clinical practice. When these assays are used to screen healthy cats for infection, confirmation of positive results is recommended because of the low prevalence of infection in this population of cats and the higher possibility that false-positive test results may occur. Confirmation can be done using an assay from a different manufacturer or Western blotting. However, Western blotting is technically demanding, subject to interoperator variability in interpretation, and it may be less sensitive than ELISA assays when performed by some laboratories.[72]

Positive ELISA assay results in the absence of FIV infection can occur in cats that have been vaccinated for FIV, or kittens less than 6 months of age that possess maternal antibody (because of infection or vaccination of the queen). No currently available serologic test, including Western immunoblotting, distinguishes between natural infection and vaccination or the presence of maternal antibody. Kittens that test positive should be retested after 6 months of age (the Advisory Bureau on Cat Diseases recommends retesting after 4 months of age).[66,73] Nevertheless, kittens less than 6 months of age should still be tested, because the vast majority of negative kittens will be declared free of infection. Molecular testing could be considered to confirm infection in kittens that test positive at less than 6 months of age (see later discussion). Cats with a history of FIV vaccination may remain antibody-positive for more than 4 years.[66] Because infection can occur in the face of vaccination, positive test results in a vaccinated cat may represent infection and/or historical vaccination. Currently, molecular testing with PCR assays is required to identify infection in these cats, but some infected cats test PCR-negative. An ELISA assay has been developed that can distinguish naturally infected from vaccinated cats, but this assay is not commercially available. The assay was used to test blood samples from 73 uninfected, unvaccinated cats; 89 uninfected, FIV-vaccinated cats; and 102 FIV-infected cats, including 3 cats that had been vaccinated.[9] The assay had a sensitivity of 97% and a specificity of 100% for detection of FIV infection in these cats.

False-negative ELISA assay results occur early in the course of illness, because cats may take up to 60 days to develop an antibody response.[66] Rarely, antibody production is delayed for 6 months or longer. Thus when recent exposure is possible, testing should be repeated a minimum of 2 months later. False-negative test results also occur in cats in the terminal phase of disease, as a result of impaired antibody production, or in kittens with rapidly progressive infections. These cats often have high plasma viral loads. Thus, if advanced FIV infection is suspected, negative test results should be followed by virus detection using PCR. When serology is used as a *screening test,* negative results are considered to be highly reliable because of the high sensitivity of the test and the low prevalence of infection in most populations of healthy cats.[66]

Immunofluorescent antibody (IFA) assays that detect antibodies to FIV have also been described. When performed by experience laboratory personnel, these have sensitivities and specificities that range from 95% to 100% when compared with Western immunoblotting.[71]

Molecular Diagnosis Using the Polymerase Chain Reaction

A variety of PCR assays have been developed for diagnosis of FIV infection. Assays may detect viral RNA (reverse transcriptase [RT]-PCR), proviral DNA, or both RNA and proviral DNA in peripheral blood. Because the FIV vaccine is inactivated and

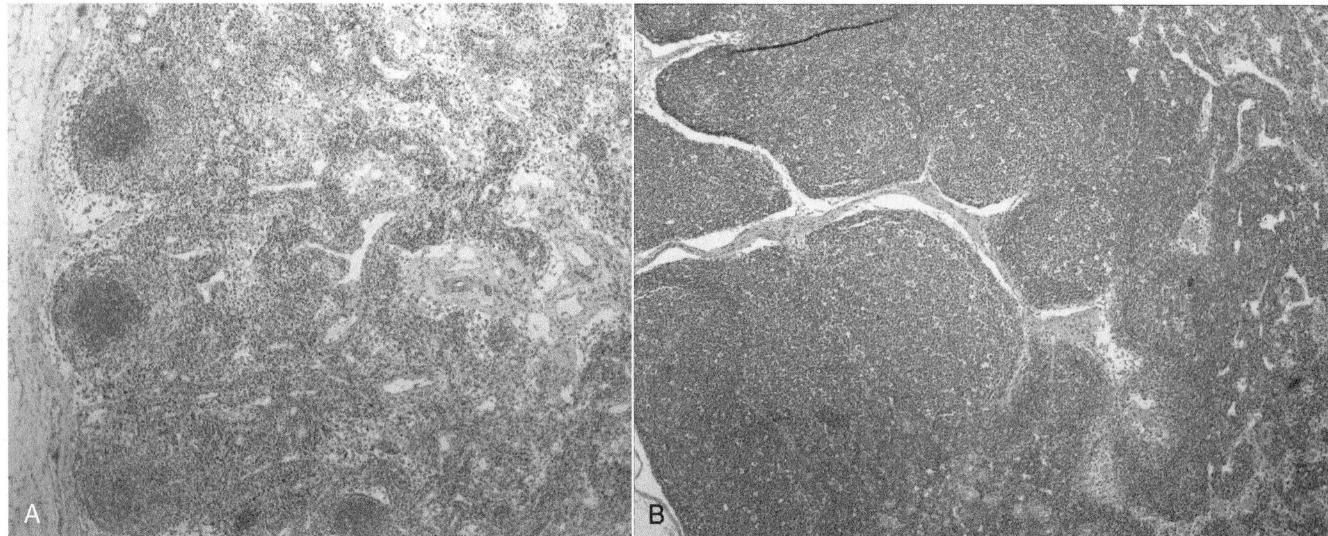

FIGURE 21-5 **A,** Depletion of paracortical areas in the mesenteric lymph node of an 8-year-old female spayed domestic shorthair with FIV infection that was euthanized as a result of the development of progressive neurologic signs. **B,** Normal feline lymph node for comparison purposes.

does not replicate or integrate into the host genome, PCR assays should not detect vaccine virus in cats that have been vaccinated for FIV. Compared with serology, PCR can be insensitive (sensitivity <80%), because viral loads in healthy cats are often extremely low, and some strains may not be detected because of variability in the sequence of the viral genome among FIV isolates. Sensitivity is likely to be higher in cats in the acute and terminal phases of disease when viral loads are higher, but this requires further study. False-positive test results have the potential to occur as a result of laboratory contamination; in some commercial laboratories, unacceptable sensitivities and specificities have been reported (as low as 41% and 44%, respectively).[74,75] In advertising materials, IDEXX Laboratories report an assay sensitivity and specificity of 80.5% and 99.9%, respectively, among 36 FIV-infected cats, 96 uninfected vaccinated cats and 92 uninfected unvaccinated cats, with no difference in specificity in the latter two groups.[76] A FRET real-time PCR assay directed at the *gag* gene has been described that differentiates between FIV subtypes (see Chapter 5 for an explanation of FRET PCR assays).[11] The assay was positive in 60% of 101 cats with positive antibody tests for FIV. A history of vaccination with the FIV vaccine was present in 13 of the cats, and all these cats tested negative. The vaccination history of the remaining cats was unknown. Given their limitations, PCR assays should not be used for diagnosis of FIV infection in the absence of concurrent serologic testing, and the results of PCR assays should not be used to decide whether vaccination should be performed. Cats that are seronegative that test positive with PCR may be in the terminal phase of disease and unable to produce antibody, or the PCR assay result may be a false positive. Latently infected cats have rarely been described that test positive for proviral DNA but negative for antibody.[76] These cats lack any immunologic or clinical abnormalities that occur with active infection.[76] Whether these cats are likely to develop productive infection (as reported in humans with latent HIV infection) is unknown.[77]

Virus Isolation

FIV can be isolated from peripheral blood lymphocytes in primary feline T cell cultures, but this is technically demanding and expensive and can take 2 to 3 weeks, so it is not used for routine diagnostic purposes.

Pathologic Findings

Gross pathologic findings in cats with FIV infection include emaciation, stomatitis, lymphadenopathy, and evidence of secondary neoplasia or opportunistic infections. Evidence of disorders of aged cats, such as hyperthyroidism, cardiomyopathy, and interstitial nephritis, may also be present. Histopathologic changes in cats with FIV infection include follicular hyperplasia or, in the chronic phase, lymphoid depletion in the paracortical regions and plasma cell infiltration of lymph nodes (Figure 21-5); lymphoplasmacytic ulcerative stomatitis (see Figure 21-4, *B*); and bone marrow pathology as described previously in this chapter. Evidence of chronic interstitial nephritis, sometimes with membranous glomerulonephritis and glomerulosclerosis, may be present. Inflammatory changes may be seen within skeletal muscle and/or the gastrointestinal tract. Histopathology of the CNS in cats infected with neurovirulent FIV strains may show mild lymphoplasmacytic meningitis, perivascular lymphocytic infiltrates, diffuse gliosis, microglial nodules, and mild neuronal degeneration and apoptosis.[59,78] Neuronal dysfunction may be more important than neuronal loss.[59]

Treatment and Prognosis

Supportive Care

Cats in the terminal phase of FIV infection may require fluid therapy, nutritional support, regular dental prophylaxis, dilute chlorhexidine-based mouth washes or oral gels, and dental extractions and antimicrobial drugs with activity against anaerobes for severe stomatitis (Table 21-5). Whole mouth extractions have been beneficial for some cats with severe stomatitis, but it is critical that all tooth roots be removed. Referral to a board-certified veterinary dentist should be considered. Topical glucocorticoids (e.g., 1% prednisolone acetate, every 4 to 12 hours depending on severity) and topical atropine are indicated for cats with anterior uveitis. Systemic glucocorticoids should only be used if absolutely necessary, because their use

TABLE 21-5

Suggested Medications for Treatment of Cats in the Terminal Phase of Feline Immunodeficiency Virus Infection

Drug	Dose	Route	Interval (hours)	Comments
Zidovudine (AZT)	5 to 15 mg/kg	PO	12	May have benefit for cats with neurologic signs or stomatitis. Monitor CBC (see text). Toxicity may be more likely at doses above 5 mg/kg.
Human recombinant interferon alpha	1 to 50 U/cat	PO	24	For stomatitis
0.12% Chlorhexidine plus zinc gluconate oral gel	1 mL	Topical	12 to 48	For stomatitis
Clavulanic acid–amoxicillin	12.5 to 25 mg/kg	PO	12	For stomatitis
Lactoferrin	200 mg powder or 40 mg/kg solution	Topical	24	For refractory gingivitis and stomatitis. Must be purchased from chemical suppliers.
Prednisolone	5 mg	PO	24	For refractory stomatitis or advanced neurologic disease. May also be required for lymphoma or other CNS neoplasms. Use only if absolutely necessary.

is associated with increased plasma viremia. Some cats with advanced neurologic signs show clinical improvement after treatment with glucocorticoids. Opportunistic infections may respond to appropriate antimicrobial treatment, but prolonged or lifelong treatment may be required. Griseofulvin should not be used to treat dermatophytosis, because it has been associated with bone marrow suppression in FIV-positive cats.[79] Recombinant human erythropoietin or darbepoetin may be useful for some cats with nonregenerative anemia and does not appear to increase viral load through activation of transcription of latent virus.[80] Although recombinant human granulocyte colony stimulating factor (G-CSF) can increase neutrophil counts in cats infected with FIV, antibodies can develop within a few weeks that cross-react with endogenous G-CSF. When recombinant human granulocyte-macrophage colony stimulating factor (GM-CSF) was used, an increase in virus load occurred, so the use of these drugs is not recommended.

Antiviral and Immunomodulator Drugs

Topical lactoferrin administration has been associated with clinical improvement in some FIV-infected cats with stomatitis (see Chapter 7). Cats with stomatitis or neurologic disease may benefit from oral or subcutaneous treatment with zidovudine (AZT), but AZT can cause bone marrow suppression, so the CBC must be monitored weekly for the first month and monthly thereafter. Treatment is not recommended for cats with myelosuppressive disease.[73] AZT should be discontinued if the hematocrit drops below 20%, after which anemia usually resolves in a few days.[73] AZT-resistant FIV mutants can develop as early as 6 months after the start of treatment. Fozivudine (45 mg/kg PO q12h) reduces viremia in cats with acute FIV infection and may be less likely to produce hematologic adverse effects.[81] Plerixafor (AMD3100), a selective antagonist of the CXCR4 receptor, is active against FIV in vitro.[82] When used in 40 naturally infected cats for 6 weeks in a placebo-controlled double-blind study, a decreased proviral load was reported without evidence of adverse effects, but there was no improvement in clinical or immunologic variables.[73,83]

Results of treatment with human recombinant IFN-α have been mixed, but prolonged survival was reported in 24 FIV-infected cats after oral administration of a low dose of the drug when compared with 6 untreated control cats.[83] Clinical scores and laboratory parameters improved in some sick, naturally infected cats that were treated with recombinant feline IFN-ω, despite no significant changes in viral load.[84]

Management of FIV-Infected Cats

Cats that test positive for FIV should be housed indoors to prevent transmission to other cats, as well as to protect them from other infections. The latter is important even in subclinically infected cats, as other infections have the potential to activate viral transcription and accelerate disease progression. The feeding of raw foods and hunting behavior should be avoided. Cats should be neutered to reduce the chance of roaming and aggressive interactions with other cats. Minimally, FIV-positive cats should be rechecked every 6 months in order to monitor body weight, assess for periodontal disease, and discuss the need for routine laboratory testing and vaccination with core vaccines. A complete physical examination, CBC, serum biochemistry panel, and urinalysis are recommended on an annual basis.[66] At least during acute FIV infection, cats can mount an immune response to vaccines,[85,86] but because vaccination with core vaccines may activate viral transcription, vaccination should be performed only for FIV-positive cats that are likely to be exposed to other cats. The use of inactivated vaccines is recommended, because of the potential for vaccine-induced disease in immunosuppressed cats.[73] When hospitalized, FIV-infected cats should be kept in separate cages *away from* isolation, where there may be other cats with transmissible infectious diseases. Perioperative antimicrobial drug treatment could be considered for cats that undergo invasive surgery or dental treatments.[66,73]

Prognosis

A limited number of studies have shown no significant difference in life span between FIV-infected cats and uninfected cats.[42,87] In one study, the median survival times of these two groups after testing for FIV infection were 3.9 (39 cats) and 5.9 (22 cats) years, respectively.[87] In a larger study of more than 1000 FIV-infected cats and more than 8000 age- and sex-matched control cats, the median survival times of the two groups were 4.9 years and 6.0 years, respectively.[66] The progression and severity of disease is related to virus strain and host immunity. Infection of geriatric and neonatal cats is associated with more rapid progression and severity of disease than infection of young adult cats.[84,88] For example, progression to terminal immunodeficiency can occur within 2 months in kittens.[89] Because the life span of FIV-infected cats may not differ greatly from that of uninfected cats, no cat should be euthanized on the basis of a positive FIV test alone.[66,73] However, other factors, such as control of the infection in group-housed or breeding cats, may necessitate euthanasia or rehoming of some cats that test positive. Once terminal FIV-related disease occurs, life spans are typically less than 1 year.

Immunity and Vaccination

The FIV vaccine first became available in the United States in July 2002 (Fel-O-Vax FIV, Fort Dodge Animal Health) and is an inactivated, adjuvanted, whole-virus vaccine that contains FIV Petaluma (subtype A) and FIV Shizuoka (subtype D). The vaccine has been available in New Zealand and Australia since 2004. It is licensed for the vaccination of healthy cats that are 8 weeks of age or older as an aid in the prevention of FIV, and in experimental challenge studies, protected 60% to 80% of cats from infection. The introduction of the vaccine generated controversy, because (1) existing serologic assays cannot differentiate between natural infection and vaccination, (2) vaccination provides only partial protection from infection, and (3) PCR assay results cannot be relied upon in vaccinated cats. Although concerns exist that the vaccine may only protect against infection with strains from homologous subtypes, studies have shown moderate protection against infection with subtype B strains.[90,91] In one study, 10 of 14 cats were protected from subtype B infection when challenged 1 year after vaccination compared with none of 5 control cats.[90] However, 13-week-old vaccinated cats were not protected from challenge with FIV subtype A strain Glasgow-8; all vaccinated and control cats were infected.[92]

Because of diagnostic test interference, uncertain efficacy in the field, and the increased risk of sarcoma formation associated with adjuvanted vaccines, the FIV vaccine is considered a noncore vaccine that should only be used for cats at high risk of infection, such as outdoor cats that fight with other cats. The initial vaccine should only be given to cats that test negative with FIV ELISA assays. Cat owners should be informed that protection is incomplete and that identification of subsequent infection may be impossible in some cats with the available diagnostic tests. The initial vaccine dose is followed by two booster doses at 3- to 4-week intervals, followed by annual boosters so long as risk persists. An identification microchip should be placed that links FIV vaccination to the microchip number, so should the cat escape or be relinquished to a shelter, a positive antibody test result is not interpreted as FIV infection.

Prevention

Transmission of FIV is reduced when cats are housed indoors. When one positive cat is identified in a household, all other cats should be tested and no new cats should be introduced, as this may lead to conflict and increased fighting behavior. Isolation of positive cats in a household should be considered. In breeding catteries, infection can be prevented by screening all new introductions, preferably with a 2-month quarantine period for introductions followed by retesting, and removal of all infected queens and toms from the cattery. Transmission in shelters can be reduced by testing on intake or housing cats singly in cages, and testing at or shortly after adoption, together with education of adopters in regard to the need to retest for infection.

Surgical needles, endotracheal tubes, breathing circuits, and instruments should never be shared between cats without proper cleaning and disinfection, and all cats used as blood donors should test negative for FIV antibodies with ELISA and, if possible, PCR assays offered by a diagnostic laboratory that has a high level of quality control. Fluid lines and multidose vials should not be shared between cats, because they can become contaminated with body fluids.

Public Health Aspects

Despite its similarities to HIV, no evidence of natural infection of humans with FIV exists.

CASE EXAMPLE

Signalment: "Arthur" an 11-year-old male neutered domestic shorthair from northern California

History: Arthur was initially brought to his veterinarian for a 2-day history of lethargy and decreased appetite. Physical examination was unremarkable. Blood work showed a hematocrit of 28% (reference range, 29% to 38%), a white cell count of 6400 cells/μL with a normal differential, clumped platelets, mild hyperbilirubinemia (0.5 mg/dL), mild hypoalbuminemia (2.4 g/dL), and hyperglobulinemia (5.5 g/dL). He was treated with amoxicillin and mirtazapine, but lethargy and inappetence persisted. Serial hemograms performed over the subsequent 3 months showed progressive leukopenia due to a neutropenia and lymphopenia (Table 21-6), during which time Arthur was treated with orbifloxacin, with some improvement in his appetite and attitude. A bone marrow aspirate performed 5 weeks after the onset of illness showed myeloid hyperplasia with a left shift. Serology for FIV and FeLV was performed 11 weeks after onset of illness, and the cat was negative for FeLV antigen and had an equivocal test result for FIV antibody. Serum thyroxine concentration was low (0.7 mcg/dL, reference range 1.1 to 3.3 mcg/dL). The cat was referred for further evaluation.

Arthur was an indoor and outdoor cat and had a history of predation (mice and birds) and fighting with other cats in the neighborhood. His diet otherwise consisted of a commercial wet cat food. He was vaccinated regularly for rabies, FeLV, feline herpesvirus-1, feline calicivirus, and feline panleukopenia virus infections.

Current Medications: Orbifloxacin, 7 mg/kg PO q12h

Other Medical History: Routine blood work had been performed 3 years previously, which showed a normal CBC, a globulin of 5 g/dL, a urine specific gravity of 1.069, and a T4 of 1.3. At that time, Arthur tested negative for FeLV antigen and positive for FIV antibody.

Physical Examination:

Body Weight: 3.1 kg

General: Quiet, alert, responsive, estimated to be 5% to 7% dehydrated, T = 103.9°F (39.9°C), HR = 144 beats/min, RR = 50 breaths/min, mucous membranes pale pink, CRT < 2 s. A dry haircoat with moderate amounts of scale was present. There was no evidence of ectoparasites.

Eyes, Ears, Nose, and Throat (with Dilated Fundoscopic Examination): Moderate gingivitis and absent mandibular canine teeth. No other clinically significant abnormalities were detected.

Musculoskeletal: Body condition score 2/9. Generalized muscle atrophy was noted. Ambulatory in all four limbs.

Cardiovascular: Aside from an intermittent gallop rhythm, no abnormalities were noted.

Respiratory: No abnormalities were detected.

Gastrointestinal and Urogenital: Abdomen soft and nonpainful on palpation, mild hepatomegaly. Urinary bladder was small and soft.

Lymph Nodes: All lymph nodes less than 1 cm in diameter.

Laboratory Findings:

CBC:

HCT 22.5% (30%-50%)
MCV 47.5 fL (42-53 fL)
MCHC 32.9 g/dL (30-33.5 g/dL)
Reticulocytes 7400 cells/μL
WBC 1100 cells/μL (4500-14,000 cells/μL)
Neutrophils 704 cells/μL (2000-9000 cells/μL)
Band neutrophils 99 cells/μL
Lymphocytes 220 cells/μL (1000-7000 cells/μL)
Monocytes 77 cells/μL (50-600 cells/μL)
32,000 platelets/μL (180,000-500,000 platelets/μL).
Neutrophils showed moderate toxicity with many Döhle bodies, and there were many macroplatelets.

Serum Chemistry Profile:

Sodium 149 mmol/L (151-158 mmol/L)
Potassium 3.1 mmol/L (3.6-4.9 mmol/L)
Chloride 115 mmol/L (117-126 mmol/L)
Bicarbonate 17 mmol/L (15-21 mmol/L)
Phosphorus 4.3 mg/dL (3.2-6.3 mg/dL)
Calcium 8.8 mg/dL (9.0-10.9 mg/dl)
BUN 17 mg/dL (18-33 mg/dL)
Creatinine 1.1 mg/dL (1.1-2.2 mg/dL)
Glucose 158 mg/dL (63-118 mg/dL)
Total protein 8.1 g/dL (6.6-8.4 g/dL)
Albumin 3.0 g/dL (2.2-4.6 g/dL)
Globulin 5.1 g/dL (2.8-5.4 g/dL)
ALT 121 U/L (27-101 U/L)
AST 113 U/L (17-58 U/L)
ALP 10 U/L (14-71 U/L)
Creatine kinase 278 U/L (73-260 U/L)
Gamma GT <3 U/L (0-4 U/L)
Cholesterol 204 mg/dL (89-258 mg/dL)
Total bilirubin 0.8 mg/dL (0-0.2 mg/dL)
Magnesium 2.4 mg/dL (1.5-2.5 mg/dL).

Anti-nuclear Antibody Serology: Positive at 1:32

Microbiologic and Virologic Testing: Point-of-care ELISA serology for FeLV antigen and FIV antibody: negative

Feline coronavirus antibody serology: negative at 1:25

Aerobic and anaerobic blood cultures (three specimens): negative

PCR for FIV proviral DNA: positive (cycle threshold value = 30, values <40 are positive)

Imaging Findings:

Abdominal Ultrasound: Hepatomegaly was identified and the spleen had a mottled echotexture. There was mild enlargement of the ileocecal lymph nodes and mild diffuse thickening of the small intestinal submucosal layer.

Thoracic Radiographs: Cardiopulmonary structures were within normal limits.

Cytologic Findings:

Liver Aspiration Cytology: A moderately bloody background contained scattered, variably sized clusters of uniform hepatocytes and low numbers of nucleated cells. The nucleated cells consisted of a mixture of nondegenerate neutrophils, lymphocytes, macrophages, and rare myeloid precursors. Several macrophages were erythrophagic. Interpretation: Possible mild myeloid extramedullary hematopoiesis.

Spleen Aspiration Cytology: The specimen was highly cellular with a pink background that contained a moderate amount of blood and scattered clumps of hemosiderin. A mixed population of lymphocytes was admixed with variable numbers of hematopoietic precursor cells. Hematopoietic precursors were primarily granulocytic precursors, with many progranulocytes. A few erythroid precursors, including erythroblasts, were noted. Plasma cells were moderately increased in number, and both immature and mature forms were seen. Several binucleated and rare trinucleated plasma cells and scattered immature lymphocytes were noted. Vacuolated macrophages were increased in number and often contained phagocytized erythrocytes or blue-green pigment consistent with hemosiderin. Scattered mitotic figures were noted. Interpretation: Moderate plasmacytosis, extramedullary hematopoiesis, and histiocytic hyperplasia with erythrophagocytosis and increased iron. The large number of immature plasma cells raised the possibility of plasma cell neoplasia; however, reactive plasmacytosis could not be ruled out.

Bone Marrow Aspiration Cytology: Numerous hypercellular unit particles were present. A few mature megakaryocytes were noted. Hematopoietic cells consisted largely of myeloid precursors, with an estimated myeloid to erythroid ratio greater than 10. Myeloid cells showed orderly maturation to the band neutrophil stage, with few segmented neutrophils. Few erythroid precursors were noted, which included rare prorubricytes, rubricytes, and metarubricytes. Scattered well-differentiated plasma cells and a small amount of hemosiderin were noted. Interpretation: Marked myeloid hyperplasia, marked erythroid hypoplasia, and moderate megakaryocytic hypoplasia. The myeloid hyperplasia together with persistent neutropenia suggested myelodysplasia.

Serum Protein Electrophoresis: A mild increase in α_2 globulins was present (1.34 g/dL, reference range, 0.4-0.9 g/dL) together with a broad-based gamma region. This was consistent with an acute-phase inflammatory response.

Diagnosis: Terminal phase of FIV infection, characterized by pancytopenia secondary to myelodysplasia; hepatopathy (open diagnosis).

Comments: The progression of FIV infection was apparent in this cat, which transitioned from a seropositive to a seronegative, PCR-positive state as a result of progressive decline in immune function and, ultimately, failure to produce antibodies. The cause of the hepatopathy was not identified. Blood cultures were negative, and spleen and liver aspiration cytology failed to reveal evidence of underlying neoplasia. Because of the plasmacytosis in the spleen, serum protein electrophoresis was performed to assist diagnosis of a plasma cell tumor (as supported by a monoclonal gammopathy), but this was not apparent. The cat was treated with clavulanic acid–amoxicillin without clinical improvement. Treatment with glucocorticoids was also offered because of the possibility of undiagnosed round cell neoplasia or immune-mediated neutropenia (in light of the myeloid hyperplasia combined with a positive antinuclear antibody test). The cat died at home 1 month later, and necropsy was not performed.

TABLE 21-6

Progression of Laboratory Abnormalities in an 11-Year-old Male Neutered Domestic Shorthair That Tested Positive for Antibodies to FIV 3 Years Earlier, at Which Time a CBC was Normal

	Days after Onset of Illness					
	39	47	56	74	83	Reference Range
Hematocrit (%)	29	29	33	27	22	30-50
White blood cells/μL	2000	2100	1000	1100	1100	4500-14,000
Neutrophils/μL	1180	1407	610	572	704	2000-9000
Lymphocytes/μL	700	588	340	462	220	1000-7000
Platelets/μL	191,000	196,000	Clumped	Clumped	32,000	180,000-500,000
FIV/FeLV serology*				Equivocal/ negative	Negative/ negative	

*SNAP FIV/FeLV Combo Test, IDEXX Laboratories.

SUGGESTED READINGS

Goldkamp CE, Levy JK, Edinboro CH, et al. Seroprevalences of feline leukemia virus and feline immunodeficiency virus in cats with abscesses or bite wounds and rate of veterinarian compliance with current guidelines for retrovirus testing. J Am Vet Med Assoc. 2008;232:1152-1158.

Hartmann K. Clinical aspects of feline immunodeficiency and feline leukemia virus infection. Vet Immunol Immunopathol. 2011;143(3-4):190-201 (for a review of molecular pathogenetic mechanisms of disease).

Hosie MJ, Addie D, Belak S, et al. Feline immunodeficiency. ABCD guidelines on prevention and management. J Feline Med Surg. 2009;11:575-584.

Levy J, Crawford C, Hartmann K, et al. 2008 American Association of Feline Practitioners' feline retrovirus management guidelines. J Feline Med Surg. 2008;10:300-316.

REFERENCES

1. Pedersen NC, Ho EW, Brown ML, et al. Isolation of a T-lymphotropic virus from domestic cats with an immunodeficiency-like syndrome. Science. 1987;235:790-793.
2. Gruffydd-Jones TJ, Hopper CD, Harbour DA, et al. Serological evidence of feline immunodeficiency virus infection in UK cats from 1975-76. Vet Rec. 1988;123:569-570.

3. Reid RW, Barr MC, Scott FW. Retrospective serologic survey for the presence of feline immunodeficiency virus antibody: a comparison of ELISA and IFA techniques. Cornell Vet. 1992;82:359-369.
4. Troyer JL, Pecon-Slattery J, Roelke ME, et al. Seroprevalence and genomic divergence of circulating strains of feline immunodeficiency virus among Felidae and Hyaenidae species. J Virol. 2005;79:8282-8294.
5. Elder JH, Lin YC, Fink E, et al. Feline immunodeficiency virus (FIV) as a model for study of lentivirus infections: parallels with HIV. Curr HIV Res. 2010;8:73-80.
6. de Parseval A, Chatterji U, Sun P, et al. Feline immunodeficiency virus targets activated CD4+ T cells by using CD134 as a binding receptor. Proc Natl Acad Sci U S A. 2004;101:13044-13049.
7. Shimojima M, Miyazawa T, Ikeda Y, et al. Use of CD134 as a primary receptor by the feline immunodeficiency virus. Science. 2004;303:1192-1195.
8. Samman A, McMonagle EL, Logan N, et al. Phylogenetic characterisation of naturally occurring feline immunodeficiency virus in the United Kingdom. Vet Microbiol. 2011;150:239-247.
9. Hayward JJ, Rodrigo AG. Molecular epidemiology of feline immunodeficiency virus in the domestic cat (Felis catus). Vet Immunol Immunopathol. 2010;134:68-74.
10. Weaver EA. A detailed phylogenetic analysis of FIV in the United States. PLoS One. 2010;5:e12004.
11. Wang C, Johnson CM, Ahluwalia SK, et al. Dual-emission fluorescence resonance energy transfer (FRET) real-time PCR differentiates feline immunodeficiency virus subtypes and discriminates infected from vaccinated cats. J Clin Microbiol. 2010;48:1667-1672.
12. Nakamura Y, Ura A, Hirata M, et al. An updated nation-wide epidemiological survey of feline immunodeficiency virus (FIV) infection in Japan. J Vet Med Sci. 2010;72:1051-1056.
13. Bachmann MH, Mathiason-Dubard C, Learn GH, et al. Genetic diversity of feline immunodeficiency virus: dual infection, recombination, and distinct evolutionary rates among envelope sequence clades. J Virol. 1997;71:4241-4253.
14. Steinrigl A, Klein D. Phylogenetic analysis of feline immunodeficiency virus in Central Europe: a prerequisite for vaccination and molecular diagnostics. J Gen Virol. 2003;84:1301-1307.
15. Kann R, Seddon J, Kyaw-Tanner M, et al. Phylogenetic analysis to define feline immunodeficiency virus subtypes in 31 domestic cats in South Africa. J S Afr Vet Assoc. 2006;77:108-113.
16. Kann RK, Kyaw-Tanner MT, Seddon JM, et al. Molecular subtyping of feline immunodeficiency virus from domestic cats in Australia. Aust Vet J. 2006;84:112-116.
17. Kann RK, Seddon JM, Meers J, et al. Feline immunodeficiency virus subtypes in domestic cats in New Zealand. N Z Vet J. 2007;55:358-360.
18. Kann R, Seddon J, Kyaw-Tanner M, et al. Co-infection with different subtypes of feline immunodeficiency virus can complicate subtype assignment by phylogenetic analysis. Arch Virol. 2007;152:1187-1193.
19. Iwata D, Holloway SA. Molecular subtyping of feline immunodeficiency virus from cats in Melbourne. Aust Vet J. 2008;86:385-389.
20. Sodora DL, Shpaer EG, Kitchell BE, et al. Identification of three feline immunodeficiency virus (FIV) env gene subtypes and comparison of the FIV and human immunodeficiency virus type 1 evolutionary patterns. J Virol. 1994;68:2230-2238.
21. Kakinuma S, Motokawa K, Hohdatsu T, et al. Nucleotide sequence of feline immunodeficiency virus: classification of Japanese isolates into two subtypes which are distinct from non-Japanese subtypes. J Virol. 1995;69:3639-3646.
22. Pistello M, Cammarota G, Nicoletti E, et al. Analysis of the genetic diversity and phylogenetic relationship of Italian isolates of feline immunodeficiency virus indicates a high prevalence and heterogeneity of subtype B. J Gen Virol. 1997;78(Pt 9):2247-2257.
23. Nishimura Y, Goto Y, Pang H, et al. Genetic heterogeneity of env gene of feline immunodeficiency virus obtained from multiple districts in Japan. Virus Res. 1998;57:101-112.
24. Martins AN, Medeiros SO, Simonetti JP, et al. Phylogenetic and genetic analysis of feline immunodeficiency virus gag, pol, and env genes from domestic cats undergoing nucleoside reverse transcriptase inhibitor treatment or treatment-naive cats in Rio de Janeiro, Brazil. J Virol. 2008;82:7863-7874.
25. Kelly PJ, Stocking R, Gao D, et al. Identification of feline immunodeficiency virus subtype-B on St. Kitts, West Indies by quantitative PCR. J Infect Dev Ctries. 2011;5:480-483.
26. Hayward JJ, Taylor J, Rodrigo AG. Phylogenetic analysis of feline immunodeficiency virus in feral and companion domestic cats of New Zealand. J Virol. 2007;81:2999-3004.
27. Nakamura K, Suzuki Y, Ikeo K, et al. Phylogenetic analysis of Vietnamese isolates of feline immunodeficiency virus: genetic diversity of subtype C. Arch Virol. 2003;148:783-791.
28. Uema M, Ikeda Y, Miyazawa T, et al. Feline immunodeficiency virus subtype C is prevalent in northern part of Taiwan. J Vet Med Sci. 1999;61:197-199.
29. Reggeti F, Bienzle D. Feline immunodeficiency virus subtypes A, B and C and intersubtype recombinants in Ontario, Canada. J Gen Virol. 2004;85:1843-1852.
30. Pecoraro MR, Tomonaga K, Miyazawa T, et al. Genetic diversity of Argentine isolates of feline immunodeficiency virus. J Gen Virol. 1996;77(Pt 9):2031-2035.
31. Nichols J, Litster A, Leutenegger C. Relationship between viral subgroup, viral load and health status in a population of cats naturally infected with feline immunodeficiency virus. Proceedings of the 2nd Symposium of the International Society for Companion Animal Infectious Diseases. 2012:Abstract 07.
32. Ueland K, Nesse LL. No evidence of vertical transmission of naturally acquired feline immunodeficiency virus infection. Vet Immunol Immunopathol. 1992;33:301-308.
33. Allison RW, Hoover EA. Covert vertical transmission of feline immunodeficiency virus. AIDS Res Hum Retroviruses. 2003;19:421-434.
34. Jordan HL, Howard J, Barr MC, et al. Feline immunodeficiency virus is shed in semen from experimentally and naturally infected cats. AIDS Res Hum Retroviruses. 1998;14:1087-1092.
35. Jordan HL, Howard JG, Bucci JG, et al. Horizontal transmission of feline immunodeficiency virus with semen from seropositive cats. J Reprod Immunol. 1998;41:341-357.
36. Little S, Sears W, Lachtara J, et al. Seroprevalence of feline leukemia virus and feline immunodeficiency virus infection among cats in Canada. Can Vet J. 2009;50:644-648.
37. Gleich SE, Krieger S, Hartmann K. Prevalence of feline immunodeficiency virus and feline leukaemia virus among client-owned cats and risk factors for infection in Germany. J Feline Med Surg. 2009;11:985-992.
38. Goldkamp CE, Levy JK, Edinboro CH, et al. Seroprevalences of feline leukemia virus and feline immunodeficiency virus in cats with abscesses or bite wounds and rate of veterinarian compliance with current guidelines for retrovirus testing. J Am Vet Med Assoc. 2008;232:1152-1158.
39. Levy JK, Edinboro CH, Glotfelty CS, et al. Seroprevalence of Dirofilaria immitis, feline leukemia virus, and feline immunodeficiency virus infection among dogs and cats exported from the 2005 Gulf Coast hurricane disaster area. J Am Vet Med Assoc. 2007;231:218-225.
40. Levy JK, Scott HM, Lachtara JL, et al. Seroprevalence of feline leukemia virus and feline immunodeficiency virus infection among cats in North America and risk factors for seropositivity. J Am Vet Med Assoc. 2006;228:371-376.
41. Yamamoto JK, Hansen H, Ho EW, et al. Epidemiologic and clinical aspects of feline immunodeficiency virus infection in cats from the continental United States and Canada and possible mode of transmission. J Am Vet Med Assoc. 1989;194:213-220.
42. Addie DD, Dennis JM, Toth S, et al. Long-term impact on a closed household of pet cats of natural infection with feline coronavirus, feline leukaemia virus and feline immunodeficiency virus. Vet Rec. 2000;146:419-424.

43. Hellard E, Fouchet D, Santin-Janin H, et al. When cats' ways of life interact with their viruses: a study in 15 natural populations of owned and unowned cats (Felis silvestris catus). Prev Vet Med. 2011;101:250-264.
44. Yamamoto JK, Sparger E, Ho EW, et al. Pathogenesis of experimentally induced feline immunodeficiency virus infection in cats. Am J Vet Res. 1988;49:1246-1258.
45. Tompkins MB, Tompkins WA. Lentivirus-induced immune dysregulation. Vet Immunol Immunopathol. 2008;123:45-55.
46. Mexas AM, Fogle JE, Tompkins WA, et al. CD4+CD25+ regulatory T cells are infected and activated during acute FIV infection. Vet Immunol Immunopathol. 2008;126:263-272.
47. Vahlenkamp TW, Tompkins MB, Tompkins WA. Feline immunodeficiency virus infection phenotypically and functionally activates immunosuppressive CD4+CD25+ T regulatory cells. J Immunol. 2004;172:4752-4761.
48. Dean GA, LaVoy A, Yearley J, et al. Cytokine modulation of the innate immune response in feline immunodeficiency virus-infected cats. J Infect Dis. 2006;193:1520-1527.
49. Lehman TL, O'Halloran KP, Hoover EA, et al. Utilizing the FIV model to understand dendritic cell dysfunction and the potential role of dendritic cell immunization in HIV infection. Vet Immunol Immunopathol. 2010;134:75-81.
50. Levy JK, Liang Y, Ritchey JW, et al. Failure of FIV-infected cats to control *Toxoplasma gondii* correlates with reduced IL2, IL6, and IL12 and elevated IL10 expression by lymph node T cells. Vet Immunol Immunopathol. 2004;98:101-111.
51. Fletcher NF, Meeker RB, Hudson LC, et al. The neuropathogenesis of feline immunodeficiency virus infection: barriers to overcome. Vet J. 2011;188:260-269.
52. Hofmann-Lehmann R, Berger M, Sigrist B, et al. Feline immunodeficiency virus (FIV) infection leads to increased incidence of feline odontoclastic resorptive lesions (FORL). Vet Immunol Immunopathol. 1998;65:299-308.
53. Beatty JA, Troyer RM, Brewester C, et al. Feline immunodeficiency virus (FIV)-associated lymphoma. Is a gammaherpesvirus involved?. Proceedings of the 2nd Symposium of the International Society for Companion Animal Infectious Diseases. 2012:Abstract 03.
54. Magden E, Quackenbush SL, VandeWoude S. FIV associated neoplasms—a mini-review. Vet Immunol Immunopathol. 2011;143:227-234.
55. Beatty JA, Callanan JJ, Terry A, et al. Molecular and immunophenotypical characterization of a feline immunodeficiency virus (FIV)-associated lymphoma: a direct role for FIV in B-lymphocyte transformation?. J Virol. 1998;72:767-771.
56. Matsumoto H, Takemura N, Sako T, et al. Serum concentration of circulating immune complexes in cats infected with feline immunodeficiency virus detected by immune adherence hemagglutination method. J Vet Med Sci. 1997;59:395-396.
57. Fujino Y, Horiuchi H, Mizukoshi F, et al. Prevalence of hematological abnormalities and detection of infected bone marrow cells in asymptomatic cats with feline immunodeficiency virus infection. Vet Microbiol. 2009;136:217-225.
58. Shelton GH, Linenberger ML, Grant CK, et al. Hematologic manifestations of feline immunodeficiency virus infection. Blood. 1990;76:1104-1109.
59. Meeker RB. Feline immunodeficiency virus neuropathogenesis: from cats to calcium. J Neuroimmune Pharmacol. 2007;2:154-170.
60. Podell M, Chen E, Shelton GD. Feline immunodeficiency virus associated myopathy in the adult cat. Muscle Nerve. 1998;21:1680-1685.
61. Maingat F, Halloran B, Acharjee S, et al. Inflammation and epithelial cell injury in AIDS enteropathy: involvement of endoplasmic reticulum stress. FASEB J. 2011;25:2211-2220.
62. O'Neil LL, Burkhard MJ, Diehl LJ, et al. Vertical transmission of feline immunodeficiency virus. Semin Vet Med Surg (Small Anim). 1995;10:266-278.
63. O'Neil LL, Burkhard MJ, Hoover EA. Frequent perinatal transmission of feline immunodeficiency virus by chronically infected cats. J Virol. 1996;70:2894-2901.
64. Weaver CC, Burgess SC, Nelson PD, et al. Placental immunopathology and pregnancy failure in the FIV-infected cat. Placenta. 2005;26:138-147.
65. English RV, Davidson MG, Nasisse MP, et al. Intraocular disease associated with feline immunodeficiency virus infection in cats. J Am Vet Med Assoc. 1990;196:1116-1119.
66. Levy J, Crawford C, Hartmann K, et al. 2008 American Association of Feline Practitioners' feline retrovirus management guidelines. J Feline Med Surg. 2008;10:300-316.
67. Goto Y, Nishimura Y, Baba K, et al. Association of plasma viral RNA load with prognosis in cats naturally infected with feline immunodeficiency virus. J Virol. 2002;76:10079-10083.
68. Gleich S, Hartmann K. Hematology and serum biochemistry of feline immunodeficiency virus-infected and feline leukemia virus-infected cats. J Vet Intern Med. 2009;23:552-558.
69. Hart SW, Nolte I. Hemostatic disorders in feline immunodeficiency virus-seropositive cats. J Vet Intern Med. 1994;8:355-362.
70. Hartmann K, Griessmayr P, Schulz B, et al. Quality of different in-clinic test systems for feline immunodeficiency virus and feline leukaemia virus infection. J Feline Med Surg. 2007;9:439-445.
71. Barr MC, Pough MB, Jacobson RH, et al. Comparison and interpretation of diagnostic tests for feline immunodeficiency virus infection. J Am Vet Med Assoc. 1991;199:1377-1381.
72. Levy JK, Crawford PC, Slater MR. Effect of vaccination against feline immunodeficiency virus on results of serologic testing in cats. J Am Vet Med Assoc. 2004;225:1558-1561.
73. Hosie MJ, Addie D, Belak S, et al. Feline immunodeficiency. ABCD guidelines on prevention and management. J Feline Med Surg. 2009;11:575-584.
74. Bienzle D, Reggeti F, Wen X, et al. The variability of serological and molecular diagnosis of feline immunodeficiency virus infection. Can Vet J. 2004;45:753-757.
75. Crawford PC, Slater MR, Levy JK. Accuracy of polymerase chain reaction assays for diagnosis of feline immunodeficiency virus infection in cats. J Am Vet Med Assoc. 2005;226:1503-1507.
76. Dandekar S, Beebe AM, Barlough J, et al. Detection of feline immunodeficiency virus (FIV) nucleic acids in FIV-seronegative cats. J Virol. 1992;66:4040-4049.
77. IDEXX Reference Laboratories Diagnostic Update. 2009. http://www.idexx.com/view/xhtml/en_us/smallanimal/reference-laboratories/testmenu/innovative-tests/real-pcr.jsf?SSOTOKEN=0. Last accessed May 18, 2012.
78. Maingat F, Vivithanaporn P, Zhu Y, et al. Neurobehavioral performance in feline immunodeficiency virus infection: integrated analysis of viral burden, neuroinflammation, and neuronal injury in cortex. J Neurosci. 2009;29:8429-8437.
79. Shelton GH, Grant CK, Linenberger ML, et al. Severe neutropenia associated with griseofulvin therapy in cats with feline immunodeficiency virus infection. J Vet Intern Med. 1990;4:317-319.
80. Arai M, Darman J, Lewis A, et al. The use of human hematopoietic growth factors (rhGM-CSF and rhEPO) as a supportive therapy for FIV-infected cats. Vet Immunol Immunopathol. 2000;77:71-92.
81. Fogle JE, Tompkins WA, Campbell B, et al. Fozivudine tidoxil as single-agent therapy decreases plasma and cell-associated viremia during acute feline immunodeficiency virus infection. J Vet Intern Med. 2011;25:413-418.
82. Egberink HF, De Clercq E, Van Vliet AL, et al. Bicyclams, selective antagonists of the human chemokine receptor CXCR4, potently inhibit feline immunodeficiency virus replication. J Virol. 1999;73:6346-6352.
83. Hartmann K, Stengel C, Klein D, et al. Efficacy and adverse effects of the antiviral compound pleraxifor in feline immunodeficiency virus-infected cats. J Vet Intern Med. 2012;26(3):483-490.

84. Pedersen NC, Leutenegger CM, Woo J, et al. Virulence differences between two field isolates of feline immunodeficiency virus (FIV-APetaluma and FIV-CPGammar) in young adult specific pathogen free cats. Vet Immunol Immunopathol. 2001;79:53-67.
85. Doménech A, Miró G, Collado VM, et al. Use of recombinant interferon omega in feline retrovirosis: from theory to practice. Vet Immunol Immunopathol. 2011;143(3-4):301-306.
86. Dawson S, Smyth NR, Bennett M, et al. Effect of primary-stage feline immunodeficiency virus infection on subsequent feline calicivirus vaccination and challenge in cats. AIDS. 1991;5:747-750.
87. Ravi M, Wobeser GA, Taylor SM, et al. Naturally acquired feline immunodeficiency virus (FIV) infection in cats from western Canada: Prevalence, disease associations, and survival analysis. Can Vet J. 2010;51:271-276.
88. George JW, Pedersen NC, Higgins J. The effect of age on the course of experimental feline immunodeficiency virus infection in cats. AIDS Res Hum Retroviruses. 1993;9:897-905.
89. O'Neil LL, Burkhard MJ, Obert LA, et al. Regression of feline immunodeficiency virus infection. AIDS Res Hum Retroviruses. 1997;13:713-718.
90. Huang C, Conlee D, Gill M, et al. Dual-subtype feline immunodeficiency virus vaccine provides 12 months of protective immunity against heterologous challenge. J Feline Med Surg. 2010;12:451-457.
91. Kusuhara H, Hohdatsu T, Okumura M, et al. Dual-subtype vaccine (Fel-O-Vax FIV) protects cats against contact challenge with heterologous subtype B FIV infected cats. Vet Microbiol. 2005;108:155-165.
92. Dunham SP, Bruce J, MacKay S, et al. Limited efficacy of an inactivated feline immunodeficiency virus vaccine. Vet Rec. 2006;158:561-562.

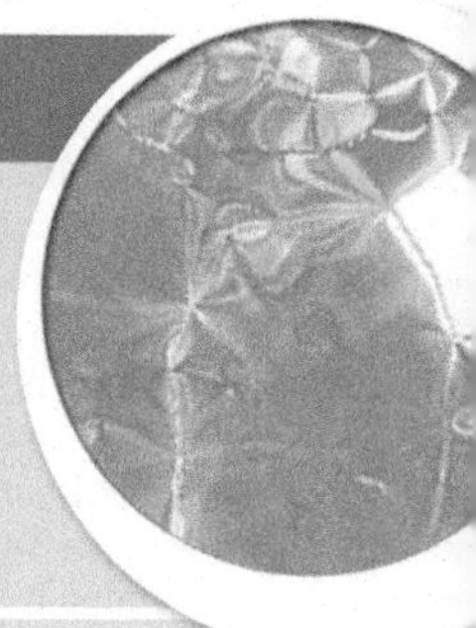

Feline Leukemia Virus Infection

Jane E. Sykes and Katrin Hartmann

Overview of Feline Leukemia Virus Infection

First Described: Scotland, 1964 (Jarrett et al.)[1]

Cause: Feline leukemia virus (family Retroviridae, subfamily Orthoretrovirinae, genus *Gammaretrovirus*)

Affected Hosts: Domestic and some wild Felidae

Geographic Distribution: Worldwide

Mode of Transmission: Prolonged close contact with salivary secretions; to a lesser extent biting, transplacental transmission, transmission through milk, and through blood transfusion

Major Clinical Signs: Lethargy, fever, pallor, stomatitis, signs of underlying lymphoma or leukemia, signs of immune-mediated disorders or opportunistic infections

Differential Diagnoses: FIV infection is the primary differential diagnosis for cats with signs of immunosuppression; feline calicivirus infection, or FIV infection are differential diagnoses for cats with stomatitis; primary immune-mediated disease and other bone marrow diseases are differential diagnoses for cats with immune-mediated diseases and cytopenias

Human Health Significance: FeLV does not infect humans.

Etiology and Epidemiology

FeLV is an enveloped RNA virus that belongs to the genus *Gammaretrovirus* of the family Retroviridae. FeLV infection remains an important cause of mortality in domestic cats through its ability to cause immune suppression, bone marrow disorders, and hematopoietic neoplasia. FeLV also causes disease in wild felids such as the highly endangered Iberian lynx.[2]

FeLV infection progresses more rapidly than FIV infection and is more pathogenic, so most cats that develop progressive infections ultimately die of FeLV-related disease. However, in contrast to FIV infection, many cats in the early state of FeLV infection regress to a permanent state of viral latency ("regressive infection"). It is possible that some cats, after exposure to a low dose of FeLV, may eliminate the infection altogether ("abortive infection"), although this appears to be a rare outcome. Regardless, a positive test result for FeLV infection in an apparently healthy cat does not always imply that FeLV-related disease and mortality will occur.

The structure of FeLV is similar to that of FIV, except that the capsid is icosahedral rather than cone shaped (Figure 22-1). There are three main subtypes of FeLV: FeLV-A, FeLV-B, and FeLV-C. Each subtype uses a different receptor to enter cells (Table 22-1). All cats infected with FeLV-B and FeLV-C are co-infected with FeLV-A, and only FeLV-A is transmitted between animals. FeLV-B and FeLV-C are more pathogenic than FeLV-A. FeLV-B arises through recombination of FeLV-A proviral DNA with endogenous FeLV sequences present in host cellular DNA.[3] FeLV-C arises from accumulation of mutations or insertions in the *env* (SU) gene of FeLV-A.[4,5] The FeLV subtype influences the clinical expression of disease (see Table 22-1). For example, FeLV-C is associated with nonregenerative anemia. Even within an FeLV subtype, mutations in the SU and the LTR regions of the viral genome affect disease outcome.[6,7] An additional subtype, FeLV-T, has been associated with immunodeficiency.

Transmission of FeLV-A primarily results from close contact with salivary secretions, such as through licking, mutual grooming, and shared food and water dishes. Other routes of transmission, such as by biting, blood transfusion, in milk, and possibly by fleas, can also occur.[8-10] The virus survives poorly outside the cat and is readily inactivated by disinfectants, soap, and desiccation. The overall prevalence of FeLV infection has declined over the past two decades with more extensive testing and vaccination. Before the institution of widespread testing and vaccination, more than 30% of cats in some catteries were infected.[11] In the early 1990s, the overall prevalence of infection was 13% in nearly 28,000 sick cats from North

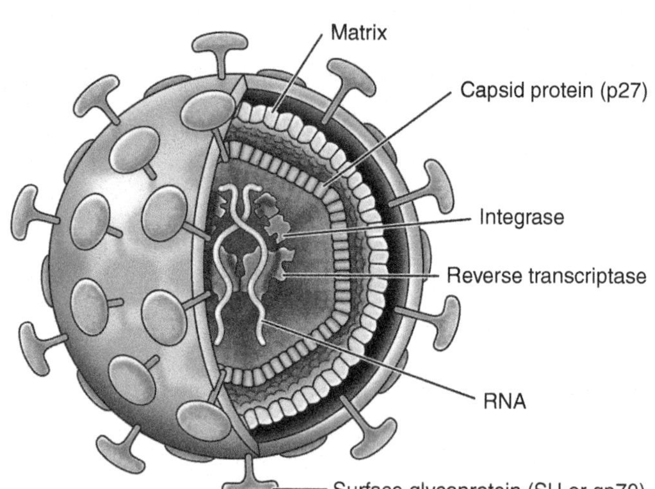

FIGURE 22-1 Structure of feline leukemia virus. Gammaretroviruses contain two identical strands of RNA and associated enzymes, which include reverse transcriptase, integrase, and protease, packaged into a core composed of the capsid protein (p27) with a surrounding matrix, all enclosed by a phospholipid membrane envelope derived from the host cell. The envelope contains a gp70 glycoprotein and the transmembrane protein p15E.

TABLE 22-1

Host Cellular Receptors Involved in FeLV Infection

FeLV Subtype	Receptor	Receptor Function	Comments
FeLV-A	FeTHTR1*	Thiamine transporter protein	Present in all cats with FeLV; transmitted exogenously
FeLV-B	FePit1 or FePit2†	Inorganic phosphate transporter protein	Results from recombination between FeLV-A and feline endogenous FeLV-related retrovirus sequences; may accelerate development of lymphoma or enhance neuropathogenicity
FeLV-C	FLVCR‡	Heme transporter protein	Arises from point mutations in FeLV-A *env* gene; associated with nonregenerative anemia

*Mendoza R, Anderson MM, Overbaugh J. A putative thiamine transport protein is a receptor for feline leukemia virus subgroup A. J Virol 2006;80(7):3378-3385.

†Anderson MM, Lauring AS, Robertson S, et al. Feline Pit2 functions as a receptor for subgroup B feline leukemia viruses. J Virol 2001;75(22):10563-10572.

‡Keel SB, Doty RT, Yang Z, et al. A heme export protein is required for red blood cell differentiation and iron homeostasis. Science 2008;319(5864):825-828.

America that were at risk for exposure.[12] The prevalence was just 7% in a similar population of approximately 1400 cats in 2006.[13] The prevalence of FeLV infection in European cats has also declined markedly.[14] Currently, the overall prevalence of infection in mixed populations of cats is 1% to 6%.[13,15-19] Cats with access to the outdoors; those that have contact with other cats; cats that are male, aggressive, or intact; and cats that are co-infected with FIV are at increased risk of FeLV infection.[12,13,15,17] Male cats are less strongly predisposed to FeLV infection than to FIV infection, and in some studies,[20] no male predisposition has been recognized. Adult cats are more likely to be infected with FeLV than cats aged less than 6 months,[13,17] but the median age of cats infected with FeLV is 3 years,[15] which is lower than that for FIV. This reflects a) the greater degree of pathogenicity of FeLV than FIV and its ability to significantly reduce lifespan; and b) the phenomenon of age-related resistance to FeLV, whereby exposure of cats that are less than 4 months of age to the virus is much more likely to lead to progressive infection than exposure of adults.[21] When 12- to 16-week old kittens are exposed to a multicat household with endemic FeLV infection, between 60% and 70% of kittens will become infected within a 5-month time period. In contrast, less than 5% of cats aged 6 months or older will become infected over the same time period; over a 2-year period, 40% to 50% of these adult cats will become infected. Infection of adult cats can also still occur with exposure to high doses of the virus or when there is underlying host immune compromise.

Clinical Features

Signs and Their Pathogenesis

The outcome of FeLV infection is extremely variable and depends strongly on the virus strain involved, the challenge dose, the route of inoculation, and factors that influence host immune function such as age, genetics, co-infections, stress, and treatment with immunosuppressive drugs. After oronasal exposure to the virus, the virus replicates in oral lymphoid tissue and then circulates in a few monocytes and lymphocytes within peripheral blood. Some cats develop systemic signs, such as fever, lethargy, and/or lymphadenopathy, during this period. A small number of infected lymphocytes then travel to the bone marrow, where the virus infects rapidly dividing precursor cells and subsequently lymphoid and epithelial cells throughout the body. This infection of the bone marrow is considered a critical step in the pathogenesis of FeLV infection. Once infection of epithelial cells in the salivary glands occurs, the virus is shed in massive quantities in saliva; low quantities of virus can also be shed in urine and feces.

Possible outcomes of infection with FeLV are shown in Figure 22-2. The immune system of some infected cats suppresses viral replication within a few weeks after infection, before significant infection of the marrow occurs. These cats develop a *regressive infection,* whereby proviral DNA is present in the host cell genome but production and shedding of virus no longer occurs (see Chapter 21). This may occur after the initial period of viremia, or viremia may never be detectable.[22] Regressive infection can persist for life and may be reactivated with immunosuppression, such as might occur during pregnancy or following treatment with immunosuppressive drugs.[23] Later in life, an unknown percentage of cats with regressive infections may develop FeLV-negative malignancies as a result of integration of viral DNA within host cellular oncogenes. Most cats with regressive infection, however, never develop clinical signs related to FeLV infection. Viral genome sequences may eventually be incompletely replicated, and as a consequence, reactivation of virus replication will become impossible in some cats over time. In *abortive infections*, no viremia occurs after infection, and virus cannot be detected using any method. Cats with abortive infections have been exposed to low doses of FeLV, and although they fail to develop viremia, they will develop antibodies to the virus.[24] Some cats that never test antigen-positive may have *focal infections*, that is, evidence of proviral DNA in some tissues but not in blood or bone marrow.[9] Cats develop *progressive infection* once involvement of the marrow is established and cellular destruction by the virus exceeds the ability of the host's immune system to suppress viral replication. Persistent viremia and progressive FeLV-related disease result (Box 22-1).

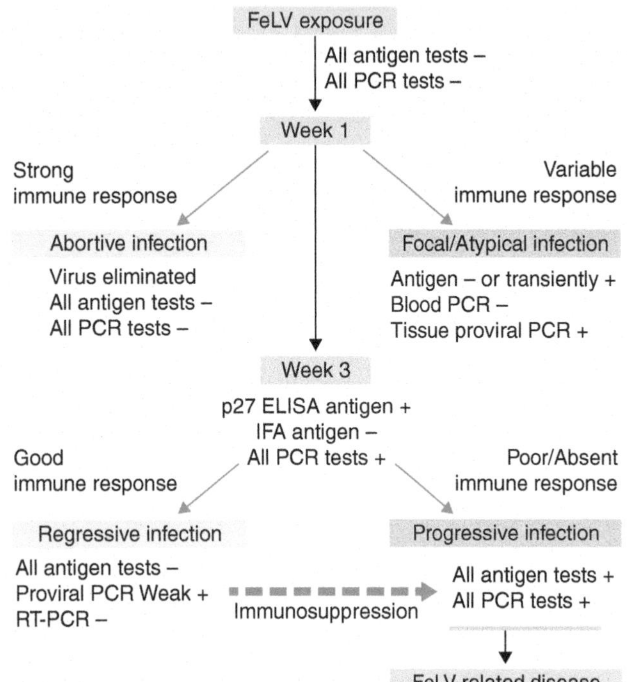

FIGURE 22-2 Outcomes of infection with FeLV. In the first week of infection, cats test negative with all antigen assays (i.e., p27 ELISA and IFA assays), RT-PCR for viral RNA, and PCR for proviral DNA. Rarely, cats exposed to low levels of virus eliminate the infection before or at this time point *(abortive infection)*. Soluble antigen assays and proviral PCR assays become positive from about the third week after infection, and virus is shed in saliva, tears, urine, and feces. After this time point, productive viral infection is suppressed by the host immune response *(regressive infection)* or the virus multiplies rapidly in the bone marrow and a progressive infection occurs, which is characterized by persistently positive antigen ELISA, IFA, viral RNA, and proviral DNA assay results. Cats with *focal or atypical infection* are never or transiently antigen positive and test negative using PCR assays on blood or bone marrow, but some tissues (such as the mammary gland or bladder) are positive with proviral PCR. The latter occurs in only a small percentage (e.g., < 5%) of infected cats.

Opportunistic Infections

Opportunistic infections may develop in FeLV infections as a result of myelo suppression or an acquired cell-mediated immunodeficiency. The immunosuppressive properties of FeLV are not fully understood but have been linked in part to the viral envelope peptide, p15E, which inhibits T and B cell function, inhibits cytotoxic lymphocyte responses, alters monocyte morphology and distribution, and has been associated with impaired cytokine production and responsiveness.[25-28] Kittens with progressive FeLV infection have impaired T cell and, to a lesser extent, B cell function.[29-32] Infected cats may develop lymphopenia, thymic atrophy, and depletion of lymphocytes within lymph node paracortical zones. CD4+ T cell malfunction may contribute to a decreased humoral and cell-mediated immune response in affected cats,[33,34] and the response to vaccination may also be impaired. Impaired neutrophil function compounds the effect of neutropenia in some infected cats.[35-37] Opportunistic infections that result include bacterial infections of the upper and lower urinary tract, hemoplasmosis, upper respiratory tract infections, feline infectious peritonitis, chronic stomatitis, toxoplasmosis, dermatophytosis, and cryptococcosis (Figure 22-3). The prevalence of some of these infections in cats with FeLV infection does not differ significantly from that in cats not infected with FeLV, but clinical signs are more severe and refractory to therapy. Infection with FeLV is an established risk factor for hemoplasma infection. In one study, it was also a risk factor for *Bartonella henselae* infection, but no evidence of clinical disease was identified in the cats infected with *B. henselae*.[38]

BOX 22-1

Clinical Outcomes of Progressive FeLV Infection

- Neoplasia, especially lymphoma, leukemia and fibrosarcomas (with FeSV)
- Opportunistic infections
- Pure red cell aplasia
- Aplastic anemia, myelodysplasia, or myelofibrosis
- Immune-mediated disease (immune-mediated hemolytic anemia, thrombocytopenia, glomerulonephritis, polyarthritis, uveitis)
- Peripheral lymphadenopathy
- Neurologic disease (e.g., anisocoria, urinary incontinence)
- Reproductive failure
- Gastrointestinal disease (uncommon)
- Other (e.g., osteochondromatosis, cutaneous horns)

FeSV, feline sarcoma virus.

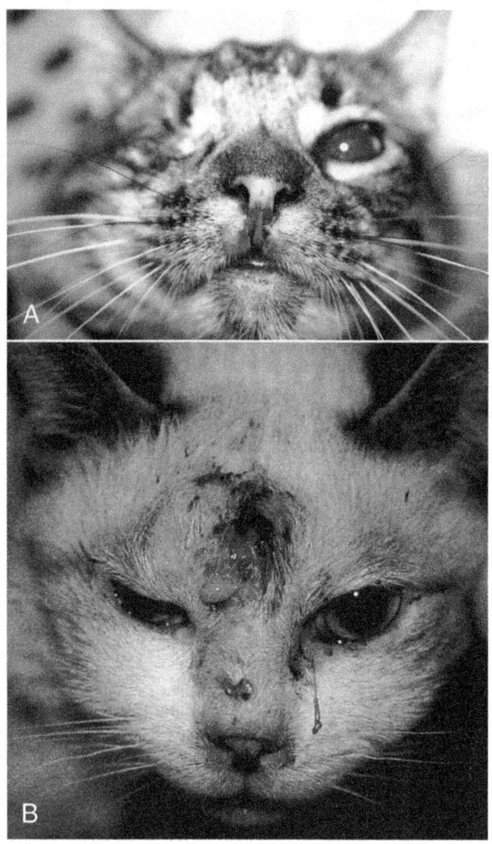

FIGURE 22-3 Opportunistic infections in cats with progressive FeLV infection. **A,** Ulceration of the nasal planum in a 6-month-old male neutered domestic medium hair cat with progressive FeLV infection as defined by positive ELISA antigen and IFA assays on peripheral blood. Stomatitis was also present, and feline calicivirus infection was suspected. **B,** Severe nasal cryptococcosis in a Siamese cat from a cattery with endemic FeLV infection.

Neoplasia

FeLV causes neoplasia in cats primarily as a result of insertional mutagenesis, by which the virus activates proto-oncogenes (especially *c-myc*, but also others such as *flit-1*) or disrupts tumor suppressor genes.[39] The most common types of neoplasia in cats infected with FeLV are lymphoma and leukemia. Cats infected with FeLV are more than 60-fold more likely to develop lymphoma than cats not infected with FeLV; this compares with approximately 5-fold for FIV.[40] Lymphoma or leukemia can be detected in nearly one quarter of cats with progressive FeLV infection at necropsy.[41] In the 1980s, as many as 70% of cases of feline lymphoma were associated with FeLV infection, but with improved control measures and vaccination, the vast majority of cats (more than 80% to 90%) seen at veterinary clinics with lymphoma now test negative for FeLV antigen.[42-44] The most common types of lymphoma in cats infected with FeLV are thymic (mediastinal), multicentric, spinal, renal, or ocular lymphoma. FeLV-associated lymphomas are mostly of T-cell origin, but B cell lymphoma can also occur. In contrast, FIV-associated lymphomas tend to be of B-cell origin.[42] Approximately 80% of cats with thymic lymphoma test positive for FeLV antigen, whereas fewer than 10% of cats with gastrointestinal lymphoma are FeLV antigen-positive. Large granular lymphoma is rarely associated with FeLV infection.[45] Cats with thymic lymphoma typically develop clinical signs of lethargy, tachypnea, and sometimes regurgitation. Most FeLV-positive cats with lymphoma are less than 4 years of age.[14]

Cats with regressive infection appear to be at greater risk for development of lymphoma than cats that were never exposed to FeLV. FeLV-negative cats that live with cats that test positive for FeLV antigen have a more than 40-fold increased risk of lymphoma compared to that expected without exposure to FeLV.[46] Several studies have investigated the prevalence of FeLV proviral DNA in tumor cells from cats that test negative for FeLV antigen. Some studies (including more recent studies that used real-time PCR assays) found no evidence of FeLV proviral DNA in feline lymphomas.[14,47,48] In older studies that used conventional PCR, more than 20% of antigen-negative lymphomas tested positive.[49,50] Additional studies from a variety of geographic locations that use multiple real-time PCR assays are required to clarify the role that FeLV plays in lymphomas and leukemias that develop in cats that test negative for FeLV antigen.

FeLV is responsible for the majority of myelogenous leukemias, erythroleukemias, megakaryocytic, and lymphoid leukemias in cats, although not all cats with these tumors test positive for FeLV antigen. Most FeLV-associated leukemias are acute. FeLV infection can underlie chronic eosinophilic leukemia,[51] chronic myelomonocytic leukemia,[52] and chronic lymphocytic leukemia. However, most cats with chronic lymphocytic leukemia are seronegative for FeLV antigen.

FeLV infection can result in the development of multiple fibrosarcomas in young cats. These occur when FeLV-A recombines with cellular oncogenes (such as *c-fes*, *c-fms*, or *c-fgr*) to form feline sarcoma viruses (FeSV). These viruses then develop mutations in these oncogenes that, when reinserted into cellular DNA, cause malignant transformation.[53,54] To replicate, FeSV requires the presence of FeLV-A, which supplies proteins such as those encoded by the *env* gene. Thus, all cats infected with FeSV test positive for FeLV antigen. FeSV-associated fibrosarcomas are characterized by multifocal, locally invasive, often ulcerated cutaneous masses that metastasize readily to the lung and other sites with a poor prognosis. FeLV-FeSV DNA sequences have been detected in some uveal melanomas from cats,[55] but other studies have failed to identify an association between FeSV and ocular melanomas or sarcomas in cats.[56,57] FeLV infection does not appear to be important in the pathogenesis of solitary fibrosarcomas or injection-site sarcomas in cats.[58,59]

Other tumor types that are variably associated with FeLV infection are feline olfactory neuroblastomas, cutaneous horns, and osteochondromatosis (multiple cartilaginous exostoses).[60] Feline olfactory neuroblastomas are rare and aggressive tumors of the nasal cavity that can lead to signs of rhinosinusitis and neurologic signs. Osteochondromatosis is characterized by benign cartilage-capped exostotic growths that arise from the surface of a bone, which can cause pain, lameness, disfigurement, and paresis due to spinal cord compression. Cutaneous horns occur as a result of benign keratinocyte hyperplasia.

BOX 22-2

Mechanisms of Anemia in Cats Infected with FeLV

Decreased RBC Production

- Pure red cell aplasia (FeLV-C)
- Aplastic anemia
- Leukemia (myelophthisis)
- Myelofibrosis
- Anemia of inflammatory disease

RBC Loss

- Thrombocytopenia secondary to immune-mediated or bone marrow disease

Increased RBC Destruction

- FeLV-associated IMHA
- Co-infection with hemoplasmas

IMHA, immune-mediated hemolytic anemia.

Anemia and Bone Marrow Disorders

Multiple mechanisms can lead to anemia in cats infected with FeLV (Box 22-2). Approximately 90% of FeLV-associated anemias are nonregenerative.[61] A variety of bone marrow disorders lead to decreased red blood cell production. FeLV-C infection results in pure red cell aplasia, a severe nonregenerative anemia associated with erythrocyte macrocytosis and depletion of erythroid precursors in the bone marrow. This occurs because FeLV-C binds to and interferes with a heme exporter protein, which results in subsequent heme toxicosis to the developing erythrocyte.[62] The presence of macrocytosis in the absence of reticulocytosis should thus raise suspicion for FeLV infection. FeLV infection can also lead to aplastic anemia in some cats, which is a deficiency in all cell lineages (platelets, myeloid, and erythroid) in the bone marrow, and replacement of the bone marrow space by adipose tissue. Anemia and bone marrow dysfunction may also result from myelophthisis secondary to leukemia, myeloid and/or erythroid dysplasia, or myelofibrosis (progressive replacement of the marrow with collagenous connective tissue) (Figure 22-4). Myelodysplasia is characterized by disordered maturation of marrow precursors, which in some

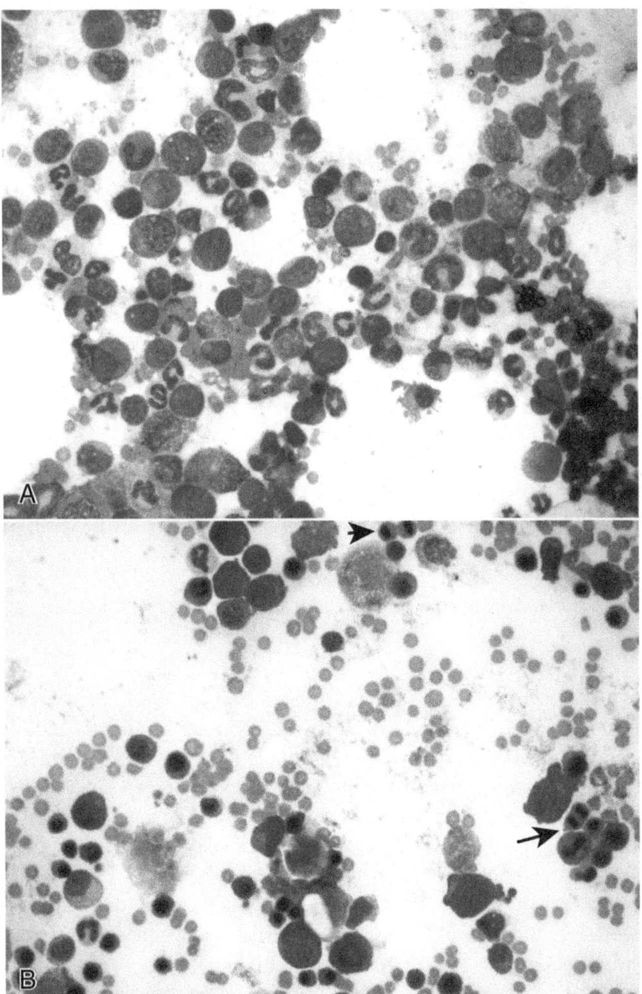

FIGURE 22-4 Bone marrow abnormalities in cats with FeLV infection. **A,** Bone marrow aspirate cytology from a 6-month old male neutered domestic shorthair cat that was evaluated for lethargy and fever. Acute leukemia, marked erythroid aplasia, marked granulocytic dysplasia, and increased eosinophilopoiesis is present. Megakaryocytic dysplasia was also identified. The G:E ratio was approximately 2950:1 with marked erythroid aplasia. Wright's stain. **B,** Bone marrow aspirate cytology from a 1-year-old male neutered domestic shorthair. Severe megaloblastic erythrodysplasia and mild megakaryocytic dysplasia were identified. The myeloid series is present but markedly decreased in all stages; the myeloid to erythroid ratio was estimated at 1:6.5 *(compare with A).* Nuclear to cytoplasmic asynchrony (megaloblastic change) is present, with immature nuclei in cytoplasm with hemoglobinization. Mitotic figures are present in moderate numbers and are seen in the late stages of the erythroid series *(arrows).*

cases precedes emergence of leukemia. FeLV infection underlies many myelodysplastic syndromes (MDS) and leukemia in cats.[63] However, over the past two decades, 50% of 28 cats with myelodysplasia and 44% of 41 cats with leukemia seen at the University of California, Davis, tested negative for FeLV antigen in peripheral blood, and only 36% of 34 cats with dysmyelopoiesis seen at the University of Minnesota were positive for FeLV antigen.[64] Several different classification systems have been used to describe feline MDS.[64] The French-American-British (FAB) classification scheme used for humans has been modified for dogs and cats. This divides MDS into 2 groups: 1) MDS with refractory cytopenia (less than 6% myeloblasts in the bone marrow, MDS-RC) and 2) MDS with excessive numbers of myeloblasts (6% to 30% myeloblasts, MDS-EB). The presence of more than 30% blasts indicates leukemia. The most common form of MDS in cats is MDS-EB.[64] Regressive FeLV infections have been detected by proviral DNA PCR in some cats with bone marrow disorders,[65] but the relationship between the presence of proviral DNA and the pathogenesis of disordered marrow function is unclear.

Anemia in cats with FeLV infection may also result from anemia of inflammatory disease, which can be triggered by opportunistic infections or neoplastic disease. Erythrocyte destruction occurs in some FeLV-infected cats as a result of secondary immune-mediated hemolytic anemia (IMHA) or co-infection with hemoplasmas (see Chapter 41). Hemorrhage as a result of thrombocytopenia or defective platelet function may also contribute to anemia. Mechanisms of thrombocytopenia include immune-mediated thrombocytopenia (ITP) and bone marrow dysfunction. Similarly, neutropenia can result from myeloid hypoplasia, myelofibrosis, myelodysplasia, myelophthisis, or maturation arrest at the myelocyte or metamyelocyte stages. In some cases, peripheral neutropenia accompanied by myeloid hyperplasia reflects underlying immune-mediated neutropenia.

Immune-Mediated Disorders

In addition to immune-mediated cytopenias, other immune-mediated disorders that can occur in association with progressive FeLV infection are glomerulonephritis,[66] uveitis,[67] and polyarthritis.[68] Circulating immune complexes have been detected in infected cats.[69-71] Because primary immune-mediated disorders are otherwise rare in cats, retrovirus testing is essential in cats that are diagnosed with these conditions before immunosuppressive drug treatment is initiated.

Neurologic Disorders

Neurologic disorders in cats with progressive FeLV infections may occur secondary to central nervous system (CNS) neoplasia, opportunistic infections, or FeLV infection itself. The envelope protein of FeLV may be neurotoxic.[72,73] Anisocoria, mydriasis, Horner's syndrome, and urinary incontinence can occur. FeLV infection may be one of the most frequent causes of urinary incontinence in cats, an otherwise uncommon condition. A myelopathy has been described in FeLV-infected cats that showed various neurologic signs such as disorientation, lethargy, increased vocalization, progressive ataxia, paresis, paralysis, hyperesthesia, urinary incontinence, recurrent constipation, and anisocoria with diminished pupillary light reflexes.[74] At necropsy, abundant FeLV antigen was detectable within neurons, endothelial cells, oligodendroglia, and astrocytes within the spinal cord.[74]

Gastrointestinal Disease

Uncommonly, FeLV causes enteritis that clinically and histologically resembles that caused by feline panleukopenia virus (FPV), except that lymphoid depletion is absent.[75] Clinical signs include vomiting, acute or chronic diarrhea that may be hemorrhagic, inappetence, weight loss, and dehydration. FeLV-infected cats with "panleukopenia-like syndrome" have intestinal crypt destruction and pancytopenia that results from myeloid destruction (Figure 22-5).[76] Although now very rare, co-infections with FeLV and FPV can also occur, and the 2 viruses may enhance each other's pathogenicity.[77] Co-infections with FeLV and other enteric viruses, such as feline coronavirus, also occur.[78] In most cases, diarrhea in cats infected by FeLV results from an etiology other than FeLV alone.

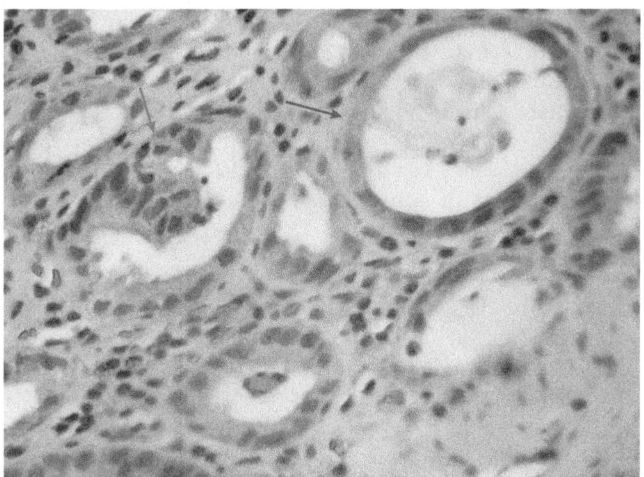

FIGURE 22-5 Histopathology of a colonic biopsy specimen from a 6-year-old intact male FeLV+ domestic shorthair with a 1-week history of anorexia, weight loss, lethargy, fever, and bloody mucoid diarrhea. Severe, diffuse, plasmacytic colitis was present with crypt epithelial necrosis and regeneration. One crypt is dilated, lined with attenuated epithelium, and contains necrotic debris *(red arrow)*. An adjacent crypt shows evidence of regeneration *(blue arrow)*. A tissue gram stain showed a mixed population of bacteria on the luminal surface, but not within crypts. A CBC showed thrombocytopenia (22,000 platelets/μL) and neutropenia (2700 neutrophils/μL) with neutrophil toxicity. A fecal parvovirus antigen test was negative, and bone marrow aspirate cytology showed evidence of myelodysplasia. Remarkably, this cat lived another 3 years with transfusion support, but ultimately was euthanized because of acute granulocytic leukemia with secondary sepsis.

Reproductive Disorders

Transplacental spread of FeLV can lead to fetal resorption, abortion, neonatal death, and fading kitten syndrome.[76] Fetal loss may also result from secondary endometritis. Kittens infected in late gestation or after birth develop thymic atrophy, failure to nurse, dehydration, lethargy, and death within the first 2 weeks of life.

Physical Examination Findings

Physical examination findings in cats with progressive FeLV infection vary dramatically depending on the stage of infection and the secondary disease process present. There may be no abnormalities, or cats may show signs of lethargy, pyrexia, mucosal pallor, petechial hemorrhages, dehydration, peripheral lymphadenomegaly, thin body condition, stomatitis, subcutaneous abscesses, or upper respiratory tract disease. Anemic cats may have a hemic murmur, tachypnea, or tachycardia, or they may be icteric. Cats with severe anemia can be laterally recumbent or comatose and hypothermic. Cats with thymic lymphoma may be tachypneic and have decreased lung and cardiac sounds on thoracic auscultation as a result of malignant pleural effusion, or heart sounds may be displaced caudally. Decreased compressibility of the cranial thorax may also be detected. Splenomegaly, hepatomegaly, renomegaly, intestinal masses, and/or abdominal lymph node enlargement may be detected on abdominal palpation of cats with multicentric lymphoma. Neurologic signs are detected infrequently when compared with signs of anemia or thoracic or abdominal lymphoma and include ataxia, anisocoria, and mydriasis. Although also relatively uncommon, uveitis may be identified, or there may be other ocular abnormalities as a result of intraocular lymphoma or co-infections with other pathogens.

Diagnosis

Infection with FeLV is often diagnosed when healthy cats are screened for infection. Screening should be performed with ELISA or related immunochromatographic in-house assays for free FeLV antigen in serum, because these assays are sensitive, specific, rapid, widely available, and most well understood. The retrovirus status of all cats should be known regardless of the presence of absence of illness.[79] The indications for retrovirus testing are described in Chapter 21 (see Box 21-1).

Even though many cats that test positive for FeLV antigen have no clinical signs or physical examination abnormalities, a CBC, chemistry panel, and urinalysis should be obtained from these cats (and at a minimum, a complete CBC with blood smear evaluation) to assess for underlying abnormalities that could signal the presence of FeLV-related disorders. Subtle hematologic abnormalities, such as erythroid macrocytosis or monocytopenia, may be present in the absence of overt clinical signs and can signify a poorer long-term outcome. Additional diagnostic tests indicated in infected cats that are anemic include a reticulocyte count, Coombs' test, and PCR assay for hemoplasmas. Bone marrow aspiration and core biopsy are indicated in cats with pancytopenia or persistent nonregenerative anemias.

Laboratory Abnormalities

Complete Blood Count

The CBC may be normal or show regenerative or nonregenerative anemia, neutropenia, lymphopenia, monocytopenia, and/or thrombocytopenia. Evidence of agglutination may be present in cats with IMHA. Moderate to marked leukocytosis and increased band neutrophils may also be present. Large numbers of circulating blasts, megakaryocytes or dysplastic cells (such as erythrocytes with giant Howell-Jolly bodies) can be found in cats with leukemia or MDS. When compared with uninfected cats, FeLV-infected cats were nearly 3.8-fold more likely to be anemic, 5-fold more likely to be thrombocytopenic, 3.6-fold more likely to be neutropenic, and 2.8-fold more likely to have lymphocytosis.[80]

Serum Biochemical Tests and Urinalysis

Findings on serum biochemistry analysis and urinalysis are nonspecific and reflect underlying disease processes. Hyperbilirubinemia and bilirubinuria may be present in cats with immune-mediated hemolytic anemia or hemoplasmosis. Cats with glomerulonephritis may be proteinuric. Some cats have evidence of bacterial urinary tract infections. Urine culture and susceptibility testing of a urine specimen obtained via cystocentesis are indicated in cats with suspected urinary tract infection.

Bone Marrow Cytology and Histopathology

Both bone marrow aspirate and core biopsy specimens should be obtained in cats with pancytopenia or nonregenerative anemia. If aspirate results are not diagnostic, the core biopsy should be submitted for interpretation. This is because bone marrow aspirates from cats with aplastic anemia or myelofibrosis are typically of low cellularity. Bone marrow findings in cats with FeLV infection include evidence of neoplastic lymphoid, erythroid, or myeloid cells (which circulate in the peripheral blood of cats with leukemia); myelodysplasia; hypoplasia or aplasia of erythroid, myeloid, or megakaryocyte cell lines; erythroid, myeloid, and megakaryocyte hyperplasia despite peripheral cytopenias; and megakaryocyte hypoplasia. Cytochemical stains that identify cells of the myeloid lineage (such as alkaline phosphatase, peroxidase, Sudan black B, and nonspecific esterase), immunocytochemistry, or flow cytometry using antibodies that target cell surface cluster of differentiation (CD) molecules may be needed to definitively identify the cell type involved in some acute undifferentiated leukemias.

Diagnostic Imaging

Imaging findings in cats with FeLV infection reflect the underlying disease process and are extremely variable. Cats with FeLV-associated thymic lymphosarcoma have a mediastinal mass on thoracic radiography that may be accompanied by mild to severe pleural effusion (Figure 22-6). Abdominal sonography in cats with multicentric lymphoma may reveal hypoechoic and enlarged abdominal lymph nodes and enlargement, hypoechogenicity, or mottling of the spleen, liver, or kidneys. Increased hepatic echogenicity can also occur with lymphoma. Intestinal masses with loss of normal bowel wall layering may also be detected. Splenomegaly may be detected in cats with immune-mediated cytopenias.

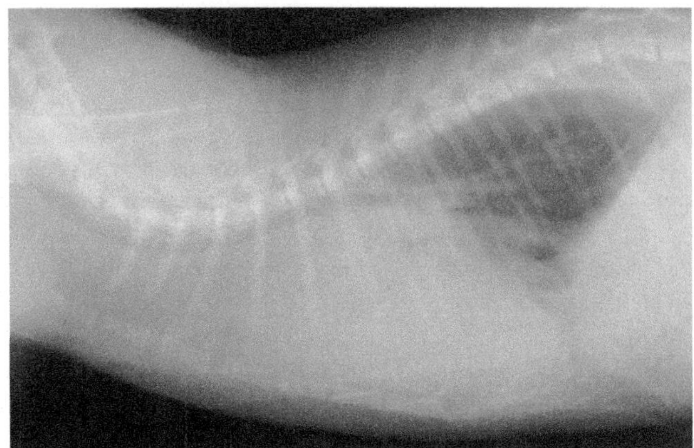

FIGURE 22-6 Lateral thoracic radiograph from a 5-year-old male neutered domestic shorthair cat with mediastinal lymphoma 11 months after it tested positive for circulating FeLV antigen. The cat was tachypneic and had muffled heart sounds that were displaced caudally. There is evidence of pleural effusion and dorsal displacement of the trachea. Cytologic examination of pleural fluid revealed large numbers of malignant lymphocytes.

Microbiologic Tests

Diagnostic assays available for FeLV infection are listed in Table 22-2.

Antigen Assays

The initial assay of choice for diagnosis of FeLV infection is an ELISA or a similar immunochromatographic test that detects soluble p27 capsid protein antigen in blood. The term *soluble* is used to distinguish these assays from assays such as IFA, which detect fixed antigen within cells. In most cats, the presence of circulating antigen correlates with viremia, although a few cats have viremia in the absence of detectable antigen or antigenemia in the absence of detectable viremia.[79] In-practice lateral flow assays are available that detect antigen in anticoagulated whole blood, plasma, or serum. In the past, the use of whole blood generated less reliable results than when plasma or serum was used, but with new-generation tests, whole blood is considered an acceptable alternative.[79] When a choice is available, serum is the preferred specimen. The use of tears or saliva is not recommended, because errors are more likely to occur. When virus isolation in culture was used as the gold standard, the sensitivity of seven different assays ranged from 92.1% to 96.8%, and the specificity ranged from 95.4% to 99.2%.[81]

TABLE 22-2

Diagnostic Assays Available for Feline Leukemia Virus Infection

Assay	Specimen Type	Target	Performance
ELISA or similar immunochromatographic tests for soluble FeLV antigen	Serum, plasma, whole blood	FeLV p27 antigen	Confirmation of positive results is recommended in healthy cats with a second test from a different manufacturer. Positive antigen test results do not signify progressive infection, and the assay must be repeated in 1 to 3 months or an IFA performed. False negatives can occur in the first month of infection.
IFA	Serum, bone marrow	FeLV antigen in blood cells	Less sensitive than ELISA. Positive results indicate infection of the bone marrow and therefore progressive infection. False positives may occur if nonspecific fluorescence is interpreted as a positive result.
PCR	Blood, bone marrow, saliva (RT-PCR); bone marrow, tissue, lymph node aspirates (PCR)	FeLV RNA (RT-PCR) or proviral DNA	Sensitivity and specificity may vary between laboratories. Never use in the absence of antigen testing. Assays that have demonstrated sensitivity and specificity may be useful to detect cats with regressive infection for elimination from blood donor programs, or to resolve the results of discordant ELISA and IFA assays. False-negative test results may occur when variant strains are present.
Virus isolation	Blood, bone marrow	Replication-competent FeLV virus	Difficult, not widely available. Requires a specialized laboratory. Used primarily as a research tool.

IFA, immunofluorescent antibody; RT, reverse transcriptase.

When ELISAs are used as screening tests, confirmation of positive test results is recommended because of the low prevalence of infection in healthy cats and the higher possibility that false-positive test results may occur. Positive test results in the absence of FeLV antigen have the potential to occur rarely as a result of operator error or nonspecific reactivity.[82] As for FIV infection, it is especially important to immediately confirm positive test results if they are likely to result in euthanasia or rehoming for disease control purposes. There are several options to confirm a positive test result:

- Perform another ELISA antigen test using an assay from a different manufacturer. However, it should be remembered that in contrast to FIV infection, cats that test truly positive for FeLV antigen early in the course of infection (i.e., before involvement of the bone marrow) may ultimately control the infection. Thus a single positive test result does not imply progressive infection, even if it is immediately repeatable using a test from a different manufacturer. If the cat has signs consistent with FeLV-related disease, a single positive test result is more likely to mean that progressive infection is present.
- Perform an IFA assay on peripheral blood smears, because cats with positive IFA results have infection of the bone marrow and, with rare exceptions, are almost always progressively infected. Cats that test negative with IFA assays may be in a transient viremic phase that may result in either progressive or regressive infection, or they may have progressive infection but the sensitivity of IFA is too low to detect it. In this case, both ELISA and IFA assays, or the ELISA assay alone, could be repeated in 1 to 4 months.
- Retest with ELISA 6 months later. If the antigen test remains positive, progressive infection is likely. In some cats, antigenemia persists for 16 weeks before regression occurs, so the test could be repeated earlier than 6 months (e.g., 12 weeks later) or monthly if client finances permit so long as the cat remains healthy.
- Perform a full CBC. If hematologic abnormalities are present, progressive infection is likely.

Negative ELISA results can occur in the first month after exposure to FeLV, before sufficient antigen is detectable in the peripheral blood. Cats that test negative within 30 days of possible exposure to the virus should be retested 1 to 2 months later. Because development of antibodies to FIV can take up to 2 months, it is usually most practical to retest for both viral infections 2 months after possible exposure. Kittens can be tested at any time, because maternal antibody does not interfere with FeLV testing.

Immunofluorescent Antibody or Immunoperoxidase Staining

IFA assays are widely offered by veterinary diagnostic laboratories and can be performed on fresh peripheral blood or bone marrow. At least two fresh smears (without anticoagulant) should be air-dried and mailed to the laboratory. IFA is less sensitive than ELISA and, depending on the laboratory, is more prone to false-negative and false-positive results and so is not recommended for screening purposes. The presence of detectable virus using IFA in circulating blood cells indicates progressive infection more than 90% of the time. Cats with early viremia (before the bone marrow is infected) test IFA-negative but ELISA-positive. Cats with regressive infection test negative with both IFA and ELISA assays (see Figure 22-2). Negative IFA test results can occur in cats with progressive infection when there are inadequate blood cells in the periphery, such as in neutropenic cats. Performing IFA on bone marrow rather than peripheral blood may help to overcome this problem. False-positive results can occur when inexperienced laboratory personnel interpret nonspecific fluorescence as a positive test result. They also have the potential to occur when the antibody conjugates bind nonspecifically to eosinophil granules, so eosinophils must be excluded in interpretation of fluorescing cells.[83]

Some cats with clinical abnormalities that strongly suggest FeLV-related disease (such as leukemia or myelodysplasia) test negative for circulating antigen using ELISA but have bone marrow cells that test positive for FeLV antigen using IFA. For example, at the author's teaching hospital, 8 of 18 cats with leukemia or MDS that tested negative for soluble FeLV antigen had bone marrow smears that were positive using IFA; the remainder tested IFA negative. This phenomenon may reflect either false-positive IFA assay results, or true infection with undetectable levels of antigen in the peripheral blood. The use of PCR on bone marrow may help to resolve the FeLV status in at least some of these cats.

Immunohistochemistry can also be used to detect viral antigen in tissue specimens or bone marrow core biopsies, although it may be less sensitive than IFA.

Molecular Diagnosis Using the Polymerase Chain Reaction

Several different PCR assays have been developed for detection of FeLV nucleic acid. Currently the major clinical indications for PCR are (1) to screen potential blood donors in conjunction with antigen testing or (2) to test for regressive infection when FeLV is strongly suspected as the cause of neoplasia but antigen tests are negative.

PCR assays may detect FeLV RNA (reverse transcriptase–polymerase chain reaction [RT-PCR]) or proviral DNA and must be carefully designed so that they do not detect endogenous FeLV sequences. At the current time, PCR assays should *never* be used in the absence of antigen testing in order to screen for or diagnose FeLV infection. The clinician needs to understand if the assay used detects proviral DNA, viral RNA, or both (some laboratories run both assays), because the clinical significance of a positive viral RNA assay (i.e., productive viral infection) differs from that of a positive proviral DNA assay (which suggests nonproductive viral infection for cats with negative antigen tests). After infection, RT-PCR assays may be positive several weeks before antigen tests or virus isolation become positive,[84] and depending on the assay, PCR for viral RNA can be more sensitive than soluble antigen tests. High viral RNA loads in blood and saliva appear to be associated with progressive infection, whereas low loads may be associated with regressive infection (Figure 22-7).[84]

PCR assays for proviral DNA can be used on blood, buffy coats, bone marrow, or tissues of cats that test negative for FeLV antigen. Cats with a positive proviral PCR test result but negative soluble antigen test, which in one study represented about 10% of cats with negative antigen test results, have regressive infection.[85,86] These cats are probably not infectious to other cats but may reactivate virus shedding with severe stress or immunosuppression, or transmit the virus through blood transfusion or vertical transmission. Proviral DNA appears to be present at much lower levels in cats with regressive infection than in those with progressive infection.[86,87] The cell types that contain FeLV proviral DNA also may differ for antigen-negative and antigen-positive cats. The proviral DNA of one FeLV strain was

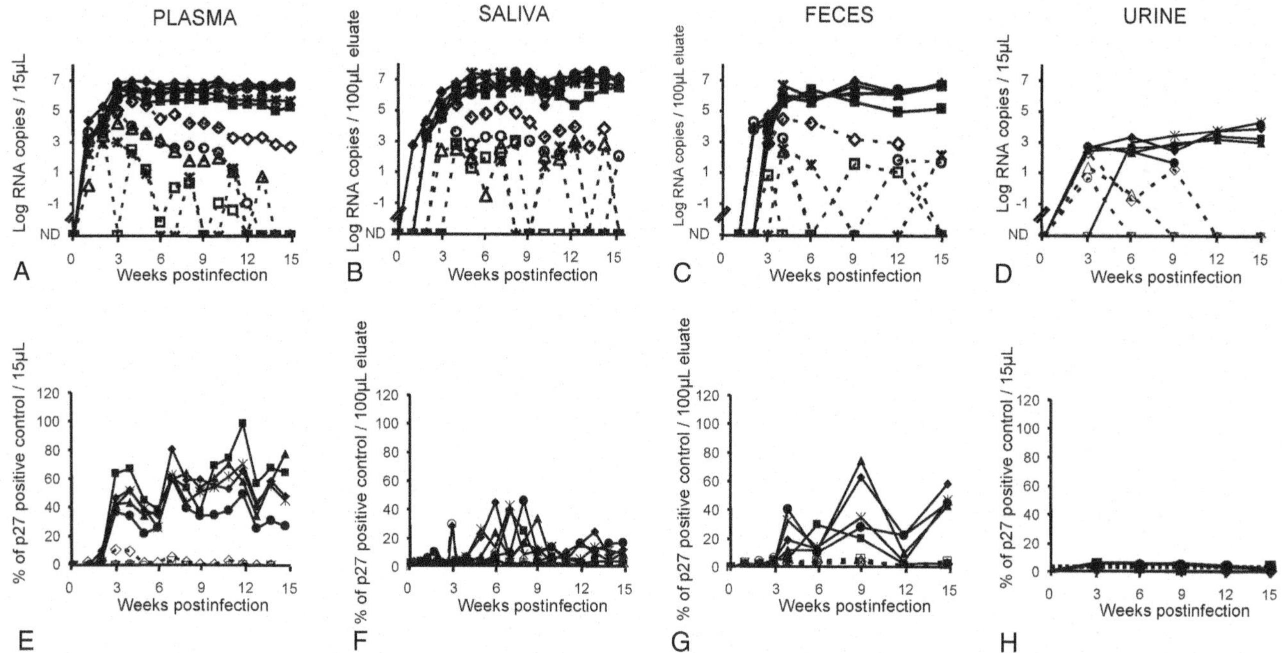

FIGURE 22-7 Viral RNA (**A-D**) and p27 antigen (**E-H**) loads in plasma (**A** and **E**), saliva (**B** and **F**), feces (**C** and **G**), and urine (**D** and **H**) in 10 cats experimentally infected with FeLV. Each line represents observations for a single cat. Continuous lines represent data from cats with progressive infection, and broken lines represent data from cats with regressive infection. (Modified from Cattori V, Randon R, Riond B, et al. The kinetics of feline leukemia virus shedding in experimentally infected cats are associated with outcome. Vet Microbiol 2009;133(3):292-296, Figure 1.)

found only in the lymphocytes of antigen-negative cats, whereas antigen-positive cats had high loads within all leukocyte types, including lymphocytes, monocytes, and granulocytes.[86,87] The use of bone marrow or tissue specimens, rather than whole blood, may increase sensitivity for detection of proviral DNA.

The sensitivity and specificity of commercially available PCR assays are likely to vary with assay design, and the usefulness of assays offered commercially has not been published, so until more information is available, great caution is warranted when interpreting the results of PCR assays for FeLV infection. Retroviruses have high rates of mutation, and the presence of sequence variations may lead to false-negative results. False-positive results occur in some PCR laboratories as a result of contamination or manual loading errors, or poor assay design. Because FeLV vaccine virus is inactivated or recombinant, it does not replicate or integrate into the host genome, so vaccination should not lead to false-positive PCR results.

Virus Isolation

FeLV can be readily isolated in cell culture. The cell culture supernatant can then be tested for production of FeLV using antigen assays or viral RNA PCR. Because growth requires several days and specialized techniques, cell culture is not routinely used for clinical diagnosis.

Antibody Assays

Although not useful for diagnosis of FeLV infection, detection of antibody responses to FeLV infection is performed on a clinical research basis with virus neutralization assays and IFA assays that detect antibodies against feline oncornavirus cell membrane–associated antigen (FOCMA).[24,48,84,88,89] Positive antibody test results in cats that test negative for FeLV antigen indicate previous exposure followed by abortive or regressive infection. Cats with progressive infections and high viral loads usually fail to develop antibody responses.[24,48,88] Antibody responses may occur after vaccination with FeLV vaccines.

Pathologic Findings

Gross and histopathologic findings in cats with FeLV infection usually reflect secondary disease processes. Lymphoma and evidence of myelodysplasia or leukemias are the most common findings, but opportunistic infections may also be detected. The intestinal tracts of cats with FeLV-associated enteritis reveal crypt cell necrosis and regeneration, lymphoplasmacytic infiltrates, and blunting and fusion of villi (See Figure 22-5).[90] Reactive lymphoid hyperplasia is also a common finding. CNS lesions include loss of axons and dilated myelin sheaths within the spinal cord.[74] Immunohistochemical stains may be applied to tissue sections to confirm the presence of FeLV antigen in association with lesions.

Treatment and Prognosis

Cats with opportunistic infections and lymphoma can be successfully treated using the same medications and supportive treatments used for FeLV negative cats with these problems. Opportunistic infections may require longer periods of treatment or, in some cases, lifelong treatment with antimicrobial drugs. Hemoplasma infections should be treated with doxycycline (see Chapter 41). Cats with nonregenerative anemias may require periodic blood transfusions. Serum erythropoietin concentrations are already high in these cats, and in many cases, treatment with darbepoetin or human recombinant erythropoietin is unsuccessful but could be attempted. The efficacy of treatments such as filgrastim is not known and may be complicated by the formation of antibodies (see Chapter 7). The management of cats with stomatitis is discussed in Chapter 21. In general, glucocorticoids and other immunosuppressive drugs

TABLE 22-3

Suggested Medications for Treatment of Cats with Feline Leukemia Virus Infection

Drug	Dose	Route	Interval (hours)	Comments
Zidovudine (AZT)	5 mg/kg	PO	12	Monitor CBC weekly during treatment for the first month, then monthly.
Feline recombinant interferon omega	1 million U/kg	SC	q24h for 5 consecutive days starting on days 0, 14, and 60	
Human recombinant interferon alpha	1 to 50 U/cat	PO	24	

should be avoided unless immune-mediated cytopenias are suspected. Some cats with FeLV-associated IMHA respond well to treatment with glucocorticoids, and glucocorticoid treatment may be unavoidable.

Antiviral agents and immunomodulators are of limited benefit for treatment of cats with FeLV infections (see Chapter 7 for more information) (Table 22-3). The use of feline recombinant IFN-ω improved clinical scores and survival times in cats with FeLV infection over a short time period (2 months) in one study.[91] Beneficial outcomes have also been described after treatment with low-dose oral human recombinant IFN-α. Zidovudine (AZT) has not performed as well for treatment of sick cats with FeLV infections as it has for those with FIV infections, and the results of some studies have shown minimal benefit. In other studies, AZT improved oral cavity inflammation, reduced antigenemia, and prolonged life span in naturally and experimentally infected cats with FeLV infection.[92,93] Controlled studies of the efficacy of other treatments, such as lymphocyte T-cell immunomodulator (T-cyte Therapeutics, Inc.) and acemannan, are required. Antivirals that show promise for treatment of FeLV infection include fozivudine (which is closely related to AZT) and the integrase inhibitor raltegravir, which has been used to treat gammaretrovirus infections in humans and inhibits FeLV replication in cell culture.[94] The safety of these drugs in cats remains to be determined.

Cats infected with FeLV should be housed indoors to prevent spread of infection to other cats. Indoor housing also minimizes exposure of infected cats to other opportunistic pathogens. Raw food diets should not be fed. Survival may be prolonged in low-stress environments, so provision of space, adequate litter boxes, management of co-infections, and a proper diet are important. Vaccines administered for prevention of respiratory viruses and FPV should be inactivated. Some FeLV-infected cats may not respond as well to vaccination as noninfected cats.

Prognosis

Survival times vary considerably depending on the stage of infection, host immunity, and the strain of FeLV involved. Nevertheless, virtually all cats that are progressively infected with FeLV go on to develop FeLV-related disease within 5 years of diagnosis.[95] A comparison of more than 800 FeLV-infected cats and 8000 controls revealed a median survival time of 2.4 years for FeLV-infected cats versus 6.3 years for controls.[79] Many progressively infected cats, especially adult cats, may live for several years with a good quality of life, and so euthanasia is not recommended on the basis of a positive FeLV test alone. Some cats with FeLV-associated lymphoma may have long-term remissions when treated with standard chemotherapy protocols. Some, but not all, studies suggest that FeLV infection is a negative prognostic indicator in cats with lymphoma.[96] One of the authors has treated a cat that initially tested positive for FeLV antigen using ELISA and had evidence of IFA-positive, severe megaloblastic erythroid dysplasia in the marrow and IMHA, yet subsequently became ELISA-negative and remained in clinical remission while being treated with glucocorticoids more than 4 years later.[97] The prognosis is least favorable for cats with leukemia, which generally survive less than a few weeks.

Immunity and Vaccination

Several parenteral vaccines are available for prevention of FeLV infection, which include adjuvanted inactivated whole virus vaccines; nonadjuvanted canarypox vectored virus vaccines that incorporate the *env* and *gag* genes of FeLV (Purevax and Eurifel, Merial); and a recombinant subunit vaccine that contains p45, the nonglycosylated form of gp70 (Leucogen, Virbac). The recombinant canarypox vaccine available in Europe is a different product than that licensed for use in the United States. Studies that have used highly sensitive PCR assays have shown that vaccination does not produce sterilizing immunity (that is, complete absence of viral RNA, DNA, antigenemia, and viremia after challenge).[98] In other words, cats develop regressive or even progressive infections, but not abortive infections after challenge.[98] Nevertheless, vaccination with recombinant subunit, canarypox vectored, and whole virus vaccine prevented progressive infection in 87%, 78%, and 44% of cats when compared with controls, respectively. One vaccine protected 83% of cats against antigenemia after challenge as long as 2 years after vaccination.[99]

In summary, no vaccine provides 100% protection against FeLV infection, and even when protection against progressive infection occurs, regressive infections still occur. However, because vaccination protects cats from progressive infection, it is indicated for all at-risk cats, such as those with outdoor exposure or those that reside in households with other FeLV antigen-positive cats. The American Association of Feline Practitioners (AAFP) highly recommends that all FeLV antigen-negative kittens be vaccinated for FeLV, because of the potential that some of these kittens may escape or become outdoor cats, even when the intention of the owner is to keep the kitten indoors.[100] Vaccination is also recommended for cats entering shelters that are likely to be housed with other cats.[79] Two doses are given in the left pelvic limb as distally as possible, 3 to 4 weeks apart from 8 to 9 weeks of age, followed by a booster at 1 year and then every 1 to 3 years thereafter, although more information is required on the duration of immunity for FeLV vaccines. The European Advisory Bureau on Cat Diseases (ABCD) suggests a booster every 2 to 3 years for cats older than 3 to 4 years of age, in light of the lower susceptibility of adult cats to infection.[101] Annual boosters are required for recombinant vaccines. Acutely ill cats should not be vaccinated, but it is acceptable to vaccinate cats with chronic diseases, such as chronic kidney disease. Testing for FeLV should be performed before each booster if exposure to FeLV was likely before the booster was required (which should apply for most cats vaccinated for FeLV). Vaccination with FeLV vaccines has been associated with injection-site sarcomas, so only cats that are likely to be exposed should be vaccinated.

Prevention

Prevention of FeLV infection involves indoor housing of cats away from other cats infected with FeLV, testing and removal (or separation) of cats that test antigen-positive from other cats, vaccination, and proper screening of blood donor cats with soluble antigen assays *and* PCR. Routine hand-washing precautions are indicated for hospitalized cats, and precautions should be taken (such as the wearing of gloves) to protect FeLV-infected cats from nosocomial pathogens. Fomites such as food and water bowls and litter boxes should not be shared between FeLV antigen-negative cats and cats with unknown or antigen-positive FeLV status. Neutering can prevent roaming and reduce the likelihood of FeLV infection. When a cat from a multicat household tests antigen-positive, all cats should be tested and retested and positive cats should be separated from other cats if possible. Euthanasia is recommended for sick, FeLV-positive cats that enter shelters.[101] People who adopt cats that have unknown retrovirus status from shelters should be educated about the disease and the need for quarantine and testing after adoption.

Public Health Aspects

Although FeLV can replicate in human cell culture lines, no conclusive evidence of natural infection with FeLV has ever been detected in humans.

CASE EXAMPLE

Signalment: "Hamster" a 6-year-old female spayed domestic shorthair from Fairfield, CA.

History: Hamster was brought to the University of California, Davis, Veterinary Medical Teaching Hospital for the problems of fever, lethargy, anorexia, diarrhea, and vomiting. The diarrhea had been present for 3 days and was greenish, mucoid, and occurred once to twice daily. The owner reported that Hamster had vomited yellow fluid at least three times during this period and was completely inappetent. Her urination habits had not changed. Hamster was taken to a local veterinary clinic on the first day of illness, where a physical examination revealed pyrexia (105.1°F or 40.6°C). She was treated with clavulanic acid–amoxicillin and a single intramuscular injection of enrofloxacin but there was no clinical improvement. Hamster had tested positive for FeLV antigen 1.5 years ago, after which time she had been housed exclusively indoors. She lived with some caged birds and three other FeLV-positive cats. None of the other cats were ill. Hamster played with elastic bands, but there was no known toxin exposure and no recent changes in her environment. Her diet usually consisted of a commercial dry cat food.

Physical Examination:

Body Weight: 6.9 kg

General: Quiet, alert, responsive, hydrated, T = 104.4°F (40.2°C), HR = 220 beats/min, RR = 36 breaths/min, mucous membranes pink, CRT = 1 s. Haircoat unkempt.

Eyes, Ears, Nose, and Throat (with Dilated Fundoscopic Examination): The only abnormality noted was mild gingivitis.

Musculoskeletal: Body condition score 7/9. Normal ambulation was present.

Cardiovascular and Respiratory: No clinically significant abnormalities were detected.

Gastrointestinal and Urogenital: The cat resented palpation of her cranial abdomen. The perianal region was stained with green fecal material.

Lymph Nodes: All lymph nodes were <1 cm in diameter.

Laboratory Findings:

CBC:

HCT 24.6% (30%-50%).
MCV 48.4 fL (42-53 fL), MCHC 32.1 g/dL (30-33.5 g/dL)
Reticulocytes 7800 cells/μL
WBC 11,470 cells/μL (4500-14,000 cells/μL)
Neutrophils 10,438 cells/μL (2000-9000 cells/μL)
Band neutrophils 459 cells/μL
Lymphocytes 344 cells/μL (1000-7000 cells/μL)
Monocytes 229 cells/μL (50-600 cells/μL)
Platelets 122,000 platelets/μL (180,000-500,000 platelets/μL). The neutrophils showed slight toxicity, and there were a few macroplatelets

Serum Chemistry Profile:

Sodium 148 mmol/L (151-158 mmol/L)
Potassium 3.8 mmol/L (3.6-4.9 mmol/L)
Chloride 110 mmol/L (117-126 mmol/L)
Bicarbonate 18 mmol/L (15-21 mmol/L)
Phosphorus 2.9 mg/dL (3.2-6.3 mg/dL)
Calcium 9.5 mg/dL (9.0-10.9 mg/dL)
BUN 15 mg/dL (18-33 mg/dL)
Creatinine 1.2 mg/dL (1.1-2.2 mg/dL)
Glucose 169 mg/dL (63-118 mg/dL)
Total protein 7.0 g/dL (6.6-8.4 g/dL)
Albumin 2.6 g/dL (2.2-4.6 g/dL)
Globulin 4.4 g/dL (2.8-5.4 g/dL)
ALT 72 U/L (27-101 U/L), AST 121 U/L (17-58 U/L)
ALP 12 U/L (14-71 U/L), γ- GGT 0 U/L (0-4 U/L)
Cholesterol 104 mg/dL (89-258 mg/dL)
Total bilirubin 0.2 mg/dL (0-0.2 mg/dL).

Urinalysis (Cystocentesis): SGr 1.020; pH 7.0, 1+ protein, 2+ hemoprotein, 0-1 WBC/HPF, 0-2 RBC/HPF, rare rods, few amorphous crystals.

Imaging Findings:

Plain Abdominal Radiographs: The small bowel was diffusely gas- and fluid-filled with normal intestinal diameter. The colon was relatively empty with a small amount of fluid. No masses were identified. There was renal asymmetry with poor visualization of the right kidney. Abdominal serosal detail appeared normal.

Abdominal Sonography: The right kidney could not be identified. The left kidney appeared normal and measured 4.2 cm in length. A small amount of fluid was present in the colon. The remainder of the abdomen was unremarkable.

Microbiologic and Virologic Testing: Aerobic bacterial urine culture: negative

Point-of-care ELISA serology for FeLV antigen and FIV antibody: positive for FeLV antigen

PCR for *Mycoplasma haemofelis* and *Candidatus* Mycoplasma haemominutum (whole blood): negative

Diagnosis: Progressive FeLV infection with suspected acute pyelonephritis (characterized by fever, gastrointestinal signs, bacteriuria, neutrophilia with a left shift, and mild thrombocytopenia). Right renal agenesis (likely congenital).

Treatment: Hamster was hospitalized and treated with intravenous fluids, enrofloxacin (5 mg/kg, slow IV, q24h) and ampicillin (20 mg/kg, IV, q8h) (note that the parenteral use of enrofloxacin in this cat was off-label and has the potential to cause irreversible blindness). Her temperature normalized within 24 hours, and there was no more vomiting or diarrhea. After 48 hours, the hematocrit was 27.6%, neutrophil count was 5759 cells/μL with no bands or toxicity, and lymphocyte count was 917 cells/μL. She was discharged from the hospital with instructions to continue antibiotic treatment for 1 month. Two weeks after the antibiotics had been discontinued, she was apparently healthy and a physical examination, CBC, kidney panel, urinalysis, and aerobic bacterial urine culture showed no abnormalities. Her hematocrit was 38.9%, white cell count was 4620 cells/μL, and platelet count was 220,000/μL. One year later, she remained clinically healthy and a CBC showed a hematocrit of 38.2%, white cell count of 4500 cells/μL, neutrophil count of 3362 cells/μL, lymphocyte count of 905 cells/μL, and a monocyte count of 45 cells/μL. Despite the mild cytopenias present, Hamster remained alive and well with a normal CBC 4 years after she was initially seen for gastrointestinal signs. She died 2 years after that, 7.5 years after she first tested positive for FeLV infection.

One of the other cats in the household, a 5-year-old, male neutered domestic medium hair cat, was euthanized 1.5 years after Hamster was initially evaluated. He developed severe normocytic, normochromic nonregenerative anemia (HCT 10.5%, with 5200 reticulocytes and 11 nucleated RBC/HPF) with neutropenia (1320 cells/μL) in association with circulating blast cells.

Comments: Even though this cat was initially seen for moderately severe illness in association with progressive FeLV infection, she made a full recovery with treatment and remained alive and well for 6 additional years. The nonregenerative anemia likely resulted from inflammatory disease. The negative urine culture may have resulted from recent treatment with antimicrobial drugs, and renal ultrasound is insensitive for diagnosis of pyelonephritis. The age of this cat, the strain of FeLV involved, and the challenge dose, as well as other environmental and genetic factors, probably all played a role in the course of disease. This case clearly demonstrates that other treatable diseases may be present in FeLV-infected cats and that search for the underlying cause of clinical signs and adequate treatment is always recommended. The second cat in the household likely also had progressive FeLV infection; the development of anemia suggested infection with FeLV-C.

SUGGESTED READINGS

Hartmann K. Clinical aspects of feline immunodeficiency and feline leukemia virus infection. Vet Immunol Immunopathol. 2011;143:190-201.

Levy J, Crawford C, Hartmann K, et al. 2008 American Association of Feline Practitioners' feline retrovirus management guidelines. J Feline Med Surg. 2008;10:300-316.

Lutz H, Addie D, Belak S, et al. Feline leukaemia. ABCD guidelines on prevention and management. J Feline Med Surg. 2009;11:565-574.

REFERENCES

1. Jarrett WFH, Crawford EM, Martin WB, et al. A virus-like particle associated with leukemia (lymphosarcoma). Nature. 1964;202:567-569.
2. Meli ML, Cattori V, Martinez F, et al. Feline leukemia virus and other pathogens as important threats to the survival of the critically endangered Iberian lynx (Lynx pardinus). PLoS One. 2009;4:e4744.
3. Stewart MA, Warnock M, Wheeler A, et al. Nucleotide sequences of a feline leukemia virus subgroup A envelope gene and long terminal repeat and evidence for the recombinational origin of subgroup B viruses. J Virol. 1986;58:825-834.
4. Lauring AS, Anderson MM, Overbaugh J. Specificity in receptor usage by T-cell-tropic feline leukemia viruses: implications for the in vivo tropism of immunodeficiency-inducing variants. J Virol. 2001;75:8888-8898.
5. Brojatsch J, Kristal BS, Viglianti GA, et al. Feline leukemia virus subgroup C phenotype evolves through distinct alterations near the N terminus of the envelope surface glycoprotein. Proc Natl Acad Sci U S A. 1992;89:8457-8461.
6. Chandhasin C, Coan PN, Levy LS. Subtle mutational changes in the SU protein of a natural feline leukemia virus subgroup A isolate alter disease spectrum. J Virol. 2005;79:1351-1360.
7. Chandhasin C, Coan PN, Pandrea I, et al. Unique long terminal repeat and surface glycoprotein gene sequences of feline leukemia virus as determinants of disease outcome. J Virol. 2005;79:5278-5287.
8. Vobis M, D'Haese J, Mehlhorn H, et al. Evidence of horizontal transmission of feline leukemia virus by the cat flea (*Ctenocephalides felis*). Parasitol Res. 2003;91:467-470.
9. Gomes-Keller MA, Gonczi E, Grenacher B, et al. Fecal shedding of infectious feline leukemia virus and its nucleic acids: a transmission potential. Vet Microbiol. 2009;134:208-217.
10. Pacitti AM, Jarrett O, Hay D. Transmission of feline leukaemia virus in the milk of a non-viraemic cat. Vet Rec. 1986;118:381-384.

11. Tenorio AP, Franti CE, Madewell BR, et al. Chronic oral infections of cats and their relationship to persistent oral carriage of feline calici-, immunodeficiency, or leukemia viruses. Vet Immunol Immunopathol. 1991;29:1-14.
12. O'Connor Jr TP, Tonelli QJ, Scarlett JM. Report of the National FeLV/FIV Awareness Project. J Am Vet Med Assoc. 1991;199:1348-1353.
13. Levy JK, Scott HM, Lachtara JL, et al. Seroprevalence of feline leukemia virus and feline immunodeficiency virus infection among cats in North America and risk factors for seropositivity. J Am Vet Med Assoc. 2006;228:371-376.
14. Stutzer B, Simon K, Lutz H, et al. Incidence of persistent viraemia and latent feline leukaemia virus infection in cats with lymphoma. J Feline Med Surg. 2011;13:81-87.
15. Gleich SE, Krieger S, Hartmann K. Prevalence of feline immunodeficiency virus and feline leukaemia virus among client-owned cats and risk factors for infection in Germany. J Feline Med Surg. 2009;11:985-992.
16. Ravi M, Wobeser GA, Taylor SM, et al. Naturally acquired feline immunodeficiency virus (FIV) infection in cats from western Canada: Prevalence, disease associations, and survival analysis. Can Vet J. 2010;51:271-276.
17. Little S, Sears W, Lachtara J, et al. Seroprevalence of feline leukemia virus and feline immunodeficiency virus infection among cats in Canada. Can Vet J. 2009;50:644-648.
18. Hellard E, Fouchet D, Santin-Janin H, et al. When cats' ways of life interact with their viruses: a study in 15 natural populations of owned and unowned cats (*Felis silvestris catus*). Prev Vet Med. 2011;101:250-264.
19. Al-Kappany YM, Lappin MR, Kwok OC, et al. Seroprevalence of *Toxoplasma gondii* and concurrent *Bartonella* spp., feline immunodeficiency virus, feline leukemia virus, and *Dirofilaria immitis* infections in Egyptian cats. J Parasitol. 2011;97: 256-258.
20. Hosie MJ, Robertson C, Jarrett O. Prevalence of feline leukaemia virus and antibodies to feline immunodeficiency virus in cats in the United Kingdom. Vet Rec. 1989;125:293-297.
21. Grant CK, Essex M, Gardner MB, et al. Natural feline leukemia virus infection and the immune response of cats of different ages. Cancer Res. 1980;40:823-829.
22. Hofmann-Lehmann R, Tandon R, Boretti FS, et al. Reassessment of feline leukaemia virus (FeLV) vaccines with novel sensitive molecular assays. Vaccine. 2006;24:1087-1094.
23. Kadar E, Sykes JE, Kass PH, et al. Evaluation of the prevalence of infections in cats after renal transplantation: 169 cases (1987-2003). J Am Vet Med Assoc. 2005;227:948-953.
24. Major A, Cattori V, Boenzli E, et al. Exposure of cats to low doses of FeLV: seroconversion as the sole parameter of infection. Vet Res. 2010;41:17.
25. Good RA, Ogasawara M, Liu WT, et al. Immunosuppressive actions of retroviruses. Lymphology. 1990;23:56-59.
26. Cianciolo GJ, Copeland TD, Oroszlan S, et al. Inhibition of lymphocyte proliferation by a synthetic peptide homologous to retroviral envelope proteins. Science. 1985;230:453-455.
27. Mitani M, Cianciolo GJ, Snyderman R, et al. Suppressive effect on polyclonal B-cell activation of a synthetic peptide homologous to a transmembrane component of oncogenic retroviruses. Proc Natl Acad Sci U S A. 1987;84:237-240.
28. Haraguchi S, Good RA, Day-Good NK. A potent immunosuppressive retroviral peptide: cytokine patterns and signaling pathways. Immunol Res. 2008;41:46-55.
29. Cockerell GL, Hoover EA, Krakowka S, et al. Lymphocyte mitogen reactivity and enumeration of circulating B- and T-cells during feline leukemia virus infection in the cat. J Natl Cancer Inst. 1976;57:1095-1099.
30. Hebebrand LC, Mathes LE, Olsen RG. Inhibition of concanavalin A stimulation of feline lymphocytes by inactivated feline leukemia virus. Cancer Res. 1977;37:4532-4533.
31. Mathes LE, Olsen RG, Hebebrand LC, et al. Abrogation of lymphocyte blastogenesis by a feline leukaemia virus protein. Nature. 1978;274:687-689.
32. Perryman LE, Hoover EA, Yohn DS. Immunologic reactivity of the cat: immunosuppression in experimental feline leukemia. J Natl Cancer Inst. 1972;49:1357-1365.
33. Trainin Z, Wernicke D, Ungar-Waron H, et al. Suppression of the humoral antibody response in natural retrovirus infections. Science. 1983;220:858-859.
34. Wernicke D, Trainin Z, Ungar-Waron H, et al. Humoral immune response of asymptomatic cats naturally infected with feline leukemia virus. J Virol. 1986;60:669-673.
35. Lafrado LJ, Olsen RG. Demonstration of depressed polymorphonuclear leukocyte function in nonviremic FeLV-infected cats. Cancer Invest. 1986;4:297-300.
36. Hoffmann-Jagielska M, Winnicka A, Jagielski D, et al. Influence of naturally acquired feline leukemia virus (FeLV) infection on the phagocytic and respiratory burst activity of neutrophils and monocytes of peripheral blood. Pol J Vet Sci. 2005;8:93-97.
37. Wardini AB, Guimaraes-Costa AB, Nascimento MT, et al. Characterization of neutrophil extracellular traps in cats naturally infected with feline leukemia virus. J Gen Virol. 2010;91:259-264.
38. Buchmann AU, Kershaw O, Kempf VA, et al. Does a feline leukemia virus infection pave the way for *Bartonella henselae* infection in cats?. J Clin Microbiol. 2010;48:3295-3300.
39. Fujino Y, Ohno K, Tsujimoto H. Molecular pathogenesis of feline leukemia virus-induced malignancies: insertional mutagenesis. Vet Immunol Immunopathol. 2008;123:138-143.
40. Shelton GH, Grant CK, Cotter SM, et al. Feline immunodeficiency virus and feline leukemia virus infections and their relationships to lymphoid malignancies in cats: a retrospective study (1968-1988). J Acquir Immune Defic Syndr. 1990;3:623-630.
41. Reinacher M. Diseases associated with spontaneous feline leukemia virus (FeLV) infection in cats. Vet Immunol Immunopathol. 1989;21:85-95.
42. Louwerens M, London CA, Pedersen NC, et al. Feline lymphoma in the post-feline leukemia virus era. J Vet Intern Med. 2005;19:329-335.
43. Teske E, van Straten G, van Noort R, et al. Chemotherapy with cyclophosphamide, vincristine, and prednisolone (COP) in cats with malignant lymphoma: new results with an old protocol. J Vet Intern Med. 2002;16:179-186.
44. Taylor SS, Goodfellow MR, Browne WJ, et al. Feline extranodal lymphoma: response to chemotherapy and survival in 110 cats. J Small Anim Pract. 2009;50:584-592.
45. Krick EL, Little L, Patel R, et al. Description of clinical and pathological findings, treatment and outcome of feline large granular lymphocyte lymphoma (1996-2004). Vet Comp Oncol. 2008;6:102-110.
46. Francis DP, Essex M, Cotter SM, et al. Epidemiologic association between virus-negative feline leukemia and the horizontally transmitted feline leukemia virus. Cancer Lett. 1981;12:37-42.
47. Wang J, Kyaw-Tanner M, Lee C, et al. Characterisation of lymphosarcomas in Australian cats using polymerase chain reaction and immunohistochemical examination. Aust Vet J. 2001;79:41-46.
48. Beatty JA, Tasker S, Jarrett O, et al. Markers of feline leukaemia virus infection or exposure in cats from a region of low seroprevalence. J Feline Med Surg. 2011;13:927-933.
49. Jackson ML, Haines DM, Meric SM, et al. Feline leukemia virus detection by immunohistochemistry and polymerase chain reaction in formalin-fixed, paraffin-embedded tumor tissue from cats with lymphosarcoma. Can J Vet Res. 1993;57:269-276.
50. Gabor LJ, Jackson ML, Trask B, et al. Feline leukaemia virus status of Australian cats with lymphosarcoma. Aust Vet J. 2001;79:476-481.
51. Gelain ME, Antoniazzi E, Bertazzolo W, et al. Chronic eosinophilic leukemia in a cat: cytochemical and immunophenotypical features. Vet Clin Pathol. 2006;35:454-459.
52. Shimoda T, Shiranaga N, Mashita T, et al. Chronic myelomonocytic leukemia in a cat. J Vet Med Sci. 2000;62:195-197.

53. Besmer P, Lader E, George PC, et al. A new acute transforming feline retrovirus with fms homology specifies a C-terminally truncated version of the c-fms protein that is different from SM-feline sarcoma virus v-fms protein. J Virol. 1986;60:194-203.
54. Donner L, Fedele LA, Garon CF, et al. McDonough feline sarcoma virus: characterization of the molecularly cloned provirus and its feline oncogene (*v-fms*). J Virol. 1982;41:489-500.
55. Stiles J, Bienzle D, Render JA, et al. Use of nested polymerase chain reaction (PCR) for detection of retroviruses from formalin-fixed, paraffin-embedded uveal melanomas in cats. Vet Ophthalmol. 1999;2:113-116.
56. Cullen CL, Haines DM, Jackson ML, et al. The use of immunohistochemistry and the polymerase chain reaction for detection of feline leukemia virus and feline sarcoma virus in six cases of feline ocular sarcoma. Vet Ophthalmol. 1998;1:189-193.
57. Cullen CL, Haines DM, Jackson ML, et al. Lack of detection of feline leukemia and feline sarcoma viruses in diffuse iris melanomas of cats by immunohistochemistry and polymerase chain reaction. J Vet Diagn Invest. 2002;14:340-343.
58. Ellis JA, Jackson ML, Bartsch RC, et al. Use of immunohistochemistry and polymerase chain reaction for detection of oncornaviruses in formalin-fixed, paraffin-embedded fibrosarcomas from cats. J Am Vet Med Assoc. 1996;209:767-771.
59. Kidney BA, Ellis JA, Haines DM, et al. Comparison of endogenous feline leukemia virus RNA content in feline vaccine and nonvaccine site-associated sarcomas. Am J Vet Res. 2001;62:1990-1994.
60. Hartmann K. Clinical aspects of feline immunodeficiency and feline leukemia virus infection. Vet Immunol Immunopathol. 2011;143:190-201.
61. Shelton GH, Linenberger ML. Hematologic abnormalities associated with retroviral infections in the cat. Semin Vet Med Surg (Small Anim). 1995;10:220-233.
62. Quigley JG, Yang Z, Worthington MT, et al. Identification of a human heme exporter that is essential for erythropoiesis. Cell. 2004;118:757-766.
63. Hisasue M, Okayama H, Okayama T, et al. Hematologic abnormalities and outcome of 16 cats with myelodysplastic syndromes. J Vet Intern Med. 2001;15:471-477.
64. Weiss DJ. Evaluation of dysmyelopoiesis in cats: 34 cases (1996-2005). J Am Vet Med Assoc. 2006;228:893-897.
65. Stutzer B, Muller F, Majzoub M, et al. Role of latent feline leukemia virus infection in nonregenerative cytopenias of cats. J Vet Intern Med. 2010;24:192-197.
66. Anderson LJ, Jarrett WF. Membranous glomerulonephritis associated with leukaemia in cats. Res Vet Sci. 1971;12:179-180.
67. Brightman 2nd AH, Ogilvie GK, Tompkins M. Ocular disease in FeLV-positive cats: 11 cases (1981-1986). J Am Vet Med Assoc. 1991;198:1049-1051.
68. Pedersen NC, Pool RR, O'Brien T. Feline chronic progressive polyarthritis. Am J Vet Res. 1980;41:522-535.
69. Tuomari DL, Olsen RG, Singh VK, et al. Detection of circulating immune complexes by a Clq/protein A-ELISA during the preneoplastic stages of feline leukemia virus infection. Vet Immunol Immunopathol. 1984;7:227-238.
70. Day NK, O'Reilly-Felice C, Hardy Jr WD, et al. Circulating immune complexes associated with naturally occurring lymphosarcoma in pet cats. J Immunol. 1980;125:2363-2366.
71. Snyder Jr HW, Jones FR, Day NK, et al. Isolation and characterization of circulating feline leukemia virus-immune complexes from plasma of persistently infected pet cats removed by ex vivo immunosorption. J Immunol. 1982;128:2726-2730.
72. Fails AD, Mitchell TW, Rojko JL, et al. An oligopeptide of the feline leukemia virus envelope glycoprotein is associated with morphological changes and calcium dysregulation in neuronal growth cones. J Neurovirol. 1997;3:179-191.
73. Mitchell TW, Rojko JL, Hartke JR, et al. FeLV envelope protein (gp70) variable region 5 causes alterations in calcium homeostasis and toxicity of neurons. J Acquir Immune Defic Syndr Hum Retrovirol. 1997;14:307-320.
74. Carmichael KP, Bienzle D, McDonnell JJ. Feline leukemia virus-associated myelopathy in cats. Vet Pathol. 2002;39:536-545.
75. Kipar A, Kremendahl J, Jackson ML, et al. Comparative examination of cats with feline leukemia virus-associated enteritis and other relevant forms of feline enteritis. Vet Pathol. 2001;38:359-371.
76. Hardy Jr WD, Hess PW, MacEwen EG, et al. Biology of feline leukemia virus in the natural environment. Cancer Res. 1976;36:582-588.
77. Lutz H, Castelli I, Ehrensperger F, et al. Panleukopenia-like syndrome of FeLV caused by co-infection with FeLV and feline panleukopenia virus. Vet Immunol Immunopathol. 1995;46:21-33.
78. Kipar A, Kremendahl J, Addie DD, et al. Fatal enteritis associated with coronavirus infection in cats. J Comp Pathol. 1998;119:1-14.
79. Levy J, Crawford C, Hartmann K, et al. 2008 American Association of Feline Practitioners' feline retrovirus management guidelines. J Feline Med Surg. 2008;10:300-316.
80. Gleich S, Hartmann K. Hematology and serum biochemistry of feline immunodeficiency virus-infected and feline leukemia virus-infected cats. J Vet Intern Med. 2009;23:552-558.
81. Hartmann K, Griessmayr P, Schulz B, et al. Quality of different in-clinic test systems for feline immunodeficiency virus and feline leukaemia virus infection. J Feline Med Surg. 2007;9:439-445.
82. Barr MC, Pough MB, Jacobson RH, et al. Comparison and interpretation of diagnostic tests for feline immunodeficiency virus infection. J Am Vet Med Assoc. 1991;199:1377-1381.
83. Floyd K, Suter PF, Lutz H. Granules of blood eosinophils are stained directly by anti-immunoglobulin fluorescein isothiocyanate conjugates. Am J Vet Res. 1983;44:2060-2063.
84. Cattori V, Tandon R, Riond B, et al. The kinetics of feline leukaemia virus shedding in experimentally infected cats are associated with infection outcome. Vet Microbiol. 2009;133:292-296.
85. Gomes-Keller MA, Gonczi E, Tandon R, et al. Detection of feline leukemia virus RNA in saliva from naturally infected cats and correlation of PCR results with those of current diagnostic methods. J Clin Microbiol. 2006;44:916-922.
86. Hofmann-Lehmann R, Huder JB, Gruber S, et al. Feline leukaemia provirus load during the course of experimental infection and in naturally infected cats. J Gen Virol. 2001;82:1589-1596.
87. Pepin AC, Tandon R, Cattori V, et al. Cellular segregation of feline leukemia provirus and viral RNA in leukocyte subsets of long-term experimentally infected cats. Virus Res. 2007;127:9-16.
88. Harbour DA, Gunn-Moore DA, Gruffydd-Jones TJ, et al. Protection against oronasal challenge with virulent feline leukaemia virus lasts for at least 12 months following a primary course of immunisation with Leukocell 2 vaccine. Vaccine. 2002;20:2866-2872.
89. Torres AN, O'Halloran KP, Larson LJ, et al. Feline leukemia virus immunity induced by whole inactivated virus vaccination. Vet Immunol Immunopathol. 2010;134:122-131.
90. Reinacher M. Feline leukemia virus-associated enteritis—a condition with features of feline panleukopenia. Vet Pathol. 1987;24:1-4.
91. de Mari K, Maynard L, Sanquer A, et al. Therapeutic effects of recombinant feline interferon-omega on feline leukemia virus (FeLV)-infected and FeLV/feline immunodeficiency virus (FIV)-coinfected symptomatic cats. J Vet Intern Med. 2004;18:477-482.
92. Hartmann K, Donath A, Beer B, et al. Use of two virustatics (AZT, PMEA) in the treatment of FIV and of FeLV seropositive cats with clinical symptoms. Vet Immunol Immunopathol. 1992;35:167-175.
93. Nelson P, Sellon R, Novotney C, et al. Therapeutic effects of diethylcarbamazine and 3′-azido-3′-deoxythymidine on feline leukemia virus lymphoma formation. Vet Immunol Immunopathol. 1995;46:181-194.
94. Cattori V, Weibel B, Lutz H. Inhibition of feline leukemia virus replication by the integrase inhibitor raltegravir. Vet Microbiol. 2011;152:165-168.

95. Addie DD, Dennis JM, Toth S, et al. Long-term impact on a closed household of pet cats of natural infection with feline coronavirus, feline leukaemia virus and feline immunodeficiency virus. Vet Rec. 2000;146:419-424.
96. Vail DM, Moore AS, Ogilvie GK, et al. Feline lymphoma (145 cases): proliferation indices, cluster of differentiation 3 immunoreactivity, and their association with prognosis in 90 cats. J Vet Intern Med. 1998;12:349-354.
97. Sykes JE, et al, unpublished observations. 2012.
98. Hofmann-Lehmann R, Cattori V, Tandon R, et al. Vaccination against the feline leukaemia virus: outcome and response categories and long-term follow-up. Vaccine. 2007;25:5531-5539.
99. Jirjis F, Davis T, Lane J, et al. Protection against feline leukemia virus challenge for at least 2 years after vaccination with an inactivated feline leukemia virus vaccine. Vet Ther. 2010;11:E1-E6.
100. Richards JR, Elston TH, Ford RB, et al. The 2006 American Association of Feline Practitioners Feline Vaccine Advisory Panel report. J Am Vet Med Assoc. 2006;229:1405-1441.
101. Lutz H, Addie D, Belak S, et al. Feline leukaemia. ABCD guidelines on prevention and management. J Feline Med Surg. 2009;11:565-574.

CHAPTER 23

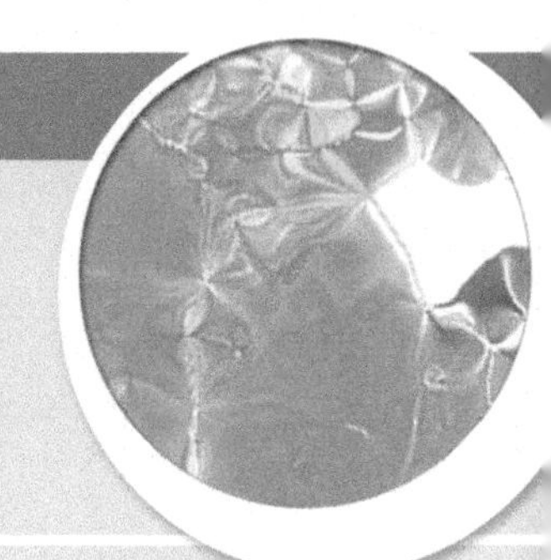

Feline Respiratory Viral Infections

Jane E. Sykes

Overview of Feline Viral Respiratory Disease

First Described in Cats: Feline herpesvirus-1 (FHV-1), 1958 (United States)[1]; feline calicivirus (FCV), 1957 (New Zealand)[2]; H5N1 influenza virus, 2006 (Thailand)[3]; pandemic H1N1 influenza virus, 2010 (United States).[4]

Causes: Feline herpesvirus-1, feline calicivirus, avian and human origin influenza A viruses

Geographic Distribution: Worldwide

Mode of Transmission: Close contact, fomite spread, to a lesser extent aerosols

Major Clinical Signs: Serous to mucopurulent nasal and ocular discharge, sneezing, stertor, conjunctivitis, lingual or facial ulceration, fever, inappetence, tachypnea, cough, rarely death. Keratitis occurs with FHV-1 infection.

Differential Diagnoses: Infections with bacteria such as *Bordetella bronchiseptica, Streptococcus* spp., or *Chlamydia felis;* other causes of rhinitis such as cryptococcosis, aspergillosis, neoplasia, foreign bodies, chronic idiopathic feline rhinosinusitis, nasopharyngeal stenosis, or nasopharyngeal polyps; feline chronic airway disease.

Human Health Significance: Influenza virus infections have been transmitted from humans to cats, and the potential for zoonotic transmission exists. FHV-1 and FCV do not infect humans.

Etiology and Epidemiology

Infectious feline upper respiratory tract disease (URTD) is a widespread and important cause of morbidity and mortality where large numbers of cats are housed together, especially in overcrowded or stressful conditions.[5] Multiple pathogens are involved and co-infections are common (Table 23-1). The most prevalent viral causes of URTD are feline herpesvirus-1 (FHV-1) and feline calicivirus (FCV). Influenza viruses also cause respiratory disease in cats but are relatively rarely identified. Bacterial causes of respiratory disease in cats include *Bordetella bronchiseptica*, *Chlamydia felis*, and *Mycoplasma* species. *Streptococcus canis* and *Streptococcus equi* subspecies *zooepidemicus* can also play a role in shelter situations and catteries. More information on the bacterial causes of feline URTD can be found in Chapters 33, 34, 38, and 40.

Feline Herpesvirus-1

FHV-1 is a large, enveloped DNA virus that has a worldwide distribution. Most cats are exposed to FHV-1 during their lifetime. FHV-1 is an alphaherpesvirus that is closely related to canine herpesvirus-1, and to a lesser extent, herpes simplex virus. There is only a single serotype of FHV-1. Isolates are also genetically similar, yet some variation in strain virulence exists.[6]

Using culture, FHV-1 has been detected in 0% to 39% of cats with URTD, although in some catteries and shelters with endemic FHV-1 infection, the prevalence may be much higher. When sensitive PCR assays are used to detect FHV-1, prevalences of infection that approach 100% have been detected in some groups of cats with acute URTD.[7] The prevalence of shedding by apparently healthy cats has ranged from 0% to 10% and most often has been lower than 2%.[5,8-14] Virtually all infected cats develop latent infection, which primarily occurs in the trigeminal ganglia. FHV-1 DNA can also be detected in other tissues of the head, such as the cornea and nasal cavity, but whether this is a true state of latency or just chronic persistent infection is not clear. Reactivation of shedding, with or without concurrent clinical signs of URTD, occurs in less than half of latently infected cats 4 to 12 days after stress.[15] Examples of stressors include transportation (such as to a veterinary clinic, boarding or breeding facility, shelter, or cat show), lactation, exposure to new cats, concurrent illness, or treatment with immunosuppressive drugs such as glucocorticoids. The duration of shedding after reactivation ranges from 1 to 13 days (mean, 7 days).[16,17] Shedding that coincides with lactation results in infection of susceptible kittens.

FHV-1 survives a maximum of 18 hours at room temperature and is readily inactivated by drying and most disinfectants. Because of this, transmission occurs primarily through close contact, although fomites remain a very important mode of transmission in crowded environments. Aerosol transmission is of lesser importance.[15,18] Aerosols generated by sneezing cats typically travel no further than a distance of 4 to 5 feet.

Feline Calicivirus

Feline calicivirus (FCV) is a non-enveloped, single-stranded RNA virus with a spherical capsid that is studded with cup-shaped depressions (*calici* = "cup") (Figure 23-1). Like FHV-1, FCV commonly causes feline URTD, accounting for 10% to over 50% of cases. The highest prevalences occur in large multicat environments. Natural infection of dogs by FCV-like strains has been reported.[19] Like other RNA viruses, the genome of FCV continually undergoes rapid mutation, which increases the diversity of strains over time. Although considerable antigenic diversity exists among FCV isolates, the degree of antigenic cross-reactivity between them is sufficient for them to be classified as a single serotype. Nucleotide sequence analysis also suggests that isolates worldwide are a single, but highly diverse, group. No correlations have been found between the genetic composition of FCV strains, different clinical manifestations of disease, or geographical location.

TABLE 23-1

Viral Causes of Transmissible Respiratory Disease in Cats

Organism	Incubation Period (days)*	Shedding Period*	Environmental Survival
Feline herpesvirus-1	2 to 6	1 to 2 weeks, with intermittent reactivation of shedding with stress	Less than a day
Feline calicivirus	2 to 6	Most <30 days, may be lifelong	Up to 1 month
Influenza viruses	Few days	<2 weeks	Hours

*Incubation and shedding periods are approximate and may differ when co-infections or immune suppression operate.

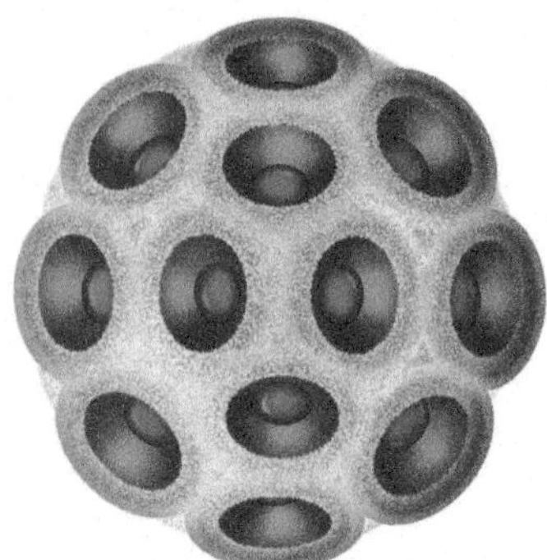

FIGURE 23-1 Schematic of the structure of the capsid of feline calicivirus.

Infected cats can develop a persistent oropharyngeal infection (>1 month in duration) in the absence of obvious clinical signs. This is termed the carrier state for FCV, and may result from immune evasion through antigenic variation of the capsid protein.[20] FCV is shed continuously from the oropharynx, and the magnitude of shedding varies with time and between individual cats.[21] Carrier cats serve as a source of infection for other cats. In many cats, shedding terminates weeks to months after infection, but in a few cats, shedding is lifelong. A single cat can be simultaneously infected with multiple variants of FCV, each derived from the original infecting strain as a result of genetic mutation, drift, and selection pressures.[20] Because of the chronic carrier state, the prevalence of FCV infection in healthy cats is high and ranged from 8% of household cats to 24% of show cats.[12]

Environmental persistence of FCV is considerably more prolonged than that of FHV-1, and FCV resists routine disinfection with quaternary ammonium compounds. Susceptibility to disinfectants may vary between FCV strains.[22] Survival in the environment has been demonstrated for as long as 28 days,[23] and related caliciviruses persist in a dried state for several months.[24] As a result, fomites are a very important means of transmission. FCV is also transmitted through direct contact with respiratory secretions and through aerosols. Fleas may spread FCV through their feces or when cats ingest fleas while grooming.[25]

Highly virulent FCV strains have been isolated from outbreaks of severe systemic febrile illness in cats in the United States and Europe known as *virulent systemic disease* (VSD),[26-31] which was first described in California in 1998. Shelter cats that were hospitalized in veterinary clinics have been a source of infection in many outbreaks, and for each outbreak, the FCV strain involved has differed. VSD has also been described in one cat from a multiple-cat household, that is, in the absence of an outbreak.[32] Otherwise healthy, adult, vaccinated cats are often affected, whereas kittens tend to show less severe signs. Although infections typically spread rapidly in outbreaks, including through fomites to pet cats of hospital staff, spread of disease has been limited to affected clinics or shelters, with no further spread within the community, and outbreaks resolve within approximately 2 months once appropriate control measures are instituted.

Influenza Viruses

Pandemic H1N1 influenza viruses originated from pigs and have caused widespread illness in humans. Natural infection with these strains has been reported in cats from the United States and Europe. Affected cats had signs of fever and respiratory and gastrointestinal tract disease and, in some cases, death.[4,33-35] Transmission from sick humans who were in contact with the cats was suspected. Cat-to-cat transmission may also have occurred.[34]

Highly pathogenic avian origin H5N1 influenza virus infection, which emerged as a cause of human illness in Hong Kong in 1997 and subsequently spread worldwide,[36] has been detected in sick and apparently healthy domestic cats and wild felids from southeast Asia[3,37,38] and central Europe.[39,40] Nevertheless, no evidence of infection was found in more than 170 cats where infected birds had been identified in Germany and Austria.[41] Infection of cats follows direct or indirect contact with infected birds, especially consumption of raw poultry; cat-to-cat transmission may also occur.[37]

Canine H3N2 virus infection was associated with bronchopneumonia in shelter-housed cats in China and Korea.[42] Experimentally, cats can also be infected with other influenza viruses, including human H2N2 and H3N2, and avian origin H7N7 and H7N3 viruses.[43,44] Widespread evidence of exposure to pandemic H1N1, seasonal H1N1, and seasonal H3N2 was found in 400 cats from Ohio in the United States.[45] Seropositive cats were 7.4 times more likely to have had respiratory illness than seronegative cats, and twice as likely to have had nonrespiratory illness than seronegative cats. More information on influenza viruses can be found in Chapter 17.

Clinical Features

Signs and Their Pathogenesis

After direct or indirect contact with virus in respiratory secretions from the conjunctiva, nasal cavity and oropharynx, FCV and FHV-1 replicate within lymphoid and epithelial cells in the upper respiratory tract and cause cytolysis. FHV-1 also replicates in corneal epithelial cells.[46] Although FHV-1 prefers to replicate in the cooler tissues of the upper respiratory tract, systemic infection with viremia occurs in some cats infected with FHV-1 and may be more likely to occur in neonates and debilitated cats. FCV and influenza viruses also replicate systemically. FCV is shed in the urine and feces of infected cats, in addition to respiratory secretions. Influenza viruses are shed in both respiratory secretions and the feces. Avian origin H5N1 influenza viruses replicate initially in the lower respiratory tract (type II pneumocytes and alveolar macrophages) or gastrointestinal tract (for example, after ingestion of an infected bird), which is followed by severe systemic infection with necrosis and inflammation in multiple organs.[38] In contrast, severe systemic infection is not a feature of H1N1 influenza virus infections in cats.[47]

Clinical signs of viral URTD occur after an incubation period of 2 to 6 days, although longer incubation periods are also possible, and incubation periods as short as 1 to 2 days can occur in cats infected with influenza viruses.[47] Viral shedding occurs as early as 24 hours after infection, and often before the onset of clinical signs. Clinical signs range considerably in severity from no signs or mild serous ocular discharge to pneumonia and death. The most severe signs tend to occur in very young or elderly debilitated cats. Concurrent immunosuppressive illness or infection with other respiratory pathogens and opportunistic bacteria also profoundly influences disease severity. Clinical signs include conjunctivitis, serous or mucopurulent ocular and nasal discharge and sneezing, and, less commonly, cough or tachypnea (Figure 23-2, *A*). Mucopurulent discharges result from secondary bacterial infections with opportunistic pathogens such as *Streptococcus* spp., *Staphylococcus* spp., *Pasteurella multocida*, and *Escherichia coli*. Ocular and nasal discharges may become crusted, and kittens' eyes may not open as a result of the sticky exudates; when severe this can be followed by extensive corneal damage and rupture of the globe. Lethargy, inappetence, hypersalivation, and fever may be present in acute infections. FCV and FHV-1 infections may also lead to pharyngitis and laryngitis, which can be accompanied by clinical signs of gagging or obstructive respiratory patterns. Ulcerative glossitis and ulceration of the nasal planum, conjunctiva, and skin is more common and severe with FCV infection but can also be associated with FHV-1 infection (see Figure 23-2, *B*). Clinical features unique to each infection are outlined next.

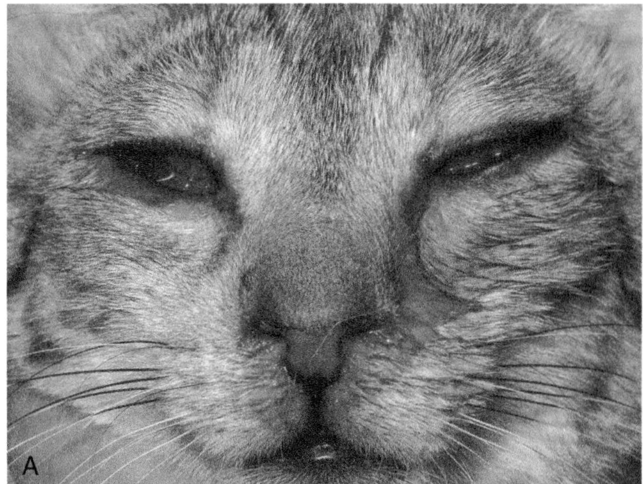

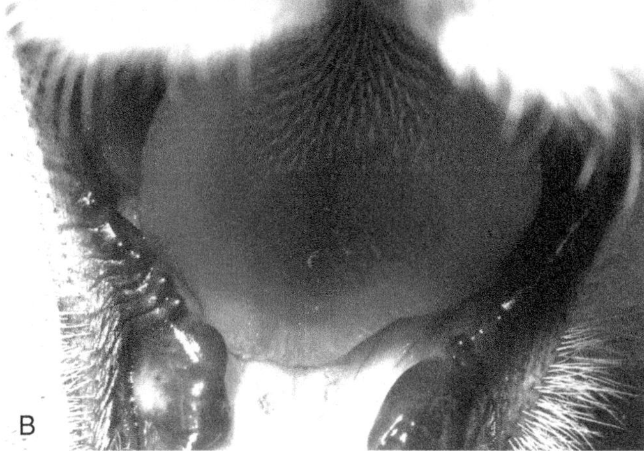

FIGURE 23-2 Chemosis, mucopurulent ocular and nasal discharge **(A)** and lingual ulceration **(B)** in a 6-month-old intact male domestic medium-hair cat with chronic nasal discharge and conjunctivitis. A conjunctival swab specimen tested positive with a PCR assay for FCV RNA and negative for FHV-1, *Chlamydia felis*, and *Mycoplasma* spp. DNA. (Courtesy of the University of California, Davis Veterinary Ophthalmology Service.)

Feline Herpesvirus-1

In neonatal infections caused by FHV-1, damage to upper respiratory epithelium may lead to osteolysis of the nasal turbinates and persistent or recurrent sinusitis and rhinitis. Rarely, neurologic signs and reproductive complications such as abortion and fetal resorption have been observed in infected cats, although it is unclear what role FHV-1 itself plays in the pathogenesis of these clinical manifestations. FHV-1 is an important cause of corneal disease in cats, and has been implicated as a cause of acute and chronic ulcerative (epithelial) keratitis, stromal keratitis, eosinophilic keratitis, corneal sequestra, and uveitis. Stromal keratitis is thought to be an immunopathologic response to persistent viral antigens. The presence of dendritic corneal ulcers is thought to be pathognomonic for FHV-1 infection. However, the role that FHV-1 plays as a cause of eosinophilic keratitis, corneal sequestra, and uveitis requires further study, because a clear association between these abnormalities and the detection of FHV-1 within corneal tissues has not always been present.[48] Consequences of ocular disease due to FHV-1 include symblepharon (adhesion of an ulcerated conjunctiva to itself or the cornea) and keratoconjunctivitis sicca. FHV-1 can also cause a severe ulcerative and eosinophilic facial dermatitis (Figure 23-3). Lesions have also been described elsewhere on the body in the absence of facial lesions.[49]

Feline Calicivirus

FCV infection has been most strongly associated with erosive or ulcerative lesions, which can occur on the nasal planum, tongue, lips, and occasionally the conjunctiva and heal over a period of 2 to 3 weeks.[50] Persistent infection with FCV has also been linked to chronic ulceroproliferative and lymphoplasmacytic stomatitis, which involves the mucosa lateral to the palatoglossal arches (caudal stomatitis), the alveolar mucosa in the premolar and molar area, and sometimes the buccal mucosa (alveolar/buccal mucositis) (Figure 23-4).[51-53] Some persistently infected cats have isolated hyperemia of the buccal mucosa along the length of the dental arcade in the absence of significant periodontal disease. There is no age predisposition for this condition.[53] Pyrexia and transient lameness due to synovitis has been described days to weeks after clinical signs of acute FCV infection and after vaccination with certain FCV vaccines. FCV has been investigated as a possible cause of feline lower urinary tract disease (feline interstitial cystitis) and enteritis in cats. Because

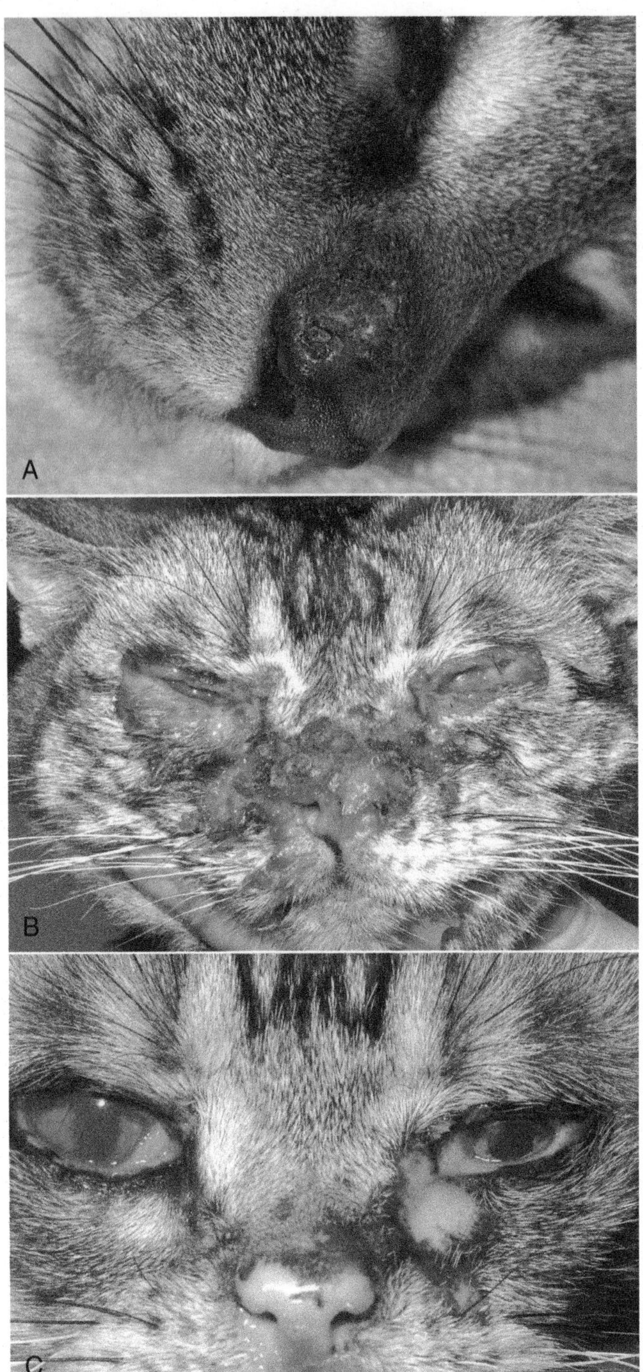

FIGURE 23-3 Ulcerative and eosinophilic facial dermatitis secondary to FHV-1 infection. **A,** 3-year-old female spayed domestic shorthair with a 2-month history of a crusted lesion on the right dorsal muzzle. **B,** Fourteen-year-old female spayed domestic shorthair with blepharokeratoconjunctivitis and severe ulcerative facial dermatitis. **C,** Same cat as in **B** after 4 months of treatment with famciclovir. Fluorescein stain is present. Biopsy in both cats showed severe, diffuse, necrotizing, and eosinophilic dermatitis with a few intranuclear inclusions bodies. A PCR assay for FHV-1 DNA on a biopsy from the cat in **B** was positive. (Courtesy of the University of California, Davis Veterinary Dermatology and Ophthalmology Services.)

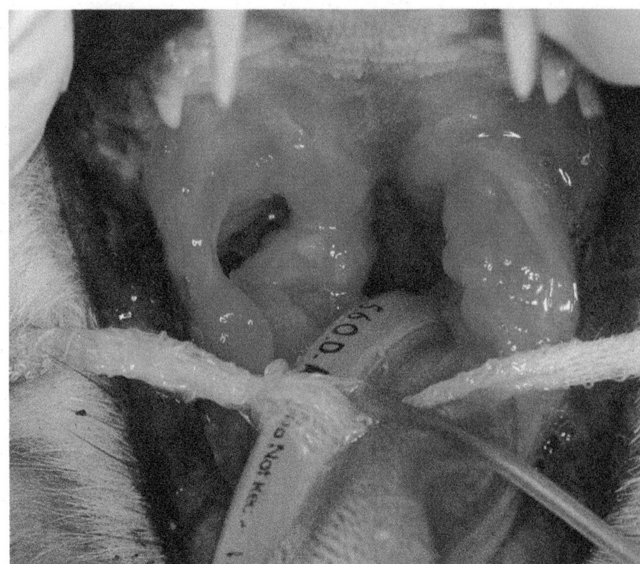

FIGURE 23-4 Severe caudal stomatitis in a retrovirus-negative, 8-year-old female spayed domestic shorthair cat that was evaluated for ptyalism. The cat lived with 12 other cats. Histopathology revealed severe plasmacytic and neutrophilic inflammation with multifocal epithelial ulceration and hyperplasia.

FCV can be shed in the urine and feces of apparently healthy cats, the significance of the virus in the pathogenesis of these conditions remains unclear.

Cats with VSD show severe signs of caliciviral URTD, including anorexia, fever (often >105°F [40.6°C]), weight loss, oral and footpad ulceration, and nasal and/or ocular discharge. VSD strains infect not only epithelial cells of the upper respiratory tract and oral cavity, but a variety of other cell types, such as endothelial cells, hepatocytes, pneumocytes, and pancreatic acinar cells.[54] FCV uses feline junctional adhesion molecule A (JAM-A) as a receptor, a member of the immunoglobulin superfamily. The lesions that develop are thought to result from disruption of intercellular tight junctions and vasculitis. Distinctive clinical signs of VSD include cutaneous edema, alopecia, crusting, and ulceration. Edema occurs most commonly on the head and limbs but may become generalized. Crusting and ulceration are most prominent on the nose, lips, pinnae, periocular regions, and distal limbs. Severe respiratory distress due to pulmonary edema or pleural effusion, or icterus as a result of hepatic necrosis or pancreatitis, develop in some cats and have been associated with a poor prognosis. Involvement of the gastrointestinal tract, liver, and pancreas may also result in vomiting and/or diarrhea. Cats also develop a coagulopathy, which can be manifested by petechial and ecchymotic hemorrhages and, rarely, epistaxis and hematochezia. In peracute infections, cats die as a result of cardiovascular arrest with few preceding signs apart from fever.

Influenza Virus Infections

In addition to fever, anorexia, lethargy, conjunctivitis, nasal and ocular discharges, and tachypnea as a result of viral pneumonia, highly pathogenic H5N1 avian origin influenza virus infections have been associated with neurologic signs such as seizures and ataxia, which result from nonsuppurative meningoencephalitis and vasculitis.[36] Diarrhea and vomiting have not been observed in cats infected with H5N1 viruses. Vomiting has been reported in cats infected with pandemic H1N1 influenza viruses, which may have a predilection for the gastrointestinal tract.[33,34]

Physical Examination Findings

Physical examination findings in cats with acute viral URTD vary from mild serous ocular discharge and conjunctivitis through to fever, severe mucopurulent ocular and nasal discharges, chemosis, dehydration, thin body condition, stertorous or stridorous respiration, tachypnea, increased breath sounds on thoracic auscultation, hypersalivation, and ulceration of the nasal planum, tongue, and lips. Because ulcerative lesions can occur at the base of the tongue near the larynx, examination of the entire tongue should be performed in cats that are febrile and inappetent, which may require sedation. Cats with VSD can have edema of the face and lips, icterus, cutaneous ulceration, evidence of petechial hemorrhages, and abdominal pain. Ulcerative keratitis with dendritic or geographical corneal ulceration may be seen in cats with acute FHV-1 infection; chronic FHV-1 infection may be manifested as stromal keratitis with neovascularization, pigmentation and fibrosis of the cornea, symblepharon, and conjunctivalization of the cornea (Figure 23-5). Eosinophilic keratitis manifests as superficial, pink to white vascularized proliferative lesions on the cornea or conjunctiva; abundant eosinophils are present in smears of corneal scrapings. Herpetic facial dermatitis is manifested as cutaneous ulceration, erythema, exudation, and adherent crusts, most commonly around the nose and eyes but occasionally on the trunk and limbs.[55] Cats with persistent FCV infection may have ulceroproliferative caudal stomatitis or buccal/alveolar mucositis, and exhibit pain on examination of the oral cavity.

Diagnosis

It is not always possible to identify the cause of transmissible respiratory disease in cats based on clinical signs alone, because each pathogen produces a similar spectrum of signs. The presence of corneal ulceration raises suspicion for FHV-1 infection, and severe lingual ulceration or facial edema and crusting raises suspicion for FCV infection, but mixed infections occur and complicate diagnosis. A history of exposure to other cats provides support for a diagnosis of viral respiratory disease, but because FHV-1 infections can recrudesce with stress, potential or known exposure to other cats is not essential to implicate respiratory viruses as a cause of disease. Previous immunization for feline respiratory viruses does not rule out the possibility of viral URTD. All cats with signs of URTD should have known retrovirus infection status, because viral URTD is common in retrovirus-infected cats. When signs such as chronic nasal discharge are present, other etiologies should also be considered, such as fungal infections, neoplasia, and foreign bodies. Diagnosis of eosinophilic keratitis and ulcerative facial dermatitis may require corneal scrapings or skin biopsy, respectively.

Laboratory Abnormalities

There are no specific CBC, biochemistry profile, or urinalysis abnormalities that aid in a diagnosis of feline viral respiratory disease. The CBC can be normal or show a mild to moderate neutrophilia, sometimes with band neutrophils or neutrophil toxicity. Lymphopenia may be present in severely affected cats. Serum biochemistry findings in cats with viral respiratory disease are usually unremarkable unless disease is severe or chronic. In cats with VSD, hematologic abnormalities include mild to severe anemia, thrombocytopenia, neutrophilia, and lymphopenia. Cats with VSD may also have hypoalbuminemia, hyperbilirubinemia, mildly increased serum activities of ALT and AST, and increased serum CK activity. Serum CK activities up to 11,000 U/L can occur.[26] Cats with chronic stomatitis may have hyperglobulinemia due to a polyclonal gammopathy.

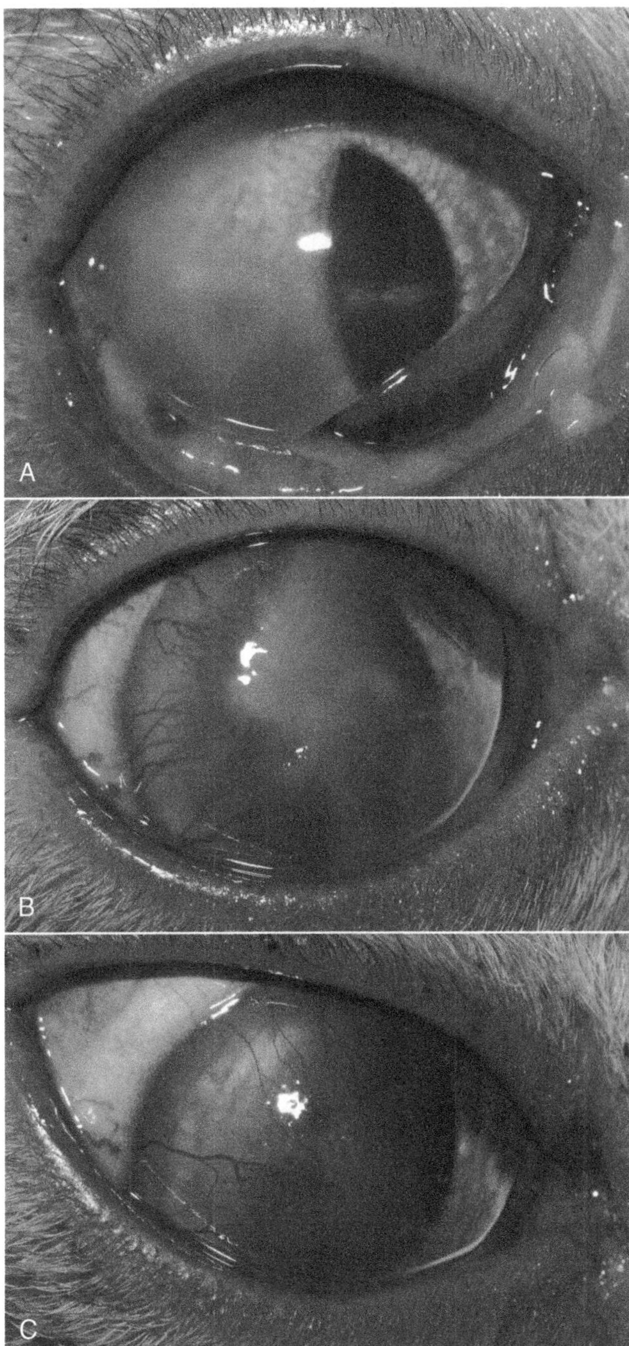

FIGURE 23-5 **A,** Ulcerative and stromal keratitis in a 2-year-old male neutered rex cat. FHV-1 infection was suspected. Treatment with famciclovir (375 mg PO q8h), L-lysine (500 mg PO q12h), and cidofovir (0.5%; one drop OD q12h) was associated with clinical improvement over a 1 month period (**B** and **C**). The cat had a history of a corneal sequestrum and subsequently developed eosinophilic keratitis. (Courtesy of the University of California, Davis Veterinary Ophthalmology Service.)

Tracheobronchial lavage specimens from cats with pneumonia may show a suppurative or mixed exudate, sometimes with evidence of secondary bacterial infection. Aerobic bacterial culture and susceptibility testing and culture for *Mycoplasma* spp. are indicated on wash specimens. Organisms such as *Pasteurella* spp., *Staphylococcus pseudintermedius*, *Streptococcus* spp., *Escherichia coli*, *Klebsiella pneumoniae*, and some *Mycoplasma* spp. infect the airways as opportunists. Bacterial culture of nasal swabs is generally not recommended because it often

TABLE 23-2

Diagnostic Assays Available for Respiratory Virus Infections in Cats

Assay	Specimen Type	Target	Performance
Virus isolation	Conjunctival, nasal, and caudal pharyngeal swabs, transtracheal and bronchoalveolar wash specimens, airway and lung specimens collected at necropsy	Virus	Negative results can occur if specimens contain no or low numbers of virus particles. May take several days and requires specialized techniques and expertise. May be the most sensitive assay for detection of FCV infections.
PCR	See Virus isolation	Viral nucleic acid	Sensitivity and specificity may vary depending on assay design. Sensitivity may be low because of brief shedding for some viruses or low-level shedding in chronic infections. Assays may not detect all virus strains. Testing specimens from multiple different anatomic sites or combining PCR with other diagnostic tests can increase sensitivity. Attenuated live vaccine virus may be detected after vaccination. Because of subclinical shedding, the significance of a positive result may be difficult to interpret. False-negative results may occur as a result of degradation of viral nucleic acid during specimen transport.
Serology	Serum	Antibodies against respiratory viral antigens	Interpretation complicated by previous vaccination and exposure. Acute and convalescent serology may be useful in outbreak situations that involve a novel strain of FCV or influenza A virus.
Histopathology	Necropsy or biopsy specimens	FHV-1 inclusions; immunostaining	Detection of FHV-1 inclusions has low sensitivity, and immunostaining and/or PCR is required to definitively identify the infecting virus.

FCV, Feline calicivirus; FHV-1, feline herpesvirus-1.

leads to growth of normal flora, which has no clinical relevance. However, resistant *Pseudomonas aeruginosa* infections can develop in some cats with chronic URTD that have been treated repeatedly with antimicrobial drugs.

Diagnostic Imaging

In uncomplicated feline URTD viral infections, plain thoracic radiographs may be unremarkable or show a mild diffuse interstitial to bronchointerstitial pattern. Alveolar patterns or lung lobe consolidation can occur with secondary bacterial pneumonia.

Microbiologic Tests

Because many cats experience self-limiting disease, attempts to obtain an etiologic diagnosis should be made when disease persists for longer than 7 to 10 days or is complicated by pneumonia, with lethargy and inappetence. When outbreaks occur in shelters or the pattern of endemic respiratory disease changes, attempts to make an etiologic diagnosis are also indicated and strongly encouraged. Because FCV and FHV-1 can be detected in apparently healthy cats, it may be difficult to know the significance of a positive test result in a single cat with signs of respiratory disease. In an outbreak situation, collection of multiple specimen types from several cats with and without clinical signs can facilitate diagnosis and allow interpretation of the significance of test results. In shelter situations or outbreaks of severe disease, necropsies can provide valuable information and should be performed by a veterinary pathologist as soon as possible after death or euthanasia. Tissues should be submitted for histopathology (in formalin), bacterial and virus isolation (fresh tissue), and PCR for respiratory viruses and bacteria (fresh or frozen tissue; see Chapter 5). There is currently no way to distinguish FCV strains that cause VSD from other FCV strains.

Assays available to detect feline respiratory viruses include virus isolation, direct immunofluorescence, and PCR assays (Table 23-2). Point-of-care ELISA assays developed for use in humans have been evaluated for detection of H5N1 influenza virus antigen in cats[56] but have low sensitivity and will not be discussed further. Because influenza viruses and FCV are RNA viruses that exhibit considerable sequence diversity, virus isolation may offer the greatest sensitivity for detection of these viruses and enables typing for influenza viruses. In contrast, FHV-1 loses infectivity more rapidly than FCV and has little sequence diversity, so PCR is more useful. The use of both PCR and culture together offers the greatest sensitivity when it is important to obtain a diagnosis. Serology may be of use for investigation of outbreaks that involve novel FCV strains or influenza virus types.

Virus Isolation

FCV, FHV-1, and influenza viruses are readily isolated in cell culture. Virus isolation for diagnosis of feline respiratory viral infections is offered to veterinarians by some commercial veterinary diagnostic laboratories that specialize in virology. The laboratory should be notified if influenza virus infection is a possibility. Suitable specimens for isolation of respiratory viruses include conjunctival, nasal, and oropharyngeal swabs, transtracheal or bronchoalveolar lavage specimens, or upper airway tissue or lung obtained at necropsy. Influenza viruses may also be isolated from feces or rectal swabs. If swabs are used for specimen collection, polyester-tipped swabs and specific virus transport media should be used, which are available from commercial testing laboratories. Cotton swabs should be avoided, because influenza viruses adhere to the cotton, which may lead to reduced sensitivity.[57] When conjunctival swabs are collected, the use of topical anesthetics should also be avoided, because they have the potential to reduce the sensitivity of virus isolation.[58] Isolation may take several days. Sensitivity can be very low in cats with chronic manifestations of infection (for example, more than 1 week after the onset of clinical signs), because shedding of respiratory viruses can be transient. In cats with mixed FCV and FHV-1 infections, FCV may obscure the presence of FHV-1, because it produces cytopathic effects more rapidly.

Fluorescent Antibody Testing

Fluorescent antibody that specifically detects FHV-1 or FCV can be applied to conjunctival smears or impression smears from lung tissue collected at necropsy. The effect of vaccination with attenuated live vaccines on fluorescent antibody test results has not been reported. The sensitivity of fluorescent antibody testing is lower than that of PCR and virus isolation,[59] and inexperienced laboratory personnel may misinterpret nonspecific fluorescence as a positive result.

Molecular Diagnosis Using the Polymerase Chain Reaction

Panels of real-time PCR assays that detect feline respiratory pathogens are offered by some commercial veterinary diagnostic laboratories and are rapid and relatively inexpensive. These can include assays for FHV-1 and FCV, as well as bacteria such as *Mycoplasma* spp., *B. bronchiseptica*, and *C. felis*. RT-PCR assays for the detection of influenza viruses are also available. The sensitivity and specificity of PCR assays can vary considerably between laboratories. Swabs of the nasal cavity, conjunctival sac, or caudal pharynx; tracheobronchial lavage specimens; skin biopsies; or upper respiratory tract and lung tissue collected at necropsy are suitable specimens for testing. Topical anesthetics and fluorescein can reduce the sensitivity of PCR assays for human herpesviral infections,[60] and so they should be avoided, although one study showed no inhibitory effect of topical fluorescein or proxymetacaine in cats on FHV-1 or *C. felis* PCR results.[61] False-negative PCR results can occur in cats with chronic infections that shed at low levels. Because FCV and influenza viruses are RNA viruses, false negatives may also result from degradation of viral RNA during specimen transport or as a result of strain variation.

Positive PCR assay results for FCV and FHV-1 should be interpreted with caution, because apparently healthy cats can shed these viruses and, although controversial, FHV-1 DNA detected in corneal, conjunctival, or nasal biopsy tissue may represent latent virus. In one shelter, a correlation between the quantity of FHV-1 present in pooled oropharyngeal and conjunctival swabs as determined using quantitative real-time PCR and the severity of histologic lesions within the nasal cavity was detected, with cycle threshold values less than 29 correlating with the most severe histologic lesions.[62] In the future, quantitation of viral nucleic acid within swabs may assist interpretation of the clinical significance of positive PCR results. PCR can also detect attenuated live vaccine virus that is shed after routine vaccination. However, this appeared to be an uncommon phenomenon in one study that used PCR to detect FHV-1 and FCV in 12 cats over a 3-week period after vaccination with intranasal or parenteral attenuated live FHV-1 and FCV vaccines. [14] The cats in this study had been previously exposed to FHV-1, and two had been vaccinated with FHV-1 and FCV vaccines, which may have reduced shedding after vaccination. Additional studies are required to determine the prevalence of positive assay results after vaccination and their relationship to vaccine virus. In outbreak situations, false-positive PCR results have the potential to occur if swabs become contaminated with virus from the environment or the hands of personnel. Clean examination gloves should be worn for each cat, and the swab should touch only the anatomic site to be tested.

Serologic Diagnosis

Serologic assays (such as ELISA or serum neutralization assays) that detect antibodies to FHV-1 and/or FCV are offered on a commercial basis to veterinarians. Unfortunately, serology is not useful for diagnosis, because of vaccine titer interference and the high prevalence of subclinical exposure to these viruses in the cat population. Titers to FCV may vary depending on the degree of homology between the infecting virus and the FCV strain used in the assay. Nevertheless, serology has been useful to investigate some outbreaks of VSD. Serology has also been used to predict protection from infection, although cats with negative titers can still have some degree of immunity, and cats with positive titers may develop illness after challenge.

Serologic assays for influenza virus exposure are based on serum neutralization or hemagglutination-inhibition (see Chapter 2) and are specific for the influenza virus strain of interest (i.e., H5N1, H1N1).

Pathologic Findings

Gross lesions in cats with viral URTD include cutaneous and lingual ulcerations, evidence of keratitis in cats infected with FHV-1, submandibular or retropharyngeal lymph node enlargement, mucosal hyperemia, and mucopurulent exudate within the nasal cavity and trachea. In cats with pneumonia, the lungs may be edematous with diffuse or multifocal consolidated areas. Histopathology may show fibrinosuppurative and necrotizing stomatitis, rhinitis, tracheitis, and/or alveolitis. When FHV-1 is present, intranuclear viral inclusions may be found within epithelial cells of the upper respiratory tract (Figure 23-6). Osteolytic changes within the nasal turbinates may also be identified in cats infected with FHV-1. Virus can be detected in epithelial cells using immunohistochemistry or fluorescent antibody staining. Skin biopsies from cats with ulcerative herpesviral dermatitis show epidermal ulceration and necrosis that extends into the superficial dermis, and infiltration with degenerated neutrophils, eosinophils, and fewer numbers of histiocytes, plasma cells, and lymphocytes. In some skin biopsies, intranuclear viral inclusions are identified.[55]

Necropsy findings in cats with VSD are variable. Frequently reported findings include individual hepatocellular necrosis and dissociation with minimal inflammation, acute interstitial pneumonia, and free pleural and abdominal fluid.[26-28,31] Acute necrotizing vasculitis of subcutaneous and oral submucosal vessels has been described.[32] Intestinal crypt necrosis and pancreatitis have been reported in experimentally infected cats.

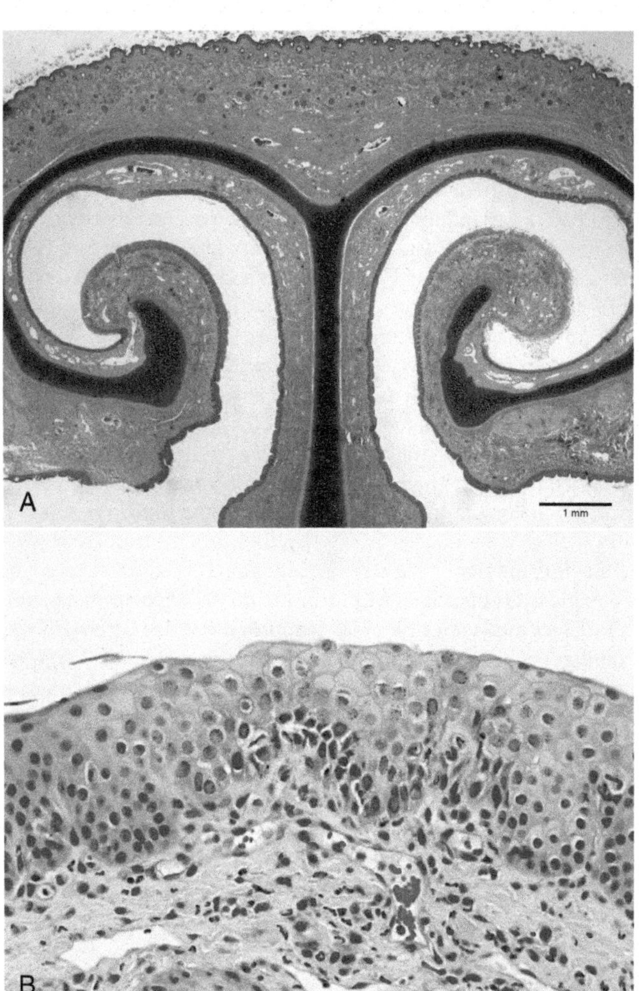

FIGURE 23-6 **A,** Cross-section of the nares of a shelter cat with rhinitis due to infection by FHV-1. Ulceration is most severe on the right side. Hematoxylin and eosin stain. **B,** Higher magnification of the nasal epithelium that shows rhinitis and the presence of intraepithelial, intranuclear inclusion bodies. (From Burns RE, Wagner DC, Leutenegger CM, et al. Histologic and molecular correlation in shelter cats with acute upper respiratory infection. J Clin Microbiol 2011;49(7):2454-2460. Images courtesy Dr. Patricia Pesavento, University of California, Davis Veterinary Anatomic Pathology Service.)

In addition to acute respiratory lesions, cats infected with H5N1 influenza viruses can have widespread necrosis and inflammation in many organs.

Treatment and Prognosis

Acute Upper Respiratory Disease

Supportive care is the mainstay of treatment for acute feline URTD and includes subcutaneous fluid therapy, antimicrobial drugs for secondary bacterial infections, and enteral nutrition. Appetite stimulants such as diazepam may be useful in some cats, but if inappetence persists for longer than 3 days, feeding tube placement is indicated. Severely affected cats may require hospitalization in isolation and treatment with parenteral fluids, nebulization, and supplemental oxygen. Acute signs generally resolve within 2 to 3 weeks with supportive care, but some cats experience frequent disease relapses and chronic complications such as keratitis and persistent stomatitis. Cats with VSD may require treatment with colloids. Mortality rates that exceed 50% can occur in outbreaks of VSD.[31]

Herpetic Keratoconjunctivitis and Facial Dermatitis

The use of antiviral drugs should be considered for cats with severe and recurrent or persistent manifestations of FHV-1 infection such as keratitis, severe conjunctivitis, and ulcerative facial dermatitis. Antiviral drugs are discussed in more depth in Chapter 7 (see Table 7-2 for dosages). Referral to a veterinary specialist for assessment of an underlying cause should be considered for cats with signs of chronic URTD. Acyclovir and its prodrug, valacyclovir, cause unacceptable toxicity when administered systemically to cats, and so their use is not recommended. In contrast, oral famciclovir is well tolerated by adult cats and kittens and results in significant clinical improvement and decreased viral shedding in cats with acute and chronic herpesviral disease (see Figure 23-3, *B* and *C*).[63,64] The prodrug of famciclovir, penciclovir, also has potential to be a useful drug for treatment of feline herpesviral infections. Because FHV-1 infection can deplete conjunctival goblet cells,[64a] frequent application of a topical mucinomimetic that contains hyaluronic acid is recommended in conjunction with famciclovir.

Topical ophthalmic preparations that contain idoxuridine, trifluridine, vidarabine, or acyclovir can be used to treat herpesviral keratitis, although the true efficacy of these drugs has not been well studied. Frequent topical application is required (5 to 6 times daily), and prolonged use can cause corneal irritation or ulceration. Idoxuridine and vidarabine are better tolerated by cats than trifluridine; vidarabine is effective against idoxuridine-resistant strains. Cidofovir and ganciclovir show greater promise as topical treatments and are highly active against FHV-1 in vitro. Topical cidofovir decreases disease severity and viral shedding in experimentally infected cats,[65] and has the advantage of requiring only twice daily administration.

Human recombinant IFN-α and recombinant feline IFN-ω inhibit FHV-1 replication in vitro and have been administered parenterally, topically (for keratitis), and orally to cats with FHV-1 infection. Obvious clinical responses to treatment have not been uniformly observed, but controlled clinical trials that involve large numbers of cats are lacking. Improvement was noted when IFN-α was given subcutaneously 2 days before inoculation of cats with FHV-1,[66] but the effect of parenteral IFN-α after the onset of clinical signs requires further investigation. Parenteral administration may be followed by the development of neutralizing antibodies beyond 3 weeks of treatment.

Lysine has shown efficacy for treatment of herpesviral conjunctivitis in cats when administered as tablets[67] and can reduce reactivated shedding by latently infected cats.[68] However, when administered to shelter cats, there was no reduction in URTD, possibly because of the stress of tablet administration.[69] Dietary formulation with lysine has also not been effective for management of URTD in shelters and in fact may contribute to a worsened outcome.[70] Administration of lysine tablets or paste could be considered for client-owned cats with chronic herpesviral disease but is not recommended in shelter situations.

The use of glucocorticoids to treat refractory keratitis is controversial, because it may reactivate virus and worsen disease. However, eosinophilic keratitis may require treatment with topical glucocorticoids. Because the role of FHV-1 in this condition is unclear, topical antiviral medications such as cidofovir are often given concurrently. Topical glucocorticoids are contraindicated when corneal ulceration is present, so the eyes should first be carefully examined after staining with fluorescein. Cats with ulcerative eosinophilic keratitis may require systemic glucocorticoid treatment until the ulcers heal. Referral to a veterinary ophthalmologist is recommended.

Chronic Gingivostomatitis

Caudal stomatitis in cats infected with FCV is often refractory to medical treatment. Clinical cure occurs in 50% to 60% of cats and there is significant improvement in 30% to 40% of cats after 1) extraction of teeth in the vicinity of lesions, 2) treatment with antimicrobial drugs with activity against anaerobic and gram-positive aerobic bacteria, and 3) the use of antiseptic mouthwashes (see Chapter 21). Cats that fail to respond to this treatment may require long-term treatment with antimicrobial and antiinflammatory drugs, although one study showed minimal improvement in cats with refractory stomatitis that were treated with prednisolone.[53] Recombinant feline IFN-ω has also been used subcutaneously and orally to treat caudal stomatitis. In a randomized, multicenter, controlled, double-blinded study of cats with refractory caudal stomatitis and alveolar/buccal mucositis, oromucosal treatment with rfIFN-ω (0.1 million units q24h) was associated with significant improvement in lesions and decreased pain scores from day 0 to day 90.[53]

Influenza Virus Infections

Oseltamivir has been used to treat captive wild and domestic cats with influenza virus infections,[33,71] but it was not effective. The optimal dose of this drug in cats is not known. Therefore, cats with suspected influenza virus infections should be treated supportively.

Immunity and Vaccination

Immunity to respiratory viruses depends on cell-mediated and systemic and local (mucosal IgA) humoral immune responses. Maternal antibody to respiratory viruses can persist until 14 weeks of age,[15] although other kittens may be susceptible to infection at 6 weeks of age.

Vaccines for FHV-1 and FCV have been available for decades, but these do not provide complete protection, and disease continues to be widespread in the cat population. Infection of kittens before completion of the primary vaccine series contributes to this problem. Both inactivated and attenuated live FHV-1 and FCV vaccines are available, and attenuated live vaccines are available for parenteral or intranasal administration. Inactivated vaccines contain adjuvant, and their use should be reserved for immunosuppressed cats (such as retrovirus-infected cats) or pregnant cats, if deemed necessary. When infections are a problem in kittens in breeding catteries, vaccination of the queen before mating is preferable to vaccination during pregnancy and may prolong the duration of maternal antibody persistence.[50] Vaccination as early as 4 weeks of age (but not before) could be considered in catteries with high rates of viral URTD. The primary series should consist of vaccines administered every 3 to 4 weeks of age until no earlier than 16 weeks of age.

No respiratory viral vaccine prevents infection, the carrier state, or reactivation of FHV-1 infection with stress, but they can reduce disease severity. Whether a cat contracts feline viral URTD after vaccination depends on factors such as virus strain virulence, the challenge dose, environmental temperature and humidity, and the presence of underlying immunosuppressive disease or other concurrent disease.

For FHV-1 infections, vaccination can reduce the duration of shedding, viral infectivity (presumably as a result of complexing of virus by antibody), and the load of latent virus in the trigeminal ganglia.[15,72,73] It is unclear if the frequency of reactivation is reduced, although this is the case for herpesviral vaccines in other species (such as the shingles vaccine for humans). The intranasal FHV-1 vaccine virus can itself become latent, but whether parenteral FHV-1 vaccine virus becomes latent is unknown. Most FCV vaccines do not prevent shedding, and virus shedding from the oropharynx can actually increase after FCV vaccination, because of shedding of attenuated live vaccine virus.

Because FHV-1 strains are antigenically similar, the immune response to one FHV-1 strain cross protects against other FHV-1 strains. Greater variability in cross protection occurs for FCV strains. Vaccines that contain F9, the most widely used FCV vaccine strain, provide partial protection against aerosol challenge with heterologous strains.[74] Cross-neutralization studies have shown that the antigenic composition of current field FCV strains may differ enough from the original F9 strain that the level of cross-protection induced by F9 vaccines may be suboptimal. As a result, it has been suggested that new FCV strains should be incorporated into FCV vaccines. However, vaccines that contain F9 still appear to generate cross-reactive antibody to a large number of currently circulating strains.[75] A nonadjuvanted, inactivated vaccine that contains two FCV strains (G1 and 431) is available in Europe, which provided greater reduction in clinical scores after challenge with a heterologous strain that the use of either strain alone and also reduced shedding.[76] Exposure of vaccinated cats to field strains of FCV may also serve to boost immune responses and ultimately broaden protection. Cats that are not exposed to field strains, such as isolated indoor cats, may be more susceptible to severe disease when hypervirulent strains appear. An adjuvanted, inactivated vaccine for VSD that contains a single hypervirulent strain was introduced in the United States in 2007. However, the degree to which this vaccine cross-protects against other hypervirulent strains is unknown, and outbreaks cease when infection control measures are implemented. Because of this and the increased risk of sarcoma formation with adjuvanted vaccines, the usefulness of the vaccine has been questioned.

Parenteral vaccines that contain FCV and FHV-1 are generally safe, although mild signs of URTD have the potential to occur if the cat licks the site of vaccination or aerosolization of vaccine occurs during administration. Intranasal vaccines are less well tolerated by cats and can be occasionally be followed by mild to moderate postvaccinal signs of URTD. This may be problematic in shelter environments where clinical signs of URTD warrant the need for separate housing. On the other hand, intranasal vaccines are advantageous in this situation because of rapid onset of immunity, with partial protection after 2 days and significant protection after 4 days.[15] They can also overcome maternal antibody at a young age, although some injectable vaccines may also still be effective at an early age. Because vaccine virus is propagated in feline kidney cells, there has been concern that parenteral administration of feline vaccines might lead to chronic renal inflammation when immune responses to vaccine components cross-react with endogenous renal antigens.[77] Further studies are required to determine whether this is clinically important.

Vaccine boosters are recommended 1 year after completion of the primary series, and at 3-yearly intervals thereafter in cats with low levels of exposure to respiratory viruses. For cats in contaminated environments such as catteries, boarding facilities, or large multicat households with frequent introductions, annual vaccination may be more appropriate. The duration of immunity after vaccination remains incompletely understood. Although partial protection persists for several years after vaccination,[78] the degree of protection does wane with time, at least for cats that receive no natural boostering in the interim (i.e., from exposure to field virus). In one report, relative FHV-1 and FCV vaccine efficacies were 95% and 85%, respectively, when challenge occurred a few weeks after primary vaccination with an inactivated vaccine.[79] This compared with 52% and 63%, respectively, when challenge occurred after 7.5 years.[80] In another study, a 50% reduction in clinical scores occurred after challenge 1 year after administration of an attenuated live FHV-1 vaccine, compared with around 75% after challenge 4 weeks after vaccination.[81] Similar results were observed for an inactivated FCV vaccine. In the field, natural boostering as a result of contact with virus shed by other cats or subclinical reactivation may maintain immunity for longer periods of time.

Prevention

In addition to vaccination, reduction of stress and overcrowding is critical for prevention of URTD, especially that due to FHV-1. Proper hand washing and disinfection in shelters, boarding facilities, and veterinary hospitals to prevent fomite transmission is also very important, and dedicated food and water bowls should be used. Inactivation of FCV requires the use of disinfectants such as sodium hypochlorite (household bleach diluted 1:30), potassium peroxymonosulfate (Trifectant, Virkon S), or accelerated hydrogen peroxide. Veterinarians should remember that all cats, whether apparently healthy or sick, can be a source of FHV-1 or FCV infection, and cats examined for routine vaccination purposes may be susceptible to nosocomial infection with these viruses. Cats should be housed individually (unless they are from the same household and tolerate close proximity to one another). Barriers between cats should be impermeable, and cats with URTD should be separated by at least 4 to 5 feet to prevent aerosol transmission. If possible, cats that enter large multicat environments and shelters should be quarantined for 3 weeks to identify cats that are incubating disease. When all other control measures fail in breeding catteries, early weaning and isolation of kittens from 4 weeks could be considered.

In regions where highly pathogenic H5N1 avian influenza virus infections have been identified in birds, cats should be kept indoors. Restriction zones defined for this purpose consist of an area within a 10-km radius of an outbreak of influenza in birds for 30 days after the discovery of infected birds.[36] Cats should also not be fed raw poultry. Separation of cats from avian species in shelters and hospital situations should be maintained.

Public Health Aspects

FHV-1 and FCV do not infect humans. Although cats can acquire influenza virus infections from humans, the risk of transmission from cats back to humans is unknown. Nevertheless, cats suspected to have influenza virus infections (such as during a recognized outbreak) should be isolated, the handling of these cats should be minimized, and appropriate protective attire should be worn, which should ideally include properly fitted high-density surgical masks.

CASE EXAMPLE

Signalment: "Boris", a 7-year-old male neutered Burmese cat from northern California.

History: Boris was brought to the University of California, Davis, Veterinary Medical Teaching Hospital for a 3-day history of inappetence, head-shaking, gagging, hypersalivation, coughing, and sneezing. The gagging occurred throughout the day and occasionally was followed by vomiting. The vomit consisted of bile-stained fluid. Boris had not been drinking. He was taken to a local emergency clinic where bilateral serous nasal discharge was noted, and he was treated for 24 hours with intravenous crystalloid fluids and amoxicillin. Blood work showed hypokalemia (4.0 mEq/L, reference range 4.5 to 5.3 mEq/L), hyperglycemia (292 mg/dL, reference range 70 to 150 mg/dL), neutrophilia (12,920 cells/μL, reference range 2500 to 12,500) and lymphopenia (136, reference range 1500 to 7000). FeLV and FIV serology was negative. A urinalysis showed a specific gravity of 1.050, pH of 7, and 1+ proteinuria and glucosuria. Lateral and dorsoventral radiographs of the thorax and abdomen showed moderate to severe gas distention of the proximal esophagus and stomach. Profuse salivation and gagging continued, and he was referred to a specialty clinic because of concerns for a possible gastrointestinal foreign body. There had been no diarrhea, no history of travel or trauma, and no recent surgical procedures. A new indoor plant was brought into the house 2 days before the onset of clinical signs. He was last immunized for FHV-1, FCV, FPV, and rabies 1 year previously. Boris was housed completely indoors and was exposed to one other cat that only occasionally had access to the outdoors. His diet consisted of a commercial dry cat food.

Physical Examination:

Body Weight: 4.8 kg

General: Lethargic, but responsive, 5% to 7% dehydrated. Held head extended and gagged and hypersalivated throughout the examination; seemed unable to swallow. Vomited bile-stained fluid once during the examination. T = 100.8°F (38.2°C), HR >240 beats/min, respiratory rate = 24 breaths/min, mucous membranes pink, CRT = 1 s. The cat's haircoat was unkempt.

Eyes, Ears, Nose, and Throat: Bilateral serous nasal discharge was present. A linear ulcer was identified on the right lateral aspect of the tongue.

Musculoskeletal: Body condition score 4/9. Ambulatory.

Cardiovascular and Respiratory: Other than tachycardia, no other abnormalities were detected.

Gastrointestinal and Genitourinary: Mild abdominal distention was present.

Lymph Nodes: All lymph nodes were < 1 cm in diameter.

Laboratory Findings:

CBC:

HCT 34.2% (30%-50%)
MCV 51.0 fL (42-53 fL)
MCHC 32.5 g/dL (30-33.5 g/dL)
WBC 12,600 cells/μL (4500-14,000 cells/μL)
Neutrophils 11,844 cells/μL (2000-9000 cells/μL)

Band neutrophils 126 cells/μL
Lymphocytes 126 cells/μL (1000-7000 cells/μL)
Monocytes 252 cells/μL (50-600 cells/μL)
Eosinophils 126 cells/μL (150-1100 cells/μL)
Platelets 989,000 platelets/μL (180,000-500,000 platelets/μL). The neutrophils showed slight toxicity, and there were a few Heinz bodies

Serum Chemistry Profile:
Sodium 141 mmol/L (151-158 mmol/L)
Potassium 4.0 mmol/L (3.6-4.9 mmol/L)
Chloride 108 mmol/L (117-126 mmol/L)
Bicarbonate 27 mmol/L (15-21 mmol/L)
Phosphorus 4.5 mg/dL (3.2-6.3 mg/dL)
Calcium 8.1 mg/dL (9.0-10.9 mg/dl)
BUN 21 mg/dL (18-33 mg/dL)
Creatinine 1.1 mg/dL (1.1-2.2 mg/dL)
Glucose 212 mg/dL (63-118 mg/dL)
Total protein 5.1 g/dL (6.6-8.4 g/dL)
Albumin 2.2 g/dL (2.2-4.6 g/dL)
Globulin 2.9 g/dL (2.8-5.4 g/dL)
ALT 83 U/L (27-101 U/L)
AST 50 U/L (17-58 U/L)
ALP 16 U/L (14-71 U/L)
Cholesterol 147 mg/dL (89-258 mg/dL)
Total bilirubin 0 mg/dL (0-0.2 mg/dL)

Endoscopy: Boris was anesthetized and an oral examination performed, which showed only mild dorsal pharyngeal lymphoid hyperplasia. Rhinoscopy showed a moderate amount of mucus and mild diffuse erythema of the nasal mucosa. Gastroduodenoscopy revealed focal areas of gastric erosion with hemorrhage.

Treatment: Boris was treated with IV crystalloid fluids (LRS with 20 mEq/L KCl at 20 mL/h), ampicillin (23 mg/kg IV q8h), enrofloxacin (2.6 mg/kg IV q24h), sucralfate (0.25 g PO q8h), and famotidine (0.25 mg/kg IV q12h). He continued to hypersalivate, and he vomited approximately 100 mL of fluid twice daily. After the first day of hospitalization, the owners reported that their other cat had developed signs of URTD, with sneezing and nasal discharge. Enteral or parenteral nutrition was discussed with the owner, but on the evening of the second day of hospitalization, Boris was found gagging and cyanotic. He was taken to the intensive care unit but developed cardiorespiratory arrest. CPR was instituted and tracheal suction revealed yellow fluid consistent with possible aspiration. Although CPR was initially successful, Boris arrested again and died shortly afterward.

Necropsy Examination: Gross necropsy examination showed numerous lingual ulcerations, mostly pinpoint but some coalescing into larger ulcers up to 1 cm long and 0.5 cm wide. Both lungs were diffusely dark red, poorly collapsed, and oozed large amounts of clear fluid on cut surface. There was a small amount of yellow ascites fluid. Histopathology revealed marked, multifocal, acute to subacute necrotizing stomatitis, rhinitis, tracheitis, bronchiolitis, and alveolitis with intranuclear herpesviral inclusions in the bronchiolar epithelium. Immunofluorescent antibody testing on lung tissue was positive for FHV-1. Virus isolation was negative. Histopathology of gastrointestinal biopsies collected at endoscopy and tissues collected at necropsy was unremarkable.

Comments: This cat died of a severe and overwhelming FHV-1 infection, despite the fact that he was an adult cat that had been vaccinated regularly. Clinical signs of anorexia, gagging and hypersalivation likely resulted from stomatitis, pharyngitis, and tracheitis. Histopathology with immunofluorescent antibody staining confirmed the involvement of FHV-1. The negative virus isolation result may have been because of an insufficient sample size, inactivation of virus by antibody, or lack of viable virus in the specimen. Because FHV-1 survives poorly in the environment, it may deteriorate in clinical specimens during transport to the laboratory.

SUGGESTED READINGS

Ali A, Daniels JB, Zhang Y, et al. Pandemic and seasonal human influenza virus infections in domestic cats: Prevalence, association with respiratory disease, and seasonality pattern. J Clin Microbiol. 2011;49:4101-4105.

Gaskell R, Dawson S, Radford A, et al. Feline herpesvirus. Vet Res. 2007;38:337-354.

Marschall J, Hartmann K. Avian influenza A H5N1 infections in cats. J Feline Med Surg. 2008;10:359-365.

Radford AD, Coyne KP, Dawson S, et al. Feline calicivirus. Vet Res. 2007;38:319-335.

REFERENCES

1. Crandell RA, Maurer FD. Isolation of a feline virus associated with intranuclear inclusion bodies. Proc Soc Exp Biol Med. 1958;97:487-490.
2. Fastier LB. A new feline virus isolated in tissue culture. Am J Vet Res. 1957;18:382-389.
3. Songserm T, Amonsin A, Jam-on R, et al. Avian influenza H5N1 in naturally infected domestic cat. Emerg Infect Dis. 2006;12:681-683.
4. Sponseller BA, Strait E, Jergens A, et al. Influenza A pandemic (H1N1) 2009 virus infection in domestic cat. Emerg Infect Dis. 2010;16:534-537.
5. Helps CR, Lait P, Damhuis A, et al. Factors associated with upper respiratory tract disease caused by feline herpesvirus, feline calicivirus, *Chlamydophila felis* and *Bordetella bronchiseptica* in cats: experience from 218 European catteries. Vet Rec. 2005;156:669-673.
6. Hamano M, Maeda K, Mizukoshi F, et al. Experimental infection of recent field isolates of feline herpesvirus type 1. J Vet Med Sci. 2003;65:939-943.
7. Veir JK, Ruch-Gallie R, Spindel ME, et al. Prevalence of selected infectious organisms and comparison of two anatomic sampling sites in shelter cats with upper respiratory tract disease. J Feline Med Surg. 2008;10:551-557.
8. Bech-Nielsen S, Fulton RW, Cox HU, et al. Feline respiratory tract disease in Louisiana. Am J Vet Res. 1980;41:1293-1298.
9. Ellis TM. Feline respiratory virus carriers in clinically healthy cats. Aust Vet J. 1981;57:115-118.
10. Harbour DA, Howard PE, Gaskell RM. Isolation of feline calicivirus and feline herpesvirus from domestic cats 1980 to 1989. Vet Rec. 1991;128:77-80.
11. Shewen PE, Povey RC, Wilson MR. A survey of the conjunctival flora of clinically normal cats and cats with conjunctivitis. Can Vet J. 1980;21:231-233.
12. Wardley RC, Gaskell RM, Povey RC. Feline respiratory viruses—their prevalence in clinically healthy cats. J Small Anim Pract. 1974;15:579-586.

13. Coutts AJ, Dawson S, Willoughby K, et al. Isolation of feline respiratory viruses from clinically healthy cats at UK cat shows. Vet Rec. 1994;135:555-556.
14. Ruch-Gallie RA, Veir JK, Hawley JR, et al. Results of molecular diagnostic assays targeting feline herpesvirus-1 and feline calicivirus in adult cats administered modified live vaccines. J Feline Med Surg. 2011;13:541-545.
15. Gaskell R, Dawson S, Radford A, et al. Feline herpesvirus. Vet Res. 2007;38:337-354.
16. Gaskell RM, Povey RC. Re-excretion of feline viral rhinotracheitis virus following corticosteroid treatment. Vet Rec. 1973;93:204-205.
17. Gaskell RM, Povey RC. Experimental induction of feline viral rhinotracheitis virus re-excretion in FVR-recovered cats. Vet Rec. 1977;100:128-133.
18. Gaskell RM, Povey RC. Transmission of feline viral rhinotracheitis. Vet Rec. 1982;111:359-362.
19. Di Martino B, Di Rocco C, Ceci C, et al. Characterization of a strain of feline calicivirus isolated from a dog faecal sample. Vet Microbiol. 2009;139:52-57.
20. Radford AD, Turner PC, Bennett M, et al. Quasispecies evolution of a hypervariable region of the feline calicivirus capsid gene in cell culture and in persistently infected cats. J Gen Virol. 1998;79 (Pt 1):1-10.
21. Wardley RC. Feline calicivirus carrier state. A study of the host/virus relationship. Arch Virol. 1976;52:243-249.
22. Di Martino B, Ceci C, Di Profio F, et al. In vitro inactivation of feline calicivirus (FCV) by chemical disinfectants: resistance variation among field strains. Arch Virol. 2010;155:2047-2051.
23. Doultree JC, Druce JD, Birch CJ, et al. Inactivation of feline calicivirus, a Norwalk virus surrogate. J Hosp Infect. 1999;41:51-57.
24. Smid B, Valicek L, Rodak L, et al. Rabbit haemorrhagic disease: an investigation of some properties of the virus and evaluation of an inactivated vaccine. Vet Microbiol. 1991;26:77-85.
25. Mencke N, Vobis M, Mehlhorn H, et al. Transmission of feline calicivirus via the cat flea (*Ctenocephalides felis*). Parasitol Res. 2009;105:185-189.
26. Hurley KE, Pesavento PA, Pedersen NC, et al. An outbreak of virulent systemic feline calicivirus disease. J Am Vet Med Assoc. 2004;224:241-249.
27. Pedersen NC, Elliott JB, Glasgow A, et al. An isolated epizootic of hemorrhagic-like fever in cats caused by a novel and highly virulent strain of feline calicivirus. Vet Microbiol. 2000;73:281-300.
28. Reynolds BS, Poulet H, Pingret JL, et al. A nosocomial outbreak of feline calicivirus associated virulent systemic disease in France. J Feline Med Surg. 2009;11:633-644.
29. Schulz BS, Hartmann K, Unterer S, et al. Two outbreaks of virulent systemic feline calicivirus infection in cats in Germany. Berl Munch Tierarztl Wochenschr. 2011;124:186-193.
30. Radford AD, Gaskell RM. Dealing with a potential case of FCV-associated virulent systemic disease. Vet Rec. 2011;168:585-586.
31. Coyne KP, Jones BR, Kipar A, et al. Lethal outbreak of disease associated with feline calicivirus infection in cats. Vet Rec. 2006;158:544-550.
32. Meyer A, Kershaw O, Klopfleisch R. Feline calicivirus-associated virulent systemic disease: not necessarily a local epizootic problem. Vet Rec. 2011;168:589.
33. Lohr CV, DeBess EE, Baker RJ, et al. Pathology and viral antigen distribution of lethal pneumonia in domestic cats due to pandemic (H1N1) 2009 influenza A virus. Vet Pathol. 2010;47:378-386.
34. Fiorentini L, Taddei R, Moreno A, et al. Influenza A pandemic (H1N1) 2009 virus outbreak in a cat colony in Italy. Zoonoses Public Health. 2011;58:573-581.
35. Ali A, Daniels JB, Zhang Y, et al. Pandemic and seasonal human influenza virus infections in domestic cats: prevalence, association with respiratory disease, and seasonality patterns. J Clin Microbiol. 2011;49:4101-4105.
36. Marschall J, Hartmann K. Avian influenza A H5N1 infections in cats. J Feline Med Surg. 2008;10:359-365.
37. Kuiken T, Rimmelzwaan G, van Riel D, et al. Avian H5N1 influenza in cats. Science. 2004;306:241.
38. Rimmelzwaan GF, van Riel D, Baars M, et al. Influenza A virus (H5N1) infection in cats causes systemic disease with potential novel routes of virus spread within and between hosts. Am J Pathol. 2006;168:176-183;quiz 364.
39. Klopfleisch R, Wolf PU, Uhl W, et al. Distribution of lesions and antigen of highly pathogenic avian influenza virus A/Swan/Germany/R65/06 (H5N1) in domestic cats after presumptive infection by wild birds. Vet Pathol. 2007;44:261-268.
40. Leschnik M, Weikel J, Mostl K, et al. Subclinical infection with avian influenza A (H5N1) virus in cats. Emerg Infect Dis. 2007;13:243-247.
41. Marschall J, Schulz B, Harder Priv-Doz TC, et al. Prevalence of influenza A H5N1 virus in cats from areas with occurrence of highly pathogenic avian influenza in birds. J Feline Med Surg. 2008;10:355-358.
42. Song DS, An DJ, Moon HJ, et al. Interspecies transmission of the canine influenza H3N2 virus to domestic cats in South Korea, 2010. J Gen Virol. 2011;92:2350-2355.
43. Harder TC, Vahlenkamp TW. Influenza virus infections in dogs and cats. Vet Immunol Immunopathol. 2010;134:54-60.
44. van Riel D, Rimmelzwaan GF, van Amerongen G, et al. Highly pathogenic avian influenza virus H7N7 isolated from a fatal human case causes respiratory disease in cats but does not spread systemically. Am J Pathol. 2010;177:2185-2190.
45. Ali A, Daniels JB, Zhang Y, et al. Pandemic and seasonal human influenza virus infections in domestic cats: Prevalence, association with respiratory disease, and seasonality pattern. J Clin Microbiol. 2011;49:4101-4105.
46. Nasisse MP, Guy JS, Davidson MG, et al. Experimental ocular herpesvirus infection in the cat. Sites of virus replication, clinical features and effects of corticosteroid administration. Invest Ophthalmol Vis Sci. 1989;30:1758-1768.
47. van den Brand JM, Stittelaar KJ, van Amerongen G, et al. Experimental pandemic (H1N1) 2009 virus infection of cats. Emerg Infect Dis. 2010;16:1745-1747.
48. Volopich S, Benetka V, Schwendenwein I, et al. Cytologic findings, and feline herpesvirus DNA and *Chlamydophila felis* antigen detection rates in normal cats and cats with conjunctival and corneal lesions. Vet Ophthalmol. 2005;8:25-32.
49. Sanchez MD, Goldschmidt MH, Mauldin EA. Herpesvirus dermatitis in two cats without facial lesions. Vet Dermatol. 2012;23:171-173, e135.
50. Radford AD, Addie D, Belak S, et al. Feline calicivirus infection. ABCD guidelines on prevention and management. J Feline Med Surg. 2009;11:556-564.
51. Belgard S, Truyen U, Thibault JC, et al. Relevance of feline calicivirus, feline immunodeficiency virus, feline leukemia virus, feline herpesvirus and *Bartonella henselae* in cats with chronic gingivostomatitis. Berl Munch Tierarztl Wochenschr. 2010;123:369-376.
52. Dowers KL, Hawley JR, Brewer MM, et al. Association of *Bartonella* species, feline calicivirus, and feline herpesvirus 1 infection with gingivostomatitis in cats. J Feline Med Surg. 2010;12:314-321.
53. Hennet PR, Camy GA, McGahie DM, et al. Comparative efficacy of a recombinant feline interferon omega in refractory cases of calicivirus-positive cats with caudal stomatitis: a randomised, multicentre, controlled, double-blind study in 39 cats. J Feline Med Surg. 2011;13:577-587.
54. Pesavento PA, Stokol T, Liu H, et al. Distribution of the feline calicivirus receptor junctional adhesion molecule A in feline tissues. Vet Pathol. 2011;48:361-368.
55. Lee M, Bosward KL, Norris JM. Immunohistological evaluation of feline herpesvirus-1 infection in feline eosinophilic dermatoses or stomatitis. J Feline Med Surg. 2010;12:72-79.
56. Marschall J, Schulz B, Hartmann K. Evaluation of a point-of-care influenza antigen test for the detection of highly pathogenic avian influenza H5N1 virus in cats. Transbound Emerg Dis. 2008;55:315-317.

57. Crawford C, Spindel M. Canine influenza. In: Miller L, Hurley K, eds. Infectious Disease Management in Animal Shelters. Ames, IA: Wiley-Blackwell; 2009:173-180.
58. Storey ES, Gerding PA, Scherba G, et al. Survival of equine herpesvirus-4, feline herpesvirus-1, and feline calicivirus in multidose ophthalmic solutions. Vet Ophthalmol. 2002;5:263-267.
59. Burgesser KM, Hotaling S, Schiebel A, et al. Comparison of PCR, virus isolation, and indirect fluorescent antibody staining in the detection of naturally occurring feline herpesvirus infections. J Vet Diagn Invest. 1999;11:122-126.
60. Goldschmidt P, Rostane H, Saint-Jean C, et al. Effects of topical anaesthetics and fluorescein on the real-time PCR used for the diagnosis of herpesviruses and *Acanthamoeba* keratitis. Br J Ophthalmol. 2006;90:1354-1356.
61. Segarra S, Papasouliotis K, Helps C. The in vitro effects of proxymetacaine, fluorescein, and fusidic acid on real-time PCR assays used for the diagnosis of feline herpesvirus-1 and *Chlamydophila felis* infections. Vet Ophthalmol. 2011;14(Suppl. 1):5-8.
62. Burns RE, Wagner DC, Leutenegger CM, et al. Histologic and molecular correlation in shelter cats with acute upper respiratory infection. J Clin Microbiol. 2011;49:2454-2460.
63. Malik R, Lessels NS, Webb S, et al. Treatment of feline herpesvirus-1 associated disease in cats with famciclovir and related drugs. J Feline Med Surg. 2009;11:40-48.
64. Thomasy SM, Lim CC, Reilly CM, et al. Evaluation of orally administered famciclovir in cats experimentally infected with feline herpesvirus type-1. Am J Vet Res. 2011;72:85-95.
64a. Lim CC, Reilly CM, Thomasy SM, et al. Effects of feline herpesvirus type 1 on tear film break-up time, Schirmer tear test results, and conjunctival goblet cell density in experimentally infected cats. Am J Vet Res. 2009;70:394-403.
65. Fontenelle JP, Powell CC, Veir JK, et al. Effect of topical ophthalmic application of cidofovir on experimentally induced primary ocular feline herpesvirus-1 infection in cats. Am J Vet Res. 2008;69:289-293.
66. Cocker FM, Howard PE, Harbour DA. Effect of human alpha-hybrid interferon on the course of feline viral rhinotracheitis. Vet Rec. 1987;120:391-393.
67. Stiles J, Townsend WM, Rogers QR, et al. Effect of oral administration of L-lysine on conjunctivitis caused by feline herpesvirus in cats. Am J Vet Res. 2002;63:99-103.
68. Maggs DJ, Nasisse MP, Kass PH. Efficacy of oral supplementation with L-lysine in cats latently infected with feline herpesvirus. Am J Vet Res. 2003;64:37-42.
69. Rees TM, Lubinski JL. Oral supplementation with L-lysine did not prevent upper respiratory infection in a shelter population of cats. J Feline Med Surg. 2008;10:510-513.
70. Drazenovich TL, Fascetti AJ, Westermeyer HD, et al. Effects of dietary lysine supplementation on upper respiratory and ocular disease and detection of infectious organisms in cats within an animal shelter. Am J Vet Res. 2009;70(11):1391-1400.
71. Thanawongnuwech R, Amonsin A, Tantilertcharoen R, et al. Probable tiger-to-tiger transmission of avian influenza H5N1. Emerg Infect Dis. 2005;11:699-701.
72. Sykes JE, Browning GF, Anderson G, et al. Differential sensitivity of culture and the polymerase chain reaction for detection of feline herpesvirus 1 in vaccinated and unvaccinated cats. Arch Virol. 1997;142:65-74.
73. Sussman MD, Maes RK, Kruger JM. Vaccination of cats for feline rhinotracheitis results in a quantitative reduction of virulent feline herpesvirus-1 latency load after challenge. Virology. 1997;228:379-382.
74. Kahn DE, Hoover EA, Bittle JL. Induction of immunity to feline caliciviral disease. Infect Immun. 1975;11:1003-1009.
75. Porter CJ, Radford AD, Gaskell RM, et al. Comparison of the ability of feline calicivirus (FCV) vaccines to neutralise a panel of current UK FCV isolates. J Feline Med Surg. 2008;10:32-40.
76. Poulet H, Brunet S, Leroy V, et al. Immunisation with a combination of two complementary feline calicivirus strains induces a broad cross-protection against heterologous challenges. Vet Microbiol. 2005;106:17-31.
77. Whittemore JC, Hawley JR, Jensen WA, et al. Antibodies against Crandell Rees feline kidney (CRFK) cell line antigens, alpha-enolase, and annexin A2 in vaccinated and CRFK hyperinoculated cats. J Vet Intern Med. 2010;24:306-313.
78. Gore TC, Lakshmanan N, Williams JR, et al. Three-year duration of immunity in cats following vaccination against feline rhinotracheitis virus, feline calicivirus, and feline panleukopenia virus. Vet Ther. 2006;7:213-222.
79. Povey RC, Koonse H, Hays MB. Immunogenicity and safety of an inactivated vaccine for the prevention of rhinotracheitis, caliciviral disease, and panleukopenia in cats. J Am Vet Med Assoc. 1980;177:347-350.
80. Scott FW, Geissinger CM. Long-term immunity in cats vaccinated with an inactivated trivalent vaccine. Am J Vet Res. 1999;60:652-658.
81. Poulet H. Alternative early life vaccination programs for companion animals. J Comp Pathol. 2007;137(Suppl. 1):S67-S71.

CHAPTER 24

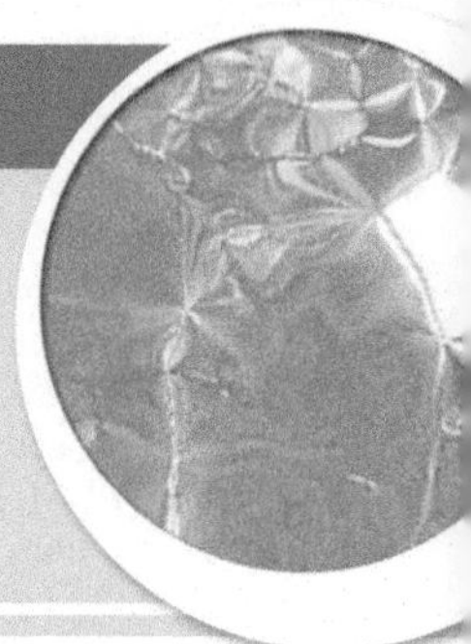

Feline Poxvirus Infections

Malcolm Bennett

Overview of Feline Poxvirus Infections

First Described: Feline poxvirus infection was first described in 1978[1]

Causes: Poxviruses (family Poxviridae). Cowpox virus infection is by far the most frequently reported poxviral infection of both cats and dogs. Other poxvirus infections, including parapoxvirus (assumed to be orf virus) and raccoonpox virus infections, have also been described in pets. Other poxviruses are also likely to infect cats and dogs but go unreported.

Affected Hosts: Cats, less often dogs, and a variety of other mammalian host species

Geographic Distribution: Cowpox virus is limited to Europe and Asia. Infections with other poxviruses have been described in North America.

Mode of Transmission: Entry through a break in the skin

Major Clinical Signs: Single or multiple, papular, and crusted skin lesions. Fever, lethargy, inappetence, and signs of pneumonia can also occur in affected cats.

Differential Diagnoses: Allergic dermatitis, facial dermatitis caused by feline herpesvirus-1, nocardiosis, mycobacteriosis, cutaneous lymphoma, autoimmune dermatoses such as pemphigus foliaceus, cutaneous drug reactions

Human Health Significance: Many poxviruses, including cowpox and orf viruses, are zoonotic, and owners of affected animals need to be advised of the threat to their health.

Etiology and Epidemiology

Cowpox Virus

Cowpox virus is a member of the *Orthopoxvirus* genus within the family Poxviridae, which are large, enveloped, double-stranded DNA viruses.[2] Other orthopoxviruses include the viruses of smallpox (now eradicated), vaccinia (the smallpox vaccine), monkeypox (which is endemic to central Africa but was recently introduced to, and eradicated from, North America), and a range of other mammalian orthopoxviruses. All orthopoxviruses are closely related genetically and antigenically; therefore, vaccinia virus can be used to immunize against all orthopoxvirus infections. Cowpox virus has the largest genome of all the orthopoxviruses. Different strains of cowpox virus exist, as determined by both biologic characteristics and nucleotide sequence. Whether these merely reflect geographic variation of the virus (and therefore its main hosts and pathogenicity) or a range of independent virus species is still to be determined. For the purpose of this account, however, they are regarded as a single viral species.

Despite its name, cowpox is rarely described in cattle; cowpox virus circulates primarily in wild rodents. It has a wide host range that includes not only rodents, cats, dogs, cattle, and human beings, but a variety of captive wildlife mammals. The main route of transmission among rodents is not known, although, as for many orthopoxviruses, the respiratory route is probably important. In most accidental hosts, which include domestic animals and human beings, the most frequent source of infection is through a break in the skin. This gives rise to the "primary" lesion. The main reservoirs of cowpox virus are voles and, to a slightly lesser extent, *Apodemus* mice. As these rodent species undergo annual population cycles, breeding mainly in the summer and fall months, viral transmission and prevalence has strong seasonality. Transmission to accidental hosts such as cats, dogs, people, and zoo animals therefore also occurs mainly (but not exclusively) in the late summer, fall, and early winter. Cats probably become infected directly from rodent hunting, whereas infection in other species is often acquired from a "liaison" or "amplifying" host. These are accidental hosts in which the virus replicates to higher titers than in the reservoir rodent hosts; thus they bridge the epidemiologic gap between the reservoir and the host of interest. The main liaison hosts for human cowpox are the domestic cat (and, in the past, possibly cattle), followed by peridomestic rodent species such as rats. Rats can also be a source of infection for captive wildlife species. The virus is very hardy and survives in scabs for weeks or months, including in the environment, where it may be a source of human infection.

Raccoonpox Virus

Raccoonpox virus is also an orthopoxvirus. Remarkably little is known about its epidemiology, or indeed about the other known North American orthopoxviruses, skunkpox, and volepox viruses, which together form a distinct clade. Raccoonpox virus appears to be fairly host specific but was isolated from a cat with cowpox-like disease in Canada.[3]

Raccoonpox virus was originally isolated from the lungs of apparently healthy raccoons in the northeastern United States, and serologic surveys in the same area suggested that more than 20% of wild raccoons had antibody to the virus. Experimental infection of raccoons also caused no obvious disease.[4] The narrow host range, low zoonotic and pathogenic potential, and endemicity of raccoonpox virus to North America has led to its development as a vector for recombinant vaccines for use in American wildlife species.

Parapoxviruses

The parapoxviruses comprise a different genus from the orthopoxviruses in the family Poxviridae. Parapoxviruses are genetically very similar to each other (but significantly different antigenically and genetically from the orthopoxviruses), and differentiation of individual species is difficult.[5] Parapoxvirus infections have been described in cats in several countries, and when characterized, the causative virus has been shown to be orf virus.[6] Orf occurs worldwide, mainly in sheep and goats, and is readily transmissible to human beings.

Parapoxviruses, like many other poxviruses, survive in the environment for long periods—possibly months or even years under the right conditions. So although cats can become infected through direct contact with sheep or goats, it is more likely that infection occurs through contact with a contaminated fomite—perhaps a piece of barbed wire or fencing that contacts a preexisting wound. The rarity of parapoxvirus infection in cats makes its study very difficult.

Clinical Features

Signs and Their Pathogenesis

Cowpox Virus

In many hosts, such as human beings, dogs, and cattle, the primary lesion of cowpox virus infection, plus perhaps some virus replication in draining lymph nodes, may be as far as disease progresses. In cats and many captive wild mammalian species, however, the virus replicates in monocytes and macrophages and spreads to multiple organs, particularly the lungs and the spleen. Here, the virus replicates further, giving rise to a secondary viremia, which is often associated with pyrexia and mild or occasionally severe systemic signs. Pneumonia can itself be fatal, but usually the secondary viremia leads to a "secondary rash" of lesions distributed across the skin and mucosae.

The signs of cowpox vary according to the host species. The classical presentation in cats is of a primary skin lesion, often with secondary bacterial infection, usually on a forelimb or the face, thought to arise from the inoculation of virus into a wound—perhaps a bite wound—while hunting infected wild rodents. In some cases, severe necrotizing facial dermatitis develops. The primary lesion may be followed by lethargy and possibly pyrexia for up to 10 days, after which multifocal skin lesions appear. These first develop as papules (Figure 24-1), which become ulcers up to 1-cm in diameter that crust over and heal over 4 to 6 weeks. This leaves small patches of alopecia until the hair regrows. In cats such as Siamese, the hair can grow back a darker color, and scars are often visible for years in cats if their hair is clipped. Infection of dogs is less common, and in dogs, lesions are usually more localized and the systemic disease much less severe.[6-8]

In many captive wild Felidae, pneumonia is more common than in domestic cats, and mortality is high. Similarly, elephants and rhinoceroses in central European zoos develop severe systemic disease and often die—indeed, this can be such a severe disease that many European zoological parks vaccinate their elephants. There are few reports of fatal cowpox in captive primates,[9] but there are anecdotal reports of high rates of subclinical seroconversion in other primate populations. Other affected zoo-kept species include giant anteater, beavers, okapi, banded mongoose, jaguarondi, and the cavy. In wild rodent reservoir hosts, clinical signs are absent or, at least, subtle. Population-level studies of naturally infected voles and mice show that infection may be associated with decreased fecundity and decreased survival.[10] When lesions are seen in rodents, they are often in "accidental" rodent hosts such as rats.

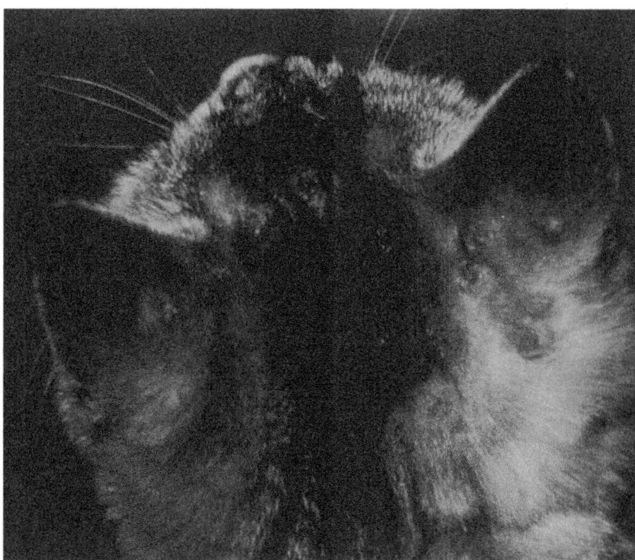

FIGURE 24-1 Secondary papules and crusted skin lesions in a cat with cowpox virus infection.

Other Poxviruses

Raccoonpox has only been reported once in a domestic cat,[3] in which it caused a disease that resembled the primary lesion of cowpox. The cat was initially evaluated for a swollen, crusty lesion on a thoracic limb digit, and 4 weeks later infection of the neighboring digit developed. Widespread secondary lesions did not develop, and the cat recovered completely. Human infection with a raccoonpox recombinant vaccine led to a single lesion on the inoculated finger, which became swollen and painful and was accompanied by axillary lymphadenopathy. Complete recovery occurred within 4 weeks.

Parapoxvirus infections have been described in cats in the United Kingdom and New Zealand.[5,10] The British cat developed multiple crusted lesions on its face and dorsum that healed within a few weeks. Two cats from farms in New Zealand had more severe clinical signs. One had a recurrent lesion on the paw of a pelvic limb. The other had a nonhealing lesion on the paw of a thoracic limb that progressed, despite surgery, over four months. Both cats were euthanized.

Diagnosis

Definitive diagnosis of poxvirus infections requires laboratory identification of the causative virus. In Europe, where cowpox virus is endemic, clinical signs combined with identification of an orthopoxvirus probably suffice to make a diagnosis. Elsewhere, however, more extensive laboratory tests are required to identify the causative virus more precisely.

Microbiologic Tests

Diagnostic assays available for poxvirus infections are shown in Table 24-1.

Cell Culture

The best specimens to collect for virus isolation are fresh skin lesions, although virus can be found in crusts from healing lesions for several weeks.[11] No special transport media are

TABLE 24-1

Diagnostic Assays Available for Poxvirus Infections

Assay	Specimen Type	Target	Performance
Virus isolation	Skin biopsies, crusts	Poxviruses	May not be widely available in some regions. Sensitive for diagnosis of orthopoxviruses, but parapoxviruses are difficult to culture.
Polymerase chain reaction (PCR)	Skin biopsies, crusts	Poxvirus DNA	Sensitivity and specificity may vary depending on assay design; assays may not differentiate between orthopoxviruses. Availability on a commercial basis may be limited in some regions. Assays for parapoxviruses are not widely available.
Histopathology	Skin biopsies, necropsy specimens	Poxvirus inclusions	Histopathology is similar for cowpox virus and raccoonpox virus. Confirmation of poxvirus infection requires immunohistochemistry or PCR.
Electron microscopy	Skin crusts	Virus particles	May not be widely available, turnaround time can be slow, and may be expensive. Orthopoxviruses and parapoxviruses can be differentiated based on their morphology.

needed. Lesions can be placed into a dry container for shipping to the laboratory at room temperature. The virus replicates in a variety of cell lines, in which it causes an obvious cytopathic effect (CPE) that resembles that of feline herpesvirus-1. Unlike most feline viruses, however, cowpox virus grows easily in cell lines derived from other mammalian species, including primates. Lesion material is ground or finely chopped and freeze-thawed several times to release virus particles. CPE usually appears within 24 to 76 hours and comprises plaques of syncytia followed by rounding and loss of cells from the center of the plaque. Staining with hematoxylin and eosin reveals large, intracytoplasmic, eosinophilic inclusion bodies. Further confirmation can be by immunostaining (e.g., immunofluorescence) to identify the virus as an orthopoxvirus, or PCR assay and sequencing.

Although raccoonpox virus grows in a variety of cell lines, diagnosis is more likely to be made by histopathology and PCR assays. This is because the virus is unlikely to be suspected initially, and biopsy and histology would be the first response of most veterinarians. Parapoxviruses are notoriously difficult to grow in cell culture, requiring primary cell cultures.

Molecular Diagnosis Using the Polymerase Chain Reaction

Some diagnostic laboratories offer PCR assays for diagnosis of poxvirus infection, which can be both sensitive and, if combined with sequencing, specific. Orthopoxviruses are so similar genetically that PCRs targeted at many orthopoxvirus genes only identify orthopoxviruses to the genus level. PCRs that differentiate between orthopoxvirus species have been described, but such assays tend to be available through research or other specialist laboratories. Of course, in much of Europe, cowpox virus is the only orthopoxvirus known to infect cats and dogs, so identification to the species level is often not necessary. Unlike orthopoxviruses, for which worries over bioterrorism have led to the development of several sensitive and specific PCR assays, molecular assays for parapoxviruses are not widely available.

Direct Electron Microscopy

Electron microscopy of skin lesions is a more rapid approach to diagnosis than cell culture and is fairly sensitive. Negative-stained suspensions of skin lesion material allow typical orthopoxvirus particles to be seen in most cases (Figure 24-2). The diagnosis of parapoxvirus infection usually relies on electron microscopy and visualization of the characteristic parapoxvirus morphology, which resembles a "ball of yarn."

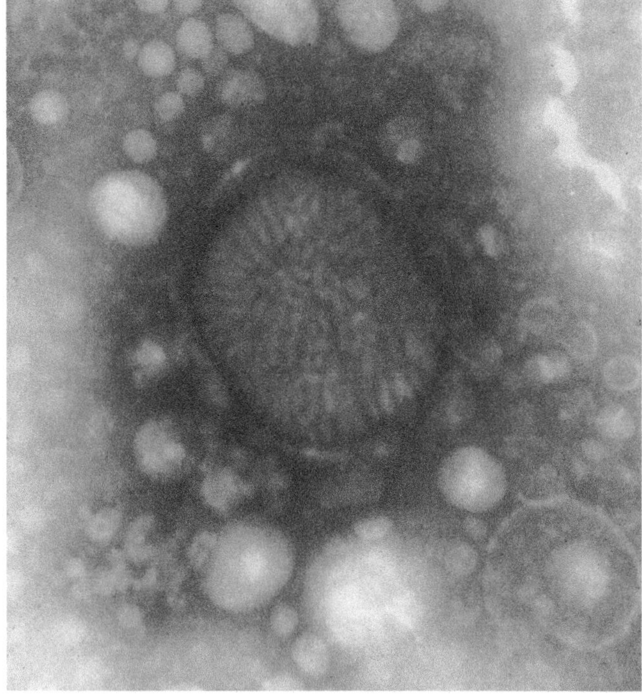

FIGURE 24-2 Electron micrograph of a cowpox virus particle. In contrast, parapoxviruses have the appearance of a new ball of yarn, with threadlike surface tubules arranged in a crisscross fashion.

Serologic Diagnosis

Previous cowpox virus infection can be diagnosed by various serologic assays including immunofluorescent antibody, ELISA, and virus neutralization assays. The prevalence of orthopoxvirus antibodies in domestic cats in Europe is usually only 1% to 2%, so a consistent clinical history combined with an antibody titer is reasonably specific.

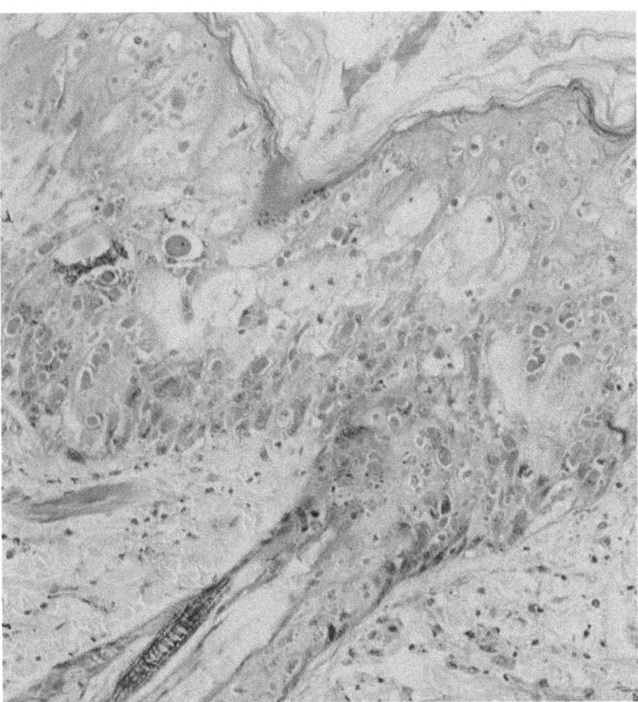

FIGURE 24-3 Histopathology of a feline poxvirus lesion that shows epithelial hyperplasia and large numbers of eosinophilic intracytoplasmic inclusion bodies.

Pathologic Findings

Many cases of cowpox in cats, dogs, and humans are diagnosed by histopathology.[6,12,13] The histology of cowpox is quite characteristic; the virus causes hyperplasia and hypertrophy of the epithelium, with infected cells often containing eosinophilic, intracytoplasmic inclusions that can be readily observed in routine hematoxylin and eosin–stained sections (Figure 24-3). These A-type inclusions comprise virus-encoded protein that forms a protective mass around newly formed virus particles. As the epithelium thickens, cells in the middle layers lyse, which gives rise to fluid-filled lacunae that, when large enough, can be seen with the naked eye as the vesicles (or pocks/pox) from which these viruses get their name. Usually the vesicles quickly ulcerate in cats. Older lesions undergo secondary bacterial infection and subsequent neutrophil infiltration before healing. Immunostaining is useful in histopathologic diagnosis, especially in older lesions or those with secondary bacterial infection.

The histopathology of raccoonpox resembles that of cowpox.[3] Hyperplastic, hypertrophic epithelium is present with eosinophilic, intracytoplasmic A-type inclusion bodies. Because North American orthopoxviruses are quite distinct from "old world" (Eurasian) orthopoxviruses, PCR assays and sequencing can readily characterize the virus, even from fixed material.[11]

Histologic examination of parapoxvirus lesions from the New Zealand cats revealed epithelial hyperplasia giving rise to multiple papillary projections from the skin surface, covered in a thick layer of compacted keratin.[5] Orf virus does not produce the A-type inclusions often seen with orthopoxviruses, but occasional basophilic or amphophilic inclusion bodies may be present (so-called B-type inclusions, which consist of condensed areas of virus replication).

Treatment and Prognosis

Treatment of poxvirus infections is supportive. There are no specific antiviral agents available. Most cats with cowpox recover completely, but some, particularly if immunosuppressed by concurrent infection or treatment with, for example, glucocorticoids, develop larger, persistent skin lesions, and/or pneumonia. Cats that develop pneumonia often die despite supportive care.

Prevention

Housing cats indoors should help to prevent poxvirus infection in cats. No vaccine is available. However, canarypox-vectored vaccines are used to prevent rabies virus and FeLV infection in cats and distemper in dogs.

Public Health Aspects

Cowpox virus infection in humans is usually limited to a skin lesion at the site of inoculation (often on the hand or face) accompanied by local lymphadenopathy and flu-like symptoms. The lesions can be painful, and an important differential diagnosis is cutaneous anthrax. In Europe, most human cases can be traced to contact with an infected cat; infection from rodents or dogs is a much less frequent event. Although most patients recover uneventfully, immunosuppression can lead to more extensive lesions and, rarely, even death.[12,14-16] Although thought not to be zoonotic, a recombinant raccoonpox vaccine caused lesions in a laboratory worker.[17] Orf is readily transmissible to humans, usually from contact with sheep and goats. Although transmission from an infected cat to a human being has not been reported, human orf associated with a cat scratch was reported from Utah in the United States.[13]

SUGGESTED READINGS

Fairley RA, Whelan EM, Pesavento PA, et al. Recurrent localised cutaneous parapoxvirus infection in three cats. N Z Vet J. 2008;56:196-201.

Glatz M, Richter S, Ginter-Hanselmayer G, et al. Human cowpox in a veterinary student. Lancet Infect Dis. 2010;10:288.

Yager JA, Hutchison L, Barrett JW. Raccoonpox in a Canadian cat. Vet Dermatol. 2006;17:443-448.

REFERENCES

1. Thomsett LR, Baxby D, Denham EM. Cowpox in the domestic cat. Vet Rec. 1978;103:567.
2. Bennett M, Smith GL, Baxby D. Cowpox virus. In: Mahy BWJ, Regenmortel MHVV, eds. Encyclopedia of Virology. 3rd ed. Oxford: Academic Press; 2008.
3. Yager JA, Hutchison L, Barrett JW. Raccoonpox in a Canadian cat. Vet Dermatol. 2006;17:443-448.
4. Thomas EK, Palmer EL, Obijeski JF, et al. Further characterization of Raccoonpox virus. Arch Virol. 1975;49:217-227.
5. Fairley RA, Whelan EM, Pesavento PA, et al. Recurrent localised cutaneous parapoxvirus infection in three cats. N Z Vet J. 2008;56:196-201.
6. Bennett M, Gaskell CJ, Gaskell RM, et al. Poxvirus infection in the domestic cat: some clinical and epidemiological observations. Vet Rec. 1986;118:387-390.
7. Kaysser P, von Bomhard W, Dobrzykowski L, et al. Genetic diversity of feline cowpox virus, Germany 2000-2008. Vet Microbiol. 2010;141:282-288.
8. von Bomhard W, Mauldin EA, Breuer W, et al. Localized cowpox infection in a 5-month-old Rottweiler. Vet Dermatol. 2011;22:111-114.

9. Girling SJ, Pizzi R, Cox A, et al. Fatal cowpox virus infection in two squirrel monkeys (*Saimiri sciureus*). Vet Rec. 2011;169:156.
10. Hamblet CN. Parapoxvirus in a cat. Vet Rec. 1993;132:144.
11. Bennett M, Baxby D, Gaskell RM, et al. The laboratory diagnosis of Orthopoxvirus infection in the domestic cat. J Small Anim Pract. 1985;26:653-661.
12. Baxby D, Bennett M, Getty B. Human cowpox 1969-93: a review based on 54 cases. Br J Dermatol. 1994;131:598-607.
13. Frandsen J, Enslow M, Bowen AR. Orf parapoxvirus infection from a cat scratch. Dermatol Online J. 2011;17:9.
14. Baxby D, Bennett M. Poxvirus zoonoses. J Med Microbiol. 1997;46:17-20:28-33.
15. Favier AL, Flusin O, Lepreux S, et al. Necrotic ulcerated lesion in a young boy caused by cowpox virus infection. Case Rep Dermatol. 2011;3:186-194.
16. Glatz M, Richter S, Ginter-Hanselmayer G, et al. Human cowpox in a veterinary student. Lancet Infect Dis. 2010;10:288.
17. Rocke TE, Dein FJ, Fuchsberger M, et al. Limited infection upon human exposure to a recombinant raccoon pox vaccine vector. Vaccine. 2004;22:2757-2760.

CHAPTER 25

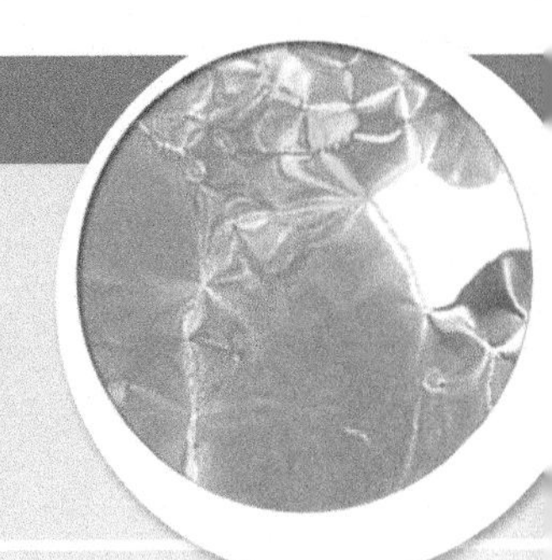

Pseudorabies

Jane E. Sykes and Sarah D. Cramer

Overview of Pseudorabies

First Described: 1902 (Hungary, Aujeszky)[1]

Cause: Suid herpesvirus-1 (Family Herpesviridae, subfamily Alphaherpesvirinae, genus *Varicellovirus*)

Affected Hosts: Domestic and feral swine, cattle, horses, sheep, goats, dogs, cats, bears, raccoons, foxes, hedgehogs, opossums, deer, Florida panther, jackals, coyotes, nonhuman primates (macaques, marmosets), chickens, pigeons, geese, ducks, buzzards, sparrow hawks, rabbits, guinea pigs, rats, and mice

Geographic Distribution: Worldwide

Mode of Transmission: Most often ingestion of uncooked pork by-products or pig carcasses

Major Clinical Signs (Dogs): Variable, but may include fever, lethargy, hypersalivation, muscle stiffness, variable facial pruritus, ataxia, behavioral changes, vomiting, diarrhea, and/or respiratory distress

Differential Diagnoses: Rabies, canine distemper, toxicoses (e.g., organophosphates, heavy metals, ethylene glycol, strychnine)

Human Health Significance: Humans appear to be resistant to infection with suid herpesvirus-1.

Etiology and Epidemiology

Pseudorabies (Aujeszky's disease) is a notifiable disease caused by the alphaherpesvirus suid herpesvirus-1 (SuHV-1). Swine are the natural hosts for SuHV-1, but other domestic and wild mammals, including ruminants, dogs, cats, raccoons, rabbits, and rodents, are susceptible to infection and fatal encephalitis. The name *pseudorabies* was applied because the clinical signs caused by the virus in rabbits resemble those of rabies. SuHV-1 has been eradicated from domestic swine through use of vaccination programs in many countries, including Finland, Sweden, Norway, the Netherlands, Denmark, Austria, Switzerland, Germany, Hungary, Slovakia, the United Kingdom, Canada, the United States, and New Zealand. The virus continues to circulate among wild boar and feral swine, which act as a reservoir for the virus.[2] Australia is also free of pseudorabies. Aujeszky's disease is a widespread problem in domestic swine herds in Asia, Latin America, and some parts of Europe.[2]

SuHV-1 is shed in the saliva and nasal discharges of swine, and transmission can occur by direct contact with these discharges or aerosols, or ingestion of infected swine carcasses or other infected animals, especially wildlife. The virus can survive on fomites and in carcasses for several weeks. In swine, clinical signs depend on the age at exposure and virus strain. Subclinical infections and shedding occur commonly. When older pigs do develop signs, they typically develop respiratory disease. Encephalitis occurs in piglets or in adult pigs that are infected with virulent strains. Reproductive disease and fetal loss can occur in pregnant sows. Recovered pigs develop latent infection of neuronal tissues with reactivation and shedding of virus in semen and nasal, oral, or vaginal secretions following stress.

Disease in dogs is uncommonly reported. However, clusters of affected dogs have been described over the past decade, primarily in hunting dogs that contact wild swine from parts of Europe (France, Germany, Belgium) and the southern United States (Florida and Oklahoma).[2-7] This has followed global expansion of wild swine populations. Disease in dogs may be more likely to occur in regions that are densely populated with wild swine, such as the southern United States (Figure 25-1) and parts of Europe such as Germany, France, Spain, Poland, and the Czech Republic.[2] Dogs that reside on swine farms may also become infected.[8] In some reports, packs of dogs have been infected after consumption of uncooked offal from infected pigs or pig carcasses.[9,10] Dogs of any age, sex, and breed can develop disease, but dog-to-dog transmission does not occur. Cats can be infected after ingestion of pork waste or infected rodents, but reports of naturally occurring Aujeszky's disease in cats are extremely rare.[11] Because subclinical infections and nonspecific signs are common in swine, identification of pseudorabies in dogs may be the first indication that disease is present in a swine herd or wild swine population.

Clinical Features

Signs and Their Pathogenesis

After inhalation or ingestion, SuHV-1 replicates in the oropharynx and is taken up by sensory nerve endings. It then travels by retrograde axonal transport to the sensory nerve ganglia and then to the central nervous system (CNS), which results in ganglioneuritis and encephalitis, especially within the brainstem. Infection can also lead to ganglioneuritis of the cardiac autonomic plexuses with associated myocardial degeneration,[12] as well as degeneration of intestinal myenteric ganglia.[10] Clinical signs appear after a short incubation period that typically ranges from 1 to 6 days, but incubation periods up to 10 days have been reported.[9] The duration of signs ranges from 6 to 96 hours.[13] The most commonly reported sign is hypersalivation. This occurs in most affected dogs, although it may not be present early in the course of illness.[10,13,14] Other signs include lethargy, fever, dysphagia, gastrointestinal signs, muscle stiffness, ataxia, head-pressing, vestibular signs (circling, head tilt,

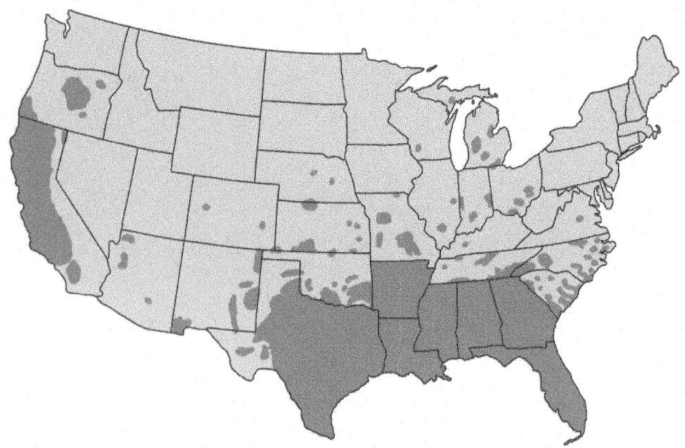

FIGURE 25-1 Geographic distribution of feral swine in the United States. (From Southeastern Cooperative Wildlife Disease Study, College of Veterinary Medicine, The University of Georgia. http://128.192.20.53/nfsms. Last accessed May 2, 2012.)

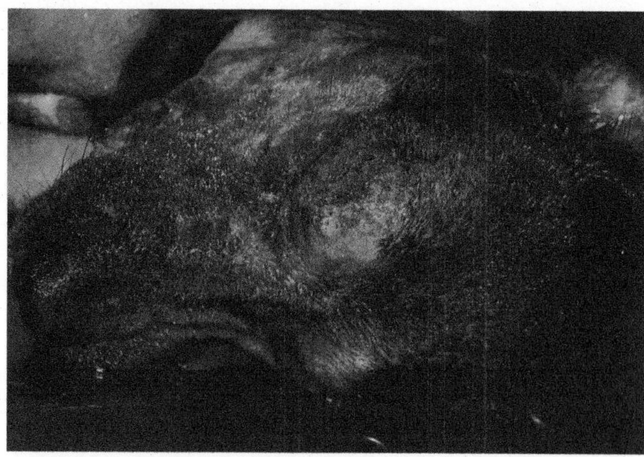

FIGURE 25-2 Evidence of facial self-mutilation in a 2-year-old intact male Catahoula hunting dog with pseudorabies. Severe exudative dermatitis is present over the right eye, external ear canal and muzzle. (Reprinted from Cramer SD, Campbell GA, Njaa BL, et al. Pseudorabies virus infection in Oklahoma hunting dogs. J Vet Diagn Invest 2011;23:915-923.)

BOX 25-1

Clinical Signs in 25 Dogs with Pseudorabies from the United States

Ptyalism: 100%
Anorexia: 84%
Ataxia: 76%
Wandering: 64%
Tachypnea: 64%
Dyspnea: 60%
Vocalization: 56%
Pruritus: 52%
Neck stiffness: 48%
Vomiting: 36%
Muscle spasms: 36%
Aggression: 36%
Trismus: 28%
Dysphagia: 24%
Abnormal pupillary light responses: 20%
Seizures: 16%
Mydriasis: 12%

Monroe WE. Clinical signs associated with pseudorabies in dogs. J Am Vet Med Assoc 1989;195:599-602.

nystagmus), recumbency, intense pruritus and self-mutilation, vocalization, behavior changes such as pacing and aggression, and tachypnea or respiratory distress (Box 25-1). Uncommonly, apparent blindness, facial paralysis, ptosis, photophobia, abnormal facial sensation, and lacrimation occur. Pruritus generally occurs on the face but can also occur on the shoulder and forelimbs.[10,13] The pruritus may result from infection of neurons that innervate those regions.[15] Gastrointestinal signs are common and include vomiting and diarrhea, which may be hemorrhagic (e.g., hematemesis or melena).[6] Seizures and coma may also occur. A variety of cardiac arrhythmias have been reported in experimentally infected dogs, which include ventricular premature complexes, ventricular tachycardia, sinus arrest, atrial tachycardia, atrial fibrillation, wandering pacemaker, second-degree heart block, T- and P-wave abnormalities, and atrioventricular dissociation.[12] Although facial pruritus is considered a classic clinical sign, in one case series, it was present in only 18% of dogs.[14] Death occurs within 96 hours (and usually 48 hours) after the onset of clinical signs. Sudden death may occur, possibly as a result of acute myocarditis.[9,14]

Physical Examination Findings

Physical examination findings in dogs with pseudorabies include mental obtundation, hypersalivation, dehydration, muscle stiffness, tachypnea or respiratory difficulty, and facial pruritus. Cutaneous excoriations and edema due to self-trauma may be identified (Figure 25-2). Other neurologic signs include ataxia, head tilt, circling, hyperesthesia, behavioral abnormalities, anisocoria, mydriasis, nystagmus, slow or absent pupillary light responses, recumbency, and coma. Fever may be present early in the course of infection (up to 108°F or 42°C),[13] but terminally, hypothermia can occur. A variety of cardiac arrhythmias may also be identified.

Diagnosis

Diagnosis of pseudorabies in dogs and cats is based on a compatible history (i.e., exposure to domestic or wild swine in regions where the virus is present), suggestive clinical signs, and histopathology and/or virus detection methods such as immunofluorescent antibody staining, immunohistochemistry, virus isolation, or PCR assay on tissues collected at necropsy (Table 25-1). Antemortem diagnosis of pseudorabies in dogs and cats using virus detection methods has not yet been described.

Laboratory Abnormalities

Laboratory abnormalities in dogs with pseudorabies are nonspecific. Mild anemia and moderate leukocytosis due to a neutrophilia may be present. Affected hunting dogs have also had eosinophilia, hyperglobulinemia, hypoalbuminemia, and hyperglycemia.[7] In these dogs, concurrent gastrointestinal parasitism may have explained the eosinophilia, hypoalbuminemia, and hyperglobulinemia. Analysis of the CSF may reveal increased CSF protein concentration and mononuclear pleocytosis.

TABLE 25-1

Diagnostic Assays Available for Pseudorabies in Dogs and Cats

Assay	Specimen Type	Target	Performance
Histopathology	Necropsy specimens, especially brainstem or ganglia	Meningoencephalitis with eosinophilic intranuclear inclusions; SuHV-1 antigen with IHC, IFA or DNA with in situ hybridization	Necropsy diagnosis
PCR	CNS, tonsils, possibly biopsies of self-traumatized skin or tonsillar swabs	SuHV-1 DNA	Unknown whether PCR could be used for antemortem diagnosis. Not widely available.
Virus isolation	CNS, tonsils, occasionally other tissues such as skin biopsies or lung tissue	SuHV-1	Specialized procedure. False negatives occur commonly.

CNS, Central nervous system; IFA, immunofluorescent antibody; IHC, immunohistochemistry; SuHV-1, suid herpesvirus-1.

Microbiologic Tests

Serologic Diagnosis

Although serology using a variety of antibody detection methods (such as ELISA and virus neutralization) is used to identify exposure in swine herds, it has not been useful for antemortem diagnosis in dogs and cats. This likely reflects the rapid course of disease and insufficient time before death for antibody responses to develop.

Virus Isolation

Although not always successful, SuHV-1 can be isolated from tissues (such as the CNS and tonsils) in pig kidney or Crandell-Rees feline kidney cell monolayers. Immunofluorescent antibody can then be used to confirm the presence of the virus in cells. The sensitivity of virus isolation as an antemortem test (e.g., on saliva or oropharyngeal swabs) is not known. Haired skin from regions of pruritus may also be suitable.

Molecular Diagnosis Using the Polymerase Chain Reaction

Conventional and real-time PCR assays have been described for detection of SuHV-1 in brain tissue collected at necropsy.[7] Whether PCR assays are useful for antemortem diagnosis is not known, but PCR could be attempted on biopsies of pruritic regions or tonsillar swab specimens.

Pathologic Findings

Abnormalities seen on gross postmortem examination in dogs with pseudorabies include facial excoriations, tonsillar enlargement, gastrointestinal mucosal hyperemia and ulceration, myocardial hemorrhage, and pulmonary edema and congestion. On histopathologic examination, perivascular infiltrates of lymphocytes, neutrophils, and macrophages may be present in the brainstem and medulla oblongata, with neuronophagia, neuronal degeneration and necrosis, focal gliosis, and eosinophilic intranuclear inclusion bodies within neurons and astrocytes (Figure 25-3). Involvement of the spinal cord was reported in a cat.[11] Other changes in dogs include suppurative tonsillar inflammation with necrosis, myocardial degeneration, fibrinoid vasculitis, and pulmonary edema. Immunohistochemistry, immunofluorescence, or in situ hybridization can be used to identify virus within neurons.[8]

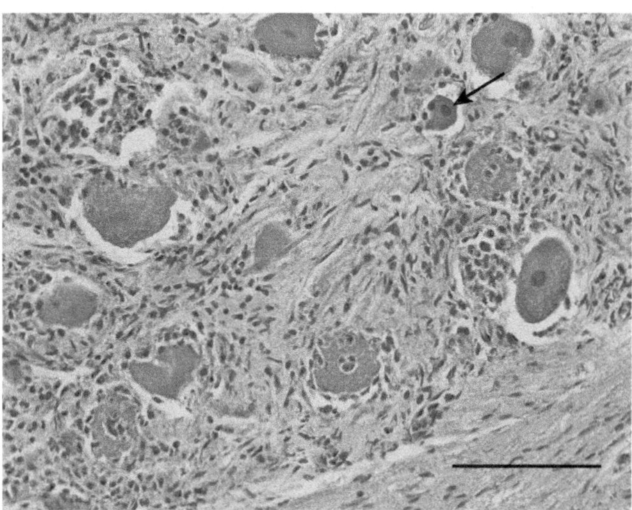

FIGURE 25-3 Histopathology in pseudorabies encephalitis. Trigeminal ganglion of the dog in Figure 25-2. Neutrophilic, lymphocytic, and histiocytic infiltrates are present. Ganglion cells are admixed with necrotic cellular debris, and neuronophagia is prominent. Within a single ganglion cell is an equivocal intracytoplasmic inclusion *(arrow)*. Bar = 50 μm. (From Cramer SD, Campbell GA, Njaa BL, et al. Pseudorabies virus infection in Oklahoma hunting dogs. J Vet Diagn Invest 2011;23:915-923.)

Treatment and Prognosis

Other than supportive care, there is no known treatment for pseudorabies in dogs and cats. Disease is almost always rapidly progressive and fatal.

Immunity and Vaccination

Although vaccines are used in swine to reduce losses where the disease is enzootic, vaccines are not available for dogs and cats, because of the sporadic incidence of the disease.

Prevention

Pseudorabies can be prevented by cooking pork by-products fed to dogs and cats, preventing contact between infected swine and dogs in regions where the disease is enzootic, and possibly through control of rodents.

Public Health Aspects

Humans appear to be refractory to infection with suid herpesvirus-1.

SUGGESTED READINGS

Cramer SD, Campbell GA, Njaa BL, et al. Pseudorabies virus infection in Oklahoma hunting dogs. J Vet Diagn Invest. 2011;23:915-923.

Muller T, Hahn EC, Tottewitz F, et al. Pseudorabies virus in wild swine: a global perspective. Arch Virol. 2011;156:1691-1705.

REFERENCES

1. Aujeszky A. Über eine neue Infektienkrankheit bei Haustieren. Zentralbl Bakteriol I Orig. 1902;32:353-357.
2. Muller T, Hahn EC, Tottewitz F, et al. Pseudorabies virus in wild swine: a global perspective. Arch Virol. 2011;156:1691-1705.
3. Thaller D, Bilek A, Revilla-Fernandez S, et al. Diagnosis of Aujeszky's disease in a dog in Austria. Wien Tierarztl Monatsschr. 2006;93:62-67.
4. Cay AB, Letellier C. Isolation of Aujeszky's disease virus from two hunting dogs in Belgium after hunting wild boars. Vlaam Diergeneeskd Tijdschr. 2009;78:194-195.
5. Toma B, Dufour B. Transmission de la maladie d'Aujeszky des sangliers aux suides domestiques. Epidemiol Sante Anim. 2004;45:115-119.
6. Buergelt CD, Romero CH, Chrisman CL. Pseudorabies in two dogs. Vet Med. 2000;95:439-442.
7. Cramer SD, Campbell GA, Njaa BL, et al. Pseudorabies virus infection in Oklahoma hunting dogs. J Vet Diagn Invest. 2011;23:915-923.
8. Quiroga MI, Nieto JM, Sur J, et al. Diagnosis of Aujeszky's disease virus infection in dogs by use of immunohistochemistry and in-situ hybridization. Zentralbl Veterinarmed A. 1998;45:75-81.
9. Hugoson G, Rockborn G. On the occurrence of pseudorabies in Sweden. II. An outbreak in dogs caused by feeding abattoir offal. Zentralbl Veterinarmed B. 1972;19:641-645.
10. Gore R, Osborne AD, Darke PG, et al. Aujeszky's disease in a pack of hounds. Vet Rec. 1977;101:93-95.
11. Hara M, Shimizu T, Nemoto S, et al. A natural case of Aujeszky's disease in the cat in Japan. J Vet Med Sci. 1991;53:947-949.
12. Olson GR, Miller LD. Studies on the pathogenesis of heart lesions in dogs infected with pseudorabies virus. Can J Vet Res. 1986;50:245-250.
13. Monroe WE. Clinical signs associated with pseudorabies in dogs. J Am Vet Med Assoc. 1989;195:599-602.
14. Hawkins BA, Olson GR. Clinical signs of pseudorabies in the dog and cat: a review of 40 cases. Iowa State Univ Vet. 1985;47:116-119.
15. Takahashi H, Yoshikawa Y, Kai C, et al. Mechanism of pruritus and peracute death in mice induced by pseudorabies virus (PRV) infection. J Vet Med Sci. 1993;55:913-920.

CHAPTER 26

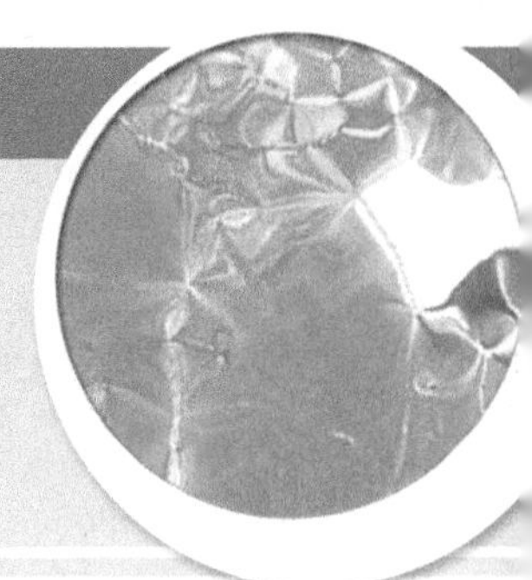

Viral Papillomatosis

Jane E. Sykes and Jennifer A. Luff

Overview of Papillomatosis in Dogs and Cats

First Described: The transmissibility of canine papillomaviruses was described in the late 1800s; electron microscopic descriptions occurred in the late 1960s[1,2]

Cause: Papillomaviruses (family Papillomaviridae)

Affected Hosts: A variety of animal species, but papillomavirus types are relatively species specific

Geographic Distribution: Worldwide

Mode of Transmission: Cutaneous or mucosal inoculation through trauma

Major Clinical Signs: Exophytic or endophytic papillomas, pigmented plaques, in situ or invasive squamous cell carcinomas

Human Health Significance: Canine and feline papillomavirus types do not appear to infect humans, although some feline papillomavirus types resemble some human papillomavirus types

Etiology and Epidemiology

Papillomaviruses cause warts, or papillomas, in a variety of animal species (Figure 26-1). They are non-enveloped, icosahedral viruses with a circular double-stranded DNA genome. Papillomaviruses have also been associated with malignant transformations within the skin and mucous membranes (Box 26-1).[3] In humans, certain papillomavirus types are more likely than others to induce malignant transformation. Papillomavirus DNA has been detected using PCR assays on the skin of dogs and cats and in the oral cavity of dogs with no signs of papillomas[4-6]; it is not clear whether this represents subclinical infection or just carriage of papillomaviruses.[7] Because of this, the association of papillomaviruses with disease in dogs and cats, especially squamous cell carcinomas (SCCs), remains somewhat unclear. Papillomaviruses are resistant in the environment and survive detergents and high temperatures. Exposure to papillomaviruses is widespread in the dog population based on serologic studies.[8] Congenital or acquired deficiencies in cell-mediated immunity may predispose to papilloma formation.[9-13]

Papillomaviruses are relatively host species specific. The number of different papillomavirus types identified in dogs and cats has expanded dramatically in recent years as a result of the use of molecular techniques. Correlations appear to exist between papillomavirus types and clinical manifestations and progression of disease, although host immune status is also important. Papillomaviruses are classified on the basis of the L1 capsid protein gene sequence. At least nine types occur in dogs; an additional five novel types have been described that are not fully classified (Table 26-1).[14-21] *Canis familiaris* papillomavirus (canine papillomavirus 1) is associated with oral papillomas and rarely with cutaneous endophytic (inverted) papillomas and invasive cutaneous SCCs.[10,22,23] Other canine papillomavirus types have been associated with cutaneous inverted and exophytic papillomas, cutaneous pigmented plaques, or cutaneous in situ SCCs. Papillomavirus DNA has been detected in a few canine oral SCCs.[23,24] However, most oral and cutaneous SCCs in dogs are negative for papillomavirus DNA. The eight canine papillomavirus types have been allocated to three different genera, Lambda, Tau, and Chi.[7,17] Chi papillomaviruses have been associated with cutaneous plaque formation. Cocker spaniels and Kerry blue terriers may be predisposed to cutaneous papillomas, and pug dogs are predisposed to pigmented plaques. Breed predispositions to papillomavirus infections may reflect the presence of congenital defects in cell-mediated immunity; however, this is not yet proven.

Papillomavirus infections are uncommonly reported in cats when compared with dogs. They have been associated with plaque-like lesions (hereafter referred to as feline plaques), dysplastic skin lesions, multicentric Bowenoid in situ SCCs (BISC), cutaneous invasive SCCs, and feline sarcoids (also known as fibropapillomas). The complete viral genome sequence for two feline papillomaviruses types has been described, as well as several stretches of additional novel feline papillomavirus sequences. Feline sarcoids have been associated with *feline sarcoid-associated papillomavirus* (FeSarPV) infection, for which cattle may be a reservoir.[25] Sarcoids have been described in cats from North America, New Zealand, the United Kingdom, Sweden, and Australia, and affected cats are often young (<5 years), male, outdoor cats from rural environments. *Felis domesticus papillomavirus 1* (FdPV-1) has been detected in feline viral plaques.[26,27] *Felis domesticus papillomavirus 2* (FdPV-2)

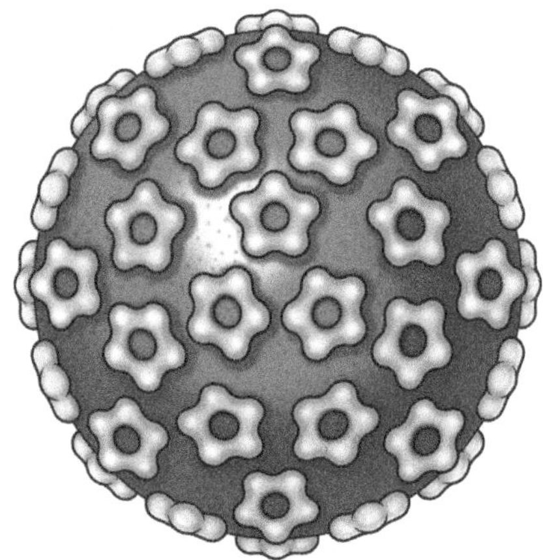

FIGURE 26-1 Structure of a papillomavirus. The virus is non-enveloped and has a icosahedral capsid composed of two different capsid proteins (L1 and L2).

BOX 26-1

Spectrum of Clinical Manifestations Associated with Papillomavirus Infections in Dogs and Cats

Dogs

Oral papillomatosis
Cutaneous exophytic papillomas (warts)
Cutaneous endophytic papillomas (inverted warts)
Pigmented cutaneous plaques
Cutaneous in situ SCCs*
Invasive cutaneous SCCs
Oral SCCs

Cats

Feline viral plaques
Bowenoid in situ carcinomas
Invasive cutaneous SCCs
Feline sarcoids

*SCCs, squamous cell carcinomas. The majority of SCCs in dogs and cats have not been associated with papillomavirus infection.

TABLE 26-1

Spectrum of Papillomavirus Types and Disease Associations in Dogs

CPV Type*	Genus	Clinical Manifestation
1	Lambda	Oral papillomas, cutaneous endophytic papillomas, invasive SCCs
2	Tau	Cutaneous endophytic and exophytic papillomas (warts)
3	Chi	Cutaneous pigmented plaques, in situ and invasive SCCs
4, 5	Chi	Cutaneous pigmented plaques
6	Lambda	Endophytic papillomas
7	Tau	Exophytic papillomas and in situ SCC
8	Chi	Cutaneous pigmented plaques
9		Cutaneous pigmented plaques

*CPV, Canine papillomavirus. Five additional types associated with cutaneous pigmented plaques exist that have not yet been definitively classified at the time of writing. (Luff JA, Affolter VK, Yeargan B, et al. Detection of six novel papillomavirus sequences in canine pigmented plaques. J Vet Diagn Invest 2012;24[3]:576-580.)

and other papillomaviruses, including papillomaviruses with homology to human papillomaviruses, have been detected in cats with plaques, BISCs, and invasive SCCs.[27-31] FdPV-2 is strongly associated with feline plaque formation.[32] The finding of papillomavirus DNA with homology to the DNA of human papillomaviruses in cats suggests the possibility of transmission of papillomaviruses between humans and cats; however, additional studies are needed.[30,31] Although papillomavirus DNA has been detected in a feline oral SCC,[33] papillomaviruses do not seem to be responsible for most oral SCCs in cats.[34]

Clinical Features

Signs and Their Pathogenesis

Infection with papillomaviruses follows inoculation of the virus through microabrasions in the skin caused by physical trauma. Initial infection and viral amplification occurs within keratinocytes of the stratum basale.[35] As basal keratinocytes undergo differentiation, early viral proteins (E proteins) are expressed and associate with regulators of the cell cycle to stimulate cell cycle progression.[35] This leads to enhanced proliferation of cells in the stratum spinosum and stratum granulosum, with accumulation of infected cells and papilloma formation (Figure 26-2). With the exception of feline sarcoids, which remain as latent (or nonproductive) infections, late viral products, including the virus capsid proteins (L1 and L2), are first expressed in cells of the stratum spinosum. Papillomaviruses are nonlytic viruses, and mature virions are shed with cells that exfoliate from the stratum corneum or the nonkeratinized cells of the mucous membranes. Infected cells develop a characteristic cytopathic effect, which consists of cytoplasmic vacuolization. Tens of thousands of virus particles are produced by each infected cell. Malignant transformation occurs as a result of the effect of certain viral products (also known as oncoproteins) on host cellular signals that are responsible for regulation of the cell cycle and/or apoptosis.[36] For example, some papillomavirus types produce proteins that degrade p53 and retinoblastoma protein (RB), which are important tumor suppressors.[37] In human papillomavirus infections, accidental integration of the human papillomavirus (HPV) genome can occur into host cell DNA, although this does not seem to be necessary for oncogenesis.[36]

Oral papillomas most commonly occur in young dogs and often regress spontaneously over a 4- to 6-week period.[7] They can also occur as a result of immunosuppression, such as after treatment with cyclosporin, less commonly chronic glucocorticoid treatment, or chronic infection with *Ehrlichia canis*. Rarely, papillomas in the caudal oropharynx obstruct respiration (Figure 26-3). Cutaneous pigmented plaques, to which pugs and miniature schnauzers are predisposed, are generally not of clinical significance but in some situations can progress to SCCs.[19,38,39] *Cutaneous exophytic* and *endophytic papillomas* usually occur as solitary masses.[7] Exophytic papillomas are proliferative nodules, whereas endophytic papillomas are cup-shaped lesions with a central, keratin-filled pore (Figure 26-4). *Feline plaques* are flat, often pigmented lesions that resemble canine papillomas histologically. *Feline sarcoids* are tumors that resemble equine sarcoids. *Multicentric BISCs* appear as multiple, hyperpigmented plaquelike lesions.

Physical Examination

Canine Oral Papillomatosis

Oral papillomas can occur on the lips, mucocutaneous junctions, tongue, pharynx, eyelids, and infrequently haired skin[7] (see Figure 26-3; Figure 26-5). They may be accompanied by halitosis, ptyalism, and oral discomfort. Early lesions are smooth and raised, but as they enlarge they may become cauliflower-like. They may be pigmented or nonpigmented.

Canine Cutaneous Exophytic Papillomas

Cutaneous exophytic papillomas are wartlike projections that appear anywhere on the body, but especially the lower limbs and footpads.

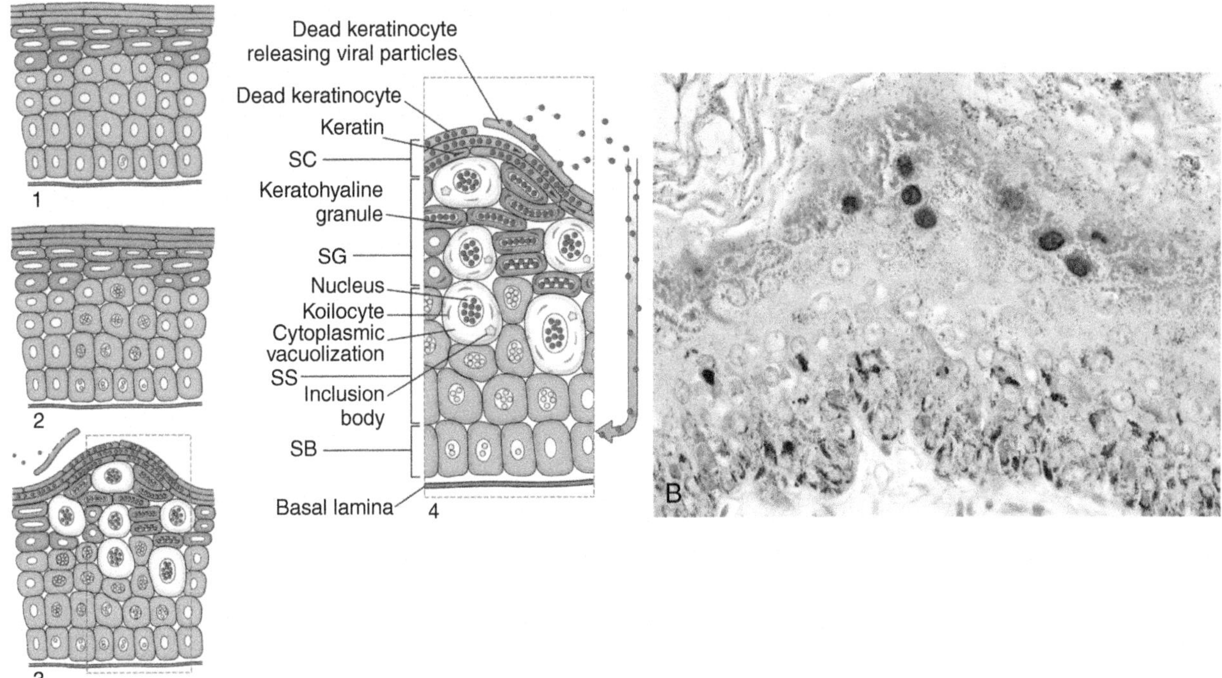

FIGURE 26-2 Schematic representation of the events of papillomavirus infection in the epidermis. **A,** (1) The primary infection occurs in a cell of the stratum basale (SB) after the virus gains entry via a microabrasion. The virus replicates and produces only early proteins, which leads to increased cellular proliferation. (2) Progeny of the initial infected cells migrate laterally and move upwards, where they accumulate in the stratum spinosum (SS) and stratum granulosum (SG). (3) Cellular differentiation ultimately occurs, and large numbers of virions are produced in association with papilloma development. Virions are shed with exfoliating keratinocytes of the stratum corneum (SC). (4) Detail from 3. **B,** Immunoperoxidase staining of papillomavirus antigen in a cutaneous plaque from a dog. (**B** courtesy of Luff J, University of California, Davis. In MacLachlan NJ, Dubovi EJ, eds. Fenner's Veterinary Virology, 4 ed. Burlington, MA: Academic Press [Elsevier]; 2011.)

Canine Endophytic Papillomas

Endophytic (or inverted) papillomas are cup-shaped cutaneous nodules that range in size from 2 mm to 2 cm in diameter with a central depression (see Figure 26-4). Several different variations have been described, but they are rare and poorly understood.[7] Single or multiple lesions can occur anywhere on the body. They have also been described in the interdigital space.[9]

Canine Pigmented Plaques

Pigmented plaques usually range in size from 1 mm to 1 cm, but in one dog progressed to larger sizes (up to 8 cm). Multiple dark, hyperkeratotic flat lesions are typically present on the ventrum or medial aspects of the limbs.[39]

Squamous Cell Carcinomas

SCCs are often ulcerated, nodular masses that may be found alongside pigmented plaques or cutaneous papillomas when malignant transformation occurs (Figure 26-6).

Feline Sarcoids

Feline sarcoids are solitary, firm, ulcerated, or nonulcerated nodules that occur most commonly on the nasal philtrum, nares, upper lip, digits, or tail tip, but have also been reported at other locations such as the eyelids and pinnae (Figure 26-7).[25,40]

Feline Plaques and BISC

In cats, plaques are usually a few millimeters in diameter or linear lesions. They are usually pigmented and occur on the head, neck, dorsal thorax, or abdomen. They can be ulcerated.[41] It may be difficult to differentiate plaques from BISCs, which also appear as pigmented plaques with crusting and ulceration. The two may occur together simultaneously.

Diagnosis

The history and gross appearance of oral papillomas in dogs is generally sufficient for diagnosis. For other papillomas and plaques, the diagnosis can be confirmed with biopsy and histopathology. A full-thickness biopsy that includes adjacent normal skin should be collected. The presence of papillomaviruses can be identified using PCR assays, immunohistochemistry, in situ hybridization, or electron microscopy, although these techniques are primarily used on a research basis. Caution should be used when interpreting the results of PCR assays because papillomaviruses can be detected on normal skin, so results should be interpreted in association with clinical signs. Identification of virus within lesions using immunohistochemistry, in situ hybridization, or electron microscopy is more supportive of causality.

Microbiologic Tests

Molecular Diagnosis Using the Polymerase Chain Reaction

PCR assays can be used to detect papillomaviruses within biopsy or cytobrush specimens from dogs and cats. Rolling circle amplification has been used on fresh biopsy specimens to amplify whole circular genomic DNA from papillomavirus lesions.[7]

Pathologic Findings

Histopathology of canine exophytic papillomas generally reveals epidermal hyperplasia (acanthosis), extensive hyperkeratosis, and clumped keratohyalin granules in the stratum spinosum. The term *koilocytosis* is used to describe cells with papillomavirus-induced cytopathic effects, which consist of extensive cytoplasmic vacuolation and nuclear pyknosis. Intranuclear inclusion bodies may also be present; these occur in the

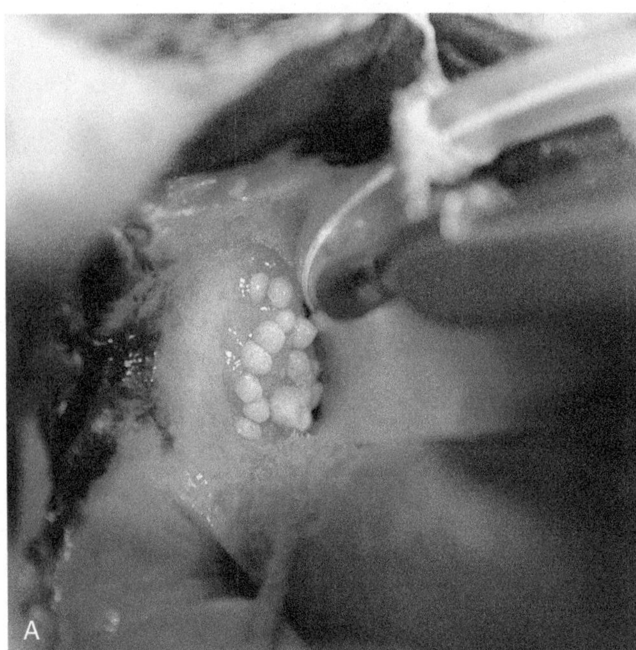

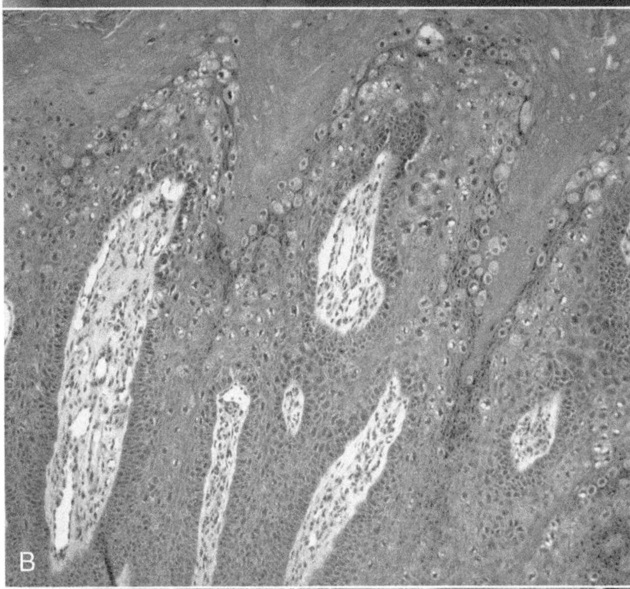

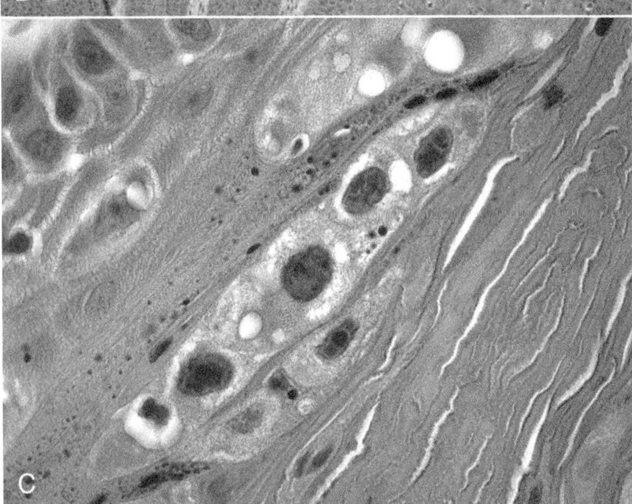

FIGURE 26-3 **A,** Oral papillomas in the pharyngeal region of a 5-year-old male neutered Boston terrier that was receiving chronic glucocorticoid treatment for a temporal lobe glioma. **B** and **C,** Histopathology of the lesions revealed hyperkeratosis with increased keratohyalin granules and multifocal intracytoplasmic inclusion bodies, as well as secondary bacterial infection (not shown). (Courtesy of the University of California, Davis Veterinary Dermatology and Neurology Services.)

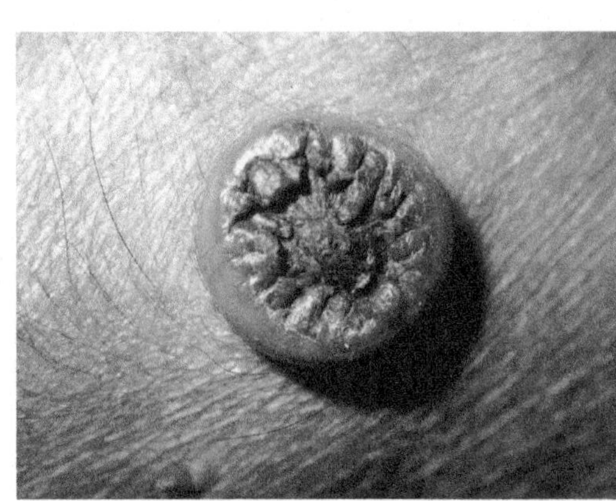

FIGURE 26-4 Inverted papilloma on the abdomen of a flat-coated retriever. (From Lange CE, Favrot C. Canine papillomaviruses. Vet Clin North Am Small Anim Pract 2011;41:1183-1195.)

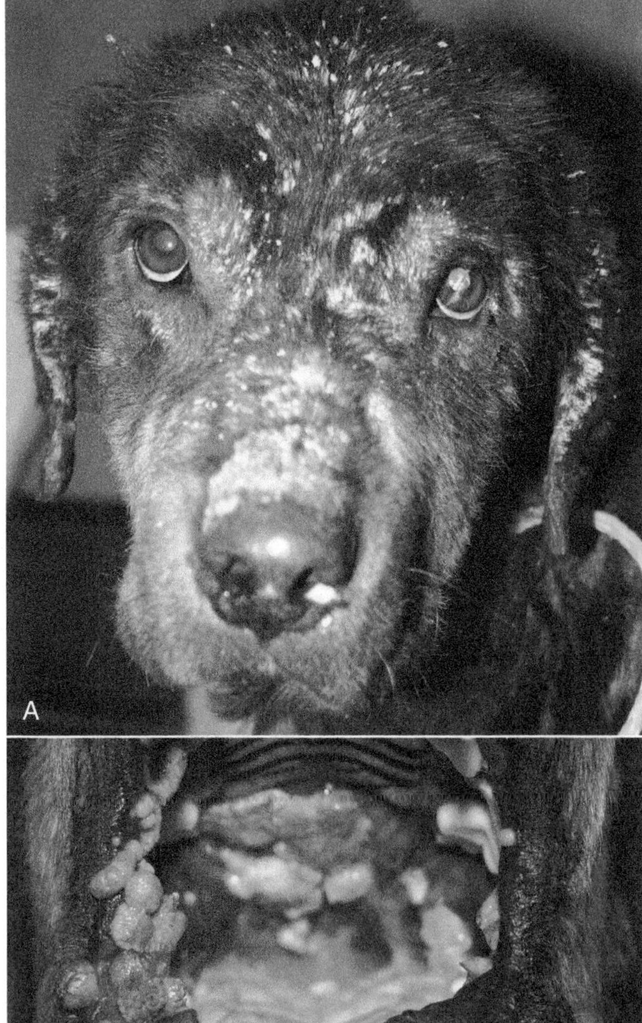

FIGURE 26-5 **A,** Adult male neutered Rottweiler with a high antibody titer to *Ehrlichia canis*, malnutrition, gastrointestinal parasitism, and sarcoptic mange. **B,** Oral papillomatosis was present on oral examination and involved the hard and soft palates, buccal mucosa, and lips.

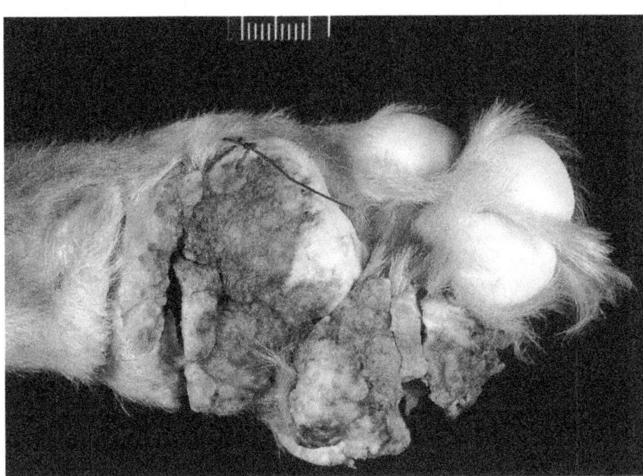

FIGURE 26-6 Right thoracic limb digital squamous cell carcinoma in a male neutered Australian shepherd after amputation. A large, 4 cm × 5 cm ulcerated mass is present. Immunohistochemistry for papillomavirus was negative, but *Canis familiaris* papillomavirus 2 was detected with PCR and sequencing. (Courtesy of the University of California, Davis Veterinary Anatomic Pathology Service.)

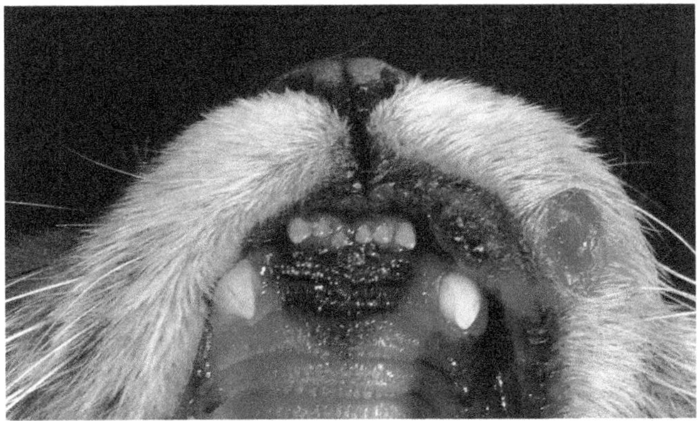

FIGURE 26-7 Sarcoid of the lip in an 8 year-old female spayed domestic longhair at necropsy. The cat was euthanized because of oral pain and inability to eat and drink. (Courtesy of the University of California, Davis Veterinary Anatomic Pathology Service.)

upper layers of the epidermis (see Figure 26-3, C). Endophytic papillomas are cup-shaped masses of epithelial hyperplasia that occur below the level of the surrounding normal skin. Koilocytosis and intranuclear inclusions are often prominent. Histopathology of pigmented plaques are characterized by locally extensive epidermal hyperplasia, hyperkeratosis, hyperpigmentation, and clumped keratohyalin granules; koilocytes and viral inclusions are generally not observed.[7] Feline sarcoids have dermal fibroplastic proliferations with overlying epithelial hyperplasia that includes long, thin rete ridges that extend into the tumor; they may be confused with sarcomas.[40] Feline plaques exhibit moderate to marked epidermal hyperplasia and koilocytosis. Intranuclear inclusions are sometimes present. In situ SCCs are characterized by epithelial hyperplasia, dysplasia, and increased numbers of mitotic figures, with an intact basement membrane. Loss of the basement membrane and invasion of the dermis indicates invasive SCC.

With the exception of feline sarcoids, immunohistochemistry using antibodies that detect conserved papillomavirus antigens (i.e., group-specific papillomavirus antigens) can confirm the presence of papillomaviruses within lesions. Canine and feline papillomavirus-specific reagents are not widely available. In situ hybridization techniques can also be used. Crystalline arrays of virus can also be identified within lesions with electron microscopy.

Treatment and Prognosis

The outcome of papillomavirus infection depends on the virus strain and host immunity. Oral and cutaneous papillomas in young dogs generally regress spontaneously 4 to 8 weeks, and sometimes 3 months after the onset of clinical signs. However, they may persist in older dogs, or when there is underlying immune compromise, and occasionally progress to malignancy. If possible, underlying immunosuppression should be treated (for example, through removal or tapering of immunosuppressive drug treatment). Lesions can be removed surgically if they cause physical obstruction or for cosmetic reasons, but surgical treatment may be followed by recurrence. Treatment with azithromycin (10 mg/kg PO q24h for 10 days) appeared to be effective in a prospective, randomized, double-blinded placebo-controlled clinical trial that included 12 dogs with oral papillomatosis and 5 dogs with cutaneous papillomatosis.[42] The use of topical or intralesional immunomodulators (such as imiquimod cream) and antiviral drugs (such as cidofovir) has shown promise for treatment of persistent papillomas in humans, but these treatments have not been evaluated in dogs and cats.

Pigmented plaques tend to persist, but most are not associated with malignant transformation. Transformation to a well-differentiated SCC was reported in an affected miniature schnauzer.[43] Feline viral plaques have the potential to transform to Bowenoid SCC in situ and invasive SCCs.[32] Feline sarcoids often recur locally after surgical removal, but metastasis does not occur. As more information becomes available, certain papillomavirus types may be more firmly linked to the presence or absence of malignant transformation, which may aid prognostication.

Immunity and Vaccination

Recovery from oral papillomatosis is associated with papillomavirus type-specific resistance to reinfection. Immunity to papillomaviruses comprises (1) the host immune response to the virus and (2) a cell-mediated immune response to the tumor, which is ultimately responsible for tumor regression. This explains why new tumors may not occur, but old tumors persist and continue to grow in the face of an immune response to the virus, and immunization with the virus does not induce tumor regression. Papillomaviruses can evade the host immune response because infection is limited to the skin, and the immunogenic capsid protein is not expressed until the virus reaches the terminally differentiated outer layer. A variety of other mechanisms of immune evasion have been identified in human papillomavirus infections, such as interference with interferons and inhibition of chemokines such as Il-8 and Il-18 by papillomavirus proteins.[44] Viral persistence is necessary for malignant transformation.

Prevention

No vaccines are available for prevention of papillomatosis in dogs and cats. Prevention of immunosuppressive conditions, such as retrovirus infections in cats, and cautious use of potent immunosuppressive drugs such as cyclosporin can also reduce the chance of papillomatosis.

Public Health Aspects

More than 100 papillomavirus types infect humans. Papillomaviruses are relatively species specific, and there is no evidence that canine papillomaviruses infect humans. However, the DNA of more than one different human papillomavirus type has been detected in epithelial lesions in cats.[30,31] Further work, including whole viral genome sequencing, is required to determine whether cats can be a source of some papillomavirus infections for humans and vice versa.

CASE EXAMPLE

Signalment: "Oscar," an adult male neutered Rottweiler mix (see Figure 26-5)

History: Oscar was brought to the University of California, Davis, Veterinary Medical Teaching Hospital for examination after adoption by a veterinary student as a stray from an Indian reservation in Arizona. The student was concerned about the possibility of malnourishment, a painful mouth, and pruritic skin disease. Since his rescue 5 days previously, the student had been feeding him four times daily with maintenance commercial wet and dry dog foods. His appetite had been ravenous and tapeworm segments had been observed in his feces. He had been isolated from other pets in the household.

Physical Examination:

Body Weight: 25.5 kg

General: Bright and alert with normal mentation, nervous. T = 100.8°F (38.2°C), HR = 90 beats/min, RR = 18 breaths/min, mucous membranes pink, CRT = 1 s.

Integument: A dull haircoat was present. Patchy generalized alopecia with severe scaling, crusting, hyperpigmentation, ulceration, and lichenification was present on the face, pinnae and pinnal margins, shoulders, trunk, and extremities.

Eyes, Ears, Nose, and Throat: Moderate mucoid discharge was present from both eyes. The incisor teeth were severely worn. Oral examination also revealed pain on opening the mouth and multiple pink to gray pedunculated masses that ranged from a few millimeters to over 1 cm in diameter on the buccal mucosa and gingiva, lateral aspect of the tongue, and on the hard and soft palates (see Figure 26-5, *B*). These were consistent with oral papillomatosis.

Musculoskeletal: Body condition score 1/9. Normal gait. No other musculoskeletal abnormalities were noted.

Cardiovascular and Respiratory: No clinically significant abnormalities were detected.

Gastrointestinal and Genitourinary: Abdominal palpation was within normal limits. Intact male with soft, symmetrical testes. Soft feces were noted on rectal examination.

Lymph Nodes: Mandibular and superficial cervical nodes were enlarged (approximately 3 cm); the popliteal nodes were sized within normal limits.

Laboratory Findings:

CBC:

HCT 32.3% (40%-55%)
MCV 64.3 fL (65-75 fL)
MCHC 36.2 g/dL (33-36 g/dL)
WBC 10,390 cells/μL (6000-13,000 cells/μL)
Neutrophils 5995 cells/μL (3000-10,500 cells/μL)
Lymphocytes 1891 cells/μL (1000-4,000 cells/μL)
Monocytes 758 cells/μL (150-1200 cells/μL)
Eosinophils 1704 cells/μL (0-1500 cells/μL)
Platelets 322,000 platelets/μL (150,000-400,000 platelets/μL)
Rare macroplatelets observed.

Serum Chemistry Profile:

Sodium 144 mmol/L (145-154 mmol/L)
Potassium 4.8 mmol/L (3.6-5.3 mmol/L)
Chloride 108 mmol/L (108-118 mmol/L)
Bicarbonate 26 mmol/L (16-26 mmol/L)
Phosphorus 5.1 mg/dL (3.0-6.2 mg/dL)
Calcium 10.1 mg/dL (9.7-11.5 mg/dl)
BUN 26 mg/dL (5-21 mg/dL)
Creatinine 0.7 mg/dL (0.3-1.2 mg/dL)
Glucose 108 mg/dL (64-123 mg/dL)
Total protein 7.7 g/dL (5.4-7.6 g/dL)
Albumin 2.9 g/dL (3.0-4.4 g/dL)
Globulin 4.8 g/dL (1.8-3.9 g/dL)
ALT 48 U/L (19-67 U/L)
AST 30 U/L (19-42 U/L)
ALP 117 U/L (21-170 U/L)
Gamma GT <3 U/L (0-6 U/L)
Cholesterol 210 mg/dL (135-361 mg/dL)
Total bilirubin 0.1 mg/dL (0-0.2 mg/dL).

Urinalysis: SGr 1.048; pH 5.0, negative protein (SSA), 1+ bilirubin; no hemoprotein, ketones or glucose; 1-2 WBC/HPF, rare RBC/HPF, rare bilirubin crystals, moderate sperm.

Cytology of Superficial and Deep Skin Scrapings: *Sarcoptes* mites were seen.

Imaging Findings: Lateral and dorsoventral thoracic radiographs were unremarkable. Abdominal ultrasonography revealed a small, 1 cm hypoechoic nodule in the body of the spleen. The remainder of the abdominal structures was within normal limits.

Microbiologic Testing: Lateral flow ELISA assay for antibodies to *Ehrlichia canis, Anaplasma phagocytophilum,* and *Borrelia burgdorferi* and *Dirofilaria immitis* antigen (4Dx SNAP, IDEXX Laboratories, ME, USA): Positive for antibodies to *E. canis*.

Vector-borne disease serology panel (*Babesia canis, A. phagocytophilum, E. canis, Rickettsia* spp. IFA): Positive for antibodies to *E. canis* (1:655,360) and *Rickettsia* spp. (1:40,960).

Fecal flotation: *Giardia* spp. cysts (<1 per 40× field), *Sarcoptes* mites (1 to 10 per 10× field).

Diagnosis: Canine oral papillomatosis; malnutrition; sarcoptic mange; suspected chronic canine monocytic ehrlichiosis; previous exposure to spotted fever group rickettsias; giardiasis; cestodiasis.

Treatment: Oscar was treated with doxycycline (5 mg/kg PO q12h for 6 weeks) for ehrlichiosis, topical selamectin (every 2 weeks for a total of 6 weeks) for sarcoptic mange, praziquantel (5 mg/kg, once) for cestodiasis, cephalexin (22 mg/kg q12h for 4 weeks) for secondary bacterial pyoderma, and fenbendazole (50 mg/kg PO q24h for 3 days) for giardiasis. The owner was instructed to bathe him with an oatmeal shampoo twice weekly. At a recheck appointment 4 weeks later, Oscar weighed 31.5 kg. The skin lesions had improved, and new hair growth was noted. Pruritus was still present. More oral papillomas were present, and the owner described worsened halitosis. Mandibular lymph nodes remained enlarged. Treatment with cephalexin and doxycycline was continued for an additional 3 weeks. Three weeks later, the dog's bodyweight was 33.4 kg, the oral papillomas and mandibular lymphadenomegaly had resolved, and Oscar was vaccinated with canine distemper virus, canine parvovirus, canine adenovirus, parainfluenza virus, and rabies virus vaccines and neutered.

Comments: The gross appearance of the oral lesions in this dog was sufficient to make a diagnosis of oral papillomatosis. Papillomatosis has been reported in other dogs with chronic *E. canis* infection, but the extent to which ehrlichiosis contributed to papillomatosis in this dog is unknown. The immunosuppression associated with malnutrition may also have played a role. Resolution of lesions occurred within 7 weeks after treatment of the immunosuppressive disorders, but papillomatosis can also resolve spontaneously over the same time period.

SUGGESTED READING

Lange CE, Favrot C. Canine papillomaviruses. Vet Clin North Am Small Anim Pract. 2011;41:1183-1195.

REFERENCES

1. Watrach AM. The ultrastructure of canine cutaneous papilloma. Cancer Res. 1969;29:2079-2084.
2. Watrach AM, Hanson LE, Meyer RC. Canine papilloma: the structural characterization of oral papilloma virus. J Natl Cancer Inst. 1969;43:453-458.
3. Munday JS, Kiupel M. Papillomavirus-associated cutaneous neoplasia in mammals. Vet Pathol. 2010;47:254-264.
4. Lange CE, Zollinger S, Tobler K, et al. Clinically healthy skin of dogs is a potential reservoir for canine papillomaviruses. J Clin Microbiol. 2011;49:707-709.
5. Munday JS, Kiupel M, French AF, et al. Amplification of papillomaviral DNA sequences from a high proportion of feline cutaneous in situ and invasive squamous cell carcinomas using a nested polymerase chain reaction. Vet Dermatol. 2008;19:259-263.
6. Munday JS, Witham AI. Frequent detection of papillomavirus DNA in clinically normal skin of cats infected and noninfected with feline immunodeficiency virus. Vet Dermatol. 2010;21:307-310.
7. Lange CE, Favrot C. Canine papillomaviruses. Vet Clin North Am Small Anim Pract. 2011;41:1183-1195.
8. Lange CE, Tobler K, Favrot C, et al. Detection of antibodies against epidermodysplasia verruciformis-associated canine papillomavirus 3 in sera of dogs from Europe and Africa by enzyme-linked immunosorbent assay. Clin Vaccine Immunol. 2009;16:66-72.
9. Goldschmidt MH, Kennedy JS, Kennedy DR, et al. Severe papillomavirus infection progressing to metastatic squamous cell carcinoma in bone marrow-transplanted X-linked SCID dogs. J Virol. 2006;80:6621-6628.
10. Sundberg JP, Smith EK, Herron AJ, et al. Involvement of canine oral papillomavirus in generalized oral and cutaneous verrucosis in a Chinese Shar Pei dog. Vet Pathol. 1994;31:183-187.
11. Le Net JL, Orth G, Sundberg JP, et al. Multiple pigmented cutaneous papules associated with a novel canine papillomavirus in an immunosuppressed dog. Vet Pathol. 1997;34:8-14.
12. Callan MB, Preziosi D, Mauldin E. Multiple papillomavirus-associated epidermal hamartomas and squamous cell carcinomas in situ in a dog following chronic treatment with prednisone and cyclosporine. Vet Dermatol. 2005;16:338-345.
13. Favrot C, Olivry T, Werner AH, et al. Evaluation of papillomaviruses associated with cyclosporine-induced hyperplastic verrucous lesions in dogs. Am J Vet Res. 2005;66:1764-1769.
14. Yuan H, Luff J, Zhou D, et al. Complete genome sequence of canine papillomavirus type 9. J Virol. 2012;86:5966.
15. Luff JA, Affolter VK, Yeargan B, et al. Detection of six novel papillomavirus sequences within canine pigmented plaques. J Vet Diagn Invest. 2012;24:576-580.
16. Delius H, Van Ranst MA, Jenson AB, et al. Canine oral papillomavirus genomic sequence: a unique 1.5-kb intervening sequence between the E2 and L2 open reading frames. Virology. 1994;204:447-452.
17. Lange CE, Tobler K, Ackermann M, et al. Three novel canine papillomaviruses support taxonomic clade formation. J Gen Virol. 2009;90:2615-2621.
18. Lange CE, Tobler K, Lehner A, et al. A case of a canine pigmented plaque associated with the presence of a Chi-papillomavirus. Vet Dermatol. 2012;23(1):76-80:e18-e19.
19. Tobler K, Favrot C, Nespeca G, et al. Detection of the prototype of a potential novel genus in the family Papillomaviridae in association with canine epidermodysplasia verruciformis. J Gen Virol. 2006;87:3551-3557.
20. Tobler K, Lange C, Carlotti DN, et al. Detection of a novel papillomavirus in pigmented plaques of four pugs. Vet Dermatol. 2008;19:21-25.
21. Yuan H, Ghim S, Newsome J, et al. An epidermotropic canine papillomavirus with malignant potential contains an E5 gene and establishes a unique genus. Virology. 2007;359:28-36.
22. Bregman CL, Hirth RS, Sundberg JP, et al. Cutaneous neoplasms in dogs associated with canine oral papillomavirus vaccine. Vet Pathol. 1987;24:477-487.
23. Teifke JP, Lohr CV, Shirasawa H. Detection of canine oral papillomavirus-DNA in canine oral squamous cell carcinomas and p53 overexpressing skin papillomas of the dog using the polymerase chain reaction and non-radioactive in situ hybridization. Vet Microbiol. 1998;60:119-130.
24. Zaugg N, Nespeca G, Hauser B, et al. Detection of novel papillomaviruses in canine mucosal, cutaneous and in situ squamous cell carcinomas. Vet Dermatol. 2005;16:290-298.
25. Munday JS, Knight CG. Amplification of feline sarcoid-associated papillomavirus DNA sequences from bovine skin. Vet Dermatol. 2010.
26. Terai M, Burk RD. *Felis domesticus* papillomavirus, isolated from a skin lesion, is related to canine oral papillomavirus and contains a 1.3 kb non-coding region between the E2 and L2 open reading frames. J Gen Virol. 2002;83:2303-2307.
27. Munday JS, Willis KA, Kiupel M, et al. Amplification of three different papillomaviral DNA sequences from a cat with viral plaques. Vet Dermatol. 2008;19:400-404.
28. Nespeca G, Grest P, Rosenkrantz WS, et al. Detection of novel papillomaviruslike sequences in paraffin-embedded specimens of invasive and in situ squamous cell carcinomas from cats. Am J Vet Res. 2006;67:2036-2041.

29. Schwittlick U, Bock P, Lapp S, et al. [Feline papillomavirus infection in a cat with Bowen-like disease and cutaneous squamous cell carcinoma]. Schweiz Arch Tierheilkd. 2011;153:573-577.
30. Munday JS, Kiupel M, French AF, et al. Detection of papillomaviral sequences in feline Bowenoid in situ carcinoma using consensus primers. Vet Dermatol. 2007;18:241-245.
31. Anis EA, O'Neill SH, Newkirk KM, et al. Molecular characterization of the L1 gene of papillomaviruses in epithelial lesions of cats and comparative analysis with corresponding gene sequences of human and feline papillomaviruses. Am J Vet Res. 2010;71:1457-1461.
32. Munday JS, Peters-Kennedy J. Consistent detection of Felis domesticus papillomavirus 2 DNA sequences within feline viral plaques. J Vet Diagn Invest. 2010;22:946-949.
33. Munday JS, Howe L, French A, et al. Detection of papillomaviral DNA sequences in a feline oral squamous cell carcinoma. Res Vet Sci. 2009;86:359-361.
34. Munday JS, Knight CG, French AF. Evaluation of feline oral squamous cell carcinomas for p16CDKN2A protein immunoreactivity and the presence of papillomaviral DNA. Res Vet Sci. 2011;90:280-283.
35. Doorbar J. The papillomavirus life cycle. J Clin Virol. 2005;32(suppl 1):S7-15.
36. Moody CA, Laimins LA. Human papillomavirus oncoproteins: pathways to transformation. Nat Rev Cancer. 2010;10:550-560.
37. Munday JS, Aberdein D. Loss of retinoblastoma protein, but not p53, is associated with the presence of papillomaviral DNA in feline viral plaques, Bowenoid in situ carcinomas, and squamous cell carcinomas. Vet Pathol. 2012;49(3):538-545.
38. Stokking LB, Ehrhart EJ, Lichtensteiger CA, et al. Pigmented epidermal plaques in three dogs. J Am Anim Hosp Assoc. 2004;40:411-417.
39. Munday JS, O'Connor KI, Smits B. Development of multiple pigmented viral plaques and squamous cell carcinomas in a dog infected by a novel papillomavirus. Vet Dermatol. 2011;22:104-110.
40. Schulman FY, Krafft AE, Janczewski T. Feline cutaneous fibropapillomas: clinicopathologic findings and association with papillomavirus infection. Vet Pathol. 2001;38:291-296.
41. Wilhelm S, Degorce-Rubiales F, Godson D, et al. Clinical, histological and immunohistochemical study of feline viral plaques and Bowenoid in situ carcinomas. Vet Dermatol. 2006;17:424-431.
42. Yagci BB, Ural K, Ocal N, et al. Azithromycin therapy of papillomatosis in dogs: a prospective, randomized, double-blinded, placebo-controlled clinical trial. Vet Dermatol. 2008;19:194-198.
43. Nagata M, Nanko H, Moriyama A, et al. Pigmented plaques associated with papillomavirus infection in dogs: is this epidermodysplasia verruciformis?. Vet Dermatol. 1995;6:179-186.
44. Kanodia S, Fahey LM, Kast WM. Mechanisms used by human papillomaviruses to escape the host immune response. Curr Cancer Drug Targets. 2007;7:79-89.

CHAPTER 27

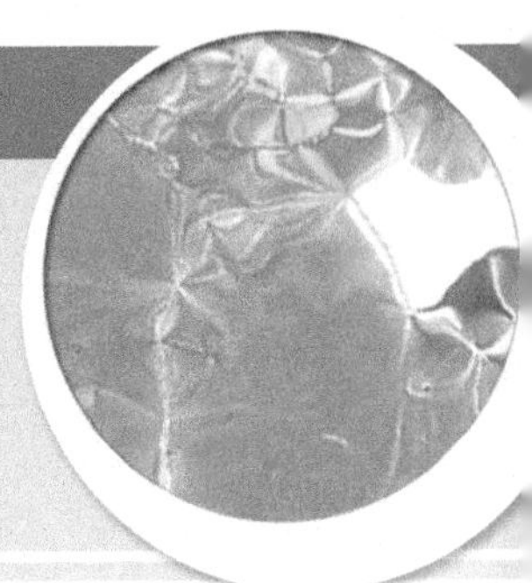

Vector-borne and Other Viral Encephalitides

Jane E. Sykes

> **Overview of Vector-borne Encephalitides in Dogs and Cats**
>
> First Described: Eastern equine encephalitis, 1831 (horses, Massachusetts)[1]; West Nile virus infection, 1937 (human, Uganda)[2]; tick-borne encephalitis virus, 1931 (humans, Austria)[3]
>
> Causes: RNA viruses that belong to the families Togaviridae (genus *Alphavirus*), such as eastern equine encephalitis virus; Bunyaviridae, such as La Crosse virus; and Flaviviridae, such as West Nile virus and tick-borne encephalitis virus
>
> Affected Hosts: A variety of animal species including horses, humans, and dogs
>
> Geographic Distribution: Follows that of the vector host. Eastern equine encephalitis virus is found in the eastern and southeastern United States, as well as Central and South America; West Nile virus is found in Africa, Asia, Middle East, Europe, and the United States; tick-borne encephalitis virus is found in continental Europe and Asia
>
> Mode of Transmission: Primarily mosquitos and for tick-borne encephalitis virus, *Ixodes* ticks.
>
> Major Clinical Signs (Dogs): Fever (sometimes >105°F [40.6°C]), lethargy, neurologic signs, and sometimes systemic signs such as anorexia and diarrhea
>
> Differential Diagnoses: Rabies, distemper, pseudorabies; bacterial, protozoal, or fungal meningitis; granulomatous meningoencephalitis; hemic neoplasia with central nervous system involvement
>
> Human Health Significance: Humans are susceptible to disease caused by many arboviruses. Dogs and cats are dead-end hosts and do not serve as reservoirs for human infection. Blood and tissues of affected dogs and cats should be handled with caution.

Etiology, Epidemiology, and Clinical Features

A large number of viruses that are spread by arthropod vectors (sometimes referred to as *arboviruses*, for *ar*thropod-*bo*rne *viruses*) can infect and cause encephalitis in dogs and cats (Box 27-1 and Table 27-1). These viruses are all enveloped RNA viruses that are unstable in the environment and readily inactivated with routine disinfectants. Disease is sporadic and most infected dogs and cats show no clinical signs of illness. For many arboviruses, only subclinical infections have been documented in dogs and cats. Arboviruses are maintained in vectors and small rodent and/or avian reservoir hosts, and some of these reservoir hosts can develop illness in association with infection. Dogs and cats, as well as other domestic animal and human hosts, are generally considered "dead end" hosts and do not maintain sufficient viremia to infect arthropods (Figure 27-1). Arboviruses replicate within the arthropod vector and are transmitted to vertebrate hosts when the vector feeds; this is followed by viremia and, in some cases, viral spread to the central nervous system (CNS) and infection of neurons (neuroinvasion), with subsequent neuronal necrosis and inflammation. When disease occurs, it has important public health significance, because the clinical signs can mimic those of rabies. Because humans have the potential to be infected with these viruses, serologic evidence of infection of dogs and cats can also have public health significance.

Alphavirus Infections (Family Togaviridae)

Alphaviruses are mosquito-borne viruses that belong to the family Togaviridae. Members of this group that are of importance to human and animal health include Eastern, Western, and Venezuelan encephalitis viruses, which primarily cause disease in humans and horses in the Americas; and Ross River virus, which causes disease in humans in Australia and the Pacific islands. Although there is one possible report of encephalitis in a dog due to Venezuelan equine encephalitis virus,[4] only eastern equine encephalitis virus (EEEV) is a significant cause of disease in dogs. Other alphaviruses cause subclinical seroconversion when they infect dogs; in some reports, seropositive cats have also been identified.[5] Dogs have been used as sentinels for the presence of the virus in epidemiologic serosurveys.[6]

EEEV is endemic in swampy areas of the southeastern United States,[7] where it is maintained in a variety of avian reservoir hosts. It causes disease in humans, horses, dogs, and other domestic animal species. Different viral lineages exist that vary in pathogenicity for humans and horses. Human cases occur in the southeastern, eastern, and Great Lakes regions of the United States, but especially Florida, Georgia, Massachusetts, and New Jersey (Figure 27-2, *A*).[8] Most affected dogs are from Georgia, but one affected dog was from New York state.[9] Dogs with signs of encephalitis have always been young (<7 months of age). Disease usually occurs in late spring or summer. Clinical signs include fever, lethargy, inappetence, and diarrhea, with rapid progression (within 1 to 2 days) to recumbency, tachypnea, miosis, nystagmus, tremors, seizures, and death.[7]

Bunyavirus Infections

Important bunyaviruses for animal and human health are the mosquito-borne viruses Rift Valley fever (genus *Phlebovirus*) and La Crosse (genus *Bunyavirus*) viruses; the tick-borne virus

TABLE 27-1

Potential Causes of Vector-borne Viral and Other Viral Encephalitides in Dogs and Cats

Virus	Classification	Vector	Affected Hosts	Geographic Distribution
Eastern equine encephalitis virus	Family Togaviridae, genus *Alphavirus*	Mosquitos	Horses, humans, dogs, other domestic farm animal species	Southeastern (especially Georgia and Florida), eastern, and Great Lakes regions of the United States
Venezuelan equine encephalitis virus	Family Togaviridae, genus *Alphavirus*	Mosquitos	Horses, humans, possibly dogs	Southern United States (Florida), Central and South America (especially Colombia, Venezuela, Trinidad, Peru, Ecuador, Mexico)
La Crosse virus	Family Bunyaviridae	Mosquitos	Humans, dogs	Eastern and Midwestern United States
West Nile virus	Family Flaviviridae	Mosquitos	Horses, humans, birds, dogs	North, Central, and South America; Africa, the Middle East, Europe, Asia, Australia
Tick-borne encephalitis virus	Family Flaviviridae	*Ixodes* ticks	Humans, horses, dogs; domestic animals are generally infected subclinically	Europe, Asia
Borna disease virus	Family Bornaviridae	None known	Horses, cattle, cats, dogs	Primarily Sweden, Austria, Germany, and Japan

BOX 27-1

General Features of Arbovirus Infections as They Relate to Dogs and Cats

- Vector-borne enveloped RNA viruses
- Most often mosquito-borne
- Maintained among small wild vertebrate reservoir hosts, especially birds and/or rodents
- Geographic distribution follows that of vector host
- Seasonal distribution that reflects activity of the vector host
- May cause disease in humans and other domestic animals, especially horses
- Infection of dogs and cats is most often subclinical
- Dogs and cats are "dead end" hosts
- Infection more prevalent in dogs than in cats
- Sporadic reports of disease, especially in young animals (<6 months)
- Neurologic signs accompanied by fever and sometimes other systemic signs (e.g., diarrhea)
- Histopathology shows neuronal necrosis, gliosis, and perivascular cuffing within the brain, which is predominantly nonsuppurative.

Crimean-Congo hemorrhagic fever virus (genus *Nairovirus*); and members of the genus *Hantavirus*, which are not transmitted by vectors and cause hemorrhagic febrile and respiratory illness in humans. Serologic evidence of infection with some these viruses has been documented in dogs and cats.[10,11] La Crosse virus is the only bunyavirus reported to cause disease in dogs under natural circumstances, but this appears to be rare.[12,13] La Crosse virus was named after La Crosse in Wisconsin, where it was first identified as a human pathogen, and is found mostly in the eastern and midwestern United States (see Figure 27-2, *B*). The virus is maintained in rodents, especially Eastern gray squirrels and chipmunks. It is a major cause of human pediatric encephalitis in North America, although mortality is low. Affected dogs have included an adult dog from Florida and three puppies from southern Georgia.[12,13] Mild fever, lethargy, ataxia, vestibular signs, and ultimately seizures occurred in the adult dog, and sudden death was reported in the puppies.

Flavivirus Infections

Vector-borne flaviviruses (*flavi* = "yellow," Latin) of importance to human and animal health are the mosquito-borne viruses Japanese encephalitis virus, yellow fever virus, Murray Valley encephalitis virus, St. Louis encephalitis virus, Wesselsbron virus, Dengue viruses, and West Nile virus (WNV), as well as the tick-borne viruses tick-borne encephalitis (TBE) virus, louping ill virus, and Powassan virus. Antibodies to some of these viruses have been detected in dogs and to a lesser extent, cats in serosurveys,[14-18] but serologic cross-reactivity among flaviviruses can occur. Although uncommon to rare, WNV in the United States and TBE virus in Europe have been reported to cause disease in dogs on more than one occasion. One dog from Africa with fatal encephalitis was initially thought to be infected with Wesselsbron disease virus,[19] but the isolate was later confirmed to be WNV.[20]

West Nile Virus Infection

West Nile virus was first isolated in 1937 from a woman in the West Nile region of Uganda.[21] In the 1950s, the virus was recognized in Israel as a cause of human neurologic disease in the elderly,[22] and subsequently was identified in other parts of Europe and South Africa. In 1999, it appeared in New York state, possibly by transport of infected humans, birds, or

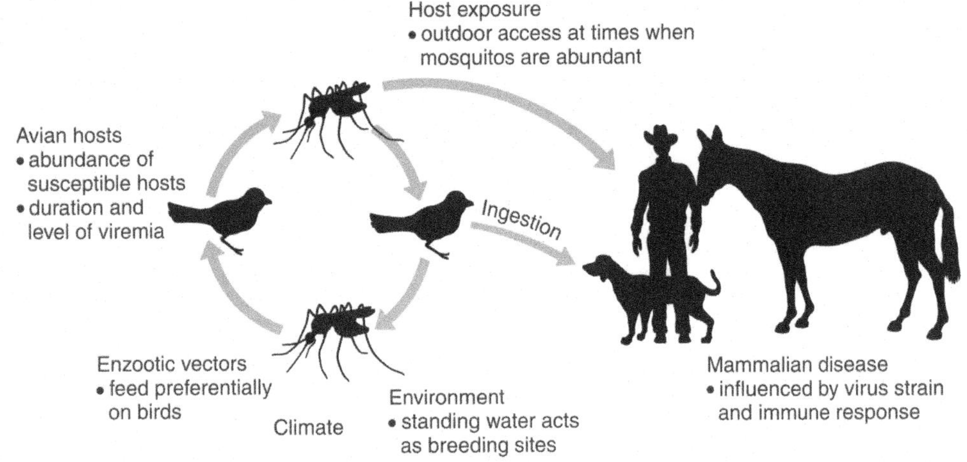

FIGURE 27-1 West Nile virus transmission cycle and factors that influence arbovirus epidemiology.

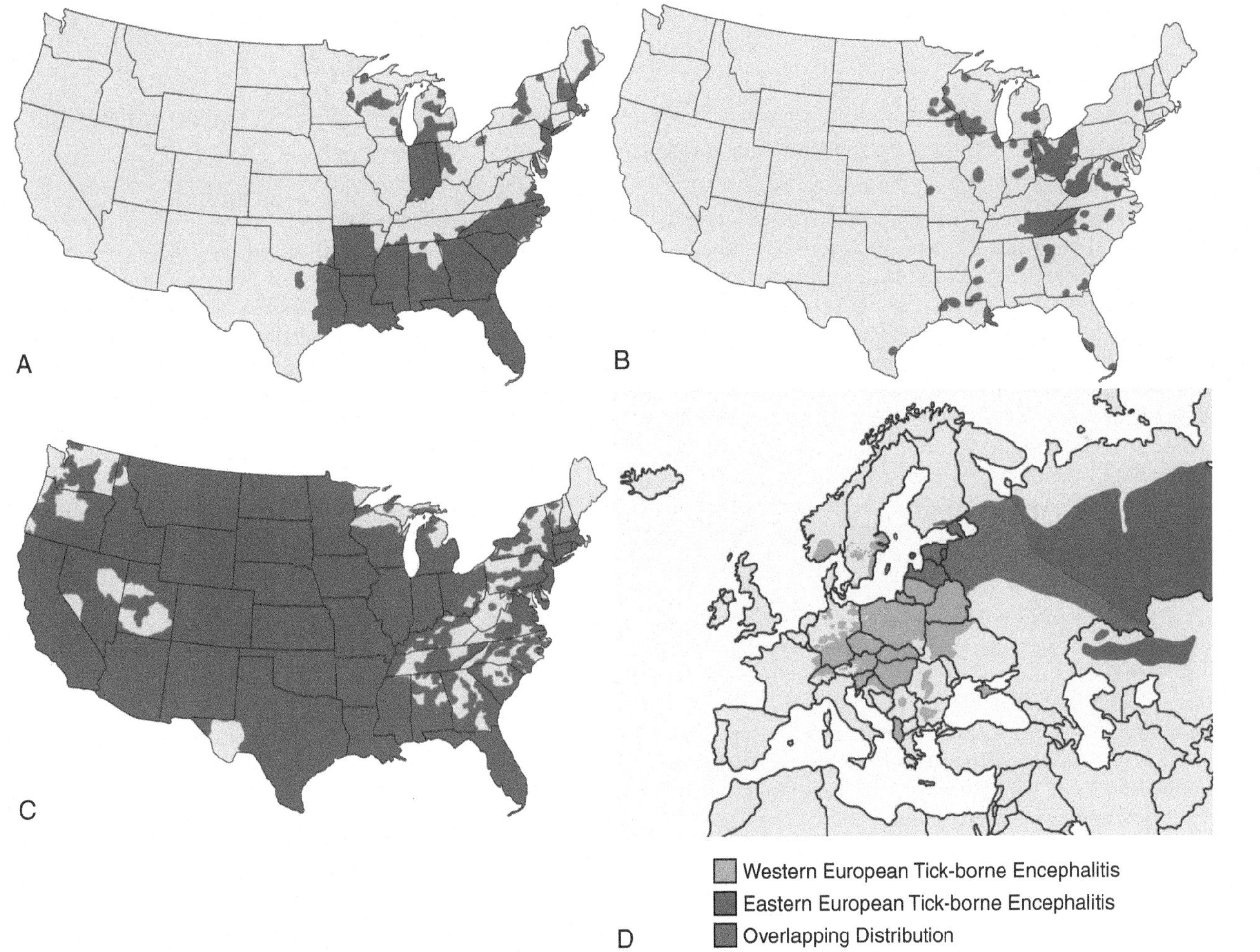

A B C D

Western European Tick-borne Encephalitis
Eastern European Tick-borne Encephalitis
Overlapping Distribution

FIGURE 27-2 Geographic distribution of some arboviruses that can cause disease in dogs and cats. **A,** Regions with eastern equine encephalitis virus transmission. **B,** Regions with La Crosse virus transmission. **C,** Regions with West Nile virus transmission. **D,** Regions with tick-borne encephalitis virus transmission.

mosquitos.[23] WNV then spread explosively westward across the United States, and by 2003, disease was detected across the United States to California (see Figure 27-2, C). WNV also spread into Canada, Mexico, the Caribbean, and Central and South America.[23,24] Several different variants of the virus exist, which differ in virulence. Strains circulating within the Western hemisphere, Europe, the Middle East, India, Africa, and Australia belong to WNV lineage 1; lineage 2 strains circulate in South Africa and Madagascar. Other lineages have also been reported.

Transmission of WNV by mosquitos increases in the warmer months, with peak activity between July and October. Birds (especially passerines such as crows, jays, and brown sparrows;

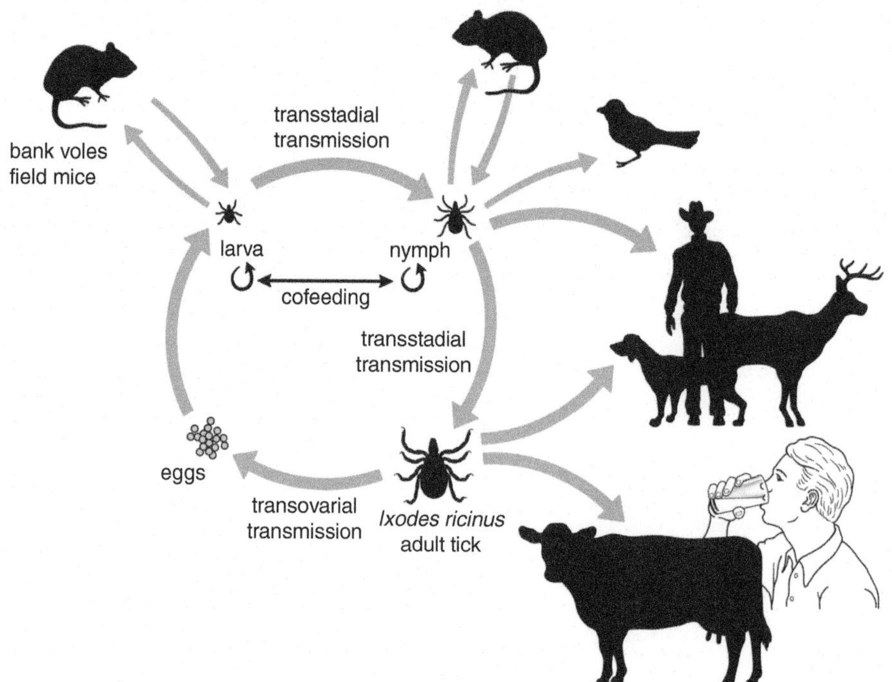

FIGURE 27-3 Transmission cycle for tick-borne encephalitis virus.

shorebirds; owls; and hawks) are important reservoir hosts (see Figure 27-1). Some avian species, such as brown sparrows, maintain high viremias in the absence of clinical signs. Other modes of transmission occur, such as ingestion through predation of infected birds or rodents, blood transfusion, needle-stick injuries, and transplacental transmission. Disease primarily occurs in birds, humans, and horses. When signs occur in humans they are often mild and self-limiting and include fever, headache, myalgia, fatigue, gastrointestinal symptoms, and a transient rash.[25] Rarely, hepatitis, pancreatitis, myocarditis, rhabdomyolysis, orchitis, uveitis, and chorioretinitis can occur. Severe, neuroinvasive disease occurs in fewer than 1% of cases, is most common in the elderly and results in high fever, cervical rigidity, muscle weakness, seizures, and flaccid paralysis. Neurologic signs result from viral invasion of neurons in the brainstem, deep nuclei, and anterior horns within the spinal cord. Clinical signs in horses result from polioencephalomyelitis and include fever and neurologic signs such as ataxia, weakness, and muscle tremors.[26] Approximately two thirds of horses recover. Infected wild birds can exhibit neurologic disease but are usually found dead. Myocarditis and meningoencephalitis are common necropsy findings in these birds.[27]

In dogs, there is widespread serologic evidence of infection, but disease is rare. Cats can become infected and seroconvert, but illness has not been described. Five clinically affected dogs have been described. All, apart from the dog from Africa, resided in various parts of the United States (Missouri, Mississippi, California, and Illinois).[28-31] All of the dogs had signs of fever and progressive neurologic disease. Neurologic signs included generalized tremors, ataxia, a head tilt, bobbing movements, altered mentation, cervical pain, abnormal placing reactions, and tetraparesis. Diarrhea, serous oculonasal discharge, conjunctivitis, abdominal pain, cardiac arrhythmias due to myocarditis, tachypnea, tachycardia, and a stiff gait associated with mild neutrophilic polyarthritis have been reported. For all dogs, diagnosis was made at necropsy.

Tick-Borne Encephalitis Viruses

TBE virus is a notifiable disease that causes potentially fatal neurologic disease in humans in Europe and Asia, where it is the most important tick-borne viral disease of humans.[32] The virus is transmitted transstadially and to a lesser extent transovarially within infected ticks, and ticks can transmit the disease to each other while co-feeding, independent of systemic viremia in vertebrate hosts.[33] Consumption of raw milk from infected ruminants is a lesser mode of transmission to humans (Figure 27-3).

Three subtypes of TBE virus exist, which vary in virulence and geographic distribution. These are designated the European, Siberian, and far-eastern subtypes.[34] The far-eastern subtype occurs in far eastern Russia, Japan, Korea, and China and is the most virulent subtype, with mortality rates in humans that may exceed 20%. In much of Europe, *Ixodes ricinus* ticks spread the European subtype (Western European TBE) whereas *Ixodes persulcatus* ticks transmit the other viral subtypes in northeastern Europe and Asia (Eastern European TBE) (Figure 27-2, *D*).[35] Both Siberian and European subtypes may be found in eastern Europe. The disease was originally detected in 1937 in Austria, but its geographic distribution has expanded rapidly so that the European subtype now occurs throughout Europe as far west as France and possibly Belgium.[17] In Europe, some of the highest incidence rates have occurred in central European countries, especially the Czech Republic.[36] Disease seasonality correlates with the activity of the tick in various parts of Europe. TBE has not been reported in the United Kingdom, but a related tick-borne flavivirus that mainly causes disease in sheep, Louping ill virus, is present. This virus rarely causes encephalitis in dogs.[37,38]

In humans, signs of TBE occur in fewer than 0.5% of infected individuals 4 to 28 days after a tick bite and are biphasic. In the first, viremic phase, fever, malaise, headache, myalgia, and vomiting occur, which resolve within 1 week. In some individuals, after an asymptomatic period that lasts 2 to 10 days, clinical signs return and are accompanied by signs of meningitis, meningoencephalitis, meningoencephalomyelitis, or meningoencephaloradiculitis. About 1% of cases are fatal, most often in the elderly,[39] but neurologic signs can persist for months or longer than a year. Co-infections with *Borrelia burgdorferi* can occur. Vaccines are currently recommended for prevention of TBE in humans, and national vaccination programs in Austria have greatly reduced the incidence of disease.[40]

Subclinical infection of dogs with TBE virus is widespread, and so dogs have been important sentinels for the presence of the virus in new regions of Europe. Rarely, illness that resembles that in humans can occur in dogs. Affected dogs have been described from Sweden, Switzerland, Austria, Germany, and Italy.[32,41] Several reports have described disease in Rottweilers, but it is not clear whether this represents a true breed predisposition. Signs in dogs include high fever, lethargy, anorexia, and neurologic signs such as decreased mentation, behavioral changes such as aggression, delayed placing reactions, ataxia, flaccid paralysis, reduced segmental reflexes, neck pain, vestibular signs, tremors, tetraparesis, miosis, anisocoria, and generalized seizures.[32,35] These signs progress rapidly over several days to a week, usually culminating in death or euthanasia. Recovery has been described rarely.

Bornaviridae

Borna disease virus (BDV) is an enveloped RNA virus that causes meningoencephalitis primarily in horses in Europe, but also in sheep, cattle, and a variety of other domestic and wild animal species. On rare occasions, cats and dogs are affected.[42,43] BDV has been suggested as a possible but unconfirmed cause of neuropsychiatric illness in humans.[44] The epidemiology of BDV remains mysterious. There is some evidence that small mammals (rodents) act as reservoir hosts. In one study, cats at risk were intact male cats, cats that hunted, and cats that resided in a rural habitat.[45] BDV can be transmitted horizontally among laboratory rodents via urine.[46] Because of seasonal disease occurrence in the spring and summer, an arthropod vector has been suspected, but like rabies virus, BDV is thought to enter the CNS principally via axonal transport from mucosal surfaces, which suggests that direct transmission may be more important. Entrance via the olfactory system has been suggested based on lesions found in horses.[44]

Feline infection was first recognized in Sweden in the early 1970s. The virus has also been detected in cats with neurologic disease from Austria, Switzerland, the United Kingdom, and Japan.[47-49] Some studies have shown a higher prevalence of antibodies to BDV in cats with neurologic signs than in cats without neurologic signs. Affected dogs have been reported from Japan and Austria.[42,43] Serologic evidence of infection has been detected in a low percentage (3.7%) of cats that lacked neurologic disease from the western United States.[50]

The clinical signs of BDV infection can be explained by the predilection of the virus for the limbic system, brainstem, and basal ganglia. In cats, the disease has been referred to as "staggering disease" and is manifested by behavioral changes and increased vocalization, anorexia, lethargy, fever, ataxia, posterior paresis, inability to retract the claws, hypersalivation, and seizures. Clinical signs generally progress over 1 to 6 weeks, which is followed by death or euthanasia or permanent residual neurologic dysfunction. Affected dogs have had anorexia, lethargy, tremors, salivation, mydriasis, circling, and seizures.[42,43]

Diagnosis

Laboratory Abnormalities

Laboratory abnormalities in dogs with vector-borne viral encephalitis are nonspecific. No or minimal abnormalities may be detected in some dogs. Mild anemia, leukopenia, lymphopenia, or leukocytosis due to a neutrophilia (sometimes with a left shift) may occur. The CSF may also be unremarkable, or there may be increased protein concentration and mononuclear pleocytosis.

Microbiologic Tests

Serologic Diagnosis

Serologic assays such as ELISAs are available for detection of antibodies to arboviruses through specialized veterinary diagnostic or research laboratories, and have primarily been used for epidemiologic serosurveys of dogs and cats. Serologic assays have, in general, not been very useful for diagnosis of acute viral encephalitis in dogs and cats. First, because disease is rare, arbovirus infections are often not suspected before death or euthanasia, and euthanasia is often performed early because of suspicion for rabies. Second, incubation periods are often short and disease in dogs progresses rapidly with a high mortality rate, so there is insufficient time for an antibody response to develop. Serologic assays have mainly been used to detect IgG and IgM in dogs with TBE from Europe.[32]

Virus Isolation

Arboviruses can be isolated in a variety of cell lines, and virus isolation has been used to detect WNV, TBE virus, and La Crosse virus in naturally infected dogs with encephalitis and BDV in cats.[12,28,47,51] Fresh or fresh-frozen brain or spinal cord homogenates are suitable specimens. Because viremia occurs, blood, CSF, lung, spleen, and liver might also be useful specimens for isolation.[28,32] Immunofluorescent antibody staining and reverse transcriptase–PCR (RT-PCR) assays are used to confirm the presence of the virus in cell cultures.[7,28,47] Because these viruses can infect humans, specialized biosafety level 3 facilities are generally required. This limits the availability and practicality of virus isolation for routine diagnostic purposes.

Molecular Diagnosis Using the Polymerase Chain Reaction

Conventional and real-time RT-PCR assays have been described for many different arboviral pathogens and BDV. Specialized veterinary diagnostic and research laboratories generally perform these assays. In dogs, RT-PCR assays have been used to detect EEEV, WNV, and BDV in clinical specimens.[7,28,42,43] Because BDV can be detected using PCR assays in tissues in the absence of clinical signs, other methods that localize virus to sites of inflammation, such as immunohistochemistry or in situ hybridization, are necessary for diagnosis of BDV encephalitis.

Pathologic Findings

In general, histopathology of the CNS in dogs with vector-borne viral infections, and cats and dogs with Borna disease, reveals nonsuppurative meningoencephalitis or meningoencephalomyelitis, with multifocal mild to moderate gliosis, neuronal necrosis, and perivascular cuffing with lymphocytes, histiocytes, and plasma cells within Virchow-Robin spaces.[12,32,43] Neutrophils predominate within the meninges of dogs infected with EEEV.[7] Within brain tissue, inflammatory infiltrates in dogs infected with EEEV have been most prominent in the gray

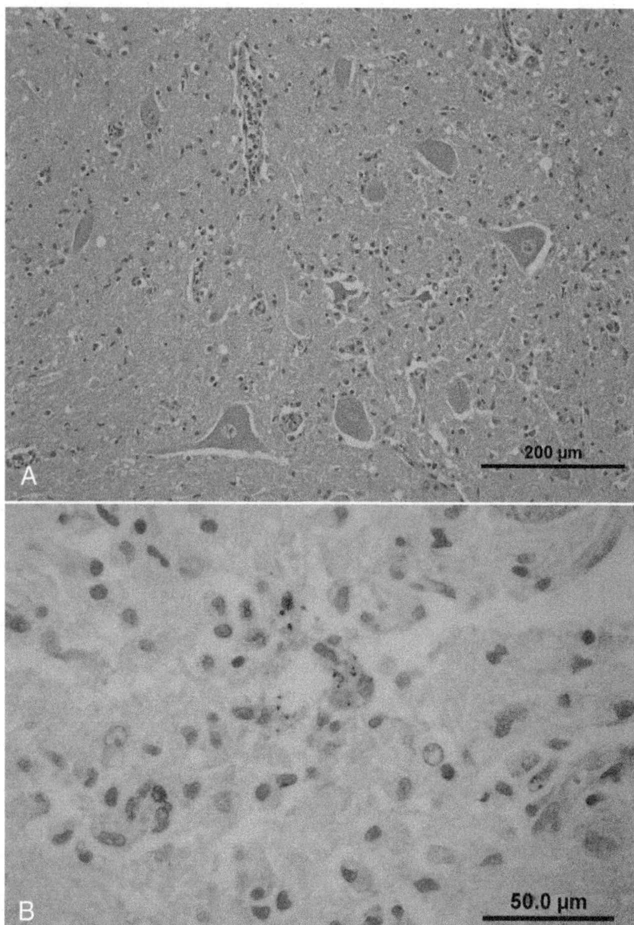

FIGURE 27-4 Spinal cord segment of a dog with WNV encephalitis that shows gliosis and multiple degenerate neurons. **A,** H&E stain. **B,** Immunohistochemical stain showing WNV immunoreactivity *(brown)*. (From Cannon AB, Luff J, Brault C, et al. Acute encephalitis, polyarthritis and myocarditis associated with West Nile virus infection in a dog. J Vet Internal Med 2006;20:1219-1223.)

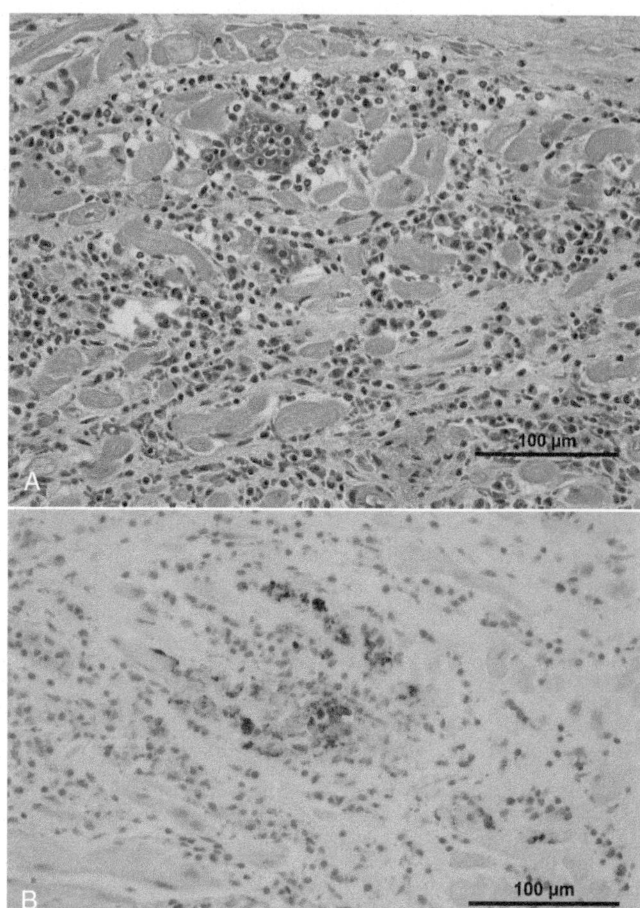

FIGURE 27-5 Severe lymphocytic and neutrophilic myocarditis and vasculitis due to WNV infection with focally extensive hemorrhage and myonecrosis. **A,** H&E stain. **B,** Immunohistochemical stain showing WNV immunoreactivity within neutrophils and histiocytes *(brown)*. (From Cannon AB, Luff J, Brault C, et al. Acute encephalitis, polyarthritis and myocarditis associated with West Nile virus infection in a dog. J Vet Internal Med 2006;20:1219-1223.)

matter of the cerebral cortices and midbrains. Gray matter has also been preferentially infected in dogs with WNV encephalitis.[28] Pathologic changes in dogs with TBE are most severe in the brainstem and the cerebellum; meningitis and spinal cord involvement have also been described.[32] BDV preferentially infects the limbic system and brainstem, although the cerebral cortex may also be involved, and one dog had diffuse disease.[39,40,44] Immunohistochemistry has been used to detect antigen of WNV, La Crosse virus, and TBE virus in CNS and other tissues of dogs, and to detect BDV antigen in the CNS of cats and dogs at necropsy (Figure 27-4).[13,28,41-43,47] In situ hybridization has been used to detect BDV RNA in the CNS of dogs and cats.[43,48]

Extraneural lesions have mainly been reported in dogs infected with WNV. Lymphocytic and necrotizing myocarditis was present in several dogs (Figure 27-5). Other findings in dogs with WNV infection have included evidence of hepatic and renal tubular epithelial cell necrosis, neutrophilic pancreatitis, and mild plasmacytic synovitis.[28-31]

Treatment and Prognosis

Treatment of dogs with vector-borne viral encephalitis is supportive only. The prognosis appears to be poor, but because only a handful of infected dogs have been reported, the true prognosis is poorly understood. In virtually all dogs with neurologic signs, diagnosis has been made at necropsy. Some dogs with TBE recover with supportive care.[32] Glucocorticoids have been used to treat some dogs and cats with viral encephalitides, but their use is controversial because of immunosuppression, and controlled studies are not available.

Immunity and Vaccination

Exposure to vector-borne viruses appears to confer immunity to future infections with the same virus. Vaccines are not available for dogs because disease is uncommon to rare. However, vaccines are available and used widely in endemic areas to prevent flavivirus infections in humans (such as TBE, yellow fever, and Japanese encephalitis) and WNV encephalitis in horses.

Prevention

The risk of arboviral infections in dogs and cats can be reduced through control of mosquito and tick vectors. Keeping pets indoors, especially at dawn and dusk when mosquitos are most active, can also reduce exposure, provided mosquitos are excluded through the use of proper screens and windows.

For viruses such as WNV and BDV, prevention of predation on dead birds or rodents may also reduce the risk of infection. Drainage of standing water and removal of containers (tin cans, old tires, flower pots, clogged gutters, bunched tarpaulins) that act as breeding sites are important for mosquito control. Water in birdbaths should be changed at least weekly. Weeds and brush should be reduced. Human mosquito repellents that contain DEET are not recommended for pets, because they can be toxic.[52] Some products labeled for tick prevention in dogs and cats may help to repel mosquitos but are not likely to completely protect against mosquito bites. More information on tick prevention can be found in Chapter 28. Only products specifically labeled for cats should be used on cats or on dogs that are in contact with cats, because of the sensitivity of cats to permethrin toxicosis.[53]

Public Health Aspects

Many arboviruses that cause disease in humans also infect dogs and cats. Dogs and cats are generally not considered reservoirs for transmission of virus to humans because they do not develop high-level or sustained viremia. As noted previously, dogs have been used as sentinels for the presence of these viruses in epidemiologic studies.

CASE EXAMPLE

Signalment: "Paloma," a 13-year-old female spayed golden retriever–Irish setter mix from Vacaville in northern California.

History: Paloma was evaluated at the University of California, Davis, Veterinary Medical Teaching Hospital in September for a 3-day history of inappetence and lethargy. Two days before, physical examination by the referring veterinarian had revealed tachycardia (96 beats/min) and pyrexia (103.1°F or 39.5°C). Results of routine CBC, biochemistry tests, and a urinalysis did not reveal clinically significant abnormalities. The dog was treated with amoxicillin (20 mg/kg PO q12h) and enrofloxacin (10 mg/kg PO q12h), without improvement.

Physical Examination:

Body Weight: 28.6 kg

General: Obtunded, 5% dehydrated. T = 106°F (41.1°C), HR = 140 beats/min, RR = 92 breaths/min, mucous membranes pink, CRT = 1 s.

Integument: No clinically significant abnormalities.

Eyes, Ears, Nose, and Throat: Bilateral enophthalmos, mild serous ocular discharge, conjunctivitis, and nuclear sclerosis were present. Moderate to severe dental disease was present. Examination of the ocular fundus showed no abnormalities.

Musculoskeletal: Body condition score 4/9. Ambulatory on all four limbs, but generalized weakness was noted. Moderate atrophy of the temporalis, quadriceps, and gastrocnemius muscles was present.

Cardiovascular, Respiratory, Gastrointestinal, Urogenital and Lymphoid Systems: Tachypnea and tachycardia were identified. There was mild cranial abdominal discomfort on palpation. All peripheral lymph nodes were normal sized.

Neurologic Examination: Decreased placing reactions were noted in all four limbs, and there was pain on manipulation of the neck.

Laboratory Findings:

CBC:

HCT 37.5% (40%-55%)
MCV 67.3 fL (65-75 fL)
MCHC 34.4 g/dL (33-36 g/dL)
WBC 6050 cells/μL (6000-13,000 cells/μL)
Neutrophils 5627 cells/μL (3000-10,500 cells/μL)
Lymphocytes 363 cells/μL (1000-4000 cells/μL)
Monocytes 61 cells/μL (150-1200 cells/μL)
Adequate platelet numbers (clumped on smear).

Serum Chemistry Profile:

Sodium 144 mmol/L (145-154 mmol/L)
Potassium 4.0 mmol/L (3.6-5.3 mmol/L)
Chloride 110 mmol/L (108-118 mmol/L)
Bicarbonate 16 mmol/L (16-26 mmol/L)
Phosphorus 3.1 mg/dL (3.0-6.2 mg/dL)
Calcium 9.1 mg/dL (9.7-11.5 mg/dl)
BUN 8 mg/dL (5-21 mg/dL)
Creatinine 0.6 mg/dL (0.3-1.2 mg/dL)
Glucose 86 mg/dL (64-123 mg/dL)
Total protein 5.7 g/dL (5.4-7.6 g/dL)
Albumin 2.3 g/dL (3.0-4.4 g/dL)
Globulin 3.4 g/dL (1.8-3.9 g/dL)
ALT 25 U/L (19-67 U/L)
AST 34 U/L (19-42 U/L)
ALP 53 U/L (21-170 U/L)
Gamma GT 3 U/L (0-6 U/L)
Cholesterol 236 mg/dL (135-361 mg/dL)
Total bilirubin 0.3 mg/dL (0-0.2 mg/dL).

Imaging Findings:

Thoracic, Abdominal, Spinal, and Joint Radiographs: No significant abnormalities were noted.

Abdominal Ultrasound: Mild mesenteric and moderate sublumbar lymphadenomegaly was identified. The dog exhibited pain on ultrasound of the right cranial abdomen, but no abnormalities in this region were identified. Impressions: mesenteric and sublumbar lymphadenomegaly.

Microbiologic Testing: Aerobic and anaerobic blood cultures (five sequentially collected specimens): negative

Serology for *Ehrlichia canis*, *Anaplasma phagocytophilum*, and *Borrelia burgdorferi* antibodies (lateral flow ELISA): negative

Treatment: Paloma was treated with lactated Ringer's solution (3 mL/kg/h IV) with potassium chloride supplementation (20 mEq/L), amoxicillin (22 mg/kg PO q8h), enrofloxacin (10 mg/kg PO q24h), and doxycycline (5 mg/kg PO q12h). Physical examination on day 2 revealed persistent pyrexia (105.6°F), tachycardia (108 beats/min), and a stiff gait, but there was no evidence of joint pain or swelling on palpation. Cytologic analysis of synovial fluid collected from both carpal and tibiotarsal joints using arthrocentesis revealed mild suppurative and mononuclear inflammation.

On day 3, the dog became tetraparetic and was unable to stand for longer than a few seconds. Pyrexia (104.5°F) persisted, and treatment with dexamethasone sodium phosphate (0.2 mg/kg IV once) and hydromorphone (0.05 mg/kg IV once) was initiated. Neurologic examination disclosed mental dullness, decreased placing reactions in all four limbs, and normal segmental reflexes. Further evaluation for neurologic disease, such as imaging of the brain, CSF analysis, or both, was offered, but declined by the owner because of financial limitations. On day 4, the dog was normothermic, and sternally recumbent. Prednisone (1 mg/kg PO q12h) and metronidazole (10 mg/kg PO q8h) were added to the treatment regime. Despite this treatment, by day 5, Paloma was laterally recumbent and obtunded. The owner elected euthanasia.

Necropsy Findings: Histopathologic findings at necropsy consisted of severe acute multifocal necrotizing perivascular and random neutrophilic pancreatitis; severe lymphocytic and neutrophilic myocarditis and vasculitis with myonecrosis; and mild, multifocal gliosis and perivascular to random lymphoplasmacytic and neutrophilic polioencephalomyelitis. The cervical spinal cord was the most severely affected. Mild perivascular plasmacytic synovitis was also present. Aerobic and anaerobic cultures of the liver, spleen, spleen, lung, and synovial fluid were negative. West Nile virus antigen was detected with immunohistochemical stains within foci of encephalomyelitis and myocarditis. The virus was isolated from fresh frozen lung tissue, and WNV RNA was detected using RT-PCR in the synovium, synovial fluid, spinal cord, heart, and kidney tissue.[25]

Diagnosis: Encephalitis, myocarditis, and polyarthritis associated with WNV infection

Comments: This was a rare case of encephalitis and myocarditis associated with WNV infection in a dog. Disease occurred in September, the time of peak activity for virus transmission by mosquitos (July to October).

(From Cannon AB, Luff JA, Brault AC, et al. Acute encephalitis, polyarthritis, and myocarditis associated with West Nile virus infection in a dog. J Vet Intern Med 2006;20:1219-1223.)

SUGGESTED READINGS

Cannon AB, Luff JA, Brault AC, et al. Acute encephalitis, polyarthritis, and myocarditis associated with West Nile virus infection in a dog. J Vet Intern Med. 2006;20:1219-1223.

Farrar MD, Miller DL, Baldwin CA, et al. Eastern equine encephalitis in dogs. J Vet Diagn Invest. 2005;17:614-617.

Murray KO, Mertens E, Despres P. West Nile virus and its emergence in the United States of America. Vet Res. 2010;41:67.

Pfeffer M, Dobler G. Tick-borne encephalitis virus in dogs—is this an issue? Parasit Vectors. 2011;4:59.

REFERENCES

1. Hanson RP. An epizootic of equine encephalomyelitis that occurred in Massachusetts in 1831. Am J Trop Med Hyg. 1957;6(5):858-862.
2. Smithburn KC, Hughes TP, Burke AW, et al. A neurotropic virus isolated from the blood of a native of Uganda. Am J Trop Med Hyg. 1940;20:471-472.
3. Schneider H. Über epidemische Meningitis serosa. Wien Klin Wochenschr. 1931;44:350.
4. Habluetzel JE, Grimes JE, Pigott Jr MB. Serologic evidence of naturally occurring Venezuelan equine encephalomyelitis virus infection in a dog. J Am Vet Med Assoc. 1973;162:461-462.
5. Kay BH, Boyd AM, Ryan PA, et al. Mosquito feeding patterns and natural infection of vertebrates with Ross River and Barmah Forest viruses in Brisbane, Australia. Am J Trop Med Hyg. 2007;76:417-423.
6. Coffey LL, Crawford C, Dee J, et al. Serologic evidence of widespread Everglades virus activity in dogs, Florida. Emerg Infect Dis. 2006;12:1873-1879.
7. Farrar MD, Miller DL, Baldwin CA, et al. Eastern equine encephalitis in dogs. J Vet Diagn Invest. 2005;17:614-617.
8. Eastern Equine Encephalitis. 2011. http://www.cdc.gov/eastern equineencephalitis/tech/epi.html.Last accessed December 7, 2011.
9. Cornell University College of Veterinary Medicine EEE found in dog first case in New York state. 2011. http://ahdc.vet.cornell.edu/news/eee.cfm. Last accessed January 29, 2013.
10. Dobly A, Cochez C, Goossens E, et al. Sero-epidemiological study of the presence of hantaviruses in domestic dogs and cats from Belgium. Res Vet Sci. 2012;92(2):221-224.
11. Shepherd AJ, Swanepoel R, Shepherd SP, et al. Antibody to Crimean-Congo hemorrhagic fever virus in wild mammals from southern Africa. Am J Trop Med Hyg. 1987;36:133-142.
12. Black SS, Harrison LR, Pursell AR, et al. Necrotizing panencephalitis in puppies infected with La Crosse virus. J Vet Diagn Invest. 1994;6:250-254.
13. Tatum LM, Pacy JM, Frazier KS, et al. Canine La Crosse viral meningoencephalomyelitis with possible public health implications. J Vet Diagn Invest. 1999;11:184-188.
14. Chang HC, Takashima I, Arikawa J, et al. Biotin-labeled protein-A enzyme-linked immunosorbent assay for the detection of Japanese encephalitis antibody in sera from humans, swine and several animal species. J Virol Methods. 1984;9:143-151.
15. Kokernot RH, Hayes J, Will RL, et al. Arbovirus studies in the Ohio-Mississippi Basin, 1964-1967. II. St. Louis encephalitis virus. Am J Trop Med Hyg. 1969;18:750-761.
16. Resnick MP, Grunenwald P, Blackmar D, et al. Juvenile dogs as potential sentinels for West Nile virus surveillance. Zoonoses Public Health. 2008;55:443-447.
17. Roelandt S, Heyman P, De Filette M, et al. Tick-borne encephalitis virus seropositive dog detected in Belgium: screening of the canine population as sentinels for public health. Vector Borne Zoonotic Dis. 2011;11:1371-1376.
18. Lindhe KE, Meldgaard DS, Jensen PM, et al. Prevalence of tick-borne encephalitis virus antibodies in dogs from Denmark. Acta Vet Scand. 2009;51:56.
19. Simpson VR, Kuebart G, Barnard B. A fatal case of Wesselsbron disease in a dog. Vet Rec. 1979;105:329.
20. Burt FJ, Grobbelaar AA, Leman PA, et al. Phylogenetic relationships of southern African West Nile virus isolates. Emerg Infect Dis. 2002;8:820-826.
21. Smithburn KC, Hughs TP, Burke AW, et al. A neurotropic virus isolated from the blood of a native of Uganda. Am J Trop Med Hyg. 1940;20:471-492.
22. Bernkopf H, Levine S, Nerson R. Isolation of West Nile virus in Israel. J Infect Dis. 1953;93:207-218.
23. Murray KO, Mertens E, Despres P. West Nile virus and its emergence in the United States of America. Vet Res. 2010;41:67.
24. Morshed M, Tang P, Petric M, et al. West Nile virus finally debuts in British Columbia 10 years after its introduction to North America. Vector Borne Zoonotic Dis. 2011;11:1221-1224.
25. Hayes EB, Gubler DJ. West Nile virus: epidemiology and clinical features of an emerging epidemic in the United States. Annu Rev Med. 2006;57:181-194.
26. Schuler LA, Khaitsa ML, Dyer NW, et al. Evaluation of an outbreak of West Nile virus infection in horses: 569 cases (2002). J Am Vet Med Assoc. 2004;225:1084-1089.
27. Steele KE, Linn MJ, Schoepp RJ, et al. Pathology of fatal West Nile virus infections in native and exotic birds during the 1999 outbreak in New York City, New York. Vet Pathol. 2000;37:208-224.

28. Cannon AB, Luff JA, Brault AC, et al. Acute encephalitis, polyarthritis, and myocarditis associated with West Nile virus infection in a dog. J Vet Intern Med. 2006;20:1219-1223.
29. Buckweitz S, Kleiboeker S, Marioni K, et al. Serological, reverse transcriptase-polymerase chain reaction, and immunohistochemical detection of West Nile virus in a clinically affected dog. J Vet Diagn Invest. 2003;15:324-329.
30. Lichtensteiger CA, Heinz-Taheny K, Osborne TS, et al. West Nile virus encephalitis and myocarditis in wolf and dog. Emerg Infect Dis. 2003;9:1303-1306.
31. Read RW, Rodriguez DB, Summers BA. West Nile virus encephalitis in a dog. Vet Pathol. 2005;42:219-222.
32. Pfeffer M, Dobler G. Tick-borne encephalitis virus in dogs—is this an issue? Parasit Vectors. 2011;4:59.
33. Randolph SE. Transmission of tick-borne pathogens between co-feeding ticks: Milan Labuda's enduring paradigm. Ticks Tick Borne Dis. 2011;2:179-182.
34. Ecker M, Allison SL, Meixner T, et al. Sequence analysis and genetic classification of tick-borne encephalitis viruses from Europe and Asia. J Gen Virol. 1999;80(Pt 1):179-185.
35. Leschnik MW, Kirtz GC, Thalhammer JG. Tick-borne encephalitis (TBE) in dogs. Int J Med Microbiol. 2002;291(suppl 33):66-69.
36. Mansfield KL, Johnson N, Phipps LP, et al. Tick-borne encephalitis virus—a review of an emerging zoonosis. J Gen Virol. 2009;90:1781-1794.
37. MacKenzie CP. Recovery of a dog from louping-ill. J Small Anim Pract. 1982;23:233-236.
38. MacKenzie CP, Lewis ND, Smith ST, et al. Louping-ill in a working collie. Vet Rec. 1973;92:354-356.
39. Vaughn DW, Barrett A, Solomon T. Flaviviruses. In: Mandell GL, Bennett JE, Dolin R, eds. Principles and Practice of Infectious Diseases. 7th ed. Philadelphia, PA: Churchill Livingstone, Elsevier; 2010:2133-2156.
40. Kunz C, Heinz FX. Tick-borne encephalitis. Vaccine. 2003;21(suppl 1): S1-2.
41. Weissenbock H, Suchy A, Holzmann H. Tick-borne encephalitis in dogs: neuropathological findings and distribution of antigen. Acta Neuropathol. 1998;95:361-366.
42. Weissenbock H, Nowotny N, Caplazi P, et al. Borna disease in a dog with lethal meningoencephalitis. J Clin Microbiol. 1998;36:2127-2130.
43. Okamoto M, Kagawa Y, Kamitani W, et al. Borna disease in a dog in Japan. J Comp Pathol. 2002;126:312-317.
44. Lipkin WI, Briese T, Hornig M. Borna disease virus—Fact and fantasy. Virus Res. 2011;162:162-172.
45. Berg AL, Reid-Smith R, Larsson M, et al. Case control study of feline Borna disease in Sweden. Vet Rec. 1998;142:715-717.
46. Sauder C, Staeheli P. Rat model of Borna disease virus transmission: epidemiological implications. J Virol. 2003; 77:12886-12890.
47. Lundgren AL, Zimmermann W, Bode L, et al. Staggering disease in cats: isolation and characterization of the feline Borna disease virus. J Gen Virol. 1995;76(Pt 9):2215-2222.
48. Nakamura Y, Watanabe M, Kamitani W, et al. High prevalence of Borna disease virus in domestic cats with neurological disorders in Japan. Vet Microbiol. 1999;70:153-169.
49. Reeves NA, Helps CR, Gunn-Moore DA, et al. Natural Borna disease virus infection in cats in the United Kingdom. Vet Rec. 1998;143:523-526.
50. Abamaku M, Yee JL, Sykes JE, et al. Borna virus-specific antibodies in sera from domestic cats in California. 2012:Submitted for publication.
51. Gresikova M, Sekeyova M, Weidnerova K, et al. Isolation of tick-borne encephalitis virus from the brain of a sick dog in Switzerland. Acta Virol. 1972;16:88.
52. Dorman DC. Diethyltoluamide (DEET) insect repellent toxicosis. Vet Clin North Am Small Anim Pract. 1990;20:387-391.
53. Malik R, Ward MP, Seavers A, et al. Permethrin spot-on intoxication of cats Literature review and survey of veterinary practitioners in Australia. J Feline Med Surg. 2010;12:5-14.

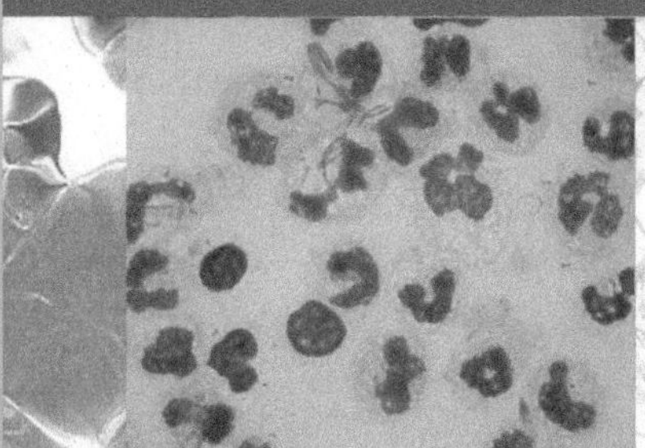

SECTION 2

Bacterial Diseases

CHAPTER 28

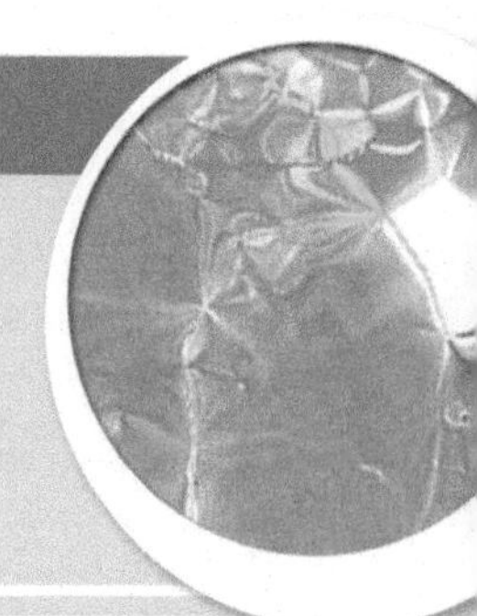

Ehrlichiosis

Jane E. Sykes

Overview of Ehrlichiosis

First Described: *Ehrlichia canis* was first described in 1935 (Algeria).[1] *Ehrlichia ewingii* was described in 1992 (United States).[2] *Ehrlichia chaffeensis* was described in 1991 (United States).[3]

Cause: *E. canis* (canine monocytic ehrlichiosis), *E. ewingii* (canine granulocytic ehrlichiosis), and *E. chaffeensis* (human monocytic ehrlichiosis); an *E. muris*-like organism also may infect dogs in the United States.[4]

Affected Hosts: *E. canis* causes disease in dogs. *E. canis* or a closely related organism may cause disease in cats and humans. *E. ewingii* causes disease in dogs, humans, and goats. *E. chaffeensis* causes disease in humans, possibly dogs and goats. The *E. muris*-like agent causes disease in humans and possibly dogs.

Geographic Distribution: *E. canis* is present worldwide, but especially in tropical and subtropical regions. *E. ewingii* is primarily found in the south-central and southeastern United States. Most reports of *E. chaffeensis* infection are from the southern and south-central United States. The *E. muris*-like agent has been found in the upper Midwest.

Mode of Transmission: *Rhipicephalus sanguineus* ticks (*E. canis*), *Amblyomma americanum* ticks (*E. ewingii* and *E. chaffeensis*).

Major Clinical Signs: The major clinical signs of *E. canis* infection are fever, lethargy, inappetence, weight loss, mucosal hemorrhages, uveitis, pallor, edema, and sometimes neurologic signs. *E. ewingii* primarily causes fever, lethargy, inappetence, and signs of polyarthritis.

Differential Diagnoses: Other tick-borne diseases (such as granulocytic anaplasmosis, Lyme borreliosis and babesiosis), bartonellosis, leptospirosis, lymphoma, multiple myeloma, systemic primary immune-mediated disease

Human Health Significance: All four ehrlichial species can infect and cause disease in humans. The most important human pathogen is *E. chaffeensis*, but the *E. muris*-like agent may also be important.

The ehrlichioses are a group of tick-transmitted diseases caused by intracellular, gram-negative bacteria that include *Ehrlichia canis, Ehrlichia ewingii,* and *Ehrlichia chaffeensis*. An organism related to *Ehrlichia ruminantium*, the cause of heartwater disease in cattle, has also been detected in ill dogs from South Africa,[5] and an organism that resembles *E. muris* has been detected in an ill dog and humans from the upper Midwest of the United States.[4] These organisms form morulae (Latin for "mulberry"), a cluster of bacteria, within phagosomes of circulating leukocytes. *Ehrlichia canis* infects monocytes and causes canine monocytic ehrlichiosis (CME), one of the most important infectious diseases of domestic dogs that are exposed to ticks worldwide. *Ehrlichia ewingii* is an unculturable bacterium that infects granulocytes and causes canine granulocytic ehrlichiosis. *Ehrlichia chaffeensis* causes human monocytic ehrlichiosis; dogs are a proposed reservoir for this organism. The geographic distribution of each pathogen is generally restricted to that of their vectors and mammalian reservoir hosts.

Organisms from the genus *Ehrlichia* are grouped within the family Anaplasmataceae. Also within this family are the bacteria *Anaplasma platys* and *Anaplasma phagocytophilum*, which cause canine thrombocytic and granulocytic anaplasmosis, respectively (see Chapter 29); and organisms belonging to the genera *Neorickettsia* (see Chapter 31). *Rickettsia rickettsii*, the cause of Rocky Mountain spotted fever (RMSF), and other spotted fever group rickettsiae belong to a separate family, the Rickettsiaceae (Chapter 30). The families Rickettsiaceae and Anaplasmataceae are phylogenetically related through the order Rickettsiales (Table 28-1). The recent availability of complete genome sequences for these organisms has helped

TABLE 28-1

Members of the Order Rickettsiales of Clinical Importance in Dogs and Cats

Family	Anaplasmataceae			Rickettsiaceae
Genus	*Ehrlichia*	*Anaplasma*	*Neorickettsia*	*Rickettsia*
Species	*E. canis* *E. chaffeensis* *E. ewingii*	*A. phagocytophilum* *A. platys*	*N. helminthoeca* *N. risticii*	*R. rickettsii*

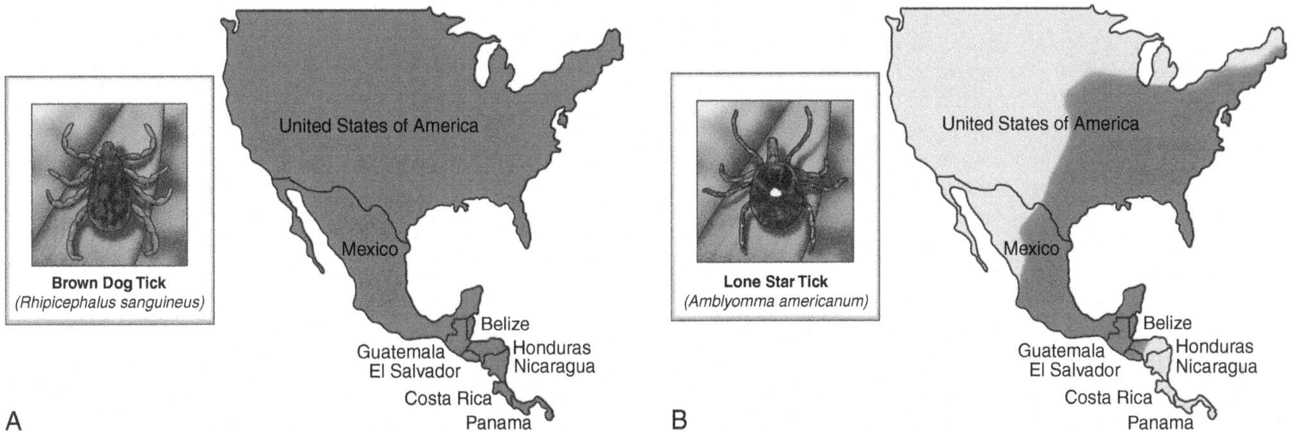

FIGURE 28-1 **A,** Distribution of *Rhipicephalus sanguineus*, which transmits *Ehrlichia canis,* in the United States, Mexico and Central America. **B,** Distribution of *Amblyomma americanum*, which transmits *Ehrlichia ewingii* and *Ehrlichia chaffeensis*. The distribution of *E. ewingii* infections in dogs more closely matches that of *A. americanum* than the distribution of *E. canis* matches that of *R. sanguineus* (highest prevalence in the southern states). This is because of chronic *E. canis* infections that occur in dogs with travel histories to southern states, where the climate is warmer and *R. sanguineus* is more prevalent.

to elucidate mechanisms of pathogenesis and host-pathogen interactions.[5-7]

The severity of clinical signs in animals with ehrlichial infections depends on factors such as the size of the inoculum, host immunity, and organism species and strain. Because of shared arthropod vectors and/or concurrent exposure to multiple vector ticks, co-infections with more than one rickettsial pathogen, as well as other arthropod-borne pathogens such as *Babesia* spp., and *Bartonella* spp., occur commonly in dogs and may complicate the clinical picture.

Ehrlichia canis Infection

Etiology and Epidemiology

E. canis is transmitted primarily by the brown dog tick (*Rhipicephalus sanguineus*), one of the most widely distributed ticks worldwide. Infection has been reported in dogs from Asia, Africa, Europe, and the Americas. Australia appears to be free of *E. canis* infection although occasionally seroreactivity to *E. canis* has been identified in dogs. The DNA of *E. canis* has been detected in other tick species, which include other *Rhipicephalus* species,[8,9] *Ixodes ricinus*,[10] *Haemaphysalis* spp. ticks,[11] and *Dermacentor* spp. ticks[11]; experimental transmission has been accomplished with *Dermacentor variabilis* ticks.[12] Different strains of *E. canis* exist that may vary in virulence. Although *R. sanguineus* is found throughout the United States, it prefers warm climates, and so disease is diagnosed most frequently in dogs living in the southeastern and southwestern states (Figure 28-1). In Europe, *R. sanguineus* is primarily found in Mediterranean regions, but its

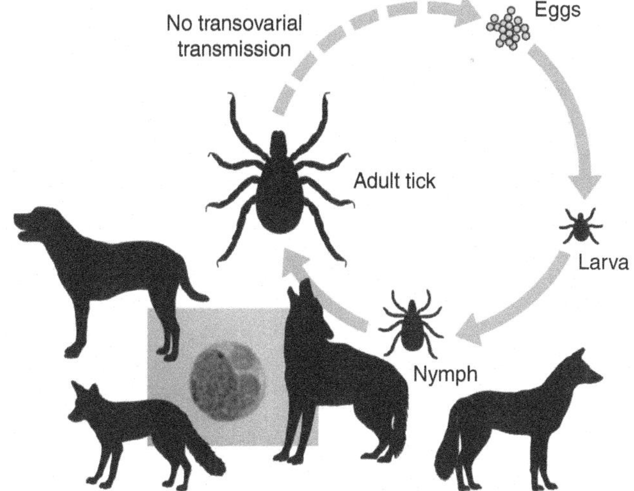

FIGURE 28-2 Life cycle of *Ehrlichia canis*. The organism is transmitted only transstadially (from larva to nymph to adult) within the tick. Jackals, foxes, and possibly coyotes also act as reservoir hosts. A morula is shown within the cytoplasm of a monocyte as seen on a blood smear.

distribution appears to be moving northward, and CME has been reported in dogs that lack travel history as far north as the Netherlands.[13] *E. canis* is the most common pathogen detected in ticks in Israel.[8] Because of chronic, subclinical infection, dogs can be transported to non-endemic regions and subsequently develop disease years later. Tick larvae or nymphs acquire infection when they feed on infected dogs. Jackals, foxes, and possibly coyotes may also act as reservoir hosts. *E. canis* is transmitted transstadially (i.e., from larva to nymph to adult) within the tick (Figure 28-2).[14] No clear age or sex predilection for CME exists, but German shepherds are reportedly more susceptible, and prognosis may be poorer in this breed. Cross-bred dogs may be less likely to develop disease.[15] Although natural infection of cats with *E. canis* (or one or more closely related organisms) has been described in North and South America,[16-18] clinical ehrlichiosis is rarely reported.

Clinical Features

Signs and Their Pathogenesis

The course of CME has been divided into acute, subclinical, and chronic phases, although in naturally infected dogs, these phases may not be readily distinguishable. Clinical signs of acute disease occur 8 to 20 days after infection. The organism multiplies by binary fission within vacuoles of mononuclear phagocytes; rupture of infected host cells leads to infection of new cells. Immune-mediated mechanisms are important in the pathogenesis of disease, and the presence of the spleen appears to contribute to disease severity.[19] The clinical manifestations vary considerably among dogs, which may reflect factors such as *E. canis* strain variation, host immune response, stage of disease, and concurrent infections. Lethargy, inappetence, fever, and weight loss are most common. Replication of the organism in reticuloendothelial tissues is associated with generalized lymphadenopathy and splenomegaly. Ocular and nasal discharges, peripheral edema, and, less commonly, mucosal and cutaneous petechial and ecchymotic hemorrhages can also occur. Bleeding tendencies result from thrombocytopenia and platelet dysfunction,[20] which may reflect immune-mediated platelet damage.[21] Neurologic signs may result from meningeal inflammation or hemorrhage. Dogs can recover spontaneously from the acute phase within 2 to 4 weeks, after which time they may eliminate the infection or remain subclinically infected. Sequestration of organisms within the spleen may occur, and the organisms may evade the host immune system through antigenic variation.[5] This subclinical phase may persist for months to years.

Chronic CME develops in only some infected dogs. Factors that influence the development of chronic disease are unclear, but genetics may play a role. The presence of pancytopenia typifies the severe chronic form of ehrlichiosis, and results from hypoplasia of all bone marrow cells.[22] Clinical signs range in severity and include lethargy, inappetence, bleeding tendencies, mucosal pallor, fever, weight loss, lymphadenopathy, splenomegaly, dyspnea, anterior uveitis, retinal hemorrhage and detachment, polyuria/polydipsia, and edema.[15,22-24] Polymyositis occurs in some dogs, which can be manifested by diffuse muscle wasting and tetraparesis.[25] Secondary opportunistic infections such as viral papillomatosis, protozoal infections, and bacterial urinary tract infections can also develop, although the precise underlying mechanism of immunosuppression, and how it relates to successful persistence of *E. canis*, has not yet been elucidated (see Figure 26-5).[26,27] Marked granular lymphocytosis and bone marrow plasmacytosis may occur, sometimes accompanied by a monoclonal gammopathy, which may lead to misdiagnosis of lymphocytic leukemia or multiple myeloma, respectively. This has led to the recommendation that all dogs with well-differentiated lymphocytosis or otherwise unexplained monoclonal gammopathy be tested for *E. canis* infection.[28] Protein-losing nephropathy may develop as a result of immune-complex glomerulonephritis.

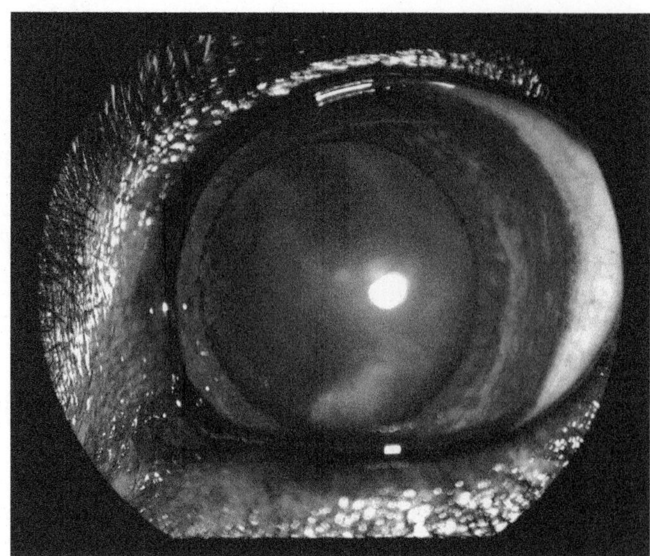

FIGURE 28-3 Retinal hemorrhage and detachment in a 4-year old female spayed Rhodesian ridgeback mix with canine monocytic ehrlichiosis. The dog also had moderate to severe, poorly regenerative, macrocytic hypochromic anemia (16.4% with a reticulocyte count of 49,000), lymphopenia (94 cells/μL), thrombocytopenia (26,000 platelets/μL), and large numbers of circulating nucleated red blood cells (75/100 WBC). Systolic blood pressure was within normal limits. (Courtesy of University of California, Davis Veterinary Ophthalmology Service.)

In reports of feline ehrlichiosis, clinical and laboratory findings have generally been similar to those in dogs; one cat had polyarthritis.[16]

Physical Examination Findings

Common physical examination findings in dogs with CME are lethargy, fever, peripheral lymphadenopathy, and splenomegaly. Ocular and nasal discharge, mucosal petechial hemorrhages, epistaxis, peripheral edema, and/or neurologic signs may be evident. Ocular abnormalities include anterior uveitis, hyphema, retinal hemorrhage, retinal detachment, and optic neuritis, with anterior uveitis being most common (Figure 28-3).[24,29] Neurologic signs include twitching, ataxia, seizures, vestibular signs, hyperesthesia, and cranial nerve defects. Dogs with chronic ehrlichiosis may have thin body condition or diffuse muscle atrophy and mucosal pallor. Findings in cats with ehrlichiosis have been similar to those in dogs, and include lethargy, splenomegaly, lymphadenopathy, petechial hemorrhages, and retinal detachment.[16,17]

Diagnosis

Laboratory Abnormalities

Complete Blood Count

Thrombocytopenia and occasionally mild leukopenia and a nonregenerative anemia occur 1 to 4 weeks after infection with *E. canis*. Mild thrombocytopenia, with increased mean platelet volume, may persist during the subclinical phase. Classically, dogs with chronic CME are pancytopenic, but more commonly, nonregenerative anemia and thrombocytopenia are noted. In some dogs, regenerative anemia or leukocytosis due to a neutrophilia and band neutrophils are present. Lymphopenia occurs in most affected dogs, but in some dogs, moderate to marked granular lymphocytosis (up to 17,000/μL) can occur. Normoblastosis, that can exceed 50 nucleated RBC per 100 WBC, may be present.

In some dogs, morulae are visualized within circulating monocytes (Figure 28-2). The finding of morulae within monocytes using cytologic evaluation of blood smears is insensitive, especially in dogs with chronic infection, and does not distinguish between *E. canis* and *E. chaffeensis* infection. Use of buffy coat smears, thin smears of blood collected from the margin of the pinna, or splenic aspirates increases the sensitivity for detection of morulae. In one study, after careful searching, morulae were found in only 2 of 19 dogs with CME.[22]

Serum Biochemical Tests

Serum chemistry abnormalities in chronic ehrlichiosis include variable hypoalbuminemia, hyperglobulinemia, and elevated ALT and ALP activities. Most often the hyperglobulinemia is due to a polyclonal gammopathy.[15] Monoclonal gammopathy can also develop. Less commonly, increases in serum urea nitrogen and creatinine concentrations are present.[22]

Urinalysis

Transient proteinuria, with urine protein:creatinine ratios that exceed 20 (reference range, <1) have been reported in dogs with acute CME. This can resolve by 6 weeks after infection.[30,31] Dogs with chronic CME may also have evidence of proteinuria. Pyuria, hematuria, and cylindruria may also be present.

Coagulation Profile

In addition to thrombocytopenia, coagulation abnormalities in dogs with CME include prolongation of the buccal mucosal bleeding time (BMBT), decreased platelet aggregation, and prolongation of the APTT.[32,33]

Cerebrospinal Fluid Analysis

Dogs with central nervous system (CNS) involvement may have increased CSF protein concentrations and lymphocytic pleocytosis.[24] Although rarely found, morulae may be detected in cells within the CSF.[34]

Bone Marrow Analysis

In dogs with chronic CME, bone marrow findings include hypoplasia or aplasia of all bone marrow elements, decreased iron stores and marrow plasmacytosis (Figure 28-4). Bone marrow mastocytosis has also been described.[35] Myelofibrosis does not typically develop in chronic CME.[36] Some dogs have normal or hypercellular marrows.

Diagnostic Imaging

Plain Radiography

Thoracic radiographs in dogs with CME often show no significant abnormalities, but sometimes bronchointerstitial infiltrates are present. This may reflect an underlying interstitial pneumonia.

Sonographic Findings

Findings on abdominal ultrasonography are nonspecific and include splenomegaly, alterations in splenic echotexture, enlargement and hypoechogenicity of the abdominal lymph nodes, and scant peritoneal effusion. Increased renal echogenicity and decreased corticomedullary definition may occur in dogs with glomerulonephritis.

Microbiologic Tests

Available diagnostic assays for ehrlichiosis in dogs and cats are listed in Table 28-2.

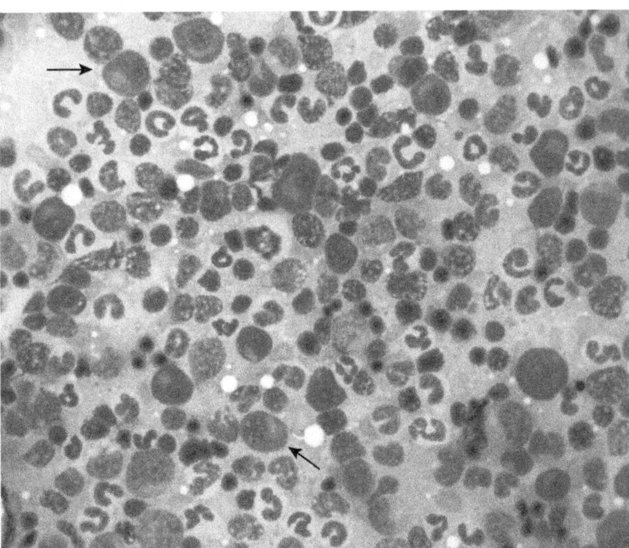

FIGURE 28-4 Bone marrow plasmacytosis in an 8-year-old female spayed Labrador retriever with canine monocytic ehrlichiosis. Serum globulin was 12.1 g/dL (reference range, 2.3-4.4 g/dL), and serum protein electrophoresis revealed a polyclonal gammopathy. Plasma cells have a clock-faced nucleus and a clear area adjacent to the nucleus; two plasma cells are identified with arrows. Mild to moderate megakaryocyte hyperplasia, mild erythroid hypoplasia, and mild mature granular lymphocytosis were also present. Romanowsky stain.

Serologic Diagnosis

Most often, the diagnosis of CME is made using serology, which may be performed using indirect immunofluorescent antibody (IFA) testing, ELISA technology, or Western blotting. Using IFA testing, which is considered the gold standard, antibodies can be detected between 7 and 28 days after initial infection. Dogs with acute ehrlichiosis may have false-negative test results if sufficient time has not elapsed for antibody production to occur. PCR assays may be helpful for diagnosis in this situation. A positive initial serum antibody titer may reflect previous exposure, and not necessarily ehrlichial disease. Retesting should be performed 2 to 3 weeks later to demonstrate seroconversion, and results of serology should be interpreted in light of a dog's clinical signs and the results of testing for other potential causes of the dog's illness. Dogs with chronic *E. canis* infection frequently have extremely high IFA titers, sometimes greater than 1:600,000, and these antibodies may persist in the face of treatment, suggesting persistence of the organism.[22] Seroconversion does not generally occur in dogs with chronic disease, although antibody titers may decline in some dogs with treatment. High titers do not correlate with the severity of hyperglobulinemia, disease in general, or duration of illness. Because of variability of reporting between laboratories, there is no standard "cutoff" titer that is used to separate positive and negative results. Serologic cross-reactivity to other *Ehrlichia* species occurs, which includes *E. ewingii* and especially *E. chaffeensis*. Cross-reactivity to *A. phagocytophilum* antigens can occur to a lesser extent. In areas where other rickettsial agents are endemic, Western blotting has been used in an attempt to confirm that positive antibody titers on IFA are truly to *E. canis* antigens. However, Western blotting is laborious to perform and interpret and not routinely available, and when *E. canis* antigens are the target used, it may be difficult to distinguish between *E. canis* and *E. chaffeensis* infection.[37] As a result, Western blotting has predominantly been used on a research basis.

TABLE 28-2

Diagnostic Assays Available for Ehrlichiosis in Dogs and Cats

Assay	Specimen Type	Target	Performance
Cell culture	Whole blood	*Ehrlichia canis*; *Ehrlichia ewingii* cannot be cultured	Not widely offered or utilized for routine diagnostic purposes. Requires several weeks' incubation.
Morula detection	Whole blood, buffy coat smears, body fluids, tissue aspirates	*E. canis* or *E. ewingii* morulae	Low sensitivity (especially for chronic *E. canis* infection). *E. canis* morulae cannot be distinguished from those of *E. chaffeensis*, and *E. ewingii* morulae cannot be differentiated from those of *A. phagocytophilum*. Morulae may be confused with platelets, cytoplasmic granules, phagocytized nuclear material, and lymphoglandular bodies.
IFA serology	Serum	Antibodies to *E. canis*	Acute and convalescent serology is required for diagnosis of acute infection, because initial results may be negative in dogs with acute disease, and positive results can reflect previous exposure rather than active infection. Dogs with chronic infection generally do not seroconvert. Cross-reactivity occurs to other ehrlichial species and occasionally to *Anaplasma* spp.
ELISA serology	Serum	Antibodies to *E. canis* or *E. ewingii* antigens	Rapid, inexpensive, can be performed as an in-practice test. Similar limitations as for IFA. Lack of quantitation limits ability to document seroconversion.
Western immunoblotting	Serum	Antibodies to specific *E. canis* or *E. ewingii* antigens	Technically difficult; primarily used on a research basis to identify serologic responses to specific ehrlichial species. May be difficult to distinguish antibody responses to *E. canis* and *E. ewingii*.
PCR	Whole blood; spleen, lymph node or bone marrow aspirates; buffy coat or tissue specimens	*E. canis*, *E. muris*, or *E. ewingii* DNA	Confirms active infection. Sensitivity and specificity may vary depending on assay design and specimen type. Sensitivity for diagnosis of chronic CME may be low. Assays that specifically detect *E. muris* are not widely available on a commercial basis.

CME, Canine monocytic ehrlichiosis; IFA, immunofluorescent antibody.

A variety of ELISA assays have been developed for detection of antibodies to *E. canis*. A point-of-care lateral-flow ELISA device for the simultaneous detection of canine heartworm antigen, antibodies to *E. canis* or *E. ewingii*, antibodies to *Borrelia burgdorferi*, and antibodies to *Anaplasma* spp. in canine serum, plasma, or whole blood has been marketed for use in companion animals (SNAP 4Dx Plus, IDEXX Laboratories, Westbrook, ME), which includes recombinant surface proteins of *E. canis* and *E. ewingii* on a single spot. According to the manufacturer, when IFA and Western blotting were used as the gold standard, the sensitivity and specificity of the *E. canis* antigen for detection of *E. canis* antibodies in 104 samples positive for *E. canis* antibodies and 236 samples negative for *E. canis* antibodies was found to be 96.2% and 100%, respectively. Other point-of-care ELISA assays for detection of *E. canis* antibodies have also been developed. A silicon disc-based assay is available in the United States through Antech Diagnostic laboratories that detects *Dirofilaria immitis* antigen and antibodies to *E. canis*, *Anaplasma* spp., and *B. burgdorferi* (Accuplex 4, Antech Diagnostics, Irvine, CA). The performance of this assay for diagnosis of ehrlichiosis has not been thoroughly investigated at the time of writing. The incidental finding of *E. canis* seroreactivity in dogs screened using these assays for heartworm antigenemia should prompt performance of a thorough physical examination and basic laboratory testing (CBC, chemistry panel, and urinalysis) to evaluate for thrombocytopenia, hyperglobulinemia, and proteinuria. When sick dogs test positive, quantitative serology should be performed so that a titer can be obtained as a baseline for acute and convalescent serologic testing or, for dogs suspected to have chronic CME, to evaluate for titers of very high magnitude that might be consistent with a dysregulated immune response to the organism.

Molecular Diagnosis Using the Polymerase Chain Reaction

Whole-blood PCR assays for *E. canis* DNA is more sensitive for early diagnosis of CME than IFA or ELISA in dogs with acute disease. PCR assays are widely available for routine diagnosis of *E. canis* infection. Several laboratories offer panels that include PCR assays for a variety of different vector-borne pathogens. The results of these assays should be interpreted in light of a dog's history, clinical signs, and the results of appropriate serologic assays; the last should be performed to support the results of PCR testing. PCR assays for *E. canis* may be performed on blood, lymph node aspirates, splenic aspirates, or bone marrow. Convalescent IFA or ELISA testing is much more sensitive than PCR assays for diagnosis of chronic CME.[22,38,39] The sensitivity of PCR assays for diagnosis of CME when performed on bone marrow in dogs with chronic ehrlichiosis can range from 25% to 68%, depending on the laboratory.[22] The use of PCR assays in the absence of serology is currently not suitable for screening potential blood donors for infection. PCR assays may be useful to confirm infection in the first week of illness, when serologic assays are often negative. Depending on the assay used, when positive, PCR can also be used to confirm the *Ehrlichia* species involved.

Blood Culture

E. canis can be cultured in certain cell lines, such as DH82 cells. This is time-consuming and generally performed only on a research basis.

Pathologic Findings

Gross pathologic findings in CME include widespread petechial and ecchymotic hemorrhages, generalized pallor, edema, lymphadenopathy, and splenomegaly.[40,41] Ascites may also be present. On histopathology, lymphoid and plasma cell hyperplasia, lymphoplasmacytic infiltrates, and vasculitis may be present in numerous organs, such as the brain, eye, spinal cord, spleen, liver, kidneys, lymph nodes, bone marrow, and lungs. Histiocytic infiltrates may be found in lymph nodes. With chronicity, the proportion of plasma cells increases. Non-suppurative meningitis and perivascular cuffing within the CNS can also occur.[40-42] Glomerulonephritis may be evident,[40] although dogs with acute CME have had interstitial nephritis and electron microscopic abnormalities that are more consistent with minimal-change glomerulonephritis, with fusion of podocyte processes.[30] Little information is available in regard to the prevalence and type(s) of glomerulonephritis that develop in dogs with chronic CME.

Treatment and Prognosis

Antimicrobial Treatment

The treatment of choice for CME is doxycycline (10 mg/kg PO q24h) (Table 28-3). It was the consensus of the ACVIM Infectious Disease Study Group that dogs and cats should be treated for a minimum of 28 days.[28] Mixed results have been obtained in studies that have evaluated the efficacy of doxycycline for treatment of *E. canis* infection. One study suggested that acute infection can be eliminated after treatment for just 16 days.[43] Another study that used ticks to infect dogs showed a failure of doxycycline, when given for 14 days, to eliminate the organism from subclinically infected dogs.[44] In another study, dogs with acute and subclinical infections became negative by PCR assay on blood after 28 days of doxycycline treatment, but dogs with chronic infections remained intermittently positive. However, ticks still became PCR positive after they fed on treated dogs, regardless of the stage of disease when treatment was initiated.[45]

Whether or not persistence of infection occurs, most dogs with acute disease show clinical improvement within 24 to 48 hours. Dogs with severe chronic disease may not respond to therapy, or cytopenias may resolve over a period of several months. Strong risk factors for mortality in one study were severe leukopenia (WBC <930 cells/μL), severe anemia (HCT <11.5%),

TABLE 28-3

Antimicrobial Drug Doses Used for Treatment of Ehrlichiosis in Dogs and Cats

Drug	Dose	Route	Interval (hours)	Minimum Duration (days)
Doxycycline	5 mg/kg	PO, IV	12*	*E. canis* 28 days; *E. ewingii* 14 days
Oxytetracycline	7.5-10 mg/kg	IV	12	Until gastrointestinal signs abate, and then change to oral doxycycline as above

*Or 10 mg/kg PO q24h.

hypokalemia (<3.7 mmol/L), and prolonged APTT (>18.25 s).[46] Platelet counts generally improve and normalize by 2 weeks following institution of therapy. After treatment, titers can decline and become negative in 6 to 9 months. Some dogs retain high titers for several years. Treatment for these dogs should be based on resolution of platelet counts and improvement of hyperglobulinemia, although hyperglobulinemia can resolve over several months after treatment is discontinued. The use of PCR assays on splenic aspirates could be considered to determine if persistent infection is present in these dogs, but whether ongoing treatment with doxycycline changes the outcome for these dogs is unknown. Platelet counts should be reassessed 1 and 3 months after discontinuation of therapy, because of the potential for relapse or reinfection. Other causes of illness (especially other vector-borne diseases such as babesiosis or bartonellosis) should also be considered in dogs that fail to respond to treatment.

Other drugs used to treat CME with variable success are chloramphenicol, imidocarb dipropionate, and enrofloxacin.[47-50] *Ehrlichia canis* appears to have intrinsic gyrase-mediated resistance to fluoroquinolones,[51] so although their use can be associated with clinical improvement, it is not recommended. The antiprotozoal drug imidocarb dipropionate appeared efficacious for treatment of *E. canis* infection in some studies but not others.[48,49]

At this time, treatment of seroreactive but otherwise healthy dogs that have normal routine bloodwork results is controversial, because it is unknown if treatment changes outcome for these dogs and has the potential to lead to antimicrobial resistance or adverse effects of drug therapy.

Supportive Care

For dogs with CME that are dehydrated or anemic, IV fluids or blood products may be required. Use of erythropoietin and granulocyte colony-stimulating factor together with prednisone was associated with treatment success in a dog with severe chronic ehrlichiosis in one case report.[52] Desmopressin acetate (DDAVP) (1 mcg/kg SC q24h) for 3 days appeared to be efficacious to treat bleeding disorders in a few dogs with CME,[33] and treatment resulted in reduction of the BMBT and APTT. If thrombocytopenia fails to resolve with doxycycline administration, a short course (up to a week) of therapy with immunosuppressive doses of glucocorticoids could be considered in addition to ongoing therapy with doxycycline.

Immunity and Vaccination

A vaccine for *E. canis* infection is currently not available, but in one study vaccination of dogs with an attenuated strain dramatically reduced disease in dogs challenged with a virulent strain of *E. canis*.[53] The immune response to *E. canis* infection is not well understood. Because *E. canis* is an intracellular pathogen, cell-mediated immune responses are required for pathogen elimination. In one study, dogs with acute infection developed CD8+ lymphocytosis that subsided after several weeks, despite organism persistence.[27] Cytokine studies suggest that the immune response may vary with the strain of *E. canis* involved.[54,55] Genetic factors are also likely to be important determinants of the immune response and outcome of infection.

Prevention

Avoidance of tick-infested areas and routine inspection of dogs for ticks after outdoor activities can help to prevent ehrlichiosis. Early removal of ticks may help to reduce transmission, because of the 24- to 36-hour delay that occurs between tick attachment and feeding. Clients should be instructed to remove ticks properly and avoid handling ticks with bare hands or crushing them, to prevent exposure to infected hemolymph. A variety of devices are available to assist tick removal, which are placed around the area where the mouthparts enter the skin to avoid crushing or squeezing the tick and leaving the mouthparts behind. Fine-tipped tweezers can be used to grasp the tick as close to the skin as possible, followed by steady retraction to remove the tick. The bite wound should then be thoroughly cleaned with a suitable antiseptic solution (such as iodine or chlorhexidine-based antiseptics) or soap and water. Ticks can be disposed in alcohol or tested for vector-borne pathogens using PCR assays.

Topical ectoparasiticides with activity against ticks also prevent tick-borne infectious diseases. Examples of canine ectoparasiticides with activity against ticks include those that contain amitraz, fipronil, pyrethroids (permethrin, etofenprox, pyrethrin, deltamethrin, flumethrin), and selamectin. In one field study, the use of monthly permethrin effectively prevented infection with *E. canis* by kenneled dogs.[56] Products that contain pyrethroids and amitraz have the most potent activity against ticks. Permethrin, deltamethrin, and amitraz cannot be used in cats, and use of these products should be avoided on dogs that co-habitate with cats. Flumethrin collars are available for use on cats (and on dogs) because unlike the other pyrethroids, flumethrin does not require hepatic glucaronidation for metabolism.[57] Products that contain amitraz, a monoamine oxidase inhibitor, should not be used in dogs treated with selective serotonin reuptake inhibitors (SSRIs) such as fluoxetine, and pet owners that are receiving SSRIs should also use alternative preventatives for their dogs. Preventatives should be applied consistently at the recommended interval for optimum activity. No preventatives completely protect dogs or cats from tick attachment, especially where tick infestation rates are high. Unfortunately, acaricide-resistant strains of *R. sanguineus* have been reported as a result of indiscriminate use of these drugs.[58]

Low dose doxycycline (6.6 mg/kg q24h PO) has also been used to prevent infection in dogs residing in kennels in which E. canis infection is a problem. Resistance to doxycycline remains a theoretical concern in this situation.

Because of chronic, subclinical infection, blood donor dogs should be screened with serology (or serology and PCR assays) for evidence of *E. canis* exposure or infection. All seropositive dogs should be excluded as donors. Transport of chronically infected dogs to non-endemic regions has the potential to introduce the infection or new strains of *E. canis* to these regions if the appropriate tick vectors are present.

Public Health Aspects

E. canis DNA has been detected in some human patients with clinical signs of human monocytic ehrlichiosis,[59] suggesting that *E. canis* might be a cause of monocytic ehrlichiosis in people. Appropriate precautions should be taken to prevent transmission when handling engorged ticks as well as blood and tissue specimens from infected dogs, and care should be taken to prevent needle-stick injuries.

Ehrlichia ewingii Infection

Etiology and Epidemiology

Ehrlichia ewingii is an unculturable bacterium that causes granulocytic ehrlichiosis in humans and in dogs. It was first recognized in dogs[2] and occurs in North America and more recently has been detected in dogs from Africa and Brazil.[60,61] Infection occurs in the south-central and southeastern parts of the United States, which reflects the distribution of the primary tick vector, *Amblyomma americanum*. Transmission within the tick is transstadial. More than 40% of dogs from an endemic area in Oklahoma and Arkansas were seropositive.[62] In another large study the overall seroprevalence was 14.5% in the central states (Oklahoma, Arkansas, Missouri, and Kansas) and 5.9% in the southeast.[63] In one study, most cases occurred from May through July,[64] but in another, cases occurred throughout the year.[65] In the study from the south-central United States, dogs were more likely to test positive with a PCR assay in August.[62] *E. ewingii* is maintained in white-tailed deer.[66] The DNA of *E. ewingii* has also been found in *Dermacentor variabilis* and *R. sanguineus* ticks,[67] but *A. americanum* is the only proven vector.

Clinical Features

Signs and Their Pathogenesis

In contrast to *E. canis* infection, *E. ewingii* infection appears to cause only acute disease; a chronic phase of disease has not been described. Like *A. phagocytophilum*, *E. ewingii* replicates in neutrophils and delays neutrophil apoptosis, which prolongs the life span of the host cell.[68]

Dogs with *E. ewingii* infection may show no signs, or fever, lethargy, anorexia, and neutrophilic polyarthritis may occur. After experimental infection, signs develop after an incubation period of 3 to 4 weeks.[69-71] Vomiting and diarrhea occur uncommonly. Neurologic signs have been described in some naturally infected dogs,[65] but the possibility of concurrent infections with other pathogens such as *Rickettsia rickettsii* was not ruled out in these dogs. *E. ewingii* can be found in apparently healthy dogs, so dogs may act as a reservoir for infection.

Physical Examination Findings

On physical examination, dogs with *E. ewingii* infection may have evidence of lethargy, fever, lameness, reluctance to move, a stiff gait, joint effusion, and pain on joint palpation. Reported neurologic signs include anisocoria, tremors, and a head tilt.[65]

Diagnosis

Laboratory Abnormalities

Common laboratory findings in dogs with *E. ewingii* infection are nonregenerative anemia and thrombocytopenia.[65,72] Reactive lymphocytosis can also occur.[65] The biochemistry panel may be unremarkable or show mild nonspecific abnormalities. Synovial fluid analysis reveals neutrophilic polyarthritis. Morulae may be detected within granulocytes in the peripheral blood or synovial fluid, but are indistinguishable from those of *A. phagocytophilum*. Nevertheless, the finding of morulae in granulocytes in *E. ewingii* endemic areas and where *A. phagocytophilum* infection is uncommon or absent is strongly suggestive of *E. ewingii* infection. In experimental infections, morulae are visible in the peripheral blood of some dogs before the onset of clinical signs, around 2 to 3 weeks postinfection.[71]

Microbiologic Tests

Serologic Diagnosis

Serologic diagnosis of *E. ewingii* infection is currently limited to a point-of-care ELISA assay that detects the presence of antibodies to a specific peptide of *E. ewingii* (SNAP 4Dx Plus, IDEXX Laboratories, Westbrook, ME). Because this peptide is combined on a spot with a peptide that detects antibodies to *E. canis*, the antibody response to these pathogens cannot be distinguished from one another. Cross-reactions may also occur to other ehrlichial species such as *E. chaffeensis*. Antibodies appear approximately 1 month after infection.[71] Dogs with acute illness may initially test negative with this assay, and positive test results may reflect the presence of antibodies from previous exposure or subclinical infection. A change from a negative to a positive result over a 2- to 4-week time period may help support a diagnosis of *E. ewingii* infection in endemic areas.

Molecular Diagnosis Using the Polymerase Chain Reaction

Whole-blood PCR assays are available for specific diagnosis of *E. ewingii* infection through some veterinary diagnostic laboratories. The sensitivity of these assays may vary between laboratories. Currently *E. ewingii*–specific PCR assays are the only means to confirm active infection with *E. ewingii* (as opposed to infection with *A. phagocytophilum* or other *Ehrlichia* species). In experimental studies, PCR becomes positive as early as 4 days after inoculation.[71]

Treatment and Prognosis

Antimicrobial Treatment

For *E. ewingii* infection, treatment with doxycycline results in rapid (within 24 to 48 hours) clinical improvement. Treatment for 2 to 4 weeks may be sufficient to eliminate infection. Subclinically infected dogs that test positive with whole-blood PCR assays may spontaneously clear infection within weeks to months. Treatment may not be required for these dogs.

Prevention

Prevention of *E. ewingii* infection involves avoidance of tick exposure and use of tick preventatives (see previously). Early tick removal also has the potential to reduce transmission. Potential blood donor dogs could be screened for infection with *E. ewingii*–specific ELISA and PCR assays. PCR assays alone (i.e., without serology) should not be used to screen blood donors.

Public Health Aspects

Human infection with *E. ewingii* has been rarely described in endemic regions of the United States.[73] Affected people have had headache, fever, and thrombocytopenia, with or without leukopenia, and responded to doxycycline treatment. Most were receiving immunosuppressive drug therapy. Although direct dog-to-human transmission does not occur, blood from affected dogs should be handled with caution.

Ehrlichia chaffeensis Infection

Ehrlichia chaffeensis causes human monocytic ehrlichiosis in North America, an emerging disease that is characterized in human patients by fever, headache, myalgia, thrombocytopenia and leukopenia, and elevations in hepatic transaminases.[74] Gastrointestinal signs, neurologic involvement, and a toxic shock–like syndrome also occur in some infected people. In the United States, it occurs primarily in the south-central, southeastern, and mid-Atlantic states, which reflects the distribution of *A. americanum* and the concurrent presence of white-tailed deer, which are reservoirs for the organism (as for *E. ewingii*). Evidence of *E. chaffeensis* DNA has also been found in humans, dogs, other animal species (including cats[18]), and ticks in Africa, Israel, Central and South America, and Asia. The organism is transmitted transstadially within the tick,[75] which feeds aggressively on humans. In naturally infected dogs, *E. chaffeensis* infection has been associated with clinical signs of lymphadenopathy, anterior uveitis, and epistaxis,[76] but the clinical implications of this infection for dogs are still unclear. Dogs maintain high antibody titers and are PCR positive for months after infection, which supports a possible role of the dog as a reservoir.[77]

Ehrlichia muris-like Infection

Ehrlichia muris was first described in a wild mouse from Japan in the mid-1990s[78,79] and *E. muris* DNA was detected in a febrile person in Russia for the first time in 2008.[80] In 2009, the DNA with strong homology to that of *Ehrlichia muris* was detected in four humans from Minnesota and Wisconsin.[80] These individuals had clinical signs and laboratory abnormalities that resembled those of granulocytic anaplasmosis (see Chapter 29), were seronegative to *A. phagocytophilum*, and showed variable seroreactivity to *E. chaffeensis*. Two of the individuals were solid-organ transplant recipients and the other two people were apparently immunocompetent. Morulae were not seen, but in mice *E. muris* forms morulae in monocytes.[78] In 2012, DNA with homology to *E. muris* was detected in an ill dog from northern Minnesota that was seronegative for *E. canis* and seroreactive to *A. phagocytophilum*,[4] although the extent to which this organism contributed to the dog's clinical signs was unclear. Because of the geographic distribution of infection, *Ixodes scapularis* is the suspected tick vector (see Chapter 29). *E. muris* DNA has been detected in *I. scapularis* ticks from northern Wisconsin.[81] The extent to which *E. muris* causes disease in dogs and humans in the United States and other countries requires further investigation but it should be considered as a possible cause of unexplained febrile illness in dogs, whether or not they have evidence of antibodies to *E. canis*.

CASE EXAMPLE

Signalment: "Ditto" a 13-year old male neutered border collie mix from Dixon, CA

History: Ditto was brought to the University of California, Davis, because of a 4-day history of lethargy and inappetence. Ditto had been drinking and there was no vomiting or diarrhea. There was no history of exposure to ticks, toxins, or trauma. Ditto was mainly confined to the backyard and did not have access to standing water. The dog had been adopted in Guam and brought to the United States several years ago. There was no other significant travel history. Ditto's diet consisted of a commercial senior dry dog food.

Current Medications: Prednisolone (0.45 mg/kg PO q48h) for allergic skin disease; this had been administered over the preceding 10 days.

Physical Examination:

Body Weight: 22.3 kg

General: Quiet, reluctant to stand. T = 102.2°F (39.0°C), HR = 152 beats/min, panting, mucous membranes pale pink, CRT <2 s. Approximately 5% to 7% dehydrated.

Integument: A sparse hair coat was present; there were no other clinically significant abnormalities. No ectoparasites were noted.

Eyes, Ears, Nose, and Throat: Severe dental calculus was present.

Musculoskeletal: Body condition score was 6/9. The dog would stand but was reluctant to walk.

Cardiovascular and Respiratory Systems: No clinically significant findings were present.

Gastrointestinal and Urogenital Systems: Cranial organomegaly was noted on abdominal palpation. Rectal examination revealed no significant abnormalities.

Lymph Nodes: All peripheral lymph nodes were normal sized.

Laboratory Findings:

CBC:

HCT 28.0% (40%-55%)
MCV 72.4 fL (65-75 fL)
MCHC 30.4 g/dL (33-36 g/dL)
Reticulocyte count 7600 cells/μL (7000-65,000 cells/μL)
Nucleated RBC 1/100 WBC
WBC 19,600 cells/μL (6000-13,000 cells/μL)
Neutrophils 15,876 cells/μL (3000-10,500 cells/μL)
Lymphocytes 392 cells/μL (1000-4000 cells/μL)
Monocytes 1568 cells/μL (150-1200 cells/μL)
Eosinophils 392 cells/μL (0-1500 cells/μL)
Basophils 392 cells/μL (0-50 cells/μL)
Platelets 127,000 platelets/μL (150,000-400,000 platelets/μL)
MPV 20.5 fL (7-13 fL).

Serum Chemistry Profile:

Sodium 141 mmol/L (145-154 mmol/L)
Potassium 4.2 mmol/L (3.6-5.3 mmol/L)
Chloride 105 mmol/L (108-118 mmol/L)
Bicarbonate 18 mmol/L (16-26 mmol/L)
Phosphorus 6.1 mg/dL (3.0-6.2 mg/dL)
Calcium 8.6 mg/dL (9.7-11.5 mg/dl)
BUN 55 mg/dL (5-21 mg/dL)
Creatinine 1.9 mg/dL (0.3-1.2 mg/dL)
Glucose 66 mg/dL (64-123 mg/dL)
Total protein 6.1 g/dL (5.4-7.6 g/dL)
Albumin 2.2 g/dL (3.0-4.4 g/dL)
Globulin 3.9 g/dL (1.8-3.9 g/dL)
ALT 49 U/L (19-67 U/L)
AST 153 U/L (19-42 U/L)
ALP 98 U/L (21-170 U/L)
Creatine kinase 341 U/L (51-399 U/L)
Gamma GT 4 U/L (0-6 U/L)
Cholesterol 282 mg/dL (135-361 mg/dL)
Total bilirubin 0.2 mg/dL (0-0.2 mg/dL)
Magnesium 2.6 mg/dL (1.5-2.6 mg/dL).

Urinalysis: SGr 1.018; pH 7.0, protein 75 mg/dL, no bilirubin, no glucose, hemoprotein 25 erythrocytes/μL, 0-2 WBC/HPF, 0-2 RBC/HPF, rare granular casts

Urine Protein: Creatinine Ratio: 19.3 (reference range, <1)

Plasma Antithrombin: 64% (reference range, 80%-120%)

Imaging Findings:

Thoracic Radiographs: The right cranial mainstem bronchus was slightly widened throughout its visible length and bronchiectasis was suspected. The cardiovascular and remaining pulmonary structures were within normal limits for the age of the patient.

Abdominal Radiographs: An ill-defined soft tissue structure was present that displaced the caudal border of the stomach cranially. The cecum was not well visualized. The liver extended past the costochondral arches with mildly rounded borders, which was interpreted as mild hepatomegaly. The soft tissue structure was thought to represent an enlarged lymph node, pancreas, or spleen.

Abdominal Ultrasound: The liver had normal parenchymal architecture. The gallbladder contained hyperechoic sludge. The spleen was enlarged with rounded edges and a heterogenous, more hypoechoic parenchyma. Both kidneys showed a somewhat thickened cortex with a good distinction between cortex and medulla. The left renal pelvis was mildly dilated, and the papilla was blunted. There were several cystic lesions within the abdomen that measured up to 3.6 cm × 5.4 cm. Septa were visualized within the cystic lesions. The cystic lesions appeared to arise from lymph nodes.

Cytologic Findings: Cytology of ultrasound-guided lymph node aspirate: There was a moderate amorphous basophilic proteinaceous background with low numbers of nucleated cells and erythrocytes. Nucleated cells were composed primarily of a mixed lymphocyte population with lower numbers of macrophages and nondegenerate. neutrophils.

Microbiologic Testing: 4Dx SNAP test serology (IDEXX Laboratories, ME): Positive for antibodies to *Ehrlichia canis*. Weakly positive for antibodies to *Anaplasma* species. Negative for antibodies to *Borrelia burgdorferi* and antigen of *Dirofilaria immitis*.

Vector-borne disease serology (IFA): Positive for antibodies to *Ehrlichia canis* at 1:163,840 and *Anaplasma phagocytophilum* at 1:2560. Negative for antibody to *Rickettsia rickettsii* at <1:40.

Vector-borne real-time PCR panel (whole blood): Positive for *Ehrlichia canis* DNA. Negative for *Anaplasma phagocytophilum, Anaplasma platys, Bartonella* spp., *Rickettsia* spp., and *Borrelia burgdorferi* DNA.

Diagnosis: Canine monocytic ehrlichiosis, characterized by thrombocytopenia, abdominal lymphadenopathy, and protein-losing nephropathy.

Treatment: Ditto was initially treated with IV crystalloids (lactated Ringer's solution supplemented with 20 mEq/L KCl), famotidine (0.5 mg/kg IV q12h), and ampicillin (20 mg/kg IV q8h). The hematocrit dropped to 18%, and 1 unit of packed RBC was administered, which was followed by a transfusion reaction, characterized by hemoglobinuria, vomiting, and icterus. Systolic blood pressure remained within normal limits throughout hospitalization. When the results of serology for *E. canis* were obtained, antimicrobial drug treatment was changed to doxycycline (5 mg/kg PO q12h). Enalapril (0.25 mg/kg PO q24h) and aspirin (0.5 mg/kg PO q24h) were used to manage the protein-losing nephropathy. Two days after initiation of doxycycline treatment, the dog's attitude and appetite improved. At discharge (day 9 of hospitalization), the hematocrit was 26.6%, reticulocytes 150,000 cells/μL, platelet count 496,000/μL, BUN 31 mg/dL, creatinine 1.5 mg/dL, albumin 1.8 g/dL, globulin 5 g/dL, and urine protein:creatinine ratio was 4. At a recheck examination 1 week after discharge, the hematocrit was stable, the platelet count was 635,000 platelets/μL, BUN 41 mg/dL, creatinine 1.3 mg/dL, and albumin 2.2 mg/dL. A kidney biopsy was not performed. Ditto was subsequently managed for protein-losing nephropathy with enalapril and a reduced protein diet for nearly 2 years, at which time hematocrit was 38.9%, platelet count 561,000 platelets/μL, BUN 27, creatinine 1.2 mg/dL, albumin 3.2 g/dL, globulin 3.6 g/dL, and the urine protein:creatinine ratio was 1.6. The spleen had returned to a sonographically normal appearance, and the cystic lymph nodes were markedly reduced in size. Additional serology or follow-up PCR was not performed. He was subsequently lost to follow-up.

Comments: In this dog, active infection with *E. canis* was confirmed through the use of whole-blood PCR assay. Where the dog became infected with *E. canis* was unclear, but infection was most likely acquired many years earlier in Guam, where ticks are abundant and *R. sanguineus* and *E. canis* are present. It is also unclear whether the glucocorticoid treatment played any role in reactivation of chronic infection. The improvement in hematologic and biochemical parameters in association with doxycycline treatment supported a role for *E. canis* in the disease. Hyperglobulinemia may have been initially masked by renal protein loss. In this case, treatment was continued for several months at the owner's request while laboratory parameters and ultrasound findings showed signs of progressive improvement. The seropositivity to *A. phagocytophilum* may have reflected previous exposure to this organism, *Anaplasma platys*, or serologic cross-reactivity between antibodies to *E. canis* and the *A. phagocytophilum* antigen used in the test kit.

SUGGESTED READINGS

Komnenou AA, Mylonakis ME, Kouti V, et al. Ocular manifestations of natural canine monocytic ehrlichiosis (*Ehrlichia canis*): a retrospective study of 90 cases. Vet Ophthalmol. 2007;10:137-142.

Mylonakis ME, Koutinas AF, Breitschwerdt EB, et al. Chronic canine ehrlichiosis (*Ehrlichia canis*): a retrospective study of 19 natural cases. J Am Anim Hosp Assoc. 2004;40:174-184.

REFERENCES

1. Donatien A, Lestoquard F. Existence en Algerie d'une *Rickettsia* du chien. Bull Soc Pathol Exot. 1935;28:418-419.
2. Anderson BE, Greene CE, Jones DC, et al. *Ehrlichia ewingii* sp. nov., the etiologic agent of canine granulocytic ehrlichiosis. Int J Syst Bacteriol. 1992;42:299-302.
3. Anderson BE, Dawson JE, Jones DC, et al. *Ehrlichia chaffeensis*, a new species associated with human ehrlichiosis. J Clin Microbiol. 1991;29:2838-2842.
4. Hegarty BC, Maggi RG, Koskinen P, et al. *Ehrlichia muris* infection in a dog from Minnesota. J Vet Intern Med. 2012;26:1217-1220.
5. Mavromatis K, Doyle CK, Lykidis A, et al. The genome of the obligately intracellular bacterium *Ehrlichia canis* reveals themes of complex membrane structure and immune evasion strategies. J Bacteriol. 2006;188:4015-4023.
6. Dunning Hotopp JC, Lin M, Madupu R, et al. Comparative genomics of emerging human ehrlichiosis agents. PLoS Genet. 2006;2:e21.
7. Felsheim RF, Kurtti TJ, Munderloh UG. Genome sequence of the endosymbiont *Rickettsia peacockii* and comparison with virulent *Rickettsia rickettsii*: identification of virulence factors. PLoS One. 2009;4:e8361.
8. Harrus S, Perlman-Avrahami A, Mumcuoglu KY, et al. Molecular detection of *Ehrlichia canis, Anaplasma bovis, Anaplasma platys, Candidatus* Midichloria mitochondrii and *Babesia canis vogeli* in ticks from Israel. Clin Microbiol Infect. 2011;17:459-463.
9. Masala G, Chisu V, Foxi C, et al. First detection of *Ehrlichia canis* in *Rhipicephalus bursa* ticks in Sardinia, Italy. Ticks Tick Borne Dis. 2012;3:396-397.
10. Wielinga PR, Gaasenbeek C, Fonville M, et al. Longitudinal analysis of tick densities and *Borrelia, Anaplasma*, and *Ehrlichia* infections of *Ixodes ricinus* ticks in different habitat areas in The Netherlands. Appl Environ Microbiol. 2006;72:7594-7601.
11. Satta G, Chisu V, Cabras P, et al. Pathogens and symbionts in ticks: a survey on tick species distribution and presence of tick-transmitted micro-organisms in Sardinia. Italy. J Med Microbiol. 2011;60:63-68.
12. Johnson EM, Ewing SA, Barker RW, et al. Experimental transmission of *Ehrlichia canis* (Rickettsiales: Ehrlichieae) by *Dermacentor variabilis* (Acari: Ixodidae). Vet Parasitol. 1998;74:277-288.
13. Beugnet F, Marie JL. Emerging arthropod-borne diseases of companion animals in Europe. Vet Parasitol. 2009;163:298-305.
14. Groves MG, Dennis GL, Amyx HL, et al. Transmission of *Ehrlichia canis* to dogs by ticks (*Rhipicephalus sanguineus*). Am J Vet Res. 1975;36:937-940.

15. Harrus S, Kass PH, Klement E, et al. Canine monocytic ehrlichiosis: a retrospective study of 100 cases, and an epidemiological investigation of prognostic indicators for the disease. Vet Rec. 1997;141:360-363.
16. Breitschwerdt EB, Abrams-Ogg AC, Lappin MR, et al. Molecular evidence supporting *Ehrlichia canis*-like infection in cats. J Vet Intern Med. 2002;16:642-649.
17. de Oliveira LS, Mourao LC, Oliveira KA, et al. Molecular detection of *Ehrlichia canis* in cats in Brazil. Clin Microbiol Infect. 2009;15(suppl 2):53-54.
18. Braga Mdo S, André MR, Freschi CR, et al. Molecular and serological detection of *Ehrlichia* spp. in cats on São Luís Island, Maranhão. Brazil. Rev Bras Parasitol Vet. 2012;21:37-41.
19. Harrus S, Waner T, Keysary A, et al. Investigation of splenic functions in canine monocytic ehrlichiosis. Vet Immunol Immunopathol. 1998;62:15-27.
20. Brandao LP, Hasegawa MY, Hagiwara MK, et al. Platelet aggregation studies in acute experimental canine ehrlichiosis. Vet Clin Pathol. 2006;35:78-81.
21. Cortese L, Terrazzano G, Piantedosi D, et al. Prevalence of anti-platelet antibodies in dogs naturally co-infected by *Leishmania infantum* and *Ehrlichia canis*. Vet J. 2011;188:118-121.
22. Mylonakis ME, Koutinas AF, Breitschwerdt EB, et al. Chronic canine ehrlichiosis (*Ehrlichia canis*): a retrospective study of 19 natural cases. J Am Anim Hosp Assoc. 2004;40:174-184.
23. Gould DJ, Murphy K, Rudorf H, et al. Canine monocytic ehrlichiosis presenting as acute blindness 36 months after importation into the UK. J Small Anim Pract. 2000;41:263-265.
24. Komnenou AA, Mylonakis ME, Kouti V, et al. Ocular manifestations of natural canine monocytic ehrlichiosis (*Ehrlichia canis*): a retrospective study of 90 cases. Vet Ophthalmol. 2007;10:137-142.
25. Buoro IBJ, Kanui TI, Atwell RB, et al. Polymyositis associated with *Ehrlichia canis* infection in two dogs. J Small Anim Pract. 1990:31.
26. Dubey JP, Pimenta AL, Abboud LC, et al. Dermatitis in a dog associated with an unidentified *Toxoplasma gondii*-like parasite. Vet Parasitol. 2003;116:51-59.
27. Hess PR, English RV, Hegarty BC, et al. Experimental *Ehrlichia canis* infection in the dog does not cause immunosuppression. Vet Immunol Immunopathol. 2006;109:117-125.
28. Neer TM, Breitschwerdt EB, Greene RT, et al. Consensus statement on ehrlichial disease of small animals from the infectious disease study group of the ACVIM. American College of Veterinary Internal Medicine. J Vet Intern Med. 2002;16:309-315.
29. Leiva M, Naranjo C, Pena MT. Ocular signs of canine monocytic ehrlichiosis: a retrospective study in dogs from Barcelona, Spain. Vet Ophthalmol. 2005;8:387-393.
30. Codner EC, Caceci T, Saunders GK, et al. Investigation of glomerular lesions in dogs with acute experimentally induced *Ehrlichia canis* infection. Am J Vet Res. 1992;53:2286-2291.
31. Codner EC, Maslin WR. Investigation of renal protein loss in dogs with acute experimentally induced *Ehrlichia canis* infection. Am J Vet Res. 1992;53:294-299.
32. Cortese L, Pelagalli A, Piantedosi D, et al. Platelet aggregation and haemostatic response in dogs naturally co-infected by *Leishmania infantum* and *Ehrlichia canis*. J Vet Med A Physiol Pathol Clin Med. 2006;53:546-548.
33. Giudice E, Giannetto C, Gianesella M. Effect of desmopressin on immune-mediated haemorrhagic disorders due to canine monocytic ehrlichiosis: a preliminary study. J Vet Pharmacol Ther. 2010;33:610-614.
34. Meinkoth JH, Hoover JP, Cowell RL, et al. Ehrlichiosis in a dog with seizures and nonregenerative anemia. J Am Vet Med Assoc. 1989;195:1754-1755.
35. Mylonakis ME, Koutinas AF, Leontides LS. Bone marrow mastocytosis in dogs with myelosuppressive monocytic ehrlichiosis (*Ehrlichia canis*): a retrospective study. Vet Clin Pathol. 2006;35:311-314.
36. Mylonakis ME, Day MJ, Siarkou V, et al. Absence of myelofibrosis in dogs with myelosuppression induced by *Ehrlichia canis* infection. J Comp Pathol. 2010;142:328-331.
37. Rikihisa Y, Ewing SA, Fox JC. Western immunoblot analysis of *Ehrlichia chaffeensis, E. canis*, or *E. ewingii* infections in dogs and humans. J Clin Microbiol. 1994;32:2107-2112.
38. Seaman RL, Kania SA, Hegarty BC, et al. Comparison of results for serologic testing and a polymerase chain reaction assay to determine the prevalence of stray dogs in eastern Tennessee seropositive to *Ehrlichia canis*. Am J Vet Res. 2004;65:1200-1203.
39. Gal A, Loeb E, Yisaschar-Mekuzas Y, et al. Detection of *Ehrlichia canis* by PCR in different tissues obtained during necropsy from dogs surveyed for naturally occurring canine monocytic ehrlichiosis. Vet J. 2008;175:212-217.
40. de Castro MB, Machado RZ, de Aquino LP, et al. Experimental acute canine monocytic ehrlichiosis: clinicopathological and immunopathological findings. Vet Parasitol. 2004;119:73-86.
41. Hildebrandt PK, Huxsoll DL, Walker JS, et al. Pathology of canine ehrlichiosis (tropical canine pancytopenia). Am J Vet Res. 1973;34:1309-1320.
42. Reardon MJ, Pierce KR. Acute experimental canine ehrlichiosis. I. Sequential reaction of the hemic and lymphoreticular systems. Vet Pathol. 1981;18:48-61.
43. Harrus S, Kenny M, Miara L, et al. Comparison of simultaneous splenic sample PCR with blood sample PCR for diagnosis and treatment of experimental *Ehrlichia canis* infection. Antimicrob Agents Chemother. 2004;48:4488-4490.
44. Schaefer JJ, Needham GR, Bremer WG, et al. Tick acquisition of *Ehrlichia canis* from dogs treated with doxycycline hyclate. Antimicrob Agents Chemother. 2007;51:3394-3396.
45. McClure JC, Crothers ML, Schaefer JJ, et al. Efficacy of a doxycycline treatment regimen initiated during three different phases of experimental ehrlichiosis. Antimicrob Agents Chemother. 2010;54:5012-5020.
46. Shipov A, Klement E, Reuveni-Tager L, et al. Prognostic indicators for canine monocytic ehrlichiosis. Vet Parasitol. 2008;153:131-138.
47. Harrus S, Waner T, Neer TM. *Ehrlichia and Anaplasma* infections. In: Greene CE, ed. Infectious Diseases of the Dog and Cat. 4th ed. St. Louis, MO: Elsevier Saunders; 2012:227-238.
48. Matthewman LA, Kelly PJ, Brouqui P, et al. Further evidence for the efficacy of imidocarb dipropionate in the treatment of *Ehrlichia canis* infection. J S Afr Vet Assoc. 1994;65:104-107.
49. Eddlestone SM, Neer TM, Gaunt SD, et al. Failure of imidocarb dipropionate to clear experimentally induced *Ehrlichia canis* infection in dogs. J Vet Intern Med. 2006;20:840-844.
50. Neer TM, Eddlestone SM, Gaunt SD, et al. Efficacy of enrofloxacin for the treatment of experimentally induced *Ehrlichia canis* infection. J Vet Intern Med. 1999;13:501-504.
51. Maurin M, Abergel C, Raoult D. DNA gyrase-mediated natural resistance to fluoroquinolones in *Ehrlichia* spp. Antimicrob Agents Chemother. 2001;45:2098-2105.
52. Aroch I, Harrus S. The use of hemopoietic growth factors: recombinant human granulocyte colony stimulating factor and recombinant human erythropoietin in severe pancytopenia due to canine monocytic ehrlichiosis. Israel J Vet Med. 2001;56:65-69.
53. Rudoler N, Baneth G, Eyal O, et al. Evaluation of an attenuated strain of *Ehrlichia canis* as a vaccine for canine monocytic ehrlichiosis. Vaccine. 2012;31:226-233.
54. Tajima T, Rikihisa Y. Cytokine responses in dogs infected with *Ehrlichia canis* Oklahoma strain. Ann N Y Acad Sci. 2005;1063:429-432.
55. Unver A, Huang H, Rikihisa Y. Cytokine gene expression by peripheral blood leukocytes in dogs experimentally infected with a new virulent strain of *Ehrlichia canis*. Ann N Y Acad Sci. 2006;1078:482-486.
56. Otranto D, Paradies P, Testini G, et al. Application of 10% imidacloprid/50% permethrin to prevent *Ehrlichia canis* exposure in dogs under natural conditions. Vet Parasitol. 2008;153:320-328.

57. Stanneck D, Rass J, Radeloff I, et al. Evaluation of the long-term efficacy and safety of an imidacloprid 10%/flumethrin 4.5% polymer matrix collar (Seresto®) in dogs and cats naturally infested with fleas and/or ticks in multicentre clinical field studies in Europe. Parasit Vectors. 2012;5:66.
58. Dantas-Torres F. The brown dog tick, *Rhipicephalus sanguineus* (Latreille, 1806) (Acari: Ixodidae): from taxonomy to control. Vet Parasitol. 2008;152:173-185.
59. Perez M, Bodor M, Zhang C, et al. Human infection with *Ehrlichia canis* accompanied by clinical signs in Venezuela. Ann N Y Acad Sci. 2006;1078:110-117.
60. Ndip LM, Ndip RN, Esemu SN, et al. Ehrlichial infection in Cameroonian canines by *Ehrlichia canis* and *Ehrlichia ewingii*. Vet Microbiol. 2005;111:59-66.
61. Oliveira LS, Oliveira KA, Mourao LC, et al. First report of *Ehrlichia ewingii* detected by molecular investigation in dogs from Brazil. Clin Microbiol Infect. 2009;15(suppl 2):55-56.
62. Little SE, O'Connor TP, Hempstead J, et al. *Ehrlichia ewingii* infection and exposure rates in dogs from the south central United States. Vet Parasitol. 2010;172:355-360.
63. Beall MJ, Alleman AR, Breitschwerdt EB, et al. Seroprevalence of *Ehrlichia canis, Ehrlichia chaffeensis* and *Ehrlichia ewingii* in dogs from North America. Parasit Vectors. 2012;5:29.
64. Liddell AM, Stockham SL, Scott MA, et al. Predominance of *Ehrlichia ewingii* in Missouri dogs. J Clin Microbiol. 2003;41:4617-4622.
65. Goodman RA, Hawkins EC, Olby NJ, et al. Molecular identification of *Ehrlichia ewingii* infection in dogs: 15 cases (1997-2001). J Am Vet Med Assoc. 2003;222:1102-1107.
66. Paddock CD, Yabsley MJ. Ecological havoc, the rise of white-tailed deer, and the emergence of *Amblyomma americanum*-associated zoonoses in the United States. Curr Top Microbiol Immunol. 2007;315:289-324.
67. Murphy GL, Ewing SA, Whitworth LC, et al. A molecular and serologic survey of *Ehrlichia canis, E. chaffeensis*, and *E. ewingii* in dogs and ticks from Oklahoma. Vet Parasitol. 1998;79:325-339.
68. Xiong Q, Bao W, Ge Y, et al. *Ehrlichia ewingii* infection delays spontaneous neutrophil apoptosis through stabilization of mitochondria. J Infect Dis. 2008;197:1110-1118.
69. Stockham SL, Tyler JW, Schmidt DA, et al. Experimental transmission of granulocytic ehrlichial organisms in dogs. Vet Clin Pathol. 1990;19:99-104.
70. Anziani OS, Ewing SA, Barker RW. Experimental transmission of a granulocytic form of the tribe Ehrlichieae by *Dermacentor variabilis* and *Amblyomma americanum* to dogs. Am J Vet Res. 1990;51:929-931.
71. Yabsley MJ, Adams DS, O'Connor TP, et al. Experimental primary and secondary infections of domestic dogs with *Ehrlichia ewingii*. Vet Microbiol. 2011;150:315-321.
72. Goldman EE, Breitschwerdt EB, Grindem CB, et al. Granulocytic ehrlichiosis in dogs from North Carolina and Virginia. J Vet Intern Med. 1998;12:61-70.
73. Buller RS, Arens M, Hmiel SP, et al. *Ehrlichia ewingii*, a newly recognized agent of human ehrlichiosis. N Engl J Med. 1999;341:148-155.
74. Dumler JS, Madigan JE, Pusterla N, et al. Ehrlichioses in humans: epidemiology, clinical presentation, diagnosis, and treatment. Clin Infect Dis. 2007;45(suppl 1):S45-S51.
75. Long SW, Zhang X, Zhang J, et al. Evaluation of transovarial transmission and transmissibility of *Ehrlichia chaffeensis* (Rickettsiales: Anaplasmataceae) in *Amblyomma americanum* (Acari: Ixodidae). J Med Entomol. 2003;40:1000-1004.
76. Breitschwerdt EB, Hegarty BC, Hancock SI. Sequential evaluation of dogs naturally infected with *Ehrlichia canis, Ehrlichia chaffeensis, Ehrlichia equi, Ehrlichia ewingii*, or *Bartonella vinsonii*. J Clin Microbiol. 1998;36:2645-2651.
77. Zhang XF, Zhang JZ, Long SW, et al. Experimental *Ehrlichia chaffeensis* infection in beagles. J Med Microbiol. 2003;52:1021-1026.
78. Kawahara M, Suto C, Rikihisa Y, et al. Characterization of ehrlichial organisms isolated from a wild mouse. J Clin Microbiol. 1993;31:89-96.
79. Wen B, Rikihisa Y, Mott J, et al. *Ehrlichia muris* sp. nov., identified on the basis of 16S rRNA base sequences and serological, morphological, and biological characteristics. J Bacteriol. 1995;45:250-254.
80. Pritt BS, Sloan LM, Johnson DK, et al. Emergence of a new pathogenic *Ehrlichia* species, Wisconsin and Minnesota, 2009. N Engl J Med. 2011;365:422-429.
81. Telford III SR, Goethert HK, Cunningham JA. Prevalence of *Ehrlichia muris* in Wisconsin deer ticks collected during the mid 1990s. Open Microbiol J. 2011;5:18-20.

CHAPTER 29

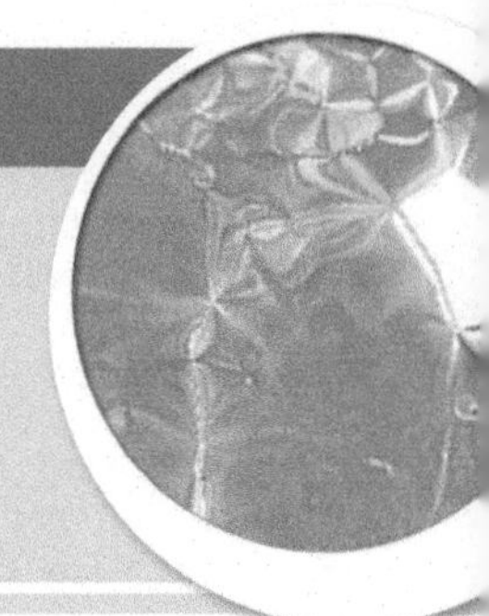

Anaplasmosis

Jane E. Sykes and Janet E. Foley

Overview of Anaplasmosis

First Described: First reports of *Anaplasma phagocytophilum* came from sheep in 1951 (Scotland).[1] Canine infection was first reported in the United States (California) in 1982.[2] *Anaplasma platys* was first reported in the United States (Florida) in 1978.[3]

Cause: *Anaplasma phagocytophilum* (granulocytic anaplasmosis), *Anaplasma platys* (thrombocytotropic anaplasmosis)

Affected Hosts: *A. phagocytophilum* causes disease in dogs, cats, humans, ruminants (European strains), horses, and camelids. *A. platys* causes thrombocytopenia in dogs.

Geographic Distribution: In the United States, *A. phagocytophilum* is most prevalent in the upper Midwest, northeast and western states. Infection also occurs throughout continental Europe and the United Kingdom, Asia, and Russia. The organism has been detected in dogs from Africa and South America. *A. platys* occurs throughout the Americas, Europe, Asia, Australia, the Middle East, and Africa.

Mode of Transmission: Tick vectors, primarily *Ixodes ricinus-persulcatus* complex ticks transmit *A. phagocytophilum*. Although unconfirmed, *Rhipicephalus sanguineus* is suspected to be the major vector of *A. platys*.

Major Clinical Signs: The major clinical signs of *A. phagocytophilum* infection are fever, lethargy, inappetence, and lameness due to polyarthritis, although vomiting, diarrhea, cough, and neck pain may occur. *A. platys* usually causes no signs, but fever and lethargy are possible.

Differential Diagnoses: Major differential diagnoses include other tick-borne diseases (such as the ehrlichioses, rickettsioses, Lyme borreliosis and babesiosis), bartonellosis, leptospirosis, primary immune-mediated disease, and lymphoma.

Human Health Significance: *A. phagocytophilum* causes human granulocytic anaplasmosis. Dogs act as a sentinel for human infection and may carry unfed ticks to humans on their coats.

Canine anaplasmosis is caused by *Anaplasma phagocytophilum* (formerly *Ehrlichia equi*, *Ehrlichia phagocytophila*, and, in humans, the human granulocytic ehrlichiosis [HGE] agent) and *Anaplasma platys*. These are tick-borne, gram-negative, obligately intracellular bacteria that belong to the family Anaplasmataceae. *A. phagocytophilum* predominantly infects neutrophils but also eosinophils, where it forms host membrane-enclosed morulae. Ticks that belong to the *Ixodes ricinus-persulcatus* complex are the major vectors for *A. phagocytophilum*. *Anaplasma platys* forms morulae within platelets. The vector of *A. platys* is probably *Rhipicephalus sanguineus*. As with the ehrlichioses, co-infections with other pathogens that are transmitted by the same or other tick species may occur and influence the clinical manifestations of disease.

Anaplasma phagocytophilum Infection

Etiology and Epidemiology

A. phagocytophilum causes granulocytic anaplasmosis in dogs, humans, horses, and, in Europe, domestic ruminants that include sheep, cattle, goats, and deer. Cats and camelids may also be affected. A variety of wild animal species, which include rodents and deer, act as reservoir hosts. For the midwestern and eastern United States, white-footed mice *(Peromyscus leucopus)* and eastern chipmunks may act as reservoirs, whereas in the western states, dusky-footed woodrats, gray squirrels, and chipmunks have been implicated. In Europe, bank voles, wood mice, shrews, and deer are likely reservoirs. Many strains of *A. phagocytophilum* exist that differ in pathogenicity and host tropism. For example, strains that infect domestic ruminants in Europe and white-tailed deer in the United States appear to be distinct from those that infect horses, humans, and dogs. Dogs, cats, and humans are accidental hosts and are not important in the transmission of infection to other host species.

The geographic distribution of the disease follows that of the tick vectors (Figure 29-1). In North America, the tick vectors of *A. phagocytophilum* are *Ixodes scapularis* in the northeastern and upper midwestern states, and *Ixodes pacificus* in the West. In Europe, the primary vector is *Ixodes ricinus*, and the disease has been described in dogs throughout continental Europe and in the UK. *Ixodes persulcatus* and *Dermacentor silvarum* ticks transmit the organism in Asia and Russia. Other *Ixodes* spp. ticks have also been implicated in transmission. Evidence of *A. phagocytophilum* infection has been found in dogs from Brazil and Tunisia, and a closely related organism was found in dogs from South Africa.[4-6] In humans, rare reports exist of direct transmission that followed close contact with blood or respiratory secretions, transplacental spread, or transmission through blood transfusion.

Many seroprevalence studies of dogs have been reported worldwide.[7] The seroprevalence varies with geographic location and whether the dogs studied were sick or healthy. The prevalence of positive antibody titers in dogs from some regions of Europe and North America exceeds 50%. A study that used a commercially available ELISA assay to determine the prevalence

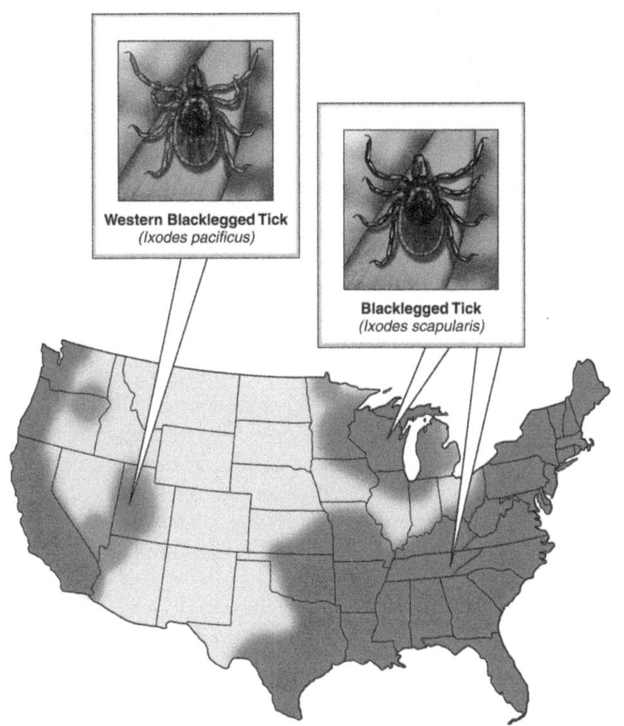

FIGURE 29-1 Distribution of *Ixodes scapularis* and *Ixodes pacificus*, the vectors of *Anaplasma phagocytophilum*, in the United States. The distribution of granulocytic anaplasmosis follows that of the tick vectors.

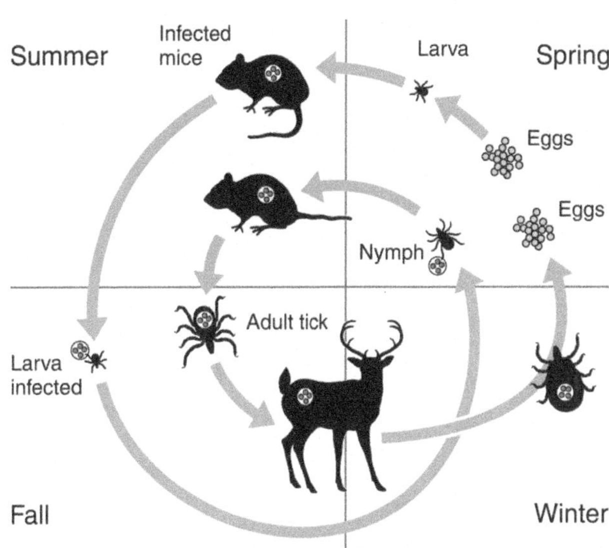

FIGURE 29-2 Life cycle of *Ixodes scapularis* ticks and *Anaplasma phagocytophilum* infection. Uninfected larvae (top right) hatch in the late spring and acquire infection from small rodents in the summer. They then over-winter (often in protected mouse burrows) and then molt into nymphs the following spring. The nymphs feed in the late spring or early summer on a variety of animal species including rodents, humans, deer, and dogs. Nymphs molt into adults in the late summer to fall, which subsequently feed on large mammals such as deer, where they mate and drop off. The females then lay eggs and die. Dogs, cats and humans become infected by nymphs or adult ticks.

of seroreactivity to *A. phagocytophilum* in more than 400,000 dogs from the United States revealed wide variation in seroprevalences. Some counties in the upper Midwest and northeastern United States had seroprevalences that exceeded 40%, although the overall seroprevalence in these regions were 6.7% and 5.5%, respectively.[8] Serologic cross-reactivity with *A. platys* may also influence these data.

The seasonal pattern of disease reflects times of peak nymphal and adult tick activities, as well as periods when humans and their dogs are active outdoors. In the western United States, *A. phagocytophilum* infection occurs most frequently in dogs between April and July, when nymphal ticks are abundant. Some infections occur in October, during early questing of adult ticks. In Minnesota and Wisconsin, most cases are diagnosed in late spring (May, June) and fall (October, November).[9-11] In a study from Berlin, most cases occurred between April and September.[12] The median age of clinically affected dogs is 6 to 8 years (range, 6 months to 14 years).[9,10,12-14] In the upper Midwest of the United States, a bimodal age distribution has been recognized, with 25% of dogs 1 year of age or less, and 50% of dogs at least 8 years of age.[10] Affected cats in the northeastern United States have ranged from 4 months to 13 years of age (mean, 3.7 years).[15] Although no breed predispositions are recognized, in one study, golden retrievers comprised almost half of affected dogs; this may reflect the popularity of these dogs for outdoor activities.[14] Infection with other tick-borne pathogens is a risk factor for *A. phagocytophilum* infection. Co-infection with *Borrelia burgdorferi,* the cause of Lyme disease, is common because *B. burgdorferi* is transmitted by the same *Ixodes* tick species.[8,10,11] In northern California, dogs seroreacted to *A. phagocytophilum* were 18 times more likely to be seropositive for *Bartonella vinsonii* subspecies *berkhoffii* than dogs that were seronegative.[16]

Clinical Features

Signs and Their Pathogenesis

A. phagocytophilum is transmitted transstadially within the tick (i.e., from larva to nymph to adult), and not transovarially (from adult to egg). Dogs and cats thus become infected after exposure to infected nymphs or adult ticks, which acquire infection when they feed on wild animal reservoir hosts as larvae or nymphs (Figure 29-2). Ticks must attach for 36 to 48 hours for transmission to occur. Once *A. phagocytophilum* enters the bloodstream, it attaches to the sialylated ligands on the surface of neutrophils, such as P-selectin glycoprotein ligand-1.[7] The organism then enters the neutrophil through caveolae-mediated endocytosis. *A. phagocytophilum* survives in the harsh neutrophil environment through dysregulation of neutrophil function and by bypassing phagolysosomal pathways. It inhibits neutrophil superoxide production and can reduce neutrophil motility and phagocytosis. *A. phagocytophilum* also reduces neutrophil adherence to endothelium and inhibits neutrophil transmigration into tissues, possibly through downregulation of selectin molecule expression.[7] This may promote its survival in peripheral blood.

Normally, neutrophils circulate for 10 to 12 hours before they enter tissues and undergo death through apoptosis. *A. phagocytophilum* delays neutrophil apoptosis, which allows it to survive longer periods of time within the neutrophil.[7] *A. phagocytophilum* may also infect other cell types, such as bone marrow cells, endothelial cells, and megakaryocytes, although the importance of these cells in the pathogenesis of infection is not clear.

The clinical signs and laboratory abnormalities that occur in dogs and cats with granulocytic anaplasmosis probably vary somewhat in different geographic locations as a result of local strain variation. The vast majority of dogs infected with

A. phagocytophilum show no clinical signs. Some dogs and cats develop a self-limiting febrile illness, which in dogs occurs after an incubation period of 1 to 2 weeks. Lethargy occurs in almost all clinically affected cats and dogs. Fever and inappetence are also common findings. Lameness, reluctance to move, polydipsia, vomiting, diarrhea, and a soft cough can also occur. Generalized lymphadenopathy and splenomegaly develop as a result of reactive lymphoid hyperplasia and, in the spleen, concurrent extramedullary hematopoiesis.[17] Uncommonly, hemorrhage, manifested as mucosal petechiae, melena, or epistaxis, has been reported in naturally infected dogs, but co-infections with other tick-borne pathogens may contribute to these signs in some dogs.[9,12,13,18] Neurologic signs such as seizures, circling, cervical pain, and decreased placing reactions have been described in a few dogs from the upper Midwest with granulocytic anaplasmosis, but one dog with seizures had a history of idiopathic epilepsy.[9,18] Neurologic signs and detection of the organism in the CSF have been uncommonly reported in humans.[19]

Infection with *A. phagocytophilum* results in mild to moderate thrombocytopenia, although other cytopenias may also occur (Table 29-1). The mechanism(s) of these hematologic abnormalities remain unclear. Anti-platelet antibodies occur in serum from humans and dogs with granulocytic anaplasmosis,[12,20] and so immune-mediated mechanisms may contribute to thrombocytopenia. However, thrombocytopenia occurs in acute disease, before antibodies are noted, so other mechanisms may be important. The bone marrow of infected dogs shows megakaryocyte hyperplasia, so platelet destruction may be involved.[21]

Impaired neutrophil function as a result of *A. phagocytophilum* infection may predispose to development of secondary opportunistic infections or influence the outcome of co-infections with other tick-borne pathogens such as *B. burgdorferi*. Although uncommon, opportunistic infections have been occasionally documented in humans and dogs with granulocytic anaplasmosis and are well in small ruminants.[22]

Infection with *A. phagocytophilum* may be self-limiting in dogs and cats, with minimal fatality or chronic disease manifestations. The extent to which *A. phagocytophilum* can persist in tissues and contribute to chronic disease manifestations in humans and dogs has been controversial, and may be dependent on the infecting strain and host immune response to infection. In one study, treatment of dogs that had been experimentally inoculated with *A. phagocytophilum* with prednisolone up to 6 months after infection was followed by the development of positive PCR results for the organism and, in some dogs, thrombocytopenia and reappearance of morulae on blood smears.[23] One dog infected with a California strain of *A. phagocytophilum* was persistently PCR-positive through day 60 postinfection, the last time point evaluated.[23]

Physical Examination Findings

The most common findings on physical examination in dogs include lethargy, fever (up to 106.7°F [41.5°C]), dehydration, tachypnea, mild peripheral lymphadenopathy, and splenomegaly.[7,10] Scleral injection may be noted. Lameness, reluctance to move, swollen joints, and pain on joint manipulation may also be detected in some dogs. Increased lung sounds, abdominal pain, epistaxis, petechial hemorrhages, and neurologic signs such as circling, cervical pain, and decreased placing reactions occur uncommonly.

Physical examination findings reported in cats have been similar to those described in dogs, and include fever, lethargy, tachypnea, increased lung sounds, mild abdominal pain, hepatomegaly, splenomegaly, vomiting, ataxia, hyperesthesia, muscle and joint pain, lameness, conjunctivitis, and ocular discharge.[15,24,25]

Diagnosis

Granulocytic anaplasmosis should be suspected in dogs and cats with acute febrile illness and thrombocytopenia that reside in endemic areas, regardless of tick exposure history. Diagnosis relies on detection of morulae within granulocytes, results of acute and convalescent serology, or molecular testing using PCR assays. The diagnostic criteria for confirmed human granulocytic anaplasmosis are clinical signs and laboratory findings suggestive of granulocytic anaplasmosis together with (1) detection of morulae within neutrophils combined with a single positive reciprocal antibody titer to *A. phagocytophilum* of at least 80; (2) a fourfold increase or decrease in the antibody

TABLE 29-1

Hematologic Abnormalities in Nine Dogs with Granulocytic Anaplasmosis in Northern California*

Test	Reference Range	Number below the Reference Range	Number within the Reference Range	Number above the Reference Range	Range for dogs with Granulocytic Anaplasmosis
Hematocrit (%)	40-55	6	3	0	19-45
Neutrophils (cells/μL)	3000-10,500	0	6	3	3513-18,592
Band neutrophils (cells/μL)	Rare	0	1	8	0-1282
Monocytes (cells/μL)	150-1200	1	7	1	142-1346
Lymphocytes (cells/μL)	1,000-4000	7	2	0	71-2693
Eosinophils (cells/μL)	0-1500	0	9	0	0-328
Platelets (cells/μL)†	150,000-400,000	6	2	0	37,000-262,000

*Diagnosis was based on compatible clinical signs and either morulae within circulating neutrophils and/or a positive real-time PCR assay result for *A. phagocytophilum*.

†Platelets were clumped for one dog.

titer within 4 weeks; (3) a positive PCR test result using specific *A. phagocytophilum* primers; or (4) isolation of *A. phagocytophilum* from blood.[22] These criteria could also be applied to dogs. The use of multiple diagnostic modalities may be needed to confirm the diagnosis of granulocytic anaplasmosis in some dogs.

Laboratory Abnormalities

Complete Blood Count

Thrombocytopenia occurs in approximately 90% of dogs with granulocytic anaplasmosis.[9,10,12,13] The platelet count in thrombocytopenic dogs may occasionally be as low as 5000 platelets/μL, although more often it is mild to moderately decreased (see Table 29-1).[9,10,12-14] The majority of affected dogs are lymphopenic, but lymphocytosis can occur.[9,12,13] Circulating reactive lymphocytes may be present. Anemia is common and typically mild and nonregenerative. Both neutrophilia and neutropenia occur, but most dogs have neutrophil counts that lie in the lower half of the reference range. Low numbers of band neutrophils, as well as mild neutrophil toxicity, are often present. Monocytopenia or monocytosis can occur.[9,12,13] Cytologic examination of blood smears often reveals morulae within granulocytes (Figure 29-3). Morulae were detected in neutrophils from 36%, 56%, 67%, and 100% of dogs in four respective case series.[9,12-14] Morulae appear as early as 4 days after experimental inoculation of dogs and persist for 4 to 8 days.[17] The morulae are indistinguishable from those of *Ehrlichia ewingii*, so serology or PCR assays are needed to confirm *A. phagocytophilum* infection.

In contrast to dogs, thrombocytopenia appears uncommon in cats infected with *A. phagocytophilum*. None of 15 sick, PCR-positive cats from the northeastern United States were thrombocytopenic.[15] The most common hematologic abnormality in cats has been lymphopenia. Morulae have been detected in some cats with granulocytic anaplasmosis.

Serum Biochemical Tests

The most frequent serum biochemistry finding in dogs with granulocytic anaplasmosis is mild to moderate hypoalbuminemia (Table 29-2). Mild hyperglobulinemia, mild electrolyte abnormalities (hypokalemia, hyponatremia, and metabolic acidosis), and a mild increase in the activities of serum ALP and to a lesser extent ALT may occur.[9,10,13,14]

Urinalysis

Urinalysis in dogs with granulocytic anaplasmosis may reveal isosthenuria, hyposthenuria, and proteinuria. Urine protein-to-creatinine ratios in two affected dogs from the United States were

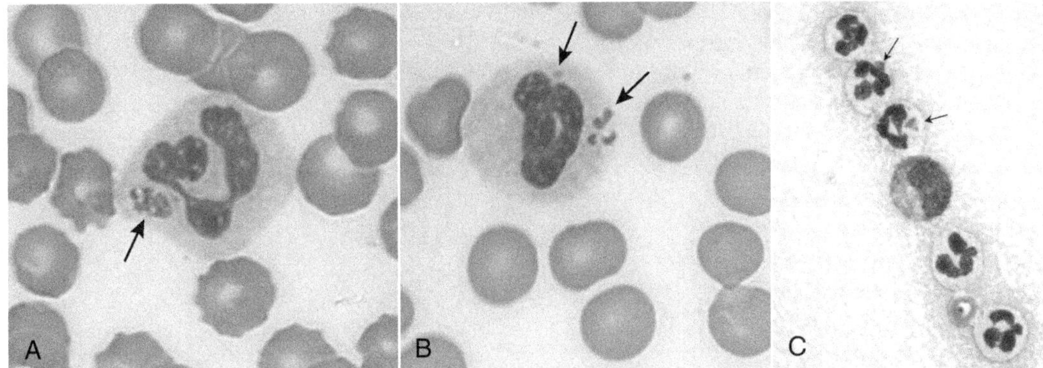

FIGURE 29-3 Intracytoplasmic morula **(A)** and cocci **(B)** of *Anaplasma phagocytophilum (arrows)* within neutrophils of an 8-year-old male neutered golden retriever with granulocytic anaplasmosis; in **(C)**, morulae are present in neutrophils within the synovial fluid of a 5-year-old curly-coated retriever that had polyarthritis.

TABLE 29-2

Findings on Serum Biochemistry Analysis in Nine Dogs with Granulocytic Anaplasmosis in Northern California*

Test	Reference Range	Number below the Reference Range	Number within the Reference Range	Number above the Reference Range	Range for dogs with Granulocytic Anaplasmosis
Sodium (mmol/L)	145-154	4	5	0	142-147
Potassium (mmol/L)	4.1-5.3	2	7	0	3.3-4.9
Bicarbonate (mmol/L)	16-26	3	6	0	11-18
Albumin (g/dL)	2.9-4.2	6	3	0	1.5-3.4
Globulin (g/dL)	2.3-4.4	0	8	1	2.7-6.0
Total bilirubin (mg/dL)	0-0.4	0	8	1	0-1.0
Alanine aminotransferase (U/L)	19-70	0	8	1	26-122
Alkaline phosphatase (U/L)	15-127	0	7	2	26-653

*Diagnosis was based on compatible clinical signs and either morulae within circulating neutrophils and/or a positive real-time PCR assay result for *A. phagocytophilum*.

1.5 and 2.2,[10] but there is no evidence that *A. phagocytophilum* infection causes severe glomerulonephritis in dogs.

Synovial Fluid Analysis

Dogs with granulocytic anaplasmosis can develop neutrophilic polyarthritis. Cytologic examination of synovial fluid in these dogs reveals increased numbers of nondegenerate neutrophils. In some affected dogs, morulae are found within these cells and the synovial fluid can be PCR positive (Figure 29-3,C).

Diagnostic Imaging

Plain Radiography

Thoracic radiographs are usually normal in dogs with granulocytic anaplasmosis but may show a mild interstitial infiltrate. Focal alveolar infiltrates occur as well.[26]

Sonographic Findings

Abdominal ultrasound may reveal splenomegaly, with a hypoechoic spleen, or mild abdominal lymphadenopathy.

Microbiologic Tests

Diagnostic assays available for anaplasmosis in dogs and cats are shown in Table 29-3.

Serologic Diagnosis

Diagnosis of granulocytic anaplasmosis can be accomplished with acute and convalescent serology. Many veterinary laboratories perform serologic testing using immunofluorescent antibody (IFA) techniques. IgG antibodies are first detectable approximately 8 days after exposure, 2 to 5 days after morulae appear. As a result, early in the course of illness, antibodies may be undetectable, so PCR assays may be more useful for diagnosis of acute infection in the absence of detectable morulae. Because positive titers can reflect previous exposure, demonstration of a fourfold rise in titer is required. Antibody titers may persist for many months.[14,23] In some human patients, antibody titers have persisted as long as 3 years.[22] In the United States, a silicon disc-based ELISA assay is available commercially for detection of antibodies to *A. phagocytophilum* (Accuplex 4, Antech Diagnostics, Irvine, CA). The performance of this assay when compared with IFA requires further study. An in-clinic lateral-flow ELISA device (IDEXX SNAP 4Dx Plus), which uses a recombinant Msp2/p44 protein, is also available for the detection of antibodies to *Anaplasma* species in dog serum. Positive results obtained with these ELISA assays do not imply that *A. phagocytophilum* is the cause of illness, and as with IFA testing, negative results can occur in dogs with acute illness due to the lag in antibody production relative to the onset of clinical signs.

Serologic cross-reactivity between *Anaplasma* species occurs. Dogs infected with *A. platys* also seroreact to *A. phagocytophilum* antigen; this includes the recombinant Msp2 assay.[8] Serologic cross-reactivity between *A. phagocytophilum* and *E. canis* also occurs, but is relatively uncommon and minor.[13,26,27] Dogs diagnosed with granulocytic anaplasmosis that have antibodies to *A. phagocytophilum* generally lack antibodies to *E. canis* using IFA testing.[7,10]

Molecular Diagnosis Using the Polymerase Chain Reaction

Several conventional and real-time PCR assays for *A. phagocytophilum* exist for detection of *A. phagocytophilum*

TABLE 29-3

Diagnostic Assays Available for Anaplasmosis in Dogs and Cats

Assay	Specimen Type	Target	Performance
Cell culture	Whole blood	*Anaplasma phagocytophilum*; *Anaplasma platys* cannot be cultured	Not widely offered or utilized for routine diagnostic purposes. Requires several weeks' incubation.
Cytology	Whole blood, buffy coat smears, body fluids, tissue aspirates	*A. phagocytophilum* or *A. platys* morulae	Low sensitivity (especially for *A. platys* infection). Morulae of *A. phagocytophilum* cannot be distinguished from those of *Ehrlichia ewingii*. Morulae may be confused with cytoplasmic granules or stain precipitate.
IFA serology	Serum	Antibodies to *Anaplasma* spp.	Acute and convalescent serology is required for diagnosis of acute infection, because initial results may be negative in dogs with acute disease and positive results may reflect previous exposure rather than active infection. Cross-reactivity occurs between *Anaplasma* spp.
ELISA serology	Serum	Antibodies to *Anaplasma* spp. antigens	Rapid, inexpensive, can be performed as an in-practice test. Similar limitations as IFA. Lack of quantitation limits ability to document seroconversion.
PCR	Whole blood, splenic or lymph node aspirates, bone marrow aspirates, buffy coat specimens, tissue specimens	*A. phagocytophilum* or *A. platys* DNA	Confirms active infection. Sensitivity and specificity may vary depending on assay design and specimen type. Because healthy animals may be PCR positive, positive PCR results must be interpreted in light of the clinical signs.

IFA, Immunofluorescent antibody.

DNA in peripheral blood, buffy coat, bone marrow, or splenic tissue. These can be useful for early diagnosis of granulocytic anaplasmosis in dogs and cats. The sensitivity and specificity of PCR assays may vary depending on the assay design and the laboratory used. Most, but not all, assays detect either the 16S rRNA gene or the outer surface protein gene *msp2* (p44). Assays that detect the *msp2* gene are usually specific for *A. phagocytophilum*, whereas assays that detect the 16S rRNA gene may detect other *Anaplasma* species, and even other bacteria. *A. phagocytophilum* DNA has occasionally been amplified from healthy dogs, so results must be interpreted in light of the clinical signs.[11] In experimentally infected dogs, whole-blood PCR becomes positive several days before and after morulae appear on blood smears.[17,23]

Culture

A. phagocytophilum can be isolated in human promyelocytic leukemia cell lines (HL-60) and tick embryo cell lines. Culture is highly sensitive for diagnosis of acute infection in human patients,[28] but it is not routinely used in dogs for diagnostic purposes because it requires special facilities, technical expertise, and prolonged incubation.

Pathologic Findings

Little information is available regarding the pathology of granulocytic anaplasmosis in dogs. Tissue injury appears to result from the host inflammatory response, rather than the bacterial infection itself.[29] In people, splenic lymphoid depletion, macrophage aggregates and apoptosis within the liver, paracortical lymphoid hyperplasia, and hemophagocytic cells within reticuloendothelial tissues have been described.[30]

Treatment and Prognosis

The treatment of choice for granulocytic anaplasmosis in dogs is doxycycline (5 mg/kg PO q12h). The optimum duration is unknown, but 2 weeks may be sufficient. The prognosis is excellent. Most dogs show clinical improvement within 24 to 48 hours of treatment, although some dogs require more than 1 week of treatment before clinical signs resolve.[10,13] Platelet counts normalize 2 to 14 days after treatment is initiated.[10] In one study, 30% of 23 owners reported that their dog returned to normal activities in 1 to 2 days after treatment was initiated, 30% reported this took 3 to 5 days, 21% 1 to 3 weeks, and 17% reported that it took a month or longer for their dogs to return to normal activity.[10] Death due to granulocytic anaplasmosis has not been described in dogs. Intravenous crystalloid fluids and antiemetics may be required for supportive care until clinical signs improve.

Immunity and Vaccination

The immune response to *A. phagocytophilum* infection is not fully characterized. Both humoral and cell-mediated immune responses appear to be important in clearance of infection. Host cytokines such as IFN-γ may play a role in the initial control of *A. phagocytophilum* infection[31,32] but may also contribute to the inflammatory process associated with disease.[33] In lambs, *A. phagocytophilum* evades the host immune response through differential expression of MSP2, an outer surface protein involved in immune recognition.[34] Variation in MSP2 also occurs in chronically infected woodrats.[35] Further research is required to document whether persistence occurs through similar mechanisms in other host species. It is possible that recovery from natural infection confers long-term protection against development of disease. Reinfection has not been reported in dogs, but was described in one human patient.[36] A vaccine for granulocytic anaplasmosis is not available for companion animals.

Prevention

Infection may be prevented by avoidance of tick exposure, prompt tick removal, and use of topical ectoparasiticides (see Chapter 28). Although not a guaranteed protection, combinations of topical imidacloprid and permethrin, or fipronil, amitraz and (*S*)-methoprene, prevent transmission of *A. phagocytophilum* to dogs from infected ticks.[37,37a]

Public Health Aspects

A. phagocytophilum infection was first recognized in humans in the upper Midwest of the United States in the early 1990s and has since been increasingly recognized in humans from the United States, Europe, and Asia. Human granulocytic anaplasmosis closely resembles the disease in dogs, which has been described as an "influenza-like illness after a tick bite."[38] Men are affected slightly more frequently than women. In Europe, the disease is most commonly reported in from Sweden and Slovenia, where it was first reported in 1997.[39] Morulae are observed less often in humans with granulocytic anaplasmosis in Europe, and the disease may be milder than that described in humans from the United States.

The most common clinical signs reported in human patients are myalgia, headache (which is often severe), malaise, and chills. Anorexia, nausea, arthralgias, and cough may also occur.[22,38,40] The disease typically resolves within 2 months in the absence of appropriate antibiotic treatment. Occasionally more severe disease may occur. In one study, up to 17% of affected humans required admission to an intensive care unit.[38] Death occurs in 1% or fewer clinically affected humans, usually as a result of complications such as a septic or toxic shock–like syndrome, respiratory insufficiency, opportunistic fungal or viral infections, rhabdomyolysis, acute renal failure, hemorrhage, or neurologic disease.[22] Severe illness tends to occur in humans of advanced age or with concurrent immunosuppressive illness or drug therapy. Laboratory testing of peripheral blood typically reveals normal or slightly decreased white blood cell and platelet counts, sometimes with a neutrophilic left shift, and mild to moderate elevation of hepatic transaminase activities. In the United States, the disease is reportable to the Centers for Disease Control and Prevention (CDC). Dogs act as sentinels for human exposure and may be a source of infection through mechanical carriage of infected ticks to humans. Blood from affected dogs should be handled with caution, and needle-stick injuries should be avoided.

Anaplasma platys Infection

Etiologic Agent and Epidemiology

Anaplasma platys infects and forms inclusions within platelets and is the cause of canine cyclic thrombocytopenia, or thrombocytotropic anaplasmosis. It does not appear to infect cats. The organism is very widespread, and infections occur throughout the Americas, Europe, Asia, Australia, the Middle East, and

Africa. *R. sanguineus* ticks are believed to transmit *A. platys*, because the DNA of *A. platys* has frequently been found in *R. sanguineus* ticks worldwide, and dogs infected with *A. platys* are often co-infected with *E. canis*. However, in a single attempt, experimental transmission of *A. platys* by *R. sanguineus* ticks failed.[41] *A. platys* DNA has been found in other tick species, such as *Dermacentor auratus* ticks in Thailand,[42] *Rhipicephalus turanicus* ticks from Israel,[43] and *Haemaphysalis* spp. and *Ixodes nipponensis* ticks from Korea.[44] Different strains of *A. platys* exist that appear to vary in pathogenicity. The organism has never been isolated in cell culture.

Clinical Features

Signs and Their Pathogenesis

Anaplasma platys causes thrombocytopenia in dogs, most often in the absence of other clinical signs, although fever, lethargy, lymphadenopathy, uveitis, pallor, and mucosal hemorrhages have been described.[45,46] Co-infections with other vector-borne pathogens may contribute to clinical signs in some dogs. Thrombocytopenia occurs 1 to 2 weeks after experimental inoculation. This initial episode is associated with the highest number of organisms in platelets, as detected using light microscopic examination of stained blood smears.[47] The platelet count nadir occurs 2 to 3 weeks postinfection and in some dogs may be lower than 20,000 platelets/μL. Visible organisms then disappear from platelets, and the platelet count returns to normal or near-normal limits within 3 to 4 days. This also corresponds with a decrease in organism load and failure to detect the organism in peripheral blood with real-time PCR, although bone marrow and splenic aspirates may remain positive.[48] Cycles of thrombocytopenia and bacteremia then occur at intervals of 7 to 14 days, after which infection and thrombocytopenia persist in some dogs but morulae or inclusions become more difficult to detect within platelets.[47] The mechanism of thrombocytopenia is unknown, but direct damage to platelets, sequestration of platelets in the spleen, and immune-mediated destruction have been hypothesized to play a role.

Co-infection of dogs with *A. platys* and *E. canis* may lead to more severe anemia than occurs with isolated *E. canis* infection.[49] The duration of *A. platys* infection may also be prolonged.

Physical Examination Findings

Most dogs with *A. platys* infection show no clinical signs. Fever, petechial hemorrhages, and uveitis have been reported, but co-infections with other vector-borne pathogens may have contributed to these signs.

Diagnosis

Laboratory Abnormalities

Usually, the only abnormality present on the CBC, biochemistry panel, and urinalysis in dogs with *A. platys* infection is thrombocytopenia. A mild, nonregenerative anemia may be found. The diagnosis can be made when morulae are seen within platelets on blood smears, but this is insensitive, and other inclusions or stain precipitate may be mistaken for organisms.

Microbiologic Tests

Direct Fluorescent Antibody

Direct fluorescent antibody techniques can be used to identify *A. platys* in platelets, but these are not widely available for routine diagnostic purposes. Molecular diagnostic assays have overcome the need for direct fluorescent antibody or immunocytochemical staining.

Serologic Diagnosis

Recent infection with an *Anaplasma* species can be detected through the use of acute and convalescent serology with IFA. Because antibodies to *A. phagocytophilum* bind to *A. platys* antigens it is not possible to distinguish the immune response to each of these pathogens with currently available assays. This can be problematic in geographic regions where both *A. platys* and *A. phagocytophilum* are found. A positive result on commercially available ELISA assays also only indicates previous exposure to an *Anaplasma* species. Dogs with recent infection may be seronegative, because antibodies to *A. platys* are not detectable for 1 to 2 weeks after inoculation. Because a single positive test result only indicates previous exposure, and seroprevalence rates in endemic areas are high, thrombocytopenia in a seropositive dog may be due to an etiology other than *Anaplasma* infection. Cross-reactivity to *E. canis* antigens does not occur in dogs with *A. platys* infections, so positive titers to *E. canis* and *A. platys* may represent previous exposure to both pathogens, or to other *Ehrlichia* or *Anaplasma* species.

Molecular Diagnosis Using the Polymerase Chain Reaction

Several conventional and real-time PCR assays have been described for detection of *A. platys* DNA. In the absence of clearly identifiable morulae within platelets, molecular diagnostic testing with reliable PCR assays that specifically detect *A. platys* DNA (as opposed to *A. phagocytophilum* DNA or *Anaplasma* species DNA) is the only way to confirm active infection. Real-time PCR assays that detect *A. platys* DNA are available commercially and in combination with assays for other vector-borne pathogens. Suitable specimens include whole blood, buffy coats, or bone marrow and splenic aspirates,[48] although it is not clear which of these specimens is optimal. When buffy coats were used, PCR assays for *A. platys* became positive as early 3 to 5 days after experimental infection, but by day 21, negative results occurred in some dogs.[48,49] The use of splenic or bone marrow aspirates may yield positive results when whole blood or buffy coat PCR for *A. platys* is negative yet infection is still suspected.

Pathologic Findings

Pathologic findings have been described in a small number of dogs that were experimentally infected with *A. platys*, and necropsied early in the course of infection.[50] The only gross necropsy finding was generalized lymphadenomegaly. Lesions consisted of reactive lymphoid hyperplasia and erythrophagocytosis by sinusoidal macrophages within lymph nodes and the spleen, crescent-shaped regions of perifollicular hemorrhage in the spleen, mild lymphoplasmacytic infiltrates in the renal interstitium, and multifocal hyperplasia of Kupffer's cells in the liver. Megakaryocyte numbers in the bone marrow were increased in some dogs.

Treatment and Prognosis

The recommended treatment for thrombocytopenic dogs infected with *A. platys* is doxycycline. The optimum dose and duration of treatment is unknown, but it is apparently eliminated using regimens effective for treatment of *E. canis* infection.

Infection could not be detected with PCR for a 3-week follow-up period after just 8 days of doxycycline treatment (10 mg/kg PO q24h), which was initiated in the acute phase of infection.[51] However, one dog remained infected after 2 weeks of treatment with tetracycline. In another study, doxycycline treatment was administered for 28 days, and infection could not be detected after this time point, even after pharmacologic immunosuppression with dexamethasone several months later.[49] Whether the duration of infection at the time of treatment affects treatment efficacy is unknown.

Prevention

See the previous discussion of *Anaplasma phagocytophilum* infection.

Public Health Aspects

Infection with *A. platys* has not been confirmed in humans.

CASE EXAMPLE

Signalment: "Copper," an 8-year old male neutered Labrador retriever from Napa, CA

History: Copper was brought to the University of California, Davis, VMTH emergency service for the problems of lethargy, inappetence, apparent neck pain of 1 week's duration, and fever. The dog had been taken to a local veterinary clinic on the day the illness began, and thrombocytopenia (113,000 platelets/μL) was detected on a CBC. ELISA serology for antibodies to *E. canis*, *B. burgdorferi*, and *A. phagocytophilum* and *Dirofilaria immitis* antigen (4Dx SNAP test, IDEXX Laboratories) was negative. Treatment with enrofloxacin (2.4 mg/kg PO q12h) and metronidazole was instituted, during which time the dog improved clinically, but when the metronidazole was discontinued after 5 days, lethargy, inappetence, and signs of neck pain returned 2 days later. A CBC at that time showed no clinically significant abnormalities. Treatment with enrofloxacin was continued, and methocarbamol (11.6 mg/kg PO q8h) and meloxicam (0.1 mg/kg PO q24h) were instituted for the neck pain. The owner took Copper's rectal temperature at home on the morning he was brought to the VMTH, and it was 105.6°F (40.9°C). Copper lived on a 20-acre winery with a reservoir and had access to wildlife and frequent tick exposure. There had been no known exposure to toxins and no travel history. The dog received monthly heartworm preventative, and flea and tick preventative was used, but only when the owner found ticks. He was normally fed a commercially available dry dog food.

Current Medications: Enrofloxacin (2.4 mg/kg PO q12h), methocarbamol (11.6 mg/kg PO q8h), and meloxicam (0.1 mg/kg PO q24h).

Other Medical History: Nine months previously, Copper was seen by the local veterinary clinic for neck pain. The dog was treated with methocarbamol, a nonsteroidal antiinflammatory drug, and rest, and the pain resolved after 7 days. The owners also reported that Copper had exhibited some weakness of his left pelvic limb for several years.

Physical Examination:

Body weight: 43.1 kg

General: Quiet, alert, responsive, adequately hydrated. T = 103.7°F (39.8°C), HR = 110 beats/min, panting, mucous membranes pink, CRT <2 s.

Integument: No clinically significant abnormalities were identified. No ectoparasites were noted.

Eyes, Ears, Nose, and Throat: Mild gingivitis and dental calculus were present. No other significant abnormalities were noted.

Musculoskeletal: Body condition score 4/9. The dog was ambulatory but had a slightly stiff thoracic limb gait. A decreased range of motion of coxofemoral joints was detected, with the left worst than the right. There was no evidence of joint pain or effusion.

Cardiovascular, Respiratory Systems, Gastrointestinal and Urogenital Systems: No clinically significant findings were identified. Rectal examination revealed no significant abnormalities.

Lymph Nodes: All peripheral lymph nodes were normal sized but slightly firm on palpation.

Neurologic Examination: Mentation and cranial nerve function were within normal limits. The dog was reluctant to move his neck on manipulation, especially to the right side, and palpation of the cervical spine elicited pain. Decreased placing reactions were noted in the left pelvic limb.

Laboratory Findings:

CBC:

HCT 35.8% (40%-55%)
MCV 64 fL (65-75 fL)
MCHC 35.8 g/dL (33-36 g/dL)
Reticulocyte count 10,200 cells/μL (7000-65,000 cells/μL)
WBC 7100 cells/μL (6000-13,000 cells/μL)
Neutrophils 6603 cells/μL (3000-10,500 cells/μL)
Band neutrophils 284 cells/μL
Lymphocytes 71 cells/μL (1000-4000 cells/μL)
Monocytes 142 cells/μL (150-1200 cells/μL)
Platelets 37,000/μL (150,000-400,000 platelets/μL)
MPV 17.2 fL (7-13 fL).

Slight toxicity was detected in neutrophils and band neutrophils, and multiple neutrophils contained basophilic intracytoplasmic inclusions (morulae) (see Figure 29-3).

Serum Chemistry Profile:

Anion gap 23 mmol/L (10-24 mmol/L)
Sodium 145 mmol/L (145-154 mmol/L)
Potassium 3.7 mmol/L (3.6-5.3 mmol/L)
Chloride 115 mmol/L (108-118 mmol/L)
Bicarbonate 11 mmol/L (16-26 mmol/L)
Phosphorus 3.9 mg/dL (3.0-6.2 mg/dL)
Calcium 10.2 mg/dL (9.7-11.5 mg/dl)
BUN 12 mg/dL (5-21 mg/dL)
Creatinine 0.7 mg/dL (0.3-1.2 mg/dL)
Glucose 61 mg/dL (64-123 mg/dL)
Total protein 6.8 g/dL (5.4-7.6 g/dL)

Albumin 3.1 g/dL (3.0-4.4 g/dL)
Globulin 3.7 g/dL (1.8-3.9 g/dL)
ALT 54 U/L (19-67 U/L)
AST 26 U/L (19-42 U/L)
ALP 106 U/L (21-170 U/L)
Creatine kinase 79 U/L (51-399 U/L)
GGT < 3 U/L (0-6 U/L)
Cholesterol 255 mg/dL (135-361 mg/dL)
Total bilirubin 0.1 mg/dL (0-0.2 mg/dL)
Magnesium 2.1 mg/dL (1.5-2.6 mg/dL).

Urinalysis: SGr 1.031; pH 8.0, 25 mg/dL protein, no bilirubin, 25 erythrocytes/μL hemoprotein, no glucose, 0-3 WBC/HPF, 15-25 RBC/HPF, no other significant abnormalities were detected.

Imaging Findings:

Spinal Radiographs: Multiple right lateral projections of the spine were reviewed. There were multiple sites of mild ventral spondylosis deformans throughout the thoracolumbar spine. Severe spondylosis was seen at the lumbosacral space with sclerosis of the endplates either side, most likely due to degenerative change. There was severe osseous remodeling of the lumbar articular facets, which was consistent with osteoarthrosis. Small areas of intervertebral disc mineralization were seen at the L2-3 and L4-5 spaces.

Thoracic Radiographs: The cardiovascular and pulmonary structures were within normal limits. There was slightly increased soft tissue opacity in the region of the sternal lymph node on the right lateral projection.

Abdominal Ultrasound: The liver was mildly hypoechoic but normal in size. The spleen was markedly enlarged but had normal echogenicity. The rest of the abdominal organs were within normal limits.

Microbiologic Testing: Aerobic bacterial urine culture: No growth

ELISA serology for vector-borne pathogens (IDEXX 4Dx SNAP test): Positive for antibodies to *A. phagocytophilum*. Negative for antibodies to *E. canis* and *B. burgdorferi*. Negative for *D. immitis* antigen.

IFA serology for vector-borne pathogens: Positive for antibody to *A. phagocytophilum* (1:2560). Negative for antibodies to *R. rickettsia* at <1:40. Negative for antibodies to *Babesia canis* at <1:40. Weak positive for antibody to *E. canis* at 1:40.

Vector-borne real-time PCR panel (whole blood): Positive for *A. phagocytophilum* (Msp gene PCR). Negative for *Anaplasma platys, Bartonella* spp., *Borrelia burgdorferi, Ehrlichia canis*, and *Rickettsia* spp. DNA.

Diagnosis: Granulocytic anaplasmosis

Treatment: Copper was treated with doxycycline (5 mg/kg PO q12h) the day after admission, when results of the CBC were available. In the interim, pain was managed with meloxicam and hydromorphone, and IV crystalloid fluids were administered. A day later, the fever had resolved and the dog's appetite and neck pain had improved, but thrombocytopenia persisted (36,000 platelets/μL). Two days after initiation of doxycycline treatment, the platelet count was 302,000 platelets/μL, and all other hematologic variables that were abnormal had returned to the reference range. At a recheck examination, 2 weeks after discharge, Copper was doing well, with no evidence of pain or stiffness. A CBC showed a platelet count of 487,000 platelets/μL.

Comments: This was an unusual case of granulocytic anaplasmosis in a dog that developed apparent cervical pain in association with infection. The dog also had osteoarthritis, but clinical signs resolved almost completely once doxycycline was instituted. Although the dog's joints did not appear painful or swollen on physical examination, it is possible that polyarthritis may have contributed to the clinical signs of stiffness. Serology was initially negative because infection was too recent for an antibody response to have developed. The diagnosis of granulocytic anaplasmosis was confirmed with molecular diagnostic testing and supported by seroconversion to *A. phagocytophilum* and identification of morulae within neutrophils. The weak positive IFA test result to *E. canis* may have reflected serologic cross-reactivity. Treatment with enrofloxacin was apparently ineffective. The need for more consistent application of tick preventatives was discussed with the owners.

SUGGESTED READING

Carrade DD, Foley JE, Borjesson DL, et al. Canine granulocytic anaplasmosis: a review. J Vet Intern Med. 2009;23:1129-1141.

REFERENCES

1. Foggie A. Studies on the infectious agent of tick-borne fever in sheep. J Pathol Bacteriol. 1951;63:1-15.
2. Madewell BR, Gribble DH. Infection in two dogs with an agent resembling *Ehrlichia equi*. J Am Vet Med Assoc. 1982;180:512-514.
3. Harvey JW, Simpson CF, Gaskin JM. Cyclic thrombocytopenia induced by a *Rickettsia*-like agent in dogs. J Infect Dis. 1978;137:182-188.
4. M'Ghirbi Y, Ghorbel A, Amouri M, et al. Clinical, serological, and molecular evidence of ehrlichiosis and anaplasmosis in dogs in Tunisia. Parasitol Res. 2009;104:767-774.
5. Inokuma H, Oyamada M, Kelly PJ, et al. Molecular detection of a new *Anaplasma* species closely related to *Anaplasma phagocytophilum* in canine blood from South Africa. J Clin Microbiol. 2005;43:2934-2937.
6. Santos HA, Pires MS, Vilela JA, et al. Detection of *Anaplasma phagocytophilum* in Brazilian dogs by real-time polymerase chain reaction. J Vet Diagn Invest. 2011;23:770-774.
7. Carrade DD, Foley JE, Borjesson DL, et al. Canine granulocytic anaplasmosis: a review. J Vet Intern Med. 2009;23:1129-1141.
8. Bowman D, Little SE, Lorentzen L, et al. Prevalence and geographic distribution of *Dirofilaria immitis, Borrelia burgdorferi, Ehrlichia canis*, and *Anaplasma phagocytophilum* in dogs in the United States: results of a national clinic-based serologic survey. Vet Parasitol. 2009;160:138-148.
9. Greig B, Asanovich KM, Armstrong PJ, et al. Geographic, clinical, serologic, and molecular evidence of granulocytic ehrlichiosis, a likely zoonotic disease, in Minnesota and Wisconsin dogs. J Clin Microbiol. 1996;34:44-48.
10. Granick JL, Armstrong PJ, Bender JB. *Anaplasma phagocytophilum* infection in dogs: 34 cases (2000-2007). J Am Vet Med Assoc. 2009;234:1559-1565.
11. Beall MJ, Chandrashekar R, Eberts MD, et al. Serological and molecular prevalence of *Borrelia burgdorferi, Anaplasma phagocytophilum*, and *Ehrlichia* species in dogs from Minnesota. Vector Borne Zoonotic Dis. 2008;8:455-464.

12. Kohn B, Galke D, Beelitz P, et al. Clinical features of canine granulocytic anaplasmosis in 18 naturally infected dogs. J Vet Intern Med. 2008;22:1289-1295.
13. Poitout FM, Shinozaki JK, Stockwell PJ, et al. Genetic variants of *Anaplasma phagocytophilum* infecting dogs in western Washington state. J Clin Microbiol. 2005;43:796-801.
14. Egenvall AE, Hedhammar AA, Bjoersdorff AI. Clinical features and serology of 14 dogs affected by granulocytic ehrlichiosis in Sweden. Vet Rec. 1997;140:222-226.
15. Savidge C, Ewing P, Andrews J, et al. *Anaplasma phagocytophilum* in cats: a retrospective analysis and clinical evaluation of fifteen cases from the north eastern United States. J Vet Intern Med. 2011;25:706:(abst).
16. Foley JE, Brown RN, Gabriel MW, et al. Spatial analysis of the exposure of dogs in rural north-coastal California to vectorborne pathogens. Vet Rec. 2007;161:653-657.
17. Egenvall A, Bjoersdorff A, Lilliehook I, et al. Early manifestations of granulocytic ehrlichiosis in dogs inoculated experimentally with a Swedish *Ehrlichia* species isolate. Vet Rec. 1998;143:412-417.
18. Eberts MD, Vissotto de Paiva Diniz PP, Beall MJ, et al. Typical and atypical manifestations of *Anaplasma phagocytophilum* infection in dogs. J Am Anim Hosp Assoc. 2011;47:e86-e94.
19. Lee FS, Chu FK, Tackley M, et al. Human granulocytic ehrlichiosis presenting as facial diplegia in a 42-year-old woman. Clin Infect Dis. 2000;31:1288-1291.
20. Wong SJ, Thomas JA. Cytoplasmic, nuclear, and platelet autoantibodies in human granulocytic ehrlichiosis patients. J Clin Microbiol. 1998;36:1959-1963.
21. Lilliehook I, Egenvall A, Tvedten HW. Hematopathology in dogs experimentally infected with a Swedish granulocytic *Ehrlichia* species. Vet Clin Pathol. 1998;27:116-122.
22. Bakken JS, Dumler S. Human granulocytic anaplasmosis. Infect Dis Clin North Am. 2008;22:433-448:viii.
23. Egenvall A, Lilliehook I, Bjoersdorff A, et al. Detection of granulocytic *Ehrlichia* species DNA by PCR in persistently infected dogs. Vet Rec. 2000;146:186-190.
24. Heikkila HM, Bondarenko A, Mihalkov A, et al. *Anaplasma phagocytophilum* infection in a domestic cat in Finland: Case report. Acta Vet Scand. 2010;52:62.
25. Tarello W. Microscopic and clinical evidence for *Anaplasma (Ehrlichia) phagocytophilum* infection in Italian cats. Vet Rec. 2005;156:772-774.
26. Plier ML, Breitschwerdt EB, Hegarty BC, et al. Lack of evidence for perinatal transmission of canine granulocytic anaplasmosis from a bitch to her offspring. J Am Anim Hosp Assoc. 2009;45:232-238.
27. Breitschwerdt EB, Hegarty BC, Hancock SI. Sequential evaluation of dogs naturally infected with *Ehrlichia canis, Ehrlichia chaffeensis, Ehrlichia equi, Ehrlichia ewingii,* or *Bartonella vinsonii*. J Clin Microbiol. 1998;36:2645-2651.
28. Aguero-Rosenfeld ME. Diagnosis of human granulocytic ehrlichiosis: state of the art. Vector Borne Zoonotic Dis. 2002;2:233-239.
29. Dumler JS, Barat NC, Barat CE, et al. Human granulocytic anaplasmosis and macrophage activation. Clin Infect Dis. 2007;45:199-204.
30. Lepidi H, Bunnell JE, Martin ME, et al. Comparative pathology, and immunohistology associated with clinical illness after *Ehrlichia phagocytophila*-group infections. Am J Trop Med Hyg. 2000;62:29-37.
31. Akkoyunlu M, Fikrig E. Gamma interferon dominates the murine cytokine response to the agent of human granulocytic ehrlichiosis and helps to control the degree of early rickettsemia. Infect Immun. 2000;68:1827-1833.
32. Birkner K, Steiner B, Rinkler C, et al. The elimination of *Anaplasma phagocytophilum* requires CD4+ T cells, but is independent of Th1 cytokines and a wide spectrum of effector mechanisms. Eur J Immunol. 2008;38:3395-3410.
33. Martin ME, Caspersen K, Dumler JS. Immunopathology and ehrlichial propagation are regulated by interferon-gamma and interleukin-10 in a murine model of human granulocytic ehrlichiosis. Am J Pathol. 2001;158:1881-1888.
34. Granquist EG, Stuen S, Lundgren AM, et al. Outer membrane protein sequence variation in lambs experimentally infected with *Anaplasma phagocytophilum*. Infect Immun. 2008;76:120-126.
35. Rejmanek D, Foley P, Barbet A, et al. Antigen variability in *Anaplasma phagocytophilum* during chronic infection of a reservoir host. Microbiology. 2012;158:2632-2641.
36. Horowitz HW, Aguero-Rosenfeld M, Dumler JS, et al. Reinfection with the agent of human granulocytic ehrlichiosis. Ann Intern Med. 1998;129:461-463.
37. Blagburn BL, Spencer JA, Billeter SA, et al. Use of imidacloprid-permethrin to prevent transmission of *Anaplasma phagocytophilum* from naturally infected *Ixodes scapularis* ticks to dogs. Vet Ther. 2004;5:212-217.
37a. McCall JW, Baker CF, Mather TN, et al. The ability of a topical novel combination of fipronil, amitraz and (S)-methoprene to protect dogs from *Borrelia burgdorferi* and *Anaplasma phagocytophilum* infections transmitted by *Ixodes scapularis*. Vet Parasitol. 2011;179:335-342.
38. Bakken JS, Krueth J, Wilson-Nordskog C, et al. Clinical and laboratory characteristics of human granulocytic ehrlichiosis. JAMA. 1996;275:199-205.
39. Strle F. Human granulocytic ehrlichiosis in Europe. Int J Med Microbiol. 2004;293(suppl 37):27-35.
40. Dumler JS, Madigan JE, Pusterla N, et al. Ehrlichioses in humans: epidemiology, clinical presentation, diagnosis, and treatment. Clin Infect Dis. 2007;45(suppl 1):S45-S51.
41. Simpson RM, Gaunt SD, Hair JA, et al. Evaluation of *Rhipicephalus sanguineus* as a potential biologic vector of *Ehrlichia platys*. Am J Vet Res. 1991;52:1537-1541.
42. Parola P, Cornet JP, Sanogo YO, et al. Detection of *Ehrlichia* spp., *Anaplasma* spp., *Rickettsia* spp., and other eubacteria in ticks from the Thai-Myanmar border and Vietnam. J Clin Microbiol. 2003;41:1600-1608.
43. Harrus S, Perlman-Avrahami A, Mumcuoglu KY, et al. Molecular detection of *Ehrlichia canis, Anaplasma bovis, Anaplasma platys, Candidatus* Midichloria mitochondrii and *Babesia canis vogeli* in ticks from Israel. Clin Microbiol Infect. 2011;17:459-463.
44. Chae JS, Yu do H, Shringi S, et al. Microbial pathogens in ticks, rodents and a shrew in northern Gyeonggi-do near the DMZ, Korea. J Vet Sci. 2008;9:285-293.
45. Harrus S, Aroch I, Lavy E, et al. Clinical manifestations of infectious canine cyclic thrombocytopenia. Vet Rec. 1997;141:247-250.
46. Glaze MB, Gaunt SD. Uveitis associated with *Ehrlichia platys* infection in a dog. J Am Vet Med Assoc. 1986;189:916-917.
47. Harvey JW. *Anaplasma platys* infection. In: Greene CE, ed. Infectious diseases of the dog and cat. 4th ed. St. Louis, MO: Elsevier Saunders; 2012:256-258.
48. Eddlestone SM, Gaunt SD, Neer TM, et al. PCR detection of *Anaplasma platys* in blood and tissue of dogs during acute phase of experimental infection. Exp Parasitol. 2007;115:205-210.
49. Gaunt S, Beall M, Stillman B, et al. Experimental infection and co-infection of dogs with *Anaplasma platys* and *Ehrlichia canis*: hematologic, serologic and molecular findings. Parasit Vectors. 2010;3:33.
50. Baker DC, Simpson M, Gaunt SD, et al. Acute *Ehrlichia platys* infection in the dog. Vet Pathol. 1987;24:449-453.
51. Chang WL, Su WL, Pan MJ. Two-step PCR in the evaluation of antibiotic treatment for *Ehrlichia platys* infection. J Vet Med Sci. 1997;59:849-851.

CHAPTER 30

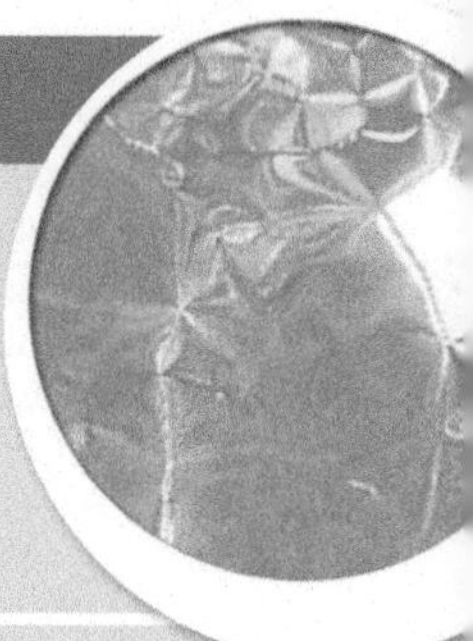

Rocky Mountain Spotted Fever

Linda Kidd and Edward B. Breitschwerdt

Overview of Rocky Mountain Spotted Fever

First Described: *R. rickettsii* was first described in Montana, United States, 1909[1] (by Ricketts)

Cause: *Rickettsia rickettsii*, a gram-negative, obligately intracellular bacteria

Affected Hosts: Humans and dogs

Geographic Distribution: North, Central, and South America

Primary Mode of Transmission: Ticks (*Dermacentor* spp., *Rhipicephalus sanguineus, Amblyomma* spp.). Most affected dogs lack a history of a tick bite.

Major Clinical Signs: Rocky Mountain spotted fever (RMSF) is an *acute*, generally febrile illness. Clinical signs are consistent with a vasculitis because *R. rickettsii* infects endothelial cells. Major clinical signs include fever, vomiting, ocular signs, lymphadenomegaly, splenomegaly, peripheral edema, cutaneous hyperemia and necrosis, polyarthritis, and neurologic signs. Signs may be complicated by simultaneous infection with other tick-borne pathogens.

Differential Diagnoses: Infection with other tick-borne agents such as *A. phagocytophilum, Ehrlichia* spp., *Bartonella* spp., *Babesia* spp., and *Borrelia burgdorferi* should be considered. Other causes of severe systemic decompensation and vasculitis, such as sepsis and SIRS due to other causes may mimic RMSF. Leptospirosis and other causes of vasculitis and thrombocytopenia may also mimic RMSF. Other differential diagnoses for the neurologic signs seen in RMSF must also be considered. Appropriate antimicrobial treatment with doxycycline must begin before the diagnosis is confirmed by laboratory testing. Misdiagnosis and delayed or inappropriate antimicrobial drug therapy increase morbidity and mortality.

Human Health Significance: Owners and their physicians should be contacted whenever RMSF is diagnosed in any canine patient, because illness in dogs can coincide with or precede illness in humans.

Etiologic Agent

Rocky Mountain spotted fever (RMSF) is caused by *Rickettsia rickettsii*, an obligately intracellular bacteria in the alphaproteobacteria (genus *Rickettsia*, family Rickettsiaceae, order Rickettsiales).[2] The terminology used to describe rickettsial disease is confusing and inconsistent due to multiple changes in the taxonomic classification of organisms in recent years.[3] The terms "rickettsial disease," "rickettsioses," and even the term "*Rickettsia*" have been used to refer to several obligately intracellular organisms including *Rickettsia, Bartonella, Ehrlichia, Anaplasma, Coxiella,* and *Neorickettsia*. Previously, all of these organisms belonged to the order Rickettsiales and most were in the family Rickettsiaceae, based on their fastidious or intracellular nature and other characteristics. Therefore, collectively members of these diverse genera were referred to as "rickettsial organisms."[4,5] Recent advances in molecular biologic techniques have resulted in the reclassification of several of these organisms. Many have been moved out of the family Rickettsiaceae, and others have been moved out of the order Rickettsiales. Now the order Rickettsiales includes only two families, the family Anaplasmataceae, which contains the genera *Anaplasma, Ehrlichia, Wolbachia,* and *Neorickettsia*; and the family Rickettsieaceae, which includes the genera *Rickettsia* and *Orientia*.[2,3,5] Currently, "rickettsial" refers to diseases caused by organisms in the genera *Anaplasma, Ehrlichia, Rickettsia, Neorickettsia,* and *Orientia*, "rickettsioses" refers to diseases caused by organisms in the family Rickettsiaceae (*Rickettsia* and *Orientia*), and the term "*Rickettsia*" refers specifically to members of the genus *Rickettsia*.[3-5]

The genus *Rickettsia* is currently divided into the spotted fever group (SFG) and the typhus group based on phenotypic and, more recently, genotypic characteristics.[3,5] Some of the phenotypic characteristics that have historically been used to group the organisms include the types of vectors that transmit them and the pathophysiologic manifestations of the disease.[3] The SFG rickettsial species are transmitted by arthropod (primarily tick) vectors and infect endothelial cells in mammalian hosts.[5] The two most pathogenic and well-studied SFG rickettsiae are *Rickettsia rickettsii*, the cause of RMSF in the Western Hemisphere, and *Rickettsia conorii*, the cause of Mediterranean spotted fever (MSF) in other areas of the world. The first case of RMSF was described in the late 1800s and the first case of MSF was described in the 1920s.[6] Therefore, these organisms and their associated diseases are the most well characterized among the SFG rickettsiae.[3] Currently, there are 20 or more species of SFG rickettsiae.[3,6] Some species appear to be nonpathogenic endosymbionts of ticks.[6] However, some SFG rickettsiae previously thought to be nonpathogenic, such as *R. parkerii* and *R. massiliae*, have recently been associated with disease in people.[7-9] Previously thought to have rather limited geographic boundaries, many SFG rickettsiae have also been detected in expanding geographic locales around the world.[6] For example, RMSF, originally described in the Bitterroot Valley of Montana, was subsequently found to be a frequent tick-transmitted infection in the eastern United States, but only recently has transmission via the brown dog tick been documented in the southwestern

United States.[10,11] Increasing travel and the effects of climate change on tick populations and habitat are thought to be in part responsible for this phenomenon.[12,13]

Epidemiology

Hosts, Life Cycle, and Transmission

Dogs are sentinels for SFG rickettsioses in people. Both *R. rickettsii* and *R. conorii* infect and cause disease in dogs.[14-20] *Rickettsia rickettsii* infection in dogs can occur before, or coincide with, outbreaks of RMSF in people in the same household or community.[21-24] Several serosurveys in endemic areas have shown an increased risk of MSF in people who live near dogs that are seropositive for SFG rickettsiae.[25-27] Other SFG rickettsial species likely infect dogs, but the extent to which they cause clinical disease has not yet been established. Species implicated in natural infection in dogs include *R. massiliae, R. japonica,* and *R. australis*.[28-31]

Young and purebred dogs are overrepresented in some but not other studies.[17,18] Although some studies suggest male dogs are at increased risk, no sex predilection has been definitively documented.[17,18,32] Severe disease has been reported in English springer spaniels with phosphofructokinase (PFK) deficiency and German shepherd dogs.[18,32] Although antibodies to SFG rickettsiae can be detected in cats that live in endemic areas, the ability of SFG rickettsiae to actively infect and cause disease in cats has not been well characterized.[33] Similarly, the ability of typhus group *Rickettsia* to cause disease both in dogs and cats has also not been well characterized and will not be discussed here.

Rickettsia rickettsii is transmitted by several hard (ixodid) ticks including *Dermacentor variabilis* (the American dog tick) (Figure 30-1, *A*), *Dermacentor andersoni* (the Rocky Mountain wood tick) (Figure 30-1, *B*), *Amblyomma americanum, Amblyomma cajennense, Amblyomma aureolatum,* and *Rhipicephalus sanguineus*.[34-38] *Amblyomma cajennense* and to a lesser extent, *A. aureolatum* transmit the rickettsia in South America. Ticks that transmit *R. rickettsii* feed once during each life stage (Figure 30-2). Both transstadial and transovarial transmission occurs in *Dermacentor* spp. infected with *R. rickettsii,* so these ticks serve as a reservoir of infection.[39,40] *Dermacentor* spp. and *Amblyomma* spp. are three-host ticks. Infection is transmitted among mammalian hosts and ticks when the tick feeds on different hosts during each stage of molting. The sylvatic cycle for *Dermacentor* ticks involves small mammals, such as chipmunks, pine voles, mice, and ground squirrels. After organisms are ingested by the tick, SFG rickettsiae initially replicate in the epithelial cells of the tick midgut, enter the hemolymph and hemocytes, and then multiply in tissues.[40] Once in the salivary glands, the organism is transmitted to a naïve mammalian host on feeding. Transmission can occur within hours of attachment. However, this may be prolonged (up to 48 hours) when changes in virulence occur under conditions such as starvation of the tick. These "dormant" rickettsiae undergo a process called reactivation after the tick begins feeding.[41] Therefore, rapid tick removal can decrease the risk of transmission in many, but not all, circumstances.

Rhipicephalus sanguineus is a one-host tick, with dogs being the preferred host.[42] *Rh. sanguineus* can adapt to hot environments and commonly resides in walls of housing structures in close proximity to humans.[42] It occasionally feeds on humans, especially when ambient temperatures are high.[12] The role of this tick as a reservoir for *R. rickettsii* in nature has yet to be elucidated.

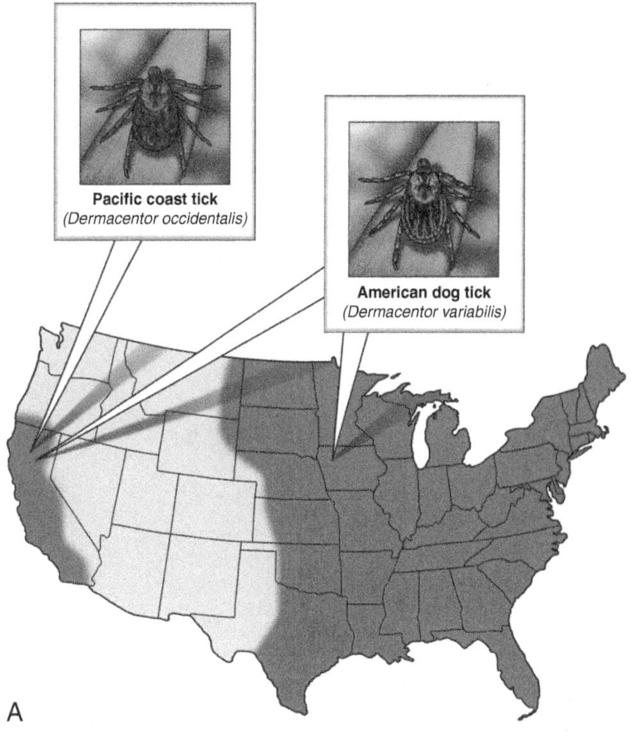

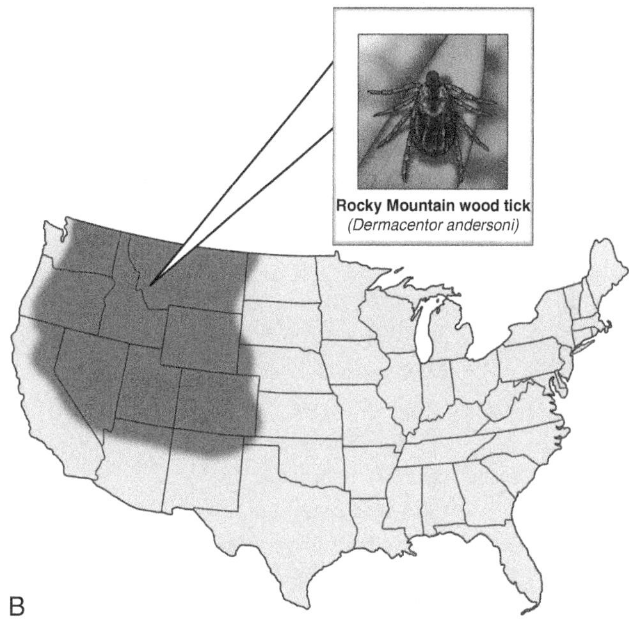

FIGURE 30-1 **A,** Distribution of *Dermacentor variabilis* and *Dermacentor occidentalis* ticks in the United States. **B,** Distribution of *Dermacentor andersoni* ticks in the United States.

The role of dogs as a natural reservoir of infection for *R. rickettsii* is also unknown.[39] Dogs are thought to act as incidental hosts when *Dermacentor* ticks are the vectors, because ticks rarely acquire the organism from rickettsemic dogs.[43] In contrast, all stages of *Rh. sanguineus* acquired infection at a high rate from experimentally infected dogs in one study, but this may have been related to the virulence of the rickettsial strain used.[38] A relatively high infection rate with SFG rickettsiae in naturally infected *Rh. sanguineus* has also been described.[37,44] Therefore, dogs may play a role in maintenance of a reservoir

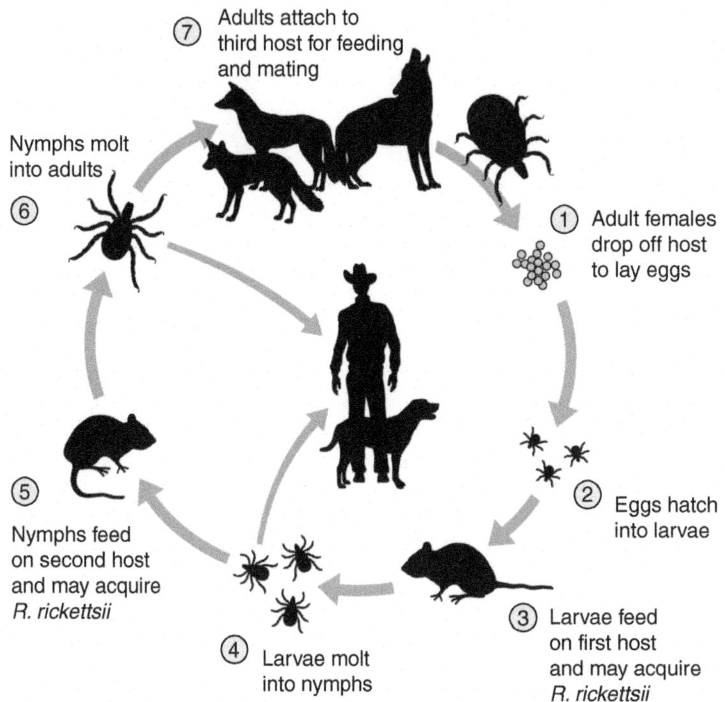

FIGURE 30-2 Transmission cycle of *Rickettsia rickettsii* in tick populations, people, and dogs. After adult female ticks lay eggs and they hatch (1 and 2), *Dermacentor* spp. ticks acquire *R. rickettsii* upon feeding as larvae or nymphs on rodents (3); they then transmit during subsequent feeding as nymphs or adults (4 and 6). Adult ticks feed on a variety of canid species, such as foxes and possibly wolves and coyotes. In addition, *R. rickettsii* infection can be maintained transovarially in *Dermacentor* ticks, so some larvae that hatch from the egg mass already harbor an infection. (Redrawn from Nicholson WL, Allen KE, McQuiston JH, et al. The increasing recognition of rickettsial pathogens in dogs and people. Trends Parasitol 2010;26[4]:205-212.)

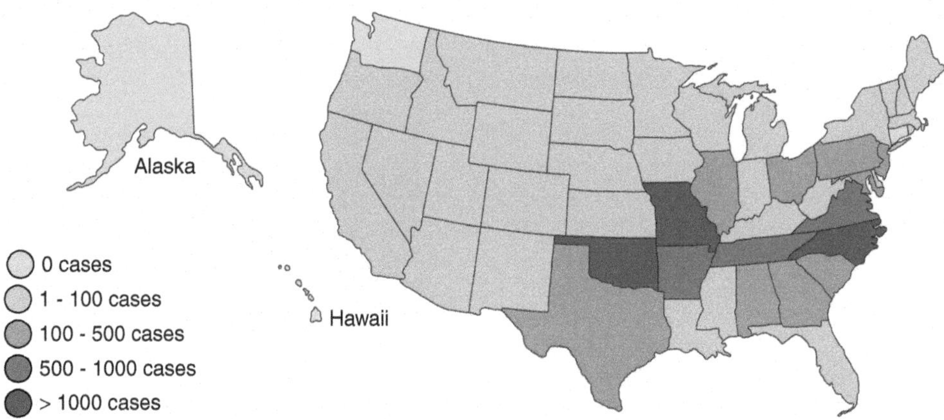

FIGURE 30-3 Geographic distribution of the incidence of spotted fever group rickettsioses in people in the United States, 2005-2009. (Compiled from data from the Centers for Disease Control and Prevention, Morbidity and Mortality Weekly Reports.)

of *R. rickettsii* infection in endemic foci where *Rh. sanguineus* is the primary vector.

Direct transmission of *R. rickettsii* to people has been described in laboratory settings through aerosolization. Direct transmission from blood or other contaminated biologic products also has the potential to occur.

Incidence and Geographic Distribution

Rocky Mountain spotted fever occurs in North, Central, and South America (where it is known as Brazilian spotted fever). In North America, most cases of RMSF occur in the southeastern and south central states (Figure 30-3). Disease distribution in the United States primarily follows the distribution of the primary vectors, *D. variabilis* and *D. andersoni,* although the importance of *D. variabilis* as vectors in endemic areas has recently been questioned.[45] Although disease can occur any time of year, most cases of canine and human RMSF are reported from April through October, months of peak tick activity.[17,46,47] Dogs that live outdoors, particularly those with access to shrubs and high grass, are at increased risk.[17]

In recent years the incidence of RMSF in people has increased.[47] Some of the increase may be due to misdiagnosis of disease caused by species of SFG rickettsiae other than *R. rickettsii.*[48,49] A similar increase in seroprevalence rates has been documented in dogs suspected to have a tick-borne infection in the United States.[50] The geographic distribution of RMSF in the United States has also increased beyond the distribution of *D. variabilis* and *D. andersoni. Rhipicephalus sanguineus* is the main vector for *R. rickettsii* in some parts of the Western Hemisphere, including Mexico and now the southwestern United States. In South America, *Amblyomma* species are the main tick vector. Tick species other than *D. variabilis, D. andersoni,* and *Rh. sanguineus* are also infected with *R. rickettsii* in the United States.[44] For example, *A. americanum* transmitted RMSF to a person in North Carolina.[36] An outbreak in Mexicali, Mexico, was attributed to *R. rickettsii* transmitted by *Rh. sanguineus* ticks associated with dogs.[51] This prompted ongoing surveillance efforts in ticks, dogs, and people in southern California, a nonendemic area for RMSF. Thus far, no *R. rickettsii* has been found in *Rh. sanguineus* ticks from dogs residing in animal shelters located just across the U.S. border from the outbreak.[52,53] This may be due to subtle differences in microenvironment or other factors that affect regional infection rates in ticks.[54]

Clinical Features

Signs and Their Pathogenesis

The endotheliotropism associated with these bacteria results in the characteristic clinical sign of infection, which is disseminated vasculitis. In people, cutaneous macules, papules, and petechiation that occur in association with vasculitis form a rash that looks like "spots," hence the name Rocky Mountain spotted fever.[6] The clinical signs, time course of illness, and response to therapy for RMSF in dogs are very similar, if not identical, to those associated with RMSF in people.[17-20,34] However, cutaneous lesions are not always present in dogs or people ("Rocky Mountain spotless fever"). In people, spotted fever rickettsioses caused by organisms other than *R. rickettsii* are often associated with eschar (an area of cutaneous necrosis) formation.[2,13] Clinicians should keep in mind that dogs from nonendemic areas that have classic signs of RMSF, or those that present with atypical clinical signs, may be infected with *R. rickettsii* or other SFG rickettsial species.

Once the organism is inoculated, it spreads through lymphatics or directly into the bloodstream to the small capillaries. *R. rickettsii* primarily infects endothelial cells, although smooth muscles and monocytes may also be infected.[2,55] The bacterial outer membrane protein A (OmpA) and outer membrane protein B (OmpB) are important for attachment, adhesion, and virulence.[56,57] These proteins are also responsible for differences in serotype, and antibodies to OmpB confer immunity to infection in experimental settings. SFG rickettsiae enter cells by inducing phagocytosis and are released into the cytoplasm through the action of enzymes such as phospholipase D and hemolysin C.[57] The bacteria live in the cytoplasm and the nucleus, deriving nutrients and energy from the host cell.[2,56] They spread from cell to cell by inducing actin to polymerize, which pushes the bacteria directly into adjacent cells.[57,58] This helps them evade the immune response and to disseminate without rupturing the cell. They are also released into circulation when they exit the luminal surface of the cell membrane or when endothelial cell death or detachment occurs.[57] Spotted fever group rickettsiae activate the transcription factor NFκB, which inhibits apoptosis and fosters further growth of the organism.[56,57]

Damage to endothelial cells leads to vasculitis and an increase in microvascular permeability. Mechanisms of cellular damage include oxidative injury through the production of reactive oxygen species, cellular necrosis, and induction of endothelial apoptosis by CD8+ T cells.[55-57,59] Activation of PFK may be important in maintaining vascular integrity and energy metabolism in endothelial cells under hypoxic or oxidative stress,[60,61] which may explain the predisposition of English springer spaniels with PFK deficiency to severe disease. Vasculitis associated with *R. rickettsii* infection manifests as disordered primary hemostasis, tissue edema, hypovolemia, and microthrombosis.

Increased vascular permeability and the associated edema and hypovolemia results from disruption of adherens junctions, endothelial cell death, expression of inflammatory cytokines such as Il1-β, IFN-γ, and TNF-α, and induction of COX-2 with subsequent prostaglandin production.[55] Microthrombosis results from altered platelet adherence to endothelium, increased tissue factor expression, increased plasminogen activator inhibitor, and the release of von Willebrand's factor.[55]

Low numbers of organisms circulate in blood for approximately 13 days after infection, which includes the time that clinical signs are observed.[19,62,63] Organisms are free and also contained within circulating endothelial cells, which are thought to be released from the vessels because of decreased adhesion after rickettsial invasion.[57] Thus, RMSF is an *acute* disease. Chronic infection has not been documented in dogs or people. Co-infection with other vector-borne agents is common and should be considered if the clinical signs are atypical, if there is an incomplete response to doxycycline therapy, or if clinical signs have been present for a week before the time of evaluation.[17,64]

Because of variation in the extent and severity of vascular injury among dogs, a range of signs can occur, and importantly, disease manifestations are initially mild and nonspecific.[15,17,18] Often, there is no known history of a tick bite. Therefore, the clinician (physician and veterinarian) must have a high index of suspicion in order to correctly diagnose and treat this disease. This is very important because a delay in diagnosis and appropriate antimicrobial therapy dramatically increases morbidity and mortality in people and in dogs.[17,46] A "One Health" approach to the management of canine and human RMSF is clearly logical. Lethargy and anorexia are common and may be the only clinical signs. Vomiting and diarrhea occur frequently in dogs and people with RMSF. Melena may be observed, as may a variety of CNS abnormalities including vestibular disease and seizures.[17,18,20] Dramatic and rapid weight loss has been described.[20]

Physical Examination Findings

Fever is present in approximately 80% of naturally infected dogs. Ocular signs are also frequently observed and may include a mucopurulent discharge, scleral and conjunctival injection and hemorrhage, conjunctivitis, uveitis, retinal hemorrhage, and retinitis (Figure 30-4). Lymphadenomegaly and splenomegaly also occur. Respiratory abnormalities include nasal discharge, epistaxis, and tachypnea. Mucocutaneous and cutaneous abnormalities include petechiae, ecchymosis, peripheral edema (which can be localized over a joint, the prepuce, or the mammary chain), hyperemia, and necrosis. Gangrenous necrosis can be so severe as to require reconstructive surgery after successful treatment of the acute febrile illness.[15-18,20,65,66] Orchitis and scrotal edema, hyperemia, and epididymal pain are common in intact male dogs and should prompt consideration of RMSF when present. Generalized myalgia and arthralgia can be observed. Arrhythmias may also be detected. CNS abnormalities can be focal or generalized and include paraparesis, tetraparesis, ataxia, hyperesthesia, ataxia, central or peripheral vestibular signs, stupor, seizures, and/or coma. Neurologic signs are more common in dogs with a high *R. rickettsii* antibody titer, which suggests a longer duration of illness or a delay in diagnosis.[17] Residual neurologic deficits may occur after infection in severely affected individuals. Microvascular hemorrhage, thrombosis, hypotension, oliguric renal failure, cardiovascular collapse, and coma can occur terminally.

Diagnosis

A combination of diagnostic testing is often necessary to confirm infection by SFG rickettsiae. Active infection is confirmed in a patient with compatible acute clinical signs and demonstration of the organism using PCR assays or immunohistochemistry (IHC), or documentation of seroconversion (Figure 30-5). Importantly, a high index of suspicion based on clinical signs is necessary, because treatment must be instituted before the results of diagnostic tests (including rapid PCR assays) confirm infection.[17,20] Co-infection with other vector-borne disease agents should be considered in patients who fail to respond rapidly to treatment (within the first 24 to 48 hours after initiation of doxycycline treatment).[64] Because direct inoculation into blood or aerosolization can cause infection, all specimens should be handled with care and marked clearly as biohazards. Needle-stick injuries, contact with cuts in the skin, and aerosolization of rickettsemic blood should be avoided.

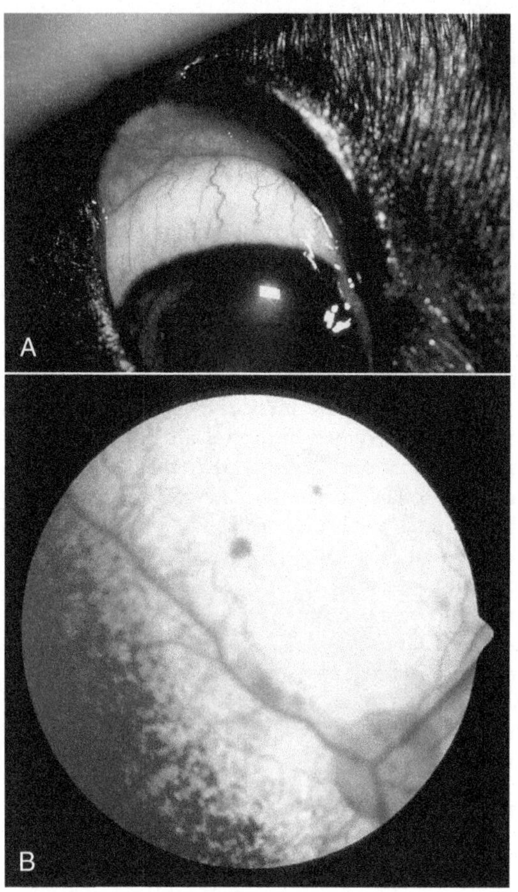

FIGURE 30-4 Ocular complications in dogs with RMSF. **A,** Conjunctival hyperemia and scleral injection. **B,** Retinal hemorrhages.

Laboratory Abnormalities

Complete Blood Count

Thrombocytopenia is common in RMSF and occurs due to vasculitis and immune-mediated platelet destruction.[67] However, it does not occur in all dogs with RMSF.[17,20] The white blood cell count may initially decrease and then tends to increase with duration of illness.[18-20] Neutrophils may have toxic change.[17] Despite the acute nature of this severe illness, a nonregenerative anemia may be present and persist until the dog is treated appropriately and begins to recover.[15,17,20]

Serum Biochemical Tests

Serum biochemical abnormalities can include hypoalbuminemia (due to vasculitis or protein-losing nephropathy), increased ALP activity, hyponatremia, and mild hyperbilirubinemia.[15,17,20,65] Hyponatremia has been associated with the syndrome of inappropriate antidiuretic hormone secretion (SIADH) in people with RMSF.

Urinalysis

Urinalysis results in dogs with RMSF are variable and may include proteinuria, hematuria and bilirubinuria, and pyuria. Granular casts can be observed.[17,18]

Coagulation Profile

Coagulation abnormalities include prolonged APTT and increased serum fibrinogen concentration. Less commonly, prolonged PT and increased fibrin degradation products are observed. Although a prothrombotic state can occur during fulminant disease, disseminated intravascular coagulation is uncommon.[15,17]

Body Fluid Cytology

Cytologic examination of aspirates from enlarged lymph nodes in dogs with RMSF is consistent with reactive lymphoid hyperplasia.[17,18] Arthrocentesis may reveal neutrophilic

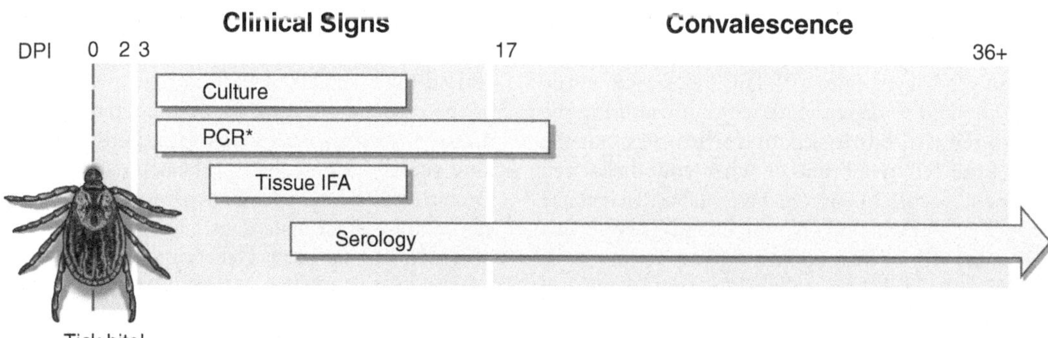

FIGURE 30-5 Timing in relation to day postinfection (DPI) that clinical signs and diagnostic tests for *Rickettsia rickettsii* may be positive in an infected dog[16,62,63,70,76] Further studies are needed to determine exactly how DNA can be detected in peripheral blood after infection.[62,63]

polyarthritis.[17,18] Cerebrospinal fluid analysis in dogs with neurologic signs may reveal a mixed cellular, neutrophilic, or lymphocytic pleocytosis.[17,18,20,68]

Diagnostic Imaging

Thoracic radiographs in dogs with RMSF may show an unstructured interstitial pattern.[18,69] Testicular ultrasound findings may be consistent with orchitis in intact males.[66]

Microbiologic Tests

Diagnostic assays available for RMSF in dogs are shown in Table 30-1. Because of the pathogenesis of the infection, laboratory diagnostics (including serology and PCR assays) may not indicate infection is present at the time that clinical signs manifest (see Figure 30-5). In addition, most diagnostic tests do not differentiate among species of SFG rickettsiae.

Culture

Because of the obligately intracellular and extremely pathogenic nature of *R. rickettsii,* culture is difficult to perform and processing of specimens for isolation is limited to BSL 3 facilities (see Table 1-4). Therefore, culture is not commonly used for routine diagnosis. Currently, *R. rickettsii* is listed as a Category A Bioterrorism agent, so all isolates must be reported to the Centers for Disease Control and Prevention or destroyed immediately.

Serologic Diagnosis

Indirect microimmunofluorescence (MIF) assays that detect IgM and IgG antibodies are most commonly used to document seroconversion in dogs infected with *R. rickettsii.*[19] Because of a lack of specificity, assays that detect IgM alone cannot be used to accurately diagnose acute RMSF.[70] There is extensive serologic cross-reactivity among SFG rickettsiae, and thus a positive titer only indicates exposure to a SFG rickettsial species. In general, the infecting species is presumed based on geographic locale, so RMSF is the presumptive diagnosis in dogs that seroconvert in the southeastern United States. However, other species of SFG rickettsiae may also be present and induce disease.[28,71] Exposure to nonpathogenic SFG rickettsiae, some of which are common endosymbionts in ticks, may be a common cause of positive titers, particularly low and persistent titers, to *R. rickettsii* in healthy people and dogs.[49,72] Serologic cross-reactivity with SFG rickettsiae also may occur in dogs and people infected with *Bartonella henselae.*[73] In addition, previous infection with *R. rickettsii* may result in persistent antibody titers.[70] Thus, infection with *R. rickettsii* cannot be definitively diagnosed based on a single positive titer. However, a single high titer in the context of acute and compatible clinical signs and an appropriate response to therapy suggests infection.[17] Titers are commonly negative early in the course of infection, because clinical signs often occur before seroconversion in naturally and experimentally infected dogs.[20,70,74] Thus, acute and convalescent serology (run in the same laboratory and ideally in the same batch) and documentation of a fourfold change in titer is necessary to confirm acute SFG rickettsiae infection. The convalescent serum specimen should be drawn 2 to 3 weeks after the acute specimen.

TABLE 30-1

Diagnostic Assays Available for Rocky Mountain Spotted Fever in Dogs

Assay	Specimen Type	Target	Performance
Indirect microimmuno-fluorescence assay (MIF)	Serum	IgM and IgG antibodies against *R. rickettsii*	Demonstration of a fourfold change in titer (seroconversion) is very sensitive. False-negative results are common during the acute phase of infection. A positive antibody response may reflect prior exposure to a nonpathogenic SFG rickettsia, or long-lived circulating antibody from previous infection with SFG rickettsiae. Cross-reactivity to other SFG rickettsiae and to *B. henselae* occurs.
PCR	Whole blood	Gene target varies with testing laboratories	In vitro sensitivity may approach 100%; however, absolute (clinical) sensitivity is lower, approximately 60%, because organisms circulate in blood in low numbers and transiently during the acute phase of infection. Sensitivity is further reduced by antimicrobial drug treatment. Specificity approaches 100%, particularly if the laboratory sequences all PCR amplicons. PCR testing for other tick-borne organisms that cause similar clinical signs is available as PCR panels from some testing laboratories. Only a few PCR assays differentiate among *Rickettsia* species. Negative PCR assay results do not rule out infection.
Histopathology with direct IFA or Gimenez staining	Cutaneous biopsy (inguinal or flank targeting areas with lesions) or necropsy specimens	Characteristic perivascular inflammation and vasculitis with necrosis and presence of the organism	Direct IFA sensitivity is approximately 80% during acute infection. Biopsy of a petechial or ecchymotic lesion may increase sensitivity. False negatives occur if organisms are absent from the lesion because of random chance, timing of specimen collection, or prior antimicrobial treatment. Does not differentiate among species of SFG *Rickettsia.*

Molecular Diagnosis Using Polymerase Chain Reaction

PCR testing of whole blood can be used to confirm infection in seronegative dogs during the acute phase of disease.[62,63,74] A sensitive PCR assay that detects and differentiates among SFG rickettsiae that infect dog blood has been described, and a variety of PCR assays are available through commercial veterinary diagnostic laboratories.[74] However, because *R. rickettsii* circulates in blood in low numbers and only transiently, the sensitivity of any diagnostic assay to detect infection in the bloodstream is limited. One real-time PCR assay, which could detect as few as five copies of organism DNA, had a sensitivity of only 53% for detection of *R. rickettsii* in acute samples from naturally infected dogs with signs of RMSF.[74] The sensitivity of another *R. rickettsii* PCR assay for detection of *R. rickettsii* in experimentally infected dogs ranged from 33% to 100% depending on the day of sampling.[63] Furthermore, false negatives can occur after initiation of appropriate antimicrobial treatment. Therefore, although a positive PCR assay result confirms infection, a negative result does not exclude the diagnosis. Some PCR assays can differentiate among infecting *Rickettsia* species, whereas others only amplify conserved rickettsial DNA targets.[62,74] Clinicians should consult with laboratories to determine the in vitro (analytical) and in vivo (clinical) sensitivity of a PCR assay and its ability to differentiate among infecting *Rickettsia* species.

Pathologic Findings

Gross Pathologic Findings

Gross pathologic findings in dogs with RMSF are consistent with vasculitis and may include edema, particularly of the ears, muzzle, and scrotum, and ecchymosis, petechiae, and/or focal hemorrhages of the skin, mucous membranes, and viscera (including the brain). Lymphadenomegaly and splenomegaly are also common findings.[15,16,20,22]

Histopathologic Findings

Microscopically, the predominant lesion is vasculitis. Neutrophils, monocytes, and/or lymphoreticular cells predominate in the inflammatory lesions. The inflammation may surround and invade large small and medium-size vessels of multiple organs and tissues and is frequently accompanied by focal necrosis and hemorrhage. Meningoencephalitis, splenitis, myocardial necrosis, glomerulonephritis, and renal vasculitis have been described.[15,20,22]

Direct IFA can be used to detect organisms in skin and other organs. Identification of abundant SFG rickettsiae within and around small to medium-size vessels and vascular endothelial cells can confirm infection.[20] In experimentally infected dogs, the sensitivity of IHC was 78.3%, and organisms could be visualized between days 7 and 12 of infection (days 3 to 8 of fever).[75] In that study, specimens collected from areas other than the central focus of vasculitis were negative. However, in naturally infected dogs, the sensitivity was 80% for skin specimens from the inguinal region. Half of those specimens lacked gross lesions.[18] Thus, the diagnostic sensitivity of IHC is most likely enhanced by obtaining lesional biopsies, but may not be decreased when a lesion is not biopsied. The sensitivity of direct IHC is decreased by antibiotic therapy. IHC does not differentiate between SFG rickettsial species. Gimenez stain can also be used to visualize rickettsial organisms in tissues or tissue culture isolation attempts, but this stain is not rickettsia specific and does not allow for differentiation among species.

Treatment

Antimicrobial Treatment

Appropriate antibiotic therapy must be immediately instituted based on clinical suspicion, and before diagnostic tests confirm infection. Inappropriate or delayed antibiotic therapy may increase morbidity and mortality.[17,46] Some antimicrobial drugs such as trimethoprim sulfonamides may actually worsen disease progression in human patients.[46] Doxycycline is the treatment of choice (Table 30-2). It effectively eliminates infection and is active against *A. phagocytophilum, Ehrlichia* spp., and *B. burgdorferi,* which may be present in co-infections or cause disease that resembles RMSF. Seven days of treatment is adequate in most cases. Treatment a few days past defervescence is recommended. A longer course of treatment is recommended for dogs that are co-infected with *Ehrlichia* spp. or *B. burgdorferi.* Chloramphenicol was effective in experimentally infected dogs.[76] However, it may be less effective than doxycycline for treating RMSF in people and has less activity in vitro against *Ehrlichia chaffeensis* and *A. phagocytophilum.*[46] Enrofloxacin was effective for treatment of RMSF in experimentally infected dogs.[76] However, enrofloxacin is not effective for treatment of *E. canis* infections.[77] Use of parenteral antimicrobial drugs may be necessary in severely debilitated or vomiting patients.

Supportive Care

Many dogs require hospitalization.[20] Aggressive supportive care for complications such as thrombosis, CNS deficits, and gastrointestinal signs may be necessary. Because of the loss of vascular integrity, fluids should be administered with caution, and colloids may be warranted in some cases. The clinician should avoid exacerbation of interstitial edema, which can contribute to cerebral edema and death. The use of glucocorticoids in dogs with RMSF is controversial. Antiinflammatory and immunosuppressive doses did not affect overall outcome experimentally infected dogs, but rickettsemia was prolonged in dogs concurrently treated with immunosuppressive doses of glucocorticoids and doxycycline.[78] Antiinflammatory doses of glucocorticoids have been used in dogs with severe CNS manifestations and may be necessary topically or systemically for treatment of ocular abnormalities.[68,79]

Prognosis

The response to appropriate antibiotic therapy in dogs with RMSF is rapid (24 to 48 hours). Co-infection with

TABLE 30-2

Antimicrobials Used to Treat Rocky Mountain Spotted Fever in Dogs

Drug	Dose (mg/kg)	Route	Interval (hours)	Duration (days)
Doxycycline	5	PO, IV	12	7 to 14
Chloramphenicol*	30	PO, IV	8	7 to 14
Enrofloxacin	3† to 5	PO, IV	12	7 to 14

*May cause aplastic anemia in humans (wear gloves); may be less effective than doxycycline.

†Dose used in experimentally infected dogs.[76] Caution required in young animals (see Chapter 8).

B. burgdorferi, *Ehrlichia* spp., *Babesia* spp., and *Bartonella* spp. should be considered in dogs with severe or prolonged clinical signs or dogs that fail to respond to doxycycline. Residual CNS and other deficits may occur in severely affected patients.[17] The prognosis is good to excellent if the disease is diagnosed and treated with appropriate antibiotics and supportive care early in the course of illness.[17,68]

Immunity and Vaccination

Cell-mediated and innate immunity is important in the clearance of rickettsial infections. CD4+ and CD8+ cells, along with macrophages and dendritic cells, are believed to be sources of inflammatory cytokines such as IFN-γ, TNF-α, Il-1β, and RANTES (CCL5). These cytokines increase production of nitric oxide synthetase and hydrogen peroxide by the endothelial cell, which helps to eliminate the organisms.[56,57] The endothelial cells themselves also produce cytokines such as IL-6, Il-8, and MCP-1 (CCL2) that recruit immune cells and combat infection. Antibodies are not thought to be important initially for clearance of infection because they form after the fulminant stages of disease.[57] However, antibodies are long-lived and together with cell-mediated immunity may prevent subsequent infection. Immunity to reinfection is thought to be lifelong in people, and experimentally infected dogs did not develop illness following rechallenge at 6 months and 3 years after the initial infection. Vaccination is not available for dogs or people currently, but may be in the future.[80]

Prevention

Avoidance of tick-infested areas and routine inspection of dogs for ticks after outdoor activities can help to prevent RMSF. The reader is referred to Chapter 28 for information on tick prevention and safe tick removal. Safe tick removal is especially critical when exposure to *R. rickettsii* is a possibility. In cases where *Rh. sanguineus* is the vector, environmental control of ticks is particularly important.

Public Health Aspects

People living near dogs and with dogs in endemic areas are at increased risk for acquiring RMSF. This is likely due to increased human contact with ticks through interaction with tick-infested dogs. Also, because of transovarial transmission, dogs and people can independently acquire the infection from different ticks questing in the same environment. Because dogs have higher exposure to ticks than their human counterparts, they serve as excellent environmental sentinels for RMSF.[21,22,24,71] In the United States, the diagnosis of SFG rickettsioses in humans is notifiable to public health authorities. Some counties in certain states also require reporting for dogs, particularly during suspected outbreaks.[81] From a public health standpoint, it is important for veterinarians to confirm a diagnosis of RMSF in a dog whenever possible, and to warn the family of the increased risk of acquiring a *R. rickettsii*–infected tick in the same location as the dog acquired the disease. Veterinarians must communicate with owners and physicians that infection in a dog may precede tick-transmitted infection to owners or neighbors. Clients should be instructed to remove ticks properly. Education of owners with regard to the importance of tick control and prevention for both people and pets and the environment is critical. Novel and well-characterized species of SFG rickettsiae are important causes of emerging infectious disease in humans. Furthermore, *R. rickettsii* is considered a potential bioterrorist agent.[80] Because dogs are sentinels for infection, veterinarians play an important role in detecting, defining, and preventing illness in their canine patients and their human companions.

CASE EXAMPLES

Rocky Mountain Spotted Fever in a Dog

Signalment: A 5-year-old MC Australian shepherd from North Carolina

History: The dog was examined by the North Carolina State University veterinary emergency service on April 11 because of recent onset of lethargy, fever, tachypnea, and a stiff gait when walking. Historically the dog had been healthy, had received routine vaccinations, heartworm preventive, and a flea acaricide, and ran approximately 3 miles each evening with the owner, who was a veterinarian. On the day of presentation and several hours after the evening run, the dog became lethargic, refused to eat dog food or treats, and seemed painful upon manipulation. The owner noticed that the dog's heart rate, which was normally 50 to 60 beats/min, was 120 beats/min at rest. Rectal temperature at home just prior to presentation was 104.4°F (40.2°C). Three days before the dog was evaluated, the owner had removed a non-engorged tick from the dog.

Physical Examination: Physical examination findings included a body weight of 21.3 kg, 3%-5% dehydration, pain score of 1 out of 4, rectal temperature of 103.7°F (39.8°C), HR 130 beats/min, tachypnea (42 breaths/min), and a normal CRT. The body condition score was 5/9. The dog stood in a hunched position and had a stiff gait, but localizing pain was not elicited on palpation of the spine, joints, or long bones. There was no nasal or ocular discharge, no petechiae or rash, and no obvious swelling or joint effusion. Popliteal lymph nodes were prominent, but there were no other abnormalities noted on physical examination. Systolic blood pressure was 153 mm Hg, and diastolic and mean blood pressures were 93 mm Hg and 111 mm Hg, respectively.

Laboratory Findings: The hematocrit was 42%, total plasma protein was 6.2 mg/dL, and the platelet count was 120,000/μL. A serum biochemical profile showed only hypoglobulinemia (1.7 g/dL).

Microbiologic Testing: A SNAP 4Dx (IDEXX Laboratories) in-house ELISA assay was negative. Indirect IFA assays for *Babesia canis, Bartonella henselae, Bartonella vinsonii* subsp. *berkhoffii*, and *Ehrlichia canis* were negative (no detectable antibodies at a 1:16 screening dilution). The dog was seroreactive to *Rickettsia rickettsii* antigens at a titer of 1:64. A PCR panel capable of detecting *Anaplasma* spp., *Babesia* spp., *Ehrlichia* spp., and *Rickettsia* spp. was negative on whole blood. A convalescent *R. rickettsii* antibody titer was 1:256, which supported a diagnosis of SFG rickettsiosis, most likely RMSF.

Treatment: Because of the acute onset of lethargy and fever, the history of recent tick attachment, the documentation of thrombocytopenia, and the relatively high frequency of RMSF in dogs and people in North Carolina, doxycycline (4.8 mg/kg PO q12h) was prescribed for 3 weeks before the results of microbiologic testing became available. The dog responded rapidly after doxycycline treatment, with appetite and behaviors normalizing within 24 to 48 hours after the first dose.

Comment: Although the clinical signs in this dog were relatively nonspecific, the clinical presentation was very typical of RMSF. Because *R. rickettsii* causes generalized vascular injury resulting in increased vascular permeability, fluid and protein leakage out of the intravascular space, and an acute neutrophilic inflammatory response throughout tissue sites within the body, pain that appears to shift in location (back pain, joint pain, abdominal pain, neck pain) is a typical disease manifestation. Also, the hunched appearance reported in this dog is commonly observed in dogs with RMSF. As this dog was owned by veterinarian and a tick had been removed a few days earlier, a clinical diagnosis and appropriate treatment were initiated earlier in the course of illness than is typical of most dogs with RMSF. The rapid initiation of doxycycline may have blunted the humoral antibody response and decreased the convalescent antibody titer to a level that is lower than expected in most cases of RMSF in dogs. It is important to note that PCR assay is insensitive in the early stages of RMSF, as there are often inadequate numbers of organisms in the blood to achieve successful amplification of rickettsial DNA. A very rapid response to doxycycline is expected, unless there has been a delay in diagnosis, accompanied by the onset of neurologic abnormalities. Dogs that develop neurologic complications experience a more prolonged recovery and can have residual neurologic deficits.

Rocky Mountain Spotted Fever in a Human Patient

On May 9, a 61-year-old man, who resided on a farm in Wake County, North Carolina, removed an embedded tick from the hairy portion of his right armpit. Although duration of attachment was unknown, it was likely that the tick was acquired 2 to 3 days earlier while pulling weeds from a hay field. Using a tick identification key, an experienced research technician classified the tick as a male *Amblyomma americanum* and stored the tick in a vial containing alcohol. On May 16, while working on the farm, the patient experienced mild nausea after drinking water and became transiently dizzy. The next morning chills developed, and by the mid-afternoon the patient became febrile (101.2°F [38.4°C]), developed muscle pain, a mild headache and remained in bed until the next morning. These symptoms became progressively more severe during the day and the tick attachment site had developed into an erythematous, circular lesion with induration and a necrotic center, consistent with a rickettsial eschar. Due to the history of tick attachment and fever (maximum temperature 102.9°F [39.4°C]), a spotted fever rickettsiosis, such as RMSF, or neutrophilic or monocytic ehrlichiosis, caused by *Ehrlichia ewingii* and *Ehrlichia chaffeensis*, respectively, was suspected. Neutropenia (2553 cells/μL) was accompanied by a left shift (5% band neutrophils) and thrombocytopenia (148,000/μL). Doxycycline was dispensed with instructions to take 100 mg q12h for 7 days. That evening, after sleeping for 6 hours, the patient ate a small quantity of food, after which he became severely nauseated and fainted, and impact with the floor was associated with a severe blow to the back of the head. The next day (May 19) a maculopapular rash appeared that predominantly involved the inferior portions of the arms and legs. Throughout the day the distribution of the rash spread and the severity progressed from barely visible to obvious over most of the body. At no time did the rash involve the palms or plantar surface of the feet. Fever resolved within 36 hours after the initiation of doxycycline, and the rash began to fade gradually after 48 hours of treatment. Within a week after starting doxycycline, the patient was experiencing no symptoms and had no sequelae as a result of the infection or the fall. A repeat CBC (May 25) identified a normal neutrophil count (4378 cells/μL), no band neutrophils, and a normal platelet count (320,000/μL). Acute-phase serum was collected and stored until the convalescent sample was obtained. *Rickettsia* and *Ehrlichia* spp. PCR was performed immediately. PCR amplicons, obtained from the patient's blood and from the tick, were sequenced, confirming the presence of *R. rickettsii* DNA. PCR for *Ehrlichia* spp. DNA was negative from both the tick and the patient. Subsequently, seroconversion to *R. rickettsii* antigens was identified (1:64 acute titer, convalescent titer 1:512 after 4 weeks). The patient did not seroconvert to *Ehrlichia* spp. antigens.

Comment: Historically, transmission of *R. rickettsii* in North America was attributed solely to *Dermacentor variabilis* in the eastern United States and to *Dermacentor andersoni* in the western United States. However, between 2002 and 2004, researchers at the Centers for Disease Control and Prevention documented *Rh. sanguineus* transmission of *R. rickettsii* to people residing in Arizona. Although this is most likely an infrequent occurrence, this patient was infected with *R. rickettsii* by *A. americanum*. It is important to note the similarities between the historical, physical examination and laboratory findings for the dog discussed previously and the human patient. In several published case reports, dogs develop RMSF before a family member contracts the infection from a tick. Thus, it is important for veterinarians to recognize and confirm a diagnosis of RMSF in dogs and to educate the client as to the risk of tick exposure within their local environment.

SUGGESTED READINGS

Gasser AM, Birkenheuer AJ, Breitschwerdt EB. Canine Rocky Mountain spotted fever: a retrospective study of 30 cases. J Am Anim Hosp Assoc. 2001;37(1):41-48.

Elchos BN, Goddard J. Implications of presumptive fatal Rocky Mountain spotted fever in two dogs and their owner. J Am Vet Med Assoc. 2003;223(10):1450-1452:1433.

Nicholson WL, Allen KE, McQuiston JH, et al. The increasing recognition of rickettsial pathogens in dogs and people. Trends Parasitol. 2010;26(4):205-212.

REFERENCES

1. Ricketts HE. Some aspects of Rocky Mountain spotted fever as shown by recent investigations, 1909. Rev Infect Dis. 1991;13(6): 1227-1240.
2. Bechah Y, Capo C, Mege JL, Raoult D. Rickettsial diseases: from *Rickettsia*-arthropod relationships to pathophysiology and animal models. Future Microbiol. 2008;3(2):223-236.
3. Raoult D, Fournier PE, Eremeeva M, et al. Naming of Rickettsiae and rickettsial diseases. Ann N Y Acad Sci. 2005;1063:1-12.
4. Jensenius M, Davis X, von Sonnenburg F, et al. Multicenter GeoSentinel analysis of rickettsial diseases in international travelers, 1996-2008. Emerg Infect Dis. 2009;15(11):1791-1798.
5. Fournier PE, Raoult D. Current knowledge on phylogeny and taxonomy of *Rickettsia* spp. Ann N Y Acad Sci. 2009;1166:1-11.
6. Parola P, Paddock CD, Raoult D. Tick-borne rickettsioses around the world: emerging diseases challenging old concepts. Clin Microbiol Rev. 2005;18(4):719-756.
7. Goddard J. Historical and recent evidence for close relationships among *Rickettsia parkeri, R. conorii, R. africae, and R. sibirica*: implications for rickettsial taxonomy. J Vector Ecol. 2009;34(2):238-242.
8. Garcia-Garcia JC, Portillo A, Nunez MJ, et al. A patient from Argentina infected with *Rickettsia massiliae*. Am J Trop Med Hyg. 2010;82(4):691-692.
9. Cragun WC, Bartlett BL, Ellis MW, et al. The expanding spectrum of eschar-associated rickettsioses in the United States. Arch Dermatol. 2010;146(6):641-648.
10. Nicholson WL, Paddock CD, Demma L, et al. Rocky Mountain spotted fever in Arizona: documentation of heavy environmental infestations of *Rhipicephalus sanguineus* at an endemic site. Ann N Y Acad Sci. 2006;1078:338-341.
11. Demma LJ, Eremeeva M, Nicholson WL, et al. An outbreak of Rocky Mountain spotted fever associated with a novel tick vector, *Rhipicephalus sanguineus*, in Arizona, 2004: preliminary report. Ann N Y Acad Sci. 2006;1078:342-343.
12. Parola P, Socolovschi C, Jeanjean L, et al. Warmer weather linked to tick attack and emergence of severe rickettsioses. PLoS Negl Trop Dis. 2008;2(11):e338.
13. Parola P, Labruna MB, Raoult D. Tick-borne rickettsioses in America: unanswered questions and emerging diseases. Curr Infect Dis Rep. 2009;11(1):40-50.
14. Solano-Gallego L, Kidd L, Trotta M, et al. Febrile illness associated with *Rickettsia conorii* infection in dogs from Sicily. Emerg Infect Dis. 2006;12(12):1985-1988.
15. Keenan KP, Buhles Jr WC, Huxsoll DL, et al. Studies on the pathogenesis of *Rickettsia rickettsii* in the dog: clinical and clinicopathologic changes of experimental infection. Am J Vet Res. 1977;38(6):851-856.
16. Keenan KP, Buhles Jr WC, Huxsoll DL, et al. Pathogenesis of infection with *Rickettsia rickettsii* in the dog: a disease model for Rocky Mountain spotted fever. J Infect Dis. 1977;135(6):911-917.
17. Gasser AM, Birkenheuer AJ, Breitschwerdt EB. Canine Rocky Mountain spotted fever: a retrospective study of 30 cases. J Am Anim Hosp Assoc. 2001;37(1):41-48.
18. Greene CE, Burgdorfer W, Cavagnolo R, et al. Rocky Mountain spotted fever in dogs and its differentiation from canine ehrlichiosis. J Am Vet Med Assoc. 1985;186(5):465-472.
19. Breitschwerdt EB, Walker DH, Levy MG, et al. Clinical, hematologic, and humoral immune response in female dogs inoculated with *Rickettsia rickettsii* and *Rickettsia montana*. Am J Vet Res. 1988;49(1):70-76.
20. Breitschwerdt EB, Meuten DJ, Walker DH, et al. Canine Rocky Mountain spotted fever: a kennel epizootic. Am J Vet Res. 1985;46(10):2124-2128.
21. Elchos BN, Goddard J. Implications of presumptive fatal Rocky Mountain spotted fever in two dogs and their owner. J Am Vet Med Assoc. 2003;223(10):1450-1452:1433.
22. Paddock CD, Brenner O, Vaid C, et al. Short report: concurrent Rocky Mountain spotted fever in a dog and its owner. Am J Trop Med Hyg. 2002;66(2):197-199.
23. Demma LJ, Traeger M, Blau D, et al. Serologic evidence for exposure to *Rickettsia rickettsii* in eastern Arizona and recent emergence of Rocky Mountain spotted fever in this region. Vector Borne Zoonotic Dis. 2006;6(4):423-429.
24. Nicholson WL, Gordon R, Demma LJ. Spotted fever group rickettsial infection in dogs from eastern Arizona: how long has it been there? Ann N Y Acad Sci. 2006;1078:519-522.
25. Raoult D, Toga B, Dunan S, et al. Mediterranean spotted fever in the South of France; serosurvey of dogs. Trop Geogr Med. 1985;37(3):258-260.
26. Mannelli A, Mandola ML, Pedri P, et al. Associations between dogs that were serologically positive for *Rickettsia conorii* relative to the residences of two human cases of Mediterranean spotted fever in Piemonte (Italy). Prev Vet Med. Jul 30 2003;60(1):13-26.
27. Segura-Porta F, Diestre-Ortin G, Ortuno-Romero A, et al. Prevalence of antibodies to spotted fever group rickettsiae in human beings and dogs from an endemic area of Mediterranean spotted fever in Catalonia, Spain. Eur J Epidemiol. 1998;14(4):395-398.
28. Beeler E, Abramowicz KF, Zambrano ML, et al. A focus of dogs and *Rickettsia massiliae*–infected *Rhipicephalus sanguineus* in California. Am J Trop Med Hyg. 2011;84(2):244-249.
29. Sexton DJ, Banks J, Graves S, et al. Prevalence of antibodies to spotted fever group rickettsiae in dogs from southeastern Australia. Am J Trop Med Hyg. 1991;45(2):243-248.
30. Satoh H, Tsuneki A, Inokuma H, et al. Seroprevalence of antibodies against spotted fever group *Rickettsia* among dogs and humans in Okinawa, Japan. Microbiol Immunol. 2001;45(1):85-87.
31. Inokuma H, Matsuda H, Sakamoto L, et al. Evaluation of *Rickettsia japonica* pathogenesis and reservoir potential in dogs by experimental inoculation and epidemiologic survey. Clin Vaccine Immunol. 2011;18(1):161-166.
32. Greene CE, Breitschwerdt EB. Rocky Mountain spotted fever, murine typhus-like disease, rickettsialpox, typhus, and Q fever. In: Greene CE, ed. Infectious Diseases of the Dog and Cat. 6th ed. Philadelphia, PA: Saunders Elsevier; 2006:232-241.
33. Bayliss DB, Morris AK, Horta MC, et al. Prevalence of *Rickettsia* species antibodies and *Rickettsia* species DNA in the blood of cats with and without fever. J Feline Med Surg. 2009;11(4):266-270.
34. Warner RD, Marsh WW. Rocky Mountain spotted fever. J Am Vet Med Assoc. 2002;221(10):1413-1417.
35. Guedes E, Leite RC, Prata MC, et al. Detection of *Rickettsia rickettsii* in the tick *Amblyomma cajennense* in a new Brazilian spotted fever-endemic area in the state of Minas Gerais. Mem Inst Oswaldo Cruz. 2005;100(8):841-845.
36. Breitschwerdt EB, Hegarty BC, Maggi RG, Lantos PM, Aslett DM, Bradley JM. *Rickettsia rickettsii* Transmission by a Lone Star Tick, North Carolina. Emerg Infect Dis. 2011;17(5):873-875.
37. Demma LJ, Traeger MS, Nicholson WL, et al. Rocky Mountain spotted fever from an unexpected tick vector in Arizona. N Engl J Med. 2005;353(6):587-594.
38. Piranda EM, Faccini JL, Pinter A, et al. Experimental infection of *Rhipicephalus sanguineus* ticks with the bacterium *Rickettsia rickettsii*, using experimentally infected dogs. Vector Borne Zoonotic Dis. 2011;11(1):29-36.

39. Chen LF, Sexton DJ. What's new in Rocky Mountain spotted fever? Infect Dis Clin North Am. 2008;22(3):415-432:vii-viii.
40. Dantas-Torres F. Rocky Mountain spotted fever. Lancet Infect Dis. 2007;7(11):724-732.
41. Kidd LB. Transmission times and prevention of tick-borne diseases in dogs. Compend Contin Educ Pract Vet. 2003;25(10):742-751.
42. Dantas-Torres F. Biology and ecology of the brown dog tick. Rhipicephalus sanguineus. Parasit Vectors. 2010;3:26.
43. Norment BR, Burgdorfer W. Susceptibility and reservoir potential of the dog to spotted fever-group rickettsiae. Am J Vet Res. 1984;45(9):1706-1710.
44. Wikswo ME, Hu R, Metzger ME, Eremeeva ME. Detection of *Rickettsia rickettsii* and *Bartonella henselae* in *Rhipicephalus sanguineus* ticks from California. J Med Entomol. 2007;44(1):158-162.
45. Stromdahl EY, Jiang J, Vince M, Richards AL. Infrequency of *Rickettsia rickettsii* in *Dermacentor variabilis* removed from humans, with comments on the role of other human-biting ticks associated with spotted fever group Rickettsiae in the United States. Vector Borne Zoonotic Dis. 2011;11(7):969-977.
46. Chapman AS, Bakken JS, Folk SM, et al. Diagnosis and management of tickborne rickettsial diseases: Rocky Mountain spotted fever, ehrlichioses, and anaplasmosis—United States: a practical guide for physicians and other health-care and public health professionals. MMWR Recomm Rep. 2006;55(RR-4):1-27.
47. Centers for Disease Control and Prevention. Rocky Mountain Spotted Fever, Statistics and Epidemiology. http://www.cdc.gov/rmsf/stats:Last accessed May 27, 2012.
48. Moncayo AC, Cohen SB, Fritzen CM, et al. Absence of *Rickettsia rickettsii* and occurrence of other spotted fever group rickettsiae in ticks from Tennessee. Am J Trop Med Hyg. 2010;83(3):653-657.
49. Raoult D, Parola P. Rocky Mountain spotted fever in the USA: a benign disease or a common diagnostic error? Lancet Infect Dis. 2008;8(10):587-589.
50. Diniz PPVP, unpublished data. 2012.
51. Eremeeva ME, Zambrano ML, Anaya L, et al. *Rickettsia rickettsii* in *Rhipicephalus* ticks, Mexicali. Mexico. J Med Entomol. 2011;48(2):418-421.
52. Tinoco-Gracia L, Quiroz-Romero H, Quintero-Martinez MT, et al. Prevalence of *Rhipicephalus sanguineus* ticks on dogs in a region on the Mexico-USA border. Vet Rec. 2009;164(2):59-61.
53. Fritz CL, Kriner P, Garcia D, et al. Tick infestation and spotted fever group *Rickettsia* in shelter dogs, California, 2009. Zoonoses Public Health. 2012;59(1):4-7.
54. Telford SR. Status of the "East Side hypothesis" (transovarial interference) 25 years later. Ann N Y Acad Sci. 2009;1166:144-150.
55. Sahni SK, Rydkina E. Host-cell interactions with pathogenic *Rickettsia* species. Future Microbiol. 2009;4(3):323-339.
56. Walker DH, Valbuena GA, Olano JP. Pathogenic mechanisms of diseases caused by *Rickettsia.* Ann N Y Acad Sci. 2003;990:1-11.
57. Walker DH. Rickettsiae and rickettsial infections: the current state of knowledge. Clin Infect Dis. 2007;45(suppl 1):S39-S44.
58. Balraj P, Renesto P, Raoult D. Advances in rickettsia pathogenicity. Ann N Y Acad Sci. 2009;1166:94-105.
59. Eremeeva ME, Liang Z, Paddock C, et al. *Rickettsia rickettsii* infection in the pine vole, *Microtus pinetorum*: kinetics of infection and quantitation of antioxidant enzyme gene expression by RT-PCR. Ann N Y Acad Sci. 2003;990:468-473.
60. Cummiskey JM, Simon LM, Theodore J, Ryan US, Robin ED. Bioenergetic alterations in cultivated pulmonary artery and aortic endothelial cells exposed to normoxia and hypoxia. Exp Lung Res. 1981;2(3):155-163.
61. Asahina T, Kashiwagi A, Nishio Y, et al. Impaired activation of glucose oxidation and NADPH supply in human endothelial cells exposed to H_2O_2 in high-glucose medium. Diabetes. 1995;44(5):520-526.
62. Breitschwerdt EB, Papich MG, Hegarty BC, et al. Efficacy of doxycycline, azithromycin, or trovafloxacin for treatment of experimental Rocky Mountain spotted fever in dogs. Antimicrob Agents Chemother. 1999;43(4):813-821.
63. Piranda EM, Faccini JL, Pinter A, et al. Experimental infection of dogs with a Brazilian strain of *Rickettsia rickettsii*: clinical and laboratory findings. Mem Inst Oswaldo Cruz. 2008;103(7):696-701.
64. Kordick SK, Breitschwerdt EB, Hegarty BC, et al. Coinfection with multiple tick-borne pathogens in a Walker Hound kennel in North Carolina. J Clin Microbiol. 1999;37(8):2631-2638.
65. Greene CE. Infectious Diseases of the Dog and Cat. 3rd ed. St. Louis, MO: Saunders Elsevier; 2006.
66. Ober CP, Spaulding K, Breitschwerdt EB, et al. Orchitis in two dogs with Rocky Mountain spotted fever. Vet Radiol Ultrasound. 2004;45(5):458-465.
67. Grindem CB, Breitschwerdt EB, Perkins PC, et al. Platelet-associated immunoglobulin (antiplatelet antibody) in canine Rocky Mountain spotted fever and ehrlichiosis. J Am Anim Hosp Assoc. 1999;35(1):56-61.
68. Mikszewski JS, Vite CH. Central nervous system dysfunction associated with Rocky Mountain spotted fever infection in five dogs. J Am Anim Hosp Assoc. 2005;41(4):259-266.
69. Drost WT, Berry CR, Breitschwerdt EB, Davidson MG. Thoracic radiographic findings in dogs infected with *Rickettsia rickettsii.* Vet Radiol Ultrasound. 1997;38(4):260-266.
70. Breitschwerdt EB, Levy MG, Davidson MG, et al. Kinetics of IgM and IgG responses to experimental and naturally acquired *Rickettsia rickettsii* infection in dogs. Am J Vet Res. 1990;51(8):1312-1316.
71. Nicholson WL, Allen KE, McQuiston JH, et al. The increasing recognition of rickettsial pathogens in dogs and people. Trends Parasitol. 2010;26(4):205-212.
72. Breitschwerdt EB, Moncol DJ, Corbett WT, et al. Antibodies to spotted fever-group rickettsiae in dogs in North Carolina. Am J Vet Res. 1987;48(10):1436-1440.
73. Solano-Gallego L, Bradley J, Hegarty B, et al. *Bartonella henselae* IgG antibodies are prevalent in dogs from southeastern USA. Vet Res. 2004;35(5):585-595.
74. Kidd L, Maggi R, Diniz PP, et al. Evaluation of conventional and real-time PCR assays for detection and differentiation of spotted fever group *Rickettsia* in dog blood. Vet Microbiol. 2008;129(3-4):294-303.
75. Davidson MG, Breitschwerdt EB, Walker DH, et al. Identification of rickettsiae in cutaneous biopsy specimens from dogs with experimental Rocky Mountain spotted fever. J Vet Intern Med. 1989;3(1):8-11.
76. Breitschwerdt EB, Davidson MG, Aucoin DP, et al. Efficacy of chloramphenicol, enrofloxacin, and tetracycline for treatment of experimental Rocky Mountain spotted fever in dogs. Antimicrob Agents Chemother. 1991;35(11):2375-2381.
77. Neer TM, Eddlestone SM, Gaunt SD, Corstvet RE. Efficacy of enrofloxacin for the treatment of experimentally induced *Ehrlichia canis* infection. J Vet Intern Med. 1999;13(5):501-504.
78. Breitschwerdt EB, Davidson MG, Hegarty BC, et al. Prednisolone at anti-inflammatory or immunosuppressive dosages in conjunction with doxycycline does not potentiate the severity of *Rickettsia rickettsii* infection in dogs. Antimicrob Agents Chemother. 1997;41(1):141-147.
79. Low RM, Holm JL. Canine Rocky Mountain spotted fever. Compend Contin Educ Pract Vet. 2005;27(7):530-538.
80. Walker DH. The realities of biodefense vaccines against *Rickettsia.* Vaccine. 2009;27(suppl 4):D52-D55.
81. Bonilla D. Tick borne disease surveillance: spotted fever group *Rickettsia.* Calif Dept Public Health Vector Borne Dis Bull. 2009;3(2):4.

CHAPTER 31

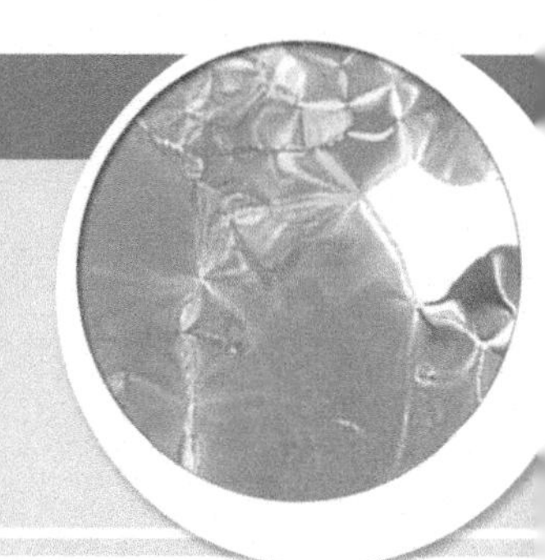

Salmon Poisoning Disease

Jane E. Sykes

Overview of Salmon Poisoning Disease

First Described: Northwestern Oregon, United States, 1814 (Astoria)[1]

Cause: *Neorickettsia helminthoeca,* a gram-negative, obligately intracellular bacteria that belongs to the family Anaplasmataceae

Affected Hosts: Dogs, foxes, coyotes, raccoons, captive bears

Intermediate Hosts: Aquatic snails, fish (especially salmonids)

Geographic Distribution: Coastal areas of Washington, Oregon, northern California, British Columbia, Brazil (2004)

Route of Transmission: Ingestion of the infected trematode vector *Nanophyetus salmincola*, most often in salmonid fish

Major Clinical Signs: Fever, lethargy, anorexia, vomiting, diarrhea, lymphadenomegaly

Differential Diagnoses: Lymphoma, canine parvovirus infection, canine distemper virus infection, granulocytic anaplasmosis, ehrlichiosis, leptospirosis, septic shock, disseminated fungal disease (especially cryptococcosis), hemorrhagic gastroenteritis, dietary indiscretion, gastrointestinal foreign body, pancreatitis, hypoadrenocorticism, inflammatory bowel disease. Appropriate antimicrobial treatment with doxycycline must begin before the diagnosis is confirmed by laboratory testing. Misdiagnosis and delayed or inappropriate antimicrobial drug therapy increase morbidity and mortality.

Human Health Significance: *Nanophyetus salmincola* can cause gastrointestinal disturbances and eosinophilia in humans, but *N. helminthoeca* does not cause human disease.

Etiologic Agent and Epidemiology

Salmon poisoning disease (SPD) is caused by the rickettsial pathogen *Neorickettsia helminthoeca,* which, like other *Neorickettsia* spp., resides within a trematode (fluke) vector for the course of the trematode's life cycle. The trematode vector of *N. helminthoeca* is *Nanophyetus salmincola,* thought to be the most common trematode species endemic to the United States.[2] The disease occurs in dogs, foxes, and coyotes and has also been reported in captive bears, but does not occur in domestic cats.[3-5] SPD is geographically restricted to coastal regions of northern California, Oregon, and Washington in the United States, and southern British Columbia in Canada (Figure 31-1). This reflects the distribution of an aquatic snail, *Oxytrema silicula* (also known as *Juga silicula*), which is an intermediate host of the trematode (Figure 31-1). The snail is prevalent in coastal streams. A similar disease has been described in dogs from Brazil.[6,7] Two related yet antigenically distinct organisms have been isolated from dogs with SPD, *N. helminthoeca* and the Elokomin fluke fever (EFF) agent.[8-12] The EFF agent may be a less pathogenic strain of *N. helminthoeca*.

Dogs usually become infected with *N. helminthoeca* when they ingest encysted trematode metacercariae within uncooked or undercooked freshwater fish, most commonly salmonid fish. The Pacific giant salamander is also a competent second intermediate host. Ingestion of encysted metacercariae is followed by maturation of the trematode, which feeds on the intestinal mucosa and inoculates the rickettsia into the host. The fluke has an oral sucker and a ventral sucker, which are used to grasp host intestinal tissue, although the fluke itself does not cause extensive damage to the intestinal wall.[13] Infected trematode ova are shed in the stool for 60 to 250 days.[14] After several months, miracidia develop within the eggs, hatch, swim away, and penetrate the snail. They then develop into rediae, each of which give rise to many free-swimming cercariae. Thousands of cercariae are released intermittently from the snail. These rapidly penetrate the skin of a fish (or are ingested by the fish), and encyst throughout the fish as metacercariae

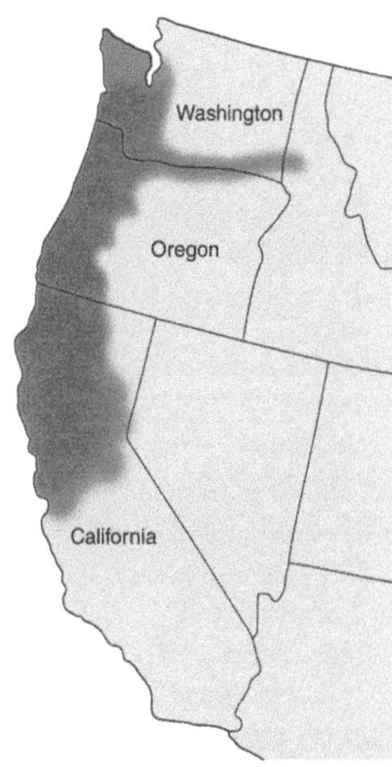

FIGURE 31-1 Geographic distribution of salmon poisoning disease in dogs from the United States. The distribution also extends into the southern portion of British Columbia.

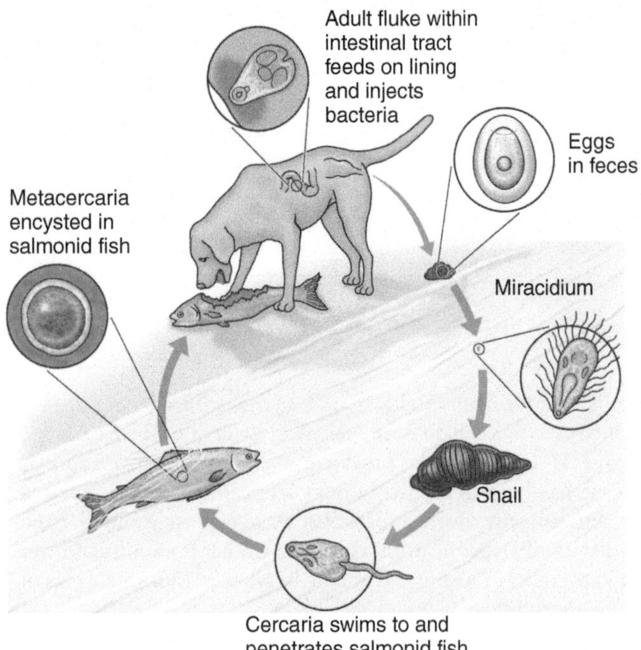

FIGURE 31-2 Life cycle of *Nanophyetus salmincola*, the trematode vector of salmon poisoning disease. The fluke harbors the rickettsial organism throughout its lifecycle.

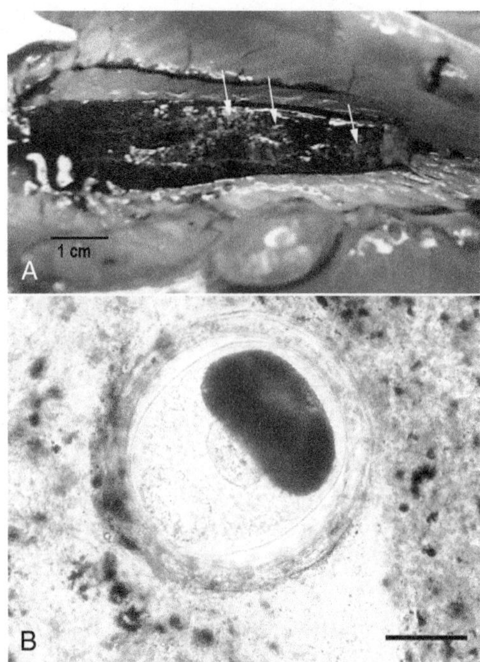

FIGURE 31-3 **A,** "Salt grain" appearance of metacercariae of *Nanophyetus salmincola* *(arrows)* in the kidneys of a Chinook salmon. (Courtesy Craig Banner, Oregon Department of Fish and Wildlife.) **B,** Wet mount squash of fresh kidney material from a Chinook salmon showing a metacercaria of *N. salmincola*. Bar = 100 μm. (Courtesy Dr. Ronald Hedrick, University of California, Davis.)

(Figures 31-2 and 31-3). Infected fish may contain more than 1000 metacercariae. Infected fish may have visible damage to their skin, and the infection may also interfere with their swimming activity.[15] Dog-to-dog transmission of *N. helminthoeca* has been demonstrated experimentally by mechanical aerosolization or rectal administration of lymph node suspensions or homogenates of rectal mucosa.[16]

Intact male dogs and Labrador retrievers appear to be overrepresented among dogs with SPD,[17] possibly because they are popular with individuals engaged in fishing activities, although dogs of any sex and breed can be affected. Dogs of any age are affected; the median age in one study was 3 years.[17] Dogs develop SPD at any time of year. Occasionally dogs from areas not endemic for SPD develop disease after they ingest fish that is imported from endemic areas.[18]

Most but not all infected dogs have a history of access to or consumption of raw or improperly cooked fish.[17,19] Consumption of any part of the fish, including the entrails and skin, may result in SPD. Supermarket-bought salmon may also be infected.[17] Infection has also been reported after swimming activity, without apparent exposure to fish.[17]

Clinical Features

Signs and Their Pathogenesis

N. helminthoeca replicates within macrophages. This results in a granulomatous inflammatory response within the stomach, intestines, lymph nodes, and spleen. Granulomatous meningitis has also been detected in dogs with SPD.[20,21] The incubation period ranges from 2 to 14 days (median, 7 days), but may be as long as 33 days.[22] The severity of illness varies considerably (Box 31-1). Dogs with peracute infection may be found dead.[17] A marked febrile response is commonly detected (>70% of cases) (Box 31-2) and may reach 107.6°F (42°C).[17] A median rectal temperature of 105°F (40.6°C) was reported in one series of naturally infected dogs.[17] Terminally ill dogs may be hypothermic. Virtually all dogs develop inappetence or anorexia, and lethargy is also common. Vomiting occurs in more than 80% of dogs, and rarely, hematemesis is present.[17] Diarrhea is also common (>70% of dogs) and may be semiformed to liquid in consistency, sometimes containing frank blood, melena, and, less commonly, mucus.[17] Occasionally, a history of diarrhea and vomiting is absent. Other signs include weight loss and increased thirst and urination. Neurologic signs that include mental obtundation, myoclonic twitching, seizures, and apparent neck pain have been reported in fewer than 20% of affected dogs, a primary differential diagnosis being canine distemper virus infection.[17]

BOX 31-1

Signs in the Clinical History of 29 Dogs with Salmon Poisoning Disease

Inappetence or anorexia: 100%
Lethargy: 86%
Vomiting: 86%
Diarrhea: 72%
Hematochezia: 38%
Weight loss: 28%
Melena: 21%
Polyuria and polydipsia: 3%

Physical Examination Findings

Dehydration is frequently noted on physical examination and may be severe. More than 70% of dogs have peripheral lymphadenomegaly, which may be generalized or involve only some peripheral lymph nodes (see Box 31-2). Lymph nodes may be up to 4 cm in diameter and firm on palpation. Lymphadenomegaly may be absent occasionally, sometimes as a result of lymph node necrosis. Abdominal palpation may reveal pain, and splenomegaly may also be detected. Other abnormalities include tachypnea or labored respirations, tachycardia, scleral or conjunctival injection, and edema that involves the limbs, face, or cervical region.[17] Mucosal pallor, tachycardia, and weak pulses may be present in dogs with hypovolemic shock. Cardiac arrhythmias such as ventricular premature contractions have also been noted, and there may be signs of hemorrhage such as epistaxis and hyphema. Rectal examination may indicate the presence of liquid stool, sometimes accompanied by fresh blood or melena.

Diagnosis

Laboratory Abnormalities

Complete Blood Count

Thrombocytopenia is present in 90% of affected dogs. Anemia is present in up to 40% of dogs with SPD and generally occurs as a result of gastrointestinal hemorrhage. More commonly, the CBC shows evidence of lymphopenia, thrombocytopenia, or neutrophilia, frequently with bandemia (Table 31-1). Uncommonly, neutropenia occurs.[17] Toxic changes may be present within neutrophils, and immature monocytes may occasionally be found in the peripheral blood. Despite the association with helminthiasis, eosinophilia has not been documented.

BOX 31-2

Physical Examination Findings in 29 Dogs with Salmon Poisoning Disease

Peripheral lymphadenomegaly: 74%
Fever: 73%
Dehydration: 65%
Abdominal pain: 28%
Tachypnea or labored respirations: 24%
Tachycardia: 24%
Neurologic signs: 17%
Weak pulses: 17%
Splenomegaly: 14%
Scleral injection: 14%
Mucosal pallor: 10%
Hypothermia: 5%

Serum Chemistry Profile

Hyponatremia and hypokalemia are the most common electrolyte abnormalities in dogs with SPD and result from gastrointestinal losses that occur with vomiting and diarrhea (Table 31-2). Low ionized calcium concentrations may be detected in some dogs, possibly as a result of decreased intestinal absorption. Hypoalbuminemia is present in most (>80%) dogs. Hypoglobulinemia and hypocholesterolemia occur in fewer than 25% of dogs with SPD, but may become profound. Abnormal liver enzyme activities may be present, the most common of which is increased ALP activity,[17,20] but increases in the activity of ALT and AST may also occur. Hyperbilirubinemia is present in fewer than 20% of dogs. Azotemia can be evident in dogs with severe dehydration.

Urinalysis

Bilirubinuria and proteinuria are frequently detected on urinalysis in dogs with SPD.[17] Uncommonly, cylindruria and glucosuria are present, perhaps as a result of renal injury secondary to impaired renal perfusion. Microscopic hematuria occurs in some dogs, possibly reflecting underlying coagulopathies that can occur in dogs with SPD.

Clotting Function

Evaluation of clotting function in some dogs with SPD shows evidence of disseminated intravascular coagulation. Abnormalities include increased PT or APTT, increased fibrin degradation products, and decreased antithrombin activity.[17]

Diagnostic Imaging

Plain Radiography

Abdominal radiographs may be unremarkable or reveal fluid-filled small intestines; decreased serosal detail; and less frequently, hepatomegaly or splenomegaly. Thoracic radiographs

TABLE 31-1

Hematologic Findings in 29 Dogs with Salmon Poisoning Disease

Test	Reference Range	Percent below the Reference Range	Percent within the Reference Range	Percent above the Reference Range	Range for Dogs with Salmon Poisoning Disease	Number of Dogs Tested
Hematocrit (%)	40-55	39	61	0	22-53	23
Neutrophils (cells/μL)	3000-10,500	4	53	43	728-26,224	23
Band neutrophils (cells/μL)	Rare	0	40	60	0-6825	20
Monocytes (cells/μL)	150-1200	9	61	30	42-3290	23
Lymphocytes (cells/μL)	1000-4000	78	22	0	0-2070	23
Eosinophils (cells/μL)	0-1500	0	100	0	0-690	21
Platelets (cells/μL)	150,000-400,000	90	0	10	10,000-446,000	20

TABLE 31-2

Findings on Serum Biochemistry Analysis in 29 Dogs with Salmon Poisoning Disease

Test	Reference Range	Percent below the Reference Range	Percent within the Reference Range	Percent above the Reference Range	Range for Dogs with Salmon Poisoning Disease	Number of Dogs Tested
Sodium (mmol/L)	145-154	59	36	5	133-161	22
Potassium (mmol/L)	4.1-5.3	41	59	0	3.7-5.0	22
Chloride (mmol/L)	105-116	9	77	14	98-118	22
Bicarbonate (mmol/L)	16-26	20	15	65	11-28	20
Calcium (mg/dL)	9.9-11.4	83	17	0	7.2-10.9	23
Phosphorus (mg/dL)	3.0-6.2	9	74	17	2.7-13.0	23
Creatinine (mg/dL)	0.5-1.6	4	4	13	0.4-3.3	23
BUN (mg/dL)	8-31	0	83	17	8-110	23
Albumin (g/dL)	2.9-4.2	83	17	0	0.9-3.8	23
Globulin (g/dL)	2.3-4.4	26	70	4	1.6-4.7	23
Cholesterol (mg/dL)	135-345	22	69	9	79-408	23
Total bilirubin (mg/dL)	0-0.4	0	83	17	0-3.1	23
ALT (U/L)	19-70	4	74	22	17-1,443	23
ALP (U/L)	15-127	0	39	61	29-985	23

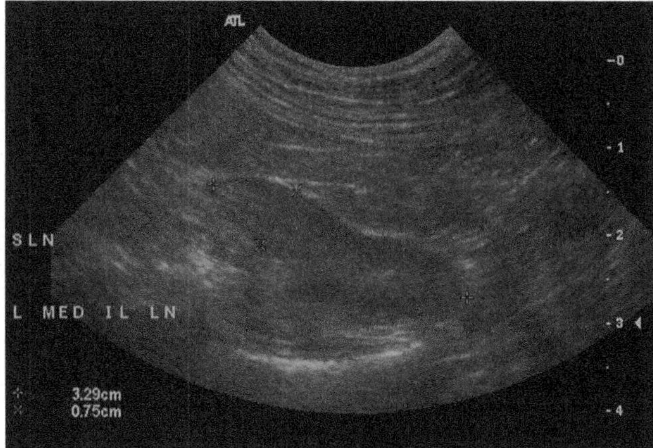

FIGURE 31-4 Enlarged and hypoechoic abdominal (medial iliac) lymph nodes as detected using abdominal sonographic examination in a 9-year-old male German shepherd dog with salmon poisoning disease.

are typically unremarkable or show reduction in size of the intrathoracic vasculature, consistent with hypovolemia.

Sonographic Findings

Abdominal ultrasound examination of dogs with SPD often shows mild or moderate generalized abdominal or mesenteric lymphadenomegaly, as well as splenomegaly with a mottled splenic echotexture. Some dogs that lack peripheral lymphadenomegaly have abdominal lymphadenomegaly on ultrasound examination,[17] and ultrasound-guided aspiration of enlarged abdominal lymph nodes can be helpful for diagnosis in dogs that lack peripheral lymphadenomegaly. Lymph nodes develop a rounded appearance with a hypoechoic or hypoechoic mottled echogenicity (Figure 31-4). Fluid-distended intestinal loops, sometimes with wall thickening, corrugation, hypermotility, or hypomotility, may be documented. Uncommonly, hepatomegaly or a small amount of free peritoneal fluid is identified.

Microbiologic Tests

Diagnostic assays for SPD are summarized in Table 31-3.

Diagnosis Using Fecal Examination

SPD can be diagnosed when operculated trematode eggs are found in fecal specimens of dogs with consistent clinical signs, which appear within 5 to 8 days after the ingestion of infected fish. Although the sensitivity of centrifugal zinc sulfate fecal flotation for detection of *N. salmincola* ova in dogs with SPD is similar to that of fecal sedimentation, some dogs that test negative by one method test positive using the other, so the sensitivity of fecal examination for diagnosis is maximized by performing both centrifugal zinc sulfate fecal flotations and fecal sedimentation together. In one study, 93% of dogs with SPD tested positive for *N. salmincola* ova using a combination of fecal flotation and fecal sedimentation.[17] False negatives may occur when the duration of illness is shorter than the prepatent period of *N. salmincola* or when light fluke burdens are present. The finding of fluke ova on fecal examination may not be diagnostic of SPD, because dogs may be infected with trematodes that do not harbor the rickettsia, and ova may be shed for months after recovery. Nevertheless, *N. salmincola* ova were detected in only 0.2% of more than 1800 fecal flotations in dogs seen at a teaching hospital in an endemic area, and all positive test results were in dogs suspected to have SPD. Thus, the specificity of fecal examination for a diagnosis of SPD appears to be extremely high.[17]

Centrifugal zinc sulfate fecal flotation may reveal co-infections with other gastrointestinal parasites, which can complicate the clinical picture. Co-infections with *Dipylidium caninum* and *Trichuris vulpis* have been reported in dogs with SPD.[17]

Cytologic Diagnosis

In addition to fecal examination for trematode ova, SPD can be diagnosed following cytologic examination of peripheral lymph node aspirates, or ultrasound-guided aspirates of abdominal lymph nodes or the spleen. Cytologic findings consist of histiocytic hyperplasia and lymphoid reactivity. Rickettsial organisms are 0.3–µm cocci or coccobacilli and may be seen in large numbers within the cytoplasm of macrophages. They resemble granular to amorphous material of a uniform blue color using Wright's stain, occasionally forming loose clusters of organisms (morulae) (Figure 31-5).[17,22,23] In as many as one quarter to one third of dogs, rickettsial organisms are not identified. The presence of histiocytic hyperplasia should alert the clinician to the possibility of SPD. Organisms may also be absent in dogs with a recent history of antimicrobial therapy.

Serologic Diagnosis

Serologic tests for *N. helminthoeca* antibodies or antigen are not available on a commercial basis for veterinary practitioners. Antibodies to *N. helminthoeca* can cross-react serologically with those of *Ehrlichia* spp., so it is possible that dogs with SPD might test positive using serologic tests for *Ehrlichia* spp. (provided enough time had elapsed for antibody formation to occur).[24] In one study, most dogs with SPD that were tested for antibodies against other rickettsial pathogens did not seroreact to *Ehrlichia canis* or *Anaplasma phagocytophilum*.[17]

Molecular Diagnosis Using the Polymerase Chain Reaction

Specific PCR assays have been used to detect the DNA of *Neorickettsia helminthoeca* in clinical specimens from affected dogs.[17] Real-time PCR assays for *N. helminthoeca* are available from some veterinary molecular diagnostic laboratories and can be performed on blood, lymph-node, or splenic aspirates and possibly fecal specimens from dogs with SPD in order to confirm the diagnosis. More research is required to understand the sensitivity and specificity of PCR assays for diagnosing SPD in dogs, including the optimum specimen type for testing.

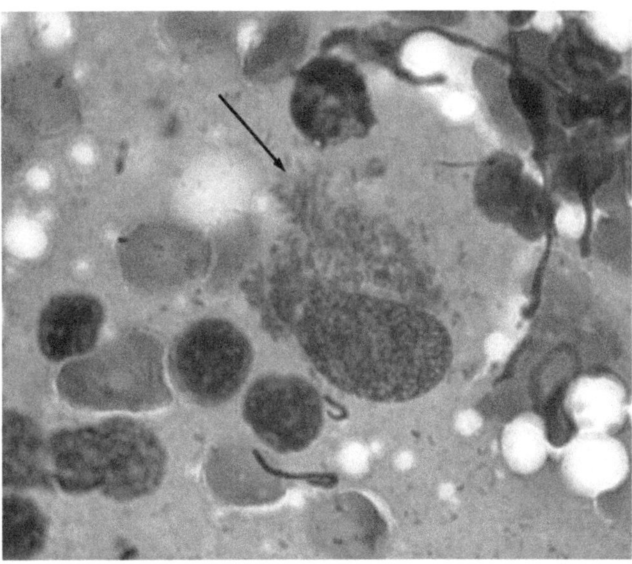

FIGURE 31-5 Lymph node aspirate from a dog with salmon poisoning disease. Note the large histiocyte that contains granular coccoid organisms consistent with *Neorickettsia helminthoeca*.

TABLE 31-3

Diagnostic Assays Available for Salmon Poisoning Disease in Dogs

Assay	Specimen Type	Target	Performance
Fecal sedimentation combined with zinc sulfate centrifugal fecal flotation	Feces	*Nanophyetus salmincola* ova	Specificity nears 100% when performed by a parasitologist. Sensitivity probably >90%. Eggs are light brown, ovoid, operculate at one end and measure 0.087 to 0.097 mm × 0.038 to 0.055 mm.
Cytology	Lymph-node or splenic aspirates	Detection of *Neorickettsia helminthoeca* within macrophages	Sensitivity >70% when performed by a veterinary clinical pathologist. Sensitivity may be improved by examination of aspirates from multiple lymph node. Organisms within macrophages may be confused with debris or hemosiderin. Other changes include lymphocytic reactivity and histiocytic hyperplasia.
Histopathology	Biopsy or necropsy specimens, especially lymph nodes, spleen, gastrointestinal tissues	*N. helminthoeca* within macrophages	Organisms may be stained with Giemsa. Antimicrobial therapy can lead to false-negative results.
PCR	Blood, lymph-node or splenic aspirates, tissue specimens, feces	*N. helminthoeca* DNA	Well validated assays that are specific for *N. helminthoeca* are not available commercially. Optimum specimen type unknown. Antimicrobial therapy may lead to negative PCR results.

Pathologic Findings

Gross Pathologic Findings

Gross necropsy findings in dogs with SPD consist of enlargement of lymphoid tissues, including the tonsils, thymus, lymph nodes, and spleen. Lymph nodes may be yellowish and edematous and may contain white foci that represent foci of granulomatous inflammation. Petechial hemorrhages may be noted on the lymph nodes, the gastrointestinal tract, pancreas, gallbladder, and urinary bladder. The gastrointestinal tract may be thickened and contain white foci. The lumen of the intestinal tract may contain free blood (Figure 31-6, *A*). Flukes are only 0.8 to 1.1 mm long and 0.3 to 0.5 mm wide[25] and may not always be visible grossly.

Histopathologic Findings

Lymphoid tissues show marked depletion of lymphoid follicles, and subcapsular and medullary sinuses are filled with histiocytes, the cytoplasm of which can contain numerous rickettsial organisms, which occasionally form clusters within vacuoles. Organisms are readily appreciated using Giemsa stain (see Figure 31-6, *C*). Lymph node and splenic necrosis may also be present.[17,22] Inflammatory nodules that contain lymphocytes, plasma cells, and infected histiocytes expand the lamina propria of the gastrointestinal tract and extend into the submucosa. Parasites consistent with *N. salmincola* may be found embedded in the mucosa, primarily within the duodenum (see Figure 31-6, *B*).[16,21] Nevertheless, flukes are not always found using histopathology in dogs that die from SPD, even in the absence of anthelmintic therapy.

One dog that died of SPD had widespread and multiple thromboses involving numerous organs with associated tissue infarction. Granulomatous meningitis has been described at necropsy in dogs that were experimentally infected with *N. helminthoeca*.[20]

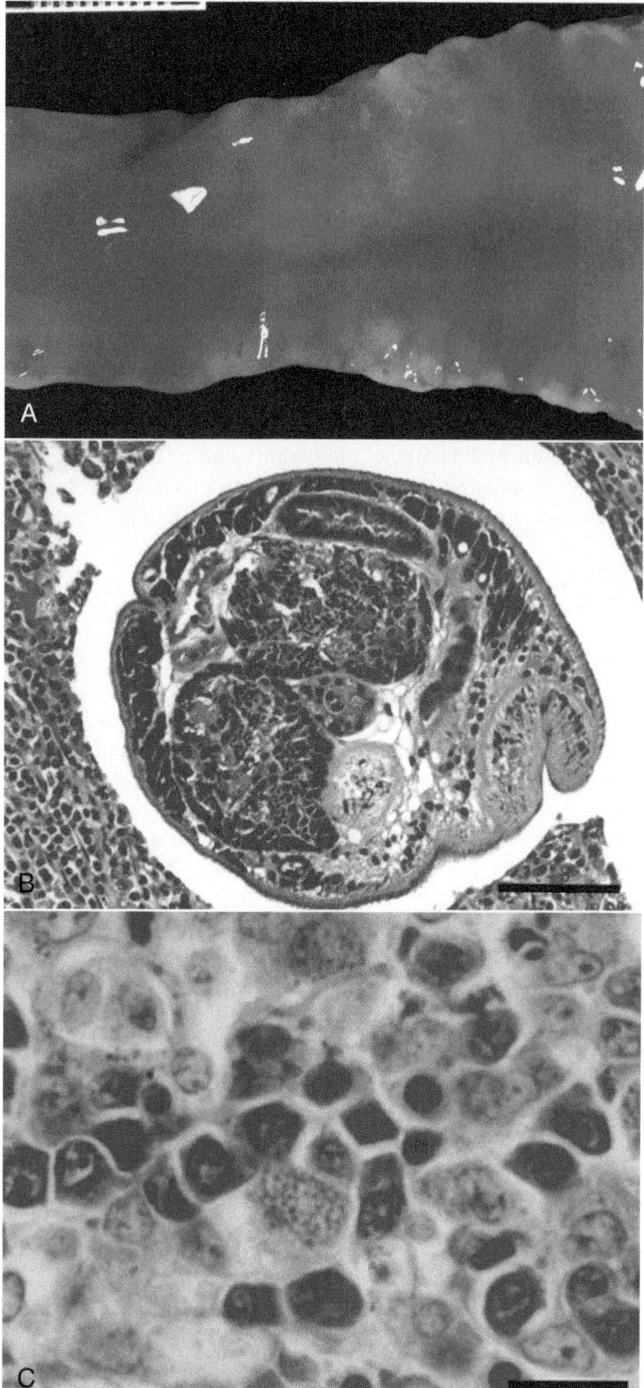

FIGURE 31-6 **A,** Intestinal mucosa of an 8-month-old female spayed Maltese mix dog that died of salmon poisoning disease. The intestinal wall was thickened and the contents were dark red and mucoid. (Courtesy University of California, Davis Veterinary Anatomic Pathology Service.) **B,** Duodenum. A transverse section of an adult *Nanophyetus* fluke is embedded within the intestinal villi. H&E stain. Bar = 200 μm. **C,** Lymph node, medullary sinus from a dog with salmon poisoning disease. Many histiocytes have intracytoplasmic clusters of coccobacilli less than 1 μm in diameter. Giemsa. Bar = 5 μm. (B and C from Sykes JE, Marks SL, Mapes S, et al. Salmon poisoning disease in dogs: 29 cases. *J Vet Intern Med* 2010;24[3]:504-513, 2010.)

Treatment and Prognosis

The treatment of choice for SPD is doxycycline, tetracycline, or oxytetracycline, which should be given for a minimum of 7 days. Administration of tetracyclines is generally associated with clinical improvement within 24 hours, and signs resolve within 1 to 4 days.[17] Dogs that are vomiting may require treatment with parenteral tetracyclines. Clinical improvement has also been reported following treatment with enrofloxacin and parenteral trimethoprim-sulfamethoxazole. Antimicrobials that do not appear to be effective include first-generation cephalosporins, penicillins, aminoglycosides, chloramphenicol, and metronidazole.[17] Although complete clinical recovery may occur without anthelmintic treatment, the fluke infection should be treated with praziquantel after initial recovery from SPD (Table 31-4).

Dogs with mild signs or infrequent vomiting may respond well to treatment with oral tetracyclines alone, whereas those with more severe disease often require hospitalization for IV antimicrobial and crystalloid fluid therapy (see Table 31-4). Oral antimicrobial therapy can be continued once vomiting ceases. The presence of severe hypovolemia or hypoalbuminemia may necessitate treatment with colloids such as fresh frozen plasma, dextrans, or hetastarch. Packed RBC or whole blood may be required for dogs with severe anemia. Treatment with total or partial parenteral nutrition may also be required if vomiting is persistent and does not respond to antiemetics such as metoclopramide, maropitant, or ondansetron. Close monitoring of hematocrit, albumin, electrolytes, acid-base status, renal parameters, and coagulation parameters may be required in some severely affected dogs. Blood cultures should be considered in dogs with severe hemorrhagic diarrhea and

TABLE 31-4

Antimicrobials Used to Treat Salmon Poisoning Disease in Dogs

Drug	Dose (mg/kg)	Route	Interval (hours)	Duration (days)
Doxycycline	5	PO, IV	12	7-14
Tetracycline	22*	PO	8	7
	7	IV	8	7
Oxytetracycline	7-10*	PO, IV	8	7
Praziquantel†	10-30	PO	24	1-2

*Reduce dose in renal failure; may cause teeth discoloration in young animals. Monitor for nephrotoxicity (cylindruria).
†For treatment of fluke infection.

abnormal perfusion parameters, after which treatment with broad-spectrum parenteral antimicrobial drugs should be commenced.

Prolonged hospitalization may be required for dogs that develop complications such as cardiac arrhythmias, intussusceptions, adverse reactions to tetracyclines, disseminated intravascular coagulation, or septicemia.[17,19] In a study of dogs evaluated at a tertiary referral hospital, death or euthanasia occurred in 14% of 29 dogs with SPD.[17] The mortality may be lower in dogs seen in primary care practice, providing appropriate treatment can be administered. In general, early treatment is associated with an excellent prognosis. Without treatment, death can occur within 5 to 10 days.

Immunity and Vaccination

Animals that recover from SPD are immune to reinfection with the same strain of *N. helminthoeca*,[22,26,27] but challenge with an alternate strain (then the EFF agent) results in disease, and antibodies fail to cross react with the alternate strain. This may explain why SPD has been reported to occur more than once in some dogs.[17,22] No vaccine is available.

Prevention

N. helminthoeca metacercariae are effectively destroyed by proper cooking or freezing of infected fish. Ingestion of raw fish by dogs in endemic areas should be discouraged, and dog owners in endemic areas should be educated about the disease. Dogs that have eaten raw fish from an endemic area, or those swimming in rivers or lakes in these areas, should be watched carefully for signs of lethargy, vomiting, or decreased appetite that occur within 2 weeks of exposure. If multiple dogs are simultaneously exposed to a source of *N. helminthoeca*, and one dog develops SPD, treatment of the other dogs in the group with 7 days of doxycycline should be considered. Medical equipment used in the treatment of dogs with SPD should not be reused on other patients without proper sterilization.

Public Health Aspects

Human infection with *N. helminthoeca* has not been reported. However, humans may become infected with the fluke, *N. salmincola,* after consumption of poorly cooked fish. Most humans are subclinically infected, although abdominal discomfort, diarrhea, vomiting, weight loss, nausea, and peripheral eosinophilia may occur.[28]

CASE EXAMPLE

Signalment: "Herman," 9-year-old male German shepherd dog from Sacramento, CA (Figure 31-7).

History: Herman's owner reported a 2-day history of inappetence, lethargy, and one episode of vomiting. The dog had been drinking normally. There had been no diarrhea, coughing, sneezing, or increased thirst and urination. The owner also reported that Herman ate turkey and chicken that contained bones 3 days before the onset of illness. He was normally fed a strict diet of rabbit- and potato-based prescription dog food and grilled salmon because of atopic dermatitis. Herman was sometimes fed salmon scraps from the local supermarket, which the owner grilled briefly. He had not traveled out of his local area. He was up to date on vaccinations, which included vaccines for distemper, hepatitis, parvovirus, and rabies.

Current Medications: Lincomycin 29 mg/kg PO q12h; trimeprazine tartrate 0.2 mg/kg PO q48h; prednisolone 0.1 mg/kg q48h for atopic dermatitis.

Other Medical History: Herman had been diagnosed with hip osteoarthritis using pelvic radiography 8 months earlier. Controlled weight loss was the recommended treatment. He was cryptorchid, and the abdominal testicle had been removed when he was a young dog. The descended testicle was still present.

Physical Examination:

Body Weight: 51.5 kg

General: Quiet, alert and responsive. Ambulatory on all four limbs. T = 104.3°F (40.2°C), HR = 108 beats/min, RR = 60 breaths/min, mucous membranes pink, CRT = 1 s.

Integument: A full, shiny haircoat was present and there was no evidence of ectoparasites.

Eyes, Ears, Nose, and Throat: No significant abnormalities were noted. A mild amount of brown waxy debris was present within both ear canals.

Musculoskeletal: A body condition score of 6/9 with symmetrical muscling was noted. Mild to moderate pelvic limb weakness was identified.

Cardiovascular: Strong femoral pulses were noted. No murmurs or arrhythmias were detected on thoracic auscultation.

Respiratory: An increased respiratory rate with increased abdominal effort was present.

Gastrointestinal and Genitourinary: Abdominal palpation revealed a tense abdomen, with abdominal splinting, and splenomegaly. There was one descended testicle, which was smooth with no masses. No abnormalities were detected on

Continued

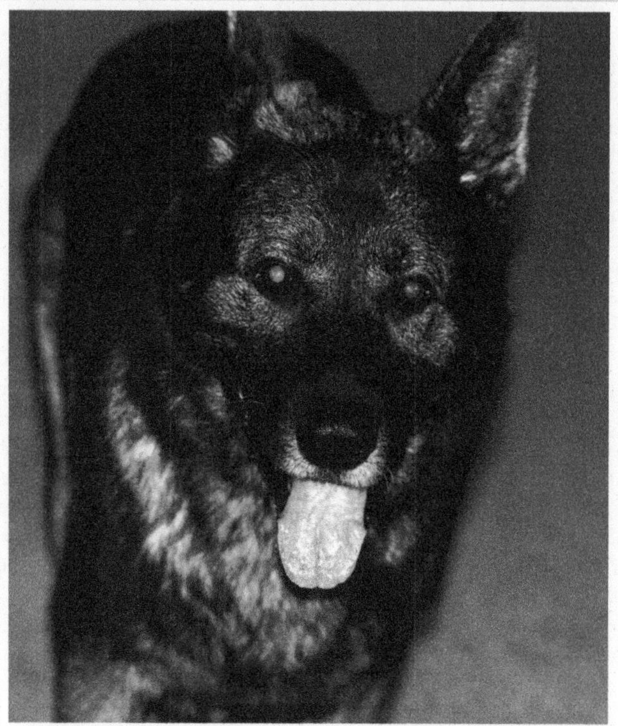
FIGURE 31-7 "Herman," a 9-year-old male German shepherd dog with salmon poisoning disease.

rectal examination. Soft feces were present in the rectum, and the prostate was palpable and symmetrical.

Lymph Nodes: Marked peripheral lymphadenopathy was present. Mandibular, superficial cervical, and popliteal lymph nodes were all 3-4 cm in diameter and firm.

Laboratory Findings:

CBC:

HCT 40.4% (40-55%)
MCV 65 fL (65-75 fL)
MCHC 36.6 g/dL (33-36 g/dL)
WBC 4240 cells/μL (6000-13,000 cells/μL)
Neutrophils 3689 cells/μL (3000-10,500 cells/μL)
Lymphocytes 466 cells/μL (1000-4000 cells/μL)
Monocytes 42 cells/μL (150-1200 cells/μL)
Platelets 74,000 platelets/μL (150,000-400,000 platelets/μL).

Serum Chemistry Profile:

Sodium 141 mmol/L (145-154 mmol/L)
Potassium 4.0 mmol/L (3.6-5.3 mmol/L)
Chloride 112 mmol/L (108-118 mmol/L)
Bicarbonate 13 mmol/L (16-26 mmol/L)
Phosphorus 2.8 mg/dL (3.0-6.2 mg/dL)
Calcium 9.9 mg/dL (9.7-11.5 mg/dl)
BUN 15 mg/dL (5-21 mg/dL)
Creatinine 1.1 mg/dL (0.3-1.2 mg/dL)
Glucose 86 mg/dL (64-123 mg/dL)
Total protein 6.9 g/dL (5.4-7.6 g/dL)
Albumin 3.6 g/dL (3.0-4.4 g/dL)
Globulin 3.3 g/dL (1.8-3.9 g/dL)
ALT 108 U/L (19-67 U/L)
AST 109 U/L (19-42 U/L)
ALP 105 U/L (21-170 U/L)
Creatine kinase 381 U/L (51-399 U/L)
GGT < 3 U/L (0-6 U/L)
Cholesterol 296 mg/dL (135-361 mg/dL)
Total bilirubin 0.4 mg/dL (0-0.2 mg/dL)
Magnesium 1.7 mg/dL (1.5-2.6 mg/dL).

Urinalysis: SGr 1.048; pH 6.0, 2+ protein (SSA), 1+ bilirubin, 1+ hemoprotein, no glucose, 0-1 WBC/HPF, 20-30 RBC/HPF, rare ammonium biurate crystals, many lipid droplets

Imaging Findings:

Thoracic Radiographs: The cardiovascular and pulmonary structures appeared within normal limits. A mild diffuse bronchial pattern throughout all lung fields was considered consistent with the age of the patient. Marked spondylosis deformans was present throughout the thoracic spine.

Abdominal Ultrasound: The liver had a diffuse, coarse echotexture. The spleen was markedly, diffusely enlarged and had a diffuse hypoechoic, mottled echotexture. The prostate gland was enlarged and had multiple small anechoic cysts within its parenchyma. One testicle was present in the scrotum and had a striated, heterogenous echotexture. A second inguinal or intra-abdominal testis was not observed. Multiple enlarged, hypoechoic inguinal lymph nodes were present (see Figure 31-3). A large (2.5 cm), round, hypoechoic mass with a focal area of mineralization was present in the cranial abdomen caudal to the liver and most likely represented a lymph node. Multiple enlarged, hypoechoic sublumbar lymph nodes were observed. The splenic lymph nodes were enlarged and mildly hypoechoic.

Cytology Findings: Cytology of ultrasound-guided splenic aspirate: splenic stromal clumps contained increased numbers of plump histiocytes and many large clumps of hemosiderin. Histiocytes were also present in moderate numbers throughout the smear, often in clumps, and often mildly vacuolated. They were occasionally erythrophagocytic and often contain hemosiderin. Interpretation: moderate to marked histiocytic inflammation.

Cytology of popliteal lymph node aspirate (see Figure 31-5): moderate reactive lymphoid hyperplasia with pyogranulomatous inflammation was identified. Rare histiocytes were present that contained intracellular small coccoid purple-blue structures that were organized individually and in clusters. These were consistent with *Neorickettsia helminthoeca* organisms.

Fecal examination: Fecal flotation: Negative for parasites.

Fecal sedimentation: *Nanophyetus salmincola* ova, <1 per 10× field

Diagnosis: Salmon poisoning disease

Treatment: Doxycycline, 5 mg/kg PO q12h for 14 days. This was associated with resolution of fever and inappetence within 24 hours of starting treatment. By 7 days after diagnosis, Herman's owner reported that Herman was completely back to his normal self.

Comments: This dog was diagnosed with SPD based on the presence of characteristic cytologic findings on examination of a lymph node aspirate, together with the detection of *N. salmincola* ova in the stool. The case was unusual because the dog was infected after ingestion of incompletely cooked supermarket-bought salmon, which the dog had been fed for years without developing illness. Although the splenic aspirate contained inflammatory cells typical of those seen in SPD, organisms could not be convincingly documented.

SUGGESTED READINGS

Mack RE, Bercovitch MG, Ling GV, et al. Salmon poisoning disease complex in dogs—a review of 45 cases. Calif Vet. 1990;44:42-45.

Sykes JE, Marks SL, Mapes S, et al. Salmon poisoning disease in dogs: 29 cases. J Vet Intern Med. 2010;24(3):504-513.

REFERENCES

1. Millemann RE, Knapp SE. Biology of *Nanophyetus salmincola* and "salmon poisoning disease." In: Dawes B, ed. Advances in Parasitology. vol. 8. New York, NY: Academic Press; 1970:1-39.
2. Harrell LW, Deardoff TL. Human nanophyetiasis: transmission by handling naturally infected coho salmon (*Oncorhynchus kisutch*). J Infect Dis. 1990;161(1):146-148.
3. Foreyt WJ, Thorson S, Gorham JR. Experimental salmon poisoning disease in juvenile coyotes (*Canis latrans*). J Wildl Dis. 1982;18(2):159-162.
4. Hedrick RP, Arnandi A, Manzer D. *Nanophyetus salmincola:* the trematode vector of *Neorickettsia helmintheca*. California Veterinarian. 1990;44:18-22.
5. Gai JJ, Marks SL. Salmon poisoning disease in two Malayan sun bears. J Am Vet Med Assoc. 2008;232(4):586-588.
6. Headley SA, Scorpio DG, Barat NC, et al. *Neorickettsia helminthoeca* in dog. Brazil. Emerg Infect Dis. 2006;12:1303-1304.
7. Headley SA, Kano FS, Scorpio DG, et al. *Neorickettsia helminthoeca* in Brazilian dogs: a cytopathological, histopathological and immunohistochemical study. Clin Microbiol Infect. 2009;15(suppl 2):21-23.
8. Cordy DR, Gorham JR. The pathology and etiology of salmon disease in the dog and fox. Am J Pathol. 1950;26:617-637.
9. Farrell RK. Transmission of two rickettsia-like disease agents of dogs by endoparasites in northwestern USA. Proc 1st Int Congr Parasitol. 1966:438.
10. Farrell RK, Leader RW, Johnston SD. Differentiation of salmon poisoning disease and Elokomin fluke fever: studies with the black bear (*Ursus americanus*). Am J Vet Res. 1973;34:919-922.
11. Kitao T, Farrell RK, Fukuda T. Differentiation of salmon poisoning disease and Elokomin fluke fever: fluorescent antibody studies with *Rickettsia sennetsu*? Am J Vet Res. 1973;34:927-928.
12. Frank DW, McGuire TC, Gorham JR, et al. Cultivation of two species of *Neorickettsia* in canine monocytes. J Infect Dis. 1974;129:257-262.
13. Bennington E, Pratt I. The life history of the salmon-poisoning fluke, *Nanophyetus salmincola* (Chapin). J Parasitol. 1960;46(1):91-100.
14. Foreyt WJ, Gorham JR, Green JS, et al. Salmon poisoning disease in juvenile coyotes: clinical evaluation and infectivity of metacercariae and rickettsiae. J Wild Dis. 1987;23(3):412-417.
15. Baldwin NL, Milleman RE, Knapp SE. "Salmon poisoning" disease. 3. Effect of experimental *Nanophyetus salmincola* infection of the fish host. J Parasitol. 1967;53(3):556-564.
16. Bosman DD, Farrell RK, Gorham JR. Non-endoparasite transmission of salmon poisoning disease of dogs. J Am Vet Med Assoc. 1970;156:1907-1910.
17. Sykes JE, Marks SL, Mapes S, et al. Salmon poisoning disease in dogs: 29 cases. J Vet Intern Med. 2010;24(3):504-513.
18. Farrell RK, Dee JF, Ott RL. Salmon poisoning in a dog fed kippered salmon. J Am Vet Med Assoc. 1968;152:370-371.
19. Mack RE, Bercovitch MG, Ling GV, et al. Salmon poisoning disease complex in dogs—a review of 45 cases. Calif Vet. 1990;44:42-45.
20. Philip CB, Hadlow WJ, Hughes LE. *Neorickettsia helminthoeca*, a new rickettsialike disease agent of dogs in western United States transmitted by a helminth. Proc 6th Int Congr Microbiol. 1953;4:70-82:Rome.
21. Hadlow WJ. Neuropathology of experimental salmon poisoning of dogs. Am J Vet Res. 1957;18:898-908.
22. Gorham JR, Foreyt WJ. Salmon poisoning disease. In: Greene CE, ed. Clinical Microbiology and Infectious Diseases of the Dog and Cat. 1st ed. Philadelphia, PA: WB Saunders; 1984:538-544.
23. Johns JL, Strasser JL, Zinkl JG, et al. Lymph node aspirate from a California wine-country dog. Vet Clin Pathol. 2006;35:243-246.
24. Rikihisa Y. Cross-reacting antigens between *Neorickettsia helminthoeca* and *Ehrlichia* species, shown by immunofluorescence and Western immunoblotting. J Clin Microbiol. 1991;29:2024-2029.
25. Witenburg G. On the anatomy and systematic position of the causative agent of so-called salmon poisoning. J Parasitol. 1932;18:258-263.
26. Donham CR, Simms BT, Miller FW. So-called salmon poisoning in dogs (progress report). J Am Vet Med Assoc. 1926;68:701-715.
27. Sakawa H, Farrell RK, Mori M. Differentiation of salmon poisoning disease and Elokomin fluke fever: complement fixation. Am J Vet Res. 1973;34:923-925.
28. Eastburn RL, Fritsche TR, Terhune Jr CA. Human intestinal infection with *Nanophyetus salmincola* from salmonid fishes. Am J Trop Med Hyg. 1987;36(3):586-591.

CHAPTER 32

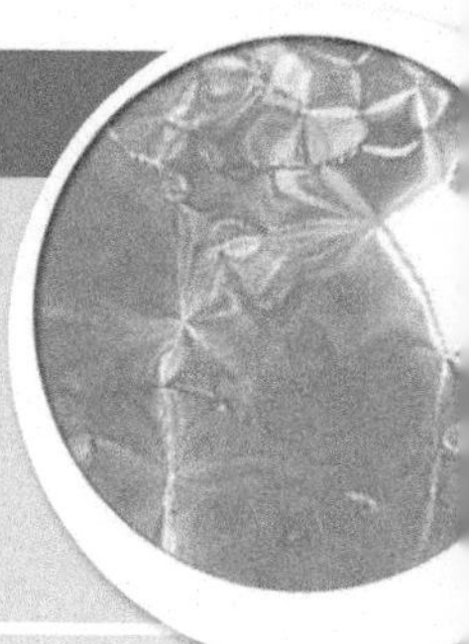

Coxiellosis and Q Fever

Jane E. Sykes and Jacqueline M. Norris

Overview of Coxiellosis and Q Fever

First Described: mid 1930s, Queensland, Australia, in slaughterhouse workers (Derrick)[1]

Cause: *Coxiella burnetii*, an obligately intracellular gram-negative bacteria that belongs to the Family Coxiellaceae

Affected Hosts: Humans are most susceptible; reproductive disease can occur in farm animal species such as sheep, goats, cattle, and horses, as well as cats and dogs

Geographic Distribution: Worldwide, with the exception of New Zealand

Major Clinical Signs: Dogs and cats are usually subclinically infected. Abortion, premature birth, and stillbirth may occur.

Differential Diagnoses: Brucellosis, bartonellosis, herpesviral infections, leptospirosis, neosporosis, canine distemper, and canine parvovirus infection. Noninfectious causes of pregnancy loss such as endocrinopathies, genetic disorders, and nutritional deficiency should also be considered.

Human Health Significance: Q fever in people results primarily from contact with infected sheep, goats, and cattle, or indirect contact with surfaces contaminated with secretions or excretions of these animals. However, contact with infected companion animals can also lead to transmission. Q fever in people is most commonly an acute febrile illness, but pneumonia and chronic complications such as endocarditis, granulomatous hepatitis, and chronic fatigue can occur.

Etiology and Epidemiology

Coxiella burnetii is a gram-negative, obligately intracellular, small, pleomorphic rod that causes Q fever in humans, a significant zoonosis worldwide. Sheep, cattle, and goats are the most commonly reported reservoirs for the organism, but infected cats and less commonly dogs have also been implicated in transmission to people.[2-5] Animals other than humans are often subclinically infected, although reproductive complications such as premature birth, abortion, and stillbirth may also occur. Reservoir hosts shed organisms in urine, feces, saliva, and/or milk, and especially in vaginal secretions and the products of parturition because of recrudescence of infection during pregnancy. The placentas of infected animals are heavily infected (up to 10^9 organisms per gram of tissue). At parturition, aerosols are created, which are subsequently inhaled by other animals and humans (Figure 32-1). Ingestion of unpasteurized contaminated milk is a less common and more controversial mode of transmission.[6,7] The term *Q fever* stands for *query* fever, the name it was given when it first emerged in Queensland, Australia, and the underlying cause had not yet been identified. In humans, acute Q fever is characterized by a febrile "flulike" illness, with headaches, and sometimes pulmonary and hepatic involvement. However, infection is initially asymptomatic in 60% of those infected.[8] Chronic Q fever can follow acute Q fever or asymptomatic infection and can be characterized by cardiac disease (endocarditis, pericarditis, myocarditis), fatigue syndromes, skin rash, and neurologic, pulmonary, and hepatic disease. In avian species, systemic illness has been associated with infection by other *Coxiella*-like organisms.[9-11]

Unlike other obligate intracellular pathogens, *C. burnetii* survives prolonged periods in the environment, where it resists high temperature, a variety of disinfectants, and ultraviolet light. The organism exists in two forms: a small cell variant, which survives in the environment, and a large cell variant, which replicates within cells. Survival of the organism for up to 10 months on wool at 15°C to 20°C (59°F to 68°F) has been reported, and it can also survive in tissues that have been stored in formalin for several months. It is inactivated by 5% hydrogen peroxide.[12] Although originally classified within the order Rickettsiales, the availability of sequence information led to its reclassification as a gammaproteobacterium in the order Legionellales, which also includes *Legionella* species. *C. burnetii* undergoes phase variation, which is associated with alterations in its cell wall components. The variants have nominally been called phase 1 and phase 2.[13] The changes in cell surface antigens and the creation of phase variants has clinical implications for serologic testing due to the production of phase 1 and phase 2 antibodies to the bacterium at different stages of natural infection (see Diagnosis, later). The whole genome of *C. burnetii* has been sequenced.[14]

C. burnetii is extremely contagious, and only small numbers of organisms are required to cause disease in people. The epidemiology of Q fever varies geographically. Because of its predilection for domestic ruminant species, Q fever is most commonly reported from rural areas. *C. burnetii* has been detected within a huge variety of different tick and other arthropod species. Within ticks, it replicates in the midgut and it is shed in large quantities in tick feces. Although ticks have the potential to transmit the organism to domestic animal species, the most significant role of ticks appears to be in transmission to wildlife.[15] *C. burnetii* has been identified in fish, wild birds, rodents, marsupials, horses, swine, camels, marine mammals, ducks, turkeys, geese, cats, dogs, and rabbits. Although the mechanism is not clearly defined, cats and dogs may become infected through exposure to infected sheep, cattle, and goats—possibly through ingestion of unpasteurized milk from these species—and

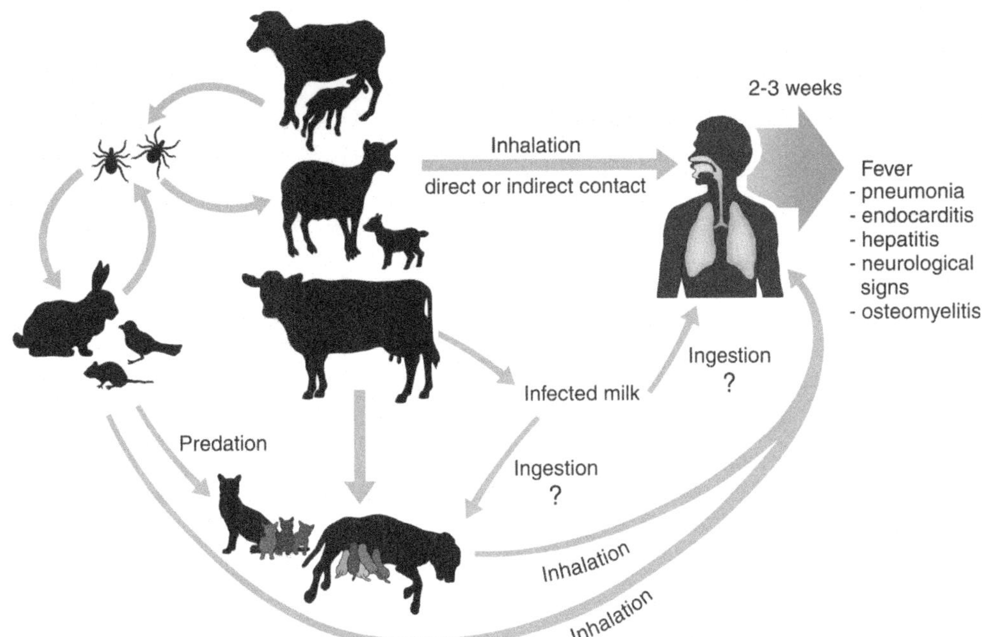

FIGURE 32-1 Transmission of *Coxiella burnetii*. The organism is most often transmitted to humans when animals give birth. People become infected by inhalation when they directly contact the products of parturition or as a result of indirect contact with organisms that survive in the environment. Sheep, cattle, and goats are the most common reservoirs of the organism for human infection, but infected cats and less commonly dogs can also transmit the infection to humans. Ticks also harbor the organism and are thought to maintain transmission to wildlife species, especially rodents (such as small mice) and rabbits, but also birds. Dogs and cats and humans can also become infected when they contact (or ingest) wildlife species. Ingestion of infected milk may be a lesser mode of transmission.

through contact with, or predation of, infected wildlife reservoir hosts such as rodents, birds, and rabbits.

Exposure to stillborn kittens or apparently healthy newborn kittens has been a risk factor for human infection in Africa, Japan, Korea, Canada, and the United States. In a study of intact female cats from Colorado, *C. burnetii* DNA was not detected in vaginal swab specimens or uterine biopsies from 50 shelter cats using a PCR assay, but 4 of 47 uterine biopsies from client-owned cats were positive.[16] Seroprevalence studies suggest that infection is more common in stray cats and dogs than client-owned animals, but further research is required to determine risk factors for exposure in dogs and cats.[17,18] No association has been found between prevalence of Q fever in people and cat or dog ownership.[19] Laboratory-acquired infections have been described in people, and infection can occur as a result of exposure to straw, manure, or dust, such as that from contaminated farm vehicles and contaminated clothing. Q fever has emerged as a disease of U.S. combat arms military personnel who are deployed to Iraq.[20] Studies of a large, 2-year outbreak in the Netherlands showed that dust-accumulating surfaces contained higher levels of *C. burnetii* DNA than vaginal swabs from sheep and goats.[21] The organism can travel for miles as a result of windborne transmission.

Clinical Features

Signs and Their Pathogenesis

After inhalation (and to a lesser extent, ingestion), *C. burnetii* enters mononuclear phagocytes and survives within the harsh environment of the phagolysosome.[22] Remarkably, the acid conditions of the lysosome appear to be a requirement for the metabolic functions of *C. burnetii*. Replication is prolonged, and minimal cytopathic effects occur in infected cells. The organism appears to modulate apoptosis in order to inhibit cell death and promote its own replication.[23] Subsequently, infected cells enter the bloodstream. After experimental infection, bacteremia may be prolonged (up to 1 month) in cats.[24] The organism can persist in a variety of tissues, and in human patients, this contributes to chronic disease manifestations, such as prolonged fever, endocarditis, vasculitis, chronic fatigue, and immune-mediated consequences such as demyelinating polyradiculoneuritis.[25] Appropriate diagnosis and treatment at the acute stage of clinical illness is important in reducing the risk of postacute Q-fever sequelae and development of chronic disease. Reactivation of shedding has been described during pregnancy in humans.[12] Infected cats and dogs usually show no clinical signs of infection, but stillbirth, abortion, and prolonged vaginal bleeding for 3 weeks before delivery have been reported in cats.[4,26] The organism replicates in trophoblasts, and in experimentally infected goats, massive bacterial replication occurs in the placenta just before abortion.[27] An infected rabbit hound dog that transmitted *C. burnetii* to a family in Nova Scotia gave birth to four puppies, all of which died within 24 hours of birth.[5] The importance of *C. burnetii* in reproductive tract disease and chronic disease manifestations such as endocarditis in cats and dogs requires further investigation.

Diagnosis

Microbiologic Tests

Diagnostic assays available for Q fever are listed in Table 32-1.

Culture

C. burnetii can be isolated in a variety of different cell lines. It has also been isolated in a cell-free medium that mimics the phagolysosome environment.[28] Because it is highly infectious

TABLE 32-1

Diagnostic Assays Available for Q Fever

Assay	Specimen Type	Target	Performance
Cell culture	Placental materials, vaginal swabs, blood, urine, feces, milk	*C. burnetii*	Not widely offered or utilized for routine diagnostic purposes. Requires special facilities.
Histopathology	Placental materials	*C. burnetii*	Organisms may be seen when present in large numbers and stain with Gimenez stain. Immunohistochemistry and fluorescence in situ hybridization can be used to identify the organisms as *C. burnetii*.
Serology	Serum	Antibodies to phase 1 or phase 2 *C. burnetii*	Acute and convalescent serology is required for diagnosis of acute infection. At least 1 month may be required for seroconversion. Cross-reactivity may occur to related bacteria. IFA is considered the serologic test of choice in human patients. CFT is the OIE standard in animals but is less sensitive.
PCR	Whole blood, tissue specimens, vaginal swabs, milk, feces	*C. burnetii* DNA	Confirms active infection. Sensitivity and specificity may vary depending on stage of infection, assay design, and specimen type. PCR is most sensitive in acute infections (in the first 2 weeks of illness in humans), but is usually negative in humans with chronic infections. Subclinical shedding in animals is variable but is greatest during parturition.

CFT, Complement fixation test; IFA, immunofluorescent antibody; OIE, World Organization for Animal Health.

to humans, most laboratories do not have the special facilities required to isolate *C. burnetii*. Thus diagnosis of infection is usually performed using immunohistochemistry, serology, or PCR.

Serologic Diagnosis

The World Organization for Animal Health (OIE) reference test for serologic diagnosis of *C. burnetii* infection in animals remains the complement fixation test (CFT),[20] despite the availability of more sensitive serologic tests. A variety of serologic assays have been used to detect antibodies to phase 1 or phase 2 *C. burnetii* antigens in humans and other animals, including immunofluorescent antibody (IFA) assays, ELISA, and the CFT. The CFT is considered the least sensitive and specific method. In human patients, anti–phase 2 antibodies (IgG and IgM) are present in acute Q fever, whereas anti–phase 1 IgG antibodies predominate in chronic infection.[15,29] In humans, the use of IFA assays has been recommended for diagnosis of Q fever.[12] Acute and convalescent serology is required for diagnosis of acute Q fever in people. It can take at least a month before seroconversion occurs; titers peak around 8 weeks after infection.[15] Because infection is usually not clinically detected in dogs and cats, serologic assays have primarily been used in dogs and cats for epidemiologic studies or as part of import requirements to Q fever–free countries such as New Zealand. Low-level cross-reactivity with other bacteria such as *Bartonella* spp. and chlamydiae has been described in some studies, which highlights the need for animal species-specific cutoff values for all serologic methods.[30,31] The concurrent performance of serology for *Bartonella* and *Chlamydia* (i.e., to determine if titers are higher or lower to these organisms than to *Coxiella*) may assist in interpretation of the results.

Molecular Diagnosis Using the Polymerase Chain Reaction

Both conventional and real-time PCR assays have been described for detection of *C. burnetii* DNA. PCR assays are the diagnostic test of choice for organism detection and have revolutionized knowledge of the epidemiology of *C. burnetii* infections. In animals, PCR assays have primarily been used on a research basis. Negative results can occur with PCR assays in chronic infections or even as early as 2 weeks after onset of acute illness in humans, because of undetectable levels of the infection or absence of bacteremia. Because *C. burnetii* is highly infectious to humans, special handling (BSL 3) conditions are required for fresh specimens that are submitted for *C. burnetii* PCR assays (see Table 1-4). When *C. burnetii* is suspected (such as in placentas or aborted material), the laboratory should be contacted in advance, and specimens should be labeled and transported appropriately.

Pathologic Findings

Little information is available about the pathology of *C. burnetii* infection in dogs and cats. In affected livestock, *C. burnetii* causes a necrotizing placentitis with mixed inflammatory cell infiltrate and nonsuppurative vasculitis. In some cases, small, basophilic intracytoplasmic organisms can be seen (Figure 32-2). The organisms stain with Gimenez, Giemsa, and modified acid-fast stains, but not Gram, silver, or periodic acid–Schiff stains.[32] Immunohistochemistry and fluorescent in situ hybridization[33] can be used to identify *C. burnetii* antigen within lesions.

Treatment

Many acute infections in people are self-limiting (or even subclinical), and symptoms respond to nonspecific therapy such as antipyretics and rehydration. However, because of concerns that relate to the development of chronic Q fever, specific antimicrobial therapy is recommended regardless of the severity of acute Q fever. When antimicrobials agents are required, doxycycline for 14 to 21 days, azithromycin for 3 to 5 days,

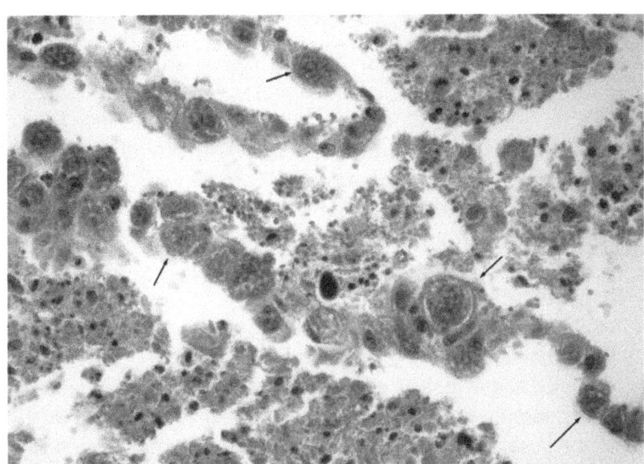

FIGURE 32-2 Histopathology showing severe, acute necrotizing placentitis in the placenta of a goat from which dead fetuses were removed by caesarian section. Trophoblasts are distended with abundant basophilic bacterial organisms *(arrows)*. The organisms were subsequently identified as *Coxiella burnetii* with immunohistochemistry.

or quinolones have been used successfully to treat pneumonia and hepatitis in human patients with *C. burnetii* infection. Combination therapy, such as doxycycline, ciprofloxacin, and rifampin for prolonged periods (e.g., 2 years) or doxycycline and hydroxychloroquine (which alkalinizes phagolysosomes) has been required for treatment of Q fever endocarditis, and valve replacement is frequently needed.[12,15] Antibody titers decrease with successful treatment. Q fever during pregnancy, which may result in abortion when infection occurs in the first trimester, is treated with trimethoprim-sulfamethoxazole for the duration of the pregnancy.[34] Treatment of an infected sheep herd with oxytetracycline on days 100 and 120 of gestation did not prevent shedding of *C. burnetii* in milk, vaginal swabs, or feces as assessed with PCR, nor did it affect the duration of shedding.[35]

Public Health Aspects

In humans, asymptomatic infections with *C. burnetii* are probably widespread. When it occurs, Q fever is most often a systemic febrile illness. Because it mimics a variety of other illnesses, and confirmatory diagnostic tests require a specific index of suspicion by the medical clinician, Q fever is most likely underrecognized. Veterinarians involved in mixed or farm animal practice, slaughterhouse workers, and workers in the livestock industry (farmers, shearers, transporters of animals) are most likely to develop Q fever as a result of direct contact with infected livestock. Person-to-person spread of Q fever is rarely reported, but humans can shed organisms during parturition, and infection of an obstetrician during delivery was described.[36] Transmission during postmortem examinations has also been reported. Between 2005 and 2008, approximately 140 to 170 cases of Q fever were reported to the Centers for Disease Control and Prevention each year, and rates of hospitalization for these cases were around 50%.[37] However, severe cases are more likely to be reported, so actual hospitalization rates are likely much lower. In Australia, 300 to 400 cases are reported annually.[38]

In humans, acute Q fever occurs after an incubation period that ranges from 9 to 39 days, although shorter incubation periods are possible with exposure to high doses of the agent.[12] The incubation period after exposure to an infected cat has ranged from 9 days to 4 weeks.[3,4] Males are predisposed, which relates to an increased likelihood of exposure. Patients who develop pneumonia may also develop severe headache, as well as sweats, chills, fatigue, and myalgia. Other signs include cough, chest pain, nausea and vomiting, sore throat, diarrhea, a rash, and abdominal pain and hematuria.[4] Myocarditis and pericarditis can occur rarely. Blood work often shows a normal white cell count, and thrombocytopenia or marked thrombocytosis can occur. Serum biochemistry testing reveals mild to moderate increases in the activity of hepatic transaminases in almost all patients.[12] Pulmonary infiltrates are present on thoracic radiographs, and in some cases, pleural effusion.[12,15] Q fever pneumonia is rarely fatal. Chronic Q fever may be manifested as endocarditis, optic neuritis, osteomyelitis, granulomatous hepatitis, interstitial pulmonary fibrosis, prolonged fever, and a chronic fatigue syndrome, which has been described in up to 20% of patients who develop acute infection with *C. burnetii*.[39] Endocarditis follows acute Q fever in fewer than 1% of cases,[29] and it may not become apparent for several years after acute illness. Approximately 3% to 5% of human endocarditis cases have been attributed to *C. burnetii*. Host factors seem to be important in whether chronic manifestations of Q fever occur. Cellular immunity and the production of IFN-γ appear to be required for resolution of infection.[29]

Because treatment with tetracyclines does not seem to reduce shedding by reservoir hosts, an emphasis has been placed on the development of effective vaccines for public health purposes. A phase 1 inactivated vaccine (Coxevac) has been used in Europe on an investigational basis to prevent shedding by reservoir livestock species, such as sheep and goats. Vaccination of sheep flocks led to a reduced number of abortions and decreased shedding, but did not completely prevent infection.[29] Vaccination was ineffective in previously infected cattle or naïve pregnant cattle.[40] Another phase 1 whole cell vaccine (Q-VAX, Commonwealth Serum Laboratories, Parkville, Australia) has also been used to protect naïve but at-risk humans, such as livestock workers (farmers, shearers, slaughterhouse workers, animal transporters), veterinarians, and laboratory workers, from infection. A Q-VAX skin test as well as serologic assays are performed as a prescreening of potential vaccine recipients for prior sensitization to Q fever antigens to minimize adverse vaccine reactions; humans with prior exposure to *C. burnetii* should never be vaccinated. It has been recommended that humans not drink raw milk from infected farms. When Q fever is discovered on a farm, sale of milk is forbidden for the year after initial diagnosis. Aborted material and placentas must be buried with lime or incinerated.[29]

CASE EXAMPLE

Signalments: 50-year-old female veterinarian and a 23-year-old female veterinary technician from southeastern Australia

History: A 3-year-old female British shorthair cat with dystocia was brought to a veterinary clinic by the breeder/owner at 8 o'clock in the morning. One kitten was stillborn in the home environment overnight. Safe delivery of the two remaining kittens required a cesarean section. Surgery was performed immediately, and the kittens were delivered and revived by vigorous rubbing with dry towels. The kittens were discolored by yellow-green placental material and were slow to revive. They were able to successfully to suckle once the queen had recovered from general anesthesia. The queen and kittens were returned to the breeder's cattery the same afternoon.

Two weeks after the surgery, the veterinarian and the veterinary technician who had been involved in the cesarean section developed fever, severe headache, neck pain, chills, night sweats, myalgia, and stiffness. The veterinarian sought medical attention. Psittacosis was considered the most likely diagnosis by the attending physician, because psittacine birds were frequently treated in the clinic. A serologic test for chlamydiosis was negative, but nevertheless treatment with doxycycline was commenced. The veterinary technician's clinical signs were more severe and included cough, chest pain, nausea, and vomiting. As a result, she was hospitalized for 3 weeks for further diagnostic testing, treatment, and convalescence. When the technician tested positive by PCR assay for *Coxiella burnetii* DNA on day 10 after the onset of illness, serial diagnostic tests for Q fever were also performed on the veterinarian (Table 32-2).

Comments: Determination of the date of onset of illness is essential in any diagnostic investigation of Q fever in people for correct interpretation of diagnostic test results. In the first 8 to 10 days after the onset of illness, patients are frequently (80%) bacteremic (and therefore PCR positive) but still antibody negative. IgM class antibody to phase 2 antigens, as measured via IFA or ELISA assays, appear as early as 10 to 12 days after the onset of illness, but this may also be delayed, as occurred in the veterinarian in this example. IgM class antibody to phase 1 and IgG class antibody to phase 2 antigens often appear on day 15 to 20, but again this can be delayed. Small animal veterinarians and veterinary technicians or nurses who are exposed to kittens and placental secretions and subsequently develop illness should inform their practitioner of the possibility of exposure to *C. burnetii* because diagnosis requires a high index of suspicion and specific diagnostic assays. Fatigue often persists in patients for months after the onset of illness (as was the case for the veterinary technician in this example) and does not necessarily mean that chronic Q fever has developed.

TABLE 32-2

Results of Diagnostic Assays for Q fever in a Veterinarian and Veterinary Technician after Exposure to an Infected Cat's Reproductive Secretions

Days after the Onset of Illness	Real-Time PCR on Whole Blood		Serology for IgM and IgG to Phase 1 and Phase 2 Antigens*	
	Veterinarian	Technician	Veterinarian	Technician
10	ND	Positive	ND	Negative for IgG and IgM to phase 2 antigen
14	Negative	ND	Negative	ND
20	Negative	Negative	Negative	Positive for IgM to phase 1 and phase 2 antigens, positive for IgG to phase 2 antigen. Positive CFT for antibodies to phase 2 antigen
35	ND	ND	Positive for IgM and IgG to phase 2 antigen. Positive CFT for antibodies to phase 2 antigens	ND

CFT, Complement fixation test; ND, not determined.
*Performed by immunofluorescent antibody unless otherwise specified.

SUGGESTED READINGS

Angelakis E, Raoult D. Q Fever. Vet Microbiol. 2010;140:297-309.

Porter SR, Czaplicki G, Mainil J, et al. Q Fever: current state of knowledge and perspectives of research of a neglected zoonosis. Int J Microbiol. 2011;2011:248-418.

REFERENCES

1. Derrick EH. "Q" fever, a new fever entity: clinical features, diagnosis and laboratory investigation. Med J Aust. 1937;2:281-299.
2. Marrie TJ, Langille D, Papukna V, et al. Truckin' pneumonia—an outbreak of Q fever in a truck repair plant probably due to aerosols from clothing contaminated by contact with newborn kittens. Epidemiol Infect. 1989;102:119-127.
3. Kosatsky T. Household outbreak of Q-fever pneumonia related to a parturient cat. Lancet. 1984;2:1447-1449.
4. Marrie TJ, MacDonald A, Durant H, et al. An outbreak of Q fever probably due to contact with a parturient cat. Chest. 1988;93:98-103.
5. Buhariwalla F, Cann B, Marrie TJ. A dog-related outbreak of Q fever. Clin Infect Dis. 1996;23:753-755.
6. Fishbein DB, Raoult D. A cluster of *Coxiella burnetii* infections associated with exposure to vaccinated goats and their unpasteurized dairy products. Am J Trop Med Hyg. 1992;47:35-40.
7. Benson WW, Brock DW, Mather J. Serologic analysis of a penitentiary group using raw milk from a Q fever infected herd. Public Health Rep. 1963;78:707-710.
8. Raoult D, Marrie T, Mege J. Natural history and pathophysiology of Q fever. Lancet Infect Dis. 2005;5:219-226.
9. Vapniarsky N, Barr BC, Murphy B. Systemic *Coxiella*-like infection with myocarditis and hepatitis in an eclectus parrot (*Eclectus roratus*). Vet Pathol. 2012;49(4):717-722.
10. Shivaprasad HL, Cadenas MB, Diab SS, et al. *Coxiella*-like infection in psittacines and a toucan. Avian Dis. 2008;52:426-432.
11. Woc-Colburn AM, Gamer MM, Bradway D, et al. Fatal coxiellosis in Swainson's Blue Mountain rainbow lorikeets (*Trichoglossus haematodus moluccanus*). Vet Pathol. 2008;45:247-254.
12. Marrie TJ, Raoult D. *Coxiella burnetii* (Q fever). In: Mandell GL, Bennett JE, Dolin R, eds. Mandell, Douglas and Bennett's Principles and Practice of Infectious Diseases. 7th ed. Philadelphia, PA: Churchill Livingstone Elsevier; 2011:2511-2519.
13. Jerrells TR, Hinrichs DJ, Mallavia LP. Cell envelope analysis of *Coxiella burneti* phase I and phase II.. Can J Microbiol. 1974;20:1465-1470.
14. Seshadri R, Paulsen IT, Eisen JA, et al. Complete genome sequence of the Q-fever pathogen *Coxiella burnetii*. Proc Natl Acad Sci U S A. 2003;100:5455-5460.
15. Angelakis E, Raoult D. Q Fever. Vet Microbiol. 2010;140:297-309.
16. Cairns K, Brewer M, Lappin MR. Prevalence of *Coxiella burnetii* DNA in vaginal and uterine samples from healthy cats of north-central Colorado. J Feline Med Surg. 2007;9:196-201.
17. Komiya T, Sadamasu K, Kang MI, et al. Seroprevalence of *Coxiella burnetii* infections among cats in different living environments. J Vet Med Sci. 2003;65:1047-1048.
18. Willeberg P, Ruppanner R, Behymer DE, et al. Environmental exposure to *Coxiella burnetii*: a sero-epidemiologic survey among domestic animals. Am J Epidemiol. 1980;111:437-443.
19. Skerget M, Wenisch C, Daxboeck F, et al. Cat or dog ownership and seroprevalence of ehrlichiosis, Q fever, and cat-scratch disease. Emerg Infect Dis. 2003;9:1337-1340.
20. Anderson AD, Baker TR, Littrell AC, et al. Seroepidemiologic survey for *Coxiella burnetii* among hospitalized U.S. troops deployed to Iraq. Zoonoses Public Health. 2011;58:276-283.
21. de Bruin A, de Groot A, de Heer L, et al. Detection of *Coxiella burnetii* in complex matrices by using multiplex quantitative PCR during a major Q fever outbreak in The Netherlands. Appl Environ Microbiol. 2011;77:6516-6523.
22. Voth DE, Heinzen RA. Lounging in a lysosome: the intracellular lifestyle of *Coxiella burnetii*. Cell Microbiol. 2007;9:829-840.
23. Voth DE, Howe D, Heinzen RA. *Coxiella burnetii* inhibits apoptosis in human THP-1 cells and monkey primary alveolar macrophages. Infect Immun. 2007;75:4263-4271.
24. Gillespie JH, Baker JA. Experimental Q fever in cats. Am J Vet Res. 1952;13:91-94.
25. Lefebvre M, Grossi O, Agard C, et al. Systemic immune presentations of *Coxiella burnetii* infection (Q fever). Semin Arthritis Rheum. 2010;39:405-409.
26. Nagaoka H, Sugieda M, Akiyama M, et al. Isolation of *Coxiella burnetii* from the vagina of feline clients at veterinary clinics. J Vet Med Sci. 1998;60:251-252.
27. Sanchez J, Souriau A, Buendia AJ, et al. Experimental *Coxiella burnetii* infection in pregnant goats: a histopathological and immunohistochemical study. J Comp Pathol. 2006;135:108-115.
28. Omsland A, Cockrell DC, Howe D, et al. Host cell-free growth of the Q fever bacterium *Coxiella burnetii*. Proc Natl Acad Sci U S A. 2009;106:4430-4434.
29. Porter SR, Czaplicki G, Mainil J, et al. Q Fever: current state of knowledge and perspectives of research of a neglected zoonosis. Int J Microbiol. 2011;2011:248-418.
30. La Scola B, Raoult D. Serological cross-reactions between *Bartonella quintana, Bartonella henselae*, and *Coxiella burnetii*. J Clin Microbiol. 1996;34:2270-2274.
31. Lukacova M, Melnicakova J, Kazar J. Cross-reactivity between *Coxiella burnetii* and chlamydiae. Folia Microbiol (Praha). 1999;44:579-584.
32. Moore JD, Barr BC, Daft BM, et al. Pathology and diagnosis of *Coxiella burnetii* infection in a goat herd. Vet Pathol. 1991;28:81-84.
33. Jensen TK, Montgomery DL, Jaeger PT, et al. Application of fluorescent in situ hybridisation for demonstration of *Coxiella burnetii* in placentas from ruminant abortions. APMIS. 2007;115:347-353.
34. Carcopino X, Raoult D, Bretelle F, et al. Managing Q fever during pregnancy: the benefits of long-term cotrimoxazole therapy. Clin Infect Dis. 2007;45:548-555.
35. Astobiza I, Barandika JF, Hurtado A, et al. Kinetics of *Coxiella burnetii* excretion in a commercial dairy sheep flock after treatment with oxytetracycline. Vet J. 2010;184:172-175.
36. Racult D, Stein A. Q fever during pregnancy—a risk for women, fetuses, and obstetricians. N Engl J Med. 1994;330:371.
37. Centers for Disease Control and Prevention. http://www.cdc.gov/qfever/stats/index.html. Last accessed December 13, 2012.
38. Australian Government Department of Health and Aging. http://www.health.gov.au/internet/publications/publishing.nsf/Content/cda-cdi34suppl.htm. Last accessed December 13, 2012.
39. Marmion BP, Shannon M, Maddocks I, et al. Protracted debility and fatigue after acute Q fever. Lancet. 1996;347:977-978.
40. Guatteo R, Seegers H, Joly A, et al. Prevention of *Coxiella burnetii* shedding in infected dairy herds using a phase I *C. burnetii* inactivated vaccine. Vaccine. 2008;26:4320-4328.

CHAPTER 33

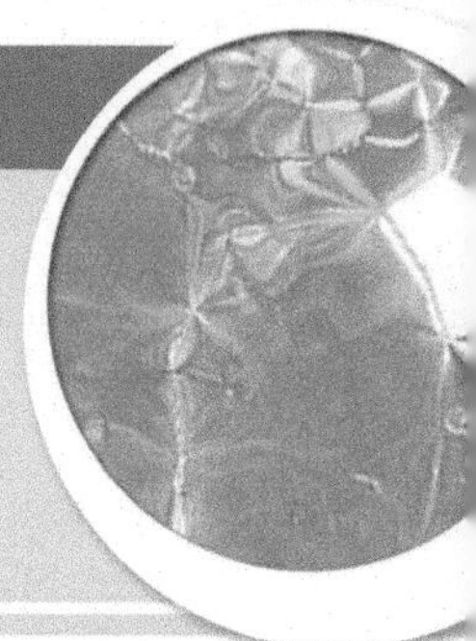

Chlamydial Infections

Jane E. Sykes

Overview of Chlamydial Infections in Dogs and Cats

First Described in Cats: 1944, United States (Baker)[1]

Causes: *Chlamydia felis* (and possibly other chlamydiae such as *Chlamydia pneumoniae*) causes ocular disease in cats; *Chlamydia psittaci* and *Chlamydia abortus* have rarely been detected in association with ocular and respiratory disease in dogs. These are obligately intracellular bacteria that belong to the family Chlamydiaceae.

Geographic Distribution: Worldwide

Mode of Transmission: Direct contact with respiratory secretions and possibly also vaginal secretions and feces

Major Clinical Signs (Cats): Acute and chronic conjunctivitis, chemosis, serous to mucopurulent ocular discharge, and blepharospasm, with or without sneezing and nasal discharge

Differential Diagnoses: The primary differential diagnoses in cats are infections with feline herpesvirus 1, feline calicivirus, *Mycoplasma* spp., and/or *Bordetella bronchiseptica*

Human Health Significance: *C. felis* has rarely been documented as a cause of human conjunctivitis. The importance of cats and dogs as a source of other human chlamydial infections is unclear. *C. psittaci* is generally acquired from avian species and not dogs and cats.

Etiology Agent and Epidemiology

Chlamydiae are obligately intracellular bacteria that belong to the order Chlamydiales. They primarily cause conjunctivitis in cats, but may also play a role in other systemic and reproductive disorders in dogs and cats that remain poorly characterized. Most knowledge of chlamydial infections results from research on human chlamydial pathogens such as *Chlamydia trachomatis, Chlamydia pneumoniae,* and *Chlamydia psittaci,* which have significant clinical and public health importance (see Public Health Significance). Chlamydiae structurally resemble gram-negative bacteria, lack peptidoglycan, and have extremely small genomes; they depend on the host cell for many amino acids and nucleotides. They exist in two forms, an infectious elementary body (EB), which is 0.2 to 0.6 µm in diameter and exists outside the cell, and the reticulate body (RB), which is larger (0.5 to 1.5 µm), is noninfectious, and replicates within the cytoplasm of host cells, before it matures and forms EBs (Figure 33-1). The EBs survive only a few days in the environment at room temperature and they are readily inactivated by most disinfectants. Transmission occurs via direct contact or, to a lesser extent, aerosols. Fomites are also likely to be an important means of transmission among group-housed cats in heavily contaminated environments. The chlamydiae at one time were separated into two genera, *Chlamydia* and *Chlamydophila,* based on sequence analysis of the 16S rRNA and 23S rRNA genes. However, there has been disagreement in the field regarding this classification, and reversion to the single genus *Chlamydia* has since been recommended based on the availability of complete genome sequence information.[2]

Chlamydiae persistently infect epithelial cells of the ocular, respiratory, gastrointestinal, and genitourinary systems; chlamydial infections of the synovium have also been reported in a number of different host species. Different chlamydial species tend to associate with certain host species, although evidence has accumulated that some chlamydial species can cause disease in more than one host species (Table 33-1). In addition, more than one chlamydial species can cause similar disease manifestations in a single host species. For example, although the human ocular disease trachoma is caused primarily by *C. trachomatis,* it has now also been associated with infection by *C. pneumoniae* and *C. psittaci*.[3] *Chlamydia felis* is an important cause of conjunctivitis and possibly reproductive disease in cats, but DNA that resembles that of the human pathogen *C. pneumoniae* has now also been detected in ocular swabs from European cats with conjunctivitis.[4] *Chlamydia abortus* DNA was detected in histopathology specimens from 1 of 13 cats with arteriosclerosis.[5] There are rare reports of chlamydial infections in dogs, in association with ocular and respiratory disease, polyarthritis, and atherosclerosis.[6-11] However, chlamydiae were not detected by PCR assay in atherosclerotic lesions from 16 dogs in one study, so the role of chlamydiae in this otherwise rare condition in dogs is uncertain.[5] Respiratory disease associated with *C. psittaci* infection has been reported most frequently among dogs.

The most significant pathogen of cats is *C. felis*, which causes acute and chronic conjunctivitis in cats worldwide. The results of genetic analysis (by multilocus variable-number tandem-repeat and multilocus sequence typing) have revealed that as many as 25 different genotypes of *C. felis* exist, and more than one genotype may circulate in some catteries.[12] Co-infections with more than one strain can occur. The prevalence of infection varies from one group of cats to another and with geographic location, age of the cat population sampled, and presence or absence of clinical illness. Infection occurs most often in multiple-cat households, especially breeding catteries. *C. felis* DNA is uncommonly detected in conjunctival swabs from healthy cats. For example, in clinically healthy household cats, those with a history of past conjunctivitis, and those with active conjunctivitis, 0%, 4.6%,

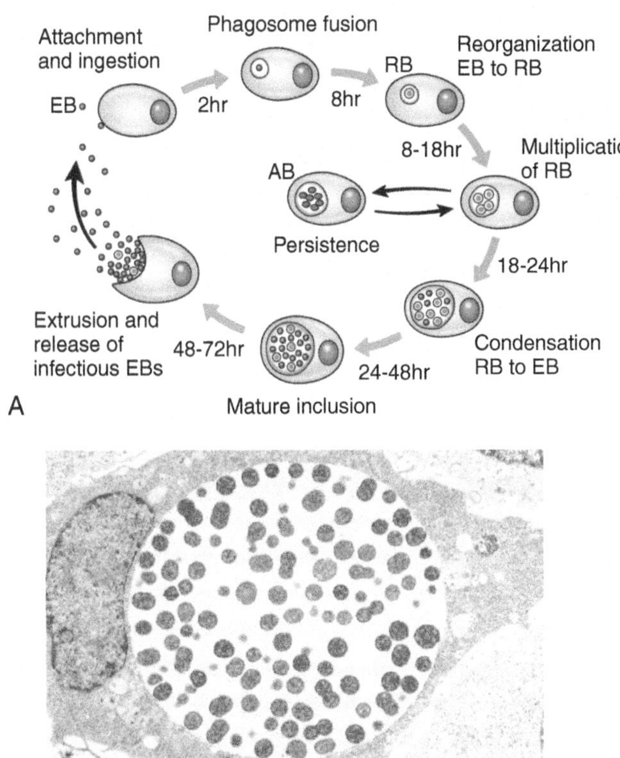

FIGURE 33-1 **A**, Life cycle of chlamydiae. From top left. Electron-dense elementary bodies (EBs) attach to and are taken up by epithelial cells. EBs then differentiate into reticulate bodies (RBs), and RBs divide by binary fission. RBs condense into EBs, and also have the potential to persist in the form of aberrant bodies (AB). EBs are released by cell lysis and infect other cells. **B**, Electron micrograph of chlamydial organisms growing in an inclusion in tissue culture. The larger reticulate bodies (RBs) have more diffuse chromatin. One of the RBs appears to be dividing. The smaller dense bodies are elementary bodies. (B from Mandell GL, Bennett JE, Dolin R. Principles and Practice of Infectious Diseases. Ed 7. Philadelphia, PA: Elsevier, 2012; 2:2440)

and 7.3% had positive PCR assay results, respectively.[13] Isolation rates of up to 30% in household cats with conjunctivitis have been reported.[14] In shelter cats, the prevalence of *C. felis* infection has ranged from 0% to 15%.[15-18] In cats from 218 European rescue shelters, breeding establishments, and private households, the prevalence of infection in cats without respiratory disease was 3%, versus 10% in those with evidence of respiratory disease.[19] Infection with *C. felis* in this European study was associated with suboptimal hygiene. Infection with *C. felis* is more often present in young cats, especially those aged 2 to 12 months; kittens less than 2 months of age may be protected by maternal antibody, although neonatal infections have been described. Cats older than 5 years of age are very unlikely to be infected with *C. felis*. Co-infections with other respiratory pathogens, such as feline herpesvirus 1 (FHV-1) and feline calicivirus (FCV), are common.

The DNA of organisms that belong to the family Parachlamydiaceae has recently been detected in cats with ocular disease. These organisms resemble *Chlamydia* and reside symbiotically within amoebae. Parachlamydial species include *Neochlamydia, Parachlamydia, Protochlamydia, Rhabdochlamydia, Criblamydia, Simkania,* and *Waddlia* species. DNA that resembles that of *Neochlamydia hartmanellae* has been detected in feline conjunctival brush specimens.[20] This organism is an endosymbiont of the amoeba *Hartmannella vermiformis*, which has been identified as a cause of ocular surface infection in people and may play some role in feline ocular infections. The DNA of *Parachlamydia acanthamoebae* has also been detected with PCR in cats with keratitis and conjunctivitis.[21] As yet, co-infections with amoebae have not been detected in cats. Further studies are required to determine the prevalence and clinical significance of these organisms.

Clinical Features

Signs and Their Pathogenesis

C. felis infection is acquired by cats primarily through close contact, fomites, or to a lesser extent, aerosol transmission. Kittens may be infected from the mother at birth. Whether venereal

TABLE 33-1

Chlamydial Species That Infect Animals and Humans

Species	Major Host(s)*	Major Clinical Manifestations
Chlamydia trachomatis	Humans	Conjunctivitis (serovars A-C); urethritis, cervicitis, proctitis (serovars D-K); lymphogranuloma venereum (serovars L1, L2, and L3)
Chlamydia pneumoniae	Humans	Upper respiratory infection, community-acquired pneumonia, possibly atherosclerosis and asthma
Chlamydia psittaci	Humans, a variety of bird species (e.g., parrots, finches, poultry, pigeons, pheasants, seagulls, egrets, puffins)	Pneumonia, systemic infection
Chlamydia felis	Cats	Conjunctivitis, upper respiratory infection, arthritis?, reproductive disease?
Chlamydia abortus	Sheep, cows, goats, other mammals	Reproductive disease
Chlamydia pecorum	Cattle and sheep	Encephalomyelitis, pneumonia, reproductive tract disease, conjunctivitis, polyarthritis
Chlamydia caviae	Guinea pigs	Keratoconjunctivitis

*Infection may occasionally extend to other host species.

transmission occurs, as reported for other chlamydial species, is unknown, but in some infected cats, the organism is shed in vaginal discharges and from the rectum as well as in ocular discharges. After uptake of EBs, the EB transitions into the RB, which replicates by binary fission in a membrane-enclosed vacuole called an inclusion and avoids lysosomal fusion. The RBs then transition back to the EB form, which is released into the extracellular milieu after cell lysis occurs and subsequently infect other host cells. The entire replication cycle takes about 2 days to complete (see Figure 33-1).[22]

Chlamydiae primarily infect epithelial cells, but they can also infect a variety of other cell types including endothelial cells, smooth muscle cells, lymphocytes, monocytes, and macrophages. *C. felis* replicates in the cytoplasm of conjunctival epithelial cells, but also spreads via the bloodstream to a variety of other tissues, such as the tonsil, lung, liver, spleen, gastrointestinal tract, and kidney.[23] Infection is typically followed 2 to 5 days later by the development of acute, chronic, or recurrent conjunctivitis, with or without signs of rhinitis such as nasal discharge and sneezing. Most cats remain otherwise well and appetent. Lower respiratory tract signs such as cough and dyspnea rarely, if ever, occur. Corneal disease such as keratitis or corneal ulceration is rare and, if present, is likely caused by other or co-infecting pathogens such as FHV-1. Experimental inoculations have also been followed by signs of fever, lethargy, lameness and joint pain (possibly due to polyarthritis), and weight loss, in addition to conjunctivitis.[24] There are also rare reports of gastritis and peritonitis in association with the detection of chlamydia-like organisms in cats.[25,26]

After the initial episode of acute conjunctivitis, infection may persist for many months. This may be accompanied by mild conjunctivitis or, in some cases, no clinical signs of disease. Organisms can be isolated from the conjunctiva for up to 215 days after experimental infection.[27,28] Whether chronic disease is the result of repeated reinfection or the presence of persistent chlamydiae is unclear. Co-infections with other agents such as FCV, FHV-1, *Bordetella,* or *Mycoplasma* may increase the severity of disease and duration of shedding. Other bacteria, including those that normally colonize the healthy conjunctival sac, also act as secondary invaders and worsen disease.

Whether *C. felis* causes reproductive disease in cats remains unclear. The stage of pregnancy at which infection occurs, co-infection with other organisms such as FHV-1, concurrent immunosuppression, route of infection, and the strain involved may be important in determining the ability of *C. felis* to cause reproductive dysfunction, if this indeed occurs in cats.

Chlamydial infections are infrequently described in dogs. *Chlamydia psittaci* has been detected in dogs with respiratory disease, such as pneumonia and pleural effusion, and/or keratoconjunctivitis.[6-8] One group of bitches that had ocular and lower respiratory signs as well as stillbirths and low litter size had nasal, conjunctival, and pharyngeal swab specimens that tested positive for *C. psittaci* with a PCR assay.[6] *Chlamydia abortus* was detected in a dog with keratoconjunctivitis.[9] The DNA of *C. pneumoniae* was detected in atherosclerotic lesions from dogs in Japan,[10] and chlamydia-like organisms were found in a dog from South Africa with polyarthritis.[11]

Physical Examination Findings

Physical examination findings in cats with chlamydiosis include conjunctivitis, chemosis, serous to mucopurulent ocular discharge, and blepharospasm (Figure 33-2). Signs of nasal involvement, such as stertorous respiration, serous or mucopurulent nasal discharge, and sneezing, may accompany conjunctivitis. Mucopurulent vaginal discharge has been reported in some cats that were experimentally infected by topical ophthalmic inoculation.

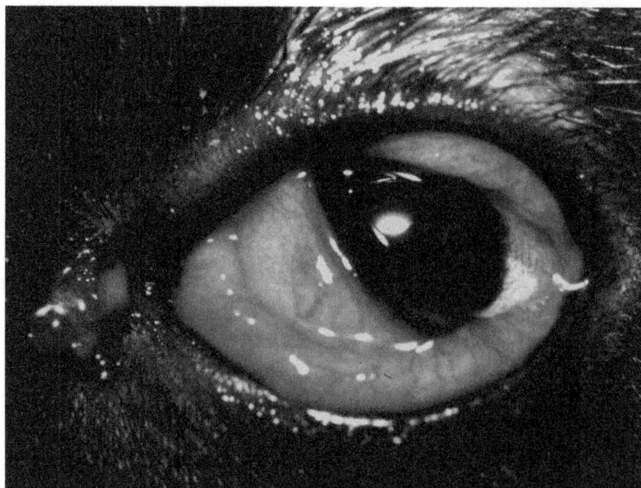

FIGURE 33-2 Domestic shorthair cat with acute chlamydial conjunctivitis. Marked hyperemia and chemosis are present, as well as serous to mucopurulent ocular discharge.

Physical examination findings described in dogs with chlamydiosis have included fever, tachypnea, keratoconjunctivitis with mucopurulent ocular discharge, shifting leg lameness, and lymphadenopathy.[6-9,11]

Diagnosis

There are no clinically significant laboratory abnormalities in cats with chlamydiosis, and there is insufficient information on laboratory abnormalities that might occur in affected dogs. Diagnosis of chlamydiosis is most often based on the results of molecular testing using PCR assays (Table 33-2). For all diagnostic tests that detect chlamydial organisms, sufficient numbers of infected epithelial cells must be collected. This generally involves vigorous swabbing of infected mucosal sites such as the conjunctiva.

Microbiologic Tests

Cytologic Examination for Inclusions

Using light microscopy, chlamydial intracytoplasmic inclusions may be seen in epithelial cells that are present in smears of conjunctival scrapings. Inclusions are made up of basophilic clusters of coccoid bacteria and are up to 10 μm in diameter (Figure 33-3). Giemsa is the preferred staining method. Inclusions are only generally visible early, if at all, during the course of infection, so this method is insensitive. Also, melanin granules in the cytoplasm of conjunctival epithelial cells can yield false-positive results. The use of direct fluorescent antibody staining or immunocytochemical stains that detect *Chlamydia* increases sensitivity and specificity.

Enzyme-Linked Immunosorbent Assay Antigen Detection

A variety of commercial antigen detection enzyme immunoassay kits have been developed and marketed for diagnosis of human chlamydial infections. Nucleic acid amplification tests have now

TABLE 33-2

Diagnostic Assays Available for Chlamydiosis in Dogs and Cats

Assay	Specimen Type	Target	Performance
Cell culture	Conjunctival swabs	*Chlamydia* spp.	Not widely offered or utilized for routine diagnostic purposes. Requires special chlamydial transport media. False negatives occur when organisms lose viability during transport or in chronic infections, when organism numbers are very low.
Cytology	Conjunctival smears	Chlamydial inclusions	Low sensitivity. Inclusions are most likely to be seen early in infection. False positives can occur when cytoplasmic granules are mistaken for inclusions. Fluorescent or immunoperoxidase antibody techniques may increase sensitivity and specificity.
Serology	Serum	Antibodies to *Chlamydia* spp.	Acute and convalescent serology is required for diagnosis of acute infection. Vaccination may interfere with interpretation of results. Not widely available or utilized worldwide.
PCR	Conjunctival swabs, scrapings, or biopsies	*Chlamydia felis* DNA or *Chlamydia* spp. DNA	Confirms active infection. Assays may be genus or species specific. Sensitivity and specificity may vary depending on assay design and specimen type. Because healthy animals occasionally test PCR positive, positive PCR results must be interpreted in light of the clinical signs. Vaccination with attenuated live chlamydial vaccines has the potential to interfere with results.

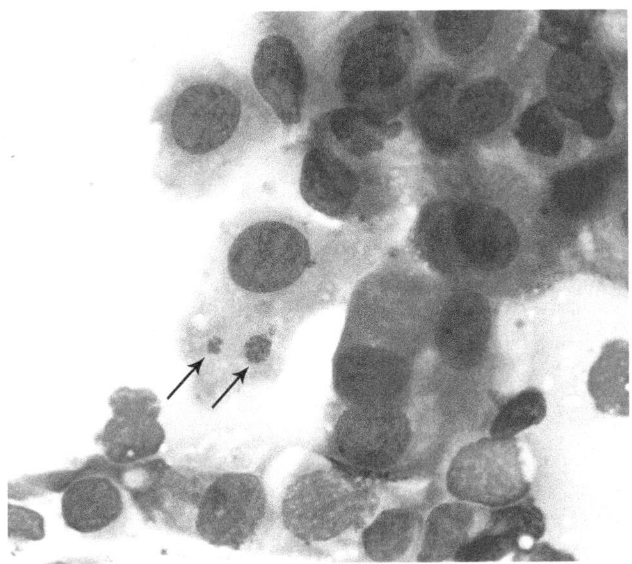

FIGURE 33-3 Conjunctival scraping from a cat with chlamydial conjunctivitis. Inclusions of *Chlamydia felis* are found in an epithelial cell *(arrows)*. Wright's stain, original magnification 1000×. (Courtesy of Judith Taylor, LabVet Consultations, Inc., Guelph, Ontario, Canada and Karen M. Young, University of Wisconsin-Madison. In Young KM, Taylor JJ: Laboratory medicine: yesterday today tomorrow: eye on the cytoplasm, Vet Clin Pathol 35:141, 2006.)

largely replaced the use of these assays for diagnosis of human infections. Antibodies used in ELISA assays that are designed to detect human chlamydial pathogens in swab specimens (such as conjunctival swabs) cross-react with *C. felis* antigen and so have also been used for diagnosis of feline chlamydiosis. Unfortunately, the kits have varied considerably in their sensitivity and specificity. In general, ELISA methods that detect chlamydial antigen have lower sensitivity and specificity than cell culture, direct fluorescent antibody methods, or PCR assays for detection of *C. felis*.

Cell Culture

Cell culture has traditionally been considered the gold standard for chlamydial diagnosis, but is now mostly performed on a research basis. Isolations from cats are usually highest from conjunctival swabs, although nasal and pharyngeal swab specimens may also contain infectious organisms. To enhance organism survival, swabs should be placed immediately in a chlamydial transport medium such as 2SP (0.2 M sucrose and 0.02 M phosphate), which can be obtained from laboratories that perform chlamydial culture. Routine viral transport media should not be used, because it contains antibiotics that inactivate the organisms. The specimen should be refrigerated (4°C) if it is not immediately sent to the laboratory and ideally should reach the laboratory within 24 hours of specimen collection. In the laboratory, organisms are readily grown in the yolk sacs of embryonating eggs or in cell lines such as McCoy or HeLa cells over a period of 2 to 3 days. Fluorescent antibody is then used to identify chlamydial inclusions within the infected cell culture (Figure 33-4).

Molecular Diagnosis Using the Polymerase Chain Reaction

The use of PCR-based assays has revolutionized diagnosis of chlamydial infections in animals and humans, because these assays are rapid, sensitive, and specific and do not require special transport conditions. Sequence analysis of PCR products can be used to differentiate between species of Chlamydiaceae. Both conventional and real-time PCR assays have been used to detect *C. felis* in conjunctival swab specimens from cats,[29-31] and real-time PCR assays that detect *C. felis* are now offered by several commercial veterinary diagnostic laboratories worldwide.

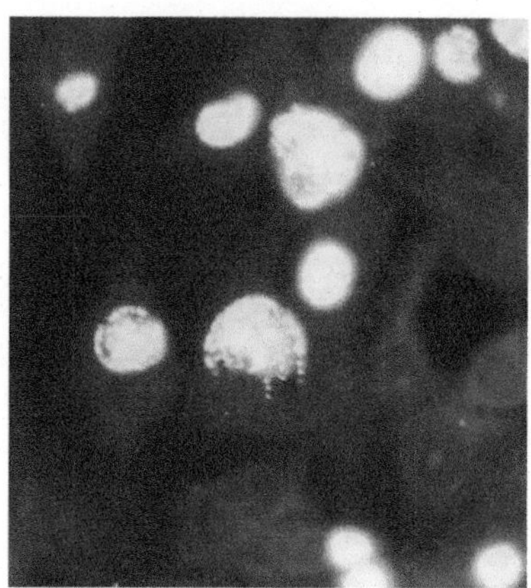

FIGURE 33-4 Chlamydial inclusions stained with fluorescent antibody in a mccoy cell monolayer. (Courtesy of Robert Suchland, Seattle, In Stamm WE, Batteiger BE. Introduction to *Chlamydia* and *Chlamydophila*. In: Mandell GL, Bennett JE, Dolin R, eds. Mandell, Douglas and Bennett's Principles and Practice of Infectious Diseases, 7 ed. Philadelphia, PA: Churchill Livingstone Elsevier; 2011.)

Unfortunately, considerable interlaboratory variation in assay performance still exists.[32] In addition, PCR assays for *C. felis* may not detect other chlamydial species, such as *C. pneumoniae*. Genus- or family-specific chlamydial PCR assays must be used to detect these organisms. The laboratory should be consulted to determine the specificity of the assay used. The use of a DNA microarray assay for detection and identification of chlamydiae in cats has also been reported.[5] The microarray assay consists of a chip that carries chlamydial species- and genus-specific probes. DNA within the specimen is first amplified and biotin labeled with PCR, and then reacted with the microarray probes.[33]

PCR assays for *C. felis* are usually more sensitive compared with cell culture for diagnosis of infection in naturally infected cats (see Table 33-1).[29] During antimicrobial treatment of infected cats, PCR assay results continue to be positive for several days.[29,30] Topical ophthalmic solutions such as proxymetacaine and fluorescein did not interfere with the ability of real-time PCR to detect *C. felis*, but there was a slight inhibitory effect when fusidic acid was used.[34] Because cats without signs of conjunctivitis occasionally test PCR positive for *C. felis*, the results of PCR must be interpreted in light of the history, clinical signs present, and response to appropriate treatment.

Serologic Testing

Serologic tests are not widely available for routine diagnosis of chlamydial infections. Assays that detect serum antibodies to chlamydiae, such as IFA or ELISA assays, are of limited benefit for detection of active infection because the IgG antibody titer increase is variable or prolonged, and IgM antibody titers are inconsistently increased. However, very high antibody titers (≥1:512) have been associated with clinical illness and/or chlamydial shedding, and high antibody titers among group-housed cats with conjunctivitis can suggest a role for *C. felis* in disease.[13,23,35] Chlamydial infections persist in the presence of high serum antibody titers, so positive antibody titers after vaccination do not imply protection. Serial titers may be needed to document active infections, and recent vaccination may interfere with interpretation of positive titer results. An ELISA assay that discriminates between the antibody response from vaccination and that from natural infection has been described but is not widely available on a commercial basis.[36]

TABLE 33-3

Suggested Medications for Treatment of Cats with Ocular Chlamydiosis

Drug	Dose	Route	Interval (hours)	Duration
Doxycycline*	10 mg/kg	PO	24	At least 4 weeks, or 2 weeks after resolution of clinical signs
Amoxicillin-clavulanate	12.5	PO	12	4 weeks
Pradofloxacin	5-7.5†	PO	24	6 weeks

*Doxycycline is the treatment of choice. For cats that fail to tolerate doxycycline, amoxicillin-clavulanate should be used. Fluoroquinolones are an option for cats that do not tolerate doxycycline or amoxicillin-clavulanate.

†Dose is for the oral suspension; if tablets are used, the dose is lower (3 mg/kg).

Treatment and Prognosis

Chlamydial infections are generally treated with tetracycline antibiotics. Oral administration of doxycycline at 5 to 10 mg/kg q12h for 3 to 4 weeks results in clinical resolution in most cats. A dose of 10 mg/kg q24h can also be used (Table 33-3).[23] Clinical improvement occurs within 24 to 48 hours after treatment is initiated. In colonies of cats, all cats should be treated for 4 weeks: in one study that used real-time PCR to detect infection, a 3-week course of treatment was insufficient to clear infection in some cats, but treatment for 28 days subsequently cleared infection in all cats.[30] Treatment for up to 6 to 8 weeks may be required. Regardless, treatment should continue for at least 2 weeks after the resolution of clinical signs.

Failure to respond completely to treatment may reflect the concurrent presence of viral upper respiratory tract pathogens. Because administration of doxycycline hyclate can result in esophagitis and esophageal stricture formation, the administration of doxycycline hyclate tablets should be followed by a bolus of water or food (see Chapter 8 for additional information on doxycycline). Ocular infections may initially respond to tetracycline eye ointment applied two or three times daily,[37] but recurrent infections have been documented,[38] likely because systemic infection with chlamydiae can occur in cats with conjunctivitis.

For cats that do not tolerate doxycycline, 4 weeks of amoxicillin-clavulanate is a suitable alternative.[39] In experimentally infected cats, the efficacy of enrofloxacin (5 mg/kg PO q24h for 14 days) was similar to that of doxycycline as determined with direct fluorescent antibody on conjunctival swabs, although a few cats in both the doxycycline and enrofloxacin groups had evidence of persistent infection at the end of the treatment period.[40] Doxycycline is preferred because of concerns that relate to the possibility of retinal toxicity in cats treated with enrofloxacin. Doxycycline was more efficacious than pradofloxacin in experimentally infected cats that were monitored with a PCR assay.[41] Sulfonamides or chloramphenicol are ineffective, and in vitro, penicillin is only inhibitory at higher doses. Treatment with azithromycin is also incompletely effective when compared with doxycycline.[42]

Immunity and Vaccination

Kittens acquire maternal antibodies to *C. felis* that usually protect them from infection until 7 to 9 weeks of age. Both humoral and cell-mediated mechanisms provide protective immunity in chlamydial infections of other host species. Natural infection seems to confer little protection against reinfection, and this protection appears to be short-lived. However, given the low prevalence of chlamydiosis in older cats, an age-related resistance to chlamydiosis appears to exist. Both inactivated and attenuated live vaccines are available to protect cats from chlamydial respiratory disease. These vaccines do not entirely prevent infection and shedding of chlamydiae after challenge, but they minimize the replication of the organism and hence reduce the severity of clinical signs. Transient fever, anorexia, lethargy, and lameness has been described 1 to 3 weeks after use of combined vaccines containing attenuated live *C. felis* in a low percentage of cats. Chlamydial vaccines are noncore vaccines that are recommended for cats with a high risk of acquiring infection, such as those introduced to or that reside in catteries with documented endemic chlamydiosis. These cats should be vaccinated regularly after initial treatment of all cats with appropriate antimicrobial drugs.

Prevention

Given that chlamydiae survive poorly in the environment and the major route of transmission is close contact, transmission can be minimized by good hygiene, quarantine, single housing, and disinfection practices in cattery situations. Chlamydiae are readily inactivated by detergent solutions.

Public Health Aspects

The most significant chlamydial pathogens of humans are *C. trachomatis*, *C. pneumoniae*, and *C. psittaci*. *C. trachomatis* causes trachoma, the leading cause of infectious blindness worldwide, and it also is the most common bacterial cause of sexually transmitted diseases in humans.[22] *C. pneumoniae* may infect nearly all humans, and is an important cause of community-acquired pneumonia worldwide. It has also been implicated in atherosclerotic cardiovascular disease, although its role in this condition remains unclear. *C. psittaci* causes psittacosis in birds and humans, a potentially life-threatening zoonosis.

C. felis has long been suspected as a cause of conjunctivitis in humans. However, many of the reports of human infection with *C. felis* before the advent of genetic detection methods remain unconfirmed, because diagnosis was based either on culture, without identification to the species level, or on serologic testing, which has the potential to cross-react with other chlamydiae and organisms such as *Bartonella*. More recently, molecular assays have been used to confirm *C. felis* infection in humans. *C. felis* was detected in the conjunctiva of a person with conjunctivitis.[24] The organism was genetically indistinguishable from an isolate later recovered from the patient's cat. Although these associations have been difficult to document, routine precautions should be taken when handling cats with conjunctivitis, especially young cats with chronic conjunctivitis. Proper hand washing and routine cleaning and disinfection are likely to be sufficient to prevent transmission.

The identification of *C. psittaci* in dogs with respiratory disease and *C. pneumoniae* in cats with ocular disease suggests that dogs and cats may have the potential to be a source of these pathogens for humans, although avian species and other infected people, respectively, are likely to be much more significant sources of infection.

CASE EXAMPLE

Signalment: "Sam," a 3-year-old male neutered domestic shorthair cat from Davis, CA

History: Sam was brought to the University of California, Davis, by a veterinary student for evaluation of fever, right thoracic limb lameness, and bilateral conjunctivitis with mucopurulent ocular discharge of 2 days' duration. No coughing, sneezing, vomiting, diarrhea, or abnormal thirst or urination had been noted. Sam lived indoors with 5 other cats, 3 of which had also had severe conjunctivitis, ocular discharge, fever, lethargy, and lameness for the last week. These 3 cats ranged from 8 months to 2.5 years of age. All of the cats had been vaccinated regularly for FHV-1, FCV, and feline panleukopenia virus and tested retrovirus-negative as kittens. They were all fed a commercial dry cat food.

Physical Examination:

Body Weight: 6.7 kg

General: Bright, alert and responsive, hydrated. T = 103.6°F (39.7°C), P = 240 beats/min, respiratory rate 66 breaths/min, mucous membranes pink, CRT = 1 s.

Eyes, Ears, Nose, and Throat: There was no evidence of ocular discharge, but mild conjunctival hyperemia was present. The nasal planum was clean and moist with no discharge; no oral erosions or ulcerations were seen.

Musculoskeletal: Body condition score 7/9. Decreased weight bearing on the left thoracic limb was noted, and the cat sometimes held his left thoracic limb up when sitting. There was possible mild effusion in the left elbow and resentment on flexion of the left carpus and both elbows.

All Other Systems: No clinically significant abnormalities were detected.

Laboratory Findings:

CBC:

HCT 46.3% (30%-50%)
MCV 46.9 fL (42-53 fL)
MCHC 30.7 g/dL (30-33.5 g/dL)
WBC 10,500 cells/μL (4500-14,000 cells/μL)
Neutrophils 7455 cells/μL (2000-9000 cells/μL)
Lymphocytes 2310 cells/μL (1000-7000 cells/μL)
Monocytes 525 cells/μL (50-600 cells/μL)
Eosinophils 210 cells/μL (150-1100 cells/μL)
Basophils 0 cells/μL (0-50 cells/μL)
Platelets 174,000/μL (180,000-500,000 platelets/μL), with moderate macroplatelets.

Serum Chemistry Profile:
Sodium 152 mmol/L (151-158 mmol/L)
Potassium 4.4 mmol/L (3.6-4.9 mmol/L)
Chloride 117 mmol/L (117-126 mmol/L)
Bicarbonate 18 mmol/L (15-21 mmol/L)
Phosphorus 4.0 mg/dL (3.2-6.3 mg/dL)
Calcium 9.5 mg/dL (9.0-10.9 mg/dl)
BUN 21 mg/dL (18-33 mg/dL)
Creatinine 1.6 mg/dL (1.1-2.2 mg/dL)
Glucose 151 mg/dL (63-118 mg/dL)
Total protein 7.1 g/dL (6.6-8.4 g/dL)
Albumin 3.1 g/dL (2.2-4.6 g/dL)
Globulin 4.0 g/dL (2.8-5.4 g/dL)
ALT 48 U/L (27-101 U/L)
AST 8 U/L (17-58 U/L)
ALP 31 U/L (14-71 U/L)
Gamma GT 0 U/L (0-4 U/L)
Cholesterol 154 mg/dL (89-258 mg/dL)
Total bilirubin 0.2 mg/dL (0-0.2 mg/dL).

Urinalysis: SGr 1.055; pH 6.5, trace protein, no hemoprotein, glucose, ketones or bilirubin, 0-1 WBC/HPF, 0-2 RBC/HPF, few lipid droplets.

Synovial Fluid Cytology: Synovial fluid from the right stifle, right carpus, left carpus, and right tarsus was examined. All specimens apart from that from the left carpus were markedly blood contaminated and so could not be properly evaluated. The cell counts in those specimens ranged from 2000 to 4000 nucleated cells/μL and consisted predominantly of neutrophils (66%-80%) and small mononuclear cells (7%-18%). The specimen from the left carpus had 2000 nucleated cells/μL, of which 14% were neutrophils, 85% large mononuclear cells, and 1% small mononuclear cells. There were moderate numbers of erythrocytes and blood-associated leukocytes, as well as low numbers of large mononuclear cells of normal morphology, which was consistent with mild blood contamination.

Conjunctival Smear Cytology: Chlamydial inclusions were visualized within several epithelial cells.

Imaging Findings: Radiographs of the left radius and ulna, including carpus and elbow joints: no radiographic abnormalities.

Microbiologic Testing: FeLV antigen and FIV antibody serology: negative
PCR for FCV (oropharyngeal swab specimens): negative
Mycoplasma culture (conjunctival swab specimen): negative

Diagnosis: A tentative diagnosis of chlamydial conjunctivitis and arthritis was made.

Treatment and Outcome: Treatment of all cats in the household with doxycycline (10 mg/kg PO q24h) was initiated. This was associated with rapid resolution of fever, ocular signs, and lameness.

Comments: The cats in this household had conjunctivitis and possibly arthritis in association with chlamydial infection. The major differential diagnosis was FCV infection, which is more widespread than chlamydiosis and for which an association between lameness and infection has been described. Infection with *Mycoplasma* spp. has also been associated with conjunctivitis as well as synovitis in cats (see Chapter 40). Lameness has developed in cats that were experimentally infected with *C. felis*, but there are no reports of lameness in association with natural infection. The negative PCR and culture results for FCV and *Mycoplasma* spp., respectively, could not definitively rule out infection with these agents. The presence of chlamydial inclusions in the conjunctival smear supported a diagnosis of chlamydiosis, but false positives can occur, and unfortunately PCR was not performed to confirm the presence of a chlamydial agent. Nevertheless, the rapid response to doxycycline supported the possibility of a bacterial cause of the arthritis. Interestingly, thrombocytopenia was present (and confirmed on smear evaluation), which has been reported in humans with chlamydial infections.[43]

SUGGESTED READINGS

Gruffydd-Jones T, Addie D, Belak S, et al. *Chlamydophila felis* infection. ABCD guidelines on prevention and management. J Feline Med Surg. 2009;11:605-609.

Laroucau K, Di Francesco A, Vorimore F, et al. Multilocus variable-number tandem-repeat analysis scheme for *Chlamydia felis* genotyping: comparison with multilocus sequence typing. J Clin Microbiol. 2012;50(6):1860-1866.

Sibitz C, Rudnay EC, Wabnegger L, et al. Detection of *Chlamydophila pneumoniae* in cats with conjunctivitis. Vet Ophthalmol. 2011;14(suppl 1):67-74.

REFERENCES

1. Baker JA. A virus causing pneumonia in cats and producing elementary bodies. J Exp Med. 1944;79(2):159-172.
2. Stephens RS, Myers G, Eppinger M, et al. Divergence without difference: phylogenetics and taxonomy of *Chlamydia* resolved. FEMS Immunol Med Microbiol. 2009;55:115-119.
3. Dean D, Kandel RP, Adhikari HK, et al. Multiple Chlamydiaceae species in trachoma: implications for disease pathogenesis and control. PLoS Med. 2008;5:e14.
4. Sibitz C, Rudnay EC, Wabnegger L, et al. Detection of *Chlamydophila pneumoniae* in cats with conjunctivitis. Vet Ophthalmol. 2011;14(suppl 1):67-74.
5. Sostaric-Zuckermann IC, Borel N, Kaiser C, et al. *Chlamydia* in canine or feline coronary arteriosclerotic lesions. BMC Res Notes. 2011;4:350.
6. Sprague LD, Schubert E, Hotzel H, et al. The detection of *Chlamydophila psittaci* genotype C infection in dogs. Vet J. 2009;181:274-279.
7. Gresham AC, Dixon CE, Bevan BJ. Domiciliary outbreak of psittacosis in dogs: potential for zoonotic infection. Vet Rec. 1996;138:622-623.
8. Arizmendi F, Grimes JE, Relford RL. Isolation of *Chlamydia psittaci* from pleural effusion in a dog. J Vet Diagn Invest. 1992;4:460-463.
9. Hoelzle K, Wittenbrink MM, Corboz L, et al. *Chlamydophila abortus*-induced keratoconjunctivitis in a dog. Vet Rec. 2005;157:632-633.
10. Sako T, Takahashi T, Takehana K, et al. Chlamydial infection in canine atherosclerotic lesions. Atherosclerosis. 2002;162:253-259.
11. Lambrechts N, Picard J, Tustin RC. *Chlamydia*-induced septic polyarthritis in a dog. J S Afr Vet Assoc. 1999;70:40-42.
12. Laroucau K, Di Francesco A, Vorimore F, et al. Multilocus variable-number tandem-repeat analysis scheme for *Chlamydia felis* genotyping: comparison with multilocus sequence typing. J Clin Microbiol. 2012;50(6):1860-1866.

13. Low HC, Powell CC, Veir JK, et al. Prevalence of feline herpesvirus 1, *Chlamydophila felis*, and *Mycoplasma* spp. DNA in conjunctival cells collected from cats with and without conjunctivitis. Am J Vet Res. 2007;68:643-648.
14. Wills JM, Howard PE, Gruffydd-Jones TJ, et al. Prevalence of *Chlamydia psittaci* in different cat populations in Britain. J Small Anim Pract. 1988;29:327-339.
15. Kang BT, Park HM. Prevalence of feline herpesvirus 1, feline calicivirus and *Chlamydophila felis* in clinically normal cats at a Korean animal shelter. J Vet Sci. 2008;9:207-209.
16. Veir JK, Ruch-Gallie R, Spindel ME, et al. Prevalence of selected infectious organisms and comparison of two anatomic sampling sites in shelter cats with upper respiratory tract disease. J Feline Med Surg. 2008;10:551-557.
17. Maggs DJ, Sykes JE, Clarke HE, et al. Effects of dietary lysine supplementation in cats with enzootic upper respiratory disease. J Feline Med Surg. 2007;9:97-108.
18. Bannasch MJ, Foley JE. Epidemiologic evaluation of multiple respiratory pathogens in cats in animal shelters. J Feline Med Surg. 2005;7:109-119.
19. Helps CR, Lait P, Damhuis A, et al. Factors associated with upper respiratory tract disease caused by feline herpesvirus, feline calicivirus, *Chlamydophila felis* and *Bordetella bronchiseptica* in cats: experience from 218 European catteries. Vet Rec. 2005;156:669-673.
20. von Bomhard W, Polkinghorne A, Lu ZH, et al. Detection of novel chlamydiae in cats with ocular disease. Am J Vet Res. 2003;64:1421-1428.
21. Richter M, Matheis F, Gonczi E, et al. *Parachlamydia acanthamoebae* in domestic cats with and without corneal disease. Vet Ophthalmol. 2010;13:235-237.
22. Saka HA, Thompson JW, Chen YS, et al. Quantitative proteomics reveals metabolic and pathogenic properties of *Chlamydia trachomatis* developmental forms. Mol Microbiol. 2011;82:1185-1203.
23. Gruffydd-Jones T, Addie D, Belak S, et al. *Chlamydophila felis* infection. ABCD guidelines on prevention and management. J Feline Med Surg. 2009;11:605-609.
24. TerWee J, Sabara M, Kokjohn K, et al. Characterization of the systemic disease and ocular signs induced by experimental infection with *Chlamydia psittaci* in cats. Vet Microbiol. 1998;59:259-281.
25. Dickie CW, Sniff ES. *Chlamydia* infection associated with peritonitis in a cat. J Am Vet Med Assoc. 1980;176:1256-1259.
26. Hargis AM, Prieur DJ, Gaillard ET. Chlamydial infection of the gastric mucosa in twelve cats. Vet Pathol. 1983;20:170-178.
27. Wills JM. Chlamydial infection in the cat. University of Bristol: PhD Thesis; 1986.
28. O'Dair HA, Hopper CD, Gruffydd-Jones TJ, et al. Clinical aspects of *Chlamydia psittaci* infection in cats infected with feline immunodeficiency virus. Vet Rec. 1994;134:365-368.
29. Sykes JE, Studdert VP, Browning GF. Comparison of the polymerase chain reaction and culture for the detection of feline *Chlamydia psittaci* in untreated and doxycycline-treated experimentally infected cats. J Vet Intern Med. 1999;13:146-152.
30. Dean R, Harley R, Helps C, et al. Use of quantitative real-time PCR to monitor the response of *Chlamydophila felis* infection to doxycycline treatment. J Clin Microbiol. 2005;43:1858-1864.
31. Helps C, Reeves N, Tasker S, et al. Use of real-time quantitative PCR to detect *Chlamydophila felis* infection. J Clin Microbiol. 2001;39:2675-2676.
32. Sandmeyer LS, Waldner CL, Bauer BS, et al. Comparison of polymerase chain reaction tests for diagnosis of feline herpesvirus, *Chlamydophila felis*, and *Mycoplasma* spp. infection in cats with ocular disease in Canada. Can Vet J. 2010;51:629-633.
33. Borel N, Kempf E, Hotzel H, et al. Direct identification of chlamydiae from clinical samples using a DNA microarray assay: a validation study. Mol Cell Probes. 2008;22:55-64.
34. Segarra S, Papasouliotis K, Helps C. The in vitro effects of proxymetacaine, fluorescein, and fusidic acid on real-time PCR assays used for the diagnosis of feline herpesvirus 1 and *Chlamydophila felis* infections. Vet Ophthalmol. 2011;14 (suppl 1):5-8.
35. Strom Holst B, Krook L, Englund S, et al. Shedding of chlamydiae in relation to titers of serum chlamydiae-specific antibodies and serum concentrations of two acute-phase proteins in cats without conjunctivitis. Am J Vet Res. 2011;72:806-812.
36. Ohya K, Okuda H, Maeda S, et al. Using CF0218-ELISA to distinguish *Chlamydophila felis*-infected cats from vaccinated and uninfected domestic cats. Vet Microbiol. 2010;146:366-370.
37. Sparkes AH, Caney SM, Sturgess CP, et al. The clinical efficacy of topical and systemic therapy for the treatment of feline ocular chlamydiosis. J Feline Med Surg. 1999;1:31-35.
38. Donati M, Piva S, Di Francesco A, et al. Feline ocular chlamydiosis: clinical and microbiological effects of topical and systemic therapy. New Microbiol. 2005;28:369-372.
39. Sturgess CP, Gruffydd-Jones TJ, Harbour DA, et al. Controlled study of the efficacy of clavulanic acid-potentiated amoxicillin in the treatment of *Chlamydia psittaci* in cats. Vet Rec. 2001;149:73-76.
40. Gerhardt N, Schulz BS, Werckenthin C, et al. Pharmacokinetics of enrofloxacin and its efficacy in comparison with doxycycline in the treatment of *Chlamydophila felis* infection in cats with conjunctivitis. Vet Rec. 2006;159:591-594.
41. Hartmann AD, Helps CR, Lappin MR, et al. Efficacy of pradofloxacin in cats with feline upper respiratory tract disease due to *Chlamydophila felis* or *Mycoplasma* infections. J Vet Intern Med. 2008;22:44-52.
42. Owen WM, Sturgess CP, Harbour DA, et al. Efficacy of azithromycin for the treatment of feline chlamydophilosis. J Feline Med Surg. 2003;5:305-311.
43. Day CJE, Fawcett IW. Psittacosis and acute thrombocytopenic purpura. J R Soc Med. 1992;85(6):360-361.

CHAPTER 34

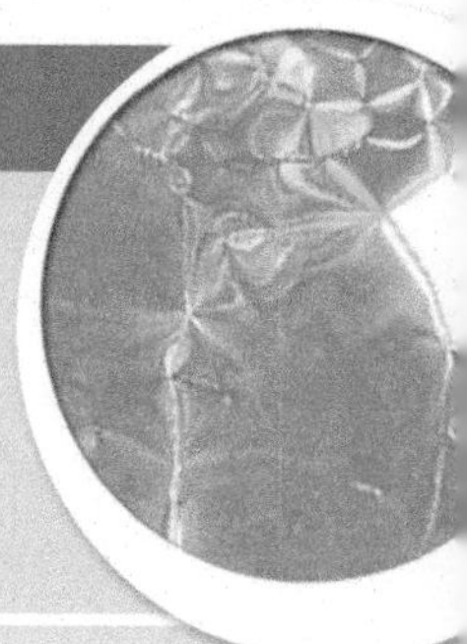

Streptococcal and Enterococcal Infections

Jane E. Sykes

> **Overview of Streptococcal and Enterococcal Infections**
>
> First Described: Streptococci were first described in Germany in 1868 by Billroth.[1] Enterococci were separated from the genus *Streptococcus* in 1984.[2]
>
> Major Causes: In dogs and cats, the most common causes are *Streptococcus canis, Streptococcus equi* subsp. *zooepidemicus, Enterococcus faecium,* and *Enterococcus faecalis,* which are gram-positive coccoid bacteria
>
> Geographic Distribution: Worldwide
>
> Mode of Transmission: Direct contact. Organisms are usually commensals that invade opportunistically.
>
> Major Clinical Signs: Neonatal septicemia, pharyngitis, cervical lymphadenitis, bacteremia and endocarditis, urinary tract infections, postoperative incision or wound infections, otitis externa, keratitis, bronchopneumonia, pyometra or metritis, meningoencephalitis, necrotizing fasciitis and toxic shock syndrome (primarily *S. canis*), rhinitis and necrotizing sinusitis, pyothorax, discospondylitis, arthritis, osteomyelitis, mastitis, cholangiohepatitis, and peritonitis
>
> Differential Diagnoses: Primarily other gram-positive and gram-negative bacterial infections
>
> Human Health Significance: Streptococcal species that infect dogs and cats occasionally infect human patients. Dogs and cats may also have the potential to serve as sources of multidrug-resistant enterococcal infections for humans.

Etiology, Epidemiology, and Clinical Features

Streptococci are catalase-negative, gram-positive cocci that divide along a single axis, forming pairs and chains of organisms (Figures 34-1 and 34-2). They are facultative to strict anaerobes that require complex media for growth, preferably supplemented with blood. More than 40 species of streptococci have been described. Species of streptococci vary in host tropism and virulence properties, and so it is important that they be discussed separately. One of the most important streptococcal pathogens of humans, *Streptococcus pyogenes,* which causes streptococcal pharyngitis ("strep throat"), does not infect dogs and cats to a significant degree (see Public Health Aspects). However, interspecies transmission has been reported for some pathogenic streptococci such as *Streptococcus pneumoniae* and *Streptococcus equi* subsp. *zooepidemicus.* As is the case in humans, streptococci that infect dogs and cats range from commensals of low virulence through to highly virulent organisms that can cause severe disease manifestations and death.

Streptococci have been classified based on their hemolytic properties into β-hemolytic streptococci, which cause complete hemolysis when they grow on blood agar; γ-hemolytic or nonhemolytic streptococci, which do not cause hemolysis; and α-hemolytic streptococci, which reduce hemoglobin, causing a greenish discoloration of the agar around bacterial colonies. Streptococci are also classified from A through W based on their surface antigens (Lancefield classification system) and classified based on phenotypic characteristics (such as pyogenic or viridans group streptococci). Major pathogenic streptococci of dogs and cats belong to Lancefield groups B, C, D, or G (Table 34-1). Pyogenic streptococci are β-hemolytic streptococci that belong to Lancefield groups A *(S. pyogenes),* B *(Streptococcus agalactiae),* C (which includes *Streptococcus dysgalactiae* and *S. equi* subsp. *zooepidemicus*), and G (which includes *Streptococcus canis*). Viridans streptococci are often nonhemolytic or α-hemolytic (*viridis* = Latin for green) and tend to be commensals that have low virulence and rarely invade tissues opportunistically. Many group D streptococci have now been classified as enterococci. Molecular typing schemes have revealed that hemolytic reactions, Lancefield antigens, and phenotypic characteristics do not necessarily predict genetic relatedness among

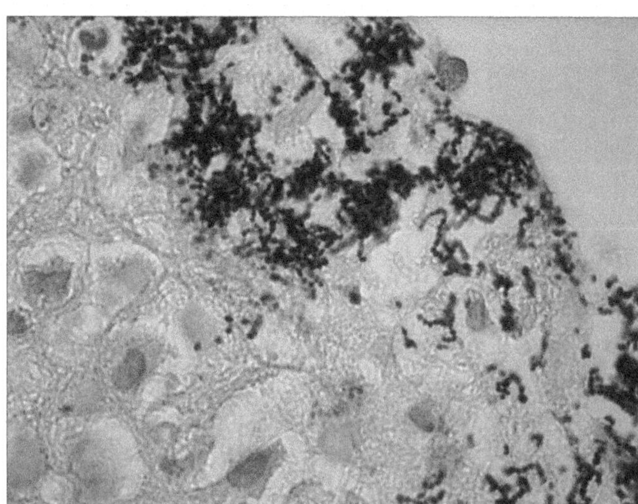

FIGURE 34-1 Histopathology of the serosal surface of the liver of a 12-day-old domestic shorthair kitten that was euthanized after it was found hypothermic and tachypneic. Severe suppurative omphalophlebitis and peritonitis was present. Lesions contained numerous chains of gram-positive cocci. Brown and Benn stain, 1000× oil magnification.

streptococcal strains. Nevertheless, these traditional classification methods are still used by laboratory staff, microbiologists, and clinicians to describe streptococci.

Streptococci invade tissues opportunistically when there is a breach in normal host barriers. This leads to a variety of clinical disease manifestations, such as pyoderma, pneumonia, endocarditis, arthritis, osteomyelitis, meningoencephalitis, cellulitis, and urinary tract infections (UTIs). Severe and life-threatening manifestations of streptococcal infection include necrotizing fasciitis (NF) and streptococcal toxic shock syndrome (STSS). Predisposing conditions for streptococcal infections in dogs and cats may include atopic dermatitis, wounds, foreign bodies (such as migrating grass awns), immunosuppressive drug treatment, and young age (especially neonates).[3] The most common clinical presentation among fetuses and neonates is streptococcal bacteremia and sepsis, which can result in abortion and death. Streptococcal pneumonia may occur in association with infections with other respiratory pathogens, such as respiratory viruses, or occur secondary to bronchitis, hematogenous spread or aspiration. In one study, streptococci were isolated from sick dogs more frequently in summer months.[3]

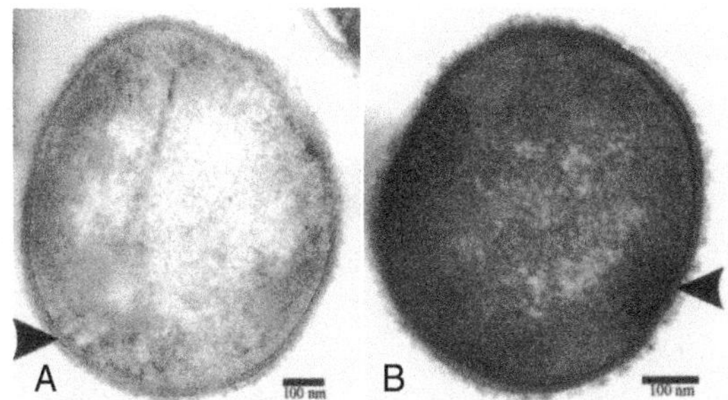

FIGURE 34-2 Electron micrograph of *Streptococcus pyogenes* **(A)** and *Streptococcus canis* **(B)**. Proteinaceous cell surface fibrillae are present on *S. canis* that resemble the M-protein surface fibrils of the human pathogen *S. pyogenes*. M-protein is a key virulence factor of *S. pyogenes*. (From DeWinter LM, Low DE, Prescott JF. Virulence of *Streptococcus canis* from canine streptococcal toxic shock syndrome and necrotizing fasciitis. Vet Microbiol 1999;70:95-110.)

Streptococcus canis

S. canis is the most frequently isolated streptococcus from dogs and cats.[3] It is a β-hemolytic, group G (pyogenic) streptococcus that colonizes the skin, genital, and gastrointestinal tracts of healthy dogs and cats. It has also been isolated from other animal species, such as rats, mice, rabbits, mink, and foxes. Infection with *S. canis* may be associated with neonatal bacteremia, pharyngitis, cervical lymphadenitis, infective endocarditis, UTIs, postoperative incision or wound infections, otitis externa, keratitis, bronchopneumonia, pyometra or metritis, meningoencephalitis, NF, STSS, rhinitis and necrotizing sinusitis, pyothorax, discospondylitis, arthritis, osteomyelitis, mastitis, cholangiohepatitis, and peritonitis. Neonatal infections can occur when organisms are transmitted from the vaginal tract during parturition. The organism can then gain access to the systemic circulation via the umbilical vein. Streptococcal meningitis results from direct extension from the sinuses or middle ear, or from bacteremia. Other embolic complications may accompany bacteremia with group G streptococci. Although opportunistic infections with *S. canis* occur sporadically, outbreaks of group G streptococcal infection have been reported in group-housed animals, which suggested spread of a virulent strain.[4-6]

Severe manifestations of *S. canis* infection, such as STSS and NF, have been increasingly described in dogs and cats in recent years, sometimes in the absence of obvious immunosuppressive underlying conditions or wounds.[6-9] Although toxic shock syndrome can also be caused by staphylococci, STSS is defined as any streptococcal infection associated with the sudden onset of shock and organ failure. Mechanisms of shock and organ failure identified in human group A streptococcal infections include elaboration of pyrogenic exotoxins by streptococci, which act as superantigens. Superantigens stimulate T cell responses through their ability to bind to, and cross-link, the MHC class II complex of antigen-presenting cells, and the T cell receptor, which bypasses normal MHC-restricted antigen processing. This leads to sudden and massive cascade of cytokine release, which in turn causes signs of fever, vomiting, and hypotension, together with tissue damage, disseminated intravascular coagulation

TABLE 34-1

Classification of Streptococci Isolated from Dogs and Cats

Species	Lancefield Antigen(s)	Hemolytic Reactions	Comments
S. canis	G	β	Most common. Dogs and cats are natural hosts. Causes a variety of clinical syndromes. Primary cause of streptococcal toxic shock syndrome and necrotizing fasciitis in dogs and cats.
S. equi subsp. *zooepidemicus*	C	β	Causes pneumonia and sinusitis, primarily in group-housed animals. Has also been associated with meningitis.
S. dysgalactiae	C	β	Uncommon. Has been isolated from dogs with septicemia, dermatitis, or pneumonia.
S. bovis group (*S. gallolyticus* and *S. infantarius*)	D	α or γ	Uncommon. Has been isolated from dogs with urinary tract infections and endocarditis.
S. agalactiae	B	β or γ	Rare. Isolated from dogs and cats with endocarditis and neonatal septicemia.

(DIC), and multiple organ dysfunction.[10] Other streptococcal virulence factors also contribute to proinflammatory cytokine release and the development of hypotension. Laboratory abnormalities include thrombocytopenia, azotemia, hypoalbuminemia, and metabolic acidosis. Death can occur within 48 hours after the onset of illness. Specific criteria are used for diagnosis of STSS in human patients, and similar definitions could be used for diagnosis of STSS in dogs and cats (Box 34-1). Because only a few dogs and cats with STSS have been described, predisposing factors have not been clearly identified. Predisposing conditions in humans include diabetes mellitus, alcoholism, surgical procedures, penetrating and nonpenetrating trauma, viral infections such as varicella, and possibly the use of nonsteroidal antiinflammatory drugs.

NF is a bacterial infection of the deep subcutaneous tissues and fascia, characterized by extensive necrosis and gangrene of the skin and underlying tissues. NF often begins as a minor wound and progresses rapidly over 24 to 72 hours, and it may be accompanied by STSS (Figure 34-3). The popular term "flesh-eating bacteria" has been used to describe the organisms involved. Streptococcal NF has been described in both dogs and cats. Lesions usually involve a limb and are intensely painful, with localized heat and swelling and accumulation of exudate along fascial planes that requires drainage and debridement. In some dogs, extensive sloughing of necrotic skin occurs.[9] Necrotizing myositis, bacteremia, and septic emboli may accompany NF.[8] Outbreaks of NF, arthritis, sinusitis, and meningitis caused by *S. canis* have been reported in cats in shelters[5] and breeding colonies.[11] Molecular typing (by pulsed-field gel electrophoresis) of isolates from one outbreak revealed that isolates were clonally related, which indicated spread of a virulent strain.[12]

Despite the recognition of severe disease manifestations in some dogs and cats, relatively little is known about virulence factors of *S. canis*. A protein analogous to M protein, a major virulence factor of *S. pyogenes,* has been identified in *S. canis* and was shown to bind plasminogen and degrade thrombi.[13] M protein has important antiphagocytic properties. Genes that encode M protein and a streptococcal hemolysin, streptolysin O, have been detected in *S. canis* isolates from dogs with NF and STSS.[14] Genes that encode other virulence factors identified in *S. pyogenes*, such as pyrogenic exotoxins (Spe genes),

BOX 34-1

Criteria Used for Diagnosis of STSS in Human Patients, with Suggested Modifications for Diagnosis of STSS in Dogs and Cats*

I Isolation of Group G streptococci (*Streptococcus canis*)

A. From a normally sterile site
B. From a nonsterile site

II Clinical signs of severity

A. Hypotension: systolic blood pressure <90 mm Hg in dogs and <80 mm Hg in cats
and
B. Two or more of the following signs:
   1. Renal impairment: creatinine above the upper limit of the reference range
   2. Coagulopathy: thrombocytopenia or DIC (prolonged clotting times, low serum fibrinogen concentration, and increased fibrin degradation products)
   3. Liver involvement: serum AST, ALT, or total bilirubin levels at least twice the upper limit of the reference range
   4. Acute respiratory distress syndrome defined as acute onset of diffuse pulmonary infiltrates and hypoxemia in the absence of cardiac failure, or evidence of diffuse capillary leak manifested as acute onset of pulmonary edema, or pleural or peritoneal effusions with hypoalbuminemia
   5. A generalized erythematous macular rash that may desquamate
   6. Soft tissue necrosis, including necrotizing fasciitis or myositis, or gangrene

*An illness that fulfills criteria IA and II is defined as a definite case. An illness that fulfills criteria IB and II is defined as a probable case if no other cause for the illness is identified.

DIC, disseminated intravascular coagulation; STSS, streptococcal toxic shock syndrome.

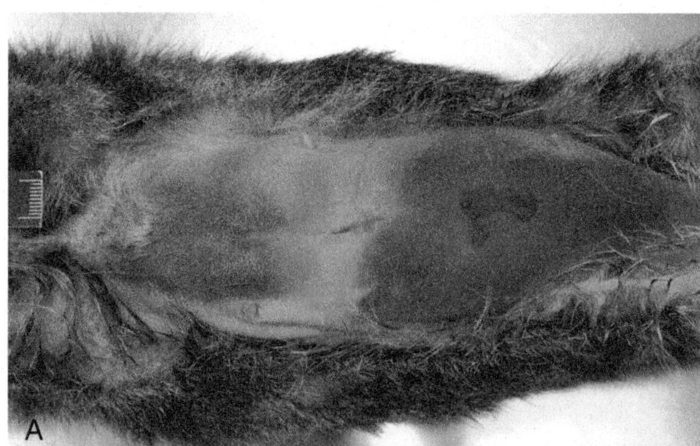

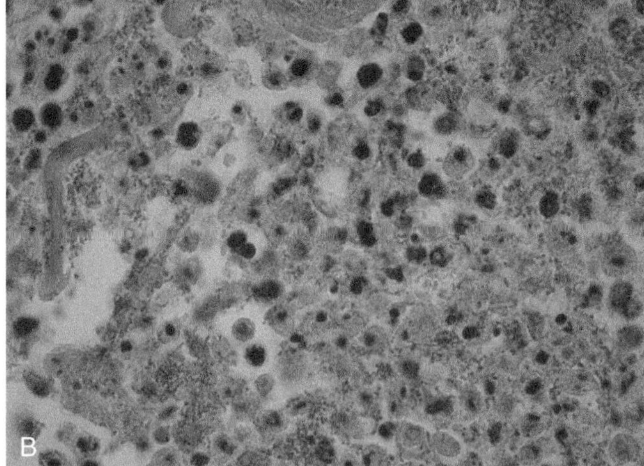

FIGURE 34-3 **A,** Two-year-old female spayed domestic shorthair that was euthanized with necrotizing cellulitis, myositis and fasciitis, and peritonitis that developed after an ovariohysterectomy site became infected with *Streptococcus canis.* **B,** Histopathology showed severe necrotizing cellulitis, myositis, and cellulitis with intralesional cocci that sometimes formed chains. H&E stain, 1000× oil magnification. (Courtesy of the University of California, Davis, Veterinary Anatomic Pathology Service.)

streptococcal superantigen (SSA), streptokinase (Ska), and C5a peptidase (Scp, which cleaves the fifth component of complement) have not been detected.

Streptococcus equi subsp. *zooepidemicus*

S. equi subsp. *zooepidemicus* is a β-hemolytic, group C streptococcus that is a commensal of the upper respiratory and lower genital tracts of horses, and appears to be an emerging pathogen of dogs and cats. Opportunistic infections such as wound infections, respiratory disease, endometritis, and abortion occur in horses. Infections have also been reported in a variety of other animal species, including cattle, sheep, pigs, monkeys, seals, ruminants, dogs, cats, and humans. Different strains of *S. equi* subsp. *zooepidemicus* exist that may vary in pathogenicity and host tropism. Infected horses may have been a source of infection for dogs in some situations,[15,16] but in other situations where infected dogs and cats have been identified, a history of horse contact was not present.

Several outbreaks of hemorrhagic, fibrinosuppurative, and necrotizing pneumonia associated with *S. equi* subsp. *zooepidemicus* infection have been described in group-housed dogs, such as those in kennels and shelter environments, from a variety of geographic locations worldwide (Figure 34-4).[17] The pneumonia progresses rapidly in some dogs can be accompanied by signs suggestive of STSS, such as fever and systemic hypovolemia. In some dogs, severe tachypnea and death occurs within 48 hours of the first signs of respiratory disease, and dogs may be found dead without any preceding clinical signs. Other infected dogs show only mild signs of respiratory disease. *S. equi* subsp. *zooepidemicus* bacteremia and sepsis has been reported in racing greyhounds.[18] Chronic lymphoplasmacytic rhinitis, sometimes with turbinate lysis, has also been described in several dogs in association with *S. equi* subsp. *zooepidemicus* infection, which resolved after specific antimicrobial treatment.[15,16] Outbreaks of pneumonia, purulent rhinosinusitis, and meningoencephalitis have been described in cats.[19,20] *S. equi* subsp. *zooepidemicus* meningoencephalitis occurred in a cat as a result of extension of otitis media/interna.[21]

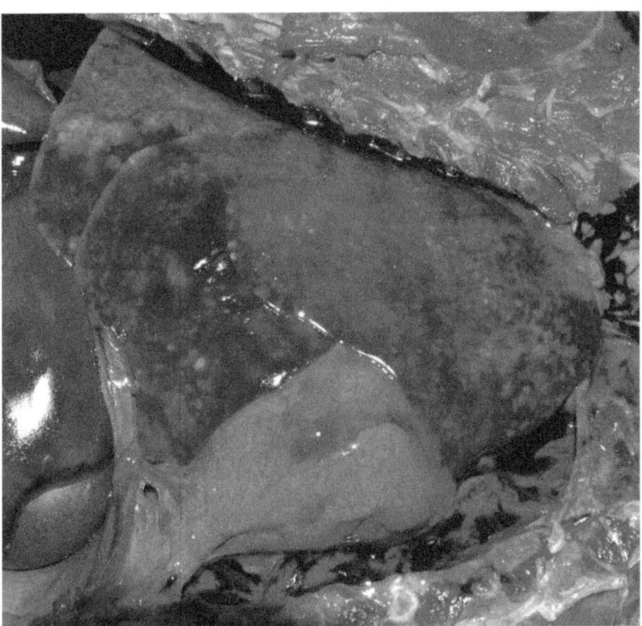

FIGURE 34-4 Pneumonia in a shelter dog caused by *Streptococcus equi* subsp. *zooepidemicus*. The lungs are consolidated and dark red. (Courtesy of Dr. Patricia Pesavento, University of California, Davis.)

The pathogenesis of infection with *S. equi* subsp. *zooepidemicus* in dogs and cats is unclear. Co-infection with other contagious respiratory pathogens can contribute to the severity of disease. Co-infections with canine distemper virus (CDV), canine adenovirus-2 (CAV-2), canine herpesvirus-1 (CHV-1), canine influenza virus (CIV), *Bordetella bronchiseptica*, or *Mycoplasma cynos* have been documented in some, but not all, affected dogs with *S. equi* subsp. *zooepidemicus* pneumonia. Experimentally, co-infection of dogs with both CIV and *S. equi* subsp. *zooepidemicus* is associated with more severe clinical manifestations of disease than when either organism is inoculated alone.[22] Other environmental factors such as overcrowding may also contribute to stress and severe disease manifestations. Superantigen genes have been detected in some isolates of *S. equi* subsp. *zooepidemicus* from dogs,[23,24] but there has been no correlation between the presence of these genes and the severity of histopathologic lesions. However, expression of proinflammatory cytokines such as TNF-α, Il-6, and Il-8 in the lungs of affected dogs suggests that a potent inflammatory response is involved in the pathogenesis of disease.[23]

Other Streptococcal Species

Like *S. equi* subsp. *zooepidemicus, S. dysgalactiae* is a β-hemolytic, group C streptococcus. There are two subspecies, *S. dysgalactiae* subsp. *equisimilis* and *S. dysgalactiae* subsp. *dysgalactiae*. After *S. canis* and *S. equi* subsp. *zooepidemicus, S. dysgalactiae* subsp. *equisimilis* was the third most common β- or γ-hemolytic streptococcal species isolated from dogs at a veterinary teaching hospital in the United States, and was detected in 13 (3.3%) of 393 dogs with streptococcal infections. Affected dogs had bacteremia and sepsis, dermatitis, or pneumonia.[3] *S. dysgalactiae* subsp. *dysgalactiae* has been reported in association with systemic neonatal infections and death in a litter of great Dane puppies.[25]

The porcine streptococcus, *Streptococcus suis,* has been isolated from cats with meningoencephalitis, pyothorax, or dermatitis.[26,27] *S. suis* was also isolated from the urine of a systemically unwell dog in Canada[28] and can be isolated from the tonsils, anus, and skin of healthy dogs and cats.[29] Although contact with pigs was not reported in the sick dogs and cats, the dog was fed commercial pig ear treats. *S. suis* has been classified into serotypes, which have epidemiologic importance. Human infections are usually serotypes 2 and 14. The cases reported in dogs and cats have not belonged to these serotypes.

Other streptococcal species isolated from dogs and cats include the human pathogen *Streptococcus constellatus* (a *Streptococcus anginosus* group organism), which was isolated from a dog with pyoderma;[30] and group B streptococci *(S. agalactiae),* which have been isolated from dogs and cats with streptococcal disease such as endocarditis and neonatal sepsis. Group B streptococci are important causes of puerperal sepsis and neonatal sepsis and meningitis in humans, as well as mastitis in cattle.

Streptococcus bovis Group (*Streptococcus gallolyticus* and *Streptococcus infantarius*)

Streptococcus bovis group organisms are α- or nonhemolytic and usually possess Lancefield group D antigens. Biotypes that belong to this group, which differ in their biochemical characteristics, have now been reclassified as distinct species, *Streptococcus gallolyticus* and *Streptococcus infantarius*.[31] *S. bovis* group organisms are commensals of the gastrointestinal tracts of humans and other animals, especially ruminants. They are important causes of bacteremia and endocarditis in humans, accounting for 11% to 17% of all endocarditis cases. They frequently affect multiple valves and are associated with embolic complications. For unknown reasons, fecal carriage of *S. bovis* group organisms by humans has been strongly associated with colorectal cancer. This especially seems to be true for *S. gallolyticus* subsp. *gallolyticus*.[32] Rarely, *S. bovis* group organisms are isolated from dogs and cats with UTIs. They have also been isolated from the blood of dogs with mitral valve endocarditis, one of which also had sternebral osteomyelitis.[33,34]

Enterococcus spp.

Enterococci are α- or nonhemolytic gram-positive bacteria that usually possess Lancefield group D antigens, are commensals of the gastrointestinal tracts of humans and other animals, and are important nosocomial pathogens. They form pairs or short chains of organisms and cannot morphologically be discriminated from streptococci. Enterococci survive harsh environmental conditions; they grow in medium that contains 6.5% NaCl, can grow at temperatures that range from 10°C to 45°C (50°F to 113°F), and hydrolyze esculin in the presence of 40% bile salts. The genus *Enterococcus* was separated from *Streptococcus* in the mid-1980s based on the results of DNA hybridization experiments.[35]

Enterococci are often resistant to a wide variety of different antimicrobial drug classes, and multiple drug resistant (MDR) enterococcal infections, especially those that are also resistant to vancomycin (vancomycin-resistant enterococci or VRE), are a significant problem in human medicine. Of great clinical importance, resistance among enterococci occurs as a result of both intrinsic and acquired resistance mechanisms. Intrinsic resistance to low levels of most β-lactam antimicrobials occurs because enterococci possess low-affinity penicillin binding proteins (PBPs). Thus penicillins are generally bacteriostatic, not bactericidal, against enterococci. Enterococci also have low-level intrinsic resistance to aminoglycosides, which results from decreased drug uptake. However, uptake of aminoglycosides is enhanced when enterococci are exposed to β-lactams, which explains the synergistic activity of this combination. Enterococci are resistant to trimethoprim-sulfamethoxazole because they utilize exogenously produced folate. Thus, even if the organisms appear sensitive to trimethoprim-sulfamethoxazole in vitro (when exogenous folate is lacking), the drug is not effective in vivo. Many laboratories therefore do not report minimum inhibitory concentrations for this organism-drug combination. Enterococcal resistance to other antimicrobials, such as macrolides and vancomycin, can result from acquired resistance mechanisms. Extensive multidrug resistance has been well documented in enterococci isolated from dogs and cats, but there are only a few reports of enterococci with acquired vancomycin resistance from dogs in the literature. These have been from the United Kingdom, New Zealand, and the United States.[36-38] All other isolates examined have been vancomycin susceptible. In contrast, VRE account for about 30% of enterococcal infections in humans from Europe and North America.[39]

Clinical microbiology laboratories often do not differentiate between *Enterococcus* species, because definitive identification can require genetic typing. Some laboratories use biochemical methods to identify *Enterococcus faecalis* and *Enterococcus faecium,* which are the most prevalent species in humans and which differ in their epidemiology, antimicrobial susceptibility, and virulence properties. *E. faecium* is more likely to show high-level resistance to penicillins and carbapenems than *E. faecalis*, and as a result, in humans, the prognosis for serious *E. faecium* infections may be worse than that for *E. faecalis* infections.[40] However, *E. faecalis* is more likely to produce biofilms than *E. faecium*.[41] Although most infections in humans have been *E. faecalis,* a worrisome increase in the prevalence of MDR *E. faecium* infections has occurred. In particular, ampicillin- and fluoroquinolone-resistant *E. faecium* strains that belong to hospital adapted strains known as clonal complex 17 (CC17) have emerged. CC17 isolates have been found in dogs, but their virulence gene profile and antimicrobial susceptibility profiles have differed from those of human isolates.[42]

In healthy dogs and cats, enterococci can be found on the skin and within the oral cavity, nasal cavity, and gastrointestinal tract. In the United States, the most prevalent species in dogs appears to be *E. faecalis,* which comprised 68% of 155 isolates.[43] In the cat, it was *Enterococcus hirae*, which comprised 52% of 121 isolates.[43] Preparations that contain *E. faecium* strain SF68 have been investigated as probiotics in dogs and cats, with mixed results.[44-46] Some studies suggest that supplementation of food with this probiotic can stimulate local and systemic immune function in dogs and cats.[47,48]

Although less pathogenic than many streptococci, important virulence factors have been identified in enterococci that enable them to invade tissues and cause disease. These include a cytolysin, gelatinase, and a serine protease, as well as several surface proteins (e.g., the Ace protein, which allows the organism to adhere to connective tissue components, such as collagen). Enterococci also possess pili that play an important role in adherence. The ability of many enterococci to form biofilms means they can be very difficult to eradicate, because they resist phagocytosis and antimicrobial drugs.[41] As in humans, the two most common species of *Enterococcus* associated with disease in dogs and cats are *E. faecalis* and *E. faecium*.[36,49] Others are shown in Box 34-2.

BOX 34-2

***Enterococcus* Species Isolated from Healthy and Sick Dogs and Cats**[36,43,50,51]

Healthy Dogs and Cats

E. faecalis
E. faecium
E. hirae
E. casseliflavus
E. durans
E. canintestini
E. avium

Sick Dogs and Cats

E. faecalis
E. faecium
E. hirae
E. casseliflavus
E. durans
E. gallinarum

Because enterococci are naturally resistant to a number of antimicrobials, treatment with broad-spectrum antibiotics (which destroy competing bacteria within the gastrointestinal tract) selects for colonization by enterococci. The development of enterococcal UTIs may be promoted by repeated use of antimicrobial drugs to treat recurrent UTIs, when the underlying cause of infection is not or cannot be resolved. Enterococci can contaminate the hospital environment and survive for long periods on fomites such as doorknobs, stethoscopes, and monitoring devices, as well as the hands, gloves, and clothing of hospital personnel. Inoculation may occur via urinary, intravenous, or other invasive devices, or organisms may enter the body from a damaged gastrointestinal tract. Severe concurrent illness and immunosuppression may predispose to infection. In addition to skin and UTIs, enterococci may be isolated from dogs and cats with UTIs, pyoderma and otitis externa, cholangiohepatitis, pancreatitis, hepatic abscesses, peritonitis, mastitis, bacteremia and endocarditis, wound infections, and discospondylitis. There have been rare reports of gastrointestinal illness in association with enterococcal infection of the gastrointestinal tract in dogs and cats. In affected cats, an association with diarrhea was supported by the presence of large mats of enterococci in association with the gastrointestinal mucosa.[52,53] Frequently, enterococci are isolated from lesions in mixed infections with other gastrointestinal microorganisms.

Physical Examination Findings

Physical examination findings in dogs and cats with *Streptococcus* or *Enterococcus* infections vary with the anatomic site(s) of infection. Streptococcal infections are an important differential diagnosis in sick or fading neonates; dogs that have physical examination findings suggestive of endocarditis; dogs and cats with severe pneumonia and pyothorax; NF; rapid onset of systemic illness in association with a wound; or outbreaks of severe purulent upper respiratory disease, hemorrhagic pneumonia, and systemic illness in group-housed animals.

Findings suggestive of streptococcal or enterococcal endocarditis include fever, lethargy, tachycardia, joint pain and swelling, systolic heart murmurs, and signs of embolic complications such as lameness, limb edema, weak or absent pulses, or neurologic signs. Animals with streptococcal pneumonia may have a fever (up to 106.3°F or 41.3°C), cough, tonsillar enlargement and hyperemia, mucopurulent nasal discharge, and/or tachypnea with increased lung sounds. Lung sounds may be decreased if pleural effusion is present. Animals with NF have variable extents of regional cutaneous erythema, sometimes in association with a wound; cutaneous ulceration, swelling, edema, intense pain, and warmth on palpation of the affected area. In some animals, extensive skin sloughing occurs. Animals with STSS may be obtunded, with weak pulses, tachycardia, tachypnea, and prolonged capillary refill time. Rectal temperatures may exceed 106°F (41.1°C), although the presence of fever is variable. Icterus may be present in animals that develop multiple organ dysfunction syndrome in association with STSS.

Diagnosis

Laboratory Abnormalities

Complete Blood Count, Biochemistry, and Urinalysis Findings

Dogs and cats with severe manifestations of streptococcal infections, such as pneumonia, NF, endocarditis, and STSS, usually have a neutrophilic leukocytosis with a left shift, toxic neutrophils, lymphopenia, and monocytosis. A degenerative left shift or circulating metamyelocytes may be present. STSS may be accompanied by thrombocytopenia as a result of DIC, azotemia and/or increased liver enzyme activities, hypoalbuminemia, and hypoglycemia. The urinalysis of dogs and cats with streptococcal or enterococcal UTIs may reveal pyuria, proteinuria, or hematuria, and cocci in pairs or chains may sometimes be evident on sediment examination.

Clotting Function

Dogs and cats with STSS that develop DIC may have clotting function abnormalities including prolonged coagulation times, increased fibrin degradation product and D-dimer concentrations, and decreased antithrombin concentrations.

Cytologic Abnormalities

Cytologic examination of specimens (respiratory lavage fluid, aspirates of affected tissues, or pus) from dogs and cats with streptococcal or enterococcal infections typically reveals large numbers of degenerate and nondegenerate neutrophils. Coccoid bacteria in pairs or chains may also be seen.

Microbiologic Tests

Isolation and Identification

Streptococci and enterococci that infect dogs and cats are readily isolated on routine bacteriologic media from aspirates, tissue biopsies, body fluids, and lavage specimens. Inoculation of complex media that contain blood is recommended. Streptococci grow well in anaerobic incubation conditions, but these are not required because of their facultative nature. The laboratory may use selective media for specimens that are heavily contaminated with other bacteria. Species are identified based on their phenotypic characteristics (such as colony morphology and hemolytic properties), biochemical reactions, and serotyping with Lancefield antisera; the last is available on a commercial basis. As noted previously, genetic typing may be required to identify some enterococci to the species level. Molecular typing methods such as pulsed-field gel electrophoresis may be required to investigate outbreaks in group-housed animals or hospital environments.

Antimicrobial susceptibility testing for streptococci is often not performed by veterinary diagnostic laboratories, because virtually all strains are penicillin susceptible. Group A streptococci (GAS) that infect humans remain universally susceptible to penicillin, but an increased prevalence of penicillin resistance, which occurs as a result of altered PBPs, has been detected in *S. pneumoniae*, which is primarily a human pathogen.[54] *S. pneumoniae* may also be resistant to other β-lactam drugs and macrolides. Evaluation of antimicrobial susceptibility is of critical importance for enterococci, because of the high prevalence of resistance in this group, and especially among *E. faecium* isolates. Susceptibility testing for aminoglycosides requires high-concentration disk diffusion or broth microdilution methods, which may not routinely be performed by some veterinary microbiology laboratories (see Treatment).

Pathologic Findings

Pathologic findings in *Streptococcus* infections vary depending on the organ system affected. Gross findings in *S. canis* sinusitis include accumulation of purulent material within the frontal sinus with osteolysis, and distortion of the nasal bridge in cats.[5] When meningitis is present, purulent material may be found in association with the meninges (Figure 34-5). Lesions of NF in dogs and cats consist of edema, ecchymoses, and necrosis that extend within the fascia and subcutis in association with

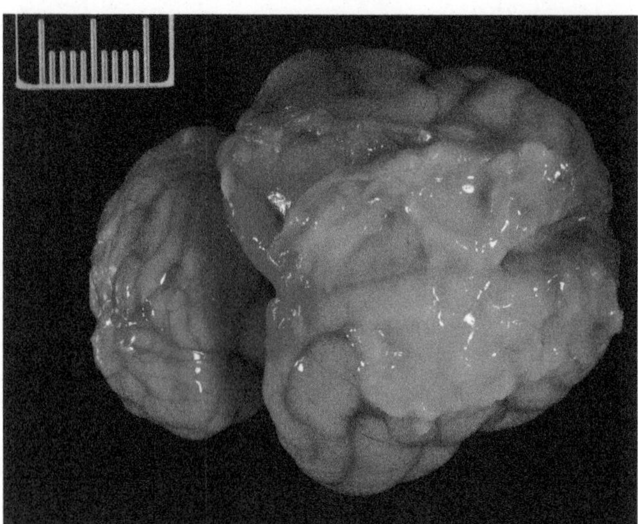

FIGURE 34-5 Accumulation of purulent exudate over the meninges in a shelter cat that died of *Streptococcus canis* meningitis. (Courtesy of Dr. Patricia Pesavento, University of California, Davis.)

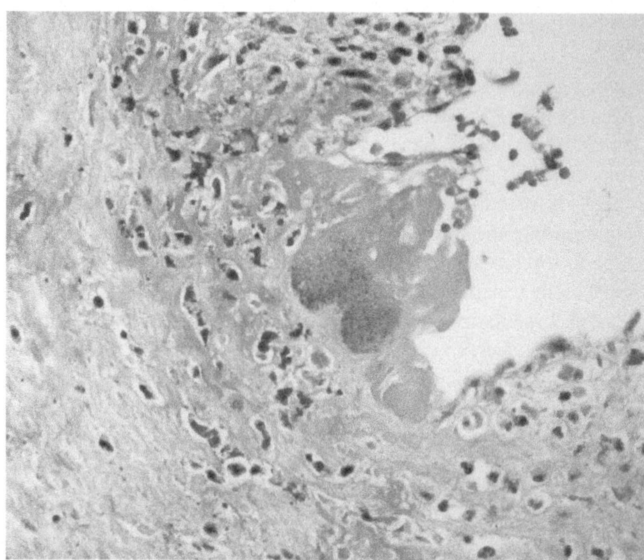

FIGURE 34-6 Histopathology of the mitral valve of an 8-year-old male neutered springer spaniel that was seen for a 1-month history of right thoracic limb lameness, anorexia, and lethargy. There is severe, subacute, fibrinonecrotic endocarditis with intralesional cocci. When the dog was first evaluated, the platelet count was 9000 platelets/μL and the dog was treated with vincristine for immune-mediated thrombocytopenia. Subsequently the dog developed vomiting and diarrhea and became obtunded. Blood cultures grew *Streptococcus canis*. At necropsy, septic emboli were present in the kidneys, spleen, and lymph nodes. Necrotizing fasciitis was also present in multiple limbs, which was thought to have developed as a result of septic embolization.

ulcerative skin lesions (see Figure 34-3). An accumulation of pus may be found between fascial planes. Congestion of a variety of organs may be present in animals that have accompanying STSS. When *S. canis* or Enterococcus endocarditis is present, adherent and friable mass lesions may be seen in association with the mitral and/or, less commonly, the aortic valves. Dogs with streptococcal endocarditis are more likely to have concurrent polyarthritis than dogs with other bacterial causes of endocarditis.[33] On histopathology, valve lesions generally contain large numbers of degenerate and nondegenerate neutrophils, hemorrhage, necrosis, fibrin thrombi, and abundant gram-positive cocci (Figure 34-6). Septic thromboemboli may be present in a variety of organs. Histopathologic lesions in neonates that die of neonatal sepsis include severe inflammation and necrosis, as well as septic emboli in a variety of tissues (see Figure 34-1).

Grossly, the lungs of dogs with *S. equi* subsp. *zooepidemicus* pneumonia may be red, consolidated, and fail to collapse (see Figure 34-4). There may be variable quantities of hemorrhagic pleural effusion, petechial and ecchymotic hemorrhages on pleural surfaces, and bloody exudate within the airways and nasal cavity.[17] Typical histopathologic changes include fibrinous, necrotizing, and/or suppurative pneumonia or bronchopneumonia; fibrin thrombi; and intralesional clusters or chains of coccoid bacteria. Within lymph nodes, marked lymphoid depletion may be present, but lymphoid hyperplasia has also been reported. Occasionally, septic thromboemboli may be present in organs such as the lymph nodes, renal glomeruli, adrenal glands, brain, and splenic sinusoids.[55,56]

Treatment and Prognosis

In general, streptococcal infections should be treated with a β-lactam drug, preferably a penicillin or a cephalosporin (Table 34-2). Early diagnosis and prompt treatment with appropriate antimicrobial drugs is essential to prevent more severe complications such as NF or STSS. In animals that present with severe signs such as septic shock or life-threatening pneumonia, initial treatment should be with a broad-spectrum antimicrobial drug combination, such as a β-lactam and an aminoglycoside, which may also have synergistic activity against some streptococci, such as group C streptococci (*S. equi* subsp. *zooepidemicus*).

Necrotizing Fasciitis, Myositis, and Toxic Shock Syndrome

Prompt surgical exploration and debridement is of critical importance in NF, because shock and organ failure will continue to progress in the face of antimicrobial treatment when necrotic tissue persists. Imaging techniques such as ultrasound may be useful to help characterize the extent of lesions before surgery. Extremely aggressive fluid resuscitation with crystalloids and blood products may also be required, while blood pressure is monitored. In human patients, deep-seated streptococcal infections (NF and STSS) are treated with *both* high-dose penicillin and clindamycin. This is because clindamycin suppresses exotoxin production by GAS, is more active than penicillin in experimental NF, and has a longer half-life than penicillin. However, clindamycin resistance exists in some GAS, whereas all GAS are susceptible to penicillin.[57] Also, penicillin may not be effective in deep-seated streptococcal infections, because stationary-phase organisms do not express PBPs. This tolerance to penicillin has also been observed in group G streptococcal infections.[58] Approximately 10% to 15% of contemporary *S. canis* isolates from dogs in Europe have demonstrated clindamycin resistance.[59,60] Given this finding, the same combination could be used to treat NF in dogs and cats.

Meningitis/Meningoencephalitis

Although high-dose penicillin has been used to treat streptococcal meningitis in human patients, penicillins typically have limited penetration of the CSF. Trimethoprim-sulfamethoxazole was used with apparent success to treat some dogs and cats with streptococcal meningitis.[21,61] See Chapter 90 for additional

TABLE 34-2

Suggested Antimicrobial Drugs for Treatment of Streptococcal Infections in Dogs and Cats

Drug	Dose (mg/kg)	Interval (hours)	Route
Penicillin G potassium or sodium*	20,000-40,000 U/kg	6-8	IV, IM
Ampicillin sodium*	10-20	6-8	IV, IM, SC
Amoxicillin	6.6-20	8-12	PO
Cefazolin sodium	20-35	8	IV, IM
Cephalexin	10-30 (dogs), 15-20 (cats)	12	PO
Trimethoprim-sulfamethoxazole†	30	12	PO, IV

*Consider use with clindamycin, 10 mg/kg q12h IV or IM for necrotizing fasciitis or myositis; consider addition of gentamicin sulfate, 9-14 mg/kg q24h IV, IM, or SC for dogs with *S. equi* subsp. *zooepidemicus* pneumonia because of synergy of this combination for group C streptococci.
†Consider use for treatment of streptococcal meningitis.

TABLE 34-3

Suggested Medications for Treatment of Enterococcal Infections in Dogs and Cats

Drug	Dose (mg/kg)	Interval (hours)	Route
Ampicillin sodium*	10-20	6-8	IV, IM, SC
Amoxicillin*	6.6-20	8-12	PO
Vancomycin†	15	8	IV
Linezolid†	10 (dogs)	8	PO
Chloramphenicol	40-50 (dogs), 12.5-20 (cats)	6-8 (dogs), 12 (cats)	PO, IV, IM
Nitrofurantoin‡	2-3	8	PO

*In human patients, used with gentamicin sulfate, 1 mg/kg q12h IV for systemic enterococcal infections caused by enterococci susceptible to high-level aminoglycosides, because of the synergy of this combination
†For enterococci that show high-level aminoglycoside resistance or when aminoglycosides cannot be used because of toxicity (animals with renal failure). Use in veterinary patients is controversial. Refer to Chapter 8 for additional information on the use of vancomycin.
‡For resistant UTIs

information on treatment of bacterial meningitis. Ceftriaxone has been used as an alternative to benzylpenicillin for treatment of human streptococcal meningitis and attains higher concentrations in the CSF.

Bacteremia and Endocarditis

The reader is referred to Chapter 86 for information on treatment of bacteremia and endocarditis.

Enterococcal Infections

Suggested medications for treatment of enterococcal infections in dogs and cats are shown in Table 34-3. Successful treatment of enterococcal infections requires knowledge of the intrinsic resistance of enterococci to low levels of β-lactams and aminoglycosides, the synergistic effect of high doses of these drugs, the lack of efficacy of trimethoprim-sulfonamide combinations in vivo, and the ability of enterococci to acquire resistance genes to a large number of other antimicrobial compounds. Aminopenicillins such as ampicillin generally have more potent activity against enterococci than does penicillin or the carbapenems. Bactericidal regimens, which consist of a β-lactam and gentamicin (or streptomycin), are used in human patients to treat systemic infections such as endocarditis or bacteremia. Enterococci are usually resistant to aminoglycosides at dilutions used in routine broth microdilution methods (low-level resistance). When the synergistic combination is indicated, but low-level resistance is present, isolates should be tested for high-level resistance (HLR) to aminoglycosides. Aminoglycoside HLR results from production of an aminoglycoside-modifying enzyme by enterococci. It emerged in the 1980s and has been a growing problem in both *E. faecium* and *E. faecalis* isolates from human patients. Aminoglycoside HLR has also been reported in *E. faecium* and *E. faecalis* isolated from dogs and cats,[36,38,62] but most isolates are susceptible to high concentrations of gentamicin. In human patients, a combination of ceftriaxone and ampicillin has been recommended to treat endocarditis caused by aminoglycoside HLR enterococci.[39] When enterococci show penicillin resistance, vancomycin can be substituted for penicillin, but this requires prolonged hospitalization for intravenous administration. Single-agent treatment with linezolid (see Chapter 8) is an oral alternative for treatment of serious penicillin-resistant enterococcal infections, but in human patients it is recommended that this only be used when combinations of β-lactams and gentamicin cannot be used because of resistance, toxicity, or treatment failure.[39] Although most strains of enterococci isolated from humans are susceptible to linezolid, resistant strains have appeared.[63] Chloramphenicol may be successful for treatment of resistant enterococcal bloodstream infections when administered orally, but it is bacteriostatic, and concerns regarding adverse effects exist (see Chapter 8).

Treatment of enterococcal UTIs with β-lactams such as ampicillin or amoxicillin may be successful even when resistance is documented in the susceptibility panel, because of the high concentrations that these drugs achieve in the urine.[39] Nitrofurantoin has also been useful for treatment of resistant enterococcal UTIs in humans, and routine treatment of subclinical bacteriuria caused by MDR enterococci is not recommended (see Chapter 89).[64] When enterococci are present with other bacteria, especially in the urinary tract, treatment of the nonenterococcal pathogen may be sufficient to resolve the infection.

Prevention

Because outbreaks of streptococcal infections in dogs and cats have been associated with overcrowding, co-infections, and other stressors, appropriate shelter and kennel management and hygiene, as well as vaccination against other respiratory pathogens, may help to prevent streptococcal infections. Proper wound care may prevent serious streptococcal infections such as bacteremia, endocarditis, NF, and STSS. Methods to reduce nosocomial infections by enterococci are outlined in Chapter 11. Resistant enterococcal infections may be prevented through restricted and appropriate use of antimicrobial drugs and proper management of underlying disorders that predispose to bacterial infections.

Public Health Aspects

Streptococci include some of the most important bacterial pathogens of humans. The β-hemolytic group A streptococcus (GAS) *S. pyogenes* causes streptococcal pharyngitis ("strep throat") and scarlet fever, as well as poststreptococcal rheumatic fever, rheumatic heart disease, and glomerulonephritis. It has been estimated that globally, GAS cause 616 million new cases of pharyngitis each year.[65] GAS has also been associated with other disease manifestations, which include NF, STSS, myositis, vaginitis, and bacteremia. As a result, *S. pyogenes* is one of the most extensively studied of all streptococci. There are more than 100 different serotypes, which are classified based on the sequence of the M protein gene (known as *emm* typing). M protein is a filamentous macromolecule that traverses the cell wall and is a key virulence factor of GAS. Transmission between humans primarily occurs through close contact, and chronic subclinical carriage of infection in the oropharynx occurs in some individuals. Although family pets have been implicated as a reservoir in households with recurrent streptococcal pharyngitis,[66,67] colonization or infection of dogs and cats with GAS appears to be rare or nonexistent when accurate streptococcal identification methods have been performed. One study found no evidence of oropharyngeal colonization by GAS in pets that were in contact with children with acute pharyngitis.[68] Even among human family members who are in contact with children with streptococcal pharyngitis, routine culture of asymptomatic individuals is not recommended, because penicillin fails to eradicate streptococcal pharyngeal carriage.[57]

The α-hemolytic streptococcus *S. pneumoniae* is a commensal of the human respiratory tract and can invade opportunistically to cause a variety of clinical manifestations that include otitis media, sinusitis, meningitis, bacteremia, and pneumonia. It possesses no Lancefield group antigens. Although extremely rare in dogs and cats, infections with *S. pneumoniae* have been reported in a dog with meningoencephalitis,[61] a cat with arthritis,[69] and a cat with cellulitis.[70] It is likely that in these reports, the dog and cats acquired the infection from humans, because humans are the natural hosts for *S. pneumoniae*.

Reports of human infection with *S. canis* and *S. equi* subsp. *zooepidemicus* exist. *S. canis* has increasingly been recognized as a cause of soft tissue infections in dog owners and has been isolated from humans with bacteremia, UTIs, osteomyelitis, and pneumonia.[71,72] Rarely, *S. equi* subsp. *zooepidemicus* has been isolated from humans with meningitis, bacteremia, endocarditis, pneumonia, osteomyelitis, septic arthritis, acute nephritis, or STSS. Most human infections with *S. equi* subsp. *zooepidemicus* have been traced to an animal source, such as contact with horses, or consumption of inadequately pasteurized milk products or pork. However, apparent transmission of *S. equi* subsp. *zooepidemicus* from a dog with *S. equi* subsp. *zooepidemicus* pneumonia to a handler, who developed severe systemic illness, has been described.[73]

Dogs and cats are also a potential source for human infection by MDR enterococci. In one study, dogs that left a veterinary intensive care unit were colonized with MDR enterococci with the capacity for biofilm formation and horizontal transfer of antimicrobial resistance genes.[74]

Because of the potential for transmission of streptococci and enterococci between dogs, cats, and humans, preventative measures such as hand washing after pets are handled, household disinfection, and avoidance of close contact (such as allowing pets to lick wounds or mucous membranes) should be considered, especially for immunocompromised pet owners.

CASE EXAMPLE

Signalment: "Jazz" a 6-year-old female spayed miniature Pinscher from Fairfield in northern California

History: Jazz was brought to the University of California, Davis, Veterinary Medical Teaching Hospital for evaluation of anorexia, lethargy, and diarrhea. Two days previously, the dog had been seen by the dermatology service for a focal area of alopecia and scaling on the dorsal midline in the thoracolumbar region that first appeared 7 months previously, enlarged to 6 × 4 cm in diameter over 2 months, and then remained static in size for the subsequent 5 months. Skin scrapings and fungal culture were performed, and four skin biopsies were obtained. An underlying vasculitis was suspected, and treatment with vitamin E (200 U PO q12h) and an oral fatty acid supplement was recommended pending the results of the diagnostic tests. The following day the owner noted edema of the right pelvic limb and discontinued the medications. Over the next 24 hours, the dog became lethargic, inappetent, and developed liquid diarrhea and polydipsia. Jazz had been vaccinated regularly for canine distemper, adenovirus and parvovirus infections and rabies and normally ate a commercial dry dog food. She was last vaccinated just after the skin lesion first appeared. The dog was mostly indoors, going outside on leash walks only, and there were no other pets in the household.

Other Medical History: Jazz had been spayed 5 weeks previously, at which time pyometra was an incidental finding and was treated with a 7-day course of amoxicillin.

Physical Examination:

Body Weight: 3.3 kg

General: Lethargic, alert and ambulatory, but weak. Vocalized on palpation of the thorax and abdomen. T = 102.2°F (39.0°C), HR = 120 beats/min, RR = 60 breaths/min, mucous membranes pink, CRT = 1 s.

Eyes, Ears, Nose, and Throat: Mild conjunctival hyperemia and bilateral serous ocular discharge were present.

Integument: There was mild subcutaneous edema and a small amount of serosanguineous fluid in the region of the skin biopsies, but sutures remained intact. There was a single, raised erythematous lesion adjacent to the skin biopsies that measured 0.5 × 0.5 cm in diameter. Severe edema was noted in the cranioventral thoracic region, which extended over an area that was 9 × 5 cm in diameter.

Other Systems, Including Peripheral Lymph Nodes: No clinically significant findings.

Laboratory Findings:

CBC:

HCT 53.1% (40%-55%)
MCV 71.2 fL (65-75 fL)
MCHC 36.7 g/dL (33-36 g/dL)
Nucleated RBC 24/100 WBC
WBC 2200 cells/μL (6000-13,000 cells/μL)
Neutrophils 792 cells/μL (3000-10,500 cells/μL)
Band neutrophils 748 cells/μL
Metamyelocytes 88 cells/μL
Myelocytes 44 cells/μL
Lymphocytes 308 cells/μL (1000-4000 cells/μL)
Monocytes 220 cells/μL (150-1200 cells/μL)
Platelets 97,000/μL (150,000-400,000 platelets/μL).
Markedly toxic band neutrophils, metamyelocytes, and myelocytes; moderately toxic neutrophils; and rare reactive lymphocytes were present.

Serum Chemistry Profile:

Sodium 128 mmol/L (145-154 mmol/L)
Potassium 4.4 mmol/L (3.6-5.3 mmol/L)
Chloride 90 mmol/L (108-118 mmol/L)
Bicarbonate 21 mmol/L (16-26 mmol/L)
Phosphorus 8.7 mg/dL (3.0-6.2 mg/dL)
Calcium 10.0 mg/dL (9.7-11.5 mg/dl)
BUN 63 mg/dL (5-21 mg/dL)
Creatinine 0.9 mg/dL (0.3-1.2 mg/dL)
Glucose 75 mg/dL (64-123 mg/dL)
Total protein 5.6 g/dL (5.4-7.6 g/dL)
Albumin 2.2 g/dL (3.0-4.4 g/dL)
Globulin 3.4 g/dL (1.8-3.9 g/dL)
ALT 185 U/L (19-67 U/L)
AST 128 U/L (19-42 U/L)
ALP 539 U/L (21-170 U/L)
Cholesterol 526 mg/dL (135-361 mg/dL)
Total bilirubin 0.5 mg/dL (0-0.2 mg/dL)

Urinalysis: SGr 1.021; pH 5.0, 1+ protein (SSA), 1+ bilirubin, 4+ hemoprotein, no glucose, no ketones, rare WBC/HPF, 0-2 RBC/HPF, few amorphous crystals, no bacteria seen

Imaging Findings: Abdominal ultrasound: Enlargement of the uterine stump was present dorsal to the bladder. There were no cystic structures within the stump and no evidence of fluid in this region or lymphadenopathy.

Cytologic Findings: Needle aspiration of edema fluid from a region adjacent to the right axilla revealed large numbers of cocci, some in pairs, in the absence of significant numbers of leukocytes.

Microbiologic Testing: Aerobic and anaerobic blood culture (three isolator specimens): One colony of coagulase-negative staphylococci was grown on one plate. The other two plates were negative. No anaerobes were cultured. The isolate was resistant to penicillin G, erythromycin, and trimethoprim-sulfamethoxazole, but susceptible to all other antimicrobials tested.

Aerobic bacterial culture (aspirate of edema fluid): Large numbers of *Streptococcus canis* colonies.

Treatment and Outcome: Treatment with IV fluids (0.9% NaCl with 20 mEq KCl/L) was initiated. Ampicillin (20 mg/kg IV q6h), enrofloxacin (5 mg/kg IV q24h), and butorphanol were administered. The dog's body temperature subsequently dropped to 98.0°F (36.7°C) and blood glucose concentration dropped to 30 mg/dL. Fluids were supplemented with dextrose and a warming pad was used, and the dog's temperature returned to normal limits. Within hours the edema had spread to the abdomen, and evidence of bruising appeared on the right thorax and ventrum. The raised erythematous lesion on the dorsum ulcerated, and dehiscence of the biopsy site adjacent to this region became apparent. Blood work showed a hematocrit of 39%, 2700 white cells/μL, 1323 band neutrophils/μL, 702 neutrophils/μL, 162 lymphocytes/μL, 513 monocytes/μL, and 37,000 platelets/μL; serum sodium concentration was 142 mmol/L, potassium 3.7 mmol/L, creatinine 0.4 mg/dL, BUN 23 mg/dL, albumin 1.2 g/dL, globulin 3.1 g/dL, cholesterol 221 mg/dL, and total bilirubin 2.3 mg/dL. The activities of ALT, AST, and ALP were 79 U/L, 136 U/L, and 292 U/L, respectively. Treatment with dextran and plasma was initiated, but systolic blood pressure dropped to 80 mm Hg, and the region adjacent to the biopsy sites became firm and painful and tore when palpated. Ampicillin was substituted with penicillin G (40,000 U/kg IV q6h). Forty-eight hours after admission, the dog was anesthetized and a large portion of necrotic skin was surgically debrided from the dog's dorsum. The debrided region was covered with a stent. During recovery the dog was tachypneic, had increased lung sounds, and systolic blood pressure dropped to 50 mm Hg. The dog developed respiratory arrest, and an endotracheal tube was placed, from which bloody fluid emanated. Cardiac arrest then ensued, and there was no response to closed cardiopulmonary resuscitation efforts.

Necropsy Findings: At necropsy, necrosis extended through the intercostal musculature of the right thoracic wall. Histopathologic lesions included severe, focally extensive, hemorrhagic and necrotizing panniculitis and fasciitis with intralesional bacteria and multifocal thrombi;

Continued

diffuse necrotizing myositis of the right thoracic wall with intralesional bacteria; severe congestion and mild, multifocal hemorrhage and thrombosis within the kidneys; centrilobular congestion and severe bile stasis within the liver; congestion and hemorrhage within the lung; and generalized lymphoid depletion and sinusoidal histiocytosis within lymph nodes. Around the uterine stump, there was focal fibrosis and mild granulomatous serositis. Very small numbers of *S. canis* were cultured from the uterine stump. Histopathology of the biopsy specimens that had been collected before the onset of systemic illness showed severe, diffuse adnexal atrophy; mild, chronic, lymphoplasmacytic mural folliculitis; focal granulomatous furunculosis with hyperkeratosis; and mild, multifocal, perivascular neutrophilic dermatitis. No microorganisms were seen, although only special staining with periodic acid–Schiff (PAS) and Gomori's methenamine silver (GMS) was performed.

Diagnosis: NF, myositis, and STSS associated with *Streptococcus canis* infection

Comments: This rare case description illustrates how rapidly NF can progress and the ineffectiveness of antibiotic treatment in the presence of devitalized tissue. Clinical findings more than satisfied the criteria for diagnosis of STSS in Box 34-1. The source of infection and the role that the uterine stump infection played was unclear. Streptococcal bacteremia was not detected in this case. It is likely that the coagulase-negative staphylococcus represented a contaminant.

SUGGESTED READINGS

Ghosh A, Dowd SE, Zurek L. Dogs leaving the ICU carry a very large multi-drug resistant enterococcal population with capacity for biofilm formation and horizontal gene transfer. PLoS One. 2011;6:e22451.

Lappin E, Ferguson AJ. Gram-positive toxic shock syndromes. Lancet Infect Dis. 2009;9:281-290.

Prescott JF, DeWinter L. Canine streptococcal toxic shock syndrome and necrotising fasciitis. Vet Rec. 1997;140:263.

Priestnall S, Erles K. *Streptococcus zooepidemicus:* an emerging canine pathogen. Vet J. 2011;188:142-148.

REFERENCES

1. Wilson LG. The early recognition of streptococci as causes of disease. Med Hist. 1987;31(4):403-414.
2. Schleifer KH, Kilpper-Balz R. Transfer of *Streptococcus faecalis* and *Streptococcus faecium* to the genus *Enterococcus faecalis* comb. nov. and *Enterococcus faecium* comb. nov. Int J Syst Bacteriol. 1984;34:31-34.
3. Lamm CG, Ferguson AC, Lehenbauer TW, et al. Streptococcal infection in dogs: a retrospective study of 393 cases. Vet Pathol. 2010;47:387-395.
4. Tillman PC, Dodson ND, Indiveri M. Group G streptococcal epizootic in a closed cat colony. J Clin Microbiol. 1982;16:1057-1060.
5. Pesavento PA, Bannasch MJ, Bachmann R, et al. Fatal *Streptococcus canis* infections in intensively housed shelter cats. Vet Pathol. 2007;44:218-221.
6. Taillefer M, Dunn M. Group G streptococcal toxic shock-like syndrome in three cats. J Am Anim Hosp Assoc. 2004;40:418-422.
7. Kulendra E, Corr S. Necrotising fasciitis with sub-periosteal *Streptococcus canis* infection in two puppies. Vet Comp Orthop Traumatol. 2008;21:474-477.
8. Sura R, Hinckley LS, Risatti GR, et al. Fatal necrotising fasciitis and myositis in a cat associated with *Streptococcus canis*. Vet Rec. 2008;162:450-453.
9. Prescott JF, DeWinter L. Canine streptococcal toxic shock syndrome and necrotising fasciitis. Vet Rec. 1997;140:263.
10. Lappin E, Ferguson AJ. Gram-positive toxic shock syndromes. Lancet Infect Dis. 2009;9:281-290.
11. Iglauer F, Kunstyr I, Morstedt R, et al. *Streptococcus canis* arthritis in a cat breeding colony. J Exp Anim Sci. 1991;34:59-65.
12. Kruger EF, Byrne BA, Pesavento P, et al. Relationship between clinical manifestations and pulsed-field gel profiles of *Streptococcus canis* isolates from dogs and cats. Vet Microbiol. 2010;146:167-171.
13. Fulde M, Rohde M, Hitzmann A, et al. SCM, a novel M-like protein from *Streptococcus canis*, binds (mini)-plasminogen with high affinity and facilitates bacterial transmigration. Biochem J. 2011;434:523-535.
14. DeWinter LM, Low DE, Prescott JF. Virulence of *Streptococcus canis* from canine streptococcal toxic shock syndrome and necrotizing fasciitis. Vet Microbiol. 1999;70:95-110.
15. Piva S, Zanoni RG, Specchi S, et al. Chronic rhinitis due to *Streptococcus equi* subspecies *zooepidemicus* in a dog. Vet Rec. 2010;167:177-178.
16. Acke E, Abbott Y, Pinilla M, et al. Isolation of *Streptococcus zooepidemicus* from three dogs in close contact with horses. Vet Rec. 2010;167:102-103.
17. Priestnall S, Erles K. *Streptococcus zooepidemicus:* an emerging canine pathogen. Vet J. 2011;188:142-148.
18. Sundberg JP, Hill D, Wyand DS, et al. *Streptococcus zooepidemicus* as the cause of septicemia in racing greyhounds. Vet Med Small Anim Clin. 1981;76:839-842.
19. Britton AP, Davies JL. Rhinitis and meningitis in two shelter cats caused by *Streptococcus equi* subspecies *zooepidemicus*. J Comp Pathol. 2010;143:70-74.
20. Blum S, Elad D, Zukin N, et al. Outbreak of *Streptococcus equi* subsp. *zooepidemicus* infections in cats. Vet Microbiol. 2010;144:236-239.
21. Martin-Vaquero P, da Costa RC, Daniels JB. Presumptive meningoencephalitis secondary to extension of otitis media/interna caused by *Streptococcus equi* subspecies *zooepidemicus* in a cat. J Feline Med Surg. 2011;13:606-609.
22. Larson LJ, Henningson J, Sharp P, et al. Efficacy of the canine influenza virus H3N8 vaccine to decrease severity of clinical disease after cochallenge with canine influenza virus and *Streptococcus equi* subsp. *zooepidemicus*. Clin Vaccine Immunol. 2011;18:559-564.
23. Priestnall SL, Erles K, Brooks HW, et al. Characterization of pneumonia due to *Streptococcus equi* subsp. *zooepidemicus* in dogs. Clin Vaccine Immunol. 2010;17:1790-1796.
24. Paillot R, Darby AC, Robinson C, et al. Identification of three novel superantigen-encoding genes in *Streptococcus equi* subsp. *zooepidemicus*, szeF, szeN, and szeP. Infect Immun. 2010;78:4817-4827.
25. Vela AI, Falsen E, Simarro I, et al. Neonatal mortality in puppies due to bacteremia by *Streptococcus dysgalactiae* subsp. *dysgalactiae*. J Clin Microbiol. 2006;44:666-668.
26. Devriese LA, Haesebrouck F. *Streptococcus suis* infections in horses and cats. Vet Rec. 1992;130:380.
27. Roels S, Devroye O, Buys H, et al. Isolation of *Streptococcus suis* from a cat with meningoencephalitis. Vet Microbiol. 2009;136:206-207.
28. Muckle A, Giles J, Lund L, et al. Isolation of *Streptococcus suis* from the urine of a clinically ill dog. Can Vet J. 2010;51:773-774.
29. Salasia SI, Lammler C, Devriese LA. Serotypes and putative virulence markers of *Streptococcus suis* isolates from cats and dogs. Res Vet Sci. 1994;57:259-261.
30. De Martino L, Nizza S, de Martinis C, et al. *Streptococcus constellatus*-associated pyoderma in a dog. J Med Microbiol. 2011.

31. Schlegel L, Grimont F, Ageron E, et al. Reappraisal of the taxonomy of the *Streptococcus bovis/Streptococcus equinus* complex and related species: description of *Streptococcus gallolyticus* subsp. *gallolyticus* subsp. nov., *S. gallolyticus* subsp. *macedonicus* subsp. nov. and *S. gallolyticus* subsp. *pasteurianus* subsp. nov. Int J Syst Evol Microbiol. 2003;53:631-645.
32. Boleij A, van Gelder MM, Swinkels DW, et al. Clinical importance of *Streptococcus gallolyticus* infection among colorectal cancer patients: systematic review and meta-analysis. Clin Infect Dis. 2011;53:870-878.
33. Sykes JE, Kittleson MD, Pesavento PA, et al. Evaluation of the relationship between causative organisms and clinical characteristics of infective endocarditis in dogs: 71 cases (1992-2005). J Am Vet Med Assoc. 2006;228:1723-1734.
34. Tou SP, Adin DB, Castleman WL. Mitral valve endocarditis after dental prophylaxis in a dog. J Vet Intern Med. 2005;19: 268-270.
35. Schleifer KH, Kilpper-Balz R. Transfer of *Streptococcus faecalis* and *Streptococcus faecium* to the genus *Enterococcus* nom. rev. as *Enterococcus faecalis* com. nov. and *Enterococcus faecium* com. nov. Int J Syst Bacteriol. 1984;34:31-34.
36. Simjee S, White DG, McDermott PF, et al. Characterization of Tn1546 in vancomycin-resistant *Enterococcus faecium* isolated from canine urinary tract infections: evidence of gene exchange between human and animal enterococci. J Clin Microbiol. 2002;40:4659-4665.
37. Manson JM, Keis S, Smith JM, et al. Characterization of a vancomycin-resistant *Enterococcus faecalis* (VREF) isolate from a dog with mastitis: further evidence of a clonal lineage of VREF in New Zealand. J Clin Microbiol. 2003;41:3331-3333.
38. Abbott Y, Kirby BM, Karczmarczyk M, et al. High-level gentamicin-resistant and vancomycin-resistant *Enterococcus faecium* isolated from a wound in a dog. J Small Anim Pract. 2009;50: 194-197.
39. Arias CA, Murray BE. *Enterococcus* species, *Streptococcus bovis* group, and *Leuconostoc* species. In: Mandell GL, Bennett JE, Dolin R, eds. Principles and Practice of Infectious Diseases. Philadelphia, PA: Churchill Livingstone, Elsevier; 2010:2643-2653.
40. Ghanem G, Hachem R, Jiang Y, et al. Outcomes for and risk factors associated with vancomycin-resistant *Enterococcus faecalis* and vancomycin-resistant *Enterococcus faecium* bacteremia in cancer patients. Infect Control Hosp Epidemiol. 2007;28:1054-1059.
41. Mohamed JA, Huang DB. Biofilm formation by enterococci. J Med Microbiol. 2007;56:1581-1588.
42. Damborg P, Top J, Hendrickx AP, et al. Dogs are a reservoir of ampicillin-resistant *Enterococcus faecium* lineages associated with human infections. Appl Environ Microbiol. 2009;75:2360-2365.
43. Jackson CR, Fedorka-Cray PJ, Davis JA, et al. Prevalence, species distribution and antimicrobial resistance of enterococci isolated from dogs and cats in the United States. J Appl Microbiol. 2009;107:1269-1278.
44. Simpson KW, Rishniw M, Bellosa M, et al. Influence of *Enterococcus faecium* SF68 probiotic on giardiasis in dogs. J Vet Intern Med. 2009;23:476-481.
45. Bybee SN, Scorza AV, Lappin MR. Effect of the probiotic *Enterococcus faecium* SF68 on presence of diarrhea in cats and dogs housed in an animal shelter. J Vet Intern Med. 2011;25: 856-860.
46. Lappin MR, Veir JK, Satyaraj E, et al. Pilot study to evaluate the effect of oral supplementation of *Enterococcus faecium* SF68 on cats with latent feline herpesvirus 1. J Feline Med Surg. 2009;11:650-654.
47. Veir JK, Knorr R, Cavadini C, et al. Effect of supplementation with *Enterococcus faecium* (SF68) on immune functions in cats. Vet Ther. 2007;8:229-238.
48. Benyacoub J, Czarnecki-Maulden GL, Cavadini C, et al. Supplementation of food with *Enterococcus faecium* (SF68) stimulates immune functions in young dogs. J Nutr. 2003;133:1158-1162.
49. Delgado M, Neto I, Correia JH, et al. Antimicrobial resistance and evaluation of susceptibility testing among pathogenic enterococci isolated from dogs and cats. Int J Antimicrob Agents. 2007;30:98-100.
50. Ossiprandi MC, Bottarelli E, Cattabiani F, et al. Susceptibility to vancomycin and other antibiotics of 165 *Enterococcus* strains isolated from dogs in Italy. Comp Immunol Microbiol Infect Dis. 2008;31:1-9.
51. Naser SM, Vancanneyt M, De Graef E, et al. *Enterococcus canintestini* sp. nov., from faecal samples of healthy dogs. Int J Syst Evol Microbiol. 2005;55:2177-2182.
52. Helie P, Higgins R. Diarrhea associated with Enterococcus faecium in an adult cat. J Vet Diagn Invest. 1999;11:457-458.
53 Nicklas JL, Moisan P, Stone MR, et al. In situ molecular diagnosis and histopathological characterization of enteroadherent *Enterococcus hirae* infection in pre-weaning-age kittens. J Clin Microbiol. 2010;48:2814-2820.
54. Rivera AM, Boucher HW. Current concepts in antimicrobial therapy against select gram-positive organisms: methicillin-resistant *Staphylococcus aureus*, penicillin-resistant pneumococci, and vancomycin-resistant enterococci. Mayo Clin Proc. 2011;86:1230-1243.
55. Garnett NL, Eydelloth RS, Swindle MM, et al. Hemorrhagic streptococcal pneumonia in newly procured research dogs. J Am Vet Med Assoc. 1982;181:1371-1374.
56. Pesavento PA, Hurley KF, Bannasch MJ, et al. A clonal outbreak of acute fatal hemorrhagic pneumonia in intensively housed (shelter) dogs caused by *Streptococcus equi* subsp. *zooepidemicus*. Vet Pathol. 2008;45:51-53.
57. Bisno AL, Stevens DL. *Streptococcus pyogenes*. In: Mandell GL, Bennett JE, Dolin R, eds. Principles and Practice of Infectious Diseases. 7th ed. Philadelphia, PA: Churchill Livingstone, Elsevier; 2010:2593-2610.
58. Pillai A, Thomas S, Williams C. Clindamycin in the treatment of group G beta-haemolytic streptococcal infections. J Infect. 2005;51:e207-e211.
59. Lyskova P, Vydrzalova M, Mazurova J. Identification and antimicrobial susceptibility of bacteria and yeasts isolated from healthy dogs and dogs with otitis externa. J Vet Med A Physiol Pathol Clin Med. 2007;54:559-563.
60. Pedersen K, Jensen H, Finster K, et al. Occurrence of antimicrobial resistance in bacteria from diagnostic samples from dogs. J Antimicrob Chemother. 2007;60:775-781.
61. Irwin PJ, Parry BW. Streptococcal meningoencephalitis in a dog. J Am Anim Hosp Assoc. 1999;35:417-422.
62. Harada T, Tsuji N, Otsuki K, et al. Detection of the esp gene in high-level gentamicin resistant *Enterococcus faecalis* strains from pet animals in Japan. Vet Microbiol. 2005;106:139-143.
63. Dowzicky MJ. Susceptibility to tigecycline and linezolid among gram-positive isolates collected in the United States as part of the tigecycline evaluation and surveillance trial (TEST) between 2004 and 2009. Clin Ther. 2011;33:1964-1973.
64. Swaminathan S, Alangaden GJ. Treatment of resistant enterococcal urinary tract infections. Curr Infect Dis Rep. 2010;12:455-464.
65. Carapetis JR, Steer AC, Mulholland EK, et al. The global burden of group A streptococcal diseases. Lancet Infect Dis. 2005;5:685-694.
66. Mayer G, Van Ore S. Recurrent pharyngitis in family of four. Household pet as reservoir of group A streptococci. Postgrad Med. 1983;74:277-279.
67. Falck G. Group A streptococci in household pets' eyes—a source of infection in humans? Scand J Infect Dis. 1997;29:469-471.
68. Wilson KS, Maroney SA, Gander RM. The family pet as an unlikely source of group A beta-hemolytic streptococcal infection in humans. Pediatr Infect Dis J. 1995;14:372-375.
69. Stallings B, Ling GV, Lagenaur LA, et al. Septicemia and septic arthritis caused by *Streptococcus pneumoniae* in a cat: possible transmission from a child. J Am Vet Med Assoc. 1987;191: 703-704.

70. Zhang S, Wilson F, Pace L. *Streptococcus pneumoniae*-associated cellulitis in a two-month-old domestic shorthair kitten. J Vet Diagn Invest. 2006;18:221-224.
71. Galperine T, Cazorla C, Blanchard E, et al. *Streptococcus canis* infections in humans: retrospective study of 54 patients. J Infect. 2007;55:23-26.
72. Lam MM, Clarridge 3rd JE, Young EJ, et al. The other group G *Streptococcus*: increased detection of *Streptococcus canis* ulcer infections in dog owners. J Clin Microbiol. 2007;45:2327-2329.
73. Abbott Y, Acke E, Khan S, et al. Zoonotic transmission of *Streptococcus equi* subsp. *zooepidemicus* from a dog to a handler. J Med Microbiol. 2010;59:120-123.
74. Ghosh A, Dowd SE, Zurek L. Dogs leaving the ICU carry a very large multi-drug resistant enterococcal population with capacity for biofilm formation and horizontal gene transfer. PLoS One. 2011;6:e22451.

CHAPTER 35

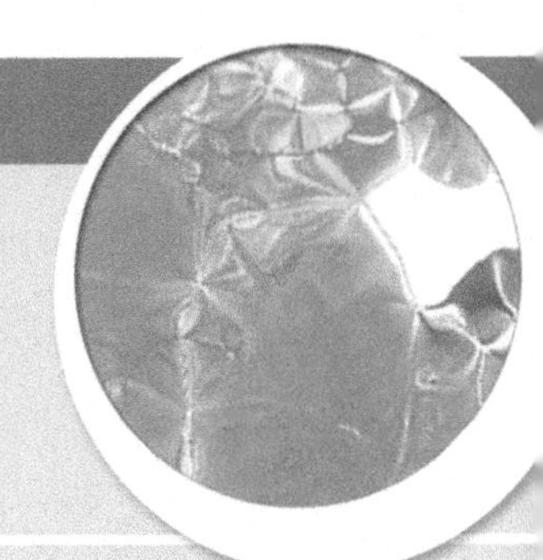

Staphylococcus Infections

Jane E. Sykes

> **Overview of Staphylococcal Infections in Dogs and Cats**
>
> First Described: 1882 in Scotland (Alexander Ogsten)[1]
>
> Causes: In dogs and cats, the most common causes are *Staphylococcus pseudintermedius, Staphylococcus schleiferi, Staphylococcus aureus,* and various coagulase-negative staphylococci, which are gram-positive coccoid bacteria.
>
> Geographic Distribution: Worldwide
>
> Mode of Transmission: Direct contact (or through fomites). Organisms are often commensals that invade opportunistically.
>
> Major Clinical Signs: Pyoderma, otitis externa, surgical site infections, osteomyelitis, bacteremia and endocarditis, bronchopneumonia, urinary tract infections, ocular surface infections, rarely necrotizing fasciitis and toxic shock syndrome, pyothorax and peritonitis, discospondylitis, arthritis
>
> Differential Diagnoses: Primarily other gram-positive and gram-negative bacterial infections
>
> Human Health Significance: Humans can become colonized with staphylococcal isolates that colonize or infect dogs and cats. Methicillin-resistant *S. aureus,* which can persistently colonize humans, is of greatest concern, although colonization of dogs with MRSA appears to be transient. *S. pseudintermedius,* which persistently colonizes dogs, has occasionally been isolated from sick and healthy people who are in contact with dogs, and is of concern because of its tendency to show a high degree of multidrug resistance.

Etiology and Epidemiology

Staphylococcus spp. are gram positive, nonmotile, non–spore forming, and usually catalase-positive cocci, which occur singly and in pairs or grapelike clusters (Figure 35-1). Most species are facultative anaerobes. Staphylococci colonize the skin and mucous membranes of an enormous variety of animal species, and disease generally follows a breakdown in normal host defenses. Staphylococci can also contaminate surfaces in the environment, where they may survive for several months.

Staphylococci are classified as *coagulase negative* or *coagulase positive* based on their ability to produce coagulase, an enzyme that cleaves fibrinogen into fibrin and results in coagulation of plasma. There are more than 40 species in the genus *Staphylococcus,*[2] many of which are adapted to live on certain host species. The major coagulase-positive staphylococci that infect dogs and cats are *Staphylococcus pseudintermedius* (previously identified as *Staphylococcus intermedius*) and *Staphylococcus aureus. Staphylococcus schleiferi* has also been isolated from dogs (and rarely cats) with pyoderma and otitis externa and has been divided into *S. schleiferi* subsp. *schleiferi,* which is coagulase-negative, and *S. schleiferi* subsp. *coagulans,* which is coagulase-positive. However, these may instead represent a single species, *S. schleiferi,* with variable coagulase production.[3] Coagulase-negative staphylococci (CoNS) tend to be of lower virulence than coagulase-positive staphylococci but occasionally cause disease in immunocompromised hosts. Examples of coagulase-negative staphylococci are *Staphylococcus felis* and *Staphylococcus epidermidis. S. felis* has been recognized as a urinary tract pathogen in cats.[4] CoNS are often not identified to the species level by microbiology laboratories.

In recent years, the prevalence of antimicrobial drug resistance has increased in *Staphylococcus* isolates obtained from canine and feline infections. A significant proportion of resistant isolates possess the *mecA* gene, which encodes an altered penicillin binding protein (PBP), known as PBP2a. The *mecA* gene is located on a large genetic element, the *staphylococcal cassette chromosome.* This PBP has low affinity for *all* β-lactam drugs (penicillins, cephalosporins, and carbapenems). As a result, staphylococci that possess this gene are also resistant to the penicillinase-resistant penicillins (oxacillin and methicillin), and so are termed *methicillin-resistant Staphylococcus* (MRS) species. Many MRS also possess resistance genes to other antimicrobial drug classes. There is no evidence that MRS are more virulent than methicillin-susceptible staphylococci, but infections with MRS are more difficult to treat with antimicrobial drugs. The prevalence of MRS isolated from dogs has ranged from 0.6% to as high as 67%, depending on the population sampled (healthy versus disease, hospitalized versus outpatients), geographic location, study dates, and sites of specimen collection. Of 89 staphylococcal isolates from dogs with superficial pyoderma seen in 2010 and 2011 by the University of California, Davis, Veterinary Dermatology service, 38.2% were MRS. This compared with 27.3% of 33 isolates from a primary care clinic in the same region.[5] Methicillin-resistant *S. pseudintermedius* (MRSP) isolates are generally resistant to more antimicrobial drug classes than methicillin-resistant *S. aureus* (MRSA) isolates from dogs and cats. Severe multidrug resistance is also prevalent among CoNS.

Staphylococcus pseudintermedius

S. pseudintermedius is the most common *Staphylococcus* species isolated from dogs. It is a commensal of the skin and mucous membranes of dogs and cats and possibly one of the most common bacterial pathogens treated by veterinarians. It primarily colonizes the anal mucosa and nares of healthy dogs and cats, but it can also be isolated from the mouth, forehead, and

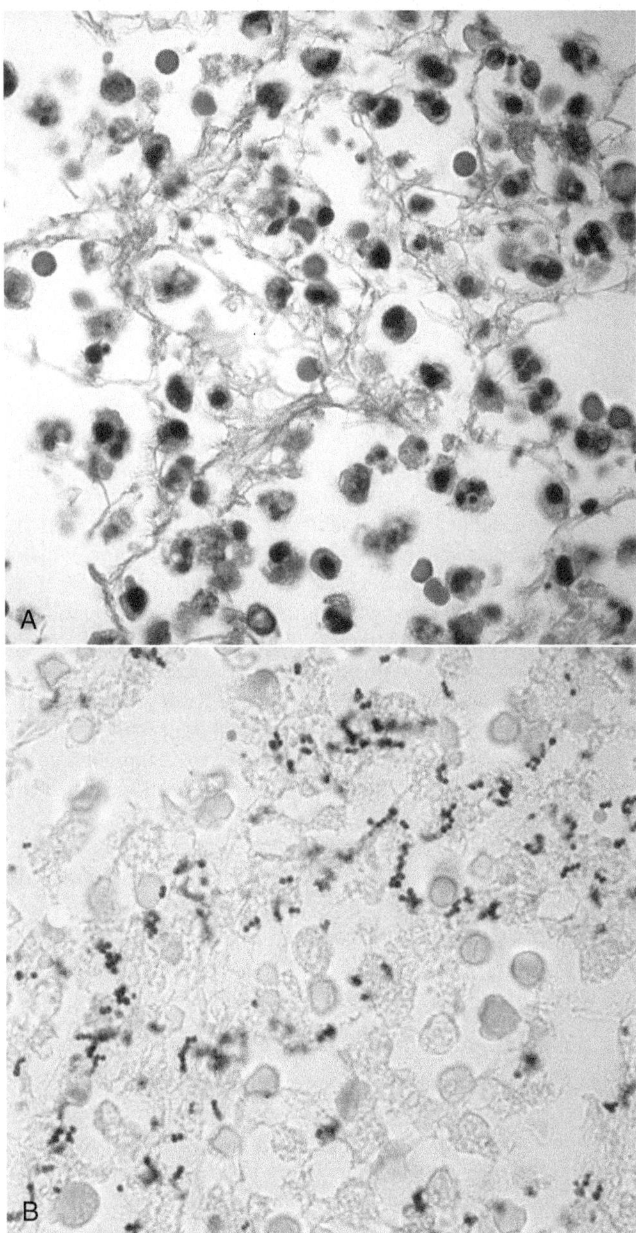

FIGURE 35-1 Histopathology of the integument from the left inguinal region and flank of an 8-year old male neutered boxer dog that had severe, regionally extensive acute neutrophilic cellulitis and panniculitis accompanied by septic shock. A methicillin susceptible *Staphylococcus pseudintermedius* was cultured from an aspirate of cellulitis fluid. The dog had also been treated with prednisone and azathioprine for 4 years to maintain remission for immune-mediated hemolytic anemia and thrombocytopenia. **A,** H&E stain. Large numbers of degenerate neutrophils are present. **B,** Staining with Brown and Benn stain reveals numerous of gram-positive coccoid bacteria, individually, in pairs, and in clusters. 1000× oil magnification.

inguinal region. It can colonize the skin transiently following grooming and licking in dogs with pruritis. Cats have a much lower prevalence of colonization with *S. pseudintermedius* than dogs. *S. pseudintermedius* invades tissues opportunistically and is a major cause of superficial and deep pyoderma, otitis externa, urinary tract infections (UTIs), and wound and surgical site infections, as well as bronchopneumonia, ocular infections, bacteremia, osteomyelitis, and infections of body cavities. An underlying immunosuppressive condition or break in host barriers is present in the majority of infections.

Before 2005, *S. pseudintermedius* were identified as *S. intermedius*. The name *S. pseudintermedius* was defined when isolates from a dog, cat, horse, and parrot were analyzed using molecular methods.[6] Subsequently, a molecular analysis of organisms from dogs and cats that had been previously identified as *S. intermedius* revealed that they were actually *S. pseudintermedius*. *S. pseudintermedius* belongs to the "*S. intermedius* group" (SIG), which comprises the three closely related species *S. intermedius*, *S. pseudintermedius*, and *S. delphini*. It is difficult to differentiate among these species with phenotypic methods alone; genetic typing methods are required. Because genetic typing methods are not available for routine identification in veterinary diagnostic laboratories, isolates from dogs with phenotypic characteristics typical of *S. intermedius* are now generally identified as *S. pseudintermedius*.[7] However, some laboratories still describe strains from dogs that have biochemical characteristics that do not quite match that typical for the type strain of *S. pseudintermedius* as "SIG organisms."

The whole genome of *S. pseudintermedius* has been sequenced, which is a major contribution to our understanding of the pathogenesis of infections caused by this organism.[8] Like *S. aureus*, *S. pseudintermedius* possesses numerous mobile genetic elements and potential virulence factors, such as toxin genes that encode for a superantigen, leukotoxin, hemolysins, and exfoliative toxins, as well as an array of proteases.

Methicillin resistance has emerged as a serious and widespread problem in *S. pseudintermedius* isolates from both healthy and sick dogs and cats. Molecular analysis has shown that among dogs, two distinct, major clones of MRSP have spread across Europe and North America, respectively.[9] Many isolates of *S. pseudintermedius* not only are methicillin resistant, but also acquire resistance genes to other classes of antimicrobials, including tetracyclines, trimethoprim-sulfonamides, fluoroquinolones, chloramphenicol, and macrolides. Isolates that are resistant to three or more different *classes* of antimicrobial drugs are defined as multiple drug resistant (MDR) isolates. Currently, many isolates remain susceptible to chloramphenicol and aminoglycosides, but the prevalence of resistance to chloramphenicol has increased among MRSP isolates. MDR *S. pseudintermedius* isolates are no more virulent or difficult to disinfect than susceptible isolates, but they are more difficult to eliminate using antimicrobial drugs. Risk factors for MRSP infection identified in dogs include previous hospitalization, living in an urban environment, older age, and, most consistently, previous antimicrobial drug treatment. Household contacts of dogs and cats with MRSP infection are also frequently colonized with MRSP.[10]

Staphylococcus aureus

S. aureus colonizes the skin and mucous membranes of humans and is one of the most common community-acquired and hospital-acquired bacterial pathogens of people. The anterior nares and the throat are preferred niches for the organism, which can be isolated from the anterior nares of up to 30% of the healthy human population. Methicillin resistance is a growing problem among isolates from humans and animals. Both hospital-acquired methicillin-resistant (HA-MRSA) and community-acquired methicillin-resistant (CA-MRSA) strains have been identified in infected human patients, and invasive *S. aureus* infections are associated with high mortality rates.

When compared with *S. pseudintermedius*, *S. aureus* tends not to colonize dogs. For example, staphylococci were isolated from 37 of 50 healthy dogs from Pennsylvania, and 6 (12%) of the dogs were colonized with *S. aureus*; 68% were colonized with *S. pseudintermedius*.[11] MRSA strains that colonize dogs may be identical to those that infect in-contact humans, but sometimes strains found on dogs differ from those found on in-contact humans.[12] The chance that a dog that is in contact with an infected human will be colonized with MRSA decreases with the time after diagnosis of human MRSA infection, which suggests transient carriage of MRSA by dogs. MRSA was not transferred between apparently healthy dogs in a kennel of dogs, and after treatment of an MRSA wound infection in one dog, all dogs tested negative for MRSA within 2 weeks.[13] Although staphylococci are isolated less commonly from cats, colonization with *S. aureus* is more prevalent and certain *S. aureus* strains may be commensals of cats; staphylococci were isolated from 17 of 50 healthy cats, 59% of which were colonized with *S. aureus* and 65% with *S. pseudintermedius*.[14]

In dogs and cats, *S. aureus* infection has been associated with clinical manifestations that include pyoderma, otitis externa, UTIs, surgical site infections, osteomyelitis, and bacteremia. Although MRSA infections are uncommonly diagnosed in dogs and cats, they have been increasingly recognized over the past 2 decades. When canine infections with MRSA do occur, they are often of human hospital origin, but human community-acquired strains have also been isolated. In one study, strong risk factors for MRSA infection (as opposed to methicillin-susceptible *S. aureus* [MSSA] infection) were the number of antimicrobial courses administered, the number of days admitted to veterinary clinics, and a history of surgical implant placement.[15] There has been concern that the use of certain antibiotics, such as cephalosporins and fluoroquinolones, may select for MRSA infections in dogs.

Staphylococcus schleiferi

Coagulase-positive and coagulase-negative *S. schleiferi* have primarily been isolated from dogs with superficial pyoderma and otitis externa, as well as from the ear canals of healthy dogs. Rarely, UTIs and respiratory infections with *S. schleiferi* have been described in dogs.[3] In dogs with pyoderma and otitis externa, *S. schleiferi* is not as prevalent as *S. pseudintermedius* but in most studies has been isolated as often, or more often, than *S. aureus*. Coagulase-negative *S. schleiferi* is a commensal of the human axilla but can cause disease in immunosuppressed humans. Coagulase-positive *S. schleiferi* may be specialized to colonize dogs.

S. schleiferi isolates from dogs with skin disease are often methicillin-resistant as a result of *mecA* gene carriage. In a study of 225 *S. schleiferi* isolates from dogs from the eastern United States, of which 52% were coagulase negative and 42% were coagulase positive, methicillin resistance was identified in 57% of the isolates.[3] Methicillin resistance was more prevalent among coagulase-negative isolates. Isolates from dogs with pyoderma may be more likely to be methicillin resistant than those from dogs with otitis externa.

Clinical Features

Signs and Their Pathophysiology

Staphylococci can cause pyoderma, otitis externa, pneumonia, UTIs, soft tissue infections, surgical site infections, bacteremia, ocular infections, and endocarditis in dogs and cats.

S. aureus and *S. pseudintermedius* possess several adhesins and produce an array of toxins. The clinical effect of these toxins is best characterized for *S. aureus* infections in humans. A number of enterotoxins have been identified in *S. aureus* and *S. pseudintermedius*; these can cause food poisoning in humans but have not been recognized as a cause of disease in dogs and cats. Staphylococcal enterotoxins are heat stable, so they are not inactivated by cooking, even when the bacteria themselves are destroyed. *Staphylococcal toxic shock syndrome* results from the expression of superantigens, which include toxic shock syndrome toxin 1, as well as a large number of enterotoxins and exotoxins that can also act as superantigens. Cellulitis, necrotizing fasciitis, and toxic shock syndrome has been rarely reported in dogs infected with *S. pseudintermedius*.[16,17] Most toxic shock syndrome and necrotizing fasciitis cases in dogs and cats are instead caused by *Streptococcus canis* (see Chapter 34). *Scalded skin syndrome* results from infection of humans with *S. aureus* strains that produce an exfoliative toxin, which hydrolyses the intercellular glycoprotein desmoglein-1. Strains of *S. pseudintermedius* that possess exfoliative toxin genes have been isolated more commonly from dogs with pyoderma than from healthy dogs, so exfoliative toxin may also play a role in canine disease. *Panton-Valentine toxin (PVL)* is a leukocidin that is found in CA-MRSA strains but only a small percentage of HA-MRSA and MSSA strains, and strains that encode PVL have been associated with skin and soft tissue infections and hemorrhagic pneumonia in children and young adults. Although a similar toxin has been identified in *S. pseudintermedius*, the role of PVL in the pathogenesis of staphylococcal infections in dogs and cats is unknown.

Some strains of *S. pseudintermedius* and *S. aureus* produce biofilm, which may contribute to the ability of these organisms to persist in the environment, cause nosocomial infections, and chronic recurrent infections that respond poorly to antimicrobial treatment.[18]

Diagnosis

Laboratory Abnormalities

Complete Blood Count, Biochemistry, and Urinalysis Findings

Dogs with staphylococcal infections of the skin and ear canal often have no clinically significant hematologic or biochemical findings. Systemic infections may be associated with neutrophilia and a left shift, toxic neutrophils, lymphopenia, and monocytosis. The urinalysis of dogs and cats with staphylococcal UTIs may reveal pyuria, proteinuria, or hematuria, and sometimes cocci in clusters may be evident on sediment examination.

Cytologic Abnormalities

Aspirates of affected tissues or pus or respiratory lavage fluid specimens from animals with staphylococcal infections may contain large numbers of degenerate and nondegenerate neutrophils. The presence of cocci in clusters suggests staphylococcal infection.

Microbiological Tests

Isolation and Identification

Staphylococci that infect dogs and cats are readily isolated on routine bacteriologic media from aspirates, tissue biopsies, body fluid, and lavage specimens. Colonies typically appear within 24 hours. Staphylococcal species are identified on the basis of phenotypic and biochemical reactions such as production of coagulase and/or clumping factor, production of hemolysins, ability to ferment carbohydrates, and acetoin production (Vogues-Proskauer reaction). PCR and sequencing of ribosomal

RNA genes (16S or 23S) may be necessary for identification of some species. CoNS are often not identified to the species level because molecular techniques are often required for accurate identification. Because CoNS are of low pathogenicity, they may be contaminants, especially if they are isolated from nonsterile sites, growth is minimal (1+), or another pathogen is present. However, they may occasionally be pathogenic. In particular, isolation of *S. felis* from urine or coagulase-negative *S. schleiferi* from dogs with pyoderma or otitis may have clinical significance.

Evaluation of antimicrobial susceptibility is of critical importance because of the high prevalence of methicillin-resistant and multidrug-resistant staphylococci in some parts of the world. Susceptibility testing for staphylococci should be performed according to recommendations of groups such as the Clinical and Laboratory Standards Institute (CLSI). Oxacillin and cefoxitin are used in the laboratory as a surrogate for detection of methicillin resistance. Laboratories should report methicillin-resistant staphylococci as resistant to all other penicillins, carbapenems, cephalosporins, and β-lactam/β-lactamase inhibitor combinations, regardless of the results of in vitro susceptibility test results for these agents.

Molecular Diagnosis Using the Polymerase Chain Reaction

Real-time PCR assays have been developed that detect and differentiate some *Staphylococcus* species, as well as identify the presence of the *mecA* gene. These assays are available in some laboratories for diagnosis of MRSA infections in humans, but to date have only been used on a research basis to characterize staphylococci isolated from dogs and cats.

Treatment and Prognosis

The approach to treatment of staphylococcal infections depends on the site of infection and the severity of disease; the reader is referred to Chapters 84 to 90 for treatment recommendations for different organ systems. Identification and management of the underlying cause (rather than repeated treatment with antimicrobial drugs) is of paramount importance to minimize selection for resistant organisms. Any foreign material (such as catheters, implants) must be removed. Bathing and topical treatments should be considered for pyoderma as an alternative to antimicrobial drug therapy (see Chapter 84). The use of topical wound treatments such as accelerated hydrogen peroxide, chlorhexidine, or silver sulfadiazine could also be considered provided infection is superficial.

When systemic antimicrobial treatment is necessary, staphylococcal infections should ideally be treated based on the results of culture and susceptibility testing and/or knowledge of the regional prevalence of methicillin resistance and multidrug resistance, because this can vary, not only between countries but also between different states or regions within a state. In regions where methicillin resistance is rare, a β-lactam drug such as cephalexin, clavulanic acid–amoxicillin, or a penicillinase-resistant penicillin could be used empirically (Table 35-1), and culture and susceptibility testing may not be necessary for uncomplicated infections such as newly diagnosed pyoderma or UTIs.

Where methicillin resistance is prevalent in the region, culture and susceptibility testing is recommended. If this is not possible, a reasonable first choice for uncomplicated infections that are not life threatening is clindamycin. Clindamycin is an attractive choice given that many infections are skin, orthopedic, or soft tissue infections (sites to which clindamycin distributes well); it is inexpensive, inhibits toxin production by staphylococci, and is available in oral and intravenous formulations. However, some MRS demonstrate *inducible clindamycin resistance*, a phenomenon whereby the organism is susceptible to clindamycin in vitro but rapidly develops resistance to clindamycin when exposed to macrolides (such as erythromycin) or lincosamides in vivo, owing to bacterial methylation of the ribosomal binding

TABLE 35-1

Suggested Antimicrobial Drugs for Treatment of Staphylococcal Infections in Dogs and Cats

Predicted/Determined Staphylococcal Susceptibility	Drug	Dose (mg/kg)	Interval (hours)	Route
Methicillin-susceptible	Ampicillin sodium	10-20	6-8	IV, IM, SC
	Cefazolin sodium	20-35	8	IV, IM
	Cephalexin	10-30 (dogs), 15-20 (cats)	12	PO
Methicillin-resistant*	Trimethoprim-sulfamethoxazole	30	12	PO, IV
	Clindamycin†	11	12	PO
	Doxycycline	10	12	PO
	Rifampin	5-10	12	PO
	Amikacin	15-30 (dogs), 10-14 (cats)	24	IV, IM, SC
	Vancomycin‡	15	6-8 (dogs), 8 (cats)	IV
	Linezolid‡	10 (dogs)	8	PO, IV
	Nitrofurantoin (macrocrystalline formulation)§	2-3	8	PO

*Susceptibility testing recommended if methicillin resistance is likely based on regional or hospital prevalence data. Many isolates are resistant to clindamycin, trimethoprim-sulfamethoxazole, doxycycline; some are resistant to chloramphenicol. Consider topical antibacterial treatment if possible.
†May not be effective if erythromycin resistance is present on the susceptibility panel due to inducible clindamycin resistance.
‡Reserve for serious infections that are resistant to all other reasonable alternatives, on the basis of culture and susceptibility testing. See Table 8-6 for vancomycin administration protocol.
§For resistant urinary tract infections only.

site for clindamycin.[19] The end result is treatment failure or relapse, although some treatment successes have been reported in human patients infected with *S. aureus* strains that have inducible clindamycin resistance. Staphylococci with inducible clindamycin resistance are resistant to macrolides such as erythromycin and susceptible to clindamycin in routine susceptibility tests. Nevertheless, not all staphylococci with this resistance pattern demonstrate inducible clindamycin resistance. Identification of inducible clindamycin resistance requires a special test known as a *D-zone test.* It involves culture of the organism on agar in the presence of an erythromycin and clindamycin disk. Organisms near to the erythromycin disk express enhanced resistance to clindamycin, which results in a D shape to the zone of inhibition around the clindamycin disk (Figure 35-2). At the time of writing, inducible clindamycin resistance appears to be prevalent in *S. aureus* isolates from dogs and cats (18% in one study of 62 isolates) but is rarely reported in *S. pseudintermedius* (0 of 46 isolates in one study, and 1 of 60 isolates in another study).[20,21] As a result, it is reasonable to assume that disease caused by *S. pseudintermedius* isolates that are susceptible to clindamycin on routine susceptibility testing is likely to respond to treatment with clindamycin. However, in some geographic locations, a high percentage of canine MRSP isolates are overtly resistant to clindamycin, which suggests that clindamycin may not be an ideal empiric treatment choice in these locations. The use of fluoroquinolones to treat staphylococcal infections has been controversial, because they have been associated with treatment failures and development of methicillin resistance in human *S. aureus* infections. In one study, a fluoroquinolone control program in a tertiary human hospital led to a significant reduction in fluoroquinolone-resistant *Pseudomonas aeruginosa* and MRSA rates over 4 years.[22]

If severe and invasive infection with an MRS is a possibility, a combination of clindamycin and an aminoglycoside could be administered parenterally, pending the results of culture and susceptibility testing. Antimicrobials that could be considered for life-threatening methicillin-resistant and multidrug-resistant staphylococcal infections include trimethoprim-sulfamethoxazole, doxycycline, aminoglycosides, rifampin, chloramphenicol, vancomycin, tigecycline, quinupristin-dalfopristin, and linezolid (see Chapter 8). Some MRS are also resistant to trimethoprim-sulfamethoxazole, doxycycline, and chloramphenicol, and toxicity may limit the usefulness of trimethoprim-sulfamethoxazole and chloramphenicol (see Chapter 8). Aminoglycosides must be given parenterally and have the potential to cause nephrotoxicity, and their activity is reduced in the presence of pus. The use of rifampin alone is controversial, because rifampin monotherapy has been associated with development of resistance in *S. aureus* infections.[23] As a result, the use of rifampin in combination with other drugs has been recommended. Minocycline has received attention as an alternative to doxycycline because some doxycycline-resistant strains (strains that possess the tetracycline efflux protein tetK) remain susceptible to minocycline. In contrast, strains that possess tetM (which protects the ribosome from tetracycline binding) are resistant to all tetracyclines. Additional information on the pharmacokinetics and definition of clinical breakpoints for minocycline are required.

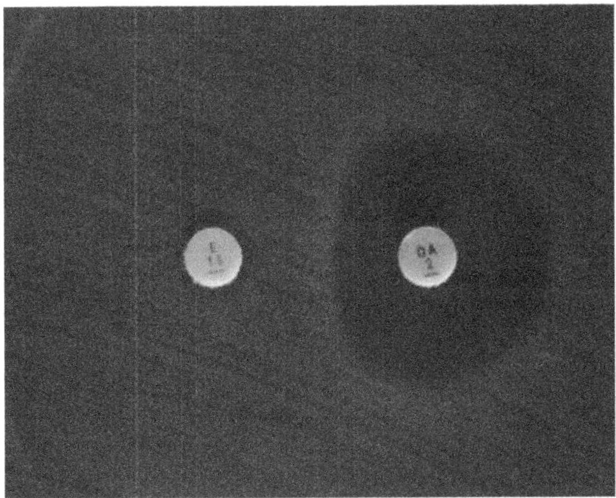

FIGURE 35-2 Positive D-zone test for inducible clindamycin resistance in staphylococci. Organisms exposed to erythromycin express enhanced resistance to clindamycin, which leads to distortion of the zone of inhibition around the clindamycin disk. (Courtesy Dr. Scott Weese, University of Guelph.)

Vancomycin, tigecycline, daptomycin, quinupristin-dalfopristin, and linezolid are important drugs for MRSA infections in humans. Whether these drugs should be used to treat companion animals has been debated, given that they are already widely used in humans and that they may be required to save the lives of companion animals. Cost and/or the need for parenteral administration (vancomycin, tigecycline, daptomycin, and quinupristin-dalfopristin) can also limit the usefulness of these drugs in companion animals. At a minimum, their use should be reserved for situations when no other treatment alternatives exist and when the infection is life threatening but has the potential to be resolved with appropriate treatment. The use of vancomycin or linezolid may be indicated in dogs with bacteremia or endocarditis due to MRSA, MRSP, or methicillin-resistant CoNS that are resistant to all options other than aminoglycosides and concerns for aminoglycoside toxicity exist.

Prevention

Prevention of staphylococcal infections involves attention to the underlying cause of disease (such as allergic dermatitis), and strict veterinary clinic and veterinary hospital infection control practices (see Chapter 11). Because canine MRSA infections may be acquired from colonized or infected humans, transmission to dogs may be reduced by hand washing and general surface cleaning and disinfection in the home environment (see Public Health Aspects, next).

Public Health Aspects

Most concern regarding the public health risk of staphylococcal infection or colonization in companion animals has related to MRSA. However, because colonization of dogs with MRSA is transient, other humans are a more significant source of human MRSA infection. Nevertheless, some studies suggest that veterinarians who work with small animals may be at increased risk for colonization with MRSA. Although around 30% of the human population is colonized with *S. aureus*, the prevalence of MRSA colonization is generally much lower than this, less than 2%. In Australia, dog and cat veterinarians had a fivefold higher risk for MRSA carriage when compared with industry and government veterinarians.[24] Small animal veterinarians in the United Kingdom were also at increased risk of colonization.[25] In a study from the United States, 17.3% of veterinarians and veterinary technicians were colonized, and the rate of colonization did not differ between small- and large-animal veterinarians.[26] In another study, only large-animal practice was associated with colonization.[27]

Regardless of the direction of transmission (human to pet versus pet to human), owners of dogs and cats diagnosed with MRSA infection should be educated about the need to wash their hands after handling their pets, clean and disinfect surfaces that might become contaminated, and not let their pet lick their face or open wounds. Infected sites should be covered with a suitable dressing to minimize contamination of the environment whenever possible. Owners should be instructed to talk to their health care providers if they have concerns about their health or the health of others in their household. In the hospital environment, transmission of MRSA may be prevented through the use of a strict hospital infection control program (see Chapter 11). Routine screening and decontamination is not recommended because dogs appear to resolve infection over time. Topical mupirocin, which has been used for decontamination in humans, is not likely to be effective in dogs and cats given the large size of their nasal cavities, and concerns have been raised regarding the need for and efficacy of decolonization with systemic antibiotics, which may only select for antimicrobial resistance.

Human infections with *S. pseudintermedius* occur occasionally in association with pet contact, although the organism generally tends not to colonize humans. However, colonization with MRSP was reported more frequently in small-animal dermatologists than colonization with MRSA.[28,29] Precautions recommended for MRSA infection are also indicated for MRSP infections.

CASE EXAMPLE

Signalment: "Elliot," a 10-year-old male neutered miniature schnauzer from San Francisco, CA

History: Elliot was seen for a possible pacemaker infection. One month after placement of a dual-chamber pacemaker for sick sinus syndrome, a fluctuant mass was noted around the generator. The seroma was aspirated, and cytologic examination of the aspirate showed many neutrophils. Treatment with clavulanic acid-amoxicillin was initiated (25 mg/kg PO q12h). One month later, there had been no apparent improvement. The wound was flushed with chlorhexidine solution and treatment with chloramphenicol was initiated, but the problem persisted. The chloramphenicol was discontinued, and the dog was referred for further evaluation. The owners reported no vomiting, diarrhea, or decreased appetite. Elliot had also been diagnosed with early myxomatous degeneration of the mitral valve based on the results of echocardiography, associated with a grade III/VI left apical systolic murmur at the time of pacemaker placement.

Physical Examination:

Body Weight: 9.8 kg

General: Quiet, alert, and responsive. Slightly tacky but pink mucous membranes, capillary refill time <2 s, approximately 5% dehydrated, T = 104°F, HR = 160 beats/min, RR = 40 breaths/min.

Eyes, Ears, Nose, and Throat: A mild crusted ocular discharge was present bilaterally, as well as mild serous nasal discharge, and moderate periodontal disease.

Integument: A 1-cm wound that discharged purulent material was present in the region of the right jugular incision, with a draining tract located along the jugular lead that extended to the pacemaker generator over the right cervical region. There was an accumulation of fluid that measured 1 cm in diameter over the generator.

Musculoskeletal: Ambulatory with normal gait, BCS 5/9

Cardiovascular: Heart rate 160 beats/min, regular rhythm, grade III/VI left apical systolic murmur, femoral pulses strong and synchronous

Respiratory: Mild crackles were auscultated in the left and right caudal lung fields.

Abdominal Palpation: Cranial organomegaly was present.

Lymph Nodes: All lymph nodes were normal in size.

Laboratory Findings:

CBC:

HCT 32.2% (40%-55%)
MCV 60.3 fL (65-75 fL)
MCHC 32.3 g/dL (33-36 g/dL)
Reticulocytes 9100 cells/μL (7000-65,000 cells/μL)
WBC 29,680 cells/μL (6000-13,000 cells/μL)
Neutrophils 22,854 cells/μL (3000-10,500 cells/μL)
Lymphocytes 4155 cells/μL (1000-4000 cells/μL)
Monocytes 594 cells/μL (150-1200 cells/μL)
Eosinophils 890 cells/μL (0-1500 cells/μL)
Platelets 446,000 platelets/μL (150,000-400,000 platelets/μL)
Slight toxicity of neutrophils and band neutrophils.

Serum Chemistry Profile:

Sodium 140 mmol/L (145-154 mmol/L)
Potassium 5.6 mmol/L (3.6-5.3 mmol/L)
Chloride 103 mmol/L (108-118 mmol/L)
Bicarbonate 16 mmol/L (16-26 mmol/L)
Phosphorus 7.5 mg/dL (3.0-6.2 mg/dL)
Calcium 11.3 mg/dL (9.7-11.5 mg/dl)
BUN 48 mg/dL (5-21 mg/dL)
Creatinine 1.8 mg/dL (0.3-1.2 mg/dL)
Glucose 81 mg/dL (64-123 mg/dL)
Total protein 7.6 g/dL (5.4-7.6 g/dL)
Albumin 2.7 g/dL (3.0-4.4 g/dL)
Globulin 4.9 g/dL (1.8-3.9 g/dL)
ALT 61 U/L (19-67 U/L)
AST 17 U/L (19-42 U/L)
ALP 190 U/L (21-170 U/L)
Creatine kinase 61 U/L (51-399 U/L)
Gamma GT 3 U/L (0-6 U/L)
Cholesterol 323 mg/dL (135-361 mg/dL)
Total bilirubin 0.1 mg/dL (0-0.2 mg/dL)
Magnesium 1.7 mg/dL (1.5-2.6 mg/dL).

Urinalysis: SGr 1.013; pH 6.0, 150 mg/dL protein, no bilirubin, 150 erythrocytes/μL hemoprotein, no glucose, no ketones, 12-18 WBC/HPF, 8-12 RBC/HPF, no other significant findings.

Coagulation Panel: PT 8.7 s (7.0-9.3 s), APTT 14.1 s (10.4-12.9 s), fibrinogen 412 mg/dL (109-311 mg/dL), D-dimers 418 ng/mL (0-186 ng/mL), antithrombin 84% (80%-120%).

Imaging Findings:

Thoracic Radiographs: See Figure 35-3. Mild cardiomegaly was present. The far caudal left pulmonary vasculature

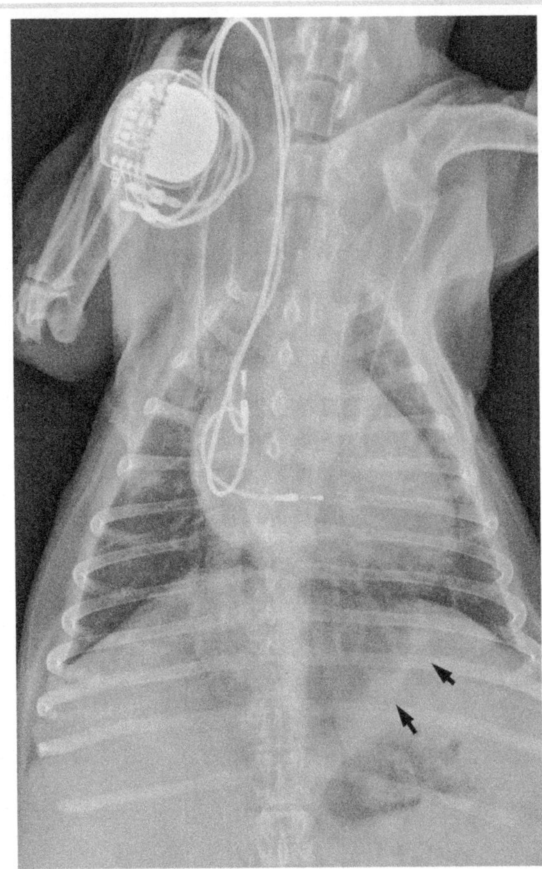

FIGURE 35-3 Dorsoventral thoracic radiograph from a 10-year-old male neutered miniature schnauzer with methicillin-resistant *Staphylococcus* bacteremia and pacemaker infection. There was a bronchointerstitial pattern and mild cardiomegaly. The caudal left pulmonary vasculature was indistinct with patchy infiltrates *(arrows)*, which raised suspicion for septic embolic pneumonia.

was indistinct with region of patchy infiltrates (arrows). The pacemaker was static in appearance with a generator embedded in the tissues dorsal to the cervical spine and two leads extending into the region of the cardiac silhouette—one terminating at the level of the right atrium and the other terminating at the level of the right ventricle. Within the viewable abdomen, the liver was persistently markedly enlarged and rounded. Given the absence of vasculature in the left caudal lung lobe, embolism in this area was suspected.

Echocardiogram (to evaluate for endocarditis): Mild mitral regurgitation was present, with no evidence of endocarditis.

Microbiologic Testing:

Aerobic Blood Culture and Susceptibility: *Bottle 1 (right cephalic catheter):* Direct smear from bottle: small numbers of gram-positive cocci and small numbers of gram-variable rods. Culture: coagulase-negative *Staphylococcus* and *Serratia marcescens*. The CoNS was methicillin resistant and resistant to clindamycin, enrofloxacin, marbofloxacin, erythromycin, trimethoprim-sulfamethoxazole; had intermediate susceptibility to gentamicin (8.00 µg/mL); and was susceptible to amikacin (≤4.00 µg/mL), chloramphenicol (8.00 µg/mL), doxycycline (4.00 µg/mL), rifampin (≤1 µg/mL), daptomycin (≤0.25 µg/mL), linezolid (≤0.5 µg/mL), and vancomycin (≤1.00 µg/mL). The *Serratia marcescens* was resistant to cefazolin, cefoxitin, cephalothin, and doxycycline; and susceptible to amikacin (≤4.00 µg/mL), amoxicillin-clavulanic acid (4.00 µg/mL), ampicillin (≤2.00 µg/mL), cefovecin (1.00 µg/mL), cefpodoxime (≤2.00 µg/mL), enrofloxacin (≤0.25 µg/mL), marbofloxacin (≤1 µg/mL), gentamicin (≤1 µg/mL), imipenem (≤1 µg/mL), ticarcillin (≤8 µg/mL), ticarcillin-clavulanate (≤8 µg/mL), and trimethoprim-sulfamethoxazole (≤0.5 µg/mL).

Bottle 2 (right lateral saphenous vein): Direct smear: small numbers of gram-positive cocci. Culture: coagulase-negative *Staphylococcus*.

Urine aerobic culture and susceptibility (cystocentesis specimen): >10^5 organisms/mL coagulase-negative *Staphylococcus*, with an identical antibiogram to that of the isolate from the blood.

Seroma Aerobic and Anaerobic Culture and Susceptibility: Small numbers of coagulase-negative *Staphylococcus*, with an identical antibiogram to that of the isolate from the blood and urine.

Diagnosis: Bacteremia and probable embolic pneumonia due to methicillin-resistant *Staphylococcus* spp. and possibly *Serratia marcescens* associated with pacemaker placement. Skin/soft tissue and urinary tract infection with methicillin-resistant *Staphylococcus* spp.

Treatment: Elliot was hospitalized with full-contact precautions that included the use of gloves and gowns and contact with a limited number of individuals. Treatment was initiated with intravenous fluids, vancomycin (10 mg/kg IV q6h) for the methicillin-resistant staphylococcal infection, and enrofloxacin (10 mg/kg IV q24h) for a possible *Serratia marcescens* infection. After 48 hours of treatment, the pacemaker was removed and replaced with a ventricular (VVIR) epicardial pacemaker, and a Penrose drain was placed at the incision site. A repeat blood culture (four bottles) performed 3 days later showed growth of the CoNS in one bottle. The pulmonary infiltrates resolved, creatinine normalized, and repeat blood and urine cultures were negative after 10 days of vancomycin treatment. The dog was discharged from the hospital. Follow-up cultures after an additional 10 days off antibiotics remained negative. Six months later, Elliot developed right-sided congestive heart failure with ascites and pleural effusion. Aerobic bacterial culture of the ascites fluid was negative. On echocardiography, the tricuspid valve was severely thickened and irregular. Endocarditis was suspected. Additional diagnostics that included blood cultures were declined by the owners, who elected euthanasia without necropsy.

Comments: Vancomycin was used to treat this severe methicillin-resistant staphylococcal infection because the dog had renal failure and there was concern for aminoglycoside toxicity. The *S. marcescens* may have represented a contaminant, but it was treated because of the severity of the dog's condition. Whether the endocarditis that developed was the result of a new infection or persistence of the original staphylococcal infection could not be determined.

SUGGESTED READING

Papich MG. Selection of antibiotics for meticillin-resistant *Staphylococcus pseudintermedius*: time to revisit some old drugs? Vet Dermatol. 2012;23(4):352-360.

REFERENCES

1. Ogsten A. Micrococcus poisoning. J Anat Physiol. 1882;16:526.
2. Ghebremedhin B, Layer F, Konig W, et al. Genetic classification and distinguishing of *Staphylococcus* species based on different partial gap, 16S rRNA, hsp60, rpoB, sodA, and tuf gene sequences. J Clin Microbiol. 2008;46:1019-1025.
3. Cain CL, Morris DO, O'Shea K, et al. Genotypic relatedness and phenotypic characterization of *Staphylococcus schleiferi* subspecies in clinical samples from dogs. Am J Vet Res. 2011;72:96-102.
4. Litster A, Moss SM, Honnery M, et al. Prevalence of bacterial species in cats with clinical signs of lower urinary tract disease: recognition of *Staphylococcus felis* as a possible feline urinary tract pathogen. Vet Microbiol. 2007;121:182-188.
5. Eckholm NG, Outerbridge CA, White SD, et al. Prevalence of and risk factors for infection with methicillin-resistant *Staphylococcus* spp. in dogs with pyoderma in northern California. Submitted. 2012.
6. Devriese LA, Vancanneyt M, Baele M, et al. *Staphylococcus pseudintermedius* sp. nov., a coagulase-positive species from animals. Int J Syst Evol Microbiol. 2005;55:1569-1573.
7. Devriese LA, Hermans K, Baele M, et al. *Staphylococcus pseudintermedius* versus *Staphylococcus intermedius*. Vet Microbiol. 2009;133:206-207.
8. Ben Zakour NL, Bannoehr J, van den Broek AH, et al. Complete genome sequence of the canine pathogen *Staphylococcus pseudintermedius*. J Bacteriol. 2011;193:2363-2364.
9. Perreten V, Kadlec K, Schwarz S, et al. Clonal spread of methicillin-resistant *Staphylococcus pseudintermedius* in Europe and North America: an international multicentre study. J Antimicrob Chemother. 2010;65:1145-1154.
10. van Duijkeren E, Kamphuis M, van der Mije IC, et al. Transmission of methicillin-resistant *Staphylococcus pseudintermedius* between infected dogs and cats and contact pets, humans and the environment in households and veterinary clinics. Vet Microbiol. 2011;150:338-343.
11. Griffeth GC, Morris DO, Abraham JL, et al. Screening for skin carriage of methicillin-resistant coagulase-positive staphylococci and *Staphylococcus schleiferi* in dogs with healthy and inflamed skin. Vet Dermatol. 2008;19:142-149.
12. Morris DO, Lautenbach E, Zaoutis T, et al. Potential for pet animals to harbour methicillin-resistant *Staphylococcus aureus* when residing with human MRSA patients. Zoonoses Public Health. 2012;59(4):286-293.
13. Loeffler A, Pfeiffer DU, Lindsay JA, et al. Lack of transmission of methicillin-resistant *Staphylococcus aureus* (MRSA) between apparently healthy dogs in a rescue kennel. Vet Microbiol. 2010;141:178-181.
14. Abraham JL, Morris DO, Griffeth GC, et al. Surveillance of healthy cats and cats with inflammatory skin disease for colonization of the skin by methicillin-resistant coagulase-positive staphylococci and *Staphylococcus schleiferi* ssp. *schleiferi*. Vet Dermatol. 2007;18:252-259.
15. Soares Magalhaes RJ, Loeffler A, Lindsay J, et al. Risk factors for methicillin-resistant *Staphylococcus aureus* (MRSA) infection in dogs and cats: a case-control study. Vet Res. 2010;41:55.
16. Girard C, Higgins R. *Staphylococcus intermedius* cellulitis and toxic shock in a dog. Can Vet J. 1999;40:501-502.
17. Weese JS, Poma R, James F, et al. *Staphylococcus pseudintermedius* necrotizing fasciitis in a dog. Can Vet J. 2009;50:655-656.
18. Osland AM, Vestby LK, Fanuelsen H, et al. Clonal diversity and biofilm-forming ability of methicillin-resistant *Staphylococcus pseudintermedius*. J Antimicrob Chemother. 2012 Apr, 67: 841-848.
19. Lewis 2nd JS, Jorgensen JH. Inducible clindamycin resistance in staphylococci: should clinicians and microbiologists be concerned? Clin Infect Dis. 2005;40:280-285.
20. Rubin JE, Ball KR, Chirino-Trejo M. Antimicrobial susceptibility of *Staphylococcus aureus* and *Staphylococcus pseudintermedius* isolated from various animals. Can Vet J. 2011;52:153-157.
21. Faires MC, Gard S, Aucoin D, et al. Inducible clindamycin-resistance in methicillin-resistant *Staphylococcus aureus* and methicillin-resistant *Staphylococcus pseudintermedius* isolates from dogs and cats. Vet Microbiol. 2009;139:419-420.
22. Lafaurie M, Porcher R, Donay JL, et al. Reduction of fluoroquinolone use is associated with a decrease in methicillin-resistant *Staphylococcus aureus* and fluoroquinolone-resistant *Pseudomonas aeruginosa* isolation rates: a 10 year study. J Antimicrob Chemother. 2012;67(4):1010-1015.
23. Falagas ME, Bliziotis IA, Fragoulis KN. Oral rifampin for eradication of *Staphylococcus aureus* carriage from healthy and sick populations: a systematic review of the evidence from comparative trials. Am J Infect Control. 2007;35:106-114.
24. Jordan D, Simon J, Fury S, et al. Carriage of methicillin-resistant *Staphylococcus aureus* by veterinarians in Australia. Aust Vet J. 2011;89:152-159.
25. Loeffler A, Pfeiffer DU, Lloyd DH, et al. Meticillin-resistant *Staphylococcus aureus* carriage in UK veterinary staff and owners of infected pets: new risk groups. J Hosp Infect. 2010;74:282-288.
26. Burstiner LC, Faires M, Weese JS. Methicillin-resistant *Staphylococcus aureus* colonization in personnel attending a veterinary surgery conference. Vet Surg. 2010;39:150-157.
27. Hanselman BA, Kruth SA, Rousseau J, et al. Methicillin-resistant *Staphylococcus aureus* colonization in veterinary personnel. Emerg Infect Dis. 2006;12:1933-1938.
28. Paul NC, Moodley A, Ghibaudo G, et al. Carriage of methicillin-resistant *Staphylococcus pseudintermedius* in small animal veterinarians: indirect evidence of zoonotic transmission. Zoonoses Public Health. 2011;58:533-539.
29. Morris DO, Boston RC, O'Shea K, et al. The prevalence of carriage of meticillin-resistant staphylococci by veterinary dermatology practice staff and their respective pets. Vet Dermatol. 2010;21(4):400-407.

CHAPTER 36

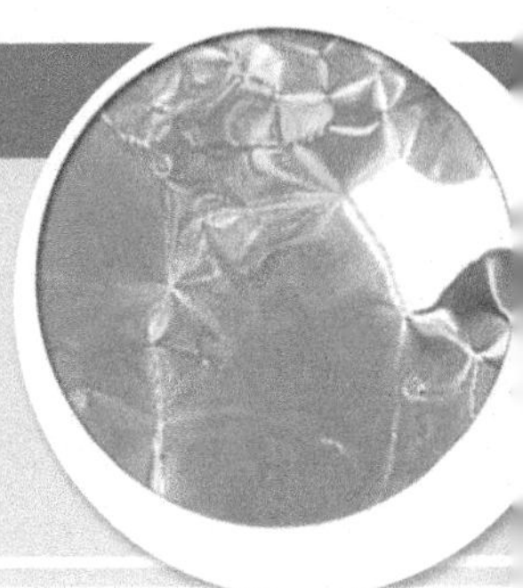

Gram-negative Bacterial Infections

Jane E. Sykes

Overview of Gram-negative Bacteria

First Described: Gram-negative bacteria were first described in Berlin by the Danish scientist Hans Christian Gram in 1884 when he used Gram stain to visualize *Klebsiella pneumoniae* in the lungs of people who died of pneumonia.[1]

Causes: Examples include *Escherichia coli, Salmonella, Enterobacter, Citrobacter, Klebsiella, Campylobacter, Pseudomonas,* and *Acinetobacter.*

Geographic Distribution: Worldwide

Mode of Transmission: Direct contact or contact with contaminated fomites; the bacteria often invade opportunistically

Major Clinical Signs: Affected sites include UTIs, wound infections, pneumonia, pyothorax, peritonitis, pyometra, ocular surface infections, otitis externa, pyoderma, bacteremia, and endocarditis, but virtually any body system can be affected.

Differential Diagnoses: Infections with gram-positive bacteria such as *Staphylococcus* spp. and *Streptococcus* spp.; to a lesser extent infections with nonbacterial pathogens such as fungi.

Human Health Significance: Gram-negative bacteria shed by dogs and cats have the potential to colonize humans, especially those with impaired host defenses. They may also be responsible for infections of dog or cat bites.

Etiology, Epidemiology, and Clinical Features

Gram-negative bacteria are widespread causes of opportunistic infections in dogs and cats and primarily cause disease when host defenses are impaired. They are important causes of nosocomial disease. In contrast to gram-positive bacteria, gram-negative bacteria have a complex outer membrane that contains lipopolysaccharide (LPS), as well as structures known as *porins* that regulate transport of molecules in and out of the cell, which includes antimicrobial drugs. Between this outer membrane and the inner (cytoplasmic) membrane is a periplasmic space, which contains the structural polymer peptidoglycan (or *murein*) (Figure 36-1). The peptidoglycan layer of gram-negative bacteria is much thinner than that of gram-positive bacteria, approximately one layer, or 7 to 8 nm thick (compared with many layers, or 20 to 80 nm thick for gram-positive bacteria). The inner cytoplasmic membrane contains many different proteins that are lipoproteins anchored into the outer lipid bilayer leaflet, transmembrane proteins, or peripheral membrane proteins that lie adjacent to the bilayer leaflets.

LPS is a large molecule that varies in composition from one bacterial species and strain to another. It contributes to the structural integrity of gram-negative bacteria and is a potent virulence factor. It consists of the *lipid A* backbone, a *core oligosaccharide,* and the *O antigen* side chain. Lipid A is a phosphorylated disaccharide to which long, hydrophobic fatty acid chains are attached, which anchor the LPS into the outer membrane (Figures 36-1 and 36-2). The lipid A component is also known as *endotoxin* because it is the biologically active portion of the molecule, in that it stimulates a potent host inflammatory response (see Chapter 86). The core oligosaccharide connects lipid A to the O antigen side chain. Its composition differs between bacterial species. The O antigen is a repeating polysaccharide that projects from the surface of the bacterial cell and varies in length from 1 to 60 repeats. It is the antigenic portion of the molecule and is responsible for serogroup classification of gram-negative bacteria.

Gram-negative cocci, such as *Moraxella* or *Neisseria,* are not widely recognized as significant pathogens of dogs and cats. However, they are commensals of the oral cavity of dogs and cats, can cause bite wound infections in humans,[2] and *Neisseria canis* was isolated in pure culture from a deep mandibular abscess from one dog.[3] Gram-negative rods are classified into Enterobacteriaceae and non-Enterobacteriaceae species. Enterobacteriaceae that cause disease in dogs and cats include *Escherichia coli, Proteus, Salmonella, Enterobacter, Citrobacter, Serratia,* and *Klebsiella.* Non-Enterobacteriaceae species include the Pasteurellaceae (*Pasteurella multocida*), as well as *Pseudomonas aeruginosa* and *Acinetobacter.* Other gram-negative bacteria are coccobacilli or spiral-shaped organisms and include *Bartonella, Bordetella, Campylobacter, Francisella, Helicobacter,* and *Brucella.*

Like gram-positive cocci, some gram-negative bacteria have tremendous ability to form biofilms, or bacterial aggregates that are embedded in a matrix of exopolysaccharide (bacterial slime), which form on living or nonliving surfaces. These protect the bacteria, and bacteria in biofilms can resist the effect of antimicrobial drugs and disinfectants.

Enterobacteriaceae

Many of the Enterobacteriaceae contribute to the normal gastrointestinal flora of animals. Organisms that belong to the Enterobacteriaceae possess a capsule (*K antigen*) and may be motile via flagella (*H antigen*). Some highly encapsulated species, such as *Klebsiella* and *Enterobacter,* have a mucoid appearance when they grow in culture. The flagella project from the bacterial cell and contain the filament-forming protein *flagellin,* which (along with LPS) can stimulate the host inflammatory response. The Enterobacteriaceae also possess fimbriae or pili, which are thinner than flagella and play a role in adhesion and sometimes bacterial aggregation. Finally, they possess a variety of complex

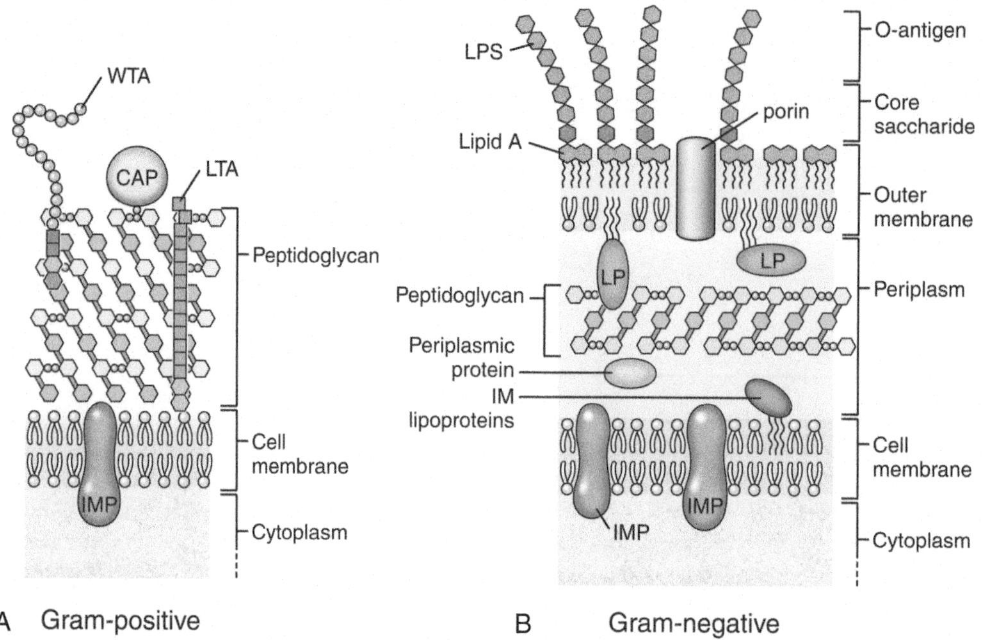

FIGURE 36-1 Structure of the envelope of gram-positive **(A)** and gram-negative **(B)** bacteria. The thickness of the peptidoglycan layer is greater in gram-positive bacteria than in gram-negative bacteria.

secretion systems (type I, II, III secretion systems). These facilitate export of toxins such as hemolysins, and molecules that are inserted into, and form pores in, host cell membranes. The bacteria then use these pores to inject toxins directly into the host cell. The Enterobacteriaceae also have a variety of iron scavenging systems, which are important virulence factors, and transmissible plasmids that contain genes for virulence factors and antimicrobial resistance factors.

Escherichia coli

Escherichia coli is the most common cause of urinary tract infections (UTIs) in dogs and cats and can also be isolated from dogs and cats with pyometra, prostatitis, peritonitis, cholangitis, cholecystitis, bacteremia and endocarditis, bronchopneumonia (such as that secondary to aspiration), and pyothorax. There is one report of necrotizing fasciitis in a dog associated with *E. coli* infection.[4]

Antibiotic resistance in *E. coli* isolates from dogs and cats is an increasing problem; 51% of 376 isolates collected from sick dogs and cats in the United States in 2005 showed resistance to at least one drug, and 29% of the 376 isolates were multiple drug resistant (MDR; defined as resistant to three or more classes of antimicrobial drugs).[5] The prevalence of resistance in 395 isolates from healthy dogs and cats from Canada was lower, 19%.[6] Extended-spectrum β-lactamase enzyme production has also been identified in *E. coli* isolates from dogs and cats in the United States,[7] and a few isolates were found to express New Dehli metallo-β-lactamase (NDM-1), which hydrolyses carbapenems.[8] Nosocomial infections with MDR *E. coli* have also been described in dogs and cats.

In humans, strains of *E. coli* that cause UTIs differ from those that cause diarrhea, and there is some evidence that this may also be true for strains that cause UTIs versus pyometra in dogs and cats.[9-11] Strains of *E. coli* that cause UTIs belong to the pathotype *extraintestinal pathogenic E. coli* (ExPEC). These strains possess a number of virulence factors, such as siderophores, type 1 and P fimbriae, hemolysin, and cytotoxic necrotizing factor. Specific virulence factors, as well as biofilm-forming capacity, have been associated with persistent or relapsing UTIs,[12,13] and uropathogenic *E. coli* can invade and persist within bladder epithelial cells. In one study, canine UTIs associated with *E. coli* were more likely to be recurrent than those associated with other uropathogens.[14] There has been concern that dogs may act as a source of *E. coli* strains that are pathogenic for humans.[11,15] In other extraintestinal *E. coli* infections, *E. coli* more closely resemble commensal strains, and host factors may be more important than bacterial virulence factors. The reader is referred to Chapter 46 for more information on intestinal *E. coli* infections.

Proteus

Proteus mirabilis is a common cause of upper and lower UTIs in dogs as well as otitis externa and uncommonly pyoderma. It produces a potent urease and so may contribute to development of struvite urolithiasis. Uroliths harbor bacteria that can emerge as the uroliths dissolve. *Proteus* has a characteristic swarming motility and may obscure the growth of other co-infecting microorganisms when grown in the laboratory on agar. *Proteus penneri,* an uncommon cause of nosocomial infections in humans, has rarely been isolated from wound infections in dogs seen at the author's hospital.

Klebsiella

The most common species of *Klebsiella* that infects dogs and cats is *K. pneumoniae. K. oxytoca* is a nosocomial pathogen in humans and has been reported in association with intravenous catheter colonization in puppies with parvoviral enteritis.[16]

K. pneumoniae primarily causes upper and lower UTIs in dogs and cats, but can also cause pneumonia, sometimes with abscessation (Figures 36-3 and 36-4). It has also been isolated from dogs with hepatic abscesses.[17] Nosocomial infections may be associated with bacteremia, endocarditis, and postoperative skin and soft tissue infections. The capsule of *K. pneumoniae* is

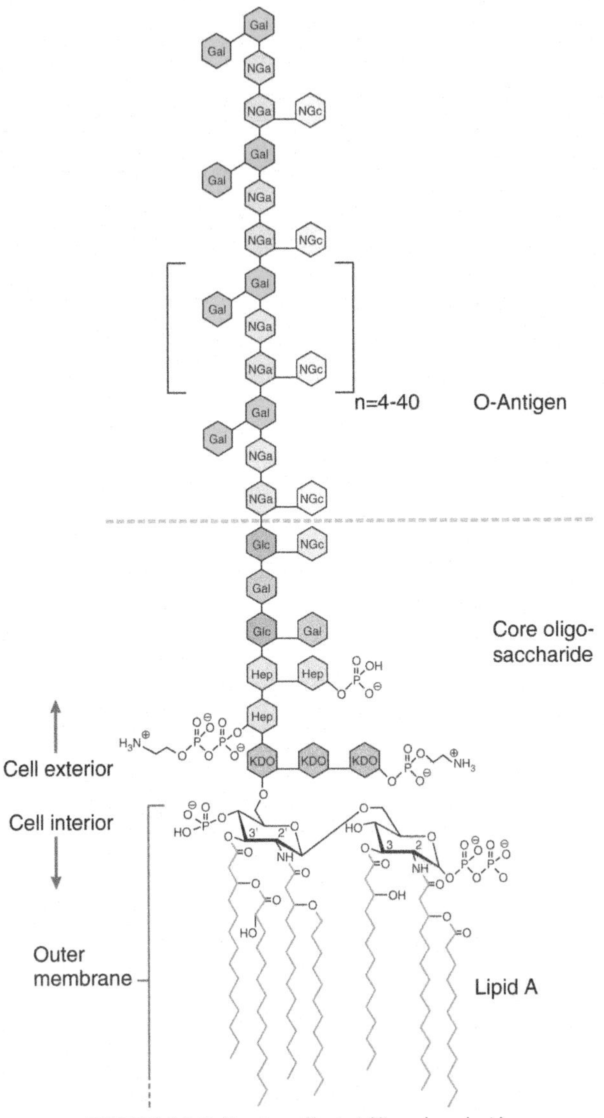

FIGURE 36-2 Structure of bacterial lipopolysaccharide.

a major virulence factor; it inhibits phagocytosis and is responsible for the mucoid appearance of the organism in culture (Figure 36-5, *A*).

All strains of *K. pneumoniae* are resistant to ampicillin, because they possess a chromosomal gene that encodes a penicillin β-lactamase. Some isolates, such as nosocomial isolates or those from persistent UTIs, possess plasmids that contain resistance genes for multiple antimicrobial drugs. Of greatest concern are *Klebsiella* isolates that express extended-spectrum β-lactamase (ESBL) enzymes, which hydrolyze third-generation cephalosporins such as cefotaxime or ceftriaxone. The genes that encode ESBLs are often located on plasmids that also contain genes for aminoglycoside resistance. Although MDR *K. pneumoniae* are not uncommonly isolated from dogs and cats, ESBL-producing *K. pneumoniae* isolates are rarely encountered. Treatment options for MDR *K. pneumoniae* may be limited to aminoglycosides, carbapenems, and sometimes trimethoprim-sulfamethoxazole.

Serratia marcescens

Serratia marcescens is an important cause of nosocomial infections in both human and veterinary medicine. In human patients it is often linked to intravenous drug use. The organism has a tremendous ability to survive in the environment and may contaminate and remain viable in disinfectant solutions.[18] It sometimes grows as a contaminant, such as in blood cultures. Some, but not all, strains of *S. marcescens* produce a red pigment when grown in culture.

In dogs, *S. marcescens* infection has been associated with UTIs, bacteremia and aortic valve endocarditis,[19] catheter-related infections in canine parvoviral enteritis,[14] and necrotizing fasciitis.[20] Contamination of blood products was linked to an outbreak of bacteremia in cats.[21] *Serratia* is resistant to ampicillin and first-generation cephalosporins as a result of a chromosomal β-lactamase. It may also acquire plasmid-mediated resistance to other antimicrobial drugs.

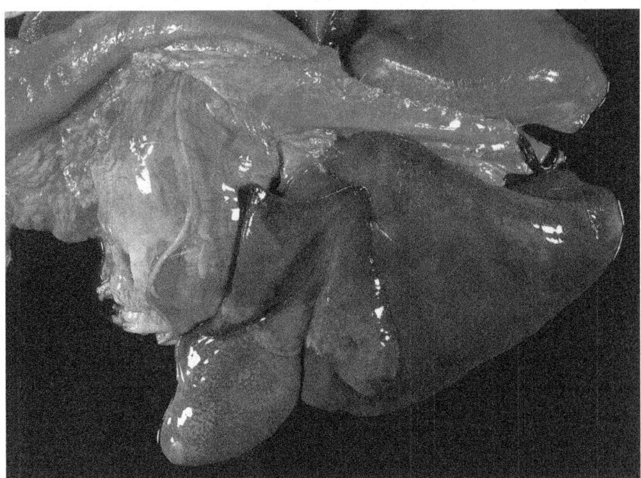

FIGURE 36-3 Lungs of an 11-year-old intact male German shepherd dog with severe, acute, suppurative, necrotizing and hemorrhagic bronchopneumonia due to *Klebsiella pneumoniae* infection. The lung lobes are severely congested. Five days before death, multiple laminectomies had been performed for intervertebral disc disease, and 2 days later the dog developed aspiration pneumonia that necessitated mechanical ventilation. Euthanasia was elected when there was further deterioration in the dog's condition, and bloody exudate was present in the endotracheal tube just before euthanasia.

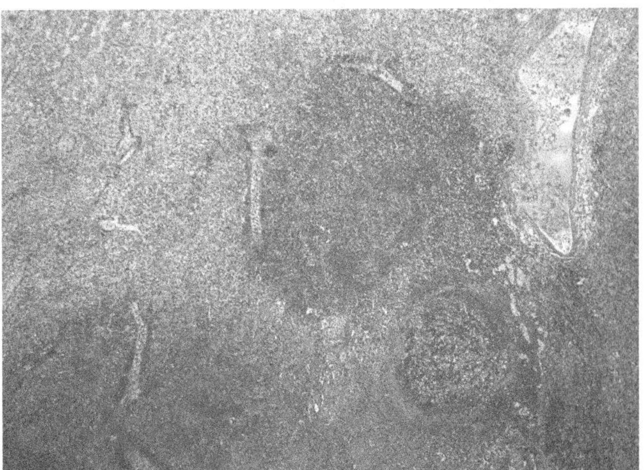

FIGURE 36-4 Histopathology of the lung from a 4-month-old intact male Newfoundland dog with severe, multifocal, necrotizing lung abscesses. Intralesional rod-shaped bacteria were also present. *Klebsiella pneumoniae* was isolated from the lesions. H&E stain, 40× magnification.

Enterobacter

Enterobacter cloacae and, to a lesser extent, *Enterobacter aerogenes* represent the majority of *Enterobacter* species isolated

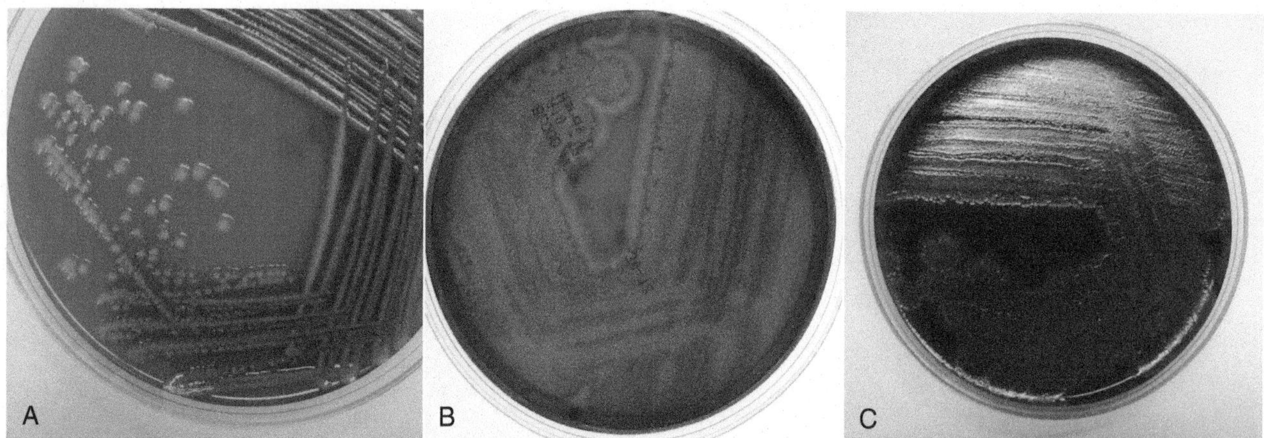

FIGURE 36-5 Gram-negative aerobic bacteria growing on blood agar. **A,** Mucoid colonies of *Klebsiella pneumoniae*. **B,** *Pseudomonas aeruginosa*. Transillumination using a light box revealed the presence of hemolysis and production of a green pigment (pyoverdin). **C,** The plate in **(B)** had a fruity odor and a "mother-of-pearl" appearance when not transilluminated.

from dogs and cats in the author's hospital. *Enterobacter* spp. are mainly isolated from dogs and cats with UTIs but occasionally cause wound or catheter-related infections. They generally are intrinsically resistant to ampicillin and first-generation cephalosporins and may also be resistant to multiple other antimicrobial drug classes.

Citrobacter

Citrobacter species are named for their ability to use citrate as a sole carbon source. *Citrobacter freundii* is most commonly isolated from dogs and cats with UTIs but can also cause catheter-related infections, bacteremia, and endocarditis.[22,23] *Citrobacter koseri* was isolated from puppies with myocarditis.[24] Like *Enterobacter* and *Serratia, Citrobacter* are usually resistant to ampicillin and first-generation cephalosporins and may acquire a number of plasmid-mediated resistance genes, including those that encode ESBLs and resistance to fluoroquinolones.

Non-Enterobacteriaceae

Pasteurella

Bacteria that belong to the family Pasteurellaceae are small, fastidious, nonmotile bacilli or coccobacilli that are commensals of the oral cavities and upper respiratory tracts of dogs and especially cats. The most common species of *Pasteurella* associated with disease in dogs and especially cats is *Pasteurella multocida*. Other species include *Pasteurella canis, Pasteurella dagmatis,* and *Pasteurella stomatis*. *Pasteurella* spp. have been associated with a wide variety of disease manifestations that include pyothorax, upper respiratory tract infections (usually secondary to viral infections or chronic rhinosinusitis), bronchopneumonia, UTIs, ocular surface infections, wound infections, cutaneous abscesses, otitis externa, bacteremia, and, rarely, infective endocarditis. They may be found in mixed infections with other bacteria, such as *Streptococcus canis*, other gram-negative bacteria, or anaerobes. In humans, they are an important cause of animal bite wound infections.[2] *Pasteurella* spp. are usually broadly susceptible to antimicrobial drugs, and the treatment of choice is a penicillin such as penicillin G, ampicillin, or amoxicillin.

Pseudomonas aeruginosa

Pseudomonas aeruginosa is the main pathogenic species in the family Pseudomonaceae. It is known for its ability to produce a variety of pigments when grown in culture, such as pyocyanin (blue), pyorubin (red), pyomelanin (black), and pyoverdin (yellow-green to yellow-brown and fluorescent), and for its characteristic "corn taco" or "grape"-like odor (see Figure 36-5, *B* and *C*). *P. aeruginosa* has one polar flagellum and is covered in thin, hairlike pili (Figure 36-6). It can also produce an extracellular

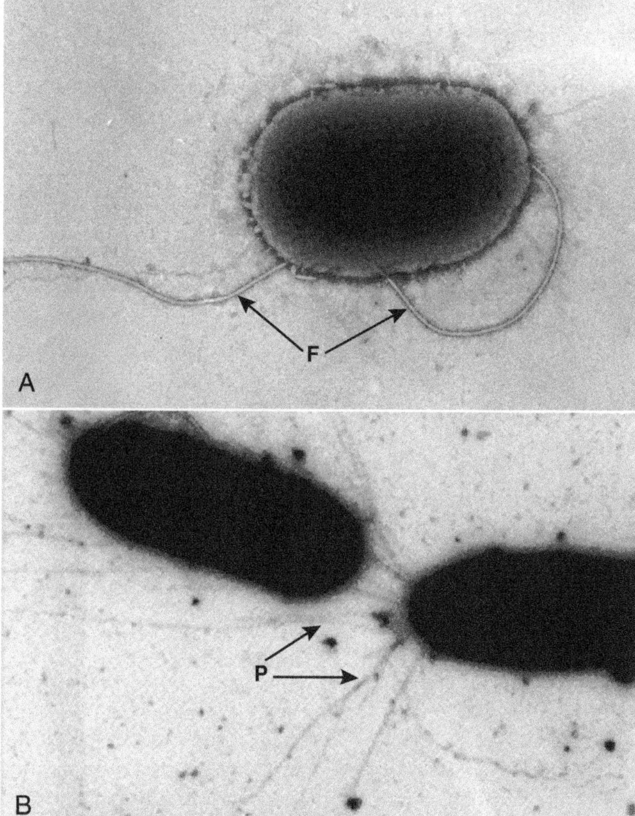

FIGURE 36-6 Electron micrograph of *Pseudomonas aeruginosa* showing ultrastructural features. **A,** Single cell with polar flagellum (*F*) with part of the flagellum running under the cell body. **B,** Two cells showing thin, hair-like pili (*P*). (**A,** Courtesy of Dr. Steve Lory. In Mandell GL, Bennett JE, Dolin R, eds. Mandell, Douglas and Bennett's principles and practice of infectious diseases, 7 ed. Philadelphia; Churchill Livingstone Elsevier; 2010:2835-2860; **B,** Courtesy of Dr. Martin Lee and Dr. Milan Bajmoczi, Harvard Medical School. In: Longo D, Fauci A, Kasper D, et al. Harrison's principles of internal medicine, 18 ed. Vol 1, New York; McGraw-Hill; 2012.)

polysaccharide known as *alginate,* which results in a mucoid colony appearance.

Pseudomonas aeruginosa is widespread in the environment and can grow in a huge variety of different conditions, reflecting its importance as a nosocomial pathogen. It is commonly found on plants, water, and soil. It can survive in disinfectants and grow in diesel and jet fuel. It is occasionally isolated from the skin, mucous membranes, and feces of healthy animals and humans. Almost any site of the body that is subject to injury can become colonized and subsequently infected. In humans, community-acquired infections can occur as a result of exposure to contaminated hot tubs, swimming pools, and contact lens solutions. In the hospital environment, *P. aeruginosa* often colonizes moist environments such as sinks, endotracheal tubes, and ventilator equipment. It also colonizes damp, macerated tissues such as the ear canals, damaged cornea, traumatized skin (such as wounds and burns), and the interdigital space. Because the organism can be resistant to a large number of different antimicrobial drugs, repeated treatment of secondary bacterial infections in sites where impaired host defenses exist with a variety of antimicrobials can select for MDR *P. aeruginosa* infection at these sites. Examples of such conditions in dogs and cats include recurrent aspiration pneumonia and/or bronchiectasis, cystitis, chronic feline rhinosinusitis, and otitis externa/media.

Pseudomonas aeruginosa possesses virtually every type of bacterial virulence factor, including exotoxins, a type III secretion system, lipopolysaccharide, pili, flagella, several proteases, phospholipases, iron-scavenging mechanisms such as pyoverdin production, and the ability to form extensive biofilms. Alginate protects the organism from phagocytosis, and the pigment pyocyanin produces reactive oxygen species, which in turn damage host cells. Multidrug resistance results from the production of specific β-lactamase enzymes (which can include ESBLs), antibiotic efflux pumps, enzymes that modify aminoglycosides or alter antibiotic binding sites (such as DNA gyrase for fluoroquinolones), and decreased bacterial permeability.

Infections with broadly susceptible *P. aeruginosa* isolates could be treated with an antipseudomonal β-lactam (e.g., ticarcillin, a carbapenem, cefepime, ceftazidime) alone or in combination with an aminoglycoside or a fluoroquinolone. The combination of an aminoglycoside and an antipseudomonal penicillin has synergistic activity against some *P. aeruginosa* infections. Currently, most MDR *P. aeruginosa* isolates from dogs and cats remain susceptible to carbapenems (such as meropenem) and aminoglycosides (especially amikacin), and so the usual treatment of choice is 1) a combination of these two drugs, 2) removal of any foreign or necrotic material and, 3) if possible, resolution or management of any other underlying cause for impaired host defenses. Because parenterally administered aminoglycosides do not effectively penetrate airway mucus, nebulized tobramycin has been used to treat resistant *P. aeruginosa* infections of the airways in human patients, but these may not adequately penetrate consolidated lung tissue.[25] Effective treatment of MDR *P. aeruginosa* infections when they occur in locations such as the feline nasal cavity may be extremely difficult, if not impossible, because of irreversible turbinate loss, the requirement for injectable antimicrobial drugs, poor penetration of aminoglycosides to the site of infection, and an inadequate ability to effectively treat all surfaces of the nasal cavity with topical aminoglycosides.

Investigation of suspected nosocomial outbreaks of *P. aeruginosa* infection generally requires typing of isolates from affected animals and the environment with molecular methods such as pulsed-field gel electrophoresis or multilocus sequence typing. Use of antibiograms alone does not adequately discriminate between strains.

Acinetobacter

Like *P. aeruginosa, Acinetobacter* is an important nosocomial opportunistic pathogen. *Acinetobacter* is present in soil and water and can be found in frozen foods, pasteurized milk, and an enormous array of inert objects in the hospital environment, where it may persist for months. It colonizes the skin and mucous membranes of healthy humans as well as those of dogs and cats.[26,27] The main species that cause disease in animals are *Acinetobacter baumannii* and, to a lesser extent, *Acinetobacter lwoffii* and *Acinetobacter calcoaceticus.* Multidrug resistant isolates of *A. baumannii* have been responsible for outbreaks of nosocomial infections in veterinary hospitals[28,29] and, like MDR *P. aeruginosa,* may be resistant to a huge variety of antimicrobial drug classes. Carbapenem-resistant *A. baumannii* have been isolated from humans as well as animals.[29,30] Clinical manifestations of *Acinetobacter* infections in dogs and cats include nosocomial UTIs (e.g., after invasive urinary procedures such as catheterization), surgical wound infections, pneumonia, catheter-related bacteremia, and, rarely, endocarditis. Necrotizing fasciitis associated with *A. baumannii* infection was described in a cat.[31] When *Acinetobacter* is grown from a specimen, care should be taken to differentiate infection from contamination. Most veterinary isolates are susceptible to aminoglycosides and carbapenems; some are susceptible to trimethoprim-sulfamethoxazole and fluoroquinolones.[28]

Diagnosis

Laboratory Abnormalities

Complete Blood Count, Biochemistry, and Urinalysis Findings

Dogs and cats with superficial gram-negative infections of sites that drain to the exterior, such as wounds, the external ear canal, the nasal cavity, and the lower urinary tract, often have no clinically significant laboratory abnormalities. Deep tissue or systemic infections with gram-negative bacteria may be associated with marked neutrophilia and a left shift, toxic neutrophils, or a degenerative left shift, sometimes with circulating metamyelocytes. Thrombocytopenia may be present in dogs and cats that develop disseminated intravascular coagulation (DIC). Anemia of inflammatory disease, lymphopenia, and monocytosis may be present. The urinalysis of dogs and cats with gram-negative bacterial UTIs may reveal pyuria, proteinuria, hematuria, and sometimes bacterial rods on sediment examination.

Coagulation Profile

Systemic gram-negative bacterial infections may be associated with evidence of DIC due to activation of the coagulation cascade by endotoxin.

Cytologic Abnormalities

Aspirates of affected tissues or pus, or transtracheal wash or bronchoalveolar lavage fluid specimens from dogs and cats with gram-negative bacterial infections may contain large numbers of degenerate and nondegenerate neutrophils, sometimes with bacterial rods.

TABLE 36-1

Examples of Systemic Antimicrobial Drugs That Could Be Selected for Treatment of Gram-Negative Bacterial Infections in Dogs and Cats (See Also Chapter 8)

Infecting Species	Drug	Dose (mg/kg)	Interval (hours)	Route
Pasteurella	Amoxicillin	20	8	PO
	Ampicillin	20	6-8	IV, IM, SC
	Penicillin G	20,000-40,000 U/kg	6-8	IV, IM
Susceptible Enterobacteriaceae	Trimethoprim-sulfamethoxazole	30	12	PO, IV
	Amoxicillin–clavulanate potassium	20	8	PO
	Ciprofloxacin	20-30	24	PO
		10	24	IV
MDR Enterobacteriaceae, *Pseudomonas*, or *Acinetobacter*	Amikacin*	15-30 (dogs), 10-14 (cats)	24	IV, IM, SC
	Gentamicin*	9-14 (dogs), 5-8 (cats)	24	IV, IM, SC
	Ticarcillin disodium, ticarcillin-clavulanate	33-50	4-6	IV
	Meropenem	12	8	SC
		25	8	IV
	Ceftazidime	30	6	IV

*Use aminoglycosides in combination with an antipseudomonal β-lactam such as ticarcillin, meropenem, or a third-generation cephalosporin.

Microbiologic Tests

Isolation and Identification

Gram-negative bacteria are readily isolated from aspirates, tissue biopsies, body fluid, blood, and lavage specimens. MacConkey and blood agar are usually used to isolate gram-negative bacteria, which usually grow within 24 to 48 hours and are subsequently differentiated on the basis of colony morphology and biochemical reactions. *Pasteurella* spp. are more fastidious, and species that infect dogs and cats do not grow on MacConkey agar. Evaluation of antimicrobial susceptibility is important for all Enterobacteriaceae, *P. aeruginosa*, and *Acinetobacter* spp., given their propensity to develop resistance to many antimicrobial drug classes.

Treatment and Prognosis

The approach to treatment of gram-negative infections depends on the site of infection and the severity of disease (Table 36-1); the reader is referred to Chapters 84 to 90 for treatment recommendations for different organ systems. Identification and management of the underlying cause are also important to minimize selection for resistant organisms. Any foreign material (such as catheters, implants) must be removed, and necrotic tissue debrided. When systemic antimicrobial drug treatment is required, it should preferably be based on the results of susceptibility testing, although *Pasteurella* spp. are generally susceptible to penicillin or aminopenicillins such as amoxicillin. Because gram-negative bacteria have higher minimum inhibitory concentrations (MICs) to penicillins than do gram-positive bacteria, the high end of the dose range and more frequent administration may be necessary. Some Enterobacteriaceae are intrinsically resistant to ampicillin and first-generation cephalosporins, and initial treatment of serious infections while awaiting the results of susceptibility testing should include an aminoglycoside, a third-generation cephalosporin, or a fluoroquinolone. Trimethoprim-sulfamethoxazole, amoxicillin, or clavulanic acid–amoxicillin are reasonable initial choices for treatment of UTIs associated with bacterial rods.[32] Treatment should also be based on knowledge of local resistance patterns among gram-negative bacteria, which may vary from region to region and practice to practice.

Prevention

Prevention of gram-negative infections involves resolution of impairment in host defenses and strict hospital infection control practices (see Chapter 11).

Public Health Aspects

Strains of *E. coli* and other MDR gram-negative bacteria harbored by dogs resemble pathogenic strains isolated from humans.[15,30] As a result, concern has been raised that companion animals may be a source of organisms for human infection, especially those that reside with humans with compromised host defenses.

Pasteurella multocida is the most commonly isolated organism from human dog and cat bite wounds.[2] *Pasteurella* spp. can also colonize the respiratory tracts of humans with underlying respiratory disease such as bronchiectasis or chronic sinusitis, and they occasionally have been reported in association with peritonitis, bacteremia, and endocarditis. Most of these humans have had contact with domestic animals in the household, and isolates from affected humans have been shown by molecular methods to be identical to those colonizing animals in the household.[33]

Thus, immunocompromised owners or those with impaired anatomic barriers should be instructed to wash their hands after handling their pet and perform regular household cleaning and disinfection. Companion animals should not be allowed to lick open wounds or the owner's face.

CASE EXAMPLE

Signalment: "Lottie", a middle-aged, female spayed domestic shorthair from northern California

History: Lottie was evaluated for chronic nasal discharge. Since her rescue as a stray 2.5 years earlier, intermittent sneezing and bilateral mucopurulent nasal discharge had been noted, and the discharge sometimes contained blood. Ten months before the evaluation, Lottie had been anesthetized for a nasal flush at a local veterinary clinic, but developed respiratory distress on recovery and was hospitalized with oxygen supplementation for 24 hours. She was ataxic, leaned to one side, and did not eat well for days, but over the subsequent months the ataxia and leaning gradually resolved. For the two weeks before the evaluation Lottie had stertorous respiration and intermittent episodes of open-mouth breathing. For the past 9 months, Lottie had been treated with marbofloxacin and prednisolone. Before that, treatments for the nasal discharge included clavulanic acid–amoxicillin, doxycycline, or azithromycin, as well as L-lysine supplementation. Lottie lived with six other cats, all of which had access to the outdoors, and she was fed commercial canned and dry cat food. The FeLV and FIV status of these cats was unknown.

Current medications: marbofloxacin (5 mg/kg PO q24h) and prednisolone (1 mg/kg PO q24h)

Physical Examination:

Body Weight: 4 kg

General: Bright, alert and responsive, hydrated. T = 100.3°F (37.9°C), P = 220 beats/min, purring, body condition score 7/9.

Eyes, Ears, Nose, and Throat: Mucopurulent nasal discharge was present that was most profuse on the left side. Nasal airflow was absent on the left side. Mild dental calculus was present, but there were no oral masses or ulceration.

Respiratory: An inspiratory stertor was present, and referred upper airway noises were detected on auscultation of the thorax.

Cardiovascular, Gastrointestinal and Genitourinary, and Lymph Nodes: No clinically significant abnormalities were detected. It was difficult to palpate abdominal structures due to the presence of abdominal fat.

Neurologic Examination: There was a mild, intermittent, left-sided head tilt. No other abnormalities were detected on full neurologic examination.

Laboratory Findings:

CBC:

HCT 39.1% (30%-50%)
MCV 44.7 fL (42-53 fL)
MCHC 29.9 g/dL (30-33.5 g/dL)
Reticulocytes 111,400 cells/μL (7000-60,000 cells/μL)
WBC 21,210 cells/μL (4500-14,000 cells/μL)
Neutrophils 16,713 cells/μL (2000-9000 cells/μL)
Lymphocytes 4115 cells/μL (1000-7000 cells/μL)
Monocytes 297 cells/μL (50-600 cells/μL)
Eosinophils 64 cells/μL (150-1100 cells/μL)
Basophils 0 cells/μL (0-50 cells/μL)
Platelets 316,000/μL (180,000-500,000 platelets/μL).

Serum Chemistry Profile:

Sodium 151 mmol/L (151-158 mmol/L)
Potassium 3.7 mmol/L (3.6-4.9 mmol/L)
Chloride 113 mmol/L (117-126 mmol/L)
Bicarbonate 19 mmol/L (15-21 mmol/L)
Phosphorus 5.8 mg/dL (3.2-6.3 mg/dL)
Calcium 10.2 mg/dL (9.0-10.9 mg/dl)
BUN 49 mg/dL (18-33 mg/dL)
Creatinine 1.4 mg/dL (1.1-2.2 mg/dL)
Glucose 128 mg/dL (63-118 mg/dL)
Total protein 8.7 g/dL (6.6-8.4 g/dL)
Albumin 3.6 g/dL (2.2-4.6 g/dL)
Globulin 5.1 g/dL (2.8-5.4 g/dL)
ALT 33 U/L (27-101 U/L)
AST 21 U/L (17-58 U/L)
ALP 36 U/L (14-71 U/L)
Gamma GT 0 U/L (0-4 U/L)
Cholesterol 192 mg/dL (89-258 mg/dL)
Total bilirubin 0.1 mg/dL (0-0.2 mg/dL).

Urinalysis: USG 1.044, pH 6, 75 mg/dL protein, no glucose, bilirubin or ketones, 250 erythrocytes/μL hemoprotein, >100 RBC/HPF (traumatic cystocentesis), 0-1 WBC/HPF.

Imaging Findings:

Thoracic Radiographs: Cardiovascular structures were within normal limits. There was a small amount of air in the cervical esophagus (likely due to aerophagia) and a mild diffuse bronchointerstitial pattern that was attributed to an obese body condition.

Skull Computed Tomography Scan: Contiguous transverse 0.6-mm collimated images of the skull were available for review without contrast administration. There was moderate turbinate destruction of both right and left nasal passages with lobular soft tissue attenuating material present along their length (Figure 36-7, *A*). There was stenosis of both frontal sinuses to the point where the left frontal sinus was completely occluded. The right frontal sinus was almost completely filled with soft tissue attenuating material. The ear canals were within normal limits bilaterally. The mandibular lymph nodes were prominent but symmetrical.

Rhinoscopy: Severe turbinate destruction with diffuse hyperemia and large accumulations of inspissated green mucus was present throughout the nasal passages (Figure 36-7, *B*). Several biopsies of the right and left nasal cavities were obtained for histopathology.

Microbiologic Testing: Aerobic bacterial culture and *Mycoplasma* culture (nasal brush specimen): a direct smear showed moderate numbers of neutrophils, but no organisms were seen. Moderate numbers of *Pseudomonas aeruginosa* were isolated. The *P. aeruginosa* was resistant to amoxicillin–clavulanic acid, ampicillin, cefazolin, cefovecin, cefoxitin, cefpodoxime, ceftiofur, chloramphenicol, doxycycline, enrofloxacin, marbofloxacin, ticarcillin, ticarcillin–clavulanic acid, and trimethoprim-sulfamethoxazole. It was susceptible only to amikacin (≤4 μg/mL), gentamicin (2 μg/mL), and imipenem (≤1 μg/mL).

Histopathology of Nasal Biopsy Specimens: The submucosa was markedly expanded and multifocally effaced by sheets of lymphocytes and plasma cells, with neutrophils and fewer numbers of mast cells surrounding irregular spicules of woven bone extending from primary turbinates. Less affected sections contain similar, predominately lymphoplasmacytic infiltrates that separated submucosal glands and elevated the superficial epithelium. Pathologic diagnosis: severe, chronic, and extensive lymphoplasmacytic and neutrophilic rhinitis with turbinate remodeling.

Continued

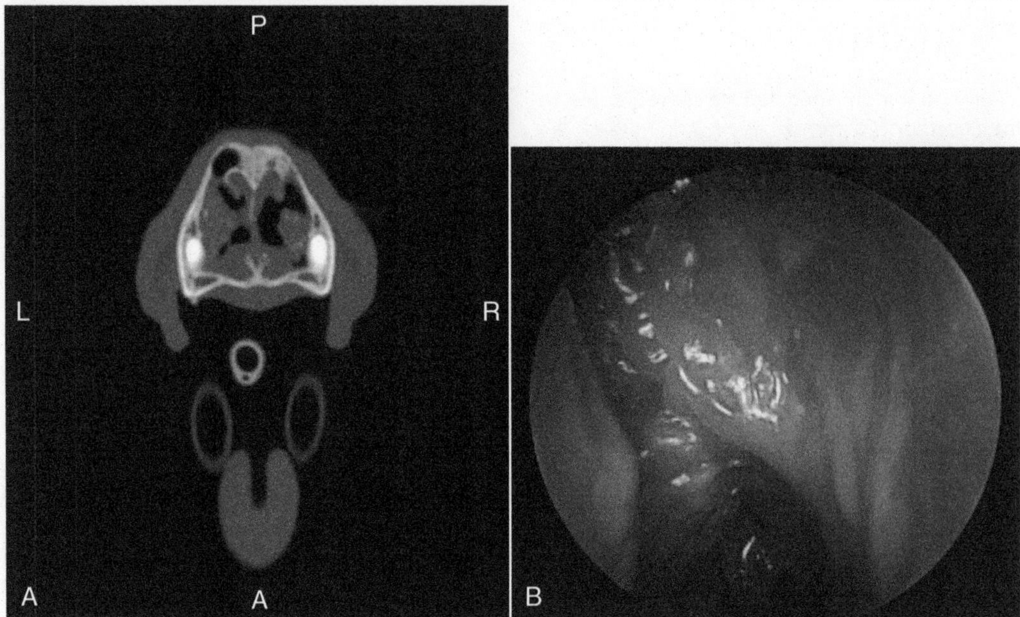

FIGURE 36-7 Nasal cavity of a middle-aged, female spayed domestic shorthair with chronic rhinosinusitis and secondary infection with multidrug-resistant *Pseudomonas aeruginosa*. **A,** Computed tomographic scan showing destruction of the turbinates of the left and right nasal passages. **B,** Rhinoscopic findings included severe turbinate destruction, hyperemia, and accumulations of thick green mucus.

Diagnosis: Feline chronic rhinosinusitis with suspected opportunistic MDR *P. aeruginosa* infection.

Treatment and Outcome: The nasal cavity was lavaged. The prednisolone was tapered over 1 week, then discontinued, and 7 days later, treatment with piroxicam was commenced (0.3 mg/kg PO q24h for 7 days, then q48h thereafter). Other medications discussed with the owner were *N*-acetylcysteine and intranasal gentamicin drops, but the prognosis given for disease resolution was poor.

Comments: The underlying cause of feline chronic rhinosinusitis is poorly defined, but infection of kittens with respiratory viruses such as feline herpesvirus 1 (FHV-1) is suspected to play a role. Severe turbinate destruction predisposes to secondary opportunistic infections with a variety of bacteria, which include staphylococci, *Bordetella bronchiseptica, Streptococcus canis, Mycoplasma* spp., *E. coli, Pasteurella multocida,* and *P. aeruginosa*. In this cat, selection for MDR *P. aeruginosa* likely resulted from repeated and chronic use of a variety of antimicrobial drugs. The reticulocytosis and increased serum BUN concentration likely was secondary to chronic epistaxis and swallowed blood. The cat's neurologic signs and head tilt were thought to be due to peripheral vestibular disease, possibly due to otitis media, but there was no evidence of middle ear disease on the CT scan.

SUGGESTED READINGS

Francey T, Gaschen F, Nicolet J, et al. The role of *Acinetobacter baumannii* as a nosocomial pathogen for dogs and cats in an intensive care unit. J Vet Intern Med. 2000;14:177-183.

Hohenhaus AE, Drusin LM, Garvey MS. *Serratia marcescens* contamination of feline whole blood in a hospital blood bank. J Am Vet Med Assoc. 1997;210:794-798.

REFERENCES

1. Gram C. Über die isolierte Färbung der Schizomyceten in Schnitt- und Trockenpräparaten [in German]. Fortschr Med. 1884;2:185-189.
2. Talan DA, Citron DM, Abrahamian FM, et al. Bacteriologic analysis of infected dog and cat bites. Emergency Medicine Animal Bite Infection Study Group. N Engl J Med. 1999;340:85-92.
3. Cantas H, Pekarkova M, Kippenes HS, et al. First reported isolation of *Neisseria canis* from a deep facial wound infection in a dog. J Clin Microbiol. 2011;49:2043-2046.
4. Worth AJ, Marshall N, Thompson KG. Necrotising fasciitis associated with *Escherichia coli* in a dog. N Z Vet J. 2005;53:257-260.
5. Shaheen BW, Boothe DM, Oyarzabal OA, et al. Antimicrobial resistance profiles and clonal relatedness of canine and feline *Escherichia coli* pathogens expressing multidrug resistance in the United States. J Vet Intern Med. 2010;24:323-330.
6. Leonard EK, Pearl DL, Finley RL, et al. Comparison of antimicrobial resistance patterns of *Salmonella* spp. and *Escherichia coli* recovered from pet dogs from volunteer households in Ontario (2005-06). J Antimicrob Chemother. 2012;67:174-181.
7. Shaheen BW, Nayak R, Foley SL, et al. Molecular characterization of resistance to extended-spectrum cephalosporins in clinical *Escherichia coli* isolates from companion animals in the United States. Antimicrob Agents Chemother. 2011;55:5666-5675.
8. Shaheen BW, Nayak R, Boothe DM. First reported case of New Delhi Metallo (NDM) carpabenem-positive gene in *Escherichia coli* from companion animals in the United States. San Francisco, USA: Proceedings of the 52nd ICAAC symposium; 2012Abstract #157.
9. Chen YM, Wright PJ, Lee CS, et al. Uropathogenic virulence factors in isolates of *Escherichia coli* from clinical cases of canine pyometra and feces of healthy bitches. Vet Microbiol. 2003;94:57-69.
10. Freitag T, Squires RA, Schmid J, et al. Feline uropathogenic *Escherichia coli* from Great Britain and New Zealand have dissimilar virulence factor genotypes. Vet Microbiol. 2005;106:79-86.
11. Siqueira AK, Ribeiro MG, Leite Dda S, et al. Virulence factors in *Escherichia coli* strains isolated from urinary tract infection and pyometra cases and from feces of healthy dogs. Res Vet Sci. 2009;86:206-210.

12. Ejrnaes K, Stegger M, Reisner A, et al. Characteristics of *Escherichia coli* causing persistence or relapse of urinary tract infections: phylogenetic groups, virulence factors and biofilm formation. Virulence. 2011;2:528-537.
13. Soto SM, Smithson A, Horcajada JP, et al. Implication of biofilm formation in the persistence of urinary tract infection caused by uropathogenic *Escherichia coli*. Clin Microbiol Infect. 2006;12:1034-1036.
14. Ball KR, Rubin JE, Chirino-Trejo M, et al. Antimicrobial resistance and prevalence of canine uropathogens at the Western College of Veterinary Medicine Veterinary Teaching Hospital, 2002-2007. Can Vet J. 2008;49:985-990.
15. Harada K, Okada E, Shimizu T, et al. Antimicrobial resistance, virulence profiles, and phylogenetic groups of fecal *Escherichia coli* isolates: a comparative analysis between dogs and their owners in Japan. Comp Immunol Microbiol Infect Dis. 2012;35:139-144.
16. Lobetti RG, Joubert KE, Picard J, et al. Bacterial colonization of intravenous catheters in young dogs suspected to have parvoviral enteritis. J Am Vet Med Assoc. 2002;220:1321-1324.
17. Farrar ET, Washabau RJ, Saunders HM. Hepatic abscesses in dogs: 14 cases (1982-1994). J Am Vet Med Assoc. 1996;208:243-247.
18. Fox JG, Beaucage CM, Folta CA, et al. Nosocomial transmission of *Serratia marcescens* in a veterinary hospital due to contamination by benzalkonium chloride. J Clin Microbiol. 1981;14:157-160.
19. Perez C, Fujii Y, Fauls M, et al. Fatal aortic endocarditis associated with community-acquired *Serratia marcescens* infection in a dog. J Am Anim Hosp Assoc. 2011;47:133-137.
20. Plavec T, Zdovc I, Juntes P, et al. Necrotizing fasciitis caused by *Serratia marcescens* after tooth extraction in a Doberman pinscher: a case report. Veterinarni Medicina. 2008;53:629-635.
21. Hohenhaus AE, Drusin LM, Garvey MS. *Serratia marcescens* contamination of feline whole blood in a hospital blood bank. J Am Vet Med Assoc. 1997;210:794-798.
22. Galarneau JR, Fortin M, Lapointe JM, et al. *Citrobacter freundii* septicemia in two dogs. J Vet Diagn Invest. 2003;15:297-299.
23. Sykes JE, Kittleson MD, Pesavento PA, et al. Evaluation of the relationship between causative organisms and clinical characteristics of infective endocarditis in dogs: 71 cases (1992-2005). J Am Vet Med Assoc. 2006;228:1723-1734.
24. Cassidy JP, Callanan JJ, McCarthy G, et al. Myocarditis in sibling boxer puppies associated with *Citrobacter koseri* infection. Vet Pathol. 2002;39:393-395.
25. Pier GB, Ramphal R. *Pseudomonas aeruginosa*. In: Mandell GL, Bennett JE, Dolin R, eds. Mandell, Douglas and Bennett's Principles and Practice of Infectious Diseases. 7th ed. Philadelphia, PA: Elsevier; 2010:2835-2860.
26. Saphir DA, Carter GR. Gingival flora of the dog with special reference to bacteria associated with bites. J Clin Microbiol. 1976;3:344-349.
27. Krogh HV, Kristensen S. A study of skin diseases in dogs and cats. II. Microflora of the normal skin of dogs and cats. Nord Vet Med. 1976;28:459-463.
28. Zordan S, Prenger-Berninghoff E, Weiss R, et al. Multidrug-resistant *Acinetobacter baumannii* in veterinary clinics. Germany. Emerg Infect Dis. 2011;17:1751-1754.
29. Francey T, Gaschen F, Nicolet J, et al. The role of *Acinetobacter baumannii* as a nosocomial pathogen for dogs and cats in an intensive care unit. J Vet Intern Med. 2000;14:177-183.
30. Endimiani A, Hujer KM, Hujer AM, et al. *Acinetobacter baumannii* isolates from pets and horses in Switzerland: molecular characterization and clinical data. J Antimicrob Chemother. 2011;66:2248-2254.
31. Brachelente C, Wiener D, Malik Y, et al. A case of necrotizing fasciitis with septic shock in a cat caused by *Acinetobacter baumannii*. Vet Dermatol. 2007;18:432-438.
32. Weese JS, Blondeau JM, Boothe D, et al. Antimicrobial use guidelines for treatment of urinary tract disease in dogs and cats: Antimicrobial Guidelines Working Group of the International Society for Companion Animal Infectious Diseases. Vet Med Int. 2011;2011:263768.
33. Sugino Y, Kato M, Yagi A, et al. *Pasteurella multocida* pneumonia with molecular evidence of zoonotic transmission. Kansenshogaku Zasshi. 2007;81:726-730.

CHAPTER 37

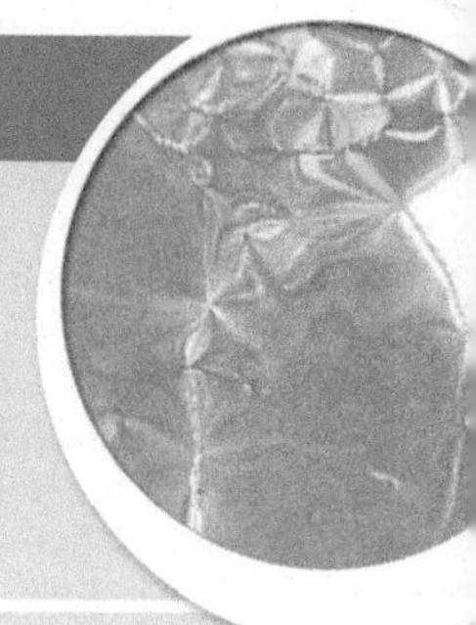

Anaerobic Bacterial Infections

Jane E. Sykes

> **Overview of Anaerobic Bacterial Infections**
>
> First Described: 1860s (Louis Pasteur)[1]
>
> Causes: *Bacteroides, Prevotella, Porphyromonas, Peptostreptococcus, Fusobacterium, Clostridium, Propionibacterium,* other species
>
> Geographic Distribution: Worldwide
>
> Mode of Transmission: Direct contact, and opportunistic invasion of tissues by commensal bacteria
>
> Major Clinical Signs: Abscess formation in a variety of tissues, pyothorax, peritonitis, pyometra, periodontal disease, osteomyelitis, bacteremia
>
> Differential Diagnoses: Primarily bacterial infections caused by gram-positive and gram-negative aerobes, but also neoplasia (when discrete abscessation is present).
>
> Human Health Significance: Anaerobes of the oral cavities of dogs and cats are an important component of animal bite wound infections in humans. Enteric clostridial infections of dogs and cats may also have public health significance (see Chapter 48).

Etiology and Epidemiology

An *anaerobe* is an organism that requires an environment that is reduced in oxygen for growth and does not grow in air. Anaerobic bacteria represent a significant component of the normal flora of the upper and lower gastrointestinal tracts of dogs and cats as well as their genital tracts; in addition, anaerobes play an important role in the regulation of the bacterial composition of the normal flora. Aerobes and facultative organisms that reside alongside anaerobes use oxygen present in these sites and reduce the local oxidation-reduction potential, which permits survival and growth of anaerobes. Sites that are protected from oxygen such as the gingival crevices also favor anaerobes. The metabolic activity of anaerobic bacteria prevents colonization of mucosal surfaces by potentially more pathogenic microbes (this is known as *colonization resistance*). Finally, anaerobes are important for the maintenance of normal mucosal barrier function.

Anaerobic bacteria can cause disease when they gain access to normally sterile sites. This occurs when mucosal barriers are disrupted, or when anaerobes gain access to subcutaneous tissues as a result of a contaminated penetrating wound. Anaerobic bacterial infections are often mixed infections owing to the concurrent presence of other anaerobes, as well as aerobes and facultative bacteria such as *Pasteurella* spp., *Escherichia coli,* streptococci, or staphylococci. Although there are hundreds of anaerobes that comprise the normal flora, the anaerobic bacterial species most often identified in disease are the gram-negative anaerobes *Fusobacterium* spp., *Bacteroides* spp., *Prevotella* spp., and *Porphyromonas* spp., and the gram-positive anaerobes *Clostridium* spp. and *Peptostreptococcus* spp. (Box 37-1).[2] An accurate understanding of the epidemiology of anaerobic bacterial infections in dogs and cats has been hampered by difficulties associated with culture of anaerobes. The use of molecular methods such as PCR has begun to shed more light on this topic. The reader is referred to Chapters 48 and 54 for information on gastrointestinal *Clostridium perfringens* and *Clostridium difficile* infections, and disease caused by the toxins of *Clostridium tetani* and *Clostridium botulinum,* respectively.

Clinical Features

Signs and Their Pathogenesis

Anaerobes can cause disease in a variety of different organs. Often, their presence is associated with abscess formation and necrosis at the site of inoculation, which contains a mixed population of anaerobic as well as facultative bacteria. The possession of virulence factors by anaerobes contributes to their ability to cause disease after host barriers are disrupted. These include capsular polysaccharides, extracellular proteases, endotoxin (gram-negative anaerobes), and a variety of other toxins. Capsular polysaccharides play an important role in the stimulation of

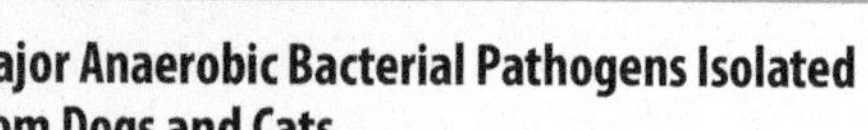

BOX 37-1

Major Anaerobic Bacterial Pathogens Isolated from Dogs and Cats

Gram-Positive Cocci

Peptostreptococcus spp. (especially *Peptostreptococcus anaerobius*)

Gram-Positive Rods

Clostridium spp.
Propionibacterium spp. (especially *Propionibacterium acnes*)

Gram-Negative Rods

Bacteroides spp. (e.g., *Bacteroides fragilis*)
Fusobacterium spp. (e.g., *Fusobacterium necrophorum* and *Fusobacterium nucleatum*)
Prevotella spp. (e.g., *Prevotella heparinolyticus*)
Porphyromonas spp.

abscess formation by certain anaerobes such as *Bacteroides, Porphyromonas, Fusobacterium,* and *Prevotella* species. Just as aerobic bacteria potentiate the survival of anaerobes through local consumption of oxygen, anaerobic bacteria produce metabolites such as short-chain fatty acids, which inhibit phagocytosis and promote survival of co-infecting facultative organisms.

Anaerobes of the oral cavity are important contributors to periodontal disease, tooth root abscesses and mandibular osteomyelitis, retrobulbar abscesses, and bite wound infections. Anaerobes are frequently isolated from the lungs and pleural cavities of dogs or cats with aspiration pneumonia and pyothorax, respectively. Intestinal anaerobes may be isolated from the abdominal cavities of animals with septic peritonitis secondary to intestinal perforation. The female genital tract is also heavily colonized with anaerobic bacteria, and pyometra may sometimes be associated with mixed aerobic and anaerobic infections that include the anaerobic species *Bacteroides, Prevotella, Fusobacterium,* and *Peptostreptococcus* species.

Plant awn migration in dogs and cats can lead to abscess formation in a variety of tissues, including retroperitoneal tissues and the brain. These abscesses usually contain a mixed population of aerobes and anaerobes, especially *Fusobacterium, Actinomyces,* and *Bacteroides* species. Brain abscessation can follow direct extension of anaerobic bacterial infection from otitis or tooth root infection. Alternatively, hematogenous spread may occur (Figure 37-1).

Periodontal Disease

Periodontal disease is one of the most common disorders seen by small animal veterinarians and may result in chronic pain, decreased appetite, and loss of teeth. It begins with formation of dental plaque as a result of poor oral hygiene and other host factors. Dental plaque is a bacterial biofilm composed primarily of gram-positive facultative anaerobes. Subsequently there is proliferation of pathogenic bacteria, which include gram-negative rods and especially anaerobes. These secrete toxins and incite an inflammatory response. Anaerobes implicated in canine and feline periodontal disease (such as *Porphyromonas gulae*) differ from those implicated in human periodontal disease *(Porphyromonas gingivalis)*.[3-6] Periodontal disease is manifested as gingival erythema, edema, gingival bleeding, and halitosis, with accumulation of calculus, gingival recession, alveolar bone loss, and sometimes the presence of purulent exudate (Figure 37-2).

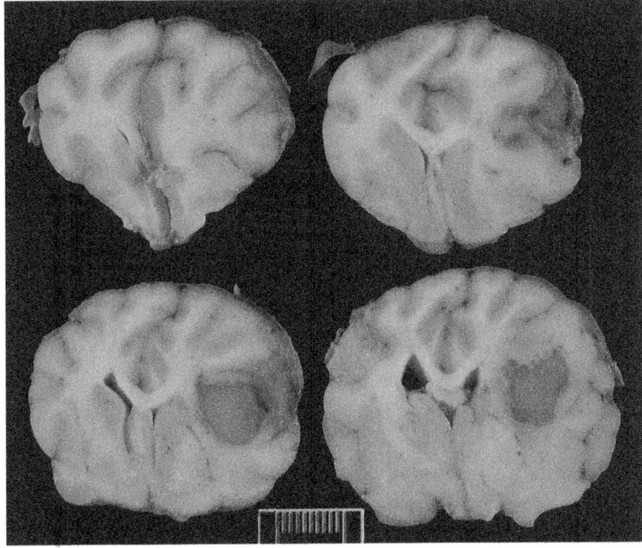

FIGURE 37-1 Abscess in the white matter of the right frontal lobe of a 2-year-old female spayed Chihuahua that had a 1-month history of difficulty chewing food and lethargy and a 3-week history of progressive obtundation, neck pain, and tetraparesis. Signs initially improved following treatment with prednisone, but then recurred as the prednisone dose was reduced. The abscess in the frontal lobe communicated with the overlying meninges, which were expanded by a chronic and fibrosing suppurative inflammatory infiltrate. Another abscess was present in the midbrain, which suggested hematogenous spread of infection. Although no bacteria were seen within the lesions with special stains, *Actinomyces canis* and *Fusobacterium nucleatum* were cultured from the lesions. (Courtesy of the University of California, Davis Veterinary Anatomic Pathology Service.)

Retrobulbar Abscesses

Retrobulbar or orbital abscesses can result from tooth root abscessation, penetrating foreign bodies such as grass awns, or penetrating trauma to the orbit. Clinical signs include unilateral exophthalmos, protrusion of the nictitans, conjunctival hyperemia, serous to mucopurulent ocular discharge, inappetence, fever, and pain on opening the mouth (Figure 37-3). A fluctuant swelling or draining tract posterior to the last ipsilateral molar may be present on examination of the oral cavity. In one study, *Bacteroides* spp. and *Clostridium* spp. were the most frequent anaerobes isolated from 34 dogs with retrobulbar abscesses; other frequently isolated bacteria were *Staphylococcus* spp., *Pasteurella* spp., and *Escherichia coli.* In cats, the most frequent anaerobe was *Bacteroides vulgatus,* and the most common non-anaerobe was *Pasteurella* spp.[7]

Skin and Soft Tissue Infections

Cat bite abscesses are one of the most common reasons that cats are brought to small animal clinics. Clinical signs include fever, lethargy, inappetence, pain, and firm or fluctuant subcutaneous swellings that may rupture and drain purulent material. Oral anaerobes and *Pasteurella multocida* are frequently isolated from these abscesses.[8] Anaerobic species involved include *Peptostreptococcus anaerobius, Porphyromonas* spp., *Clostridium villosum, Fusobacterium* spp., *Bacteroides* spp. (especially *Bacteroides tectum*), and *Prevotella* spp.[9] Despite the widespread occurrence of cat bite abscesses, studies that use molecular methods to identify the types and relative prevalences of anaerobes in cat bite abscesses are lacking.

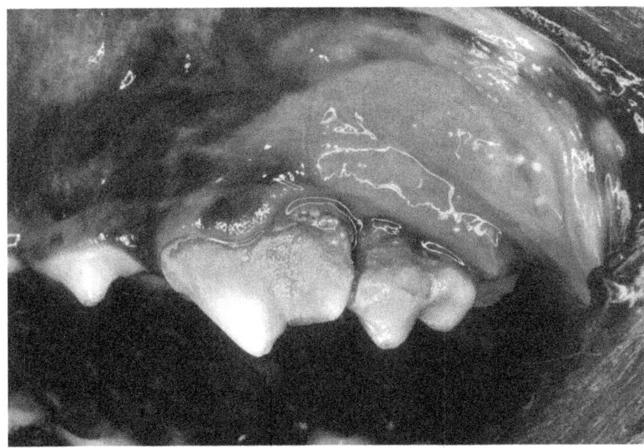

FIGURE 37-2 Periodontitis in a dog. There is significant gingival inflammation, plaque and calculus accumulation, and purulent exudate. Gingival recession and contact ulceration of the buccal mucosa are also present. (Courtesy of Dr. Frank Verstraete, University of California, Davis Dentistry and Oral Surgery Service.)

Other skin and soft tissue infections associated with a variety of anaerobes include foreign body penetrating wounds and dog bite wounds (see Chapter 57).

Pneumonia and Pyothorax

Anaerobes such as *Fusobacterium* spp., *Peptostreptococcus anaerobius, Prevotella* spp., and *Porphyromonas* spp. are frequently isolated from dogs and cats with aspiration pneumonia, foreign body pneumonia (especially that due to plant awn migration), and pyothorax.[10] Dogs with plant awn migration develop multifocal necrotizing pneumonia with abscess formation. In some cases, aspiration pneumonia is followed by lung abscess formation (Figure 37-4). In human patients, a period of 6 to 7 days is required for necrosis and abscess formation to occur after aspiration, and so aspiration pneumonia with lung abscess formation is generally a chronic disease process.

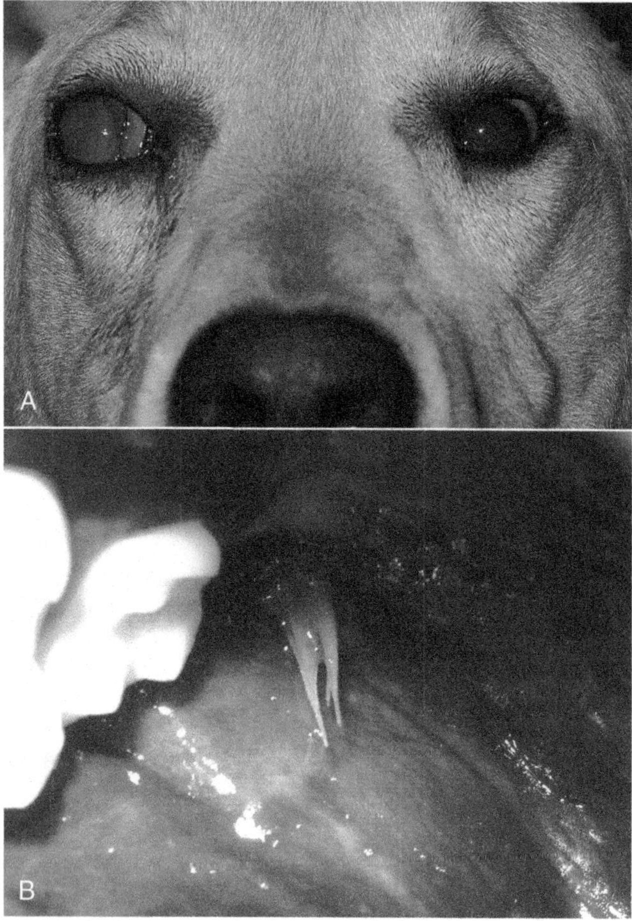

FIGURE 37-3 Retrobulbar abscess and endophthalmitis secondary to a migrating grass awn foreign body in a 10-month-old intact male Labrador retriever. **A,** Note the mucopurulent ocular discharge from the right eye, as well as buphthalmos (enlargement of the eye) and exophthalmos. The nictating membrane and conjunctiva are hyperemic, and there is diffuse corneal edema. Hypopyon and iris bombe were also present. Globe retropulsion was reduced and painful on the right side. **B,** Multiple grass awns were present all over the dog's haircoat, and an awn (shown) was removed from the gingiva posterior to the last right maxillary molar tooth. The right eye was subsequently enucleated. No additional grass awns were found. Histopathology of the globe showed severe chronic fibrinosuppurative panophthalmitis with focal, 0.3-cm scleral rupture in the caudal sclera near the optic nerve, regional orbital granulation tissue, and rupture of the lens. (Courtesy of the University of California, Davis Veterinary Ophthalmology Service.)

The reader is referred to Chapter 87 for more information on bacterial pneumonia and pyothorax.

Peritonitis

Septic peritonitis that involves anaerobes may result from perforation of the intestinal tract, especially the cecum or colon. *Bacteroides* and *Clostridium* species are most often isolated from these infections. *Fusobacterium* and *Propionibacterium* species may also be isolated.[11] Disease that results from bowel perforation often contains a population of organisms that reflect the bowel flora at the site of perforation, including anaerobes, facultative gram-positive anaerobes (especially *Enterococcus* spp.), *Candida* spp., and facultative gram-negative anaerobes such as *Escherichia coli.* Rupture of the female genital tract secondary to pyometra may also result in anaerobic bacterial peritonitis.

Bacteremia

Anaerobes are occasionally isolated from dogs and cats with bloodstream infections, usually as polymicrobial infections with aerobic bacteria. In a European study of 66 bacteremic cats, 12% of bacteria isolated from the bloodstream were obligate anaerobes.[12] In a study of 140 bacteremic dogs, anaerobes comprised 9% of the isolates.[13] Of 39 dogs and 10 cats with critical illness and bacteremia from Colorado, anaerobes were isolated from 31% of the dogs and 40% of the cats. The most common anaerobe isolated from the 39 dogs was *C. perfringens* (9 dogs), followed by *Bacteroides* species (2 dogs).[14] The cats were infected with *Bacteroides* or *Fusobacterium* species. The possibility of mixed aerobic-anaerobic bacterial bloodstream infection should be considered in dogs with systemic grass awn migration. However, anaerobic bacteria appear to be a very rare cause of endocarditis in dogs (see Chapter 86).[15]

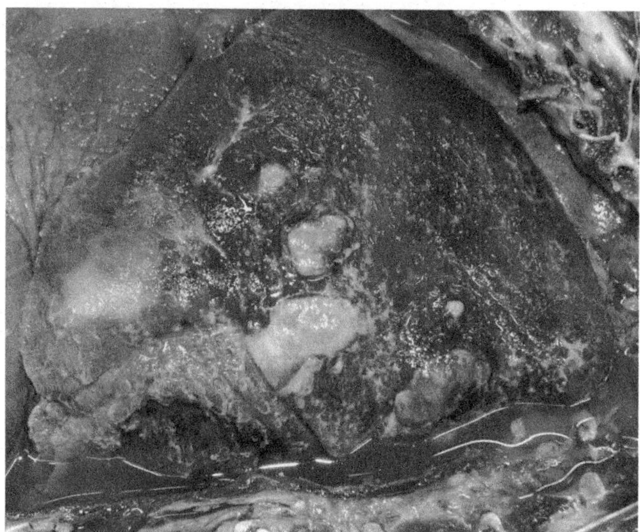

FIGURE 37-4 Necropsy findings in an 11-year-old male neutered Labrador retriever with severe aspiration pneumonia secondary to laryngeal tie-back surgery for laryngeal paralysis, which occurred 2 months before death. Aspiration led to bronchopneumonia with multifocal abscessation, pleural rupture, pyothorax, and pneumothorax. There are multiple to coalescing black to dark gray, soft, irregular foci in the lungs that measured up to 4.5 cm in diameter. On cut surface, dark gray to black material oozed from the parenchyma. Aerobic bacterial culture yielded large numbers of bacteria that included *Streptococcus canis,* nonfermenter group 3 organisms, and *Pasteurella canis.* Anaerobic culture yielded large numbers of *Peptostreptococcus anaerobius.* (Courtesy of the University of California, Davis, Veterinary Anatomic Pathology Service.)

Diagnosis

Abnormalities that suggest an anaerobic bacterial infection include a putrid odor, discolored purulent discharge, gas production within tissues (especially with *C. perfringens* infections) (Figure 37-5), a bite or puncture wound, penetrating foreign bodies, abscessation, pyothorax, aspiration pneumonia, damage to mucosal surfaces with which anaerobes are usually associated, and/or necrotic or gangrenous tissue (Box 37-2). However, absence of these features does not rule out infection with anaerobes, and some of these abnormalities occur with pure aerobic bacterial infections. For example, although anaerobes such as *Clostridium* spp. may be involved in emphysematous cystitis in humans and dogs, the most common cause of emphysematous cystitis is *E. coli*.

Laboratory Abnormalities

Complete Blood Count, Biochemistry, and Urinalysis Findings

No specific CBC, biochemistry, or urinalysis findings suggest anaerobic infection. Infections may be associated with leukocytosis due to a neutrophilia with a left shift and toxic neutrophils.

Cytologic Analysis

Cytologic analysis of exudate in aerobic bacterial infections typically reveals neutrophilic inflammation accompanied by bacteria of mixed morphology and gram staining characteristics. This and/or the presence of filamentous rod-shaped bacteria within these exudates should increase suspicion for an anaerobic infection (Figure 37-6).

Microbiologic Tests

Bacterial Isolation and Identification

Optimal techniques for isolation of anaerobic bacteria are described in Chapter 3. The decision to request anaerobic bacterial culture should be considered carefully, because anaerobes are difficult to culture, tend to have predictable susceptibility to antimicrobial drugs, and can contaminate specimens, which can lead to misleading results. If anaerobic culture is performed, the best specimens to collect are tissues or body fluids that are normally sterile. Fluids (e.g., 1 to 2 mL) or tissue specimens are preferable to swab specimens. Specimens should immediately be placed in an anaerobic transport medium and shipped to the laboratory as soon as possible, because even brief exposure to oxygen impairs isolation. Growth is often slow when compared to other facultative organisms, and cultures should be incubated for 7 days. Because most anaerobe infections also involve aerobes, aerobic bacterial culture should always be requested concurrently.

Extensive antimicrobial susceptibility testing is not routinely performed for anaerobes because it is laborious, expensive, and can have a long turnaround time. Because infections are polymicrobial (two or more anaerobe species as well as facultative organisms present), susceptibility testing for all pathogens present is often cost prohibitive to

BOX 37-2

Disease Processes That Suggest the Possibility of Anaerobic Bacterial Infection

- Abscess formation
- Putrid odor
- Necrotic tissue
- Negative cultures despite the presence of bacteria on cytologic examination
- Exposure to plant foreign bodies such as grass awns
- Interdigital or retrobulbar soft tissue involvement
- Dental infections
- Aspiration pneumonia
- Pyothorax
- Gastrointestinal perforation
- Pyometra
- Bite wound infections

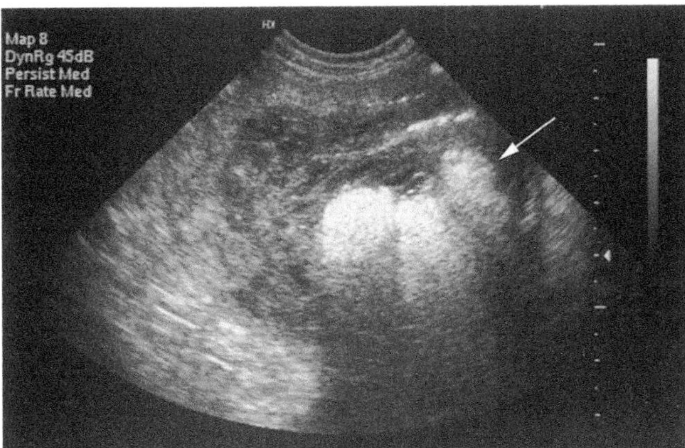

FIGURE 37-5 Splenic abscess in an 11-year-old male neutered Labrador mix that also had duodenal lymphoma. Ultrasound image of a large splenic mass that contains numerous hyperechoic foci and shadowing, consistent with the presence of gas. Necropsy showed severe, focally extensive, neutrophilic, and necrotizing splenitis. The duodenum was perforated at the site of the neoplasm. *Escherichia coli, Bacteroides tectum,* and a *Prevotella heparinolyticus*–like organism were cultured from the splenic abscess.

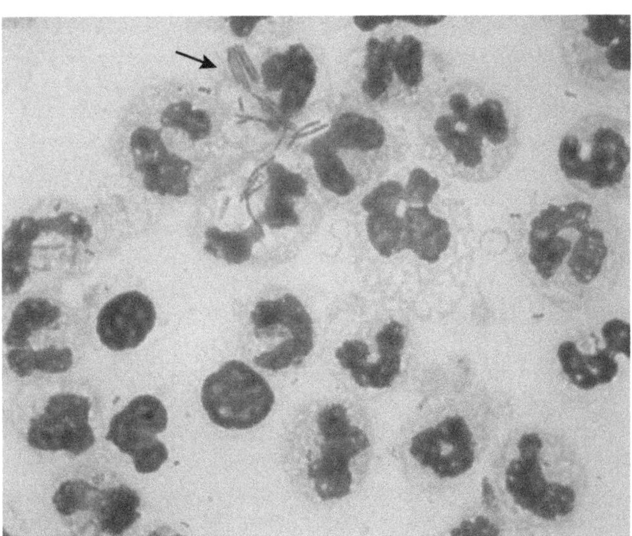

FIGURE 37-6 Cytology of pleural fluid collected using thoracocentesis from an 8-year-old female spayed domestic shorthair with pyothorax. A mixed population of bacteria that includes filamentous organisms suggestive of anaerobes *(arrow)* is present. Aerobic and anaerobic bacterial culture yielded a mixed growth of *Prevotella* spp., *Peptostreptococcus anaerobius*, *Fusobacterium* spp., and an unidentified anaerobic gram-positive rod. Wright's stain, 1600× magnification.

TABLE 37-1

Suggested Antimicrobial Drugs for Treatment of Anaerobic Bacterial Infections in Dogs or Cats*

Drug	Dose (mg/kg)	Interval (hours)	Route
Amoxicillin–clavulanate potassium	12.5-25	12	PO
Ampicillin-sulbactam	10-20†	8	IV, IM
Metronidazole	15 15	12 12 (dogs), 24 (cats)	IV PO
Clindamycin hydrochloride, clindamycin phosphate	11 10	12 (dogs), 24 (cats) 12	PO IV‡, IM
Chloramphenicol, chloramphenicol sodium succinate	40-50 (dogs), 12.5-20 (cats)	6-8 (dogs), 12 (cats)	PO, IV, IM§
Pradofloxacin	3 (dogs), 5-10 (cats)	24	PO‖

*The concurrent presence of aerobes should also be considered when selecting antimicrobial drugs.
†Dose according to ampicillin component.
‡For IV administration, dilute 1:10 in 0.9% saline and administer over 30-60 minutes.
§See Chapter 8 for warnings about chloramphenicol use.
‖Use of pradofloxacin in dogs at high doses has been associated with myelosuppression and is extra-label in the United States. Doses shown for cats are for the oral suspension; a dose of 3 mg/kg is recommended for the tablet formulation.

pet owners. In addition, anaerobes that infect dogs and cats generally have predictable drug susceptibilities. Nevertheless, because antimicrobial resistance has increased among anaerobes that infect humans, the possibility of drug resistance should be considered when infections do not respond to treatment with drainage and appropriate antimicrobial drugs. Some veterinary diagnostic laboratories perform rapid tests for β-lactamase enzyme production by anaerobes (see Case Example).

Treatment and Prognosis

Treatment of anaerobic bacterial infections involves surgical removal of necrotic tissue, drainage of abscesses through surgical or imaging-guided approaches, restoration of blood supply, and medical management with antimicrobial drugs (Table 37-1). Antimicrobial drugs with activity against most anaerobes are β-lactam/β-lactamase inhibitor drug combinations (such as clavulanic acid–amoxicillin or ampicillin-sulbactam), clindamycin, metronidazole, chloramphenicol, and carbapenems. Although penicillin and first-generation cephalosporins may be effective, some pathogenic anaerobes that infect dogs and cats (especially *Bacteroides* but also a significant percentage of *Prevotella, Porphyromonas,* and *Fusobacterium* isolates) may be resistant to these drugs through the production of β-lactamase enzymes. Approximately 20% of *Bacteroides* and *Clostridium* isolates are resistant to clindamycin, but other anaerobes are susceptible.[2] Factors such as tissue penetration should be considered when selecting antimicrobial drugs, and the concurrent presence of aerobic bacteria must also be taken into account. Thus a combination of a β-lactam/β-lactamase inhibitor drug or clindamycin and a drug with activity against gram-negative bacteria, such as a fluoroquinolone or an aminoglycoside, is a reasonable choice for initial treatment of serious infections while awaiting the results of susceptibility testing for aerobic bacteria when mixed aerobic-anaerobic infections are suspected. For infections that do not require parenteral therapy, pradofloxacin also has potent activity against a variety of aerobes, anaerobes and mycoplasmas (see Chapter 8).

With the exception of newer generation fluoroquinolones such as pradofloxacin, anaerobes are resistant to fluoroquinolones. Anaerobes are also generally resistant to trimethoprim-sulfamethoxazole and have unpredictable resistance to tetracyclines. Aminoglycosides are remarkable for their complete inactivity against anaerobes.

Prevention

Prevention of anaerobic bacterial infections involves management or prevention of underlying conditions that predispose to these infections. Vaccines for prevention of anaerobic bacterial infections are not available. An inactivated, whole-cell *Porphyromonas denticanis, Porphyromonas gulae,* and *Porphyromonas salivosa* vaccine was available for several years for prevention of periodontal disease in dogs but was withdrawn from the market because of apparent lack of efficacy.

Public Health Aspects

Anaerobes that reside in the oral cavity of dogs and cats are important causes of bite wound infections in humans, next to *Pasteurella* species. The reader is referred to Chapter 57 for more information on the public health significance of bite wound infections.

CASE EXAMPLE

Signalment: "Cocoa," a 4-month-old intact female Labrador retriever from Gonzales in northern California

History: Cocoa was brought to the University of California, Davis, Veterinary Medical Teaching Hospital for evaluation of seizures. Approximately 6 weeks before referral, the dog was seen for left ocular exophthalmos. She was treated with amoxicillin–clavulanic acid for 1 week, and the exophthalmos resolved, but subsequently right ocular exophthalmos developed. This resolved after another 1-week course of amoxicillin–clavulanic acid. One month later, Cocoa appeared painful on opening her mouth. She was treated with cephalexin and meloxicam with no apparent improvement. Two days later she became inappetent. When the owners offered her food by hand, she ate, became ataxic, fell over, her thoracic limbs stiffened, and foamy saliva was noted around her mouth. She was taken to an emergency clinic, and she vomited in the car. At the emergency clinic she had three generalized seizures that were treated with diazepam. She was also treated with enrofloxacin (5 mg/kg IV, once).

Cocoa's diet normally consisted of commercial dog food, and she had been vaccinated for distemper, hepatitis, and parvoviral enteritis at 8 and 12 weeks of age. There had been no coughing, sneezing, diarrhea, exposure to ticks or toxins, trauma, or travel outside California.

Physical Examination:

Body Weight: 15.3 kg

General: Quiet but alert and responsive. Hydrated. T = 102.8°F (39.3°C), HR = 110 beats/min, panting, mucous membranes pink, CRT = 1 second.

Eyes, Ears, Nose, and Throat: No clinically significant abnormalities were noted. There was no evidence of pain on opening the mouth provided neck movement was prevented during the examination.

Integument, Musculoskeletal, Cardiovascular, Gastrointestinal, Genitourinary Systems, and Peripheral Lymph Nodes: No clinically significant findings.

Neurologic Examination: Mild obtundation was noted. The dog held her head down and was reluctant to move her neck. There was moderate to marked ataxia that involved all four limbs, with the pelvic limbs most severely affected, and the right pelvic and thoracic limbs more severely affected than the left. Cranial nerve examination revealed only a decreased corneal reflex on the right side. Decreased placing reactions were noted in all four limbs, with the right limbs more severely affected. There was severe pain on palpation of the cervical spine and moderate pain on palpation of the lumbosacral spine. Multifocal CNS lesions were suspected.

Laboratory Findings:

CBC:

HCT 34.4% (40%-55%)
MCV 64.9 fL (65-75 fL)
MCHC 34.9 g/dL (33-36 g/dL)
Reticulocytes 22,000 cells/μL (7000-65,000 cells/μL)
WBC 17,780 cells/μL (6000-13,000 cells/μL)
Neutrophils 12,979 cells/μL (3000-10,500 cells/μL)
Band neutrophils 533 cells/μL
Lymphocytes 3023 cells/μL (1000-4000 cells/μL)
Monocytes 1245 cells/μL (150-1200 cells/μL)
Platelets 392,000 platelets/μL (150,000-400,000 platelets/μL).

Serum Chemistry Profile:

Sodium 143 mmol/L (145-154 mmol/L)
Potassium 4.6 mmol/L (3.6-5.3 mmol/L)
Chloride 102 mmol/L (108-118 mmol/L)
Bicarbonate 23 mmol/L (16-26 mmol/L)
Phosphorus 6.9 mg/dL (3.0-6.2 mg/dL)
Calcium 11.1 mg/dL (9.7-11.5 mg/dl)
BUN 7 mg/dL (5-21 mg/dL)
Creatinine 0.4 mg/dL (0.3-1.2 mg/dL)
Glucose 95 mg/dL (64-123 mg/dL)
Total protein 6.1 g/dL (5.4-7.6 g/dL)
Albumin 2.8 g/dL (3.0-4.4 g/dL)
Globulin 3.3 g/dL (1.8-3.9 g/dL)
ALT 35 U/L (19-67 U/L)
AST 52 U/L (19-42 U/L)
ALP 103 U/L (21-170 U/L)
Creatine kinase 556 U/L (51-399 U/L)
Gamma GT 4 U/L (0-6 U/L)
Cholesterol 262 mg/dL (135-361 mg/dL)
Total bilirubin 0.1 mg/dL (0-0.2 mg/dL).

Urinalysis: SGr 1.013; pH 6.5, negative for protein, glucose, ketones, bilirubin, hemoprotein, WBC, RBC, casts, and bacteria.

Imaging Findings:

Thoracic Radiographs: Cardiopulmonary structures were within normal limits.

Abdominal Ultrasound: The gastric wall was mildly thickened with bright, echogenic speckles within the muscularis layer. The submucosa of the stomach was echogenic. These changes were suggestive of gastritis. The remainder of the abdominal ultrasound was unremarkable.

Spinal Radiographs: Open physes were present within the vertebral column. No abnormalities were identified.

Brain MRI: In the precontrast brain study, a flattened, fusiform extradural structure was identified in the dorsal part of the foramen magnum that caused moderate dorsoventral compression of the spinal cord (see arrow in Figure 37-7). This structure was hypointense to brain but hyperintense to CSF on the T1-weighted images and moderately hyperintense on dual echo and fluid-attenuated inversion recovery (FLAIR) images. The postcontrast brain study showed diffuse meningeal enhancement that involved the spinal cord and brain, with the most prominent enhancement noted along the ventral brainstem and left cerebral hemisphere. This contrast enhancement pattern was consistent with meningitis. A discrete rim of enhancement surrounded the aforementioned fusiform structure, which gave it a cystic appearance. The structure had partial fluid characteristics, and, in light of the meningeal enhancement, an abscess was suspected.

Analysis of CSF (Lumbar CSF): CSF protein: 726 mg/dL (reference range, <25 mg/dL)

Total RBC: 5 cells/μL (reference range, 0 cells/μL)

Total nucleated cells: 7500 cells/μL (reference range, <2 cells/μL)

Differential: 88% neutrophils, 12% large mononuclear cells

Microscopic evaluation: The specimen was highly cellular and contained a large number of nondegenerate neutrophils. A few pyknotic forms were noted. Lower numbers of

Continued

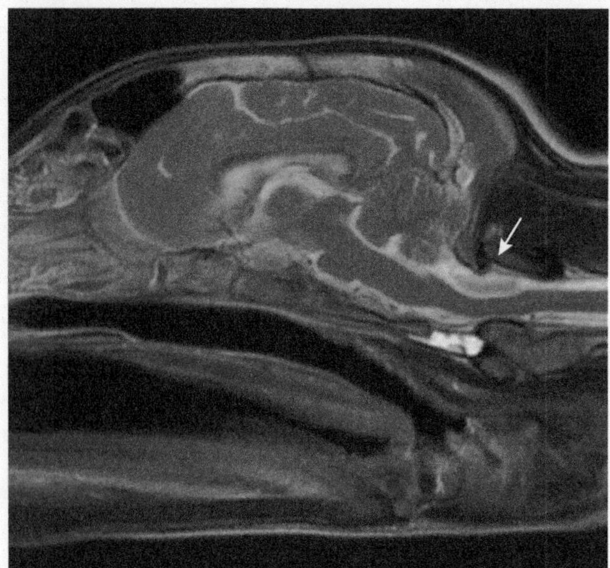

FIGURE 37-7 Postcontrast brain MRI, 4-month-old intact female Labrador retriever with *Bacteroides fragilis* meningitis and an epidural abscess located in the dorsal part of the foramen magnum. There is a flattened, fusiform structure in the dorsal part of the foramen magnum associated with moderate dorsoventral compression of the spinal cord *(arrow)*. Diffuse meningeal enhancement and a discrete rim of enhancement surrounding the fusiform structure are present.

monocytoid cells, large reactive lymphocytes, and rare eosinophils also were observed. Interpretation: Marked neutrophilic pleocytosis (purulent inflammation).

Cytologic Analysis of CSF (Cisternal): A direct smear of cisternal CSF contained disrupted cells and mildly to moderately degenerate neutrophils. These were admixed with low numbers of monocytoid cells and intermediate-sized reactive lymphocytes. Rare neutrophils were observed with intracellular rod-shaped bacteria. Few free rod-shaped bacteria were noted in the background.

Microbiologic Testing: Aerobic urine culture: No growth was detected.

Aerobic and anaerobic blood cultures: No growth was detected.

Aerobic and anaerobic CSF culture: Small numbers of *Bacteroides fragilis*, positive for β-lactamase production.

Diagnosis: *Bacteroides fragilis* meningitis with extradural abscess formation

Treatment and Outcome: Cocoa was treated with ticarcillin (50 mg/kg IV q6h), metronidazole (10 mg/kg IV q8h), and crystalloid fluids (LRS with 20 mEq/L KCl at 50 mL/h, IV). The following day her mentation improved and she became more willing to move. On day 3 after starting antibiotics, treatment was changed to clavulanic acid–amoxicillin (16 mg/kg PO q8h) and metronidazole (16 mg/kg PO q12h). On day 4, Cocoa was less ataxic and had normal placing reactions, but had a seizure while on a walk outside. The seizure lasted 45 seconds and was manifested by jaw chomping and defecation, but Cocoa did not fall over or lose consciousness. Potassium bromide (40 mg/kg PO q8h for 4 days, then 40 mg/kg PO q24h) was added to the treatment regimen, and Cocoa was discharged from the hospital.

At a recheck 3 weeks later, Cocoa's owners reported that she had shown steady clinical improvement and for the last week she had been acting like a normal puppy. There had been no seizures. She had received the final set of the puppy vaccine series 1 week earlier. No abnormalities were detected on neurologic examination. A CBC showed persistent mild nonregenerative anemia (hematocrit 34.8%), 5253 neutrophils/μL, and 228 band neutrophils/μL. A repeat MRI showed a decrease in the meningeal enhancement and marked reduction in the size of the cystic structure, although there was persistent mild spinal cord compression. Analysis of CSF revealed a CSF protein concentration of 37 mg/dL, <1 RBC/μL, 24 nucleated cells/μL, with 12% neutrophils, 51% small mononuclear cells, and 37% large mononuclear cells. Microscopic examination of the CSF revealed a heterogenous population of lymphocytes that included small mature lymphocytes, larger reactive lymphocytes, and many plasmacytoid lymphocytes along with mature plasma cells and moderately vacuolated macrophages. A few nondegenerate neutrophils were present. Antimicrobial drug treatment was continued and a recheck was recommended in 3 months, but the dog was subsequently lost to follow-up.

Comments: The history of exophthalmos increased suspicion for an anaerobic bacterial infection of the CNS in this dog and was the reason that anaerobic culture of the CSF and blood was performed. Given the young age of this dog, a migrating foreign body (e.g., plant awn) was suspected. The history, together with the distribution of lesions in the CNS and the lack of lesions elsewhere, suggested direct extension of the infection from the retrobulbar location to the meninges, rather than hematogenous spread of infection. Because the dog was treated with antibiotics before culture was performed, the concurrent presence of other facultative organisms or other anaerobic species may have been obscured. The identification of β-lactamase production by the *B. fragilis* isolate was not surprising, because of the high (>90%) prevalence of β-lactamase production by this species. *B. fragilis* is also known for its propensity to form abscesses.

SUGGESTED READING

Jang SS, Breher JE, Dabaco LA, et al. Organisms isolated from dogs and cats with anaerobic infections and susceptibility to selected antimicrobial agents. J Am Vet Med Assoc. 1997;210:1610-1614.

REFERENCES

1. Sebald M, Hauser D. Pasteur, oxygen and the anaerobes revisited. Anaerobe. 1995;1:11-16.
2. Jang SS, Breher JE, Dabaco LA, et al. Organisms isolated from dogs and cats with anaerobic infections and susceptibility to selected antimicrobial agents. J Am Vet Med Assoc. 1997;210:1610-1614.
3. Hardham J, Reed M, Wong J, et al. Evaluation of a monovalent companion animal periodontal disease vaccine in an experimental mouse periodontitis model. Vaccine. 2005;23:3148-3156.
4. Kato Y, Shirai M, Murakami M, et al. Molecular detection of human periodontal pathogens in oral swab specimens from dogs in Japan. J Vet Dent. 2011;28:84-89.
5. Perez-Salcedo L, Herrera D, Esteban-Saltiveri D, et al. Comparison of two sampling methods for microbiological evaluation of periodontal disease in cats. Vet Microbiol. 2011;149:500-503.
6. Senhorinho GN, Nakano V, Liu C, et al. Detection of *Porphyromonas gulae* from subgingival biofilms of dogs with and without periodontitis. Anaerobe. 2011;17:257-258.

7. Wang AL, Ledbetter EC, Kern TJ. Orbital abscess bacterial isolates and in vitro antimicrobial susceptibility patterns in dogs and cats. Vet Ophthalmol. 2009;12:91-96.
8. Love DN, Jones RF, Bailey M, et al. Isolation and characterisation of bacteria from abscesses in the subcutis of cats. J Med Microbiol. 1979;12:207-212.
9. Love DN, Malik R, Norris JM. Bacteriological warfare amongst cats: what have we learned about cat bite infections? Vet Microbiol. 2000;74:179-193.
10. Walker AL, Jang SS, Hirsh DC. Bacteria associated with pyothorax of dogs and cats: 98 cases (1989-1998). J Am Vet Med Assoc. 2000;216:359-363.
11. Culp WT, Zeldis TE, Reese MS, et al. Primary bacterial peritonitis in dogs and cats: 24 cases (1990-2006). J Am Vet Med Assoc. 2009;234:906-913.
12. Greiner M, Wolf G, Hartmann K. Bacteraemia in 66 cats and antimicrobial susceptibility of the isolates (1995-2004). J Feline Med Surg. 2007;9:404-410.
13. Greiner M, Wolf G, Hartmann K. A retrospective study of the clinical presentation of 140 dogs and 39 cats with bacteraemia. J Small Anim Pract. 2008;49:378-383.
14. Dow SW, Curtis CR, Jones RL, et al. Bacterial culture of blood from critically ill dogs and cats: 100 cases (1985-1987). J Am Vet Med Assoc. 1989;195:113-117.
15. Sykes JE, Kittleson MD, Pesavento PA, et al. Evaluation of the relationship between causative organisms and clinical characteristics of infective endocarditis in dogs: 71 cases (1992-2005). J Am Vet Med Assoc. 2006;228:1723-1734.

CHAPTER 38

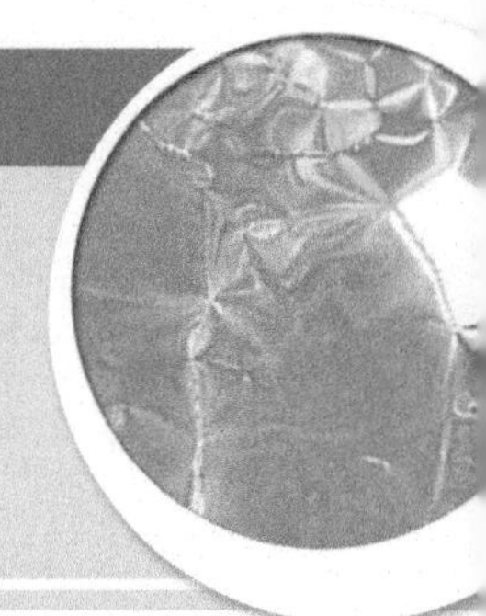

Bordetellosis

Jane E. Sykes

Overview of Canine and Feline Bordetellosis

First Described: 1911 (*Bacillus bronchicanis*, Ferry).[1] The genus *Bordetella* was named after Bordet, who first described *Bordetella pertussis* (Bordet and Gengou, 1906).[2]

Cause: *Bordetella bronchiseptica,* an aerobic gram-negative motile bacterium (family Alcaligenaceae)

Affected Hosts: Dogs, cats, wild carnivores, pigs, horses, rabbits, rodents, turkey, humans. Dogs and cats share the same strains.

Geographic Distribution: Worldwide

Mode of Transmission: Aerosol, contact with contaminated fomites and water sources

Major Clinical Signs: Sneezing, serous to mucopurulent nasal discharge, harsh or honking cough (especially dogs). Dogs and cats with bronchopneumonia can develop fever, lethargy, inappetence, tachypnea, productive cough, and mucopurulent nasal and ocular discharge.

Differential Diagnoses: Upper and lower respiratory diseases such as collapsing trachea, viral respiratory infections, fungal pneumonia, protozoal pneumonia, respiratory tract neoplasia, airway foreign bodies, chronic bronchitis, eosinophilic bronchopneumopathy or granulomatosis, parasitic infections (such as *Filaroides, Oslerus, Capillaria, Paragonimus, Dirofilaria*), bronchopneumonias secondary to conditions such as laryngeal paralysis or ciliary dyskinesia, left-sided congestive heart failure

Human Health Significance: *B. bronchiseptica* is closely related to *B. pertussis* and *Bordetella parapertussis,* which cause whooping cough in humans. Uncommonly, it has been associated with respiratory disease in humans and rarely systemic infections such as peritonitis, septicemia, and meningitis. It primarily causes disease in the immunocompromised. Contact with dogs and cats has been associated with human infections, but host specificity may also be strain related.

Etiologic Agent and Epidemiology

Bordetella spp. are small, pleomorphic, gram-negative coccobacilli. They have fimbriae (pili) and can be motile by means of flagella. There are at least nine different bacterial species in the genus *Bordetella* (Table 38-1).[3] The only species known to cause disease in dogs and cats is *Bordetella bronchiseptica,* but *B. bronchiseptica* is closely related to *B. pertussis* and *B. parapertussis,* which cause pertussis (whooping cough) in humans. In fact, there is evidence that *B. pertussis* evolved from a distinct, human-associated lineage of *B. bronchiseptica,*[4] and it has been recommended that *B. bronchiseptica, B. pertussis,* and *B. parapertussis* be reclassified as subspecies of the "*B. bronchiseptica* cluster."[5] *B. pertussis* can colonize puppies in the absence of clinical signs of respiratory disease.[6]

Worldwide, *B. bronchiseptica* is an important cause of respiratory disease in dogs and cats; it also infects and causes respiratory illness in many different animal species including wild carnivores, pigs, rabbits, and occasionally horses, other herbivores, rodents, turkeys, and humans. There are a large number of different strains of *B. bronchiseptica* that vary in virulence and host specificity. Nevertheless, the results of molecular typing efforts have shown that strains that infect dogs can be passed to cats and vice versa.[7-9] The whole genome of *B. bronchiseptica* has been sequenced.[10] Its genome is larger than that of its close relatives, and it possesses several plasmids, some of which mediate antimicrobial drug resistance.[11]

Like viral respiratory infections, bordetellosis is especially prevalent in dogs and cats in shelter, pet stores, boarding facilities, and other situations where large numbers of potentially stressed animals may have been in close contact with one another. Infections with *B. bronchiseptica* frequently occur in concert with respiratory viral and/or *Mycoplasma* spp. infections (see Chapters 17, 23, and 40). Unlike *B. pertussis* and *B. parapertussis, B. bronchiseptica* can persist in the environment for at least 10 days and can grow in natural water sources,[12] but is susceptible to most disinfectants provided they are used correctly.

The prevalence of *B. bronchiseptica* infections in group-housed animals, including shelters, varies from group to group, even in the same geographic region. *B. bronchiseptica* can be isolated from apparently healthy cats and cats with respiratory disease, but is more likely to be isolated from cats with respiratory disease. In one European study that included 1748 cats from private multicat households, shelters, and breeding catteries, the more cats in the group, the greater the chance that *B. bronchiseptica* would be detected. In rescue shelters, increased seroprevalence has been associated with poor hygiene.[13] In a study of 742 cats in the United Kingdom, *B. bronchiseptica* was isolated from 0% of pet cats, 19.5% of cats from rescue shelters, and 13.5% of cats from research colonies.[14] *B. bronchiseptica* was cultured from 3.1% of 614 cats from four shelters in Louisiana,[15] 5.1% of nasal swabs from 59 cats with acute respiratory disease in Colorado,[16] and none of 22 cats with respiratory disease in a shelter in California.[17] However, the prevalence of infection was nearly 50% in nasal

TABLE 38-1

Species That Belong to the Genus *Bordetella*

Species	Host(s)	Disease
Bordetella bronchiseptica	Dogs, cats, pigs, horses, rabbits, rodents, humans	Rhinitis, tracheobronchitis, bronchopneumonia
Bordetella pertussis	Humans	Whooping cough
Bordetella parapertussis	Humans, sheep	Whooping cough (humans); ovine-adapted strains cause respiratory disease in sheep
Bordetella holmesii	Humans	Upper respiratory tract disease, bacteremia
Bordetella trematum	Humans	Otitis media and wound infections
Bordetella avium	Poultry (especially turkey)	Rhinotracheitis
Bordetella hinzii	Birds, rarely humans	Normal flora of birds, bacteremia, cholangitis in humans
Bordetella petrii	Environment, rarely humans	None, osteomyelitis
Bordetella ansorpii	Humans	Bacteremia, skin infection

swabs from 40 cats with rhinitis from a shelter in Colorado.[18] Similarly, a high prevalence (26%) of infection was detected with a PCR assay in 100 cats with upper respiratory disease from central Italy.[19]

Only a few studies have examined the epidemiology of *B. bronchiseptica* infection in dogs. In a case review from the eastern United States, *B. bronchiseptica* was isolated from 32 (49%) of 65 pet dogs under 1 year of age with radiographic and microbiologic evidence of bacterial bronchopneumonia. Most of these dogs had originated from breeders (40%) or pet stores (41%), and only 8% were from shelters. Dogs infected with *B. bronchiseptica* were younger (7 to 35 weeks of age), had been owned for a shorter period of time (median, 18 days), were more likely to have originated from a pet store and were less likely to have originated from a breeder than dogs with pneumonia caused by other organisms. *B. bronchiseptica* was isolated from dogs with respiratory disease as well as from healthy dogs in a rehoming kennel in the United Kingdom.[20]

Clinical Features

Signs and Their Pathogenesis

Transmission of *B. bronchiseptica* occurs primarily by the airborne route, but contact with contaminated fomites and water sources may also be important. The organism is highly contagious. Much of what is known about *B. bronchiseptica* pathogenesis is based on studies of infections in host species other than the dog or cat. *B. bronchiseptica* is inhaled, adheres to respiratory cilia, evades the immune system, and secretes toxins that damage the respiratory epithelium (Figure 38-1). Adhesion of virulent strains of *B. bronchiseptica* to respiratory cilia occurs by means of fimbrial adhesins (FIM), a filamentous hemagglutinin (FHA), pertactin, and cell wall lipopolysaccharide. *Bordetella* colonization factor A (BcfA) is another outer membrane protein that appears to be important for tracheal colonization by *B. bronchiseptica*.[21] *B. bronchiseptica* possesses genes that encode for pertussis toxin, an important adhesin in *B. pertussis*. These genes are not expressed in vitro, but there is some evidence for pertussis toxin expression in vivo.[22] Evasion of host defenses is mediated by the organism's outer capsule (which is absent in *B. pertussis* and *B. parapertussis*), adenylate cyclase toxin, and pertactin. The capsule protects it from phagocytosis and destruction by complement. Adenylate cyclase toxin catalyzes the conversion of ATP to cAMP, which inhibits the migration and activation of phagocytes and T-lymphocytes. Pertactin allows the organism to resist neutrophil-mediated clearance.[23] A type VI secretion system also appears to play a key role in persistence of *B. bronchiseptica*.[24] Other virulence determinants present in the outer membrane include lipopolysaccharide and the Brk protein (*B*ordetella *r*esistance to *k*illing), which allow the organism to resist complement-mediated destruction. At least two other important exotoxins damage respiratory epithelial cells and cells of the immune system, and incite cytokine production: tracheal cytotoxin (TCT) and dermonecrotic toxin (DNT). *B. bronchiseptica* also possesses a type III secretion system that allows it to inject as-yet-undefined effector proteins into cellular targets.[5]

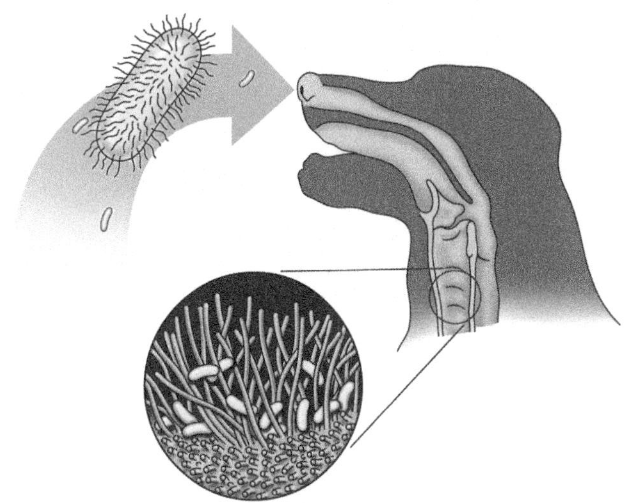

FIGURE 38-1 *Bordetella bronchiseptica* infection. *B. bronchiseptica* is inhaled, adheres to respiratory cilia by means of fimbrial adhesins, evades the immune system and secretes a variety of toxins that damage the respiratory epithelium.

The inflammation and altered cell function that occur as a result of *B. bronchiseptica* infection lead to increased fluid and mucus secretion, and impairment in host innate immune defenses predisposes to opportunistic viral and bacterial infections. Clinical signs vary in severity and may reflect factors such as the bacterial strain involved, host immunity, and the presence of co-infections. The incubation period ranges from 2 to 10 days. Rhinitis and tracheobronchitis may be associated with serous to mucopurulent nasal discharge, sneezing, stertor, and, especially in dogs, a persistent, often paroxysmal harsh cough. In some dogs, development of bronchopneumonia leads to fever, productive cough, lethargy, and decreased appetite.

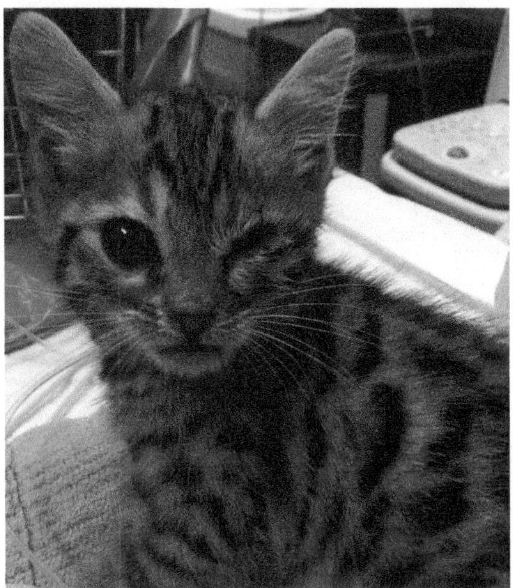

FIGURE 38-2 Kitten with *Bordetella bronchiseptica* conjunctivitis and bronchopneumonia. The kitten was tachypneic and had mucopurulent ocular discharge.

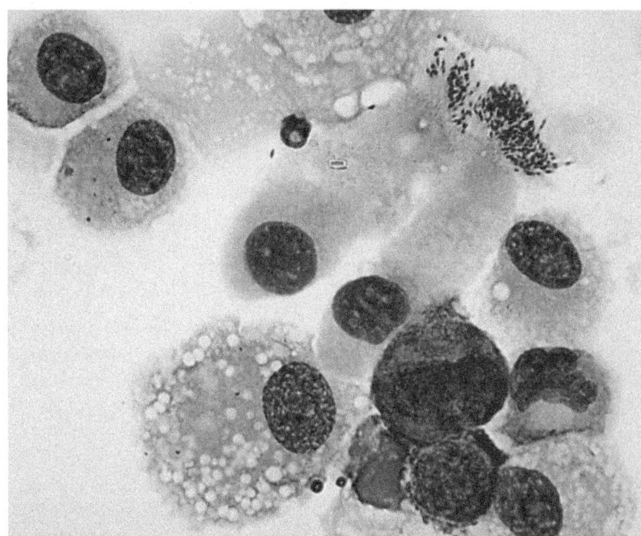

FIGURE 38-3 Bronchoalveolar lavage cytology from a dog infected with *Bordetella bronchiseptica*. Numerous coccobacilli are adhered to the cilia of columnar epithelial cells. Wright stain, 1000× oil magnification. (Courtesy of Michael Scott, Michigan State University. In Raskin RE, Meyer D, eds. Canine and Feline Cytology: A Color Atlas and Interpretative Guide, 2 ed, St. Louis, MO: Saunders; 2010.)

Bronchopneumonia may be due to *B. bronchiseptica* itself or it may result from co-infection with other respiratory pathogens, such as canine distemper virus (CDV). In cats, infection is significantly associated with sneezing, and cough is uncommon.[14] Cats with pneumonia may develop tachypnea, cyanosis, and death.

Shedding of *B. bronchiseptica* by both dogs and cats can continue intermittently for at least a month and sometimes several months after infection. Evasion of the immune system through survival inside phagocytes may explain the persistent infection that occurs. In contrast, *B. pertussis* is rapidly destroyed by macrophages.[25]

Physical Examination Findings

On physical examination, dogs with uncomplicated bordetellosis are bright, alert, and active with a paroxysmal cough that can occur throughout the examination. The cough is often easily elicited on tracheal or laryngeal palpation. Conjunctivitis and serous to mucopurulent ocular and nasal discharge may be present in affected dogs and cats (Figure 38-2). Dogs and cats with complicated *Bordetella* bronchopneumonia may be pyrexic, lethargic, and tachypneic with increased respiratory effort. There may also be increased lung sounds and/or referred upper airway noises on thoracic auscultation, and mucopurulent nasal discharge.

Diagnosis

Laboratory Abnormalities

There are no specific laboratory abnormalities in uncomplicated bordetellosis. Usually the CBC is normal. Dogs with bronchopneumonia can also have a normal CBC,[26] or a mild to moderate neutrophilia, bandemia, and toxic neutrophils may be present. Cytologic examination of transtracheal lavage (TTL) or bronchoalveolar lavage (BAL) specimens may reveal a suppurative or mixed exudate, and sometimes intracellular and extracellular coccobacilli are visible (Figure 38-3).

Diagnostic Imaging

Plain Radiography

Plain thoracic radiographs in dogs with uncomplicated bordetellosis may be unremarkable or show a mild diffuse interstitial or bronchointerstitial pattern. *Bordetella* bronchopneumonia may be characterized by development of peribronchial and alveolar infiltrates and lobar consolidation.

Microbiologic Tests

The main assays used for diagnosis of bordetellosis in dogs and cats are aerobic bacterial culture and PCR assays, which can be performed on nasal or oropharyngeal swabs, TTL or BAL specimens, or respiratory tract tissue collected at necropsy (Table 38-2). In some studies, *B. bronchiseptica* has been detected in nasal but not oropharyngeal swabs, but in other studies, the use of oropharyngeal swabs was more sensitive. Collection of swab specimens from the nasal cavity or posterior nasopharynx is preferred for diagnosis of pertussis in humans because these regions have ciliated epithelial cells, for which *B. pertussis* has affinity.[27] False-negative results occur when organism numbers in secretions are low, and depending on the sensitivity of the PCR assay used and the viability of the bacteria in the specimen, culture may be positive when PCR is negative and vice versa. Although the detection of *B. bronchiseptica* in TTL or BAL specimens is diagnostic for bordetellosis, it may be more difficult to interpret the significance of a positive culture or PCR assay result from nasal or oropharyngeal swabs, especially among group-housed dogs and cats when the background prevalence of infection is high. Co-infections with viral respiratory pathogens should always be considered when *B. bronchiseptica* is detected, as well as the presence of other comorbidities that suppress the innate or adaptive immune system that could predispose to bordetellosis (e.g., ciliary dyskinesia or brachycephalic obstructive syndrome in dogs, retroviral infections in cats).

Bacterial Culture

B. bronchiseptica can usually be isolated on routine aerobic bacterial culture media, such as MacConkey agar and blood agar.

TABLE 38-2

Diagnostic Assays Available for Bordetellosis in Dogs and Cats

Assay	Specimen Type	Target	Performance
Aerobic bacterial culture	Nasal and oropharyngeal swabs, transtracheal and bronchoalveolar lavage specimens, airway and lung specimens collected at necropsy	*B. bronchiseptica*	False negatives can occur when specimens contain no or low numbers of organisms, or after antimicrobial treatment. Allows subsequent susceptibility testing. The clinical significance of positive culture results from nasal and oropharyngeal swab specimens may be difficult to interpret.
PCR assays	See Aerobic bacterial culture	*B. bronchiseptica* DNA	Sensitivity and specificity can vary depending on assay design. False negatives can occur when specimens contain no or low numbers of organisms, or after antimicrobial treatment. Testing specimens from multiple different anatomic sites or combining PCR assays with other diagnostic tests can increase sensitivity. Avirulent live vaccine organisms may be detected for several weeks after intranasal vaccination. Because of subclinical shedding, the clinical significance of a positive result may be difficult to interpret.
Serology	Serum	Antibodies against *Bordetella* antigens	Interpretation complicated by previous vaccination and widespread exposure.

Charcoal-based medium that is supplemented with cephalexin is preferred for isolation of *B. pertussis*, which is more fastidious. For *B. bronchiseptica*, use of methicillin or oxacillin in selective media can prevent overgrowth by contaminating microflora.[5] The laboratory should be informed when bordetellosis is on the differential diagnosis list. In one study, *B. bronchiseptica* was isolated from cats using nasal swabs but not oropharyngeal swabs.[16] The use of Dacron, rayon, or calcium alginate swabs is preferred for culture of *B. pertussis*, because growth is inhibited when cotton swabs are used.[27] Unlike PCR assays, successful detection of *B. bronchiseptica* using culture allows susceptibility testing, which assists in rational antimicrobial drug selection.

Molecular Diagnosis Using the Polymerase Chain Reaction

Sensitive and specific real-time PCR assays that detect *B. bronchiseptica* DNA have been described,[13,28] and assays are available through several commercial veterinary diagnostic laboratories. Some laboratories offer panels that also detect other respiratory pathogens, which can be useful for detection of coinfections. As with culture, negative results can occur when organism numbers are low in the specimen, or when there has been recent antimicrobial drug use; however, PCR assays may be more likely to be positive than culture in these situations. Positive PCR assay results can occur for at least 3 weeks after intranasal vaccination.[29] A conventional PCR assay that differentiates between field strains and one vaccine strain of *B. bronchiseptica* has been described,[29] but commercially available real-time assays that distinguish between field and vaccine strains are needed.

Serologic Diagnosis

Antibodies to *B. bronchiseptica* can be detected using bacterial agglutination or recombinant or whole-cell ELISA assays, but serology is of limited use for diagnosis because of the high prevalence of antibodies in the dog and cat population and the influence of vaccination, which is routinely performed on entry to most shelters. Serology has primarily been used to study the epidemiology of infection and to examine immune responses as they relate to vaccination.

Pathologic Findings

Gross Pathologic Findings

Gross pathologic findings in dogs with uncomplicated bordetellosis are usually minimal. There may be an accumulation of mucopurulent exudate in the airways.

Histopathologic Findings

Microscopic findings in dogs or cats with bordetellosis consist of a suppurative inflammatory response that is usually confined to the ciliated portions of the respiratory tract. Cilia are mostly intact, but regional bronchial epithelial necrosis may be present. Mild lymphoid hyperplasia may be present. Depending on the stage and severity of infection, aggregates of bacteria may be observed in association with the cilia.[30]

Treatment and Prognosis

Antimicrobial Treatment

B. bronchiseptica isolates from dogs and cats have the propensity to exhibit multidrug resistance (i.e., resistance to three or more antimicrobial drug classes). Resistance to amoxicillin and trimethoprim-sulfamethoxazole is common. Many infections are mild or self-limiting, and so antimicrobial drug treatment should be reserved for animals with confirmed *B. bronchiseptica* infection that have persistent clinical signs (>7 to 10 days) or those with more severe clinical signs and radiographic abnormalities that suggest bronchopneumonia. Young kittens and puppies (<6 to 8 weeks of age) are candidates for early initiation of treatment because disease in neonates may progress rapidly to pneumonia and death. Treatment should be based whenever possible on the results of culture and susceptibility testing.

When susceptibility results are not available, or when they are pending and bordetellosis is strongly suspected, the initial drug of choice is doxycycline. At the time of writing, doxycycline resistance is uncommon among isolates from dogs and cats,[31-33] and doxycycline effectively penetrates lung tissue. Unfortunately, doxycycline is not the best choice for other secondary bacterial pneumonias because it is bacteriostatic and parenteral doxycycline can be expensive and difficult to administer. This reinforces the need for culture whenever feasible in animals with evidence of pneumonia. Bacterial shedding may continue despite resolution of clinical signs, so affected dogs and cats should remain in isolation from other animals whenever possible for at least 2 months after treatment.

Rarely, treatment with systemic antimicrobial drugs fails to resolve clinical signs of bordetellosis, and the organism persists despite documented susceptibility to the antimicrobial drug selected. In this situation, a short period of nebulized aminoglycosides could be considered. Because this can cause airway irritation, its use should probably be restricted for dogs with refractory bronchopneumonia, or severe and persistent tracheobronchitis (for example, >4 weeks in duration).

Supportive Care and Prognosis

The prognosis for dogs with uncomplicated bordetellosis is excellent. Cats and dogs with bronchopneumonia usually require other supportive treatments, such as IV fluid therapy, appropriate nutritional support, supplemental oxygen, and nebulization (see Chapters 17 and 23). In one study, bronchopneumonia associated with *B. bronchiseptica* infection was more severe than that associated with other bacterial agents, and affected dogs also had higher $PvCO_2$ values, were more likely to require supplemental oxygen, and had longer mean hospitalization times (7.2 days compared with 4.9 days).[26]

Immunity and Vaccination

Antibodies to outer surface molecules of *B. bronchiseptica*, especially IgA in mucosal secretions, are important for bacterial clearance. Several avirulent live, mucosal (intranasal or oral) *B. bronchiseptica* vaccines are available for dogs, some of which also contain canine parainfluenza virus with or without canine adenovirus 2. These vaccines are designed to stimulate mucosal immunity and provide protection within 3 days after a single dose of vaccine.[34] Protection with intranasal vaccines also occurs in the face of maternal antibody and can last at least 1 year.[35,36] Inactivated parenteral *B. bronchiseptica* vaccines are also available for dogs, but two doses administered 3 to 4 weeks apart are required to stimulate maximal immunity, which occurs 1 week after the second dose. The rapid onset of protection that follows the use of intranasal vaccines makes them the vaccine type of choice for puppies and animals introduced into heavily contaminated environments, such as shelters, when immunization in advance of entry is usually not possible. Mucosal vaccines should not be given to animals treated with antimicrobial drugs (because they inactivate bacteria in the vaccine), and administration of intranasal vaccines to aggressive animals without sedation may not be feasible. Transient signs of mild to moderate respiratory disease occur in a small percentage of vaccinated dogs and cats several days after mucosal vaccination. In shelters, it may not be possible to differentiate between postvaccinal disease and infectious respiratory disease due to field pathogens, which complicates decisions that relate to isolation practices. Inadvertent parenteral administration of intranasal vaccines has the potential to lead to injection site reactions, hepatic necrosis, and even death in some dogs.[37] Subcutaneous fluids should be administered at the site of vaccination, and immediate treatment with antimicrobial drugs is indicated. It has been suggested that gentamicin sulfate solution be instilled into the affected area (2 to 4 mg/kg gentamicin sulfate in 10 to 30 mL of saline), and dogs should then be treated with oral doxycycline for 5 to 7 days.[38] Special packaging has been developed by some vaccine manufacturers in an attempt to prevent inadvertent parenteral administration of the intranasal vaccine.

Concerns have been raised that intranasal *B. bronchiseptica* vaccines may cause respiratory disease in immunosuppressed humans who inhale the vaccine during administration or who contact vaccine organisms shed by recently immunized dogs.[39,40] However, as yet, there has been no molecular proof that the *B. bronchiseptica* strains isolated from affected human patients match vaccine strains. In fact, in one report of *B. bronchiseptica* pneumonia in an infant that was temporally related to intranasal vaccination of a pet dog, genetic analysis (ribotyping) showed that the vaccine was not the source of the infant's exposure.[41] The organism matched to another *B. bronchiseptica* strain that had previously been isolated from a human patient.

Intranasal *B. bronchiseptica* vaccination is followed by the development of low titers of serum IgG, whereas serum IgG responses are higher after parenteral vaccination (as might be expected). Parenteral whole-cell vaccines, and more recently acellular vaccines that include virulence factors such as pertactin, FIM, FHA, and pertussis toxin, are widely used to prevent pertussis in humans.[26] Fewer scientific data are available on the efficacy of parenteral *B. bronchiseptica* vaccines in dogs when compared with intranasal vaccines. One study showed that an intranasal vaccine was more effective than a parenteral antigen extract vaccine.[42] Additional challenge studies are required that directly compare the efficacy of intranasal and parenteral *B. bronchiseptica* vaccines for dogs.

In some countries, intranasal *B. bronchiseptica* vaccines are available for cats, which can reduce signs of disease after challenge as long as 1 year after vaccination.[43] Because disease is rarely severe in cats more than 6 weeks of age, vaccination of cats has not been recommended on a routine basis,[43] but could be considered as an adjunct to management strategies such as reduction of overcrowding and proper disinfection if outbreaks of bordetellosis are a problem in group-housed cats. Vaccination of immunocompromised cats is not recommended.[44]

Prevention

In the absence of management strategies to reduce stress, overcrowding, and comorbidities, vaccination is unlikely to completely prevent bordetellosis. The reader is referred to the sections on prevention in Chapters 17 (dogs) and 23 (cats) for more additional information on prevention and management of outbreaks of respiratory infections in group-housed animals.

Public Health Aspects

B. bronchiseptica is an uncommon cause of respiratory disease in humans, but has been isolated from humans without clinical signs and humans with mild to severe respiratory disease, including pneumonia.[45] Most, but not all, affected humans have underlying immunosuppressive conditions that predispose them to infection. *B. bronchiseptica* peritonitis has been reported in human patients receiving continuous peritoneal dialysis.[46,47] Bacteremia and meningitis have also been reported.[48] Recent exposure to cats and to dogs with signs of "kennel cough" has been noted in most human cases,[45,49] but airborne transmission between humans can occur in hospital settings.[50] At least in mouse models, human acellular pertussis vaccines appear to cross-protect against *B. bronchiseptica*.[51] Infections with *B. bronchiseptica* may be underrecognized in people, because the direct fluorescent antibody test used for diagnosis of pertussis may not distinguish between *B. pertussis* and *B. bronchiseptica*. Clinically, recognition of *B. bronchiseptica* infections in humans is important, because *B. bronchiseptica* is resistant to macrolides, which are first-line agents for pertussis.[41] Until more is understood about the risks of canine mucosal *B. bronchiseptica* vaccines for immunocompromised people, parenteral vaccination of at-risk dogs owned by seriously immunocompromised humans is probably warranted, and the owners of these dogs should be instructed to avoid or minimize situations in which their dogs could come into contact with large numbers of other dogs.

CASE EXAMPLE

Signalment: 7-week-old intact female Persian kitten from California

History: A research colony kitten was examined for a 3-day history of respiratory signs. Three days previously, sneezing was observed in this kitten and one of its littermates. A day later, the kitten developed lethargy, inappetence, and respiratory distress, and the littermate was found dead. The kitten had been treated with lactated Ringer's solution (6 mL SC q24h) and azithromycin suspension (0.7 mg/kg PO q24h) since it became unwell. Two other kittens in the litter remained unaffected, and one had mild nasal discharge. All of the cats had tested negative for FeLV antigen and FIV antibody using a commercially available in-house ELISA kit.

Physical Examination:

Body Weight: 0.37 kg

General: Alert, open-mouth breathing. T = 97.5°F (36.4°C), HR = 220 beats/min, RR = 40 breaths/min, mucous membranes pale pink.

Eyes, Ears, Nose, and Throat: No abnormalities were noted.

Musculoskeletal: Body condition score 4/9.

Respiratory: Markedly increased inspiratory and expiratory effort, tachypnea, and open-mouth breathing were noted. Increased lung sounds were detected on auscultation.

Cardiovascular, Gastrointestinal, and Genitourinary Systems and Lymph Nodes: No clinically significant abnormalities were detected.

Imaging Findings: Thoracic radiographs: There was collapse of the left cranial lung lobe and partial volume loss in the left caudal lung lobe with evidence of mediastinal shift to the left, possibly secondary to a bronchial mucus plug. A focal increase in opacity was noted in the area of the right middle lung lobe with hyperinflation of the right cranial and caudal lung lobes. There were regions of gas trapping, and the bronchi were enlarged. Emphysema was suspected, possibly congenital. Consolidation in the area of the right middle lung lobe was compatible with pneumonia.

Outcome: The kitten was treated with oxygen supplementation, terbutaline (0.01 mg/kg SC q6h), ticarcillin-clavulanate (50 mg/kg IV q8h), LRS with 5% dextrose (1 mL/hr IV), a single dose of dexamethasone (1 mg/kg IV), and a single dose of furosemide (2 mg/kg IV). Euthanasia was performed 24 hours later due to lack of improvement and the poor prognosis.

Necropsy Findings: An endotracheal wash was performed immediately after euthanasia. This revealed marked, septic, suppurative inflammation and mild to moderate epithelial hyperplasia. Bacteria were present in large numbers extracellularly, within degenerate neutrophils, and in large mats.

Gross necropsy findings consisted of diffuse lung lobe collapse with multiple firm dark red areas throughout the parenchyma. On histopathology, there was severe, multi-focal to coalescing, acute necrosuppurative bronchopneumonia with abundant clusters of gram-negative bacteria. Examination of the upper respiratory tract showed mild, multifocal neutrophilic rhinitis and mild, multifocal, lymphocytic tracheitis. The other kitten was also necropsied, with similar findings.

Microbiologic Testing (Endotracheal Wash Specimen): Culture for aerobic bacteria, *Mycoplasma* spp., and virus isolation revealed only moderate numbers of *Bordetella bronchiseptica*.

Diagnosis: *Bordetella bronchiseptica* bronchopneumonia.

Comments: This outbreak of severe bordetellosis in a research cat colony resulted in the death of several kittens, which deteriorated rapidly even in the face of supportive care. Co-infections were not detected, although PCR testing was not performed and the negative *Mycoplasma* culture and virus isolation results did not rule out the possibility of co-infection. Although susceptibility testing was not performed, resistance to the antimicrobials that were used can occur in *B. bronchiseptica*. Furthermore, the dose of azithromycin used as reported in the medical record was subtherapeutic.

SUGGESTED READINGS

Berkelman RL. Human illness associated with use of veterinary vaccines. Clin Infect Dis. 2003;37:407-414.

Mattoo S, Cherry JD. Molecular pathogenesis, epidemiology, and clinical manifestations of respiratory infections due to *Bordetella pertussis* and other *Bordetella* subspecies. Clin Microbiol Rev. 2005;18:326-382.

REFERENCES

1. Ferry NS. Further studies on the *Bacillus bronchicanis*, the cause of canine distemper. Am Vet Rev. 1912;16:77.
2. Bordet J, Gengou O. Le microbe de la coqueluche. Annales de L'Institut Pasteur. 1906;20:731-741.

3. Gross R, Keidel K, Schmitt K. Resemblance and divergence: the "new" members of the genus *Bordetella*. Med Microbiol Immunol. 2010;199:155-163.
4. Diavatopoulos DA, Cummings CA, Schouls LM, et al. *Bordetella pertussis*, the causative agent of whooping cough, evolved from a distinct, human-associated lineage of *B. bronchiseptica*. PLoS Pathog. 2005;1:e45.
5. Mattoo S, Cherry JD. Molecular pathogenesis, epidemiology, and clinical manifestations of respiratory infections due to *Bordetella pertussis* and other *Bordetella* subspecies. Clin Microbiol Rev. 2005;18:326-382.
6. Belcher KL, Wise DJ, Veit HP. Canine colonization and transmission of *Bordetella pertussis*. Ann N Y Acad Sci. 2000;916:687-690.
7. Binns SH, Speakman AJ, Dawson S, et al. The use of pulsed-field gel electrophoresis to examine the epidemiology of *Bordetella bronchiseptica* isolated from cats and other species. Epidemiol Infect. 1998;120:201-208.
8. Dawson S, Jones D, McCracken CM, et al. *Bordetella bronchiseptica* infection in cats following contact with infected dogs. Vet Rec. 2000;146:46-48.
9. Foley JE, Rand C, Bannasch MJ, et al. Molecular epidemiology of feline bordetellosis in two animal shelters in California. USA. Prev Vet Med. 2002;54:141-156.
10. Parkhill J, Sebaihia M, Preston A, et al. Comparative analysis of the genome sequences of *Bordetella pertussis, Bordetella parapertussis* and *Bordetella bronchiseptica*. Nat Genet. 2003;35:32-40.
11. Speakman AJ, Binns SH, Osborn AM, et al. Characterization of antibiotic resistance plasmids from *Bordetella bronchiseptica*. J Antimicrob Chemother. 1997;40:811-816.
12. Kirilenko NI. Survival of *Bordetella pertussis* in the air and on some objects. Zh Mikrobiol Epidemiol Immunobiol. 1965;42:39-42.
13. Helps CR, Lait P, Damhuis A, et al. Factors associated with upper respiratory tract disease caused by feline herpesvirus, feline calicivirus, *Chlamydophila felis* and *Bordetella bronchiseptica* in cats: experience from 218 European catteries. Vet Rec. 2005;156:669-673.
14. Binns SH, Dawson S, Speakman AJ, et al. Prevalence and risk factors for feline *Bordetella bronchiseptica* infection. Vet Rec. 1999;144:575-580.
15. Hoskins JD, Williams J, Roy AF, et al. Isolation and characterization of *Bordetella bronchiseptica* from cats in southern Louisiana. Vet Immunol Immunopathol. 1998;65:173-176.
16. Veir JK, Ruch-Gallie R, Spindel ME, et al. Prevalence of selected infectious organisms and comparison of two anatomic sampling sites in shelter cats with upper respiratory tract disease. J Feline Med Surg. 2008;10:551-557.
17. Burns RE, Wagner DC, Leutenegger CM, et al. Histologic and molecular correlation in shelter cats with acute upper respiratory infection. J Clin Microbiol. 2011;49:2454-2460.
18. Spindel ME, Veir JK, Radecki SV, et al. Evaluation of pradofloxacin for the treatment of feline rhinitis. J Feline Med Surg. 2008;10:472-479.
19. Di Martino B, Di Francesco CE, Meridiani I, et al. Etiological investigation of multiple respiratory infections in cats. New Microbiol. 2007;30:455-461.
20. Chalker VJ, Toomey C, Opperman S, et al. Respiratory disease in kennelled dogs: serological responses to *Bordetella bronchiseptica* lipopolysaccharide do not correlate with bacterial isolation or clinical respiratory symptoms. Clin Diagn Lab Immunol. 2003;10:352-356.
21. Sukumar N, Mishra M, Sloan GP, et al. Differential Bvg phase-dependent regulation and combinatorial role in pathogenesis of two *Bordetella* paralogs, BipA and BcfA. J Bacteriol. 2007;189:3695-3704.
22. Stefanelli P, Mastrantonio P, Hausman SZ, et al. Molecular characterization of two *Bordetella bronchiseptica* strains isolated from children with coughs. J Clin Microbiol. 1997;35:1550-1555.
23. Inatsuka CS, Xu Q, Vujkovic-Cvijin I, et al. Pertactin is required for *Bordetella* species to resist neutrophil-mediated clearance. Infect Immun. 2010;78:2901-2909.
24. Weyrich LS, Rolin OY, Muse SJ, et al. A type VI secretion system encoding locus is required for *Bordetella bronchiseptica* immunomodulation and persistence in vivo. PLoS One. 2012;7:e45892.
25. Schneider B, Gross R, Haas A. Phagosome acidification has opposite effects on intracellular survival of *Bordetella pertussis* and *B. bronchiseptica*. Infect Immun. 2000;68:7039-7048.
26. Radhakrishnan A, Drobatz KJ, Culp WT, et al. Community-acquired infectious pneumonia in puppies: 65 cases (1993-2002). J Am Vet Med Assoc. 2007;230:1493-1497.
27. Waters V, Halperin S. *Bordetella pertussis*. In: Mandell GL, Bennett JE, Dolin R, eds. Mandell, Douglas, and Bennett's Principles and Practice of Infectious Diseases. 7th ed. Philadelphia, PA: Elsevier; 2010:2955-2964.
28. Koidl C, Bozic M, Burmeister A, et al. Detection and differentiation of *Bordetella* spp. by real-time PCR. J Clin Microbiol. 2007;45:347-350.
29. Iemura R, Tsukatani R, Micallef MJ, et al. Simultaneous analysis of the nasal shedding kinetics of field and vaccine strains of *Bordetella bronchiseptica*. Vet Rec. 2009;165:747-751.
30. Bemis DA, Greisen HA, Appel MJ. Pathogenesis of canine bordetellosis. J Infect Dis. 1977;135:753-762.
31. Speakman AJ, Binns SH, Dawson S, et al. Antimicrobial susceptibility of *Bordetella bronchiseptica* isolates from cats and a comparison of the agar dilution and E-test methods. Vet Microbiol. 1997;54:63-72.
32. Speakman AJ, Dawson S, Corkill JE, et al. Antibiotic susceptibility of canine *Bordetella bronchiseptica* isolates. Vet Microbiol. 2000;71:193-200.
33. Johnson LR, Queen EV, Vernau W, et al. Microbiologic and cytologic assessment of bronchoalveolar lavage fluid from dogs with lower respiratory infection: 105 cases (2001-2011), 2012 (Submitted for publication).
34. Gore T, Headley M, Laris R, et al. Intranasal kennel cough vaccine protecting dogs from experimental *Bordetella bronchiseptica* challenge within 72 hours. Vet Rec. 2005;156:482-483.
35. Lehar C, Jayappa H, Erskine J, et al. Demonstration of 1-year duration of immunity for attenuated *Bordetella bronchiseptica* vaccines in dogs. Vet Ther. 2008;9:257-262.
36. Jacobs AA, Theelen RP, Jaspers R, et al. Protection of dogs for 13 months against *Bordetella bronchiseptica* and canine parainfluenza virus with a modified live vaccine. Vet Rec. 2005;157:19-23.
37. Toshach K, Jackson MW, Dubielzig RR. Hepatocellular necrosis associated with the subcutaneous injection of an intranasal *Bordetella bronchiseptica*-canine parainfluenza vaccine. J Am Anim Hosp Assoc. 1997;33:126-128.
38. Larson LJ, Newbury S, Schultz R. Canine and feline vaccinations and immunology. In: Miller L, Hurley K, eds. Infectious Disease Management in Animal Shelters. Ames, IA: Wiley-Blackwell; 2009:61-82.
39. Gisel JJ, Brumble LM, Johnson MM. *Bordetella bronchiseptica* pneumonia in a kidney-pancreas transplant patient after exposure to recently vaccinated dogs. Transpl Infect Dis. 2010;12:73-76.
40. Berkelman RL. Human illness associated with use of veterinary vaccines. Clin Infect Dis. 2003;37:407-414.
41. Rath BA, Register KB, Wall J, et al. Persistent *Bordetella bronchiseptica* pneumonia in an immunocompetent infant and genetic comparison of clinical isolates with kennel cough vaccine strains. Clin Infect Dis. 2008;46:905-908.
42. Davis R, Jayappa H, Abdelmagid OY, et al. Comparison of the mucosal immune response in dogs vaccinated with either an intranasal avirulent live culture or a subcutaneous antigen extract vaccine of *Bordetella bronchiseptica*. Vet Ther. 2007;8:32-40.
43. Williams J, Laris R, Gray AW, et al. Studies of the efficacy of a novel intranasal vaccine against feline bordetellosis. Vet Rec. 2002;150:439-442.

44. Egberink H, Addie D, Belak S, et al. *Bordetella bronchiseptica* infection in cats. ABCD guidelines on prevention and management. J Feline Med Surg. 2009;11:610-614.
45. Wernli D, Emonet S, Schrenzel J, et al. Evaluation of eight cases of confirmed *Bordetella bronchiseptica* infection and colonization over a 15-year period. Clin Microbiol Infect. 2011;17:201-203.
46. Hadley K, Torres AM, Moran J, et al. *Bordetella bronchiseptica* peritonitis—beware of the dog! Perit Dial Int. 2009;29:670-671.
47. Byrd LH, Anama L, Gutkin M, et al. *Bordetella bronchiseptica* peritonitis associated with continuous ambulatory peritoneal dialysis. J Clin Microbiol. 1981;14:232-233.
48. Woolfrey BF, Moody JA. Human infections associated with *Bordetella bronchiseptica*. Clin Microbiol Rev. 1991;4:243-255.
49. Goldberg JD, Kamboj M, Ford R, et al. "Kennel cough" in a patient following allogeneic hematopoietic stem cell transplant. Bone Marrow Transplant. 2009;44:381-382.
50. Huebner ES, Christman B, Dummer S, et al. Hospital-acquired *Bordetella bronchiseptica* infection following hematopoietic stem cell transplantation. J Clin Microbiol. 2006;44:2581-2583.
51. Goebel EM, Zhang X, Harvill ET. *Bordetella pertussis* infection or vaccination substantially protects mice against *B. bronchiseptica* infection. PLoS One. 2009;4:e6778.

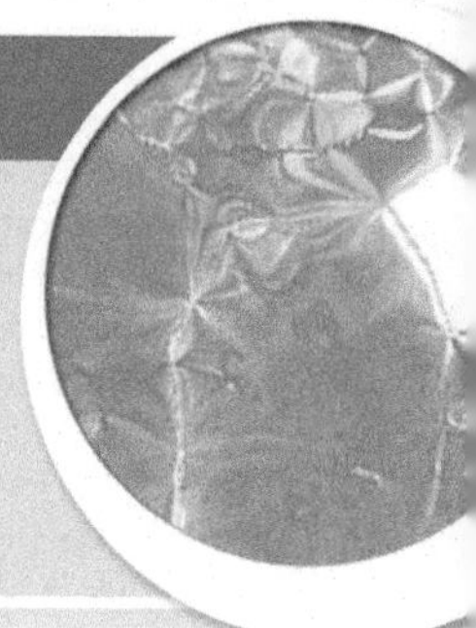

CHAPTER 39

Cell Wall–Deficient Bacterial Infections

Jane E. Sykes

Overview of Cell Wall–Deficient Bacterial Infections

First Described: 1935, London (Kleineberger)[1]

Causes: Cell wall–deficient strains of a variety of gram-positive and gram-negative bacteria

Geographic Distribution: Worldwide

Major Clinical Signs: Chronic draining or ulcerated soft tissue and skin lesions, polyarthritis, possibly other chronic pyogenic and pyogranulomatous lesions

Differential Diagnoses: Infections due to other fastidious bacteria such as *Mycoplasma, Nocardia, Mycobacterium, Bartonella, Brucella*, nutritionally variant streptococci such as *Granulicatella*, or, for animals with polyarthritis, *Borrelia burgdorferi*; fungal infections (e.g., due to *Sporothrix schenckii* or *Coccidioides immitis*); persistence of a foreign body; neoplasia; congenital immunodeficiency; primary immune-mediated disease

Human Health Significance: Likely similar to that for the corresponding walled (or "normal") variant of the bacterial species involved

Etiologic Agent and Epidemiology

Cell wall–deficient bacteria (CWDB), also known as *L-phase* or *L-form* bacteria, are bacterial variants that lack a cell wall, although they may in fact possess small amounts of peptidoglycan.[2] The name *L-form* was given to these bacteria because they were discovered at the Lister Institute in London. L-form bacteria are distinct from mycoplasmas, because *Mycoplasma* spp. do not originate from bacteria that normally possess a cell wall. A huge variety of gram-positive and gram-negative bacterial species may become CWDB when exposed to certain stressors in the laboratory (such as antimicrobial drugs) (Box 39-1). Some of these bacteria remain as CWDB (stable L-forms), whereas others revert back to possession of a cell wall (unstable L-forms). CWDB assume a spherical or pleomorphic shape, and are susceptible to osmotic lysis. However, they resist β-lactam drugs such as penicillin, and may be able to evade the innate immune response. Thus, it has been proposed that reversion to cell wall–deficient forms may be a mechanism of bacterial persistence. Although the formation of CWDB has been well documented in the laboratory, the role that CWDB play in disease remains controversial.[3]

Clinical Features

In human patients, CWDB have been implicated in culture-negative endocarditis, bacteremia, uveitis, pneumonia, osteomyelitis and arthritis, urinary tract infections, soft tissue infections, and meningitis.[3] In cats, CWDB have been implicated as a cause of subcutaneous abscesses and arthritis.[4,5] A cell wall–deficient *Nocardia* sp. was isolated from a dog with polyarthritis that was refractory to antibiotics,[6] and a *Pseudomonas aeruginosa* L-form was isolated from the blood of a dog after antibiotic treatment for *P. aeruginosa* endocarditis.[7]

Diagnosis

Physical examination and laboratory findings in cats and dogs infected with CWDB may be similar to those for other chronic, persistent bacterial infections. Infection with CWDB should be considered in cats and dogs with culture-negative pyogranulomatous or suppurative inflammatory lesions, or when a bacterial etiology is suspected on the basis of clinical signs but routine

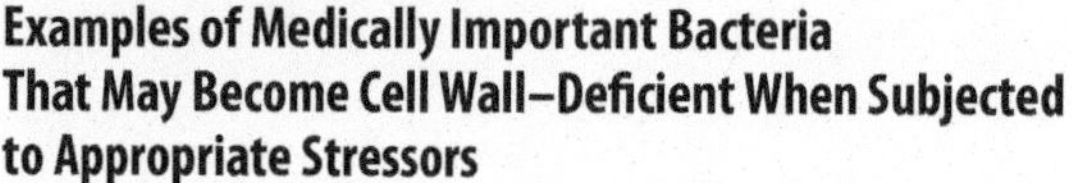

BOX 39-1

Examples of Medically Important Bacteria That May Become Cell Wall–Deficient When Subjected to Appropriate Stressors

Staphylococcus spp.
Streptococcus spp.
Enterococcus spp.
Escherichia coli
Serratia marcescens
Pasteurella multocida
Pseudomonas aeruginosa
Proteus mirabilis
Salmonella typhimurium
Lactobacillus spp.
Nocardia spp.
Actinomyces spp.
Bacillus spp.
Brucella spp.
Corynebacterium spp.
Borrelia burgdorferi
Leptospira interrogans

Adapted from Onwuamaegbu ME, Belcher RA, Soare C. Cell wall-deficient bacteria as a cause of infections: a review of the clinical significance. J Int Med Res 2005;33:1-20.

TABLE 39-1

Assays Available for Diagnosis of Cell Wall–Deficient Bacterial Infections in Dogs and Cats

Assay	Specimen Type	Target	Performance
Culture	Biopsies, body fluids, wash specimens	Cell wall–deficient bacteria (CWDB)	Requires special L-form bacterial (hyperosmolar) media
Cytology or histopathology	Biopsies, smears of affected tissues	CWDB	Organisms usually not visible owing to the lack of a cell wall, but may be gram-variable. Low sensitivity and cannot be used to identify absence of a cell wall (although the presence of organisms that stain strongly with Gram stain indicates the presence of walled bacteria).
Electron microscopy	Biopsies	CWDB	Confirms the presence of CWDB in lesions. May not distinguish CWDB from *Mycoplasma* spp. Often expensive and not readily available for routine diagnostic purposes.
Broad-range bacterial PCR assay and sequencing	Biopsies, body fluids, wash specimens	16S ribosomal subunit DNA of CWDB	Confirms presence of bacteria in lesions when culture is negative. False positives may occur if contaminating bacteria are present. Does not distinguish between CWDB and their walled counterparts. Sensitivity and specificity may vary between assays.

cultures are negative. Definitive diagnosis is difficult because the organisms are not always readily visualized using light microscopy, and passage through special hypertonic laboratory media is required for growth of CWDB in culture (Table 39-1). Electron microscopy has been used to identify the organisms in lesions. The use of broad-range bacterial PCR assays that detect bacterial 16S ribosomal subunit DNA in tissues may be useful to detect L-form bacteria in tissues in the future when routine culture methods are negative, although this method does not distinguish between CWDB and their walled counterparts. Infection with CWDB could also be suspected when lesions resolve after treatment with tetracyclines.

Treatment and Prognosis

CWDB are generally susceptible to tetracyclines such as doxycycline. Other antimicrobial drugs that act through cell wall–independent mechanisms, such as fluoroquinolones, chloramphenicol, and macrolides, may also be active against some L-form bacteria.

Public Health Aspects

The role that CWDB play in zoonotic disease is unclear, but it is reasonable to believe it is similar to that of the corresponding walled (or normal) variant of the bacterial species implicated. A single report described isolation of an L-form of *Streptococcus sanguinis* from a vascular graft of a hemodialysis patient.[8] The affected person's pet dog was reported to often lick the graft site, and *S. sanguinis* was also isolated from the dog's oral cavity. Although this was suggestive of zoonotic transmission, the identity of the isolates was not confirmed with molecular methods.

SUGGESTED READINGS

Carro T, Pedersen NC, Beaman BL, et al. Subcutaneous abscesses and arthritis caused by a probable bacterial L-form in cats. J Am Vet Med Assoc. 1989;194:1583-1588.

Chmel H. Graft infection and bacteremia with a tolerant L-form of *Streptococcus sanguis* in a patient receiving hemodialysis. J Clin Microbiol. 1986;24:294-295.

REFERENCES

1. Kleineberger E. The natural occurrence of pleuropneumonia-like organisms in apparent symbiosis with *Streptobacillus moniliformis* and other bacteria. J Pathol Bacteriol. 1935;40:93-105.
2. Joseleau-Petit D, Liebart JC, Ayala JA, et al. Unstable *Escherichia coli* L forms revisited: growth requires peptidoglycan synthesis. J Bacteriol. 2007;189:6512-6520.
3. Onwuamaegbu ME, Belcher RA, Soare C. Cell wall–deficient bacteria as a cause of infections: a review of the clinical significance. J Int Med Res. 2005;33:1-20.
4. Carro T, Pedersen NC, Beaman BL, et al. Subcutaneous abscesses and arthritis caused by a probable bacterial L-form in cats. J Am Vet Med Assoc. 1989;194:1583-1588.
5. Keane DP. Chronic abscesses in cats associated with an organism resembling *Mycoplasma*. Can Vet J. 1983;24:289-291.
6. Buchanan AM, Beaman BL, Pedersen NC, et al. *Nocardia asteroides* recovery from a dog with steroid- and antibiotic-unresponsive idiopathic polyarthritis. J Clin Microbiol. 1983;18:702-708.
7. Bone WJ. L-form of *Pseudomonas aeruginosa* the etiologic agent of bacterial endocarditis in a dog. Vet Med Small Anim Clin. 1970;65:224-227.
8. Chmel H. Graft infection and bacteremia with a tolerant L-form of *Streptococcus sanguis* in a patient receiving hemodialysis. J Clin Microbiol. 1986;24:294-295.

CHAPTER 40

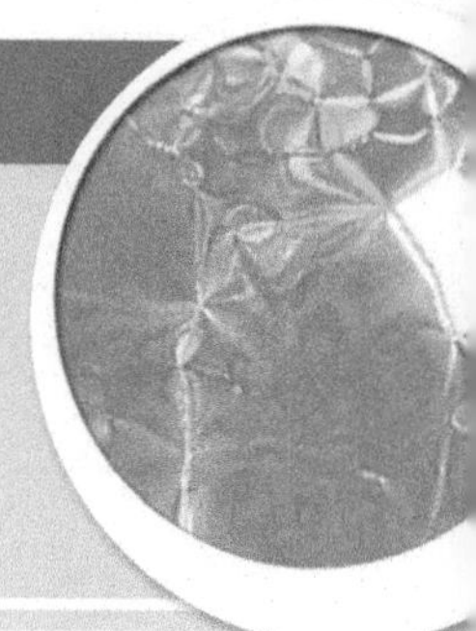

Mycoplasma Infections

Jane E. Sykes

Overview of Mycoplasma and Ureaplasma Infections

First Described: Dogs, Japan 1934 (Shoetensack).[1] Reports of human *Mycoplasma* infections also occurred around this time.[2]

Causes: *Mycoplasma cynos* and *Mycoplasma felis* have been most commonly associated with disease, but many other *Mycoplasma* species infect dogs and cats

Geographic Distribution: Worldwide

Mode of Transmission: Direct contact, fomite transmission in overcrowded environments. Opportunistic invasion of commensal mycoplasmas also occurs.

Major Clinical Signs: Conjunctivitis, sneezing and nasal discharge (cats); cough, tachypnea, fever, weight loss (lower respiratory disease); swollen, painful joints (polyarthritis); subcutaneous abscesses; neurologic signs (meningoencephalitis); prostatitis, epididymitis-orchitis, or lower urinary tract signs (dogs)

Differential Diagnoses: Primarily gram-positive and gram-negative bacterial infections. Differential diagnoses for suspected mycoplasma respiratory disease include viral infections, fungal and parasitic causes of pneumonia, aspiration pneumonia, and neoplasia.

Human Health Significance: Canine and feline mycoplasma species have rarely been detected in immunocompromised humans with mycoplasmosis who have had contact with pet cats and dogs.

Etiology and Epidemiology

Mycoplasmas are fastidious bacteria that lack a cell wall. They belong to the class Mollicutes (which translates to "soft skin"), and are the smallest known free-living organisms. Many require sterols for growth, and *Ureaplasma* species require urea for fermentation. Mycoplasmas measure only 0.3 to 0.8 μm in size. More than 120 different species of *Mycoplasma* and 7 species of *Ureaplasma* have been identified. The spectrum of mycoplasma species that infect or colonize dogs and cats is incompletely understood because precise species identification has been difficult (Box 40-1).[3-7] Additional mycoplasma species are likely to be discovered with the application of molecular methods in the future. Some *Mycoplasma* spp. infect multiple host species. Mycoplasmas are often difficult to grow on cell-free media, and some, such as the hemotropic mycoplasmas, have never been successfully cultured in the laboratory (see Chapter 41). The remainder of this chapter refers only to nonhemotropic mycoplasma species.

BOX 40-1

Nonhemotropic *Mycoplasma* and *Ureaplasma* Species Found in Dogs and Cats[3-7]

Dogs	Cats
M. cynos	*M. felis*
M. canis	*M. gateae*
M. molare	*M. arginini*
M. arginini	*M. feliminutum*
M. bovigenitalium	*M. canadense**
M. edwardii	*M. cynos**
M. feliminutum	*M. lipophilum**
M. felis	*M. hyopharyngis**
M. gateae	*U. felinum*
M. maculosum	*U. cati*
M. opalescens	*Acholeplasma laidlawii*
M. spumans	
M. sp. HRC689	
M. sp. VJC358	
U. canigenitalium	
Acholeplasma laidlawii	

*Identified on the basis of DNA sequencing of small segments of the 16S rRNA gene; sequence analysis of longer fragments may reveal these are in fact other mycoplasma species.

Mycoplasmas are commensal bacteria found widely in association with mucous membranes of all mammalian species. Simultaneous colonization with more than one *Mycoplasma* species is common. Mycoplasmas have also been associated with keratoconjunctivitis and/or upper respiratory tract disease (URTD) in cats; reproductive disease and urinary tract infections (UTIs) in dogs; and lower respiratory tract disease, skin and soft tissue infections, meningoencephalitis, and arthritis in both cats and dogs (Box 40-2).[8-18] Because mycoplasmas are commonly isolated from the upper respiratory and genital tracts of healthy dogs and cats, their role in ocular, upper respiratory tract, and urogenital tract disease has been difficult to determine. Several studies have now identified an increased prevalence of mycoplasmas in cats with conjunctivitis or URTD when compared with healthy cats.[13,19,20] Mycoplasmas can act as secondary invaders when other pathogenic viruses and bacteria are present, or when normal host defenses are impaired by factors such as underlying neoplasia or immunosuppressive drug

BOX 40-2

Diseases That May Be Associated with Mycoplasma Infections in Dogs and Cats

Cats
Conjunctivitis
Upper respiratory tract disease
Pyothorax

Dogs
Urinary tract infections
Prostatitis
Epididymitis and orchitis

Both Cats and Dogs
Bronchopneumonia
Skin and soft tissue infections (abscesses)
Meningoencephalitis
Polyarthritis

therapy. When mycoplasmas are associated with systemic disease or pneumonia, young animals (less than 1 year of age) are often involved. Some mycoplasma species appear to be more pathogenic than others. For example, evidence has accumulated that *Mycoplasma cynos* is associated with lower respiratory disease in dogs.[21,22] In one study, *M. cynos* infection was associated with increased severity of canine infectious respiratory disease, younger age, and longer time spent in a kennel.[22] Experimental infection with *M. cynos* leads to respiratory disease in dogs, but infection with *Mycoplasma gateae, Mycoplasma canis,* and *Mycoplasma spumans* does not.[23] The role of mycoplasmas in feline lower urinary tract disease and lymphoplasmacytic pododermatitis has been investigated using molecular techniques, but no association was found.[24,25]

Clinical Features

Signs and Their Pathogenesis

In order to colonize mammalian hosts, mycoplasmas must adhere to host cells. Mycoplasma species that infect humans are known to possess specific adhesins, but these have not been well characterized in mycoplasmas from dogs and cats. Invasion of deeper tissues and disease occurs as a result of immunosuppression or disruption of normal host barriers. Some mycoplasmas, such as the human pathogen *Mycoplasma pneumoniae,* produce toxins, but whether similar virulence factors are present in mycoplasmas isolated from dogs and cats is unknown. A number of pathogenic mycoplasma species of humans can invade cells, which may contribute to organism persistence and difficulties associated with isolation in the laboratory. Transmission of pathogenic mycoplasmas such as *M. cynos* may occur in overcrowded environments as a result of close contact or fomite spread. The finding of identical strains in multiple dogs from a kennel environment (using molecular typing methods) supports the concept of transmission between dogs in this environment.[26] The extent to which mycoplasmas survive in the environment varies among mycoplasma species and has not been determined for mycoplasmas that infect dogs and cats.

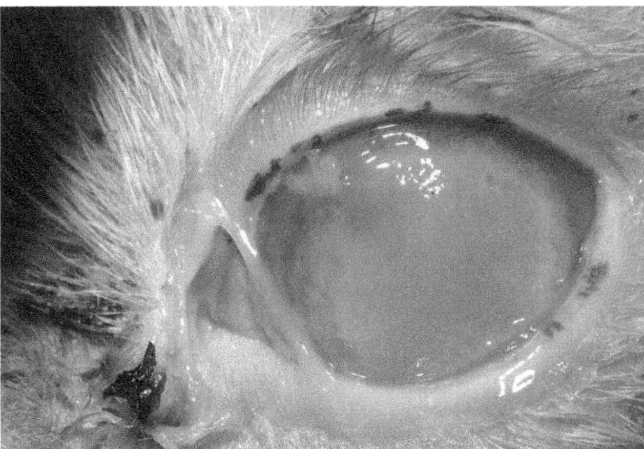

FIGURE 40-1 Ulcerative keratitis in a 4-year-old female spayed Persian. Involvement of feline herpesvirus-1 was suspected, and *Mycoplasma* spp. was isolated from a corneal swab. The significance of the *Mycoplasma* infection was unclear, but the ulcer healed after topical treatment with topical ofloxacin and azithromycin drops. (Courtesy of the University of California, Davis, Veterinary Ophthalmology Service.)

Conjunctivitis and Upper Respiratory Tract Disease

Mycoplasma spp. are commonly detected in cats in association with conjunctivitis and URTD. Concurrent infections with other upper respiratory pathogens (such as *Bordetella bronchiseptica*, *Chlamydia felis*, and feline respiratory viruses) may contribute to clinical signs. Stressors such as overcrowding and unhygienic conditions may promote proliferation of mycoplasmas and their transmission between cats. Ulcerative keratitis has been reported in association with *Mycoplasma* infection, but the presence of corneal involvement may reflect the concurrent presence of feline herpesvirus 1 (FHV-1) or other factors that predispose to secondary invasion by *Mycoplasma* spp. (Figure 40-1).

Pneumonia and Pyothorax

Virtually all dogs and cats harbor mycoplasmas in their upper respiratory tracts. Fewer than 25% of healthy dogs harbor mycoplasmas in their trachea or lungs. In one study mycoplasmas were detected in tracheobronchial lavage specimens from 21% of 28 cats with pulmonary disease, but not from 18 healthy cats.[27,28] Mycoplasmas can be isolated from the lower airways and lungs of dogs and cats with pneumonia, sometimes in pure culture.[29] Factors that predispose to the development of mycoplasma pneumonia are not always apparent.[30] Clinical signs include variable fever, cough, tachypnea, lethargy, and decreased appetite. Concurrent signs of URTD have been reported in some affected cats.[30] Rarely, mycoplasmas can be cultured from the pleural fluid of cats and dogs with pyothorax, in pure culture or in mixed infections with other organisms.[31-33]

Urogenital Tract

Mycoplasma and *Ureaplasma* spp. have been found in the semen and urine of dogs with infertility and purulent epididymitis.[34] The role of mycoplasmas in reproductive tract disease in dogs and cats is unclear because they are commonly isolated from the urogenital tract of healthy dogs and cats. Large numbers of mycoplasmas (>10^5 CFU/mL) can occasionally be isolated in pure culture from urine collected by cystocentesis from dogs with prostatitis and lower urinary tract signs.[14,34] Dogs with mycoplasma UTIs often have other comorbidities that impair normal urinary defenses, such as urinary tract neoplasia, calculi, or neurologic disease.[14]

Arthritis and Bacteremia

Isolated case reports exist of polyarthritis due to infection with *M. spumans* or *Mycoplasma edwardii* (dogs) and *M. gateae* or *M. felis* (cats). Synovial fluid analysis usually reveals the presence of large numbers of neutrophils. This may lead to diagnostic confusion with primary immune-mediated polyarthritis. Systemic signs such as lethargy, fever, and inappetence usually accompany lameness. Evidence of immune compromise, such as underlying neoplasia or surgery, young age, or a history of glucocorticoid treatment, has generally been present in dogs and cats with mycoplasma polyarthritis. *M. felis* has also been isolated from cats with monoarthritis, possibly secondary to bite wound infections.[17]

Meningoencephalitis

Mycoplasmas may gain access to the central nervous system after penetrating wounds, ascending infection from the middle ear, or hematogenous spread. Meningoencephalitis associated with *M. felis* infection was described in a 10-month-old cat that showed signs of lethargy, fever, a head tilt, nystagmus, and tetraparesis.[12] *M. felis* was isolated in pure culture from the CSF. The cat also had evidence of otitis media-interna at necropsy, but the role this played in development of the mycoplasma infection was unclear. *M. edwardii* was isolated from the brain of a 6-week-old dog with a sudden onset of seizures.[8] Suppurative and histiocytic meningitis was detected at necropsy, in conjunction with evidence of a possible penetrating wound to the skull. Recently, infection with *Mycoplasma canis* has been associated with some cases of granulomatous meningoencephalomyelitis and necrotizing meningoencephalitis in dogs,[35] which requires further study.

Physical Examination Findings

Physical examination findings in dogs and cats with mycoplasma infections depend on the organ affected, as well as underlying disease processes that facilitate opportunistic invasion by mycoplasmas. Ocular infections in cats are characterized by serous to mucopurulent ocular discharge, conjunctival hyperemia, and possibly keratitis. Upper respiratory tract infections may result in nasal discharge and sneezing, with or without conjunctivitis. Fever, tachypnea, and increased lung sounds may be present with pneumonia. Urinary tract infections may lead to clinical signs of lower urinary tract disease, such as hematuria or stranguria. *Mycoplasma* arthritis may be manifested by fever, joint pain and swelling, and sometimes local lymphadenopathy.[9-11]

Diagnosis

Laboratory Abnormalities

Complete Blood Count, Serum Biochemical Tests, and Urinalysis

Findings on the CBC, serum biochemistry panel, and urinalysis in dogs or cats with *Mycoplasma* infections are nonspecific and influenced by underlying immunocompromising disease processes. Dogs and cats with pneumonia, mycoplasma bacteremia, and polyarthritis may have a neutrophilia with a left shift and neutrophil toxicity, a degenerative left shift, mild nonregenerative anemia, hypoalbuminemia, and evidence of organ dysfunction such as increased liver enzyme activities and azotemia.[9,10,15]

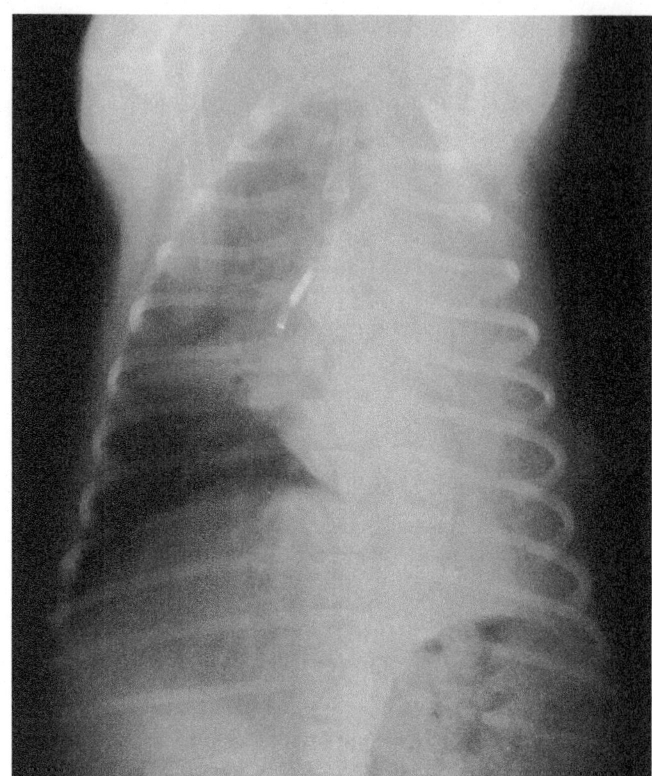

FIGURE 40-2 Ventrodorsal thoracic radiograph from a 3-month-old intact female pug with *Mycoplasma cynos* pneumonia. There is consolidation of the lung lobes associated with the left hemithorax and the right middle lung lobe. A diffuse interstitial pattern is present in the remainder of the right lung fields.

Diagnostic Imaging

Plain Radiography

Mycoplasma pneumonia may be characterized by interstitial to alveolar patterns or lung lobe consolidation (Figure 40-2); sometimes, mild pleural effusion is present. Radiographs of the joints of dogs and cats with mycoplasma polyarthritis may reveal periarticular soft tissue swelling. Erosive changes to the subchondral bone have also been described.[9]

Microbiologic Tests

Assays available for diagnosis of mycoplasma infections in dogs and cats are shown in Table 40-1.

Cytologic Examination

Mycoplasma spp. are often not visible by light microscopy because of their small size. They do not stain with Gram stain because they lack a cell wall. Cytologic examination of affected body fluids (such as bronchoalveolar lavage fluid, synovial fluid, and CSF) usually reveals a predominance of neutrophils with fewer histiocytes and lymphocytes.[9,10,12,29,30]

Isolation and Identification

Specimens suitable for mycoplasma culture include synovial fluid, blood, CSF, urine collected by cystocentesis, pleural fluid, semen, and tracheobronchial or bronchoalveolar lavage specimens. Swabs of the nasal cavity, conjunctiva, cornea, urethra, vagina, or cervix can also be submitted, but interpretation of results from these sites is difficult. If swabs are used, the swab should be rubbed vigorously on the mucosa, because mycoplasmas are cell associated. Rapid transport to the laboratory is

TABLE 40-1

Assays Available for Diagnosis of Mycoplasma Infections in Dogs and Cats

Assay	Specimen Type	Target	Performance
Culture	Swabs, body fluids, lavage specimens, tissue obtained at necropsy	Cultivable mycoplasma species	Some organisms grow on blood agar, but others require special mycoplasma media. The presence of uncultivable mycoplasmas may lead to false-negative results. Turnaround time may be slow (several days to weeks); species differentiation and antimicrobial drug susceptibility testing is often not performed. The significance of positive results from the upper respiratory and genital tract may be unclear.
PCR assays	Swabs, body fluids, lavage specimens, tissue obtained at necropsy	*Mycoplasma* DNA	Allows rapid detection of mycoplasmas. More sensitive than culture for detection of fastidious or uncultivable mycoplasmas, although sensitivity and specificity may vary between assays. Some assays are designed to only detect certain pathogenic *Mycoplasma* species, such as *Mycoplasma cynos*. Sequencing of the PCR product may permit species identification. The clinical significance of positive results may be unclear.

important, because mycoplasmas are susceptible to deterioration in the environment. The use of special transport media (e.g., Stuart's medium or Amies medium without charcoal) for swab or tissue specimens may increase yield of fastidious mycoplasma species if a delay of several hours is likely between collection of specimens and transport to the laboratory. Specimens should be refrigerated if delayed transport is unavoidable. If the delay is likely to be longer than 24 hours, specimens in transport media should ideally be frozen at −80°C. Some mycoplasma species will still grow in the laboratory if specimens are kept refrigerated for 2 to 3 days.

Some mycoplasmas grow on blood agar under routine aerobic or anaerobic conditions. Others require special mycoplasma media, and some fail to grow under any laboratory conditions. The rate of growth in culture varies from one *Mycoplasma* species to another; for some mycoplasmas, colonies are visible in 2 or 3 days, whereas others require several weeks of incubation before colonies appear. Examination of plates under the light microscope may be required for detection of *Mycoplasma* colonies, because the colonies range in size from 15 to 300 μm in diameter. The colonies of many mycoplasma species have a characteristic "fried egg" appearance (Figure 40-3). Biochemical properties can then be used to subgroup mycoplasmas, but species identification has traditionally required the use of species-specific antisera. Because cross-reactions can occur between species even when antisera are used, molecular typing methods (such as 16S rRNA gene or 16S/23S rRNA intergenic spacer region PCR assays and sequence analysis of the respective PCR products) are now the method of choice for species identification.[3] Most veterinary diagnostic laboratories currently report only growth of a *Mycoplasma* species and do not identify organisms to the species level unless specifically requested. It is difficult to interpret the significance of a positive mycoplasma culture from mucosal sites that can normally be colonized by mycoplasmas, including the lower respiratory tracts of dogs, so results must be interpreted in light of the clinical findings and the results of other diagnostic tests.

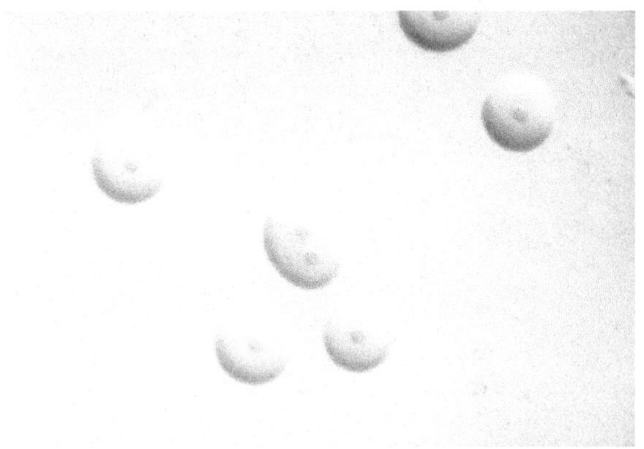

FIGURE 40-3 Colonies of *Mycoplasma bovirhinis* showing the "fried egg" appearance that is typical of the growth of some *Mycoplasma* spp. in culture. (From The genera *Mycoplasma* and *Ureaplasma*. In Songer JG Post KW, eds. Veterinary Microbiology Bacterial and Fungal Agents of Animal Disease, 2 ed, St. Louis, MO: Saunders; 2005.)

Antimicrobial susceptibility testing for mycoplasmas is labor intensive and not routinely performed, and established breakpoints are not available. When performed, the most widely used method is microbroth dilution (see Chapter 3).[36]

Molecular Diagnosis Using the Polymerase Chain Reaction

Some veterinary diagnostic laboratories offer PCR assays that directly detect mycoplasma DNA in clinical specimens, without the need for culture. Several conventional and real-time PCR assays have been used to detect mycoplasmas of dogs and cats.[37-40] These assays may be specific for certain mycoplasma species (such as *M. cynos* or *M. felis*) or they may be genus-specific assays that detect a variety of mycoplasma species. PCR assays may be more sensitive than culture for detection of fastidious mycoplasma species. Sequencing of the PCR product generated from genus-specific PCR assays may be used to identify the infecting species present, provided the PCR amplicon is sufficiently long. As with culture, the significance of a

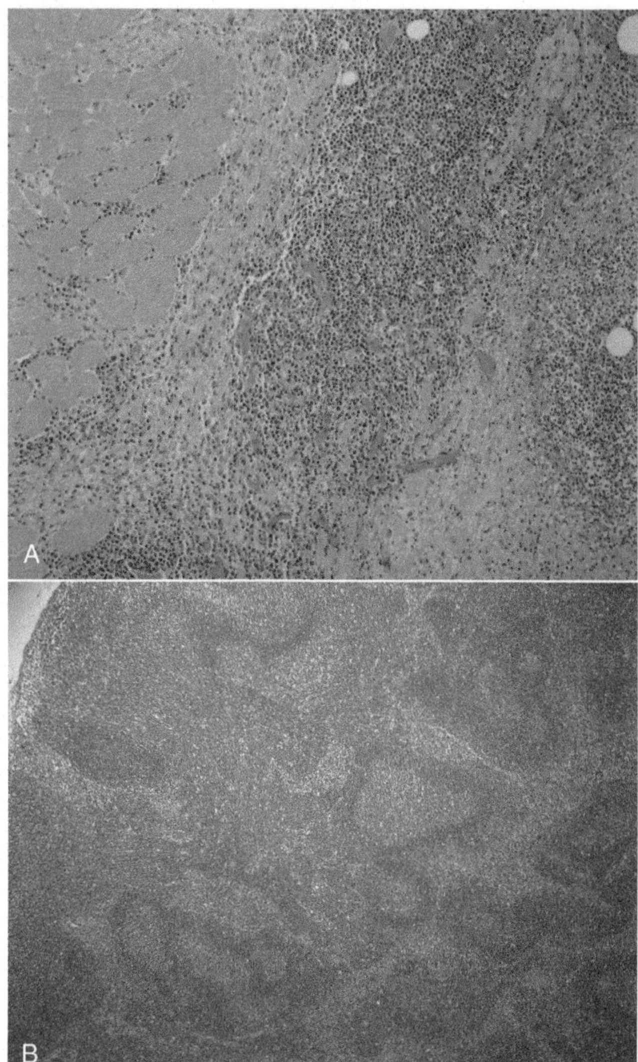

FIGURE 40-4 Histopathology of the inguinal subcutaneous tissues **(A)** and sublumbar lymph node **(B)** from a 6-month-old, retrovirus–negative, male neutered domestic shorthair with severe suppurative cellulitis, steatitis, dermatitis, and myositis of the scrotal skin and subcutaneous tissue. A pure culture of a *Mycoplasma* species was obtained from the lesion. The cat had been neutered 13 days previously and was evaluated for a 2-day history of lethargy and reluctance to move. Physical examination revealed fever (104.6°F [40.3°C]), conjunctivitis, generalized peripheral lymphadenomegaly, and firm mass lesions in the inguinal area. In addition to suppurative cellulitis and myositis, marked systemic lymph-node hyperplasia was present. Hyperplasia was most profound in the sublumbar lymph nodes, which were 4 cm in diameter.

positive PCR test result for *Mycoplasma* spp. may be unclear given the role the frequent colonization of healthy animals with mycoplasmas, so results must be interpreted with the underlying disease process and the results of other diagnostic tests.

Pathologic Findings

Gross pathology in dogs and cats with mycoplasmal diseases usually reveals purulent material in affected tissues. Histopathology shows predominantly neutrophilic inflammation, although histiocytes may also be present. Reactive lymphadenopathy may also be evident as a result of immune stimulation (Figure 40-4).

TABLE 40-2

Suggested Antimicrobial Drug Treatment for Mycoplasma Infections in Dogs and Cats

Drug	Dose (mg/kg)	Route	Interval (hours)
Doxycycline	5 to 10	PO or IV	12 to 24
Enrofloxacin*	5	PO or IV	24
Marbofloxacin	2.75 to 5.5	PO	24
Pradofloxacin†	5 to 10 (cats) 3 mg/kg (dogs)	PO	24

*For cats, use enrofloxacin only when other alternatives are not possible because of risk for irreversible blindness.

†Use of pradofloxacin is extra-label in dogs in the United States (see Chapter 8). The dose for cats is for the oral suspension. The dose for the tablet formulation is 3 mg/kg.

Treatment and Prognosis

Treatment of mycoplasma infections involves specific antimicrobial therapy (Table 40-2) as well as management of other underlying disorders that predisposed to invasion by mycoplasmas. Tetracyclines or fluoroquinolones are active against most mycoplasma isolates. The optimal duration is unknown, but treatment for at least 2 weeks is reasonable. In a prospective study of shelter cats with URTD and *M. felis* infection, a 14-day course of doxycycline was more effective in causing reduction in *M. felis* load as determined with real-time PCR than a 7-day course, but there was no overall significant difference in the reduction in clinical signs between the two groups.[41] Nevertheless, 25% of the cats treated for 14 days were still infected after that time. In another study of cats with conjunctivitis, three weeks of treatment with pradofloxacin or doxycycline was required to eliminate *Mycoplasma* DNA.[40] β-Lactam drugs are not active against mycoplasmas, because they lack any peptidoglycan. Mycoplasmas are also intrinsically resistant to trimethoprim-sulfonamide combinations and rifampin. Some species are resistant to macrolides.

Immunity and Vaccination

Mycoplasma spp. persist in tissues in the face of the immune response. Mechanisms to evade the host immune response such as antigenic variation of outer surface proteins have been identified in several mycoplasma species. Innate, humoral (especially IgA), and cell-mediated immune responses may be required to clear mycoplasma infections, with humoral mechanisms of critical importance. Vaccines to limit disease caused by pathogenic mycoplasma species such as *M. cynos* are currently not available, although mycoplasma vaccines have been used with success in food production animal species.

Prevention

Prevention of mycoplasma infections involves management or reversal of disorders that predispose to opportunistic invasion by mycoplasmas. Reduction of overcrowding and concurrent infections in shelter environments may also reduce the incidence and severity of mycoplasma infections (see Chapter 11).

Routine disinfectants are sufficient to inactivate mycoplasmas that persist in the environment.

Public Health Aspects

The vast majority of mycoplasma species associated with disease in humans are different from those found in dogs and cats. However, pharyngeal colonization with *M. canis* was reported in a family and their pet dog.[42] *Mycoplasma felis* was isolated from the joints of a woman with common variable immunodeficiency who developed septic arthritis.[43] The woman had worked in an animal shelter, lived with a cat, and had been bitten on the hand by a healthy cat 6 months before she was evaluated. A mycoplasma was also isolated from a cat scratch wound on the hand of a veterinarian.[44] Although *Staphylococcus aureus* was initially isolated from the wound, it failed to resolve completely after treatment with erythromycin. Subsequently, tenosynovitis developed, and a mycoplasma was isolated. The identity of the mycoplasma could not be determined using biochemical and serologic methods, and whether a cat was truly the source of this infection was not proven.

CASE EXAMPLE

Signalment: "Delilah", a 3-month old intact female pug dog from Reno, NV

History: Delilah was brought to the University of California, Davis, Veterinary Medical Teaching Hospital for evaluation of pneumonia. She had been purchased from a pet store 3 weeks before the date of evaluation. The owner noticed nasal and ocular discharge when the dog was brought home from the store, as well as a dry, nonproductive cough. Delilah was taken to a local veterinary clinic where a diagnosis of "kennel cough" was made. She was then treated with clavulanic acid–amoxicillin (15 mg/kg PO q12h) for 2 weeks. However, the cough persisted, and Delilah's respiratory effort increased. She was hospitalized at the local veterinary clinic and treated with ticarcillin-clavulanate (50 mg/kg IV q8h), supplemental oxygen, nebulization, and coupage. Radiographs showed infiltrates in the left lung lobes and right middle lung lobe that worsened over the course of hospitalization, so she was referred for further evaluation and treatment. There had been no decrease in appetite, vomiting, or diarrhea. She was fed a commercial puppy food and had no history of ticks, travel, trauma, or toxin exposure. The owner was not aware of previous vaccinations.

Physical Examination:

Body Weight: 2.2 kg

General: Quiet, alert, hydrated. T = 101.0°F (38.3°C), HR = 220 beats/min, RR = 60 breaths/min, slightly tacky mucous membranes with a normal capillary refill time.

Eyes, Ears, Nose, and Throat: Mild serous oculonasal discharge was present bilaterally. Conjunctival hyperemia and chemosis were present, as well as scleral injection.

Musculoskeletal: BCS 4/9. Fully ambulatory with no evidence of muscle atrophy. Poor body conformation was present, characterized by medial deviation of the tarsi and hyperextension of the carpi.

Respiratory: Tachypnea was present with marked abdominal effort. Lung sounds were markedly increased, especially on the left side. There were no crackles or wheezes. A nonproductive cough occurred several times during the examination.

All Other Systems: No clinically significant abnormalities were detected.

Laboratory Findings:

Venous Blood Gas: pH = 7.348, pCO_2 44 mm Hg, pO_2 44.7 mm Hg, HCO_3 23.2 mmol/L, base excess −1.4 mmol/L, ionized calcium 1.43 mmol/L, lactate 3.3 mmol/L.

CBC:

HCT 35.4% (40%-55%)
MCV 68.6 fL (65-75 fL)
MCHC 31.1 g/dL (33-36 g/dL)
WBC 31,580 cells/μL (6000-13,000 cells/μL)
Neutrophils 6948 cells/μL (3000-10,500 cells/μL)
Band neutrophils 9790 cells/μL
Lymphocytes 9158 cells/μL (1000-4000 cells/μL)
Monocytes 4737 cells/μL (150-1200 cells/μL)
Eosinophils 947 cells/μL (150-1100 cells/μL)
Platelets 307,000 platelets/μL (150,000-400,000 platelets/μL).
Band neutrophils and mature neutrophils had evidence of toxic changes.

Serum Chemistry Profile:

Sodium 147 mmol/L (145-154 mmol/L)
Potassium 4.9 mmol/L (3.6-5.3 mmol/L)
Chloride 104 mmol/L (108-118 mmol/L)
Bicarbonate 24 mmol/L (16-26 mmol/L)
Phosphorus 8.0 mg/dL (3.0-6.2 mg/dL)
Calcium 10.5 mg/dL (9.7-11.5 mg/dl)
BUN 10 mg/dL (5-21 mg/dL)
Creatinine 0.5 mg/dL (0.3-1.2 mg/dL)
Glucose 110 mg/dL (64-123 mg/dL)
Total protein 5.9 g/dL (5.4-7.6 g/dL)
Albumin 2.5 g/dL (3.0-4.4 g/dL)
Globulin 3.4 g/dL (1.8-3.9 g/dL)
ALT 12 U/L (19-67 U/L)
AST 38 U/L (19-42 U/L)
ALP 144 U/L (21-170 U/L)
Gamma GT 0 U/L (0-6 U/L)
Cholesterol 188 mg/dL (135-361 mg/dL)
Total bilirubin 0.0 mg/dL (0-0.2 mg/dL).

Urinalysis: SGr 1.045; pH 7.0, no protein, glucose, ketones, bilirubin, WBC, or RBC were present. Rare triple phosphate and a few sodium urate crystals were noted.

Imaging Findings:

Thoracic Radiographs: There was complete consolidation of the lung lobes associated with the left hemithorax (see Figure 40-2). Prominent air bronchogram formation was noted in these lobes and in the right middle lung lobe, which also appeared consolidated. Diffuse interstitial markings were present in the remainder of the right lung fields.

Thoracic Ultrasound: Complete consolidation of the left lung was the only abnormality detected.

Cytologic Findings: Transtracheal lavage: One direct smear was evaluated that was highly cellular and contained a minimal amount of mucus. Cells were essentially all neutrophils,

Continued

which were primarily nondegenerate but occasionally mildly to moderately degenerate. A single extracellular rod and two neutrophils with intracellular structures that resembled bacteria were found. Interpretation: Marked suppurative inflammation.

Microbiologic Testing: Gram-stained direct smear of transtracheal lavage fluid: Large numbers of neutrophils were seen.

Aerobic and anaerobic bacterial culture and *Mycoplasma* culture (transtracheal wash fluid): Large numbers of *Mycoplasma* spp.; DNA sequence analysis revealed 100% identity to *Mycoplasma cynos*. No other aerobic or anaerobic organisms were isolated.

Direct fluorescent antibody for distemper virus antigen (conjunctival smear): Negative

Centrifugal zinc sulfate fecal flotation: Negative

Diagnosis: *Mycoplasma cynos* bronchopneumonia

Treatment: Before the culture results were available, Delilah was treated with supplemental oxygen, nebulization, coupage, and IV fluids. Treatment with ticarcillin-clavulanate was continued for 3 days, then changed to enrofloxacin (5 mg/kg PO q24h) and amoxicillin-clavulanate (19 mg/kg PO q12h). Daily nebulization with gentamicin was also initiated, because there had been no improvement and persistent bordetellosis was considered possible. The following morning, lung sounds were improved and Delilah was playful. Her nasal discharge resolved and the frequency of cough reduced. The CBC showed a regenerative anemia (hematocrit 33.2%, with 95,300 reticulocytes); 14,112 slightly toxic neutrophils/μL; 1008 band neutrophils/μL; 5796 lymphocytes/μL; and 3780 monocytes/μL. Growth of *Mycoplasma* spp. was reported 5 days after specimens were submitted for culture. Oxygen supplementation was withdrawn, and Delilah was discharged on day 8 of hospitalization, although significant radiographic improvement was not yet evident and an occasional productive cough was still present. Treatment with enrofloxacin, amoxicillin-clavulanate, coupage, and exercise restriction was continued at home. At a recheck 3 weeks later, Delilah had gained weight (3.5 kg). An intermittent, moist, but nonproductive cough was present only in the morning. Her appetite was normal, and there was no evidence of exercise intolerance or oculonasal discharge. A physical examination was unremarkable. A CBC showed persistent mild regenerative anemia, with 7260 neutrophils/μL and 330 band neutrophils/μL. Thoracic radiographs showed improved aeration of the left lung lobes, and near complete resolution of the right-sided infiltrates. The amoxicillin-clavulanate was discontinued. Further improvement in the cough and pulmonary infiltrates was observed at a recheck 3 weeks later. After an additional 7 weeks of treatment, the cough had resolved, but partial atelectasis of the cranial portion of the left lung lobe persisted.

Comments: The isolation of a pure culture of *Mycoplasma cynos* from this dog's airways, the lack of response to β-lactam antibiotics, and a prompt response to enrofloxacin treatment supported a diagnosis of mycoplasma pneumonia (and possibly also URTD) in this dog. The concurrent presence of respiratory viruses remains possible because other than direct fluorescent antibody testing for canine distemper virus, diagnostic tests for respiratory viruses were not performed, and co-infection with multiple respiratory pathogens in dogs from pet stores and shelter environments is common. Resolution of the cough and radiographic changes occurred over several months. Concern existed in regard to cartilage toxicity in such a young dog due to prolonged treatment with enrofloxacin, but no adverse effects occurred. The regenerative anemia was interesting and may have reflected pulmonary hemorrhage or immune-mediated hemolysis. Reticulocytosis has been reported in human patients with community-acquired pneumonia due to *Mycoplasma pneumoniae*.

SUGGESTED READINGS

Chalker VJ, Owen WM, Paterson C, et al. Mycoplasmas associated with canine infectious respiratory disease. Microbiology. 2004;150:3491-3497.

Hartmann AD, Hawley J, Werckenthin C, et al. Detection of bacterial and viral organisms from the conjunctiva of cats with conjunctivitis and upper respiratory tract disease. J Feline Med Surg. 2010;12:775-782.

Stenske KA, Bemis DA, Hill K, et al. Acute polyarthritis and septicemia from *Mycoplasma edwardii* after surgical removal of bilateral adrenal tumors in a dog. J Vet Intern Med. 2005;19:768-771.

REFERENCES

1. Shoetensack HM. Pure cultivation of filterable virus isolated from canine distemper. Kitasako Archives Exp Med. 1934;11:227-290.
2. Baseman JB, Tully JG. Mycoplasmas: sophisticated, reemerging, and burdened by their notoriety. Emerg Infect Dis. 1997;3(1):21-32.
3. Spergser J, Rosengarten R. Identification and differentiation of canine *Mycoplasma* isolates by 16S-23S rDNA PCR-RFLP. Vet Microbiol. 2007;125:170-174.
4. Hartmann AD, Hawley J, Werckenthin C, et al. Detection of bacterial and viral organisms from the conjunctiva of cats with conjunctivitis and upper respiratory tract disease. J Feline Med Surg. 2010;12:775-782.
5. Heyward JT, Sabry MZ, Dowdle WR. Characterization of mycoplasma species of feline origin. Am J Vet Res. 1969;30:615-622.
6. Tan RJ. Susceptibility of kittens to *Mycoplasma felis* infection. Jpn J Exp Med. 1974;44:235-240.
7. Chalker VJ. Canine mycoplasmas. Res Vet Sci. 2005;79:1-8.
8. Ilha MR, Rajeev S, Watson C, et al. Meningoencephalitis caused by *Mycoplasma edwardii* in a dog. J Vet Diagn Invest. 2010;22:805-808.
9. Zeugswetter F, Hittmair KM, de Arespacochaga AG, et al. Erosive polyarthritis associated with *Mycoplasma gateae* in a cat. J Feline Med Surg. 2007;9:226-231.
10. Stenske KA, Bemis DA, Hill K, et al. Acute polyarthritis and septicemia from *Mycoplasma edwardii* after surgical removal of bilateral adrenal tumors in a dog. J Vet Intern Med. 2005;19:768-771.
11. Barton MD, Ireland L, Kirschner JL, et al. Isolation of *Mycoplasma spumans* from polyarthritis in a greyhound. Aust Vet J. 1985;62:206-207.
12. Beauchamp DJ, da Costa RC, Premanandan C, et al. *Mycoplasma felis*–associated meningoencephalomyelitis in a cat. J Feline Med Surg. 2011;13:139-143.
13. Haesebrouck F, Devriese LA, van Rijssen B, et al. Incidence and significance of isolation of *Mycoplasma felis* from conjunctival swabs of cats. Vet Microbiol. 1991;26:95-101.
14. Jang SS, Ling GV, Yamamoto R, et al. *Mycoplasma* as a cause of canine urinary tract infection. J Am Vet Med Assoc. 1984;185:45-47.

15. Moise NS, Crissman JW, Fairbrother JF, et al. *Mycoplasma gateae* arthritis and tenosynovitis in cats: case report and experimental reproduction of the disease. Am J Vet Res. 1983;44:16-21.
16. Hooper PT, Ireland LA, Carter A. *Mycoplasma* polyarthritis in a cat with probable severe immune deficiency. Aust Vet J. 1985;62:352.
17. Liehmann L, Degasperi B, Spergser J, et al. *Mycoplasma felis* arthritis in two cats. J Small Anim Pract. 2006;47:476-479.
18. Gray LD, Ketring KL, Tang YW. Clinical use of 16S rRNA gene sequencing to identify *Mycoplasma felis* and *M. gateae* associated with feline ulcerative keratitis. J Clin Microbiol. 2005;43:3431-3434.
19. Low HC, Powell CC, Veir JK, et al. Prevalence of feline herpesvirus 1, *Chlamydophila felis*, and *Mycoplasma* spp DNA in conjunctival cells collected from cats with and without conjunctivitis. Am J Vet Res. 2007;68:643-648.
20. Holst BS, Hanas S, Berndtsson LT, et al. Infectious causes for feline upper respiratory tract disease—a case-control study. J Feline Med Surg. 2010;12:783-789.
21. Rycroft AN, Tsounakou E, Chalker V. Serological evidence of *Mycoplasma cynos* infection in canine infectious respiratory disease. Vet Microbiol. 2007;120:358-362.
22. Chalker VJ, Owen WM, Paterson C, et al. Mycoplasmas associated with canine infectious respiratory disease. Microbiology. 2004;150:3491-3497.
23. Rosendal S. Canine mycoplasmas: pathogenicity of mycoplasmas associated with distemper pneumonia. J Infect Dis. 1978;138:203-210.
24. Abou N, Houwers DJ, van Dongen AM. PCR-based detection reveals no causative role for *Mycoplasma* and *Ureaplasma* in feline lower urinary tract disease. Vet Microbiol. 2006;116:246-247.
25. Bettenay SV, Lappin MR, Mueller RS. An immunohistochemical and polymerase chain reaction evaluation of feline plasmacytic pododermatitis. Vet Pathol. 2007;44:80-83.
26. Mannering SA, McAuliffe L, Lawes JR, et al. Strain typing of *Mycoplasma cynos* isolates from dogs with respiratory disease. Vet Microbiol. 2009;135:292-296.
27. Randolph JF, Moise NS, Scarlett JM, et al. Prevalence of mycoplasmal and ureaplasmal recovery from tracheobronchial lavages and of mycoplasmal recovery from pharyngeal swab specimens in cats with or without pulmonary disease. Am J Vet Res. 1993;54:897-900.
28. Randolph JF, Moise NS, Scarlett JM, et al. Prevalence of mycoplasmal and ureaplasmal recovery from tracheobronchial lavages and prevalence of mycoplasmal recovery from pharyngeal swab specimens in dogs with or without pulmonary disease. Am J Vet Res. 1993;54:387-391.
29. Chandler JC, Lappin MR. Mycoplasmal respiratory infections in small animals: 17 cases (1988-1999). J Am Anim Hosp Assoc. 2002;38:111-119.
30. Foster SF, Barrs VR, Martin P, et al. Pneumonia associated with *Mycoplasma* spp. in three cats. Aust Vet J. 1998;76:460-464.
31. Malik R, Love DN, Hunt GB, et al. Pyothorax associated with *Mycoplasma* species in a kitten. J Small Anim Pract. 1991;32:31-34.
32. Gulbahar MY, Gurturk K. Pyothorax associated with a *Mycoplasma* sp. and *Arcanobacterium pyogenes* in a kitten. Aust Vet J. 2002;80:344-345.
33. Walker AL, Jang SS, Hirsh DC. Bacteria associated with pyothorax of dogs and cats: 98 cases (1989-1998). J Am Vet Med Assoc. 2000;216:359-363.
34. L'Abee-Lund TM, Heiene R, Friis NF, et al. *Mycoplasma canis* and urogenital disease in dogs in Norway. Vet Rec. 2003;153:231-235.
35. Barber RM, Porter BF, Li Q, et al. Broadly reactive polymerase chain reaction for pathogen detection in canine granulomatous meningoencephalomyelitis and necrotizing meningoencephalitis. J Vet Intern Med. 2012;26:962-968.
36. Waites KB, Taylor-Robinson D. Mycoplasma and Ureaplasma. In: Versalovic J, Carroll KC, Funke G, Jorgensen JH, Landry ML, Warnock DW, eds. Manual of Clinical Microbiology. Washington, DC: ASM Press; 2011:970-985.
37. Rebelo AR, Parker L, Cai HY. Use of high-resolution melting curve analysis to identify *Mycoplasma* species commonly isolated from ruminant, avian, and canine samples. J Vet Diagn Invest. 2011;23:932-936.
38. Soderlund R, Bolske G, Holst BS, et al. Development and evaluation of a real-time polymerase chain reaction method for the detection of *Mycoplasma felis*. J Vet Diagn Invest. 2011;23:890-893.
39. Chalker VJ, Owen WM, Paterson CJ, et al. Development of a polymerase chain reaction for the detection of *Mycoplasma felis* in domestic cats. Vet Microbiol. 2004;100:77-82.
40. Hartmann AD, Helps CR, Lappin MR, et al. Efficacy of pradofloxacin in cats with feline upper respiratory tract disease due to *Chlamydophila felis* or *Mycoplasma* infections. J Vet Intern Med. 2008;22:44-52.
41. Kompare B, Litster AL, Leutenegger CM, et al. Randomized masked clinical trial to compare 7-day and 14-day course length of doxycycline in the treatment of *Mycoplasma felis* infection in shelter cats. Comp Immunol Microbiol Infect Dis. 2012:Dec 13 [Epub].
42. Armstrong D, Yu BH, Yagoda A, et al. Colonization of humans by *Mycoplasma canis*. J Infect Dis. 1971;124:607-609.
43. Bonilla HF, Chenoweth CE, Tully JG, et al. *Mycoplasma felis* septic arthritis in a patient with hypogammaglobulinemia. Clin Infect Dis. 1997;24:222-225.
44. McCabe SJ, Murray JF, Ruhnke HL, et al. *Mycoplasma* infection of the hand acquired from a cat. J Hand Surg Am. 1987;12:1085-1088.

CHAPTER 41

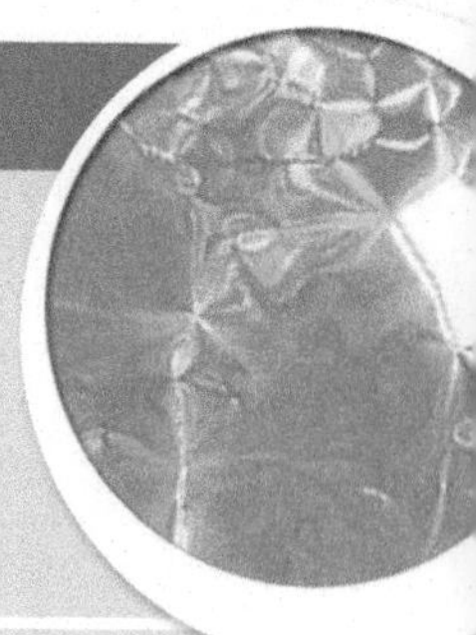

Hemoplasma Infections

Jane E. Sykes and Séverine Tasker

Overview of Hemoplasma Infections

First Described: Feline hemoplasmas, South Africa, 1942 (Clark)[1]; canine hemoplasmas, Germany, 1928 (Kikuth)[2]

Cause: *Mycoplasma haemofelis, 'Candidatus* Mycoplasma haemominutum,' '*Candidatus* Mycoplasma turicensis' (cats). The most prevalent hemoplasmas in dogs are *Mycoplasma haemocanis* and '*Candidatus* Mycoplasma haematoparvum.'

Affected Hosts: Cats and wild felids, dogs and wild canids; other hemoplasma species cause disease in a variety of other animal species.

Geographic Distribution: Worldwide

Mode of Transmission: Experimentally, transmission can occur through ingestion or injection of infected blood; the mode of transmission in the field uncertain. Biting or aggressive interactions are a suspected mode, and possibly vertical transmission. Ticks are suspected to transmit *Mycoplasma haemocanis*. Other unidentified arthropod vectors may also be involved.

Major Clinical Signs: Fever, lethargy, inappetence, weakness, pallor.

Differential Diagnoses: Cytauxzoonosis, FIV infection, FeLV infection, feline infectious peritonitis, primary immune-mediated hemolytic anemia, Heinz body hemolytic anemia, inherited erythrocyte disorders such as pyruvate kinase deficiency and the red cell fragility disorder of Abyssinian and Somali cats

Human Health Significance: DNA sequences that match those found in *Mycoplasma haemofelis* were detected in a human co-infected with HIV and *Bartonella henselae*. DNA sequences of other animal hemoplasmas have also been detected in humans.

Etiology and Epidemiology

Hemotropic mycoplasmas (hemoplasmas) are small (0.3-0.8 μm), unculturable mycoplasmas that reside on the surface of erythrocytes and can cause variable degrees of hemolytic anemia in infected hosts. Hemoplasmas infect a wide variety of mammalian species, including humans, and have a worldwide distribution. Although previously classified as *Haemobartonella* and *Eperythrozoon* spp., sequence analysis of the 16S rRNA genes of these organisms has shown that they are closely related to the pneumoniae group of mycoplasmas, which includes the human mycoplasmal pathogens *Mycoplasma pneumoniae* and *Mycoplasma genitalium*.

At least three hemoplasma species infect domestic as well as wild cats, *Mycoplasma haemofelis*, '*Candidatus* Mycoplasma haemominutum,' and '*Candidatus* Mycoplasma turicensis.' The '*Candidatus*' prefix is applied to newly discovered hemoplasmas until more information is available to support their classification. This is because hemoplasmas cannot be cultured in the laboratory, which limits full characterization of these organisms. *M. haemofelis* (previously the Ohio strain, or large form of *Haemobartonella felis*) is the most pathogenic organism and can cause moderate to severe hemolytic anemia in immunocompetent cats. The resulting disease has been referred to as *feline infectious anemia*. Using cytologic evaluation of blood smears, *M. haemofelis* organisms are cocci that sometimes form short chains of three to six organisms (Figure 41-1). *M. haemofelis* is the least prevalent of the three feline hemoplasmas. It has been found using PCR in 0.5% to 5% of sick cats at veterinary hospitals. The whole genome sequences of *M. haemofelis* and *M. haemominutum* have been determined.[3-5]

'*Ca.* M. haemominutum' (previously the California strain or small form of *H. felis*) is generally smaller than *M. haemofelis* and has not clearly been associated with disease in immunocompetent cats. Using cytologic evaluation of blood smears, '*Ca.* M. haemominutum' are small cocci, 0.3 to 0.6 μm in diameter, although *M. haemofelis* and '*Ca.* M. haemominutum' cannot

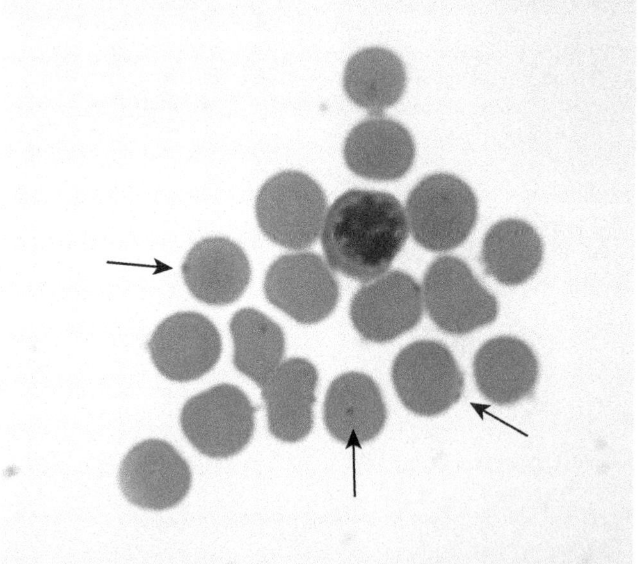

FIGURE 41-1 Romanowsky-stained blood smear from an 8-year-old male neutered domestic shorthair cat showing epierythrocytic bacteria typical of *Mycoplasma haemofelis* (arrows).

always reliably be distinguished by this method. '*Ca.* M. haemominutum' is common in the cat population worldwide, infecting as many as 20% of cats that visit veterinary hospitals.[6-8] Infection of cats with '*Ca.* M. haemominutum' results in a mild decrease in hematocrit. There is some evidence that '*Ca.* M. haemominutum' may play a role in disease. For example, cats that are co-infected with FeLV and '*Ca.* M. haemominutum' develop more significant anemia than cats infected with '*Ca.* M. haemominutum' alone, and progression to FeLV-induced myeloproliferative disease occurred more rapidly.[9] There are also descriptions of cats with hemolytic anemia in which the only recognized cause of anemia was '*Ca.* M. haemominutum.'[10] '*Ca.* M. haemominutum' is commonly found in co-infections with '*Ca.* M. turicensis' or *M. haemofelis*. Mixed infections with all three feline hemoplasma species also have been described.

'*Ca.* M. turicensis' was first described in a cat from Switzerland that had severe intravascular hemolysis (*turicensis* pertains to Turicum, the Latin name of Zurich).[11] Infections with '*Ca.* M. turicensis' have since been detected worldwide.[8,12-14] '*Ca.* M. turicensis' has never been seen using light microscopic examination of blood smears, and organism loads in infected cats are typically low. Infection with '*Ca.* M. turicensis' is slightly more prevalent in the cat population than infection with *M. haemofelis*. Most studies show a prevalence of 0.5% to 10% in sick cats that visit veterinary hospitals. The pathogenic potential of this organism is not fully understood. Inoculation of an immunosuppressed cat with '*Ca.* M. turicensis' resulted in severe anemia,[11] but little or no anemia occurs in immunocompetent cats after inoculation with '*Ca.* M. turicensis.' Cofactors, such as co-infection with other hemoplasmas or concurrent immunosuppression, may influence the development of anemia in cats infected with '*Ca.* M. turicensis.'

Infection of cats by hemoplasmas is strongly associated with male sex, nonpedigree status, and outdoor access (Box 41-1).[8,12,15,16] Infection with '*Ca.* M. haemominutum' is more prevalent in older cats, presumably because the chance of acquiring persistent subclinical infection increases over time. In contrast, young cats may be more likely to develop disease after infection by *M. haemofelis*. Some studies, but not others, have shown an association between retrovirus and hemoplasma infections. Cats infected with *M. haemofelis* in the United States were 6 times more likely to be FIV infected than cats negative for hemoplasmas.[15]

Several hemoplasma species also infect dogs. Infection with *Mycoplasma haemocanis* (previously *Haemobartonella canis*) has been associated with hemolytic anemia in splenectomized dogs, and rarely in dogs with other immunosuppressive disease or concurrent infections. The 16S rRNA gene of *M. haemocanis* has the same sequence as *M. haemofelis*, but the whole genome sequence of *M. haemocanis* distinguishes it as a different species.[17] *M. haemocanis* is a coccoid organism that often forms long chains of organisms (Figure 41-2). The prevalence of this infection is particularly high in kennel-raised dogs, which are often infected subclinically.[18] In the southwestern United States, infection was also prevalent among coyotes.[19]

Three additional hemoplasma species have been detected in dogs. '*Candidatus* Mycoplasma haematoparvum' is a small (0.3 μm) coccoid organism that resembles '*Ca.* Mycoplasma haemominutum' morphologically as well as genetically (Figure 41-3). '*Ca.* M. haemominutum' has also been detected in several dogs using PCR assays, and organisms that resemble '*Ca.* M. haematoparvum' and '*Ca.* M. haemominutum' have been detected in European wolves and bush dogs from Brazil.[20] The ovine hemoplasma *Mycoplasma ovis* was detected in the spleens of a small number of dogs from the southeastern United States, and the bovine hemoplasma '*Ca.* Mycoplasma haemobos' was detected in a dog from northern Australia.[21,22] The clinical importance of these hemoplasma species in dogs remains unclear.

The mode of transmission of hemoplasmas remains unclear. To some extent, fleas and other arthropod vectors may be capable of transmitting feline hemoplasmas,[23] but experimental evidence for vector-borne transmission of feline hemoplasmas is weak. Transmission of *M. haemocanis* by the brown dog tick, *Rhipicephalus sanguineus*, has been demonstrated experimentally, although this was before PCR assays were available to confirm infection.[24] Geographic variation in the prevalence of

BOX 41-1

Risk Factors Associated with Infection by Feline Hemotropic Mycoplasmas as Determined Using Species-Specific Real-Time PCR Assays

Mycoplasma haemofelis
Younger age
Male sex
FIV seroreactivity
FeLV seroreactivity

'*Candidatus* Mycoplasma haemominutum'
Older age
Male sex
FIV seroreactivity
Nonpedigree status
Outdoor access

'*Candidatus* Mycoplasma turicensis'
Male sex

From Ettinger SJ, Feldman EC, eds. Textbook of Veterinary Internal Medicine, 7 ed, St. Louis, MO: Saunders; 2011.

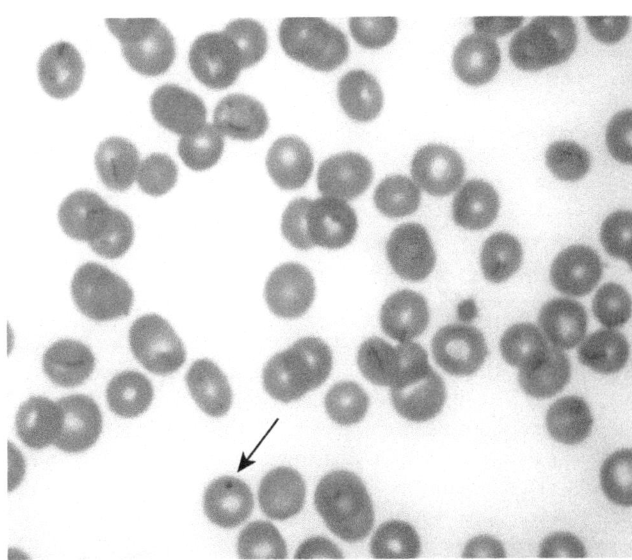

FIGURE 41-2 Romanowsky-stained blood smear showing chains of epierythrocytic bacteria typical of *Mycoplasma haemocanis*. A Howell-Jolly body is also present *(arrow)*.

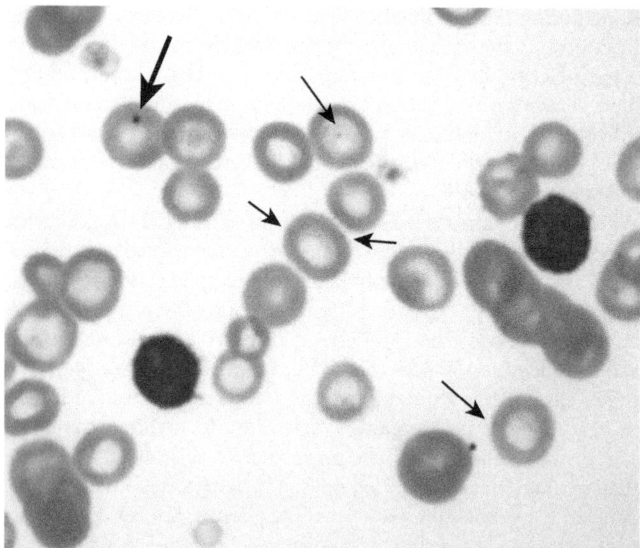

FIGURE 41-3 Blood smear from a dog showing *'Candidatus* Mycoplasma haematoparvum' *(small arrows)* and a Howell-Jolly Body *(large arrow)*.

hemoplasma infection in dogs and cats supports a role for arthropod vectors in transmission. For example, in Europe, infection with *M. haemocanis* is more prevalent in Mediterranean countries, which follows the distribution of *Rh. sanguineus*. Vertical (e.g., transplacental) spread has also been hypothesized and has been documented for bovine hemoplasmas. Biting has been suggested as a means of transmission of feline hemoplasmas, and the strong male sex predilection, recent history of cat bite abscessation in some cats, and association with FIV infection in some studies supports this mode. Additionally, studies in Switzerland found that subcutaneous inoculation of blood that contained '*Ca.* M. turicensis' resulted in transmission, whereas inoculation of saliva that contained '*Ca.* M. turicensis' did not.[25] This suggests that hemoplasma transmission by social contact (saliva via mutual grooming etc.) is less likely than transmission by aggressive interaction (blood transmission during a cat bite incident). Because infection can also be transmitted by ingestion of blood, it may be that the biting cat (rather than the bitten cat) is most at risk for acquisition of infection. Transmission of *M. haemocanis* through ingestion of infected blood has also been described,[26] so aggressive interactions between dogs may also have the potential to transmit hemoplasmas; however, this mode of transmission remains to be proven in field circumstances. Transmission can also occur following blood transfusion.

Clinical Features

Signs and Their Pathogenesis

Because only *M. haemofelis* infection is associated with significant anemia in cats, only the pathogenesis of disease induced by this species is described here. After experimental infection, there is a delay of 2 to 34 days before the onset of clinical signs. Anemia then occurs and persists for about 18 to 30 days (acute phase), although its severity and chronicity vary considerably between infected cats. Anemia predominantly results from extravascular hemolysis, and the onset of anemia is usually followed by a strong regenerative response with reticulocytosis. The organism resides in an indentation on the erythrocyte surface (Figure 41-4). Production of both cold and warm reactive erythrocyte-bound antibodies, increased osmotic fragility, and decreased erythrocyte life span have been noted in infected cats.[27-29] The organisms can also "bridge" adjacent erythrocytes, which might promote splenic trapping and removal of red blood cells. In contrast, erythrocyte-bound antibody formation and significant reticulocytosis have not been documented in cats infected with '*Ca.* M. haemominutum' or '*Ca.* M. turicensis.'

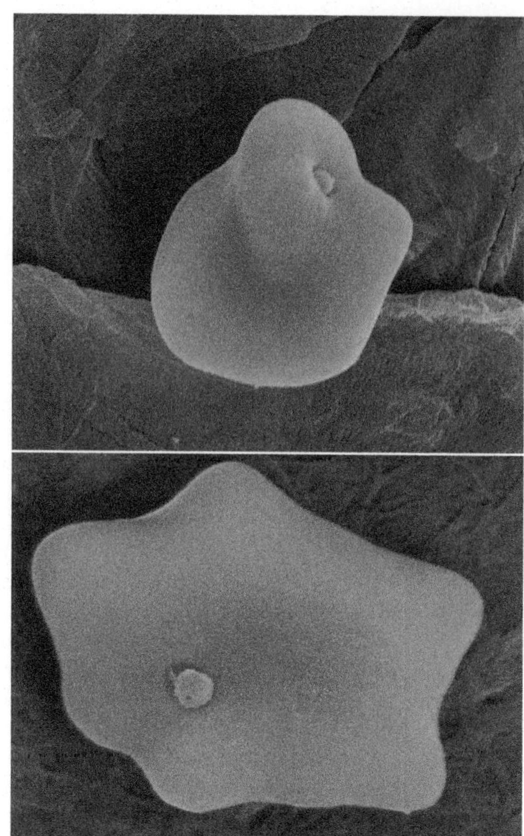

FIGURE 41-4 Electron micrographs showing epierythrocytic location of *Mycoplasma haemofelis*.

Anemia can result in signs of lethargy, inappetence, pallor, and weakness. Some owners report that their cats eat dirt or litter or lick cement (pica). Weight loss and dehydration can occur. Rapid development of anemia may result in neurologic signs, vocalization, collapse, and death. In some infected cats, cyclical changes in the hematocrit and numbers of infected erythrocytes occur, with sharp declines in the hematocrit correlating with appearance of large numbers of organisms in blood smears.[30-32] The proportion of erythrocytes associated with visible organisms on blood smears can decline from 90% to less than 1% in less than 3 hours.[33,34] These dramatic fluctuations in organism numbers appear to result from rapid replication of *M. haemofelis*, followed by rapid clearance from the blood as a result of the host's immune response. Repeated antigenic variation in *M. haemofelis* may allow the organism to again proliferate in the face of this immune response, which contributes to ongoing fluctuations in organism numbers.

In cats that survive the acute phase, the hematocrit then returns to normal or near-normal (recovery phase), and organisms can no longer be visualized in blood smears. It is possible that at least some of these recovered cats remain persistently infected, whereby the organism evades the host immune system, and that recrudescence of anemia may follow stress, pregnancy, intercurrent infection, or neoplasia.[32,33] However, evidence is accumulating that differences may exist in the ability of hemoplasmas to persist within the host, the carrier state being more frequent for '*Ca.* M. haemominutum' but less frequent for *M. haemofelis* and '*Ca.* M. turicensis.' In cats, splenectomy has a variable effect on the course of hemoplasmosis. Recrudescence of anemia and bacteremia has been documented in some chronically infected cats after splenectomy, although other studies suggest that splenectomy increases the number of visible organisms in blood smears without causing significant anemia.[32,34] Infection of splenectomized cats with '*Ca.* M. haemominutum' does not appear to enhance the pathogenicity of this organism.[35]

Dogs that develop clinical hemoplasmosis have usually had a history of splenectomy or, less commonly, concurrent immunosuppressive illness or drug treatment or co-infections with other bloodborne pathogens such as *Babesia* spp. and *Ehrlichia canis*. Clinical signs include weakness, lethargy, and pallor, and some dogs are inappetent.

Physical Examination Findings

Physical examination findings in cats with acute *M. haemofelis* infection include fever, weakness, mucosal pallor, tachypnea, tachycardia, and weak or bounding femoral pulse quality. Other physical examination abnormalities can include dehydration, cardiac murmurs, splenomegaly, and occasionally mild icterus (Figure 41-5). Moribund cats may be hypothermic.

Dogs with hemoplasmosis can show lethargy and mucosal pallor. Fever is usually absent.

Cats infected with '*Ca.* M. haemominutum' or '*Ca.* M. turicensis,' and dogs infected with '*Ca.* M. haematoparvum' generally appear healthy unless concurrent disease is present.

Diagnosis

Laboratory Abnormalities

Complete Blood Count

The most characteristic CBC abnormality in dogs and cats infected with *M. haemocanis* and *M. haemofelis*, respectively, is regenerative anemia, with macrocytosis, anisocytosis, reticulocytosis, polychromasia, Howell-Jolly bodies, and, especially in cats, sometimes marked normoblastemia. Manual reticulocyte counts should be interpreted with caution in cats infected with *M. haemofelis*, because both hemoplasma-infected erythrocytes have the same appearance as reticulocytes in blood smears stained with methylene blue. Autoagglutination may be noted in blood smears. Nonregenerative anemia can be present when sufficient time for a regenerative response has not yet elapsed, or as a result of concurrent FeLV infection or any other disease that suppresses the regenerative response. Concurrent occult hemoplasma infection should be considered in any anemic FeLV-positive cat, even in the absence of reticulocytosis. Neutrophil counts may be normal, elevated, or low, and lymphopenia may be present. Thrombocytopenia can also occur in affected dogs and cats, but often the platelet count is within the reference range.

Serum Biochemical Tests

The serum chemistry profile in cats with hemoplasmosis may reveal increased activities of ALT and AST as a result of hypoxia; metabolic acidosis; mild to moderate hyperbilirubinemia; and prerenal azotemia. Hyperproteinemia may be seen in some cats.

Urinalysis

The urinalysis is usually unremarkable; bilirubinuria may be present in hyperbilirubinemic cats.

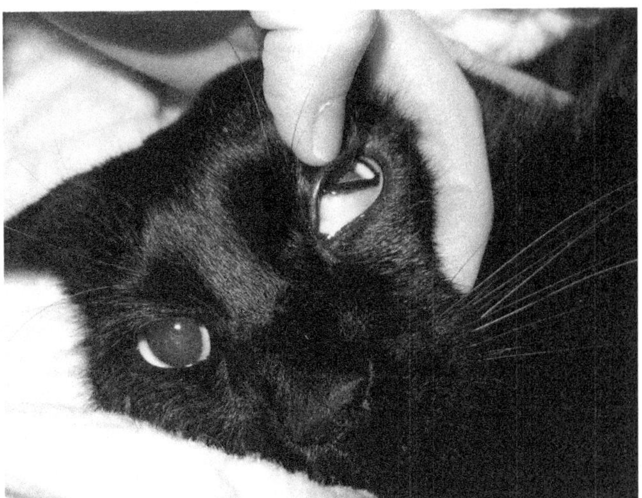

FIGURE 41-5 Mild icterus of the nictating membrane in an 8-year-old male neutered domestic shorthair with hemolytic anemia secondary to *Mycoplasma haemofelis* infection.

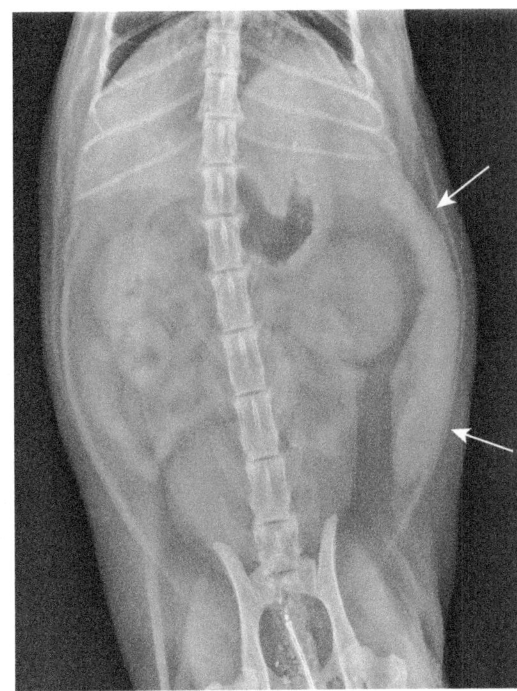

FIGURE 41-6 Ventrodorsal abdominal radiograph from an 8-year-old male neutered domestic shorthair cat with hemolytic anemia secondary to *Mycoplasma haemofelis* Infection. There is marked splenomegaly (*arrows*).

Diagnostic Imaging

The most common radiographic finding in cats with hemoplasmosis is splenomegaly (Figure 41-6). The spleen may be absent in affected dogs because of previous splenectomy.

Microbiologic Tests

Assays available for diagnosis of hemoplasmosis in dogs and cats are listed in Table 41-1.

Cytologic Examination of Blood Smears

Cytologic detection of hemoplasmas has low sensitivity and specificity, especially for diagnosis of feline infectious anemia. *M. haemofelis* is visible less than 50% of the time in acutely infected cats, because organisms can disappear for days before

TABLE 41-1

Assays Available for Diagnosis of Hemoplasmosis in Dogs and Cats

Assay	Specimen Type	Target	Performance
Cytologic examination	Blood smears	Hemoplasmas	Poor sensitivity, especially in affected cats. Organisms are seen on blood smears in fewer than 50% of sick cats. False positives can occur when stain precipitate, drying artifact, basophilic stippling, and Howell-Jolly bodies are misinterpreted as hemoplasmas.
PCR	Whole blood, blood smears	Hemoplasma DNA	Sensitivity and specificity can vary depending on assay design. Results must be interpreted in light of the species detected and the clinical findings. *Mycoplasma haemofelis* and *Mycoplasma haemocanis* are most likely to be associated with anemia.

reappearing on blood smears over the course of infection. Because organisms detach from erythrocytes within hours of blood collection, fresh blood smears should be submitted. False-positive diagnoses occur when stain artifacts such as precipitate are confused with organisms; thus, careful staining with a properly prepared, uncontaminated Romanowsky-type stain solution is essential. Organisms also need to be distinguished from basophilic stippling and Howell-Jolly bodies. '*Ca.* M. haemominutum' is small and is not usually visible in chronically infected cats. '*Ca.* M. turicensis' has never been seen on blood smears with light microscopy. Hemoplasmas are visible in many clinically affected dogs, and because *M. haemocanis* tends to form chains, it is more readily differentiated from stain artifacts and erythrocyte morphologic changes than is *M. haemofelis*. However, hemoplasmas are not usually visible in chronically infected dogs or in dogs infected with '*Ca.* M. haematoparvum.'

Culture

Attempts to isolate and grow feline hemotropic mycoplasmas in the laboratory have been unsuccessful, so blood culture cannot be used for diagnosis of hemoplasmosis.

Molecular Diagnosis Using the Polymerase Chain Reaction

PCR assays are currently the tests of choice for diagnosis of hemoplasmosis in dogs and cats. Numerous assays have been described to date, which are generally based on detection of the 16S rRNA gene. These are significantly more sensitive than blood smear evaluation, although they occasionally do not detect infection in apparently healthy carrier cats when organism numbers in the blood are below the detection limit of the PCR assay.[6,30,36,37] Both conventional and real-time PCR assays have been described. Some conventional PCR assays do not differentiate between *M. haemofelis* and '*Ca.* M. turicensis,' because the primers used in the assay generate the same-sized PCR product when either or both of these species are present. Real-time PCR assays are usually species specific. Because the pathogenic potential of each hemoplasma species differs, the laboratory should be consulted to determine the species specificity of the assay(s) offered. Alternative causes of anemia should always be considered, especially in cats that test positive for '*Ca.* M. haemominutum' or '*Ca.* M. turicensis,' because infection with these organisms is not commonly associated with anemia. Indeed, *all* PCR results should be interpreted in conjunction with the patient's clinical signs, the degree and nature of the anemia present, and any concurrent signs or diseases present that could be contributing to the clinical signs. Dried blood smears can also be tested but are less sensitive than liquid whole blood specimens.[38] PCR assays designed to detect *M. haemofelis* generally also detect *M. haemocanis* because of the high 16S rRNA gene sequence homology between these species, but a separate assay is required for detection of '*Ca.* M. haematoparvum.'

Serologic Diagnosis

The development of serologic tests for diagnosis of hemoplasmosis has been hampered by the inability to culture hemoplasmas in the laboratory. However, the application of molecular techniques has led to the identification of antigens for serologic assay development. Specifically, an ELISA that detects antibodies to an immunodominant protein of *M. haemofelis*, DnaK, has been developed. Cats produce antibodies to this antigen after infection,[39,40] and in a study that examined the immune response to '*Ca.* M. turicensis' infection, antibody titers to DnaK declined with antimicrobial drug treatment.[39] Serologic cross-reactivity occurs to this antigen for all three feline hemoplasma species[40]; therefore, the assay does not discriminate between infection with *M. haemofelis* and other hemoplasmas, but determination of acute and convalescent titers may be helpful to distinguish acute from chronic infection. Currently this assay is available only on a research basis.

Pathologic Findings

Generalized pallor, splenomegaly, and, in some cats, icterus are the main gross necropsy finding in cats that die or are euthanized as a result of hemoplasmosis. Histopathologic findings include extramedullary hematopoiesis, follicular hyperplasia, and erythrophagocytosis within the spleen.

Treatment and Prognosis

Treatment is indicated for cats and dogs with clinical signs and laboratory abnormalities consistent with hemoplasmosis. Although controversial, treatment could also be considered for apparently healthy cats that test positive for *M. haemofelis* in view of the potential for recrudescence of disease with this hemoplasma species. It may be difficult or impossible to eradicate infection with some hemoplasma species or strains, especially '*Ca.* M. haemominutum.' Indeed, no antibiotic treatment regime consistently eliminates hemoplasma infection in cats.

The treatment of choice for hemoplasmosis is doxycycline for a minimum of 2 weeks (see Chapter 8 for information on doxycycline) (Table 41-2); some have suggested using longer courses of treatment (6 to 8 weeks) to ensure that infection is

TABLE 41-2

Suggested Drug Dosages for Treatment of Hemoplasmosis in Cats

Drug	Dose (mg/kg)	Route	Interval (hours)	Duration
Doxycycline	10	PO	24	2 weeks
Marbofloxacin	2.75 to 5.5	PO	24	
Pradofloxacin*	5 to 10	PO	24	
Enrofloxacin†	5	PO	24	

*Dose listed is for the oral suspension for cats.
†Only when other alternatives are not available because of potential for irreversible blindness when enrofloxacin is used in cats.

eliminated. Real-time PCR could be used to monitor response to antibiotic treatment if quantitative information is available. Fluoroquinolones are an alternative; marbofloxacin and pradofloxacin,[41] when available, are both efficacious. Enrofloxacin is also usually effective,[42] but diffuse retinal degeneration and acute blindness have been reported following the use of this fluoroquinolone and, although this is rare, caution must be exercised with its use in cats. The response of the different hemoplasma species, and indeed different strains of the same species, to antibiotics varies. Most successful studies that have demonstrated treatment efficacy have evaluated the response of *M. haemofelis* to treatment. Affected dogs and cats may also require supportive treatment with IV crystalloids or blood products. Clinical improvement usually occurs within 2 to 3 days. The use of immunosuppressive doses of glucocorticoids to suppress the associated immune-mediated hemolytic process is controversial, given that glucocorticoids can cause reactivation of latent infection, but may be necessary in cats that fail to respond to antimicrobial therapy alone, or when the diagnosis is uncertain, especially if erythrocyte-bound antibodies are identified.

Doxycycline is the drug of choice for treatment of *M. haemocanis* infection. Treatment of a splenectomized dog with oxytetracycline for approximately 1 month was associated with clinical improvement, but infection persisted as determined with quantitative PCR, and relapse occurred when treatment was withdrawn.[43] Infection also persisted after treatment with enrofloxacin, despite eventual recovery from anemia. In contrast, in *M. haemocanis*–infected dogs with intact spleens, doxycycline treatment for 4 weeks appeared to result in resolution of infection as determined by PCR assay, whereas '*Ca.* M. haematoparvum'–infected dogs remained PCR positive.[19] A splenectomized dog was apparently cured of *M. haemocanis* infection after 12 weeks of doxycycline treatment.[44]

Immunity and Vaccination

Little information is available in regard to the immune response to hemoplasma infection, and no vaccines are available. Because co-infections with multiple hemoplasma species occur, infection with one species does not appear to protect against infection with other species.

Prevention

Inadvertent transmission of hemoplasmas by transfusion of blood from carrier cats has been documented, and so all blood donor dogs and cats should be tested for hemoplasmas with PCR assays. In the future, screening with serologic assays may also be used to identify potential donor animals. Whenever possible, cats and dogs that are PCR positive for any of the known hemoplasma species should be excluded as donors. Given the high prevalence of subclinical '*Ca.* M. haemominutum' infection among cats, in some circumstances it may not be possible to find a donor that is '*Ca.* M. haemominutum' negative. At this time, it is unclear whether transfusion of blood from cats that are infected with '*Ca.* M. haemominutum' is associated with adverse outcome, but it remains a possibility. Keeping cats indoors is also likely to prevent infection, as outdoor access has been identified as a risk factor. Control of fleas and ticks is recommended.

Public Health Aspects

Organisms that resembled hemoplasmas were identified in human blood smears decades ago. Molecular techniques that were originally designed for detection of canine and feline hemoplasmas have since been applied to human blood, and a variety of hemoplasma species have now been identified. In addition, application of these methods to archived human blood smears believed to contain hemoplasmas based on cytological evaluation yielded negative results, suggesting the possibility of historical misdiagnosis.[45] Infection with a novel hemoplasma, designated '*Ca.* Mycoplasma haemohominis,' has been identified in a person with hemolytic anemia.[46] *M. haemofelis* DNA was identified in a person from Brazil who was co-infected with HIV and *Bartonella henselae*.[47] In addition, DNA of *Mycoplasma ovis* was detected in a Texas veterinarian who was co-infected with *B. henselae*.[48] *Mycoplasma suis* DNA has been found in farm workers from China.[49] The identification of the DNA of animal hemoplasmas in humans should be viewed cautiously because only a small portion or portions of the hemoplasma genome was detected in each of these case reports. *M. haemocanis* and *M. haemofelis* have identical 16S rRNA gene sequences, but different host tropisms, and so the organisms detected in these humans may not necessarily be the same as those that infect domestic animal species. Until further information is available, veterinarians should handle blood from animals with caution.

CASE EXAMPLE

Signalment: "Shadow," an 8-year-old male neutered domestic shorthair from Fairfield, CA

History: Shadow was brought to the University of California, Davis, Veterinary Medical Teaching Hospital emergency service for treatment of severe anemia. The owners reported that he had disappeared 5 days previously. The evening that he was brought to the emergency service, he was found splayed across a fence and was unwilling to move, and vocalizing and salivating profusely. He was immediately taken to a local emergency clinic where he was found to be obtunded, pale, and severely dehydrated. His pulse was 180 beats/min, respiratory rate was 60 breaths/min, and temperature was 94.0°F (34.4°C). A systolic blood pressure was 80 mm Hg. A PCV was 12%. Shadow's condition was stabilized after treatment with supplemental oxygen, active warming, and IV crystalloid fluids (Normosol-R, 50 mL over 30 minutes, then 25 mL/hr). He tested negative for FIV antibody and FeLV antigen with an in-practice ELISA assay. Shadow was an indoor-outdoor cat that was acquired as a stray kitten from the owner's backyard. There had been no previous history of illness.

Physical Examination:

Body Weight: 6 kg

General: Obtunded, laterally recumbent. T = 97.8°F (36.6°C), HR = 150 beats/min, RR = 60 breaths/minute, purring, pale and tacky mucous membranes with no detectable capillary refill, weak pulses.

Integument: No ectoparasites were noted. The pinnae and ventral abdominal skin were icteric.

Eyes, Ears, Nose, and Throat: Moderate dental calculus was present. Pallor and mild icterus of the mucous membranes, nictitans, and sclera was noted (see Figure 41-5).

Musculoskeletal: Body condition score was 7/9.

Cardiovascular: Weak pulses. No other clinically significant abnormalities were detected. No murmurs were detected but the heart sounds were difficult to auscultate because of persistent purring.

Respiratory: Tachypneic; auscultation was limited because of purring.

Gastrointestinal and Genitourinary: Nonpainful abdomen. Moderate cranial organomegaly. Urinary bladder not palpable.

Neurologic: A full neurologic examination was not performed but no abnormalities were detected on examination of cranial nerve functions.

Lymph Nodes: No clinically significant abnormalities detected.

Laboratory Findings:

PCV/TPP: 14%/7.3 g/dL, icteric plasma.

Saline Slide Agglutination Test: Negative for autoagglutination.

Blood Smear Examination: Marked polychromasia, normoblastosis, and mild anisocytosis were present. Coccoid bodies that resembled hemoplasmas were present in association with erythrocytes (see Figure 41-1).

Electrolyte/Acid-Base Panel (Venous Blood): HCO_3 = 14 mmol/L, pH = 7.365, pCO_2 = 21.9 mm Hg, pO_2 = 35.4 mm Hg, Hb = 2.8 g/dL, O_2 = 59.5%, potassium = 4.0 mmol/L, sodium = 144 mmol/L, ionized calcium = 1.2 mmol/L, glucose = 157 mg/dL, lactate = 8.4 mmol/L, base excess = −12.2 mmol/L.

Imaging Findings:

Thoracic Radiographs: No clinically significant abnormalities were detected.

Abdominal Radiographs: The spleen was markedly enlarged (See Figure 41-6). The liver was mildly enlarged. Small mineral densities were present within ingesta and feces in the stomach and colon, respectively.

Treatment: The cat was placed on a heating pad and transfused with 1 unit of packed RBC, and supplemental oxygen was administered, after which heart rate increased to 200 beats/min and respiratory rate decreased to 40 breaths/min. Rectal temperature increased to 103.7°F (39.8°C) during the transfusion, and so dexamethasone was administered because of the concern for a transfusion reaction (0.2 mg/kg IV once). The cat was also treated with enrofloxacin (5 mg/kg IV q24h) (see comments section later) for suspected hemoplasmosis. The results of laboratory testing after transfer to the internal medicine service the day after admission are shown here.

CBC (Post Transfusion and Antimicrobial Treatment):

HCT 12.7% (30%-50%)
MCV 76.5 fL (42-53 fL)
MCHC 26.8 g/dL (30-33.5 g/dL)
Reticulocytes 155,600 cells/μL (7000-60,000 cells/μL)
Nucleated RBC 39/100 WBC (0/100 WBC)
Corrected WBC 9800 cells/μL (4500-14,000 cells/μL)
Neutrophils 8134 cells/μL (2000-9000 cells/μL)
Band neutrophils 98 cells/μL
Lymphocytes 784 cells/μL (1000-7000 cells/μL)
Monocytes 784 cells/μL (50-600 cells/μL)
Eosinophils 0 cells/μL (150-1100 cells/μL)
Basophils 0 cells/μL (0-50 cells/μL)
Platelets 142,000/μL (180,000-500,000 platelets/μL).
Cytologic examination revealed marked anisocytosis, marked polychromasia, few Howell-Jolly bodies, and many macrocytes and microcytes. No hemoplasmas were identified.

Serum Chemistry Profile:

Sodium 143 mmol/L (151-158 mmol/L)
Potassium 5.2 mmol/L (3.6-4.9 mmol/L)
Chloride 107 mmol/L (117-126 mmol/L)
Bicarbonate 11 mmol/L (15-21 mmol/L)
Phosphorus 6.6 mg/dL (3.2-6.3 mg/dL)
Calcium 9.6 mg/dL (9.0-10.9 mg/dL)
BUN 47 mg/dL (18-33 mg/dL)
Creatinine 1.2 mg/dL (1.1-2.2 mg/dL)
Glucose 98 mg/dL (63-118 mg/dL)
Total protein 7.2 g/dL (6.6-8.4 g/dL)
Albumin 3.0 g/dL (2.2-4.6 g/dL)
Globulin 4.2 g/dL (2.8-5.4 g/dL)
ALT 166 U/L (27-101 U/L)
AST 201 U/L (17-58 U/L)
ALP 24 U/L (14-71 U/L)
GGT 0 U/L (0-4 U/L)
Cholesterol 75 mg/dL (89-258 mg/dL)
Total bilirubin 6.1 mg/dL (0-0.2 mg/dL)
Magnesium 3.4 mg/dL (1.5-2.5 mg/dL)
Creatine kinase 446 U/L (73-260 U/L).

Urinalysis: USG 1.040, pH 6, 75 mg/dL protein, no glucose, 5 mg/dL ketones, 6 mg/dL bilirubin, 250 erythrocytes/µL hemoprotein, 0-1 RBC/HPF, 0 WBC/HPF, rare transitional epithelial cells.

Microbiologic Testing: Real-time PCR for *Mycoplasma haemofelis, 'Candidatus* Mycoplasma haemominutum,' and *'Candidatus* Mycoplasma turicensis' (blood smear): Positive for *M. haemofelis* DNA

Diagnosis: Feline infectious anemia (*Mycoplasma haemofelis* infection)

Additional Treatment and Outcome: Treatment was changed to doxycycline (10 mg/kg followed by 5 mL of water PO q24h for 3 weeks). Treatment with IV crystalloid fluids was continued and oxygen supplementation was discontinued. Two days after admission, the PCV was 16% and the cat became aggressive and began eating. The cat was discharged the following day with a PCV of 18%, and a recheck at the local veterinary clinic that included a CBC was recommended 1 week later. The owner subsequently elected to house Shadow indoors.

Comments: This represents a typical case of hemoplasmosis in a male neutered cat with access to the outdoors. Specific testing for hemoplasmas with PCR was performed on blood smears because treatment with packed RBC and antibiotics had been initiated immediately on admission and whole blood was not saved before treatment was instituted. Although PCR on blood smears has lower sensitivity than when whole liquid blood is used, in this case sufficient organisms were present to generate a positive result, which confirmed the diagnosis of hemoplasmosis. Because the cat was hypovolemic on admission, parenteral antimicrobial treatment was chosen. Subsequently, treatment with oral doxycycline was initiated. Although continued treatment with oral enrofloxacin may have been a suitable alternative to doxycycline, retinal degeneration was a possible adverse effect of continued treatment with enrofloxacin. Retesting for retroviruses was indicated 2 months after the first test was performed at the local veterinary clinic, as the cat may have been exposed to retroviruses but not yet have developed positive test results (see Chapters 21 and 22).

SUGGESTED READINGS

Dowers KL, Tasker S, Radecki SV, et al. Use of pradofloxacin to treat experimentally induced *Mycoplasma haemofelis* infection in cats. Am J Vet Res. 2009;70:105-111.

Tasker S, Helps CR, Day MJ, et al. Use of real-time PCR to detect and quantify *Mycoplasma haemofelis* and "*Candidatus* Mycoplasma haemominutum" DNA. J Clin Microbiol. 2003;41:439-441.

REFERENCES

1. Clark R. *Eperythrozoon felis* (sp. nov.) in a domestic cat. J S Afr Vet Med Assoc. 1942;13:15-16.
2. Kikuth W. Über einen neuen Anämeerreger: *Bartonella canis* nov. spec. Klin Wochenschr. 1928;7:1729-1730.
3. Barker EN, Darby AC, Helps CR, et al. Genome sequence for '*Candidatus* Mycoplasma haemominutum,' a low-pathogenicity hemoplasma species. J Bacteriol. 2012;194:905-906.
4. Barker EN, Helps CR, Peters IR, et al. Complete genome sequence of *Mycoplasma haemofelis*, a hemotropic mycoplasma. J Bacteriol. 2011;193:2060-2061.
5. Santos AP, Guimaraes AM, do Nascimento NC, et al. Genome of *Mycoplasma haemofelis*, unraveling its strategies for survival and persistence. Vet Res. 2011;42:102.
6. Jensen WA, Lappin MR, Kamkar S, et al. Use of a polymerase chain reaction assay to detect and differentiate two strains of *Haemobartonella felis* in naturally infected cats. Am J Vet Res. 2001;62:604-608.
7. Tasker S, Binns SH, Day MJ, et al. Use of a PCR assay to assess the prevalence and risk factors for *Mycoplasma haemofelis* and '*Candidatus* Mycoplasma haemominutum' in cats in the United Kingdom. Vet Rec. 2003;152:193-198.
8. Sykes JE, Drazenovich NL, Ball LM, et al. Use of conventional and real-time polymerase chain reaction to determine the epidemiology of hemoplasma infections in anemic and nonanemic cats. J Vet Intern Med. 2007;21:685-693.
9. George JW, Rideout BA, Griffey SM, et al. Effect of preexisting FeLV infection or FeLV and feline immunodeficiency virus coinfection on pathogenicity of the small variant of *Haemobartonella felis* in cats. Am J Vet Res. 2002;63:1172-1178.
10. Reynolds CA, Lappin MR. '*Candidatus* Mycoplasma haemominutum' infections in 21 client-owned cats. J Am Anim Hosp Assoc. 2007;43:249-257.
11. Willi B, Boretti FS, Cattori V, et al. Identification, molecular characterization, and experimental transmission of a new hemoplasma isolate from a cat with hemolytic anemia in Switzerland. J Clin Microbiol. 2005;43:2581-2585.
12. Willi B, Tasker S, Boretti FS, et al. Phylogenetic analysis of '*Candidatus* Mycoplasma turicensis' isolates from pet cats in the United Kingdom, Australia, and South Africa, with analysis of risk factors for infection. J Clin Microbiol. 2006;44:4430-4435.
13. Peters IR, Helps CR, Willi B, et al. The prevalence of three species of feline haemoplasmas in samples submitted to a diagnostics service as determined by three novel real-time duplex PCR assays. Vet Microbiol. 2008;126:142-150.
14. Tanahara M, Miyamoto S, Nishio T, et al. An epidemiological survey of feline hemoplasma infection in Japan. J Vet Med Sci. 2010;72:1575-1581.
15. Sykes JE, Terry JC, Lindsay LL, et al. Prevalences of various hemoplasma species among cats in the United States with possible hemoplasmosis. J Am Vet Med Assoc. 2008;232:372-379.
16. Willi B, Boretti FS, Baumgartner C, et al. Prevalence, risk factor analysis, and follow-up of infections caused by three feline hemoplasma species in cats in Switzerland. J Clin Microbiol. 2006;44:961-969.
17. Nascimento NC, Santos AP, Guimaraes AM, et al. *Mycoplasma haemocanis* str. Illinois chromosome, complete genome. In: National Center for Biotechnology Information, January 11, 2012 ed. Bethesda, MD: National Institutes of Health; 2012.
18. Kemming GI, Messick JB, Enders G, et al. *Mycoplasma haemocanis* infection—a kennel disease? Comp Med. 2004;54:404-409.
19. Sykes JE, unpublished data, 2012.
20. André MR, Adania CH, Allegretti SM, et al. Hemoplasmas in wild canids and felids in Brazil. J Zoo Wildl Med. 2011;42:342-347.
21. Varanat M, Maggi RG, Linder KE, et al. Molecular prevalence of *Bartonella, Babesia*, and hemotropic *Mycoplasma* sp. in dogs with splenic disease. J Vet Intern Med. 2011;25:1284-1291.
22. Hii SF, Kopp SR, Thompson MF, et al. Canine vector-borne disease pathogens in dogs from south-east Queensland and north-east Northern Territory. Aust Vet J. 2012;90(4):130-135.
23. Woods JE, Brewer MM, Hawley JR, et al. Evaluation of experimental transmission of '*Candidatus* Mycoplasma haemominutum' and *Mycoplasma haemofelis* by *Ctenocephalides felis* to cats. Am J Vet Res. 2005;66:1008-1012.

24. Seneviratna P, Weerasinghe, Ariyadasa S. Transmission of *Haemobartonella canis* by the dog tick, *Rhipicephalus sanguineus*. Res Vet Sci. 1973;14:112-114.
25. Museux K, Boretti FS, Willi B, et al. In vivo transmission studies of '*Candidatus* Mycoplasma turicensis' in the domestic cat. Vet Res. 2009;40:45.
26. Lumb WV. Haemobartonellosis in the dog. In: 8th Gaines Veterinary Symposium 1958;15–16.
27. Maede Y. Studies on feline haemobartonellosis. IV. Lifespan of erythrocytes of cats infected with *Haemobartonella felis*. Nihon Juigaku Zasshi. 1975;37:269-272.
28. Maede Y, Hata R. Studies on feline haemobartonellosis. II. The mechanism of anemia produced by infection with *Haemobartonella felis*. Nihon Juigaku Zasshi. 1975;37:49-54.
29. Zulty JC, Kociba GJ. Cold agglutinins in cats with haemobartonellosis. J Am Vet Med Assoc. 1990;196:907-910.
30. Foley JE, Harrus S, Poland A, et al. Molecular, clinical, and pathologic comparison of two distinct strains of *Haemobartonella felis* in domestic cats. Am J Vet Res. 1998;59:1581-1588.
31. Tasker S, Helps CR, Day MJ, et al. Use of real-time PCR to detect and quantify *Mycoplasma haemofelis* and '*Candidatus* Mycoplasma haemominutum' DNA. J Clin Microbiol. 2003;41:439-441.
32. Harvey DG, Gaskin JM. Feline haemobartonellosis: attempts to induce relapses of clinical disease in chronically infected cats. J Am Anim Hosp Assoc. 1978;14:453.
33. Harvey JW, Gaskin JM. Experimental feline haemobartonellosis. J Am Anim Hosp Assoc. 1977;13:28.
34. Alleman AR, Pate MG, Harvey JW, et al. Western immunoblot analysis of the antigens of *Haemobartonella felis* with sera from experimentally infected cats. J Clin Microbiol. 1999;37:1474-1479.
35. Sykes JE, Henn JB, Kasten RW, et al. *Bartonella henselae* infection in splenectomized domestic cats previously infected with hemotropic *Mycoplasma* species. Vet Immunol Immunopathol. 2007;116:104-108.
36. Berent LM, Messick JB, Cooper SK. Detection of *Haemobartonella felis* in cats with experimentally induced acute and chronic infections, using a polymerase chain reaction assay. Am J Vet Res. 1998;59:1215-1220.
37. Messick JB, Berent LM, Cooper SK. Development and evaluation of a PCR-based assay for detection of *Haemobartonella felis* in cats and differentiation of *H. felis* from related bacteria by restriction fragment length polymorphism analysis. J Clin Microbiol. 1998;36:462-466.
38. Sykes JE, Owens SD, Terry JC, et al. Use of dried blood smears for detection of feline hemoplasmas using real-time polymerase chain reaction. J Vet Diagn Invest. 2008;20:616-620.
39. Novacco M, Wolf-Jackel G, Riond B, et al. Humoral immune response to a recombinant hemoplasma antigen in experimental '*Candidatus* Mycoplasma turicensis' infection. Vet Microbiol. 2012;157:464-470.
40. Barker EN, Helps CR, Heesom KJ, et al. Detection of humoral response using a recombinant heat shock protein 70, DnaK, of *Mycoplasma haemofelis* in experimentally and naturally hemoplasma-infected cats. Clin Vaccine Immunol. 2010;17:1926-1932.
41. Dowers KL, Tasker S, Radecki SV, et al. Use of pradofloxacin to treat experimentally induced *Mycoplasma haemofelis* infection in cats. Am J Vet Res. 2009;70:105-111.
42. Tasker S, Helps CR, Day MJ, et al. Use of a Taqman PCR to determine the response of *Mycoplasma haemofelis* infection to antibiotic treatment. J Microbiol Methods. 2004;56:63-71.
43. Hulme-Moir KL, Barker EN, Stonelake A, et al. Use of real-time quantitative polymerase chain reaction to monitor antibiotic therapy in a dog with naturally acquired *Mycoplasma haemocanis* infection. J Vet Diagn Invest. 2010;22:582-587.
44. Pitorri F, Dell'Orco M, Carmichael N, et al. Use of real-time quantitative PCR to document the successful treatment of *Mycoplasma haemocanis* infection with doxycycline in a dog. Vet Clin Pathol. 2012;41:493-496.
45. Tasker S, Peters IR, Mumford AD, et al. Investigation of human haemotropic *Mycoplasma* infections using a novel generic haemoplasma qPCR assay on blood samples and blood smears. J Med Microbiol. 2010;59:1285-1292.
46. Steer JA, Tasker S, Barker EN, et al. A novel hemotropic *Mycoplasma* (hemoplasma) in a patient with hemolytic anemia and pyrexia. Clin Infect Dis. 2011;53:e147-151.
47. dos Santos AP, dos Santos RP, Biondo AW, et al. Hemoplasma infection in HIV-positive patient. Brazil. Emerg Infect Dis. 2008;14:1922-1924.
48. Sykes JE, Lindsay LL, Maggi RG, et al. Human coinfection with *Bartonella henselae* and two hemotropic mycoplasma variants resembling *Mycoplasma ovis*. J Clin Microbiol. 2010;48:3782-3785.
49. Yuan CL, Liang AB, Yao CB, et al. Prevalence of *Mycoplasma suis* (*Eperythrozoon suis*) infection in swine and swine-farm workers in Shanghai, China. Am J Vet Res. 2009;70:890-894.

CHAPTER 42

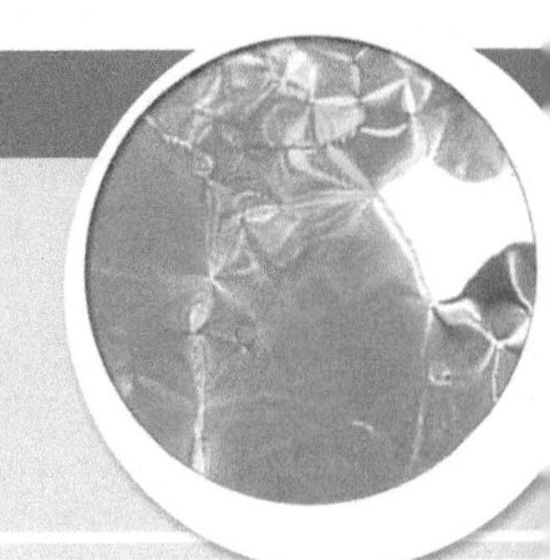

Actinomycosis

Jane E. Sykes

Overview of Actinomycosis

First Described: Actinomycosis was first described in 1877 (in cattle) (Otto Bollinger, Germany)[1]

Causes: *Actinomyces* spp. and *Arcanobacterium* spp. (order Actinomycetales, family Actinomycetaceae)

Geographic Distribution: Worldwide, but especially regions where plant awns are prevalent

Mode of Transmission: Opportunistic invasion of commensal bacteria following disruption of cutaneous or mucosal barriers

Major Clinical Signs: Subcutaneous masses and draining skin lesions (cervicofacial and cutaneous-subcutaneous disease); pulmonary nodules, masses, and/or effusion with cough and tachypnea (thoracic disease); abdominal effusion or masses (abdominal disease); thoracolumbar pain or pelvic limb paresis/paralysis (retroperitoneal disease); rarely neurologic signs due to meningitis or brain abscesses (central nervous system disease).

Differential Diagnoses: Mycobacterial infections, streptomycosis, nocardiosis, bartonellosis, fungal infections, neoplasia

Human Health Significance: Direct transmission of disease from animals to humans does not occur, but humans have developed actinomycosis after bites from healthy dogs or cats.

Etiology and Epidemiology

Actinomycosis is caused by anaerobic or microaerophilic, filamentous, gram-positive bacteria that belong to the genus *Actinomyces* (and to a lesser extent, the related genus *Arcanobacterium*). These organisms are normal inhabitants of mucous membranes, especially of the oropharynx, but also the genital and gastrointestinal tracts, and cause opportunistic infections. Together with other oral commensal bacteria, actinomycetes colonize the periodontal mucosal surfaces and adhere to the tooth surface to form plaque. Numerous *Actinomyces* species have been cultured from the mucous membranes, dental plaque, and saliva of healthy dogs and cats. Organisms isolated from ill dogs and cats with actinomycosis are shown in Box 42-1.[2-15]

Usually, actinomycosis develops when *Actinomyces* spp. are inoculated into tissues along with other bacteria, often as a result of a deeply penetrating wound or foreign body migration. Young adult to middle-age large-breed dogs that have outdoor access are often affected, especially retriever and hunting breeds.[16,17] There is no clear sex predisposition, and the median age of dogs with actinomycosis is approximately 5 years.[18] Actinomycosis in outdoor dogs is often related to exposure to penetrating plant foreign bodies such as grass awns. In cats, actinomycosis usually follows bite wounds and so is more commonly diagnosed in males.[18,19] In the author's hospital, two-thirds (11 of 17) cats with actinomycosis are male. However, underlying retrovirus infection is uncommonly present and does not appear to predispose to disease.

Because *Actinomyces* species are difficult to culture and are susceptible to antimicrobial drugs that are often used empirically, the prevalence of actinomycosis in dogs and cats is probably underestimated.

Clinical Features

Signs and Their Pathogenesis

After ingestion or inhalation, plant awns become contaminated with *Actinomyces* spp. and other bacteria from the oropharynx, and then migrate to various sites and act as a nidus of infection. Alternatively, organisms can be introduced into tissues at the time of a bite wound injury. The latter is the most common route of infection in cats, and can manifest as pyothorax, peritonitis, or cellulitis.[18,19] Other co-infecting aerobic and anaerobic bacteria

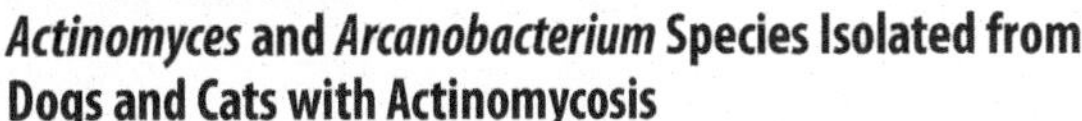

BOX 42-1

Actinomyces and _Arcanobacterium_ Species Isolated from Dogs and Cats with Actinomycosis

Dogs

Actinomyces viscosus[2-4]
Actinomyces bowdenii[5]
Actinomyces hordeovulneris[6]
Actinomyces canis[7]
Actinomyces odontolyticus[8]
Actinomyces catuli[9]
Actinomyces turicensis[10]
Actinomyces hyovaginalis[11]
Actinomyces urogenitalis[11]
Arcanobacterium pyogenes[12]

Cats

Actinomyces viscosus[13,14]
Actinomyces bowdenii[5]
Actinomyces hordeovulneris[11]
Actinomyces meyeri[15]
Actinomyces odontolyticus[14]
Arcanobacterium pyogenes[12]

from the oral cavity or intestinal tract ("companion microbes") undermine normal host defenses and reduce oxygen tension, which allows *Actinomyces* spp. to persist. *Actinomyces* spp. that possess fimbriae can bind to specific cell surface receptors on other bacteria, especially streptococci. This bacterial co-aggregation inhibits the ability of neutrophils to phagocytize the organisms.[20] Dense colonies of *Actinomyces* spp. form, and these, together with other associated bacteria, are surrounded by neutrophils, macrophages, and plasma cells, with slowly progressive pyogranulomatous inflammation (Figure 42-1). Large aggregations of organisms form "sulfur granules," which are tan to yellow colonies of actinomycetes, which can be microscopic or visible grossly. Proteolytic enzymes from the associated bacteria, macrophages, and degranulated neutrophils destroy connective tissue, which facilitates extension of the disease through normal tissue planes. Less often, organisms spread hematogenously to distant sites. In some cases, the inflammatory reaction is accompanied by mass formation and extensive fibrosis. The center of the lesions can eventually suppurate and soften, or draining tracts may develop. The tracts can close and reappear over weeks to months as infection gradually spreads through tissues.

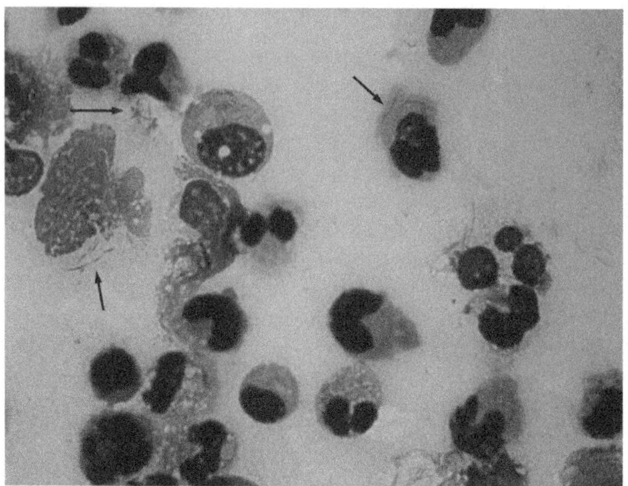

FIGURE 42-1 Abdominal fluid cytology from a 3-year-old male neutered domestic longhair cat with a 1-week history of progressive lethargy and anorexia, ascites, hyperbilirubinemia, and hypoproteinemia. Abdominal fluid analysis revealed a total protein of 2.2 g/dL, and 75,500 nucleated cells/μL, with 92% neutrophils and 8% large mononuclear cells. High numbers of moderately degenerative neutrophils were present with low numbers of macrophages. Moderate numbers of filamentous beaded bacteria were present both in the background and within phagocytes *(arrows)*. *Actinomyces* spp. and *Fusobacterium nucleatum* were isolated from the peritoneal fluid. Necropsy revealed severe, chronic peritonitis with intralesional filamentous bacteria.

The most common clinical forms of actinomycosis in cats and dogs involve the cervicofacial region, thorax, abdomen, and subcutaneous tissue, but central nervous system (CNS) infections (meningitis and meningoencephalitis) and ocular infections (keratitis and endophthalmitis) can also occur.[21,22] *Cervicofacial actinomycosis* can follow bite wounds, perforation of the oropharynx by a foreign body, or chronic periodontal disease. The mandibular, submandibular, and ventral or lateral cervical areas are most frequently affected, but infections that involve the face, retrobulbar space, and temporal area also occur (Figure 42-2, *A* and *B*). *Cutaneous-subcutaneous actinomycosis* typically involves the lateral thoracic wall, flank region, and occasionally the limbs. Lesions on the thoracic or abdominal walls may represent extensions of thoracic, abdominal, or retroperitoneal actinomycosis.

Thoracic actinomycosis may be limited to the lung parenchyma but can involve other thoracic structures, such as the mediastinum, pleura, pericardium, and thoracic wall. It usually follows aspiration of oropharyngeal material, often together with a contaminated grass awn. Alternative routes of thoracic infection include mediastinal involvement after esophageal perforation or direct extension of subcutaneous or abdominal disease. Clinical signs include cough and less commonly hemoptysis, tachypnea, respiratory distress, and subcutaneous

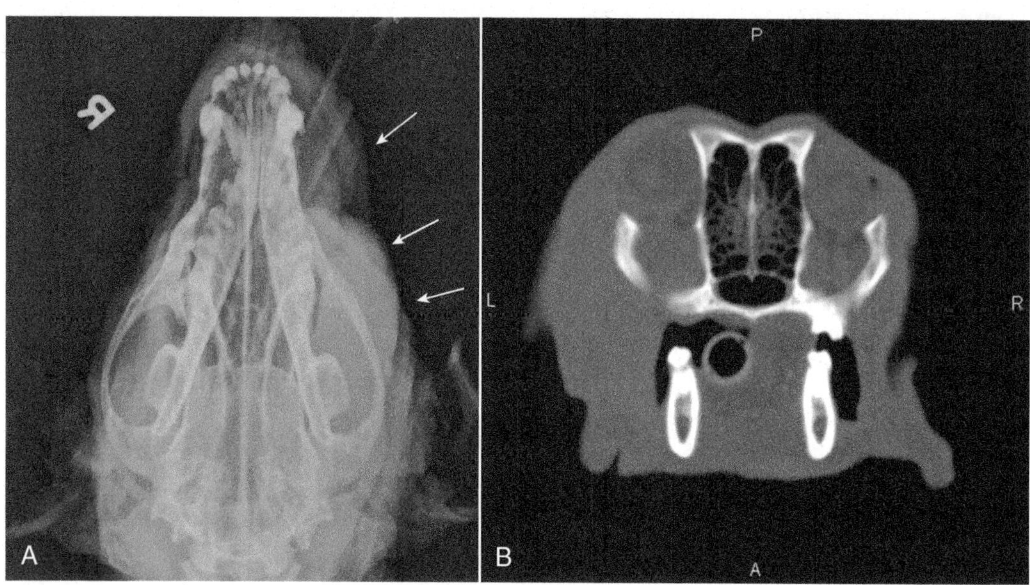

FIGURE 42-2 Cervicofacial actinomycosis in an 8-year-old female spayed Labrador retriever with slowly progressive, left-sided facial swelling. Skull radiograph **(A)** and computed tomographic scan **(B)**. There was severe, regional soft tissue swelling over the left side of the face, which involved the left masseter muscle and zygomatic salivary glands and extended into the retrobulbar space, with secondary exophthalmos. Multiple premolars and molars of the left maxillary arcade were missing. Biopsy of the lesion revealed severe, diffuse, pyogranulomatous cellulitis with intralesional gram-positive, acid-fast negative bacilli. Culture yielded *Actinomyces hordeovulneris* (based on 16S rRNA gene sequencing), *Pasteurella multocida* subsp. *multocida*, *Neisseria canis* (based on 16S rRNA gene sequencing) and an *Eikenella*-like organism.

soft tissue masses or draining skin lesions on the thoracic wall. Sometimes there is a history of neck pain, gagging, or hypersalivation before the onset of tachypnea, possibly due to passage of a penetrating foreign body.

Abdominal actinomycosis develops when ingested foreign bodies penetrate the gastrointestinal tract, which leads to the formation of intra-abdominal mass lesions and ascites.[2,16,23] Abdominal involvement may also follow direct extension from subcutaneous tissues or hematogenous spread of the organism to abdominal organs such as the liver. Although dogs are more often affected than cats, intra-abdominal actinomycotic masses can occur in cats.[24,25] *Retroperitoneal actinomycosis* in dogs often follows the migration of plant awns through the lung and up the crus of the diaphragm to its dorsal attachment. Initially, fever of unknown origin may be the only clinical sign. Ultimately, progression can lead to osteomyelitis and compression fractures of the vertebral bodies, with spinal pain and paresis or paralysis of the pelvic limbs (Figure 42-3).[3,26,27]

Although rare, actinomycosis of the brain and meninges can also occur in dogs (Figure 42-4).[28-30] Brain abscesses may follow hematogenous dissemination from a distant site, or meningitis may result from extension of infection from an adjacent site, such as the middle ear.[29,31] In humans, risk factors for CNS actinomycosis include dental disease or tooth extraction, head trauma, gastrointestinal tract surgery, and chronic otitis, mastoiditis, or sinusitis. CNS actinomycosis has been reported in dogs in association with concurrent otitis media/interna[30] and head trauma,[28] and in cats in association with retrobulbar abscesses[31] and cutaneous abscesses of the tail base.[13,32]

Rarely, *Actinomyces* infections of the urinary bladder,[12,33] gallbladder,[34,35] and heart valve[4,10,36,37] have been recognized in dogs, cats, and human patients.

Physical Examination Findings

Lesions in dogs and cats with cervicofacial or cutaneous-subcutaneous actinomycosis may fluctuant or firm, indurated, have draining sinuses, and rarely are ulcerated. Pain and fever are variable. Thoracic or abdominal actinomycosis is often accompanied by a thin body condition and fever. Dogs and cats with thoracic actinomycosis may show tachypnea or respiratory distress, and thoracic auscultation may reveal decreased lung sounds if pyothorax or intrathoracic mass lesions are present. Masses and/or ascites may be detected on abdominal palpation of dogs with abdominal actinomycosis. Dogs with retroperitoneal actinomycosis can show pain on palpation of the abdomen or spine; signs of pelvic limb paralysis or paresis may be also present, such as pelvic limb ataxia, delayed or absent placing reactions, increased segmental reflexes, and loss of pain sensation. Neurologic signs in dogs with *Actinomyces* meningitis or encephalitis include altered behavior, decreased consciousness, cervical pain, vision loss, ataxia, tetraparesis, and seizures.

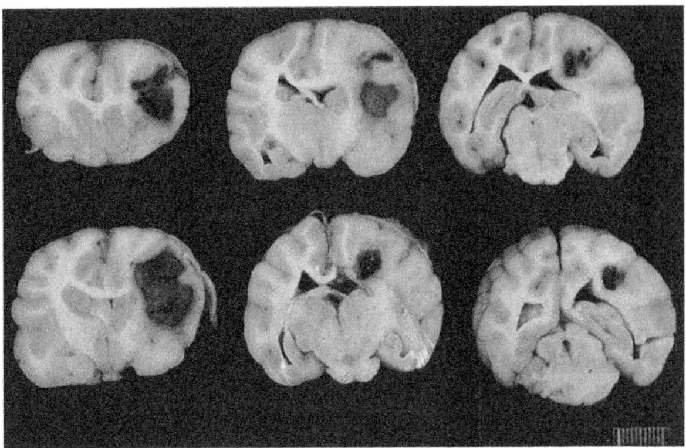

FIGURE 42-4 Necropsy findings in a 1-year-old male neutered Yorkshire terrier with suspected CNS actinomycosis. Three weeks previously, surgery to correct an extrahepatic portosystemic shunt and remove a urate cystolith had been performed. The dog's appetite and activity level did not improve after the surgery, and for the week before the dog was reexamined, disorientation and weakness was noted. The dog deteriorated rapidly after it was hospitalized, and euthanasia was performed. Three separate abscesses were found in the left cerebral cortex. Histopathology revealed neutrophilic inflammation, hemorrhage, and granular mats of material that contained gram-positive, acid-fast negative branching bacteria (consistent with *Actinomyces* spp.), as well as a dense population of gram-negative, Giemsa-positive cocci. (Courtesy University of California, Davis, Veterinary Anatomic Pathology Service.)

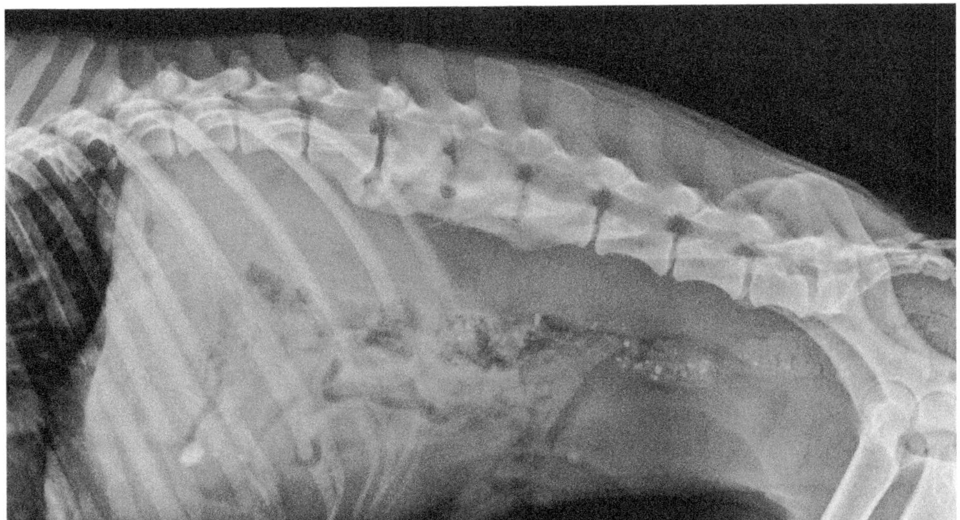

FIGURE 42-3 Left lateral spinal radiograph from a 3-year-old female Border collie with retroperitoneal actinomycosis. The dog was seen for a 3-day history of lethargy, fever, abdominal pain, and progressive pelvic limb paresis. Severe, smoothly marginated ventral spondylosis bridges the L1-L4 space. There is also marked irregular osteolysis of the 2nd, 3rd, and 4th lumbar vertebrae. There is loss of visualization, narrowing, and irregularity of the intervertebral disc spaces at L2-3 and L3-4. There is marked loss of detail within the retroperitoneal space, and the colon is displaced slightly ventrally. Irregular mineral foreign bodies are present in the stomach and colon.

Diagnosis

In the human literature, actinomycosis has been referred to as the "most misdiagnosed disease."[38] Fibrous masses are frequently mistaken for neoplastic lesions, although reports of *Actinomyces* spp. infections that complicate neoplasia exist in human medicine.[39,40] Aspiration of firm lesions is often unrewarding, organisms are often difficult to isolate from lesions, and short periods of antimicrobial drug treatment are ineffective, which all serve to further mislead the clinician to a diagnosis of neoplasia. Actinomycosis should be considered on the list of differential diagnosis in any animal with a history of penetrating plant awn foreign bodies, draining skin lesions, chronic fibrous masses, persistent bite wounds, pyothorax, retroperitoneal abscesses, or focal neurologic signs, especially when young-adult to middle-aged dogs are affected. Ultimately, diagnosis is based on clinical signs, identification of organisms with typical morphology with cytology or histopathology, and culture.

Laboratory Abnormalities

Complete Blood Count, Serum Biochemical Tests, and Urinalysis

Animals with extensive, chronic actinomycosis may have mild to moderate nonregenerative anemia, leukocytosis with a mild to moderate left shift and monocytosis, hypoalbuminemia, and hyperglobulinemia, which may be marked. Dogs with body cavity effusions may be hypoglycemic. There are usually no specific urinalysis findings.

Cytologic Examination of Body Fluids

Cytologic examination of aspirates of abscesses, effusions, or CSF from animals with actinomycosis typically reveals a suppurative to pyogranulomatous inflammatory response (>75% neutrophils). Total protein in pleural fluid is generally greater than 3.0 g/dL, with erythrocyte and nucleated cell counts often greater than 70,000 cells/μL. CSF from dogs and cats with cerebral actinomycosis can grossly resemble pus. Aspirates of firm masses may yield only a small amount of blood. Sulfur granules may be visible in effusion fluid or purulent material from cutaneous lesions, grossly as white to tan to gray granules, or microscopically as dense clusters of organisms. When bacteria are visualized, they may be filamentous rods suggestive of *Actinomyces* spp., or "companion" microorganisms. Actinomycetes are gram-positive, non-acid-fast filamentous organisms that are occasionally branched. The filaments are less than 1 μm wide, vary in length, and can stain irregularly, producing a beaded appearance (see Figure 42-1). *Nocardia* spp., *Corynebacterium* spp., and *Mycobacterium* spp. can be confused with *Actinomyces* species.

Diagnostic Imaging

Plain Radiography

Radiographs of cervicofacial or cutaneous-subcutaneous lesions may show evidence of adjacent osteomyelitis and/or periosteal new bone formation. Pulmonary involvement may manifest as interstitial or alveolar infiltrates, sometimes with consolidation (Figure 42-5, *A*). Air bronchograms may be seen within pulmonary mass lesions, which suggests the presence of a nonneoplastic

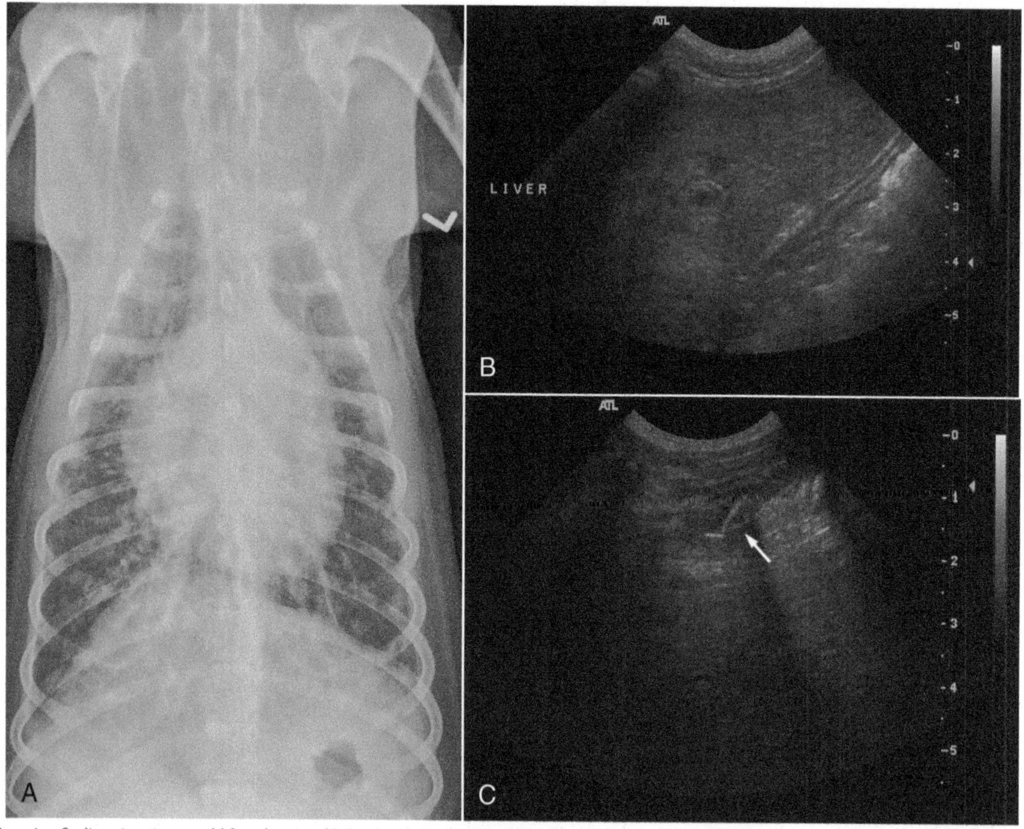

FIGURE 42-5 Imaging findings in a 1-year-old female spayed Labrador retriever with systemic actinomycosis secondary to grass awn migration. **A,** Dorsoventral thoracic radiograph. Patchy diffuse interstitial opacities were present in all lung fields. **B,** Ultrasound image of the liver. Within the left liver, there were focal, ill-defined heteroechoic or hypoechoic nodules. One of these areas (shown) had a hyperechoic rim with echogenic luminal contents. The nodules were consistent with multifocal hepatic abscesses. **C,** Ultrasound image of the thoracic wall. A linear plant awn foreign body was identified *(arrow)*.

process. Other variable findings include pleural thickening, pleural effusion, widening of the mediastinum, pleural mass lesions, enlargement of the cardiac silhouette (with pericardial involvement), and periosteal new bone formation or osteomyelitis involving adjacent ribs, vertebral bodies, or sternebrae. Dogs with retroperitoneal actinomycosis may have periosteal new bone formation on the ventral aspects of two or three adjacent vertebral bodies (usually T13 through L4) on abdominal radiography; involvement of disc spaces is uncommon (see Figure 42-3). Abdominal actinomycosis may be characterized by loss of abdominal detail due to peritoneal effusion and intra-abdominal mass lesions.

Sonographic Findings

Ultrasonography in dogs with actinomycosis can be useful to identify linear grass awn foreign bodies (see Figure 42-5).[41,42] Sonographic abnormalities in dogs with abdominal disease include variable amounts of flocculent ascites fluid, abdominal lymphadenopathy, and nodular or mass lesions that incorporate or displace adjacent structures. New bone formation may be detected on interrogation of the ventral aspects of the vertebral bodies in dogs with retroperitoneal disease.

Advanced Imaging

For animals with CNS involvement, MRI may reveal meningeal thickening, contrast enhancement, and/or intraparenchymal contrast-enhancing mass lesions.[18] MRI may also be useful for detection of grass awn foreign bodies. Advanced imaging allows assessment of the extent of actinomycosis (see Figure 42-2), which can assist with surgical planning.

Microbiologic Tests

Diagnostic assays available for *Actinomyces* infection in dogs and cats are shown in Table 42-1.

Isolation and Identification

Because *Actinomyces* is a commensal of the oral cavity, it is commonly swallowed, inhaled, and transferred by licking; therefore, culture of the organism from the airways, gastrointestinal tract, or skin does not necessarily constitute infection. Consistent cytologic or histopathologic findings (pyogranulomatous inflammation with or without the presence of filamentous bacteria) and the presence of companion microorganisms support the diagnosis of actinomycosis.

Specimens for culture can be collected through fine-needle aspiration or, if possible, biopsy. Because *Actinomyces* species are susceptible to many antimicrobial drugs, treatment of animals before obtaining specimens for culture can also prevent recovery of the organisms. Culture may be negative or yield only "companion" microorganisms, which can obscure the presence of *Actinomyces* spp. As a result, diagnosis is often based only on cytologic or histologic identification of the organism in specimens from animals with appropriate clinical signs.

Most *Actinomyces* spp. that cause disease in dogs and cats are facultative anaerobes, but a few *(A. bovis, A. israelii, A. meyeri)* are obligate anaerobes.[5,7,9,43] The facultative anaerobes can grow under aerobic conditions, and some, such as *A. viscosus,* grow best in these conditions. In addition, "companion" microorganisms are often obligate anaerobes or other aerobes. Therefore, both aerobic and anaerobic cultures should be requested when an *Actinomyces* spp. infection is suspected, and the laboratory should be notified that *Actinomyces* spp. may be present. Tissue specimens, aspirates of pus, or sulfur granules are ideal specimens for anaerobic culture.

Visible growth of *Actinomyces* spp. can occur within 48 hours but usually requires 5 to 7 days. It may be necessary to hold plates 2 to 4 weeks. Species identification using traditional biochemical tests is difficult. PCR amplification and DNA sequence analysis of the 16S rRNA gene may be necessary for precise species identification. In the future, matrix-assisted laser desorption/ionization-time of flight (MALDI-TOF) mass spectrometry may prove most useful for identification of *Actinomyces* species (see Chapter 3).[44]

In addition to actinomycetes, one to five other associated bacteria are often recovered from properly handled specimens. The most commonly isolated organisms are resident flora of the oral cavity or intestinal tract and include the anaerobes *Fusobacterium*, *Peptostreptococcus*, *Prevotella*, or *Bacteroides* spp.; and *Pasteurella multocida, Escherichia coli,* and *Streptococcus* spp. Occasionally, pure cultures of *Actinomyces* spp. are isolated, but this does not exclude the concurrent presence of other organisms, especially strict anaerobes.

TABLE 42-1

Diagnostic Assays Available for *Actinomyces* Infection in Dogs and Cats

Assay	Specimen Type	Target	Performance
Culture	Aspirates of purulent material (e.g., abscesses, pleural effusion), whole blood, CSF, tissue specimens obtained by biopsy or at necropsy (e.g., subcutaneous tissue, heart valve, lung tissue), sulfur granules	*Actinomyces* spp.	Some organisms require anaerobic conditions. Requires several weeks' incubation, and overgrowth by companion bacteria may occur. Because *Actinomyces* spp. are mucosal commensal bacteria, isolation from contaminated sites does not imply disease causation. PCR and sequencing may be required to identify the species present.
Cytology or histopathology with organism detection using special stains	Aspirates or tissue specimens	*Actinomyces* spp. organisms	Organisms are gram positive, do not take up acid-fast stain, and are often accompanied by other bacteria and sulfur granules. Definitive diagnosis requires culture because *Nocardia* can resemble *Actinomyces* spp.

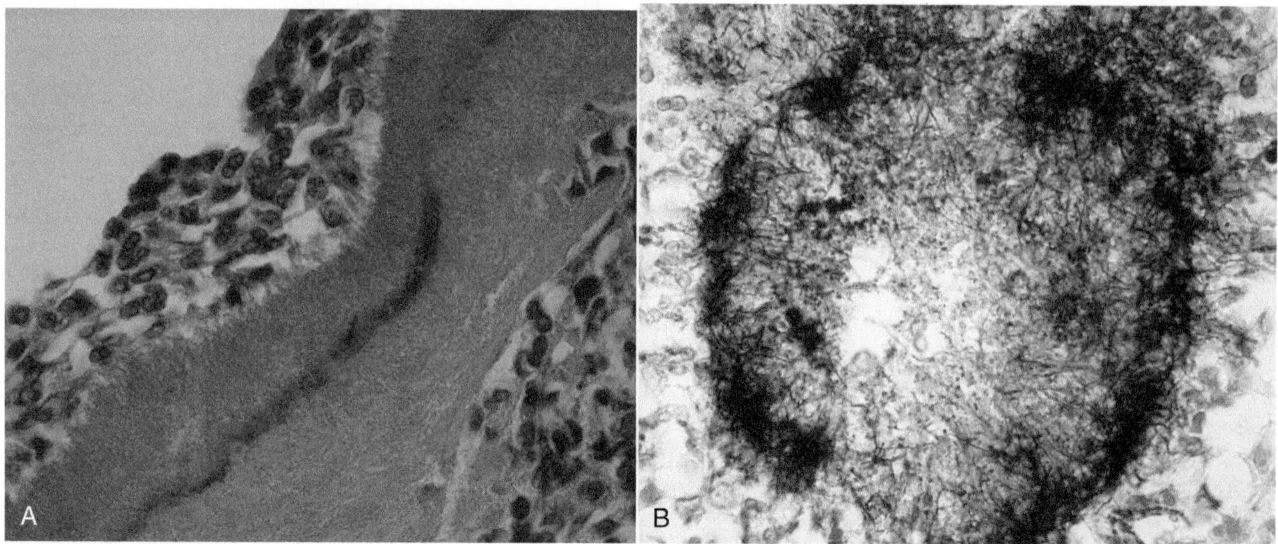

FIGURE 42-6 Histopathology of a biopsy specimen from the xiphoid of a 10-year-old intact male English pointer dog with actinomycosis due to a migrating plant awn foreign body. The dog had a 1-month history of a ventral thoracic wall mass. **A,** Dense, granular mats of branching bacteria were present in a background of extensive granulation tissue and embedded plant material (not shown). H&E stain. **B,** Brown and Benn (gram) stain revealed colonies of gram-positive, filamentous, branching bacteria. *Actinomyces bowdenii* (based on 16S rRNA gene sequencing), *Pasteurella canis, Porphyromonas canoris, Propionibacterium acnes,* a *Bacteroides gingivalis*–like organism, and a *Bacteroides ureolyticus*–like organism were isolated from the lesion.

Molecular Diagnosis Using the Polymerase Chain Reaction

Specific PCR assays for *Actinomyces* spp. have been developed and used for diagnosis of human actinomycosis[45] but are not commercially available for veterinary diagnosis.

Pathologic Findings

Gross lesions in animals with actinomycosis often consist of one or more poorly defined, indurated masses of the subcutaneous tissues, thoracic cavity, lungs, abdominal cavity, or retroperitoneal space, which incorporate adjacent structures. Masses may contain pockets of a reddish-brown exudate. Fistulas, plant material, and sulfur granules may be found. Abdominal or thoracic effusions are often reddish-brown and can contain sulfur granules. Animals with thoracic and abdominal infections may also have a diffuse, red, velvety to granular thickening of the pleura or peritoneum and omentum. Rarely, abscesses are present in the brain, or purulent meningitis is identified.

Histopathology of affected tissues reveals abscesses with a core of neutrophils encapsulated by granulation tissue that contains macrophages, plasma cells, and lymphocytes in a dense, fibrous tissue matrix. When present, sulfur granules are generally in the center of microabscesses, but multiple tissue sections may be needed to find them. In tissue sections stained with hematoxylin and eosin, the granules are round, oval, or scalloped amphophilic solid masses (Figure 42-6). They vary in size from 30 to 3000 μm in diameter and often are rimmed by partially confluent radiating eosinophilic club-shaped structures collectively known as the *Splendore-Hoeppli phenomenon.* This phenomenon can also occur with zygomycosis, sporotrichosis, parasitic infections, foreign body reactions, and hypereosinophilic syndrome.[46,47] Antigen-antibody complexes, complement, and major basic protein of eosinophils have been detected within the Splendore-Hoeppli phenomenon. Special stains (Gram stains, Giemsa and silver stains) are required to stain *Actinomyces* spp. and reveal clumps of tangled, intermittently branched, thin (<1 μm) filaments (see Figure 42-6, *B*). Other nonfilamentous bacteria and/or plant material may also be present. *Actinomyces* are not acid fast. With the rare exception of some *Nocardia* spp. that are not acid fast, other fungi and bacteria that produce tissue granules can be distinguished from *Actinomyces* based on their staining and morphologic properties.

Treatment and Prognosis

Treatment of actinomycosis usually requires prolonged antimicrobial drug treatment. Penicillin is the antimicrobial drug of choice because isolates are uniformly susceptible to penicillins (Table 42-2). High-dose therapy for weeks to months is generally required for animals with chronic infections and extensive fibrosis. In human patients with actinomycosis, high doses of penicillin are given parenterally for 2 to 6 weeks, followed by oral therapy with amoxicillin for 6 to 12 months.[48] If the animal is stable clinically, oral therapy can be tried from the outset.[8,49] Treatment must be extended for weeks to months beyond resolution of measurable disease to prevent relapse; in some cases, treatment for longer than a year may be required.[8,16] However, when actinomycosis is associated with foreign body migration, shorter durations of treatment may be possible if the foreign body is removed, drainage is established, and extensive scar tissue has not formed. Alternative antimicrobial drug choices include clindamycin, doxycycline, chloramphenicol, carbapenems, and ceftriaxone.[48] It is recommended that cephalexin, metronidazole, and aminoglycosides be avoided for treatment of human actinomycosis.[48] Infections associated with companion microbes also usually resolve with penicillin, but on occasion they require broader spectrum antibiotics during the initial treatment period followed by long-term administration of penicillin.

Excepting when foreign body material is present (Figure 42-7), surgery has a controversial role in the treatment of actinomycosis, but may be required if there is extensive fibrous tissue formation or large accumulations of purulent material to facilitate

TABLE 42-2

Medications That Could Be Used to Treat *Actinomyces* spp. Infections in Dogs and Cats with Actinomycosis

Drug	Dose	Route	Interval (hours)
Penicillin G	100,000 U/kg	IV, IM	6-8
Ampicillin sodium	20	IV, IM, SC	6-8
Amoxicillin	20	PO	8
Clindamycin*	11	PO	12 (dogs), 24 (cats)
Doxycycline†	5-10	PO	12-24

*For IV administration of clindamycin phosphate, see Chapter 8.
†10 mg/kg q12h preferred if tolerated without gastrointestinal adverse effects. Doxycycline hyclate or clindamycin should always be administered with a bolus of water to avoid esophagitis.

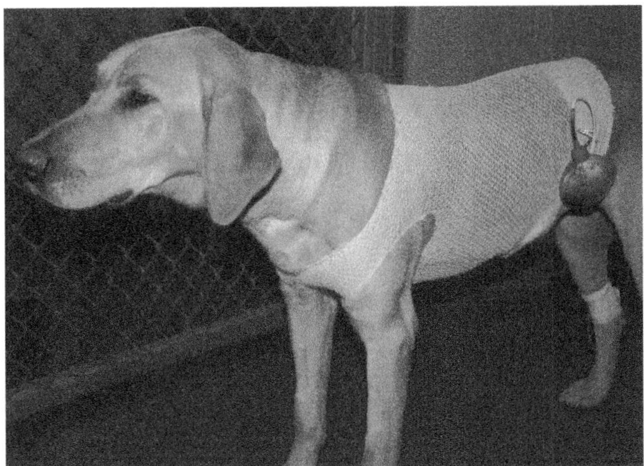

FIGURE 42-7 One-year-old female spayed Labrador retriever with systemic actinomycosis secondary to a plant awn foreign body after surgical removal of the plant awn and placement of a grenade drain.

drug penetration (see Chapter 87 for information on management of pyothorax). In human medicine, an initial attempt to control disease with aggressive medical therapy alone has been suggested, with surgical therapy if the response to treatment is inadequate.[48] In animals with pulmonary abscesses, removal of affected lung lobes may be required. Fibrotic lesions are often extensively vascularized and may obliterate tissue planes, which complicates dissection. In dogs with solitary masses that involve the thoracic and abdominal walls, radical surgical excision is often curative, but repeat surgeries may be needed. An initial period of antibiotic therapy may reduce the size of lesions and improve lesion definition, which facilitates surgery followed by continued antimicrobial drug treatment at a later date. Surgery is also required if a nidus such as a grass awn is present.

Appropriate treatment of actinomycosis results in a cure rate of greater than 90%.[8,16,50] Cure rates with meningitis/meningoencephalitis and advanced thoracic or peritoneal disease with extensive mass lesions may be lower.

Prevention

Prevention of actinomycosis involves restriction of access to areas with extensive grass awn formation and avoidance of fighting and biting activity between animals. When wounds occur, they should be carefully examined for foreign material and cleaned promptly. Plant awns found on animals' coats should be removed and discarded as soon as possible and the finding of one should prompt a thorough search for others.

Public Health Aspects

No reports exist of actinomycosis being transmitted from clinically infected animals to humans or other animals; however, humans bitten by dogs, cats, or other people can develop actinomycosis (see Chapter 57).[51] The most common species that infects humans is *A. israelii*.[48] This is a commensal of the canine oral cavity but has not been isolated from dogs or cats with actinomycosis. Nevertheless, *A. viscosus, A. odontolyticus,* and *A. meyeri* have been isolated from canine and feline as well as human actinomycosis.

CASE EXAMPLE

Signalment: "Penny", a 1-year-old, female spayed Labrador retriever from Herald in northern California

History: Penny was evaluated by the University of California, Davis, veterinary emergency service for a 1-week history of progressive inappetence, weight loss, lethargy, and fever. Two days before she was evaluated, Penny vomited up some kibble, and had not eaten anything since. The owner reported that her feces had been formed and there were no changes in thirst or urination. Earlier the same day, Penny had been evaluated at another veterinary clinic where a grade IV/VI left-sided cardiac murmur was auscultated and thoracic radiographs showed a bronchoalveolar and interstitial lung pattern. She was treated with cefazolin (27 mg/kg IV) and furosemide (1 mg/kg SC) and referred. Penny had been fully vaccinated for canine distemper virus, canine parvovirus, canine adenovirus, and rabies. She had missed some doses of heartworm prophylaxis medication recently and received no other medications. She lived with three other healthy

Labrador retrievers. She roamed on 8 acres of land, and there was a pond on the property where she swam and was known to eat crayfish and frogs. Her usual diet consisted of a commercial dry puppy food. Seven months earlier, she had been evaluated at another veterinary clinic for vomiting and inappetence. At that time she was moderately azotemic; an exploratory laparotomy was performed for a suspected foreign body, but no foreign body was found.

Physical Examination:

Body Weight: 22.5 kg

General: Quiet, alert, responsive and wagging tail. Approximately 5% dehydrated. T = 105.2°F (40.7°C), HR 160 beats/min, RR = 42 breaths/min. Pink, slightly tacky mucous membranes, CRT < 2 s.

Integument: Full clean haircoat, no evidence of ectoparasites.

Eyes, Ears, Nose, and Throat: No clinically significant abnormalities were noted.

Musculoskeletal: BCS 3/9. Generalized mild muscle atrophy was present.

Cardiovascular: A grade II/VI left systolic murmur was auscultated. Femoral pulses were strong, regular, and synchronous.

Respiratory: Increased breath sounds were present bilaterally and diffusely. There was a mild increase in respiratory effort.

All Other Systems: No clinically significant abnormalities were noted.

Laboratory Findings:

CBC:

HCT 24.0% (40%-55%),
MCV 65.6 fL (65-75 fL)
MCHC 35.0 g/dL (33-36 g/dL)
WBC 29,850 cells/μL (6000-13,000 cells/μL)
Neutrophils 16,119 cells/μL (3000-10,500 cells/μL)
Lymphocytes 2985 cells/μL (1000-4000 cells/μL)
Monocytes 7761 cells/μL (150-1200 cells/μL)
Eosinophils 0 cells/μL (0-1500 cells/μL)
Basophils 0 cells/μL (0-50 cells/μL)
Platelets 98,000 platelets/μL (150,000-400,000 platelets/μL)
MPV 20.1 fL (7-13 fL).

A few slightly toxic band neutrophils and moderate numbers of macroplatelets were present.

Serum Chemistry Profile:

Sodium 144 mmol/L (145-154 mmol/L)
Potassium 4.3 mmol/L (3.6-5.3 mmol/L)
Chloride 114 mmol/L (108-118 mmol/L)
Bicarbonate 15 mmol/L (16-26 mmol/L)
Phosphorus 5.3 mg/dL (3.0-6.2 mg/dL)
Calcium 9.6 mg/dL (9.7-11.5 mg/dL)
BUN 22 mg/dL (5-21 mg/dL)
creatinine 0.8 mg/dL (0.3-1.2 mg/dL)
Glucose 44 mg/dL (64-123 mg/dL)
Total protein 7.8 g/dL (5.4-7.6 g/dL)
Albumin 2.5 g/dL (3.0-4.4 g/dL)
Globulin 5.3 g/dL (1.8-3.9 g/dL)
ALT 31 U/L (19-67 U/L)
AST 76 U/L (19-42 U/L)
ALP 612 U/L (21-170 U/L)
Gamma GT 5 U/L (0-6 U/L)
Cholesterol 292 mg/dL (135-361 mg/dL)
Total bilirubin 0.8 mg/dL (0-0.2 mg/dL)

Urinalysis: SGr 1.016; pH 5.0, 1+ protein (SSA), 1+ bilirubin, 2+ hemoprotein, 1+ glucose, 0-1 WBC/HPF, 0-3 RBC/HPF, rare granular casts, many amorphous crystals, rare bilirubin crystals, many lipid droplets

Coagulation Panel: PT 7.7 s (7.5-10.5 s), APTT 15.2 s (9-12 s), fibrinogen 232 mg/dL (90-255 mg/dL), D-dimer 1.0-2.0 μg/mL (0-0.25 μg/mL).

Imaging Findings:

Thoracic Radiographs (3 View): There were patchy diffuse unstructured interstitial opacities in all lung lobes (see Figure 42-5, *A*). Cardiovascular structures appeared within normal limits. The liver was markedly enlarged.

Echocardiography: The left ventricle was eccentrically hypertrophied. The papillary muscles had normal shape and echogenicity. There was no enlargement of the left atrium. There was no evidence of endocarditis. Decreased fractional shortening (26%; reference range, approximately 34%-46%) and increased end systolic diameter (3.9 cm; reference range, approximately 1.8-3.5 cm) and E-point septal separation (6.8 mm) were indicative of systolic dysfunction, which could also be appreciated subjectively. There was mild tricuspid regurgitation and trivial pulmonic insufficiency. Conclusions: Moderate systolic dysfunction. It was recommended that the dog's diet and taurine blood/plasma levels be evaluated. It was also considered possible that the dog's febrile state was responsible for some of abnormalities observed on the echocardiogram.

Abdominal Ultrasound: The liver was diffusely mottled, particularly in the left caudal region (see Figure 42-5, *B*). Within the left caudal liver, there was a focal, ill-defined heteroechoic area approximately 1 cm in diameter. Other smaller, ill-defined hypoechoic nodules were also present within the left liver. One of these areas had a well-demarcated, hyperechoic rim with irregular echogenic luminal contents and measured approximately 0.5 cm in diameter. Multiple large mesenteric lymph nodes were just caudal to the liver; the largest measured 1.3 cm by 4.5 cm. There was a small amount of anechoic free abdominal fluid. The spleen was moderately enlarged, but the echotexture and echogenicity appeared within normal limits. There was mild renal pyelectasia bilaterally, but the renal papillae appeared within normal limits.

Microbiologic Testing: Aerobic and anaerobic blood cultures (five specimens): Negative

IFA serology for serum antibody to *Ehrlichia canis, Anaplasma phagocytophilum, Rickettsia rickettsii,* and *Babesia canis*: Negative

IFA serology for serum antibody to *Bartonella vinsonii* subsp. *berkhoffii, Bartonella clarridgeiae,* and *Bartonella henselae*: Negative

Bartonella culture (whole blood): Negative

Serology for *Coccidioides* serum antibodies: Negative

Cytologic Findings:

Splenic Aspirate (Ultrasound-Guided): Two smears were examined that contained a large amount of blood in the background and were highly cellular. Several small clumps of splenic stromal cells were noted. A large heterogeneous population of lymphocytes was found, with a moderate increase in plasma cells. A moderate number of hematopoietic cells was also present, including megakaryocytes, myeloid, and erythroid precursors. Interpretation: Moderate reactive lymphoid hyperplasia and extramedullary hematopoiesis.

Liver Aspirate (Ultrasound-Guided): Smears contained a diffusely stippled background with abundant nuclear debris and were highly cellular. A large population of mildly to markedly degenerate neutrophils were observed. Degenerate cells ranged from highly pyknotic to severely karyolytic. A few neutrophils contained small intracellular bacterial rods. Interpretation: Marked suppurative inflammation with bacterial sepsis.

Further Microbiologic Testing:

Aerobic and Anaerobic Culture (Ultrasound-Guided Liver Aspirate): Small numbers of suspect *Actinomyces* spp. No anaerobes cultured. Partial 16S rRNA gene PCR and sequence analysis revealed 99% identity to *Actinomyces bowdenii*.

Diagnosis: Systemic *A. bowdenii* infection with hepatic involvement

Treatment: Immediately on admission, Penny was treated with IV lactated Ringer's solution with 20 mEq/L KCl and 5% dextrose at 75 mL/hr. After the specimens for blood culture were collected, treatment with enrofloxacin (10 mg/kg IV q24h) and ampicillin (22 mg/kg IV q8h) was initiated. Within 24 hours, the dog's rectal temperature had decreased to 101.3°F (38.5°C), the blood glucose had increased from 41 mg/dL to 107 mg/dL, and Penny began eating. The liver aspirate was submitted for culture on day 2 of hospitalization. A recheck abdominal ultrasound examination on day 3 showed progressive abscessation of the left liver and further enlargement of the gastrohepatic lymph nodes. By day 4 of hospitalization, growth of an organism resembling an *Actinomyces* sp. was reported. On day 5, antimicrobial drug treatment was changed to clavulanic acid–amoxicillin (17 mg/kg q8h). However, later in the day, Penny's temperature increased to 103.6°F (39.8°C), and so the initial antimicrobial drug prescription was reinstated. The dog's hematocrit had also dropped to 19%. Thoracic radiographs were repeated and showed almost complete resolution of the patchy pulmonary infiltrates. A follow-up echocardiogram was unchanged. Abdominal ultrasound examination was again repeated and showed persistent hypoechogenicity of the left liver lobe, but during the procedure a hyperechoic lesion that was consistent with a plant awn foreign body was discovered in the subcutaneous tissue in a caudoventral intercostal space. On day 6, surgery was performed to remove the plant awn. Packed red cells were administered during the procedure, and a 16F thoracostomy tube was placed because the thoracic cavity was entered during the search for the foxtail, which, with the assistance of intraoperative ultrasound examination, was eventually located under the 13th rib just outside the pleural space. Sulfur granules were found embedded in the tissue during surgery. A closed suction grenade drain was also placed (see Figure 42-7). The thoracostomy tube was removed later in the day. Treatment with enrofloxacin and ampicillin was continued, as well as with oxymorphone (0.04 mg/kg SC q6h) to control pain. On day 7, Penny's temperature was 100.7°F (38.2°C), and the drain was removed. Aerobic and anaerobic culture of the foxtail revealed small numbers of penicillin-susceptible *Enterococcus faecalis* and an organism resembling a *Streptomyces* sp. No anaerobes were cultured. Penny was discharged on day 8 with instructions to continue treatment with clavulanic acid–amoxicillin for an additional month. The dog had no further clinical signs of illness.

Comments: This is an unusual case of disseminated *A. bowdenii* infection that led to hematogenous pneumonia and hepatic abscessation. Although there was an initial defervescence with antimicrobial drug treatment, anemia and pyrexia persisted, which led to a search for an abscess that might require drainage or a plant awn. Fortunately, a plant awn was ultimately identified with ultrasound and removed, after which the dog's illness resolved completely. *E. faecalis* was isolated from the plant awn and represented a "companion microbe," but whether dissemination of this organism occurred was unclear. The *Streptomyces* sp. may have been a contaminant, or the *Actinomyces* sp. that was misidentified. The owner was warned that additional plant awns might still be present. The cause of the cardiomyopathy was not determined; plasma and whole blood taurine concentrations were within normal limits, and follow-up examination was not performed.

SUGGESTED READINGS

Barnes LD, Grahn BH. *Actinomyces* endophthalmitis and pneumonia in a dog. Can Vet J. 2007;48:1155-1158.

Edwards DF, Nyland TG, Weigel JP. Thoracic, abdominal, and vertebral actinomycosis. Diagnosis and long-term therapy in three dogs. J Vet Intern Med. 1988;2:184-191.

Kirpensteijn J, Fingland RB. Cutaneous actinomycosis and nocardiosis in dogs: 48 cases (1980-1990). J Am Vet Med Assoc. 1992;201:917-920.

REFERENCES

1. Bollinger O. Über eine neue Pilmkrankheit beim Rinde. Zbl Med Wissensch. 1877;15:481-485.
2. Georg LK, Brown JM, Baker HJ, et al. *Actinomyces viscosus* as an agent of actinomycosis in the dog. Am J Vet Res. 1972;33:1457-1470.
3. Davenport AA, Carter GR, Schirmer RG. Canine actinomycosis due to *Actinomyces viscosus*: report of six cases. Vet Med Small Anim Clin. 1974;69:1442, 1444-1447.
4. Meurs KM, Heaney AM, Atkins CE, et al. Comparison of polymerase chain reaction with bacterial 16S primers to blood culture to identify bacteremia in dogs with suspected bacterial endocarditis. J Vet Intern Med. 2011;25:959-962.
5. Pascual C, Foster G, Falsen E, et al. *Actinomyces bowdenii* sp. nov., isolated from canine and feline clinical specimens. Int J Syst Bacteriol. 1999;49(Pt 4):1873-1877.
6. Buchanan AM, Scott JL. *Actinomyces hordeovulneris*, a canine pathogen that produces L-phase variants spontaneously with coincident calcium deposition. Am J Vet Res. 1984;45:2552-2560.
7. Hoyles L, Falsen E, Foster G, et al. *Actinomyces coleocanis* sp. nov., from the vagina of a dog. Int J Syst Evol Microbiol. 2002;52:1201-1203.
8. Edwards DF, Nyland TG, Weigel JP. Thoracic, abdominal, and vertebral actinomycosis. Diagnosis and long-term therapy in three dogs. J Vet Intern Med. 1988;2:184-191.
9. Hoyles L, Falsen E, Pascual C, et al. *Actinomyces catuli* sp. nov., from dogs. Int J Syst Evol Microbiol. 2001;51:679-682.

10. Junius G, Bavegems V, Stalpaert M, et al. Mitral valve endocarditis in a Labrador retriever caused by an actinomyces species identified as *Actinomyces turicensis*. J Vet Intern Med. 2004;18:899-901.
11. Sykes JE, Unpublished observations, 2012.
12. Billington SJ, Post KW, Jost BH. Isolation of *Arcanobacterium (Actinomyces) pyogenes* from cases of feline otitis externa and canine cystitis. J Vet Diagn Invest. 2002;14:159-162.
13. Bestetti G, Bühlman V, Nicolet J, et al. Paraplegia due to *Actinomyces viscosus* infection in a cat. Acta Neuropathol (Berl). 1977;39:231-235.
14. Love DN, Jones RF, Bailey M, et al. Isolation and characterisation of bacteria from abscesses in the subcutis of cats. J Med Microbiol. 1979;12:207-212.
15. Love DN, Jones RF, Bailey M, et al. Isolation and characterisation of bacteria from pyothorax (empyaemia) in cats. Vet Microbiol. 1982;7:455-461.
16. Hardie EM, Barsanti JA. Treatment of canine actinomycosis. J Am Vet Med Assoc. 1982;180:537-541.
17. Kirpensteijn J, Fingland RB. Cutaneous actinomycosis and nocardiosis in dogs: 48 cases (1980-1990). J Am Vet Med Assoc. 1992;201:917-920.
18. Sykes JE. Actinomycosis and nocardiosis. In: Greene CE, ed. Infectious Diseases of the Dog and Cat. 4th ed. St. Louis: Elsevier Saunders; 2012:484-495.
19. Love DN, Jones RF, Bailey M, et al. Bacteria isolated from subcutaneous abscesses in cats. Aust Vet Pract. 1978;8:87-90.
20. Ochiai K, Kurita-Ochiai T, Kamino Y, et al. Effect of co-aggregation on the pathogenicity of oral bacteria. J Med Microbiol. 1993;39:183-190.
21. Ledbetter EC, Scarlett JM. Isolation of obligate anaerobic bacteria from ulcerative keratitis in domestic animals. Vet Ophthalmol. 2008;11:114-122.
22. Barnes LD, Grahn BH. *Actinomyces* endophthalmitis and pneumonia in a dog. Can Vet J. 2007;48:1155-1158.
23. Chastain CB, Grier RL, Hogle RM, et al. Actinomycotic peritonitis in a dog. J Am Vet Med Assoc. 1976;168:499-501.
24. Kawamura N, Shimada A, Morita T, et al. Intraperitoneal actinomycosis in a cat. Vet Rec. 2005;157:593-594.
25. Sharman MJ, Goh CS, Kuipers von Lande RG, et al. Intra-abdominal actinomycetoma in a cat. J Feline Med Surg. 2009;11:701-705.
26. Frendin J, Greko C, Hellmén E, et al. Thoracic and abdominal wall swellings in dogs caused by foreign bodies. J Small Anim Pract. 1994;35:499-508.
27. Johnson DE, Summers BA. Osteomyelitis of the lumbar vertebral in dogs caused by grass-seed foreign bodies. Aust Vet J. 1971;47:289-294.
28. Anvik JO, Lewis R. *Actinomyces* encephalitis associated with hydrocephalus in a dog. Can Vet J. 1976;17:42-44.
29. Couto SS, Dickinson PJ, Jang S, et al. Pyogranulomatous meningoencephalitis due to *Actinomyces* sp. in a dog. Vet Pathol. 2000;37:650-652.
30. Sturges BK, Dickinson PJ, Kortz GD, et al. Clinical signs, magnetic resonance imaging features, and outcome after surgical and medical treatment of otogenic intracranial infection in 11 cats and 4 dogs. J Vet Intern Med. 2006;20:648-656.
31. Barrs VR, Nicoll RG, Churcher RK, et al. Intracranial empyema: literature review and two novel cases in cats. J Small Anim Pract. 2007;48:449-454.
32. Stowater JL. Actinomycosis in the spinal canal of cat. Feline Pract. 1978;8:26-27.
33. Dhamborvorn T, Tritipsatit S, Meemongkoldilok S. Actinomycosis of the urinary bladder. J Med Assoc Thai. 2001;84:109-112.
34. Ormsby AH, Bauer TW, Hall GS. Actinomycosis of the cholecystic duct: case report and review. Pathology. 1998;30:65-67.
35. Harvey AM, Holt PE, Barr FJ, et al. Treatment and long-term follow-up of extrahepatic biliary obstruction with bilirubin cholelithiasis in a Somali cat with pyruvate kinase deficiency. J Feline Med Surg. 2007;9:424-431.
36. Sykes JE, Kittleson MD, Pesavento PA, et al. Evaluation of the relationship between causative organisms and clinical characteristics of infective endocarditis in dogs: 71 cases (1992-2005). J Am Vet Med Assoc. 2006;228:1723-1734.
37. Mardis JS, Many Jr WJ. Endocarditis due to *Actinomyces viscosus*. South Med J. 2001;94:240-243.
38. Cope VZ. Visceral actinomycosis. Ann R Coll Surg Engl. 1949;5:394-410.
39. Afolabi IR, Shashidhar VM. Carcinoma of the oesophagus masquerading as actinomycosis: a case report and a review of literature. Pac Health Dialog. 2004;11:94-95.
40. Batur Calis A, Ozbal AE, Basak T, et al. Laryngeal actinomycosis accompanying laryngeal carcinoma: Report of two cases. Eur Arch Otorhinolaryngol. 2006;263:783-785.
41. Frendin J. Diagnostic imaging of back pain. J Small Anim Pract. 1999;40:278-285.
42. Sivacolundhu RK, O'Hara AJ, Read RA. Thoracic actinomycosis (arcanobacteriosis) or nocardiosis causing thoracic pyogranuloma formation in three dogs. Aust Vet J. 2001;79:398-402.
43. Hoyles L, Falsen E, Pascual C, et al. *Actinomyces catuli* sp. nov., from dogs. Int J Syst Evol Microbiol. 2001;51:679-682.
44. Ng LS, Sim JH, Eng LC, et al. Comparison of phenotypic methods and matrix-assisted laser desorption ionisation time-of-flight mass spectrometry for the identification of aero-tolerant *Actinomyces* spp. isolated from soft-tissue infections. Eur J Clin Microbiol Infect Dis. 2011.
45. Fujita Y, Iikura M, Horio Y, et al. Pulmonary *Actinomyces graevenitzii* infection presenting as organizing pneumonia diagnosed by PCR analysis. J Med Microbiol. 2012;61:1156-1158.
46. Read RW, Zhang J, Albini T, et al. Splendore-Hoeppli phenomenon in the conjunctiva: immunohistochemical analysis. Am J Ophthalmol. 2005;140:262-266.
47. Sykes JE, Weiss DJ, Buoen LC, et al. Idiopathic hypereosinophilic syndrome in 3 Rottweilers. J Vet Intern Med. 2001;15:162-166.
48. Russo TA. Agents of actinomycosis. In: Mandell GL, Bennett JE, Dolin R, eds. Principles and Practice of Infectious Diseases. 7th ed. Philadelphia, PA: Elsevier; 2010:3209-3219.
49. Nelson JD, Hermann DW. Oral penicillin therapy for thoracic actinomycosis. Pediatr Infect Dis. 1986;5:594-595.
50. Frendin J. Pyogranulomatous pleuritis with empyema in hunting dogs. Zentralbl Vet Med. 1997;44:167-178.
51. Reiner SL, Harrelson JM, Miller SE, et al. Primary actinomycosis of an extremity: a case report and review. Rev Infect Dis. 1987;9:581-589.

CHAPTER 43

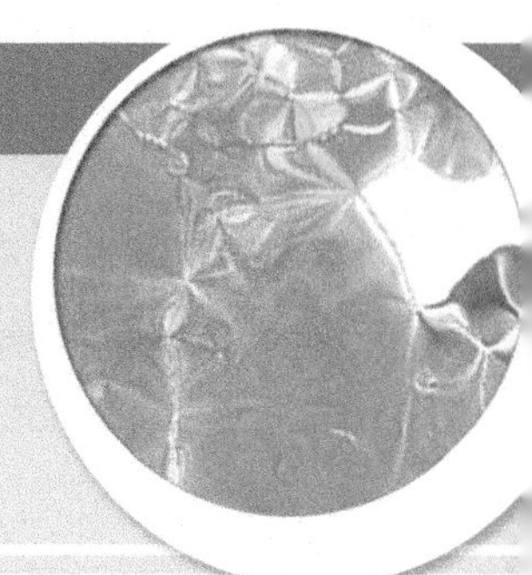

Nocardiosis

Jane E. Sykes

> **Overview of Nocardiosis**
>
> First Described: 1888, Alfort, France (Edmond Nocard)[1]
>
> Causes: *Nocardia* spp. (order Actinomycetales, family Nocardiaceae)
>
> Geographic Distribution: Worldwide, although infections in dogs and cats are most commonly reported from Brazil, the western United States, and Australia
>
> Mode of Transmission: Inhalation or cutaneous inoculation of organisms in the environment, with opportunistic proliferation in the face of impaired host immune defenses
>
> Major Clinical Signs: Lethargy, weight loss, inappetence; subcutaneous masses and nonhealing, crusted, or draining skin lesions; pulmonary nodules, masses and/or effusion with cough and tachypnea; signs of dissemination (neurologic signs, chorioretinitis, abdominal effusion or masses, lameness)
>
> Differential Diagnoses: Actinomycosis, streptomycosis, mycobacteriosis, bartonellosis, fungal infections, neoplasia, leishmaniosis
>
> Human Health Significance: Direct transmission of disease from animals to humans does not occur, but humans have developed disease after bites or scratches from healthy dogs or cats.

Etiology and Epidemiology

Nocardia are filamentous, branching, gram-positive bacteria that belong to the family Nocardiaceae (Figure 43-1). More than 50 *Nocardia* species have been recognized since the advent of molecular identification methods, approximately half of which are human and animal pathogens.[2] The advent of molecular methods has also led to extensive revision of the taxonomy of *Nocardia* spp. Species that belong to the former *N. asteroides* complex are now considered distinct species and include *Nocardia cyriacigeorgica* (formerly *N. asteroides* sensu stricto), *Nocardia abscessus, Nocardia nova, Nocardia farcinica,* and *Nocardia otitidiscaviarum*.[2] Knowledge of the species involved is clinically important, because each *Nocardia* species differs in its antimicrobial susceptibility patterns, epidemiology, and pathogenicity. They also differ in their cell wall mycolic acid content, which affects their ability to stain with acid-fast stains.

Like actinomycosis, nocardiosis is a suppurative to granulomatous, localized, or disseminated opportunistic infection caused by filamentous bacteria. However, unlike *Actinomyces* spp. (which are commensals of mucous membranes), *Nocardia* spp. are ubiquitous soil saprophytes that degrade organic matter. They are also found in fresh and salt water, in dust, and on decaying plants and fecal matter.[2] They can be carried mechanically on the claws or skin. Infections are acquired via inhalation of organisms or inoculation via puncture wounds. Transfer of infection between animals does not occur.

Nocardiosis is much less frequently reported in dogs and cats than actinomycosis, although nocardiosis is increasingly recognized in both human medicine and companion animals in association with immunocompromise, such as occurs with potent immunosuppressive drug therapy (especially cyclosporine).[3-5] Where vaccination for canine distemper virus (CDV) is inadequate or not widely instituted, nocardiosis in dogs has been associated with CDV-induced immunosuppression.[6]

The prevalence of nocardiosis and the predominant *Nocardia* species that cause disease vary geographically. For example, within the United States, human nocardiosis has been most commonly reported from the southwestern states. Dry, dusty, and windy conditions in these areas may facilitate aerosolization and dispersal of nocardiae.[7] Dogs and cats from Australia and the western United States are most commonly infected with *Nocardia nova*.[8-10] Other species isolated from dogs and cats are shown in Table 43-1.[11-16] In humans, *Nocardia brasiliensis* is the most common species isolated from patients that reside in tropical locations such as the southwestern United States, Central and South America, and Australia.

More than 60% of people with nocardiosis have underlying immunosuppressive disorders such as AIDS, chronic obstructive pulmonary disease, autoimmune diseases that require immunosuppressive drug therapy, solid organ transplantation, diabetes

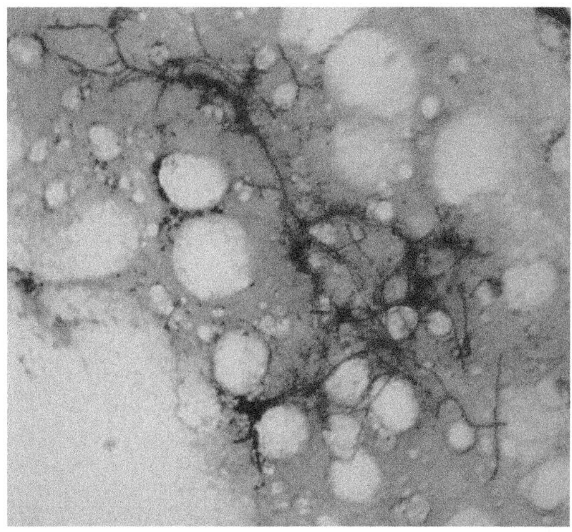

FIGURE 43-1 Gram-stained smear showing *Nocardia* spp. The organisms are gram-positive, filamentous, branching, and slightly beaded.

TABLE 43-1

Nocardia Species Isolated from Dogs and Cats with Nocardiosis

Host Species	Dogs	Country
Dogs	*N. nova*	United States, Australia[8,9]
	N. paucivorans	United States[9]
	N. asiatica	United States[9]
	N. abscessus	United States[5]
	N. otitidiscaviarum	Brazil[6]
	N. farcinica	Australia[8]
Cats	*N. nova*	United States, Australia[9]
	N. cyriacigeorgica	Australia[8]
	N. africana	Japan,[11] Brazil[12]
	N. elegans	Japan[13]
	N. brasiliensis	United States[14]
	N. otitidiscaviarum	Spain[15]
	N. tenerifensis	United States[16]

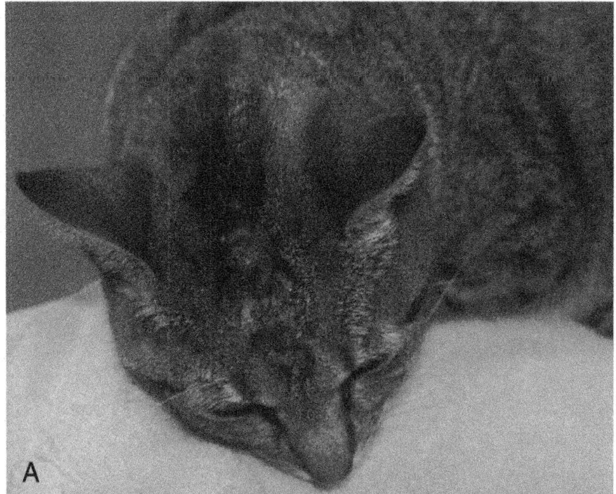

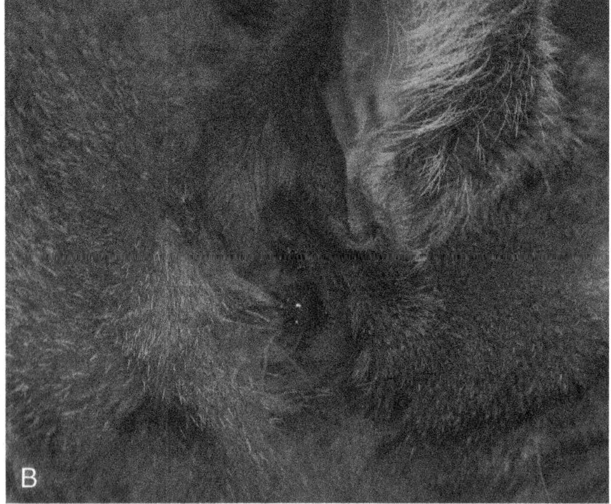

FIGURE 43-2 Six-year-old male neutered domestic shorthair cat with cutaneous-subcutaneous nocardiosis. The lesions progressed over at least a year after a cat bite abscess that was initially treated with amoxicillin-clavulanic acid. They consisted of nodular and crusted lesions on the head **(A)** and cervical region **(B)** that drained fluid and extended down the cervical region to the cranioventral thorax. The cat tested negative for retroviruses. (Courtesy University of California, Davis, Veterinary Dermatology Service.)

mellitus, and hemic neoplasia.[17] Underlying immunosuppressive disease or drug treatment also seems to predispose dogs to nocardiosis. Nocardiosis has been documented in several dogs treated with cyclosporine and in a dog with lymphoma.[3-5,9] Most affected cats have cutaneous infections that develop after scratch or bite wounds.[8,18] Accordingly, more than 75% to 80% of affected cats are male; in the author's hospital, 9 of 10 affected cats were male.[8,9,19] Cats of any age can be affected, and no breed predilection has been identified.[8] Some cats have underlying disorders that predispose them to nocardiosis, such as a history of renal transplantation, underlying retroviral infection, or glucocorticoid administration. Others have no obvious underlying immunosuppressive disease.

Clinical Features

Signs and Their Pathogenesis

The pathogenicity of *Nocardia* spp. is influenced by the strain and growth phase of the organism, and host susceptibility. Virulent *Nocardia* strains are facultative intracellular pathogens that inhibit phagosome-lysosome fusion, neutralize phagosomal acidification, resist oxidative burst, secrete superoxide dismutase, and alter lysosomal enzymes within neutrophils and macrophages.[17] These effects are partly related to the content and structure of mycolic acids within the bacterial cell wall, which vary among strains and throughout the growth phase. Filamentous log-phase cells in the environment can be highly resistant to phagocytosis. Some strains have a greater propensity to invade the central nervous system (CNS).[19,20]

The normal host response to infection is characterized by an initial pyogenic inflammatory response, but a cell-mediated immune response is necessary to destroy the organisms. Diminished host resistance, especially impaired cell-mediated immunity (CMI), is a primary factor in susceptibility to nocardiosis and the extent to which dissemination occurs.

Cutaneous-subcutaneous nocardiosis, the most common form in cats (>75% of affected cats), is characterized by slow and progressive circumferential spread of a nonhealing, draining wound (Figure 43-2). Lesions are typically subacute to chronic. Infections of feeding tube sites can also occur.[21] Mycetoma-like lesions in the inguinal area resemble those described for rapidly growing mycobacterial infections (see Chapter 44), with multiple draining sinuses. These may result from contamination of "raking" injuries inflicted by the hindlimbs during fighting behavior,[8] or contamination of traumatic wounds from penetrating plant material. Cutaneous-subcutaneous nocardiosis was documented in 8 of 9 dogs from Brazil[6] but represents the minority of canine nocardiosis cases in California and Australia.[8,9] Dogs with cutaneous involvement typically develop draining wounds and masses, often on the head and limbs. Osteomyelitis can occur in association with cutaneous lesions.

The pathogenesis of *pulmonary or disseminated nocardiosis* is similar to that of the deep mycoses. Branching nocardial filaments fragment into small, unicellular particles that are aerosolized and inhaled, possibly in dust. Once within the lung, *Nocardia* spp. proliferate in the face of immune suppression, which leads to formation of intrapulmonary masses or pneumonia, hilar lymphadenopathy, and/or extrapulmonary masses and pyothorax (Figure 43-3, *A*). Pulmonary nocardiosis is the most common form of nocardiosis in humans and also occurs in dogs and less commonly in cats. In dogs, it can have a peracute onset characterized by tachypnea, hemoptysis, hypothermia,

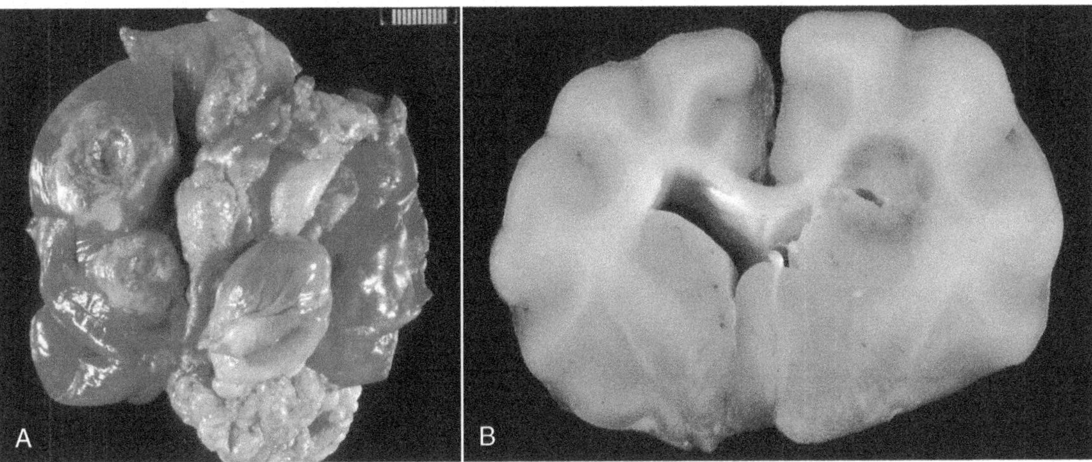

FIGURE 43-3 Gross necropsy findings in a 4-year-old male neutered domestic shorthair cat with disseminated nocardiosis caused by *Nocardia nova*. The cat was a renal transplant recipient. **A,** Multifocal to coalescing large, white to gray, caseous pulmonary masses are present within the lungs. **B,** The brain contained multifocal, white to gray foci that histologically consisted of large numbers of neutrophils and filamentous bacteria. (Courtesy University of California, Davis Veterinary Anatomic Pathology Service.)

collapse, and death; however, subacute to chronic clinical signs are more common.[22-25] Co-infection with CDV is occasionally reported.[6,26,27] Disseminated nocardiosis occurs when organisms in the lung erode into blood vessels and spread systemically, with abscess formation in a variety of organs. This results in signs of lethargy, fever, inappetence, and signs that relate to the location of the infectious process. Disseminated disease occurs in cats as well as in dogs. The most frequently involved extrathoracic organs after dissemination are skin and subcutaneous tissue, kidney, liver, spleen, lymph nodes, CNS, eye, bone, and joints. In dogs and cats, CNS lesions can result in seizures or neurologic signs that relate to the local effects of abscesses or granulomas in the brain, meninges, or spinal cord (see Figure 43-3, *B*). CNS involvement is common in human nocardiosis. Peritoneal nocardiosis has rarely been reported in cats, possibly as a result of penetrating wounds to the abdomen.[8,28]

Physical Examination Findings

Physical examination findings in animals with cutaneous-subcutaneous disease consist of chronic, sometimes crusted, ulcerated, nonhealing draining wounds, and in cats may involve the extremities, inguinal area, flank, head, bridge of the nose, and neck (see Figure 43-2). Animals with pulmonary or systemic involvement may have a thin body condition, lethargy, and fever. Tachypnea and cough may be present, and lung sounds may be increased (with bronchopneumonia) or decreased (with pyothorax). Involvement of the liver, spleen, and lymph nodes may result in hepatomegaly, splenomegaly, and/or peripheral or abdominal lymphadenomegaly. Ophthalmic examination may reveal chorioretinitis. Bone or joint infection results in focal limb swelling and lameness. Animals with CNS involvement may show mental obtundation, anisocoria, decreased menace and pupillary light responses, head tilt, nystagmus, decreased gag reflexes, and/or delayed or absent placing reactions.

Diagnosis

A diagnosis of nocardiosis is usually suspected based on the presence of persistent pyogenic to pyogranulomatous inflammatory lesions and the presence of filamentous bacteria, together with a history of immunosuppression, although the last is not always present. Confirmation of the diagnosis requires culture.

Laboratory Abnormalities

Complete Blood Count and Serum Biochemical Tests

Hematologic abnormalities in nocardiosis are similar to those with actinomycosis (nonregenerative anemia, neutrophilic leukocytosis with a left shift, monocytosis, and sometimes marked hyperglobulinemia). However, in immunosuppressed animals, lymphopenia, monocytopenia, and eosinopenia may be present. Hypercalcemia associated with granulomatous disease was reported in a cat with nocardiosis.[29]

Cytologic Examination of Body Fluids

Examination of pleural effusion, bronchoalveolar lavage fluid, and aspirates of abscesses from animals with nocardiosis typically reveals suppurative to pyogranulomatous inflammation, with large numbers of degenerate neutrophils. Gram-positive, often partially or weakly acid-fast, beaded, filamentous organisms that branch at right angles may be observed individually or in loose aggregates (see Figure 43-1). The filaments may also fragment to form rods and coccoid forms. In contrast, *Actinomyces* spp. is not acid fast, and *Mycobacterium* spp. do not branch. When the infecting *Nocardia* sp. is not acid fast, it may not be distinguishable from an *Actinomyces* sp. organism. With Romanowsky-type stains, organisms are eosinophilic or basophilic and have a beaded appearance. They are usually around 0.5 µm in diameter and up to 30 µm long, but thicker organisms were described in a dog infected with *N. abscessus* (2 µm).[5] Macroaggregates (i.e., sulfur granules) occur infrequently in effusions. In contrast to actinomycosis, mixed bacterial populations in deep tissue sites are rarely present.

Diagnostic Imaging

Plain Radiography

Radiographs of cutaneous-subcutaneous lesions can reveal soft tissue swelling with or without associated bone lysis and periosteal proliferation. The radiographic appearance of pulmonary lesions varies and includes multiple, diffuse pulmonary nodules; intrapulmonary or extrapulmonary solitary masses; focal or diffuse bronchointerstitial to alveolar infiltrates; lobar consolidations; pleural effusions; and, often, dramatic hilar lymphadenopathy (Figure 43-4).

Sonographic Findings

Abdominal ultrasound findings in dogs and cats with disseminated nocardiosis have not been described in detail because disseminated disease with abdominal organ involvement is rare. However, intraparenchymal mass lesions and flocculent ascites fluid might be expected.

Advanced Imaging

Nodular lung lesions similar to those described in humans were identified with computed tomography in one dog with disseminated nocardiosis.[5] Computed tomographic and MRI abnormalities in dogs and cats with confirmed CNS nocardiosis have not been reported. One dog with suspected nocardiosis based on histopathology had a large, T2-hyperintense circumscribed lesion in the occipital cortex that was consistent with a brain abscess, together with widespread cerebral edema and herniation of the cerebellum through the foramen magnum.[4]

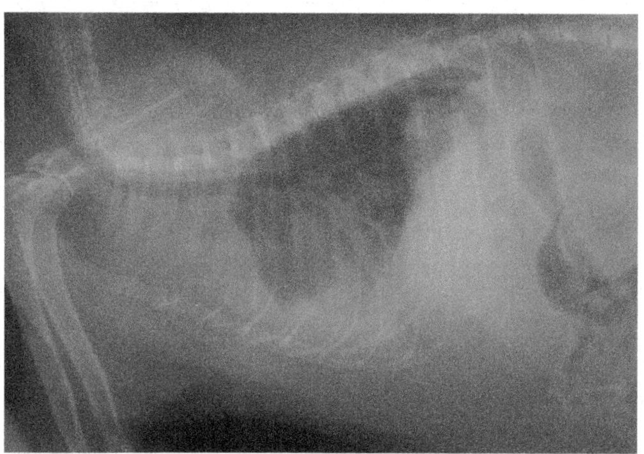

FIGURE 43-4 Lateral thoracic radiograph of a 4-year-old male neutered domestic shorthair cat with disseminated nocardiosis. Pleural effusion is present and obscures the cardiac silhouette. A mass is associated with the caudal aspect of the left caudal lung lobe.

Microbiologic Tests

Diagnostic assays available for *Nocardia* infection in dogs and cats are shown in Table 43-2.

Isolation and Identification

Nocardia spp. grow aerobically at a wide temperature range on simple media (e.g., Sabouraud's glucose agar, blood agar). Organisms are usually recovered in pure cultures, and colonies are often visible after 2 days. However, in some cases, 2 to 4 weeks of incubation may be necessary, and the organism may be overgrown by contaminating bacteria. Thus, the laboratory should be alerted if nocardiosis is suspected, so that selective media and long incubation times are used. Colonies are smooth and moist, or rugose with a powdery surface due to aerial filamentation, and may be pigmented. Organisms may then be identified based on their microscopic appearance and their ability to take up acid fast stains. However, not all pathogenic strains of *Nocardia* species are acid fast.[19,20,30] L-form *Nocardia* spp., which are cell wall–deficient variants, have been associated with disease in people and a dog.[31] These bacteria require special media for isolation and culture, similar to mycoplasmas (see Chapter 39).

Traditionally, *Nocardia* species have been distinguished based on their growth characteristics and antibiotic susceptibility patterns; however, molecular methods provide a more reliable and rapid means of speciation. Sequence analysis of PCR products from the 16S rRNA gene identifies most pathogenic *Nocardia* spp., but differentiation of closely related species may require analysis of other genes, multilocus sequence typing, or DNA-DNA hybridization.[2,17] DNA-DNA hybridization is considered the gold standard for nocardial species determination.[2] Matrix-assisted laser desorption/ionization–time of flight (MALDI-TOF) mass spectrometry shows promise for rapid and reliable identification of *Nocardia* species in clinical microbiology laboratories.[32] PCR assays have also been used to directly detect *Nocardia* spp. in clinical specimens, without prior isolation.[2]

Because *Nocardia* organisms are ubiquitous in soil and may be inhaled by healthy animals, the isolation of small numbers of organisms from ulcerated skin lesions or the respiratory tract may not be clinically significant and must be interpreted in conjunction with clinical signs and history of immune compromise. Repeated positive cultures, pure cultures, or isolation of large

TABLE 43-2

Diagnostic Assays Available for *Nocardia* Infection in Dogs and Cats

Assay	Specimen Type	Target	Performance
Culture	Aspirates of purulent material (e.g., abscesses, pleural effusion); whole blood; tissue specimens obtained by biopsy or at necropsy (e.g., subcutaneous tissue, lung tissue)	*Nocardia* spp.	Grows on most simple media. May require several weeks' incubation. Because *Nocardia* spp. are soil saprophytes, isolation from skin lesions does not imply disease causation. PCR and sequencing may be required to identify the species present.
Cytology or histopathology with organism detection using special stains	Aspirates or tissue specimens	*Nocardia* spp. organisms	Organisms are gram-positive, variably acid-fast, and are not typically accompanied by sulfur granules, other bacteria, or the Splendore-Hoeppli phenomenon. Definitive diagnosis requires culture because non–acid-fast *Nocardia* can resemble *Actinomyces* spp.

numbers of the organism also suggest nocardiosis, and isolation of a single colony from a normally sterile site is significant. Visualization of gram-positive filamentous bacteria in cytology specimens in association with acute inflammatory cells also assists in determination of clinical significance.

The susceptibility of *Nocardia* spp. to antimicrobial drugs varies considerably between different *Nocardia* species, and so species identification can be used to guide antimicrobial drug selection (see Treatment, later) (Table 43-3). Susceptibility testing for *Nocardia* spp. is difficult and should be done by laboratories with special expertise. Susceptibility testing may be helpful when there is a failure to respond to therapy or relapse occurs from drug resistance. It may also be useful if there are concerns that relate to adverse drug reactions to sulfonamides, the initial treatment of choice (e.g., in dogs with immune-mediated disease that is complicated by cyclosporine-associated nocardiosis). Testing is also indicated when *N. farcinica* is present, which tends to be highly resistant to antimicrobial drugs, or when a nocardial species with unpredictable susceptibility is isolated.

Pathologic Findings

Nocardiosis is characterized by suppurative necrosis and abscess formation and infrequently granulomas (see Figure 43-3). Gross lesions in organs such as the spleen, lung, liver, and the brain typically consist of numerous small (1 mm) to large (several centimeters), discrete or coalescing, intraparenchymal white or gray-white nodules. On cut section, nodules appear caseous to purulent. Lymph nodes are enlarged, often massively, and are firm to fluctuant with a caseous to purulent core. A reddish-brown exudate may be present in the pleural or peritoneal space or within abscesses. Although formation of sulfur granules by *Nocardia* spp. is uncommon compared with *Actinomyces* spp., small granules are occasionally found in skin lesions and pleural and peritoneal fluid.[10,22,28,33]

Histopathology usually reveals a central region of necrosis and suppuration, which, depending on the host immune response, may be surrounded by macrophages, lymphocytes, and plasma cells (Figure 43-5, *A*). In chronic cutaneous-subcutaneous infections, pyogranulomatous foci may be interspersed within dense fibrous tissue. Plant material may be observed if plants were involved in inoculation of *Nocardia* spp. into tissues, but this is more common with actinomycosis.

Nocardia filaments are usually present in abundance within regions of necrosis and suppuration. They are poorly visible in tissue sections stained with hematoxylin and eosin or with Gridley's fungal or periodic acid–Schiff. Organisms can be stained with Gram stain (see Figure 43-5, *B*) or methenamine silver preparations,[5] especially with prolonged silver nitrate exposure. They are usually partially acid fast and have the same appearance described previously in the Cytology section. In chronic skin infections, tissue granules characterized by colonies arranged in large, rosette-like arrays have been described. In contrast to actinomycosis, other bacteria and the Splendore-Hoeppli phenomenon are not generally present.

Treatment and Prognosis

Treatment

Successful treatment of nocardiosis relies on the combination of appropriate antimicrobial therapy combined with the

TABLE 43-3

Suggested Antimicrobial Drug Selection for Treatment of Pathogenic *Nocardia* spp. Based on Minimum Inhibitory Concentration Data

Nocardia Species	Appropriate Antimicrobial Drug Choices	Antimicrobial Drugs to Avoid
N. abscessus	Ampicillin, amoxicillin–clavulanic acid, ceftriaxone, linezolid, amikacin and gentamicin, sulfamethoxazole	Imipenem, ciprofloxacin, clarithromycin
N. brevicatena/paucivorans complex	Ampicillin, amoxicillin–clavulanic acid, ceftriaxone, amikacin, sulfamethoxazole, ciprofloxacin	Gentamicin, clarithromycin
N. nova complex (includes *N. nova*, *N. africana*)	Ampicillin, sulfamethoxazole, erythromycin, clarithromycin, ceftriaxone, imipenem, amikacin	Amoxicillin–clavulanic acid
N. farcinica	Amikacin, sulfamethoxazole, ciprofloxacin (most isolates), imipenem (most isolates)	Ampicillin, broad-spectrum cephalosporins, clarithromycin, aminoglycosides other than amikacin
N. cyriacigeorgica	Ceftriaxone, amikacin, imipenem	Ampicillin, amoxicillin–clavulanic acid, clarithromycin, ciprofloxacin
N. brasiliensis	Minocycline, amoxicillin–clavulanic acid, sulfamethoxazole	Ampicillin, ciprofloxacin, clarithromycin
N. otitidiscaviarum	Gentamicin, amikacin, sulfamethoxazole, ciprofloxacin	All β-lactam antibiotics

Data from Brown-Elliott BA, Brown JM, Conville PS, et al. Clinical and laboratory features of the *Nocardia* spp. based on current molecular taxonomy. Clin Microbiol Rev 2006;19:259-282.

use of surgical drainage or debridement. Chronic, extensive lesions may require surgical debridement or resection. Appropriate antimicrobial therapy that includes surgical drainage is not always effective, possibly because of an inadequate host immune response.[8] Existing immunosuppressive drug treatment should be discontinued or reduced, provided it does not cause relapse of a life-threatening underlying disease process.

The initial selection of an antimicrobial drug or drug combination should take into account the site of the infection, the host immune status, the infecting *Nocardia* species (see Table 43-3), and, if available, susceptibility test results.[17] However, in vitro susceptibilities do not always translate into a clinical response in vivo. Sulfonamides, including trimethoprim-sulfonamide combinations (TMS), are the first line antimicrobial drugs for treatment of nocardiosis (Table 43-4). Treatment durations from 1 to 3 months are recommended in people with cutaneous infections, up to 6 months for uncomplicated pulmonary infections, and 12 months or longer for systemic infections or infections in those who are immunocompromised.[17] Clinical improvement is generally observed within 7 to 10 days of starting treatment. High doses of trimethoprim-sulfas given for long periods to dogs (and to a lesser extent, cats) can produce a variety of adverse effects such as keratoconjunctivitis sicca and myelosuppression (see Chapter 8). If adverse drug reactions occur, selection of drugs other than TMS should ideally be based on susceptibility test results. If these are not available, choices should be made based on published susceptibility data for different *Nocardia* species (see Table 43-3). *Nocardia nova* is susceptible to amoxicillin but resistant to amoxicillin-clavulanic acid because of induction of chromosomal β-lactamase by clavulanic acid.[8,10] Substitution of antimicrobial drugs within a drug class may not provide effective treatment; for example, although susceptible to amikacin, *N. farcinia* isolates are resistant to gentamicin, and although susceptible to minocycline, *N. brasiliensis* isolates are mostly resistant to doxycycline.[34] Two- or three-drug combinations including TMS, amikacin, and either ceftriaxone or imipenem have been used, pending the results of susceptibility tests to treat severe nocardiosis in human patients.[2] A combination of amikacin and imipenem should be effective against all isolates. Combination treatment with amikacin and TMS was suggested for cats with *N. farcinica* infections, which generally require an aggressive, combination drug treatment.[8] After susceptibility testing, monotherapy with linezolid has consistently been used with success to treat some refractory *Nocardia* infections in humans.[35] *Nocardia* isolates from dogs and cats have high minimum inhibitory concentrations for fluoroquinolones,[36] which are not generally recommended for treatment.

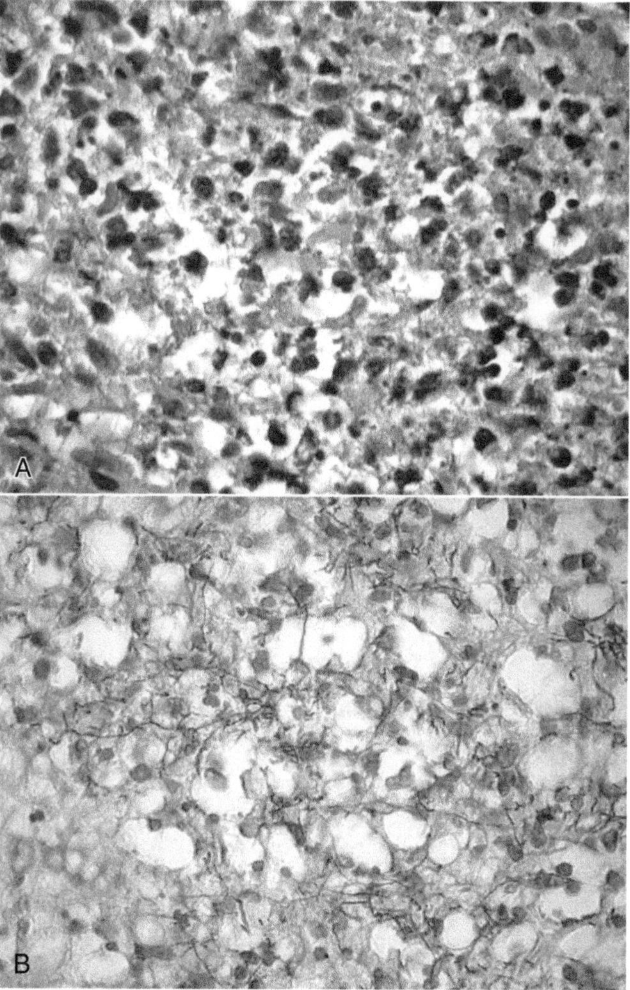

FIGURE 43-5 Histopathologic findings in nocardiosis. **A,** Severe, necrotizing pyogranulomatous inflammation is present with intralesional bacteria, which are barely visible. H&E stain. **B,** Gram staining revealed tangles of filamentous, branching gram-positive bacteria. Brown and Benn stain.

If CNS disease is present, either high doses of TMS given parenterally, or drugs with excellent CNS penetration, which include third-generation cephalosporins, carbapenems, or linezolid should be considered. The use of linezolid in veterinary patients is controversial because it is an important drug for resistant bacterial infections in humans (see Chapter 8).

Prognosis

In a review of 53 dogs with nocardiosis, 50% of the dogs died and 39% were euthanized.[24] Of 36 cats with nocardiosis, 16 were either euthanized or died.[8] The high mortality rate may relate to underlying immunosuppressive disease or immunosuppressive

TABLE 43-4

Medications That Could Be Used to Treat Dogs and Cats with Nocardiosis *

Drug	Dose (mg/kg)	Route	Interval (hours)
Trimethoprim-sulfamethoxazole	30	PO, IV	12
Amikacin†	10-14 (cat), 15-30 (dog)	IV, IM, SC	24
Imipenem-cilastatin†	2-5	IV	8

*Pending species identification with or without susceptibility testing.

†Amikacin and imipenem-cilastatin are generally used in combination with each other or with trimethoprim-sulfamethoxazole.

drug treatment, delayed diagnosis, and inappropriate treatment. With earlier diagnosis and more aggressive, multidrug therapy, mortality of nocardiosis in animals may decrease to the rate reported in people. Only 20% of humans with primary infections died, whereas 42% of patients with predisposing conditions and more than 50% of patients with systemic or CNS nocardiosis died.[19]

Immunity and Vaccination

Immunity to nocardiosis is dependent on intact CMI. There are no vaccines for nocardiosis.

Prevention

Prevention of nocardiosis in cats involves housing cats indoors and limiting their fighting or biting activity. Any wounds should be carefully examined for foreign material and cleaned promptly. Disease in both dogs and cats may be prevented by avoidance of excessive immunosuppression with potent drugs such as cyclosporine.

Public Health Aspects

No cases of human nocardiosis acquired from direct contact with an animal have been reported; however, several cases of cutaneous nocardiosis transmitted to people by cat scratches have been documented.[37-40] Humans with impaired CMI (such as those receiving immunosuppressive drug therapy or those with HIV infection) should wear gloves and practice hand washing after handling pets with nocardiosis, or another individual in the household should treat these animals.

CASE EXAMPLE

Signalment: "Bob," a 6-year-old male neutered domestic shorthair cat from San Francisco, CA

History: Bob, a renal transplant recipient, was evaluated for a 2-week history of decreased activity and progressive inappetence and lethargy. He was taken to a local emergency clinic where blood work showed only mild hyponatremia (130 mmol/L) and a white cell count of 19,000 cells/μL. No abnormalities were detected on abdominal ultrasound examination. Bob was treated overnight with IV fluids and sent home with instructions to administer amoxicillin-clavulanic acid (12.5 mg/kg PO q12h). However, the cat's condition failed to improve, and so he was taken to a local veterinary clinic 3 days later. Further laboratory testing showed hyponatremia, hypoalbuminemia, and mild hyperbilirubinemia. Urinalysis showed a specific gravity of 1.054, 3+ bilirubin, 1+ hemoprotein, 0-2 WBC/HPF, 6-10 RBC/HPF, and no bacteria or casts. Aerobic bacterial urine culture was negative. The following day Bob became tachypneic and pleural effusion was identified. In-house examination of the effusion fluid revealed cloudy fluid that contained large numbers of erythrocytes, degenerate neutrophils, and macrophages. No bacteria were seen with Gram stain. Bob was then referred to the University of California, Davis, Veterinary Medical Teaching Hospital for further evaluation.

Bob had received a renal transplant at 3.5 years of age and since then had been treated with prednisone (0.5 mg/kg PO q12h) and cyclosporine (4 mg/kg PO q12h). A recent whole blood trough cyclosporine concentration was 1100 ng/mL.

Physical Examination:

Body Weight: 5.1 kg

General: Severely obtunded, T = 100.8°F (38.2°C), HR = 240 beats/min, RR = 55 breaths/min, mild generalized icterus, mucous membranes pink to icteric, CRT = 1 s, hydrated.

Eyes, Ears, Nose, and Throat: The only clinically significant abnormalities related to the eyes. Anisocoria was present with the left pupil larger than the right. Direct and consensual pupillary light reflexes were present, and the cornea and anterior chamber were clear with no ocular discharge. Fundoscopic examination showed focal areas of tapetal hyperreflectivity and focal dark and dull lesions with peripheral hyperreflectivity.

Musculoskeletal: BCS 7/9, with generalized weakness, recumbency and unwillingness/inability to walk.

Respiratory: Tachypnea with a shallow respiratory pattern was identified. Decreased lung sounds were present ventrally.

All Other Systems: No clinically significant abnormalities were present. The transplanted kidney could be palpated in the right abdomen. The urinary bladder was small.

Neurologic Examination:

Mentation: Obtunded.

Gait/Posture: The cat had a tendency to lean to the right, but could not or would not walk more than a few steps.

Cranial Nerves: Menace responses were absent bilaterally.

Postural Reactions: Delayed placing reactions were identified in all four limbs.

Spinal Reflexes and Panniculus Reflex: Normal.

Neuroanatomic Location: Cerebrothalamic, possibly right sided.

Laboratory Findings:

CBC:

HCT 30.4% (30%-50%), MCV 46.5 fL (42-53 fL)
MCHC 32.6 g/dL (30-33.5 g/dL)
Reticulocytes 18,000 cells/μL (7000-60,000 cells/μL)
WBC 22,860 cells/μL (4500-14,000 cells/μL)
Neutrophils 19,660 cells/μL (2000-9000 cells/μL)
Band neutrophils 2286 cells/μL
Lymphocytes 457 cells/μL (1000-7000 cells/μL)
Monocytes 229 cells/μL (50-600 cells/μL)
Eosinophils 229 cells/μL (150-1100 cells/μL)
Basophils 0 cells/μL (0-50 cells/μL).

Platelets clumped but adequate. Neutrophils had slight toxic change, and band neutrophils had marked toxic change.

Serum Chemistry Profile:

Sodium 136 mmol/L (151-158 mmol/L)
Potassium 3.5 mmol/L (3.6-4.9 mmol/L)
Chloride 98 mmol/L (113-121 mmol/L)
Bicarbonate 18 mmol/L (15-21 mmol/L)

Continued

Phosphorus 4.3 mg/dL (3.2-6.3 mg/dL)
Calcium 8.3 mg/dL (9.4-11.4 mg/dl)
BUN 48 mg/dL (18-33 mg/dL)
Creatinine 0.8 mg/dL (1.1-2.2 mg/dL)
Glucose 140 mg/dL (73-134 mg/dL)
Total protein 4.8 g/dL (6.6-8.4 g/dL)
Albumin 1.4 g/dL (1.9-3.9 g/dL)
Globulin 3.4 g/dL (2.9-5.3 g/dL)
ALT 19 U/L (28-106 U/L)
AST 27 U/L (12-46 U/L)
ALP 5 U/L (14-71 U/L)
Gamma GT 0 U/L (0-4 U/L)
Cholesterol 141 mg/dL (89-258 mg/dL)
Total bilirubin 1.5 mg/dL (0-0.2 mg/dL).

Imaging Findings:

Thoracic Radiographs: See Figure 43-4. There was a moderate amount of pleural effusion. A mass was associated with the caudal aspect of the left caudal lung lobe. The cardiac silhouette was completely obscured on the lateral projection. On the ventrodorsal projection, there appeared to be a mass effect superimposed over the caudal border of the cardiac silhouette that deformed the left and right caudal lung lobes.

Abdominal Ultrasound: The native kidneys were markedly diminished in size, were irregular in contour, and had a markedly irregular parenchyma with a lack of corticomedullary distinction. The transplanted kidney appeared within normal limits. The muscularis layer of the small intestine was mildly thickened diffusely. A Y-shaped region of mineralization was identified within the right liver lobes, which was likely associated with the biliary system.

Treatment and Outcome: Thoracocentesis was performed, and 35 mL of turbid red fluid was removed. Unfortunately, the cat became progressively more agitated and tachypneic, thoracocentesis was aborted, and Bob was placed in a cage with oxygen supplementation. Preliminary cytologic examination of the fluid yielded results that were consistent with referring veterinarian's findings. Treatment with IV crystalloid fluids (0.9% NaCl with 20 mEq/L KCl at 12 mL/hr), enrofloxacin (2.5 mg/kg IV q12h), and ampicillin (22 mg/kg IV q8h) was initiated, and pleural fluid was submitted to the laboratory for cytologic examination and aerobic and anaerobic bacterial culture. The plan was to stabilize Bob with this treatment until additional thoracocentesis and chest tube placement could be performed. Differential diagnoses considered were cryptococcosis, toxoplasmosis, FIP, a systemic bacterial infection, or neoplasia. However, 10 hours after admission, Bob developed respiratory and cardiac arrest. The owner elected euthanasia.

Necropsy Findings: Gross necropsy findings consisted of 120 mL of flocculent, serosanguinous fluid within the thoracic cavity and multifocal to coalescing, variably sized, white to gray, firm to caseous nodules that largely effaced the caudal lung lobes and extended through the pleural surface, with adhesions to the thoracic diaphragm and pleura (see Figure 43-3, *A*). A 3-mm nodule was also present in the wall of the left ventricle. The peritoneal cavity contained multiple adhesions from the small intestines to the omentum and the stomach to the left abdominal wall. The right medial liver lobe contained a focal, white to gray mass that was 10 cm in diameter and oozed purulent material when cut. The spleen contained multiple, white, raised, pinpoint foci. The native kidneys were shrunken, pale, irregular, and had loss of corticomedullary definition. The right transplanted kidney contained 3-4, tan, firm, homogenous cortical nodules that ranged from 2 to 4 mm in diameter. On cut section, the brain contained multifocal, randomly distributed, soft, white to gray, homogenous foci that measured 1-4 mm in diameter (see Figure 43-3, *B*). Histopathology of the lung, pleural, myocardium, thoracic diaphragm, spleen, liver, transplanted kidney, adrenal medulla, stomach, salivary gland, brain, and meninges revealed chronic, severe, necrotizing pyogranulomatous inflammation with intralesional branching filamentous bacteria. There was also chronic, moderate, multifocal and necrotizing pyogranulomatous choroiditis and cyclitis in both eyes. The bacteria were gram positive but were not acid fast (see Figure 43-5, *B*).

Microbiologic Testing: Aerobic and anaerobic bacterial culture (liver, lung specimens collected at necropsy): Small numbers of *Nocardia nova*. No other bacteria were cultured.

Diagnosis: Disseminated *Nocardia nova* infection

Comments: In this case, nocardiosis followed a rapid clinical course, as can occur in human patients with severe immunodeficiency. The trough whole blood cyclosporine concentration was high; the goal of treatment is to obtain blood concentrations of approximately 300 to 500 ng/mL, although the optimum concentration that achieves adequate but not excessive immunosuppression in cats is not known.[18] Treatment with antimicrobial drugs was not effective given the advanced nature and severity of the disease in this cat.

SUGGESTED READINGS

Brown-Elliott BA, Brown JM, Conville PS, et al. Clinical and laboratory features of the *Nocardia* spp. based on current molecular taxonomy. Clin Microbiol Rev. 2006;19:259-282.

MacNeill AL, Steeil JC, Dossin O, et al. Disseminated nocardiosis caused by *Nocardia abscessus* in a dog. Vet Clin Pathol. 2010;39:381-385.

Malik R, Krockenberger MB, O'Brien CR, et al. *Nocardia* infections in cats: a retrospective multi-institutional study of 17 cases. Aust Vet J. 2006;84:235-245.

REFERENCES

1. Nocard ME. Note sur la maladie des boeufs de la Guadeloupe connue sous le nom de farcin. Ann Inst Pasteur (Paris). 1888;2:293-302.
2. Brown-Elliott BA, Brown JM, Conville PS, et al. Clinical and laboratory features of the *Nocardia* spp. based on current molecular taxonomy. Clin Microbiol Rev. 2006;19:259-282.
3. Paul AE, Mansfield CS, Thompson M. Presumptive *Nocardia* spp. infection in a dog treated with cyclosporin and ketoconazole. N Z Vet J. 2010;58:265-268.
4. Smith PM, Haughland SP, Jeffery ND. Brain abscess in a dog immunosuppressed using cyclosporin. Vet J. 2007;173:675-678.
5. MacNeill AL, Steeil JC, Dossin O, et al. Disseminated nocardiosis caused by *Nocardia abscessus* in a dog. Vet Clin Pathol. 2010;39:381-385.
6. Ribeiro MG, Salerno T, Mattos-Guaraldi AL, et al. Nocardiosis: an overview and additional report of 28 cases in cattle and dogs. Rev Inst Med Trop Sao Paulo. 2008;50:177-185.

7. Saubolle MA, Sussland D. Nocardiosis: review of clinical and laboratory experience. J Clin Microbiol. 2003;41:4497-4501.
8. Malik R, Krockenberger MB, O'Brien CR, et al. *Nocardia* infections in cats: a retrospective multi-institutional study of 17 cases. Aust Vet J. 2006;84:235-245.
9. Sykes JE. Unpublished observations. 2012.
10. Hirsh DC, Jang SS. Antimicrobial susceptibility of *Nocardia nova* isolated from five cats with nocardiosis. J Am Vet Med Assoc. 1999;215:815-817, 795-816.
11. Hattori Y, Kano R, Kunitani Y, et al. *Nocardia africana* isolated from a feline mycetoma. J Clin Microbiol. 2003;41:908-910.
12. de Farias MR, Werner J, Ribeiro MG, et al. Uncommon mandibular osteomyelitis in a cat caused by *Nocardia africana*. BMC Vet Res. 2012;8:239.
13. Harada H, Endo Y, Sekiguchi M, et al. Cutaneous nocardiosis in a cat. J Vet Med Sci. 2009;71:785-787.
14. Ajello L, Walker WW, Dungworth DL, et al. Isolation of *Nocardia brasiliensis* from a cat with a review of its prevalence and geographic distribution. J Am Vet Med Assoc. 1961;138:370-376.
15. Ramos-Vara JA, Wu CC, Lin TL, et al. *Nocardia tenerifensis* genome identification in a cutaneous granuloma from a cat. J Vet Diagn Invest. 2007;19:577-580.
16. Luque I, Astorga R, Tarradas C, et al. *Nocardia otitidiscaviarum* infection in a cat. Vet Rec. 2002;151:488.
17. Sorrell TC, Mitchell DH, Iredell JR, et al. *Nocardia* species. In: Mandell GL, Bennett JE, Dolin R, eds. Principles and Practice of Infectious Diseases. Philadelphia, PA: Elsevier; 2010:3199-3207.
18. Edwards DF. Actinomycosis and nocardiosis. In: Greene CE, ed. Infectious Diseases of the Dog and Cat. 3rd ed. St Louis, MO: Saunders Elsevier; 2006:451-461.
19. Beaman BL, Beaman L. *Nocardia* species: host-parasite relationships. Clin Microbiol Rev. 1994;7:213-264.
20. McNeil MM, Brown JM. The medically important aerobic actinomycetes: epidemiology and microbiology. Clin Microbiol Rev. 1994;7:357-417.
21. Kadar E, Sykes JE, Kass PH, et al. Evaluation of the prevalence of infections in cats after renal transplantation: 169 cases (1987-2003). J Am Vet Med Assoc. 2005;227:948-953.
22. Campbell B, Scott DW. Successful management of nocardial empyema in a dog and cat. J Am Anim Hosp Assoc. 1975;11:769-773.
23. Cross RF, Nagao WT, Morrison RH. Canine nocardiosis; a report of two cases. J Am Vet Med Assoc. 1953;123:535-536.
24. Marino DJ, Jaggy A. Nocardiosis. A literature review with selected case reports in two dogs. J Vet Intern Med. 1993;7:4-11.
25. Lobetti RG, Collett MG, Leisewitz A. Acute fibrinopurulent pneumonia and haemoptysis associated with *Nocardia asteroides* in three dogs. Vet Rec. 1993;133:480.
26. Ackerman N, Grain E, Castleman W. Canine nocardiosis. J Am Anim Hosp Assoc. 1982;18:147-153.
27. Beaman BL, Sugar AM. *Nocardia* in naturally acquired and experimental infections in animals. J Hyg (Lond). 1983;91:393-419.
28. Tilgner SL, Anstey SI. Nocardial peritonitis in a cat. Aust Vet J. 1996;74:430-432.
29. Mealey KL, Willard MD, Nagode LA, et al. Hypercalcemia associated with granulomatous disease in a cat. J Am Vet Med Assoc. 1999;215:959-962, 946.
30. Lerner PI. Nocardiosis. Clin Infect Dis. 1996;22:891-903; quiz 904-905.
31. Buchanan AM, Beaman BL, Pedersen NC, et al. *Nocardia asteroides* recovery from a dog with steroid- and antibiotic-unresponsive idiopathic polyarthritis. J Clin Microbiol. 1983;18:702-708.
32. Verroken A, Janssens M, Berhin C, et al. Evaluation of matrix-assisted laser desorption ionization–time of flight mass spectrometry for identification of *Nocardia* species. J Clin Microbiol. 2010;48:4015-4021.
33. Davenport DJ, Johnson GC. Cutaneous nocardiosis in a cat. J Am Vet Med Assoc. 1986;188:728-729.
34. Gomez-Flores A, Welsh O, Said-Fernandez S, et al. In vitro and in vivo activities of antimicrobials against *Nocardia brasiliensis*. Antimicrob Agents Chemother. 2004;48:832-837.
35. Kobayashi N, Sueoka-Aragane N, Naganoby N, et al. Disseminated nocardiosis caused by *Nocardia concava* with acute respiratory failure and central nervous system involvement treated with linezolid. Intern Med. 2012;51:3281-3285.
36. Govendir M, Norris JM, Hansen T, et al. Susceptibility of rapidly growing mycobacteria and *Nocardia* isolates from cats and dogs to pradofloxacin. Vet Microbiol. 2011;153:240-245.
37. Astudillo L, Dahan S, Escourrou G, et al. Cat scratch responsible for primary cutaneous *Nocardia asteroides* in an immunocompetent patient. Br J Dermatol. 2001;145:684-685.
38. Bottei E, Flaherty JP, Kaplan LJ, et al. Lymphocutaneous *Nocardia brasiliensis* infection transmitted via a cat scratch: a second case. Clin Infect Dis. 1994;18:649-650.
39. Freland C, Fur JL, Nemirovsky-Trebucq B, et al. Primary cutaneous nocardiosis caused by *Nocardia otitidiscaviarum*: two cases and a review of the literature. J Trop Med Hyg. 1995;98:395-403.
40. Sachs MK. Lymphocutaneous *Nocardia brasiliensis* infection acquired from a cat scratch: case report and review. Clin Infect Dis. 1992;15:710-711.

CHAPTER 44

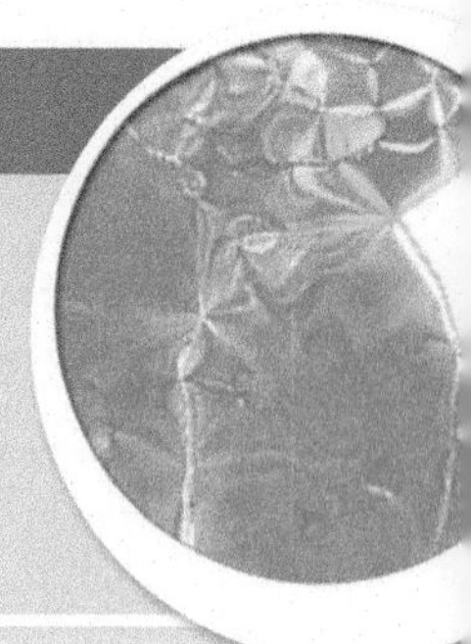

Mycobacterial Infections

Jane E. Sykes and Danièlle A. Gunn-Moore

Overview of Mycobacterial Infections in Dogs and Cats

First Described: Evidence of tuberculosis in humans dates back to 2400 to 3400 BC, but the causative agent was not demonstrated until 1882 (Robert Koch).[1]

Causes: *Mycobacterium* spp. (order Actinomycetales, family Mycobacteriaceae)

Geographic Distribution: Worldwide, but the distribution of different mycobacterial species varies.

Major Clinical Signs: Cutaneous nodular, ulcerated, or draining skin lesions; peripheral or internal lymphadenopathy; pneumonia with cough and/or tachypnea; osteomyelitis; granulomatous or pyogranulomatous infiltrates in a variety of abdominal organs and, rarely, the central nervous system and eye.

Differential Diagnoses: Neoplasia (especially lymphoma), feline infectious peritonitis (cats), tularemia, nocardiosis, actinomycosis, rhodococcosis, bartonellosis, leishmaniasis, and fungal infections

Human Health Significance: Transmission of mycobacteria from dogs or cats to humans has not been reported. However, the potential for transmission of *M. tuberculosis* and *M. bovis* to humans exists. Humans acquire infection by other mycobacteria from environmental sources.

Mycobacterium spp. are aerobic, nonmotile, non–spore-forming, gram-positive, acid-fast pleomorphic bacilli that cause chronic infections in humans and animals. *Mycobacterium* spp. have a high cell wall mycolic acid content, which causes them to retain a pink color when stained with acid-fast stains such as Ziehl-Neelsen or Kinyoun stains and examined under the microscope. As a result, the term "acid-fast bacilli" (AFB) is often associated with mycobacteria, although *Nocardia* is variably acid fast (see Chapter 43).

Mycobacterium spp. belong to the family Mycobacteriaceae and are grouped into those that belong to the *Mycobacterium tuberculosis* complex (MTBC), the *Mycobacterium avium* complex (MAC), the lepromatous mycobacteria, and nontuberculous mycobacteria other than *M. avium* (Table 44-1). Disease caused by these groups of microorganisms differs in its epidemiology, pathogenesis, clinical presentation, zoonotic potential, and response to antimicrobial treatment. Accordingly, each group is considered separately in this chapter.

Mycobacterium tuberculosis Complex

Etiology and Epidemiology

MTBC bacteria include the slowly growing, host-associated bacteria *Mycobacterium tuberculosis, Mycobacterium bovis, Mycobacterium microti, Mycobacterium africanum, Mycobacterium pinnipedii, Mycobacterium caprae,* and *Mycobacterium canettii.* These organisms cause tuberculosis in humans and animals. Only *M. tuberculosis, M. bovis,* and *M. microti* infect dogs and cats (Table 44-2). *M. africanum* and *M. canettii* are rare causes of human tuberculosis in Africa, *M. pinnipedii* infects seals, and *M. caprae* is primarily a ruminant pathogen. MTBC organisms share greater than 95% DNA-DNA homology, and so are difficult to differentiate from one another, even with many molecular methods. Unlike other mycobacterial species, MTBC bacteria do not survive well in the environment, although *M. bovis* can survive months in feces or carcasses.

Humans are the only reservoir host for *M. tuberculosis,* which is responsible for more than 90% of tuberculosis in humans. Cats are resistant to infection with *M. tuberculosis.* Disease due to *M. tuberculosis* has been reported in dogs that reside in various parts of the United States, Africa, France, and Switzerland.[2-9] Affected dogs from Europe have had travel histories; one was from western Africa and the other was a stray from southern Europe.[2,3] Dogs are usually infected after prolonged aerosol exposure to contaminated human respiratory secretions, so the disease is a "reverse zoonosis" (or *anthropozoonosis*). Thus, disease occurs in dogs where tuberculosis occurs in humans. In the United States, *M. tuberculosis* infection is most prevalent in humans from the northeast/mid-Atlantic states, southern states, Alaska, California, and Nevada (Figure 44-1). Dogs have not transmitted *M. tuberculosis* infection to humans despite prolonged close contact in some situations,[7] possibly because the pulmonary cavitary lesions that are required for transmission do not develop to the same extent in dogs as they do in humans. However, organisms have been detected in dogs' sputum, so transmission remains possible.

Cats are most often infected with *M. microti* or *M. bovis.*[10] Rodents (especially voles and shrews) are reservoir hosts for *M. microti,* and cattle and a variety of wildlife species are reservoir hosts for *M. bovis.* The overwhelming majority of feline infections with *M. microti* and *M. bovis* have been reported from the United Kingdom, where *M. microti* infection is endemic in voles, wood mice, and shrews, and *M. bovis* infection is endemic in Eurasian badgers and cattle. Infections with *M. microti* and *M. bovis* comprise a third of feline infections with culturable mycobacteria in the United Kingdom.[10] Cats infected with *M. bovis* tend to be young adult cats (median age 3 years),

TABLE 44-1

Mycobacterial Pathogens of Clinical Significance in Dogs and Cats

Group	Mycobacterial Species	Description
M. tuberculosis complex	*M. tuberculosis, M. bovis, M. microti*	Host-associated, slow-growing species. Cause cutaneous and disseminated granulomatous disease in dogs (all three species) and cats (*M. bovis* and *M. microti*)
M. avium-intracellulare complex	*M. avium* subsp. *avium, M. avium* subsp. *hominissuis*	Opportunistic, environmental, slow-growing species. Cause cutaneous and disseminated granulomatous disease in dogs (subsp. *hominissuis*) and cats (subsp. *avium*). Some may cause leprosy syndromes in cats.
Lepromatous mycobacteria	*M. lepraemurium*, the CLG organism, and other unnamed species, some with genetic resemblance to known nontuberculous mycobacteria	Highly fastidious or unculturable mycobacteria. Cause nodular granulomatous to pyogranulomatous cutaneous disease in cats (all species) or dogs (CLG organism).
Rapidly growing nontuberculous mycobacteria	*M. fortuitum, M. smegmatis, M. abscessus, M. chelonae, M. thermoresistibile, M. goodii, M. flavescens, M. alvei*	Opportunistic, environmental, rapidly growing species. Cause pyogranulomatous panniculitis, pneumonia, or disseminated infections in cats or dogs
Slowly growing nontuberculous mycobacteria other than *M. avium*	*M. kansasii, M. ulcerans, M. genavense, M. malmoense, M. celatum, M. terrae, M. simiae, 'M. visibile'**	Opportunistic, environmental, slowly growing species. Cause pyogranulomatous cutaneous or disseminated disease in dogs or cats.

CLG, Canine leproid granuloma.
*The exact position of *'M. visibile'* is not clear; it has also been grouped within the lepromatous mycobacteria.

TABLE 44-2

Organisms of the *Mycobacterium tuberculosis* Complex of Clinical Significance in Dogs and Cats

Species	Host(s)	Major Reservoir Hosts	Geographic Distribution of Reported Cases in Companion Animals	Clinical Signs	Human Health Significance
M. tuberculosis	Dogs	Humans	United States, Africa, southern Europe	Pneumonia and tracheobronchial lymphadenopathy; rarely dissemination to the CNS, liver, kidney	Primary cause of tuberculosis in humans. Reverse zoonosis. Transmission back to humans not reported but may be possible.
M. bovis	Cats, rarely dogs	Cattle, Eurasian badgers, other wildlife species	Southwestern England and Wales, New Zealand, Argentina, rarely United States	Cutaneous lesions, peripheral lymphadenopathy, occasionally dissemination to abdominal lymph nodes and other organs, osteomyelitis	Rare cause of tuberculosis in humans but transmission from animals to humans theoretically possible
M. microti	Cats, very rarely dogs	Voles, wood mice, shrews, camelids	Southwestern Scotland, northern and southern England, western Europe	Cutaneous lesions, peripheral lymphadenopathy, less often pneumonia, arthritis, osteomyelitis, ocular lesions	Very rare cause of tuberculosis in humans

whereas the median age of cats infected with *M. microti* is 8 years.[10] All affected cats have been more than 1 year of age, which likely reflects the long incubation period associated with these infections. Retroviral infection does not appear to predispose to infection.

M. bovis infections mainly occur in cats that reside in Wales and southwestern England and that have access to the outdoors (Figure 44-2).[10] Feline *M. bovis* infections also occur in New Zealand, where brushtail possums act as reservoir hosts[11]; Argentina, where stray cats are often fed raw cattle

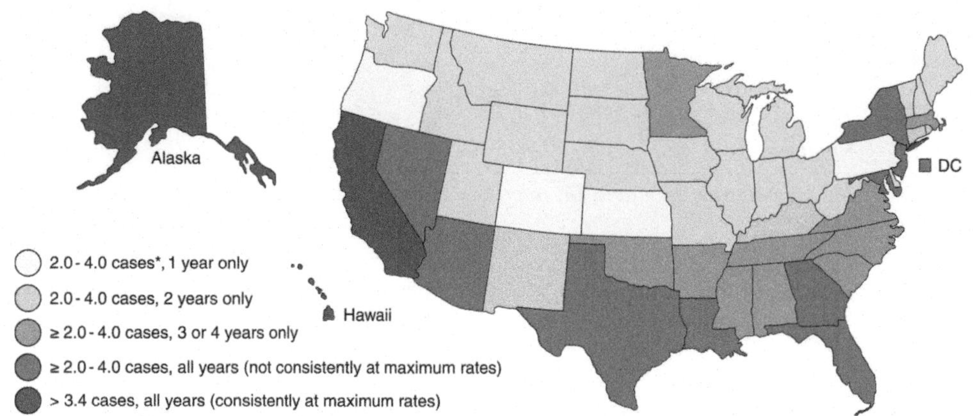

FIGURE 44-1 Geographic distribution of human cases of *Mycobacterium tuberculosis* infection in the United States, 2005-2011. Compiled from Morbidity and Mortality Weekly reports data on trends in human tuberculosis, years 2005, 2007, 2008, 2010, and 2011. *The intensity of the red color reflects the absolute number of cases/year, and whether case numbers were persistently high or varied among the 5 years evaluated. Thus the states that persistently have the highest rates of *M. tuberculosis* infection are Alaska, Hawaii, California, and New York (Long Island).

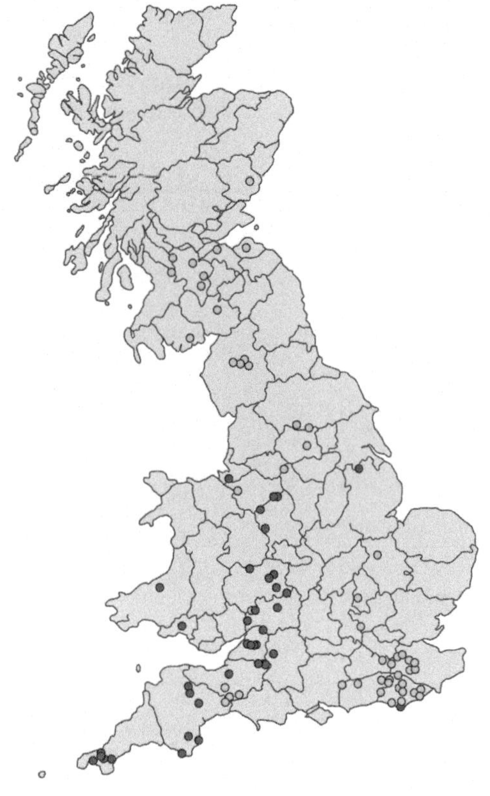

FIGURE 44-2 Geographic distribution of *Mycobacterium bovis* and *Mycobacterium microti* isolates from cats in the United Kingdom. (Redrawn from Gunn-Moore DA, McFarland SE, Brewer JI, et al. Mycobacterial disease in cats in Great Britain: I. Culture results, geographical distribution and clinical presentation of 339 cases. J Feline Med Surg 2011;13:934-944.)

lung[12]; and rarely the United States.[13] In the United Kingdom, spillover of infection from cattle, badgers, and possibly small rodents to cats is suspected. Aggressive interactions between cats and infected badgers may also be a route of transmission, especially as most cutaneous lesions occur at sites where fight and bite wounds often occur.[10,14] Ingestion of unpasteurized milk by cats is no longer a common route of transmission. A study from the United States showed no evidence of transmission of *M. bovis* to cats or dogs that lived on infected cattle farms.[15] Major wildlife reservoirs in North America, which include white-tailed deer, bison, and elk, are less likely than small mammals to interact with cats, which may explain why fewer *M. bovis* infections are reported in cats from North America when compared with the United Kingdom. Dogs are uncommonly infected with *M. bovis*.[16-18] Wounds inflicted by badgers or a squirrel have preceded disease in affected dogs.[16] In recent years, disease in dogs has been restricted to southwestern England or Ireland.

M. microti infections mainly occur in cats with outdoor access from the United Kingdom, with major clusters in southwestern Scotland/northern England and southern England (see Figure 44-2).[10,19] Spillover of disease from voles to cats is suspected.[19] Vole and llama genotypes of *M. microti* have been identified. Cats in the United Kingdom and one in Switzerland have been infected with the vole type.[20] A dog from France was infected with the llama type.[21]

Clinical Features

Signs and Their Pathogenesis

MTBC organisms are inhaled (*M. tuberculosis* and possibly *M. bovis*), ingested (*M. bovis* or *M. microti*), or inoculated into the skin (*M. bovis* or *M. microti*) and replicate locally. Organisms are then ingested by macrophages but survive and replicate within these cells. Macrophage destruction leads to recruitment of lymphocytes and additional monocytes, which initiates tubercle formation. Infected macrophages also travel to local lymph nodes, with development of a *primary complex* lesion. If cell-mediated immunity (CMI) is defective, dissemination to distant sites can occur. Delayed type hypersensitivity (DTH) responses can control the initial infection or may lead to central necrosis and calcification of the primary complex lesions, with persistence of organisms in the center of the lesions.

Clinical signs in dogs with pulmonary tuberculosis due to *M. tuberculosis* are slowly progressive. They consist of chronic, productive, or nonproductive cough, as well as inappetence, weight loss, and lethargy.[4,7] Rarely, dissemination to nonpulmonary sites such as the central nervous system (CNS), liver,

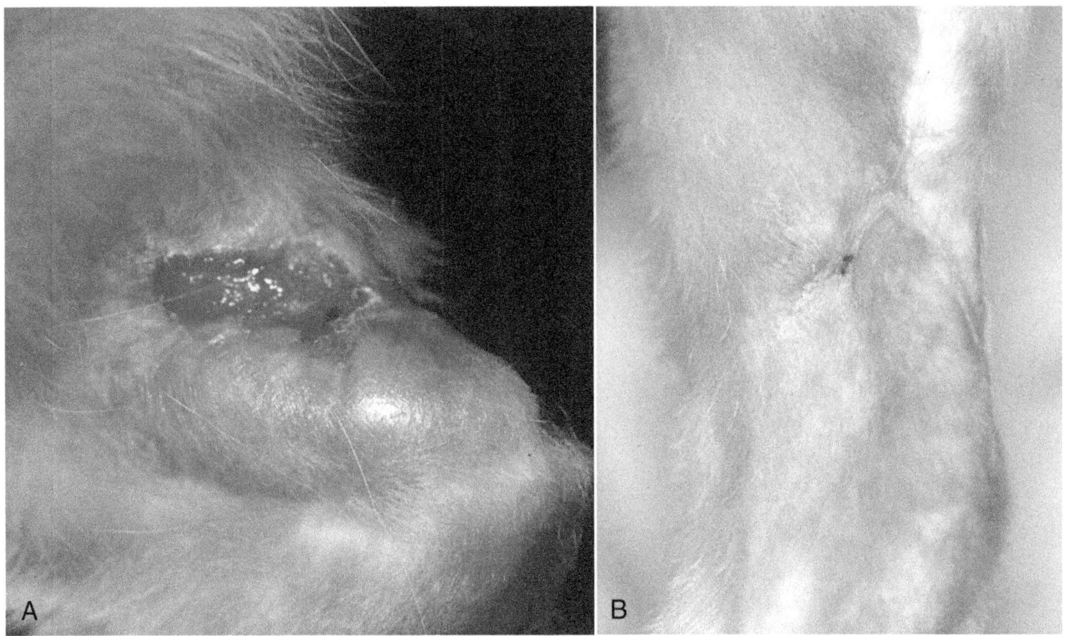

FIGURE 44-3 Ulcerative skin lesion due to *Mycobacterium microti* infection in a 6-year-old male neutered domestic shorthair. **A,** Before treatment. **B,** After 2 months of treatment with a combination of marbofloxacin, azithromycin, and rifampin.

or kidney leads to neurologic signs, weight loss, vomiting, or diarrhea.[2,3,9] Involvement of the lungs, liver, kidneys, and/or lymph nodes can occur in dogs infected with *M. bovis*.[16,18,22] Isolated lung and tracheobronchial node involvement similar to that often reported for *M. tuberculosis* was described in one dog that was infected with *M. bovis*.[18]

Most (>75%) cats infected with *M. bovis* and *M. microti* have had cutaneous nodular lesions with or without mandibular lymphadenopathy. Multifocal peripheral lymphadenopathy may be present.[23] Mesenteric lymphadenopathy, pneumonia, ocular lesions, and arthritis occur in some cats infected with *M. microti*.[20,23-25] Dissemination may result in weight loss, fever, and inappetence. Lung involvement may be associated with tachypnea, dyspnea, or cough.[18]

Physical Examination Findings

Dogs with pulmonary involvement caused by *M. tuberculosis* may show fever, increased lung sounds, and cough. Other physical examination findings that relate to dissemination of infection are present less often, such as thin body condition, neurologic signs, or hepatomegaly. Abnormal findings on examination of the respiratory tract and/or abdominal organs may also be detected in dogs with disseminated *M. bovis* or *M. microti* infection.

The most common physical examination findings in cats (and to a lesser extent, dogs) that are infected with *M. bovis* or *M. microti* are single or multiple firm cutaneous nodules, and enlargement of one or more peripheral lymph nodes (Figures 44-3 and 44-4). Cutaneous nodules may be mobile or fixed to underlying tissues (muscle and bone) and can ulcerate or drain purulent fluid. Skin lesions are most prevalent on the head but can also occur on the limbs and the trunk.[20,23] Enlarged mesenteric lymph nodes, spleen, and/or liver may be detected on abdominal palpation. Involvement of internal lymph nodes is more common with *M. bovis* infections (21% of cats) than with *M. microti* infections (9% of cats).[10] Lameness may be present in cats with skeletal involvement.

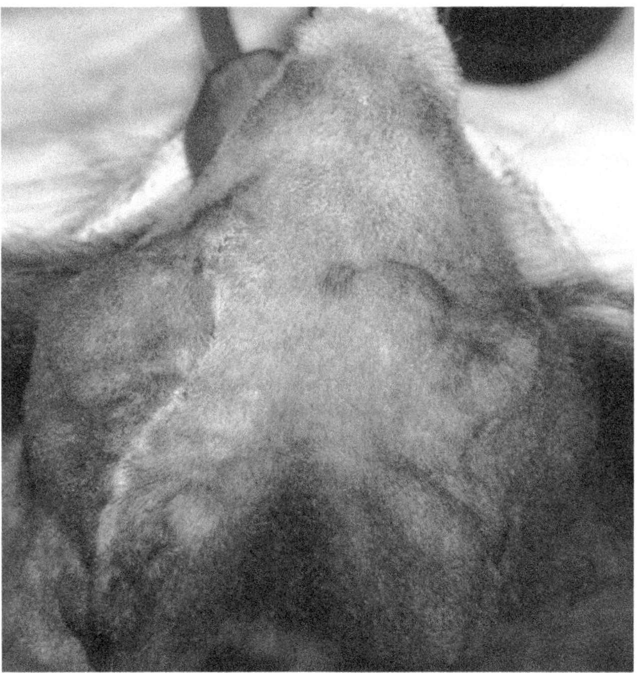

FIGURE 44-4 Mandibular lymphadenopathy in a cat infected with *Mycobacterium microti*.

Diagnosis

Diagnosis of MTBC infection relies on suggestive history, clinical signs, and radiographic abnormalities, combined with the results of histopathology, molecular tests, and culture. When mycobacterial infection is suspected, clinical specimens should be divided into portions—one for histopathology (in formalin), one for mycobacterial culture, one for routine cultures for other bacterial species, and one for mycobacterial PCR (fresh or frozen). The laboratory should be informed that mycobacterial infection is a possibility.

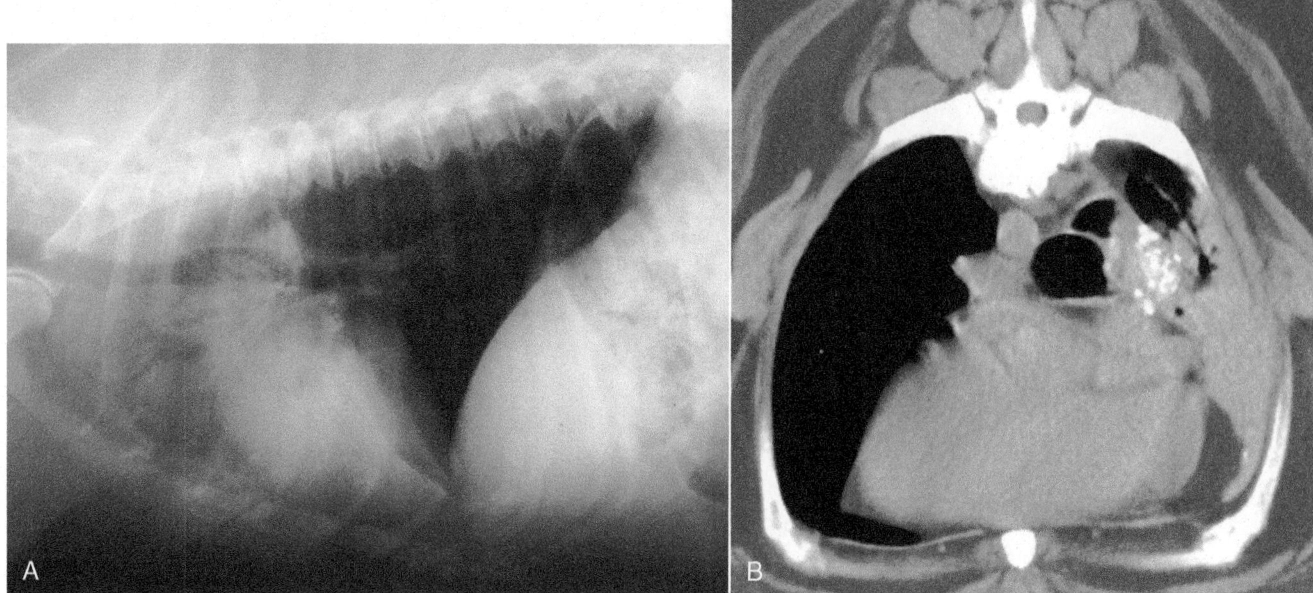

FIGURE 44-5 Lateral thoracic radiograph **(A)** and 7-mm collimated computed tomography (CT) image immediately cranial to the carina **(B)** from a 9-year-old female spayed golden retriever with pulmonary tuberculosis. **A,** Consolidation of the right cranial lung lobe is present together with interstitial to alveolar infiltrates in the right middle lung lobe. **B,** On the CT scan, the right cranial lung lobe is consolidated and markedly volume reduced. Air bronchograms are present centrally that extend dorsally toward a focal region of aerated lung. The granular mineral opacity adjacent to the right margin of the trachea represents mineralized lymphadenopathy of the right tracheobronchial lymph nodes. (From Sykes JE, Cannon AB, Norris AJ, et al. *Mycobacterium tuberculosis* complex infection in a dog. J Vet Intern Med 2007;21:1108-1112.)

Laboratory Abnormalities

Complete Blood Count, Serum Biochemical Tests, and Urinalysis

Laboratory abnormalities in dogs and cats infected with MTBC organisms are nonspecific. Mild anemia of inflammatory disease and neutrophilic leukocytosis, sometimes with a left shift, and monocytosis are often present. The serum chemistry profile may show hypoalbuminemia and hyperglobulinemia. Hypercalcemia of granulomatous disease can also occur in dogs or cats.[10,17] Increased serum liver enzyme activities have been reported in dogs with hepatic involvement.[3]

Diagnostic Imaging

Plain Radiography

Findings on plain thoracic radiography in dogs infected with *M. tuberculosis* or *M. bovis* include tracheobronchial or mediastinal lymphadenopathy,[3,4,7] interstitial to alveolar infiltrates,[22] pleural effusion,[3] and lobar consolidation (Figure 44-5, *A*).[7,22] Similar abnormalities can occur in cats infected with *M. microti* and *M. bovis* (Figure 44-6). Bronchial, alveolar, nodular interstitial, and unstructured interstitial patterns predominate in cats, and perihilar lymphadenopathy can be present.[20,26] Calcification of pulmonary lesions or lymph nodes may be evident in dogs or cats. Hepatomegaly, splenomegaly, or lymphadenopathy, with or without ascites, may be present on abdominal radiography, or abdominal radiographs may be unremarkable.[26] Radiographic evidence of osteomyelitis (especially osteolysis) can occur in cats infected with *M. microti* or *M. bovis,* often in association with overlying cutaneous lesions.[26]

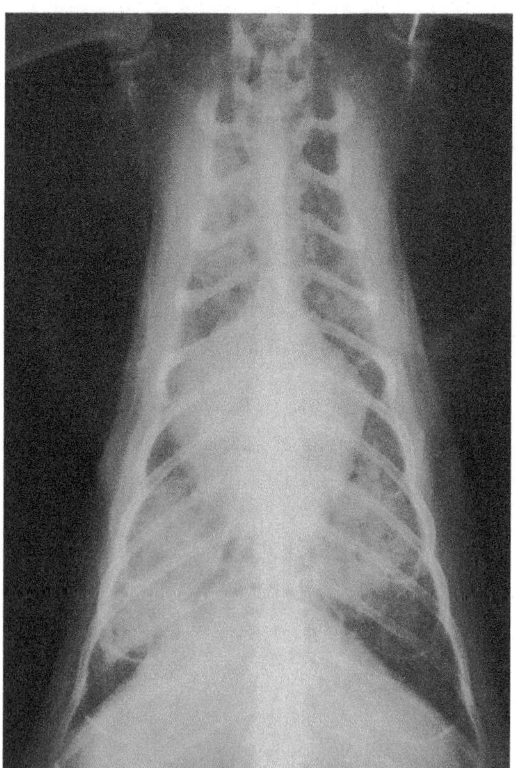

FIGURE 44-6 Pneumonia in a 6-year-old male neutered oriental shorthair with suspected *Mycobacterium microti* infection. Bronchoalveolar lavage revealed pyogranulomatous inflammation, but acid-fast stains were negative. Results of an IFN-γ assay suggested infection by *M. microti*.

Computed Tomography

Thoracic CT findings have been reported for a dog infected with *M. tuberculosis*.[7] Lung lobe consolidation, multifocal stellate opacities, bronchial stenosis, bronchiectasis,

TABLE 44-3

Assays Available for Diagnosis of Mycobacterial Infections in Dogs and Cats

Assay	Specimen Type	Target	Performance
Acid-fast staining	Tissue aspirates, buffy coat smears, body fluids, airway lavage specimens, tissues obtained at biopsy or necropsy	Acid-fast bacteria	Insensitive, especially for some mycobacterial species such as MTBC bacteria. Other bacteria, such as *Rhodococcus* and *Nocardia*, may also be acid fast, so positive results are not specific for *Mycobacterium* spp.
Gamma-interferon response assay	Whole blood (peripheral blood mononuclear cells)	Cell-mediated immune response to mycobacterial antigens	Not yet well validated, but show promise for discrimination between *M. bovis* and *M. microti* infections in the United Kingdom. Variable responses to *M. avium*.
Mycobacterial culture	See acid-fast staining; avoid use of aspirates or swabs if possible	Culturable *Mycobacterium* spp.	Some mycobacterial species are unculturable. Growth of MTBC organisms and slowly growing nontuberculous mycobacteria may take weeks to months, and identification requires special expertise. Allows detailed molecular typing and susceptibility testing.
PCR	See acid-fast staining	Mycobacterial DNA	Permits rapid identification of mycobacterial infection and differentiates MTBC from other mycobacteria, so appropriate precautions can be instituted. False-negative results can occur with insufficient specimen size, if there are very few bacteria present, or if degradation of DNA occurs. False-positive results are possible as a result of laboratory contamination.

tracheobronchial wall thickening, and partially mineralized masses consistent with enlarged mediastinal and tracheobronchial lymph nodes were present (Figure 44-5, *B*). In this dog, the mineralization was not visible on plain thoracic radiographs. CT in human patients with tuberculosis is considered more sensitive than plain radiography for detection of pulmonary lesions and enlarged lymph nodes and provides better visualization of calcifications.

Sonographic Findings

Abdominal sonography in animals with MTBC infections may be unremarkable or reveal hepatomegaly, splenomegaly, abdominal lymphadenopathy, and/or ascites. A dog with disseminated *M. tuberculosis* infection had multifocal hypoechoic masses within the kidneys and liver and mineralization of the hepatic and renal parenchyma.[4]

Cytologic Examination

Cytologic examination of aspirates, effusion, or lavage specimens from the respiratory tract of dogs with pulmonary tuberculosis typically reveals a mixed population of often heavily vacuolated histiocytes and smaller numbers of degenerate or nondegenerate neutrophils and small lymphocytes.[3,7,22] Intracytoplasmic, nonstaining bacilli were seen in macrophages in a bronchoalveolar lavage specimen from a dog infected with *M. bovis*.[22] Moderate anisocytosis or anisokaryosis of exfoliated respiratory epithelial cells can be present, which might cause suspicion for pulmonary neoplasia.[7] The presence of cholesterol crystals, caseous debris, and concentrically laminated crystalline structures known as calcospherite bodies can be a clue for the presence of MTBC infection.[7,22]

Microbiologic Tests

Assays available for diagnosis of mycobacterial infections are listed in Table 44-3.

Acid-Fast Stains

Acid-fast stains can be applied to smears or tissue sections for detection of tuberculous mycobacteria. Organisms are faintly beaded bacilli, and are often within macrophages. The presence of AFB suggests mycobacterial infection, but is not specific for infection with MTBC organisms. Acid-fast staining of smears or Cytospin preparations can be insensitive for detection of MTBC organisms, and negative results do not rule out infection.

Immunologic Assays

Intradermal inoculation of tuberculin (a purified protein derivative from *M. tuberculosis*), or the *Mantoux test,* is well validated and widely used in human medicine for diagnosis of, and screening for, infection with MTBC organisms. Infected individuals develop a cutaneous DTH reaction at the site of inoculation 48 to 72 hours later. False-negative test results can occur as a result of underlying immunosuppression. False-positive results occur as a result of nontuberculous mycobacterial infection. Cats do not respond reliably to tuberculin skin testing. In dogs, tuberculin testing has been performed on the medial surface of the pinna, but false-positive results have been documented with a variety of other bacterial infections. Tests for anti-mycobacterial antibodies are also not specific.[27] Cell-based assays (ELISA and ELISPOT), which measure IFN-γ production by patient peripheral blood mononuclear cells in response to specific mycobacterial antigens, have been used for diagnosis of tuberculosis in humans and cattle. These assays have been adapted for use in cats and have the potential to rapidly distinguish infection with

M. bovis from that with *M. microti* when responses to different mycobacterial antigens are compared.[28]

Bacterial Isolation and Identification

Routine aerobic, anaerobic, fungal, and mycoplasma cultures are negative when performed on specimens collected from animals with MTBC infections. Mycobacterial culture is required and is the gold standard for diagnosis of MTBC infection. The use of laboratories with expertise in isolation of MTBC is recommended. Respiratory specimens such as respiratory lavages are usually treated with the mucolytic *N*-acetylcysteine and a sodium hydroxide solution to destroy contaminating bacteria. Specimens from normally sterile sites, such as pleural fluid, are not decontaminated so that viable mycobacteria are preserved as much as possible. Specimens are then inoculated onto special liquid or solid media for isolation of mycobacteria, such as 7H11 agar or Lowenstein-Jensen media (an egg-based medium). Modifications to the media composition may be required on the basis of the mycobacterial species suspected, so good communication between the clinician and the microbiology laboratory can optimize the chance of successful culture. Growth is evident 1 to 3 weeks after inoculation of liquid media, and 3 to 8 weeks after inoculation of solid media. However, inoculation of solid media is still required, because some strains grow only on solid media, and growth on solid media allows assessment of colony morphology. Once growth is evident, nucleic acid–based assays, mycolic acid analysis with high-performance liquid chromatography, or mass spectrometry (MALDI-TOF)[29] can be used to determine whether the organism belongs to the MTBC. Antimicrobial drug susceptibility testing can also be performed.

Currently, performance of a series of phenotypic (biochemical) assays on cultured isolates is the gold standard method for differentiation of mycobacterial species that belong to the MTBC. Molecular techniques such as PCR-restriction endonuclease analysis, DNA probing, and 16S rRNA gene sequencing do not differentiate among MTBC species. Specialized molecular techniques for further typing of MTBC isolates include mycobacterial interspersed repetitive unit-variable-number tandem repeat (MIRU-VNTR) typing and spoligotyping. Spoligotyping is a PCR-hybridization typing method that targets the direct repeat region of MTBC strains. This region contains multiple DNA sequence repeats interspersed with nonrepetitive spacer sequences. MTBC species vary in the numbers of repeats and the presence or absence of some spacers and can be differentiated on the basis of their hybridization patterns. Spoligotyping also allows identification of prevalent *M. tuberculosis* genotypes, such as the Beijing genotype, an aggressive, highly transmissible strain that has been associated with multiple drug resistance. MIRU-VNTR is often combined with spoligotyping for identification of MTBC organisms. Spoligotyping has been performed on several MTBC isolates from dogs and cats.

Molecular Diagnosis Using the Polymerase Chain Reaction

Real-time PCR-based assays are available on a commercial basis in some countries for rapid detection of *Mycobacterium* spp. DNA in clinical specimens from dogs and cats. An understanding of the range of mycobacterial species detected by an assay is of paramount importance for proper interpretation of the results. Genus-specific *Mycobacterium* spp. assays are available, as well as assays that detect mycobacteria other than tuberculosis (MOTT) organisms. These assays can be used in combination to determine whether an MTBC organism is present. A positive result with a genus-specific assay but a negative result with an assay for MOTT organisms implies the presence of an MTBC organism. The results of mycobacterial PCR assays should be interpreted in light of clinical findings, and PCR assays should always be used with mycobacterial culture, which is the only way to confirm the mycobacterial species involved and allows antimicrobial drug susceptibility testing. The latter is important given the public health implications of MTBC infections.

Pathologic Findings

Gross Pathologic Findings

The most frequent gross pathologic findings in dogs infected with *M. tuberculosis* are pulmonary congestion, lobar consolidation, or granulomatous mass formation and sometimes massive enlargement of tracheobronchial and mediastinal nodes. Lymph nodes may contain multifocal gritty, yellow, caseous material.[4,7,22] Pleural effusion may also be present.[3] In dogs with disseminated disease, pale nodular lesions may be found in abdominal organs such the liver, peritoneal surfaces, and kidneys.[2,4,22] In one unusual case, a dog from Africa had nodular lesions that were confined to the liver and brain.[2] Dogs infected with *M. bovis* have abnormalities similar to those infected with *M. tuberculosis*.[16-18] In addition to cutaneous lesions and peripheral lymphadenomegaly, cats with disseminated *M. bovis* or *M. microti* infections may have abdominal lymphadenomegaly and multifocal tumor-like, grayish-white masses within parenchymal organs that can have hemorrhagic margins and/or a soft purulent center. Pulmonary lesions are often grayish red and may be accompanied by serosanguineous pleural effusion.

Histopathologic Findings

Histopathologic findings are similar for all MTBC diseases. Characteristic tubercles or granulomas are present in tissues, which vary in size and may coalesce (Figure 44-7). Tubercles consist of abundant epithelioid macrophages and lesser numbers of neutrophils. Multinucleated giant cells are rarely present in dogs or cats.[4,30] The inflammatory foci are surrounded by a layer of macrophages, neutrophils, lymphocytes, and plasma cells and an outer layer (or background) of granulation tissue. The center of the tubercle may be necrotic. Central mineralization and lipid accumulation occurs in some dogs infected with *M. tuberculosis*,[7,22] but mineralization is rare in cats infected with *M. microti* or *M. bovis*. Acid-fast stains reveal low numbers of AFB in tubercle centers in most cases, but a careful search may be required (Figure 44-8).[4,7]

Treatment and Prognosis

Dogs and cats with suspected MTBC infection should be placed in isolation, and aerosol precautions are indicated (see Chapter 11). Treatment of dogs and cats with MTBC infection is controversial because of concerns that relate to zoonotic potential. It should only be performed after owners have been fully educated about the potential risks of disease transmission. Most affected dogs have been euthanized without specific treatment, but occasionally euthanasia of animals with non-MTBC mycobacterial infection has occurred before a diagnosis of MTBC was confirmed. Combination drug therapy with the antimycobacterial drugs ethambutol, isoniazid, rifampin, and pyrazinamide is used to treat human patients. Ethambutol and isoniazid interfere with mycobacterial cell wall synthesis; the mechanism of action of pyrazinamide is not known, and *M. bovis* is naturally resistant

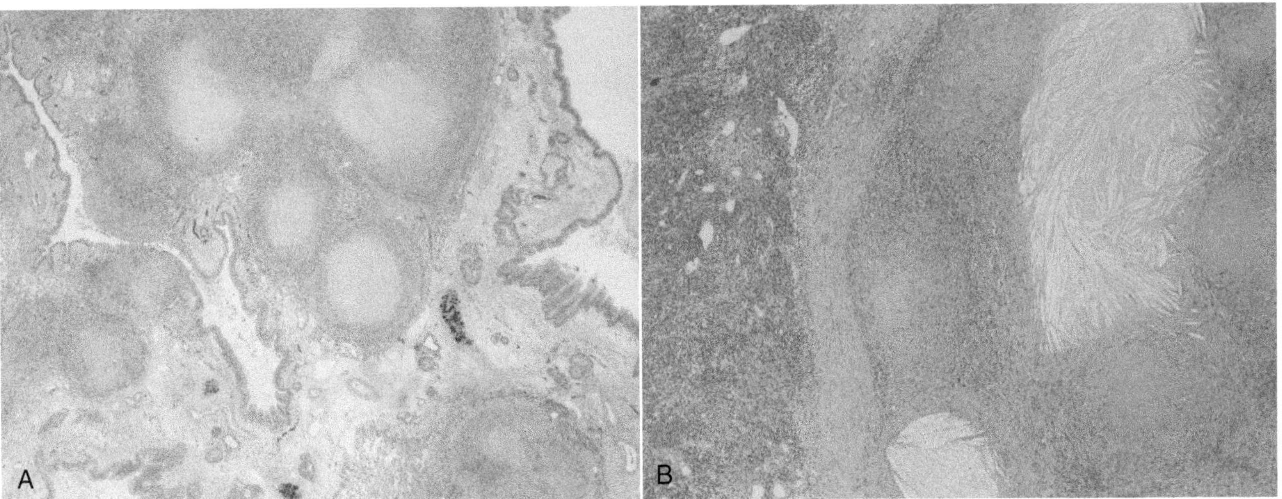

FIGURE 44-7 Multifocal granuloma formation in the lung **(A)** and thoracic lymph node **(B)** of a 9-year-old female spayed golden retriever with pulmonary tuberculosis. The granuloma within the lymph node contains a lake of lipid and necrotic cellular debris, surrounded by an internal layer of epithelioid macrophages, a thick layer of fibrosis, and an external layer of lymphocytes, plasma cells, and histiocytes. Fite and Ziehl-Neelsen acid-fast stains revealed scant numbers of acid-fast positive bacteria in areas of central necrosis (not shown).

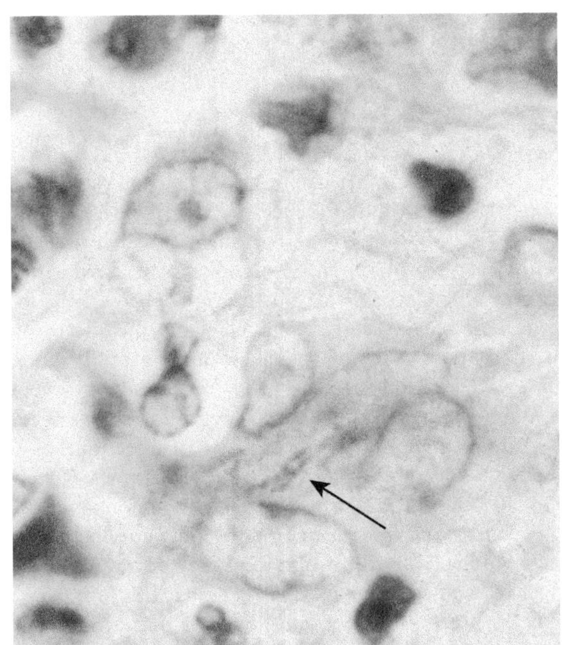

FIGURE 44-8 Rare acid-fast bacteria in a biopsy specimen from a cat infected with *M. microti*.

to it. Treatment of a dog with *M. tuberculosis* infection was attempted with rifampin, isoniazid, and clarithromycin, but the dog was euthanized after seizures developed.[7] The seizures were suspected to be an adverse effect of isoniazid administration.

Successful treatment of cats with cutaneous and/or pulmonary MTBC infections has been achieved with combinations of fluoroquinolones, clarithromycin or azithromycin, doxycycline, and a rifamycin; most successfully treated cases have received a fluoroquinolone, clarithromycin or azithromycin, and a rifamycin (Table 44-4). Surgical excision of small skin lesions can be curative if dissemination is not present, but lesions may dehisce and progress if resection is not complete, and it may not always be possible to determine whether dissemination has occurred. The use of three drugs has been recommended for the first 2 months of treatment (e.g., rifampin, clarithromycin, and a fluoroquinolone), followed by a continuation period with two drugs (usually the macrolide and the fluoroquinolone, because rifamycins are more often associated with adverse effects). Esophagostomy tube placement may be necessary to facilitate treatment and reduce the chance of exposure of the owner to the infection through bite or scratch wounds.

Immunity and Vaccination

There are no vaccines available for prevention of mycobacterial disease in animals.

Prevention

Prevention of *M. tuberculosis* infections in dogs relies on appropriate control and treatment of *M. tuberculosis* infections in affected humans that are in close contact with dogs. Prophylaxis with a single antimycobacterial drug such as isoniazid could be considered for dogs that reside with affected humans, but isoniazid has the potential to cause adverse effects such as seizures in dogs. The possibility of chronic infection by potentially zoonotic pathogens such as *M. tuberculosis* should be considered before stray dogs are adopted from underdeveloped countries.

In cats, prevention of *M. bovis* and *M. microti* infections can be achieved when cats are housed indoors and rodent populations controlled. The feeding of raw cattle or game (e.g., deer, elk) also has the potential to transmit *M. bovis* to dogs or cats and should be discouraged.

Public Health Aspects

Disease caused by MTBC bacteria is usually notifiable to public health authorities. More than 90% of human tuberculosis is caused by *M. tuberculosis*. Only 1% of cases result from *M. bovis* infection, and human infection with *M. microti* is very rare.[31] Factors such as HIV infection, homelessness, and intravenous drug use predispose humans to *M. tuberculosis* infection. Tuberculosis continues to be an important public health problem worldwide and especially in Africa. It is second only to HIV as a cause of death worldwide from a single infectious

TABLE 44-4

Suggested Drug Doses for Treatment of Mycobacterial Infections*

Drug	Dose (mg/kg)	Route	Interval (hours)	Major Adverse Effects in Dogs and Cats
Isoniazid	5-10	PO	24	Hepatotoxicity, seizures. Start at a low dose; do not exceed 300 mg/day. Monitor liver enzymes.
Ethambutol	10-25	PO	48-72	Unknown; neuropathies, especially optic neuritis with visual disturbances occur in humans.
Rifampin	5-10	PO	12-24	Gastrointestinal, hepatotoxicity, orange discoloration of urine, tears, sclera, mucous membranes, feces. Monitor liver enzymes.
Clarithromycin	7.5	PO	12	Rare; hepatotoxicity and gastrointestinal signs possible.
Doxycycline	10	PO	12	Gastrointestinal
Enrofloxacin	5-10 (dogs only)†	PO	24	Gastrointestinal
Marbofloxacin	2.75-5.5	PO	24	Gastrointestinal
Clofazimine	25 mg/cat, 4-8 mg/kg (dogs)	PO	24	Cutaneous photosensitization,‡ orange pigmentation to the skin, gastrointestinal. May be difficult to obtain in some countries.

*See text for recommended drug combinations for each mycobacterial species and additional drugs that may be useful.
†The use of other fluoroquinolones such as marbofloxacin or pradofloxacin is preferred in cats because of the risk of retinal toxicity (see Chapter 8).
‡Bennett S. Photosensitisation induced by clofazimine in a cat. Aust Vet J 2007;85:375-380.

agent,[32] and drug resistance is emerging globally. Over the past 2 decades, case numbers have decreased to the lowest levels in history in the United States.[33] In the United States, the incidence rate is highest among non-Hispanic Asians, non-Hispanic blacks, and Hispanics, which is 25, 8, and 7 times greater, respectively, than the rate for non-Hispanic whites.[33] Disease in immigrants to the United States results from reactivation of disease acquired in other countries.

Public health authorities should be notified if a diagnosis of MTBC infection is made in a dog or cat. An investigation may be performed by these authorities in order to identify the source of infection, and it may be necessary to perform one or more Mantoux tests on individuals with significant contact with infected animals. Although transmission of *M. tuberculosis* from infected dogs to humans has not been reported as a result of direct contact, veterinary staff were infected when a necropsy of an infected dog was performed, possibly following aerosolization of infected brain tissue when the skull was sectioned with an electric saw.[2] Properly fitted high-density surgical masks (N95 masks) should be worn if surgery or necropsy is performed on a dog or cat suspected to have tuberculosis.

Mycobacterium avium Complex

Etiology and Epidemiology

The *Mycobacterium avium* complex (MAC) consists of two closely related species, *M. avium* and *Mycobacterium intracellulare*. There are four subspecies of *M. avium*: *hominissuis, avium, paratuberculosis,* and *silvaticum*. *M. avium* subsp. *hominissuis* causes most human infections. The distribution of subspecies in affected dogs and cats is currently not clear, because molecular methods are required for identification at the subspecies level. *M. avium* subsp. *hominissuis* infections have been identified in several dogs from continental Europe,[34,35] whereas *M. avium* subsp. *avium* was isolated from an affected cat.[36] The DNA of *M. avium* subsp. *paratuberculosis* was detected in intestinal biopsies from dogs with chronic gastrointestinal signs, but the role of this organism in disease was not clear.[37] Unlike MTBC organisms, which are associated with reservoir hosts, MAC organisms are environmental saprophytes with a worldwide distribution. They can be found in soil, dust, and aquatic environments that include showers, faucets, household drinking water, swimming pools, and hot tub spas.[38] The organisms also infect free-living amoebae and form biofilms, which may promote environmental persistence. In the United Kingdom, a spatial cluster of infection has been identified in cats from eastern England.[10] Subclinical infections with *M. avium* subsp. *avium* are common among birds, and *M. avium* subsp. *avium* is the main cause of avian tuberculosis.[39] Ingestion of infected birds or bird feces may be a route of transmission to cats or dogs, but this requires clarification.

MAC organisms cause opportunistic infections in immunocompromised individuals. Most affected dogs and cats are 1 to 5 years of age. In dogs, disease occurs sporadically in any breed, but basset hounds, miniature schnauzers, and possibly Yorkshire terriers may be predisposed, possibly because of an inherited CMI deficiency. In cats, retrovirus infection or treatment with potent immunosuppressive drugs may predispose to MAC infection, although most cats have no identifiable immunodeficiency. Siamese cats as well as Abyssinians and Somalis may be predisposed.[40,41] Disseminated MAC infection has also been reported in feline renal transplant recipients[42,43] and in a cat treated with chemotherapy for lymphoma.[44] Infection is not transmissible from one infected individual to another, but disease may initially be indistinguishable from that caused by MTBC bacteria. In the United States, although still rare, infection of cats and dogs with MAC organisms is more common than infection with MTBC organisms. In the United Kingdom, *M. avium* accounted for only 15% of 159 culturable mycobacterial infections in cats (73% were MTBC infections).[10] The median age of affected cats is 8 years.

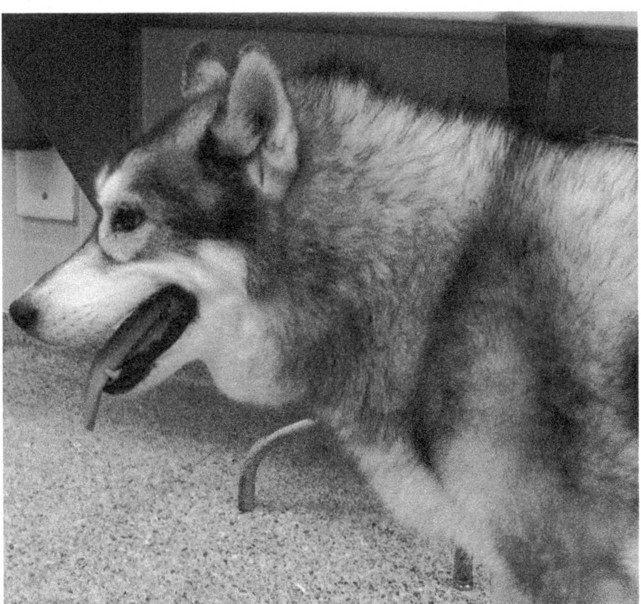

FIGURE 44-9 Five-year-old female spayed husky dog with *Mycobacterium avium* lymphadenitis. Swellings in the mandibular region are apparent.

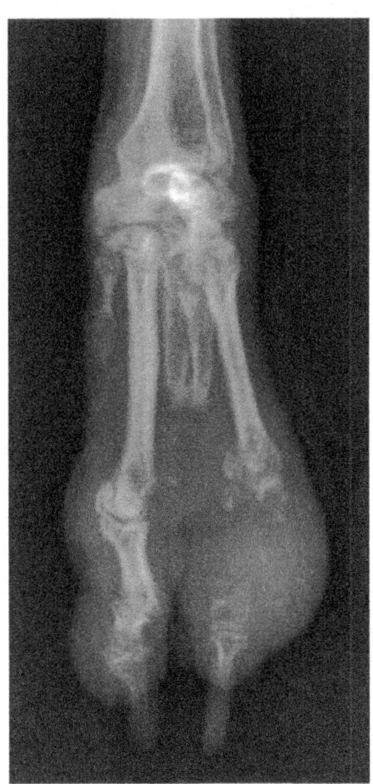

FIGURE 44-10 Digital osteomyelitis in an 8-year-old female spayed Yorkshire terrier dog with *Mycobacterium avium* infection. The first and second phalanges of the fifth digit are destroyed, and there is irregular mineralization within a large soft tissue swelling in this region. There is also moderate soft tissue swelling at the second digit. The third and fourth digits had been previously amputated at the mid-metacarpal bones, which are now fused at their distal aspect.

Clinical Features

Signs and Their Pathogenesis

Disease due to MAC organisms occurs when organisms in soil, water, or dust are inhaled, ingested, or inoculated into skin wounds in the face of host immunocompromise. Disseminated infection often leads to nonspecific signs such as fever, lethargy, inappetence, and weight loss, together with signs that relate to specific organ involvement. In cats, disease resembles that caused by *M. bovis* or *M. microti,* with cutaneous lesions (especially on the head and limbs) in some cats, osteomyelitis, pulmonary involvement with tachypnea or cough, peripheral and abdominal lymphadenomegaly, and gastrointestinal, liver, splenic, renal, omental, and uncommonly CNS or marrow involvement.[41,42,44-50] Gastrointestinal involvement may initially manifest as weight loss despite a good appetite.[41]

Dogs with MAC infections often develop marked peripheral or abdominal lymphadenopathy, tonsillar enlargement, hepatosplenomegaly, and/or osteomyelitis. In some dogs, mandibular or cervical lymphadenopathy may be so severe that respiratory distress and dysphagia occur (Figure 44-9).[51] At necropsy, AFB and associated inflammatory lesions may also be found in the small and large intestines, liver, spleen, lung and pleura, bone marrow, and rarely the spinal cord.[34,52-56] Involvement of the gastrointestinal tract may lead to chronic vomiting, diarrhea, hematochezia, melena, inappetence, and weight loss. Intestinal rupture in one dog led to bacterial peritonitis. Even though inflammatory lesions with intralesional AFB have been detected in the lung at necropsy, pulmonary involvement is not a prominent clinical feature of MAC infections in dogs, which may help to distinguish the disease from *M. tuberculosis* infection.

Physical Examination Findings

Physical examination of cats with MAC infections may reveal fever, a thin body condition, cutaneous lesions similar to those described for MTBC infection, peripheral or abdominal lymphadenopathy, renomegaly, hepatomegaly, tachypnea, and/or increased lung sounds. Rarely, neurologic signs such as nystagmus occur.[41] In dogs, low-grade fever, a thin body condition, dehydration, mucosal pallor, tonsillar enlargement, lymphadenomegaly (especially of the mandibular or abdominal nodes), hepatosplenomegaly, and/or abdominal pain may be found. Melena or hematochezia may be detected on rectal examination. Osteomyelitis may be associated with lameness or mass lesions in association with underlying bone involvement (Figure 44-10). A dog with spinal cord involvement had pelvic limb paresis.[53]

Diagnosis

Laboratory Abnormalities

Complete Blood Count, Serum Biochemical Tests, and Urinalysis

Findings on routine laboratory tests in dogs and cats with MAC infections are similar to those described for MTBC infection. Most affected dogs or cats have had mild to moderate nonregenerative anemia, neutrophilia with bandemia, lymphopenia, hypoalbuminemia, hyperglobulinemia or hypoglobulinemia, and sometimes hypercalcemia, hyperbilirubinemia, and increased liver enzyme activities.[48,54,57] An absence of hematologic or biochemical abnormalities has also been described.

Diagnostic Imaging

Plain Radiography

When radiographic abnormalities are present in cats infected with *M. avium*, they often consist of diffuse interstitial or bronchointerstitial pulmonary patterns.[41,48] Diffuse interstitial patterns may be present in the absence of clinical signs of respiratory involvement. Thoracic lymphadenopathy or mediastinal

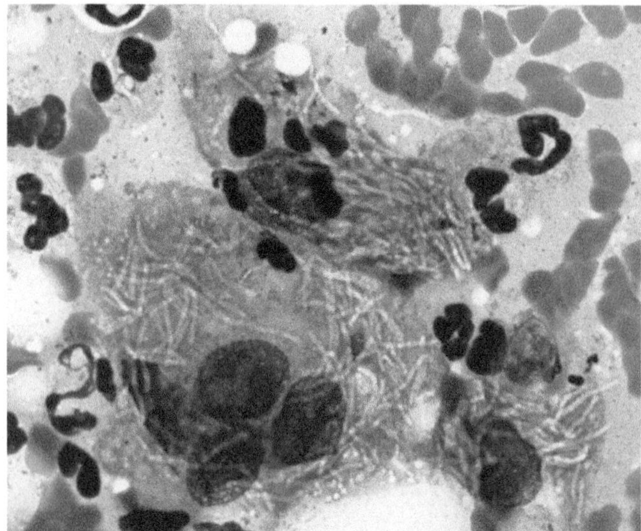

FIGURE 44-11 Aspirate cytology from a cutaneous mass in a cat that developed after prolonged (>1 year) treatment with cyclosporine. Large numbers of negatively stained mycobacterial organisms are present. (Image courtesy Dr. William Vernau, University of California, Davis Veterinary Clinical Pathology Service.)

masses may be present in dogs.[35] Abdominal radiographs may show abdominal masses or hepatosplenomegaly in both dogs and cats. Radiographs of affected bone may reveal soft tissue swelling and bony lytic lesions or periosteal proliferation (see Figure 44-10).

Sonographic Findings

Abdominal sonography in animals with MAC infections may be unremarkable or reveal hepatomegaly, splenomegaly, hypoechoic nodules within the liver or spleen, intestinal wall thickening, hyperechoic mesentery, or enlarged, hypoechoic, or heteroechoic abdominal nodes.[58]

Cytologic Examination

Cytologic examination of aspirates from lymph nodes, abdominal organs, or respiratory lavage specimens from cats or dogs with *M. avium* infection reveals large numbers of histiocytes with nonstaining intracellular bacteria (Figure 44-11) and lower numbers of neutrophils.

Microbiologic Tests

For assays available for diagnosis of mycobacterial infections in dogs and cats, see Table 44-3.

Acid-Fast Stains

Application of acid-fast stains to smears or tissue sections can be used to identify MAC organisms in clinical specimens. In general, AFB are identified more readily in MAC infections when compared with MTBC infections, and most reports of affected dogs and cats report the detection of organisms in cytology specimens stained with acid-fast stains.

Bacterial Isolation and Identification

See the previous discussion of MTBC infection for information on mycobacterial culture. Like MTBC organisms, MAC organisms grow slowly in culture. Up to 6 weeks of incubation may be required for visible growth. MAC species are then identified using commercial DNA probe-based assays or PCR analysis. Subspecies determination requires specialized typing techniques such as IS*1245* restriction fragment length polymorphism typing, MIRU-VNTR, or the use of PCR assays that detect gene fragments present in some *M. avium* subspecies but not others.[34,36,59]

Molecular Diagnosis Using the Polymerase Chain Reaction

See the previous discussion of MTBC infection for information on mycobacterial PCR assays.

Pathologic Findings

In general, pathologic findings in cats or dogs with MAC infection consist of focal, multifocal, or generalized lymphadenomegaly (up to 5 cm in diameter), and nodules in the spleen, liver, lungs, omentum, intestinal wall, and occasionally the kidneys. Nodules are white, gray, or yellow and may be caseous on cut section. Gastrointestinal mucosal hemorrhage may be evident in dogs.[54]

Histopathology in MAC infections typically reveals large numbers of histiocytes and lesser numbers of neutrophils, which in some cases surround necrotic foci. Multinucleated giant cells are rarely seen, and mineralization has not been described. Moderate to large numbers of AFB are usually present within histiocytes (Figure 44-12).

Treatment and Prognosis

Treatment of MAC infections in dogs or cats is challenging, but apparent cure has been reported in a few cats.[36,41,48] As for infection with MTBC organisms, the use of two or three drugs in combination is recommended to prevent emergence of resistance. The availability of macrolides (especially clarithromycin) has greatly improved outcome for human patients with MAC infections, so inclusion of clarithromycin or azithromycin is important. The currently recommended treatment for humans with MAC infections consists of a rifamycin, ethambutol, and a macrolide such as clarithromycin. Treatment of a dog with a combination of drugs that did not include a macrolide was unrewarding.[51] Various combinations of clarithromycin, clofazimine, doxycycline, rifamycins, and fluoroquinolones have been used to treat affected cats (see Table 44-4). Clofazimine is an antimycobacterial drug with an unknown mechanism of action. In human patients, it has primarily been used to treat lepromatous or rapidly growing opportunistic mycobacteria, but may have some activity against MAC organisms. It may be difficult or impossible to obtain in some countries.

Public Health Aspects

Like dogs and cats, humans acquire MAC infections from the environment; direct transmission from animals to people has not been described. Ownership of caged birds by immunocompromised humans has been discouraged in the past because of the potential that these birds might shed MAC organisms. However, human disease is caused by *M. avium* subsp. *hominissuis* and not the avian organism (subsp. *avium*), so the feces of caged birds may not represent a significant source of infection. Three clinical forms of MAC disease occur in people: localized pulmonary disease (which includes "hot tub lung disease," a hypersensitivity pneumonitis), cervical lymphadenitis, and disseminated disease.[60] Disseminated disease occurs most often in HIV-infected humans, but children with congenital

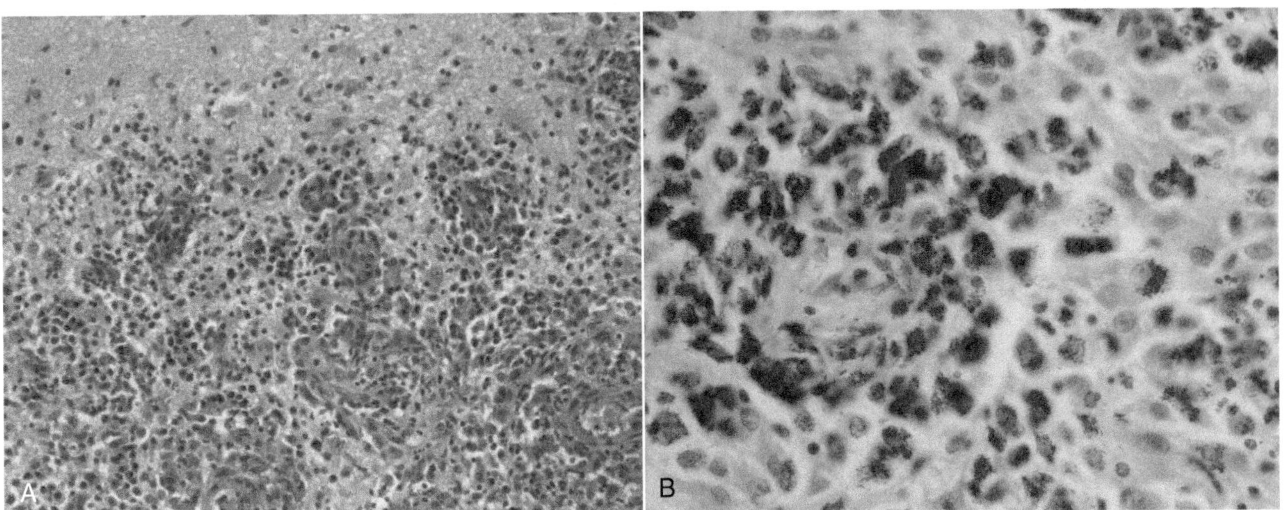

FIGURE 44-12 **A,** Granulomatous inflammation in the brain of a 10-year-old male neutered Siamese mix cat with disseminated *Mycobacterium avium* infection. H&E stain. **B,** Section from the same cat stained with Ziehl-Neelsen (acid-fast) stain. There are large numbers of intracellular acid-fast bacteria.

immunodeficiencies can also be affected. Prophylactic antimycobacterial drug treatment is recommended for HIV-infected humans with CD4+ T cell counts that are less than 50 cells/mm^3.[60] Cervical lymphadenitis is an uncommon disease of children less than 3 years of age.

Although transmission of MAC organisms from diseased dogs and cats to humans should not, in theory, occur by direct contact, it may not be possible to distinguish infection with *M. avium* from infection with MTBC organisms (especially *M. bovis*) based on clinical presentation. Thus, in regions where *M. bovis* infections occur, animals suspected to have MAC infections should be isolated until the results of PCR assays confirm MAC infection. Cytologic or histopathologic evidence of large numbers of organisms also suggests MAC as opposed to MTBC infection. Veterinary staff should take care to avoid needle-stick injuries or cutaneous inoculation when collecting specimens (such as lymph node aspirates) from dogs and cats with *M. avium* infections because of the possibility that disease might occur after cutaneous inoculation. Sedation is recommended whenever lymph node aspiration is indicated for an animal with an unknown cause of lymphadenopathy. When mycobacterial disease is suspected, care should also be taken not to aerosolize tissues at necropsy (as occurs with electric saws).

Lepromatous Mycobacteria

Etiology and Epidemiology

Lepromatous mycobacteria are highly fastidious or unculturable mycobacteria that cause nodular cutaneous lesions in dogs or cats. Feline leprosy is caused by *Mycobacterium lepraemurium* and probably several other mycobacterial species. In fact, with the recent discovery of these other mycobacterial species, localized nodular cutaneous disease in cats caused by MAC organisms, or organisms that resemble other nontuberculous mycobacteria (NTM), has fallen under the general heading of feline leprosy syndromes.[61-63]

Feline leprosy has been described in the Netherlands, the United Kingdom, the United States, western Canada, Australia, New Zealand, Italy, and Greece. Affected cats range in age from 1 year to 14 years and are often from rural or semirural environments. Inoculation of organisms into the skin through rodent bites or cat fight wounds is the suspected mode of transmission.

Disease in dogs is known as canine leproid granuloma syndrome (CLGS). It has mainly been reported from the western United States and coastal regions of Australia.[64-66] The organism that causes CLGS has only been partially characterized by the use of PCR sequencing. It has never been isolated in culture and does not yet have a Latin name, but is often referred to as the "CLG organism." A similar, and possibly the same, organism has also been detected using PCR in cats with leprosy.[63] Boxer dogs or their crosses are predisposed, and possibly also German shepherd dogs.[65,66] The mode of transmission to dogs is unknown. Transmission by biting insects has been hypothesized because most lesions occur on the pinnae and head.

Clinical Features

Lepromatous mycobacteria cause single or multiple nodular cutaneous or subcutaneous lesions, which may ulcerate. In cats, lesions are usually on the head or forelimbs, but can also occur at other body sites. Affected cats are usually systemically well. Two pathologic variants of feline disease have been described.[62,63] The first form, "tuberculoid feline leprosy," is characterized by multifocal to coalescing pyogranulomas with central caseous necrosis, as well as increased numbers of lymphocytes and plasma cells in the dermis and panniculus. Multinucleate giant cells may or may not be present, and acid-fast stains reveal variable numbers of AFB, primarily in regions of necrosis. The second form, "lepromatous feline leprosy," is characterized by pyogranulomatous dermatitis and panniculitis with sheets of epithelioid macrophages and neutrophils, moderate to abundant multinucleate giant cells, and large numbers of AFB with minimal necrosis. Organisms that resemble *M. lepraemurium* can be detected in both these clinical forms, whereas the CLG organism has only been detected in cats with the tuberculoid form.[63] The distribution of histopathologic types may vary geographically.

In dogs, CLGS is characterized by the development of firm cutaneous nodules that range in diameter from millimeters to several centimeters. Larger lesions may ulcerate. Most lesions are found on the pinnae, but they may also be found on the head, muzzle, forelimbs, and trunk (Figure 44-13). Histopathology

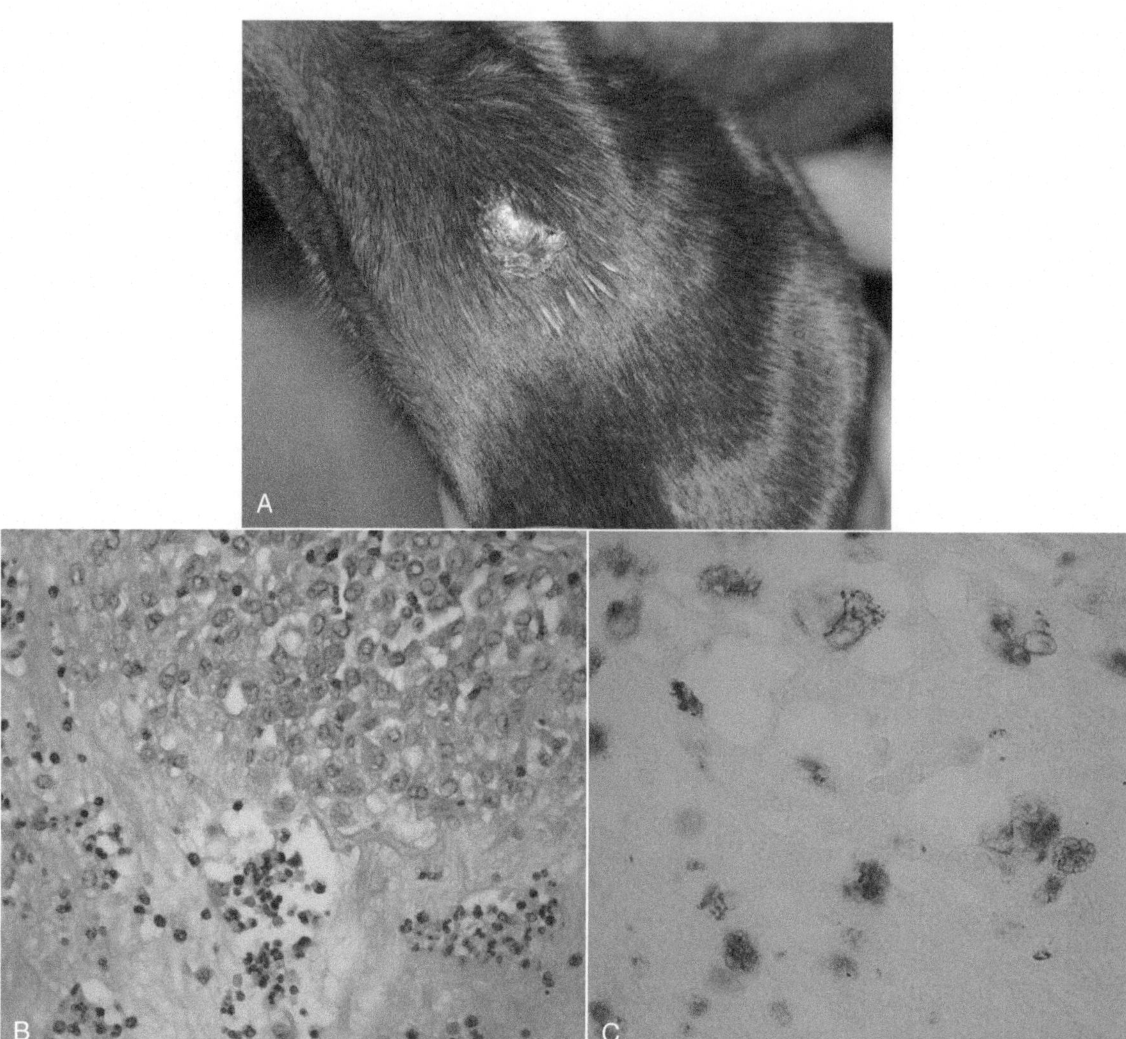

FIGURE 44-13 **A,** Pinna of a 5-year-old male neutered boxer dog with CLGS. A crusted lesion was present that measured 1 × 2 cm in diameter. **B,** Histopathology of CLGS lesions reveals pyogranulomatous inflammation. **C,** A BCG immunostain (brown) identified the presence of intracellular *Mycobacterium* spp. organisms.

reveals coalescing accumulations of histiocytes and neutrophils, with fewer numbers of lymphocytes and plasma cells.[64,66] Multinucleate giant cells may be present, and there may be large numbers of intracellular AFB.

Diagnosis

Diagnosis of leproid syndromes is based on the presence of typical skin lesions, absence of signs of dissemination or systemic illness, suggestive cytologic and histopathologic findings, negative mycobacterial culture results, and positive 16S rRNA gene PCR assay results where PCR assays are available. Cytologic examination of fine-needle aspirates usually reveals pyogranulomatous inflammation with intracellular, negatively stained bacteria, which subsequently stain with acid-fast stains. Sequence analysis of PCR products that are generated from biopsy specimens is required to determine the likely species present.

Treatment

Treatment of feline leproid lesions with a combination of clofazimine and clarithromycin is often successful (see Table 44-4). Wide surgical excision could be considered for small, localized lesions, but has the potential to be followed by dehiscence and extension of disease. If necessary, antimicrobial drug treatment for several weeks followed by surgery may be most successful. In dogs, granulomas may resolve spontaneously within 1 to 3 months. In dogs with progressive or widespread CLGS, a combination of clarithromycin and a rifamycin may be effective.[67]

Prevention and Public Health Aspects

Mycobacterial organisms that cause canine and feline lepromatous disease are not transmitted directly to humans. However, lesions may resemble those caused by *M. microti* and *M. bovis*, so where these diseases are endemic, precautions should be taken until a causative organism is identified with molecular methods.

Nontuberculous Bacteria Other Than *Mycobacterium avium-intracellulare*

Etiology and Epidemiology

NTM species include a variety of opportunistic, environmental mycobacteria that have been classified based on their rate

TABLE 44-5

Cutaneous and Disseminated Disease in Dogs and Cats Caused by Slow-Growing Opportunistic Nontuberculous Mycobacteria

Mycobacterial Species	Species Affected	Clinical Abnormalities	Geographic Location
M. kansasii	Dog	Chronic pleural effusion with pulmonary arterial and pleuroperitoneal shunt infection	North Carolina, USA[83]
M. simiae	Cat	Disseminated disease with generalized lymphadenopathy, lung and skin involvement, and granulomatous chorioretinitis	Switzerland[84]
M. genavense	Cat (FIV+)	Disseminated disease with involvement of lungs, liver, lymph nodes, skin, kidney, spleen	New South Wales, Australia[85]
	Dog	Disseminated disease with involvement of lymph nodes and possibly liver and spleen	New York, USA[86]
M. xenopi	Cat	Cutaneous lesion	Australia[87]
	Cat	Disseminated disease with kidney, lymph node, pancreatic, and marrow involvement	Florida, USA[88]
	Cat	Disseminated disease with lymphadenopathy, gastrointestinal involvement, and ascites	Wisconsin, USA[89]
M. xenopi-like	Cat (FIV+)	Tracheal granuloma	Italy[90]
M. ulcerans	Dog	Cutaneous ulcerating lesions on distal limbs or tail base	Victoria, Australia[91]
	Cat	Mass on nasal bridge	Victoria, Australia[92]
'*M. visibile*' (originally '*M. visibilis*')	Cat	Cutaneous and disseminated disease with involvement of the eyes, skeletal muscle, and a variety of other organs except the liver and kidneys	Western Canada and United States[93]
M. malmoense	Cat	Cutaneous involvement	United Kingdom[10]
M. celatum	Cat	Cutaneous involvement and fever	United Kingdom[10]
M. terrae	Cat	Cutaneous involvement	United Kingdom[94]

of growth in culture (rapid, intermediate, or slow) (see Table 44-1). They are found in soil and a variety of water sources and cause cutaneous, pulmonary, or disseminated disease in dogs and cats. Rapidly growing mycobacteria (RGM) grow in culture within 7 days and include several groups of organisms to which *M. fortuitum, M. septicum, M. abscessus, M. chelonae, M. smegmatis, M. thermoresistibile, M. goodii,* and *M. mucogenicum* belong. Slowly growing mycobacteria require more than 7 days (and sometimes many months) before significant growth occurs in culture. Other than MAC organisms, examples include *M. kansasii, M. terrae, M. xenopi, M. ulcerans, M. malmoense, M. simiae,* and *M. genavense.*

Rapidly Growing Mycobacteria

RGM are responsible for the vast majority of cutaneous mycobacterial disease in cats in the United States and Australia, but infections have also been described in the United Kingdom, Canada, western Europe, and New Zealand. The most commonly isolated species in both the United States and Australia are *M. fortuitum* and *M. smegmatis*, but infections with other RGM also occur (see Table 44-1).[68-71] These organisms have a tropism for adipose tissue, and when inoculated into the skin by means of cat fight injuries (bites or scratches) or other penetrating wounds (and rarely surgical wounds),[72] mycobacterial panniculitis develops. Most affected cats are female spayed cats. Underlying immunosuppressive disease is usually not present. Cutaneous disease occurs less often in dogs and results from infection with *M. fortuitum, M. smegmatis, M. abscessus,* or *M. goodii.*[72-75] No age, breed, or sex predisposition has been recognized, but most dogs are in good body condition or obese. Some dogs have a history of bite wounds or trauma.[73] Concurrent hyperadrenocorticism was described in one dog.[75]

M. fortuitum can cause pulmonary disease in dogs[76-79] as well as bacteremia.[72] Lipoid mycobacterial pneumonia rarely occurs in cats and may arise in association with lactulose or paraffin treatment for furballs.[80] Pneumonia was also described in a cat infected with *M. thermoresistibile.*[81] Disseminated RGM infections are very rare. Disseminated disease that resembled MAC infection was described in a basset hound infected with *M. smegmatis.*[82]

Slowly Growing Mycobacteria

A variety of slowly growing mycobacteria cause cutaneous or disseminated disease in dogs and cats that resembles disease caused by MAC organisms (Table 44-5).[83-94] These include the known human pathogens *M. kansasii, M. simiae, M. genavense, M. xenopi, M. celatum, M. malmoense, M. terrae,* and *M. ulcerans.* Some, but not all affected cats have been infected with FIV, and one cat had CD4+ lymphopenia.[88] *M. ulcerans* causes ulcerative skin lesions in humans, cats, or dogs in certain parts of Australia.

Clinical Features

Rapidly Growing Mycobacteria

In cats, mycobacterial panniculitis occurs most often in the inguinal fat pad, but lesions may also be found elsewhere on the lateral abdomen, perineum, dorsum, and pelvic limbs (Figure 44-14). The subcutis becomes thickened and adheres to the dermis, after which nodular and draining skin lesions develop. The majority of affected cats are otherwise well; the development of systemic illness is rare. In dogs, nodular lesions or nonhealing wounds with draining tracts often occur in the inguinal region, cervical region, and/or other proximal body locations.

Pneumonia due to RGM generally results in signs of fever, lethargy, decreased appetite, cough, and tachypnea, with increased lung sounds on thoracic auscultation. Thoracic radiographs frequently reveal lung lobe consolidation and alveolar patterns. In the cat with *M. thermoresistibile* pneumonia, extensive pulmonary mineralization developed.[81] The dog with disseminated *M. smegmatis* infection had granulomatous hepatitis and lymphadenitis.

Slowly Growing Mycobacteria Other Than MAC

Clinical features of slowly growing mycobacterial infections other than MAC infections have varied from one case to another and are summarized in Table 44-5. Animals with disseminated disease can have clinical abnormalities that are indistinguishable from those caused by *M. avium*.

Diagnosis

Diagnosis of RGM infection is usually based on the presence of consistent clinical abnormalities, and the results of cytology, histopathology, and mycobacterial culture (see Table 44-3). Cytologic examination of fine needle aspirates or lavage specimens generally reveals pyogranulomatous inflammation. However, airway lavage fluid from a dog with *M. fortuitum* pneumonia contained mostly neutrophils.[76] Heavily vacuolated macrophages and lipid vacuoles may be present in aspirates from animals with panniculitis. Organisms may or may not be visible with routine stains or acid-fast stains. Histopathology shows pyogranulomatous inflammation without tubercle formation or necrosis. Large lipid vacuoles that contain acid-fast bacilli may be present. Although molecular assays are often used for speciation, direct use of PCR assays on clinical specimens is often not required for diagnosis because RGM grow readily on routine culture media (blood agar). Culture also allows subsequent antimicrobial drug susceptibility testing to be performed at specialized facilities.

Cytology and histopathology findings for slow-growing NTM are similar to those for MAC infections. Diagnosis of slow-growing mycobacterial infection requires specialized mycobacterial culture or the use of PCR assays. *M. xenopi* requires culture at higher temperatures (42°C to 44°C), whereas other mycobacterial species require lower temperatures (28°C or 30°C). Organisms such as *M. genavense* and *M. ulcerans* can be difficult to grow on solid media, and so molecular methods may be required to identify these species.

Treatment and Prognosis

Treatment options for RGM infections include doxycycline, fluoroquinolones, clarithromycin, aminoglycosides, sulfonamides, or carbapenems (see Table 44-4 and Chapter 8). Many cutaneous and pulmonary infections respond well to treatment with doxycycline, aminoglycosides, and/or a fluoroquinolone.[74-78] Multidrug-resistant isolates are more difficult to treat; moxifloxacin, pradofloxacin, or linezolid could be considered when other treatment options are not possible.[95] As for lepromatous

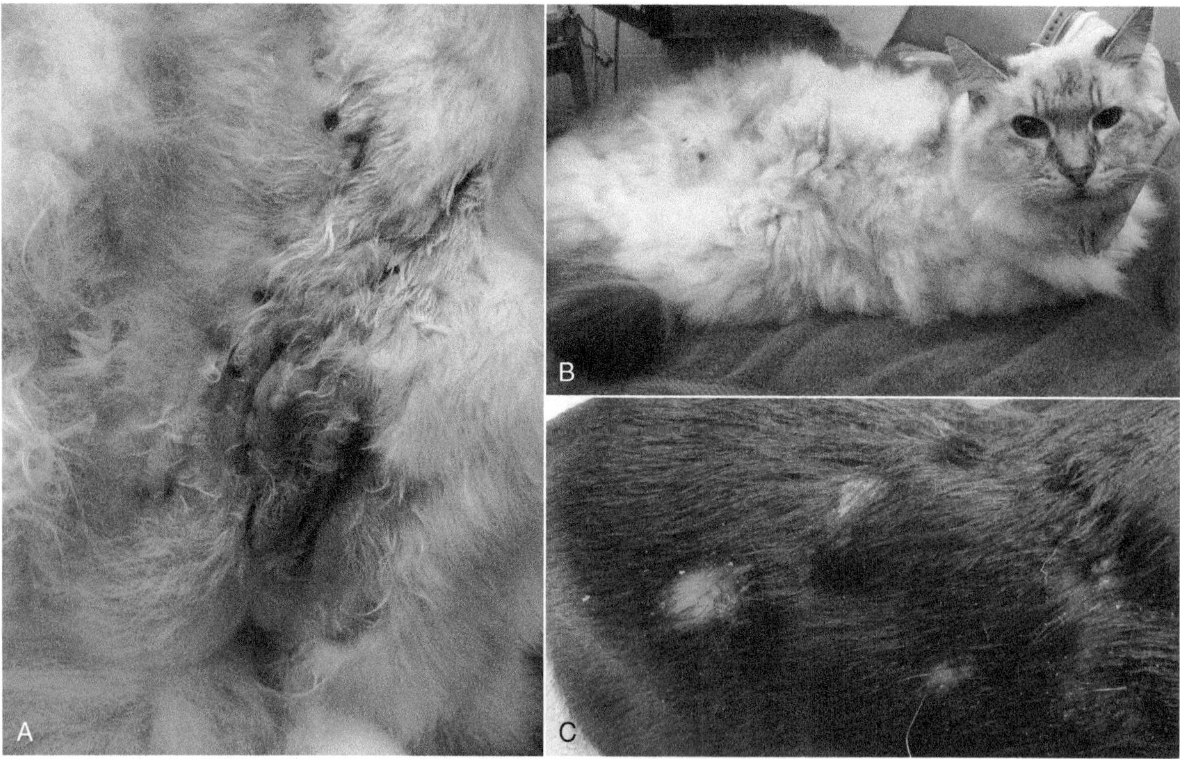

FIGURE 44-14 Cutaneous-subcutaneous infections with rapidly-growing mycobacteria. **A** and **B**, Thirteen-year-old male neutered Siamese cat with mycobacterial panniculitis. There are multiple nodular lesions in the inguinal region **(A)** and lateral flank and dorsal lumbar regions **(B)**. In this cat, lesions progressed slowly over 8 years despite treatment with antimicrobial drugs. **C**, Dorsum of an 8-year old dachshund mix with a multidrug resistant *Mycobacterium abscessus* infection. Multiple draining wounds and extensive scarring are present.

disease, surgical excision of cutaneous lesions is often followed by dehiscence and progression if resection is not complete. However, radical surgical excision by an experienced surgeon could be considered after antimicrobial drug treatment if lesions reduce in size but fail to resolve. Intraoperative treatment of affected cats with an aminoglycoside has been suggested.[96] Treatment should continue for 2 months beyond complete resolution of the lesions and is generally required for at least 4 to 12 months.

M. ulcerans infections generally respond to monotherapy with clarithromycin or a fluoroquinolone.[91,92] For animals with slowly growing mycobacterial infections, options similar to those used to treat MAC infections are indicated—that is, combinations of clarithromycin, a rifamycin, and a fluoroquinolone. In human patients, *M. kansasii* infections are treated with rifampin and ethambutol, with or without isoniazid.[97] The prognosis for disseminated infections in dogs and cats appears to be guarded to poor.

Public Health Aspects

NTM are opportunistic, environmental mycobacteria that are not usually transmitted from animals to humans. Disease in humans resembles that in dogs and cats. Localized cutaneous and soft tissue infections with NTM have occurred after traumatic wounds and lacerations, including after dog and cat bites.[98-100] Infections with RGM can occur after surgical procedures such as liposuction, LASIK surgery, and acupuncture.[97] Catheter-related infections have also been described. Disseminated disease caused by NTM almost always occurs in humans with HIV infection or other immunosuppressive illness or drug therapy.

CASE EXAMPLE

Signalment: "Sarah", a 5-year-old female spayed husky dog from Santa Cruz in coastal northern California

History: Sarah was evaluated for a 1-month history of protrusion of the anus, swelling of the neck, progressive lethargy, and inappetence. She had been diagnosed with zinc-responsive dermatitis 3 years prior, and symmetrical lupoid onychodystrophy 6 months prior. There were two other dogs and three cats in the household, none of which were unwell. The dogs lived in a suburban household and occasionally traveled to southern California, and were normally fed a commercial dry maintenance dog food. There was no known history of tick or toxin exposure or interactions with other wildlife or domestic farm animal species. The owner was a white non-Hispanic male who had been sick for some months. His doctor believed he had acquired the illness from Sarah.

Current Medications: Zinc (2.5 mg/kg q12h PO), tetracycline (25 mg/kg q12h PO), niacinamide (25 mg/kg q12h PO), fish oil capsules (1 capsule PO q12h), and vitamin E (20 IU/kg PO q12h) for the zinc-responsive dermatitis and onychodystrophy. Fipronil with S-methoprene was used for flea and tick control on a monthly basis.

Physical Examination:

Body Weight: 20 kg

General: Quiet to lethargic, hydrated, responsive, preferred to lie down but was ambulatory. T=102.9°F (39.4°C), HR = 140 beats/min, RR = 70 breaths/min

Integument: No abnormalities were detected.

Eyes, Ears, Nose, and Throat: A small amount of purulent ocular discharge was present from the left eye. A fundic examination was unremarkable. Moderate dental calculus.

Musculoskeletal: Body condition score was 4/9, with symmetrical muscling. Moderate ventral cervical and submandibular swelling was present.

Cardiovascular: No murmurs or arrhythmias, femoral pulses adequate. Mucous membranes were pale pink, with a CRT of 2 s.

Respiratory: Referred upper airway noises were auscultated.

Gastrointestinal/Genitourinary: The dog's abdomen was nonpainful. The rectal mucosa was proliferative and hyperemic and protruded from the anus. A rectal examination revealed a nodular diffusely thickened mucosa with a granular texture and prominent sublumbar lymph nodes. There was evidence of melena and frank blood on the glove. No vulvar discharge was noted.

Neurologic: Palpebral, menace, and papillary light responses were intact bilaterally. No neurologic deficits were apparent. A full neurologic examination was not performed.

Lymph Nodes: Generalized peripheral lymphadenopathy was present. The mandibular nodes were 5-6 cm in diameter, lobular and firm. The superficial cervical nodes were 3 cm in diameter, and the inguinal nodes were enlarged at 2 cm, with the left larger than the right. The popliteal nodes were enlarged at 2-3 cm bilaterally.

Laboratory Findings:

CBC:

HCT 22% (40%-55%)
MCV 52 fL (65-75 fL)
MCHC 30 g/dL (33-36 g/dL)
Reticulocyte count 25,200 cells/μL
WBC 40,510 cells/μL (6000-13,000 cells/μL)
Neutrophils 29,977 cells/μL (3000-10,500 cells/μL)
Band neutrophils 2431 cells/μL
Lymphocytes 2026 cells/μL (1000-4000 cells/μL)
Monocytes 2431 cells/μL (150-1200 cells/μL)
Eosinophils 3646 cells/μL (0-1500 cells/μL)
Platelets 387,000 platelets/μL (150,000-400,000 platelets/μL).
Band and mature neutrophils were slightly toxic.

Serum Chemistry Profile:

Sodium 132 mmol/L (145-154 mmol/L)
Potassium 3.5 mmol/L (3.6-5.3 mmol/L)
Chloride 103 mmol/L (108-118 mmol/L)
Bicarbonate 17 mmol/L (16-26 mmol/L)
Phosphorus 4.1 mg/dL (3.0-6.2 mg/dL)
Calcium 8.6 mg/dL (9.7-11.5 mg/dl)
BUN 6 mg/dL (5-21 mg/dL)

Continued

Creatinine 0.6 mg/dL (0.3-1.2 mg/dL)
Glucose 93 mg/dL (64-123 mg/dL)
Total protein 4.3 g/dL (5.4-7.6 g/dL)
Albumin 2.1 g/dL (3.0-4.4 g/dL)
Globulin 2.2 g/dL (1.8-3.9 g/dL)
ALT 43 U/L (19-67 U/L)
AST 51 U/L (19-42 U/L)
ALP 115 U/L (21-170 U/L)
Creatine kinase 202 U/L (51-399 U/L)
GGT < 3 U/L (0-6 U/L)
Cholesterol 146 mg/dL (135-361 mg/dL)
Total bilirubin 0 mg/dL (0-0.2 mg/dL)
Magnesium 2.0 mg/dL (1.5-2.6 mg/dL).

Urinalysis: SGr 1.005; pH 7.5; no protein, bilirubin, hemoprotein, or glucose; rare WBC/HPF, 0 RBC/HPF, few lipid droplets.

Imaging Findings:

Thoracic Radiographs: No abnormalities were detected.

Abdominal Ultrasound: All abdominal lymph nodes were enlarged and irregular. There were focal regions of thickening and irregularity within the small bowel. The liver and spleen were unremarkable.

Aspiration Cytology (Mandibular Lymph Node): Multiple, variably sized aggregates of macrophages were scattered along with numerous karyolytic and degenerated neutrophils and a residual lymphoid population in a light pink background that contained low numbers of erythrocytes and lysed cells. The macrophages were large and distended with intracellular, negatively staining thick, relatively short, rod-shaped bacteria. Intracellular organisms were noted within neutrophils and large multinucleated giant cells, as well as being located extracellularly. The bacilli were acid fast. Interpretation: Pyogranulomatous inflammation due to infection with *Mycobacterium* spp.

Microbiologic Testing: Real-time PCR assay for *Mycobacterium* genus organisms (lymph node aspirate): Positive

Real-time PCR assay for *M. avium* complex organisms (lymph node aspirate): Positive

Mycobacterial culture and susceptibility testing (National Jewish Laboratories, Denver, CO): Positive for *M. avium* after incubation for 26 days. The organism was identified by HPLC. The organism was tentatively designated as resistant to ciprofloxacin, rifabutin, and rifampin; of intermediate susceptibility to clofazimine, kanamycin, amikacin, ethambutol, streptomycin, and moxifloxacin; and susceptible to clarithromycin. The organism was susceptible to ethambutol and of intermediate susceptibility to rifampin when the two drugs were used in combination.

Diagnosis: Disseminated *M. avium* infection.

Treatment: Before the availability of culture results, the dog was treated with a combination of enrofloxacin, clarithromycin, and ethambutol. The tetracycline and niacinamide combination was discontinued because of the potential for underlying immunosuppression. The lymph nodes ruptured after the aspirates were collected and drained purulent exudate. Unfortunately, this was followed shortly afterward by the development of fever, lethargy, and dysphagia secondary to severe lymphadenomegaly, and the owners elected euthanasia.

Comments: This dog was suspected to have mycobacterial infection caused by an organism other than a MTBC organism from the outset, based on the dog's background, clinical presentation, and the presence of large numbers of AFB on cytology. *M. tuberculosis* most often causes pulmonary disease in dogs. *M. bovis* infections have been described in the Hispanic population in southern California and rarely in cattle from California,[101] so *M. bovis* infection was possible but seemed highly unlikely based on exposure history and the epidemiology of this disease in dogs. The use of PCR assays allowed rapid confirmation that the organism belonged to *M. avium*.

SUGGESTED READINGS

Baral RM, Metcalfe SS, Krockenberger MB, et al. Disseminated *Mycobacterium avium* infection in young cats: overrepresentation of Abyssinian cats. J Feline Med Surg. 2006;8:23-44.

Bennett S. Photosensitisation induced by clofazimine in a cat. Aust Vet J. 2007;85:375-380.

Davies JL, Sibley JA, Myers S, et al. Histological and genotypical characterization of feline cutaneous mycobacteriosis: a retrospective study of formalin-fixed paraffin-embedded tissues. Vet Dermatol. 2006;17:155-162.

Posthaus H, Bodmer T, Alves L, et al. Accidental infection of veterinary personnel with *Mycobacterium tuberculosis* at necropsy: a case study. Vet Microbiol. 2011;149:374-380.

Shrikrishna D, de la Rua-Domenech R, Smith NH, et al. Human and canine pulmonary *Mycobacterium bovis* infection in the same household: re-emergence of an old zoonotic threat? Thorax. 2009;64:89-91.

REFERENCES

1. Sakula A. Robert Koch: centenary of the discovery of the tubercle bacillus, 1882. Thorax. 1982;37:246-251.
2. Posthaus H, Bodmer T, Alves L, et al. Accidental infection of veterinary personnel with *Mycobacterium tuberculosis* at necropsy: a case study. Vet Microbiol. 2011;149:374-380.
3. Turinelli V, Ledieu D, Guilbaud L, et al. *Mycobacterium tuberculosis* infection in a dog from Africa. Vet Clin Pathol. 2004;33:177-181.
4. Hackendahl NC, Mawby DI, Bemis DA, et al. Putative transmission of *Mycobacterium tuberculosis* infection from a human to a dog. J Am Vet Med Assoc. 2004;225:1573-1577:1548.
5. Liu S, Weitzman I, Johnson GG. Canine tuberculosis. J Am Vet Med Assoc. 1980;177:164-167.
6. Foster ES, Scavelli TD, Greenlee PG, et al. Cutaneous lesion caused by *Mycobacterium tuberculosis* in a dog. J Am Vet Med Assoc. 1986;188:1188-1190.
7. Sykes JE, Cannon AB, Norris AJ, et al. *Mycobacterium tuberculosis* complex infection in a dog. J Vet Intern Med. 2007;21:1108 1112.
8. Parsons SD, Gous TA, Warren RM, et al. Pulmonary *Mycobacterium tuberculosis* (Beijing strain) infection in a stray dog. J S Afr Vet Assoc. 2008;79:95-98.
9. Erwin PC, Bemis DA, McCombs SB, et al. *Mycobacterium tuberculosis* transmission from human to canine. Emerg Infect Dis. 2004;10:2258–2260.
10. Gunn-Moore DA, McFarland SE, Brewer JI, et al. Mycobacterial disease in cats in Great Britain: I. Culture results, geographical distribution and clinical presentation of 339 cases. J Feline Med Surg. 2011;13:934-944.
11. de Lisle GW, Collins DM, Loveday AS, et al. A report of tuberculosis in cats in New Zealand, and the examination of strains of *Mycobacterium bovis* by DNA restriction endonuclease analysis. N Z Vet J. 1990;38:10-13.

12. Zumarraga MJ, Vivot MM, Marticorena D, et al. *Mycobacterium bovis* in Argentina: isolates from cats typified by spoligotyping. Rev Argent Microbiol. 2009;41:215-217.
13. Kaneene JB, Bruning-Fann CS, Dunn J, et al. Epidemiologic investigation of *Mycobacterium bovis* in a population of cats. Am J Vet Res. 2002;63:1507-1511.
14. Corner LA, Murphy D, Gormley E. *Mycobacterium bovis* infection in the Eurasian badger (*Meles meles*): the disease, pathogenesis, epidemiology and control. J Comp Pathol. 2011;144:1-24.
15. Wilkins MJ, Bartlett PC, Berry DE, et al. Absence of *Mycobacterium bovis* infection in dogs and cats residing on infected cattle farms: Michigan, 2002. Epidemiol Infect. 2008;136:1617-1623.
16. van der Burgt GM, Crawshaw T, Foster AP, et al. *Mycobacterium bovis* infection in dogs. Vet Rec. 2009;165:634.
17. Ellis MD, Davies S, McCandlish IA, et al. *Mycobacterium bovis* infection in a dog. Vet Rec. 2006;159:46-48.
18. Shrikrishna D, de la Rua-Domenech R, Smith NH, et al. Human and canine pulmonary *Mycobacterium bovis* infection in the same household: re-emergence of an old zoonotic threat? Thorax. 2009;64:89-91.
19. Smith NH, Crawshaw T, Parry J, et al. *Mycobacterium microti*: More diverse than previously thought. J Clin Microbiol. 2009;47:2551-2559.
20. Rufenacht S, Bogli-Stuber K, Bodmer T, et al. *Mycobacterium microti* infection in the cat: a case report, literature review and recent clinical experience. J Feline Med Surg. 2011;13:195-204.
21. Deforges L, Boulouis HJ, Thibaud JL, et al. First isolation of *Mycobacterium microti* (Llama-type) from a dog. Vet Microbiol. 2004;103:249-253.
22. Bauer NB, O'Neill E, Sheahan BJ, et al. Calcospherite-like bodies and caseous necrosis in tracheal mucus from a dog with tuberculosis. Vet Clin Pathol. 2004;33:168-172.
23. Gunn-Moore DA, Jenkins PA, Lucke VM. Feline tuberculosis: a literature review and discussion of 19 cases caused by an unusual mycobacterial variant. Vet Rec. 1996;138:53-58.
24. de Bolla GJ. Tuberculosis in a cat. Vet Rec. 1994;134:336.
25. Blunden AS, Smith KC. A pathological study of a mycobacterial infection in a cat caused by a variant with cultural characteristics between *Mycobacterium tuberculosis* and *M. bovis*. Vet Rec. 1996;138:87-88.
26. Bennett AD, Lalor S, Schwarz T, et al. Radiographic findings in cats with mycobacterial infections. J Feline Med Surg. 2011;13:718-724.
27. Greene CE, Gunn-Moore DA. Infections caused by slow-growing mycobacteria. In: Greene CE, ed. Infectious Diseases of the Dog and Cat. 4th ed. St. Louis, MO: Elsevier Saunders; 2012:495-510.
28. Rhodes SG, Gruffydd-Jones T, Gunn-Moore D, et al. Adaptation of IFN-gamma ELISA and ELISPOT tests for feline tuberculosis. Vet Immunol Immunopathol. 2008;124:379-384.
29. Saleeb PG, Drake SK, Murray PR, et al. Identification of mycobacteria in solid-culture media by matrix-assisted laser desorption ionization-time of flight mass spectrometry. J Clin Microbiol. 2011;49:1790-1794.
30. Gunn-Moore DA, McFarland SE, Schock A, et al. Mycobacterial disease in a population of 339 cats in Great Britain: II. Histopathology of 225 cases, and treatment and outcome of 184 cases. J Feline Med Surg. 2011;13:945-952.
31. Xavier Emmanuel F, Seagar AL, Doig C, et al. Human and animal infections with *Mycobacterium microti*. Scotland. Emerg Infect Dis. 2007;13:1924-1927.
32. World Health Organization. World Health Organization Report on the Global Tuberculosis Epidemic. Geneva; 2012. Available from http://www.who.int/tb/publications/global_report/en/. Last accessed February 2, 2013.
33. Trends in tuberculosis-United States, 2011. MMWR Morb Mortal Wkly Rep 2012;61:181–185.
34. Haist V, Seehusen F, Moser I, et al. *Mycobacterium avium* subsp. *hominissuis* infection in 2 pet dogs. Germany. Emerg Infect Dis. 2008;14:988-990.
35. Campora L, Corazza M, Zullino C, et al. *Mycobacterium avium* subspecies *hominissuis* disseminated infection in a Basset Hound dog. J Vet Diagn Invest. 2011;23:1083-1087.
36. de Groot PH, van Ingen J, de Zwaan R, et al. Disseminated *Mycobacterium avium* subsp. *avium* infection in a cat, the Netherlands. Vet Microbiol. 2010;144:527-529.
37. Glanemann B, Schonenbrucher H, Bridger N, et al. Detection of *Mycobacterium avium* subspecies *paratuberculosis*–specific DNA by PCR in intestinal biopsies of dogs. J Vet Intern Med. 2008;22:1090-1094.
38. Whiley H, Keegan A, Giglio S, et al. *Mycobacterium avium* complex—the role of potable water in disease transmission. J Appl Microbiol. 2012;113:223-232.
39. Mijs W, de Haas P, Rossau R, et al. Molecular evidence to support a proposal to reserve the designation *Mycobacterium avium* subsp. *avium* for bird-type isolates and "*M. avium* subsp. *hominissuis*" for the human/porcine type of *M. avium*. Int J Syst Evol Microbiol. 2002;52:1505-1518.
40. Jordan HL, Cohn LA, Armstrong PJ. Disseminated *Mycobacterium avium* complex infection in three Siamese cats. J Am Vet Med Assoc. 1994;204:90-93.
41. Baral RM, Metcalfe SS, Krockenberger MB, et al. Disseminated *Mycobacterium avium* infection in young cats: overrepresentation of Abyssinian cats. J Feline Med Surg. 2006;8:23-44.
42. Griffin A, Newton AL, Aronson LR, et al. Disseminated *Mycobacterium avium* complex infection following renal transplantation in a cat. J Am Vet Med Assoc. 2003;222:1097-1101:1077-1098.
43. Kadar E, Sykes JE, Kass PH, et al. Evaluation of the prevalence of infections in cats after renal transplantation: 169 cases (1987-2003). J Am Vet Med Assoc. 2005;227:948-953.
44. Malik R, Gabor L, Martin P, et al. Subcutaneous granuloma caused by *Mycobacterium avium* complex infection in a cat. Aust Vet J. 1998;76:604-607.
45. Graham KJ, Brain PH, Spielman D, et al. Concurrent infection with *Cryptococcus neoformans/gattii* species complex and *Mycobacterium avium* affecting the subcutis and bone of a pelvic limb in a cat. J Feline Med Surg. 2011;13:776-780.
46. Riviere D, Pingret JL, Etievant M, et al. Disseminated *Mycobacterium avium* subspecies infection in a cat. J Feline Med Surg. 2011;13:125-128.
47. Barry M, Taylor J, Woods JP. Disseminated *Mycobacterium avium* infection in a cat. Can Vet J. 2002;43:369-371.
48. Sieber-Ruckstuhl NS, Sessions JK, Sanchez S, et al. Long-term cure of disseminated *Mycobacterium avium* infection in a cat. Vet Rec. 2007;160:131-132.
49. Morita Y, Kimur H, Kozawa K, et al. Cutaneous infection in a cat caused by *Mycobacterium avium* complex serovar 6. Vet Rec. 2003;152:120.
50. Latimer KS, Jameson PH, Crowell WA, et al. Disseminated *Mycobacterium avium* complex infection in a cat: presumptive diagnosis by blood smear examination. Vet Clin Pathol. 1997;26: 85-89.
51. Miller MA, Greene CE, Brix AE. Disseminated *Mycobacterium avium-intracellulare* complex infection in a miniature schnauzer. J Am Anim Hosp Assoc. 1995;31:213-216.
52. Gow AG, Gow DJ. Disseminated *Mycobacterium avium* complex infection in a dog. Vet Rec. 2008;162:594-595.
53. Kim DY, Cho DY, Newton JC, et al. Granulomatous myelitis due to *Mycobacterium avium* in a dog. Vet Pathol. 1994;31:491-493.
54. Horn B, Forshaw D, Cousins D, et al. Disseminated *Mycobacterium avium* infection in a dog with chronic diarrhoea. Aust Vet J. 2000;78:320-325.
55. Bauer N, Burkhardt S, Kirsch A, et al. Lymphadenopathy and diarrhea in a Miniature Schnauzer. Vet Clin Pathol. 2002;31:61-64.
56. O'Toole D, Tharp S, Thomsen BV, et al. Fatal mycobacteriosis with hepatosplenomegaly in a young dog due to *Mycobacterium avium*. J Vet Diagn Invest. 2005;17:200-204.

57. Eggers JS, Parker GA, Braaf HA, et al. Disseminated *Mycobacterium avium* infection in three miniature schnauzer litter mates. J Vet Diagn Invest. 1997;9:424-427.
58. Naughton JF, Mealey KL, Wardrop KJ, et al. Systemic *Mycobacterium avium* infection in a dog diagnosed by polymerase chain reaction analysis of buffy coat. J Am Anim Hosp Assoc. 2005;41:128-132.
59. Radomski N, Thibault VC, Karoui C, et al. Determination of genotypic diversity of *Mycobacterium avium* subspecies from human and animal origins by mycobacterial interspersed repetitive-unit-variable-number tandem-repeat and IS1311 restriction fragment length polymorphism typing methods. J Clin Microbiol. 2010;48:1026-1034.
60. Gordin FM, Horsburgh CR. *Mycobacterium avium* complex. In: Mandell GL, Bennett JE, Dolin R, eds. Principles and Practice of Infectious Diseases. 7th ed. Philadelphia, PA: Elsevier; 2010:3177-3189.
61. Hughes MS, James G, Taylor MJ, et al. PCR studies of feline leprosy cases. J Feline Med Surg. 2004;6:235-243.
62. Malik R, Hughes MS, James G, et al. Feline leprosy: two different clinical syndromes. J Feline Med Surg. 2002;4:43-59.
63. Davies JL, Sibley JA, Myers S, et al. Histological and genotypical characterization of feline cutaneous mycobacteriosis: a retrospective study of formalin-fixed paraffin-embedded tissues. Vet Dermatol. 2006;17:155-162.
64. Charles J, Martin P, Wigney DI, et al. Cytology and histopathology of canine leproid granuloma syndrome. Aust Vet J. 1999;77:799-803.
65. Malik R, Love DN, Wigney DI, et al. Mycobacterial nodular granulomas affecting the subcutis and skin of dogs (canine leproid granuloma syndrome). Aust Vet J. 1998;76:403-407:398.
66. Foley JE, Borjesson D, Gross TL, et al. Clinical, microscopic, and molecular aspects of canine leproid granuloma in the United States. Vet Pathol. 2002;39:234-239.
67. Malik R, Martin P, Wigney D, et al. Treatment of canine leproid granuloma syndrome: preliminary findings in seven dogs. Aust Vet J. 2001;79:30-36.
68. Malik R, Wigney DI, Dawson D, et al. Infection of the subcutis and skin of cats with rapidly growing mycobacteria: a review of microbiological and clinical findings. J Feline Med Surg. 2000;2:35-48.
69. Horne KS, Kunkle GA. Clinical outcome of cutaneous rapidly growing mycobacterial infections in cats in the south-eastern United States: a review of 10 cases (1996-2006). J Feline Med Surg. 2009;11:627-632.
70. Jang SS, Hirsh DC. Rapidly growing members of the genus *Mycobacterium* affecting dogs and cats. J Am Anim Hosp Assoc. 2002;38:217-220.
71. Beccati M, Peano A, Gallo MG. Pyogranulomatous panniculitis caused by *Mycobacterium alvei* in a cat. J Small Anim Pract. 2007;48:664.
72. Sykes JE. Unpublished observations, 2012.
73. Malik R, Shaw SE, Griffin C, et al. Infections of the subcutis and skin of dogs caused by rapidly growing mycobacteria. J Small Anim Pract. 2004;45:485-494.
74. Bryden SL, Burrows AK, O'Hara AJ. *Mycobacterium goodii* infection in a dog with concurrent hyperadrenocorticism. Vet Dermatol. 2004;15:331-338.
75. Fox LE, Kunkle GA, Homer BL, et al. Disseminated subcutaneous *Mycobacterium fortuitum* infection in a dog. J Am Vet Med Assoc. 1995;206:53-55.
76. Irwin PJ, Whithear K, Lavelle RB, et al. Acute bronchopneumonia associated with *Mycobacterium fortuitum* infection in a dog. Aust Vet J. 2000;78:254-257.
77. Wylie KB, Lewis DD, Pechman RD, et al. Hypertrophic osteopathy associated with *Mycobacterium fortuitum* pneumonia in a dog. J Am Vet Med Assoc. 1993;202:1986-1988.
78. Turnwald GH, Pechman RD, Turk JR, et al. Survival of a dog with pneumonia caused by *Mycobacterium fortuitum*. J Am Vet Med Assoc. 1988;192:64-66.
79. Jang SS, Eckhaus MA, Saunders G. Pulmonary *Mycobacterium fortuitum* infection in a dog. J Am Vet Med Assoc. 1984;184:96-98.
80. Couto SS, Artacho CA. *Mycobacterium fortuitum* pneumonia in a cat and the role of lipid in the pathogenesis of atypical mycobacterial infections. Vet Pathol. 2007;44:543-546.
81. Foster SF, Martin P, Davis W, et al. Chronic pneumonia caused by *Mycobacterium thermoresistibile* in a cat. J Small Anim Pract. 1999;40:433-438.
82. Grooters AM, Couto CG, Andrews JM, et al. Systemic *Mycobacterium smegmatis* infection in a dog. J Am Vet Med Assoc. 1995;206:200-202.
83. Pressler BM, Hardie EM, Pitulle C, et al. Isolation and identification of *Mycobacterium kansasii* from pleural fluid of a dog with persistent pleural effusion. J Am Vet Med Assoc. 2002;220:1313-1334;1336-1340.
84. Dietrich U, Arnold P, Guscetti F, et al. Ocular manifestation of disseminated *Mycobacterium simiae* infection in a cat. J Small Anim Pract. 2003;44:121-125.
85. Hughes MS, Ball NW, Love DN, et al. Disseminated *Mycobacterium genavense* infection in a FIV-positive cat. J Feline Med Surg. 1999;1:23-29.
86. Kiehn TE, Hoefer H, Bottger EC, et al. *Mycobacterium genavense* infections in pet animals. J Clin Microbiol. 1996;34:1840-1842.
87. Tomasovic AA, Rac R, Purcell DA. *Mycobacterium xenopi* in a skin lesion of a cat. Aust Vet J. 1976;52:103.
88. Meeks C, Levy JK, Crawford PC, et al. Chronic disseminated *Mycobacterium xenopi* infection in a cat with idiopathic CD4+ T lymphocytopenia. J Vet Intern Med. 2008;22:1043-1047.
89. MacWilliams PS, Whitley N, Moore F. Lymphadenitis and peritonitis caused by *Mycobacterium xenopi* in a cat. Vet Clin Pathol. 1998;27:50-53.
90. De Lorenzi D, Solano-Gallego L. Tracheal granuloma because of infection with a novel mycobacterial species in an old FIV-positive cat. J Small Anim Pract. 2009;50:143-146.
91. O'Brien CR, McMillan E, Harris O, et al. Localised *Mycobacterium ulcerans* infection in four dogs. Aust Vet J. 2011;89:506-510.
92. Elsner L, Wayne J, O'Brien CR, et al. Localised *Mycobacterium ulcerans* infection in a cat in Australia. J Feline Med Surg. 2008;10:407-412.
93. Appleyard GD, Clark EG. Histologic and genotypic characterization of a novel *Mycobacterium* species found in three cats. J Clin Microbiol. 2002;40:2425-2430.
94. Henderson SM, Baker J, Williams R, et al. Opportunistic mycobacterial granuloma in a cat associated with a member of the *Mycobacterium terrae* complex. J Feline Med Surg. 2003;5:37-41.
95. Govendir M, Hansen T, Kimble B, et al. Susceptibility of rapidly growing mycobacteria isolated from cats and dogs, to ciprofloxacin, enrofloxacin and moxifloxacin. Vet Microbiol. 2011;147:113-118.
96. O'Brien CR, Fyfe JA, Malik R. Infections caused by rapidly-growing mycobacteria. In: Greene CE, ed. Infectious Diseases of the Dog and Cat. 4th ed. St. Louis, MO: Elsevier Saunders; 2012:515-521.
97. Brown-Elliott BA, Wallace RJ. Infections due to non-tuberculous mycobacteria other than *Mycobacterium avium-intracellulare*. In: Mandell GL, Bennett JE, Dolin R, eds. Principles and Practice of Infectious Diseases. Philadelphia, PA: Elsevier; 2010:3191-3198.
98. Southern Jr PM. Tenosynovitis caused by *Mycobacterium kansasii* associated with a dog bite. Am J Med Sci. 2004;327:258-261.
99. Ariel I, Haas H, Weinberg H, et al. *Mycobacterium fortuitum* granulomatous synovitis caused by a dog bite. J Hand Surg Am. 1983;8:342-343.
100. Ngan N, Morris A, de Chalain T. *Mycobacterium fortuitum* infection caused by a cat bite. N Z Med J. 2005;118:U1354.
101. Rodwell TC, Kapasi AJ, Moore M, et al. Tracing the origins of *Mycobacterium bovis* tuberculosis in humans in the USA to cattle in Mexico using spoligotyping. Int J Infect Dis. 2010;14(suppl 3):e129-e135.

CHAPTER 45

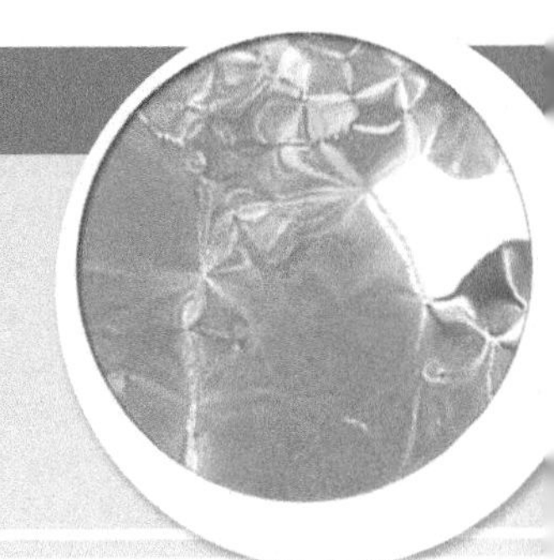

Salmonellosis

Jane E. Sykes and Stanley L. Marks

Overview of Salmonellosis

First Described: Washington, DC, United States, 1885 (Theobald Smith and Daniel Salmon)[1]

Cause: *Salmonella* spp. (gram-negative rods that belong to the Enterobacteriaceae)

Affected Hosts: A large variety of warm-blooded animals and humans; cold-blooded animals may be subclinically infected

Geographic Distribution: Worldwide

Primary Mode of Transmission: Fecal-oral

Major Clinical Signs: Fever, lethargy, anorexia, diarrhea, vomiting, and less commonly reproductive failure, neurologic and/or respiratory signs

Differential Diagnoses: Differential diagnoses for suspected *Salmonella* enterocolitis include canine and feline parvovirus infection, canine distemper virus infection, campylobacteriosis, clostridial diarrhea, salmon poisoning disease, giardiasis, tritrichomoniasis (cats), cryptosporidiosis, whipworms, leptospirosis, dietary indiscretion, gastrointestinal foreign body, pancreatitis, inflammatory bowel disease, lymphoma, hypoadrenocorticism, hyperthyroidism, toxins (including drugs)

Human Health Significance: Important zoonosis. Dogs and cats may be a source of human infection with some *Salmonella* serotypes, some of which may be resistant to multiple antimicrobial drugs.

Etiology and Epidemiology

Salmonella are gram-negative, motile, non–spore-forming facultative anaerobic rods that belong to the family Enterobacteriaceae. Most *Salmonella* exist in two phases, which differ in composition of their flagellar antigens.

Salmonella are ubiquitous organisms that can be isolated from the intestinal tracts of an enormous variety of animal species and are a major cause of enterocolitis and sometimes severe systemic illness in humans and animals. Infections can be transferred between animal species and are zoonotic. Many infections are food borne, especially in association with milk, meat, and eggs. *Salmonella* spp. have a remarkable ability to survive long periods of time (weeks to years) in the environment, and so fomite transmission is important. In addition, *Salmonella* can multiply rapidly in contaminated food left at room temperature and can survive freezing for several weeks.[2]

The genus *Salmonella* comprises two species, *Salmonella enterica* and *Salmonella bongori*, each of which contains multiple serotypes.[3] Serotypes of *S. bongori* are generally associated with cold-blooded animals and rarely have been isolated from warm-blooded animals, including a dog with diarrhea.[4] There are six subspecies of *S. enterica* (Table 45-1) and approximately 2500 different serotypes. These are identified on the basis of agglutination reactions of their O (somatic) and H (flagellar) antigens (see Chapter 36). Subspecies I serotypes, which are responsible for almost all disease in humans and warm-blooded animals worldwide, are assigned names such as *S.* ser. Typhimurium. Unless named before 1966, serotypes that belong to other subspecies are designated using antigenic formulas. The formulas describe the subspecies, O antigens: H antigens (phase 1): and if present, H antigens (phase 2) (e.g., *S.* IV 45:g,z_{51}:—).

Certain serotypes of *Salmonella* are host restricted, whereas others infect a broad range of host species. *Salmonella* serotype Typhi, for example, is adapted to humans, causing typhoid fever, and does not infect animals. Other serotypes are adapted to certain host species, with rare transmission to other hosts. *Salmonella* serotype Typhimurium is the most commonly isolated serotype from diseased humans and animals.

Infection of dogs and cats with *Salmonella* has been associated with the feeding of raw meat diets,[5-9] although commercial dry and raw dog food and pig ear pet treats have also become contaminated with the organism.[5,10-13] Occasionally, co-infections with multiple *Salmonella* serotypes occur.[14] Outbreaks of *S.* ser. Typhimurium infection in cats have been associated with seasonal bird migrations ("songbird fever").

Salmonella is generally isolated less than 1% of the time from the feces of dogs and cats that are fed processed commercial

TABLE 45-1

Classification of Salmonellae

Salmonella Species	*Salmonella* Subspecies	Example Serotypes
Salmonella enterica	*enterica* (I)	*Salmonella* ser. Typhimurium *S.* ser. Typhi *S.* ser. Choleraesuis
	salamae (II)	*S.* ser. Greenside
	arizonae (IIIa)	*S.* IIIa 18:z_4,z_{23}:—
	diarizonae (IIIb)	*S.* IIIb 60:k:z
	houtenae (IV)	*S.* ser. Marina
	indica (VI)	*S.* ser. Srinagar
Salmonella bongori	V	*S.* ser. Brookfield

pet foods,[15-19] although one study of household pet dogs in Ontario, Canada revealed a shedding prevalence of 23%.[20] The highest rates of infection have been found in group-housed dogs, especially those fed raw meat diets, such as racing sled dogs and greyhound breeding facilities, where prevalences have exceeded 75%.[8,21] *Salmonella* was isolated from the feces of 18 of 26 (69%) healthy pre-race Alaskan sled dogs, and 19 of 30 (63%) diarrheic racing Alaskan sled dogs, which underscored the lack of an association between the isolation of *Salmonella* and clinical diarrhea.[8] Coprophagic behavior may also contribute to salmonellosis in dogs. In cats, the feeding of raw poultry may increase risk for *Salmonella* infection,[22] and occasionally, high prevalences of infection have been detected in group-housed cats[18] and shelter cats. Ingestion of infected wild bird species by cats during seasonal bird migrations can also lead to salmonellosis (songbird fever). In a study of diarrheic and nondiarrheic shelter cats in Florida, the prevalence of *Salmonella* shedding as determined by PCR assay was 6% and 4%, respectively.[23] Susceptibility to shedding and disease is highest in immunosuppressed dogs and cats, including young animals, pregnant animals, those in overcrowded conditions, and those with underlying immunosuppressive illness (such as neoplasia, diabetes mellitus, retroviral infection, and immune-mediated disease) or immunosuppressive drug therapy.[24,25]

Clinical Features

Signs and Their Pathogenesis

After ingestion, salmonellae that survive the acidic environment of the stomach gain access to the intestine, where they disrupt tight junctions and actively invade (1) enterocytes; (2) M cells within the ileum (which sample luminal antigens); and (3) dendritic cells, which send protrusions into the gut lumen between intestinal epithelial cells. Interaction of *Salmonella* with immune cells and epithelial cells within the gut leads to production of cytokines and chemokines, with massive influx of lymphocytes, macrophages, and neutrophils, sometimes with severe epithelial injury and mucosal sloughing.[26] Localization in the mesenteric lymph nodes, Peyer's patches, solitary intestinal lymphoid tissues, and intestinal epithelium, along with evasion of the host immune response, is followed by persistent shedding, often for several weeks, after which animals can become latently infected. Reactivation of shedding, with or without clinical illness, may occur, sometimes as a result of stress or immunosuppression.[27,28]

If the organism has properties that allow it to spread systemically and host defenses are impaired, bacteremia and extraintestinal infection follows.[29] More virulent strains have a greater ability to multiply intracellularly in nonphagocytic cells. Fever, hypoglycemia, and leukopenia occur. The *Salmonella* lipopolysaccharide (LPS) can then induce endotoxic shock, with hypotension and activation of the complement and coagulation cascade. The coagulation cascade is also activated with exposure to *Salmonella* porins, which are hydrophobic outer membrane proteins. Disseminated intravascular coagulation (DIC) follows.

Dogs and cats infected with *Salmonella* spp. may show no signs or they may develop enterocolitis, focal suppurative infection, or severe systemic illness. The majority of dogs are chronically and subclinically infected. When disease occurs, signs often begin 3 to 5 days after infection or onset of immunosuppression. Fever (occasionally as high as 106°F [41°C]), lethargy, and anorexia may be followed by abdominal pain, vomiting, and watery to mucoid, often hemorrhagic diarrhea, and dehydration. Weight loss may be seen. Diarrhea may take several weeks to resolve. Rarely, chronic intermittent diarrhea that lasts up to 8 weeks develops.[30]

Severely affected animals develop signs of septic shock (see Chapter 86). Neurologic signs, and signs that relate to endocarditis, arthritis, pancreatitis, pneumonia, peritonitis, and cholecystitis occur in some animals. Infected cats may develop severe enterocolitis, with fever, pancytopenia, and hyperbilirubinemia. Some cats show persistent fever and anorexia with no diarrhea. Conjunctivitis has been described in cats in association with *Salmonella* infection.[31]

Occasionally salmonellae localize in a particular organ, such as the lungs or urinary tract (Figure 45-1). Signs of dysfunction of that organ system may follow, even when enteric signs or positive fecal culture results are absent.[32] Abortion and stillbirth can occur after transplacental infection, and the dam may also infect her neonates, which leads to fading puppies.[33-35]

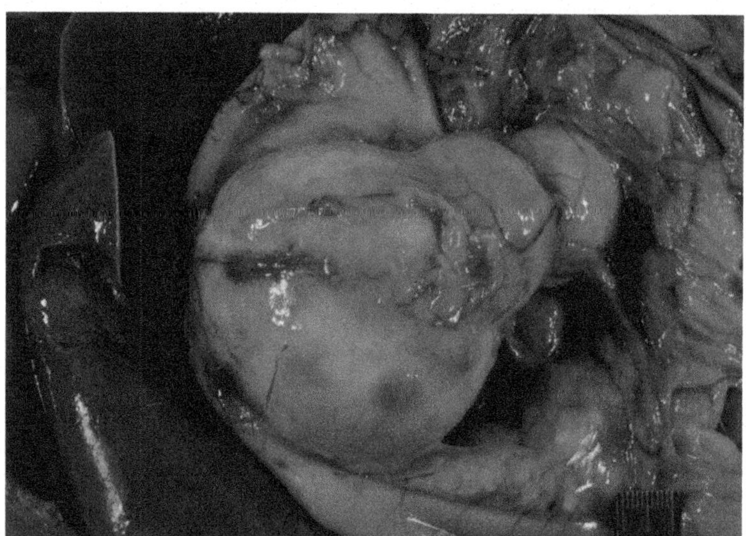

FIGURE 45-1 Large, chronic pancreatic abscess due to *Salmonella* Typhimurium associated with a pancreatic adenocarcinoma in a 15-year-old castrated male domestic shorthair cat. The mass was multicystic and fluctuant, and when cut open was filled with cloudy fluid and lined by thick tan debris. (Courtesy University of California, Davis, Veterinary Anatomic Pathology Service.)

Diagnosis

The traditional diagnosis of canine and feline salmonellosis is made based on culture of the organism in conjunction with clinical signs and assessment of potential risk factors, such as hospitalization, age, environmental exposure, and antibiotic administration. Diagnostic assays available for salmonellosis in dogs and cats are shown in Table 45-2.

Laboratory Abnormalities

Complete Blood Count

The CBC in dogs or cats with salmonellosis may be unremarkable or may show a neutrophilia with a left shift; in bacteremic animals, anemia, a degenerative left shift, toxic neutrophils, lymphopenia, and thrombocytopenia are usually present. Rarely, intracellular bacteria are seen within neutrophils.

Serum Chemistry Profile

In animals with severe salmonellosis, changes on the serum chemistry profile include elevated liver enzyme activities, hyperbilirubinemia, azotemia, hypoalbuminemia, hypocholesterolemia, hypoglycemia, and electrolyte abnormalities.

Urinalysis

Salmonella spp. occasionally localize in the kidneys, with associated isosthenuria, pyuria, proteinuria, casts, and bacteriuria.

Clotting Function

Dogs and cats that develop DIC may have clotting function abnormalities that include prolonged coagulation times, increased fibrin degradation product concentrations, and decreased antithrombin concentrations.

Diagnostic Imaging

Plain Radiography

Thoracic radiographs in animals with salmonellosis may reveal bronchointerstitial to alveolar infiltrates in animals with pneumonia, or pleural effusion with pyothorax. Abdominal radiographs can reveal fluid-filled intestines, decreased serosal detail, and/or mild hepatomegaly.

Sonographic Findings

Depending on the severity of the infection, abdominal ultrasound may be unremarkable in dogs and cats with salmonellosis, or show changes that include abdominal lymphadenomegaly, intestinal wall thickening, fluid-filled bowel segments, hepatomegaly, splenomegaly, or ascites.

Microbiologic Testing

Bacterial Isolation

A diagnosis of salmonellosis can be made when *Salmonella* is isolated from a normally sterile site, such as the blood, bronchoalveolar lavage specimens, synovial fluid, or urine specimens collected by cystocentesis. Isolation of *Salmonella* from feces does not confirm that the organism is the cause of disease, but it can raise suspicion that *Salmonella* may be playing a role in enterocolitis, and it has zoonotic significance (see Public Health Aspects, later). Isolation also allows antimicrobial susceptibility testing, which is important because many isolates of *Salmonella* are resistant to multiple antimicrobial drugs.

Salmonella grow readily at 37°C on routine bacteriologic media from specimens that have been collected from a normally sterile site. Selective media are required for specimens that are heavily contaminated with other bacteria such as feces. Examples of selective media include enrichment broths such as tetrathionate broth or Selenite F broth. After enrichment, subculturing is performed on a medium such as deoxycholate, which also favors growth of *Salmonella*. Many veterinary laboratories incorporate such protocols for isolation of *Salmonella* as part of a panel for detection of enteropathogenic bacteria. Once *Salmonella* is isolated, the organism can be identified based on biochemical reactions and serotyping, which involves agglutination testing with O and H antisera. In the future, use of whole cell matrix-assisted laser desorption ionization-time-of-flight (MALDI-TOF) mass spectrometry in veterinary clinical microbiology laboratories should allow identification of *Salmonella* at the species and subspecies level within minutes.[36] It also can identify some important *S. enterica* subsp. *enterica* to the serovar level, and could reduce the need for laborious subtyping procedures.[37]

Molecular Diagnosis Using the Polymerase Chain Reaction

Some veterinary diagnostic laboratories offer PCR assays for *Salmonella*, some of which have been shown as highly sensitive and specific when compared with culture.[38,39] PCR is more rapid than culture but currently does not provide information on antimicrobial susceptibility. It has been recommended that PCR assay after overnight enrichment in a nonselective broth be adopted as the gold standard for diagnosis, and that all specimens that test positive by PCR assay be cultured using selective

TABLE 45-2

Diagnostic Assays Available for Salmonellosis in Dogs and Cats

Assay	Specimen Type	Target	Performance
Bacterial isolation	Feces, blood, synovial fluid, tissue aspirates, bronchoalveolar lavage fluid, peritoneal or pleural effusions, urine, CSF, tissues obtained at necropsy	*Salmonella* species	Sensitive and specific. False negatives may occur, especially following antimicrobial therapy. Isolation from feces does not imply that *Salmonella* is the cause of disease. Allows subsequent antimicrobial susceptibility testing.
PCR	As for isolation	*Salmonella* DNA	Rapid (within hours); can be highly sensitive and specific. Positive results from feces do not imply that *Salmonella* is the cause of disease. Does not allow susceptibility testing or typing for epidemiologic purposes.

enrichment to isolate and identify the infecting organism.[40] As with culture, detection of the organism in feces using PCR assays does not prove that it is the cause of gastrointestinal illness.

Pathologic Findings

Gross Pathologic Findings

Gross necropsy findings in dogs and cats with severe salmonellosis include widespread petechial and ecchymotic hemorrhages, hemorrhagic enteritis, abscesses within parenchymal organs, enlarged mesenteric lymph nodes, and fibrinohemorrhagic ascites fluid. Pulmonary consolidation and edema may also be present.

Histopathologic Findings

Histopathologic lesions in dogs and cats with salmonellosis are highly variable. Changes in severely affected animals may include suppurative pneumonia, necrotizing hepatitis, and necrotizing and fibrinohemorrhagic enterocolitis, typhlitis, and cholecystitis. More chronic lesions such as chronic cholecystitis have also been described.[41,42] Sometimes, gram-negative bacilli are identified within lesions with tissue Gram stains (Figure 45-2).

Treatment and Prognosis

The movement of dogs and cats that test positive for *Salmonella* should be limited, and if possible, hospitalized animals should be isolated. The mere detection of *Salmonella* in the feces of dogs and cats with uncomplicated diarrhea does not warrant antimicrobial administration, and supportive care only is recommended. Most of these animals have self-limiting disease and shedding, and injudicious antimicrobial administration has the potential to prolong the carrier state and contribute to antimicrobial resistance. Treatment of an animal with uncomplicated diarrhea is also not advocated if the owner is immunocompromised, although appropriate husbandry recommendations and barrier control must be enforced.

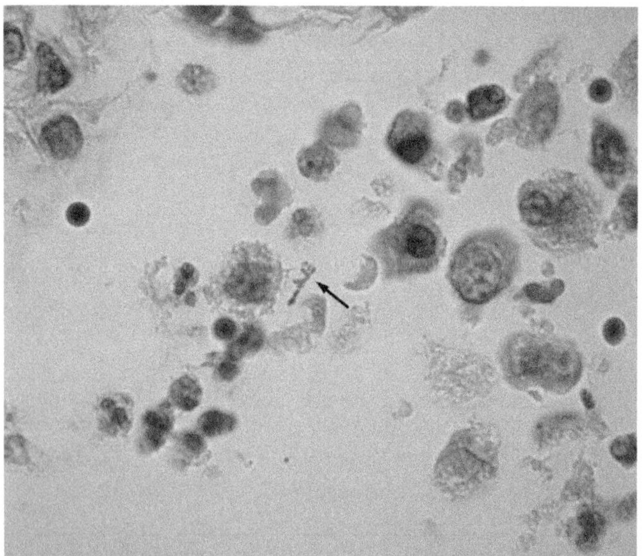

FIGURE 45-2 Gram-negative bacilli (*arrow*) in the lungs of a cat with suppurative cholecystitis and pneumonia due to *Salmonella arizonae*. The cat had been treated with prednisone and cyclosporine for immune-mediated hemolytic anemia. Brown and Benn stain, 1000× magnification.

Dogs and cats with systemic salmonellosis may require aggressive intravenous fluid therapy and colloidal support with hydroxyethyl starch or plasma, together with parenteral antimicrobial drugs. The choice of antimicrobial drugs should be based on the results of culture and susceptibility, because of the potential for resistance to multiple antimicrobial drugs through plasmid transfer. In the event of systemic disease, administration of a combination of ampicillin and a fluoroquinolone is advocated as empiric therapy while awaiting results of culture and susceptibility. Because of the importance of endotoxin in the pathogenesis of sepsis due to gram-negative bacteria such as *Salmonella*, considerable effort has been invested in development and application of drugs targeting endotoxin.[43] Clear benefit through reduction in mortality has not yet been demonstrated for these treatments, and to date they have not been widely used in dogs and cats. Most recently, investigations have been focused on antagonists of Toll-like receptor 4, which is the LPS receptor.[44] Eritoran tetrasodium (E5564) and TAK-242 are examples of TLR4 antagonists that have been used in clinical trials involving septic humans.[45]

Immunity and Vaccination

Salmonella spp. can persist in the host by interfering with dendritic cell function in the intestinal tract. The organism penetrates dendritic cells and avoids lysosomal degradation, which prevents subsequent antigen presentation by dendritic cells on molecules of the major histocompatibility complex.[46] Reduced intracellular proliferation of the organism within antigen-presenting cells may also limit antigen presentation and the development of an effective immune response.[47] Although *Salmonella* vaccines have been developed, none are available for dogs and cats.

Prevention of Enteric Bacterial Infections

Prevention of enteric bacterial infections includes feeding dogs and cats properly cooked foods, hand washing before and after handling pets and pet food, and prevention of coprophagic behavior. Proper handling and storage of pet foods can also limit the potential for food contamination during storage by rodents, insects, and human hands.

Within the hospital setting, fomites such as food dishes, endoscopes, proctoscopes, and rectal thermometers should be disinfected between uses, and single-use disposable thermometer covers should be used. Cages should be cleaned and properly disinfected (see Chapter 11) between animals. Blood donors should not be housed with the regular hospital population, as they may be a source of *Salmonella* infection.

Dogs and cats diagnosed with salmonellosis or *Salmonella* shedding should be isolated from other animals until shedding stops. Fecal cultures should be repeated every 2 weeks, and termination of shedding is identified when three successive negative cultures have been obtained.

Public Health Aspects

All enteric bacterial infections of dogs and cats have the potential to infect and cause illness in humans. Nontyphoid salmonellosis (salmonellosis other than that caused by *S.* ser. Typhi) can be transmitted from domestic animals to humans and cause serious enterocolitis, with fever, severe abdominal pain, diarrhea, nausea, inappetence, chills, and headache. Serious complications tend to occur in children, the elderly, or otherwise immunocompromised individuals such as those infected with HIV. The majority of cases result from ingestion of improperly cooked foods of animal origin, such as meat, milk, and eggs. Most, if not all, pet reptiles carry *Salmonella*, and there has been considerable effort to educate the public about the hazards of reptile-associated salmonellosis. Dogs, and to a lesser extent cats, are less commonly incriminated as a source of *Salmonella*. Of particular concern, multidrug-resistant *Salmonella* strains, such as *S.* ser. Typhimurium strain DT 104, have been isolated from dogs, cats, and reptiles.[20,48] People exposed to dogs and cats that are fed raw meat diets are at increased risk of exposure.

Proper hand washing after handling pets, pet food, and fomites such as bedding and food dishes can help prevent zoonotic transmission of *Salmonella*. Reptile ownership by families with children younger than 5 years of age or among the immunosuppressed is discouraged by public health authorities.[49] Proper food handling practices, including separating raw meat from vegetables and proper cooking of meat, can also reduce salmonellosis in humans.

CASE EXAMPLE

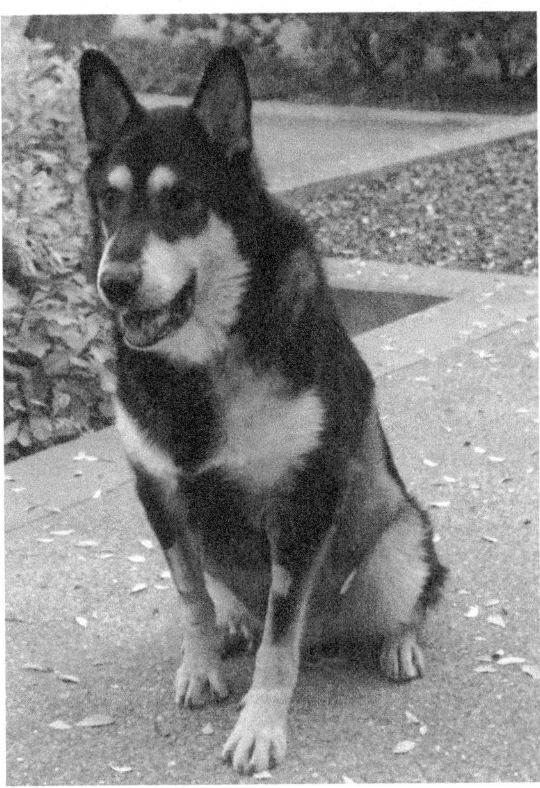

FIGURE 45-3 "Sampson", a 3-year-old male castrated shepherd mix with salmonellosis.

Signalment: "Sampson," a 3-year-old male castrated shepherd mix from Fresno in southern California (Figure 45-3).

History: Sampson was brought to a veterinarian for evaluation of a 3-month history of bilateral tarsal joint swelling. Some clinical improvement had been noted after treatment with oral tetracycline (28 mg/kg PO q8h) for 2 weeks. Subsequently, he was treated with oral prednisone (1.1 mg/kg PO q12h). Two weeks after the prednisone treatment was initiated, Sampson became nonambulatory in his pelvic limbs, and all of his peripheral joints became swollen and he was referred to the University of California, Davis, Veterinary Medical Teaching Hospital. A mass had been removed from his left dorsolateral thorax 3 weeks before referral that was assumed to be a foxtail abscess. Sampson had a good appetite. Increased thirst and urination had been noted after the prednisone treatment was initiated. There had been no coughing, sneezing, vomiting, or diarrhea. He was fed a duck- and potato-based diet for food allergy dermatitis and had been treated intermittently with prednisone, 4 mg PO q24h, for this condition since he was 6 months old. He had not traveled outside his local area, but he lived on a ranch and was known to consume horse feces and dead wild animals. There was no known tick exposure. He was up to date on vaccinations including canine distemper, adenovirus, parvovirus, and rabies vaccines.

Current medications: Prednisone 0.9 mg/kg PO q12h

Physical Examination:

Body Weight: 35.8 kg

General: Quiet, alert and responsive, 5% to 7% dehydrated. Recumbent. T = 102.9°F (39.4°C), HR = 140 beats/min, panting, mucous membranes pink and tacky, CRT = 1 s.

Integument: Multifocal epidermal collarettes were present and the haircoat was dry. A shaved area was present on the left lateral thoracic wall.

Eyes, Ears, Nose, and Throat: Moderate periodontal disease was present. A fundic examination was within normal limits.

Musculoskeletal: Body condition score was 5/9 with pelvic limb muscle atrophy. Pain and effusion of the carpi, tarsi, and stifles with decreased range of motion was noted. Spinal and pericervical pain was detected on palpation of these regions.

Cardiovascular: Weak but synchronous femoral pulses were noted. No murmurs or arrhythmias were auscultated.

Respiratory: There were moderately increased breath sounds in all lung fields.

Gastrointestinal/Genitourinary: The abdomen was tense on palpation and moderate hepatomegaly was detected. The dog urinated a large amount of odiferous urine during the examination. No abnormalities were detected on rectal examination.

Lymph Nodes: Moderate peripheral lymphadenopathy was present. Mandibular, superficial cervical, and popliteal lymph nodes were all 1.5 to 2.5 cm in diameter.

Laboratory Findings:

CBC:

HCT 35.4% (40%-55%)
MCV 67 fL (65-75 fL)
MCHC 35.6 g/dL (33-36 g/dL)

Continued

Reticulocytes 101,200 cells/μL (7000-65,000 cells/μL)
WBC 7870 cells/μL (6000-13,000 cells/μL)
Neutrophils 6139 cells/μL (3000-10,500 cells/μL)
Band neutrophils 1495 cells/μL
Metamyelocytes 79 cells/μL
Lymphocytes 0 cells/μL (1000-4000 cells/μL)
Monocytes 79 cells/μL (150-1200 cells/μL)
Platelets 419,000 platelets/μL (150,000-400,000 platelets/μL).
Neutrophils, band neutrophils, and metamyelocytes all showed moderate toxic changes.

Serum Chemistry Profile:

Sodium 148 mmol/L (145-154 mmol/L)
Potassium 4.4 mmol/L (3.6-5.3 mmol/L)
Chloride 105 mmol/L (108-118 mmol/L)
Bicarbonate 14 mmol/L (16-26 mmol/L)
Phosphorus 5.8 mg/dL (3.0-6.2 mg/dL)
Calcium 10.3 mg/dL (9.7-11.5 mg/dl)
BUN 10 mg/dL (5-21 mg/dL)
Creatinine 0.4 mg/dL (0.3-1.2 mg/dL)
Glucose 111 mg/dL (64-123 mg/dL)
Total protein 6.1 g/dL (5.4-7.6 g/dL)
Albumin 2.3 g/dL (3.0-4.4 g/dL)
globulin 3.8 g/dL (1.8-3.9 g/dL)
ALT 560 U/L (19-67 U/L)
AST 72 U/L (19-42 U/L)
ALP 3318 U/L (21-170 U/L)
Creatine kinase 197 U/L (51-399 U/L)
Gamma GT 59 U/L (0-6 U/L)
Cholesterol 212 mg/dL (135-361 mg/dL)
Total bilirubin 0.3 mg/dL (0-0.2 mg/dL).

Urinalysis: SGr 1.010; pH 8.0, 1+ protein (SSA), 3+ hemoprotein, no bilirubin or glucose, 25-35 WBC/HPF, 10-15 RBC/HPF, many rods.

Imaging Findings:

Thoracic Radiographs: The cardiovascular and pulmonary structures appeared within normal limits.

Right and Left Carpal, Stifle, and Tarsal Radiographs: Intracapsular soft tissue swelling was associated with all joints.

Spinal Radiographs: No abnormalities were detected.

Abdominal Ultrasound: The liver was enlarged and hyperechoic. There was echogenic sediment in the urinary bladder.

Echocardiogram: Thickening and hyperechogenicity of the posterior leaflet of the tricuspid valve was noted (arrowhead) which raised suspicion for endocarditis (Figure 45-4).

Cytology Findings: Arthrocentesis of right and left carpi, right tarsus and right stifle: Purulent inflammation was noted in the right tarsus, right stifle, and left carpus, with approximately 85% neutrophils and the remaining cells were a mixture of small and large mononuclear cells. In the right stifle, degenerate neutrophils are visualized, and some contained intracellular rod-shaped bacteria.

Microbiologic Testing: Serologic testing: An in-clinic ELISA for antibodies to *Borrelia burgdorferi*, *Anaplasma phagocytophilum*, and *Ehrlichia canis* was negative. Serum IFA for antibodies to *Bartonella vinsonii* subspecies *berkhoffii* was negative. Serology for *Coccidioides* spp. antibodies was also negative.

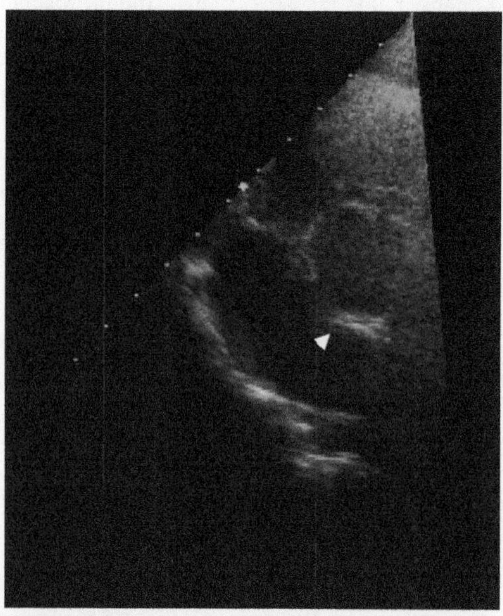

FIGURE 45-4 Thickening and hyperechogenicity of the posterior tricuspid valve leaflet (*arrowhead*) in a dog with *Salmonella arizonae* bacteremia.

Aerobic bacterial culture of blood, joint fluid, and urine collected by cystocentesis: *Salmonella arizonae*, susceptible to all antimicrobials tested.

Diagnosis: *Salmonella arizonae* septic polyarthritis, bacteremia, and possible tricuspid valve endocarditis.

Treatment: Before obtaining susceptibility results, Sampson was treated with intravenous crystalloids, opioids for pain control, enrofloxacin (5 mg/kg IV q24h), and ampicillin (30 mg/kg IV q8h). The ampicillin was discontinued when the susceptibility results became available. The prednisone was tapered over a 3-day period and discontinued. The dog was moved to an isolation ward on diagnosis of salmonellosis. During hospitalization, Sampson's appetite declined initially, and he remained very painful for 6 days. After that time, he was able to sit up, began eating, and was discharged 8 days after admission.

Comments: *Salmonella arizonae* infections in humans have been associated with direct or indirect contact with reptiles. Reptile-associated salmonellosis is an increasing problem in humans in the United States and is especially a problem in infants and immunocompromised adults in contact with snakes and iguanas, or those who eat sun-dried rattlesnake meat for medicinal purposes. Horse feces from the farm were cultured for *Salmonella* and were negative. It is possible that the infection in this dog occurred as a result of ingestion of wild reptiles. The long history of glucocorticoid therapy for atopic dermatitis in this dog may have contributed to immunosuppression and predisposition to systemic salmonellosis.

SUGGESTED READINGS

Behravesh CB, Ferraro A, Deasy M, et al. Human *Salmonella* infections linked to contaminated dry dog and cat food, 2006-2008. Pediatrics. 2010;126(3):477-483.

Grassl GA, Finlay BB. Pathogenesis of enteric *Salmonella* infections. Curr Opin Gastroenterol. 2008;24(1):22-26.

Morley PS, Strohmeyer RA, Tankson JD, et al. Evaluation of the association between feeding raw meat and *Salmonella enterica* infections at a Greyhound breeding facility. J Am Vet Med Assoc. 2006;228(10):1524-1532.

REFERENCES

1. Salmon DE, Smith T. Investigations in swine plague. USDA Bur Anim Indus Ann Rep. 1885:184.
2. Dominguez SA, Schaffner DW. Survival of salmonella in processed chicken products during frozen storage. J Food Prot. 2009;72(10):2088-2092.
3. Brenner FW, Villar RG, Angulo FJ, et al. Salmonella nomenclature. J Clin Microbiol. 2000;38(7):2465-2467.
4. Foti M, Daidone A, Aleo A, et al. *Salmonella bongori* 48:z35:— in migratory birds, Italy. Emerg Infect Dis. 2009;15(3):502-503.
5. Finley R, Ribble C, Aramini J, et al. The risk of salmonellae shedding by dogs fed *Salmonella*-contaminated commercial raw food diets. Can Vet J. 2000;48(1):69-75.
6. Lefebvre SL, Reid-Smith R, Boerlin P, et al. Evaluation of the risks of shedding salmonellae and other potential pathogens by therapy dogs fed raw diets in Ontario and Alberta. Zoonoses Public Health. 2008;55(8-10):470-480.
7. Lenz J, Joffe D, Kauffman M, et al. Perceptions, practices, and consequences associated with foodborne pathogens and the feeding of raw meat to dogs. Can Vet J. 2009;50(6):637-643.
8. McKenzie E, Riehl J, Banse H, et al. Prevalence of diarrhea and enteropathogens in racing sled dogs. J Vet Intern Med. 2010;24(1):97-103.
9. Finley R, Reid-Smith R, Ribble C, et al. The occurrence and antimicrobial susceptibility of salmonellae isolated from commercially available canine raw food diets in three Canadian cities. Zoonoses Public Health. 2008;55(8-10):462-469.
10. Centers for Disease Control and Prevention. Multistate outbreak of human *Salmonella* infections caused by contaminated dry dog food: United States, 2006-2007. MMWR Morb Mortal Wkly Rep. 2008;57(19):521-524.
11. Behravesh CB, Ferraro A, Deasy M, et al. Human *Salmonella* infections linked to contaminated dry dog and cat food, 2006-2008. Pediatrics. 2010;126(3):477-483.
12. Selmi M, Stefanelli S, Bilei S, et al. Contaminated commercial dehydrated food as source of multiple *Salmonella* serotypes outbreak in a municipal kennel in Tuscany. Vet Ital. 2011;47(2):183-190.
13. Centers for Disease Control and Prevention. Notes from the field: human *Salmonella infantis* infections linked to dry dog food—United States and Canada. MMWR Morb Mortal Wkly Rep. 2012;2012(61):436.
14. Morse EV, Duncan MA, Estep DA, et al. Canine salmonellosis: a review and report of dog to child transmission of *Salmonella enteritidis*. Am J Public Health. 1976;66(1):82-84.
15. Hill SL, Cheney JM, Taton-Allen GF, et al. Prevalence of enteric zoonotic organisms in cats. J Am Vet Med Assoc. 2000;216(5):687-692.
16. Spain CV, Scarlett JM, Wade SE, et al. Prevalence of enteric zoonotic organisms in cats less than 1 year old in central New York State. J Vet Intern Med. 2001;15(1):33-38.
17. Stavisky J, Radford AD, Gaskell R, et al. A case-control study of pathogen and lifestyle risk factors for diarrhea in dogs. Prev Vet Med. 2011;99:185-192.
18. Van Immerseel F, Pasmans F, De Buck J, et al. Cats as a risk for transmission of antimicrobial drug-resistant *Salmonella*. Emerg Infect Dis. 2004;10(12):2169-2174.
19. Murphy C, Reid-Smith RJ, Prescott JF, et al. Occurrence of antimicrobial resistant bacteria in healthy dogs and cats presented to private veterinary hospitals in southern Ontario: a preliminary study. Can Vet J. 2009;50(10):1047-1053.
20. Leonard EK, Pearl DL, Finley RL, et al. Comparison of antimicrobial resistance patterns of *Salmonella* spp. and *Escherichia coli* recovered from pet dogs from volunteer households in Ontario (2005-2006). J Antimicrob Chemother. 2012;67:174-181.
21. Morley PS, Strohmeyer RA, Tankson JD, et al. Evaluation of the association between feeding raw meat and *Salmonella enterica* infections at a Greyhound breeding facility. J Am Vet Med Assoc. 2006;228(10):1524-1532.
22. Philbey AW, Brown FM, Mather HA, et al. Salmonellosis in cats in the United Kingdom: 1955 to 2007. Vet Rec. 2009;164(4):120-122.
23. Sabshin SJ, Levy JK, Tupler T, et al. Enteropathogens identified in cats entering a Florida animal shelter with normal feces or diarrhea. J Am Vet Med Assoc. 2012;241:331-337.
24. Hohenhaus AE, Rosenberg MP, Moroff SD. Concurrent lymphoma and salmonellosis in a cat. Can Vet J. 1990;31(1):38-40.
25. Moazed TC, Deeb BJ, DiGiacomo RF. Subcutaneous abscess due to *Salmonella adelaide* in a grey collie with cyclic hematopoiesis. Lab Anim Sci. 1990;40(6):639-641.
26. Grassl GA, Finlay BB. Pathogenesis of enteric *Salmonella* infections. Curr Opin Gastroenterol. 2008;24(1):22-26.
27. Delaloye J, Merlani G, Petignat C, et al. Nosocomial nontyphoidal salmonellosis after antineoplastic chemotherapy: reactivation of asymptomatic colonization? Eur J Clin Microbiol Infect Dis. 2004;23(10):751-758.
28. Lomborg SR, Agerholm JS, Jensen AL, et al. Effects of experimental immunosuppression in cattle with persistently high antibody levels to *Salmonella dublin* lipopolysaccharide O-antigens. BMC Vet Res. 2007;3:17.
29. Fierer J, Guiney DG. Diverse virulence traits underlying different clinical outcomes of *Salmonella* infection. J Clin Invest. 2001;107(7):775-780.
30. Dow SW, Jones RL, Henik RA, et al. Clinical features of salmonellosis in cats: six cases (1981-1986). J Am Vet Med Assoc. 1989;194(10):1464-1466.
31. Fox JG, Beaucage CM, Murphy JC, et al. Experimental *Salmonella*-associated conjunctivitis in cats. Can J Comp Med. 1984;48(1):87-91.
32. Rodriguez Jr CO, Moon ML, Leib MS. *Salmonella choleraesuis* pneumonia in a cat without signs of gastrointestinal disease. J Am Vet Med Assoc. 1993;202(6):953-955.
33. Morse EV, Duncan MA. Canine salmonellosis: prevalence, epizootiology, signs, and public health significance. J Am Vet Med Assoc. 1975;167(9):817-820.
34. Caldow GL, Graham MM. Abortion in foxhounds and a ewe flock associated with *Salmonella montevideo* infection. Vet Rec. 1998;142(6):138-139.
35. Redwood DW, Bell DA. *Salmonella panama*: isolation from aborted and newborn canine fetuses. Vet Rec. 1983;112(15):362.
36. Dieckmann R, Helmuth R, Erhard M, et al. Rapid classification and identification of salmonellae by whole-cell matrix-assisted laser desorption ionization-time of flight mass spectrometry. Appl Environ Microbiol. 2008;74:7767-7778.
37. Dieckmann R, Malorny B. Rapid screening of epidemiologically important *Salmonella enterica* subsp. *enterica* serovars by whole-cell matrix-assisted laser desorption ionization-time of flight mass spectrometry. Appl Environ Microbiol. 2011;77:4136-4146.
38. Kurowski PB, Traub-Dargatz JL, Morley PS, et al. Detection of *Salmonella* spp. In fecal specimens by use of real-time polymerase chain reaction assay. Am J Vet Res. 2002;63(9):1265-1268.
39. Pusterla N, Byrne BA, Hodzic E, et al. Use of quantitative real-time PCR for the detection of *Salmonella* spp. in fecal samples from horses at a veterinary teaching hospital. Vet J. 2010;186(2):252-255.
40. Ward MP, Alinovi CA, Couëtil LL, Wu CC. Evaluation of a PCR to detect *Salmonella* in fecal samples of horses admitted to a veterinary teaching hospital. J Vet Diagn Invest. 2005;17:118-123.

41. Timbs DV, Durham PJ, Barnsley DJ. Chronic cholecystitis in a dog infected with Salmonella typhimurium. N Z Vet J. 1974;22(6):100-102.
42. Stiver SL, Frazier KS, Mauei MJ, et al. Septicemic salmonellosis in two cats fed a raw-meat diet. J Am Anim Hosp Assoc. 2003;39(6):538-542.
43. Opal SM, Glück T. Endotoxin as a drug target. Crit Care Med. 2003;31(suppl 1):S57-S64.
44. Leon CG, Tory R, Jia J, et al. Discovery and development of Toll-like receptor 4 (TLR4) antagonists: a new paradigm for treating sepsis and other diseases. Pharm Res. 2008;25(8):1751-1761.
45. Wittebole X, Castanares-Zapatero D, Laterre PF. Toll-like receptor 4 modulation as a strategy to treat sepsis. Mediators Inflamm. 2010;2010:568396.
46. Bueno SM, Gonzáles PA, Carreño LJ, et al. The capacity of *Salmonella* to survive inside dendritic cells and prevent antigen presentation to T cells is host specific. Immunology. 2008;124(4):522-533.
47. Albaghdadi H, Robinson N, Finlay B, et al. Selectively reduced intracellular proliferation of *Salmonella enterica* serovar typhimurium within APCs limits antigen presentation and development of a rapid CD8 T cell response. J Immunol. 2009;183(6):3778-3787.
48. Wright JG, Tengelsen LA, Smith KE, et al. Multidrug-resistant *Salmonella* Typhimurium in four animal facilities. Emerg Infect Dis. 2005;11(8):1235-1241.
49. Centers for Disease Control and Prevention. http://www.cdc.gov/Features/salmonellafrogturtle. Last accessed December 23, 2012.

CHAPTER 46

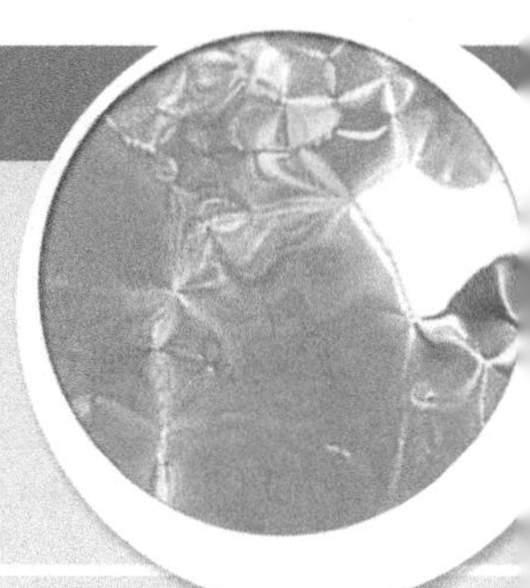

Enteric *Escherichia coli* Infections

Jane E. Sykes and Stanley L. Marks

> **Overview of Enteric *Escherichia coli* Infections**
>
> First Described: Germany, 1885 (Theodor Escherich)[1]
>
> Cause: *Escherichia coli* (gram-negative rods that belong to the Enterobacteriaceae)
>
> Affected Hosts: Humans and a large variety of animals
>
> Geographic Distribution: Worldwide
>
> Primary Mode of Transmission: Fecal-oral
>
> Major Clinical Signs: Fever, lethargy, inappetence, diarrhea, vomiting
>
> Differential Diagnoses: Differential diagnoses for suspected *E. coli* enterocolitis include canine and feline parvovirus infection, canine distemper virus infection, salmon poisoning disease, campylobacteriosis, clostridial diarrhea, salmonellosis, giardiasis, tritrichomoniasis (cats), cryptosporidiosis, whipworms, pythiosis, histoplasmosis, leptospirosis, dietary indiscretion, gastrointestinal foreign body, pancreatitis, inflammatory bowel disease, lymphoma, hypoadrenocorticism, hyperthyroidism (cats), toxins (including drugs).
>
> Human Health Significance: Dogs and cats may be a source of human infection with some *E. coli* serotypes.

Etiology and Epidemiology

Escherichia coli are pleomorphic gram-negative, non–spore-forming rods that belong to the family Enterobacteriaceae. Like *Salmonella*, *E. coli* can survive long periods of time in feces, dust, and water. They are part of the normal flora of the gastrointestinal tract but can be associated with enterocolitis in the presence of bacterial virulence factors and impaired local or systemic immunity. As with *Salmonella* infections, *E. coli* infections can be transferred between animal species and some may be zoonotic; many infections are food borne.

There are more than 170 serogroups of *E. coli* based on the identity of the bacterial O (somatic) antigen, the sugar that is on the most external portion of the bacterial lipopolysaccharide (LPS) (see Chapter 36). Organisms are also identified on the basis of their H (flagellar) antigens—for example, O157:H7 *E. coli*. Both the bacterial LPS (endotoxin) and the flagellar antigens are bacterial virulence factors. Other virulence factors in *E. coli* include adhesins, bacterial exotoxins such as cytotoxic necrotizing factor (CNF), hemolysins, heat-labile (LT) and heat-stable (ST) enterotoxins, and the capsular polysaccharide (K).

E. coli strains that cause gastrointestinal disease have been divided into seven distinct pathogenic categories (pathovars). Each pathovar is defined by a characteristic set of virulence factors that act in concert to determine the clinical, pathologic, and epidemiologic features of the disease they cause. The seven pathovars include enteropathogenic *E. coli* (EPEC), enterotoxigenic *E. coli* (ETEC), enterohemorrhagic *E. coli* (EHEC), necrotoxigenic *E. coli* (NTEC), enteroinvasive *E. coli* (EIEC), enteroaggregative *E. coli* (EAEC), and adherent-invasive *E. coli* (AIEC) (Table 46-1). Currently, the epidemiology of many of these strains and their role in disease causation is not well defined in small animals, with most work having been done in humans and farm animal species. Many strains have been isolated from both nondiarrheic and diarrheic dogs and cats. An association between EPEC and EHEC (including H7:O157) infection and diarrhea in dogs has been detected.[2,3] In addition, AIEC strains have been well associated with granulomatous colitis in boxer dogs.[4]

Clinical Features

Signs and Their Pathogenesis

EPEC strains carry the *eae*A gene on their chromosome (*E. coli* attaching effacing), which is located in a "pathogenicity island" referred to as LEE (locus of enterocyte effacement). The *eae*A gene encodes a 94-kDa protein, intimin, which allows the organism to adhere intimately to intestinal epithelial cells. This leads to local effacement of the microvilli and formation of numerous, actin-rich pedestals on which the bacteria reside (Figure 46-1).[5] The bacteria secrete their own receptor, the Tir receptor, and Tir-intimin interactions are involved in pedestal formation. The pedestals may help the bacteria to remain extracellular, and thus escape immune recognition by the host. The resulting characteristic histopathologic lesions on enterocytes have been referred to as "attaching and effacing lesions." Subsequent signal transduction events induced by EPEC may be associated with loss of tight junction integrity and altered electrolyte transport, with associated watery diarrhea. The EPEC pathovar does not produce Shiga toxin, Shiga-like toxin, or verotoxins. EPEC serotypes that have been associated with diarrhea in humans have been identified in dogs and cats.[6,7]

ETEC are a major cause of diarrhea in human infants in developing countries and are the agents most frequently responsive for traveler's diarrhea. ETEC pathovars have been associated with up to 31% of cases of canine diarrhea, particularly in young dogs.[8-10] Most of the canine ETEC strains express ST enterotoxin, whereas ETEC strains that produce LT enterotoxin are rarely found. The bacteria adhere to the proximal small intestinal mucosa and produce plasmid-encoded LT and ST enterotoxins. LT is related to cholera toxin and is taken up by enterocytes. Once within intestinal epithelial cells, it activates adenylate cyclase, which leads to increased concentrations of intracellular cyclic AMP with resultant secretion of electrolytes

TABLE 46-1

Pathogenic Strains of *Escherichia coli* That Cause Enterocolitis

Strain	Lesion	Signs	Virulence Characteristic
Enteropathogenic *E. coli* (EPEC)	Attaching and effacing lesions (effacement of microvilli and pedestal formation)	Watery diarrhea	*eaeA* gene (encodes intimin)
Enterotoxigenic *E. coli* (ETEC)	Adhere using fimbria and produce heat-labile (LT) and/or heat-stable (ST) toxins	Diarrhea	LT and ST production
Enterohemorrhagic *E. coli* (EHEC); also known as Shiga-toxin–producing *E. coli* (STEC) or verotoxin-producing *E. coli* (VTEC)	Produce Shiga-like toxins (verotoxins) that cause vascular endothelial damage, also produce attaching and effacing lesions	Diarrhea, hemorrhagic colitis, hemolytic-uremic syndrome	Shiga-like toxin production, see also EPEC
Necrotoxigenic *E. coli* (NTEC)	Produce cytotoxic necrotizing factors (CNFs)	Diarrhea, bacteremia, urinary tract infections in humans	CNFs
Enteroinvasive *E. coli* (EIEC)	Actively invade colonic epithelial cells	Large bowel diarrhea	Plasmid-encoded invasion genes such as *ipaH*
Adherent-invasive *E. coli* (AIEC)	Invade colonic epithelial cells using unknown virulence mechanisms	Granulomatous/histiocytic ulcerative colitis in dogs (especially boxers)	None known
Enteroaggregative *E. coli* (EAEC)	Adhere to intestinal epithelium via fimbriae and aggregate in bricklike fashion	Persistent watery diarrhea in humans	*aggR* gene

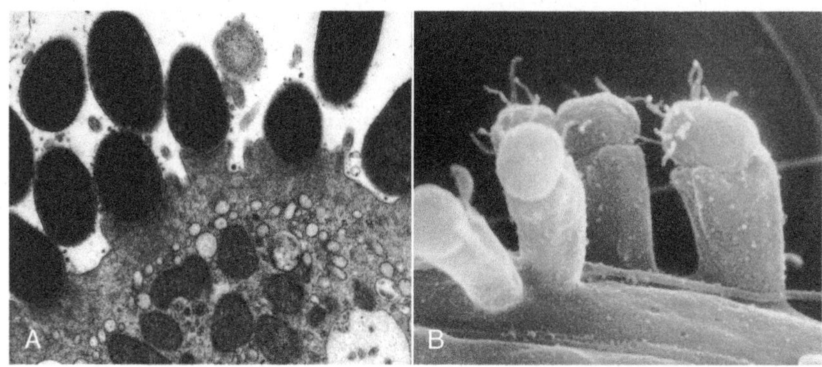

FIGURE 46-1 Scanning and transmission electron micrographs showing actin pedestals induced by enteropathogenic and enterohemorrhagic *Escherichia coli* (EPEC and EHEC). **A,** EPEC generates attaching and effacing (AE) lesions on the intestinal epithelium after infection of gnotobiotic piglets. Note the pedestal-like structures on host cells beneath attached bacteria. (From Campellone KG, Leong JM. Tails of two Tirs: actin pedestal formation by enteropathogenic *E. coli* and enterohemorrhagic *E. coli*. Curr Opin Microbiol 2003;6(1):82-90.) **B,** Actin pedestals that resemble AE lesions formed in vivo are also generated on cultured epithelial (HeLa) cells. (Courtesy of Knutton S. In: Knutton S, Rosenshine L, Pallen, MJ, et al. A novel EspA-associated surface organelle of enteropathogenic *Escherichia coli* involved in protein translocation into epithelial cells. EMBO J. 1998;17:2166-2176.)

and water that lead to diarrhea, hypovolemia, and metabolic acidosis. LT may also downregulate innate host immune responses and promote ETEC adherence. In contrast, ST binds to the extracellular domain of guanylyl cyclase C, which leads to accumulation of intracellular cyclic GMP and ultimately secretion of chloride and decreased absorption of NaCl, with resultant osmotic diarrhea. Two different ST enterotoxins have been identified, STa and STb. ST-producing ETEC have been detected in young dogs with diarrhea.[8-10]

In addition to producing attaching and effacing lesions similar to those created by EPEC, EHEC (Shiga-toxin–producing *E. coli*, or STEC) produce Shiga-like toxins (also known as verotoxins). They cause diarrhea, hemorrhagic colitis, and hemolytic-uremic syndrome (HUS) (e.g., *E. coli* strain O157:H7). Shiga-like toxins are absorbed from the intestinal lumen and cause vascular endothelial damage, which may lead to a multiorgan thrombotic process in the absence of bacteremia. EHEC can also produce other toxins that contribute to the pathogenesis of the disease. HUS in humans is characterized by renal failure, widespread microthrombotic damage to a variety of organs, hemolytic anemia, and sometimes diarrhea. Similar syndromes have been described in dogs, but an associated *E. coli* infection was not demonstrated.[11,12] HUS has been reproduced experimentally in dogs with a non-O157:H7 *E. coli* serotype.[13] Based on the similarity of renal lesions to those described in HUS, and the practice of feeding predominantly raw meat diets to greyhounds, it has been hypothesized that cutaneous and renal glomerular vasculopathy of greyhounds (also known as "Alabama rot" or "Greenetrack disease") may result from infection with EHEC strains such as O157:H7.[14] A similar condition was described in a great Dane from Germany.[15] Some dogs develop cutaneous lesions in the absence of renal failure; other dogs develop renal failure before the onset of cutaneous lesions.

NTEC produce two toxins: CNF and cytolethal distending toxin. Multiple CNF types have been identified (CNF1, CNF2, and CNF3). NTEC have been associated with diarrhea, bacteremia, and urinary tract infections in human patients, as well as with diarrhea in dogs.[16]

EIEC actively invade colonic epithelial cells. This, together with the associated inflammatory response, leads to hemorrhagic, large bowel diarrhea. In human patients, the EIEC pathovar is uncommonly detected compared with EPEC and ETEC. AIEC, which lack the virulence genes that identify EIEC, have been associated with granulomatous colitis in boxer dogs and infrequently in the French bulldog and Border collie. This infection typically affects young adult boxer dogs that show signs of severe colitis, with colonic thickening and ulceration, and weight loss that is often marked.[4,17] It has been suggested that a heritable anomaly in boxer dogs predisposes them to the infection, given the marked breed predisposition for the disease.[18]

The EAEC pathovar is considered an emerging pathogen in human patients. It adheres to epithelial cells of the terminal ileum and colon using fimbriae in a characteristic "stacked brick" pattern. Expression of these fimbriae is encoded by a plasmid gene known as *aggR*. Bacterial aggregation is followed by damage and a subsequent inflammatory response, which leads to development of persistent watery diarrhea. Occasionally, EAEC strains also produce toxins, such as verocytotoxin.[19] Their role in dogs and cats requires further investigation.

Physical Examination Findings

Physical examination may reveal dehydration and abdominal pain in puppies with *E. coli* diarrhea. Dogs with HUS have had cutaneous erythema and well-demarcated, multifocal cutaneous ulcers of the limbs. Fever and peripheral edema have also been described. Boxer dogs with granulomatous colitis may have poor body condition. A thickened and irregular rectal wall may be detected on rectal palpation, and the feces may contain fresh blood and mucus.

Diagnosis

Diagnosis of intestinal *E. coli* infections, with the exception of granulomatous colitis of boxer dogs, is difficult or impossible with currently available diagnostic assays, because of the fact that healthy dogs and cats shed *E. coli*, and it is a combination of bacterial virulence factors and host immune competence that contributes to the development of clinical signs. This section therefore focuses primarily on the more specific clinical syndromes caused by EHEC and AIEC.

Laboratory Abnormalities

Complete Blood Count

CBC changes in dogs with *E. coli* diarrhea are generally mild and nonspecific. Leukocytosis may be present. Dogs infected with EHEC may be thrombocytopenic and have evidence of microangiopathic hemolysis. Microcytic anemia may be present in boxer dogs with granulomatous colitis.

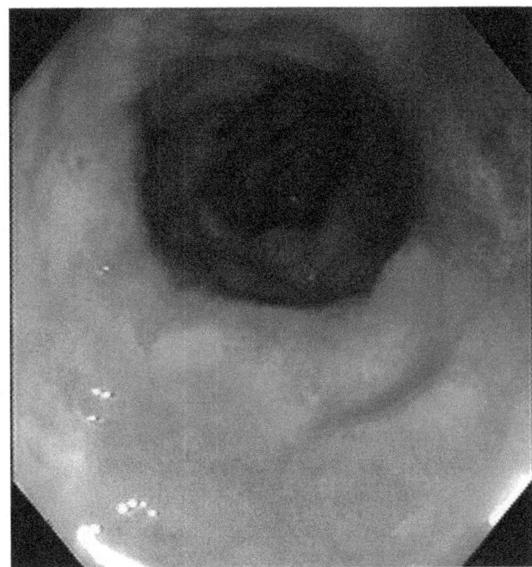

FIGURE 46-2 Ulcerated and erythematous colon of a 2-year-old intact male boxer dog with granulomatous colitis as viewed during colonoscopy. The dog had a 7-month history of marked weight loss and severe diarrhea, with increased frequency of defecation and hematochezia.

Serum Chemistry Panel and Urinalysis

Laboratory abnormalities in dogs with *E. coli* diarrhea could include electrolyte abnormalities and prerenal azotemia in dogs with severe diarrhea. Dogs infected with EHEC have had variable evidence of hypoalbuminemia, prerenal azotemia, increased activities of ALT and creatine kinase, hematuria, proteinuria, and isosthenuria. Boxer dogs with granulomatous colitis are commonly hypoalbuminemic.

Diagnostic Imaging

Findings on abdominal radiography and abdominal ultrasound are typically unremarkable or show fluid-filled intestinal loops. Abdominal ultrasound in boxer dogs with granulomatous colitis often reveals mild or moderate mesenteric or sublumbar lymphadenomegaly, and the colonic wall can appear thickened.

Endoscopic Findings

Proctoscopy or colonoscopy is usually performed in order to obtain colonic biopsies from boxer dogs suspected to have granulomatous colitis. Proctoscopy requires less fastidious colonic preparation compared to colonoscopy, can be performed under heavy sedation, and is more cost effective compared to colonoscopy. Most boxer dogs with granulomatous colitis have involvement of the descending colon, underscoring the diagnostic utility of proctoscopy. Common changes in appearance to the colonic wall include erythema, irregularity, and ulceration of the rectal wall (Figure 46-2).

Microbiologic Testing

Bacterial Isolation and Typing

E. coli is commonly isolated on routine bacteriologic media from feces of both healthy and diarrheic dogs. A differential medium such as MacConkey agar is often used. Apart from dogs with granulomatous colitis, attempts to specifically identify *E. coli* as a cause of diarrhea are generally performed only by reference or public health laboratories when an outbreak has occurred, or for research purposes. *E. coli* can be isolated from colonic biopsies of dogs with granulomatous colitis, which permits subsequent antimicrobial susceptibility testing.[20] Serologic identification, which is performed using specific O and H antisera, can be costly and is generally performed by large public health laboratories in epidemiologic investigations.

Virulence Assays

Immunoassays are available for detection of Shiga toxin, ST, and LT. A Vero cell cytotoxicity assay has been used to detect verocytotoxin. Identification of EPEC and AIEC often relies on assays that assess adherence in tissue culture. In research settings, molecular diagnostic techniques using DNA probes or PCR assays have revolutionized the ability to detect and differentiate between pathogenic and nonpathogenic strains of *E. coli*. EPEC characteristically possess the *eaeA* gene. Detection of genes that encode LT, ST, and Shiga-like toxin allows identification of ETEC and EHEC. EIEC are identified based on the presence of invasion-associated genes such as *ipaH*. The *aat* gene is a diagnostic marker for EAEC detection.[19]

Pathologic Findings

The most significant pathologic findings in intestinal *E. coli* infections occur with EHEC and AIEC infections.

EHEC

Cutaneous ulcerative lesions in dogs with suspected HUS are characterized histopathologically by fibrinoid vascular necrosis, with dermal thrombosis and leukocytoclastic vasculitis. Grossly, the kidneys may be swollen and have cortical petechiae. Histopathology reveals hyaline fibrinous thrombi in glomerular capillaries and afferent arterioles, glomerular and multifocal tubular necrosis, and leukocytoclastic vasculitis with fibrinoid necrosis.

AIEC

Histopathologic lesions in boxers and French bulldogs with granulomatous colitis are pathognomonic and include neutrophilic inflammation, epithelial ulceration, crypt hyperplasia and distortion, decreased goblet cell numbers, and abundant macrophages that stain positive with periodic acid–Schiff (PAS) stain (Figure 46-3). The presence of *E. coli* within macrophages can be confirmed using fluorescence in situ hybridization, which has been recommended as part of the diagnostic work-up of dogs suspected to have histiocytic ulcerative colitis.[5,18]

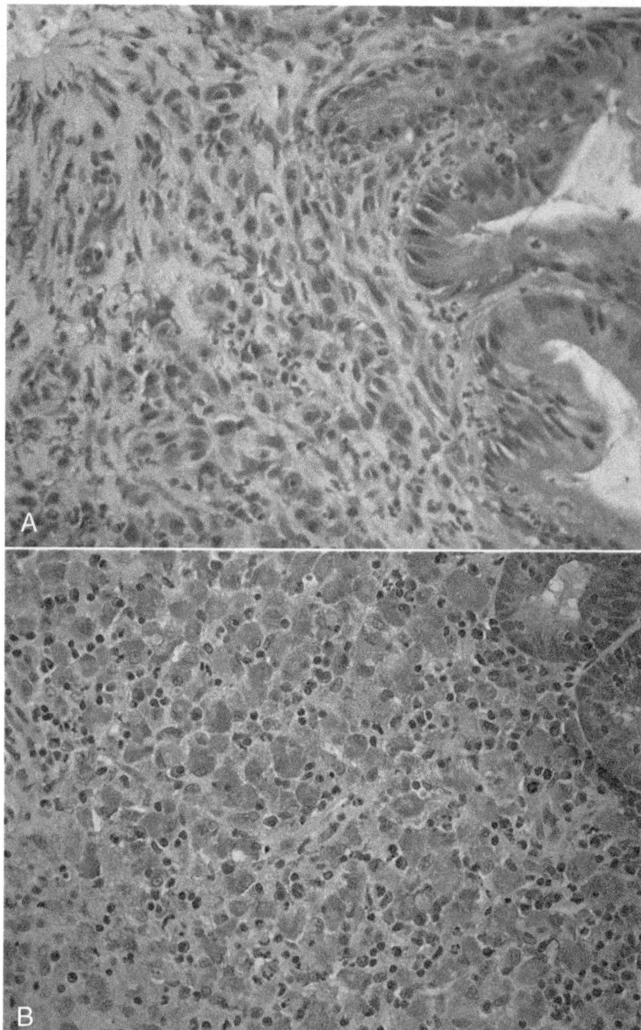

FIGURE 46-3 **A,** Histopathology showing severe, chronic, histiocytic colitis in a 2-year-old male boxer dog. The inflammatory infiltrate is comprised of large, epithelioid macrophages and lesser numbers of neutrophils, plasma cells, and lymphocytes. **B,** Histiocytes in the lamina propria contain PAS-positive material.

Treatment and Prognosis

Dogs and cats with severe diarrhea due to pathogenic *E. coli* may require intravenous fluid therapy. Dogs with granulomatous colitis can show dramatic responses to treatment with enrofloxacin (10 mg/kg PO q24h), and a minimum treatment duration of 8 weeks is recommended.[18] Administration of fluoroquinolones is usually associated with rapid resolution of clinical signs and resolves cellular infiltration characteristic of this disorder on colonic biopsy. Because enrofloxacin resistance has been documented in some isolates from dogs with granulomatous colitis, attempts to isolate *E. coli* from colonic biopsies before treatment is recommended so that antimicrobial susceptibility testing can be performed.[20] Antimicrobials that penetrate intracellularly, such as fluoroquinolones, chloramphenicol, rifampin, or trimethoprim-sulfonamides, should be chosen for treatment based on the results of susceptibility testing.

Immunity and Vaccination

Currently, no vaccines for *E. coli* infections are available for dogs and cats. Vaccines for EPEC, ETEC, and EHEC have been investigated for animals and humans on a research basis,[21-23] including a transdermal LT vaccine for prevention of travelers' diarrhea.[24]

Prevention

The reader is referred to Chapter 11 and Chapter 45 for information on prevention of enteric bacterial infections.

Public Health Aspects

Pathogenic *E. coli* that cause diarrhea have been particularly prevalent in children in developing countries and in travelers to developing countries. EHEC can be acquired following ingestion of undercooked ground hamburger meat, vegetables, and nonchlorinated drinking and swimming water that have been contaminated with fecal material. Infection has also been reported following contact with animals housed in petting zoos.[25] HUS is reported as the most common cause of acute renal failure in children. Clinical signs in humans consist of gastrointestinal signs, often with profuse, bloody diarrhea, abdominal cramps, pallor, weakness, and oliguria or anuria.[26] Dogs have been suggested as a source of human infection with EPEC and EHEC.[27,28]

The possibility of zoonotic transmission of multidrug resistant *E. coli* that are shed by dogs and cats is an emerging concern. A variety of resistance mechanisms have been identified in *E. coli* isolates from dogs and cats, which include production of efflux pumps and extended-spectrum and AmpC β-lactamase enzymes. There is some evidence that *E. coli* strains shed by healthy companion animals can be shared with humans that reside in the same household,[29-32] but more studies are required to determine the extent to which this occurs and its zoonotic significance. Transfer of plasmids that carry resistance genes from canine or feline *E. coli* isolates and those of humans also has the potential to occur.

For hospitalized animals, staff should use contact precautions for any dog or cat suspected to have enteropathogenic illness, including the use of warning signs, gloves, and gowns, hand washing, and cleaning with bleach-based or accelerated hydrogen peroxide-based disinfectants. Endoscopes should be disinfected thoroughly between uses. Veterinarians should discuss the zoonotic implications of enteropathogenic bacterial infection with pet owners, especially in relation to the presence of young children or otherwise immunocompromised individuals in the household.

CASE EXAMPLE

Signalment: "Caesar", 2-year-old male boxer dog from Tulare, CA (Figure 46-4)

History: Caesar was evaluated for chronic diarrhea, which had been present since he was 6 months of age. His feces were loose and contained a small amount of frank blood. He strained to defecate many times a day, and the owner sometimes noticed mucus in the diarrhea. Every few months, Caesar's appetite and energy level declined and the diarrhea became more severe. His signs transiently improved after treatment with subcutaneous fluids and metronidazole. The owners had tried a variety of different diets such as fiber-supplemented diets and elimination diets that contain novel, single protein sources, but these strategies did not help. His current diet was a digestible commercial diet, and his appetite was good. He was up to date on vaccinations, including those for rabies, canine distemper, canine parvovirus, canine adenovirus, and *Bordetella bronchiseptica*. He was primarily an indoor dog with access to a suburban backyard.

Physical Examination:

Body Weight: 23.4 kg

General: Bright, alert, and responsive. Ambulatory on all four limbs. T = 102.5°F (39.2°C), HR = 102 beats/min, panting, mucous membranes pink, CRT = 1 s.

Integument, Eyes, Ears, Nose, and Throat: No significant abnormalities were noted. A moderate amount of dental calculus was present.

Musculoskeletal: Body condition score was 3/9 with symmetrical muscling.

All Other Systems: On rectal examination, the walls of the rectum were smooth. There was fresh blood on the glove following palpation. No other clinically significant abnormalities were noted.

Laboratory Findings:

CBC:

HCT 54.4% (40%-55%)
MCV 76.8 fL (65-75 fL)

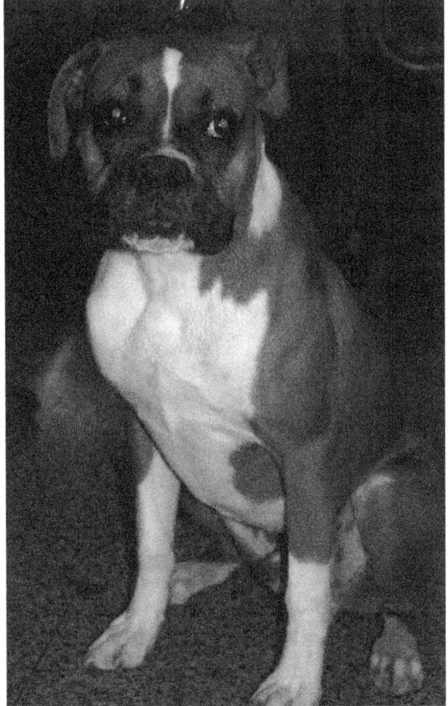

FIGURE 46-4 "Caesar," a 2-year-old male boxer dog from Tulare, CA, that was diagnosed with granulomatous colitis following colonoscopy and biopsy.

MCHC 32.9 g/dL (33-36 g/dL)
WBC 12,590 cells/μL (6000-13,000 cells/μL)
Neutrophils 9631 cells/μL (3000-10,500 cells/μL)
Lymphocytes 1674 cells/μL (1000-4000 cells/μL)
Monocytes 781 cells/μL (150-1200 cells/μL)
Platelets were clumped but appeared adequate in number.

Serum Chemistry Profile:

Sodium 155 mmol/L (145-154 mmol/L)
Potassium 4.2 mmol/L (3.6-5.3 mmol/L)
Chloride 116 mmol/L (108-118 mmol/L)
Bicarbonate 23 mmol/L (16-26 mmol/L)
Phosphorus 4.4 mg/dL (3.0-6.2 mg/dL)

Calcium 10.4 mg/dL (9.7-11.5 mg/dl)
BUN 18 mg/dL (5-21 mg/dL)
Creatinine 1.1 mg/dL (0.3-1.2 mg/dL)
Glucose 105 mg/dL (64-123 mg/dL)
Total protein 6.5 g/dL (5.4-7.6 g/dL)
Albumin 2.9 g/dL (3.0-4.4 g/dL)
Globulin 3.6 g/dL (1.8-3.9 g/dL)
ALT 68 U/L (19-67 U/L)
AST 46 U/L (19-42 U/L)
ALP 86 U/L (21-170 U/L)
GGT 5 U/L (0-6 U/L)
Cholesterol 200 mg/dL (135-361 mg/dL)
Total bilirubin 0.1 mg/dL (0-0.2 mg/dL).

Fecal Examination: Centrifugal fecal flotation: Negative for parasites.

Colonoscopy: The entire mucosal surface of the colon was erythematous and irregular, with multifocal areas of mucosal ulceration (see Figure 45-1).

Histopathology of Colonic Biopsies: Severe, chronic, histiocytic and ulcerative colitis. Histiocytes in the lamina propria contained PAS-positive material (see Figure 46-3).

Diagnosis: Granulomatous colitis of boxer dogs

Treatment: Enrofloxacin, 6 mg/kg PO q24h for 8 weeks and a commercial low-residue dry and canned dog food. This was associated with clinical improvement within a week after starting the medication. At a recheck 4 weeks later, the owner reported that Caesar's feces were completely normal in consistency and frequency.

Comments: In this dog, the diagnosis of granulomatous colitis was made solely based on histopathologic findings. Culture of a biopsy specimen could also have been performed and is now recommended given the emergence of fluoroquinolone-resistant AIEC strains of *E. coli.*

SUGGESTED READINGS

Sherman PM, Ossa JC, Wine E. Bacterial infections: new and emerging enteric pathogens. Curr Opin Gastroenterol. 2010;26(1):1-4.

Simpson KW, Dogan B, Rishniw M, et al. Adherent and invasive *Escherichia coli* is associated with granulomatous colitis in boxer dogs. Infect Immun. 2006;74(8):4778-4792.

REFERENCES

1. Escherich T. Die Darmbakterien des Neugeborenen und Säuglings. Fortschr Med. 1885;3:515-522, 547-554.
2. Sancak AA, Rutgers HC, Hart CA, et al. Prevalence of enteropathic *Escherichia coli* in dogs with acute and chronic diarrhea. Vet Rec. 2004;154(4):101-106.
3. Morato EP, Leomil L, Beutin L, et al. Domestic cats constitute a natural reservoir of human enteropathogenic *Escherichia coli* types. Zoonoses Public Health. 2009;56(5):229-237.
4. Simpson KW, Dogan B, Rishniw M, et al. Adherent and invasive *Escherichia coli* is associated with granulomatous colitis in boxer dogs. Infect Immun. 2006;74(8):4778-4792.
5. Celli J, Deng W, Finlay BB. Enteropathogenic *Escherichia coli* (EPEC) attachment to epithelial cells: exploiting the host cell cytoskeleton from the outside. Cell Microbiol. 2000;2(1):1-9.
6. Morato EP, Leomil L, Beutin L, et al. Domestic cats constitute a natural reservoir of human enteropathogenic *Escherichia coli* types. Zoonoses Public Health. 2009;56:229-237.
7. de Almeida PM, Arais LR, Andrade JR, et al. Characterization of atypical Enteropathogenic *Escherichia coli* (aEPEC) isolated from dogs. Vet Microbiol. 2012;158:420-424.
8. Drolet R, Fairbrother JM, Harel J, et al. Attaching and effacing and enterotoxigenic *Escherichia coli* associated with enteric colibacillosis in the dog. Can J Vet Res. 1994;58(2):87-92.
9. Hammermueller J, Kruth S, Prescott J, et al. Detection of toxin genes in *Escherichia coli* isolated from normal dogs and dogs with diarrhea. Can J Vet Res. 1995;59(4):265-270.
10. Beutin L. *Escherichia coli* as a pathogen in dogs and cats. Vet Res. 1999;30(2-3):285-298.
11. Chantrey J, Chapman PS, Patterson-Kan JC. Haemolytic-uraemic syndrome in a dog. J Vet Med A Physiol Pathol Clin Med. 2002;49(9):470-472.
12. Dell'Orco M, Bertazzolo W, Pagliaro L, et al. Hemolytic-uremic syndrome in a dog. Vet Clin Pathol. 2005;34(3):264-269.
13. Wang JY, Wang SS, Yin PZ. Haemolytic-uraemic syndrome caused by a non-O157:H7 *Escherichia coli* strain in experimentally inoculated dogs. J Med Microbiol. 2006;55(Pt 1):23-29.
14. Cowan LA, Hertzke DM, Fenwick BW, et al. Clinical and clinicopathologic abnormalities in greyhounds with cutaneous and renal glomerular vasculopathy: 18 cases (1992-1994). J Am Vet Med Assoc 210(6):789–793.
15. Rotermund A, Peters M, Hewicker-Trautwein M, et al. Cutaneous and renal glomerular vasculopathy in a great Dane resembling "Alabama rot" of greyhounds. Vet Rec. 2002;151(17):510-512.
16. Starcic M, Johnson JR, Stell AL, et al. Haemolytic *Escherichia coli* isolated from dogs with diarrhea have characteristics of both uropathogenic and necrotoxigenic strains. Vet Microbiol. 2002;85(4):361-377.
17. Van Kruiningen HJ, Civco IC, Cartun RW. The comparative importance of *E. coli* antigen in granulomatous colitis of Boxer dogs. APMIS. 2005;113(6):420-425.
18. Mansfield CS, James FE, Craven M, et al. Remission of histiocytic ulcerative colitis in Boxer dogs correlates with eradication of invasive intramucosal *Escherichia coli*. J Vet Intern Med. 2009;23(5):964-969.
19. Scavia G, Staffolani M, Fisichella S, et al. Enteroaggregative *Escherichia coli* associated with a foodborne outbreak of gastroenteritis. J Med Microbiol. 2008;57(Pt 9):1141-1146.
20. Craven M, Dogan B, Schukken A, et al. Antimicrobial resistance impacts clinical outcome of granulomatous colitis in boxer dogs. J Vet Intern Med. 2010;24(4):819-824.
21. Gu J, Liu Y, Yu S, et al. Enterohemorrhagic *Escherichia coli* trivalent recombinant vaccine containing EspA, intimin and Stx2 induces strong humoral immune response and confers protection in mice. Microbes Infect. 2009;11(10-11):835-841.
22. Keller R, Hilton TD, Rios H, et al. Development of a live oral attaching and effacing *Escherichia coli* vaccine candidate using *Vibrio cholerae* CVD 103-HgR as antigen vector. Microb Pathog. 2010;48(1):1-8.
23. Rojas RL, Gomes PA, Bentancor LV, et al. *Salmonella enterica* serovar Typhimurium vaccine strains expressing a nontoxic Shiga-like toxin 2 derivative induce partial protective immunity to the toxin expressed by enterohemorrhagic *Escherichia coli*. Clin Vaccine Immunol. 2010;17(4):529-536.
24. Frech SA, Dupont HL, Bourgeois AL, et al. Use of a patch containing heat-labile toxin from *Escherichia coli* against traveller's diarrhoea: a phase II, randomized, double-blind, placebo-controlled field trial. Lancet. 2008;371(9629):2019-2025.

25. Sherman PM, Ossa JC, Wine E. Bacterial infections: new and emerging enteric pathogens. Curr Opin Gastroenterol. 2010;26(1):1-4.
26. Scheiring J, Andreoli SP, Zimmerhackl LB. Treatment and outcome of Shiga-toxin-associated hemolytic-uremic syndrome. Pediatr Nephrol. 2008;23(10):1749-1760.
27. Nakazato G, Gyles C, Ziebell K, et al. Attaching and effacing *Escherichia coli* isolated from dogs in Brazil: characteristics and serotypic relationship to human enteropathogenic *E. coli* (EPEC). Vet Microbiol. 2004;101(4):269-277.
28. Hogg RA, Holmes JP, Ghebrehewet S, et al. Probable zoonotic transmission of verocytotoxigenic *Escherichia coli* O157 by dogs. Vet Rec. 2009;164(10):304-305.
29. Harada K, Okada E, Shimuzu T, et al. Antimicrobial resistance, virulence profiles and phylogenetic groups of fecal *Escherichia coli* isolates: a comparative analysis between dogs and their owners in Japan. Comp Immunol Microbiol Infect Dis. 2012;35:139-144.
30. Stenske KA, Bemis DA, Gillespie BE, et al. Comparison of clonal relatedness and antimicrobial susceptibility of *Escherichia coli* from healthy dogs and their owners. Am J Vet Res. 2009;70:1108-1116.
31. Johnson JR, Clabots C, Kuskowski MA. Multiple-host sharing, long-term persistence, and virulence of *Escherichia coli* clones from human and animal household members. J Clin Microbiol. 2008;46:4078-4082.
32. Damborg P, Nielsen SS, Guardabassi L. *Escherichia coli* shedding patterns in humans and dogs: insights into within-household transmission of phylotypes associated with urinary tract infections. Epidemiol Infect. 2012;137:1457-1464.

CHAPTER 47

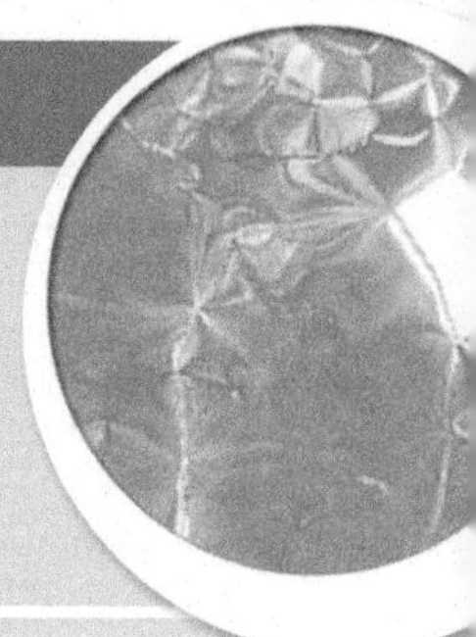

Campylobacteriosis

Jane E. Sykes and Stanley L. Marks

Overview of Campylobacteriosis

First Described: Germany, 1886 (Theodor Escherich)[1]; the organism was not isolated until the 1950s

Cause: *Campylobacter* spp. (curved to spiral gram-negative bacteria that belong to the Campylobactereaceae)

Affected Hosts: Humans and a large variety of other animal species

Geographic Distribution: Worldwide

Primary Mode of Transmission: Fecal-oral

Major Clinical Signs: Fever, lethargy, anorexia, large bowel diarrhea

Differential Diagnoses: Differential diagnoses for suspected *Campylobacter* enterocolitis include canine and feline parvovirus infection, canine distemper virus infection, salmon poisoning disease, *Escherichia coli* infection, clostridial diarrhea, salmonellosis, giardiasis, tritrichomoniasis (cats), cryptosporidiosis, whipworms, leptospirosis, dietary indiscretion, gastrointestinal foreign body, pancreatitis, inflammatory bowel disease, lymphoma, hyperthyroidism (cats), hypoadrenocorticism, toxins (including drugs).

Human Health Significance: Important zoonosis. Dogs and cats may be a source of human infection with *Campylobacter*, some of which may be resistant to antimicrobial drugs.

Etiology and Epidemiology

Campylobacter are thin, gram-negative, curved, S-shaped or spiral rods that are often motile by means of a single polar flagellum at one or both ends (Figure 47-1). They are microaerophilic (i.e., they grow best when levels of oxygen are lower than that present in the atmosphere), and are widespread in the gastrointestinal tracts of animals. *Campylobacter* spp. have the potential to be zoonotic and are an important cause of foodborne illness in humans, especially in association with poultry products. They can survive weeks to months in water. More than a dozen species have been identified in dogs and cats (Box 47-1). All species are commonly isolated from both healthy and diarrheic dogs and cats. The prevalence of shedding by clinically healthy dogs, for example, ranges from 15% to 87%,[2] and as high as 58% of non-diarrheic and diarrheic cats shed *Campylobacter* as determined by PCR assay.[3] *Campylobacter jejuni* is most commonly incriminated as a cause of diarrhea. The evidence for disease causation by other species, such as *Campylobacter upsaliensis* and *Campylobacter helveticus*, is less certain, because the isolation rates of these species are often similar in healthy and diarrheic dogs and cats. In one study, *Campylobacter* species were isolated more commonly from healthy cats than from cats with diarrhea.[3]

C. jejuni, C. helveticus, and *C. upsaliensis* are the species most frequently isolated from the stool of dogs and cats, with *C. helveticus* and *C. upsaliensis* being the predominant isolates in some studies.[3,4] Other commonly identified species in dogs and cats include *Campylobacter coli, C. helveticus,* and *Campylobacter lari*. In one study, up to 12 *Campylobacter* species were present simultaneously in dogs,[5] and coinfection with multiple *Campylobacter* species was detected in 47% of 74 cats from which *Campylobacter* was isolated.[3] The prevalence of *Campylobacter* carriage is particularly high in young dogs and cats and those housed with large numbers of other animals such as in kennels or shelters. Increased isolation rates are also observed in the spring, summer, and fall months, depending on study location.[6,7] Cats less than 1 year of age were significantly more likely to shed *Campylobacter* than cats older than a year of age, and median duration of shedding was around 6 weeks in a study from the upper Midwestern United States.[7] Young age and the feeding of homemade cooked food to dogs was associated with *Campylobacter* carriage in dogs from eastern Canada.[2] Ownership of puppies and kittens is a significant risk factor for development of campylobacteriosis by humans, especially young children.[8,9]

Clinical Features

Signs and Their Pathogenesis

Campylobacter colonize the lower intestinal tract, including the jejunum, ileum, and colon. In contrast to other enteropathogenic bacteria, *Campylobacter* possess relatively few virulence factors, and host factors are important in determining the severity of clinical signs that develop. *Campylobacter* can invade intestinal epithelial cells and produce cytolethal distending toxin, which causes cell cycle arrest and apoptosis, and in humans, stimulates Il-8 production, which leads to an inflammatory response. The organism can produce a polysaccharide capsule, which may also be a virulence factor.[10] Puppies and kittens less than 6 months of age are most likely to show diarrhea in association with *Campylobacter* infection, and stress, overcrowding, and concurrent gastrointestinal infections with other bacteria, protozoa, and helminth parasites may also contribute to clinical signs. The severity of diarrhea can range from mild diarrhea with loose stools through to watery, bloody, or mucoid diarrhea, with lethargy, inappetence, and, less commonly, vomiting. Other signs of large bowel diarrhea such as tenesmus may also be present. Fever may occur in severe acute campylobacteriosis in puppies and kittens. Diarrhea is generally self-limiting within a 1- to 2-week period, although chronic diarrhea can also occur in dogs.[11,12] Rarely, extraintestinal *Campylobacter* infections in dogs have been

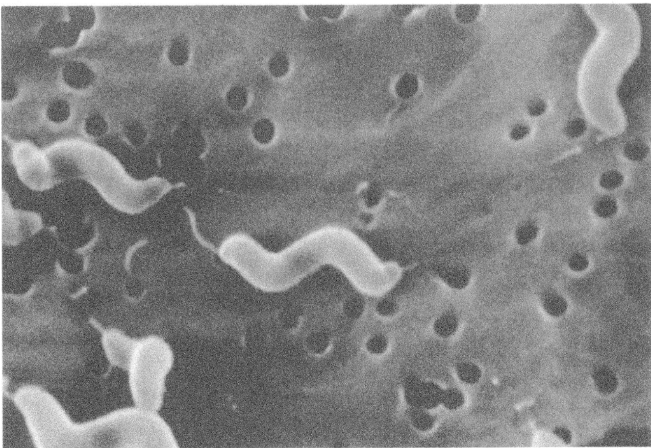

FIGURE 47-1 Scanning electron micrograph of *Campylobacter*. (From Centers for Disease Control and Prevention, Atlanta, GA.)

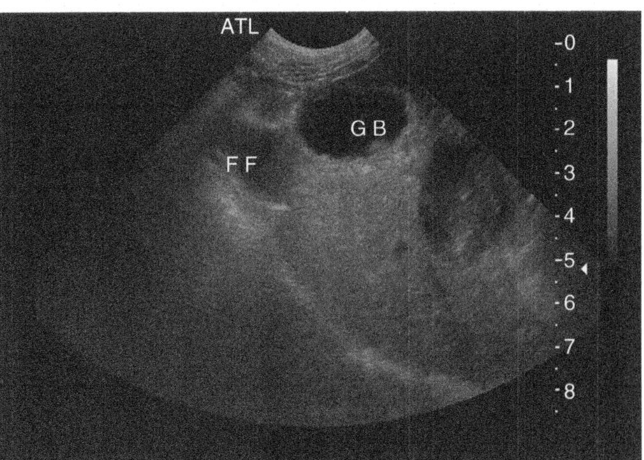

FIGURE 47-2 Abdominal ultrasound image from a 10-year-old intact male Brittany spaniel with *Campylobacter* bacteremia, gastroenteritis, and probable cholecystitis, showing thickening and irregularity of the gallbladder *(GB)* wall and free abdominal fluid *(FF)*.

***Campylobacter* Species Described in Dogs and Cats**

C. jejuni
C. upsaliensis
C. lari
C. coli
C. helveticus
C. concisus
C. fetus
C. gracilis
C. mucosalis
C. showae
C. sputorum
C. curvus
C. hyointestinalis
C. rectus

reported, specifically cholecystitis, bacteremia, and abortion.[13,14] These have also been described in humans.[15,16]

Physical Examination Findings

Physical examination findings in severely affected young animals with campylobacteriosis are variable and include lethargy, dehydration, fever, and abdominal pain. Diarrhea, sometimes with fresh blood or mucus, may be found on rectal examination in dogs.

Diagnosis

Laboratory Abnormalities

Complete Blood Count and Chemistry Panel

Basic laboratory testing in puppies and kittens with *Campylobacter* diarrhea generally reveals mild and nonspecific changes. A leukocytosis may be present. Animals with systemic campylobacteriosis and cholecystitis may show neutrophilia or neutropenia with increased circulating band neutrophils and biochemical evidence of cholestasis and hepatic dysfunction (see Case Example).

Diagnostic Imaging

Findings on plain abdominal radiography and abdominal ultrasound are typically unremarkable or show fluid-filled intestinal loops. A thickened gallbladder wall may be seen using ultrasound in animals with *Campylobacter* cholecystitis (Figure 47-2).

Microbiologic Testing

Microbiologic assays available for diagnosis of campylobacteriosis in dogs and cats include microscopic examination, culture, and PCR assays (Table 47-1). Because of the high prevalence of *Campylobacter* colonization in healthy dogs and cats, it is difficult to interpret the significance of positive test results on feces. The results must always be considered in light of the patient signalment, history, clinical signs, and exclusion of other causes of diarrhea. Specific identification of *C. jejuni*, as opposed to other *Campylobacter* species, may also add support to the role of *Campylobacter* in disease.

Microscopic Examination

Although not diagnostic for campylobacteriosis, a direct fecal smear may reveal large numbers of fine, S-shaped or gull-shaped organisms following staining with Gram or Romanowsky stains (Figure 47-3). Detection of these organisms only suggests the presence of *Campylobacter*-like organisms and should *not* be used as the sole method to diagnose campylobacteriosis because of the inability to differentiate between similar-appearing organisms such as *Arcobacter* or nonpathogenic campylobacters. Fecal leukocytes may also be present. More advanced microscopic techniques that have been used to identify *Campylobacter* in the feces include darkfield and phase-contrast microscopy, which are used on fresh fecal specimens and show the characteristic morphology and darting motility of the organism. These are generally not performed routinely in clinical situations and require significant technical expertise.

Bacterial Isolation

Campylobacter cannot be isolated on routine bacteriological media. Fecal enteric panels designed to detect bacterial enteropathogens in feces generally include isolation on selective media such as charcoal- or blood-based *Campylobacter* media, which often contain antimicrobials to eliminate other bacteria (such as cefoperazone). The inoculated medium is incubated

TABLE 47-1

Diagnostic Assays Available for Campylobacteriosis in Dogs and Cats

Assay	Specimen Type	Target	Performance
Bacterial isolation	Feces, blood, bile, intestinal tissues collected at necropsy	*Campylobacter* organism	False negatives may occur, especially following antimicrobial therapy, and some species may not grow under routine conditions used to isolate *Campylobacter*. Isolation from feces does not imply that *Campylobacter* is the cause of disease. Allows subsequent antimicrobial susceptibility testing.
Polymerase chain reaction	As for isolation	*Campylobacter* DNA	Rapid (within hours); can be highly sensitive and specific. Positive results from feces do not imply that *Campylobacter* is the cause of disease. Some assays do not differentiate between *Campylobacter* species, but others are species specific (e.g., only *Campylobacter jejuni* or only *Campylobacter coli*). Check with the laboratory to determine what assays are offered.

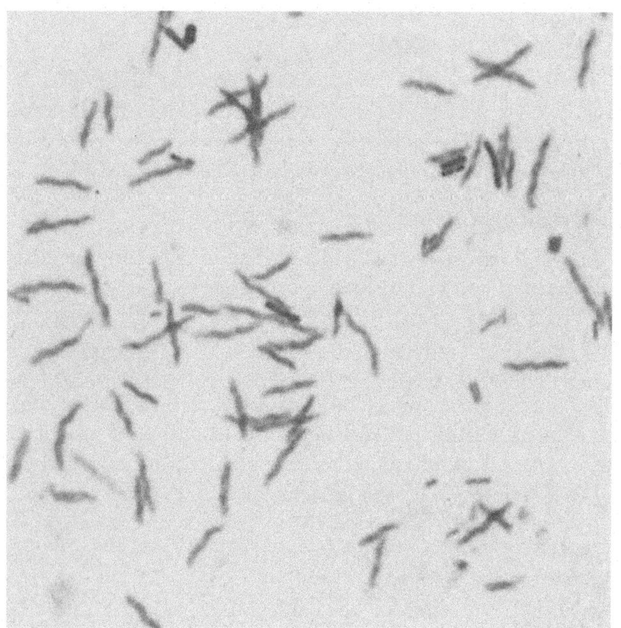

FIGURE 47-3 Cytology showing *Campylobacter* organisms. Gram stain, 1000× magnification.

in a microaerophilic environment for 72 to 96 hours. Incubation is frequently carried out at 42°C to select for thermophilic *Campylobacter*; however, a temperature of 37°C should also be used to ensure isolation of variable or nonthermophilic species. The use of direct plating onto charcoal-based media may be most sensitive for isolation of *Campylobacter* from pets, but use of a combination of isolation methods increases sensitivity further.[17] Some strains require more hydrogen than others and do not grow under routine conditions used for *Campylobacter* isolation. Species identification can then be performed on the basis of biochemical testing or the use of PCR followed by sequencing of the PCR product. Biochemical testing can be highly variable, resulting in inaccurate identification. Serotyping has been traditionally used to identify strains of *C. jejuni* for epidemiologic studies, and more recently, molecular methods such as pulsed-field gel electrophoresis and PCR-based typing methods (including multilocus sequence typing), have been used.[18-20] Techniques based on matrix-assisted laser desorption/ionization-time-of-flight (MALDI-TOF) mass spectrometry also show promise for rapid identification of *Campylobacter* species and strains (see Chapter 3).[21,22] Isolation of *Campylobacter* in culture permits subsequent antimicrobial susceptibility testing, although this is not routinely performed by most veterinary laboratories.

Molecular Diagnosis Using the Polymerase Chain Reaction

Both conventional and real-time PCR-based assays have been developed for direct detection of *Campylobacter* in stool, and some are available commercially for use in dogs and cats. An advantage of PCR is that it can detect species that grow poorly in culture, and it overcomes problems relating to overgrowth of other fecal bacteria.[3] Both *Campylobacter* genus-specific and species-specific assays (such as those that only detect *C. jejuni*) have been developed. In human patients, a real-time PCR assay for detection of *C. jejuni* was at least as sensitive as culture.[23]

Pathologic Findings

Gross Pathologic Findings

Gross necropsy findings in puppies with campylobacteriosis include fluid-filled intestinal loops with mucosal congestion and edema, especially within the distal jejunum, ileum, cecum, and colon.[12,24] Mesenteric lymphadenomegaly may also be present.

Histopathologic findings

Campylobacter infection can result in villous blunting and fusion, epithelial hyperplasia, and congestion and lymphoplasmacytic inflammation of the lamina propria. Crypts contain filamentous bacteria that stain with silver stains such as Warthin-Starry (Figure 47-4). Immunohistochemistry can be used to identify *Campylobacter* within intestinal crypts.[12]

Treatment and Prognosis

Uncomplicated campylobacteriosis is generally self-limiting and resolves with supportive therapy. Because isolation of *Campylobacter* even from diarrheic feces does not necessarily imply causation for the clinical signs, specific treatment may not be warranted and may further disrupt the intestinal microflora. Treatment could be considered for severely ill dogs and cats. Macrolides (such as erythromycin or azithromycin) and fluoroquinolones (such as enrofloxacin, 5 mg/kg q24h for 5 to 7 days) are often efficacious, although resistance to these antimicrobials has been documented in some *Campylobacter* isolates.[25,26] Treatment failures could reflect resistance to the antimicrobial used or infection with a nonpathogenic *Campylobacter* species and persistence of clinical signs from another unidentified cause. Recrudescence of infection has been documented in human patients after treatment.[27]

Immunity and Vaccination

Innate, humoral, and cell-mediated immune responses are critical for clearance of *Campylobacter* infection.[28] Short-term protection that is somewhat serotype specific can result from frequent exposure to *Campylobacter*, but immunity wanes with time, and reinfection is possible. Considerable effort has been expended into development of vaccines for humans and poultry.[29-31] No vaccine currently exists for prevention of *Campylobacter* infection in dogs and cats.

Public Health Aspects

Campylobacter is the most common bacterial cause of enteric illness in humans worldwide. Over 90% of human campylobacteriosis in industrialized countries results from consumption of contaminated chicken products, as well as beef and milk. Drinking water and swimming water may also be a source of infection. To a lesser extent, contact with other food animal species, wild birds, and pet dogs and cats has been associated with human campylobacteriosis.[32] Ingestion of as few as 500 organisms can lead to infection. When clinical signs occur, early signs develop after an incubation period of 1 to 7 days and include fever, myalgia, vomiting, and headache, which generally last 1 to 3 days, followed by up to one week of watery to bloody diarrhea and abdominal pain. Illness may be mild to severe, requiring hospitalization. Severe illness is more likely to occur in the immunosuppressed. Reactive arthritis and Guillain-Barré syndrome, an acute inflammatory demyelinating polyneuropathy, are late-onset immune-mediated consequences that can sometimes occur in association with infection and may persist for weeks or years.[32] In fact, *C. jejuni* is the most common infection that precedes Guillain-Barré syndrome, which occurs in 1 in 1000 infected individuals.[25] Extraintestinal infections that have been described include bacteremia, hepatitis, cholecystitis, pancreatitis, peritonitis, abortion and neonatal sepsis, urinary tract infections, myocarditis, and meningitis, although these are very rare in immunocompetent individuals. *Campylobacter* enteritis has also been identified as a risk factor for inflammatory bowel disease.[33]

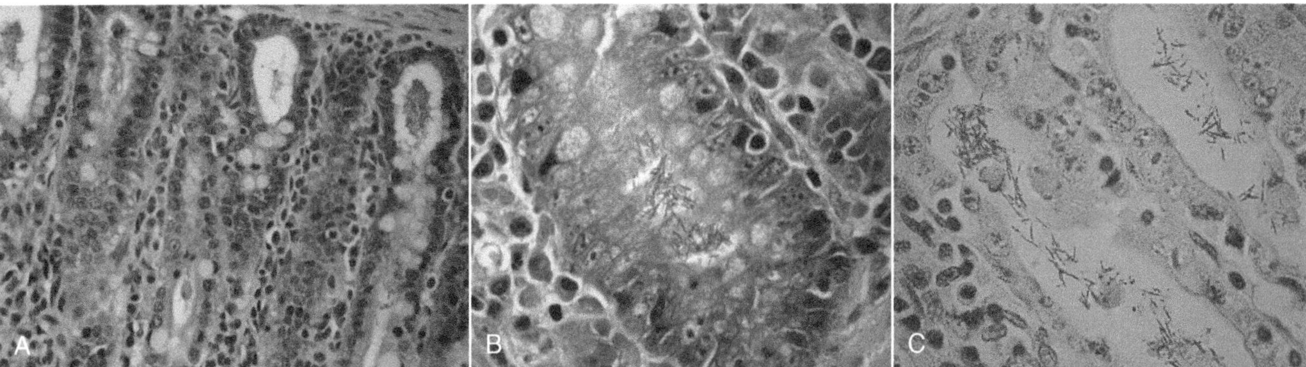

FIGURE 47-4 Histopathology of an intestinal section from a 3-month-old Chihuahua puppy with *Campylobacter jejuni*–associated diarrhea. Abundant filamentous, spiral bacteria pack the crypts and there is an associated lymphoplasmacytic enterocolitis. **A,** H&E stain; **B,** Giemsa stain; **C,** Warthin-Starry silver stain.

CASE EXAMPLE

Signalment: "Henry," a 10-year-old intact male Brittany spaniel from Dixon in northern California

History: Henry was brought to an emergency clinic for a 1-day history of anorexia, lethargy, and fever. The owner, a retired veterinarian, noted that Henry's rectal temperature was 106°F (41.1°C). There had been no vomiting or diarrhea, and the dog had been drinking normally. Henry was a field trial dog and was hunting a week before becoming ill. He was housed in an outdoor run with no access to foreign objects other than gravel. There were nine other apparently healthy dogs in the household. The dogs were fed a commercial dry and canned diet.

Physical Examination:

Body Weight: 17.8 kg

General: Quiet, alert and responsive, 5% to 7% dehydrated. Ambulatory. T = 106.4°F (41.3°C), HR = 140 beats/min, RR = 40 breaths/min, mucous membranes pale pink and tacky, CRT = 2 s.

Integument, Eyes, Ears, Nose, and Throat: A large amount of dental calculus was noted. There was moderate waxy debris in both ear canals and pinnal erythema.

Musculoskeletal: Body condition score was 4/9, and the dog was ambulatory with symmetrical muscling.

Cardiovascular: The femoral pulses were fair and synchronous. No murmurs or arrhythmias were auscultated.

Respiratory: Harsh breath sounds were bilaterally noted on thoracic auscultation, which were loudest in the ventral lung fields.

Gastrointestinal and Genitourinary: The abdomen was tense on palpation and moderate hepatomegaly was noted. The urinary bladder was large. No abnormalities were detected on rectal examination.

Lymph Nodes: All were within normal limits.

Laboratory Findings:

CBC:

HCT 42.9% (40%-55%)
MCV 70 fL (65-75 fL)
MCHC 34.5 g/dL (33-36 g/dL)

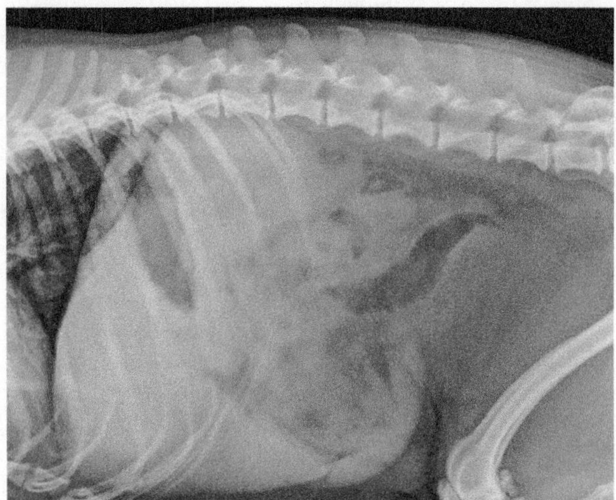

FIGURE 47-5 Abdominal radiograph from a 10-year-old intact male Brittany spaniel with *Campylobacter* bacteremia, gastroenteritis, and probable cholecystitis that shows hepatomegaly and corrugation of the colonic wall.

2 nucleated red blood cells/100 WBC
WBC 6600 cells/μL (6,000-13,000 cells/μL)
Neutrophils 2904 cells/μL (3000-10,500 cells/μL)
Band neutrophils 2838 cells/μL
Metamyelocytes 330 cells/μL
Lymphocytes 330 cells/μL (1000-4000 cells/μL)
Monocytes 198 cells/μL (150-1200 cells/μL)
Eosinophils 0 cells/μL (0-1500 cells/μL)
Platelets 144,000/μL (150,000-400,000 platelets/μL).
Neutrophils, band neutrophils, and metamyelocytes showed mild toxic changes.

Serum Chemistry Profile:
Sodium 146 mmol/L (145-154 mmol/L)
Potassium 4.1 mmol/L (3.6-5.3 mmol/L)
Chloride 116 mmol/L (108-118 mmol/L)
Bicarbonate 15 mmol/L (16-26 mmol/L)
Phosphorus 3.9 mg/dL (3.0-6.2 mg/dL)
Calcium 8.6 mg/dL (9.7-11.5 mg/dl)
BUN 21 mg/dL (5-21 mg/dL)
Creatinine 0.8 mg/dL (0.3-1.2 mg/dL)
Glucose 86 mg/dL (64-123 mg/dL)
Total protein 5.0 g/dL (5.4-7.6 g/dL)
Albumin 2.7 g/dL (3.0-4.4 g/dL)
Globulin 2.3 g/dL (1.8-3.9 g/dL)
ALT 794 U/L (19-67 U/L)
AST 275 U/L (19-42 U/L)
ALP 461 U/L (21-170 U/L)
GGT 37 U/L (0-6 U/L)
Cholesterol 273 mg/dL (135-361 mg/dL)
Total bilirubin 0.7 mg/dL (0-0.2 mg/dL).

Urinalysis: SGr 1.013 (after fluid bolus), pH 7.5, 2+ protein (SSA), 1+ bilirubin, 1+ hemoprotein, no glucose, rare WBC/HPF, rare RBC/HPF, rare granular casts.

Imaging Findings:

Thoracic and Abdominal Radiographs: The cardiovascular and pulmonary structures were within normal limits. The liver was moderately enlarged. The colon was mildly gas distended and had a corrugated appearance (Figure 47-5).

Abdominal Ultrasound: There was moderate enlargement of the liver and spleen. The gallbladder wall was thickened and mildly irregular. There was moderate peritoneal effusion. The stomach and duodenal wall were mildly thickened. Moderate mesenteric lymphadenopathy was identified, particularly around the liver and ileocolic junction. The prostate was enlarged with multiple small parenchymal cysts, but was symmetric and smoothly margined. A sample of orange, somewhat turbid abdominal fluid and an aspirate of a mesenteric lymph node were obtained using ultrasound guidance.

Cytology Findings: Abdominal fluid: Modified transudate. TP = 4.8 g/dL, 20,000 RBC/μL, 460 nucleated cells/μL, with 72% neutrophils, 21% small mononuclear cells, and 7% large mononuclear cells. The nucleated cells were primarily nondegenerate neutrophils with smaller numbers of lymphocytes and macrophages. The lymphocytes were a heterogenous population of small mature lymphocytes and scattered granular lymphocytes. Several pyknotic cells and rare erythrophagocytic macrophages were present. No infectious organisms were seen.

Mesenteric lymph node: Mild lymphoid reactivity.

Microbiologic Testing: Vector-borne disease serologic testing (IFA): Positive for serum *Babesia canis* antibodies (1:160), negative for antibodies to *Rickettsia rickettsii, Anaplasma phagocytophilum,* and *Ehrlichia canis*.

Aerobic and anaerobic bacterial culture of abdominal fluid: No growth.

Aerobic bacterial urine culture (cystocentesis specimen): No growth.

Aerobic and anaerobic blood culture (four specimens collected over 5 hours, the first inoculated into a blood culture bottle and the remainder into isolator tubes): Direct smear of blood culture bottle contents showed rare small curved gram-negative rods. Anaerobic culture of first specimen showed small curved gram-negative rods suspicious for *Campylobacter* spp. Partial sequencing of the 16S rRNA gene revealed 100% identity to *Campylobacter jejuni*. All other specimens yielded no growth.

Fecal enteric panel: *Clostridium difficile* TcdA and TcdB toxin ELISA negative. ELISA negative for *Clostridium perfringens* enterotoxin. No *Salmonella* spp. cultured. No *Clostridium difficile* cultured. Small numbers of *Campylobacter* spp. cultured (*C. jejuni* using partial 16S rRNA gene sequencing).

Diagnosis: *Campylobacter jejuni* bacteremia and probable cholangiohepatitis/cholecystitis

Treatment and Outcome: Henry was hospitalized and treated aggressively with intravenous fluids, and before culture results became available, enrofloxacin (5 mg/kg IV q12h) and ampicillin (22 mg/kg IV q8h). Shortly after admission he vomited and developed mucus-containing diarrhea, and subsequently melena was observed. Over the next 48 hours his temperature gradually normalized, but he continued to vomit intermittently. Neutropenia persisted, and his platelet count dropped to 105,000. He also became icteric, and there were progressive increases in the activities of liver enzymes (ALT 1179 U/L, AST 946 U/L, ALP 1088 U/L, GGT 15 U/L, total bilirubin 3.9 g/dL). By day 4 after presentation, vomiting and diarrhea ceased and he began eating a bland diet. Laboratory testing showed resolution of neutropenia and thrombocytopenia. He was discharged from the hospital and treated with enrofloxacin (10 mg/kg PO q24h) for 4 weeks. One week after discharge, Henry was doing well and had a normal appetite and activity level. The owner reported that another dog in the household subsequently developed vomiting and diarrhea, and *Campylobacter* spp. were cultured from the dog's feces.

Comments: This was an unusual case of *C. jejuni* bacteremia and probable cholangiohepatitis/cholecystitis in a dog that required blood culture for definitive diagnosis. Culture of bile was not performed, but might also have been helpful. Had *C. jejuni* only been isolated from the dog's feces, its clinical significance would have been less apparent. Whether or not the other dog in the household truly had campylobacteriosis is unknown.

SUGGESTED READINGS

Butzler JP. *Campylobacter*, from obscurity to celebrity. Clin Microbiol Infect. 2004;10(10):868-876.

Chaban B, Ngeleka M, Hill JE. Detection and quantification of 14 *Campylobacter* species in pet dogs reveals an increase in species richness in feces of diarrheic animals. BMC Microbiol. 2010;10:73.

Dasti JI, Tareen AM, Lugert R, et al. *Campylobacter jejuni*: a brief overview on pathogenicity-associated factors and disease-mediating mechanisms. Int J Med Microbiol. 2010;300(4):205-211.

REFERENCES

1. Escherich T. Über das Vorkommen von Vibrionen im Darmkanal und den Stuhlgängen der Säuglinge. Münch Med Wochenschr. 1886;33:815-817, 833-835.
2. Leonard EK, Pearl DL, Janecko N, et al. Factors related to *Campylobacter* spp. carriage in client-owned dogs visiting veterinary clinics in a region of Ontario, Canada. Epidemiol Infect. 2011;139:1531-1541.
3. Queen EV, Marks SL, Farver TB. Prevalence of selected bacterial and parasitic agents in feces from diarrheic and healthy control cats from northern California. J Vet Intern Med. 2012;26(1):54-60.
4. Parsons BN, Porter CJ, Ryvar R, et al. Prevalence of *Campylobacter* spp. in a cross-sectional study of dogs attending veterinary practices in the UK and risk indicators associated with shedding. Vet J. 2010;184(1):66-70.
5. Chaban B, Ngeleka M, Hill JE. Detection and quantification of 14 *Campylobacter* species in pet dogs reveals an increase in species richness in feces of diarrheic animals. BMC Microbiol. 2010;10:73.
6. Sandberg M, Bergsjo B, Hofshagen M, et al. Risk factors for *Campylobacter* infection in Norwegian cats and dogs. Prev Vet Med. 2002;55:241-253.
7. Bender JB, Shulman SA, Averbeck GA, et al. Epidemiologic features of *Campylobacter* infection among cats from the western United States. J Am Vet Med Assoc. 2005;226(4):544-547.
8. Wolfs TF, Dulm B, Geelen SP, et al. Neonatal sepsis by *Campylobacter jejuni*: genetically proven transmission from a household puppy. Clin Infect Dis. 2001;32(5):E97-E99.
9. Deming MS, Tauxe RV, Blake PA, et al. *Campylobacter* enteritis at a university: transmission from eating chicken and from cats. Am J Epidemiol. 1987;126(3):526-534.
10. Guerry P, Poly F, Riddle M, et al. *Campyobacter* polysaccharide capsules: virulence and vaccines. Front Cell Infect Microbiol. 2012;2:7.
11. Davies AP, Gebhart CJ, Meric SA. *Campylobacter*-associated chronic diarrhea in a dog. J Am Vet Med Assoc. 1984;184(4):469-471.
12. Brown C, Martin V, Chitwood S. An outbreak of enterocolitis due to *Campylobacter* spp. in a beagle colony. J Vet Diagn Invest. 1999;11(4):374-376.
13. Odendaal MW, de Cramer KG, van der Walt ML, et al. First isolation of *Campylobacter jejuni* from the vaginal discharge of three bitches after abortion in South Africa. Onderstepoort J Vet Res. 1994;61(2):193-195.
14. Bulgin MS, Ward AC, Sriranganathan N, et al. Abortion in the dog due to *Campylobacter* species. Am J Vet Res. 1984;45(3):555-556.
15. Smith JL. *Campylobacter jejuni* infection during pregnancy: long-term consequences of associated bacteremia, Guillain-Barré syndrome, and reactive arthritis. J Food Prot. 2002;65(4):696-708.
16. Udayakumar D, Sanaullah M. *Campylobacter* cholecystitis. Int J Med Sci. 2009;6(6):374-375.
17. Acke E, McGill K, Golden O, et al. A comparison of different culture methods for the recovery of *Campylobacter* species from pets. Zoonoses Public Health. 2009;56(9-10):490-495.
18. Parsons BN, Cody AJ, Porter CJ, et al. Typing of *Campylobacter jejuni* isolates from dogs by use of multilocus sequence typing and pulsed-field gel electrophoresis. J Clin Microbiol. 2009;47(11):3466-3471.
19. Cornelius AJ, Gilpin B, Carter P, et al. Comparison of PCR binary typing (P-BIT), a new approach to epidemiological subtyping of *Campylobacter jejuni*, with serotyping, pulsed-field gel electrophoresis, and multilocus sequence typing methods. Appl Environ Microbiol. 2010;76(5):1533-1544.
20. Parsons BN, Porter CJ, Stavisky JH, et al. Multilocus sequence typing of human and canine *Campylobacter upsaliensis* isolates. Vet Microbiol. 2012;157:391-397.
21. Kiehntopf M, Melcher F, Hänel I, et al. Differentiation of *Campylobacter* species by surface-enhanced laser desorption/ionization-time-of-flight mass spectrometry. Foodborne Pathog Dis. 2011;8:875-885.
22. Bessède E, Solecki O, Sifré E, et al. Identification of *Campylobacter* species and related organisms by matrix-assisted laser desorption/ionization-time-of-flight (MALDI-TOF) mass spectrometry. Clin Microbiol Infect. 2011;17:1735-1739.
23. Lin S, Wang X, Zheng H, et al. Direct detection of *Campylobacter jejuni* in human stool samples by real-time PCR. Can J Microbiol. 2008;54(9):742-747.
24. Fox JG, Maxwell KO, Ackerman JI. *Campylobacter jejuni* associated diarrhea in commercially reared beagles. Lab Anim Sci. 1984;34(2):151-155.
25. Butzler JP. *Campylobacter*, from obscurity to celebrity. Clin Microbiol Infect. 2004;10(10):868-876.
26. Lindow JC, Poly F, Tribble DR, et al. Caught in the act: in vivo development of macrolide resistance to *Campylobacter jejuni* infection. J Clin Microbiol. 2010;48(8):3012-3015.
27. Baqar S, Tribble DR, Carmolli M, et al. Recrudescent *Campylobacter jejuni* infection in an immunocompetent adult following experimental infection with a well-characterized organism. Clin Vaccine Immunol. 2010;17(1):80-86.
28. Janssen R, Krogfelt KA, Cawthraw SA, et al. Host-pathogen interactions in *Campylobacter* infections: the host perspective. Clin Microbiol Rev. 2008;21(3):505-518.
29. Jagusztyn-Krynicka EK, Łaniewski P, Wyszyńska A. Update on *Campylobacter jejuni* vaccine development for preventing human campylobacteriosis. Expert Rev Vaccines. 2009;8(5):625-645.
30. Tribble DR, Baqar S, Carmolli MP, et al. *Campylobacter jejuni* strain CG8421: a refined model for the study of campylobacteriosis and evaluation of *Campylobacter* vaccines in human subjects. Clin Infect Dis. 2009;49(10):1512-1519.
31. Buckley AM, Wang J, Hudson DL, et al. Evaluation of live-attenuated *Salmonella* vaccines expressing *Campylobacter* antigens for control of *C. jejuni* in poultry. Vaccine. 2010;28(4):1094-1105.
32. Dasti JI, Tareen AM, Lugert R, et al. *Campylobacter jejuni*: a brief overview on pathogenicity-associated factors and disease-mediating mechanisms. Int J Med Microbiol. 2010;300(4):205-211.
33. Kalischuk LD, Buret AG. A role for *Campylobacter jejuni*–induced enteritis in inflammatory bowel disease? Am J Physiol Gastrointest Liver Physiol. 2010;298(1):G1-G9.

CHAPTER 48

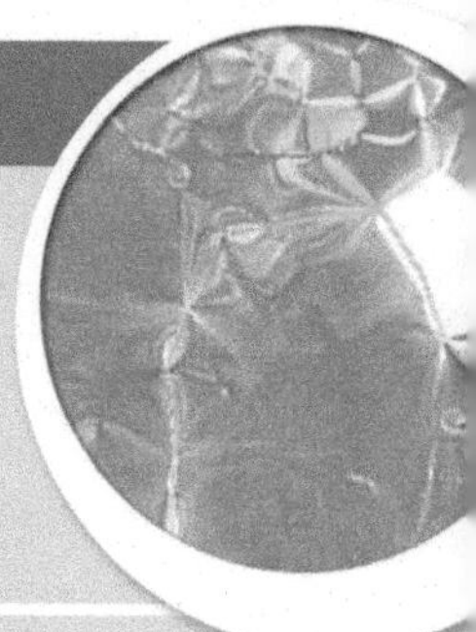

Enteric Clostridial Infections

Jane E. Sykes and Stanley L. Marks

Overview of Clostridial Diarrhea

First Described: 1978 (*C. difficile*, causative role in pseudomembranous colitis in humans)[1]; 1892 (*C. perfringens*, by Nuttall and Welch).[2] Evidence for a role of *C. perfringens* in food-borne illness was gathered over 50 years later.[3]

Cause: *Clostridium difficile* and *Clostridium perfringens* (gram-positive, spore-forming anaerobic rods)

Affected Hosts: Humans and a variety of other animals

Geographic Distribution: Worldwide

Primary Mode of Transmission: Fecal-oral; disease can result from toxin production by organisms resident in the gastrointestinal tract

Major Clinical Signs: Lethargy, anorexia, diarrhea, occasionally fever

Differential Diagnoses: Differential diagnosis for suspected clostridial enterocolitis include canine and feline parvovirus infection, canine distemper virus infection, salmon poisoning disease, campylobacteriosis, salmonellosis, giardiasis, tritrichomoniasis (cats), cryptosporidiosis, whipworms, leptospirosis, dietary indiscretion, gastrointestinal foreign body, pancreatitis, inflammatory bowel disease, lymphoma, hypoadrenocorticism, toxins (including drugs)

Human Health Significance: Dogs and cats have the potential to be a source of human infection with *C. difficile*, because they can harbor strains (ribotypes) that have been detected in humans. The role of dogs and cats as a source of *C. perfringens* infection is poorly understood.

Etiology and Epidemiology

Clostridium difficile and *Clostridium perfringens* are gram-positive, spore-forming, obligately anaerobic rods that are capable of toxin production. Clostridial spores are spherical to oval and distend the bacterial cells when they form within them (Figure 48-1). *Clostridium* species are found in soil and the intestinal tracts of a variety of different animal species, including those of healthy dogs and cats. Their spores are very resistant to disinfection and can persist in the environment, including within hospitals, for years. Despite their similarities, many differences exist between *C. difficile* and *C. perfringens* that relate to epidemiology, interpretation of diagnostic test results, and treatment.

C. difficile is the most common cause of hospital and antimicrobial-associated diarrhea in humans and has also been associated with nosocomial diarrhea in dogs and cats in veterinary hospitals.[4,5] In one study, living with an immunocompromised human was a risk factor for *C. difficile* infection in dogs, but strains present in dogs differed from those in the household environment.[6] Dogs that visit human health care facilities are also at risk of acquiring *C. difficile* infections.[7] The emergence of "hypervirulent" *C. difficile* strains in people has resulted in an increased incidence of disease, increased mortality rates, increased relapse rates, and recognition of community-associated disease.[8] A similar change has not been observed in animals; however, a hypervirulent strain (North American pulsotype 1 or NAP1) was identified in a dog.[9] *C. difficile* strains have been classified on the basis of PCR-based typing of their ribosomal RNA genes (PCR-ribotyping). In one study, multiple animals in shelter environments were colonized with a single PCR-ribotype (SLO 066, 045, and 010 in three different shelters, respectively).[10] More detailed genetic analysis of the *C. difficile* strains isolated by multilocus variable number of tandem repeat analysis (MLVA) suggested that horizontal transmission of strains 045 and 010 occurred within the shelter.

C. perfringens is especially widespread in soil and dust and consists of five biotypes, A to E, based on the possession of one or more of four major toxin genes (encoding alpha, beta, epsilon, and iota toxins). Each biotype can also express a subset of at least 10 other established toxins, including *C. perfringens* enterotoxin (CPE). Almost all infections in dogs and cats are *C. perfringens* biotype A, which also causes the majority of clostridial food-borne illness in humans. The zoonotic potential of *C. difficile* and *C. perfringens* is still incompletely understood.

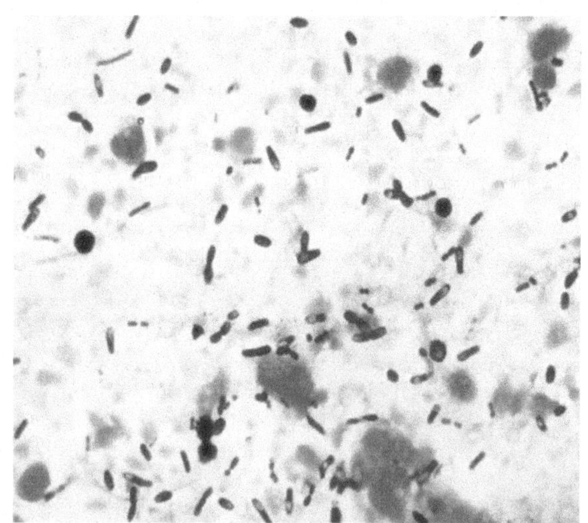

FIGURE 48-1 Fecal smear from a dog with diarrhea showing spore-distended clostridial rods, leading to a characteristic "safety pin" and "tennis racquet" appearance.

The importance of *C. perfringens* and *C. difficile* as causes of diarrhea in dogs and cats has been controversial, because they can be isolated from both diarrheic and healthy animals. For example, *C. perfringens* can be isolated using culture from the feces of more than 70% of both diarrheic and nondiarrheic dogs.[11,12] The prevalence of *C. perfringens* colonization of healthy cats appears to be lower than that in dogs, with isolation rates of 43% to 63%.[13] Similarly, toxin production can be detected in both healthy and diarrheic dogs and cats, although most studies have shown a correlation between production of certain clostridial toxins and diarrhea.[11]

Clinical Features

Signs and Their Pathogenesis

Both *C. difficile* and *C. perfringens* cause diarrhea by producing toxins. The diarrhea can be mild and self-limiting or severe, acute, and hemorrhagic, with life-threatening consequences that relate to dehydration and hypovolemic shock. Inappetence, vomiting, fever, and abdominal pain have also been described in cats with *C. difficile*-associated diarrhea.[14] Vomiting can also occur in dogs. Although clostridial diarrhea is often described as a large bowel–type diarrhea, clinical manifestations of both small and large bowel diarrhea have been well documented.

C. difficile can produce up to five toxins, the most well studied being toxin A (TcdA), toxin B (TcdB), and *C. difficile* binary toxin (CDT, an ADP-ribosyltransferase that is made up of two components). CDT-positive strains have not been reported in dogs and cats. In contrast to humans, a history of antibiotic use does not always seem to be necessary for colonization and disease in dogs and cats, although in one study administration of antimicrobials before admission and the use of immunosuppressive drugs during hospitalization were risk factors for nosocomial colonization.[4] Toxins A and B are thought to be most important in the pathogenesis of diarrhea.[15] These are large toxins that inactivate the Rho family of GTPases, which regulate intracellular actin dynamics. The result is a disruption of the cell cytoskeleton, with subsequent rounding and death of intestinal epithelial cells, and loss of tight junctions. The two toxins also cause release of inflammatory cytokines from mast cells, macrophages, and epithelial cells.[15]

In dogs, *C. perfringens* infection has been associated with nosocomial diarrhea,[16] hemorrhagic enteritis,[17-19] and acute and chronic large bowel diarrhea. *C. perfringens* diarrhea in dogs and cats is thought to occur subsequent to massive proliferation and sporulation of resident clostridial organisms in the intestinal lumen following an alteration in local intestinal conditions. Decreased peristalsis, the effects of antimicrobial drugs on the resident intestinal microflora, diet changes, and/or co-infections with other intestinal pathogens has the potential to trigger sporulation. *C. perfringens* produces CPE on sporulation, but other toxins and bacterial virulence factors may also be involved in the pathogenesis of diarrhea, because diarrhea can occur in the absence of CPE production. CPE is a pore-forming protein toxin that is released when vegetative clostridial cells lyse and release their spores. It binds primarily to claudin, a component of epithelial tight junctions, which leads to increased paracellular permeability.[20] The role of CPE in the development of diarrhea in dogs and cats is unclear, because CPE is detected in 34% of diarrheic dogs, and in 5% to 14% of nondiarrheic dogs.[11,12] There may be an association between the detection of CPE in dogs with acute hemorrhagic diarrheal syndrome (AHDS), as CPE was detected in 8 of 12 dogs (67%) with AHDS.[18]

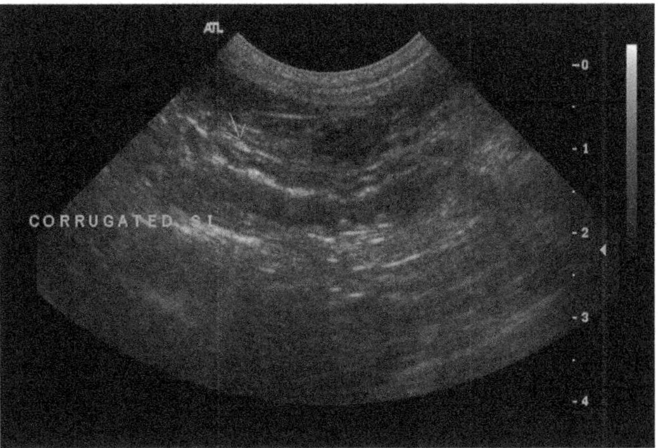

FIGURE 48-2 Abdominal ultrasound image showing thickening and corrugation of the small intestinal wall of a 2-year-old intact male chihuahua with *Clostridium perfringens*–associated vomiting, hematemesis, diarrhea, and hematochezia. Large numbers of spore-forming gram-positive rods were seen on a fecal smear. *C. perfringens* enterotoxin was detected in the feces using an ELISA assay.

The prevalence of *C. perfringens*–associated diarrhea in cats is much lower than in dogs, and CPE has been detected at a similar rate in diarrheic and nondiarrheic cats (2% to 4.1%).[13] In another study, CPE was detected with ELISA in 19.6% of 46 diarrheic dogs versus 2.1% of 48 healthy dogs, and in 8.3% of 48 diarrheic cats versus 0% of 39 healthy cats.[21] In a PCR-based study of cats and dogs in an animal shelter in Florida, the *C. perfringens* alpha toxin gene was detected in 64% of 50 diarrheic dogs and 40% of 50 nondiarrheic dogs, which was significantly different.[22] In contrast, it was detected in 42% of 50 diarrheic and 50% of 50 nondiarrheic cats in the same shelter.[23] Thus the role that *C. perfringens* plays in feline diarrhea, if any, remains unclear.

Physical Examination Findings

Physical examination findings in dogs and cats with severe clostridial diarrhea include dehydration, fever, and abdominal pain, with or without signs of hypovolemic shock. Rectal examination may reveal loose or watery stools, sometimes with fresh blood and mucus.

Diagnosis

Laboratory Abnormalities

Complete Blood Count and Chemistry Panel

Basic laboratory testing in dogs and cats with clostridial diarrhea usually reveals mild and nonspecific changes. A neutrophilic leukocytosis with a left shift and toxic changes may be present in dogs and cats with acute clostridial gastroenteritis. In addition, a discordant hematocrit and serum total protein concentration can be identified in some dogs with *C. perfringens* and *C. difficile*-associated diarrhea. The hematocrit can be markedly increased in the face of a normal or low-normal total protein.

Diagnostic Imaging

Findings on plain abdominal radiography and abdominal ultrasound examination in animals with clostridial diarrhea are typically unremarkable or show fluid-filled intestinal loops. Mild thickening and corrugation of the small intestinal or colonic wall may be detected on ultrasound examination (Figure 48-2).

TABLE 48-1

Diagnostic Assays Available for Clostridial Enterocolitis in Dogs and Cats

Assay	Specimen Type	Target	Performance
Bacterial isolation	Feces	*C. perfringens* and *C. difficile*	Isolation from feces does not imply that *Clostridium* is the cause of disease. Allows genotyping and subsequent antimicrobial susceptibility testing if needed. False negatives may occur, especially for *C. difficile*, which requires strict anaerobic conditions.
Common antigen test	Feces	*C. difficile*	Excellent negative predictive value for *C. difficile* (i.e., a negative test result suggests *C. difficile* is not present). A positive test result does not imply that *C. difficile* is the cause of disease.
Toxin immunoassays	Feces	*C. perfringens* enterotoxin (CPE); *C. difficile* toxin A and toxin B	Positive test results may occur in dogs and cats that do not have diarrhea; negative results do not rule out clostridial diarrhea, as other toxins may be involved and CPE is relatively labile.
PCR	Feces	*Clostridium* toxin gene DNA	Rapid (within hours). Positive results from feces do not imply that *Clostridium* is the cause of disease. Toxin gene PCR assays may be useful for diagnosis in conjunction with positive ELISA results for toxin production. Negative results may occur if other toxin genes are important or if inhibitors of PCR are present.

Microbiologic Testing

Diagnostic assays available for clostridial enterocolitis in dogs and cats are shown in Table 48-1. Because organisms and their toxins can be found in healthy and diarrheic animals, the results must be interpreted in light of the history, clinical signs, and diagnostic testing to rule out other causes of disease.

Microscopic Examination

Spore-forming rods may be identified on microscopic examination of fecal smears that have been stained with Wright stains (see Figure 48-1). Rods that contain endospores have the appearance of "tennis racquets" or "safety pins." However, there is no association between fecal endospore counts and the presence of diarrhea, or between endospore counts and the detection of CPE in fecal specimens. Detection of fecal endospores is thus an unreliable test for diagnosis of *C. perfringens* diarrhea in dogs and cats and should not be used as a stand-alone test to make clinical inferences in diarrheic dogs and cats.[11,24]

Bacterial isolation. Both *C. difficile* and *C. perfringens* can be isolated from feces of dogs and cats using strict anaerobic conditions for incubation. *C. perfringens* is more tolerant of oxygen than *C. difficile* and therefore may be easier to isolate (hence the name *difficile*, because of its difficulty to isolate in the laboratory).

C. difficile can be isolated from 0% to 40% of diarrheic and healthy dogs. When fecal culture for *C. difficile* is performed on a viable fecal specimen by a reputable laboratory, a negative result suggests that *C. difficile* is not present. However, a positive culture does not differentiate between toxigenic and nontoxigenic strains, and further testing for toxin is warranted.

Because of the high carriage rate of *C. perfringens* in both healthy and diarrheic dogs (>70% in both groups), routine isolation of *C. perfringens* is not recommended for diagnosis, unless epidemiologic studies that require genetic typing are undertaken in outbreak situations. Quantitative stool spore counts have been used to aid diagnosis of *C. perfringens* diarrhea in humans. The stool is treated with heat or alcohol after which it is cultured anaerobically and colonies are counted. Median spore counts of greater than 10^6 per gram of feces collected within 48 hours after the onset of illness are suggestive of infection.[25] Such counts can still be detected in humans with no signs of illness, and the method, when used without assessment of toxin production, has not proven useful for diagnosis of *C. perfringens* diarrhea in dogs.[12]

ELISA for *C. difficile* Antigen

C. difficile antigen ELISA is easy to perform, rapid, and highly sensitive. The antigen test detects "common antigen" (glutamate dehydrogenase; GDH) that is predominantly present in toxigenic and nontoxigenic *C. difficile* strains and a few uncommon *Clostridium* spp. This test has the same limitations as culture in terms of detection of nontoxigenic strains, although a negative test for GDH can virtually rule out infection with *C. difficile.*

Assays for Toxin Production

Several commercial serologic assays are available for detection of *C. difficile* toxin A and toxin B in feces. Fecal swab specimens generally do not contain a sufficient quantity of stool for these assays. Even when performed on larger volumes of stool, the sensitivities and specificities of these assays vary considerably, and the etiologic predictive values are relatively low for all tests. In other words, a positive result does not prove that a clostridial infection is the cause of a dog or cat's diarrhea. Currently, assays based on ELISA methodology have shown the best correlation in dogs between clostridial toxin detection and the presence of diarrhea in dogs.[11,16,24] Panels should include assays for both *C. difficile* toxin A and toxin B, because TcdA-negative, TcdB-positive strains have been documented in dogs, and production of both toxins is not needed for disease causation.[26] The reference standard in human medicine for *C. difficile* toxin production is a cell culture cytotoxicity assay, which uses Vero cells and neutralizing antibody to inhibit cytopathic effects.[27,28] However, culture followed by molecular detection of toxin genes within the isolated strains (also known as "toxigenic culture") appears to be a more sensitive reference standard.[28] Both of these assays are time consuming and expensive, require specific technical expertise, and are of limited availability. The use of multiple assays in sequence has been advocated for diagnosis of *C. difficile* infection in humans.[29] Specifically, fecal isolation of *C. difficile* or detection of common antigen should be followed with ELISA testing for toxin A and toxin B. Detection of toxin but failure to identify *C. difficile* should be interpreted with caution, considering the relatively high sensitivity of organism or common antigen detection methods compared to toxin ELISA.

Detection of *C. perfringens* enterotoxin in stool is the most widely used diagnostic tool for *C. perfringens* infection in both humans and animals. Two commercially available immunoassays are currently used in veterinary diagnostic laboratories: a reverse passive latex agglutination assay (RPLA) and an ELISA. The assays have not been validated in animals to date. In addition, the RPLA has been associated with false-positive results when compared to several different ELISA methods.

Molecular Diagnosis Using the Polymerase Chain Reaction

Real-time PCR assays are commercially available for detection of *C. perfringens* and *C. difficile* toxin genes in the feces of dogs and cats. It is important to recognize that the presence of clostridial toxin genes within fecal specimens does not prove that clostridia are the cause of an animal's diarrhea, because they do not prove that the organism is actively producing toxin within the intestinal tract of a patient. Conversely, a negative PCR result for clostridial toxin genes does not rule out clostridial diarrhea, as clostridia may be present that possess other virulence factors, and inhibitors of PCR are common in fecal specimens. Real-time PCR assays for *C. difficile* toxin genes have been developed for diagnosis of *C. difficile* diarrhea in humans.[30] Some assays can detect mutations within the toxin gene that correlate with increased toxin production. However, it is still not well understood how well the results of these assays correlate with clinical illness. Similarly, detection of the *cpe* gene has been used to diagnose *C. perfringens* diarrhea in humans.[31] In one study, fecal specimens from diarrheic dogs were more likely to be positive for CPE as detected using ELISA and PCR for the *cpe* gene (28%) when compared with nondiarrheic dogs (4%). Such a combination of testing for the toxin (CPE) via ELISA and the enterotoxin gene (*cpe*) via PCR is likely superior to either test alone.[12] At the time of writing, real-time PCR assays that provide quantitative information on toxin gene copy numbers are available through some veterinary diagnostic laboratories. The degree to which toxin gene copy numbers correlate with clinical signs requires further study.

Treatment and Prognosis

Animals with suspected clostridial enterocolitis that are systemically ill (fever, hemorrhagic gastroenteritis, inflammatory or toxic leukogram) merit appropriate antimicrobial therapy (Table 48-2). There is no documented evidence for a benefit of antimicrobial therapy in dogs with uncomplicated *Clostridium*-associated diarrhea, and most of these animals can be managed supportively to ensure adequate hydration status without antimicrobial therapy. In fact, a prospective, blinded study that randomized dogs with hemorrhagic gastroenteritis that showed no signs of sepsis to two groups, one treated with clavulanic acid–amoxicillin for 7 days and one treated with placebo, showed no difference in mortality rate, dropout rate, duration of hospitalization, or severity of clinical signs, either on any individual day or over the course of disease.[32]

Metronidazole is the drug of choice for treatment of complicated *C. difficile* infections. Oral vancomycin (which is not absorbed from the gastrointestinal tract) is occasionally used in human medicine to treat metronidazole-resistant isolates. The vast majority of *C. perfringens* isolates from dogs are sensitive to metronidazole, ampicillin, amoxicillin, tylosin, and macrolides such as erythromycin.[33] Because of the infrequency of resistance to these drugs, the lack of known breakpoints for veterinary anaerobes, and the lack of relationship between positive stool cultures and disease, antimicrobial susceptibilities are not performed on a routine basis for these organisms when isolated from dogs and cats. Most animals with complicated clostridial enterocolitis can be successfully treated with antimicrobials for 5 to 7 days, and appropriate treatment is generally associated with clinical improvement within 24 to 36 hours.

Immunity and Vaccination

No vaccines are available to prevent clostridial diarrhea in dogs and cats.

Public Health Aspects

C. difficile is increasingly recognized as an important cause of nosocomial diarrhea and pseudomembranous colitis in humans, especially the elderly, which is induced by antimicrobial treatment (especially ampicillin, amoxicillin, clindamycin, cephalosporins, and fluoroquinolones)[34] or disruption of the normal gastrointestinal flora. Humans with *C. difficile* infection develop bloating, and often foul-smelling diarrhea with abdominal pain, usually 5 to 10 days after starting antibiotics.

TABLE 48-2

Antimicrobials That Can Be Used to Treat Complicated Clostridial Diarrhea in Dogs and Cats*

Drug	Dose (mg/kg)	Route	Interval (hours)	Duration (days)
Metronidazole	10	PO	12	5-7
Ampicillin	22	PO	8-12	5-7
Amoxicillin	22	PO	12	5-7
Tylosin	5 to 10	PO	24	5-7
Erythromycin	15	PO	8	5-7

*Antimicrobial treatment of uncomplicated clostridial diarrhea is not recommended.

Other signs include fever, nausea, anorexia, and malaise. Rare and life-threatening complications of pseudomembranous colitis include acute toxic megacolon, an acute dilatation of the colon with signs of obstruction, and colonic perforation. Hypervirulent strains (such as PCR-ribotype 027) that produce CDT, toxin A, and toxin B have been increasingly identified recently that cause a more severe disease, higher relapse rates, and increased mortality.[35] Efforts are underway to develop vaccines for *C. difficile* infections in humans.[36] There is evidence that dogs may shed *C. difficile* strains similar to those that infect humans. Human colonization and disease usually occurs in hospital situations, and community-acquired infection is uncommon, although concerns have been raised regarding the role of meat and companion animal food products in transmission of the organism.[6,37]

C. perfringens infections are associated with sporadic and antimicrobial-associated diarrhea in humans and CPE is one of the most commonly identified causes of food poisoning in the industrialized world.[38] Clinical signs of infection include foul-smelling, frothy diarrhea, cramping and abdominal pain, and occasionally nausea and vomiting, usually 7 to 15 hours after eating suspected food, especially meat products that have been cooked with improper cooling and reheating.[39] Vegetative cells are then ingested, and this can be followed by massive sporulation with toxin production in the intestinal tract. The zoonotic potential of *C. perfringens* isolates from dogs and cats requires further investigation.

CASE EXAMPLE

Signalment: "Bradley", 2-year old male Chihuahua from Grass Valley in northern California

History: Bradley was brought to an emergency clinic for evaluation of a 12-hour history of hematemesis and diarrhea. He initially vomited up dog food, after which he continued to vomit hourly, and the vomiting progressed to hematemesis. He also developed bloody diarrhea. He had been inappetent and not drinking, and the owner felt he was much quieter than usual. He primarily resided indoors and in the owner's backyard, and there was no history of travel or access to toxins. There were two other apparently healthy dogs in the household. He was up to date on vaccinations for canine parvovirus, distemper virus, canine adenovirus, and rabies. His diet consisted of commercial dry dog food, dog bones, and table scraps.

Physical Examination:

Body Weight: 3.4 kg

General: Quiet, alert and responsive, ambulatory, 5% to 7% dehydrated. Recumbent. T = 100.0°F (37.8°C), HR = 100 beats/min, RR = 30 breaths/min, mucous membranes pink and tacky, CRT = 2 s.

Integument: A full coat with a small amount of flea excrement was present. Bloody diarrhea contaminated the hair in the perianal region.

Eyes, Ears, Nose, and Throat: No abnormalities were noted.

Musculoskeletal: Body condition score was 4/9.

Cardiovascular: The femoral pulses were fair and synchronous. No murmurs or arrhythmias were auscultated.

Respiratory: Normal breath sounds were present in all lung fields.

Gastrointestinal and Genitourinary: The dog was nonpainful on abdominal palpation, but defecated red, jelly-like material several times in the room following the examination. He also urinated a large amount of odiferous urine during the examination. No abnormalities were detected on rectal examination apart from the abnormal stool color and consistency.

Lymph Nodes: All lymph nodes were within normal limits on palpation.

Laboratory Findings:

CBC:

HCT 46% (40%-55%)
MCV 68 fL (65-75 fL)
MCHC 36.3 g/dL (33-36 g/dL)
WBC 11,030 cells/μL (6000-13,000 cells/μL)
Neutrophils 7280 cells/μL (3000-10,500 cells/μL)
Band neutrophils 1324 cells/μL
Lymphocytes 1655 cells/μL (1000-4000 cells/μL)
Monocytes 772 cells/μL (150-1200 cells/μL)
Eosinophils 0 cells/μL (0-1500 cells/μL)
Platelets 273,000/μL (150,000-400,000 platelets/μL).
Neutrophils and band neutrophils showed mild to moderate toxic changes.

Serum Chemistry Profile:

Sodium 147 mmol/L (145-154 mmol/L)
Potassium 4.5 mmol/L (3.6-5.3 mmol/L)
Chloride 111 mmol/L (108-118 mmol/L)
Bicarbonate 29 mmol/L (16-26 mmol/L)
Phosphorus 3.9 mg/dL (3.0-6.2 mg/dL)
Calcium 9.6 mg/dL (9.7-11.5 mg/dl)
BUN 15 mg/dL (5-21 mg/dL)
Creatinine 0.4 mg/dL (0.3-1.2 mg/dL)
Glucose 123 mg/dL (64-123 mg/dL)
Total protein 5.1 g/dL (5.4-7.6 g/dL)
Albumin 3.1 g/dL (3.0-4.4 g/dL)
Globulin 2.0 g/dL (1.8-3.9 g/dL)
ALT 68 U/L (19-67 U/L)
AST 31 U/L (19-42 U/L)
ALP 30 U/L (21-170 U/L)
GGT < 3 U/L (0-6 U/L)
Cholesterol 168 mg/dL (135-361 mg/dL)
Total bilirubin 0.1 mg/dL (0-0.2 mg/dL).

Urinalysis: SGr 1.042, pH 6.0, 1+ protein (SSA), 1+ bilirubin, no hemoprotein, no glucose, 1-2 WBC/HPF, 0 RBC/HPF, rare granular casts.

Coagulation Panel: PT 8.9 s (7.5-10.5 s), APTT 18.1 s (9-12 s); fibrinogen 349 mg/dL (90-255 mg/dL).

Imaging Findings: Abdominal ultrasound: Mild mesenteric and sublumbar lymphadenopathy was identified. The small intestines had mild wall thickening and a corrugated appearance (see Figure 48-2). The colon was fluid filled.

Fecal Examination: Fecal flotation: Negative for parasites.
Fecal sedimentation: Negative for parasites.

Microbiologic Testing: Parvovirus fecal antigen ELISA: Negative.
Fecal direct smear: Large numbers of gram positive rods were present, some with spores.
Fecal enteric panel: *Clostridium difficile* toxin A and toxin B antigen ELISA negative. ELISA positive for *Clostridium perfringens* enterotoxin. No *Salmonella* spp. cultured. No *Clostridium difficile* cultured. No *Campylobacter* spp. cultured.

Diagnosis: Suspected *C. perfringens*–associated gastroenteritis.

Treatment: Bradley was initially hospitalized and treated with intravenous fluids, nothing by mouth, and metronidazole (7.5 mg/kg IV q12h). Vomiting did not continue, but red gelatinous diarrhea continued every hour for the next 12 hours. Within 24 hours, he had become bright and alert and was offered a bland diet, which he ate well. He was discharged and treated with metronidazole for an additional 5 days, with gradual reintroduction of his regular food.

Comments: Infection by *C. perfringens* was strongly suspected in this case based on the combination of consistent clinical signs, negative assay results for other pathogens, a positive toxin ELISA assay, and response to treatment with metronidazole. However, because the feces of healthy dogs can contain *C. perfringens* enterotoxin, a definitive diagnosis of *C. perfringens* enterocolitis could not be made.

SUGGESTED READINGS

Marks SL, Kather EJ, Kass PH, et al. Genotypic and phenotypic characterization of *Clostridium perfringens* and *Clostridium difficile* in diarrheic and healthy dogs. J Vet Intern Med. 2002;16(5):533-540.

Weese JS, Armstrong J. Outbreak of *Clostridium difficile*–associated disease in a small animal veterinary teaching hospital. J Vet Intern Med. 2003;17(6):813-816.

Weese JS, Staempfli HR, Prescott JF, et al. The roles of *Clostridium difficile* and enterotoxigenic *Clostridium perfringens* in diarrhea in dogs. J Vet Intern Med. 2001;15(4):374-378.

REFERENCES

1. George RH, Symonds JM, Dimock F. Identification of C. *difficile* as a cause of pseudomembranous colitis. Br Med J. 1978;i:695.
2. Welch WH, Nuttall GHF. A gas-producing bacillus (*Bacillus aerogenes capsulatus*, nov. spec.) capable of rapid development in blood vessels after death. Bull Johns Hopkins Hosp. 1892;3:81-91.
3. Hobbs BC, Smith ME, Oakley CL, et al. *Clostridium welchii* food poisoning. J Hyg. 1953;51(1):75-101.
4. Weese JS, Armstrong J. Outbreak of *Clostridium difficile*–-associated disease in a small animal veterinary teaching hospital. J Vet Intern Med. 2003;17(6):813-816.
5. Clooten J, Kruth S, Arroyo L, et al. Prevalence and risk factors for *Clostridium difficile* colonization in dogs and cats hospitalized in an intensive care unit. Vet Microbiol. 2008;129(1-2):209-214.
6. Weese JS, Finley R, Reid-Smith RJ, et al. Evaluation of *Clostridium difficile* in dogs and the household environment. Epidemiol Infect. 2010;138(8):1100-1104.
7. Lefebvre SL, Reid-Smith RJ, Waltner-Toews D, et al. Incidence of acquisition of methicillin-resistant *Staphylococcus aureus, Clostridium difficile*, and other health-care-associated pathogens by dogs that participate in animal-assisted interventions. J Am Vet Med Assoc. 2009;234(11):1404-1417.
8. Pepin J, Alary M, Valiquette L, et al. Increasing risk of relapse after treatment of *Clostridium difficile* colitis in Quebec, Canada. Clin Infect Dis. 2005;40:1591-1597.
9. Lefebvre S, Arroyo L, Weese J. Epidemic *Clostridium difficile* strain in hospital visitation dog. Emerging Infect Dis. 2006;12:1036-1037.
10. Schneedberg A, Rupnik M, Neubauer H, et al. Prevalence and distribution of *Clostridium difficile* PCR ribotypes in cats and dogs from animal shelters in Thuringia, Germany. Anaerobe. 2012;18:484-488.
11. Weese JS, Staempfli HR, Prescott JF, et al. The roles of *Clostridium difficile* and enterotoxigenic *Clostridium perfringens* in diarrhea in dogs. J Vet Intern Med. 2001;15(4):374-378.
12. Marks SL, Kather EJ, Kass PH, et al. Genotypic and phenotypic characterization of *Clostridium perfringens* and *Clostridium difficile* in diarrheic and healthy dogs. J Vet Intern Med. 2002;16(5):533-540.
13. Marks SL, unpublished observations, 2011.
14. Weese JS, Weese HE, Bourdeau TL, et al. Suspected *Clostridium difficile*–associated diarrhea in two cats. J Am Vet Med Assoc. 2001;218(9):1436-1439,1421.
15. Carter GP, Rood JI, Lyras D. The role of toxin A and toxin B in *Clostridium difficile*–associated disease: past and present perspectives. Gut Microbes. 2010;1(1):58-64.
16. Kruth SA, Prescott JF, Welch MK, et al. Nosocomial diarrhea associated with enterotoxigenic *Clostridium perfringens* infection in dogs. J Am Vet Med Assoc. 1989;195(3):331-334.
17. Sasaki J, Goryo M, Asahina M, et al. Hemorrhagic enteritis associated with *Clostridium perfringens* type A in a dog. J Vet Med Sci. 1999;61(2):175-177.
18. Cave NJ, Marks SL, Kass PH, et al. Evaluation of a routine diagnostic fecal enteric panel for dogs with diarrhea. J Am Vet Med Assoc. 2002;221:52-59.
19. Schlegel BJ, Van Dreumel T, Slavić D, et al. *Clostridium perfringens* type A fatal acute hemorrhagic gastroenteritis in a dog. Can Vet J. 2012;53:555-557.
20. McClane BA. The complex interactions between *Clostridium perfringens* enterotoxin and epithelial tight junctions. Toxicon. 2001;39(11):1781-1791.
21. Leutenegger CM, Marks SL, Robertson J. Toxin quantification of *Clostridium perfringens* is a predictor for diarrhea in dogs and cats [Abstract]. J Vet Intern Med. 2012;26:794.
22. Tupler T, Levy JK, Sabshin SJ, et al. Enteropathogens identified in dogs entering a Florida animal shelter with normal feces or diarrhea. J Am Vet Med Assoc. 2012;241:338-343.
23. Sabshin SJ, Levy JK, Tupler R, et al. Enteropathogens identified in cats entering a Florida animal shelter with normal feces or diarrhea. J Am Vet Med Assoc. 2012;241:331-337.
24. Marks SL, Melli A, Kass PH, et al. Evaluation of methods to diagnose *Clostridium perfringens*–associated diarrhea in dogs. J Am Vet Med Assoc. 1999;214(3):357-360.
25. Birkhead G, Vogt RL, Heun EM, et al. Characterization of an outbreak of *Clostridium perfringens* food poisoning by quantitative fecal culture and fecal enterotoxin measurement. J Clin Microbiol. 1988;26(3):471-474.
26. Kuehne SA, Cartman ST, Heap JT, et al. The role of toxin A and toxin B in *Clostridium difficile* infection. Nature. 2010;467(7316):711-713.
27. Meer RR, Songer JG, Park DL. Human disease associated with *Clostridium perfringens* enterotoxin. Rev Environ Contam Toxicol. 1997;150:75-94.
28. Crobach MJ, Dekkers OM, Wilcox MH, et al. European Society of Clinical Microbiology and Infectious Diseases (ESCMID): data review and recommendations for diagnosing *Clostridium difficile*-infection (CDI). Clin Microbiol Infect. 2009;15(12):1053-1066.

29. Schmidt ML, Gilligan PH. *Clostridium difficile* testing algorithms: what is practical and feasible? Anaerobe. 2009;15(6):270-273.
30. Sloan LM, Duresko BJ, Gustafson DR, et al. Comparison of real-time PCR for detection of the *tcdC* gene with four toxin immunoassays and culture in diagnosis of *Clostridium difficile* infection. J Clin Microbiol. 2008;46(6):1996-2001.
31. Loh JP, Liu YC, Chew SW, et al. The rapid identification of *Clostridium perfringens* as the possible aetiology of a diarrhoeal outbreak using PCR. Epidemiol Infect. 2008;136(8):1142-1146.
32. Unterer S, Strohmeyer K, Kruse BD, et al. Treatment of aseptic dogs with hemorrhagic gastroenteritis with amoxicillin/clavulanic acid: a prospective blinded study. J Vet Intern Med. 2011;25(5):973-979.
33. Marks SL, Kather EJ. Antimicrobial susceptibilities of canine *Clostridium difficile* and *Clostridium perfringens* isolates to commonly utilized antimicrobial drugs. Vet Microbiol. 2003;94(1):39-45.
34. Pépin J, Saheb N, Coulombe MA, et al. Emergence of fluoroquinolones as the predominant risk factor for *Clostridium difficile*–associated diarrhea: a cohort study during an epidemic in Quebec. Clin Infect Dis. 2005;41(9):1254-1260.
35. Cartman ST, Heap JT, Kuehne SA, et al. The emergence of "hypervirulence" in *Clostridium difficile*. Int J Med Microbiol. 2010;300(6):387-395.
36. Lee BY, Popovich MJ, Tian Y, et al. The potential value of *Clostridium difficile* vaccine: an economic computer simulation model. Vaccine. 2010;28(32):5245-5253.
37. Gould LH, Limbago B. *Clostridium difficile* in food and domestic animals: a new foodborne pathogen? Clin Infect Dis. 2010;51(5):577-582.
38. Brynestad S, Granum PE. *Clostridium perfringens* and food-borne infections. Int J Food Microbiol. 2002;74(3):195-202.
39. Shandera WX, Tacket CO, Blake PA. Food poisoning due to *Clostridium perfringens* in the United States. J Infect Dis. 1983;147(1):167-170.

CHAPTER 49

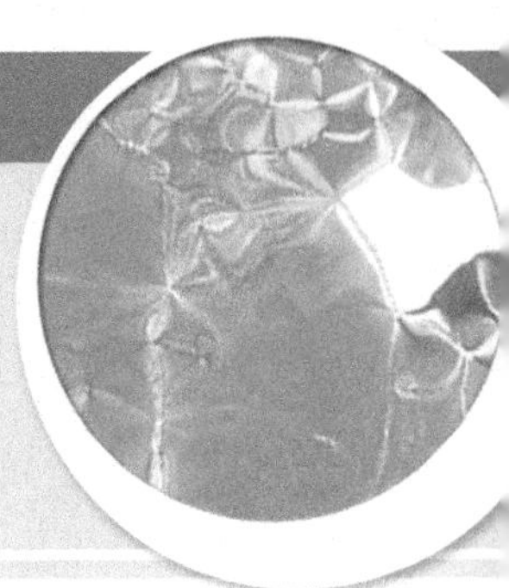

Gastric *Helicobacter*-like Infections

Jane E. Sykes and Stanley L. Marks

Overview of *Helicobacter* Infections in Dogs and Cats

First Described: 1881 by Rappin (France),[1] who observed spiral bacteria in a dog's stomach; the association between *H. pylori* infection and disease in humans was made in 1983 by Warren and Marshall (Australia).[2]

Cause: Various species of non–*H. pylori* helicobacters, rarely *H. pylori* in cats (gram-negative spiral-shaped bacteria that belong to the family Helicobacteraceae)

Primary Mode of Transmission: Fecal-oral and oral-oral transmission proposed, possibly water-borne. Transmission through contact with vomitus may also occur.

Affected Hosts: Humans and a variety of other animals are colonized by helicobacters; an association with disease is clearest for humans and ferrets

Geographic Distribution: Worldwide

Major Clinical Signs (Dogs and Cats): Possibly chronic vomiting (gastric helicobacters) or diarrhea (intestinal helicobacters), although evidence for a causative role in disease is weak

Differential Diagnoses: Dietary indiscretion, gastrointestinal foreign body, chronic pancreatitis, inflammatory bowel disease, food-responsive enteropathy, eosinophilic fibrosing gastritis (cats), bilious vomiting syndrome, gastrointestinal neoplasia (lymphoma, mast cell neoplasia, gastric adenocarcinoma), chronic infiltrative infectious diseases of the gastrointestinal tract (including feline infectious peritonitis, mycobacteriosis, canine cryptococcosis, pythiosis), hypoadrenocorticism, hyperthyroidism, toxins (including drugs), gastric helminthiasis (e.g., *Physaloptera* and *Ollulanus* spp.)

Human Health Significance: Dogs and cats may be a source of human infection with non–*H. pylori* helicobacters that have been associated with gastritis, gastroduodenal ulceration, and low-grade mucosa-associated lymphoid tissue (MALT) lymphoma in humans.

Etiology and Epidemiology

Helicobacter spp. are flagellate, gram-negative, microaerophilic, curved to spiral-shaped motile bacteria. They are grouped into gastric, hepatic, and intestinal *Helicobacter* species, with intestinal species residing primarily in the large intestine.[3,4] In humans, gastric *Helicobacter* spp. are an important cause of gastritis and gastroduodenal ulceration and increase the risk for development of gastric adenocarcinoma and lymphoma. In contrast, the extent to which *Helicobacter* spp. cause disease in dogs and cats is not fully understood, and newly discovered organisms in dogs and cats have drawn most attention in regard to their zoonotic potential.[5]

Helicobacter pylori, the type organism, is the most important species infecting humans. *H. pylori* infection is extremely rare in cats and has only been identified in one colony of cats to date.[6] It has not been described in dogs. Dogs and cats are generally infected with gastric non–*H. pylori* helicobacters (also referred to as gastric helicobacter-like organisms, or GHLOs).[5] These are much larger than *H. pylori* (5 to 10 µm long versus 1.5 to 3 µm long for *H. pylori*), and species cannot be differentiated from one another based on their light or electron microscopic appearance alone (Figure 49-1). The nomenclature of non–*H. pylori* helicobacters is complicated. Species identified in dogs and cats are listed in Table 49-1.[4,7-16] Before their genetic characterization, non–*H. pylori* helicobacters were originally referred to as "*Gastrospirillum hominis*" and later "*Helicobacter heilmannii.*" Subsequent analysis of multiple gene sequences from a variety of "*H. heilmannii*" from dogs and cats has revealed that "*H. heilmannii*" is not one but a group of organisms that includes *H. felis, H. bizzozeronii, H. salomonis,* and an organism that has been confusingly named *H. heilmannii.* These organisms have also been implicated in human disease, albeit less commonly than *H. pylori.*[5]

Depending on the study, between 60% and 100% of dogs and cats carry non–*H. pylori* helicobacters, and gastric *Helicobacter* spp. can be found in apparently healthy animals and dogs and cats without signs of vomiting.[5,17-22] *H. felis* infection has been associated with gastric pathology in dogs in some studies[23] but not others.[24] Dogs and cats are probably colonized shortly after birth, as a result of fecal-oral and oral-oral transmission.[25] Transmission through contact with vomitus may also occur. Water-borne transmission may play a role in spread of *H. pylori* to humans.[26] Shelter and colony dogs and cats may have a higher prevalence of colonization, most likely due to the close proximity of animals to one another. One *Helicobacter* species may be able to suppress the presence of another, so that dogs and cats are primarily colonized with a single species, although in some animals, the simultaneous presence of multiple species has been found.[27-30] The organisms have a remarkable ability to survive the low pH of the stomach, which they resist by living deep in the mucus glands of the stomach and through production of the enzyme urease. The urease catalyzes the hydrolysis of urea to carbon dioxide and ammonia, which raises the pH of the organism's milieu. In dogs and cats, the organisms are also found within the canaliculi and the cytoplasm of parietal cells.[25,30,31]

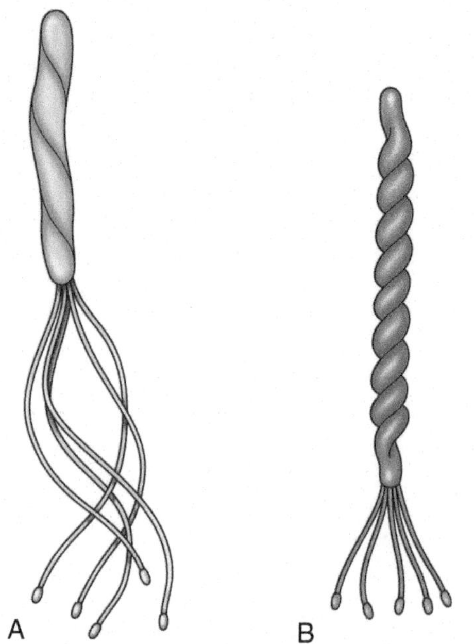

FIGURE 49-1 Structure of gastric *Helicobacter* species. Note the terminal bunches of flagellar filaments. **A,** *Helicobacter pylori*. **B,** Gastric helicobacter-like organism.

TABLE 49-1

***Helicobacter* Species Identified in Dogs, Cats, and Humans[4,7-16]**

Species	Location	Host
H. bizzozeronii	Stomach	Dog, humans
H. salomonis	Stomach	Dog
H. cynogastricus	Stomach	Dog
H. heilmannii	Stomach	Dog, cat, humans
H. felis	Stomach	Dog, cat, humans
H. pametensis	Stomach	Cat
H. baculiformis	Stomach	Cat
H. pylori	Stomach	Cat
"*Flexispira rappini*"	Stomach, intestine	Dog, cat
H. bilis	Stomach, intestine	Dog, cat
H. cinaedi	Intestine	Dog, cat
H. fennelliae	Intestine	Dog, cat
"*H. colifelis*"	Intestine	Cat
H. marmotae	Intestine	Cat
H. canis	Intestine, liver	Dog, cat, humans

Clinical Features

Signs and Their Pathogenesis

The majority of dogs and cats infected with *Helicobacter* spp. show no clinical signs. *Helicobacter* infection of some dogs and cats has been hypothesized to cause chronic intermittent vomiting, inappetence, pica, belching, weight loss, fever, and polyphagia.[31] Unfortunately, strong evidence that supports an association with such disease in dogs and cats is lacking. Clinical signs in some animals with biopsy-confirmed infection resolve following specific therapy for gastric helicobacter infection,[31-33] although the results of one study were difficult to interpret because an elimination diet was administered concurrently.[31] Experimental and natural infection of dogs and cats with non–*H. pylori* helicobacters has been associated with chronic lymphoplasmacytic gastritis and lymphoid follicular hyperplasia. Gastroduodenal ulceration and marked alterations in the gastric acid secretory axis, as occur in humans, have not been observed in dogs and cats.[24,33,34] However, not all animals infected with non–*H. pylori* helicobacters have histopathologic evidence of gastritis, and no correlation has been observed between the severity of gastric pathology and the degree of colonization by helicobacters. More severe gastritis with marked lymphoid follicular hyperplasia and neutrophilic inflammatory infiltrates has been reported in cats and acutely in puppies experimentally infected with *H. pylori*.[35,36] The puppies developed gastrointestinal signs, including vomiting and loose stool, shortly after inoculation. It is possible that the degree of bacterial invasion and gastritis in dogs and cats varies with the infecting *Helicobacter* species or even strain.[30] In humans, gastric pathology has been associated with possession of a number of pathogenicity genes by *H. pylori,* including *cag*A (cytotoxin-associated gene A), *vac*A (vacuolating cytotoxin), and *ice*A (induced by contact with epithelium).[37] The degree of vacuolating cytotoxin production can also vary among strains.[38]

In human patients, *H. pylori* infection has been well associated with gastric low-grade, B-cell, mucosa-associated lymphoid tissue (MALT) lymphoma. Eradication of *H. pylori* achieves complete remission in some patients with *H. pylori*–positive early-stage gastric MALT lymphoma.[39] One study suggested a possible association between *Helicobacter* spp. infection and gastric lymphoma in cats,[40] but additional studies are required to determine the role of *Helicobacter* spp. infection in feline gastric disease.

Non–*H. pylori* helicobacters have been detected in the hepatobiliary system of cats with neutrophilic cholangitis[41] and lymphocytic cholangitis,[42] although this may reflect ascending bacterial infection secondary to an underlying disease process. *H. canis* was detected in the liver of a 2-month-old puppy with multifocal necrotizing hepatitis that had acute weakness and vomiting, and died within hours.[43] *H. canis* was also detected in a colony of Bengal cats with diarrhea, but its role as a causative agent was uncertain.[44] Abundant organisms that genetically resembled *H. canis* were detected microscopically throughout the large intestine of a 2-month-old kitten with severe diarrhea, vomiting, dehydration, weight loss, and inappetence.[3] In one study, the presence of heavy colonic infection with enterohepatic *Helicobacter* spp. infection in a group of laboratory dogs was associated with the presence of mucosal atrophy and fibrosis, and a possible role of *Helicobacter* spp. infection in canine inflammatory bowel disease was suggested.[29]

Diagnosis

Microbiologic Testing

Clinical diagnosis of *Helicobacter* infection in dogs and cats has most commonly been based on histopathology, cytology, rapid urease testing, and, to a lesser extent, PCR on gastric biopsies (Table 49-2). Other tests such as the urea breath and blood tests, fecal PCR, and serologic tests are primarily used in human patients and in the research arena.

Diagnosis Using Cytology and Histopathology

Spiral organisms can be readily detected in touch impression smears of gastric tissue obtained following biopsy or necropsy,

TABLE 49-2

Diagnostic Assays Available for Gastric *Helicobacter* Infection in Dogs and Cats*

Assay	Specimen Type	Target	Performance
Bacterial isolation	Gastric biopsies	*Helicobacter* organisms	Can take up to 10 days. Low sensitivity for non–*H. pylori* helicobacters, which can be difficult to culture. Patchy distribution may also lead to false negatives. Allows typing and antimicrobial susceptibility testing.
Cytology	Impression smears of gastric biopsies or cytology brush specimens	*Helicobacter* organisms	Rapid and sensitive, but false negatives can occur. Patchy distribution may also lead to false negatives. Does not provide information on inflammatory or architectural changes in underlying tissue.
Histopathology	Gastric biopsies	*Helicobacter* organisms	Less sensitive than cytologic examination. Patchy distribution may also lead to false negatives. Use of silver stains increases sensitivity when organism numbers are low. Allows determination of associated gastric histopathology.
Rapid urease testing	Gastric biopsies	*Helicobacter* urease	Rapid and very sensitive. Patchy distribution and low organism loads may lead to false negatives. Very rare false positives with other urease-producing organisms.
PCR	Gastric biopsies	*Helicobacter* DNA	Rapid (within hours); can be highly sensitive and specific. Sequence analysis can determine the species involved. Primarily used on a research basis.
Serology	Serum	Antibodies to *Helicobacter* spp.	Moderate sensitivity in dogs and cats. Results do not correlate well with gastric histopathology and do not always correlate with active infection. Primarily used in research settings.
Urea breath and blood testing	Breath, blood	Radiolabeled carbon dioxide derived from the activity of *Helicobacter* urease	Requires specialized detection equipment. Although sensitive, false negatives may occur, such as following acid suppression. In dogs and cats, has been primarily used in research settings to date.

*For all tests, positive results do not imply that *Helicobacter* is the cause of disease.

after staining with Gram or Diff Quik stains (Figure 49-2). A cytology brush can also be used to obtain a specimen during endoscopy. Several biopsies or brush specimens may need to be evaluated from different regions of the stomach (fundus, cardia, antrum/pylorus) when the distribution of organisms is patchy. When organism burdens are high, the organisms can be detected using histopathology, which allows assessment of concurrent gastric pathology (Figures 49-3 and 49-4). The use of silver stains (such as Warthin-Starry stain or Steiner stain), Giemsa, or toluidine blue stain, as well as immunostaining, dramatically increases sensitivity for organism detection (see Figures 49-3, *C*, and 49-4, *C*).[45]

Bacterial Isolation

Isolation of gastric helicobacters is difficult and has low sensitivity. Growth typically requires incubation on selective media in microaerobic conditions for 5 to 10 days. Isolation is advantageous in research settings because it allows subsequent identification of the organism using conventional biochemical testing, whole-cell protein profiling, and DNA analysis.[21,46] It also allows antimicrobial susceptibility testing, which has recently been recommended before treating humans for *H. pylori* infection because of the increasing prevalence of antimicrobial resistance.[47] Resistance to antimicrobials has also been documented in non–*H. pylori* helicobacters isolated from dogs and cats.[48]

Rapid Urease Testing

The rapid urease test involves incubating a gastric biopsy in a urea broth that contains the pH indicator phenol red. If gastric helicobacters are present, helicobacter urease breaks down the urea; with the release of ammonia, a rise in pH and a color change occur. The change in color can occur within 1 to 3 hours, although the broth is generally incubated at room temperature for 24 hours. The test is very sensitive, but false-negative results can occur if the distribution within the stomach is patchy or if organism loads are low. False-positive results have rarely been reported when other urease-producing bacteria are present in the stomach, such as *Proteus* spp.

Detection of *Helicobacter* DNA

PCR assays have been extensively used to detect *Helicobacter* species in tissues on a research basis, including those from dogs and cats. Sequence analysis of the PCR products can allow identification of the *Helicobacter* species present. Fluorescent in situ hybridization (FISH) has also been used to detect, localize, and identify *Helicobacter* species infection in tissues from dogs and cats.[4,32,40,49]

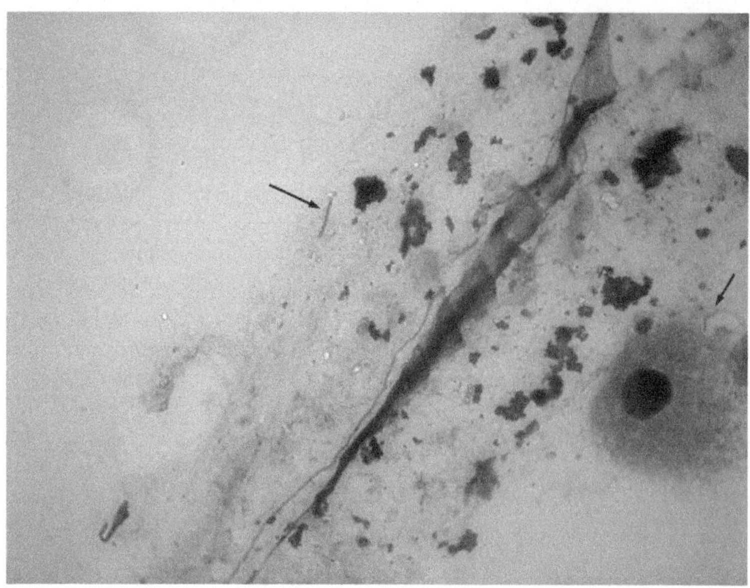

FIGURE 49-2 Spiral-shaped gastric *Helicobacter*-like organisms visible in a Diff Quik–stained smear *(arrows)* of a gastric biopsy from a 2-year-old male neutered Cavalier King Charles spaniel with chronic vomiting and regurgitation for which no other cause was apparent (1000× magnification).

Serology

A variety of serum ELISA and immunoblotting assays have been used in humans to detect antibodies and screen for *H. pylori* infection, and some can be used to some extent to monitor the success of therapy.[50,51] Serologic assays have been used on a research basis to noninvasively detect non–*H. pylori* helicobacter infection in dogs and cats, in some studies demonstrating moderate sensitivity and good specificity.[52-54]

Urea Breath and Blood Testing

Diagnosis and monitoring of the extent of *H. pylori* infection in human patients can also be accomplished noninvasively using urea breath and blood testing, which involves oral administration of urea containing ^{14}C or the stable isotope ^{13}C. After ingestion, the labeled urea is converted to ammonia by *Helicobacter* urease, and the released carbon is absorbed systemically, where it can be measured in the blood. Subsequently, the labeled carbon dioxide is exhaled and can be measured in the breath. Acid suppression interferes with test results by decreasing *Helicobacter* urease activity, and so testing is generally performed several days after discontinuing treatment. False positives can also occur.[55] Urea breath and blood testing has been used with success in dogs,[56] and breath testing has been used in cats[20,57] both before and following specific treatment for *Helicobacter* infection.

Stool Antigen Assays

Assays that detect *H. pylori* antigen in feces have been used in human patients,[55] but their use in dogs and cats has not been described.

Pathologic Findings

Infection with non–*H. pylori* helicobacters in dogs and cats has primarily been associated with chronic lymphocytic or lymphoplasmacytic gastritis, with lymphoid follicular hyperplasia (see Figures 49-3, *A*, and 49-4, *A*), although the extent of inflammation varies dramatically from absent to severe.[19,58,59] An eosinophilic inflammatory component has been described in some cats.[58] Neutrophil and eosinophil infiltrates can accompany mononuclear inflammation in some cats infected with *H. pylori*.[58,60] Organisms may be found in the superficial mucus and crypts, and sometimes within parietal cells see Figures 49-3 and 49-4).

Histopathologic findings in a cat infected with an intestinal helicobacter included large numbers of densely packed spiral bacteria covering the intestinal mucosa and present within the crypts, and minimal inflammatory changes. Hepatic changes in a dog with *H. canis* infection consisted of randomly distributed and coalescing hepatocellular necrosis with associated neutrophilic and mononuclear infiltrates.[43]

Treatment and Prognosis

Whether antimicrobial treatment should be used for *Helicobacter* infections in dogs and cats is unknown. Humans with *H. pylori* infections are typically treated with a combination of a proton pump inhibitor, amoxicillin, and clarithromycin, with or without bismuth subsalicylate. Treatment of humans is reserved for symptomatic individuals; the development of antimicrobial resistance by *H. pylori* is increasingly of concern.[61] Treatment should be reserved for dogs and cats with gastrointestinal signs that have no other identifiable cause of illness, after a diagnosis of gastritis and *Helicobacter* infection has been confirmed using biopsy. A 2-week course of combination therapy with antimicrobials and a proton pump inhibitor or an H_2 antagonist does not reliably eliminate gastric helicobacters in dogs and cats, although clinical signs often resolve.[33,56,62,63] Reinfection can occur in some animals after treatment. This theory is underscored by a study of 20 dogs that were naturally infected with *Helicobacter* spp. and treated with triple therapy (clarithromycin, amoxicillin, and lansoprazole) for 7 days. The dogs were then randomized into a control group kept in isolation, and an experimental group, which was placed in contact with *Helicobacter*-positive dogs for 60 days. Triple therapy was effective in 100% of the dogs; however, recurrence of infection occurred in 80% of dogs in

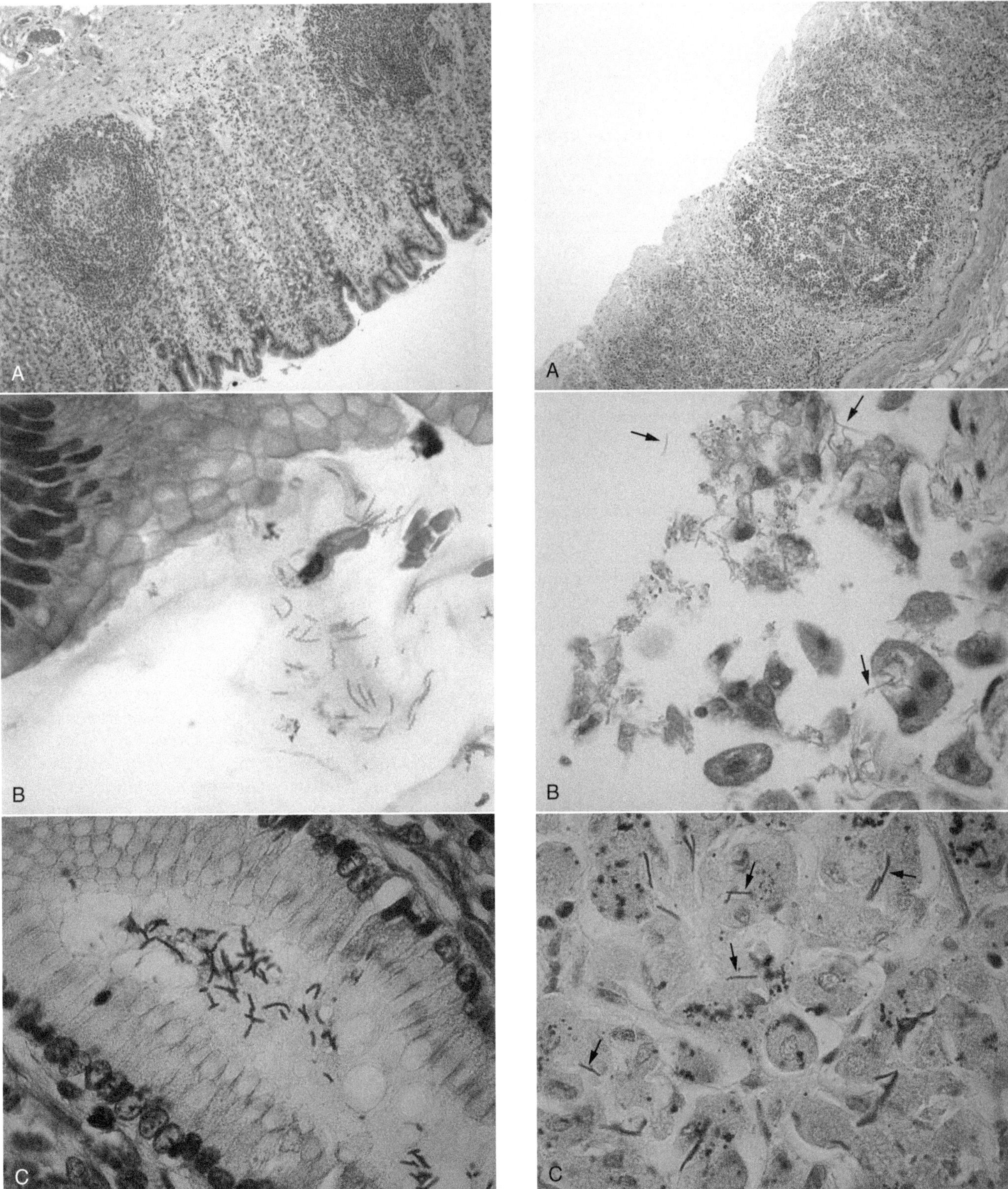

FIGURE 49-3 Histopathology of the stomach of a 2-year-old female spayed Maltese terrier with chronic vomiting and regurgitation. **A,** Lymphoid follicular nodules. The remaining lamina propria is infiltrated by small numbers of eosinophils, neutrophils, lymphocytes, and plasma cells. H&E stain, 40× magnification. **B,** Large numbers of spiral-shaped bacteria are visible in the superficial mucous and gastric glands. H&E stain, 1000× magnification. **C,** Agyrophilic intralesional spiral-shaped bacteria within the gastric glands. Warthin-Starry stain, 1000× magnification.

FIGURE 49-4 Histopathology of the stomach of a 14-year-old male neutered domestic shorthair that was infected with FIV and was euthanized because of squamous cell carcinoma. Gastrointestinal signs were not reported. **A,** Severe, chronic, lymphofollicular gastritis. H&E stain, 40× magnification. **B,** Abundant fine, spiral-shaped bacteria were visualized in the superficial mucous and within parietal cells *(arrows)*. H&E stain. **C,** Warthin-Starry stain showing intracellular agyrophilic spiral-shaped bacteria *(arrows)*; 1000x magnification.

TABLE 49-3

Antimicrobials Used with Success to Treat *Helicobacter* spp. Infection in Dogs and Cats

Drug	Dose (mg/kg)	Route	Interval (hours)	Duration (days)
Metronidazole	10-15	PO	12	14-21
Amoxicillin	22	PO	12	14-21
Bismuth subsalicylate	0.22 mL/kg	PO	6-8	14-21
Clarithromycin	5-10	PO	12	14-21
Omeprazole	0.7-1.0	PO	24	14-21
Famotidine	0.5-1.0	PO	12	14-21

The first three drugs are administered as a combination. Alternatively, clarithromycin can be combined with amoxicillin and administered with either omeprazole or famotidine. Bismuth compounds should be avoided in cats. Omeprazole should be given on an empty stomach 30 minutes before a meal.

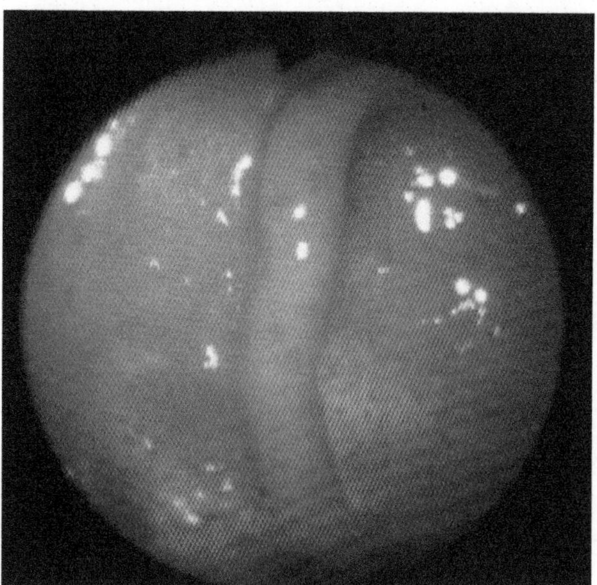

FIGURE 49-5 Endoscopic image of lymphoid follicular gastritis in a 2-year-old maltese terrier with chronic vomiting and regurgitation that was associated with the presence of large numbers of gastric helicobacter like-organisms. Note the 'goose pimple' appearance of the mucosa.

the experimental group, and in none of the dogs in the control group after 60 days.[64] A 3-week course of amoxicillin, metronidazole, and bismuth subsalicylate (Table 49-3) cleared gastric helicobacters in dogs and cats, with resolution of vomiting, but histopathologic evidence of gastritis did not resolve.[32] Metronidazole could be substituted with clarithromycin.[21] One study showed that concurrent use of an H_2 antagonist in dogs did not change outcome.[33] This is consistent with the lack of abnormalities in the gastric acid secretory axis in dogs infected with non–*H. pylori* helicobacters.[24,34]

Immunity and Vaccination

Gastric helicobacters persist in the stomach despite a vigorous humoral immune response. Research has been underway to develop an effective vaccine for *H. pylori* infection in humans, and a variety of *H. pylori* antigens induce protection in healthy human volunteers or mouse models.[65] No vaccine is available for *Helicobacter* infection in dogs and cats, and a greater understanding of the role of gastric helicobacters in canine and feline disease will be required in order to assess the need for effective vaccines against these organisms.

Public Health Aspects

At least 50% of the world's human population is infected with *H. pylori*, although the prevalence of infection has decreased in developed countries.[66] In the Western world, 1% to 10% of people develop gastroduodenal ulceration as a result of chronic *H. pylori* infection. A smaller percentage of infected people (<3%) develop gastric adenocarcinoma or MALT lymphoma in association with infection. Duodenal ulceration results from increased gastrin release in response to *H. pylori*–induced gastric antral inflammation. Factors that influence outcome are not well understood, but an individual's immune response to the organism, as well as the possession of virulence factors by *H. pylori* strains, appears to play an important role.[66] Eradication of infection using antimicrobial therapy can cure gastroduodenal ulceration and MALT lymphoma, but gastric adenocarcinoma generally persists despite treatment.[67] Although *H. pylori* has been documented to infect a colony of cats, infection of cats with this species is extremely rare, and exposure to pets is not a risk factor for *H. pylori* infection in humans.

Non–*H. pylori* gastric helicobacter infection is uncommon in humans compared with *H. pylori* infection. Nevertheless, these helicobacters have also been associated with chronic active gastritis, gastroduodenal ulceration, and MALT lymphomas in people. Disease is generally less severe than that caused by *H. pylori*.[5] Clinical signs in humans may be absent or consist of nausea, epigastric pain, vomiting, hematemesis, heartburn, and decreased appetite. Treatment with triple antibiotic therapy and bismuth subsalicylate can resolve infection and gastritis. Pets have been suggested as a source of these helicobacters for humans,[5,7,68-71] and close contact with dogs and cats is a risk factor for infection.[72] Licking has been suggested as a mode of transmission, based on the presence of non–*H. pylori* helicobacter DNA in the oral cavity of dogs.[25] Pigs play an even more important role in zoonotic transmission of non–*H. pylori* gastric helicobacters, the swine helicobacter *H. suis* being the most prevalent species identified in humans.[5]

Intestinal helicobacters found in dogs and cats, especially *H. cinaedi*, have been associated with enteric disease and bacteremia in immunocompromised humans.[73] The relative role of dogs and cats in transmission of these organisms to humans is unknown. Nosocomial spread of *H. cinaedi* was suggested among immunocompromised humans in one report.[74]

CASE EXAMPLE

Signalment: "Mochi," a 2-year-old female spayed Maltese terrier from Dixon, CA

History: Mochi had been vomiting and regurgitating intermittently since she was 1 year of age. As a puppy, the owner (a veterinary student) reported intermittent episodes of "burping." The vomiting occurred 2 to 5 times throughout the day and was not associated with eating, drinking, or exercise. The vomitus usually consisted of brown fluid with no recognizable food particles. Dietary changes that included a digestible elimination diet containing a novel, single protein source followed by a fat-restricted prescription diet had not resulted in improvement in her clinical signs. Therapy with cisapride (3 mg PO q8h) and famotidine (2.5 mg PO q24h) or omeprazole (3.5 mg PO q24h) resulted in only slight improvement in the frequency of vomiting. Her appetite was appropriate, and there had been no weight loss or diarrhea. She primarily lived indoors with one cat. She was up to date on vaccinations, which included those for rabies, distemper, parvovirus, and canine adenovirus.

Physical Examination:

Body Weight: 3 kg

General: Bright, alert and responsive, hydrated, nervous. Ambulatory on all 4 limbs. T = 100.4°F (38.0°C), HR = 120 beats/min, RR = 28 breaths/min, mucous membranes pink and moist, CRT = 1 s.

Integument, Eyes, Ears, Nose, and Throat: No clinically significant abnormalities were noted.

Musculoskeletal: The dog's body condition score was 4/9 with symmetrical muscling.

Cardiovascular, Respiratory, and Lymph Nodes: No clinically significant abnormalities were noted.

Gastrointestinal and Genitourinary: Abdominal palpation was unremarkable. "Burping" behavior was observed in the room, which occurred without any prodromal signs or abdominal effort. Lip-smacking behavior occurred immediately afterwards. Rectal examination was normal.

Laboratory Findings:

CBC:

HCT 46.5% (40%-55%)
MCV 64.4 fL (65-75 fL)
MCHC 35.9 g/dL (33-36 g/dL)
WBC 5700 cells/μL (6000-13,000 cells/μL)
Neutrophils 3112 cells/μL (3000-10,500 cells/μL)
Lymphocytes 1830 cells/μL (1000-4000 cells/μL)
Monocytes 257 cells/μL (150-1200 cells/μL)
Eosinophils 479 cells/μL (0-1500 cells/μL)
Platelets 277,000/μL (150,000-400,000 platelets/μL).

Serum Chemistry Profile:

Sodium 147 mmol/L (145-154 mmol/L)
Potassium 4.4 mmol/L (3.6-5.3 mmol/L)
Chloride 111 mmol/L (108-118 mmol/L)
Bicarbonate 23 mmol/L (16-26 mmol/L)
Phosphorus 5.3 mg/dL (3.0-6.2 mg/dL)
Calcium 10.6 mg/dL (9.7-11.5 mg/dl)
BUN 22 mg/dL (5-21 mg/dL)
Creatinine 1.1 mg/dL (0.3-1.2 mg/dL)
Glucose 95 mg/dL (64-123 mg/dL)
Total protein 5.7 g/dL (5.4-7.6 g/dL)
Albumin 4.0 g/dL (3.0-4.4 g/dL)
Globulin 1.7 g/dL (1.8-3.9 g/dL)
ALT 42 U/L (19-67 U/L)
AST 45 U/L (19-42 U/L)
ALP 52 U/L (21-170 U/L)
GGT < 3 U/L (0-6 U/L)
Cholesterol 241 mg/dL (135-361 mg/dL)
Total bilirubin 0.2 mg/dL (0-0.2 mg/dL).

Urinalysis: SGr 1.040, pH 7.0, no protein, glucose, or ketones, trace hemoprotein, 0-1 WBC/HPF, 0-1 RBC/HPF, moderate lipid droplets.

Serum Pancreatic Lipase Immunoreactivity: <30 μg/L (reference range 0-200 μg/L)

Imaging Findings:

Abdominal Radiographs: A moderate amount of gas was identified within multiple small intestinal loops, but an obstructive pattern was not identified.

Thoracic Radiographs: The cardiopulmonary structures were within normal limits. A small amount of gas was visualized within the esophagus on the left lateral projections.

Esophagram: Unremarkable study.

Abdominal Ultrasound: No abnormalities were identified.

Gastroduodenoscopy: Gross findings were suggestive of diffuse lymphoid follicular hyperplasia, with a mild "goose pimple" appearance to the gastric mucosa (Figure 49-5). Multiple biopsies of all regions of the stomach and multiple duodenal biopsies were obtained and submitted for histopathology.

Histopathology: Stomach: Moderate, lymphofollicular, eosinophilic, and lymphoplasmacytic gastritis with intralesional spiral bacteria (see Figure 49-3). Duodenum: Mild, chronic, lymphofollicular, eosinophilic, and lymphoplasmacytic duodenitis and ileitis. Jejunum: Diffuse, mild, eosinophilic, and lymphoplasmacytic enteritis.

Diagnosis: Chronic gastritis associated with *Helicobacter* spp. infection; mild eosinophilic and lymphoplasmacytic enteritis.

Treatment: Treatment for the *Helicobacter* infection was initiated with metronidazole (30 mg PO q12h), amoxicillin (60 mg PO q12h), and bismuth subsalicylate for 2 weeks. The owner reported almost complete resolution of the vomiting following treatment, but signs returned after treatment was discontinued, and an additional course of treatment was instituted. Treatment with a fat-restricted prescription diet was continued. The frequency of vomiting then decreased to once a week.

Comments: Whether the *Helicobacter* spp. infection in this dog contributed to clinical signs or was an incidental finding in a dog with underlying enteritis was not clear. The failure to respond to multiple diet changes, including an elimination diet, and the dramatic response to triple therapy supported a possible role for *Helicobacter* spp. infection, or a diagnosis of antibiotic-responsive gastroenteropathy that was unrelated to *Helicobacter* spp. infection.

SUGGESTED READING

Haesebrouck F, Pasmans F, Flahou B, et al. Gastric helicobacters in domestic animals and nonhuman primates and their significance for human health. Clin Microbiol Rev. 2009;22(2):202-223.

REFERENCES

1. Rappin JP. Contre l'etude de bacterium de la bouche etat normal. In: College de France, Nantes; 1881.
2. Warren JR, Marshall BJ. Unidentified curved bacilli on gastric epithelium in active chronic gastritis. Lancet. 1983;1:1273-1275.
3. Foley JE, Solnick JV, Lapointe JM, et al. Identification of a novel enteric *Helicobacter* species in a kitten with severe diarrhea. J Clin Microbiol. 1998;36:908-912.
4. Recordati C, Gualdi V, Craven M, et al. Spatial distribution of *Helicobacter* spp. in the gastrointestinal tract of dogs. Helicobacter. 2009;14:180-191.
5. Haesebrouck F, Pasmans F, Flahou B, et al. Gastric helicobacters in domestic animals and nonhuman primates and their significance for human health. Clin Microbiol Rev. 2009;22:202-223.
6. Handt LK, Fox JG, Dewhirst FE, et al. *Helicobacter pylori* isolated from the domestic cat: public health implications. Infect Immun. 1994;62:2367-2374.
7. Alon D, Paitan Y, Ben-Nissan Y, et al. Persistent *Helicobacter canis* bacteremia in a patient with gastric lymphoma. Infection. 2010;38:62-64.
8. Baele M, Decostere A, Vandamme P, et al. *Helicobacter baculiformis* sp. nov., isolated from feline stomach mucosa. Int J Syst Evol Microbiol. 2008;58:357-364.
9. De Groote D, Van Doorn LJ, Van den Bulck K, et al. Detection of non-*pylori Helicobacter* species in "*Helicobacter heilmannii*"-infected humans. Helicobacter. 2005;10:398-406.
10. Fox JG, Shen Z, Xu S, et al. *Helicobacter marmotae* sp. nov. isolated from livers of woodchucks and intestines of cats. J Clin Microbiol. 2002;40:2513-2519.
11. Hanninen ML, Happonen I, Saari S, et al. Culture and characteristics of *Helicobacter bizzozeronii*, a new canine gastric *Helicobacter* sp. Int J Syst Bacteriol. 1996;46:160-166.
12. Jalava K, Kaartinen M, Utriainen M, et al. *Helicobacter salomonis* sp. nov., a canine gastric *Helicobacter* sp. related to *Helicobacter felis* and *Helicobacter bizzozeronii*. Int J Syst Bacteriol. 1997; 47:975-982.
13. Kiehlbauch JA, Brenner DJ, Cameron DN, et al. Genotypic and phenotypic characterization of *Helicobacter cinaedi* and *Helicobacter fennelliae* strains isolated from humans and animals. J Clin Microbiol. 1995;33:2940-2947.
14. Kivisto R, Linros J, Rossi M, et al. Characterization of multiple *Helicobacter bizzozeronii* isolates from a Finnish patient with severe dyspeptic symptoms and chronic active gastritis. Helicobacter. 2010;15:58-66.
15. Rossi M, Hanninen ML, Revez J, et al. Occurrence and species level diagnostics of *Campylobacter* spp., enteric *Helicobacter* spp. and *Anaerobiospirillum* spp. in healthy and diarrheic dogs and cats. Vet Microbiol. 2008;129:304-314.
16. Van den Bulck K, Decostere A, Baele M, et al. *Helicobacter cynogastricus* sp. nov., isolated from the canine gastric mucosa. Int J Syst Evol Microbiol. 2006;56:1559-1564.
17. Eaton KA, Dewhirst FE, Paster BJ, et al. Prevalence and varieties of *Helicobacter* species in dogs from random sources and pet dogs: animal and public health implications. J Clin Microbiol. 1996;34:3165-3170.
18. Happonen I, Linden J, Saari S, et al. Detection and effects of helicobacters in healthy dogs and dogs with signs of gastritis. J Am Vet Med Assoc. 1998;213:1767-1774.
19. Hermanns W, Kregel K, Breuer W, et al. Helicobacter-like organisms: histopathological examination of gastric biopsies from dogs and cats. J Comp Pathol. 1995;112:307-318.
20. Neiger R, Dieterich C, Burnens A, et al. Detection and prevalence of *Helicobacter* infection in pet cats. J Clin Microbiol. 1998;36:634-637.
21. Neiger R, Simpson KW. *Helicobacter* infection in dogs and cats: facts and fiction. J Vet Intern Med. 2000;14:125-133.
22. Otto G, Hazell SH, Fox JG, et al. Animal and public health implications of gastric colonization of cats by helicobacter-like organisms. J Clin Microbiol. 1994;32:1043-1049.
23. Lee A, Krakowka S, Fox JG, et al. Role of *Helicobacter felis* in chronic canine gastritis. Vet Pathol. 1992;29:487-494.
24. Simpson KW, McDonough PL, Strauss-Ayali D, et al. *Helicobacter felis* infection in dogs: effect on gastric structure and function. Vet Pathol. 1999;36:237-248.
25. Recordati C, Gualdi V, Tosi S, et al. Detection of *Helicobacter* spp. DNA in the oral cavity of dogs. Vet Microbiol. 2007;119:346-351.
26. Travis PB, Goodman KJ, O'Rourke KM, et al. The association of drinking water quality and sewage disposal with *Helicobacter pylori* incidence in infants: the potential role of water-borne transmission. J Water Health. 2010;8:192-203.
27. Wiinberg B, Spohr A, Dietz HH, et al. Quantitative analysis of inflammatory and immune responses in dogs with gastritis and their relationship to *Helicobacter* spp. infection. J Vet Intern Med. 2005;19:4-14.
28. Ekman E, Fredriksson M, Trowald-Wigh G, et al. *Helicobacter* spp. in the saliva, stomach, duodenum and faeces of colony dogs. Vet J. 2013;195:127-129.
29. Castiglioni V, Vailati Facchini R, Mattiello S, et al. Enterohepatic *Helicobacter* spp. in colonic biopsies of dogs: molecular, histopathological and immunohistochemical investigations. Vet Microbiol. 2012;159:107-114.
30. Lanzoni A, Faustinelli I, Cristofori P, et al. Localization of *Helicobacter* spp. in the fundic mucosa of laboratory Beagle dogs: an ultrastructural study. Vet Res. 2011;42:42.
31. Lecoindre P, Chevallier M, Peyrol S, et al. Gastric helicobacters in cats. J Feline Med Surg. 2000;2:19-27.
32. Jergens AE, Pressel M, Crandell J, et al. Fluorescence in situ hybridization confirms clearance of visible *Helicobacter* spp. associated with gastritis in dogs and cats. J Vet Intern Med. 2009;23:16-23.
33. Leib MS, Duncan RB, Ward DL. Triple antimicrobial therapy and acid suppression in dogs with chronic vomiting and gastric *Helicobacter* spp. J Vet Intern Med. 2007;21:1185-1192.
34. Simpson KW, Strauss-Ayali D, McDonough PL, et al. Gastric function in dogs with naturally acquired gastric *Helicobacter* spp. infection. J Vet Intern Med. 1999;13:507-515.
35. Perkins SE, Fox JG, Marini RP, et al. Experimental infection in cats with a cagA+ human isolate of *Helicobacter pylori*. Helicobacter. 1998;3:225-235.
36. Rossi G, Rossi M, Vitali CG, et al. A conventional beagle dog model for acute and chronic infection with *Helicobacter pylori*. Infect Immun. 1999;67:3112-3120.
37. Ramis IB, Fonseca TL, de Moraes EP, et al. Molecular basis of pathogenicity in *Helicobacter pylori* clinical isolates. J Clin Microbiol. 2010;48:3776-3778.
38. Atherton JC, Cao P, Peek Jr RM, et al. Mosaicism in vacuolating cytotoxin alleles of *Helicobacter pylori*. Association of specific vacA types with cytotoxin production and peptic ulceration. J Biol Chem. 1995;270:17771-17777.
39. Chen LT, Lin JT, Tai JJ, et al. Long-term results of anti–*Helicobacter pylori* therapy in early-stage gastric high-grade transformed MALT lymphoma. J Natl Cancer Inst. 2005;97:1345-1353.
40. Bridgeford EC, Marini RP, Feng Y, et al. Gastric *Helicobacter* species as a cause of feline gastric lymphoma: a viable hypothesis. Vet Immunol Immunopathol. 2008;123:106-113.
41. Greiter-Wilke A, Scanziani E, Soldati S, et al. Association of *Helicobacter* with cholangiohepatitis in cats. J Vet Intern Med. 2006;20:822-827.

42. Otte CMA, Perez Gutierrez O, Favier RP, et al. Detection of bacterial DNA in bile of cats with lymphocytic cholangitis. Vet Microbiol. 2012;156:217-221.
43. Fox JG, Drolet R, Higgins R, et al. *Helicobacter canis* isolated from a dog liver with multifocal necrotizing hepatitis. J Clin Microbiol. 1996;34:2479-2482.
44. Foley JE, Marks SL, Munson L, et al. Isolation of *Helicobacter canis* from a colony of Bengal cats with endemic diarrhea. J Clin Microbiol. 1999;37:3271-3275.
45. Prachasilpchai W, Nuanualsuwan S, Chatsuwan T, et al. Diagnosis of *Helicobacter* spp. infection in canine stomach. J Vet Sci. 2007;8:139-145.
46. Jalava K, On SL, Vandamme PA, et al. Isolation and identification of *Helicobacter* spp. from canine and feline gastric mucosa. Appl Environ Microbiol. 1998;64:3998-4006.
47. Wenzhen Y, Yumin L, Quanlin G, et al. Is antimicrobial susceptibility testing necessary before first-line treatment for *Helicobacter pylori* infection? Meta-analysis of randomized controlled trials. Intern Med. 2010;49:1103-1109.
48. Van den Bulck K, Decostere A, Gruntar I, et al. In vitro antimicrobial susceptibility testing of *Helicobacter felis, H. bizzozeronii*, and *H. salomonis*. Antimicrob Agents Chemother. 2005;49:2997-3000.
49. Priestnall SL, Wiinberg B, Spohr A, et al. Evaluation of "*Helicobacter heilmannii*" subtypes in the gastric mucosas of cats and dogs. J Clin Microbiol. 2004;42:2144-2151.
50. Herbrink P, van Doorn LJ. Serological methods for diagnosis of *Helicobacter pylori* infection and monitoring of eradication therapy. Eur J Clin Microbiol Infect Dis. 2000;19:164-173.
51. Talebkhan Y, Ebrahimzadeh F, Esmaeili M, et al. *Helicobacter pylori* Omp18 and its application in serologic screening of infection. Curr Microbiol. 2011;62:325-330.
52. Seidel KE, Stolte M, Lehn N, et al. Antibodies against *Helicobacter felis* in sera of cats and dogs. Zentralbl Veterinarmed B. 1999;46:181-188.
53. Strauss-Ayali D, Scanziani E, Deng D, et al. *Helicobacter* spp. infection in cats: evaluation of the humoral immune response and prevalence of gastric *Helicobacter* spp. Vet Microbiol. 2001;79:253-265.
54. Strauss-Ayali D, Simpson KW, Schein AH, et al. Serological discrimination of dogs infected with gastric *Helicobacter* spp. and uninfected dogs. J Clin Microbiol. 1999;37:1280-1287.
55. Calvet X, Sanchez-Delgado J, Montserrat A, et al. Accuracy of diagnostic tests for *Helicobacter pylori*: a reappraisal. Clin Infect Dis. 2009;48:1385-1391.
56. Cornetta AM, Simpson KW, Strauss-Ayali D, et al. Use of a [^{13}C] urea breath test for detection of gastric infection with *Helicobacter* spp in dogs. Am J Vet Res. 1998;59:1364-1369.
57. Neiger R, Seiler G, Schmassmann A. Use of a urea breath test to evaluate short-term treatments for cats naturally infected with *Helicobacter heilmannii*. Am J Vet Res. 1999;60:880-883.
58. Scanziani E, Simpson KW, Monestiroli S, et al. Histological and immunohistochemical detection of different *Helicobacter* species in the gastric mucosa of cats. J Vet Diagn Invest. 2001;13:3-12.
59. Simpson KW, Strauss-Ayali D, Scanziani E, et al. *Helicobacter felis* infection is associated with lymphoid follicular hyperplasia and mild gastritis but normal gastric secretory function in cats. Infect Immun. 2000;68:779-790.
60. Simpson KW, Strauss-Ayali D, Straubinger RK, et al. *Helicobacter pylori* infection in the cat: evaluation of gastric colonization, inflammation and function. Helicobacter. 2001;6:1-14.
61. Graham DY, Fischbach L. *Helicobacter pylori* treatment in the era of increasing antibiotic resistance. Gut. 2010;59:1143-1153.
62. Happonen I, Linden J, Westermarck E. Effect of triple therapy on eradication of canine gastric helicobacters and gastric disease. J Small Anim Pract. 2000;41:1-6.
63. Perkins SE, Yan LL, Shen Z, et al. Use of PCR and culture to detect *Helicobacter pylori* in naturally infected cats following triple antimicrobial therapy. Antimicrob Agents Chemother. 1996;40:1486-1490.
64. Anacleto TP, Lopes LR, Andreollo NA, et al. Studies of distribution and recurrence of *Helicobacter* spp. gastric mucosa of dogs after triple therapy. Acta Cir Bras. 2011;26:82-87.
65. Velin D, Michetti P. Advances in vaccination against *Helicobacter pylori*. Expert Rev Gastroenterol Hepatol. 2010;4:157-166.
66. Herrera V, Parsonnet J. *Helicobacter pylori* and gastric adenocarcinoma. Clin Microbiol Infect. 2009;15:971-976.
67. McColl KE. Clinical practice. *Helicobacter pylori* infection. N Engl J Med. 2010;362:1597-1604.
68. Dieterich C, Wiesel P, Neiger R, et al. Presence of multiple "*Helicobacter heilmannii*" strains in an individual suffering from ulcers and in his two cats. J Clin Microbiol. 1998;36:1366-1370.
69. Lavelle JP, Landas S, Mitros FA, et al. Acute gastritis associated with spiral organisms from cats. Dig Dis Sci. 1994;39:744-750.
70. Thomson MA, Storey P, Greer R, et al. Canine-human transmission of *Gastrospirillum hominis*. Lancet. 1994;344:1097-1098.
71. van Loon S, Bart A, den Hertog EJ, et al. *Helicobacter heilmannii* gastritis caused by cat to child transmission. J Pediatr Gastroenterol Nutr. 2003;36:407-409.
72. Meining A, Kroher G, Stolte M. Animal reservoirs in the transmission of *Helicobacter heilmannii*. Results of a questionnaire-based study. Scand J Gastroenterol. 1998;33:795-798.
73. De Groote D, Ducatelle R, Haesebrouck F. Helicobacters of possible zoonotic origin: a review. Acta Gastroenterol Belg. 2000;63:380-387.
74. Minauchi K, Takahashi S, Sakai T, et al. The nosocomial transmission of *Helicobacter cinaedi* infections in immunocompromised patients. Intern Med. 2010;49:1733-1739.

CHAPTER 50

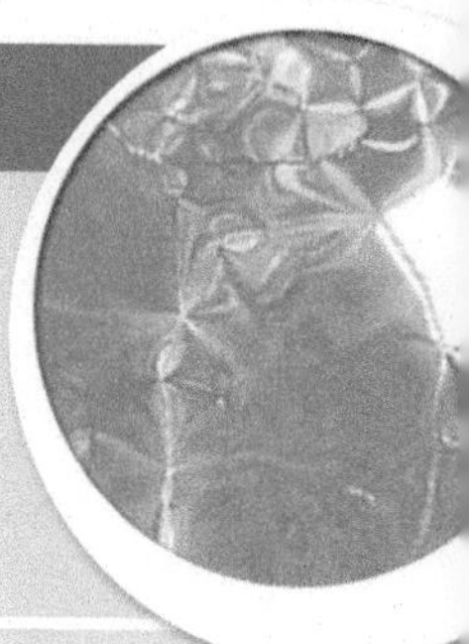

Leptospirosis

Jane E. Sykes

Overview of Leptospirosis

First Described: Heidelberg, Germany, 1886 (Adolf Weil)[1]

Cause: *Leptospira* spp. (a spirochete)

Affected Hosts: Dogs, rarely cats, more than 150 other mammalian species

Geographic Distribution: Worldwide

Major Clinical Signs: Fever, lethargy, reluctance to move, anorexia, polyuria and polydipsia, vomiting, diarrhea, icterus, respiratory difficulty

Major Differential Diagnoses: Nephrotoxicoses (e.g., NSAIDs, grapes and raisins, ethylene glycol), Lyme nephritis, acute glomerulonephritides, bacterial pyelonephritis, acute pancreatitis, canine monocytic ehrlichiosis, Rocky Mountain Spotted Fever, bacterial sepsis, leishmaniosis

Human Health Significance: Zoonosis. Human infection results from direct or indirect contact with contaminated urine. No signs, a mild influenza-like illness, or severe illness with multiorgan failure (Weil's disease) have the potential to occur.

Etiologic Agent and Epidemiology

Leptospirosis is a widespread zoonotic disease caused by systemic infection by pathogenic spirochetes of the genus *Leptospira*. *Leptospira* spp. are thin (0.1 μm in diameter), flexible, motile, spiral-shaped bacteria that have a hook-shaped end (*leptos* = "thin," *spira* = "coiled"). A huge variety of different mammalian species may be infected by leptospires. These hosts can shed the organism in their urine and contaminate the environment. Infection of incidental hosts results in disease that varies in severity from a mild febrile illness to severe multisystemic disease. Both dogs and cats can develop leptospirosis, but cats appear to be relatively resistant to development of clinical illness. As a result, leptospirosis is uncommonly described in cats.[2-5]

Both pathogenic and saprophyte *Leptospira* species exist in nature. Saprophytic species, such as *Leptospira biflexa,* live in water and soil and do not infect animal hosts. Disease in dogs is primarily caused by the pathogenic species *Leptospira interrogans* and *Leptospira kirschneri.* Within the genus *Leptospira*, more than 250 different serovars of pathogenic leptospires are recognized, which are distinguished based on differences in their lipopolysaccharide (LPS) O antigens. The serovars are grouped into more than 20 antigenically related serogroups (Table 50-1). At least 10 serovars have been associated with disease in dogs worldwide. Each serovar is adapted to one or more wild or domestic animal reservoir host species (see Table 50-1).

Recently, PCR-based DNA typing methods have been used to identify *Leptospira* strains on the basis of their genotype, instead of using the serovar classification method. Specific genotypes appear to associate more strongly with particular reservoir hosts and disease manifestations than has been found for serovars.[6,7] Multiple different leptospiral serovars have been isolated from single outbreaks of human leptospirosis associated with specific clinical manifestations (such as pulmonary hemorrhage).[8] Therefore, virulence factors other than outer surface antigens (which define serovars) may more important determinants of clinical manifestations of disease than the identity of the infecting serovar.

Pathogenic *Leptospira* species do not replicate outside the host and are readily inactivated in the environment when exposed to excessive heat, ultraviolet irradiation, a variety of disinfectants, and freezing conditions. However, when conditions are optimal, pathogenic leptospires can survive in water and wet soil for weeks to months.[9] Dogs that drink from, swim, or wade in environmental water sources can become infected; exposure to wildlife or farm animals and their urine is also a risk factor. In developing countries, dogs may be infected as a result of access to sewage.[10] Although the "classic" signalment for a dog with leptospirosis is a large-breed, outdoor, intact male dog, dogs of any age, breed, and sex may be affected. For example, geriatric, small-breed dogs that live in urban or suburban areas and that contact rodents or rodent urine can develop the disease. Indeed, over the past decade, residence in urban areas has emerged as a risk factor for *Leptospira* infection in dogs in some parts of North America, possibly due to exposure to urban wildlife species.[11] Cats may be infected after ingestion of infected prey, so outdoor exposure and hunting behavior may be risk factors for cats.[2]

Outbreaks of disease in dogs have been correlated with periods of high annual rainfall and may occur approximately 3 months after wet weather.[12-14] The peak seasonal distribution in parts of North America where freezing winters occur is late fall,[11,15,16] but in more temperate regions, peak seasonal distribution occurs after months of high rainfall (such as in the winter in northern California).[13] Leptospirosis is most prevalent in parts of the world where there is higher annual rainfall and a warm climate, but the presence of infected reservoir hosts also influences the geographic distribution of leptospirosis. Within North America, dogs that live in or travel to Hawaii, northern California, Oregon, Washington, the upper Midwest and Midwest, parts of Texas, Colorado, and the northeastern and mid-Atlantic coastal regions may be more likely to develop infection.[17] Leptospirosis also occurs in dogs in the southeastern United States,[18] and the disease has been widely reported in dogs from Ontario in Canada.[16] Numerous reports describe leptospirosis in dogs from across Europe.[19] Major disease foci among people include the Caribbean, Central and South America, India, Southeast Asia, South America, and Oceania.

TABLE 50-1

Selected Serovars of *Leptospira interrogans* and *Leptospira kirschneri* that Infect Dogs*

Species	Serogroup	Serovar	Potential Reservoir Hosts	Country
Leptospira interrogans	Icterohaemorrhagiae	Icterohaemorrhagiae	Rats	United States, France
	Canicola	Canicola	Dogs	India, United States
	Pomona	Pomona	Horses, cattle, sea lions	United States
	Australis	Bratislava	Pigs, hedgehogs, horses	United States
	Sejroe	ND	Mice	Germany
	Ballum	Ballum	Mice, gray squirrels, muskrats, opossums	United States
Leptospira kirschneri	Grippotyphosa	Grippotyphosa	Raccoons, fox squirrels, muskrats, bobcats, voles, mice, rats, cattle, horses	United States

*Isolated from dogs with naturally-occurring leptospirosis, or that induce disease in dogs after experimental inoculation.

Worldwide, the most common serovars thought to infect dogs before the introduction of canine *Leptospira* vaccines several decades ago were Icterohaemorrhagiae and Canicola.[20] Since that time, widespread seroconversion to other serovars, especially Grippotyphosa and Pomona in North America, has been noted in sick dogs. Increased testing for these serovars may have contributed to this phenomenon, as well as increased contact between dogs and wildlife and farm animal reservoir hosts for these serovars.[21] Serovars that currently cause disease in the dog population are poorly understood, because the results of serology do not accurately predict the infecting serovar,[22] and culture and identification of leptospiral serovars is insensitive, requires significant technical expertise, and is not widely available (see Diagnosis, later).[23]

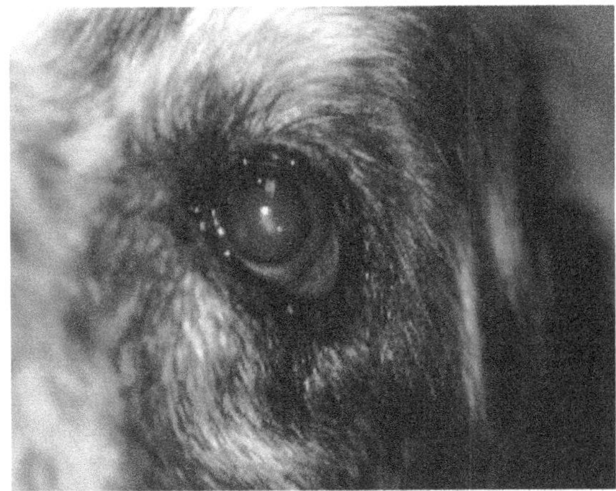

FIGURE 50-1 Uveitis in an Australian shepherd with leptospirosis with leakage of serum bilirubin into the aqueous humor.

Clinical Features

Signs and Their Pathogenesis

Pathogenic leptospires penetrate intact mucous membranes or abraded skin. They multiply rapidly in the bloodstream as early as 1 day postinfection, which may be followed by the development of vasculitis and multiorgan failure. The spirochetes can produce a variety of toxins, including phospholipases, sphingomyelinases, and pore-forming proteins. Infection follows direct contact with infected urine or, more commonly, contact with soil, water, food, or other fomites that have been contaminated with infected urine. Transmission has also occurred as a result of bite wound inoculation (such as from infected rodents), ingestion of infected tissues, and venereal and placental transfer.

The incubation period for acute leptospirosis is approximately 7 days, but may be shorter or longer depending on the dose and strain virulence of the leptospires involved, and the host immune response.[24] Dogs can also develop signs of chronic kidney disease months or more than a year after acute kidney injury. Early renal damage in this situation may be associated with transient or undetected clinical signs, which are subsequently followed by either clearance or persistence of infection and progression of renal damage. Longer incubation periods might occur in cats,[2] but further study is required.

Leptospirosis varies considerably in severity, which may contribute to underrecognition of the disease. Many dogs probably show no signs of illness or develop only a mild, transient febrile illness. Severe clinical signs and death result from renal failure and/or injury to the liver and lungs. Leptospirosis should be suspected in dogs that develop signs of acute febrile illness, kidney and hepatic injury, uveitis, or pulmonary hemorrhage; it should also be suspected in breeding dogs with abortion, stillbirths, or neonatal deaths.[20] Clinical signs in affected cats resemble those in dogs, although some cats have lacked evidence of hepatic injury.[2]

Fever occurs only at the onset of illness and is often accompanied by shivering, reluctance to move, and generalized muscle tenderness that may result from myositis. This may be followed by signs of lethargy, polyuria and polydipsia, inappetence, vomiting, and diarrhea.[24-27] Gastrointestinal signs in some dogs may result from pancreatitis and enteritis, in addition to acute renal and liver damage. Polyuria and polydipsia may result from a decreased responsiveness of the inner medullary connecting ducts to antidiuretic hormone (acquired nephrogenic diabetes insipidus). However, some dogs show decreased thirst and urination. Liver involvement leads to icterus in some dogs (Figure 50-1). Components of leptospiral endotoxin such as oleic and linoleic acid are thought to interfere with hepatic transport pumps, which leads to functional hepatic impairment.[28] Hepatocyte apoptosis and injury to hepatocyte membranes is also suspected

TABLE 50-2

Complete Blood Count Findings at Admission in Dogs with Leptospirosis from Northern California*

Test	Reference Range	Percent Below the Reference Range	Percent Within the Reference Range	Percent Above the Reference Range	Range for Dogs with Leptospirosis	Number Tested
Hematocrit (%)	40-55	78	22	0	12-48	54
Neutrophils (cells/µL)	3000-10,500	0	35	65	3474-14,311	54
Band neutrophils (cells/µL)	Rare	0	63	37	0-2954	54
Monocytes (cells/µL)	150-1200	0	65	35	162-4594	54
Lymphocytes (cells/µL)	1000-4000	30	70	0	162-3769	54
Eosinophils (cells/µL)	0-1500	0	100	0	0-970	54
Platelets (cells/µL)	150,000-400,000	28	61	11	40,000-522,000	53

*Diagnosis based on results of acute and convalescent phase serology together with consistent clinical signs.

to occur; leptospirosis in humans and guinea pig models is associated with loss of the cellular adhesion molecule E-cadherin on hepatocytes.[20]

Less commonly, uveitis, myocardial damage, or reproductive complications occur. Leptospiral DNA can be detected in the aqueous humor of human patients with leptospiral uveitis, and the development of uveitis may be delayed up to 18 months after the onset of acute illness.[29] ECG alterations can occur in dogs that suggest myocardial damage.[30] Abortion can occur during pregnancy.[31] Stillbirth and neonatal deaths have also been described.

Bleeding tendencies in dogs with leptospirosis may be manifested as petechial hemorrhages, hematuria, hematemesis, epistaxis, hematochezia, or melena.[25,30,32] Although the precise mechanisms are unknown, bleeding tendencies may reflect the presence of endothelial damage and disordered coagulation. In human patients, thrombocytopenia (≤100,000 platelets/µL) and prolonged PT have been associated with bleeding.[33,34] Tachypnea may be noted as a result of severe pulmonary hemorrhage syndrome (SPHS).[35,36] SPHS is recognized commonly in humans with severe leptospirosis, is not associated with significant lung colonization by the spirochete, and seems to have an immune-mediated pathogenesis.[37] The prevalence of SPHS in dogs appears to be particularly high in continental Europe. For example, pulmonary complications occurred in more than two thirds of dogs with leptospirosis in Berlin.[36] Vasculitis can also contribute to the development of peripheral edema and mild pleural and peritoneal effusions. In human patients, aseptic meningitis is a common complication of leptospirosis and results in signs of severe headache, delirium, and less commonly seizures and altered sensory perception.[38] Whether meningitis occurs in dogs is unknown.

The extent to which leptospires can cause chronic hepatic injury in dogs is also unknown. In one report from France, leptospires were detected in bile canaliculi of young dogs with chronic hepatitis using immunohistochemistry and electron microscopy. These dogs showed signs of poor growth, weight loss, and ascites.[39,40] Attempts to detect *Leptospira* DNA in liver tissue from dogs with chronic active hepatitis have been unrewarding.

Physical Examination Findings

Findings on physical examination of dogs with leptospirosis vary with disease severity, chronicity, and the infecting leptospiral strain. Severely affected dogs may show fever, dull mentation, dehydration, mild generalized peripheral lymphadenopathy, diffuse muscle pain, and pain on palpation of the abdomen or kidneys. Fever is typically only present early in the course of infection. In oliguric or anuric dogs that have been treated aggressively with intravenous fluids, evidence of overhydration may be present. Rarely, arrhythmias are detected on cardiac auscultation. Careful ophthalmologic examination may reveal conjunctivitis, scleral injection, and occasionally uveitis. Mild pallor, petechial or ecchymotic hemorrhages, and, less commonly, epistaxis may be present. Respiratory difficulty, tachypnea, and harsh lung sounds may be evident in dogs that develop pulmonary complications. Dogs with liver involvement may be icteric. Rectal examination occasionally reveals melena or hematochezia.

Diagnosis

Laboratory Abnormalities

Complete Blood Count

The hemogram in dogs with leptospirosis may reveal neutrophilia, sometimes with bandemia; nonregenerative anemia; lymphopenia; and/or thrombocytopenia (Table 50-2). Thrombocytopenia occurs in up to 53% of dogs.[25,26,30,41] The mechanism is unclear; disseminated intravascular coagulation (DIC) or immune-mediated mechanisms may be involved.

Serum Biochemical Tests

Findings on the serum chemistry panel vary depending on leptospiral strains that circulate in a particular geographic region (Table 50-3). In all geographic locations, a combination of azotemia and elevated liver enzyme activities, especially when thrombocytopenia is present, should raise suspicion for leptospirosis. Azotemia is generally present in more than 80% to 90% of dogs,[25,26,30,42] although in one European study, increased serum creatinine concentration was present in only 57% of affected dogs.[41] Uncommonly, dogs exhibit increased liver enzyme activities in the absence of azotemia. Signs of hepatic dysfunction are associated with minimal histologic damage to the liver and include variable, and generally mild to moderate, increases in serum ALT, AST, and ALP activities and total bilirubin concentration.

TABLE 50-3

Serum Biochemistry Findings at Admission in Dogs with Leptospirosis from Northern California*

Test (Number of Dogs Tested)	Reference Range	Percent Below the Reference Range	Percent Within the Reference Range	Percent Above the Reference Range	Range for Dogs with Leptospirosis	Number of Dogs Tested
Sodium (mmol/L)	145-154	33	61	6	134-162	54
Potassium (mmol/L)	4.1-5.3	35	44	20	2.8-7.6	54
Chloride (mmol/L)	105-116	57	37	6	98-118	54
Bicarbonate (mmol/L)	16-26	33	61	6	11-28	54
Calcium (mg/dL)	9.9-11.4	39	44	17	7.2-10.9	54
Phosphorus (mg/dL)	3.0-6.2	0	9	91	2.7-13.0	54
Creatinine (mg/dL)	0.5-1.6	0	0	100	0.4-3.3	54
BUN (mg/dL)	8-31	0	2	98	8-110	54
Albumin (g/dL)	2.9-4.2	96	4	0	0.9-3.8	54
Globulin (g/dL)	2.3-4.4	9	78	13	1.6-4.7	54
Cholesterol (mg/dL)	135-345	4	91		79-408	54
Total bilirubin (mg/dL)	0-0.4	0	69	32	0-3.1	54
ALT (U/L)	19-70	0	43	48	17-1443	54
ALP (U/L)	15-127	0	67	33	29-985	54
CK (U/L)	46-320	31	8	62	5-258,720	13

*Diagnosis based on results of acute and convalescent phase serology together with consistent clinical signs.

Other findings on the serum chemistry panel include hypoalbuminemia and a variety of electrolyte abnormalities. Hyponatremia, hypochloremia, or hyperphosphatemia occur in most dogs. Decreased expression of sodium transporters by proximal convoluted tubule cells contributes to impaired sodium resorption, increased distal sodium delivery, and potassium wasting.[43] As a result, dogs with acute oliguric renal failure may have paradoxical hypokalemia.

Moderately and occasionally markedly increased serum CK activity is present in some dogs due to myositis. Increased serum troponin concentrations have been found in some dogs with leptospirosis, which suggests myocardial damage.[30] Increased serum pancreatic lipase immunoreactivity may occur, probably as a result of pancreatitis.

Urinalysis

Findings on urinalysis in dogs with leptospirosis include isosthenuria, occasionally hyposthenuria, and variable glucosuria, proteinuria, pyuria, cylindruria, and bilirubinuria.[20,26,30,42] Urine protein to creatinine (UPC) ratios may be increased. Glucosuria was present in 77% of 44 dogs with leptospirosis at the author's institution, and in 21 dogs that had UPC ratios measured, the ratios ranged from 0.4 to 11.6 (median, 3, reference range less than 0.5). Most proteins in the urine are of low molecular weight, which supports a tubular rather than glomerular origin of these proteins.[30,44] Leptospires are not visible in urine sediment by routine light microscopy.

Coagulation Function

Aside from thrombocytopenia, analysis of hemostatic function in dogs with leptospirosis shows variable increases in fibrinogen, D-dimer, and fibrinogen degradation product concentrations. Antithrombin activity may be decreased. Prolongations in PT and PTT have been present in up to 15% of tested dogs.[20,26,30] PT prolongations are associated with mortality in human patients.[34] In some dogs, a shortened PT is present,[42] possibly because of DIC. In human patients, leptospirosis has been associated with an imbalance between coagulation and fibrinolysis.[34]

Diagnostic Imaging

Plain Radiography

Plain thoracic radiography in dogs with leptospirosis may show no abnormalities, or mild to severe, diffuse interstitial pulmonary patterns may be present. Thoracic radiographs from dogs with SPHS can show severe nodular to diffuse interstitial and alveolar patterns (Figure 50-2). Uncommonly, mild pleural effusion is present.

Sonographic Findings

Findings on abdominal sonography include mild renomegaly, increased renal cortical echogenicity, mild pyelectasia, perirenal fluid accumulation or mild ascites, and a medullary band of increased echogenicity within the kidneys (Figure 50-3).[45] None of these signs are specific for leptospirosis. Ultrasonographic changes suggestive of pancreatitis are occasionally present, such as enlargement and hypoechogenicity of the pancreas. Thickening of the gastric, and less commonly small intestinal wall may also be present. Mild to moderate hepatomegaly and splenomegaly with mottling of the splenic echotexture may be detected, with or without evidence of mild abdominal lymphadenomegaly.

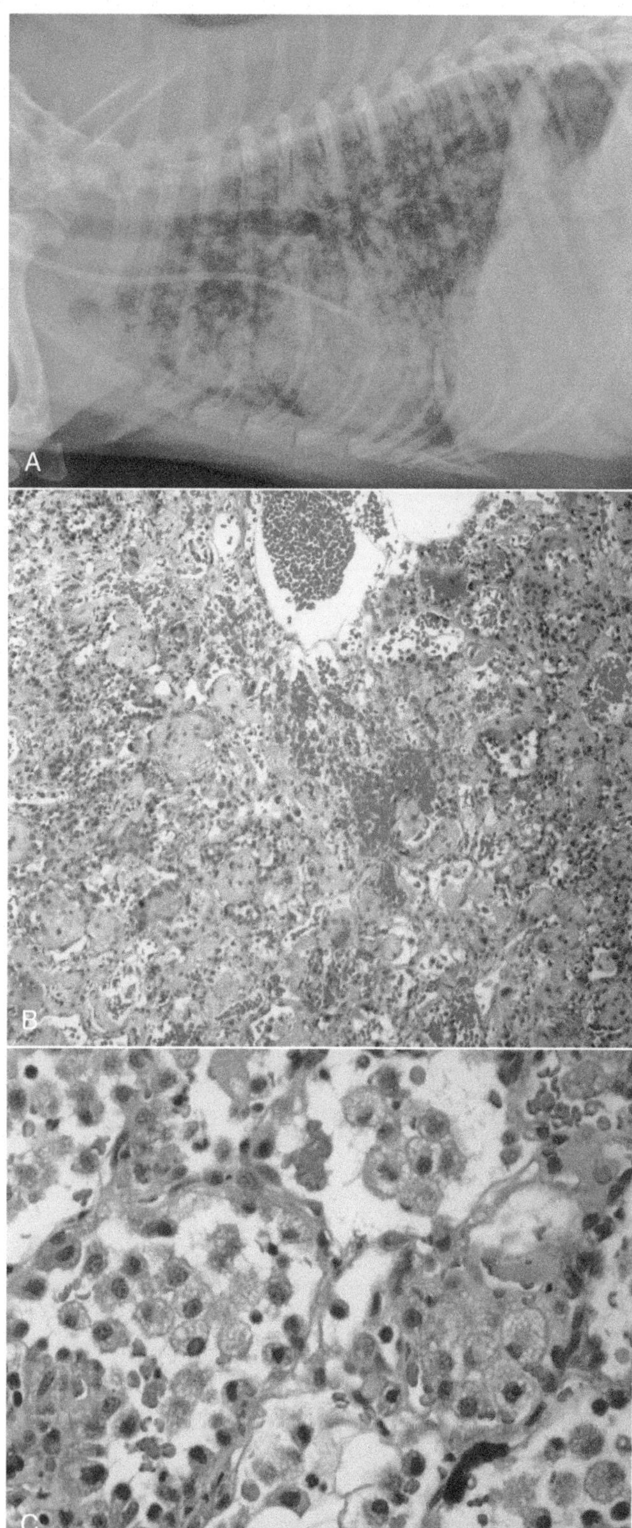

FIGURE 50-2 Clinical images from a 4-year-old male neutered Havanese terrier with severe leptospiral pulmonary hemorrhage syndrome and anuric renal failure. **A,** Right lateral thoracic radiograph. A severe, diffuse alveolar pattern is present. Mechanical ventilation was needed and ultimately euthanasia was performed because of respiratory failure. Histopathology of a lung biopsy showed severe pulmonary hemorrhage **(B)** and marked alveolar histiocytosis **(C)**.

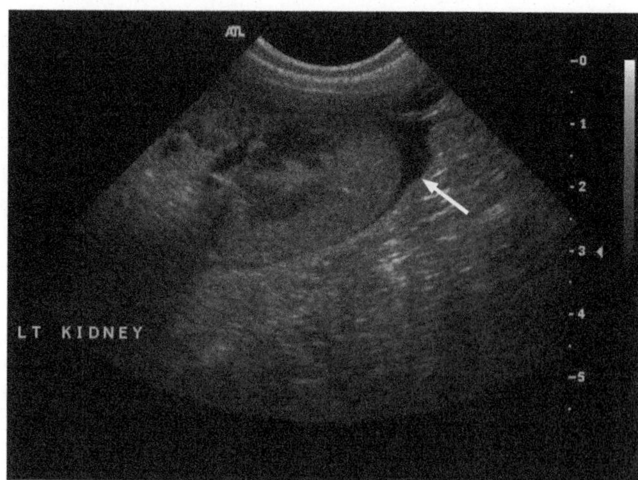

FIGURE 50-3 Abdominal sonogram image showing perirenal fluid accumulation in a 1.5-year-old male neutered kelpie with renal failure due to acute leptospirosis.

Microbiologic Tests

Diagnostic assays available for leptospirosis in dogs are described in Table 50-4. Most often, diagnosis is based on acute and convalescent phase serology.

Darkfield Microscopy

Examination of urine sediment using darkfield microscopy is insensitive for diagnosis of leptospirosis. Considerable experience is required to accurately identify the spirochetes, so false positives also have the potential to occur.

Culture

Culture of leptospires is not routinely performed, because it is slow, can be insensitive, and is not widely available. Special leptospira growth media is required, such as Ellinghausen-McCullough-Johnson-Harris (EMJH) medium. Cultures must be incubated for up to 3 to 6 months, and overgrowth with other bacteria can occur if cultures become contaminated. Venous blood and/or urine should be collected using aseptic technique before initiating antimicrobial drug treatment. Ideally, a few drops of blood or urine are inoculated directly into culture medium alongside the patient. In humans, blood is optimally collected during the initial febrile period; urine can be collected after the first week of illness. Because the exact time of infection may be unknown, submission of both blood and urine can increase the chance of a positive test result.

Only certain reference laboratories have expertise in culture of leptospires and the ability to identify leptospires to the serovar level, which is performed using a cross agglutinin absorption test. Genetic typing methods such as pulsed field gel electrophoresis can also be performed.[23] Despite the difficulties associated with culture and identification of leptospires, a proper understanding of the epidemiology of leptospirosis depends on the use of these methods.

Serologic Diagnosis

Currently the test of choice for diagnosis of leptospirosis is serology using the microscopic agglutination test (MAT).[20] In this assay, the laboratory mixes serial dilutions of patient sera with a panel of live leptospiral serovars. The laboratory then reports the agglutinating antibody titer for each of the serovars tested,

TABLE 50-4

Diagnostic Assays Available for Leptospirosis in Dogs

Assay	Specimen Type	Target	Performance
Darkfield microscopy	Urine	*Leptospira* organisms	Low sensitivity and specificity. Requires considerable technical expertise to interpret correctly.
Culture	Whole blood, urine	Leptospires	Low sensitivity. Special media and prolonged incubation times required. Difficult and not widely available. Antimicrobial therapy may lead to false-negative results. Currently the only method that permits accurate serovar identification.
Serology (MAT)	Serum	Antibodies against various leptospiral serovars	False negatives can occur early in the course of illness or with immunosuppression. False positives can occur with a history of vaccination or with previous exposure. Paired titers performed at the same laboratory generally required for diagnosis. Interlaboratory variation in results may occur.
Histopathology	Kidney tissue collected via biopsy or necropsy	Leptospires	Organisms may be visualized with silver stains, immunohistochemistry, or fluorescence in situ hybridization. Antimicrobial therapy may lead to false-negative results.
PCR	Blood, urine, tissue specimens	*Leptospira* DNA	Sensitivity and specificity unclear and may vary between assays offered by different laboratories. Antimicrobial therapy may lead to negative PCR results.

which is the highest dilution of serum that causes the organisms to agglutinate as assessed using darkfield microscopy. Seropositive dogs can have high titers to multiple serovars tested because of serologic cross-reactivity. The highest titer does not necessarily predict the infecting serovar.[22] The serovar that produces the highest titer may also change when serology is repeated over the course of illness.[20]

Documentation of a fourfold or greater increase in titer to at least one serovar over time is usually required for diagnosis using the MAT, because titers are often low or negative in the first few days of illness, and a single high titer can result from previous exposure or a history of vaccination for leptospirosis. Later in the course of illness, a fourfold decrease in titer may also be appropriate for diagnosis. Traditionally, convalescent titers are performed 2 to 4 weeks after the acute titer, although seroconversion can sometimes occur as early as 3 to 5 days after the initial titer is obtained. Nevertheless, successive titers should be spaced at least 1 week apart, and it is critically important to use the same laboratory for each set of titers.[20] Antimicrobial treatment has the potential to blunt a rise in titer, but dogs usually seroconvert despite antimicrobial treatment.[42] Titers that result from previous vaccination, previous exposure or chronic infection generally change by one dilution over time (e.g., from 1:400 to 1:800) or remain static. Titers persist for at least 1 year after natural infection, although they often decline by 4 months after vaccination.[46] Nevertheless, postvaccinal titers can persist for longer than a year and be maintained at high levels (≥1600), especially if ongoing exposure to field strains occurs. Thus, although single positive titers can raise suspicion for the disease, they cannot be used to confirm the diagnosis of leptospirosis. After immunization, paradoxical cross-reactivity to serogroups other than those used in the vaccine can occur,[46] so titers to non-vaccinal serovars in vaccinated dogs do not necessarily imply natural exposure to field strains.

False-negative titers have the potential to occur if the infecting serovar (or a related serovar) is not included in the panel of serovars used to perform the test. Assays for diagnosis of human leptospirosis generally include a larger panel of serovars (>20) than those used routinely in veterinary diagnostics (5 to 7 serovars). Assays should optimally include serovars from serogroups that are known to circulate in the local dog population, although this information is not often readily available.

The MAT is widely available and relatively inexpensive, but is complex to perform and interpret. Performance of the test is hazardous to laboratory workers because live pathogenic serovars are used, and the test is difficult to standardize. Considerable interlaboratory variation in results can occur, in terms of both the magnitude of the titers reported and the pattern of seroreactivity to each serovar included in the test.[47] The identity of serovars used in the assay must be verified periodically to ensure that cross-contamination or culture deterioration has not occurred. A leptospirosis proficiency testing scheme is offered by the International Leptospirosis Society (ILS) to assist laboratories in the maintenance of quality assurance for the MAT.[48,49] Veterinarians should strive to use laboratories that participate in this quality assurance scheme.

Other serologic assays under investigation for diagnosis of leptospirosis include ELISA assays for IgG and IgM antibodies that are directed against leptospiral surface antigens.[50-53] The performance of such assays have the potential to vary geographically based on the serogroups that are prevalent in the region. In Europe, a lateral-flow assay that detects IgM (Test-it, Royal Tropical Institute/Life Assay Diagnostics) is available for diagnosis of acute canine leptospirosis.[50] This assay appeared to have high clinical sensitivity for diagnosis of leptospirosis in dogs in the Netherlands (100%) and the West Indies (78%), with a low rate of false positives in healthy dogs from the Netherlands, the West Indies, and Mexico (<5%).

Molecular Diagnosis Using the Polymerase Chain Reaction

Several veterinary diagnostic laboratories in the United States and Europe offer PCR assays for the detection of the DNA of pathogenic leptospires in blood and/or urine. The sensitivity and specificity of these assays in dogs with leptospirosis has not been thoroughly assessed and have the potential to vary geographically, because of differences in shedding patterns for different serovars. Assay performance also is likely to vary from one laboratory to another. PCR assays have the potential to be advantageous for diagnosis early in the course of illness, when serologic tests are negative, or in dogs that possess residual antibody after vaccination. Specimens for PCR testing are best obtained before initiation of antimicrobial drug treatment, and both blood and urine should be submitted in order to optimize sensitivity. Negative results do not rule out a diagnosis of leptospirosis. Because subclinically infected dogs can shed leptospires, a positive PCR test result on urine may not necessarily correlate with illness. Vaccination of healthy dogs with inactivated *Leptospira* vaccines should not lead to positive PCR assay results,[54] so a history of *Leptospira* vaccination should not interfere with PCR diagnosis. Currently available PCR assays do not provide information on the infecting serovar or serogroup.

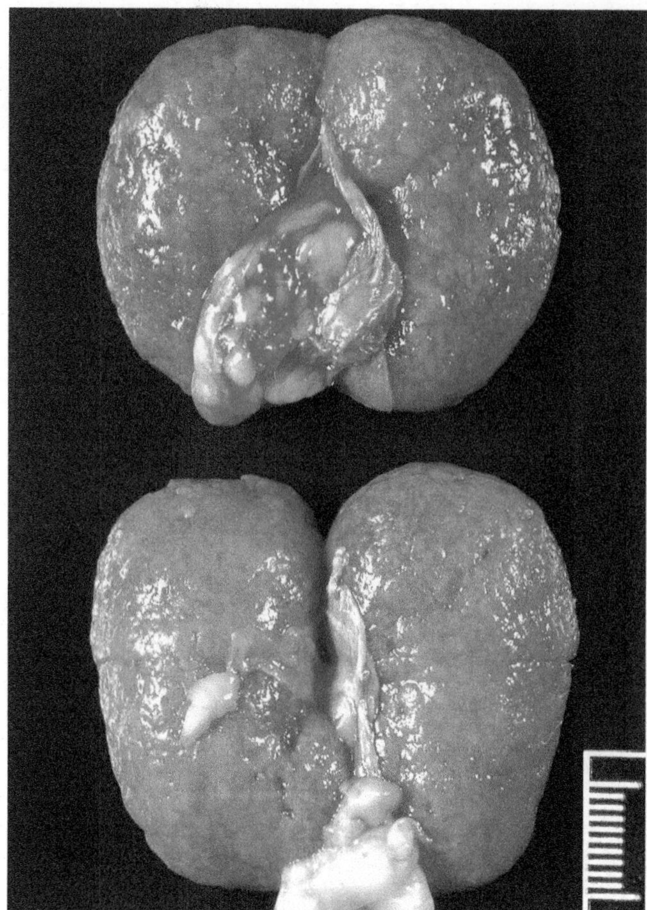

FIGURE 50-4 Shrunken, irregular kidneys from a 16-year-old male neutered Jack Russell terrier. The dog was treated for severe acute leptospirosis at 12 years of age. At that time, after six dialysis treatments, the dog was discharged from the hospital with a creatinine of 4.2 mg/dL. Four years later, the dog died for reasons unrelated to renal injury but had evidence of chronic renal injury at necropsy. (Image courtesy UC Davis Veterinary Anatomic Pathology Service.)

Pathologic Findings

Gross Pathologic Findings

Gross pathologic findings in dogs with leptospirosis include jaundice, petechial and ecchymotic hemorrhages, and sometimes fibrin thrombi throughout the body. The lungs of dogs with SPHS may be wet, mottled, heavy, and dark-pink to red in color.[36] Ascites and/or pleural or pericardial effusion may be present, and the intestinal lumen may be filled with blood or contain melena. The kidneys of dogs with acute disease may be mildly enlarged, pale and sometimes mottled or petechiated; they may also contain infarcts. Dogs with chronic renal injury secondary to the infection can have kidneys that are shrunken and irregular (Figure 50-4).

Histopathologic Findings

Infection of the kidneys by leptospires leads to an interstitial nephritis, with mixed inflammatory infiltrates. Acute tubular necrosis can also occur as a result of vasculitis and renal ischemia (Figure 50-5, *A*).[36] Histopathologic changes in the liver are often mild and include mild random hepatic necrosis, mild neutrophilic periportal hepatitis, cholestasis, or liver plate disarray (Figure 50-6). Multifocal, random, neutrophilic, and necrotizing myocarditis can also occur; myonecrosis is occasionally described in skeletal muscle. Lung pathology in dogs with SPHS resembles that described in human patients and consists of intra-alveolar hemorrhage, pneumocyte necrosis, and hyaline membrane formation, in the absence of significant inflammation.

Silver stains such as Warthin-Starry stain and immunohistochemistry can be used to visualize bacteria within tissue specimens (see Figure 50-5, *B*). Fluorescence in situ hybridization has also been used to identify and localize leptospires within the kidneys (see Figure 5-1).

Treatment and Prognosis

Antimicrobial Drugs

Penicillins or doxycycline are recommended for initial treatment of humans and dogs with leptospirosis. Treatment should be initiated as early as possible, before the results of diagnostic assays become available. In hamster models, doxycycline clears spirochetes from all tissues, including the kidney, within 3 days of infection; ampicillin is less effective at clearing organisms from the kidney.[55] Based on current evidence, the ACVIM Consensus Statement on leptospirosis in dogs

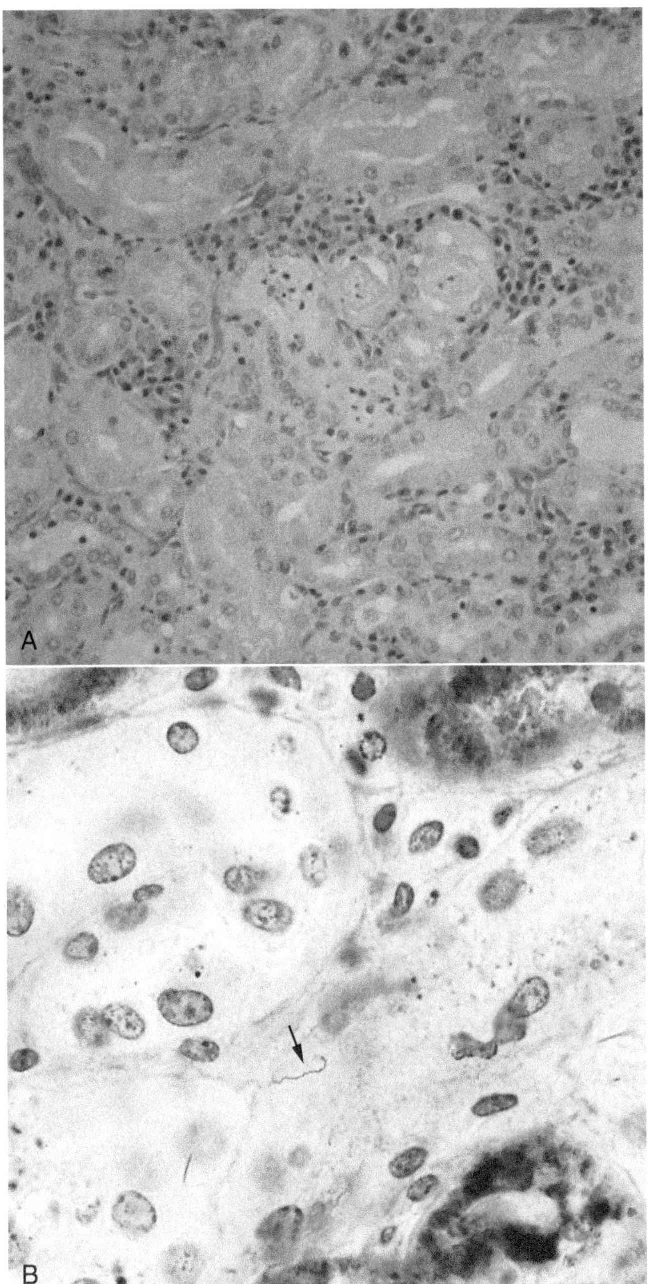

FIGURE 50-5 **A,** Histopathology of the kidney of a dog that died of leptospirosis. Acute tubular necrosis and interstitial nephritis is present. H&E stain. **B,** Warthin-Starry showing low numbers of leptospires in the renal interstitium *(arrow)*. (Images courtesy Dr. Patricia Pesavento, University of California, Davis Veterinary Anatomic Pathology Service.)

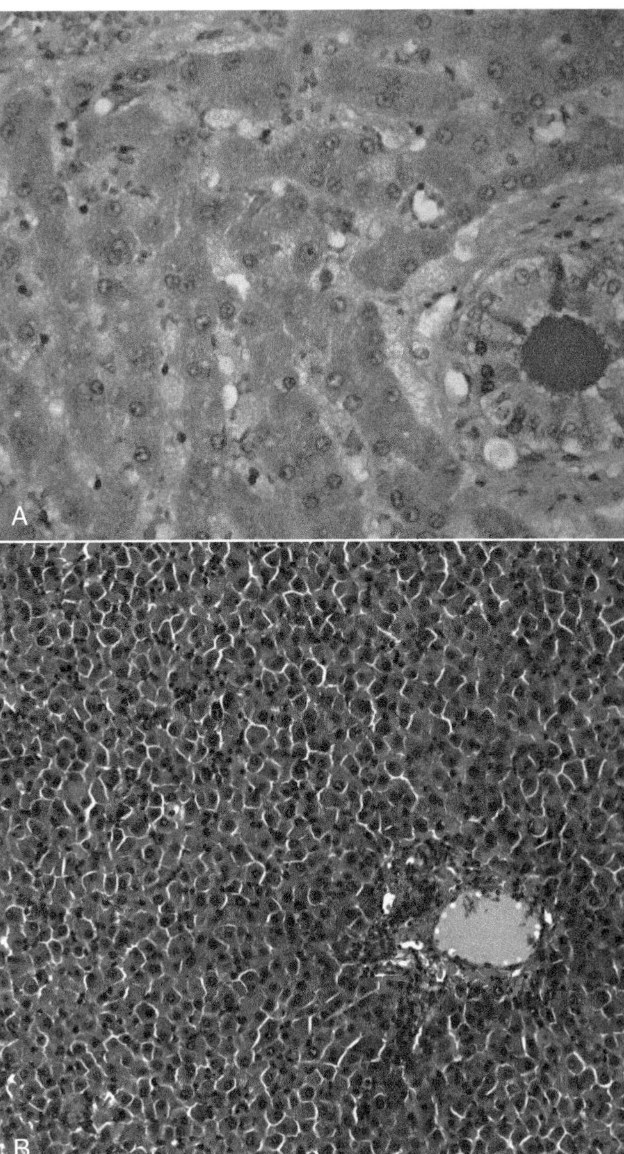

FIGURE 50-6 Histopathology of the liver in leptospirosis. **A,** Minimal hepatic changes and severe cholestasis in an 8-year-old male neutered Australian shepherd mix that was euthanized because of anuric leptospirosis. The activity of serum ALP and the serum total bilirubin concentration were mildly increased, and the dog seroconverted with the highest titer to serovar Pomona (1:400 to >1:3200 12 days later). **B,** Liver plate disarray with hepatocellular dissociation in a dog with leptospirosis. (B, Image courtesy John Cullen, North Carolina State University and Jean-Jacques Fontaine, École Nationale Vétérinaire d'Alfort)

recommends that all dogs with leptospirosis should be treated with doxycycline, 5 mg/kg q12h PO or IV for 2 weeks.[20] If vomiting or other adverse reactions preclude the use of doxycycline, parenteral ampicillin or penicillin G can be used (Table 50-5). Dogs initially treated with a penicillin derivative should be treated with doxycycline for 2 weeks after gastrointestinal signs resolve. Fluoroquinolones are not highly efficacious for clearance of leptospires from tissues.[56] Other antimicrobials that have been efficacious in clinical trials involving human patients with leptospirosis include ceftriaxone, cefotaxime, and azithromycin.[57,58]

TABLE 50-5

Antimicrobials Recommended for Treatment of Leptospirosis in Dogs

Drug	Dose	Route	Interval (hours)	Duration (days)
Doxycycline	5 mg/kg	PO, IV	12	14
Ampicillin	20 mg/kg*	IV	6	Variable
Penicillin	25,000-40,000 U/kg	IV	12	Variable

*Reduce dose in renal failure.

Supportive Care

Dogs with severe disease require aggressive treatment with IV crystalloids, potassium supplementation, antiemetics, antihypertensives, antacids, blood products, and parenteral or enteral nutrition, with attention to precautions to minimize zoonotic transmission (see Public Health Aspects, later). Referral to a 24-hour care facility, ideally with access to dialysis, should be considered for severely ill dogs because of the need for intensive monitoring and close observation. Electrolyte and acid-base status may require frequent monitoring.

Fluid therapy is critical and should be calculated based on measurement of "outs and ins," together with careful attention to body weight, respiratory rate, lung sounds, blood pressure, and if possible, central venous pressure. Dogs with polyuric renal failure may require extremely high fluid rates. For dogs with oliguric or anuric renal failure, high fluid rates can lead to overhydration and respiratory failure. Urine output in dogs with oliguria or anuria should be closely monitored through use of a closed, indwelling urinary catheter and collection bag system. Diuretics such as furosemide and mannitol may be indicated. Failure of urine production after adequate hydration is achieved is an indication for dialysis (see Renal Replacement Therapy, next). Once recovery of kidney values has occurred, fluids should be tapered slowly before they are discontinued to ensure that proper hydration status is maintained. In some dogs, possibly because of enteritis or pancreatitis, inappetence persists for several days after kidney and liver values normalize. Continued nutritional support is required during this period.

Dogs with SPHS may require oxygen therapy and, rarely, mechanical ventilation. The optimum treatment for dogs with SPHS is unknown. Human patients with SPHS have had improved outcome following cyclophosphamide therapy and plasma exchange.[59]

Renal Replacement Therapy

Early hemodialysis results in improved survival and shorter hospital stays in human patients with leptospirosis.[60] Renal replacement therapy is indicated for dogs with inadequate urine output that develop volume overload, hyperkalemia, a BUN greater than 80 mg/dL, or signs of uremia that do not respond to medical management.[20] Approximately 50% of 89 dogs with leptospirosis at the University of California, Davis, VMTH in the past 10 years received hemodialysis; the median number of hemodialysis treatments required was 3 (range, 1 to 14). Recovery of adequate renal function usually occurs within 2 to 4 weeks of starting dialysis.

Prognosis

When the treatment is initiated early and aggressively, the prognosis for recovery from acute leptospirosis is excellent. Survival rates are in excess of 50%,[41] and in centers where hemodialysis is available, survival rates can exceed 80%. Precise survival rates for dogs with SPHS are unknown but may be lower. Successful treatment is associated with normalization of the platelet count, serum BUN and creatinine concentrations, and serum liver enzyme activities within 10 to 14 days. Icterus may be slow to resolve, and urine-concentrating ability may not return for at least 4 weeks. Some dogs have residual permanent renal damage after recovery.

Immunity and Vaccination

Recurrence of leptospirosis in dogs after recovery from natural infection appears to be rare, but the duration of immunity after natural infection is unknown. Immunity after vaccination with inactivated vaccines is serogroup specific and possibly serovar specific, although partial immunity to heterologous serogroups was shown in one report.[61] A live attenuated LPS mutant *L. interrogans* serovar Manilae vaccine was shown to induce strong protection in hamsters against challenge either with the same or a serologically unrelated (Pomona) serovar.[62] After challenge with serovar Pomona, survival rates were 100% in hamsters immunized with the attenuated live vaccine, compared with only 40% for those immunized with an inactivated serovar Manilae vaccine.

Current vaccines for dogs are inactivated bacterins. Bivalent vaccines that contained only serovars Icterohaemorrhagiae and Canicola were first introduced for prevention of leptospirosis in dogs. In the United States, these have now been replaced with four-serovar vaccines that contain serovars Icterohaemorrhagiae, Canicola, Grippotyphosa, and Pomona. In Europe, serovar Icterohaemorrhagiae and Canicola vaccines are still available, but vaccines that contain serovar Icterohaemorrhagiae, Canicola, and Grippotyphosa (Pfizer Animal Health) and serovar Copenhageni (serogroup Icterohaemorrhagiae), Portland-vere (serogroup Canicola), Bratislava (serogroup Australis), and Dadas (serogroup Grippotyphosa) (MSD Animal Health) have been introduced. Leptospiral vaccines effectively prevent disease and reduce shedding after challenge with the serovar included in the vaccine. The duration of immunity following vaccination is at least 12 months.[32,63,64] Leptospirosis has occurred in North American dogs immunized with bivalent vaccines; however, disease is rare in dogs immunized with four-serovar vaccines.[13]

In the past, vaccination for with *Leptospira* vaccines has been associated with type I hypersensitivity reactions such as anaphylaxis, especially in small-breed dogs. Anecdotal evidence from industry and veterinary practitioners in North America suggests that the prevalence of these reactions has considerably reduced in recent years (to <1%) following efforts from industry to remove constituents that have been associated with vaccine reactivity.[20]

Immunization is recommended for dogs at risk of exposure. In some regions, this may be dogs that contact wildlife or farm animals, or dogs that swim, wade, or drink from environmental water sources. In other regions, dogs in urban or suburban backyards may be at risk if there is significant exposure to wildlife or rodents in the immediate home environment. Immunization may be optimally performed a few months before the onset of the peak season for leptospirosis in a given geographic region. There is no evidence that the initial series needs to be readministered to dogs that are over due for an annual booster. For dogs that experience natural infection, immunization could commence a year after recovery, although the duration of immunity after natural infection and the degree and duration of cross-protection to heterologous serovars that follows natural infection requires further investigation.

Prevention

Leptospirosis can be prevented by restricting dogs' access to potential reservoir host species or environmental water sources. Access to wildlife and farm animals can be reduced through fencing and rodent control. Where this is not possible, immunization is recommended.

Public Health Aspects

In humans, leptospirosis occurs after an incubation period of 2 to 20 days (mean, 10 days). In 90% of infections, it is a mild, influenza-like illness. Less commonly, it is manifested by severe multiorgan failure, with renal failure, hepatic failure, or SPHS. Abortion can occur during pregnancy. Weil's disease, which is characterized by impaired renal and hepatic function, usually occurs a week after an initial illness characterized by fever, myalgia, headache, chills, and conjunctivitis.[1]

In developed countries, most human leptospirosis cases follow recreational activities that involve water, such as houseboating or participation in triathlons, caving, or white-water rafting.[65,66] Individuals who contact farm animals can also develop leptospirosis. Contact with wild rodents adopted as pets has also led to human disease.[67] In developing countries, stray dogs may be a source of human infection, although rodents are also important in this situation.[68] The extent to which domestic cats might serve as reservoir hosts is not understood.

Reports of transmission from clinically affected incidental hosts (as opposed to subclinically infected reservoir hosts) to other animals are rare, and there are no reports that document transmission of leptospires from pet dogs to humans with the support of molecular typing methods. Appropriate antimicrobial therapy may also reduce the possibility of transmission to humans. Nevertheless, precautions should be taken in the hospital environment to minimize zoonotic transmission (see Chapter 11). All dogs with acute renal failure should be handled as leptospirosis suspects until an alternative diagnosis is established. Suggested precautions are shown in Box 50-1. Urine from dogs with leptospirosis can be inactivated with a variety of disinfectant solutions, including iodine-based disinfectants, quaternary ammonium solutions, and accelerated hydrogen peroxide. Large volumes of urine can be inactivated by 1:1 dilution with a 10% solution of household bleach. In dogs with indwelling urinary catheters, 10% bleach should be injected directly into the collection bag before disposal. All blood, urine, and tissues from dogs should be treated as medical waste. If a dog dies or is euthanized, individuals who are to handle the remains should be alerted of the possibility of leptospirosis.

Owners of affected dogs should be educated in regard to the zoonotic nature of the disease. The risk of infection to owners is probably low, because urinary shedding generally does not occur until 7 to 10 days after the onset of illness, and doxycycline treatment likely results in clearance of bacteria from the kidneys and urine within 2 to 3 days. Nevertheless, until antimicrobial therapy is completed, owners should avoid contact with their dog's urine. Routine household disinfectants and gloved hands should be used to clean up urinary accidents that occur indoors. Dogs should be taken to urinate in a place that is away from water and away from other pets and people, especially children. Owners should wash their hands after they handle their pets. Veterinarians should recommend that owners seek medical attention if illness occurs around the time their dog is diagnosed with leptospirosis, or if they have any questions about the disease in humans. Immunocompromised humans should be referred to their medical practitioners for advice. Owners should also be informed that environmental sources of infection may represent an ongoing risk, not only to other dogs in the household but also to humans. If other dogs in the household may have been exposed at the same time as the dog diagnosed with leptospirosis, those dogs should be treated with doxycycline for 2 weeks, because subclinical infection and shedding may have occurred.[20]

Veterinarians should contact their local or state health department or the Centers for Disease Control and Prevention if additional questions arise regarding the public health risks and zoonotic transmission of leptospirosis.[20]

BOX 50-1

Suggested In-Hospital Precautions for Dogs with Known or Suspected Leptospirosis

- Warning signage on the cage or run
- Minimize movement around the hospital, avoiding transport along common hallways
- Gloves and disposable gowns
- Protective eyewear and face shields if aerosolization of urine likely
- Handwashing before and after handling
- No pregnant or immunocompromised staff to work with the patient
- Prompt disinfection of urine and urine spills
- Treatment with appropriate antimicrobial drugs
- Indwelling rather than intermittent urinary catheterization for monitoring urine output
- Dogs walked or gurneyed outside to urinate frequently if urinary catheter not in place
- Urination outside in a designated area that can be easily disinfected
- Warnings to others who handle the dog or specimens from the dog

CASE EXAMPLE

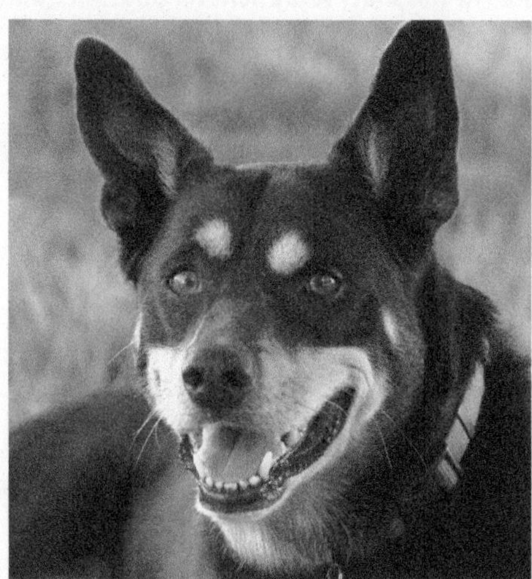

FIGURE 50-7 "Makalu," a 1.5-year-old male neutered kelpie dog that developed leptospirosis.

Signalment: "Makalu," a 1.5-year-old male neutered kelpie dog from Dixon in northern California (Figure 50-7).

History: Makalu had a 1-day history of lethargy and inappetence. The owner, a veterinarian, took his temperature at home and it was >104°F (40°C). There had been no vomiting, diarrhea, coughing, sneezing, or increased thirst and urination. Makalu lived on a property with another dog, three cats, sheep, goats, and a pot-bellied pig. He normally ate a commercial dry dog food; he consumed a rawhide the day before he became ill. There was no history of previous travel, toxins, trauma, medications, or tick exposure. He was 3 months overdue for vaccination but had been vaccinated as a puppy for distemper, hepatitis, parvovirus, rabies, and leptospirosis. The owner did not recall which *Leptospira* vaccines he received.

Physical Examination:

Body Weight: 22.4 kg

General: Quiet, alert and responsive. Ambulatory on all four limbs, T = 103.7°F (39.8°C), HR = 80 beats/min, RR = 20 breaths/min, mucous membranes pink, CRT = 1 s. Estimated to be 7% to 8% dehydrated based on skin turgor.

Integument, Eyes, Ears, Nose, and Throat: Mild scleral injection and chemosis were present bilaterally.

Musculoskeletal: Appeared stiff, but there was no evidence of synovial effusion. Vocalized on flexion of the right thoracic limb.

Cardiovascular: Strong femoral pulses. No murmurs or arrhythmias auscultated. Systolic blood pressure was 145 mm Hg.

Respiratory: Quiet bronchovesicular sounds were present in all lung fields.

Gastrointestinal and Genitourinary: A tense abdomen was noted, with abdominal splinting noted on palpation. No abnormalities were detected on rectal examination.

Lymph Nodes: No abnormalities were detected.

Laboratory Findings:

CBC:

HCT 41.4% (40%-55%)
MCV 70.2 fL (65-75 fL)
MCHC 36.0 g/dL (33-36 g/dL)
WBC 8820 cells/μL (6000-13,000 cells/μL)
Neutrophils 7673 cells/μL (3000-10,500 cells/μL)
Lymphocytes 353 cells/μL (1000-4000 cells/μL)
Monocytes 441 cells/μL (150-1200 cells/μL)
Platelets 74,000 platelets/μL (150,000-400,000 platelets/μL).

Serum Chemistry Profile:

Sodium 143 mmol/L (145-154 mmol/L)
Potassium 3.7 mmol/L (4.1-5.3 mmol/L)
Chloride 104 mmol/L (105-116 mmol/L)
Bicarbonate 17 mmol/L (16-26 mmol/L)
Phosphorus 5.1 mg/dL (3.0-6.2 mg/dL)
Calcium 9.6 mg/dL (9.9-11.4 mg/dl)
BUN 90 mg/dL (8-31 mg/dL)
Creatinine 4.6 mg/dL (0.5-1.6 mg/dL)
Glucose 110 mg/dL (70-118 mg/dL)
Total protein 5.1 g/dL (5.4-7.4 g/dL)
Albumin 2.4 g/dL (2.9-4.2 g/dL)
Globulin 2.7 g/dL (2.3-4.4 g/dL)
ALT 42 U/L (19-67 U/L)
AST 146 U/L (21-54 U/L)
ALP 73 U/L (15-127 U/L)
Creatine kinase 1387 U/L (46-320 U/L)
GGT 2 U/L (0-6 U/L)
Cholesterol 189 mg/dL (135-345 mg/dL)
Total bilirubin 0.4 mg/dL (0-0.4 mg/dL).

Urinalysis: SGr 1.013; pH 7.5, 2+ protein (SSA), 1+ bilirubin, 3+ hemoprotein, 2+ glucose, 0 WBC/HPF, 20-30 RBC/HPF, rare transitional epithelial cells.

Coagulation Profile: PT 8.8 (7.5-10.5), APTT 16.8 (9-12), fibrinogen 280 (90-255).

Serum Ethylene Glycol Assay: Negative.

Imaging Findings:

Thoracic Radiographs: The cardiovascular and pulmonary structures appeared within normal limits.

Abdominal Ultrasound: The liver and spleen were both enlarged. The tail of the spleen had a mildly mottled echotexture. Both kidneys were mildly enlarged, and measured approximately 8 cm in length. The renal cortices were mildly echogenic. A small amount of subcapsular and retroperitoneal fluid was noted in association with both kidneys. The mesenteric lymph nodes were prominent.

Microbiologic Testing: Aerobic bacterial culture of blood and urine: No growth.

Leptospira serology (MAT): Day 2 after the onset of illness, negative for antibodies to serovars Canicola, Grippotyphosa, Hardjo, Icterohaemorrhagiae, and Pomona at 1:100. Positive for antibodies to serovar Bratislava at 1:100. Day 10 after the onset of illness, negative for antibodies to serovar Canicola. Positive for antibodies to serovars Grippotyphosa (1:400), Hardjo (1:100), Icterohaemorrhagiae (1:800), Pomona (1:12,800), and Bratislava (1:3200).

Diagnosis: Leptospirosis.

Treatment: Makalu was aggressively treated with intravenous fluids, mannitol, famotidine, a metoclopramide, and ampicillin (20 mg/kg IV q6h). Despite this treatment and administration of furosemide, urine output remained at <0.8 mL/kg/hr. After 18 hours of hospitalization, dialysis was initiated. After a second dialysis treatment 2 days later, polyuria ensued (Table 50-6). On day 3, DIC developed, with further prolongation of the PT (14.3 s) and APTT (21.1 s), hypofibrinogenemia (<90 mg/dL), and a positive D-dimer assay. The dog was treated with multiple units of fresh frozen plasma. Treatment with ondansetron was also initiated on day 3 because of persistent vomiting, and total parenteral nutrition was instituted on day 4. Makalu's mentation improved on day 5 and he began eating on day 8.

Comments: Antibody titers in this dog were very low or negative initially because insufficient time had elapsed for antibody production to occur. The diagnosis of leptospirosis was based on consistent clinical signs together with seroconversion on day 10. Liver enzyme activities were not increased in this dog on admission, but increased subsequently. Without dialysis, this dog would have died from the disease.

TABLE 50-6

Serial Changes in Clinicopathologic Variables in a Hospitalized Dog with Leptospirosis That Was Treated with Hemodialysis

Variable	Day 1	Day 3	Day 4	Day 5	Day 8	Day 10
ALT (U/L)	62	ND	105	110	82	71
ALP (U/L)	83	ND	97	97	79	75
Bilirubin (mg/dL)	0.4	ND	0.5	0.8	0.3	0.3
BUN (mg/dL)	105 (27)*	144 (30)	54	47	35	27
Creatinine (mg/dL)	5.6 (2.2)	12.9 (3.1)	4.8	3.3	2.1	1.6
Albumin (g/dL)	2.2	2.4	2.5	2.9	3.0	3.1
Platelets (x1000/μL)	74	ND	26	91	92	clumped
Urine output (mL/kg/hr)	<0.8	0.25	10	10	7	ND

*Values in parentheses are postdialysis values. ND, not done.

SUGGESTED READINGS

Araujo ER, Seguro AC, Spichler A, et al. Acute kidney injury in human leptospirosis: an immunohistochemical study with pathophysiological correlation. Virchows Arch. 2010;456(4):367-375.

Sykes JE, Hartmann K, Lunn KF, et al. 2010 ACVIM small animal consensus statement on leptospirosis: diagnosis, epidemiology, treatment and prevention. J Vet Intern Med. 2011;25(1):1-13.

REFERENCES

1. Levett PN. Leptospirosis. Clin Microbiol Rev. 2001;14:296-326.
2. Arbour J, Blais M, Carioto L, et al. Clinical leptospirosis in three cats (2001-2009). J Am Anim Hosp Assoc. 2012;48:256-260.
3. Bryson DG, Ellis WA. Leptospirosis in a British domestic cat. J Small Anim Pract. 1976;17:459-465.
4. Mason RW, King SJ, McLachlan NM. Suspected leptospirosis in two cats. Aust Vet J. 1972;48:622-623.
5. Rees HG. Leptospirosis in a cat. New Zealand Vet J. 1964;12:64.
6. Zuerner RL, Alt DP. Variable nucleotide tandem-repeat analysis revealing a unique group of *Leptospira interrogans* serovar Pomona isolates associated with California sea lions. J Clin Microbiol. 2009;47:1202-1205.
7. Timoney JF, Kalimuthusamy N, Velineni S, et al. A unique genotype of *Leptospira interrogans* serovar Pomona type kennewicki is associated with equine abortion. Vet Microbiol. 2011;150:349-353.
8. Trevejo RT, Rigau-Perez JG, Ashford DA, et al. Epidemic leptospirosis associated with pulmonary hemorrhage—Nicaragua, 1995. J Infect Dis. 1998;178:1457-1463.
9. Zaitsev SV, Chernukha Iu G, Evdokimova OA, et al. Survival rate of *Leptospira* pomona in the soil at a natural leptospirosis focus. Zh Mikrobiol Epidemiol Immunobiol. 1989:64-68.
10. Meeyam T, Tablerk P, Petchanok B, et al. Seroprevalence and risk factors associated with leptospirosis in dogs. Southeast Asian J Trop Med Public Health. 2006;37:148-153.
11. Raghavan R, Brenner K, Higgins J, et al. Evaluations of land cover risk factors for canine leptospirosis: 94 cases (2002-2009). Prev Vet Med. 2011;101:241-249.
12. Adin CA, Cowgill LD. Treatment and outcome of dogs with leptospirosis: 36 cases (1990-1998). J Am Vet Med Assoc. 2000;216:371-375.
13. Hennebelle J, Sykes JE, Carpenter T, et al. Spatial and temporal patterns of *Leptospira* spp. seroreactivity in dogs from northern California. J Am Vet Med Assoc. 2012.
14. Ward MP. Seasonality of canine leptospirosis in the United States and Canada and its association with rainfall. Prev Vet Med. 2002;56:203-213.
15. Gautam R, Guptill LF, Wu CC, et al. Spatial and spatio-temporal clustering of overall and serovar-specific *Leptospira* microscopic agglutination test (MAT) seropositivity among dogs in the United States from 2000 through 2007. Prev Vet Med. 2010;96:122-131.
16. Prescott J. Canine leptospirosis in Canada: a veterinarian's perspective. CMAJ. 2008;178:397-398.
17. Moore GE, Guptill LF, Glickman NW, et al. Canine leptospirosis, United States, 2002-2004. Emerg Infect Dis. 2006;12:501-503.
18. Brown CA, Roberts AW, Miller MA, et al. *Leptospira interrogans* serovar grippotyphosa infection in dogs. J Am Vet Med Assoc. 1996;209:1265-1267.
19. Ellis WA. Control of canine leptospirosis in Europe: time for a change? Vet Rec. 2010;167:602-605.
20. Sykes JE, Hartmann K, Lunn KF, et al. 2010 ACVIM small animal consensus statement on leptospirosis: diagnosis, epidemiology, treatment, and prevention. J Vet Intern Med. 2011;25:1-13.
21. Rentko VT, Clark N, Ross LA, et al. Canine leptospirosis. A retrospective study of 17 cases. J Vet Intern Med. 1992;6:235-244.
22. Levett PN. Usefulness of serologic analysis as a predictor of the infecting serovar in patients with severe leptospirosis. Clin Infect Dis. 2003;36:447-452.
23. Galloway RL, Levett PN. Application and validation of PFGE for serovar identification of *Leptospira* clinical isolates. PLoS Negl Trop Dis. 2010;4:e824.
24. Greenlee JJ, Alt DP, Bolin CA, et al. Experimental canine leptospirosis caused by *Leptospira interrogans* serovars pomona and bratislava. Am J Vet Res. 2005;66:1816-1822.

25. Birnbaum N, Barr SC, Center SA, et al. Naturally acquired leptospirosis in 36 dogs: serological and clinicopathological features. J Small Anim Pract. 1998;39:231-236.
26. Goldstein RE, Lin RC, Langston CE, et al. Influence of infecting serogroup on clinical features of leptospirosis in dogs. J Vet Intern Med. 2006;20:489-494.
27. Greenlee JJ, Bolin CA, Alt DP, et al. Clinical and pathologic comparison of acute leptospirosis in dogs caused by two strains of *Leptospira kirschneri* serovar grippotyphosa. Am J Vet Res. 2004;65:1100-1107.
28. Burth P, Younes-Ibrahim M, Santos MC, et al. Role of nonesterified unsaturated fatty acids in the pathophysiological processes of leptospiral infection. J Infect Dis. 2005;191:51-57.
29. Chu KM, Rathinam R, Namperumalsamy P, et al. Identification of *Leptospira* species in the pathogenesis of uveitis and determination of clinical ocular characteristics in south India. J Infect Dis. 1998;177:1314-1321.
30. Mastrorilli C, Dondi F, Agnoli C, et al. Clinicopathologic features and outcome predictors of *Leptospira interrogans* Australis serogroup infection in dogs: a retrospective study of 20 cases (2001-2004). J Vet Intern Med. 2007;21:3-10.
31. Rossetti CA, Liem M, Samartino LE, et al. Buenos Aires, a new *Leptospira* serovar of serogroup Djasiman, isolated from an aborted dog fetus in Argentina. Vet Microbiol. 2005;107:241-248.
32. Minke JM, Bey R, Tronel JP, et al. Onset and duration of protective immunity against clinical disease and renal carriage in dogs provided by a bi-valent inactivated leptospirosis vaccine. Vet Microbiol. 2009;137:137-145.
33. Chierakul W, Tientadakul P, Suputtamongkol Y, et al. Activation of the coagulation cascade in patients with leptospirosis. Clin Infect Dis. 2008;46:254-260.
34. Wagenaar JF, Goris MG, Partiningrum DL, et al. Coagulation disorders in patients with severe leptospirosis are associated with severe bleeding and mortality. Trop Med Int Health. 2010;15:152-159.
35. Kohn B, Steinicke K, Arndt G, et al. Pulmonary abnormalities in dogs with leptospirosis. J Vet Intern Med. 2010;24:1277-1282.
36. Klopfleisch R, Kohn B, Plog S, et al. An emerging pulmonary haemorrhagic syndrome in dogs: similar to the human leptospiral pulmonary haemorrhagic syndrome? Vet Med Int. 2010;2010:928541.
37. Croda J, Neto AN, Brasil RA, et al. Leptospirosis pulmonary haemorrhage syndrome is associated with linear deposition of immunoglobulin and complement on the alveolar surface. Clin Microbiol Infect. 2010;16:593-599.
38. Jha S, Ansari MK. Leptospirosis presenting as acute meningoencephalitis. J Infect Dev Ctries. 2010;4:179-182.
39. Adamus C, Buggin-Daubie M, Izembart A, et al. Chronic hepatitis associated with leptospiral infection in vaccinated beagles. J Comp Pathol. 1997;117:311-328.
40. Bishop L, Strandberg JD, Adams RJ, et al. Chronic active hepatitis in dogs associated with leptospires. Am J Vet Res. 1979;40:839-844.
41. Geisen V, Stengel C, Brem S, et al. Canine leptospirosis infections—clinical signs and outcome with different suspected *Leptospira* serogroups (42 cases). J Small Anim Pract. 2007;48:324-328.
42. Sykes JE. Unpublished observations, 2012.
43. Araujo ER, Seguro AC, Spichler A, et al. Acute kidney injury in human leptospirosis: an immunohistochemical study with pathophysiological correlation. Virchows Arch. 2010;456:367-375.
44. Zaragoza C, Barrera R, Centeno F, et al. Characterization of renal damage in canine leptospirosis by sodium dodecyl sulphate–polyacrylamide gel electrophoresis (SDS-PAGE) and Western blotting of the urinary proteins. J Comp Pathol. 2003;129:169-178.
45. Forrest LJ, O'Brien RT, Tremelling MS, et al. Sonographic renal findings in 20 dogs with leptospirosis. Vet Radiol Ultrasound. 1998;39:337-340.
46. Barr SC, McDonough PL, Scipioni-Ball RL, et al. Serologic responses of dogs given a commercial vaccine against *Leptospira interrogans* serovar pomona and *Leptospira kirschneri* serovar grippotyphosa. Am J Vet Res. 2005;66:1780-1784.
47. Miller MD, Annis KM, Lappin MR, et al. Variability in results of the microscopic agglutination test in dogs with clinical leptospirosis and dogs vaccinated against leptospirosis. J Vet Intern Med. 2011;25:426-432.
48. Chappel RJ, Goris M, Palmer MF, et al. Impact of proficiency testing on results of the microscopic agglutination test for diagnosis of leptospirosis. J Clin Microbiol. 2004;42:5484-5488.
49. International Leptospirosis MAT Proficiency Testing Scheme. 2013. http://www.med.monash.edu.au/microbiology/staff/adler/proftemp.html. Last accessed February 3, 2013.
50. Abdoel TH, Houwers DJ, van Dongen AM, et al. Rapid test for the serodiagnosis of acute canine leptospirosis. Vet Microbiol. 2011;150:211-213.
51. Chalayon P, Chanket P, Boonchawalit T, et al. Leptospirosis serodiagnosis by ELISA based on recombinant outer membrane protein. Trans R Soc Trop Med Hyg. 2011;105:289-297.
52. La-Ard A, Amavisit P, Sukpuaram T, et al. Evaluation of recombinant Lig antigen-based ELISA for detection of leptospiral antibodies in canine sera. Southeast Asian J Trop Med Public Health. 2011;42:128-137.
53. Sun A, Wang Y, Du P, et al. A sensitive and specific IgM-ELISA for the serological diagnosis of human leptospirosis using a rLipL32/1-LipL21-OmpL1/2 fusion protein. Biomed Environ Sci. 2011;24:291-299.
54. Midence JN, Leutenegger CM, Chandler AM, et al. Effects of recent *Leptospira* vaccination on whole blood real-time PCR testing in healthy client-owned dogs. J Vet Intern Med. 2011;26:149-152.
55. Truccolo J, Charavay F, Merien F, et al. Quantitative PCR assay to evaluate ampicillin, ofloxacin, and doxycycline for treatment of experimental leptospirosis. Antimicrob Agents Chemother. 2002;46:848-853.
56. Griffith ME, Moon JE, Johnson EN, et al. Efficacy of fluoroquinolones against *Leptospira interrogans* in a hamster model. Antimicrob Agents Chemother. 2007;51:2615-2617.
57. Panaphut T, Domrongkitchaiporn S, Vibhagool A, et al. Ceftriaxone compared with sodium penicillin G for treatment of severe leptospirosis. Clin Infect Dis. 2003;36:1507-1513.
58. Phimda K, Hoontrakul S, Suttinont C, et al. Doxycycline versus azithromycin for treatment of leptospirosis and scrub typhus. Antimicrob Agents Chemother. 2007;51:3259-3263.
59. Trivedi SV, Vasava AH, Bhatia LC, et al. Plasma exchange with immunosuppression in pulmonary alveolar haemorrhage due to leptospirosis. Indian J Med Res. 2010;131:429-433.
60. Cerqueira TB, Athanazio DA, Spichler AS, et al. Renal involvement in leptospirosis—new insights into pathophysiology and treatment. Braz J Infect Dis. 2008;12:248-252.
61. Sonrier C, Branger C, Michel V, et al. Evidence of cross-protection within *Leptospira interrogans* in an experimental model. Vaccine. 2000;19:86-94.
62. Srikram A, Zhang K, Bartpho T, et al. Cross-protective immunity against leptospirosis elicited by a live, attenuated lipopolysaccharide mutant. J Infect Dis. 2011;203:870-879.
63. Chandler AM, Goldstein RE. Assessing renal colonization in dogs 15 months after receiving a multi-serovar bacterin based on vaccine, vs unvaccinated dogs, all experimentally infected with *Leptospira kirschneri* serovar Grippotyphosa [Abstract]. J Vet Intern Med. 2010;24:764.
64. Klaasen HL, Molkenboer MJ, Vrijenhoek MP, et al. Duration of immunity in dogs vaccinated against leptospirosis with a bivalent inactivated vaccine. Vet Microbiol. 2003;95:121-132.
65. Monahan AM, Miller IS, Nally JE. Leptospirosis: risks during recreational activities. J Appl Microbiol. 2009;107:707-716.
66. Stern EJ, Galloway R, Shadomy SV, et al. Outbreak of leptospirosis among adventure race participants in Florida, 2005. Clin Infect Dis. 2010;50:843-849.
67. Strugnell BW, Featherstone C, Gent M, et al. Weil's disease associated with the adoption of a feral rat. Vet Rec. 2009;164:186.
68. Martins G, Penna B, Lilenbaum W. The dog in the transmission of human leptospirosis under tropical conditions: victim or villain? Epidemiol Infect. 2012;140:207-208.

CHAPTER 51

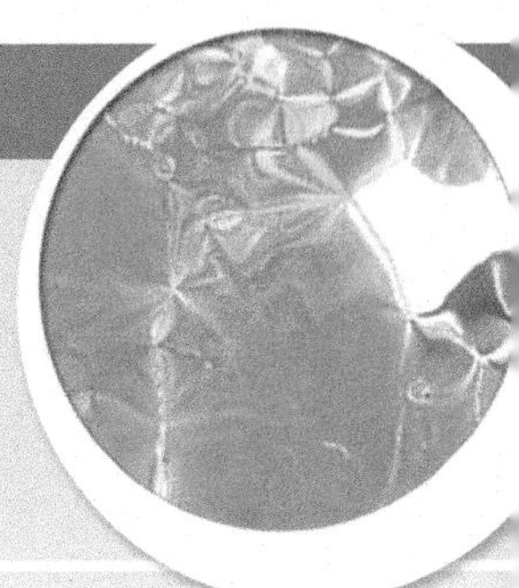

Lyme Borreliosis

Jane E. Sykes

Overview of Lyme Borreliosis

First Described: Connecticut, USA, 1982 (Burgdorfer)[1]

Cause: *Borrelia burgdorferi* sensu lato (a spirochete)

Primary Mode of Transmission: *Ixodes* spp. ticks

Affected Hosts: Humans and a large variety of animals; disease occurs in dogs, humans, horses, cattle

Geographic Distribution: North America, Europe, Asia

Major Clinical Signs: Fever, lethargy, inappetence, lameness due to polyarthritis. Signs of Lyme nephropathy include vomiting, weight loss, and polyuria and polydipsia.

Differential Diagnoses: Differential diagnoses for suspected Lyme polyarthritis includes bilateral cruciate ligament rupture, primary immune-mediated polyarthritis, septic polyarthritis, and polyarthritis secondary to infection with other pathogens such as *Ehrlichia ewingii*, *Bartonella* spp., *Ehrlichia canis*, *Anaplasma phagocytophilum*, *Rickettsia rickettsii*, and fungal organisms. Differential diagnosis for suspected Lyme nephritis include leptospirosis, bacterial pyelonephritis, primary immune-mediated glomerulonephritis, familial nephropathies, amyloidosis, and glomerulonephritis secondary to other chronic infections such as *Dirofilaria immitis*, *Babesia canis*, *E. canis*, and *Leishmania* spp. infections.

Human Health Significance: Dogs and cats are not a direct source of human infection but may bring unfed infected ticks into the house. Evidence of canine exposure to *B. burgdorferi* is a sentinel for human exposure.

Etiologic Agent and Epidemiology

Lyme borreliosis, or Lyme disease, is a vector-borne spirochetosis caused by the motile, corkscrew-shaped bacterium *Borrelia burgdorferi* sensu lato. Lyme disease occurs in North America, Europe, and Asia. It was named after Old Lyme in Connecticut, where clusters of the disease were first recognized in children with juvenile rheumatoid arthritis in 1976.[2] However, chronic cutaneous manifestations of infection were recognized in human patients in Germany as far back as 1883.[3] The spirochete was first detected in ticks by Burgdorfer in 1982.[1] A variety of different mammalian hosts and humans may be infected. The disease has been increasingly recognized and is now the most common vector-borne infectious disease of humans in the United States and Europe. Reforestation of farmland and proliferation of deer and tick populations may have contributed to emergence of the disease in humans.[4] Cats can be infected and seroconvert, but appear to be relatively resistant to development of disease.[5] Dogs can develop fever, arthritis, and renal disease, but most infected dogs show no signs of illness.

More than 15 different species of *B. burgdorferi* sensu lato have been described, some of which are nonpathogenic (Table 51-1). *Borrelia turicatae,* the cause of tick-borne relapsing fever in humans, has been detected in sick dogs from Texas.[6] The DNA of *Borrelia lonestari,* which is thought to be nonpathogenic, has been detected in dogs from Arkansas.[7] In North America, Lyme disease is caused by *Borrelia burgdorferi* sensu stricto, whereas in Europe and Asia, other species that belong to *Borrelia burgdorferi* sensu lato are more important, specifically *Borrelia afzelii* and *Borrelia garinii.* This may account for differences in clinical manifestations that occur in human patients in Europe compared with those in North America (see Public Health Significance, later). Some strains of *B. burgdorferi* appear to have increased virulence, such as *B. burgdorferi* OspC type A within the United States.[8]

B. burgdorferi sensu lato is transmitted by *Ixodes ricinus-persulcatus* complex ticks (Table 51-2). The geographic distribution of Lyme disease reflects that of the vector ticks as well as the competency of the reservoir hosts involved. In the United States, the vectors are *Ixodes scapularis* in the east and upper Midwest, and *Ixodes pacificus* in the West (see Chapter 29). Major foci of infection exist in the upper Midwest, Northeast, mid-Atlantic, and parts of northern California (Figure 51-1).[9] In some endemic areas, seroprevalence in dogs is nearly 90%,[10] although seroprevalence in a study that used a C6 ELISA assay (see Diagnosis, later) was lower than this in endemic areas such as Connecticut and Massachusetts, around 20%.[11] Infection is passed transstadially within the tick (i.e., from larva to nymph to adult), and not transovarially (from adult to egg). Reservoirs for the spirochete in the Northeast and the upper Midwest are *Peromyscus leucopus,* the white-footed mouse, which can harbor large numbers of the organism without overt signs of illness,[12] as well as shrews and chipmunks.[13] In the western United States, the western gray squirrel is the primary reservoir host.[14] Lyme disease is less prevalent in the western United States because *I. pacificus* prefers to feed on the western fence lizard, a poor reservoir for the spirochete. Similarly, the low prevalence of Lyme disease in the southeastern United States, is because *I. scapularis* ticks feed primarily on lizards in this region.[15] *B. burgdorferi* is primarily transmitted to humans by nymphal ticks, because they are extremely small and often enough go unnoticed. Adult ticks may be more important for transmission of infection to dogs.[16] The nymphs of *I. scapularis* quest in the late spring and summer, when humans and dogs are often outdoors and become exposed. The peak questing times for *I. scapularis* adult ticks are in the spring and fall. Other

TABLE 51-1

Pathogenic and Nonpathogenic Species That Belong to *Borrelia burgdorferi* sensu lato and Their Geographic Distributions

	United States	Europe	Asia
Pathogenic	*B. burgdorferi* sensu stricto	*B. burgdorferi* sensu stricto *B. afzelii* *B. garinii*	*B. afzelii* *B. garinii*
Non-pathogenic or questionable pathogenicity	*B. bissettii* *B. andersonii* *B. californiensis* *B. carolinensis* *B. americana* *B. kurtenbachii*	*B. valaisiana** *B. bissettii** *B. spielmanii** *B. lusitaniae* *B. bavariensis*	*B. bissettii** *B. japonica* *B. turdi* *B. tanukii* *B. sinica* *B. yangtze*

**B. valaisiana* and *B. bissettii* have been isolated from single cases of Lyme borreliosis; *B. spielmanii* has been detected in early skin lesions (Stanek G, Reiter M. The expanding Lyme *Borrelia* complex—clinical significance of genomic species? Clin Microbiol Infect 2011;17:487-493).

TABLE 51-2

Vectors of Lyme Disease Worldwide

Geographic Location	Tick Species	Common Name	Reservoir host for *Borrelia*
Western United States	*Ixodes pacificus*	Pacific black-legged tick	Western gray squirrel
Northeastern and upper Midwestern United States	*Ixodes scapularis*	Black-legged tick	White-footed mouse, shrews, chipmunks
Europe	*Ixodes ricinus*	Castor bean or sheep tick	Squirrels, thrushes, chipmunks, mice, shrews, hedgehogs, rats, hares, pheasants, voles
Asia	*Ixodes persulcatus*	Taiga tick	Voles

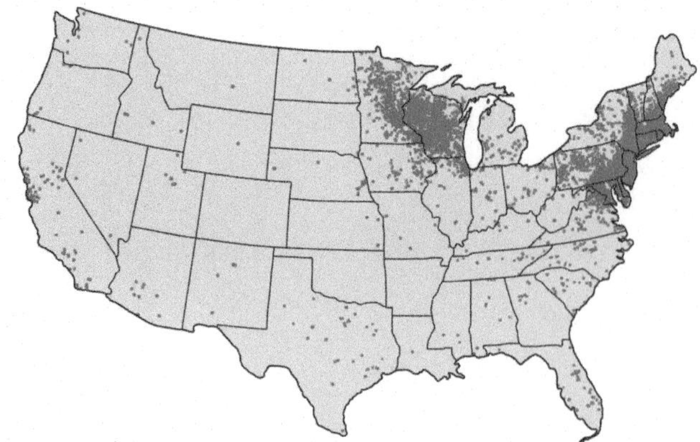

FIGURE 51-1 Approximate geographic distribution of Lyme borreliosis in humans (and dogs) in the United States.

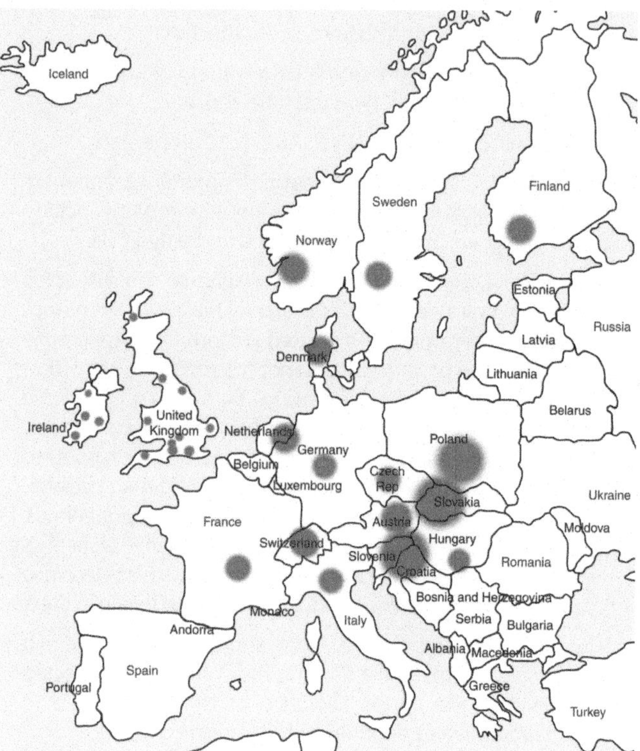

FIGURE 51-2 Countries and regions where Lyme borreliosis occurs in Europe. The size of the red dot correlates with the relative prevalence of the infection in those areas.

vector-borne pathogens, such as *Anaplasma phagocytophilum*, may be co-transmitted and complicate the clinical picture. There is some evidence that co-infection with *A. phagocytophilum* can enhance the pathogenicity of *B. burgdorferi*.[17]

In continental Europe, Lyme disease is most prevalent in central and eastern Europe, especially Poland, Slovakia, and Slovenia, but also Germany, Switzerland, Austria, and southern Scandinavia (Figure 51-2). *B. garinii* was detected in a dog from the Czech republic with meningoencephalitis,[18] and *B. afzelii* has been detected in dogs from Poland.[19] Evidence of infection has also been found in dogs from the British Isles,[20] where endemic areas include the Scottish Highlands, Ireland, Wales, the Lake District, the Yorkshire Moors, Exmoor, Wiltshire, Berkshire, and particularly the New Forest, the South Downs, and the Thetford Forest region. A huge variety of reservoir hosts appear to be involved in Europe. Small rodents such as squirrels appear to be an important reservoir host for *B. afzelii*, and birds such as blackbirds and song thrushes are important reservoir hosts for *B. garinii*.[21]

The complete genome of *B. burgdorferi* has been sequenced. The organism expresses different outer-surface lipoproteins at different stages of infection, which allows it to adapt to dramatically different environments within the arthropod vector and the mammalian host. This property of the organism has been exploited for the purpose of diagnostic assay and vaccine development. Outer surface proteins of importance include OspA, OspC, and VlsE. Over the fall, winter, and spring, the spirochete remains dormant within the nymphal tick and expresses OspA, which allows it to adhere to the tick midgut. When the tick ingests mammalian blood in the late spring and summer, OspA expression is downregulated by the spirochete, and OspC expression is upregulated.[22] The spirochete then moves to the tick hemolymph and salivary glands. OspC binds a tick salivary gland protein, which may help the organism evade the host immune response. OspC also binds to mammalian plasminogen and helps the spirochete to disseminate within the mammalian host.[23] VlsE undergoes recombinational shuffling of its genetic code, which further allows the spirochete to evade the immune response.[24] Finally, *B. burgdorferi* may undergo metamorphosis into a spherical shape when it encounters unfavorable conditions within the host, such as when it is exposed to antibiotics, nutrient deprivation, and changes in pH.[25] This may also contribute to its ability to evade the immune system and resist antimicrobial drug treatment.

Clinical Features

Signs and Their Pathogenesis

Transmission is thought to require tick attachment for a minimum of 24 hours,[26] but in some cases transmission may occur at earlier time points.[27] The spirochete replicates at the site of tick attachment, then disseminates to multiple locations. Although it can be transiently found in blood, the organism primarily replicates and spreads through connective tissue (Figure 51-3). It binds proteins such as plasminogen, β_3 integrins such as the platelet integrin $\alpha_{IIb}\beta_3$, glycosaminoglycans, fibronectin, laminin, and decorin (a collagen proteoglycan).[28] After invasion, the organism can persist in dogs for over a year, through evasion of host immune responses.[29]

In contrast to human Lyme disease, dogs do not develop an early skin rash (erythema migrans). It has been estimated that only 10% of affected dogs show overt signs of illness. Initial signs in dogs occur 2 to 5 months after a tick bite and consist of variable fever, inappetence, thrombocytopenia, and lameness due to neutrophilic polyarthritis. In a study of experimentally infected dogs, the first joint to be affected was the joint closest to the site of the tick bite, which supports the notion that spirochetes reach the joints as a result of spread through connective tissue.[29,30] Subsequently, other joints can be affected, and dogs may develop shifting lameness. It is not clear whether dogs develop other clinical manifestations seen in humans such as persistent, antibiotic-refractory Lyme arthritis; uveitis; carditis; or encephalopathy. Complete heart block was described in a seropositive dog from Connecticut that had pathologic changes at necropsy consistent with Lyme carditis.[31]

Lyme nephritis is a syndrome of membranoproliferative glomerulonephritis that has been recognized in dogs in association with exposure to *B. burgdorferi*. Rare reports of a similar disease in human patients exist.[32] Golden and Labrador retriever breeds appear to be overrepresented,[33] and it has been suggested that Shetland sheepdogs and Bernese mountain dogs might also be predisposed.[34-36] Dogs with Lyme nephritis are younger than dogs with other glomerular diseases. In one study, more than 50% of dogs with Lyme nephritis were 5 years of age or younger.[33] Many affected dogs are also thrombocytopenic, and some also have polyarthritis.[33] The pathogenesis of Lyme nephritis is uncertain; immune-mediated mechanisms have been proposed.[37] The DNA or antigen of the spirochete cannot be consistently detected within renal biopsies.[37,38] Subendothelial deposits of IgM, IgG, and C3 can be detected within the glomeruli.[33] Clinical signs result from proteinuria and renal failure and include inappetence, lethargy, weight loss, vomiting, and polyuria and polydipsia.

Physical Examination Findings

Physical examination findings in dogs with Lyme arthritis include lethargy, fever, lameness, and swollen, warm, painful joints. Mild generalized peripheral lymphadenopathy may be present. Dogs with Lyme nephritis may have a thin body condition, dehydration, and show evidence of peripheral edema, pleural effusion, or ascites, especially after crystalloid fluid administration. Complications of hypertension can sometimes occur, such as retinal detachment.

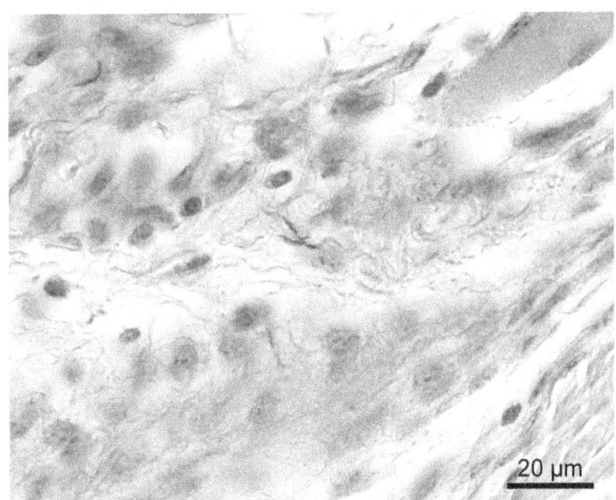

FIGURE 51-3 *Borrelia burgdorferi* in the metatarsal tendon sheath of a mouse with severe combined immunodeficiency. (Courtesy Dr. Stephen Barthold, Center for Comparative Medicine, University of California, Davis.)

Diagnosis

Diagnosis of Lyme disease is notoriously difficult. The overwhelming majority of infected dogs experience subclinical infection, after which positive antibody titers may persist for months or years. Because only a small percentage (e.g., <10%) of infections result in disease, it is important to distinguish between diagnosis of *infection* or previous exposure to the spirochete and diagnosis of Lyme *disease*. Dogs with positive antibody titers may develop unrelated illnesses, which results in diagnostic confusion. As in human patients, the diagnosis must be established based on characteristic clinical signs, a history of exposure in an endemic area, and a positive antibody response to *B. burgdorferi*.[39] A history of tick exposure may not always be present.

Laboratory Abnormalities

Complete Blood Count

The most common finding on the CBC of dogs with Lyme polyarthritis or nephritis is mild to moderate thrombocytopenia. The mechanism of thrombocytopenia is not known, but it may be immune mediated, because treatment of dogs with Lyme nephritis with immunosuppressive drugs can result in normalization of the platelet count. Mild to moderate anemia and leukocytosis due to a mature neutrophilia may be present in dogs with Lyme nephritis, but white cell counts may also be normal. Lymphopenia and mild neutropenia can also occur.

Serum Biochemical Tests

Dogs with polyarthritis typically have minimal changes on serum biochemistry testing. Dogs with Lyme nephritis may show azotemia, mild to marked hypoalbuminemia, metabolic acidosis, and electrolyte changes such as hyperphosphatemia, hypochloremia, and mild hyperkalemia or hypokalemia. Uncommonly, hypercholesterolemia is present.

Urinalysis

The urinalysis in dogs with Lyme nephritis generally reveals isosthenuria and proteinuria. Pyuria and microscopic hematuria may also be present. Urine protein to creatinine ratios are often greater than 5 and may be above 15 in some dogs.

Coagulation Profile

Dogs with Lyme nephritis may have low antithrombin activities as a result of glomerular antithrombin loss, which may lead to hypercoagulability syndromes. Sometimes, abnormalities such as a shortened PT, prolonged APTT, and increased fibrinogen and D-dimer concentrations are present.[40]

Synovial Fluid Cytology

Dogs with Lyme arthritis may have normal synovial fluid cytology,[30] or there may be markedly increased numbers of nondegenerate neutrophils within the synovial fluid of distal joints (>5000 and frequently >10,000 cells/μL). Because not all joints may be affected, synovial fluid should be collected from at least three and preferably four peripheral joints.

Diagnostic Imaging

Plain Radiography

Lyme arthritis is a nonerosive polyarthritis, so the only changes visible on plain radiography of the joints are increased periarticular soft tissue opacity. Thoracic radiography is generally unremarkable, but pleural effusion is occasionally identified in severely hypoalbuminemic dogs with Lyme nephritis.

Sonographic Findings

Abdominal sonographic examination is normal in dogs with Lyme arthritis. In dogs with nephritis, thickening and increased echogenicity of the renal cortices, decreased renal corticomedullary distinction, and peritoneal effusion may be seen.

Microbiologic Tests

Specific diagnostic assays available for Lyme borreliosis in dogs are described in Table 51-3.

TABLE 51-3

Diagnostic Assays Available for Lyme Borreliosis in Dogs

Assay	Specimen Type	Target	Performance
Bacterial isolation	Skin biopsy close to the tick bite site; synovial fluid	*B. burgdorferi* spirochete	Low sensitivity, requires special media, and may take several weeks. Isolation does not imply that *B. burgdorferi* is the cause of disease.
Serology (C6 assay)	Serum	Antibodies against *B. burgdorferi* C6 protein	Positive serology does not equate with Lyme disease, so test results must be interpreted in light of clinical findings. False positives can occur in regions of low prevalence. False negatives are rare, because antibodies are present by the time dogs develop illness. Cross-reactivity with vaccine antibodies does not occur.
Serology (whole cell IFA and ELISA)	Serum	Antibodies against *B. burgdorferi* antigens	As for C6 serology except that cross-reactivity with vaccine antibodies occurs, and false positives may also occur with other inflammatory diseases, and other spirochete infections.
Serology (Western immunoblot)	Serum	Antibodies against *B. burgdorferi* antigens	Used to confirm the serological response to natural infection in dogs that test positive with whole-cell ELISA and IFA. Technically difficult to perform and requires expertise to interpret. Positive serology does not equate with Lyme disease, so test results must be interpreted in light of clinical findings.
Serology (multiplex fluorescent bead assay)	Serum	Antibodies against *B. burgdorferi* OspA, OspC, and OspF	Antibodies to OspC appear only early in infection, whereas those to OspF reflect chronic infection and appear to correlate with the C6 antibody response. Sensitivity and specificity in dogs with naturally occurring Lyme disease unknown. Positive serology does not equate with Lyme disease, so test results must be interpreted in light of clinical findings.
Serology (multi-target silicon disc–based assay)	Serum	Antibodies against *B. burgdorferi* OspA, OspC, and OspF, SLP, and P39	Sensitivity and specificity in dogs with naturally occurring Lyme disease requires further study. Positive serology does not equate with Lyme disease, so test results must be interpreted in light of clinical findings.
PCR	As for isolation	*B. burgdorferi* DNA	Rapid but insensitive. Synovial fluid from dogs with polyarthritis may be the best specimen, but further study is needed. Assay performance can vary between laboratories.

Culture

B. burgdorferi can be isolated from tissue specimens in Barbour-Stoenner-Kelly medium. The optimal specimen for culture is a skin biopsy collected from a site adjacent to the tick bite, which is rarely identifiable in affected dogs. Incubation of cultures for several weeks may be required. Because of these factors, culture is not generally used on a routine basis for diagnosis.

Serologic Diagnosis

Serologic tests for antibody are the main assays used for diagnosis of Lyme disease in humans and also in dogs, but it is critical to recognize that positive serology does not necessarily equate with the presence of Lyme disease. In Europe, infection with nonpathogenic variants of *B. burgdorferi* sensu lato can result in positive serologic results, which further complicates diagnosis. Because the infection is chronic and persistent, and the incubation period is long, paired serology is generally not performed, because seroconversion may not occur. However, paired serology using serologic panels that include *B. burgdorferi* may be required for diagnosis of other vector-borne diseases that might be present. Positive test results in regions of low prevalence are more likely to be false positives than in regions of high prevalence, so interpretation of positive results should be performed with care in low-prevalence regions.

Currently, one of the most widely used serodiagnostic tests for canine Lyme disease is based on a C6 ELISA, which detects antibodies against a portion of the VlsE lipoprotein. The advantages of the C6 ELISA assay are that (1) it detects IgG antibodies 3 to 5 weeks after the time of infection, so by the time dogs develop clinical signs they are virtually always seropositive,[41] and (2) it is negative in dogs that have been vaccinated for Lyme disease, because the antigen is not expressed by organisms used in Lyme vaccines. The C6 ELISA is available as an in-practice lateral-flow assay, in combination with serodiagnostic spots for *Ehrlichia canis/Ehrlichia ewingii* antibody, *Anaplasma* spp. antibody, and *Dirofilaria immitis* antigen (SNAP 4Dx Plus, IDEXX Laboratories, ME) and as a quantitative ELISA (Quant C6), which is performed at IDEXX central veterinary diagnostic laboratories. There is no correlation between the magnitude of the C6 ELISA titer and disease severity. In a study from Europe, positive test results did not correlate with disease.[36] Another rapid immunochromatographic ELISA assay has recently become available in the United States (Abaxis VetScan Canine Lyme Rapid Test) that detects antibodies to a different portion of the VlsE lipoprotein, OspC and p41; these are combined on a single line.

Other serologic assays that are available include whole-cell ELISA or immunofluorescent antibody (IFA) assays and Western blotting (WB; see Chapter 2 for a description of these techniques). WB has traditionally been considered the gold standard assay. False positives using whole-cell ELISA and IFA have the potential to occur in patients with other spirochete infections, with other inflammatory disorders, and in vaccinated dogs. In human patients, a two-tiered approach is recommended for diagnosis.[39] Serum from patients who test positive for IgM or IgG with ELISA is then subjected to WB, because WB has increased specificity. WB has been used to differentiate the response to immunization and natural infection in dogs (Figure 51-4).[42] It has also been used to identify "dual status" dogs, that is, dogs that have been both immunized and naturally infected. WB is more time-consuming to perform than ELISA and IFA and experience is required to interpret it correctly.[43]

A multiplex fluorescent bead assay has been marketed in North America for detection of antibodies to three antigens of *B. burgdorferi:* OspA, OspC, and OspF.[43] The assay uses tiny beads to which OspA, OspC, and OspF are coupled. Dog serum is added to the beads, and if present, antibodies in the serum bind to the antigens and can be detected using a fluorescent conjugate. The pattern of reactivity to each antigen can be used to differentiate among the response to vaccination, early infection, and chronic infection. The presence of anti-OspA antibodies suggests previous vaccination, because vaccines contain OspA, and the spirochete rarely expresses OspA within

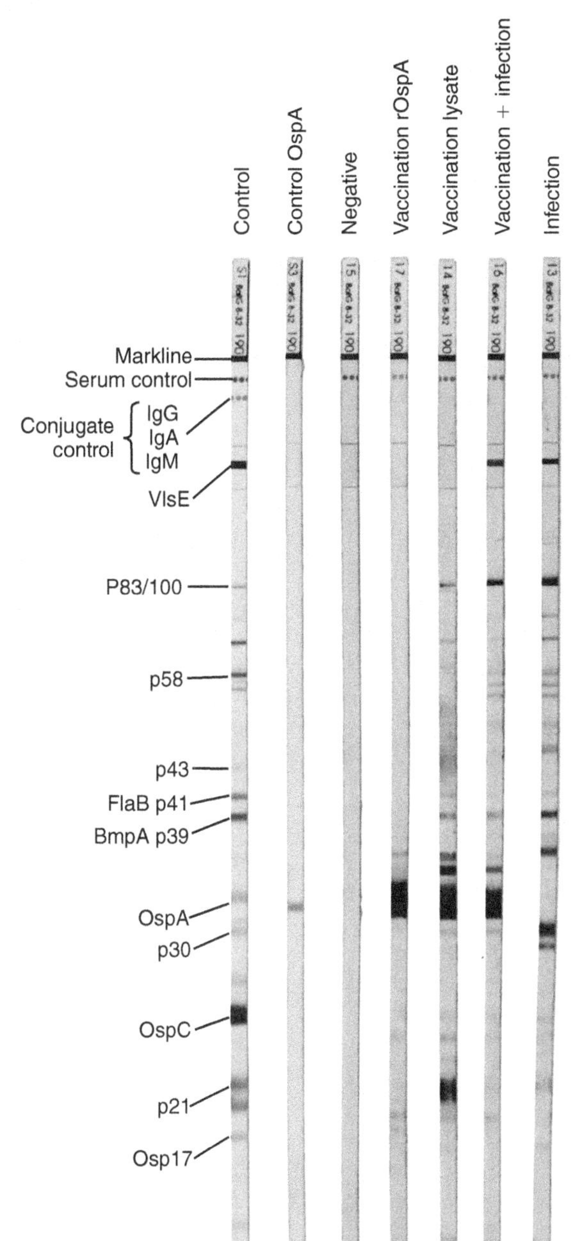

FIGURE 51-4 Western immunoblots of sera from dogs not infected with *B. burgdorferi* (Negative); immunized with recombinant OspA (vaccination rOspA); Immunized with a whole cell lysate vaccine (vaccination lysate); immunized and infected with *B. burgdorferi* (vaccination + infection); and infected only with *B. burgdorferi* (infection). The left strip shows all major signals available on the blot (control); the second strip from the left is stained with a monoclonal antibody against OspA (control OspA). (Courtesy R. Straubinger, Ludwig-Maximillians-Universitat, Munich, Germany. In: Greene CE: Infection Diseases of the Dog and Cat. 4th ed. St. Louis: Elsevier/Saunders; 2012.)

the host. OspC is expressed as the spirochete moves to the tick salivary glands and shortly after it enters the host. Thus an antibody response to OspC may suggest recent infection; titers decline and become undetectable beyond 3 months after infection.[44] Antibodies to OspC appear as early as 3 weeks after experimental infection of dogs, and OspF as early as 5 weeks.[44] OspF is expressed in more chronic infections, and can be detected together with the C6 antibody response in naturally exposed dogs (Figure 51-5).[44,45] In dogs, when WB was used as the gold standard, the sensitivities of the OspA, OspC, and OspF assays were 83%, 62%, and 82%, and the specificities were 90%, 89%, and 86%, respectively. The use of WB as the gold standard was questioned, and it was suggested that in fact, the fluorescent bead assay may have greater sensitivity and specificity than WB. The performance of the fluorescent bead assay is yet to be thoroughly evaluated in dogs with naturally occurring Lyme disease.

A novel silicon disc–based serologic assay is available in the United States for detection of antibodies to *B. burgdorferi, E. canis,* and *A. phagocytophilum* and antigen to *Dirofilaria immitis* (Accuplex 4, Antech Diagnostics, Irvine, CA). The assay for *B. burgdorferi* detects antibodies to the spirochete proteins OspA, OspC, OspF, P39, and SLP and is performed at central veterinary diagnostic laboratories. Preliminary data suggests that laboratory analysis of the response to these proteins correlates with the results of WB and can differentiate between the responses to natural infection and vaccination, and acute and chronic infection.[46]

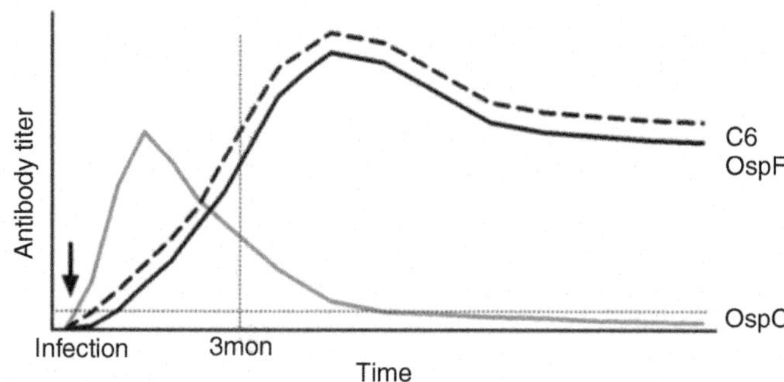

FIGURE 51-5 Proposed canine antibody response to OspC, OspF, and C6 antigens of *B. burgdorferi* during early and late infection. Data were obtained by fluorescent bead multiplex analysis. The lines for the first 3 months after infection are based on multiplex results from experimentally infected dogs. After 3 months the lines are projected from data obtained from patient sera. The horizontal dotted line shows the cutoff value for the multiplex assay. The vertical dotted line indicates 3 months after infection. (Modified from Wagner B, Freer H, Rollins A, et al. Antibodies to *Borrelia burgdorferi* OspA, OspC, OspF, and C6 antigens as markers for early and late infection in dogs. Clin Vaccine Immunol 2012;19:527-535.)

Molecular Diagnosis Using the Polymerase Chain Reaction

As with culture, PCR assays are best performed on skin biopsy specimens collected from a region adjacent to the tick bite site. In human patients, the use of PCR assays for diagnosis of Lyme borreliosis on blood has low sensitivity, and so false negatives are common when *B. burgdorferi* PCR assay is used as part of a whole-blood vector-borne infection PCR panel. Synovial fluid or synovial membrane biopsies may be the optimum specimen for diagnosis of Lyme arthritis in dogs. This is also true in human patients.[47] However, in a study of experimentally infected dogs, PCR assay of the synovial fluid was insensitive.[30] The sensitivity and specificity of PCR assays when used on specimens such as synovial fluid for diagnosis of canine Lyme borreliosis requires further study.

Pathologic Findings

Gross Pathologic Findings

Gross pathologic findings in dogs with Lyme arthritis include peripheral lymphadenomegaly, joint swelling, and synovial effusion.[29] The synovial fluid may be yellow-tinged and cloudy, with decreased viscosity. In dogs with nephritis, the kidneys are diffusely light tan and may have pinpoint red foci over the cortical surfaces.[33] In addition, evidence of systemic edema, thrombosis and infarction, and uremia (such as parathyroid hyperplasia, ulcerative stomatitis, and gastritis) may be present.

Histopathologic Findings

Histopathology of the joints of dogs that have been experimentally infected with *B. burgdorferi* reveals fibrinosuppurative or lymphoplasmacytic inflammation of the synovial membranes, joint capsules, and tendon sheaths.[29,30] Inflammation can sometimes be found in the joints even when a history of lameness is not present.[29] In human patients, organisms have been demonstrated in the synovium using immunostains and electron microscopy.[48] Other findings in experimentally infected dogs include periarteritis and perineuritis, especially within joint capsules and the skin, as well as lymphoid hyperplasia within peripheral lymph nodes. Mild, focal meningitis and encephalitis was identified in dogs that were infected with *B. burgdorferi* and immunosuppressed with dexamethasone.[49]

Renal histopathology in dogs with Lyme nephritis reveals diffuse membranoproliferative glomerulonephritis (Figure 51-6), dilation of the cortical renal tubules, tubular necrosis and regeneration, and mild to moderate, diffuse interstitial lymphoplasmacytic inflammation.[33] Periglomerular or diffuse interstitial fibrosis may be present in dogs with end-stage disease.

Treatment and Prognosis

Antimicrobial Treatment

Antibiotic treatment is recommended for seropositive dogs that have clinical illness consistent with Lyme disease. There is no evidence that treatment of healthy seropositive dogs is beneficial and it may lead to drug adverse effects and contribute to antimicrobial resistance in other bacteria and antimicrobial shortages. The antibiotic of choice for Lyme arthritis is doxycycline. The optimal dose and duration of treatment is unknown. Recommended doses have included 5 mg/kg PO q12h and 10 mg/kg PO q12h or 10 mg/kg PO q24h.[34,50] Four weeks of treatment has been recommended[34] because the clinical manifestations of disease resemble those of late-stage disease in human patients, for which relapses occur when treatment durations of less than 30 days are used.[39] Dogs with polyarthritis generally respond clinically to doxycycline treatment within 24 to 48 hours. Other differential diagnoses for polyarthritis should be considered if an inadequate response to treatment occurs. On the other hand, a clinical response to doxycycline treatment is not sufficient to make a diagnosis of Lyme arthritis. This is because there are other doxycycline-responsive causes of infectious polyarthritis in dogs; signs of primary immune-mediated polyarthritis can wax and wane; and doxycycline has antiinflammatory properties that may contribute to clinical improvement. For dogs that do not tolerate doxycycline, amoxicillin can be used, which also has activity against *B. burgdorferi* (Table 51-4). Azithromycin and third-generation cephalosporins have also been used to treat Lyme disease in human patients.[39] Doxycycline treatment

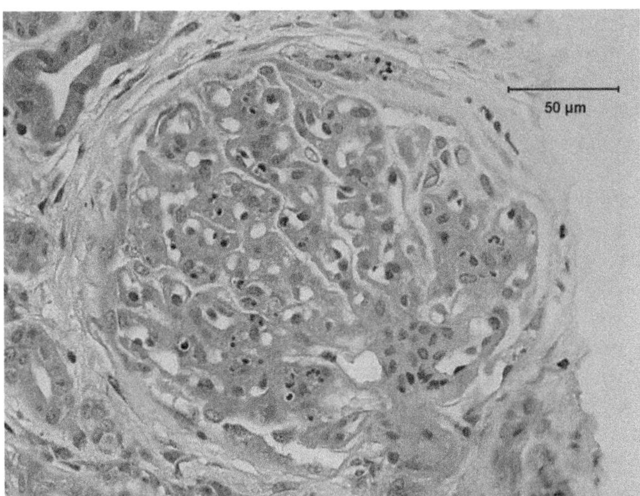

FIGURE 51-6 Membranoproliferative glomerulonephritis in a 6-year-old, intact male golden retriever dog that was seropositive for *B. burgdorferi* C6 protein antibodies and had clinical and biochemical evidence of protein-losing nephropathy. The morphologic diagnosis was moderate to severe, diffuse, global membranoproliferative glomerulonephritis with moderate chronic-active tubulointerstitial nephritis. The capillary walls are thickened and there is mesangial cell proliferation. There was also evidence of focal arteriolar mural disorganization, lamination, and sclerosis in this biopsy specimen. (Image courtesy Dr. George Lees, Texas A&M University.)

is also recommended for dogs with Lyme nephritis, although clinical improvement generally does not occur with antimicrobial treatment alone (see Supportive Care).

Although treatment leads to clinical improvement and a reduction in antibody titers, *B. burgdorferi* can persist in tissues after treatment is discontinued. Studies in mouse and primate models have shown that despite negative cultures after treatment, PCR assays remain positive, and infection can be transmitted from PCR-positive to naïve animals.[51,52] Regardless of the serologic test used, antibody titers can persist for months or years after resolution of clinical signs and antimicrobial drug treatment, so the results of antibody testing are not consistently useful to guide further treatment when clinical resolution of arthritis has occurred.

Supportive Care

Dogs with arthritis usually respond rapidly to treatment with antibiotics, and additional treatment may not be necessary. Severe pain associated with arthritis may be treated with nonsteroidal antiinflammatory drugs or opiate analgesics such as tramadol. Because Lyme arthritis can be reactivated in some dogs by administration of glucocorticoids more than a year after exposure,[53] glucocorticoids are not recommended for their antiinflammatory effects.

Dogs with Lyme nephritis require management for protein-losing nephropathy, which may include treatment with intravenous crystalloids and colloids, angiotensin-converting enzyme inhibitors such as enalapril or benazepril, low-dose aspirin in an attempt to reduce thrombotic events, and nutritional support with a reduced protein diet. Placement of an esophagostomy or gastrostomy tube for feeding purposes may be required. Blood pressure should be monitored and if necessary, antihypertensive drugs such as amlodipine should be administered and titrated to effect. Anecdotally, improved outcomes have been noted in dogs with Lyme nephritis after immunosuppressive drug treatment (Table 51-5). The optimum protocol is yet to be determined. Dogs treated with immunosuppressive drugs should be carefully monitored for adverse effects of drug therapy.

TABLE 51-4

Suitable Antimicrobials for Treatment of Lyme Disease in Dogs

Drug	Dose	Route	Interval (hours)	Duration (days)
Doxycycline	5 to 10 mg/kg	PO	12	28
Amoxicillin	20 mg/kg	PO	8	28

TABLE 51-5

Immunosuppressive Drug Protocols That Could Be Considered for Treatment of Lyme Nephritis in Dogs in Conjunction with Antimicrobial Drug Treatment

Drug	Dose	Route	Interval and Duration
Methylprednisolone sodium succinate with either cyclophosphamide, mycophenolate mofetil, or azathioprine below	5 mg/kg	IV	24 hours for 2 days
Cyclophosphamide	200 mg/m^2	IV	Every 14 days for a maximum of 6 cycles. Recheck CBC 1 week after each treatment.
Mycophenolate mofetil	10 mg/kg	IV or PO	12 hours until remission occurs, then consider tapering
Azathioprine	1-2 mg/kg	PO	24 hours for 7 days, then every 48 hours until remission occurs, then consider tapering

Prognosis

It is estimated that more than 90% of dogs that are infected with *B. burgdorferi* show no signs of illness. Dogs with Lyme arthritis generally recover rapidly with antimicrobial treatment and do not develop relapse of disease. It is not clear whether the "antibiotic-refractory arthritis" that occurs in a small percentage of genetically predisposed human patients also occurs in dogs. Seropositive dogs with antibiotic-refractory polyarthritis may have other unrelated causes of their disease, such as primary immune-mediated polyarthritis.

The prognosis for dogs with Lyme nephritis is guarded to poor. In the past, it was noted that most dogs die or are euthanized within days to weeks.[34] Death often results from systemic thrombosis or oliguric or anuric renal failure. Anecdotally, longer survival times of months to over a year have been noted in some dogs treated with immunosuppressive drugs in addition to doxycycline and other supportive treatments.

Immunity and Vaccination

Borrelia spp. can evade the host immune response through modification of outer surface proteins and possibly metamorphosis to a resistant spherical form.[54] Interference with B-cell responses by the spirochete also seems to occur.[55] Humoral immunity is most critical for resolution of infection, although T-cell responses may be important for resolution of cell-mediated consequences of infection, such as carditis in human patients.[56]

Several vaccines are available in North America for reduction of Lyme disease in dogs. Lyme vaccines stimulate the formation of borreliacidal antibodies that are directed against the surface proteins normally expressed by the spirochete when it resides within the tick. When the tick ingests dog blood that contains these antibodies, complement-mediated lysis of the bacteria occurs *within the tick*. Thus, bacteria are inactivated before they invade the host. A canine recombinant OspA vaccine is available that induces the formation of antibodies only against OspA. This subunit vaccine is similar to a Lyme disease vaccine that was previously available for prevention of human Lyme borreliosis (LYMErix, GlaxoSmithKline). In humans, the vaccine was shown to be safe and efficacious, conferring immunity on 76% of adults and 100% of children with a low prevalence of local injection site reactions and flu-like symptoms.[57] However, this vaccine was withdrawn in February 2002 because of concerns that it may trigger autoimmune disease as a result of molecular mimicry in sensitive individuals, despite a lack of scientific justification for these concerns.[58,59]

Two inactivated whole spirochete vaccines are also available for dogs. One contains two strains of *B. burgdorferi*, one of which expresses high levels of OspC. The other vaccine is a single-strain vaccine. The potential advantage of these vaccines is that they stimulate immunity not only to OspA, but also to other surface proteins expressed by the spirochete. This may provide the opportunity to neutralize *B. burgdorferi* when OspA is downregulated, such as when the organism is in the salivary glands and after it enters the host. Concern has been expressed that whole-cell vaccines may be more likely to trigger autoimmune consequences in dogs than the subunit vaccine, especially in dogs that have been previously exposed to *B. burgdorferi*.[34] However, no strong evidence exists that these types of adverse reactions occur. Both OspA and whole-cell vaccines provide protection against infection and disease that results from experimental challenge.[60,61] A study in an endemic area for Lyme disease found a reduced prevalence of C6 seropositivity in dogs that had been vaccinated with a whole-cell bacterin when compared with dogs that had not been vaccinated, suggesting the possibility of protection from natural infection.[62] The dual-strain bacterin has been shown to have a 1-year duration of immunity.[63] Although no Lyme vaccine can be relied on to provide complete protection, side-by-side comparisons of canine Lyme vaccines that are available on the market have not been performed. In addition, whether Lyme vaccination protects against, or contributes to, the most severe consequence of infection, Lyme nephritis, is unknown. Finally, whether there are any advantages or disadvantages of vaccinating dogs that are already seropositive as a result of natural infection remains to be elucidated. The recent identification of reinfection (as opposed to relapse) as a cause of recurrent clinical signs of borreliosis in human patients[64] suggests that vaccination of previously exposed individuals may offer some benefit, because the protection induced by vaccination (anti-OspA antibodies) differs from that induced by natural infection (no anti-OspA antibodies). However, whether recurrent Lyme disease occurs in dogs as a result of reinfection is not known.

Prevention

Avoidance of tick-infested areas, use of topical ectoparasiticides, and routine inspection of dogs for ticks after outdoor activities can help to prevent Lyme disease. Ticks should be removed within 24 hours of attachment, before transmission of the spirochete can occur, but removal up to 60 hours after attachment may still reduce the chance of transmission.[65] Refer to Chapter 28 for general information on tick prevention and removal. Although treatment with a single dose of doxycycline after a known *Ixodes* tick bite can prevent Lyme disease in humans[66] and mice,[67] it is controversial because of the very low risk of infection after a tick bite.[68] A study in mice showed that treatment 2 or more days after tick removal was ineffective.[67]

For healthy dogs that test positive for antibodies to *B. burgdorferi* during a heartworm screen with assays that include a *B. burgdorferi* ELISA, a urinalysis could be offered in order to assess for proteinuria.[34] If proteinuria is detected, further work-up that includes a urine protein to creatinine ratio, aerobic bacterial culture of the urine, serum biochemistry panel, and imaging may be indicated. However, whether treatment of seropositive, proteinuric dogs with doxycycline influences the progression of Lyme nephropathy is not known, so this is controversial. Similarly, a CBC or platelet count could be performed, but whether treatment of thrombocytopenic dogs is necessary is also unknown. At a minimum, tick control for seropositive, apparently healthy dogs should be recommended.

Public Health Aspects

Lyme disease is the most common vector-borne disease of humans in the Northern Hemisphere, and the prevalence of the disease has increased progressively.[69] In humans, the first sign of disease in 80% to 90% of infected individuals is erythema migrans, which is a characteristic "bull's-eye" rash that occurs 3 to 30 days after a tick bite and moves outward from the bite site at a rate of approximately 1 cm/day. In some people, the rash is pruritic or painful, and it may be accompanied by headache and malaise. Early disseminated disease can appear as multiple erythema migrans rashes; myocardial disease that is usually characterized by atrioventricular block; or neuroborreliosis. Neuroborreliosis is more common in Europe and may be characterized by the development of cranial nerve palsies or signs of meningitis and polyradiculoneuritis. Arthritis is a manifestation of late Lyme disease. A small percentage of infected individuals, especially those of certain human leukocyte antigen (HLA) types, can develop chronic, antibiotic-refractory arthritis, which may result from persistence of spirochete residues in tissues.[70] European strains, particularly *B. afzelii*, can also induce a chronic skin manifestation known as acrodermatitis chronica atrophicans.[71]

Dogs do not pose a direct zoonotic risk to humans in the household. However, they may carry infected, unfed ticks into the household that could subsequently attach to humans. The presence of antibodies in dogs can also indicate increased human risk as a result of common exposure to infected ticks in the environment (sentinel exposure).

CASE EXAMPLE

Signalment: "Dako", a 7-year-old MC Doberman Pinscher dog from Amador County in northern California

History: Dako was evaluated for a 2-day history of lethargy, apparent blindness, inappetence, and inability to walk. He was taken to a local emergency clinic within 24 hours of illness, where a neurologic examination was considered abnormal and an intracranial lesion was suspected. He was treated with intravenous fluids and given a single dose of ampicillin (1 g). The following day his mentation and thoracic limb strength had improved, but he remained unable to walk and developed urinary incontinence. He lived on a farm and had contact with sheep, horses, llamas, chickens, geese, cats, and four other dogs, all of which were currently healthy, although an additional dog had died of acute renal failure 1 month earlier. There was no travel history or toxin exposure, but frequent exposure to ticks occurred. Dako's diet consisted of commercial dry dog food, and occasionally pieces of cooked steak and raw goose eggs. He had not received a Lyme vaccine in the past but had been vaccinated regularly for distemper, adenovirus, parvovirus, parainfluenza, and rabies. Dako had been diagnosed several years previously with color dilution alopecia.

Current Medications: Monthly topical flea and tick preventative (fipronil and *S*-methoprene), monthly oral heartworm preventative (ivermectin and pyrantel).

Physical Examination:

Body Weight: 43.1 kg

General: Quiet, alert, and responsive. Hydrated. Ambulatory on all four limbs but appeared very painful. T = 101.9°F (38.8°C), HR = 78 beats/min, RR = 24 breaths/min, mucous membranes pink, CRT = 1 s.

Integument, Eyes, Ears, Nose, and Throat: A thin haircoat with scaling was noted. Mild episcleral injection was present bilaterally. Moderate dental calculus and gingivitis were also present.

Musculoskeletal: Body condition score was 5/9 and the dog was symmetrically well muscled. Multiple distal joints were severely swollen and painful on palpation, including both carpi, tarsi, stifle, and elbow joints. The dog appeared painful when rising from recumbency and when walked, with pronounced right pelvic limb lameness.

Cardiovascular, Respiratory, Gastrointestinal, and Genitourinary: No clinically significant abnormalities were detected. The dog had a large bladder, and actively urinated a large amount during the examination. Rectal examination was unremarkable.

Lymph Nodes: Bilateral popliteal lymphadenomegaly (3 cm in diameter) was noted. The remaining peripheral lymph nodes measured 2 cm in diameter. All nodes were soft on palpation.

Neurologic Examination: No neurologic abnormalities were detected.

Laboratory Findings:

CBC:

HCT 48.4% (40%-55%)
MCV 69.6 fL (65-75 fL)
MCHC 34.9 g/dL (33-36 g/dL)
WBC 17,100 cells/μL (6000-13,000 cells/μL)
Neutrophils 15,561 cells/μL (3000-10,500 cells/μL)
Lymphocytes 171 cells/μL (1000-4000 cells/μL)
Monocytes 1026 cells/μL (150-1200 cells/μL)
Eosinophils 342 cells/μL (0-1500 cells/μL), platelets clumped.

Serum Chemistry Profile:

Sodium 148 mmol/L (143-151 mmol/L)
Potassium 3.5 mmol/L (3.6-4.8 mmol/L)
Chloride 115 mmol/L (108-116 mmol/L)
Bicarbonate 20 mmol/L (20-29 mmol/L)
Phosphorus 3.1 mg/dL (2.6-5.2 mg/dL)
Calcium 10.0 mg/dL (9.6-11.2 mg/dL)
BUN 11 mg/dL (11-33 mg/dL)
Creatinine 0.8 mg/dL (0.8-1.5 mg/dL)
Glucose 102 mg/dL (86-118 mg/dL)
Total protein 6.1 g/dL (5.4-6.9 g/dL)
Albumin 3.6 g/dL (3.4-4.3 g/dL)
Globulin 2.5 g/dL (1.7-3.1 g/dL)
ALT 17 U/L (21-72 U/L)
AST 36 U/L (20-49 U/L)
ALP 60 U/L (14-91 U/L)
Creatine kinase 217 U/L (55-257 U/L)
GGT 1 U/L (0-6 U/L)
Cholesterol 167 mg/dL (139-353 mg/dL)
Total bilirubin 0.1 mg/dL (0-0.2 mg/dL)
Magnesium 1.8 mg/dL (1.9-2.5 mg/dL).

Urinalysis: SGr 1.018; pH 8.0, negative protein (SSA), negative bilirubin, negative glucose, 0-1 WBC/HPF, 0-2 RBC/HPF.

Imaging Findings:

Thoracic Radiographs: Unremarkable.

Abdominal Ultrasound: The liver was diffusely hypoechoic but was normal in size. There was mild bilateral adrenomegaly (0.9 cm). The urinary bladder was very large and was in a pelvic location.

Microbiologic Testing: 4Dx SNAP test (IDEXX Laboratories): Positive for *B. burgdorferi* antibodies; negative for antibodies to *Anaplasma* spp. and *E. canis*; negative for *Dirofilaria immitis* antigen.

Cytology of Synovial Fluid Obtained via Arthrocentesis

	Right Carpus	Left Carpus	Right Tarsus	Left Stifle
Cell count (cells/μL)	23,730	29,370	ND	1020
Neutrophils (%)	85	94	76	12
Small mononuclear cells (%)	2	0	1	41
Large mononuclear cells (%)	13	6	23	47
Interpretation	Marked purulent inflammation with nondegenerate neutrophils			Very mild purulent inflammation with nondegenerate neutrophils

ND, not done.

Lyme C6 Quant antibody ELISA (IDEXX Laboratories): 153 U/mL (normal, <30 U/mL).

PCR for *B. burgdorferi* on synovial fluid: Negative.

Diagnosis: Neutrophilic polyarthritis; possibly secondary to *B. burgdorferi* infection.

Treatment: Dako was treated with doxycycline (5 mg/kg PO q12h) and tramadol (2 mg/kg PO q8h) and showed dramatic clinical improvement within 24 hours of initiating treatment. A physical examination was normal 2 weeks later.

Comments: The positive serology and response to doxycycline suggested the possibility of Lyme arthritis, although it is possible there was some other cause that was not identified and the presence of C6 antibodies was not related to this dog's illness. It may have been too early in the course of illness for this dog to have seroconverted to other vector-borne pathogens such as *A. phagocytophilum*. Other diagnostic assays that might have been useful in this dog (and in this geographic location) include serology for *Bartonella* spp.; PCR on blood for vector-borne pathogens such as *A. phagocytophilum, Rickettsia* spp., and *Ehrlichia canis;* aerobic bacterial culture of the synovial fluid; and convalescent serology for vector-borne pathogens. The negative synovial fluid PCR result did not rule out the possibility of Lyme arthritis, because organism numbers within the synovial fluid of animals with Lyme arthritis may be extremely low. The dog had been treated with ampicillin before it was seen, which also may have reduced organism numbers further.

SUGGESTED READINGS

Little SE, Heise SR, Blagburn BL, et al. Lyme borreliosis in dogs and humans in the USA. Trends Parasitol. 2010;26(4):213-218.

Littman MP, Goldstein RE, Labato MA, et al. ACVIM small animal consensus statement on Lyme disease in dogs: diagnosis, treatment, and prevention. J Vet Intern Med. 2006;20(2):422-434.

Radolf JD, Caimano MJ, Stevenson B, et al. Of ticks, mice and men: understanding the dual-host lifestyle of Lyme disease spirochaetes. Nat Rev Microbiol. 2012;10(2):87-99.

REFERENCES

1. Burgdorfer W, Barbour AG, Hayes SF, et al. Lyme disease—a tick-borne spirochetosis? Science. 1982;216:1317-1319.
2. Steere AC, Malawista SE, Snydman DR, et al. Lyme arthritis: an epidemic of oligoarticular arthritis in children and adults in three Connecticut communities. Arthritis Rheum. 1977;20:7-17.
3. Buchwald A. Ein Fall von diffuser idiopathischer haut Atrophie. Arch Derm Syph. 1883;15:553-556.
4. Barbour AG. Fall and rise of Lyme disease and other *Ixodes* tick-borne infections in North America and Europe. Br Med Bull. 1998;54:647-658.
5. Burgess EC. Experimentally induced infection of cats with *Borrelia burgdorferi.* Am J Vet Res. 1992;53:1507-1511.
6. Whitney MS, Schwan TG, Sultemeier KB, et al. Spirochetemia caused by *Borrelia turicatae* infection in 3 dogs in Texas. Vet Clin Pathol. 2007;36:212-216.
7. Fryxell RT, Steelman CD, Szalanski AL, et al. Survey of *Borreliae* in ticks, canines, and white-tailed deer from Arkansas. U.S.A. Parasit Vectors. 2012;5:139.
8. Strle K, Jones KL, Drouin EE, et al. *Borrelia burgdorferi* RST1 (OspC type A) genotype is associated with greater inflammation and more severe Lyme disease. Am J Pathol. 2011;178:2726-2739.
9. Carrade D, Foley J, Sullivan M, et al. Spatial distribution of seroprevalence for *Anaplasma phagocytophilum, Borrelia burgdorferi, Ehrlichia canis,* and *Dirofilaria immitis* in dogs in Washington, Oregon, and California. Vet Clin Pathol. 2011;40:293-302.
10. Magnarelli LA, Anderson JF, Schreier AB. Persistence of antibodies to *Borrelia burgdorferi* in dogs of New York and Connecticut. J Am Vet Med Assoc. 1990;196:1064-1068.
11. Bowman D, Little SE, Lorentzen L, et al. Prevalence and geographic distribution of *Dirofilaria immitis, Borrelia burgdorferi, Ehrlichia canis,* and *Anaplasma phagocytophilum* in dogs in the United States: results of a national clinic-based serologic survey. Vet Parasitol. 2009;160:138-148.
12. Levine JF, Wilson ML, Spielman A. Mice as reservoirs of the Lyme disease spirochete. Am J Trop Med Hyg. 1985;34:355-360.
13. Brisson D, Dykhuizen DE, Ostfeld RS. Conspicuous impacts of inconspicuous hosts on the Lyme disease epidemic. Proc Biol Sci. 2008;275:227-235.
14. Salkeld DJ, Lane RS. Community ecology and disease risk: lizards, squirrels, and the Lyme disease spirochete in California, USA. Ecology. 2010;91:293-298.
15. Oliver Jr JH, Lin T, Gao L, et al. An enzootic transmission cycle of Lyme borreliosis spirochetes in the southeastern United States. Proc Natl Acad Sci U S A. 2003;100:11642-11645.
16. Little SE, Heise SR, Blagburn BL, et al. Lyme borreliosis in dogs and humans in the USA. Trends Parasitol. 2010;26:213-218.
17. Nyarko E, Grab DJ, Dumler JS. *Anaplasma phagocytophilum*–infected neutrophils enhance transmigration of *Borrelia burgdorferi* across the human blood brain barrier in vitro. Int J Parasitol. 2006;36:601-605.
18. Kybicova K, Schanilec P, Hulinska D, et al. Detection of *Anaplasma phagocytophilum* and *Borrelia burgdorferi* sensu lato in dogs in the Czech Republic. Vector Borne Zoonotic Dis. 2009;9:655-661.
19. Zygner W, Gorski P, Wedrychowicz H. Detection of the DNA of *Borrelia afzelii, Anaplasma phagocytophilum* and *Babesia canis* in blood samples from dogs in Warsaw. Vet Rec. 2009;164:465-467.
20. Shaw SE, Binns SH, Birtles RJ, et al. Molecular evidence of tick-transmitted infections in dogs and cats in the United Kingdom. Vet Rec. 2005;157:645-648.
21. Hanincová K, Taragelová V, Koci J, et al. Association of *Borrelia garinii* and *B. valaisiana* with songbirds in Slovakia. Appl Environ Microbiol. 2003;69:2825-2830.
22. Pal U, Yang X, Chen M, et al. OspC facilitates *Borrelia burgdorferi* invasion of *Ixodes scapularis* salivary glands. J Clin Invest. 2004;113:220-230.
23. Lagal V, Portnoi D, Faure G, et al. *Borrelia burgdorferi* sensu stricto invasiveness is correlated with OspC-plasminogen affinity. Microbes Infect. 2006;8:645-652.
24. Dresser AR, Hardy PO, Chaconas G. Investigation of the genes involved in antigenic switching at the vlsE locus in *Borrelia burgdorferi*: an essential role for the RuvAB branch migrase. PLoS Pathog. 2009;5:e1000680.
25. Al-Robaiy S, Dihazi H, Kacza J, et al. Metamorphosis of *Borrelia burgdorferi* organisms—RNA, lipid and protein composition in context with the spirochetes' shape. J Basic Microbiol. 2010;50(suppl 1):S5-S17.
26. Berger BW, Johnson RC, Kodner C, et al. Cultivation of *Borrelia burgdorferi* from human tick bite sites: a guide to the risk of infection. J Am Acad Dermatol. 1995;32:184-187.
27. Hynote ED, Mervine PC, Stricker RB. Clinical evidence for rapid transmission of Lyme disease following a tickbite. Diagn Microbiol Infect Dis. 2012;72:188-192.

28. Antonara S, Ristow L, Coburn J. Adhesion mechanisms of *Borrelia burgdorferi*. Adv Exp Med Biol. 2011;715:35-49.
29. Summers BA, Straubinger AF, Jacobson RH, et al. Histopathological studies of experimental Lyme disease in the dog. J Comp Pathol. 2005;133:1-13.
30. Susta L, Uhl EW, Grosenbaugh DA, et al. Synovial lesions in experimental canine Lyme borreliosis. Vet Pathol. 2012;49:453-461.
31. Levy SA, Duray PH. Complete heart block in a dog seropositive for *Borrelia burgdorferi*. Similarity to human Lyme carditis. J Vet Intern Med. 1988;2:138-144.
32. Kirmizis D, Efstratiadis G, Economidou D, et al. MPGN secondary to Lyme disease. Am J Kidney Dis. 2004;43:544-551.
33. Dambach DM, Smith CA, Lewis RM, et al. Morphologic, immunohistochemical, and ultrastructural characterization of a distinctive renal lesion in dogs putatively associated with *Borrelia burgdorferi* infection: 49 cases (1987-1992). Vet Pathol. 1997;34:85-96.
34. Littman MP, Goldstein RE, Labato MA, et al. ACVIM small animal consensus statement on Lyme disease in dogs: diagnosis, treatment, and prevention. J Vet Intern Med. 2006;20:422-434.
35. Gerber B, Eichenberger S, Wittenbrink MM, et al. Increased prevalence of *Borrelia burgdorferi* infections in Bernese Mountain Dogs: a possible breed predisposition. BMC Vet Res. 2007;3:15.
36. Barth C, Straubinger RK, Sauter-Louis C, et al. Prevalence of antibodies against *Borrelia burgdorferi* sensu lato and *Anaplasma phagocytophilum* and their clinical relevance in dogs in Munich, Germany. Berl Munch Tierarztl Wochenschr. 2012;125:337-344.
37. Hutton TA, Goldstein RE, Njaa BL, et al. Search for *Borrelia burgdorferi* in kidneys of dogs with suspected "Lyme nephritis." J Vet Intern Med. 2008;22:860-865.
38. Chou J, Wunschmann A, Hodzic E, et al. Detection of *Borrelia burgdorferi* DNA in tissues from dogs with presumptive Lyme borreliosis. J Am Vet Med Assoc. 2006;229:1260-1265.
39. Steere AC. *Borrelia burgdorferi* (Lyme disease, Lyme borreliosis). In: Mandell GL, Bennett JE, Dolin R, eds. Principles and Practice of Infectious Diseases. 7th ed. Philadelphia, PA: Elsevier; 2010:3071-3081.
40. Sykes JE. Unpublished observations. 2012.
41. Liang FT, Jacobson RH, Straubinger RK, et al. Characterization of a *Borrelia burgdorferi* VlsE invariable region useful in canine Lyme disease serodiagnosis by enzyme-linked immunosorbent assay. J Clin Microbiol. 2000;38:4160-4166.
42. Leschnik MW, Kirtz G, Khanakah G, et al. Humoral immune response in dogs naturally infected with *Borrelia burgdorferi* sensu lato and in dogs after immunization with a *Borrelia* vaccine. Clin Vaccine Immunol. 2010;17:828-835.
43. Wagner B, Freer H, Rollins A, et al. A fluorescent bead-based multiplex assay for the simultaneous detection of antibodies to B. *burgdorferi* outer surface proteins in canine serum. Vet Immunol Immunopathol. 2011;140:190-198.
44. Wagner B, Freer H, Rollins A, et al. Antibodies to *Borrelia burgdorferi* OspA, OspC, OspF, and C6 antigens as markers for early and late infection in dogs. Clin Vaccine Immunol. 2012;19:527-535.
45. Magnarelli LA, Levy SA, Ijdo JW, et al. Reactivity of dog sera to whole-cell or recombinant antigens of *Borrelia burgdorferi* by ELISA and immunoblot analysis. J Med Microbiol. 2001;50:889-895.
46. Moroff S, Sokolchik I, Woodring T, et al. Classification of *Borrelia burgdorferi* infection using results of 5 antibody targets in an automated system [Abstract]. J Vet Intern Med. 2012;26:792.
47. Schwaiger M, Peter O, Cassinotti P. Routine diagnosis of *Borrelia burgdorferi* (sensu lato) infections using a real-time PCR assay. Clin Microbiol Infect. 2001;7:461-469.
48. Nanagara R, Duray PH, Schumacher Jr HR. Ultrastructural demonstration of spirochetal antigens in synovial fluid and synovial membrane in chronic Lyme disease: possible factors contributing to persistence of organisms. Hum Pathol. 1996;27:1025-1034.
49. Chang YF, Novosel V, Chang CF, et al. Experimental induction of chronic borreliosis in adult dogs exposed to *Borrelia burgdorferi*–infected ticks and treated with dexamethasone. Am J Vet Res. 2001;62:1104-1112.
50. Greene CE, Straubinger RK, Levy SA. Borreliosis. In: Greene CE, ed. Infectious Diseases of the Dog and Cat. 4th ed. St Louis, MO: Saunders Elsevier; 2012.
51. Embers ME, Barthold SW, Borda JT, et al. Persistence of *Borrelia burgdorferi* in rhesus macaques following antibiotic treatment of disseminated infection. PLoS One. 2012;7:e29914.
52. Hodzic E, Feng S, Holden K, et al. Persistence of *Borrelia burgdorferi* following antibiotic treatment in mice. Antimicrob Agents Chemother. 2008;52:1728-1736.
53. Straubinger RK, Straubinger AF, Summers BA, et al. Status of *Borrelia burgdorferi* infection after antibiotic treatment and the effects of corticosteroids: an experimental study. J Infect Dis. 2000;181:1069-1081.
54. Singh SK, Girschick HJ. Molecular survival strategies of the Lyme disease spirochete *Borrelia burgdorferi*. Lancet Infect Dis. 2004;4:575-583.
55. Hastey CJ, Elsner RA, Barthold SW, et al. Delays and diversions mark the development of B cell responses to *Borrelia burgdorferi* infection. J Immunol. 2012;188:5612-5622.
56. Bockenstedt LK, Kang I, Chang C, et al. CD4+ T helper 1 cells facilitate regression of murine Lyme carditis. Infect Immun. 2001;69:5264-5269.
57. Poland GA, Jacobson RM. The prevention of Lyme disease with vaccine. Vaccine. 2001;19:2303-2308.
58. Poland GA. Vaccines against Lyme disease: what happened and what lessons can we learn? Clin Infect Dis. 2011;52(suppl 3):s253-s258.
59. Abbott A. Lyme disease: uphill struggle. Nature. 2006;439:524-525.
60. LaFleur RL, Dant JC, Wasmoen TL, et al. Bacterin that induces anti-OspA and anti-OspC borreliacidal antibodies provides a high level of protection against canine Lyme disease. Clin Vaccine Immunol. 2009;16:253-259.
61. Conlon JA, Mather TN, Tanner P, et al. Efficacy of a nonadjuvanted, outer surface protein A, recombinant vaccine in dogs after challenge by ticks naturally infected with *Borrelia burgdorferi*. Vet Ther. 2000;1:96-107.
62. Levy SA. Use of a C6 ELISA test to evaluate the efficacy of a whole-cell bacterin for the prevention of naturally transmitted canine *Borrelia burgdorferi* infection. Vet Ther. 2002;3:420-424.
63. LaFleur RL, Callister SM, Dant JC, et al. One-year duration of immunity induced by vaccination with a canine Lyme disease bacterin. Clin Vaccine Immunol. 2010;17:870-874.
64. Nadelman RB, Hanincova K, Mukherjee P, et al. Differentiation of relapse from reinfection in recurrent Lyme disease. N Engl J Med. 2012;367:1883-1890.
65. Piesman J, Dolan MC. Protection against Lyme disease spirochete transmission provided by prompt removal of nymphal *Ixodes scapularis* (Acari: Ixodidae). J Med Entomol. 2002;39:509-512.
66. Nadelman RB, Nowakowski J, Fish D, et al. Prophylaxis with single-dose doxycycline for the prevention of Lyme disease after an *Ixodes scapularis* tick bite. N Engl J Med. 2001;345:79-84.
67. Piesman J, Hojgaard A. Protective value of prophylactic antibiotic treatment of tick bite for Lyme disease prevention: an animal model. Ticks Tick Borne Dis. 2012;3:193-196.
68. Shapiro ED. Doxycycline for tick bites—not for everyone. N Engl J Med. 2001;345:133-134.
69. Centers for Disease Control and Prevention. 2012. http://www.cdc.gov/lyme/stats/chartstables/casesbyyear.html. Last accessed December 30, 2012.
70. Bockenstedt LK, Gonzalez DG, Haberman AM, et al. Spirochete antigens persist near cartilage after murine Lyme borreliosis therapy. J Clin Invest. 2012;122:2652-2660.
71. Mullegger RR. Dermatological manifestations of Lyme borreliosis. Eur J Dermatol. 2004;14:296-309.

CHAPTER 52

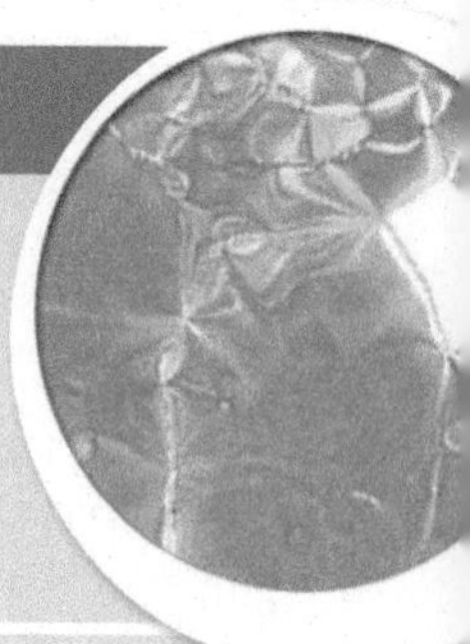

Bartonellosis

Jane E. Sykes and Bruno B. Chomel

Overview of Bartonellosis in Dogs and Cats

First Described: Peru, 1905 (Alberto Barton Thompson) (*Bartonella bacilliformis*).[1] Identification of *Bartonella* as the cause of cat scratch disease in humans did not occur until 1983.[2]

Causes: The most common species in cats are *Bartonella henselae* and *Bartonella clarridgeiae*; in dogs, they are *Bartonella vinsonii* subsp. *berkhoffii* and *B. henselae*.

Geographic Distribution: Worldwide, with highest prevalence in subtropical and tropical regions

Major Mode of Transmission: Fleas (*Ctenocephalides felis*); possibly other flea species (such as *Pulex* spp.) and vectors such as ticks, lice, biting flies

Major Clinical Signs: Signs that relate to infective endocarditis (lethargy, fever, cardiac murmur, cough, tachypnea, lameness, neurologic signs) are the most frequent and well understood manifestations of bartonellosis in dogs. *Bartonella* can also cause endocarditis and myocarditis in cats and is suspected to cause (or contribute to) caudal stomatitis and possibly other systemic inflammatory disorders such as uveitis.

Differential Diagnoses: Cats: major differential diagnoses are other bacterial causes of endocarditis and feline infectious peritonitis. Dogs: other bacterial causes of endocarditis, other vector-borne diseases such as ehrlichiosis, anaplasmosis, borreliosis and babesiosis, and immune-mediated inflammatory diseases.

Human Health Significance: *Bartonella* causes cat scratch disease in immunocompetent humans as well as vasculoproliferative disorders in immunocompromised humans.

Etiology and Epidemiology

Bartonella spp. are fastidious, intraerythrocytic gram-negative bacteria that infect a wide range of domestic and wild mammalian host species. Different *Bartonella* species have adapted to specific mammalian reservoir hosts and can infect and occasionally cause disease in alternative, incidental hosts. More than 10 species of *Bartonella* infect cats or dogs worldwide (Tables 52-1 and 52-2). *Bartonella* infections are important because cats are the principal reservoir host for *Bartonella henselae*, the main cause of cat scratch disease (CSD) in humans, and subclinical bacteremia in cats is widespread (8% to 56% of healthy cats worldwide).[3]

Cat fleas *(Ctenocephalides felis)* play a major role in the transmission of feline *Bartonella* infections. The presence of cat fleas is essential for maintenance of the infection within the cat population.[4] *B. henselae* can multiply in the digestive system of the flea and survive several days in flea feces.[5] The main source of infection appears to be flea feces that are inoculated by contaminated cat claws.[6] There is some evidence that *Bartonella* is present in the saliva of cats, but shedding of *B. henselae* in cat saliva has not been clearly documented. Other potential vectors, such as *Pulex* flea species, ticks, lice, and biting flies, also harbor *Bartonella* DNA, and experimental transmission of *Bartonella birtlesii* has been accomplished with *Ixodes ricinus* ticks.[7] There is epidemiologic evidence that ticks may transmit *Bartonella* to dogs.

Because *Bartonella* infections are often subclinical in dogs and cats, the full extent to which *Bartonella* spp. cause *disease* in naturally infected dogs and cats remains unclear. *Bartonella* spp. have been widely studied for their role in a number of idiopathic inflammatory disorders of cats, including uveitis, lymphadenopathy, caudal stomatitis, and rhinitis, without definitive evidence of disease causation. Without doubt, they are important causes of endocarditis in dogs and occasionally cause endocarditis and myocarditis in cats (Table 52-3 and Box 52-1).

Epidemiology of *Bartonella* in Cats

The most common *Bartonella* species isolated from cats is *B. henselae*. Less commonly, cats are infected with *Bartonella clarridgeiae* or *Bartonella koehlerae*, which also have been linked to human disease.[5,8] Young cats (≤1 year) are more likely than older cats to be bacteremic, and stray or feral cats are more likely to be bacteremic than pet cats.[5,9,10] Older cats are more likely to be seropositive than young cats, which likely reflects the increased chance of exposure over time. The prevalence of *Bartonella* bacteremia in cats is also highest in warm, humid climates (e.g., 68% in the Philippines), whereas it is low in colder climates (e.g., 0% in Norway).[5] At least two genotypes of *B. henselae* infect cats, type Houston-1 (type I) and type Marseille (type II). *B. henselae* type Marseille predominates among cats in the western United States, western continental Europe, the United Kingdom, and Australia; type Houston-1 is dominant in Asia (Japan and the Philippines).[5] However, within a given country, the prevalence of these types varies among cat populations, and type Houston-1 is more often isolated from humans with bartonellosis, even when type Marseille is more prevalent in the cat population. Some molecular typing methods reveal an even broader genetic diversity among feline strains, and most of the strains that infect humans cluster in a limited number of groups.

TABLE 52-1

Species of *Bartonella* Known to Infect Cats

Bartonella Species	Primary Reservoir	Primary Vector
B. henselae	Cats	Cat flea (*Ctenocephalides felis*)
B. clarridgeiae	Cats	Cat flea
B. koehlerae	Probably cats	Cat flea?
B. quintana	Humans	Human body louse (*Pediculus humanus*)
B. bovis	Ruminants (cattle, deer)	Biting flies?
B. vinsonii subspecies *berkhoffii*	Coyotes, domestic dogs	Unknown (fleas, ticks?)

TABLE 52-2

Species of *Bartonella* Known to Infect Dogs

Bartonella Species	Primary Reservoir	Primary Vector
B. henselae	Domestic cats	Cat flea (*Ctenocephalides felis*)
B. vinsonii subsp. *berkhoffii*	Coyotes, domestic dogs, foxes	Unknown (fleas, ticks?)
B. rochalimae	Wild carnivores, domestic dogs	Fleas (*Pulex irritans*)
B. clarridgeiae	Domestic cats	Cat flea
B. koehlerae	Domestic cats	Unknown
B. quintana	Human	Body louse (*Pediculus humanus*) (in humans)
B. washoensis	California ground squirrel	Unknown
B. bovis	Ruminants (cattle, deer)	Unknown
B. elizabethae	Rats	Oriental rat flea (*Xenopsylla cheopis*)
B. grahamii	Wild mice	Rodent fleas (*Ctenophthalmus nobilis*)
B. taylorii	Wild mice	Rodent fleas (*Ctenophthalmus nobilis*)
B. vinsonii subsp. *arupensis*	White-footed mouse	Unknown
B. volans–like	Southern flying squirrel	Unknown
"*Candidatus B. merieuxii*" (strain HMD)	Dogs, jackals	Unknown

TABLE 52-3

Examples of Clinical Manifestations That May, in Some Circumstances, Be Associated with *Bartonella* Infection in Naturally Infected Cats

Strength of Association	Clinical Manifestation	*Bartonella* Species
Definite	Endocarditis[26]	*B. henselae*
	Myocarditis and diaphragmatic myositis[27]	
Probable	Osteomyelitis[28]	*B. v. berkhoffii*
	Systemic reactive angioendotheliomatosis[29]	
Possible*	Caudal stomatitis[32-37]	Unknown
	Lower urinary tract disease[32,36]	
	Uveitis[30,31]	
	Lymphadenopathy[37]	
	Fever[38]	

*Results of experimental studies are conflicting or there is insufficient evidence to prove an association with disease.

Epidemiology of *Bartonella* in Dogs

Dogs are most commonly infected with *Bartonella vinsonii* subsp. *berkhoffii* or *B. henselae*. Domestic and wild dogs are thought to be the natural reservoir for *B. v. berkhoffii*, because *B. v. berkhoffii* establishes prolonged bacteremia in dogs. In California, 35% of coyotes *(Canis latrans)* tested were seropositive, and 28% of coyotes from a highly endemic region were bacteremic.[5] Other *Bartonella* species have also been detected in dogs (see Table 52-2). Novel species also have been identified in dogs from Thailand, Sri Lanka, and the Mediterranean.[11-13]

Because it is often difficult to culture *Bartonella* from domestic dog blood, prevalence studies in dogs are usually based on antibody detection. Unfortunately, this correlates poorly with bacteremia. In addition, serologic cross-reactivity occurs among *Bartonella* species so seroprevalence studies cannot be *Bartonella* species-specific. The prevalence of antibodies to *B. v. berkhoffii* in dogs is highest in tropical or subtropical regions. For example, seroprevalences as high as 47% were detected in stray dogs from Morocco.[14] In the southeastern United States, the prevalence of *B. henselae* antibodies in healthy dogs was 10%; a higher prevalence (27%) was found in sick dogs.[15] Risk factors identified in dogs in the southeastern United States were tick exposure, residence in a rural environment, roaming, and outdoor exposure.[16] The prevalence of *B. henselae* antibodies in sick dogs from the western United States is less than 2%.[17]

Clinical Features

Signs and Their Pathogenesis

After infection, *Bartonella* replicates in erythrocytes and can also infect endothelial cells and bone marrow progenitor cells.[18] It then establishes chronic, often subclinical bacteremia, which can last for weeks, months, or even more than a year and may be a specific adaptation to a mode of transmission by blood-sucking

BOX 52-1

Descriptive Case Reports or Small Case Series Where *Bartonella* Has Been Detected within Lesions in Dogs using Culture or PCR

Endocarditis
B. v. berkhoffii[45-47]
B. henselae[45,48]
B. clarridgeiae[46]
B. koehlerae[48]
B. quintana[49]
B. rochalimae[50]

Chronic lymphocytic hepatitis with copper accumulation (Doberman)
B. clarridgeiae[51]

Systemic pyogranulomatous disease, hyperviscosity syndrome
Bartonella spp.[52]

Pyogranulomatous lymphadenitis
B. henselae[53]

Granulomatous hepatitis
B. henselae[51]

Peliosis hepatis
B. henselae[54]

Systemic granulomatous disease and sialometaplasia
B. henselae
B. v. berkhoffii[55]

Chronic erosive polyarthritis
B. henselae
B. v. berkhoffii[56]

Massive post-traumatic seroma
B. henselae
B. v. berkhoffii[57]

Hemangiopericytoma
B. v. berkhoffii or *B. henselae*[29]

Epistaxis
B. v. berkhoffii or *B. henselae*[58]

Meningoradiculoneuritis and pyogranulomatous dermatitis or panniculitis
B. v. berkhoffii[59]

Bacillary angiomatosis
B. v. berkhoffii[60]

arthropods.[19] Infection of endothelial cells may be more likely to occur in incidental hosts and appears to be necessary for the development of disorders such as vasculoproliferative disease and endocarditis. *Bartonella* is thought to cause vasculoproliferative disease via cytokine-induced stimulation of endothelial cell proliferation and inhibition of endothelial cell apoptosis. Virulence factors characterized in *Bartonella* species include adhesins, heme acquisition mechanisms, type IV secretion systems, and a low-potency lipopolysaccharide, among others.[20] Host immunocompromise, such as due to genetic susceptibility (e.g., breed-related immunodeficiency syndromes), poor nutrition, overcrowding, co-infections with other pathogens, immunosuppressive drug treatment, or defects in normal host barriers (such as congenital valvular disease in dogs with endocarditis), may also influence whether disease ultimately develops in infected dogs and cats.

The vast majority of infected dogs and cats show no overt clinical signs of illness when bacteremic. In some situations, disease manifestations that occur in *Bartonella* spp.–infected dogs and cats are otherwise uncommon to rare and/or known to be associated with *Bartonella* infection in human patients; organisms may also have been visualized with silver stains using light microscopy in affected tissues (e.g., endocarditis or myocarditis lesions). In other situations, nonspecific clinical signs are present (e.g., uveitis, gingivostomatitis, chylothorax, polyarthritis, chronic rhinitis, idiopathic lower urinary tract disease, lymphadenopathy, reproductive disease, or neurologic disorders), and it has been impossible to clearly assign a role to *Bartonella* in disease causation. A clear understanding of the role of *Bartonella* in disease causation has also been thwarted by limitations of diagnostic tests available for detection of infection.

Clinical Manifestations in Cats

Experimental infections of specific pathogen free cats with *Bartonella* have shed light on disease processes that can follow infection of cats with *Bartonella*. Cats infected with *B. henselae* develop a small papule at the site of inoculation, and transient fever and lymphadenopathy.[21-24] Transient neurologic signs (such as staring and behavioral abnormalities) and reproductive disorders can also occur. Some cats infected with *B. henselae* and/or *B. clarridgeiae* show no clinical signs, and gross lesions are lacking at necropsy. However, histopathology reveals peripheral lymph node hyperplasia, splenic follicular hyperplasia, lymphocytic cholangitis/pericholangitis, lymphocytic hepatitis, lymphoplasmacytic myocarditis, and/or interstitial lymphocytic nephritis.[21,23]

In naturally infected cats, *Bartonella* can rarely cause endocarditis and myocarditis. Generally speaking, infective endocarditis is rare in cats, but a few of the reported cases have been associated with *Bartonella* infection. *B. henselae* DNA has been amplified from aortic valvular vegetative lesions of cats, with visualization of the organism in lesions using silver stains.[25,26] Dramatic pyogranulomatous myocarditis and diaphragmatic myositis were associated with *B. henselae* infection in two cats that died in a North Carolina shelter, and organisms were detected in lesions with silver stains and immunohistochemistry (IHC) (Figure 52-1).[27] Carpal and metacarpal osteomyelitis was also associated with a *B. v. berkhoffii* infection in a cat; *Bartonella* DNA was detected in bone lesions as well as in the blood.[28] The DNA of *B. v. berkhoffii* and *B. henselae* was also detected in cardiac tissues of several cats with systemic reactive angioendotheliomatosis.[29]

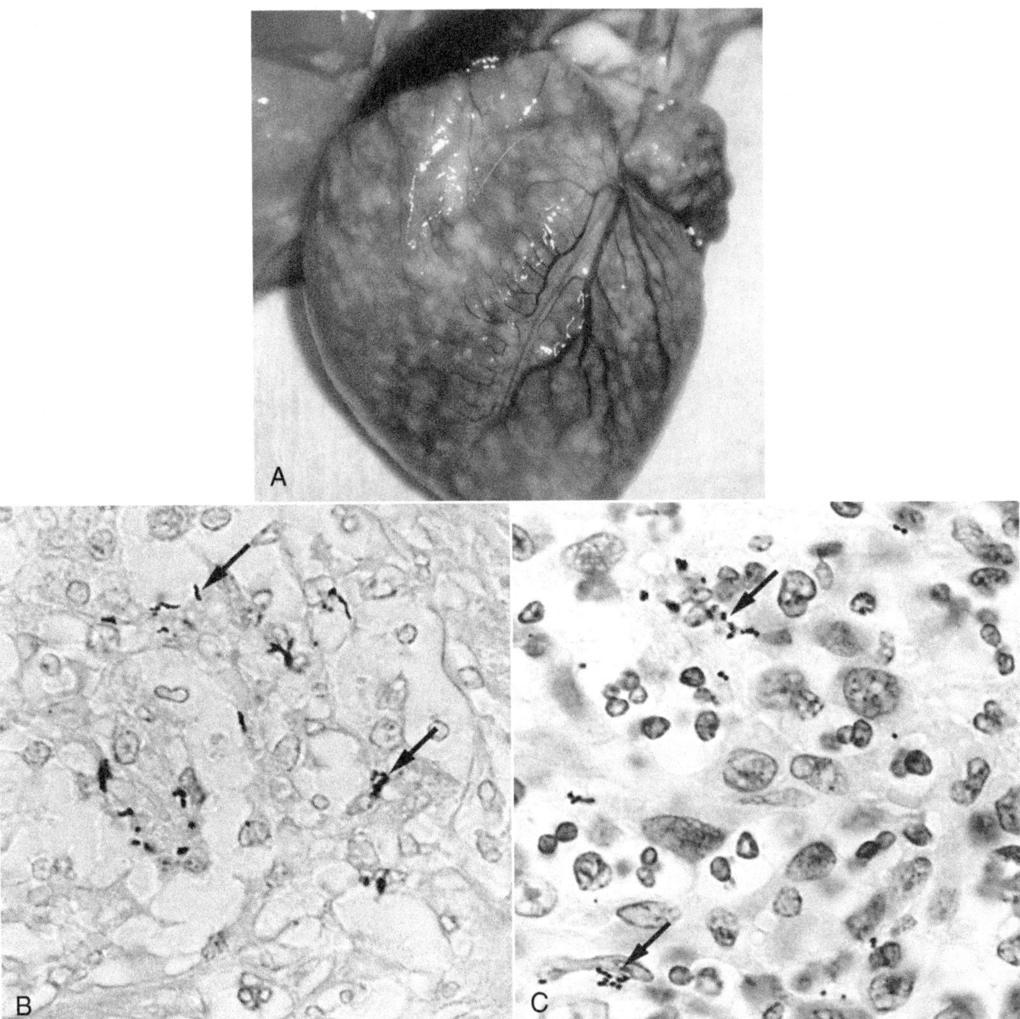

FIGURE 52-1 **A,** Granulomatous myocarditis associated with *Bartonella henselae* infection in an 8-week-old female domestic shorthair introduced to a shelter that was ridden with fleas. **B,** Histopathology of the heart of the affected cat showing intralesional agyrophilic bacteria *(arrows)*. Warthin-Starry stain. **C,** Short bacilli *(arrows)* in an inflammatory focus are immunoreactive *(brown)* for *Bartonella henselae*–specific monoclonal antibody. Immunohistochemistry with diaminobenzidine chromogen, hematoxylin counterstain. (**A,** Courtesy Drs. Jack Broadhurst and Edward Breitschwerdt. From Varanat M, Broadhurst J, Linder KE, et al. Identification of *Bartonella henselae* in 2 cats with pyogranulomatous myocarditis and diaphragmatic myositis. Vet Pathol 2012;49:608-611.)

Bartonella has been investigated for its role in a large number of idiopathic conditions in cats (see Table 52-3).[26-38] These include uveitis,[30-32] caudal gingivostomatitis,[32-37] fever of unknown origin,[38] lower urinary tract disease,[32,36,39] chronic kidney disease,[32,36] pancreatitis,[40] lymphadenopathy (Figure 52-2),[37] neurologic disease,[32,41,42] pododermatitis,[43] and chronic idiopathic rhinosinusitis.[44] There is currently no convincing and repeatable scientific evidence that *Bartonella* infection causes any of these conditions. Studies have varied in the methodology used to detect infection (serology, culture, and/or PCR assays), and many of the conditions investigated likely have multifactorial etiologies. An understanding of the significance of *Bartonella* in these conditions will probably require prospective study of large numbers of cats with clearly defined clinical illness using *Bartonella* culture and/or PCR assays.

Clinical Manifestations in Dogs

Bartonella spp. are important causes of blood-culture–negative endocarditis in dogs (see Box 52-1).[25,29,45-60] Infection with *Bartonella* was identified in 6 (19%) of 31 dogs with culture-negative endocarditis in California.[61] Worldwide, the DNA of several *Bartonella* species has been detected in the heart valves of dogs with endocarditis. The most common species identified has been *B. v. berkhoffii*. In dogs, *Bartonella* endocarditis usually involves the aortic valve, although the mitral valve is occasionally affected, so the possibility of bartonellosis should not be ruled out in dogs with mitral valve endocarditis. Dogs with *Bartonella* endocarditis are more likely to be afebrile and more likely to have congestive heart failure than dogs with other causes of endocarditis, and their median survival time is shorter (Figure 52-3).[61] Complications of *Bartonella* endocarditis include thromboembolic disease and neutrophilic polyarthritis.

Bartonella, or *Bartonella* DNA, has been detected in lesions from dogs with a variety of chronic pyogranulomatous or granulomatous inflammatory and vasculoproliferative diseases (see Box 52-1). *Bartonella* was detected in a dog with peliosis hepatis and a dog with bacillary angiomatosis, rare conditions that are strongly associated with *Bartonella* infection in humans.[54,60] Peliosis hepatis and bacillary angiomatosis are vasculoproliferative diseases characterized by the presence of blood-filled proliferations of vascular tissue in the liver and skin, respectively. Based on case reports and seroprevalence studies, *Bartonella* is suspected to cause polyarthritis, epistaxis, thrombocytopenia,

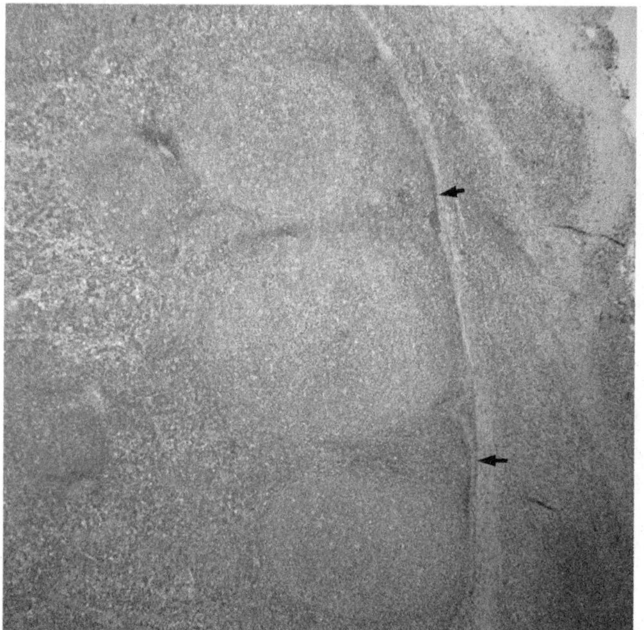

FIGURE 52-2 Lymph node of a 1-year-old, retrovirus-negative, flea-ridden cat with a 3-month history of fever, mild lethargy, and generalized peripheral lymphadenopathy but a normal appetite. The right axillary and both mandibular lymph nodes measured 3 cm in diameter; the remaining peripheral lymph nodes were 2 cm in diameter. A serum chemistry profile revealed hyperglobulinemia (6.5 g/dL). Serum protein electrophoresis revealed a polyclonal gammopathy. Histopathology of the right axillary, right mandibular and right popliteal lymph node showed lymphofollicular hyperplasia and marked neutrophilic, lymphocytic, and histiocytic capsulitis and perilymphadenitis. Note the florid capsulitis to the right of the arrows, which indicate the outer extent of the lymph node parenchyma. Silver stains (Warthin-Starry and Steiner stains) showed a small amount of granular staining within cells, which possibly represented intracellular agyrophilic bacteria. The DNA of *Bartonella henselae* and *Bartonella clarridgeiae* was detected in the lymph node using PCR, and blood cultures were positive for *B. henselae*. Interestingly, the cat was seronegative to *B. henselae* and *B. clarridgeiae*.

and/or splenomegaly in dogs.[17] However, these associations could also reflect the presence of other detected or undetected, co-transmitted vector-borne pathogens that cause these disorders. *Bartonella* has been investigated for its role in canine lymphoma[62]; neurologic disease[63]; splenic disorders including lymphoid nodular hyperplasia, hemangiosarcoma, and fibrohistiocytic nodules[64]; idiopathic cavitary effusion[65]; and idiopathic rhinitis.[66] As for cats, the role that *Bartonella* plays in these conditions, if any, is unclear and requires further study.

Physical Examination Findings

In dogs with *Bartonella* endocarditis, physical examination findings include lethargy, inappetence and thin body condition; lameness or recumbency due to thromboembolic complications, weakness, or polyarthritis; joint effusion; and, uncommonly, fever (as high as 104.9°F [41°C]). Evidence of cardiac disease and congestive heart failure is often present, including respiratory distress, cough, increased lung sounds, and systolic and/or diastolic heart murmurs, cardiac arrhythmias, and pulse deficits. Neurologic signs such as anisocoria and obtundation can occur in dogs with thromboembolism that involves the central nervous system. There may also be evidence of flea or tick infestations in some dogs. Other physical examination findings that might be present in dogs with other manifestations of bartonellosis are mass lesions that involve the nasal cavity, lymph nodes, or salivary glands; splenomegaly or hepatomegaly; cavitary effusions; peripheral edema; epistaxis; or nodular skin lesions.

Physical examination findings in cats with *Bartonella* endocarditis or myocarditis have included fever, lethargy, respiratory distress, cardiac murmurs, and arrhythmias.[26,27]

Diagnosis

Diagnosis of bartonellosis is based on the presence of consistent clinical abnormalities (especially endocarditis or myocarditis, but also other systemic inflammatory or vasculoproliferative diseases), histopathologic findings, and positive culture or PCR

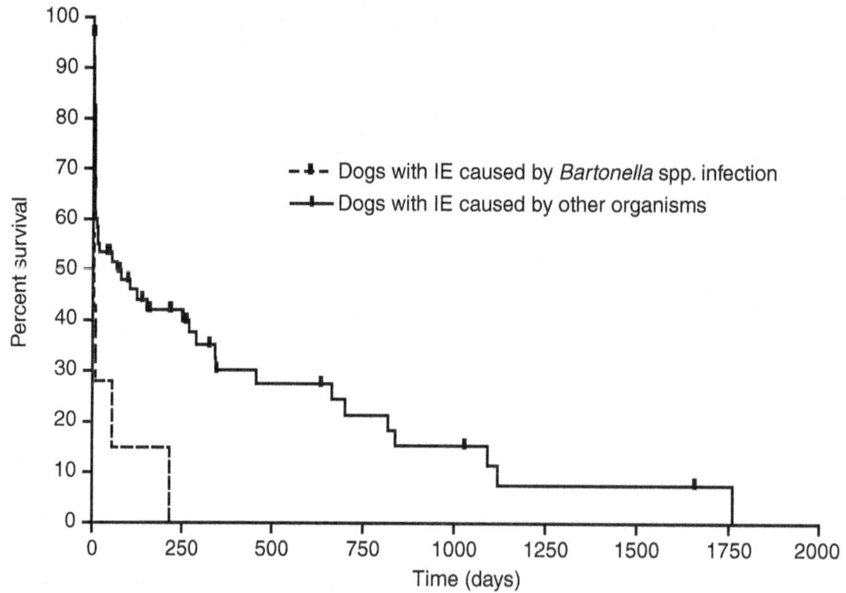

FIGURE 52-3 Kaplan-Meier survival curve comparing survival of dogs with *Bartonella* infectious endocarditis (IE) with that of dogs with IE caused by other pathogens. (From Sykes JE, Kittleson MD, Pesavento PA, et al. Evaluation of the relationship between causative organisms and clinical characteristics of infective endocarditis in dogs: 71 cases (1992-2005). J Am Vet Med Assoc 2006;228:1723-1734.)

TABLE 52-4

Diagnostic Assays Available for *Bartonella* Infection in Dogs and Cats

Assay	Specimen Type	Target	Performance
Culture	Whole blood, tissue specimens obtained at necropsy (e.g., heart valve, myocardium) or by biopsy (e.g., liver biopsy, skin biopsy)	*Bartonella* spp.	Confirms infection and allows species identification. Specialized culture conditions required; best performed in laboratories with special expertise. Requires several weeks' incubation. Sensitivity is especially low in dogs because of low-level or intermittent bacteremia. Use of BAPGM enrichment media followed by PCR may increase sensitivity but may increase the chance of false-positive results due to PCR-related contamination. Positive culture results alone do not apply disease causation, because healthy dogs and cats can have *Bartonella* in their blood.
Histopathology with organism detecting using silver stains or IHC	Tissue specimens obtained by biopsy or necropsy	*Bartonella* spp. organisms	Low sensitivity, but supports disease causation when positive and properly performed and interpreted.
Serology	Serum	Antibodies to *Bartonella* spp.	Variable cross-reactivity between *Bartonella* species; species-specific assays are required. Immunofluorescent antibody, ELISA, and Western immunoblot assays are available. Results correlate poorly with bacteremia. Positive results do not imply disease causation, because a significant proportion of healthy dogs and cats are seropositive. Positive titers are usually present in dogs and cats with endocarditis.
PCR	Whole blood, splenic or lymph node aspirates, tissue specimens obtained at necropsy or biopsy	*Bartonella* spp. DNA	Confirms active infection more rapidly than culture. Sensitivity and specificity may vary depending on assay design and specimen type; may not necessarily be more sensitive than culture. Because healthy animals may be PCR positive, positive PCR results must be interpreted in light of the clinical signs. False positive results may occur as a result of PCR-related contamination.

assay results on blood and affected tissues (Table 52-4). It may be impossible to identify *Bartonella* as the cause of disease if the organism is detected only in the blood and if affected tissues (e.g., valvular vegetations) cannot be obtained for analysis, because healthy dogs and especially cats can be bacteremic. Other possible causes of disease must also be investigated, and a response to antibiotic treatment could be evaluated (see Case Example).[67] It is even more difficult to establish a definitive diagnosis based on serology, but when culture and PCR assay results are negative, positive serologic test results *in dogs* may be of some value in the presence of consistent clinical abnormalities. More specifically (and as occurs in humans), dogs with *Bartonella* endocarditis usually have high antibody titers to *Bartonella* spp. Organism detection tests are insensitive in dogs because dogs tend to have very low levels of bacteremia when compared with cats.

Laboratory Abnormalities

Hematologic and biochemistry abnormalities in dogs and cats with *Bartonella* endocarditis are nonspecific and often mild. The CBC may show a mild nonregenerative anemia (31% to 39%), variable leukocytosis primarily due to neutrophilia (up to 43,000 neutrophils/μL), and mild thrombocytopenia (usually above 100,000 platelets/μL). In a few dogs, low to moderate numbers of circulating band neutrophils, lymphocytosis, and/or monocytosis are present.[49,68,69] The biochemistry panel may reveal mild azotemia (creatinine <3 mg/dL), mild hypoalbuminemia, and, less often, hyperglobulinemia. Isosthenuria, proteinuria, cylindruria, and slightly increased urine protein-to-creatinine ratios have been present in the urine of some affected dogs. Dogs with hepatic disorders associated with *Bartonella* infection have had moderately increased activities of serum ALT and/or ALP.[51,54]

Diagnostic Imaging

Plain Radiography

Thoracic radiographs in dogs with *Bartonella* endocarditis often show evidence of congestive heart failure, with venous engorgement and pulmonary edema (Figure 52-4). Lung lobe consolidation and hilar lymphadenopathy were described in a dog with systemic granulomatous disease and sialometaplasia.[55]

Abdominal Ultrasound

Ultrasound of dogs with systemic granulomatous or pyogranulomatous disease may reveal lymphadenomegaly and organomegaly,[52] and mixed echogenic patterns within the liver.[51] The dog with peliosis hepatis had ascites and multiple, small nodular masses and hypoechoic cystic lesions within the liver.[54]

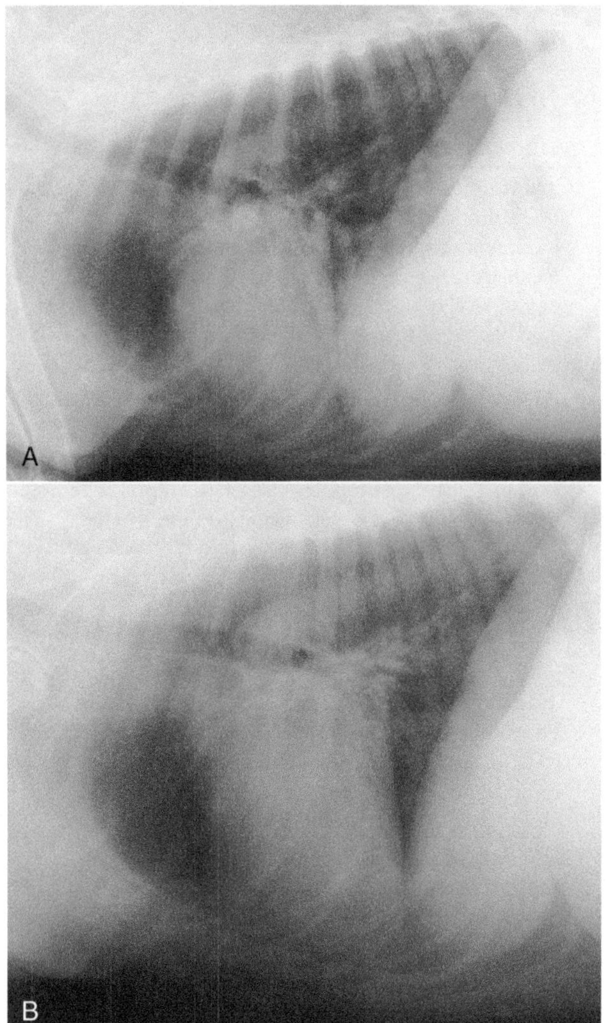

FIGURE 52-4 Lateral thoracic radiograph from a 3-year-old female spayed Doberman pinscher with early congestive heart failure due to endocarditis, before (A) and after (B) treatment with furosemide. The dog was seroreactive to *Bartonella vinsonii* subsp. *berkhoffii* with a titer of 1:256 and *Bartonella henselae* with a titer of 1:64. **A,** There is mild cardiomegaly with left atrial enlargement. There is increased pulmonary interstitial opacity that is most pronounced in the accessory lung lobe, as well as cranial to the heart. **B,** Pulmonary infiltrates have significantly resolved.

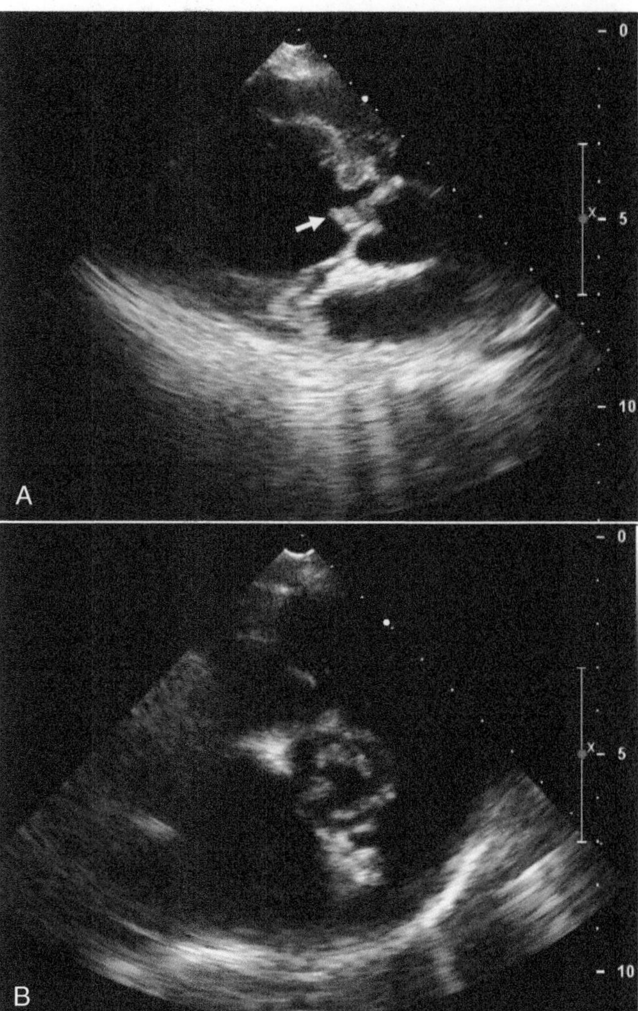

FIGURE 52-5 Echocardiogram images from a 13-year old German shepherd dog with blood culture–negative endocarditis. The dog also had biopsy-confirmed glomerulonephritis. IFA serology for *Bartonella vinsonii* subsp. *berkhoffii*, *Bartonella clarridgeiae*, and *Bartonella henselae* were positive at titers of 1:512, 1:1024, and 1:128, respectively. On the long-axis view **(A)** there is an irregular hyperechoic lesion attached to the aortic valve cusps *(arrow)*, and the cusps appear thickened. On the short-axis view **(B)**, the normal "Mercedes Benz" sign has been destroyed by the aortic valvular thickenings.

Echocardiography

Echocardiography in dogs and cats with *Bartonella* endocarditis reveals oscillating valvular vegetations or thickened and hyperechoic valve leaflets, which usually involve the aortic valve (Figure 52-5). There may be evidence of aortic regurgitation or insufficiency and eccentric hypertrophy of the left ventricle in some dogs.

Microbiologic Tests

Culture

Culture of blood or other tissues for *Bartonella* allows definitive diagnosis of infection. However, blood culture requires special techniques and can be insensitive because of the relapsing nature of bacteremia. In contrast to the situation in cats, culture has especially low sensitivity in dogs because of the low level of bacteremia in dogs (especially when they act as incidental hosts and develop disease). Blood for culture should be obtained using sterile technique and the blood placed in EDTA-containing tubes, and then chilled or frozen during shipment. Collection of blood into plastic EDTA tubes allows the tubes to be frozen directly, which releases organisms from erythrocytes after which they are plated onto special media. Blood should be sent to laboratories familiar with the culture of these fastidious organisms, and the laboratories should be contacted for specific instructions regarding specimen collection and submission. Special media (such as fresh chocolate agar, or brain-heart infusion agar enriched with 5% to 10% blood) and culture conditions (5% CO_2, temperatures of 35°C to 37°C) are used to enhance the likelihood of isolation of *Bartonella*.[62] Extended incubation times of up to 6 to 8 weeks are often required. Serial *Bartonella* blood cultures may enhance the chance of a positive result. The use of an insect growth medium (*Bartonella* Alpha Proteobacteria Growth Medium, or BAPGM) that is enriched with multiple micronutrients and defibrinated sheep blood for pre-enrichment culture of blood and potentially other tissues, followed by PCR assay of the liquid culture and subinoculation of the liquid culture onto agar plates, may enhance the sensitivity of culture for diagnosis of *Bartonella* infections of dogs. It also has the potential to yield other fastidious organisms not cultured under routine conditions that may play a role in endocarditis.[70]

Molecular Diagnosis Using the Polymerase Chain Reaction

A variety of PCR-based assays have been developed for rapid detection of *Bartonella* DNA in blood or other tissues. Some veterinary diagnostic laboratories offer real-time PCR assays for detection of *Bartonella* species as a component of vector-borne PCR panels. Some assays detect all species of *Bartonella*, whereas others are species-specific. Genetic analysis of the resultant PCR products can also be performed to identify the infecting species. The clinical performance of many of these assays when compared with culture has not been well studied. When used directly on blood specimens, PCR assays may be no more sensitive than culture for detection of *Bartonella*, and detection of DNA does not always equate to detection of living organisms. False-positive PCR assay results due to laboratory contamination have the potential to occur.

Serologic Diagnosis

Immunofluorescent antibody (IFA), ELISA, and Western immunoblot assays are available for detection of antibodies to *Bartonella* species. Some degree of cross-reactivity occurs among *Bartonella* species, but multiple species-specific assays still should be performed to increase the chance of antibody detection. Paired titers are not valuable because disease typically results from chronic and persistent infection. If serologic testing is performed in dogs, at a minimum it should include testing for *B. henselae, B. v. berkhoffii, B. rochalimae,* and *B. clarridgeiae.* Measurement of serum antibodies to *Bartonella* has a limited ability to help determine whether a sick animal has an active *Bartonella* infection. In both cats and dogs, bacteremia can occur in the absence of detectable antibodies (see Figure 52-2), and seropositive cats and dogs are not always bacteremic. Fewer than half of antibody-positive cats are bacteremic, and 3% to 15% of antibody-negative cats are bacteremic.[67] Because of this, serology is not recommended for routine diagnosis of *Bartonella* infection in cats. Because of the low sensitivity of PCR and culture in dogs, serology could be considered when these assays and routine blood cultures are negative (or in conjunction with PCR and culture) to support a diagnosis of *Bartonella* endocarditis (which is usually associated with high antibody titers).

Pathologic Findings

Gross necropsy of dogs and cats with *Bartonella* endocarditis may reveal evidence of congestive heart failure, with lung congestion and edema. Single or multiple, variably sized nodules are typically present on the periphery of valvular leaflets, which may be small and firm or large, granular, and friable (Figure 52-6). White plaques may be found adherent to the adjacent endocardial surfaces. Histopathology reveals chronic inflammation, with fibrous tissue and extensive mineral deposits. The presence of valvular mineralization should raise suspicion for *Bartonella* endocarditis, because mineralization is uncommonly associated with endocarditis caused by other bacteria.[61] Small bacilli may be seen within lesions with silver stains or immunohistochemical stains for *B. henselae*.[26,27,60] Silver stains must be interpreted with caution, because necrotic debris and nuclear material can mimic positive staining. Gross lesions in the dog with peliosis hepatis consisted of multiple, 0.1- to 0.3-cm cysts in the liver that were filled with cloudy, serosanguineous fluid.[54] The cysts were lined with endothelial cells, and there was evidence of telangiectasia

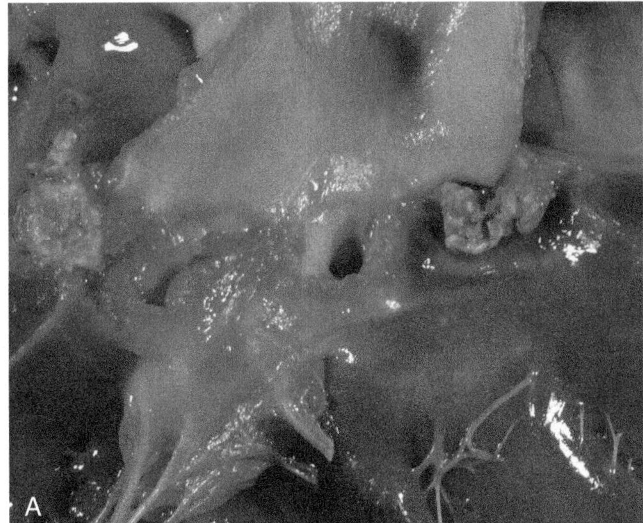

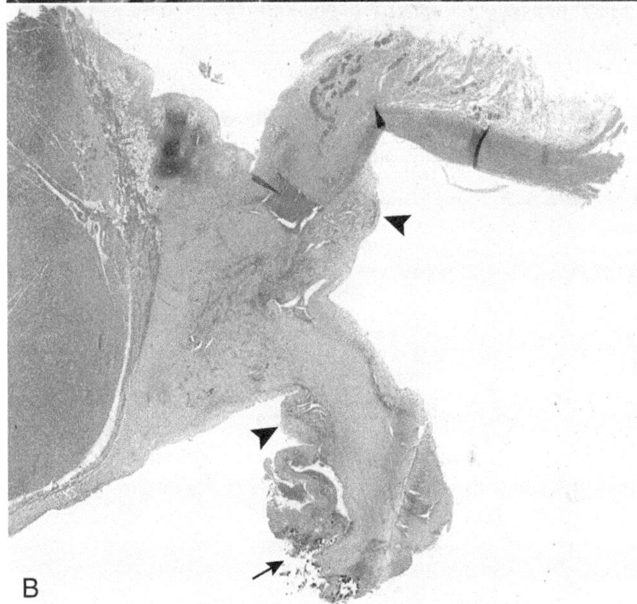

FIGURE 52-6 Gross pathologic findings (A) and histopathology (B) of the aortic valve from a dog with *Bartonella* endocarditis. **A,** The periphery of the valve is eroded. Variably sized, mineralized nodules expand the valve leaflet. There are multifocal, slightly raised, dull white plaques on the surface of the adjacent aorta and ventricular endocardium. **B,** Aortic valve, aorta, and ventricular septum. The distal leaflet is fragmented and contains mineral deposits *(arrow)* and hemorrhage. At the base of the valve, the endothelial surface is lifted and there are broad bands of loose connective tissue, small vessels, and endothelial-lined clefts *(arrowheads)*. H&E stain. Bar = 180 μm. (Reprinted from Pesavento PA, Chomel BB, Kasten RW, et al. Pathology of *Bartonella* endocarditis in six dogs. Vet Pathol 2005;3:370-373.)

scattered through other parts of the liver. Nodular granulomatous or pyogranulomatous lesions in lymphoid or other tissues (such as the liver, lymph nodes, and nasal cavity) have also been described in dogs with bartonellosis,[47,51,71] and nodular pyogranulomatous inflammatory lesions with intralesional bacteria were described in the myocardium and diaphragm of cats with *Bartonella* myocarditis and diaphragmatic myositis.[27]

Treatment and Prognosis

Efficacy has not been established for any antimicrobial that could be used to eliminate *Bartonella* bacteremia in cats or dogs. In humans, doxycycline, erythromycin, and rifampin are the most

TABLE 52-5

Medications That Could Be Used to treat *Bartonella* spp. Infections in Sick Dogs and Cats Suspected to have Bartonellosis

Drug	Dose (mg/kg)	Route	Interval (hours)
Ampicillin sodium	10-20	IV	6-8
Gentamicin sulfate*	9-14 (dogs), 5-8 (cats)	IV, IM, SC	24
Amoxicillin-clavulanate	12.5-25	PO	8
Doxycycline	10	PO	12
Rifampin†	5	PO	12
Azithromycin	5-10	PO	24
Marbofloxacin	2.75-5.5	PO	24
Enrofloxacin‡	5 (cats), 5-20 (dogs)	PO	24

*Use in combination with ampicillin for initial treatment of endocarditis; other aminoglycosides could be substituted for gentamicin (such as amikacin). Monitor renal values during treatment.

†Use in combination with doxycycline; avoid monotherapy with rifampin because of the potential for rapid selection for resistant bacteria. May cause gastrointestinal adverse effects.

‡Other fluoroquinolones are preferred in cats due to the higher risk of retinal toxicity with enrofloxacin. Doses of 5 mg/kg q24h should never be exceeded in cats.

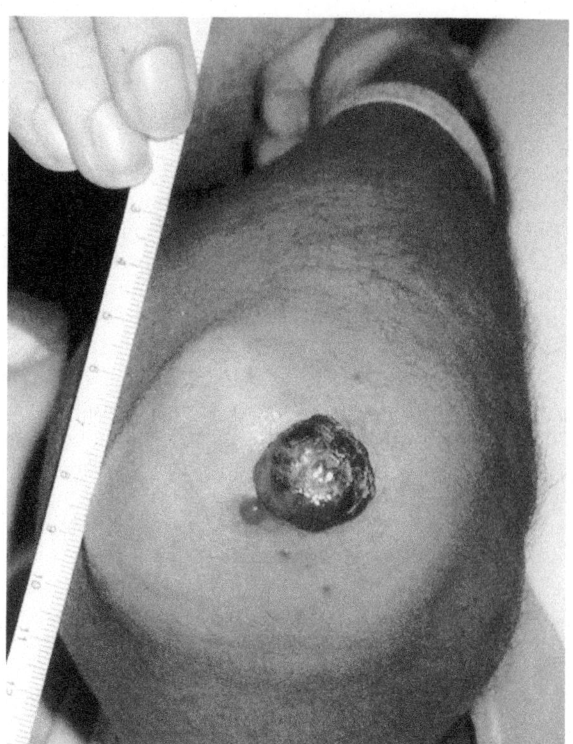

FIGURE 52-7 A crop of cutaneous bacillary angiomatosis lesions on the elbow of an AIDS patient. All lesions involuted with doxycycline treatment. (From Slater LN, Welch DF. *Bartonella*, including cat-scratch disease. In: Mandell GL, Bennett JE, Dolin R, eds. Mandell, Douglas and Bennett's Principles and Practice of Infectious Diseases, 7 ed. Philadelphia, PA: Churchill Livingstone Elsevier; 2010:2995-3009.)

frequently recommended antimicrobials for treatment of *Bartonella* infection, but clinical improvement has been reported after the use of penicillin, gentamicin, ceftriaxone, ciprofloxacin, or azithromycin. Treatment for 2 weeks is recommended for immunocompetent patients (e.g., for CSD), and for a minimum of 6 weeks in immunocompromised humans. Relapses in bacteremia, fever, or other disease manifestations have been reported in immunocompromised humans, despite a 6-week treatment regimen.

The prognosis for *Bartonella* endocarditis in dogs and cats is generally poor. Supportive care and medications such as furosemide to manage congestive heart failure are often required. A combination of a β-lactam and an aminoglycoside or doxycycline is recommended for treatment of *Bartonella* endocarditis in human patients, and valve replacement is usually indicated (see Chapter 86).[72] Oral antimicrobial alternatives for dogs that are stable include high-dose doxycycline, alone or in combination with rifampin; azithromycin; or fluoroquinolones, alone or in combination with amoxicillin (Table 52-5). Resistance of *B. henselae* to azithromycin and fluoroquinolones has been documented.[73] Data from experimentally or naturally infected cats indicate that a high dose of doxycycline may be necessary to eliminate *Bartonella* infection in cats. Amoxicillin–clavulanic acid may also be an appropriate choice for treatment of infected cats when a definitive diagnosis is not known. If there is no response after 7 days, a change to a fluoroquinolone or azithromycin could be considered.[67] Extreme care should be taken to avoid scratches or bites when administering drugs to bacteremic cats.

Immunity and Vaccination

There are no vaccines for prevention of bartonellosis in cats or dogs. *Bartonella* evades the host immune system and establishes a persistent intracellular infection. Dogs and cats can be co-infected with multiple different *Bartonella* species and genotypes. Vaccination and challenge with the same or different *Bartonella* species results in variable protection, and protection is generally species specific.[74-76]

Prevention

Prevention of *Bartonella* infections in cats and dogs is best accomplished by avoiding exposure to arthropod vectors. Flea control measures, such as use of ectoparasiticides, can interrupt transmission of *B. henselae* among cats and should be maintained year-round.[67,77] Housing cats indoors may also reduce exposure to fleas. *B. henselae* and *B. clarridgeiae* have been transmitted through inoculation of infected cat blood; therefore, cats of unknown *Bartonella* status or cats that are positive by culture, serology, and/or PCR for *Bartonella* should be excluded as blood donor cats.

Public Health Aspects

Cats are the major reservoirs for *B. henselae*, the principal cause of CSD in immunocompetent humans. CSD is characterized by formation of a pustule at the site of inoculation (a cat scratch) within 14 days, followed by development of local lymphadenopathy and malaise 1 to 3 weeks after the scratch (or bite), which can persist for weeks to months. Most cases of CSD are self-limiting after several months and respond minimally to antimicrobial drug treatment. Occasionally CSD is complicated by other disorders such as encephalopathy, relapsing bacteremia, osteomyelitis, neuroretinitis, or endocarditis, which require antimicrobial drug treatment. Vasculoproliferative diseases such as bacillary peliosis (e.g., peliosis hepatis) and bacillary angiomatosis (Figure 52-7) are among the most common complications in immunocompromised humans.[20] Young cats are most often implicated in transmission to humans, because young cats are more likely to be bacteremic than older cats. Dogs are less likely to act as reservoirs for human disease when compared with cats, because the prevalence of *Bartonella* infection and the magnitude of bacteremia in dogs are lower than that in cats. Nevertheless, dogs have occasionally been implicated in transmission of *Bartonella* to humans through bite wounds or scratches, and to date, all *Bartonella* species identified in sick dogs are also pathogenic or potentially pathogenic in humans. Immunocompromised humans should preferably choose adult, well-socialized cats over kittens as pets and should be properly educated in regard to the need for flea prevention. Cats' claws should be trimmed regularly, but there is no evidence that declawing prevents transmission. Animal scratches or bites should be avoided, and if they occur, they should be washed thoroughly with soap and water, after which prompt medical attention should be sought. The Guidelines for Preventing Opportunistic Infections among HIV-Infected Persons (United States Public Health Service and Infectious Diseases Society of America) state "No evidence indicates any benefits to cats or their owners from routine culture or serologic testing of the pet for *Bartonella* infection."[78] There is also no antimicrobial drug treatment that reliably eliminates bacteremia from cats, and administration of antimicrobial drugs to cats may result in unnecessary bites, scratches, and contact with cat saliva. Pros and cons for the testing of healthy cats for *Bartonella* infection are shown in Box 52-2.[67]

Bartonella has the potential to be transmitted to veterinarians as a result of scratches or bite wounds as well as needlestick injuries.[79,80] Because of the high prevalence of *Bartonella* bacteremia in stray and young cats, veterinarians should take care to avoid these injuries (consider use of sedation whenever possible if necessary), thoroughly wash wounds that occur, and seek medical attention early if necessary. Gloves should be worn if skin contact with animal blood or saliva is anticipated.

Although cats and dogs are important reservoirs of *Bartonella*, humans can also develop bartonellosis through other routes of transmission, such as via other arthropods and possibly through blood transfusions.[81] Human body lice primarily transmit *B. quintana* among humans (especially the homeless), which causes relapsing fever (trench fever) and endocarditis.

BOX 52-2

Advantages and Disadvantages of Routine Testing of Healthy Cats for *Bartonella* spp. Infection

Advantages

Cats with positive *Bartonella* test results can be eliminated as blood donors or breeding animals

Cats with negative *Bartonella* test results (serology *and* culture or PCR) may be safer pets than cats that test positive

Testing cats for *Bartonella* spp. may allow veterinarians to avoid claims or litigation

Disadvantages

Bartonella serology and PCR can be falsely positive

Some cats with positive serologic test results may have eliminated infection and be immune to reinfection

Cats with negative test results may still be bacteremic, or become bacteremic within the near future

Detection of positive *Bartonella* spp. test results in some situations may lead to needless euthanasia

A focus on testing may lead to underappreciation of the need for other relevant health care such as flea control

There is no treatment that reliably eliminates bacteremia in healthy cats, and antimicrobial drug treatment of cats has not been shown to prevent human infection

Treatment of positive cats may increase the risk of human infection due to an increased risk of bites and scratches

Treatment of positive cats may lead to unnecessary life-threatening adverse drug reactions such as esophageal strictures (doxycycline) or blindness (fluoroquinolones); it also selects for antimicrobial-resistant bacteria

CASE EXAMPLE

Signalment: "Pesto," a 16-month-old female spayed domestic medium hair cat from Rio Vista in northern California

History: Pesto was evaluated at the University of California, Davis, Veterinary Medical Teaching Hospital for progressive lethargy over the previous month. Since obtained as a kitten, she had shown intermittent signs of upper respiratory tract disease, characterized by sneezing, serous to mucopurulent nasal and ocular discharges, inappetence, blepharospasm, tachypnea, and a cough, for which she had been treated with amoxicillin or doxycycline on at least three separate occasions. Between episodes she appeared healthy, but she had always been thin. There had been no vomiting, diarrhea, or changes in thirst or urination. Pesto was obtained as a stray kitten, tested negative for FeLV and FIV, and had been housed indoors ever since. She was neutered at 8 months of age without complication. Five months earlier, she traveled briefly to Oregon with the owner. She lived with a dog and a retrovirus-negative kitten that was introduced 5 months ago. One other sibling had died of FIP, which was confirmed on necropsy. Pesto was up to date on vaccinations for respiratory viruses, panleukopenia virus, and rabies. She was not receiving any medications.

Physical Examination:

Body Weight: 2.9 kg.

General: Quiet, alert, responsive, and hydrated. T = 103°F (39.5°C), HR = 240 beats/min, RR = 40 breaths/minute, moist and pink mucous membranes, CRT <2 s.

Integument: No ectoparasites were noted. The haircoat was full and lustrous.

Eyes, Ears, Nose, and Throat: In the left eye, mild conjunctivitis with moderate serous ocular discharge was

Continued

present. Mild corneal opacity was present in the right eye. No abnormalities detected on examination of the oral cavity. There was no evidence of nasal discharge or abnormal nasal airflow.

Musculoskeletal: Body condition score 4.5/9, ambulatory, adequate muscle mass.

All Other Systems: No clinically significant abnormalities were detected. A full neurologic examination was not performed.

Ophthalmologic Examination: Pesto behaved as if visual and was relatively comfortable with mild blepharospasm. The menace response, palpebral reflexes, and pupillary light reflexes were normal. There was no evidence of eyelid abnormalities or episcleral or conjunctival injection. Mild chemosis was present bilaterally. There was no aqueous flare, the lenses were normal, and a fundic examination was normal. The dorsal third of the right cornea had superficial vessels that extended from the limbus and a 2- to 3-mm central area where ghost vessels were present, which may have represented a previous dendritic ulcer. A rose Bengal stain was negative for ulceration.

Laboratory Findings:

CBC:

HCT 31% (30%-50%)
MCV 37.8 fL (42-53 fL)
MCHC 34.2 g/dL (30-33.5 g/dL)
Reticulocytes 29,000 cells/μL (7000-60,000 cells/μL)
WBC 7030 cells/μL (4500-14,000 cells/μL)
Neutrophils 4570 cells/μL (2000-9000 cells/μL)
Lymphocytes 2179 cells/μL (1000-7000 cells/μL)
Monocytes 141 cells/μL (50-600 cells/μL)
Eosinophils 70 cells/μL (150-1100 cells/μL)
Basophils 70 cells/μL (0-50 cells/μL)
Platelets clumped but adequate. A few Dohle bodies were seen within neutrophils.

Serum Chemistry Profile:

Sodium 146 mmol/L (151-158 mmol/L)
Potassium 4.5 mmol/L (3.6-4.9 mmol/L)
Chloride 110 mmol/L (117-126 mmol/L)
Bicarbonate 18 mmol/L (15-21 mmol/L)
Phosphorus 5.1 mg/dL (3.2-6.3 mg/dL)
Calcium 9.8 mg/dL (9.0-10.9 mg/dl)
BUN 20 mg/dL (18-33 mg/dL)
Creatinine 1.0 mg/dL (1.1-2.2 mg/dL)
Glucose 119 mg/dL (63-118 mg/dL)
Total protein 12.0 g/dL (6.6-8.4 g/dL)
Albumin 2.4 g/dL (2.2-4.6 g/dL)
Globulin 9.6 g/dL (2.8-5.4 g/dL)
ALT 42 U/L (27-101 U/L)
AST 25 U/L (17-58 U/L)
ALP 8 U/L (14-71 U/L)
GGT 9 U/L (0-4 U/L)
Cholesterol 134 mg/dL (89-258 mg/dL)
Total bilirubin 0.2 mg/dL (0-0.2 mg/dL).

Serum Protein Electrophoresis: Results were consistent with a polyclonal gammopathy.

Imaging Findings:

Thoracic Radiographs: No clinically significant abnormalities were noted.

Abdominal Ultrasound: Lymph nodes were moderately enlarged throughout the abdomen, including the gastric, splenic, and jejunal nodes. Hepatic and sublumbar nodes were enlarged to a lesser degree. The echotexture of the enlarged nodes was homogeneous. The left adrenal gland was moderately enlarged, measuring 0.66 cm in thickness. The right adrenal gland could not be differentiated from multiple enlarged nodes. No free fluid was identified.

Microbiologic Testing: In-clinic FeLV antigen and FIV antibody ELISA assay: Negative.

Feline coronavirus serum antibody IFA assay: Positive at 1:25,600.

Treatment: Pesto was treated with L-lysine (500 mg PO q12h), for possible FHV-1 infection, and doxycycline (10 mg/kg PO q24h, immediately followed by a bolus of water), for possible chlamydiosis or mycoplasmosis. The owner could not administer the L-lysine, only the doxycycline, and reported improvement in Pesto's activity level and appetite several days after starting the doxycycline.

Additional Diagnostics and Outcome: Pesto was evaluated again 2 weeks later for possible lymph node aspiration or biopsy under sedation. Abdominal ultrasound showed persistent abdominal lymphadenomegaly. Cytologic examination of an ultrasound-guided aspirate of a mesenteric lymph node revealed mild to moderate lymphoid reactivity. Plasma cells were increased in number and were admixed throughout the specimen with rare mast cells and eosinophils. Low numbers of vacuolated macrophages and nondegenerate neutrophils were also observed. RT-PCR for feline coronavirus RNA on the lymph node aspirate was negative. IFA serology for antibodies to *B. clarridgeiae* was negative, whereas serology for antibodies to *B. henselae* was positive at 1:64. *B. henselae* was cultured from the blood. Treatment was changed from doxycycline to azithromycin, and again there was mild improvement in Pesto's attitude. However, several days later the cat became lethargic again, and her appetite decreased further. After 3 weeks of treatment with azithromycin, Pesto was reexamined. Because of the cat's fractious temperament, sedation was required. No abnormalities were detected on physical examination. A CBC showed a hematocrit of 23%, MCV of 39.2 fL, MCHC of 32.6 g/dL, reticulocyte count of 23,200 cells/μL, 8220 slightly toxic neutrophils/μL, 788 band neutrophils/μL, 1239 lymphocytes/μL, 788 eosinophils/μL, and 298,000 platelets/μL. A biochemistry panel showed similar abnormalities to those previously present (mild hyponatremia, hypochloremia, and hyperglycemia and low creatinine), and the globulin had increased to 12.4 mg/dL, with a total protein of 14.4 mg/dL. IFA serology and culture for *Bartonella* were repeated and showed a titer of 1:1024 to *B. clarridgeiae* and 1:4096 to *B. henselae*; *Bartonella* spp. culture was negative. An ultrasound-guided biopsy of an enlarged mesenteric lymph node was obtained. Histopathology showed a mixed, dense inflammatory infiltrate composed of neutrophils, lymphocytes, and plasma cells. Some of the macrophages present stained positive using immunohistochemistry for feline coronavirus antigen. Treatment with prednisone (1 mg/kg PO q12h for 5 days, then 1 mg/kg PO q24h thereafter) was initiated. Four days later, the cat became anorectic and tachypneic and was euthanized. A necropsy was not performed.

Diagnosis: Feline infectious peritonitis and concurrent *B. henselae* bacteremia

Comments: *Bartonella* infection in this cat was initially suspected because of fever and lymphadenopathy, and infection with *B. henselae* was confirmed with *Bartonella* culture. Ultimately, an alternate diagnosis (FIP) was made based on the presence of the combination of marked hyperglobulinemia, a very high feline coronavirus titer, and histopathology of a mesenteric lymph node and IHC for coronavirus antigen. There was also minimal response to antimicrobial drugs with activity against *Bartonella*. Thus, the *Bartonella* bacteremia was an incidental finding. *Bartonella* bacteremia was detected in the face of doxycycline treatment, which highlights the fact that antimicrobial drug treatment does not always clear bacteremia. The cat was fractious and the owner could not effectively administer the L-lysine twice daily, but assured the veterinarian that Pesto had received the doxycycline. The owner may have been exposed to *Bartonella* during treatment. Treatment with azithromycin was followed by a single negative culture, but antibody titers increased, so the *Bartonella* infection may have been relatively recent.

SUGGESTED READINGS

Breitschwerdt EB. Feline bartonellosis and cat scratch disease. Vet Immunol Immunopathol. 2008;123:167-171.

Brunt J, Guptill L, Kordick DL, et al. American Association of Feline Practitioners 2006 Panel report on diagnosis, treatment, and prevention of *Bartonella* spp. infections. J Feline Med Surg. 2006;8:213-226.

REFERENCES

1. Barton AL. Descripcion de elementos endoglobulares hallados en los enfermos de fiebre verrucoca. Cron Med Lima. 1909;26:7-10.
2. Wear DJ, Margileth AM, Hadfield TL, et al. Cat scratch disease: a bacterial infection. Science. 1983;221:1403-1405.
3. Breitschwerdt EB. Feline bartonellosis and cat scratch disease. Vet Immunol Immunopathol. 2008;123:167-171.
4. Chomel BB, Kasten RW, Floyd-Hawkins K, et al. Experimental transmission of *Bartonella henselae* by the cat flea. J Clin Microbiol. 1996;34:1952-1956.
5. Boulouis HJ, Chang CC, Henn JB, et al. Factors associated with the rapid emergence of zoonotic *Bartonella* infections. Vet Res. 2005;36:383-410.
6. Foil L, Andress E, Freeland RL, et al. Experimental infection of domestic cats with *Bartonella henselae* by inoculation of *Ctenocephalides felis* (Siphonaptera: Pulicidae) feces. J Med Entomol. 1998;35:625-628.
7. Reis C, Cote M, Le Rhun D, et al. Vector competence of the tick *Ixodes ricinus* for transmission of *Bartonella birtlesii*. PLoS Negl Trop Dis. 2011;5:e1186.
8. Chomel BB, Boulouis HJ, Breitschwerdt EB. Cat scratch disease and other zoonotic *Bartonella* infections. J Am Vet Med Assoc. 2004;224:1270-1279.
9. Chomel BB, Abbott RC, Kasten RW, et al. *Bartonella henselae* prevalence in domestic cats in California: risk factors and association between bacteremia and antibody titers. J Clin Microbiol. 1995;33:2445-2450.
10. Chomel BB, Boulouis HJ, Maruyama S, et al. *Bartonella* spp. in pets and effect on human health. Emerg Infect Dis. 2006;12:389-394.
11. Bai Y, Kosoy MY, Boonmar S, et al. Enrichment culture and molecular identification of diverse *Bartonella* species in stray dogs. Vet Microbiol. 2010;146:314-319.
12. Diniz PP, Billeter SA, Otranto D, et al. Molecular documentation of *Bartonella* infection in dogs in Greece and Italy. J Clin Microbiol. 2009;47:1565-1567.
13. Brenner EC, Chomel BB, Singhasivanon OU, et al. *Bartonella* infection in urban and rural dogs from the tropics: Brazil, Colombia, Sri Lanka, and Vietnam. Epidemiol Infect. 2012:1-8.
14. Henn JB, Vanhorn BA, Kasten RW, et al. Antibodies to *Bartonella vinsonii* subsp. *berkhoffii* in Moroccan dogs. Am J Trop Med Hyg. 2006;74:222-223.
15. Solano-Gallego L, Bradley J, Hegarty B, et al. *Bartonella henselae* IgG antibodies are prevalent in dogs from southeastern USA. Vet Res. 2004;35:585-595.
16. Pappalardo BL, Correa MT, York CC, et al. Epidemiologic evaluation of the risk factors associated with exposure and seroreactivity to *Bartonella vinsonii* in dogs. Am J Vet Res. 1997;58:467-471.
17. Henn JB, Liu CH, Kasten RW, et al. Seroprevalence of antibodies against *Bartonella* species and evaluation of risk factors and clinical signs associated with seropositivity in dogs. Am J Vet Res. 2005;66:688-694.
18. Mandle T, Einsele H, Schaller M, et al. Infection of human CD34+ progenitor cells with *Bartonella henselae* results in intraerythrocytic presence of *B. henselae*. Blood. 2005;106:1215-1222.
19. Chomel BB, Boulouis HJ, Breitschwerdt EB, et al. Ecological fitness and strategies of adaptation of *Bartonella* species to their hosts and vectors. Vet Res. 2009;40:29.
20. Pulliainen AT, Dehio C. Persistence of *Bartonella* spp. stealth pathogens: from subclinical infections to vasoproliferative tumor formation. FEMS Microbiol Rev. 2012;36:563-599.
21. Kordick DL, Brown TT, Shin K, et al. Clinical and pathologic evaluation of chronic *Bartonella henselae* or *Bartonella clarridgeiae* infection in cats. J Clin Microbiol. 1999;37:1536-1547.
22. Guptill L, Slater LN, Wu CC, et al. Evidence of reproductive failure and lack of perinatal transmission of *Bartonella henselae* in experimentally infected cats. Vet Immunol Immunopathol. 1998;65:177-189.
23. Guptill L, Slater L, Wu CC, et al. Experimental infection of young specific pathogen-free cats with *Bartonella henselae*. J Infect Dis. 1997;176:206-216.
24. Mikolajczyk MG, O'Reilly KL. Clinical disease in kittens inoculated with a pathogenic strain of *Bartonella henselae*. Am J Vet Res. 2000;61:375-379.
25. Chomel BB, Kasten RW, Williams C, et al. *Bartonella* endocarditis: a pathology shared by animal reservoirs and patients. Ann N Y Acad Sci. 2009;1166:120-126.
26. Chomel BB, Wey AC, Kasten RW, et al. Fatal case of endocarditis associated with *Bartonella henselae* type I infection in a domestic cat. J Clin Microbiol. 2003;41:5337-5339.
27. Varanat M, Broadhurst J, Linder KE, et al. Identification of *Bartonella henselae* in 2 cats with pyogranulomatous myocarditis and diaphragmatic myositis. Vet Pathol. 2012;49:608-611.
28. Varanat M, Travis A, Lee W, et al. Recurrent osteomyelitis in a cat due to infection with *Bartonella vinsonii* subsp. *berkhoffii* genotype II. J Vet Intern Med. 2009;23:1273-1277.
29. Beerlage C, Varanat M, Linder K, et al. *Bartonella vinsonii* subsp. *berkhoffii* and *Bartonella henselae* as potential causes of proliferative vascular diseases in animals. Med Microbiol Immunol. 2012;201:319-326.
30. Lappin MR, Kordick DL, Breitschwerdt EB. *Bartonella* spp antibodies and DNA in aqueous humour of cats. J Feline Med Surg. 2000;2:61-68.
31. Fontenelle JP, Powell CC, Hill AE, et al. Prevalence of serum antibodies against *Bartonella* species in the serum of cats with or without uveitis. J Feline Med Surg. 2008;10:41-46.
32. Sykes JE, Westropp JL, Kasten RW, et al. Association between *Bartonella* species infection and disease in pet cats as determined using serology and culture. J Feline Med Surg. 2010;12:631-636.

33. Dowers KL, Hawley JR, Brewer MM, et al. Association of *Bartonella* species, feline calicivirus, and feline herpesvirus 1 infection with gingivostomatitis in cats. J Feline Med Surg. 2010;12:314-321.
34. Belgard S, Truyen U, Thibault JC, et al. Relevance of feline calicivirus, feline immunodeficiency virus, feline leukemia virus, feline herpesvirus and *Bartonella henselae* in cats with chronic gingivostomatitis. Berl Munch Tierarztl Wochenschr. 2010;123:369-376.
35. Quimby JM, Elston T, Hawley J, et al. Evaluation of the association of *Bartonella* species, feline herpesvirus 1, feline calicivirus, feline leukemia virus and feline immunodeficiency virus with chronic feline gingivostomatitis. J Feline Med Surg. 2008;10:66-72.
36. Glaus T, Hofmann-Lehmann R, Greene C, et al. Seroprevalence of *Bartonella henselae* infection and correlation with disease status in cats in Switzerland. J Clin Microbiol. 1997;35:2883-2885.
37. Ueno H, Hohdatsu T, Muramatsu Y, et al. Does coinfection of *Bartonella henselae* and FIV induce clinical disorders in cats? Microbiol Immunol. 1996;40:617-620.
38. Lappin MR, Breitschwerdt E, Brewer M, et al. Prevalence of *Bartonella* species antibodies and *Bartonella* species DNA in the blood of cats with and without fever. J Feline Med Surg. 2009;11:141-148.
39. Breitschwerdt EB, Levine JF, Radulovic S, et al. *Bartonella henselae* and *Rickettsia* seroreactivity in a sick cat population from North Carolina. Int J Appl Res Vet Med. 2005;3:287-302.
40. Bayliss DB, Steiner JM, Sucholdolski JS, et al. Serum feline pancreatic lipase immunoreactivity concentration and seroprevalences of antibodies against *Toxoplasma gondii* and *Bartonella* species in client-owned cats. J Feline Med Surg. 2009;11:663-667.
41. Pearce LK, Radecki SV, Brewer M, et al. Prevalence of *Bartonella henselae* antibodies in serum of cats with and without clinical signs of central nervous system disease. J Feline Med Surg. 2006;8:315-320.
42. Leibovitz K, Pearce L, Brewer M, et al. *Bartonella* species antibodies and DNA in cerebral spinal fluid of cats with central nervous system disease. J Feline Med Surg. 2008;10:332-337.
43. Bettenay SV, Lappin MR, Mueller RS. An immunohistochemical and polymerase chain reaction evaluation of feline plasmacytic pododermatitis. Vet Pathol. 2007;44:80-83.
44. Berryessa NA, Johnson LR, Kasten RW, et al. Microbial culture of blood samples and serologic testing for bartonellosis in cats with chronic rhinosinusitis. J Am Vet Med Assoc. 2008;233:1084-1089.
45. Fenimore A, Varanat M, Maggi R, et al. *Bartonella* spp. DNA in cardiac tissues from dogs in Colorado and Wyoming. J Vet Intern Med. 2011;25:613-616.
46. MacDonald KA, Chomel BB, Kittleson MD, et al. A prospective study of canine infective endocarditis in northern California (1999-2001): emergence of *Bartonella* as a prevalent etiologic agent. J Vet Intern Med. 2004;18:56-64.
47. Breitschwerdt EB, Kordick DL, Malarkey DE, et al. Endocarditis in a dog due to infection with a novel *Bartonella* subspecies. J Clin Microbiol. 1995;33:154-160.
48. Ohad DG, Morick D, Avidor B, et al. Molecular detection of *Bartonella henselae* and *Bartonella koehlerae* from aortic valves of Boxer dogs with infective endocarditis. Vet Microbiol. 2010;141:182-185.
49. Kelly P, Rolain JM, Maggi R, et al. *Bartonella quintana* endocarditis in dogs. Emerg Infect Dis. 2006;12:1869-1872.
50. Henn JB, Gabriel MW, Kasten RW, et al. Infective endocarditis in a dog and the phylogenetic relationship of the associated "*Bartonella rochalimae*" strain with isolates from dogs, gray foxes, and a human. J Clin Microbiol. 2009;47:787-790.
51. Gillespie TN, Washabau RJ, Goldschmidt MH, et al. Detection of *Bartonella henselae* and *Bartonella clarridgeiae* DNA in hepatic specimens from two dogs with hepatic disease. J Am Vet Med Assoc. 2003;222:35:47-51.
52. Tabar MD, Maggi RG, Altet L, et al. Gammopathy in a Spanish dog infected with *Bartonella henselae*. J Small Anim Pract. 2011;52:209-212.
53. Morales SC, Breitschwerdt EB, Washabau RJ, et al. Detection of *Bartonella henselae* DNA in two dogs with pyogranulomatous lymphadenitis. J Am Vet Med Assoc. 2007;230:681-685.
54. Kitchell BE, Fan TM, Kordick D, et al. Peliosis hepatis in a dog infected with *Bartonella henselae*. J Am Vet Med Assoc. 2000;216:519-523:517.
55. Saunders GK, Monroe WE. Systemic granulomatous disease and sialometaplasia in a dog with *Bartonella* infection. Vet Pathol. 2006;43:391-392.
56. Cadenas MB, Maggi RG, Diniz PP, et al. Identification of bacteria from clinical samples using *Bartonella* alpha-Proteobacteria growth medium. J Microbiol Methods. 2007;71:147-155.
57. Diniz PP, Wood M, Maggi RG, et al. Co-isolation of *Bartonella henselae* and *Bartonella vinsonii* subsp. *berkhoffii* from blood, joint and subcutaneous seroma fluids from two naturally infected dogs. Vet Microbiol. 2009;138:368-372.
58. Breitschwerdt EB, Hegarty BC, Maggi R, et al. *Bartonella* species as a potential cause of epistaxis in dogs. J Clin Microbiol. 2005;43:2529-2533.
59. Cross JR, Rossmeisl JH, Maggi RG, et al. *Bartonella*-associated meningoradiculoneuritis and dermatitis or panniculitis in 3 dogs. J Vet Intern Med. 2008;22:674-678.
60. Yager JA, Best SJ, Maggi RG, et al. Bacillary angiomatosis in an immunosuppressed dog. Vet Dermatol. 2010;21:420-428.
61. Sykes JE, Kittleson MD, Pesavento PA, et al. Evaluation of the relationship between causative organisms and clinical characteristics of infective endocarditis in dogs: 71 cases (1992-2005). J Am Vet Med Assoc. 2006;228:1723-1734.
62. Duncan AW, Marr HS, Birkenheuer AJ, et al. *Bartonella* DNA in the blood and lymph nodes of Golden Retrievers with lymphoma and in healthy controls. J Vet Intern Med. 2008;22:89-95.
63. Barber RM, Li Q, Diniz PP, et al. Evaluation of brain tissue or cerebrospinal fluid with broadly reactive polymerase chain reaction for *Ehrlichia*, *Anaplasma*, spotted fever group *Rickettsia*, *Bartonella*, and *Borrelia* species in canine neurological diseases (109 cases). J Vet Intern Med. 2010;24:372-378.
64. Varanat M, Maggi RG, Linder KE, et al. Molecular prevalence of *Bartonella*, *Babesia*, and hemotropic *Mycoplasma* sp. in dogs with splenic disease. J Vet Intern Med. 2011;25:1284-1291.
65. Cherry NA, Diniz PP, Maggi RG, et al. Isolation or molecular detection of *Bartonella henselae* and *Bartonella vinsonii* subsp. *berkhoffii* from dogs with idiopathic cavitary effusions. J Vet Intern Med. 2009;23:186-189.
66. Hawkins EC, Johnson LR, Guptill L, et al. Failure to identify an association between serologic or molecular evidence of *Bartonella* infection and idiopathic rhinitis in dogs. J Am Vet Med Assoc. 2008;233:597-599.
67. Brunt J, Guptill L, Kordick DL, et al. American Association of Feline Practitioners 2006 Panel report on diagnosis, treatment, and prevention of *Bartonella* spp. infections. J Feline Med Surg. 2006;8:213-226.
68. Cockwill KR, Taylor SM, Philibert HM, et al. *Bartonella vinsonii* subsp. *berkhoffii* endocarditis in a dog from Saskatchewan. Can Vet J. 2007;48:839-844.
69. Chomel BB, Mac Donald KA, Kasten RW, et al. Aortic valve endocarditis in a dog due to *Bartonella clarridgeiae*. J Clin Microbiol. 2001;39:3548-3554.
70. Davenport AC, Mascarelli PE, Maggi RG, et al. Phylogenetic diversity of bacteria isolated from sick dogs using the BAPGM enrichment culture platform [Abstract]. J Vet Intern Med. 2012;26:786-787.
71. Pappalardo BL, Brown T, Gookin JL, et al. Granulomatous disease associated with *Bartonella* infection in 2 dogs. J Vet Intern Med. 2000;14:37-42.
72. Gould FK, Denning DW, Elliott TS, et al. Guidelines for the diagnosis and antibiotic treatment of endocarditis in adults: a report of the Working Party of the British Society for Antimicrobial Chemotherapy. J Antimicrob Chemother. 2012;67:269-289.

73. Biswas S, Maggi RG, Papich MG, et al. Molecular mechanisms of *Bartonella henselae* resistance to azithromycin, pradofloxacin and enrofloxacin. J Antimicrob Chemother. 2010;65:581-582.
74. Yamamoto K, Chomel BB, Kasten RW, et al. Homologous protection but lack of heterologous-protection by various species and types of *Bartonella* in specific pathogen-free cats. Vet Immunol Immunopathol. 1998;65:191-204.
75. Greene CE, McDermott M, Jameson PH, et al. *Bartonella henselae* infection in cats: evaluation during primary infection, treatment, and rechallenge infection. J Clin Microbiol. 1996;34:1682-1685.
76. Regnery RL, Rooney JA, Johnson AM, et al. Experimentally induced *Bartonella henselae* infections followed by challenge exposure and antimicrobial therapy in cats. Am J Vet Res. 1996;57:1714-1719.
77. Bradbury CA, Lappin MR. Evaluation of topical application of 10% imidacloprid–1% moxidectin to prevent *Bartonella henselae* transmission from cat fleas. J Am Vet Med Assoc. 2010;236:869-873.
78. Kaplan JE, Masur H, Holmes KK. Guidelines for preventing opportunistic infections among HIV-infected persons—2002. Recommendations of the U.S. Public Health Service and the Infectious Diseases Society of America. MMWR Recomm Rep. 2002;51:1-52.
79. Oliveira AM, Maggi RG, Woods CW, et al. Suspected needle stick transmission of *Bartonella vinsonii* subspecies *berkhoffii* to a veterinarian. J Vet Intern Med. 2010;24:1229-1232.
80. Lin JW, Chen CM, Chang CC. Unknown fever and back pain caused by *Bartonella henselae* in a veterinarian after a needle puncture: a case report and literature review. Vector Borne Zoonotic Dis. 2011;11:589-591.
81. Magalhaes RF, Urso Pitassi LH, Lania BG, et al. Bartonellosis as cause of death after red blood cell unit transfusion. Ultrastruct Pathol. 2009;33:151-154.

CHAPTER 53

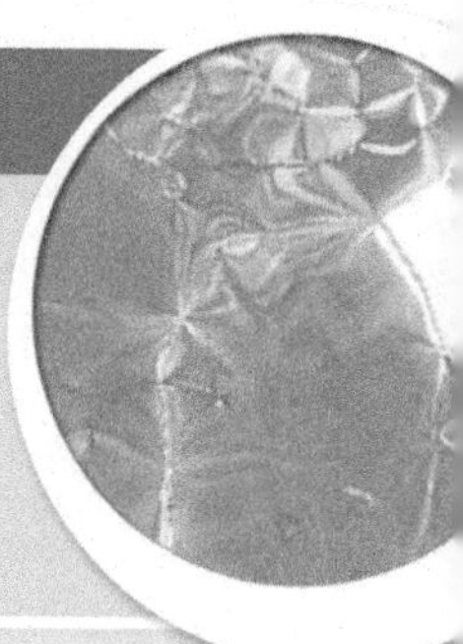

Canine Brucellosis

Autumn P. Davidson and Jane E. Sykes

> **Overview of Brucellosis in Dogs**
>
> First Described: *B. canis* was first isolated from dogs by Leland Carmichael in 1966 (USA)[1]
>
> Causes: *Brucella canis;* rarely *Brucella suis, Brucella melitensis,* or *Brucella abortus*
>
> Geographic Distribution: Worldwide, but infections are most often reported from the southwestern United States, Central and South America, China, and Japan
>
> Major Clinical Signs: No signs or infertility, abortion, nonpainful scrotal enlargement and dermatitis, testicular atrophy, lymphadenopathy, splenomegaly, signs related to discospondylitis (spinal pain, pelvic limb paresis, or paralysis), uveitis, chorioretinitis, rarely osteomyelitis and meningoencephalitis.
>
> Major Mode of Transmission: Direct exposure to contaminated body fluids (oral, nasal, conjunctival, venereal)
>
> Differential Diagnoses: Bartonellosis, mycobacterial infections, chronic vector-borne diseases associated with splenomegaly such as ehrlichiosis and babesiosis, coxiellosis, other bacterial and fungal causes of discospondylitis, intervertebral disc disease, hemic neoplasia (such as lymphoma or multiple myeloma). Additional differential diagnoses for dogs with ophthalmitis include deep mycoses, rickettsial diseases, leptospirosis, and toxoplasmosis.
>
> Human Health Significance: *B. canis* can be transmitted to humans and most often causes mild, influenza-like illness.

Etiology and Epidemiology

Canine brucellosis is caused by *Brucella canis*, a small, gram-negative, non–spore-forming aerobic coccobacillus. *Brucella abortus, Brucella melitensis,* and *Brucella suis* occasionally cause canine infections but are comparatively rare.[2,3] *B. canis* infections are zoonotic, but other species of *Brucella* present a greater risk to human health.[4,5]

Brucellosis is the primary contagious infectious venereal disease of concern in canine reproduction. *Brucella canis* causes reproductive failure in both male and female dogs. Screening for *B. canis* infection is an important part of the pre-breeding evaluation of any dog and should be included in the initial diagnostics in any case of canine abortion, orchitis, epididymitis, and apparent infertility in bitches or dogs. Because the incidence of canine brucellosis is low in many geographic locations, breeder compliance with regular screening can wane, which makes continued veterinarian vigilance important. Notably, neutered and maiden or virgin dogs can also be infected. *B. canis* can also cause systemic disease (such as discospondylitis) in dogs not used for reproduction. Dogs with *B. canis* discospondylitis are typically medium- to large-breed dogs, with body weights that range from 14 to 64 kg; dogs have ranged in age from 1 to 8 years, with a median of 4 years in one study.[6-9] Of 22 dogs with *B. canis* discospondylitis known to the authors, 18 (82%) were intact male dogs, 3 (14%) were female spayed, and 1 (4%) were male neutered.[6,8-10] Three dogs described in the literature with *B. canis* ophthalmitis did not fit this signalment; one dog was a Pomeranian and none were intact males.[11]

Transmission of *B. canis* occurs through direct exposure to body fluids that contain sufficient numbers of bacteria to cause infection (2×10^6 CFU), most often semen, lochia, aborted fetuses/placentas, milk, and/or urine. Transmission is therefore primarily oral, nasal, or conjunctival and secondarily venereal (i.e., through the mucous membranes). Oronasal and conjunctival exposure follows the ingestion or aerosolization of infectious materials. The aerosol route is especially important in crowded kennel conditions. Transplacental transmission and direct cutaneous inoculation can also occur. Although fomite-associated transmission can occur under appropriate circumstances, *B. canis* is short-lived outside the host and is readily inactivated by common disinfectants, such as quaternary ammonium compounds, 1% sodium hypochlorite, 70% ethanol, iodine/alcohol solutions, and glutaraldehyde.[12]

Members of the Canidae family are the natural hosts of *B. canis*. Canine brucellosis occurs most commonly as outbreaks in large commercial kennels, and less commonly in privately owned dogs. Although the geographic distribution of canine brucellosis is not fully understood, outbreaks of canine brucellosis have geographic orientation, with increased incidence seen in the southernmost United States and commonly in Mexico, Central and South America, the People's Republic of China, and Japan. There are sporadic reports of disease in Canada and throughout Europe.[7,13-17] Australia and New Zealand appear to be free of the disease. However, because infection with *B. canis* is chronic and subclinical, the organism can readily be imported into regions where the prevalence of disease is low through the movement of infected dogs. The increased practice and success of canine semen processing for exportation (chilling and cryopreservation) for the purpose of artificial insemination now makes canine brucellosis a concern worldwide, as direct mucosal contact among dogs is no longer necessary for transmission.

Clinical Features

Signs and Their Pathogenesis

Brucella organisms attach to and penetrate mucous membranes; the severity of disease is proportional to the infectious dose. After

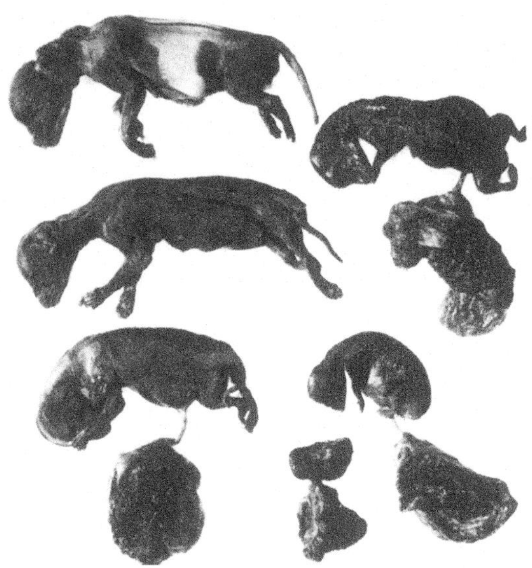

FIGURE 53-1 Midterm abortion from a *Brucella canis* affected bitch diagnosed by AGID. Note the variation in fetal development indicating that death occurred at different stages. (Courtesy Patricia Olson, DVM, PhD, DACT.)

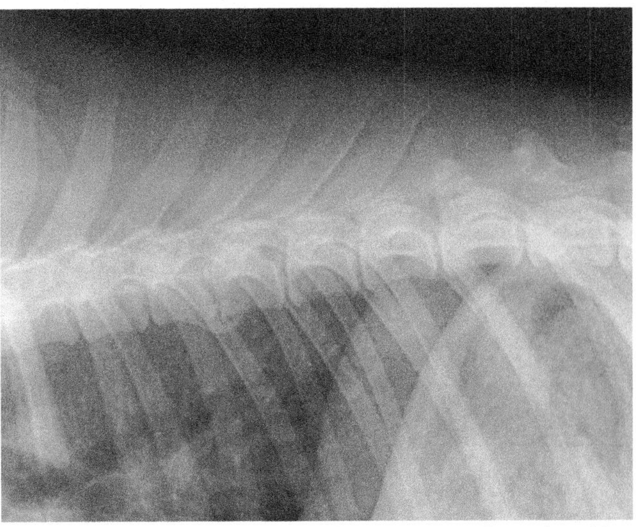

FIGURE 53-2 *Brucella* discospondylitis at the T7-T8 junction with ventral spondylosis and collapse of the intervertebral disc space. (Courtesy Anna Park, DVM, and James Lavely, DVM, DACVIM [Neurology].)

replication in regional lymph nodes, bacteremia occurs within 7 to 30 days after exposure with subsequent dissemination to reticuloendothelial cells, the prostate, uterus, and placenta. *B. canis* has a predilection for steroid-dependent (reproductive) tissues. The organism survives facultatively within monocytes and macrophages of the reticuloendothelial system. *Brucella* organisms can survive and multiply in reticuloendothelial cells because they inhibit the bactericidal myeloperoxidase-peroxide-halide system through the release of 5′-guanosine and adenine. Early in infection, polymorphonuclear cells and macrophages kill intracellular *B. canis* relatively ineffectually.[18]

Brucella organisms can be found in the rough endoplasmic reticulum of placental trophoblastic giant cells in an infected bitch's gravid uterus. Severe necrotizing placentitis with infarction of the labyrinth region, coagulation necrosis of the chorionic villi, and necrotizing arteritis result in fetal death. The organism can be found in the gastric contents of aborted fetuses. Necrotizing vasculitis and granulomatous inflammation results in epididymal and subsequent testicular and prostatic pathology.[3,19]

Brucellosis in dogs is associated with a high morbidity but low mortality. The clinical systemic signs are often subtle and include suboptimal athletic performance, lumbar pain, lameness, weight loss, and lethargy. The primary clinical sign of canine brucellosis in the breeding bitch is pregnancy loss, which can occur early (day 20) in gestation resulting in fetal resorption, or more commonly (75% of dogs) later in gestation (generally 4 to 59 days), which results in abortion (Figure 53-1). Bitches with pregnancy loss early in gestation can appear to be infertile (fail to conceive) unless early ultrasonographic pregnancy evaluation is performed to identify pregnancy. Nongravid bitches can show no signs or can show regional lymphadenopathy (pharyngeal if orally acquired, inguinal and pelvic if venereally acquired).

The primary acute clinical signs of canine brucellosis in the male dog involve the portions of the reproductive tract that participate in the maturation, transport, and storage of spermatozoa. Epididymitis is common, with associated orchitis and scrotal dermatitis, and resultant deterioration of semen quality and fertility. Chronically, testicular atrophy and infertility can occur. The organism can be found in the prostate gland and urethra and is shed intermittently in the urine. Anti-sperm antibodies develop in association with brucellosis-induced epididymal granulomas and further contribute to infertility. Pyospermia develops 3 to 4 months postinfection. Chronic infections in either sex can result in uveitis or endophthalmitis, lymphadenitis, splenomegaly, or discospondylitis; occasionally, dermatitis and meningoencephalitis have been reported (Figure 53-2).[3,8,11,20] Owners of dogs with discospondylitis most often describe episodic neck pain or lameness, which can occasionally be accompanied by lethargy or decreased activity. Bacteremia can persist for years, and subclinically infected dogs can remain infectious for long intervals. Infection of the bone that surrounded a total hip replacement was described in two dogs 9 and 12 months after surgery.[21]

Large numbers of organisms are shed in the vulvar discharge of bitches 4 to 6 weeks postabortion. The highest concentration of organisms is shed in the semen of infected dogs 2 to 3 months postinfection, with lesser amounts for years. Urine can serve as a contaminated vehicle because of the proximity of the urinary and genital tracts in the dog, with shedding present for months to years, and is more prevalent in males. Organisms can also be shed in milk.[22-24]

Spontaneous apparent recovery can occur 1 to 5 years postinfection, but true clearance of the organism is difficult to document. Bitches that have been treated with antimicrobial drugs can produce normal litters after multiple abortions, but can remain infectious to their offspring. Dogs may remain infertile because of irreparable damage to the spermatogenic apparatus.[3,23]

Physical Examination Findings

For dogs with clinical *B. canis* infections, fever is rarely present. Affected male dogs may have an enlarged but nonpainful scrotum and secondary scrotal pyoderma, which results from excessive licking. Enlargement of the epididymis is often present. Some chronically infected male dogs have small, soft testicles due to testicular atrophy. Other dogs have generalized peripheral lymphadenomegaly, and splenomegaly may be detected on abdominal palpation. The most common finding in dogs with discospondylitis is spinal pain.[8,9] Other findings

TABLE 53-1

Diagnostic Assays Available for *Brucella* Infection in Dogs

Assay	Specimen Type	Target	Performance
Culture	Whole blood, urine, disc aspirates or bone fragments, tissue specimens obtained at necropsy (e.g., spleen, uterus, prostate), aborted fetuses and placental tissue, seminal fluid	*Brucella* spp.	Confirms infection but is insensitive. Antibiotic treatment can lead to false-negative results.
Histopathology with organism detection using IHC	Tissue specimens obtained by biopsy or at necropsy	*Brucella* spp. organisms	IHC may have low sensitivity depending on the tissue examined, but supports disease causation when positive and properly performed and interpreted.
Serology, rapid slide agglutination test (RSAT), and mercaptoethanol RSAT	Serum	Antibodies to *Brucella* spp.	Rapid and inexpensive. False positives are common as a result of cross-reactivity with other bacterial species and require confirmation with an alternative test. Positive results do not imply active infection. False-negative results with RSAT can occur in dogs with discospondylitis. The sensitivity of the RSAT may be higher than that of the ME-RSAT.
Serology, tube agglutination test	Serum	Antibodies to *Brucella* spp.	See RSAT. Usually positive by 2 weeks after infection. Titers ≥ 1:200 tend to correlate with bacteremia.
Serology, agar gel immunodiffusion	Serum	Antibodies to *Brucella* spp.	See RSAT. Requires special expertise and is time-consuming to perform. May not be positive until 12 weeks after infection. Cytoplasmic antigen assays are more specific for *Brucella* spp. antigens.
Serology, indirect immunofluorescent antibody (IFA)	Serum	Antibodies to *Brucella* spp.	See RSAT. Requires expertise to perform and interpret. May have lower specificity and sensitivity when compared with ELISA assays or the tube agglutination test.
Serology, ELISA	Serum	Antibodies to *Brucella* spp.	Has the potential to be sensitive and specific, but assays vary in performance. A standard, accepted assay is not currently available.
PCR	Whole blood, splenic or lymph node aspirates, disc aspirates, tissue specimens obtained at necropsy, vaginal swabs, seminal fluid, urine, placental materials, or fetuses	*Brucella* spp. DNA	Confirms active infection and has the potential to be more sensitive than culture. Sensitivity and specificity may vary depending on assay design, specimen type, and quality assurance practices in the laboratory. Results should be interpreted with caution and in light of the clinical picture and the results of serologic tests and/or culture.

IHC, immunohistochemistry.

include lameness, delayed placing reactions, ataxia, pelvic limb hyperreflexia, and, uncommonly, pelvic limb paresis or tetraparesis. Meningoencephalitis may result in behavioral changes, anisocoria, ataxia, circling, or a head tilt. For unknown reasons, ocular abnormalities are often unilateral and include blepharospasm, conjunctival hyperemia, and evidence of uveitis, such as aqueous flare, miosis, iris hyperpigmentation, loss of the normal contour of the iris surface, hypopyon, posterior synechiae, and secondary glaucoma.[11] Corneal edema, vitreous opacities, swelling and hyperemia of the optic disc, and evidence of multifocal granulomatous chorioretinitis have also been described. Ocular abnormalities and discospondylitis are frequently present in the absence of other systemic signs of illness. However, some, but not all dogs with discospondylitis have other, subtle physical examination abnormalities that suggest brucellosis, such as dermatitis, uveitis, small testicles, or lymphadenopathy.[8]

Diagnosis

The diagnosis of canine brucellosis is based on suggestive clinical signs and the results of serology; culture of blood, urine, or tissues; histopathology; and/or PCR assays. Because no single antemortem test has 100% sensitivity, and serologic assays lack specificity, a combination of diagnostic assays is often required to make a diagnosis (Table 53-1). When multiple dogs with infertility problems are present in a household or kennel, as many dogs as possible should be tested with serology and blood culture to increase the chance of a reliable diagnosis.

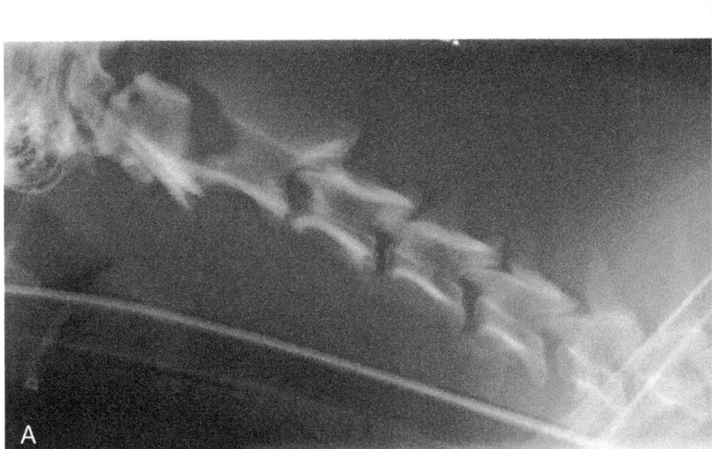

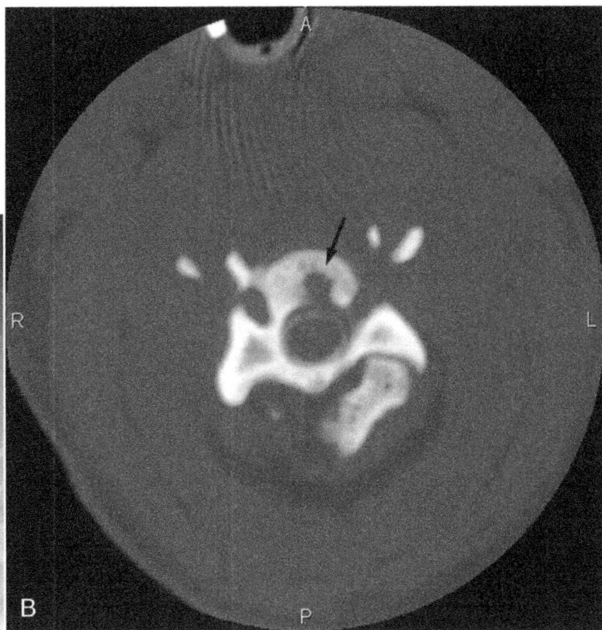

FIGURE 53-3 Radiographic images from a 1-year-old female spayed labradoodle with *Brucella canis* discospondylitis that was evaluated for cervical pain. CSF analysis revealed a CSF protein concentration of 31 g/dL, with 3 nucleated cells/μL, 89% of which were small mononuclear cells and 11% of which were large mononuclear cells (marginal lymphocytic pleocytosis). *Brucella canis* was isolated from 5 of 5 blood culture specimens. Urine culture was negative. Of significance, a *B. canis* rapid slide agglutination test was negative. The dog was treated successfully with antimicrobial drugs (doxycycline and clavulanic acid–amoxicillin) and lesions resolved radiographically. **A,** Plain lateral radiograph of the cervical spine. There is endplate lucency associated with cranial endplate of C3 at the C2-3 articulation. The C2-3 disc space appears narrowed. **B,** Computed tomography image. Central lysis of the end plates at C2-3 is present *(arrow)*, compatible with discospondylitis at C2-3.

Laboratory Abnormalities

Complete Blood Count, Serum Biochemical Tests, and Urinalysis

The results of routine laboratory tests are often within reference ranges in dogs with brucellosis. The CBC may show leukocytosis due to a neutrophilia.[11] Degenerate left shifts, monocytosis, and/or lymphopenia have been uncommonly reported.[9,20] The chemistry panel is often normal, but hyperglobulinemia and hypoalbuminemia may be present. A lack of abnormalities on routine laboratory testing or the presence of splenomegaly or abdominal lymphadenomegaly in dogs with discospondylitis should raise suspicion for *B. canis* infection. Urinalysis is generally within normal limits, even when *B. canis* bacteriuria is present.

Cytologic Analysis of Tissue Aspirates

Aspirates of the spleen or lymph nodes of dogs with brucellosis reveal lymphoid reactivity, sometimes with plasmacytosis. Prostatic aspirates in one dog with prostatitis showed granulomatous inflammation with intracellular gram-negative coccobacilli.[7]

Cytologic Analysis of Body Fluids

CSF analysis in dogs with *Brucella* discospondylitis is usually unremarkable. A dog with meningoencephalitis had neutrophilic pleocytosis and increased CSF protein concentration.[3] Aspirates of ocular fluids (aqueous or vitreous humor) from a dog with panophthalmitis revealed pyogranulomatous inflammation with extracellular and intracellular small gram-negative cocci.[11]

Semen Examination

Diminished sperm counts (oligospermia), poor motility (asthenospermia), and increased morphologic abnormalities (teratospermia) are characteristic of semen in dogs infected with *Brucella*. Detached sperm heads, proximal and distal cytoplasmic droplets, and acrosomal deformities are the most common morphologic abnormalities. Sperm head-to-head agglutination suggests the presence of anti-sperm antibodies. An absence of sperm in the ejaculate (azoospermia) can also be found.

Diagnostic Imaging

Plain Radiography and Advanced Imaging

Plain radiography may show evidence of either multifocal or focal discospondylitis (see Figure 53-2; Figure 53-3, *A*). Advanced imaging (CT or MRI) may be more sensitive than plain radiographs for detection of endplate lucency (see Figure 53-3, *B*; see also Chapter 85).

Sonographic Findings

Abdominal ultrasound examination of dogs with brucellosis may show no abnormalities, or abdominal lymphadenomegaly and splenomegaly may be present. Ultrasound of the prostate may reveal prostatic irregularity, hyperechogenicity, and cavitation.[7]

Microbiologic Tests

Serologic Diagnosis

There are two reasons to perform serologic tests for brucellosis in dogs: (1) as part of a routine screening program in breeding kennels, whereby healthy dogs are screened for infection, and (2) for diagnosis of active infection in sick dogs that are suspected to have brucellosis because of infertility, reproductive losses, epididymitis, discospondylitis, osteomyelitis, or ophthalmitis.

Assays used for screening purposes are usually rapid and inexpensive, but can suffer from low specificity (a high rate of false-positive test results) due to strong cross-reactivity between surface lipopolysaccharide (LPS) antigens of *B. canis* and those of other nonpathogenic infectious agents. Up to 50% to 60% of dogs can have false-positive test results because of cross-reacting antibodies to microorganisms such as *Bordetella, Pseudomonas, Escherichia coli,* and *Moraxella* spp. Even when the antibodies detected truly represent anti-*Brucella* antibodies, the presence of these antibodies does not indicate active infection with *Brucella* because dogs can remain seropositive for months after they clear the infection. Antibodies to *Brucella* do not become detectable until 2 to 12 weeks after infection, so a window of time exists in which an infected dog eludes serologic diagnosis with any assay used. False negatives also occasionally occur in dogs with chronic sequestered infections. Beyond the first 3 months of infection, the sensitivity of screening assays is generally believed to be high, but in some scenarios it might be lower than previously thought.[25] Examples of screening assays include the rapid slide agglutination test (RSAT); the semiquantitative 2-mercaptoethanol modified RSAT (ME-RSAT); the semiquantitative tube agglutination test (TAT); agar gel immunodiffusion (AGID) assays; and indirect IFA or ELISA assays. Veterinarians need to understand the limitations of the assays available to them through local veterinary diagnostic laboratories. The RSAT uses *Brucella ovis* as the antigen, whereas the ME-RSAT uses *B. canis* antigen, which may improve specificity. However, in one study, the sensitivity of the ME-RSAT was only 32%, when compared with 71% for the RSAT, so the RSAT may be preferable for screening.[25] In the TAT, a titer of more than 1:200 correlates well with positive blood cultures, but lower titers are more difficult to interpret. The performance of AGID assays requires trained laboratory personnel and special media. Two types of AGID assay are available: an assay that uses cell wall antigens as the substrate (cell wall AGID assay) and an assay that uses cytoplasmic antigens of *Brucella* as the substrate (cytoplasmic AGID assay). The cell wall assay has from the same low specificity as other assays that detect antibodies to *Brucella* LPS, and the sensitivity may be lower than that of the RSAT.[25] In contrast, the cytoplasmic assay is specific for antibodies to *Brucella*, so, when available, it is a useful confirmatory assay for dogs that test positive with other rapid serologic assays. Indirect IFA has lower sensitivity than many other serologic assays. A number of ELISA assays have been developed to overcome difficulties that relate to the low specificity of serologic assays for *B. canis* and the limited availability of other assays. The performance of these ELISA assays has varied, but sensitive and specific ELISA assays have been developed that may prove useful for rapid serologic testing in the future.[26]

In practice, for screening purposes, healthy bitches are tested at least 1 month before a planned breeding or introduction to a breeding kennel with a serologic assay of low specificity such as the RSAT because these assays are rapid, readily available, and inexpensive. Healthy, fertile stud dogs should be tested annually with the RSAT. If the test result is negative, in cases of subfertility or if recent exposure is suspected, a second test is performed a month later, to assess for seroconversion (which would be expected if the dog was early in the course of infection when first tested). If the test result is positive, a confirmatory assay should be performed. This could include the TAT or a more specific assay, such as the cytoplasmic AGID assay, a specific ELISA assay, blood culture, or a reliable PCR assay, although blood culture can lack sensitivity.[13,15] Usually the assay(s) selected is based on test availability and financial resources of the owner. Positive serologic test results for dogs with discospondylitis or other disease manifestations suggestive of brucellosis should be confirmed using culture or a reliable PCR assay whenever possible. Although false-negative serologic test results are uncommon in dogs with discospondylitis, negative serologic test results in dogs with discospondylitis do not rule out infection with *Brucella* spp., and attempts should also be made to detect the organism with culture or PCR assays. Of various dogs with *B. canis* discospondylitis or ophthalmitis, 15 of 18 were positive with the RSAT, 16 of 16 were positive with the TAT, and 6 of 7 were positive with AGID assays.[6,8-11] The 3 dogs that were negative with the RSAT had discospondylitis. One was positive by blood culture, and the other 2 dogs tested positive with the TAT at a later date.[8,10]

Isolation and Identification

Despite improvements in serologic diagnostic methods, confirmatory blood cultures are still indicated when brucellosis is suspected. *B. canis* is readily isolated from the blood of bacteremic individuals for several months after infection. Specimens for blood culture should be collected as detailed in Chapter 3. A positive *B. canis* culture has been advocated as the best diagnostic test in the first 2 months of the disease; however, dogs can become abacteremic 27 to 64 months after infection but remain infected. Occasionally *B. canis* can be isolated from urine, tissue specimens such as aborted fetuses or placental material, necropsy specimens (especially spleen, prostate, and uterus), vaginal swabs, or disc aspirates. Of dogs with *Brucella* discospondylitis or ophthalmitis, 6 of 15 dogs tested positive by blood culture, 3 of 13 by urine culture, and 4 of 6 by culture of disc material or bone chips from the intervertebral disc space obtained at surgery.[6,8-10]

B. canis is an aerobe, but unlike other *Brucella* species, added CO_2 (5% to 10%) can be inhibitory. Multiplication is slow at the optimum temperature of 37°C, and enriched medium (tryptose or trypticase soy media) is occasionally needed to support adequate growth. *Brucella* colonies become visible in 2 to 3 days. Growth of *Brucella* can be identified on the basis of rough (as opposed to smooth) colony morphology, staining characteristics, and slide agglutination with anti-*Brucella* serum. Identification to the species level is best done in a specialized laboratory. Differentiation between *B. canis* and *B. suis* can be difficult.[13] In the United States, the New York State Diagnostic Laboratory at Cornell University, the Tifton Veterinary Diagnostic and Investigational Laboratory in Georgia, and the University of Florida are recognized to be reliable for definitive testing made necessary by positive *B. canis* screening tests in dogs intended for breeding, or for clinically affected dogs undergoing evaluation for infertility or abortion, or when outbreaks are being managed.[3,27] Susceptibility testing can be performed, but in vitro test results may not correlate well to the in vivo treatment response.

Molecular Diagnosis Using the Polymerase Chain Reaction

PCR assays have been used to successfully identify *B. canis* in semen from dogs with negative culture results, which suggests that this may ultimately be the most sensitive method of testing as part of the male dog pre-breeding evaluation, especially in cases where management of an outbreak is the concern.[28] PCR assays were also used to detect *B. canis* in the aqueous humor of dogs with endophthalmitis[11] and in lymph node aspirates.[29] Assays have been designed that differentiate between the *Brucella* species present.[30] A real-time PCR assay was used to detect *B. canis* in tissue specimens, urine, buffy coat, and intervertebral disc material of a dog with discospondylitis when culture of intervertebral disc material, blood, and urine was negative.[7] Some veterinary diagnostic laboratories in the United States now offer real-time PCR assays for detection of *B. canis* on a commercial basis.

Pathologic Findings

The main pathologic findings of *B. canis* infections consist of lymphoplasmacytic to lymphohistiocytic follicular hyperplasia in lymphoid tissues, lymphohistiocytic to neutrophilic endophthalmitis, and mild lymphohistiocytic meningitis. Occasionally, mild lymphoid and histiocytic infiltrates are present in other tissues, such as the liver and lung.[15] A mixed lymphohistiocytic inflammatory response is also present in the uterus (endometritis) of females and the testicles, epididymis and spermatic cord, and prostate of male dogs. Prostatic and testicular fibrosis may be found. Placental trophoblasts can contain large numbers of gram-negative bacteria, and coagulative necrosis may be present. In male dogs, lesions are more likely to be restricted to the reproductive system. Immunohistochemistry has been used to confirm the presence of *Brucella* spp. in placental tissues.[13]

Treatment and Prognosis

In certain jurisdictions, brucellosis is a reportable disease in dogs or in humans. Infected dogs and bitches should be removed from breeding programs and quarantined. Eradication of the disease in kennel situations has not been successful without removal (culling) of all current or historically infected dogs. Because of the zoonotic potential of the disease and difficulty in eradicating the infection, euthanasia of affected dogs has been recommended. Infection in household or small hobby kennel dogs often results in client requests for alternatives to euthanasia. Neutering decreases the amount of organism shed in semen and uterine discharge, but does not eradicate infection. Urine shedding can persist, and the organism can be found in internal organs and the bloodstream.

Antibiotic therapy has historically not been rewarding, likely because the organism is intracellular and bacteremia is periodic. Antimicrobial drug treatment can reduce antibody titers without clearing infection. Relapses are common. Combination therapy should be used whenever possible, preferably with tetracyclines (high-dose doxycycline or minocycline) for at least 1 to 2 months and an aminoglycoside (streptomycin or gentamicin) for the first 1 to 2 weeks of treatment (Table 53-2). Some also advocate use of two 1-week courses of aminoglycoside treatment spaced 1 month apart, or treatment with streptomycin every other week for 8 weeks.[11] Combination therapy with tetracyclines and streptomycin is thought to be the most successful treatment, but unavailability of streptomycin, nephrotoxicity, parenteral therapy requirements, and expense may be problematic.[31-33] In addition, aminoglycosides do not provide adequate ocular or CNS penetration for dogs with ophthalmitis or meningitis. A combination of doxycycline and rifampin has been used to treat human brucellosis but may not be well tolerated by dogs because of gastrointestinal adverse effects. The use of three or four drugs in combination (e.g., streptomycin, enrofloxacin, doxycycline with or without rifampin) was efficacious for treatment of ophthalmitis in dogs.[11] Topical 1% prednisolone acetate and atropine ointment may be required for management of uveitis.[11]

One study reported a possible benefit of therapy with enrofloxacin (5 mg/kg q12h PO for 4 weeks, often for multiple courses) in a small group of infected dogs and bitches. Enrofloxacin did not completely eliminate *B. canis*, but it maintained fertility and avoided the recurrence of abortions, transmission of the disease to subsequently whelped puppies, and dissemination of microorganisms during parturition. Ultimately, however, most treated individuals remained culture positive.[34] Combinations of enrofloxacin and doxycycline may be a more effective alternative for dogs unable to tolerate aminoglycoside or rifampin treatment and for dogs that have ocular or CNS involvement, but studies are lacking.

TABLE 53-2

Medications That Could Be Used to Treat *Brucella* spp. Infections in Dogs

Drug	Dose (mg/kg)	Route	Interval (hours)
Doxycycline*	10-15	PO	12
Streptomycin	20	IM	24
Gentamicin sulfate	9-14	IV, IM, SC	24
Rifampin	5	PO	12
Enrofloxacin	5-10	PO	24

*Use in combination with one of the other drugs listed. Combinations of drugs are preferred for treatment where possible.

Vaccination and Immunity

Serum agglutinating antibodies do not protect against infection in the dog, and immunity likely depends on cell-mediated immunity. Presently, the development of a vaccine is considered undesirable because the *Brucella* vaccines evaluated have offered only moderate protection, and immunized dogs develop antibodies that confound serodiagnosis.

Prevention

Prevention of infection and elimination of infected dogs should be the principal control strategy in kennels. Prevention requires at least yearly testing of all breeding stock and the testing of all dogs to be introduced into a kennel. Ideally, two negative screening tests performed at least a month apart should occur before a dog or bitch is introduced into a breeding facility. *Confirmed* positive dogs should be isolated (euthanasia is advised by many authors), neutered, treated, and tested monthly (AGID, culture, or reliable PCR assay) until two consecutive negative tests occur, although occult infection can still be present.

Private breeders should require serologic screening of all bitches offered for breeding and confirmatory negative test results if positive results occur during screening before they accept a bitch into their kennel. Stud dogs should be screened at least annually. Because of the potential for nonvenereal transmission, screening of maiden dogs and bitches before breeding is also recommended.[35,36]

Public Health Aspects

Humans can become infected with *B. canis*, although they are relatively resistant to infection and other *Brucella* species account for the majority of human disease. Approximately 40 cases of human infection have been reported worldwide; however, the actual number is unknown. Serologic assays used for diagnosis of brucellosis in humans often do not detect antibodies to *B. canis*, so the disease may be overlooked. Transmission to humans most commonly occurs through contact with an infected dog's semen, vulvar discharge from an infected bitch, or aborted fetuses or placentas, or through direct, accidental laboratory exposure.[8] Thus, disease is more likely to occur in people who are in contact with breeding dogs, but disease occasionally occurs in the owners of pet dogs with discospondylitis.[10] Immunocompromised humans, children, and those who are pregnant may be at greater risk for development of disease. Infection of humans with *B. canis* typically results in nonspecific, persistent clinical signs of fever, muscle aches, night sweats, and general malaise. Rarely, granulomatous hepatitis, hepatosplenomegaly, osteomyelitis, pulmonary disease, and endocarditis have been reported. In one case report, disease occurred in an HIV-infected dachshund dog breeder who reported infertility in one of the dogs, which had been tested by a veterinarian and was seropositive with a screening assay. Confirmatory testing with AGID performed at a university veterinary diagnostic laboratory yielded a negative result, so brucellosis was not thought to be present. However, subsequent blood culture of all of the dogs in the household was positive in one other dog.[37] Affected humans are typically treated successfully with combinations of doxycycline and either aminoglycosides (for the first week) or rifampin, but monotherapy has been associated with unacceptable rates of relapse.

Prevention of human disease involves eradication of the disease in dog kennels; precautions such as the wearing of gloves and protective clothing when in contact with aborted material; and hand washing after handling dogs and before eating. Although it is preferable that immunocompromised individuals do not participate in dog breeding activities, if necessary, these individuals should take special care if they interact with breeding dogs. Contact with dogs with reproductive problems or their secretions should be avoided whenever possible, and if aborted material must be handled, gloves, gowns, and face protection should be worn, all protective wear should be disposed of properly, and hands should be washed thoroughly.

CASE EXAMPLE

Signalment: "Sadie", a 6-year-old female spayed Border collie mix from northern California

History: Sadie was brought to her local veterinarian for listlessness and reluctance to jump noted during the previous 48 hours. She had been adopted from a local humane shelter as an ovariohysterectomized 11-month-old. She lived in a rural agricultural area in northern California and was the only dog in the household.

Physical Examination: Sadie's vital signs were within normal limits, mucous membrane color was pink, and she was quiet and alert on physical examination. Body weight was 25 kg. Mild dental tartar was evident. Thoracic auscultation and abdominal palpation were normal, pulses were synchronous, and no peripheral lymphadenomegaly was evident. Palpable dorsal thoracolumbar pain was demonstrated. She was reluctant to rise but was ambulatory. The neurologic examination including a fundoscopic examination was normal.

Laboratory Findings: A complete blood count, chemistry panel, and urinalysis were performed. Mild neutropenia (2958 cells/μL; reference range, 3000-11,500 cells/μL) was found, and the chemistries and urinalysis were normal with no proteinuria.

Imaging Findings: Radiographs of the spine revealed evidence of disc space collapse, spondylosis, and discospondylitis at the T7-T8 disc space (see Figure 53-2).

Microbiologic Testing: A SNAP 4DX test (IDEXX Laboratories) for antigen of *Dirofilaria immitis* and antibodies to *Ehrlichia canis*, *Anaplasma phagocytophilum*, and *Borrelia burgdorferi* was negative. Aerobic bacterial urine culture was negative. Serum was submitted for a *Brucella canis* IFA, which was positive at a titer of 1:200. A *B. canis* AGID was submitted and was also positive.

Treatment: Sadie was treated with tramadol (1-2 mg/kg PO q8h) and carprofen (3 mg/kg PO q12h). Once the serologic test results were available, a tentative diagnosis of *B. canis* discospondylitis was made, and she was treated with enrofloxacin (5.5 mg/kg PO q12h). Clinical improvement was reported in 2 weeks, and repeat radiographs were performed in 1 and 5 months. Equivocal change was reported in the appearance of T7-T8 at 1 month, but the 5-month radiograph showed no progression, suggesting the lesion was no longer active. The owners were advised of the zoonotic potential of this disease and the potential hazard of transmission to other dogs. The potential need for lifelong antibiotic therapy with risk of relapse was also discussed.

Comments: Dogs with *Brucella* discospondylitis frequently are brought to their veterinarian for clinical signs of spinal pain or lameness that resemble common musculoskeletal injuries such as intervertebral disc disease or rupture of the cranial cruciate ligament. Although not typical, this case illustrates the fact that *B. canis* disease can occur in female spayed, nonbreeding dogs and often occurs in the absence of fever or significant abnormalities on routine laboratory testing. A diagnosis of *Brucella* discospondylitis was strongly suspected based on positive serologic test results with multiple assays. Blood culture was not performed, but urine culture was negative. Monotherapy with fluoroquinolones has been associated with high rates of relapse in human patients once antimicrobial drug treatment has been discontinued, so it is generally not recommended. Nevertheless, it can occasionally be successful.

SUGGESTED READINGS

Hollett RB. Update on canine brucellosis. Theriogenology. 2010;1: 287-295.

Lawaczeck E, Toporek J, Cwikla J, et al. *Brucella canis* in a HIV-infected patient. Zoonoses Public Health. 2011;58:150-152.

Wanke MM. Canine brucellosis. Anim Reprod Sci. 2004;82-83:195-207.

REFERENCES

1. Carmichael LE. Abortion in 200 beagles. J Am Vet Med Assoc. 1966;149:1126.
2. Barr SC, Eilts BE, Roy AF, et al. *Brucella suis* biotype 1 infection in a dog. J Am Vet Med Assoc. 1986;189:686-687.
3. Greene CE, Carmichael LE. Canine brucellosis. In: Greene CE, ed. Infectious Diseases of the Dog and Cat. 4th ed. St. Louis, MO: Elsevier Saunders; 2012:398-411.
4. Blankenship RM, Sanford JP. *Brucella canis.* A cause of undulant fever. Am J Med. 1975;59:424-426.
5. Lucero NE, Escobar GI, Ayala SM, et al. Diagnosis of human brucellosis caused by *Brucella canis.* J Med Microbiol. 2005;54:457-461.
6. Anderson GI, Binnington AG. Discospondylitis and orchitis associated with high *Brucella* titre in a dog. Can Vet J. 1983;24:249-252.
7. Corrente M, Franchini D, Decaro N, et al. Detection of *Brucella canis* in a dog in Italy. New Microbiol. 2010;33:337-341.
8. Kerwin SC, Lewis DD, Hribernik TN, et al. Diskospondylitis associated with *Brucella canis* infection in dogs: 14 cases (1980-1991). J Am Vet Med Assoc. 1992;201:1253-1257.
9. Henderson RA, Hoerlein BF, Kramer TT, et al. Discospondylitis in three dogs infected with *Brucella canis.* J Am Vet Med Assoc. 1974;165:451-455.
10. Sykes JE. Unpublished observations, 2012.
11. Ledbetter EC, Landry MP, Stokol T, et al. *Brucella canis* endophthalmitis in 3 dogs: clinical features, diagnosis, and treatment. Vet Ophthalmol. 2009;12:183-191.
12. Carmichael LE, Joubert JC. Transmission of *Brucella canis* by contact exposure. Cornell Vet. 1988;78:63-73.
13. Brennan SJ, Ngeleka M, Philibert HM, et al. Canine brucellosis in a Saskatchewan kennel. Can Vet J. 2008;49:703-708.
14. Dunne J, Sehgal K, McMillan A, et al. Canine brucellosis in a dog imported into the UK. Vet Rec. 2002;151:247.
15. Gyuranecz M, Szeredi L, Ronai Z, et al. Detection of *Brucella canis*–induced reproductive diseases in a kennel. J Vet Diagn Invest. 2011;23:143-147.
16. Nockler K, Kutzer P, Reif S, et al. Canine brucellosis—a case report. Berl Munch Tierarztl Wochenschr. 2003;116:368-372.
17. Strom Holst B, Lofqvist K, Ernholm L, et al. The first case of *Brucella canis* in Sweden: background, case report and recommendations from a Northern European perspective. Acta Vet Scand. 2012;54:18.
18. Shin SJ, Carmichael LE. Canine brucellosis caused by *Brucella canis.* In: Carmichael LE, ed. Recent Advances in Canine Infectious Diseases. Ithaca, NY: International Veterinary Information Service; 1999.
19. Moore JA, Kakuk TJ. Male dogs naturally infected with *Brucella canis.* J Am Vet Med Assoc. 1969;155:1352-1358.
20. Dawkins BG, Machotka SV, Suchmann D, et al. Pyogranulomatous dermatitis associated with *Brucella canis* infection in a dog. J Am Vet Med Assoc. 1982;181:1432-1433.
21. Smeak DD, Olmstead ML, Hohn RB. *Brucella canis* osteomyelitis in two dogs with total hip replacements. J Am Vet Med Assoc. 1987;191:986-990.
22. Carmichael LE, Kenney RM. Canine abortion caused by *Brucella canis.* J Am Vet Med Assoc. 1968;152:605-616.
23. Johnson CA, Walker RD. Clinical signs and diagnosis of *Brucella canis* infection. Compend Cont Educ Pract Vet. 1992;14:763-772.
24. Schoeb TR, Morton R. Scrotal and testicular changes in canine brucellosis: a case report. J Am Vet Med Assoc. 1978;172:598-600.
25. Keid LB, Soares RM, Vasconcellos SA, et al. Comparison of agar gel immunodiffusion test, rapid slide agglutination test, microbiological culture, and PCR for the diagnosis of canine brucellosis. Res Vet Sci. 2009;86:22-26.
26. de Oliveira MZ, Vale V, Keid L, et al. Validation of an ELISA method for the serological diagnosis of canine brucellosis due to *Brucella canis.* Res Vet Sci. 2011;90:425-431.
27. Wooley RE, Hitchcock PL, Blue JL, et al. Isolation of *Brucella canis* from a dog seronegative for brucellosis. J Am Vet Med Assoc. 1978;173:387-388.
28. Keid LB, Soares RM, Vasconcellos SA, et al. A polymerase chain reaction for the detection of *Brucella canis* in semen of naturally infected dogs. Theriogenology. 2007;67:1203-1210.
29. Aras Z, Ucan US. Detection of *Brucella canis* from inguinal lymph nodes of naturally infected dogs by PCR. Theriogenology. 2010;74:658-662.
30. Kang SI, Her M, Kim JW, et al. Advanced multiplex PCR assay for differentiation of *Brucella* species. Appl Environ Microbiol. 2011;77:6726-6728.
31. Jennings PB, Crumrine MH, Lewis Jr GE, et al. The effect of a two-stage antibiotic regimen on dogs infected with *Brucella canis.* J Am Vet Med Assoc. 1974;164:513-514.
32. Johnson CA, Bennett M, Jensen RK, et al. Effect of combined antibiotic therapy on fertility in brood bitches infected with *Brucella canis.* J Am Vet Med Assoc. 1982;180:1330-1333.
33. Nicoletti P. Further studies on the use of antibiotics in canine brucellosis. Compend Cont Educ Pract Vet. 1991;13:944.
34. Wanke MM, Delpino MV, Baldi PC. Use of enrofloxacin in the treatment of canine brucellosis in a dog kennel (clinical trial). Theriogenology. 2006;66:1573-1578.
35. Hollett RB. Canine brucellosis: outbreaks and compliance. Theriogenology. 2006;66:575-587.
36. Jones RL, Emerson JK. Canine brucellosis in a commercial breeding kennel. J Am Vet Med Assoc. 1984;184:834-835.
37. Lawaczeck E, Toporek J, Cwikla J, et al. *Brucella canis* in a HIV-infected patient. Zoonoses Public Health. 2011;58:150-152.

CHAPTER 54

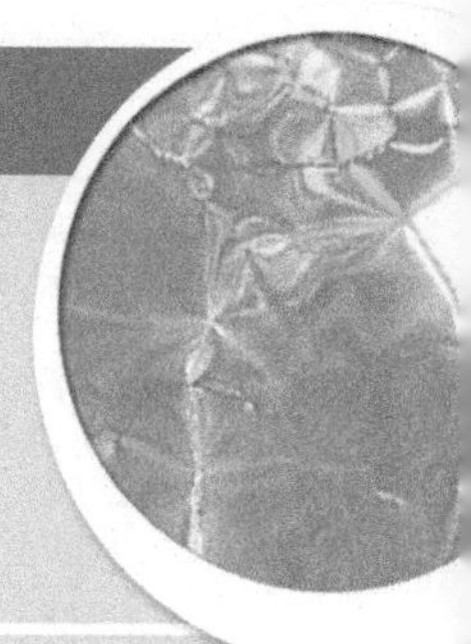

Tetanus and Botulism

Jane E. Sykes

> **Overview of Tetanus and Botulism**
>
> First Described: The etiology of tetanus was identified in the late 1800s in Germany (Nicolaier).[1] *C. botulinum* and its toxin were first described in Belgium in 1897 (van Ermengem).[2] Before that, descriptions of both diseases had been recorded; tetanus was described by Hippocrates more than 2000 years ago.
>
> Causes: Toxins of *Clostridium botulinum* (botulism) or *Clostridium tetani* (tetanus)
>
> Geographic Distribution: Worldwide
>
> Major Mode of Transmission: Ingestion of preformed toxin (botulism) or cutaneous inoculation of spores into a wound (tetanus)
>
> Major Clinical Signs: Spastic paralysis (tetanus) or flaccid paralysis (botulism)
>
> Differential Diagnoses: Differential diagnoses for suspected botulism include polyradiculoneuritis, paralytic rabies, tick paralysis, coral snake poisoning, myasthenia gravis, and ionophore toxicity. For tetanus they include strychnine toxicosis, hypocalcemia, metaldehyde toxicity, and extraocular myositis
>
> Human Health Significance: Botulism and tetanus are not directly transmissible from animals to humans, but care should be taken when handling specimens from animals with botulism.

Etiology and Epidemiology

Tetanus and botulism are neurologic diseases caused by the toxins of *Clostridium tetani* and *Clostridium botulinum* that occur worldwide. These organisms are gram-positive, sluggishly motile, anaerobic spore-forming bacilli. The spores of *C. tetani* and *C. botulinum* are extremely resistant in the environment and resist boiling and disinfection with alcohol or formalin.

Botulism

In dogs and especially cats, botulism is rare and usually follows ingestion of preformed neurotoxin within carrion, especially waterfowl or poultry carrion. Disease in dogs can coincide with outbreaks of botulism in waterfowl. Botulism outbreaks in dogs have been reported in hunting foxhounds.[3,4] Most affected dogs are medium- to large-breed, intact male or intact female dogs that vary in age. The only report of botulism in cats was an outbreak of disease that occurred after several cats were fed pelican carrion.[5] The relative resistance of dogs and cats to botulism has been hypothesized to reflect an adaptive response to a carnivorous lifestyle. *C. botulinum* produces seven related toxins: A, B, C, D, E, F, and G. Most human botulism is caused by types A, B, and E.[6] Botulism in dogs and cats almost always results from ingestion of toxin C,[3,5,7-9] with the exception of a few dogs in the Senegal that had type D intoxication.[10]

Tetanus

C. tetani is widespread in the soil and feces of animals. It produces two toxins, *tetanospasmin* and *tetanolysin*. Tetanolysin does not appear to have clinical significance. Humans and horses are most susceptible to tetanus, and so widespread vaccination against the disease is performed in these species. Disease occurs occasionally in dogs and is rare in cats. The development of tetanus in dogs and cats usually follows introduction of spores into a penetrating wound, but more than one third of affected dogs have no known wound history *(cryptogenic tetanus)*.[11] Traumatic wounds of the feet, claws, or head; draining tracts associated with grass awn migration; animal bite wounds; tick bite wounds; bleeding claw trim wounds; wounds that result from chronic protozoal or fungal infections of the skin; teething wounds in dogs; and surgical wounds (which include spay and neuter operations) have all been implicated.[11-14] Although dogs of any age, breed, or sex develop tetanus, disease occurs most often in young, large-breed, active, intact male dogs.[11,13,14] Disease is seen in puppies as young as 8 weeks of age; some studies describe a significant proportion of affected dogs as less than 1 year of age. Disease is also more severe in young dogs.[11] Cats are often young cats with outdoor access, but cats of any age have been affected.[15]

Clinical Features

Signs and Their Pathogenesis

The toxins of *C. tetani* and *C. botulinum* have similar structures and mechanisms of action, even though they cause diseases that contrast sharply with one another. Both toxins are among the most potent toxins known and act at femtomolar concentrations. They consist of two polypeptide chains, a heavy (H) chain and a light (L) chain, joined by a disulfide bond (Figure 54-1). The heavy chain attaches to presynaptic nerve terminal membrane receptors, although the precise receptors have not been identified because of the extremely low concentrations at which these toxins act. Variation in receptor binding affinities may explain differences in species susceptibility to clostridial neurotoxins. The toxin is then internalized via receptor-mediated endocytosis into the presynaptic nerve terminal, where it has a local impact on nerve cell function (botulinum toxin) and also travels by retrograde axonal transport to the nerve cell body

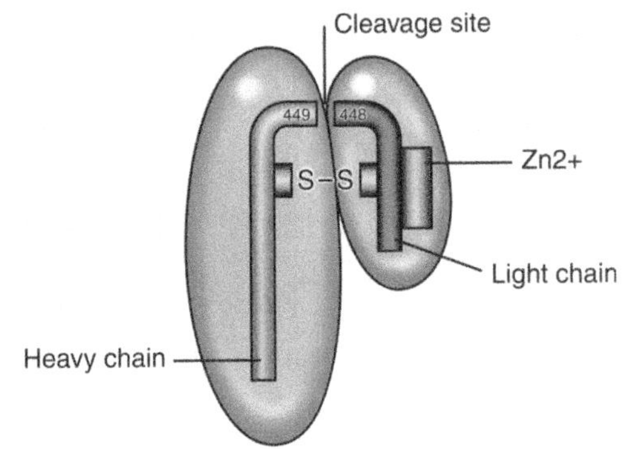

FIGURE 54-1 Schematic of the structure of *Clostridium tetani* and *Clostridium botulinum* toxins.

and diffuses into inhibitory interneurons, where it impacts inhibitory interneuron function (tetanospasmin). The L chain, a zinc-dependent matrix metalloproteinase, is released from the vesicle and subsequently cleaves one or more *docking proteins.* These proteins are critical for the release of neurotransmitters from synaptic vesicles into the synaptic cleft and are located on the membrane of synaptic vesicles *(synaptobrevin)* or the presynaptic cell membrane (*syntaxin* and *SNAP-25*). Synaptobrevin binds to the docking proteins located on the presynaptic membrane. The resulting complex (the SNARE complex) docks the synaptic vesicle at the proper location for fusion and exocytosis of neurotransmitter molecules into the synaptic space (Figure 54-2). Tetanospasmin cleaves synaptobrevin, whereas botulinum neurotoxin C cleaves syntaxin; other botulinum neurotoxins cleave synaptobrevin or SNAP-25. The process of recovery involves the sprouting of new presynaptic terminals, followed by recovery of the original synapse, after which new terminal outgrowths retract.[16]

Botulism

C. botulinum spores germinate in anaerobic conditions and produce toxin. They grow best in temperatures that range from 30°C to 37°C. The toxin is ingested, survives the acid stomach conditions, and is absorbed into the bloodstream from the small intestine. It then travels to peripheral cholinergic synapses, which include the neuromuscular junction and autonomic synapses, and inhibits release of acetylcholine (ACh). This leads to ascending symmetrical flaccid paralysis, development of megaesophagus, and signs of autonomic dysfunction. Clinical signs usually occur within 12 to 72 hours after ingestion of botulinum toxin and may be complicated by signs of dietary indiscretion, although gastrointestinal signs may also reflect the presence of autonomic dysfunction. Disease progresses rapidly over 1 or 2 days, and then begins to resolve with supportive care. Death can result from respiratory muscle paralysis or aspiration of intestinal contents. Abnormalities in affected cats were ascending flaccid paralysis, lethargy, hypothermia, tachypnea, dehydration, and urinary incontinence.[5]

Tetanus

C. tetani spores are introduced into tissues where they germinate, replicate locally, and produce toxin in anaerobic conditions. Ingestion is not a route of transmission, because tetanospasmin is destroyed by gastrointestinal secretions. The toxin is produced as a single polyprotein that is cleaved extracellularly by a bacterial protease into the L and H chains, which remain connected by the disulfide bond. It then binds to presynaptic terminals of lower motor neurons and is internalized, travels up axons by retrograde axonal flow, and enters inhibitory interneurons in the brain and spinal cord, where it interferes with release of γ-aminobutyric acid (GABA) and glycine inhibitory neurotransmitters (Figure 54-2, *B*). Toxin can also spread hematogenously to the central nervous system (CNS) from the wound site. The result is unhindered excitation of motor neurons, spastic paralysis, and dysfunction of the sympathetic and parasympathomimetic nervous systems. Clinical signs occur 3 days to 3 weeks after a wound in both cats or dogs. Shorter incubation periods occur when the wound is proximal to the CNS and when a large amount of toxin is present. Paralysis may initially be localized to the wound site but can then generalize. Involvement of the head is common in dogs, and often owners of dogs with tetanus first notice an unusual appearance to their dog's eyes, a "swollen" face, or evidence of dysphagia.[11] Regurgitation or vomiting of food occurs in less than 20% of affected dogs, and a voice change or dysuria may be noted. Death occurs in severely affected dogs due to paralysis of respiratory muscles; infectious complications such as pneumonia; upper airway obstruction; the development of severe hyperthermia with disseminated intravascular coagulation (DIC), multiple organ failure, and/or pulmonary thromboembolism; and cardiac arrhythmias.[11,13,14] Hiatal hernia and coxofemoral joint luxations have also been described as complications of tetanus in dogs.[11,14,17] Disease in cats is usually localized to the limbs, but generalized tetanus can occur.[15,18-21] Many affected cats have an initial history of disappearance for days to a week or more, after which lameness is noted.

Physical and Neurologic Examination Findings

Dogs and cats with botulism or tetanus are usually alert, afebrile, and in good body condition, but lethargy and anorexia occur in some animals. Hyperthermia can occur with severe tetanus.

Botulism

Physical examination findings in dogs with botulism depend on the severity of intoxication. Fever is absent unless aspiration pneumonia has developed. Mildly affected dogs show only ataxia or pelvic limb paresis, whereas dogs with severe intoxication are quadriplegic with absent voluntary motor activity and are unable to rise from lateral recumbency. The ability to wag the tail is often retained.[3,8,9] Neurologic examination can reveal decreased cranial nerve function, especially facial nerve function and a decreased gag reflex, sometimes accompanied by ptyalism.[3,7,9,22] A weak blink reflex can result in corneal ulceration. A mucopurulent ocular discharge may be present. Mydriasis with sluggish pupillary light reflexes has been described.[3,22] Segmental reflexes may be intact, decreased, or absent, but pain sensation is preserved. Occasionally tachycardia and tachypnea are present. Tachypnea may result from diaphragmatic muscle weakness or secondary aspiration pneumonia. Increased lung sounds may also be present on thoracic auscultation of dogs with secondary aspiration pneumonia. Physical examination findings in one affected cat consisted of hypothermia, lethargy, dehydration, quadriplegia, and decreased segmental reflexes.[5]

Tetanus

In dogs with tetanus, involvement of the head and generalized disease occurs more often than occurs in cats. A wound may or

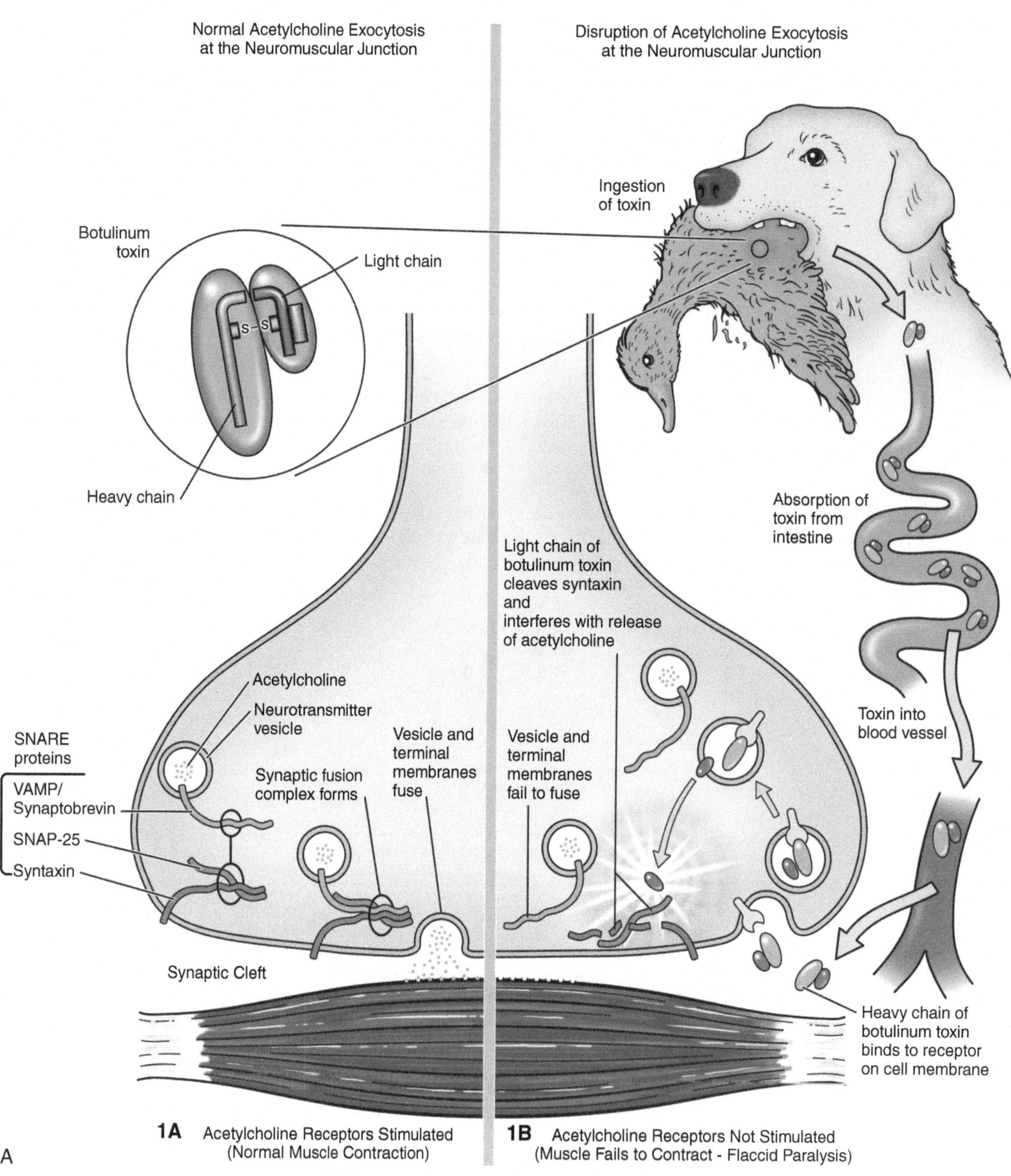

FIGURE 54-2 Action of clostridial neurotoxins. **A,** Botulism Toxin.

Continued

may not be found. Dogs with localized forelimb tetanus have caudal retraction of the limb with extension of both the elbow and carpus.[15] In dogs with generalized tetanus, a wrinkled forehead, erect ears, retracted lips *(risus sardonicus),* and prolapsed third eyelids are almost always present, usually in association with generalized muscle stiffness (see Figure 54-3, *A*). Miosis may be present. It may be difficult or impossible to open the mouth. Dogs that are ambulatory walk slowly with a stiff, stilted gait and can have a wide-based or "sawhorse" stance; voluntary movement of the head may occur slowly or appear difficult, and the tail may be erect. Laryngeal spasm and hypersalivation occur in approximately half of affected dogs.[13,14] Reflexes are exaggerated or difficult to elicit. Severely affected dogs are anxious and hypersensitive, develop opisthotonos, vocalize, tremble or

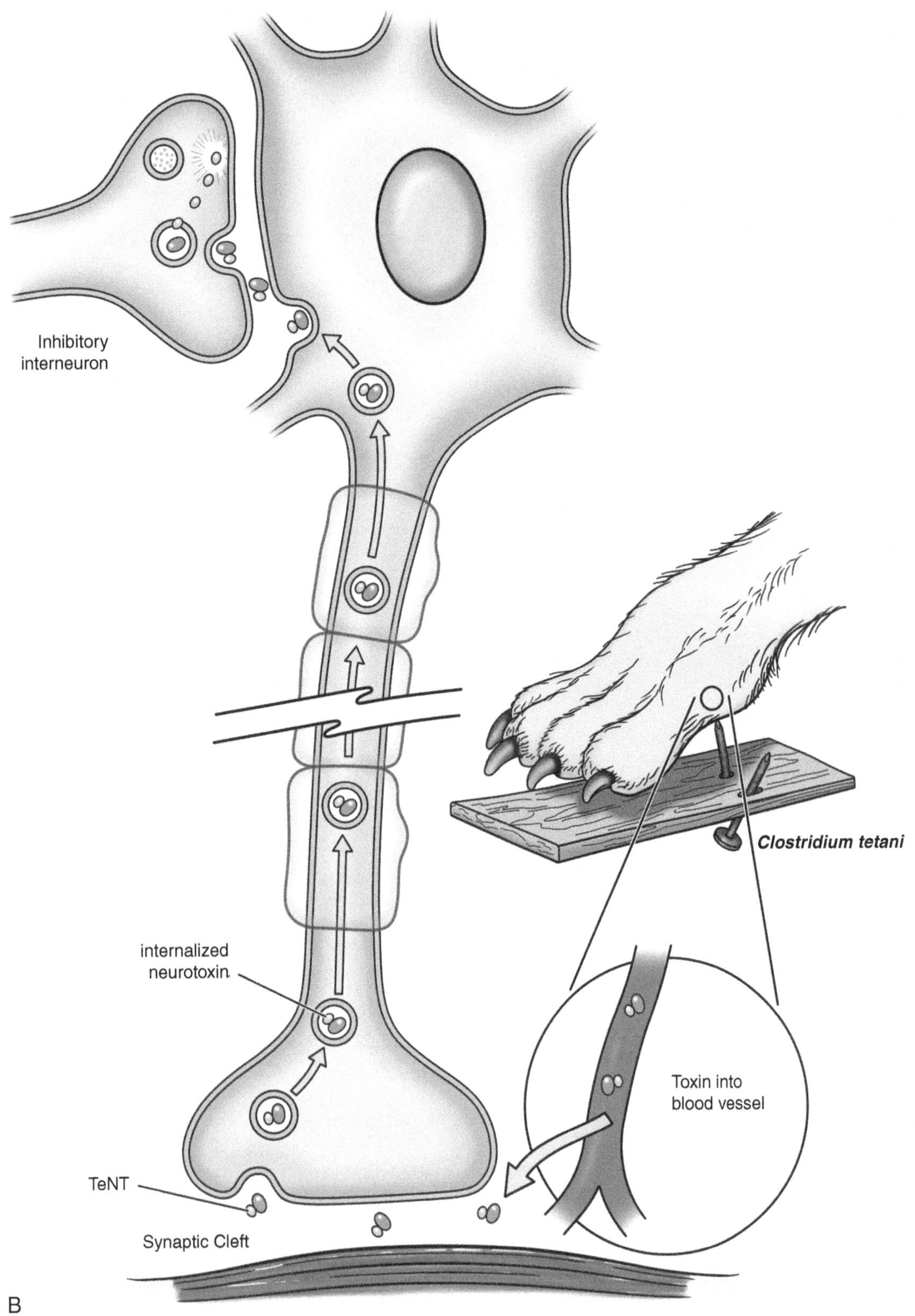

FIGURE 54-2, cont'd. **B,** Tetanospasmin.

even have a seizure when stimulated, and may be hyperthermic due to increased muscle activity (up to 111°F or 43.9°C).[11] A semicomatose state may even result. Abdominal palpation may reveal an enlarged bladder that is difficult to express, or palpation may not be possible because of abdominal muscle spasm. Hypoventilation may be present, or tetanic spasms may trigger episodes of dyspnea. At least a third of dogs are bradycardic or have bradyarrhythmias (which include atrioventricular block or sinus arrest), with heart rates that range from 40 to 60 beats/min; another third of dogs are tachycardic (>150 beats/min) or have variable heart rates, which may reflect autonomic dysfunction or pain.[11]

Cats with localized tetanus often have extensor rigidity of a single limb, on which a wound may be identified. When the forelimb is affected, spasm of the triceps muscle results in caudal extension of the limb with carpal flexion (in contrast to dogs) and elbow extension (Figure 54-3, *B*).[20,23,24] The head and neck may be deviated toward the affected limb.[15] When disease generalizes, the contralateral limb and subsequently all four limbs may be affected.[20] Affected cats may be reluctant to move or hyperesthetic. Lockjaw *(trismus)*, protrusion of the third eyelid, retracted lips *(risus sardonicus)*, wrinkling of the forehead, or opisthotonos can occur in cats with generalized tetanus. Segmental reflexes may be exaggerated, or it may not be possible to elicit reflexes because of severe muscle spasticity. Dyspnea, tachypnea, and open-mouth breathing may occur.[12] Cranial nerve responses are usually normal. Miosis may be present.

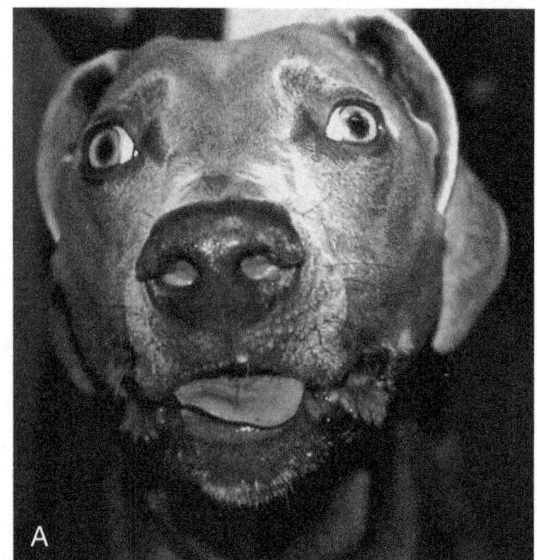

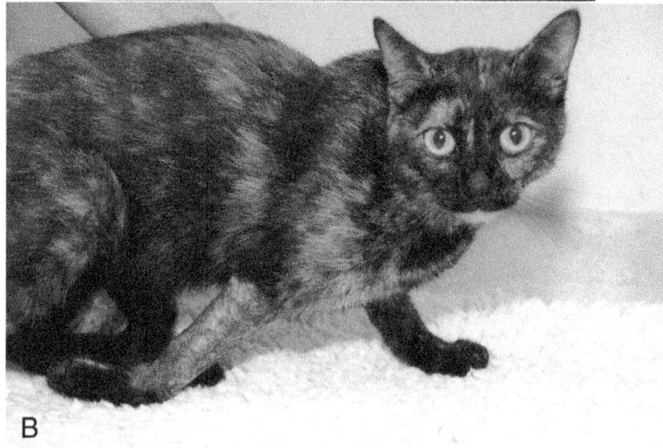

FIGURE 54-3 **A,** Image of a Weimaraner with generalized tetanus. The dog walked with a stiff gait and was salivating profusely. Risus sardonicus is evident. **B,** Three-year-old female domestic shorthair cat with localized tetanus that was seen for a 3-day history of right thoracic limb lameness. Extension of the shoulder and elbow and partial flexion of the carpal joint is present. (From Langner KFA, Schenk HC, Leithaeuser C, et al. Localised tetanus in a cat. Vet Rec 2011;169:126.)

Diagnosis

Diagnosis of tetanus and botulism in dogs and cats is most often based on a consistent history and clinical abnormalities, exclusion of the few other possible causes of disease (e.g., with assays for myasthenia gravis in dogs with botulism), and sometimes electrodiagnostic testing. The primary differential diagnoses for botulism are acute polyradiculoneuritis and myasthenia gravis; paralytic rabies should also be considered. There are few other disorders other than strychnine poisoning that truly mimic tetanus. Serologic assays have been used to detect an antibody response to botulinum toxins. Finally, specific assays that detect botulinum toxin in serum, gastrointestinal contents, or food can be performed (Table 54-1).

Laboratory Abnormalities

Complete Blood Count, Serum Biochemical Tests, and Urinalysis

Routine laboratory test results in animals with tetanus or botulism are often normal, but stress hyperglycemia, mild to severe increases in the activity of serum creatine kinase (usually <20,000 U/L but sometimes >200,000 U/L, reference range 46-320 U/L), mildly increased AST activity, and myoglobinuria may be present in animals with tetanus.[11,14] Dehydration may result in hemoconcentration or prerenal azotemia. Animals with wounds or aspiration pneumonia may have an inflammatory leukogram. Severe hyperthermia in dogs with tetanus may lead to laboratory evidence of multiple organ dysfunction, with moderate to severe hypoalbuminemia, azotemia, and/or increased liver enzyme activities and hyperbilirubinemia. Thrombocytopenia and coagulation test abnormalities consistent with DIC may also be present in these dogs.

CSF Analysis

CSF analysis in dogs and cats with botulism and tetanus typically shows no abnormalities.

TABLE 54-1

Laboratory Assays Available for Diagnosis of Botulism

Assay	Specimen Type	Target	Performance
Mouse inoculation bioassay	Feces, vomitus, intestinal contents, serum, foodstuffs	Botulinum toxin	Gold standard for diagnosis. False negatives can occur if toxin degradation occurs. Slow turnaround time means diagnosis is generally retrospective. Laborious and requires the use of laboratory animals.
ELISA toxin assays	Feces, vomitus, intestinal contents, serum, foodstuffs	Botulinum toxin	Rapid and inexpensive. Standard ELISA toxin assays have a lower sensitivity than the mouse inoculation assay.
ELISA assays that detect the antibody response to botulinum toxin	Serum	Anti–botulinum toxin antibodies	Negative antibody titers occur early in the course of disease, so acute and convalescent titers must be performed. Thus, diagnosis is retrospective.

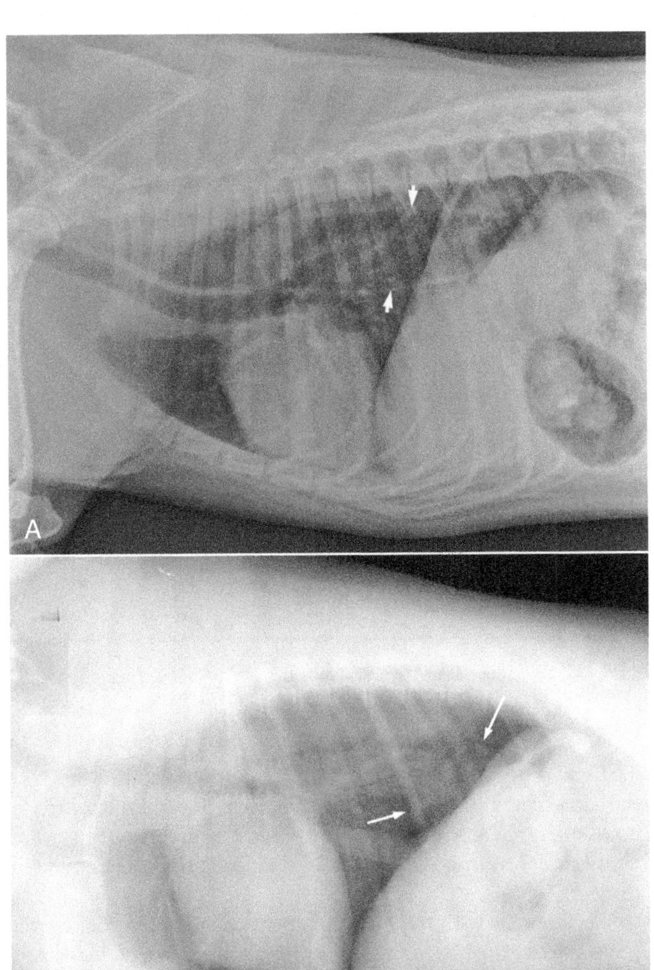

FIGURE 54-4 Radiographic findings in dogs with botulism (A) and tetanus (B). **A,** Lateral thoracic radiograph from a 6-year-old female spayed Labrador retriever with botulism. Megaesophagus is present. The *white arrows* delineate the dorsal and ventral esophageal wall. **B,** Lateral thoracic radiograph from a 3-year-old female spayed English springer spaniel with tetanus that was seen for vomiting, dysuria, respiratory distress, and a stiff gait. Pneumothorax and a hiatal hernia *(arrows)* can be appreciated. Before the radiographs were taken, an exploratory laparotomy had been performed because a foreign body was suspected. The pneumothorax developed postoperatively for reasons that were unclear. A foxtail wound was later found on the left distal pelvic limb between the digits. The dog was hospitalized for 19 days, during which time all radiographic abnormalities resolved.

Diagnostic Imaging

Thoracic radiographs in dogs with botulism may be unremarkable, or megaesophagus may be present (Figure 54-4, *A*). Evidence of carrion bones are occasionally present in the stomach. Changes consistent with aspiration pneumonia in dogs with botulism or tetanus may also be apparent.[11,22] Rarely, dogs with tetanus have evidence of a hiatal hernia on thoracic radiography, which appears as a soft tissue mass in the caudal thorax (see Figure 54-4, *B*). Abdominal ultrasound examination may be normal, or mild abdominal lymphadenopathy may be identified.

Electrodiagnostic Tests

Electromyography (EMG) and electroneurography can be useful to support a diagnosis of botulism in some dogs (Table 54-2). Sedation or anesthesia for electrophysiologic testing is generally not advisable in dogs with megaesophagus and aspiration pneumonia, although EMG can be performed without anesthesia.[3] Electroneurography studies involve electrical stimulation of one or more motor nerves and assessment of the resultant electrical activity in the innervated muscle. Electroneurography findings in dogs with botulism include normal F waves (late waves that disappear in acute polyradiculoneuritis) and decreased magnitude of the compound muscle action potential.[3,22,25] Repetitive nerve stimulation at low frequencies can result in decremental responses, but repetitive nerve stimulation at high frequencies in dogs with botulism has no effect on the muscle response.[22] In humans with botulism, an incremental response to repetitive nerve stimulation occurs at high frequencies.[26] Motor nerve conduction velocity (MNCV) is normal or decreased. On EMG, the primary finding is prolonged or increased insertional activity in botulism.[3,22] Fibrillation potentials and positive sharp waves have also been described.[3,25] Animals with tetanus have had normal EMGs and MNCVs as well as motor unit potentials and pathologic spontaneous muscle activity,[14,20,21,24] but electrodiagnostic testing is not specific for a diagnosis of tetanus and is usually not required.

Microbiologic Tests

Isolation and Identification

Attempts to culture *C. tetani* from wounds are not recommended because the presence of *C. tetani* in a wound does not necessarily imply toxin production. In addition, this is insensitive.[11,13]

Serologic Diagnosis

ELISA assays that detect the antibody response to botulinum neurotoxin are available and were used to confirm a diagnosis of botulism in one dog.[7] A convalescent specimen collected 3 weeks after the onset of illness was positive, but specimens collected at the time the dog was first evaluated and 10 days later were negative. Thus, the diagnosis is generally retrospective with this method because most dogs have recovered by the time seroconversion occurs. The antibody response to tetanospasmin is not significant.

Toxin Detection

Botulinum toxin can be detected in feces, vomitus, gastrointestinal contents collected at necropsy, carrion, or serum. Specimens should be held at 4°C, marked with a warning label, and shipped immediately to the laboratory. The most sensitive assay is a mouse inoculation assay, in which untreated mice and mice treated with serotype-specific antitoxin are inoculated with the specimen to determine if the antitoxin is protective.[27] However, several days are required to run this assay. Toxin type–specific ELISA assays are available for rapid detection of neurotoxin C, but standard ELISA assays lack sensitivity when compared with mouse inoculation. Research efforts have been focused on the development of a variety of novel, rapid, highly sensitive, and inexpensive diagnostic assays that detect minute quantities of botulinum toxins.[27]

Pathologic Findings

There are no specific gross or histopathologic findings associated with botulism or tetanus. Evidence of complications such as aspiration pneumonia, pulmonary thromboembolism, or DIC may be present in dogs with tetanus.

Treatment and Prognosis

Specific Treatment

There is no readily available specific treatment for botulism in dogs. In the United States, heptavalent equine antitoxin is

TABLE 54-2

Pathophysiologic, Clinical, and Electrophysiologic Features of Botulism, Polyradiculoneuritis, and Myasthenia Gravis

	Botulism	Polyradiculoneuritis	Acquired Myasthenia Gravis
Pathophysiology	Inhibition of acetylcholine release by botulinum toxin	Inflammatory disorder of nerve roots	Antibody formation to acetylcholine receptors at the neuromuscular junction
Neurologic abnormalities	Decreased reflexes, progressive tetraparesis, respiratory compromise, autonomic signs, dysphonia, megaesophagus	Decreased reflexes, progressive tetraparesis, facial weakness, dysphonia, respiratory compromise, with or without hyperesthesia	Normal reflexes, muscle weakness and rapid fatigue, megaesophagus
EMG	Normal/subnormal	Abnormal	Normal
Electroneurography	Decreased CMAP amplitudes, normal F-waves, decremental response to repetitive nerve stimulation at low frequency (and incremental response at high frequency in humans)	Decreased CMAP amplitudes, absent F-waves, usually normal MNCV	Usually normal CMAP amplitudes, decremental response to repetitive nerve stimulation at low frequency

Modified from Uriarte A, Thibaud JL, Blot S. Botulism in 2 urban dogs. Can Vet J 2010;51:1139-1142.
CMAP, Compound muscle action potential; MNCV, Motor nerve conduction velocity.

TABLE 54-3

Suggested Dosages of Medication for Specific Treatment of Tetanus

Drug	Dose	Route	Interval (hours)	Duration (days)
Metronidazole	15 mg/kg	IV, PO	12	10
Tetanus equine antitoxin	100-1000 units/kg	IV, IM*	NA	Once
	500 units	SC near wound site	NA	Once
Human tetanus immune globulin	500 units	IM near wound if found	IM	Once

NA, Not applicable.
*IV use is preferred. Administer 0.1 mL intradermally as a test dose before infusion. The full dose should then be given slowly over 10 minutes.

available from the Centers for Disease Control and Prevention for treatment of human botulism. However, its availability is tightly controlled, so it may be impossible to obtain for treatment of dogs or cats.[28] Tetanus antitoxin is more widely available and should be administered as a single dose IV (equine antitoxin) or IM (human antitoxin) after an initial intradermal test dose to evaluate for allergic reactions (Table 54-3). Dogs that react to the test dose should be premedicated with diphenhydramine and a low dose of dexamethasone. Adverse reactions to antitoxin include vomiting, retching, or tachypnea and may occur even in premedicated dogs.[11] Reduction in the rate of antitoxin administration or discontinuation of treatment leads to resolution of clinical signs. Administration of antitoxin does not reverse existing paralysis because it is unable to enter nerve terminals, but it may neutralize free toxin. A small amount of antitoxin can be administered locally if a wound is identified.

The efficacy of tetanus antitoxin is controversial, and the optimal dose is not known. In one study, early IV administration of equine tetanus antitoxin did not influence disease progression or mortality as opposed to administration later in the course of disease.[11]

For animals with tetanus, treatment with antimicrobials that have activity against *C. tetani* is also recommended. This is not indicated for animals with botulism, because ingested toxin is preformed. Appropriate antimicrobials for treatment of tetanus include intravenous metronidazole or penicillin G. Metronidazole is preferred because of its improved penetration into purulent material and the fact that penicillin can antagonize GABA. Studies in human patients have also shown improved outcome with metronidazole as opposed to procaine penicillin.[29] Once antitoxin has been administered and spasms are controlled (see Supportive Care), wounds should also be debrided or flushed extensively with hydrogen peroxide solution. Earlier appropriate antimicrobial treatment and wound debridement may not influence progression or mortality.[11]

Supportive Care

For both tetanus and botulism, supportive care is an essential part of management. The extent of care required depends on the severity of illness. Intravenous fluids, soft bedding, frequent turning to prevent decubital ulcers, application of ocular lubricant to prevent corneal ulceration, bladder expression or urinary catheterization (ideally intermittent), enemas to relieve constipation, and nutritional support in the form of hand feeding, feeding tubes, or total parenteral nutrition may be required. Force feeding is not recommended because it is unlikely to satisfy caloric needs and can contribute to the development of aspiration pneumonia. Occasionally (<10% of affected dogs with tetanus), mechanical ventilation is required to support respiration.[11] For dogs with botulism, antimicrobial drugs should only be used if infection develops (e.g., bacterial pneumonia or urinary tract infection). Aminoglycosides should be avoided because they may contribute to neuromuscular blockade.

Dogs or cats with generalized tetanus should be placed in a quiet, dimly lit environment away from excessive visual or auditory stimuli. Cotton balls can be used as earplugs. Sedatives and/or muscle relaxants such as acepromazine, diazepam, midazolam, or methocarbamol may be useful. Severely affected animals may require a constant-rate infusion of drugs such as pentobarbital, phenobarbital, or propofol. Barbiturates are no longer recommended for treatment of tetanus in humans; benzodiazepines are preferred. If human disease is severe, drugs that cause neuromuscular blockade such as vecuronium are used, but this necessitates mechanical ventilation.[30] Methocarbamol often appears ineffective and requires frequent administration.[11,13] Benzodiazepines are preferred to methocarbamol because they are GABA agonists and also provide some sedation. Successful control of muscle spasms relieves pain and hyperthermia. If used, opioids should be administered with caution because they may contribute to constipation or gastrointestinal adverse effects. The use of fans and cool fluids may also be beneficial for dogs with tetanus-induced heat stroke. Administration of atropine may be required for animals with bradyarrhythmias (HR <60 beats/min). Rarely, upper respiratory obstruction has necessitated tracheostomy,[14] or bradyarrhythmias have required temporary pacemaker placement.[11]

Prognosis

Provided complications do not occur, prognosis is generally good for animals with tetanus or botulism. The overall 28-day survival rate for dogs with tetanus in one study was around 80%,[11] whereas in another study of 20 dogs it was only 50%.[13] A classification system has been developed to assess the severity of tetanus in dogs for the purpose of prognostication (Table 54-4).[11] The survival rate for dogs that progressed to tetanus severity classes I or II was 100%, but it dropped to 60% for dogs that progressed to tetanus severity class III or IV.[11] However, at the time of initial evaluation, only 11% of 37 dogs were in classes III or IV, and dogs progressed to higher classes unpredictably, with 47% of the dogs categorized in class III or IV when the highest recorded class was assigned. Dogs with severe tetanus are more likely to develop complications such as aspiration pneumonia or multiple organ dysfunction than dogs with mild tetanus. In a few dogs that recover (<10% of dogs that develop tetanus), intermittent localized muscle spasm continues to occur for many months, which may be noticed by the owner during activities such as sleeping or eating.[11]

TABLE 54-4

Tetanus Severity Classification System for Dogs

Class	Clinical Signs
I	Absence of class II, III or IV signs *and* any or all of: • Miosis, enophthalmos, risus sardonicus, erect ears, or trismus • Hypersensitivity to noise, light or touch • Ambulatory
II	Absence of class III or IV signs *and* any or all of: • Dysphagia • Stiff gait, sawhorse stance, erect tail • Ambulatory
III	Class I or class II signs, absence of class IV signs, *and* any or all of: • Recumbency • Muscle fasciculations or spasms • Seizures
IV	Class I, II, or III signs *and* any or all of: • Bradycardia (HR ≤60 beats/min) or bradyarrhythmia • Sinus tachycardia (HR ≥140 beats/min) or tachyarrhythmia • Labile hypertension or hypotension (mean arterial blood pressure ≤60 mm Hg or ≥ 130 mmHg, or systolic arterial blood pressure ≤80 mm Hg or ≥150 mm Hg) • Periods of apnea or respiratory arrest

Modified from Burkitt JM, Sturges BK, Jandrey KE, et al. Risk factors associated with outcome in dogs with tetanus: 38 cases (1987-2005). J Am Vet Med Assoc 2007;230:76-83.

Immunity and Vaccination

Given the relative rarity of tetanus and botulism in dogs and cats, vaccination is not recommended for these species. Recurrent tetanus or botulism has been documented in human patients, so recovery from natural disease does not necessarily result in protection from future episodes of disease. Thus, preventative measures should be discussed with owners of pets that recover from tetanus or botulism.

Prevention

Prevention of botulism involves limiting access of cats and dogs to carrion and feeding heat-processed commercial diets that are unspoiled. Although botulinum toxin can be denatured through boiling, spores can survive this treatment. Thus, cooked food should not be allowed to stand for long periods before it is fed to pets. The spores of *C. botulinum* are inactivated by pressure-cooking foods.

For tetanus, control of (1) roaming, (2) exposure to plant awns, and (3) aggressive interactions with other animals may reduce the chance that wounds develop. If wounds are noticed, they should be cleaned promptly with soap and water. Surgical instruments should always be sterilized properly before use so that tetanus spores are inactivated, and needles should never be reused. Tetanus spores can be inactivated with iodine, glutaraldehyde, hydrogen peroxide, or autoclaving at 121°C and 15 psi for 15 minutes.

Public Health Aspects

Animals with botulism or tetanus cannot transmit these conditions directly to humans who handle them. Nevertheless, feces, tissues, or body fluids from animals with botulism should be handled with care and marked with warning labels before they are submitted to the laboratory because the toxin is so potent. The main risk that dogs with tetanus pose to humans is through bite wounds, which can occur when owners attempt to administer medications.

Three forms of botulism occur in people: infant botulism, wound botulism, and food botulism.[26] Infant botulism occurs as a result of local production of botulinum toxin within the intestinal tract by *C. botulinum* in the absence of the competing intestinal microflora that are normally found in adults. Wound botulism occurs almost exclusively as a result of injection of contaminated heroin into the skin by intravenous drug users. Botulinum toxin preparations are used to treat conditions such as strabismus, esophageal achalasia, cervical dystonia, axillary hyperhydrosis (excessive sweating), or blepharospasm. There are rare reports of iatrogenic botulism after such use.[31] Life-threatening iatrogenic botulism has also occurred after use of botulinum preparations that were unlicensed for cosmetic treatment of wrinkles.[32] Significant concerns have been raised about the possible use of botulinum toxin as an agent of bioterrorism. This has stimulated considerable research on the disease, which is otherwise very rare.

Tetanus in humans is rare in developed countries, because most children are immunized against the disease. When it occurs, it is most often in people older than 60 years of age because of waning immunity.[30] Worldwide, the vast majority of cases occur in neonates from sub-Saharan Africa because of lack of immunization.

CASE EXAMPLE

Signalment: "Jenny," a 6-year-old female spayed Labrador retriever from Winters in northern California

History: Jenny was brought to the University of California, Davis, veterinary emergency service early in the morning for a 2-hour history of inability to stand. Her owners awoke to find her in another room, unable to get up for her morning walk. She appeared anxious and was breathing with increased effort, but was still wagging her tail. She also did not want to eat breakfast. There had been no known history of travel, toxins, trauma, or tick exposure. Over the past 2 months, she had been treated with prednisone (1 mg/kg PO q24h for 5 days, followed by 0.74 mg/kg PO q24h thereafter) for allergic dermatitis. Three weeks before the onset of illness she was treated with a short course of cephalexin after an aural hematoma was repaired. Jenny had been regularly vaccinated with rabies, distemper, hepatitis, and parvovirus vaccines.

Physical Examination:

Body Weight: 27.2 kg

General: Bright, alert, responsive, and hydrated. Laterally recumbent and anxious. HR = 140 beats/min, T = 101°F, panting.

Integument, Eyes, Ears, Nose, and Throat: Sutures were present on the pinna of the right ear from the recent aural hematoma repair. Moderate dental calculus and gingivitis was present. There were no other abnormalities noted.

Musculoskeletal: BCS 5/9. The dog was unable to use the pelvic limbs to bear weight.

Cardiovascular, Respiratory, Gastrointestinal, Genitourinary, and Lymph Nodes: No clinically significant abnormalities were present.

Neurologic Examination:

Mentation: Appropriate, anxious.

Gait/Posture: The dog was nonambulatory, but voluntary movement was present in all four limbs. She was unable to stand and support weight, but could crawl and shuffle. She attempted to bear weight on her thoracic limbs and could maintain sternal recumbency. When supported to stand, the pelvic limbs collapsed and the thoracic limbs were minimally able to bear weight.

Cranial Nerves: Slightly reduced palpebral reflexes and gag reflex. Absent corneal reflexes. No other deficits were noted.

Postural Reactions: These were difficult to assess because of the dog's inability to stand, but appeared decreased.

Segmental Reflexes: Reduced muscle tone was present in the thoracic limbs. Triceps, patella, and gastrocnemius reflexes were decreased. Reduced thoracic limb withdrawal reflexes were noted, but pelvic limb withdrawal reflexes were intact. Panniculus and perineal reflexes were also intact. Pain perception remained intact.

Spinal Palpation: No apparent pain was present on palpation or cervical manipulation.

Neuroanatomic Location: Neuromuscular disease.

Laboratory Findings:

CBC:

HCT 41.0% (40%-55%)
MCV 69 fL (65-75 fL)
MCHC 36.6 g/dL (33-36 g/dL)
WBC 5800 cells/μL (6000-13,000 cells/μL)
Neutrophils 3671 cells/μL (3000-10,500 cells/μL)
Lymphocytes 1769 cells/μL (1000-4000 cells/μL)
Monocytes 197 cells/μL (150-1200 cells/μL)
Eosinophils 145 cells/μL (0-1500 cells/μL)
Platelets clumped but adequate (150,000-400,000 platelets/μL).

Serum Chemistry Profile:

Sodium 146 mmol/L (145-154 mmol/L)
Potassium 3.9 mmol/L (3.6-5.3 mmol/L)
Chloride 107 mmol/L (108-118 mmol/L)
Bicarbonate 21 mmol/L (16-26 mmol/L)
Phosphorus 2.3 mg/dL (3.0-6.2 mg/dL)
Calcium 11.4 mg/dL (9.7-11.5 mg/dl)
BUN 15 mg/dL (5-21 mg/dL)
Creatinine 0.9 mg/dL (0.3-1.2 mg/dL)
Glucose 105 mg/dL (64-123 mg/dL)
Total protein 7.1 g/dL (5.4-7.6 g/dL)
Albumin 4.2 g/dL (3.0-4.4 g/dL)
Globulin 2.9 g/dL (1.8-3.9 g/dL)
ALT 64 U/l (19-67 U/L)
AST 25 U/L (19-42 U/L)
ALP 129 U/L (21-170 U/L)
Creatine kinase 57 U/L (51-399 U/L)
GGT 4 U/L (0-6 U/L)
Cholesterol 204 mg/dL (135-361 mg/dL)
Total bilirubin 0.2 mg/dL (0-0.2 mg/dL).

Urinalysis: SGr 1.025; pH 7.0, trace protein (SSA), 1+ bilirubin, no hemoprotein, glucose, ketones, WBC/HPF, RBC/HPF, bacteria or crystals in the sediment. Many lipid droplets were present.

Imaging Findings:

Thoracic Radiographs: The cardiopulmonary structures were within normal limits. There were mineral opacities within the stomach. There was a small amount of gas in the midthoracic esophagus.

Abdominal Ultrasound Examination: Mild mesenteric lymphadenopathy was identified. No other abnormalities were present.

Neuromuscular Testing: Edrophonium response test for myasthenia gravis: negative

Treatment: Jenny was admitted to the intensive care unit and treated with supportive care that included IV fluids (lactated Ringer's solution with 20 mEq/L KCl at 75 mL/hr), soft bedding, intermittent manual bladder expression, physical therapy (massage and passive range-of-motion exercises), and frequent turning. Treatment with prednisone was discontinued. Respiratory function was monitored continuously by observation, serial examination, and serial venous pCO_2 measurements. After repeated inspections for ticks, fipronil was applied in case the signs resulted from tick paralysis. Serum was submitted for an acetylcholine receptor antibody titer, and feces were submitted for a botulinum toxin assay. Over the subsequent 12 to 18 hours, Jenny became anxious after she was fed canned food and began to retch and hypersalivate. Thoracic radiographs were repeated and showed megaesophagus (see Figure 54-4, *A*). Severe tachycardia also developed (HR = 210 beats/min). An ECG showed ventricular tachycardia followed by supraventricular tachycardia. Systolic blood pressure was 145 mm Hg. Acepromazine was administered (0.01 mg/kg IV once), after which her heart rate decreased to 90 beats/min, with a normal sinus rhythm. A second neurologic examination showed progression of disease with reduced cervical tone and an inability to hold up the head, tetraplegia with absence of all segmental reflexes, and a reduced tail wag. The owners were warned that mechanical ventilation may be needed should the disease progress. Over the course of the next day, dysphonia and a mild cough developed, and Jenny regurgitated several times. Gastrostomy or jejunostomy tube feeding or parenteral nutrition were offered to the owner, but were declined. Four days after admission, improvement in the triceps reflex was noted, and on day 5, some voluntary movement was noted in the pelvic and thoracic limbs. At that time Jenny was successfully fed meatballs of canned food by hand. She was kept in sternal recumbency for 30 minutes after eating to minimize further aspiration. On day 7, the acetylcholine receptor antibody and botulinum toxin assay results became available.

Serum acetylcholine receptor antibody titer: 0.05 nmol/L (reference range, <0.6 nmol/L)

Botulinum toxin C mouse bioassay (fecal specimen): Positive for type C botulinum toxin. An extract from the fecal specimen was lethal in the bioassay. The effects were eliminated by heating the extract at 80°C for 10 minutes, which indicated that the toxic effects were due to a heat-labile toxin. Mice were also protected from the effects by anti–type C botulinum antisera but not by anti–type A botulinum antisera.

Diagnosis: Botulism.

Outcome: On day 8 after hospitalization, thoracic radiographs showed resolution of megaesophagus and no evidence of pneumonia. By day 10, Jenny began to shuffle along the floor. All segmental reflexes had returned but remained reduced. The dog was discharged from the hospital with instructions for continuation of care in the home environment. By day 15, Jenny's owners reported that her normal bark had returned, and she could walk 20 steps and defecate and urinate unassisted. A month after discharge she was reexamined and no abnormalities were detected.

Comments: The main differential diagnoses considered for this dog were myasthenia gravis and botulism. Initially, polyradiculoneuritis was also considered, but the subsequent development of megaesophagus was not consistent with this disorder. Ultimately, a diagnosis of botulism was confirmed through assay of the stool for botulinum toxin. A history of carrion ingestion was not known, but the dog lived in a semirural area, and the presence of mineralized stomach contents suggested that it had occurred. Prednisone administration may have contributed to polyphagia and ingestion of carrion by this dog.

SUGGESTED READINGS

Burkitt JM, Sturges BK, Jandrey KE, et al. Risk factors associated with outcome in dogs with tetanus: 38 cases (1987-2005). J Am Vet Med Assoc. 2007;230:76-83.

Cai S, Singh BR, Sharma S. Botulism diagnostics: from clinical symptoms to in vitro assays. Crit Rev Microbiol. 2007;33:109-125.

Chertow DS, Tan ET, Maslanka SE, et al. Botulism in 4 adults following cosmetic injections with an unlicensed, highly concentrated botulinum preparation. JAMA. 2006;296:2476-2479.

REFERENCES

1. Nicolaier A. Über infectiösen Tetanus. Dtsch Med Wochenschr. 1884;10:842-844.
2. Van Ermengem EP. Über einen neuen anaeroben *Bacillus* und seine Beziehung zum Botulismus. Z Hyg Infektionskrankh. 1897;26:1-56.
3. Barsanti JA, Walser M, Hatheway CL, et al. Type C botulism in American Foxhounds. J Am Vet Med Assoc. 1978;172:809-813.
4. Darke PG, Roberts TA, Smart JL, et al. Suspected botulism in foxhounds. Vet Rec. 1976;99:98-99.
5. Elad D, Yas-Natan E, Aroch I, et al. Natural *Clostridium botulinum* type C toxicosis in a group of cats. J Clin Microbiol. 2004;42:5406-5408.
6. Sobel J, Tucker N, Sulka A, et al. Foodborne botulism in the United States, 1990-2000. Emerg Infect Dis. 2004;10:1606-1611.
7. Bruchim Y, Steinman A, Markovitz M, et al. Toxicological, bacteriological and serological diagnosis of botulism in a dog. Vet Rec. 2006;158:768-769.
8. Wallace V, McDowell DM. Botulism in a dog—first confirmed case in New Zealand. N Z Vet J. 1986;34:149-150.
9. Farrow BR, Murrell WG, Revington ML, et al. Type C botulism in young dogs. Aust Vet J. 1983;60:374-377.

10. Doutre MP. 2nd case of botulism type D in the dog in Senegal. Rev Elev Med Vet Pays Trop. 1983;36:131-132.
11. Burkitt JM, Sturges BK, Jandrey KE, et al. Risk factors associated with outcome in dogs with tetanus: 38 cases (1987-2005). J Am Vet Med Assoc. 2007;230:76-83.
12. Sykes JE. Unpublished observations, 2012.
13. Bandt C, Rozanski EA, Steinberg T, et al. Retrospective study of tetanus in 20 dogs: 1988-2004. J Am Anim Hosp Assoc. 2007;43:143-148.
14. Adamantos S, Boag A. Thirteen cases of tetanus in dogs. Vet Rec. 2007;161:298-302.
15. Malik R, Church DB, Maddison JE, et al. Three cases of local tetanus. J Small Anim Pract. 1989;30:469-473.
16. Meunier FA, Lisk G, Sesardic D, et al. Dynamics of motor nerve terminal remodeling unveiled using SNARE-cleaving botulinum toxins: the extent and duration are dictated by the sites of SNAP-25 truncation. Mol Cell Neurosci. 2003;22:454-466.
17. Goldhammer MA, Chapman PS, Grierson JM. Coxofemoral luxation in a Border collie as a complication of a *Clostridium tetani* infection. J Small Anim Pract. 2008;49:159-162.
18. Langner KF, Schenk HC, Leithaeuser C, et al. Localised tetanus in a cat. Vet Rec. 2011;169:126.
19. Lee EA, Jones BR. Localised tetanus in two cats after ovariohysterectomy. N Z Vet J. 1996;44:105-108.
20. Polizopoulou ZS, Kazakos G, Georgiadis G, et al. Presumed localized tetanus in two cats. J Feline Med Surg. 2002;4:209-212.
21. Tomek A, Kathmann I, Faissler D, et al. [Tetanus in cats: 3 case descriptions]. Schweiz Arch Tierheilkd. 2004;146:295-302.
22. Uriarte A, Thibaud JL, Blot S. Botulism in 2 urban dogs. Can Vet J. 2010;51:1139-1142.
23. Malik R, Simpson DJ, Church DB. What is your diagnosis? Tetanus. J Small Anim Pract. 1998;39(217):252.
24. De Risio L, Gelati A. Tetanus in the cat—an unusual presentation. J Feline Med Surg. 2003;5:237-240.
25. van Nes JJ, van der Most van Spijk D. Electrophysiological evidence of peripheral nerve dysfunction in six dogs with botulism type C. Res Vet Sci. 1986;40:372-376.
26. Reddy P, Bleck TP. *Clostridium botulinum* (botulism). In: Mandell GL, Bennett JE, Dolin R, eds. Principles and Practice of Infectious Diseases. 7th ed. Philadelphia, PA: Elsevier; 2010:3097-3102.
27. Cai S, Singh BR, Sharma S. Botulism diagnostics: from clinical symptoms to in vitro assays. Crit Rev Microbiol. 2007;33:109-125.
28. Investigational heptavalent botulinum antitoxin (HBAT) to replace licensed botulinum antitoxin AB and investigational botulinum antitoxin E. MMWR Morb Mortal Wkly Rep. 2010;59:299.
29. Ahmadsyah I, Salim A. Treatment of tetanus: an open study to compare the efficacy of procaine penicillin and metronidazole. Br Med J (Clin Res Ed). 1985;291:648-650.
30. Reddy P, Bleck TP. *Clostridium tetani* (tetanus). In: Mandell GL, Bennett JE, Dolin R, eds. Principles and Practice of Infectious Diseases. 7th ed. Philadelphia, PA: Elsevier; 2010:3091-3096.
31. Coban A, Matur Z, Hanagasi HA, et al. Iatrogenic botulism after botulinum toxin type A injections. Clin Neuropharmacol. 2010;33:158-160.
32. Chertow DS, Tan ET, Maslanka SE, et al. Botulism in 4 adults following cosmetic injections with an unlicensed, highly concentrated botulinum preparation. JAMA. 2006;296:2476-2479.

CHAPTER 55

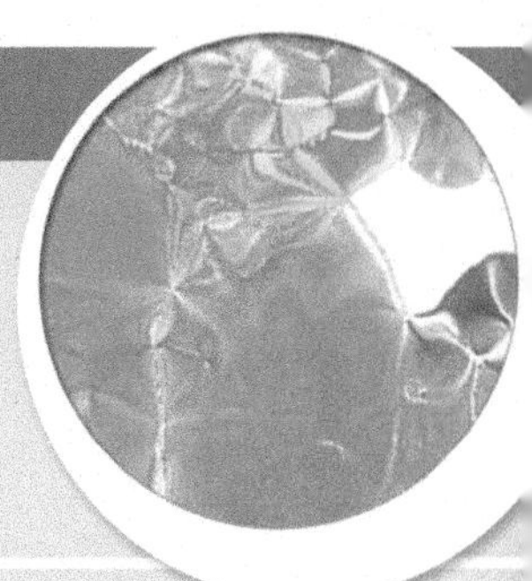

Yersinia pestis (Plague) and Other Yersinioses

Jane E. Sykes and Bruno B. Chomel

Overview of Plague

First Described: Descriptions of plague date back to around 1300 BC. The causative agent was isolated in 1894, in Hong Kong (Alexandre Yersin).[1]

Cause: *Yersinia pestis*, a gram-negative coccobacillus (family Enterobacteriaceae)

Affected Hosts: *Y. pestis* causes disease in rodents, rabbits, wild carnivores, domestic dogs and cats, and humans. Goats, deer, antelope, camelids, and nonhuman primates can also develop illness.

Geographic Distribution: Southwestern United States; foci also exist in Asia, Africa, and South America

Major Mode of Transmission: Flea-borne, via an enormous variety of rodent flea species; ingestion of infected rodents or rabbits by cats and dogs

Major Clinical Signs: Fever, lethargy, inappetence, lymphadenopathy, subcutaneous abscesses

Differential Diagnoses: Tularemia, cat bite abscesses, *Streptococcus* spp. infections, feline infectious peritonitis

Human Health Significance: A small percentage (10%) of human plague cases result from exposure to infected cats, through bites, scratches, or respiratory droplet inhalation from cats with pneumonic plague. Dogs and cats can also expose humans through the carriage of infected fleas into households (especially sleeping areas).

Etiology and Epidemiology

The genus *Yersinia* includes 11 different species, three of which are pathogenic in humans, cats, and dogs: *Yersinia pestis* and the enteropathogenic species *Yersinia pseudotuberculosis* and *Yersinia enterocolitica*. *Yersinia* spp. are nonmotile, gram-negative coccobacilli that belong to the family Enterobacteriaceae. Only *Y. pestis* is transmitted by arthropod vectors.

Yersinia pestis causes plague, which is maintained in wild burrowing rodents in rural regions of Asia, Africa, and the Americas (Figure 55-1). There is no plague in Australia, and the last case of plague in Europe was reported after World War II. The organism is transmitted between rodents by rodent fleas; humans, dogs, and cats are usually accidental and "dead-end" hosts (although direct transmission can occur through aerosols in humans and cats with pneumonic disease). Fleas become infected when they feed on heavily bacteremic rodents. The organism replicates in the flea intestine and creates a blockage of the intestinal tract, which causes the "starved" flea to repeatedly and aggressively feed and regurgitate bacteria into the bite site of a new host.[2] A large number of flea species can transmit *Y. pestis*, but some flea species, such as the Oriental rat flea (*Xenopsylla cheopis*) worldwide and the ground squirrel flea (*Oropsylla montana*) in the western United States are particularly efficient vectors. Although nowhere near as efficient as these two fleas as a vector, the cat flea (*Ctenocephalides felis*) can infest rodent reservoirs and also has the potential to transmit *Y. pestis*.[3] *Y. pestis* attains very high concentrations in rodent blood (10^8 organisms/mL) before death of the rodent occurs, which allows fleas to acquire sufficient numbers of bacteria for efficient transmission to other rodents.[4] Fleas can remain infected for more than a year, which permits transmission long after the death of an infected rodent.

Plague is transmitted to cats or dogs when they ingest infected mammals (especially rodents or rabbits) or less commonly, after the bite of a rodent flea. Humans are infected by (1) the bite of an infected flea; (2) direct contact with contaminated tissues (such as handling dead rodents, rabbits, or other dead wild mammalian carnivores); or rarely (3) inhalation of respiratory secretions by infected animals, especially cats (Figure 55-2). Death of a rodent from plague can cause the rodent's fleas to bite humans and other animals in a search for an alternative blood meal.

In the United States, plague in humans, dogs, and cats is now uncommon, although it is likely underrecognized in dogs and cats. Cats are considerably more susceptible to disease than dogs. Affected cats can be of any age, breed, and sex, with a mean age of 3 years in one case series.[5] Most plague cases in humans and cats occur in the southwestern United States, particularly northern New Mexico, but also southern Colorado, northern Arizona, and to a lesser extent California, southern Oregon, and western Nevada (especially in the Sierra Mountain ranges) (Figure 55-3). The probability of an area in the United States being a high-risk plague habitat increases with elevation up to 2300 meters and declines as elevation increases thereafter.[6] Rodent or rabbit species associated with human cases include white-tailed antelope squirrels, ground squirrels, rock squirrels, cottontail rabbits, jack rabbits, prairie dogs, deer mice, Colorado chipmunks, and wood rats.[2] The prevalence of antibodies to *Y. pestis* in a survey of 4115 dogs and 466 cats from California in the mid-1990s was less than 5% in both species.[7]

In general, plague has a seasonal distribution that correlates with the timing of epizootics that lead to a die-off of susceptible rodents. In the United States, most plague cases occur from February through August, when rodents and their fleas are most active and humans and their companion animals are more likely to be outdoors. In general, the organism does not survive well in the environment outside infected hosts, with survival less than

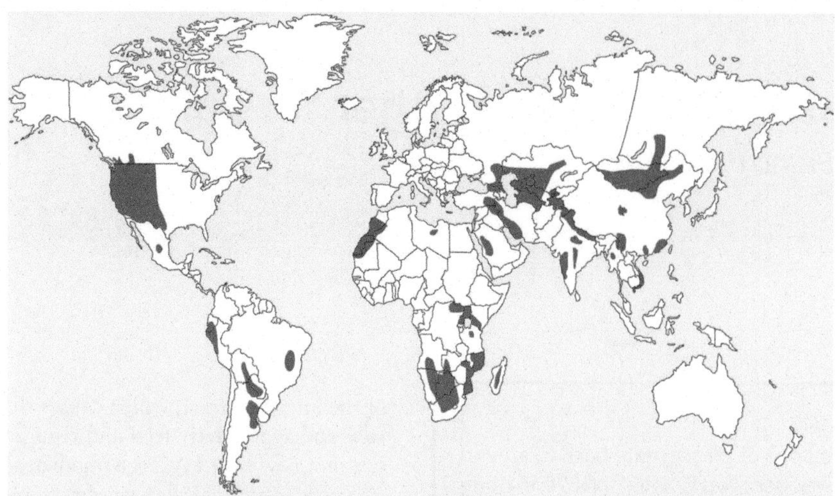

FIGURE 55-1 Worldwide distribution of plague endemic areas. (Data compiled from the World Health Organization, Centers for Disease Control and Prevention, and other sources. From Centers of Disease Control and Prevention. Prevention of plague: recommendations of the Advisory Committee on Immunization Practices (ACIP). MMWR Recomm Rep 1996;45:1-15. In: Mandell GL, Bennett JE, Dolin R, eds. Mandell, Douglas and Bennett's Principles and Practice of Infectious Diseases, 7th ed. Philadelphia, PA, Churchill Livingstone, Elsevier, 2011.)

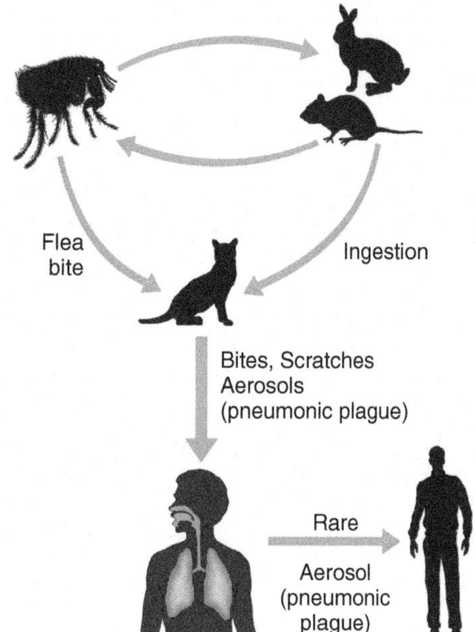

FIGURE 55-2 The role of the cat in transmission of *Yersinia pestis* to humans. Most humans are infected by direct contact with wildlife reservoir hosts or a bite from an infected flea, but infections can also occur as a result of cat bites or direct exposure to cats that have pneumonic plague. Dogs can also be infected but are less susceptible than cats to disease and shedding. Direct aerosol transmission from one human to another is rare and only occurs in humans that have terminal pneumonic plague.

72 hours on hard surfaces.[8] However, *Y. pestis* survived at least 24 days in blood-contaminated soil that was protected from UV light.[9] The extent to which environmental survival of *Y. pestis* contributes to the geographic distribution and epidemiology of the disease requires further clarification.

Clinical Features

Signs and Their Pathogenesis

After inoculation into the mammalian host by fleas, *Y. pestis* is taken up by mononuclear cells, in which it survives, replicates, and produces F1 capsular envelope antigen. The envelope allows it to further resist phagocytosis. Cats and dogs usually become infected after they ingest bacteremic rodents or other wildlife species that may have died of plague. In this situation, the organism has already produced a capsule and disseminates more rapidly than occurs after flea-borne transmission. Organisms are carried by lymphatics to regional lymph nodes. In more than half of affected cats, this results in an intense neutrophilic inflammatory response, variable fever, inappetence, and formation of the *bubo*, which is an enlarged and tender lymph node that occasionally forms an abscess and drains purulent material. This form of disease is known as *bubonic plague* and is the least fatal form of the disease. The location of the bubo(es) depends on the initial site of infection. In cats that ingest infected rodents, the mandibular or retropharyngeal lymph nodes are usually involved, and affected cats shed bacteria from the oropharynx. Less often (around 20% of cats with bubonic plague), other peripheral lymph nodes are involved; this may follow flea-borne transmission that occurs at sites distant to the head.[5]

In some cats, bubo formation is accompanied by bacteremia, with associated endotoxemia and sepsis, and formation of hemorrhagic, neutrophilic, and necrotizing lesions in many organs. Disseminated intravascular coagulation and multiple organ failure can then ensue. Signs of severe sepsis or septic shock in affected cats include tachypnea, vomiting, tachycardia or bradycardia, and weak pulse quality. In some situations, bacteremia and multiple organ involvement occurs in the absence of identifiable buboes *(septicemic form)*, which has a high mortality rate. *Pneumonic plague* occurs in about 10% of affected cats as a result of hematogenous spread of bacteria to the lungs or, less often, by inhalation of organisms and can result in dyspnea and cough. The incubation period for plague is estimated to be 1 to 6 days, with shorter incubation periods after ingestion or inhalation of the organism, and death can occur in as few as 2 to 3 days in the absence of appropriate treatment; occasionally the clinical course extends for 2 to 3 weeks. Some (<20%) of cats show no signs of illness, or there may be transient fever, decreased appetite, and recovery. Transient febrile illness is also common in dogs.

Physical Examination Findings

Physical examination in cats with plague reveals lethargy (82% of cats), fever (71% of cats; mean rectal temperature of 105.1°F [40.5°C]), dehydration, a thin body condition, and lymphadenopathy. Lymphadenopathy most often involves the mandibular nodes. In one case series, 33% of 67 cats with bubonic plague had bilateral lymphadenopathy, 32% had left-sided lymphadenopathy, and 13% had right-sided lymphadenopathy; in the remainder of cats, the location was not known.[5] Bilateral disease occurred only when the mandibular and cervical nodes were involved. Lymph nodes may be markedly enlarged (up to 8 cm, with a mean of around 4 cm); may be edematous, abscessated, and painful on palpation; and may drain purulent material. Drainage was reported in 6 (15%) of 40 cats with bubonic plague. Dyspnea or tachypnea can be present in cats with pulmonary involvement or possibly as a result of painful lymphadenopathy. Other reported physical examination abnormalities in cats with plague include ocular or nasal discharge (14% of cats) and abscesses that involve sites other than the lymph nodes, such as the sublingual region or the tongue, oral cavity, face, limbs, or trunk. Physical examination findings in dogs suspected to have plague have included fever, lethargy, mandibular or cervical bubo formation, oral ulceration and ptyalism, and cough.[10]

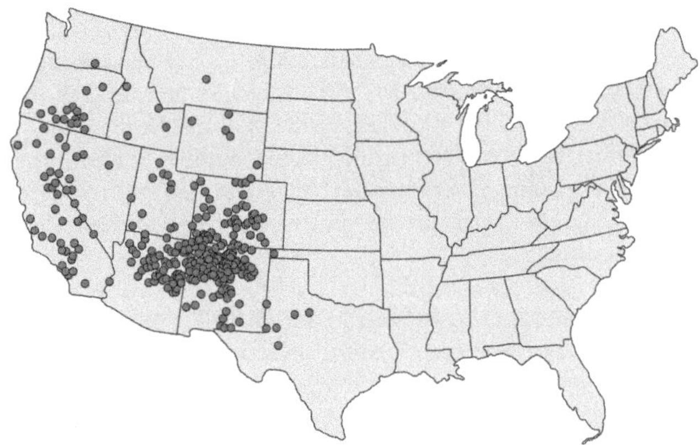

FIGURE 55-3 Approximate distribution of human plague cases in western United States, 1970 to 2012. Each dot represents a case, with the dot placed randomly in the county of exposure. (Modified from Dennis DT, Mead PS. *Yersinia* species, including plague. In: Mandell GL, Bennett JE, Dolin R, eds. Mandell, Douglas and Bennett's Principles and Practice of Infectious Diseases, 7th ed. Philadelphia, PA, Churchill Livingstone, Elsevier, 2011. Data from 2007-2012 collated from ProMed-Mail reports, http://www.promedmail.org/. Last accessed February 5, 2013).

Diagnosis

Diagnosis of plague is based on a history of residence in an endemic area as well as contact with, or predation of, wild mammals (especially rodents or lagomorphs). Duration of illness, physical examination findings, and lymph node aspirate cytology also support the diagnosis. There is a relative lack of information available on laboratory abnormalities in dogs and cats with plague because the disease is rare. Ultimately, a diagnosis of plague can only be confirmed by culture, direct fluorescent antibody testing, and/or serologic testing. Confirmation of the diagnosis may ultimately take weeks, so a high level of suspicion for the disease is needed in endemic areas.

Laboratory Abnormalities

Hematologic abnormalities in naturally infected cats most often consist of mild to moderate neutrophilia, usually with a mild to moderate left shift, and occasionally lymphopenia and monocytopenia.[5] Mild leukopenia can occur in cats with pneumonic plague. Platelet counts have not been widely reported in naturally infected cats but may be low in cats with severe sepsis. The serum biochemistry panel may show hypoalbuminemia, hyperglycemia, azotemia, electrolyte abnormalities, and increased liver enzyme activities.[11]

Diagnostic Imaging

Plain Radiography

Findings on thoracic radiography in cats with pneumonic plague have not been described in detail, but include diffuse interstitial, alveolar, and often nodular lung opacities.

Sonographic Findings

Abdominal ultrasound findings in cats with plague have not been reported. Based on pathologic findings, they might include abdominal lymphadenomegaly, splenomegaly, and hepatomegaly.

Microbiologic Tests

Diagnostic assays currently available for plague in dogs and cats are described in Table 55-1.

TABLE 55-1

Diagnostic Assays Currently Available for Plague in Dogs and Cats

Assay	Specimen Type	Target	Performance
Culture	Lymph node aspirates, blood, tissues collected at necropsy	*Yersinia pestis*	Recent antibiotic treatment may cause false-negative results. May take 48 hours for colonies to appear. Hazardous to laboratory personnel and should be sent to laboratories with appropriate expertise when possible.
Cytology	Lymph node aspirates	*Y. pestis* organisms (bipolar staining bacilli)	Low sensitivity. Recent antibiotic treatment may cause false-negative results.
Direct IFA	Lymph node aspirates, tissues collected at necropsy	*Y. pestis* F1 antigen	Increases sensitivity for detection of *Y. pestis* over cytology alone, but false negatives can still occur. Recent antibiotic treatment may cause false-negative results. Must be performed by laboratories with expertise in plague diagnosis.
Serology	Serum	Antibodies to *Yersinia pestis*	Acute and convalescent serology is required for diagnosis of acute infection, because initial results may be negative, and positive results may reflect previous exposure rather than active infection.

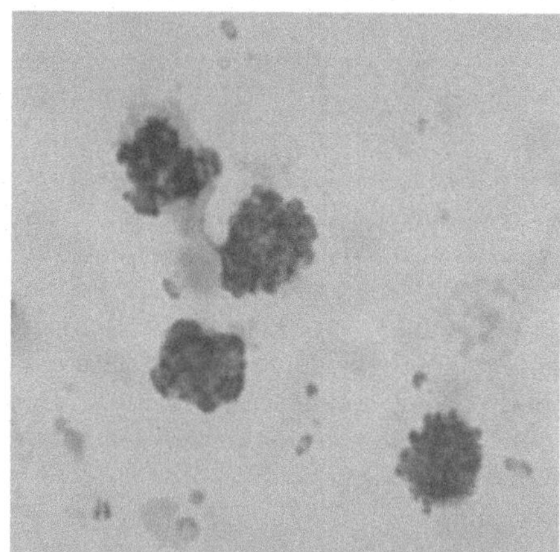

FIGURE 55-4 Lymph node aspirate cytology from a cat with bubonic plague. Bipolar rods are scattered throughout the field. (From Nelson RW, Couto CG, eds. Small Animal Internal Medicine, 4 ed. St. Louis, MO: Mosby; 2009.)

Cytologic Demonstration of Bacteria

Y. pestis is usually found in large numbers in tissues. If plague is suspected, aspirates of buboes or other affected tissues should be collected and smears prepared in isolation while wearing protective clothing, including eye protection and properly fitted high-density face masks (see Chapter 11). The smears should be heat fixed or immediately immersed in fixative solution to inactivate any organisms present. Cytologic examination shows massive numbers of neutrophils and a monomorphic population of coccobacilli with bipolar staining (Figure 55-4). This is in contrast to cat bite abscesses, where a mixture of bacteria is usually present.

Direct Immunofluorescent Antibody and Antigen ELISA Assays

Heat-fixed slides prepared from lymph node aspirates can be submitted to approved testing facilities for application of immunofluorescent antibody against the F1 envelope antigen. Local public health authorities should be contacted for information on recommended testing facilities if immunofluorescent antibody (IFA) testing is required. IFA can also be applied to impression smears from tissues obtained at necropsy. However, negative IFA results do not rule out plague, so culture and serology should also be considered.[5] A lateral-flow dipstick assay has been described for rapid (within 15 minutes), sensitive, and specific in-clinic diagnosis of plague in human patients, although false negatives may still occur.[12,13] This assay detects F1 antigen in body fluids such as sputum, lymph node aspirates, serum, and urine and has an estimated shelf life of about 2 years at room temperature. It has not been validated for diagnosis of plague in cats.

Isolation and Identification

Y. pestis can be grown from clinical specimens on routine media used for isolation of organisms that belong to the Enterobacteriaceae. The organism grows slowly, and colonies are smaller than those of other Enterobacteriaceae, so cultures must be held for at least 48 hours. If plague is suspected, specimens should never be shipped to routine veterinary diagnostic laboratories. Instead, local public health authorities should be contacted immediately for instructions regarding how and where to submit specimens for culture of *Y. pestis*.

Serology

Acute and convalescent serology is required for serologic diagnosis of plague in dogs and cats. The most widely used serologic test is a passive hemagglutination inhibition (HI) assay (see Chapter 2), which is available through public health laboratories approved for plague diagnosis. Because of the extremely short incubation period, a significant proportion of affected cats and dogs may have negative titers when they first are brought to the veterinarian, so convalescent serum should be submitted at least 10 to 14 days after the initial titer. Some cats may die before a rise in antibody titer occurs.[11] A fourfold increase in titer together with consistent clinical abnormalities confirms the diagnosis of plague. Titers in affected cats in one study ranged from less than 1:4 for acute specimens to 1:8192 for convalescent specimens.[5]

TABLE 55-2

Suggested Antimicrobial Drugs for Treatment of Plague in Cats

Drug	Dose (mg/kg)	Route	Interval (hours)	Duration
Doxycycline	10	IV or PO*	24	10 days
Gentamicin	5-8	IV, IM, SC	24	10 days

*Oral administration should be avoided for at least the first 72 hours of treatment to minimize exposure of the caregiver to *Y. pestis*. For IV doxycycline administration, dilute in 100 mL of lactated Ringer's saline and administer over 2 hours; if fluid overload is a concern, consider parenteral tetracycline or use of an aminoglycoside.

Molecular Diagnosis Using the Polymerase Chain Reaction

PCR assays have been described for detection of *Y. pestis* DNA and are an attractive means of diagnosis because of their sensitivity and rapid turnaround time. In addition, the organism can be deliberately inactivated before specimens are submitted to the laboratory for PCR testing, which reduces the risk of laboratory-acquired infection. Real-time PCR assays have been validated for use on clinical specimens from humans,[13] but to date assays have not been validated for diagnosis of the disease in cats or dogs. Real-time PCR was considerably more sensitive for diagnosis of human plague in Africa than the lateral-flow dipstick antigen assay or culture.

Pathologic Findings

Gross pathologic findings in cats with plague include enlarged lymph nodes or abscesses with associated edema and hemorrhage, focal (up to 1 cm) lung lesions, and hemorrhages in a variety of organs. Histopathology reveals hemorrhage, necrosis, neutrophilic infiltrates, and often very large numbers of small coccobacilli in tissues.

Treatment and Prognosis

Treatment of cats and dogs with plague involves supportive care, abscess drainage, and antimicrobial drug administration (Table 55-2). Animals suspected to have plague should be housed in isolation at least for the first 72 hours of antimicrobial drug therapy and handled by as few individuals as possible. Public health authorities should be notified immediately. Gowns, gloves, and suitable face protection (eye protection and a properly fited high-density surgical mask) should be worn, and protective wear should be properly removed and disposed of after handling affected cats. Cats and dogs

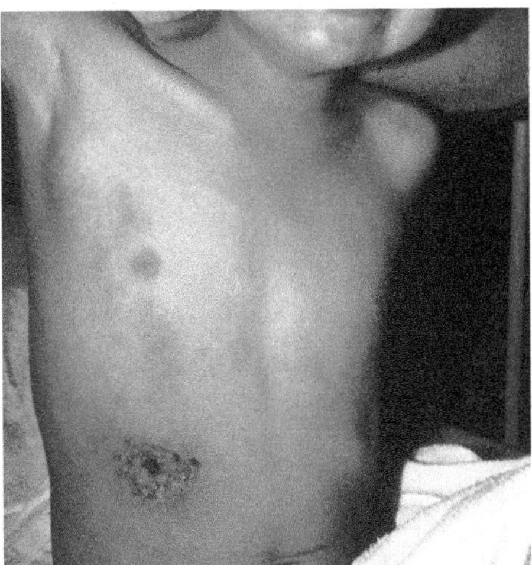

FIGURE 55-5 Axillary bubo with ulceration and eschar formation at the site of an infected flea bite. (Centers for Disease Control and Prevention.) (From Dennis DT, Mead PS. *Yersinia* species, including plague. In: Mandell GL, Bennett JE, Dolin R, eds. Mandell, Douglas and Bennett's Principles and Practice of Infectious Diseases, 7 ed, Philadelphia, PA: Churchill Livingstone, Elsevier; 2010.)

with plague should also be treated for fleas. Abscesses should be lanced and flushed with chlorhexidine solution. Any biohazardous waste should be double bagged and disposed of correctly. Routine disinfectants can be used to inactivate the organism in the environment. Antimicrobials with activity against most isolates of *Y. pestis* are aminoglycosides or tetracyclines such as doxycycline. Trimethoprim-sulfamethoxazole and chloramphenicol also have activity against *Y. pestis*. Parenteral aminoglycosides such as gentamicin are preferred for seriously ill animals. Mortality rates in naturally infected cats that are not treated with antimicrobial drugs can reach 75%, but most (>90%) of cats treated with antimicrobial drugs survive.[5] The time between antimicrobial drug treatment and recovery of affected cats ranged from 1 to 10 days in one study (mean, 4.4 days).[5]

Immunity and Vaccination

There are no plague vaccines for dogs and cats. Although vaccines have been used to prevent plague in highly at-risk humans, these did not protect against pneumonic plague. Currently there are no vaccines approved for use in the United States. Because *Y. pestis* is a potential agent of bioterrorism, efforts have been focused on development of subunit vaccines. However, *Y. pestis* has also been considered an unlikely agent of bioterrorism because in general it does not survive well in the environment, and person-to-person transmission requires close contact with a dying person, usually on the last day of life.[2,14]

Prevention

Prevention of plague in dogs and cats involves housing cats indoors in endemic areas and discouragement of predation or exposure to/consumption of wild animal carcasses. Dogs should not be allowed to dig around rodent burrows in endemic areas. Flea preventatives should reduce the chance that dogs and cats will carry infected fleas into the house. Rodent control in the environment (e.g., removal of garbage and food scraps) should also be performed.

Public Health Aspects

The clinical course of plague in humans closely resembles that in cats (Figure 55-5). Three major pandemics of plague have occurred in humans: Justinian plague, which occurred in the Mediterranean basin during the sixth century Byzantine era; the "Black Death," which began in 1347 and spread throughout Europe; and modern plague, which began in China in the 1860s and was subsequently spread by ship rats to all continents inhabited by humans. Currently, more than 95% of human plague cases reported to the WHO originate from sub-Saharan Africa and Madagascar.[15] From 1970 to 2007, 415 cases were reported in the United States, with 59 deaths.[16] In endemic regions, humans who have close contact with rodents or their canine or feline predators are at risk. The vast majority of humans are infected as a result of contact with rodent fleas. Human disease has also been reported after skinning of rabbits or contact with wild carnivores. Fewer than 10% of human plague cases result from exposure to cats, with infection transmitted from cats to humans after a bite, scratch, or inhalation of respiratory droplets from cats with pneumonic plague.[17-19] However, exposure to cats often results in pneumonic plague, which has the worst prognosis and can progress to death within as little as 24 hours after the onset of symptoms. Occasionally, dogs or cats carry rodent fleas into the house, which may then transmit the infection to humans. Sleeping with a dog may also increase the risk of infection.[20] Exposure to infected fleas carried into a household by a dog was suspected in a report of two affected humans in Oregon, one of whom slept in the same bed with the pet dog during the 2 weeks before onset of illness.[21] The dog seroconverted to *Y. pestis*.

Flea control and reduction of pet exposure to rodents also serve to reduce plague in humans. Pet owners should be made aware that pets can carry fleas (and ticks) into the house and that flea control may reduce the chance of arthropod-transmitted human disease. Adoption of wild animals should be discouraged. In the veterinary hospital situation, plague can be prevented if there is a high index of suspicion for the disease and appropriate precautions are taken (see Treatment and Prognosis). Owners of pets suspected to have plague should be advised to contact their physicians without delay. Humans with exposure to affected animals are generally treated with prophylactic doxycycline for 7 days.

Other Yersinioses

Y. pseudotuberculosis and *Y. enterocolitica* are enteropathogenic bacteria that are distributed worldwide. They are classified into serotypes based on their O antigens, with different classification systems used for the two pathogens. Enteropathogenic yersiniae are maintained in a variety of food animal and wild animal reservoirs and are well known causes of food-borne febrile gastrointestinal illness in humans. Pigs are a major reservoir for *Y. enterocolitica*, and outbreaks have followed consumption of undercooked pork products. *Y. enterocolitica* can also grow in food held at refrigeration temperatures. Affected human patients frequently exhibit right lower abdominal pain due to mesenteric adenitis or ileitis, which can mimic appendicitis. A small proportion of patients develop complications such as secondary polyarthritis and erythema nodosum (panniculitis).[16] Children are most susceptible. Immunocompromised humans (such as those with diabetes mellitus, malignancy, or immunosuppressive drug therapy) can occasionally develop bacteremia with systemic spread and abscesses in a variety of different organs. The mortality rate in this situation is at least 50%.[16]

Dogs and cats can shed *Y. enterocolitica* and *Y. pseudotuberculosis* in their feces in the absence of clinical signs.[22,23] *Y. enterocolitica* was also isolated from 19% of 144 tonsils from stray dogs in Ireland.[24] Strains found in dogs can resemble those implicated in human disease,[25] and in several reports, dogs were suspected as a source for human infection and disease. *Y. enterocolitica* infection was associated with hepatitis in a 2-year-old Pekingese dog from Korea[26] and hepatitis and myocarditis in a 4-month-old Rottweiler.[24] It has also been isolated from young dogs with hemorrhagic diarrhea. There have been several reports of *Y. pseudotuberculosis* infection in cats, with microabscess formation in a variety of abdominal organs.[27-29] A young adult dog evaluated at the authors' hospital for hemoptysis and lung consolidation had pulmonary *Y. pseudotuberculosis* infection.

Enteropathogenic *Yersinia* species are usually susceptible to doxycycline, trimethoprim-sulfamethoxazole, chloramphenicol, aminoglycosides, and fluoroquinolones. Some organisms produce β-lactamase enzymes.

In dogs and cats, prevention of enteropathogenic yersiniosis involves feeding properly cooked foods and preventing predation. Other measures to reduce zoonotic transmission include hand washing after handling dogs and cats (especially before eating), wearing gloves when contact with saliva or feces is anticipated, and preventing dogs from licking the face or open wounds.

CASE EXAMPLE

Refer to Chapter 56, Tularemia, for a case example.

SUGGESTED READINGS

Butler T. Plague into the 21st century. Clin Infect Dis. 2009;49:736-742.

Eidson M, Thilsted JP, Rollag OJ. Clinical, clinicopathologic, and pathologic features of plague in cats: 119 cases (1977-1988). J Am Vet Med Assoc. 1991;199:1191-1197.

Wilkie M, McGivern T, Skeels M, et al. Notes from the field: Two cases of human plague—Oregon, 2010. Morb Mortal Wkly Rep. 2011;60:214.

REFERENCES

1. Yersin A. La peste bubonique a Hong Kong. Ann Inst Pasteur (Paris). 1894;8:662-667.
2. Butler T. Plague into the 21st century. Clin Infect Dis. 2009;49: 736-742.
3. Eisen RJ, Borchert JN, Holmes JL, et al. Early-phase transmission of *Yersinia pestis* by cat fleas (*Ctenocephalides felis*) and their potential role as vectors in a plague-endemic region of Uganda. Am J Trop Med Hyg. 2008;78:949-956.
4. Lorange EA, Race BL, Sebbane F, et al. Poor vector competence of fleas and the evolution of hypervirulence in *Yersinia pestis*. J Infect Dis. 2005;191:1907-1912.
5. Eidson M, Thilsted JP, Rollag OJ. Clinical, clinicopathologic, and pathologic features of plague in cats: 119 cases (1977-1988). J Am Vet Med Assoc. 1991;199:1191-1197.
6. Eisen RJ, Enscore RE, Biggerstaff BJ, et al. Human plague in the southwestern United States, 1957-2004: spatial models of elevated risk of human exposure to *Yersinia pestis*. J Med Entomol. 2007;44:530-537.
7. Chomel BB, Jay MT, Smith CR, et al. Serological surveillance of plague in dogs and cats, California, 1979-1991. Comp Immunol Microbiol Infect Dis. 1994;17:111-123.
8. Rose LJ, Donlan R, Banerjee SN, et al. Survival of *Yersinia pestis* on environmental surfaces. Appl Environ Microbiol. 2003;69:2166-2171.
9. Eisen RJ, Petersen JM, Higgins CL, et al. Persistence of *Yersinia pestis* in soil under natural conditions. Emerg Infect Dis. 2008;14:941-943.
10. Orloski KA, Eidson M. *Yersinia pestis* infection in three dogs. J Am Vet Med Assoc. 1995;207:316-318.
11. Gasper PW, Barnes AM, Quan TJ, et al. Plague (*Yersinia pestis*) in cats: description of experimentally induced disease. J Med Entomol. 1993;30:20-26.
12. Chanteau S, Rahalison L, Ralafiarisoa L, et al. Development and testing of a rapid diagnostic test for bubonic and pneumonic plague. Lancet. 2003;361:211-216.
13. Riehm JM, Rahalison L, Scholz HC, et al. Detection of *Yersinia pestis* using real-time PCR in patients with suspected bubonic plague. Mol Cell Probes. 2011;25:8-12.
14. Kool JL. Risk of person-to-person transmission of pneumonic plague. Clin Infect Dis. 2005;40:1166-1172.
15. Stenseth NC, Atshabar BB, Begon M, et al. Plague: past, present, and future. PLoS Med. 2008;5:e3.
16. Dennis DT, Mead PS. *Yersinia* species, including plague. In: Mandell GL, Bennett JE, Dolin R, eds. Principles and Practice of Infectious Diseases. 7th ed. Philadelphia, PA: Elsevier; 2010:2943-2953.
17. Doll JM, Zeitz PS, Ettestad P, et al. Cat-transmitted fatal pneumonic plague in a person who traveled from Colorado to Arizona. Am J Trop Med Hyg. 1994;51:109-114.
18. Thornton DJ, Tustin RC, Pienaar BJ, et al. Cat bite transmission of *Yersinia pestis* infection to man. J S Afr Vet Assoc. 1975; 46:165-169.
19. Werner SB, Weidmer CE, Nelson BC, et al. Primary plague pneumonia contracted from a domestic cat at South Lake Tahoe. Calif. JAMA. 1984;251:929-931.
20. Gould LH, Pape J, Ettestad P, et al. Dog-associated risk factors for human plague. Zoonoses Public Health. 2008;55:448-454.
21. Wilkie M, McGivern T, Skeels M, et al. Notes from the field: Two cases of human plague—Oregon, 2010. Morb Mortal Wkly Rep. 2011;60:214.
22. Fenwick SG, Madie P, Wilks CR. Duration of carriage and transmission of *Yersinia enterocolitica* biotype 4, serotype 0:3 in dogs. Epidemiol Infect. 1994;113:471-477.
23. Fukushima H, Nakamura R, Iitsuka S, et al. Prospective systematic study of *Yersinia* spp. in dogs. J Clin Microbiol. 1984;19:616-622.
24. Murphy BP, Drummond N, Ringwood T, et al. First report: *Yersinia enterocolitica* recovered from canine tonsils. Vet Microbiol. 2010;146:336-339.
25. Wang X, Cui Z, Wang H, et al. Pathogenic strains of *Yersinia enterocolitica* isolated from domestic dogs (*Canis familiaris*) belonging to farmers are of the same subtype as pathogenic *Y. enterocolitica* strains isolated from humans and may be a source of human infection in Jiangsu Province, China. J Clin Microbiol. 2010;48:1604-1610.
26. Byun JW, Yoon SS, Lim SK, et al. Hepatic yersiniosis caused by *Yersinia enterocolitica* 4:O3 in an adult dog. J Vet Diagn Invest. 2011;23:376-378.
27. Iannibelli F, Caruso A, Castelluccio A, et al. *Yersinia pseudotuberculosis* in a Persian cat. Vet Rec. 1991;129:103-104.
28. Spearman JG, Hunt P, Nayar PS. *Yersinia pseudotuberculosis* infection in a cat. Can Vet J. 1979;20:361-364.
29. Obwolo MJ, Gruffydd-Jones TJ. *Yersinia pseudotuberculosis* in the cat. Vet Rec. 1977;100:424-425.

CHAPTER 56

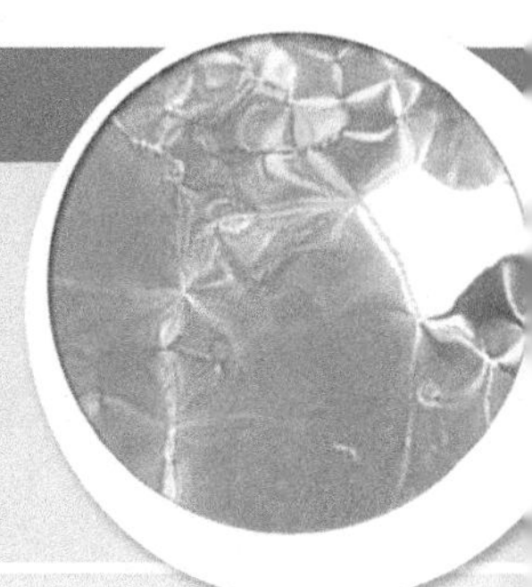

Tularemia

Jane E. Sykes and Bruno B. Chomel

Overview of Tularemia

First Described: 1911, Tulare County, California[1]

Cause: Virulent strains of *Francisella tularensis,* a gram-negative coccobacillus (family Francisellaceae)

Major Vectors: Ticks (especially *Dermacentor andersoni, Dermacentor variabilis,* and *Amblyomma americanum* in the eastern United States), biting flies (western United States), mosquitos (Scandinavia)

Affected Hosts: Some 190 mammalian species, which include rodents, rabbits, wild carnivores, domestic dogs and cats, sheep, horses, nonhuman primates, and humans

Geographic Distribution: Northern Hemisphere between 30 degrees and 71 degrees of latitude; most disease is reported from the United States, where virulent strains are most prevalent

Major Clinical Signs: Fever, lethargy, inappetence, lymphadenopathy, subcutaneous abscesses, splenomegaly, hepatomegaly

Differential Diagnoses: Plague, cat bite abscess, *Streptococcus* spp. infections, feline infectious peritonitis, mycobacterial infections, lymphoma, sepsis caused by other gram-negative bacteria

Human Health Significance: Cats and less commonly dogs can transmit tularemia to humans after they are exposed to infected rodents or rabbits. Cat bites are most commonly implicated.

Etiologic Agent and Epidemiology

Tularemia (also known as rabbit fever, hare fever, deerfly fever, and lemming fever) is an extremely infectious but uncommon zoonotic disease caused by *Francisella tularensis,* a small (0.2 × 0.2 × 0.7 μm), nonmotile, aerobic, encapsulated gram-negative coccobacillus. The name "tularemia" comes from the first isolation of the organism from sick rodents in Tulare County, California, in 1911. There are four subspecies of *F. tularensis: tularensis, holarctica, novicida,* and *mediasiatica*. Subspecies *tularensis* (also known as type A) and *holarctica* (type B) cause most disease in humans. Subspecies *mediasiatica* is only found in Asia and the former Soviet Union. Subspecies *novicida* can cause illness in severely immunosuppressed humans and is widely studied as a model for tularemia because of its low virulence to laboratory workers.

F. tularensis subsp. *tularensis* has the greatest degree of virulence for humans and predominates in North America, whereas the less virulent subspecies *holarctica* predominates in Europe. Additional genetic variation within type A and type B subpopulations of *F. tularensis* correlates with geographic distribution of cases and the severity of disease.[2] Molecular subtyping has further divided type A into subpopulations A1a, A1b, A2a, and A2b. The highest mortality in humans, 24%, results from infections by A1b.[3]

Tularemia occurs primarily in the Northern Hemisphere, especially between 30 degrees and 71 degrees of latitude (Figure 56-1). Human disease caused by a subspecies *novicida*–like organism was reported from the Northern Territory in Australia in 2003.[4] Even in North America, where *F. tularensis* subsp. *tularensis* predominates, tularemia is a rare disease, and most human cases occur in the central and north-central United States, especially Arkansas, Missouri, Kansas, South Dakota, and Oklahoma, with an additional focus in Massachusetts (especially Martha's Vineyard) (Figure 56-2). Despite its rarity, tularemia is a reportable disease in the United States because *F. tularensis* is considered a potential agent of bioterrorism. In western Europe, tularemia is endemic in Scandinavia but has emerged in new parts of Sweden and is increasingly reported in humans from more southern locations, such as Germany, France, and Spain.[5] Tularemia has been absent from the United Kingdom, with the exception of travel-related disease. It also occurs in Russia and Japan.[6]

Canine and feline disease due to *F. tularensis* has only been reported from the United States. Young adult cats and dogs are usually affected. As with plague, cats are more susceptible than dogs. Cases are reported most often from Oklahoma[7-9] and Kansas,[10] but also from other locations that include Montana,[11] Missouri,[12] Massachusetts,[13] central Virginia,[14] and eastern Oregon,[15] which mirrors the distribution in humans. Tularemia is likely underdiagnosed in cats and dogs because clinical signs

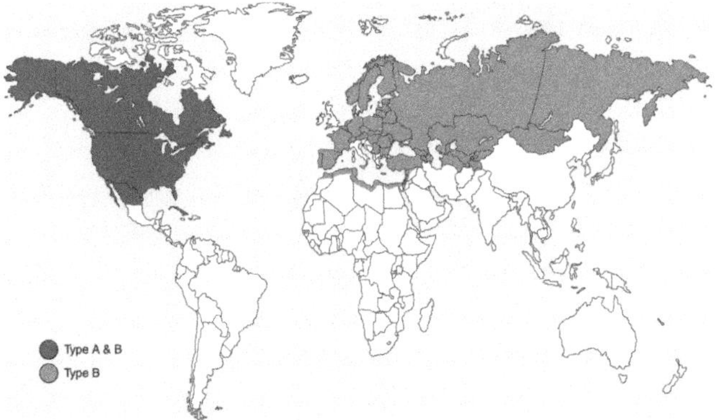

FIGURE 56-1 Global distribution of tularemia (Centers for Disease Control and Prevention).

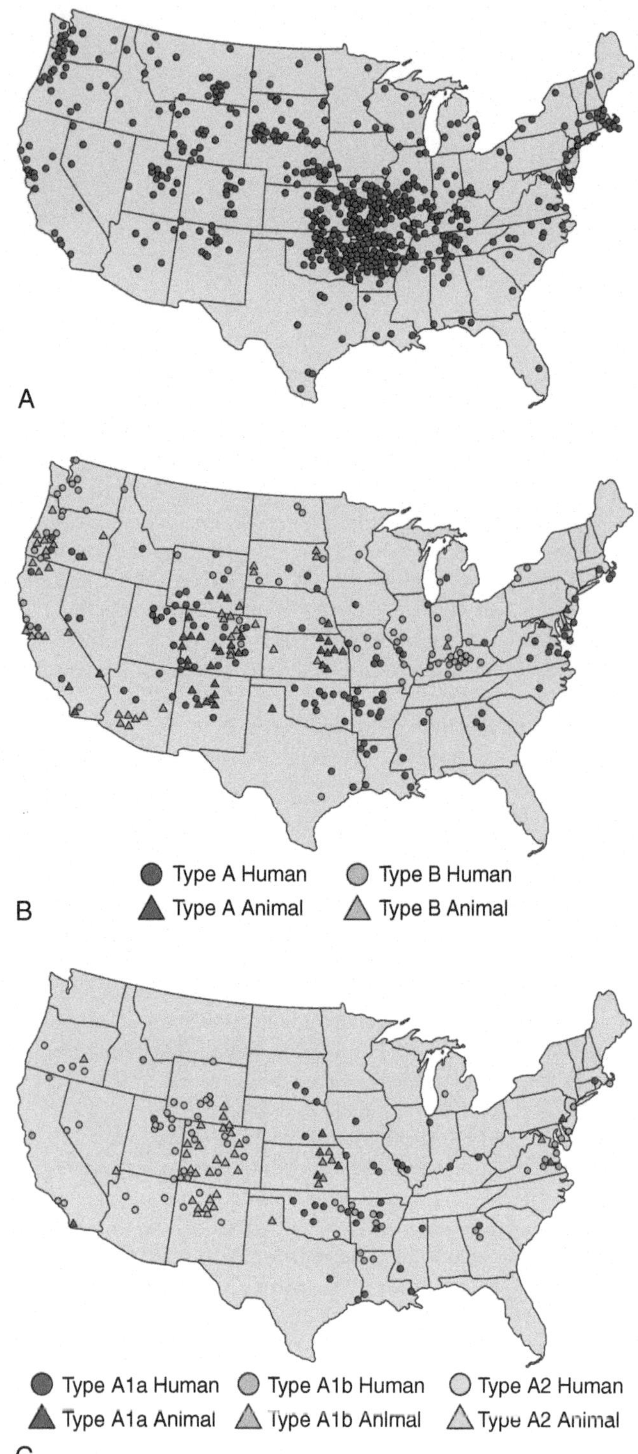

FIGURE 56-2 Geographic distribution of tularemia in the USA. Compare this with the geographic distribution of plague (Figure 55-3). **A,** Overall distribution of human tularemia cases. **B,** Distribution of type A and type B isolates from humans and animals. **C,** Distribution of isolates from humans and animals by molecular subtype. Note that the geographic distribution of human type A cases follows the distribution of subtype A1, the most virulent subtype being A1b. (**A** and **B** modified from Kugeler KJ, Mead PS, Janusz AM, et al. Molecular epidemiology of Francisella tularensis in the United States. Clin Infect Dis 2009;48:863-870.)

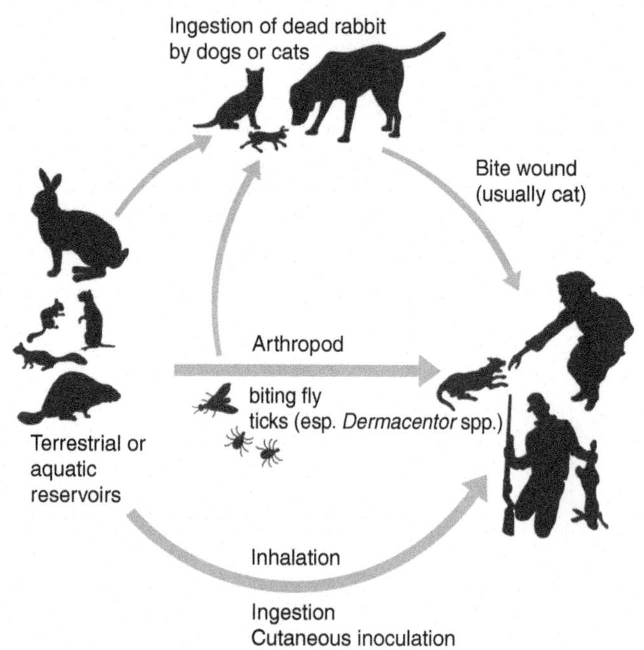

FIGURE 56-3 Transmission cycle for *Francisella tularensis*.

are nonspecific. Many cats with tularemia are diagnosed with tularemia at necropsy.[7,10] The seroprevalence in pet cats from Connecticut and New York state was 12%.[16]

F. tularensis is maintained in the environment by a huge variety of terrestrial and aquatic mammals, which include rabbits, hares, ground squirrels, prairie dogs, lemmings, voles, beavers, muskrats, water rats, and other rodents.[6] It often causes severe disease in these species, although subclinical carriage may also occur. It can be transmitted by arthropod bites, inhalation or ingestion of the organism, and direct skin contact with infected tissues (probably when there are minute breaks in the skin) (Figure 56-3). Inhalation of as few as 10 organisms can cause human disease, whereas larger numbers of organisms (10^8) must be ingested for disease to occur. Cats and dogs become infected when they hunt rodents or lagomorphs; a history of rabbit ingestion was most often described in association with the few reported feline and canine cases.[7-9] In the western United States (Utah, Nevada, and California), the most common arthropod vectors are biting flies, whereas ticks (especially *Dermacentor* ticks and *Amblyomma americanum*) are the most common vectors east of the Rocky Mountains. In Europe, *Dermacentor* ticks and *Ixodes ricinus* are the main tick vectors; mosquitos are important vectors in Scandinavia.[17] *F. tularensis* is well known for its ability to survive up to several months in fresh water sources, and survival in brackish water has also been demonstrated.[18] Survival and replication of *F. tularensis* within free-living amoebae such as *Hartmannella vermiformis* may contribute to the organism's ability to persist in water sources.[19] The organism can also survive for years in frozen rabbit meat.

Clinical Features

Signs and Their Pathogenesis

The clinical manifestations of tularemia depend on the virulence of the infecting strain, the route of inoculation, and host immunity. Although tularemia may rapidly progress to death in cats, protracted illness has also been described.[15]

F. tularensis survives in macrophages through evasion of cellular destruction by phagosomes and inhibition of the respiratory burst. Several different virulence factors of *F. tularensis* have been identified, which include bacterial lipopolysaccharide (LPS), pili, a capsule, and a series of acid phosphatase enzymes. The endotoxic activity of the LPS of *F. tularensis* is 1000-fold less potent than that of *Escherichia coli*.[20,21] Production of acid phosphatase enzymes may be key to the organism's ability to inhibit the respiratory burst and survive in macrophages.[22] Many stages of the organism's intracellular lifestyle depend on a pathogenicity island (group of virulence genes) known as the *Francisella* pathogenicity island.

For the first few days after cutaneous inoculation, *F. tularensis* replicates locally and can produce a papule that may then ulcerate. It then disseminates to local lymph nodes, which may be followed by bacteremia and sepsis, with infection of systemic, primarily reticuloendothelial tissues. The organism invades not only macrophages but also nonphagocytic cells such as hepatocytes and alveolar epithelial cells,[23] with induction of a profound inflammatory response and necrosis. Incubation periods that range from 1 to 5 days have been suspected in naturally occurring tularemia in dogs and cats, but longer incubation periods (up to 21 days) can occur in humans. Clinical signs typically manifest as a sudden onset of fever, lethargy, and inappetence. Other manifestations in affected cats have included a thin body condition, icterus, hepatomegaly, vomiting, dehydration, peripheral and/or abdominal lymphadenomegaly, splenomegaly, and oral and/or lingual ulceration. Hypothermia and bradycardia can occur in moribund cats[7]; one cat had seizures and was nonresponsive.[14] A single cat with localized cutaneous tularemia had a chronic (1-year duration) draining skin lesion in the region of (but not involving) the mandibular lymph nodes, in the absence of systemic signs.[15] In the rare reports of naturally affected dogs, clinical signs have included fever, anorexia, and peripheral lymphadenopathy.[8,24] One dog also had bilateral mucoid ocular discharge and mild conjunctival hyperemia,[8] and another had tonsillitis.[24]

Physical Examination Findings

Physical examination in cats with tularemia may reveal lethargy, fever (up to 105.1°F [40.5°C]) or hypothermia, a thin body condition, and dehydration.[7,9,11-13] Ulceration of the oral mucous membranes or tongue may be present.[7,13] Icterus may also occur.[25] Moribund cats may be hypothermic and bradycardic and may have weak pulse quality. Mild to marked peripheral lymphadenopathy is present in most but not all cats. Lymphadenopathy may be restricted to the lymph nodes of the head and neck[13] or may be generalized.[7,9] Abdominal palpation may reveal hepatomegaly or splenomegaly, or abdominal lymph nodes may be palpable. Fever, lethargy, peripheral lymphadenopathy, mucoid ocular discharge, and tonsillitis may be present in dogs.[8,24]

Diagnosis

Tularemia should be considered in cats and dogs with lymphadenopathy and fever that have a history of residence in or recent travel to an endemic area, as well as contact with or predation of wild mammals (especially lagomorphs). Plague is the major differential diagnosis of zoonotic importance in the southwestern United States (Table 56-1). Ultimately, the diagnosis can be confirmed by culture, PCR, and/or serologic testing. With the exception of PCR, access to approved laboratories that practice biosafety level 3 procedures is required to perform these tests when tularemia is suspected. Local public health authorities should be contacted to report suspicion for the disease and for information on recommended testing facilities.

Laboratory Abnormalities

Complete Blood Count, Biochemistry Profile, and Urinalysis

Leukocyte counts in a limited number of cats with tularemia have been normal, decreased (as low as 1300 cells/μL), or increased with evidence of neutrophil toxicity.[7,9,13,14] Moderate to marked bandemia may be present.[9,13] Thrombocytopenia is a common finding (as low as 41,000 platelets/μL).[7,9] The serum biochemistry panel may show hypoglycemia, azotemia, and electrolyte abnormalities, increased liver enzyme activities, and hyperbilirubinemia (up to 7.6 mg/dL).[7,9,14] Bilirubinuria and hemoglobinuria may be present.[7] Mature neutrophilia, lymphopenia, and increased serum ALP activity were present in a dog with tularemia.[8] In human patients, abnormalities include thrombocytopenia, elevated serum transaminase activities, increased serum creatine kinase activity, myoglobinuria, and pyuria.[26]

Cytologic Examination of Lymph Node Aspirates

Cytologic examination of lymph node aspirates in cats with tularemia may reveal lymph node hyperplasia.[9] Lymph nodes may also contain necrotic debris and increased numbers of macrophages and/or degenerate neutrophils.[7,13] Because *F. tularensis* is tiny and stains only faintly, organisms are less likely to be visualized than those of *Yersinia pestis* (see Chapter 55).

Diagnostic Imaging

Plain Radiography

Findings on thoracic radiography in cats with tularemia have not been well described; one cat had normal thoracic radiographs.[9] Findings on abdominal radiography have included hepatomegaly and fluid-filled intestinal loops.[9]

Sonographic Findings

Abdominal ultrasound findings in cats with tularemia could include abdominal lymphadenomegaly, splenomegaly, and/or hepatomegaly. Abdominal lymphadenomegaly was described in one cat.[9]

Microbiologic Tests

Diagnostic assays currently available for tularemia in dogs and cats are described in Table 56-2.

Direct Detection

Heat-fixed slides can be submitted to experienced laboratories for direct immunofluorescent antibody (IFA) staining for *F. tularensis*. Alternatively, IFA or immunoperoxidase stains can be applied to tissues obtained at necropsy.[10] Negative results do not rule out tularemia, but in some cases IFA may detect the organism when culture is negative.[27] Fluorescence in situ hybridization (FISH) has also been used to detect *F. tularensis* in tissues and differentiate between subspecies.[28] As for plague, lateral-flow assays have been described for rapid detection of *F. tularensis* LPS antigen in clinical specimens such as urine.[29] The use of these assays in dogs and cats has not been described.

Isolation and Identification

F. tularensis can be grown from clinical specimens, but it is very fastidious, grows slowly, is hazardous to laboratory personnel,

TABLE 56-1

Differences and Similarities between Plague and Tularemia in Cats and Dogs in the United States

	Plague	Tularemia
Organism	Gram-negative bacillus (Enterobacteriaceae). Survives relatively poorly in the environment. Grows on routine culture media used for gram-negative bacteria.	Gram-negative coccobacillus (Francisellaceae). Can persist in the environment and water sources for months. Fastidious growth in culture; often requires special media and prolonged incubation.
Major Arthropod vectors	Diverse variety of rodent and rabbit fleas	*Dermacentor* spp. and *Amblyomma americanum* ticks
Geographic location	Southwestern United States	Western, southwestern, central, and eastern United States
Affected hosts	Cats > dogs	Cats > dogs
Usual history	Rodent contact or exposure to rodent fleas	Rodent and especially rabbit contact; ingestion often reported
Clinical signs	Acute disease with high fever and lymphadenopathy, most often of the mandibular and/or retropharyngeal lymph nodes. Hyperbilirubinemia and icterus do not appear to be common in affected cats.	Acute or more chronic disease (sometimes associated with a thin body condition) with oral ulceration, lymphadenopathy of the mandibular and/or retropharyngeal lymph nodes, or generalized lymphadenopathy and abdominal organomegaly. Hyperbilirubinemia is frequent in affected cats, and icterus has been described.
Lymph node aspirate cytology	Neutrophilic inflammation; monomorphic population of bipolar staining bacilli often present	Lymphoid reactivity or neutrophilic to pyogranulomatous inflammation and necrosis; bacteria often not visualized
Antimicrobial drugs	Aminoglycosides, doxycycline, chloramphenicol, trimethoprim-sulfamethoxazole	Aminoglycosides are the treatment of choice. Doxycycline, chloramphenicol, and fluoroquinolones may be effective but may be followed by relapse.
Zoonotic potential	Exposure to cats with pneumonic plague can lead to human infection; bites and scratches have also been implicated. Human pneumonic plague usually results from exposure to infected cats and can progress to death within a few days. Exposed humans may require prophylaxis with doxycycline.	Most often follows bites from affected cats, less often scratches. Course of disease longer and mortality may be lower than occurs with pneumonic plague. Medical attention should be sought if bites or scratches occur.

TABLE 56-2

Diagnostic Assays Currently Available for Tularemia in Dogs and Cats

Assay	Specimen Type	Target	Performance
Culture	Lymph node aspirates, blood, tissues collected at necropsy	*Francisella tularensis*	Recent antibiotic treatment may cause false-negative results. May require special media and takes at least 48 hours for colonies to appear. Hazardous to laboratory personnel and should be sent to laboratories with appropriate expertise when possible.
Direct immunofluorescent antibody	Lymph node aspirates, tissues collected at necropsy	*F. tularensis* antigen	May be positive when culture is negative. False negatives can still occur. Recent antibiotic treatment may cause false-negative results.
Serology	Serum	Antibodies to *F. tularensis*	Acute and convalescent serology is required for diagnosis, because initial results may be negative and positive results may reflect previous exposure rather than active infection. Seroconversion may take up to 3 weeks.

and does not always grow on media used for routine isolation of gram-negative bacteria such as MacConkey agar (in contrast to *Y. pestis*). The use of cysteine-supplemented media (such as cysteine heart agar) and incubation in a CO_2-supplemented environment enhances recovery of the organism. Growth generally occurs 48 to 72 hours after inoculation, but cultures must be held for 7 to 10 days. Overgrowth of contaminating bacteria can occur unless the media is supplemented with antibiotics that inactivate these organisms. *F. tularensis* may grow from blood specimens after inoculation of routine blood culture media. The organism is identified on the basis of biochemical testing with or without the use of molecular methods such as 23S rRNA gene PCR sequencing (which allow subspecies determination). Whole-cell matrix-assisted laser desorption ionization–time of flight (MALDI-TOF) mass spectrometry, which measures the mass of peptides and small proteins from whole cells, has also been used for identification of *F. tularensis* isolates to the subspecies level.[30]

Serology

As for plague, acute, and convalescent serology, with a fourfold increase in titer, is required for serodiagnosis of tularemia in affected dogs and cats and is less hazardous to human health than culture. Tube agglutination and microagglutination assays are the standard methods for serodiagnosis, but ELISA assays have also been developed. Because of the extremely short incubation period, affected cats and dogs may have negative titers when they first are brought to the veterinarian, so convalescent serum should be submitted at least 2 to 3 weeks after the initial titer if the animal survives. Some cats die from the disease before a rise in antibody titer occurs. In addition, high titers may persist after recovery from infection, so a single positive titer is not diagnostic for tularemia.

Molecular Diagnosis Using the Polymerase Chain Reaction

PCR assays that detect *F. tularensis* DNA represent an attractive means of diagnosis because of their sensitivity, rapid turnaround time, low risk to laboratory personnel, and the ability of some assays to differentiate between subspecies and genotypes of *F. tularensis*.[31] A PCR assay was used to detect *F. tularensis* in tissues at necropsy in a cat.[12] A number of real-time PCR assays have been used to detect *F. tularensis* in human clinical specimens. Despite the sensitivity of PCR assays, false negatives can still occur. Real-time PCR assays for *F. tularensis* are offered on a commercial basis by some veterinary diagnostic laboratories in the United States.

Pathologic Findings

Gross pathologic findings in cats with tularemia include icterus, oral ulceration, lymphadenomegaly, splenomegaly, and hepatomegaly. Multifocal to coalescing irregular yellow, gray, or white foci (usually 1 to 5 mm in diameter) are present in these organs, and sometimes other organs such as the lung and myocardium.[7,12,13] When examined histopathologically, the nodules represent well-circumscribed but non-encapsulated masses of caseous necrosis, with abundant cellular debris, surrounded by infiltrates of degenerate neutrophils, macrophages, and/or fibroblasts. Lesions are centered on the splenic white pulp and cortical lymphoid follicles within lymph nodes. Necrosis and hemorrhage of lymphoid follicles within the gastrointestinal tract may be present.[7,11] Organisms may be discernible with silver staining as tiny coccobacilli[11] or can be demonstrated with immunoperoxidase or immunofluorescence methods.[10,27]

TABLE 56-3

Suggested Antimicrobial Drugs for Treatment of Tularemia in Cats*

Drug	Dose (mg/kg)	Route	Interval (hours)	Duration
Gentamicin	5-8	IV, IM, SC	24	14 days
Doxycycline	5	PO†	12	2-3 weeks
Marbofloxacin	2.75-5.5	PO	24	2-3 weeks

*The same antimicrobial drugs could be used to treat dogs; doses shown are for cats.

†Parenteral aminoglycosides are preferred for at least the first 72 hours of treatment to minimize exposure of the caregiver to *F. tularensis* during treatment.

Treatment and Prognosis

Treatment of cats (and, although less commonly affected, dogs) with tularemia involves supportive care and antimicrobial drug administration (Table 56-3). As for plague, animals suspected to have tularemia should be housed in isolation at least for the first 72 hours of antimicrobial drug therapy and handled by as few individuals as possible. Public health authorities should be notified. Gowns, gloves, and suitable face protection (eye protection and a properly fitted high density surgical mask) should be worn, and protective wear should be properly removed and disposed of after handling affected cats. Any biohazardous waste should be double bagged and disposed of correctly. Routine disinfectants should be used to inactivate the organism in the environment. The drug of choice for initial treatment of tularemia is a parenteral aminoglycoside such as gentamicin. Doxycycline can also be used but is associated with a higher relapse rate in humans than occurs with aminoglycosides.[26] Fluoroquinolones are active against *F. tularensis* in vitro, but like tetracyclines, they may be associated with relapse in vivo.[32] Extension of the course of treatment from 2 weeks to 3 weeks when fluoroquinolones or doxycycline is used has been effective for treatment of human tularemia.[25] Other drugs with in vitro activity against *F. tularensis* include chloramphenicol and erythromycin.[33]

Immunity and Vaccination

Natural infection by *F. tularensis* is followed by protection against reinfection. Because *F. tularensis* is facultatively intracellular, cell-mediated immune responses are required for pathogen clearance, although humoral immunity is also important.[23] As a result, inactivated vaccines have not been effective for prevention of tularemia, because they primarily induce humoral immunity. An attenuated live vaccine that contained *F. tularensis* subsp. *holarctica* (live vaccine strain, or LVS) has been available for prevention of serious disease in people at high risk of exposure. However, this remains unlicensed because of concerns regarding efficacy and the route of administration, which is by scarification.[34] Since then there has been strong interest in vaccine development for prevention of human tularemia, because of concerns that the organism will be used as a weapon of bioterrorism.[23] Vaccines are not likely to be available for dogs and cats given the rarity of disease in these species and the minor role that they play in transmission of disease to humans.

Prevention

Prevention of tularemia in dogs and cats involves housing cats indoors and discouragement of predation or exposure to dead wild rodents and rabbits. Use of tick preventatives also reduces the chance that dogs and cats will carry infected ticks into the house. Rodent control in the environment (e.g., removal of garbage) should also be performed.

Public Health Aspects

Humans are most commonly infected by *F. tularensis* after arthropod bites or handling infected wild animals. In the United States, disease is most commonly reported in late spring and summer. Occupations associated with an increased risk of tularemia include farming, hunting, landscaping, meat handling, working with sheep, veterinary practice, and laboratory work. Severe illness is most often reported in young children (5 to 9 years) and the aged (>75 years). Men are more likely to be affected than women.[26]

Several overlapping forms of disease have been described in humans, the development of which depends on the route of inoculation and the virulence of the infecting strain: ulceroglandular, glandular, oculoglandular, oropharyngeal, typhoidal, and pneumonic.[26] Ulceroglandular tularemia results from cutaneous inoculation, oropharyngeal disease follows ingestion and pneumonic tularemia can result from aerosol inhalation. Pneumonic tularemia has been described in people after activities such as lawn mowing or brush cutting in tick-infested areas. Infection of humans from dogs and cats can occur after these animals carry *F. tularensis* in their mouths after ingestion of wild prey. Human-to-human transmission does not occur.

Clinical signs in humans consist of acute onset of a flu-like illness, with fever, chills, and malaise. Sore throat, abdominal pain, vomiting, diarrhea, lymphadenopathy, and a cough may also occur. Infection with less virulent strains may result in transient flu-like illness followed by recovery. Without treatment, clinical signs can persist for several months, with chronic lymphadenopathy, weight loss, and debilitation.[26] Disease in chronically affected humans can resemble cat scratch disease.

Ulceroglandular tularemia is the most common form of tularemia seen in humans. It consists of a red and painful papule at the site of skin infection, with associated lymphadenopathy (Figure 56-4). The papule then undergoes necrosis, forming an ulcer, which can take weeks to heal. In some individuals, lymph nodes may suppurate and become fluctuant. Multiple lesions can occur on the hands when infected animals have been handled, whereas tick bites typically result in single lesions elsewhere on the body.[26] Only lymphadenopathy may be present if the ulcer heals before the time of evaluation *(glandular tularemia)*. *Oculoglandular tularemia* occurs when organisms gain access through the conjunctiva and is characterized by conjunctivitis, conjunctival ulceration, lacrimation, and associated lymphadenopathy.[26] *Oropharyngeal tularemia* is characterized by fever and severe throat pain; tonsillitis, oral ulceration, and associated lymphadenopathy may be present, which resembles the disease described in dogs and cats (which usually acquire infection via ingestion). Oropharyngeal tularemia tends to occur in children who ingest contaminated food or water and can resemble "strep throat."[26] *Typhoidal tularemia* is a febrile illness in the absence of prominent lymphadenopathy and may be associated with sore throat, abdominal pain, diarrhea, vomiting, icterus, and, with more chronic illness, hepatomegaly and splenomegaly. *Pneumonic tularemia* is the most severe form and results from inhalation of the organism or hematogenous spread of the organism to the lung, with clinical signs such as cough, chest pain, and hemoptysis. Thoracic radiographs can reveal lobar infiltrates, hilar lymphadenopathy, pleural effusion, and miliary infiltrates.[26] Changes resemble those seen in other chronic pneumonias, such as tuberculosis or fungal disease.

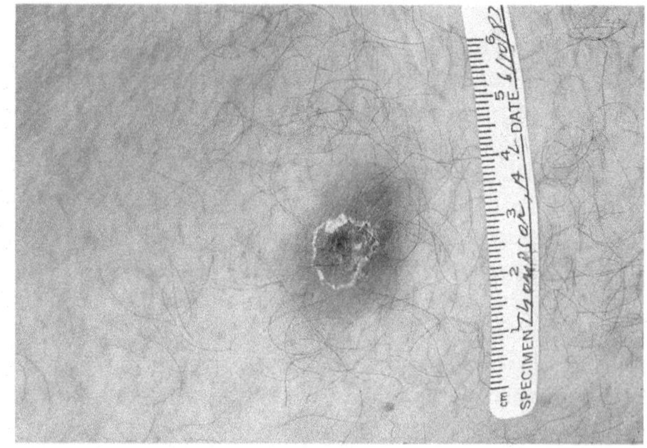

FIGURE 56-4 Papule undergoing central necrosis with desquamation on the thigh of a middle-aged man infected with *Francisella tularensis*. (Courtesy of Dr. Joseph A. Bocchini, Louisiana State University Health Sciences Center, Shreveport, LA. In: Mandell GL, Bennett JE, Dolin R, eds. Principles and Practice of Infectious Diseases, 7th ed, Philadelphia, PA: Churchill Livingstone; 2010:2927-2937.)

Although not the most common route of infection for humans, cat-bite–associated tularemia has been described (including among veterinary staff), and cats that live in rural endemic areas are important vectors of the most virulent strain of *F. tularensis*, type A1b.[25] Disease in humans can mimic *Pasteurella multocida* cellulitis, the most common bacterial infection after a cat bite, but treatment with amoxicillin or clavulanic acid–amoxicillin is ineffective. Less commonly, human disease follows cat scratches or casual contact with cats.[27] In some cases, cats had recent contact with or ingested wild rabbits or rodents. Both apparently healthy and sick cats have been involved. Aerosol exposure to organisms on the coats of dogs (such as occurs when dogs shake their coats after contact with infected rabbits) has rarely been suspected in clusters of human disease.[35-37] In summary, tularemia should especially be considered in humans who develop illness in endemic areas within 3 weeks after a bite from a cat that is a stray or that has had a recent history of wild rabbit or rodent contact.

CASE EXAMPLE

Signalment: "Sam," a 5-year-old male neutered domestic shorthair cat from Woodland in northern California

History: Sam was brought to the University of California, Davis, veterinary emergency service for evaluation of fever and inappetence. The owner first noticed he was ill 4 days previously, when he regurgitated a small amount of pink fluid about 1 hour after eating. The following day he was not eating and lethargic, and his water consumption was reduced. On day 3, he was taken to a local veterinary clinic where he was found to be febrile (105°F [40.5°C]), icteric, and had a mass on the left side of his neck. He was treated with enrofloxacin (4.5 mg/kg SC, once), ketoprofen (1.9 mg/kg SC), and clavulanic acid–amoxicillin (12 mg/kg PO q12h). The results of a CBC showed a mild neutrophilia (13,083 cells/μL; reference range, 2500-12,500 cells/μL) with slightly toxic neutrophils and a mild lymphopenia (1176 cells/μL; reference range, 1500-7000 cells/μL). A biochemistry panel showed hyponatremia (133 mEq/L; reference range, 147-156 mEq/L), hypochloremia (99 mEq/L; reference range, 111-125 mEq/L), hypokalemia (3.4 mEq/L; reference range, 3.9-5.3 mEq/L), hyperglycemia (214 mg/dL; reference range, 70-150 mg/dL), hyperbilirubinemia (3.7 mg/dL; reference range, 0-0.4 mg/dL), increased serum CK activity (1858 U/L; reference range, 64-440 U/L), and a mild metabolic acidosis (bicarbonate 12 mEq/L; reference range, 13-25 mEq/L). ELISA serology for FeLV antigen and FIV antibody and IFA serology for FCoV antibody were negative. On receipt of the laboratory test results, the local veterinarian recommended referral.

Sam had been fed commercial dry and canned cat food and was treated monthly with fipronil. He had been acquired at 6 weeks of age, at which time he was neutered. He had been vaccinated annually by the owner for feline respiratory viruses and feline panleukopenia virus, and was vaccinated for rabies for the first time 4 months earlier. He lived with three other cats, three dogs, and two rabbits, and the owner had brought home a wild mouse from the Lake Tahoe (Sierras) region several weeks before Sam became ill. The rabbits were acquired by the owner 6 months ago, were kept indoors, and did not receive flea control. The owner fostered cats and occasionally dogs for the local animal shelter and cared for a colony of feral cats, which did not interact with the household cats. The household cats lived harmoniously indoors.

Physical Examination:

Body Weight: 5.4 kg

General: Lethargic but responsive. Resented handling. T = 105.9°F [41.1°C], RR = 60 breaths/min, HR = 176 beats/min, CRT <2 s.

Integument: Mild scaling was present throughout the haircoat, but no ectoparasites were visible.

Eyes, Ears, Nose, and Throat: No clinically significant abnormalities were present.

Musculoskeletal: Body condition score 6/9. There was a 2 × 2 × 6 cm firm subcutaneous mass alongside the trachea on the left side.

Cardiovascular: There were no murmurs or arrhythmias detected on cardiac auscultation. Pulses were strong and synchronous.

Respiratory: Tachypnea was present with a shallow respiratory pattern. Normal bronchovesicular sounds were present in all lung fields.

Abdominal Palpation: No clinically significant abnormalities were identified. The urinary bladder was palpable but small.

Lymph Nodes: The left mandibular lymph node was enlarged at 2 cm. All other lymph nodes appeared to be within normal limits.

Laboratory Findings:

CBC:

HCT 20.3% (30%-50%)
MCV 42.9 fL (42-53 fL)
MCHC 33.0 g/dL (30-33.5 g/dL)
Reticulocytes 9500 cells/μL (7000-60,000 cells/μL)
WBC 23,120 cells/μL (4500-14,000 cells/μL)
Neutrophils 18,958 cells/μL (2000-9000 cells/μL)
Band neutrophils 3699 cells/μL
Lymphocytes 231 cells/μL (1000-7000 cells/μL)
Monocytes 231 cells/μL (50-600 cells/μL)
Eosinophils 0 cells/μL (150-1100 cells/μL)
Basophils 0 cells/μL (0-50 cells/μL)
Platelets 102,000/μL (180,000-500,000 platelets/μL).

Serum Chemistry Profile:

Anion gap 18 mmol/L (13-27 mmol/L)
Sodium 143 mmol/L (151-158 mmol/L)
Potassium 3.2 mmol/L (3.6-4.9 mmol/L)
Chloride 110 mmol/L (117-126 mmol/L)
Bicarbonate 18 mmol/L (15-21 mmol/L)
Phosphorus 3.0 mg/dL (3.2-6.3 mg/dL)
Calcium 8.8 mg/dL (9.0-10.9 mg/dL)
BUN 15 mg/dL (18-33 mg/dL)
Creatinine 0.8 mg/dL (1.1-2.2 mg/dL)
Glucose 151 mg/dL (63-118 mg/dL)
Total protein 6.6 g/dL (6.6-8.4 g/dL)
Albumin 2.5 g/dL (2.2-4.6 g/dL)
Globulin 4.1 g/dL (2.8-5.4 g/dL)
ALT 30 U/L (27-101 U/L)
AST 39 U/L (17-58 U/L)
ALP 5 U/L (14-71 U/L)
GGT < 3 U/L (0-4 U/L)
Cholesterol 134 mg/dL (89-258 mg/dL)
Total bilirubin 2.1 mg/dL (0-0.2 mg/dL)
Magnesium 2.0 mg/dL (1.5-2.5 mg/dL)
Creatine kinase 586 U/L (73-260 U/L).

Urinalysis: SGr 1.014; pH 8.0, trace protein (SSA), 1+ bilirubin, 2+ hemoprotein, 2+ glucose, rare WBC/HPF, 7-12 RBC/HPF, few lipid droplets.

Imaging Findings:

Thoracic Radiographs and Abdominal Ultrasound: No clinically significant abnormalities were present.

Cervical Ultrasound: There was moderate to severe enlargement of the retropharyngeal lymph nodes bilaterally and of the left mandibular salivary gland.

Microbiologic Testing: Cytologic examination of lymph node aspirates (mandibular and retropharyngeal): A slightly bloody background was admixed with markedly increased numbers of variably degenerate neutrophils. Low numbers of lymphocytes and scattered macrophages are also observed. Interpretation: marked suppurative inflammation.

Continued

Comments: Although no intracellular bacteria were seen, the number of neutrophils and their variably degenerate nature suggested sepsis as the primary differential diagnosis.

Aerobic and anaerobic bacterial culture and susceptibility (lymph node aspirate): No growth.

PCR for *Francisella tularensis* DNA (lymph node aspirate): Negative.

Diagnosis: Severe suppurative lymphadenitis and fever; suspect plague or tularemia.

Treatment: Sam was transferred to isolation, during which time he bit a clinician, and treated with intravenous fluids (lactated Ringer's solution and 20 mEq/L KCl at 15 mL/h IV) and antimicrobial drugs (ampicillin, 20 mg/kg IV q8h and gentamicin, 5 mg/kg IV q24h). Public health officials were contacted. The cat's rectal temperature initially increased to 107°F (41.6°C); dark brown diarrhea was also noted. On the second day of hospitalization, Sam's rectal temperature was 105°F (40.5°C), and by day 3 it had normalized and Sam began to eat. It increased again to 103.9°F (40.0°C) the following day, and the right mandibular and retropharyngeal lymph nodes became palpably enlarged. Subsequently, the cat's rectal temperature normalized, laboratory abnormalities improved, and the lymph nodes decreased in size and were soft on palpation. The cat was discharged with instructions to continue treatment with oral amoxicillin and subcutaneous gentamicin for 7 days, with a recheck planned at that time for an examination and convalescent *Y. pestis* and *F. tularensis* serology. The owner did not bring Sam back for a recheck examination, but a follow-up telephone conversation indicated that Sam had recovered completely.

Comments: A diagnosis of plague or tularemia was never confirmed in this cat, although strongly suspected based on the history of wild rodent and rabbit exposure (with the rodent adopted from a plague endemic region), and the clinical abnormalities that were present. The findings of hyperbilirubinemia, thrombocytopenia, and increased serum CK activity were perhaps more suggestive of tularemia than plague, although hyperbilirubinemia and thrombocytopenia can occur in human plague. The history of antibiotic treatment may have contributed to the negative cytology, culture, and PCR results. Culture was requested on site shortly after admission because plague and tularemia were initially overlooked as likely diagnoses. Once these diseases were considered, an attempt was made to send specimens out to a public health laboratory for additional testing, but this was complicated by concerns that related to the potentially hazardous nature of the specimens. Handling of the cat was limited to as few individuals as possible and was difficult because the cat was aggressive. The clinician who was bitten by the cat immediately saw her physician, who prescribed doxycycline for 7 days. Rabies quarantine was also instituted because the cat was incompletely vaccinated for rabies. The owner was educated about the possibility of plague or tularemia and the implications for human health. Although flea control was used, not all of the animals received flea prevention, and there was significant turnover of a variety of wildlife and domestic animal species in the household. Continued adoption of wild animals by the owner was discouraged.

SUGGESTED READINGS

Kugeler KJ, Mead PS, Janusz AM, et al. Molecular epidemiology of *Francisella tularensis* in the United States. Clin Infect Dis. 2009;48:863-870.

Spagnoli ST, Kuroki K, Schommer SK, et al. Pathology in practice. Francisella tularensis. J Am Vet Med Assoc. 2011;238:1271-1273.

Weinberg AN, Branda JA. Case records of the Massachusetts General Hospital. Case 31-2010. A 29-year-old woman with fever after a cat bite. N Engl J Med. 2010;363:1560-1568.

REFERENCES

1. McCoy GW, Chapin CW. *Bacterium tularense*, the cause of a plague-like disease in rodents. Public Health Bulletin. 1912;53:17-23.
2. Petersen JM, Molins CR. Subpopulations of *Francisella tularensis* ssp. *tularensis* and *holarctica*: identification and associated epidemiology. Future Microbiol. 2010;5:649-661.
3. Kugeler KJ, Mead PS, Janusz AM, et al. Molecular Epidemiology of *Francisella tularensis* in the United States. Clin Infect Dis. 2009;48:863-870.
4. Whipp MJ, Davis JM, Lum G, et al. Characterization of a *novicida*-like subspecies of *Francisella tularensis* isolated in Australia. J Med Microbiol. 2003;52:839-842.
5. Mahy S, Chavanet P, Piroth L, et al. Emergence of tularemia in France: paradigm of the Burgundy region. Int J Infect Dis. 2011;15:e882-e883.
6. Ellis J, Oyston PC, Green M, et al. Tularemia. Clin Microbiol Rev. 2002;15:631-646.
7. Baldwin CJ, Panciera RJ, Morton RJ, et al. Acute tularemia in three domestic cats. J Am Vet Med Assoc. 1991;199:1602-1605.
8. Meinkoth KR, Morton RJ, Meinkoth JH. Naturally occurring tularemia in a dog. J Am Vet Med Assoc. 2004;225:538:545-547.
9. Woods JP, Crystal MA, Morton RJ, et al. Tularemia in two cats. J Am Vet Med Assoc. 1998;212:81-83.
10. DeBey BM, Andrews GA, Chard-Bergstrom C, et al. Immunohistochemical demonstration of *Francisella tularensis* in lesions of cats with tularemia. J Vet Diagn Invest. 2002;14:162-164.
11. Rhyan JC, Gahagan T, Fales WH. Tularemia in a cat. J Vet Diagn Invest. 1990;2:239-241.
12. Spagnoli ST, Kuroki K, Schommer SK, et al. Pathology in practice. *Francisella tularensis*. J Am Vet Med Assoc. 2011;238:1271-1273.
13. Gliatto JM, Rae JF, McDonough PL, et al. Feline tularemia on Nantucket Island. Massachusetts. J Vet Diagn Invest. 1994;6:102-105.
14. Inzana TJ, Glindemann GE, Snider G, et al. Characterization of a wild-type strain of *Francisella tularensis* isolated from a cat. J Vet Diagn Invest. 2004;16:374-381.
15. Valentine BA, DeBey BM, Sonn RJ, et al. Localized cutaneous infection with *Francisella tularensis* resembling ulceroglandular tularemia in a cat. J Vet Diagn Invest. 2004;16:83-85.
16. Magnarelli L, Levy S, Koski R. Detection of antibodies to *Francisella tularensis* in cats. Res Vet Sci. 2007;82:22-26.
17. Lundstrom JO, Andersson AC, Backman S, et al. Transstadial transmission of *Francisella tularensis* holarctica in mosquitoes. Sweden. Emerg Infect Dis. 2011;17:794-799.
18. Berrada ZL, Telford Iii SR. Survival of *Francisella tularensis* Type A in brackish-water. Arch Microbiol. 2011;193:223-226.
19. Santic M, Ozanic M, Semic V, et al. Intra-vacuolar proliferation of *F. novicida* within *H. vermiformis*. Front Microbiol. 2011;2:78.
20. Ancuta P, Pedron T, Girard R, et al. Inability of the *Francisella tularensis* lipopolysaccharide to mimic or to antagonize the induction of cell activation by endotoxins. Infect Immun. 1996;64:2041-2046.
21. Gunn JS, Ernst RK. The structure and function of *Francisella* lipopolysaccharide. Ann N Y Acad Sci. 2007;1105:202-218.

22. Dai S, Mohapatra NP, Schlesinger LS, et al. The acid phosphatase AcpA is secreted in vitro and in macrophages by *Francisella* spp. Infect Immun. 2012;80:1088-1097.
23. Barry EM, Cole LE, Santiago AE. Vaccines against tularemia. Hum Vaccin. 2009;5:832-838.
24. Gustafson BW, DeBowes LJ. Tularemia in a dog. J Am Anim Hosp Assoc. 1996;32:339-341.
25. Weinberg AN, Branda JA. Case records of the Massachusetts General Hospital. Case 31-2010. A 29-year-old woman with fever after a cat bite. N Engl J Med. 2010;363:1560-1568.
26. Penn RL. *Francisella tularensis* (tularemia). In: Mandell GL, Bennett JE, Dolin R, eds. Principles and Practice of Infectious Diseases. 7th ed. Philadelphia, PA: Churchill Livingstone, Elsevier; 2010:2927-2937.
27. Capellan J, Fong IW. Tularemia from a cat bite: case report and review of feline-associated tularemia. Clin Infect Dis. 1993;16:472-475.
28. Splettstoesser WD, Seibold E, Zeman E, et al. Rapid differentiation of *Francisella* species and subspecies by fluorescent in situ hybridization targeting the 23S rRNA. BMC Microbiol. 2010;10:72.
29. Grunow R, Splettstoesser W, McDonald S, et al. Detection of *Francisella tularensis* in biological specimens using a capture enzyme-linked immunosorbent assay, an immunochromatographic handheld assay, and a PCR. Clin Diagn Lab Immunol. 2000;7:86-90.
30. Seibold E, Bogumil R, Vorderwulbecke S, et al. Optimized application of surface-enhanced laser desorption/ionization time-of-flight MS to differentiate *Francisella tularensis* at the level of subspecies and individual strains. FEMS Immunol Med Microbiol. 2007;49:364-373.
31. Molins CR, Carlson JK, Coombs J, et al. Identification of *Francisella tularensis* subsp. *tularensis* A1 and A2 infections by real-time polymerase chain reaction. Diagn Microbiol Infect Dis. 2009;64:6-12.
32. Steward J, Piercy T, Lever MS, et al. Treatment of murine pneumonic *Francisella tularensis* infection with gatifloxacin, moxifloxacin or ciprofloxacin. Int J Antimicrob Agents. 2006;27:439-443.
33. Urich SK, Petersen JM. In vitro susceptibility of isolates of *Francisella tularensis* types A and B from North America. Antimicrob Agents Chemother. 2008;52:2276-2278.
34. Conlan JW, Oyston PC. Vaccines against *Francisella tularensis*. Ann N Y Acad Sci. 2007;1105:325-350.
35. Rumble CT. Pneumonic tularemia following the shearing of a dog. J Med Assoc Ga. 1972;61:355.
36. Siret V, Barataud D, Prat M, et al. An outbreak of airborne tularaemia in France, August 2004. Euro Surveill. 2006;11:58-60.
37. Teutsch SM, Martone WJ, Brink EW, et al. Pneumonic tularemia on Martha's Vineyard. N Engl J Med. 1979;301:826-828.

CHAPTER 57

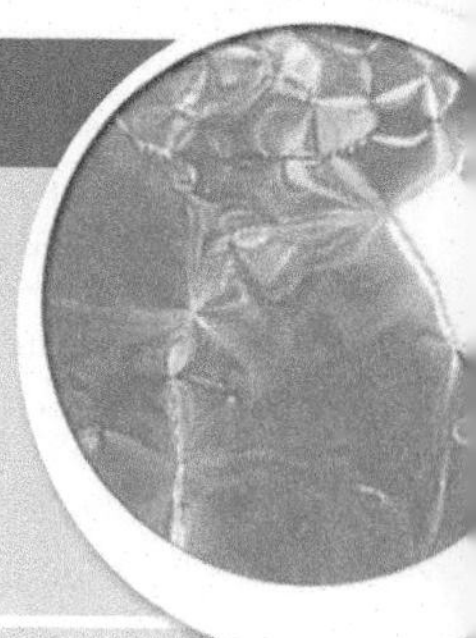

Bite and Scratch Wound Infections

Jane E. Sykes

Overview of Bacterial Bite Wound Infections

Causes: A variety of aerobic and anaerobic bacteria that include mycoplasmas and mycobacterial species. *Pasteurella* spp. are commonly isolated.

Geographic Distribution: Worldwide

Major Clinical Signs: Fever, lethargy, inappetence, hyperesthesia, puncture wounds, cutaneous swellings, lacerations, tissue avulsions, and signs that relate to damage and/or infection of other structures (such as the thorax, abdomen, and brain and spinal cord)

Differential Diagnoses: Other traumatic injuries, cutaneous neoplasia, sterile nodular panniculitis (dogs), plague, tularemia

Human Health Significance: Cat and dog bite wound infections are common in humans and may be life threatening in the immunocompromised. They also can be associated with transmission of potentially serious bloodborne bacterial diseases such as bartonellosis and tularemia.

Etiology and Epidemiology

Bite wounds are one of the most common reasons that dogs or cats are brought to veterinary hospitals for care. Despite this, there is surprisingly little information available on their epidemiology in comparison to the plethora of publications on animal bite wounds in people (see Public Health Aspects). Bite wounds often result in bacterial infection, but can also result in systemic viral infection (especially in the case of bitten cats), and less often, fungal or bloodborne protozoal infections such as babesiosis (Table 57-1).

Bacterial pathogens that cause bite wound infections are usually members of the normal oral cavity flora of the biting animal species, but organisms in the environment can also contaminate bite or scratch wounds (e.g., *Clostridium tetani, Mycobacterium* spp., or *Nocardia* spp.). Bite wounds are instantly contaminated with millions of bacterial species from the oral cavity, but only a small proportion of these species possess virulence properties that allow them to proliferate within the wound and cause disease. The degree to which proliferation occurs also depends on host factors such as underlying immunocompromise. The bacterial species that cause bite wound infections in dogs and cats differ from those that cause dog or cat bite wound infections in human patients, so data from human studies cannot be extrapolated to dog or cat bite wound infections.

Dogs

Bite wounds in dogs most often result from aggressive dog-dog interactions. The dog breeds affected depend on regional variation in dog breed popularity. Younger adult, male dogs and especially intact male dogs appear to be predisposed, but studies that compare affected dogs to a control (or "background") population have not been reported.[1-3] Bite wounds in dogs can also result from the bites of other domestic and wild animal species, but the epidemiology of infections that result from these wounds is not well described.

Approximately 20% of dog-dog bite wounds become *infected*, as opposed to *contaminated*. The likelihood that a wound becomes infected increases with the time lag between the aggressive interaction and when veterinary attention is sought.[2,3] Infection develops 8 to 24 hours after the bite occurs and is less likely to be develop if the wound is limited to the dermis.[3] The distribution of bacterial species involved varies from one study to another and may be influenced by whether infected or only contaminated wounds were evaluated. The most common bacterial species isolated from dog-dog bite wounds are *Staphylococcus pseudintermedius, Enterococcus* spp., *Pasteurella* spp., streptococci, and *Escherichia coli.*[1-3] *Staphylococcus aureus* and *Capnocytophaga canimorsus,* which are important pathogens in humans that are bitten by dogs, are rarely isolated from bitten dogs,[2,3] although the prevalence of *C. canimorsus* is probably underestimated because it is very difficult to grow in culture. In the author's hospital, *Pasteurella* spp. accounted for 17% of 41 bacterial species cultured from 33 dog bite wounds, followed by a variety of staphylococci (some methicillin-resistant) (15%), *E. coli* (12%), *Enterococcus* spp. (7%), and *Bacteroides* spp. (7%). Other organisms were *Peptostreptococcus* spp., *Clostridium* spp., and *Pseudomonas aeruginosa* (each 5%); and *Streptococcus viridans, Actinomyces* spp., *Acinetobacter* spp., *Serratia marcescens, Klebsiella pneumoniae, Myroides* spp., *Prevotella* spp., *Fusobacterium* spp., *Aeromonas* spp., *Mycobacterium smegmatis,* and *Mycoplasma* spp. (one isolate each or 2%). Obligate anaerobes were isolated from 5 dogs (15%), and in all 5 of these dogs, multiple bacterial species were isolated.

Cats

Most bite wounds in cats result from aggressive interactions with other cats, but nonfatal dog bite wounds can also occur. Occasionally, cats are bitten by a variety of other small wildlife species that vary geographically based on the local fauna present. In contrast to dogs, which often crush and tear tissues with their teeth, cats deliver deep puncture wounds that create an environment where obligate and facultative anaerobes flourish. Thus, anaerobic bacterial infections are more prevalent in cat bite abscesses than in dog bite wounds, and accordingly, polymicrobial infections are

TABLE 57-1

Pathogens That Cause Local or Systemic Infections in Dogs and Cats as a Consequence of Bite or Scratch Wounds from the Same or Another Animal Species

Organism Class	Dogs	Cats
Viruses	Rabies	Rabies FeLV FIV
Mycoplasmas	Hemotropic mycoplasmas?	Nonhemotropic *Mycoplasma* spp. Hemotropic mycoplasmas?
Gram-negative aerobes*	*Pasteurella* spp. *Escherichia coli* *Pseudomonas aeruginosa* *Acinetobacter* spp. *Proteus* spp. *Enterobacter* spp. *Serratia marcescens* *Aeromonas* spp. *Capnocytophaga canimorsus*	*Pasteurella* spp. *Escherichia coli*
Gram-positive aerobes*	*Staphylococcus* spp., especially *S. pseudintermedius* *Streptococcus* spp. *Enterococcus* spp. *Actinomyces* spp. *Corynebacterium* spp.	*Streptococcus* spp. *Enterococcus* spp. *Actinomyces* spp. *Nocardia* spp. *Lactobacillus* spp. *Corynebacterium* spp.
Anaerobes	*Bacteroides* spp. *Clostridium* spp. *Porphyromonas* spp. *Fusobacterium* spp. *Peptostreptococcus* spp. *Propionibacterium* spp. *Prevotella* spp. *Eubacterium* spp.	*Bacteroides* spp. *Prevotella* spp. *Porphyromonas* spp. *Fusobacterium* spp. *Clostridium* spp. *Propionibacterium* spp.
Mycobacteria	Tuberculous mycobacteria (e.g., *M. bovis* in the United Kingdom) Rapidly growing mycobacteria	Tuberculous mycobacteria (e.g., *M. microti* in the United Kingdom) Rapidly growing mycobacteria (e.g., *M. fortuitum*) Lepromatous mycobacteria (e.g., *M. lepraemurium*)
Fungi	*Sporothrix schenckii*	*Sporothrix schenckii* Opportunistic molds (e.g., *Paecilomyces* spp.), dematiaceous molds
Protozoa	*Babesia gibsoni* *Babesia conradae?*	None known

*The term 'aerobe' refers to facultative anaerobes and obligate aerobes.

present more often in closed cat bite abscesses than in dog bite wounds. In a study of 36 closed cat bite abscesses, 168 bacterial strains were isolated, of which 72% were obligate anaerobes and 28% were facultative anaerobes.[4] The most prevalent anaerobes isolated from cat bite abscesses include *Porphyromonas, Bacteroides, Prevotella, Peptostreptococcus,* and *Fusobacterium. Pasteurella multocida*, a commensal of the oral cavity of virtually all cats, is the most common facultative anaerobe present.[4-6] *Porphyromonas* spp. appear to be particularly prevalent; in one study of 15 abscesses in Australian cats, they accounted for 92% to 99% of all the facultative and obligate anaerobes present.[7] Less often *Actinomyces*, β-hemolytic streptococci, lactobacilli, and *Propionibacterium* spp. have been isolated.

Clinical Features

Dogs

Among dogs, dog bite wounds consist of abrasions, lacerations, avulsions (i.e., skin flaps), crushing injuries, and deep puncture wounds (Figure 57-1). Abscesses can also develop. Dog bite wounds may also penetrate body cavities and cause pneumothorax or damage the esophagus, vertebral column, or gastrointestinal tract. Pyothorax or bacterial peritonitis can also occur. Most dogs have between 1 and 5 wounds. Rarely, more than 10 wounds are present.[1-3] The majority of bite wounds occur cranial to the diaphragm, especially on the head and neck (Figure 57-2). The location of the bite wounds also depends on the size of the bitten

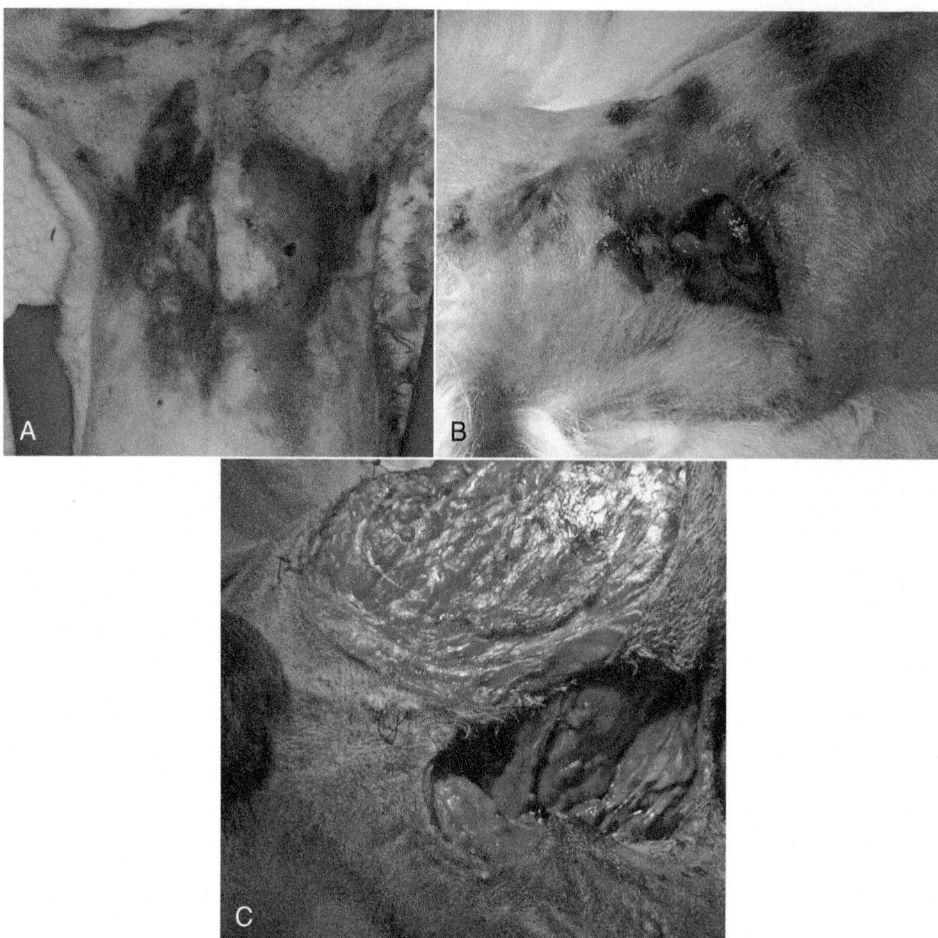

FIGURE 57-1 Dog bite wounds. **A,** Multiple puncture wounds, abrasions and lacerations to the abdomen of a 10-year-old female spayed mixed breed dog. A portion of the jejunum had perforated and had herniated into the subcutaneous tissue. The dog developed cardiac arrest after 2 days of aggressive treatment that included surgery and was euthanized. **B,** Five-year-old male neutered Pomeranian dog with a bite wound to the lateral cervical region from a pit-bull terrier dog that resulted in tissue avulsion. **C,** Inguinal region of a 6-year-old intact male German shepherd dog with severe bite wounds and tissue avulsion that resulted in extensive exposure of muscle and bone. The dog had been attacked by four other dogs. The dog survived with aggressive medical treatment and surgery that included amputation of the right pelvic limb. (Courtesy of the University of California, Davis Veterinary Emergency and Critical Care Service.)

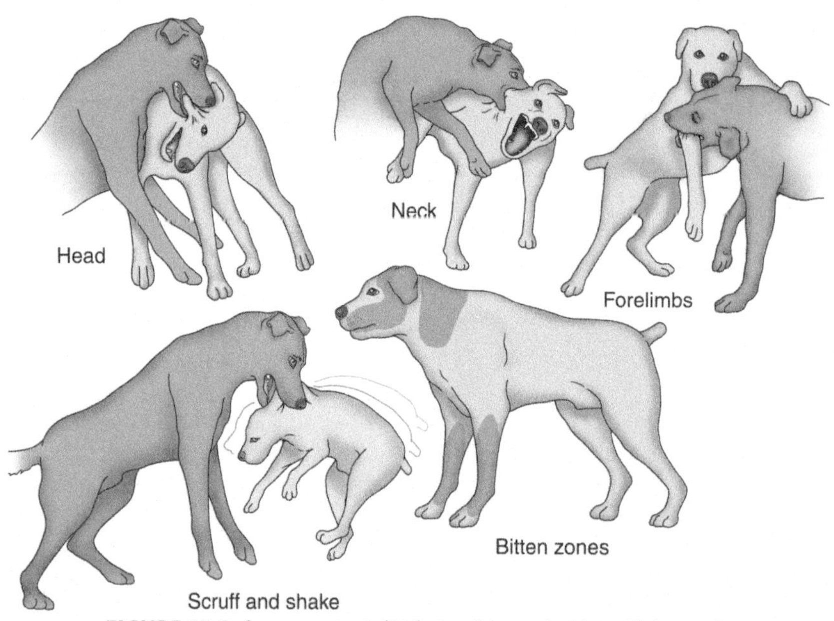

FIGURE 57-2 Common anatomic distribution of dog-to-dog bite and fight wounds.

dog; large-breed dogs are more likely to have wounds on the neck and face, but small-breed dogs often have wounds on their dorsum. Injury to underlying tissue is frequently dramatically more severe than is apparent on the surface. Classification systems have been used to describe the severity of dog-dog bite wounds based on the type of injury (laceration vs. puncture wound) and the presence or absence of dead space or abscessation.[1-3] Abscessation is rarely associated with dog bite wounds as compared with cat bite wounds.[3] The presence of pus, fever, erythema, subcutaneous emphysema, and/or a foul odor suggests that infection has occurred. Uncommonly, hematogenous spread of bacteria leads to signs of severe sepsis or septic shock (see Chapter 86).

Cats

In cats, cat bite wounds may be difficult to identify on the surface, but infection can extend to penetrate bone, joints, tendon and muscle.[5] Cat bite wounds are most often located on the forelimbs, lateral aspect of the face, and near the base of the tail (Figure 57-3).[8] In contrast, scratches are often found on the bridge of the nose, pinna, and inguinal region. Cat bite abscesses are characterized by the presence of firm or fluctuant subcutaneous swellings or masses, with or without fever, lethargy, inappetence, and hyperesthesia. Some cats are brought to the veterinarian solely because of lethargy, and a careful physical examination is required before an abscess or cellulitis is detected. One or more scabs may be found on top of the abscess, or the overlying skin may lack hair and have a gray, necrotic appearance. If the abscess ruptures, cream-colored or red-brown purulent material may be identified on the haircoat, sometimes in association with a foul odor (Figure 57-4). Alternatively, the haircoat may be matted over the site. Lameness may be apparent if the limbs are involved, and especially if there is extension to the bone or a joint. Involvement of the thoracic cavity may be associated with fever, lethargy, tachypnea, and decreased lung sounds due to pyothorax (see Chapter 87). Bite wounds to the calvarium can result in neurologic signs such as circling, disorientation, head pressing, mental obtundation, delayed or absent placing reactions, tetraparesis, anisocoria,

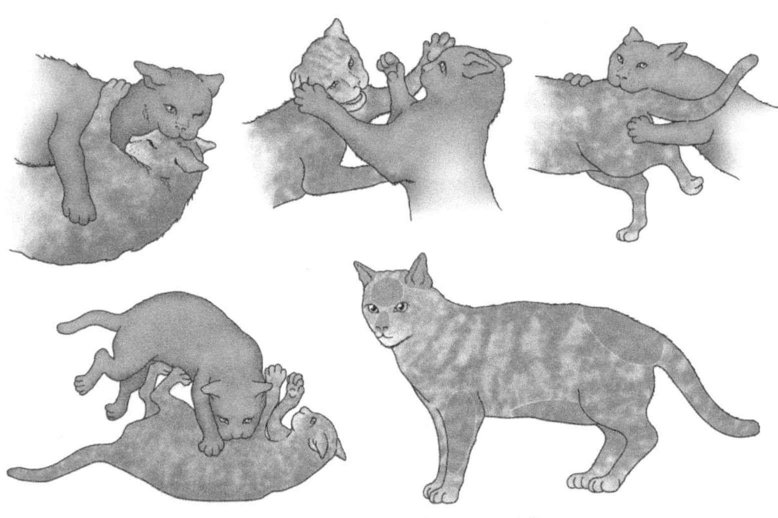

FIGURE 57-3 Common anatomic distribution of cat-to-cat bite and fight wounds ("wound cat"). (Adapted from Malik R, Norris J, White J, et al. "Wound cat." J Feline Med Surg 2006;8:135-140.)

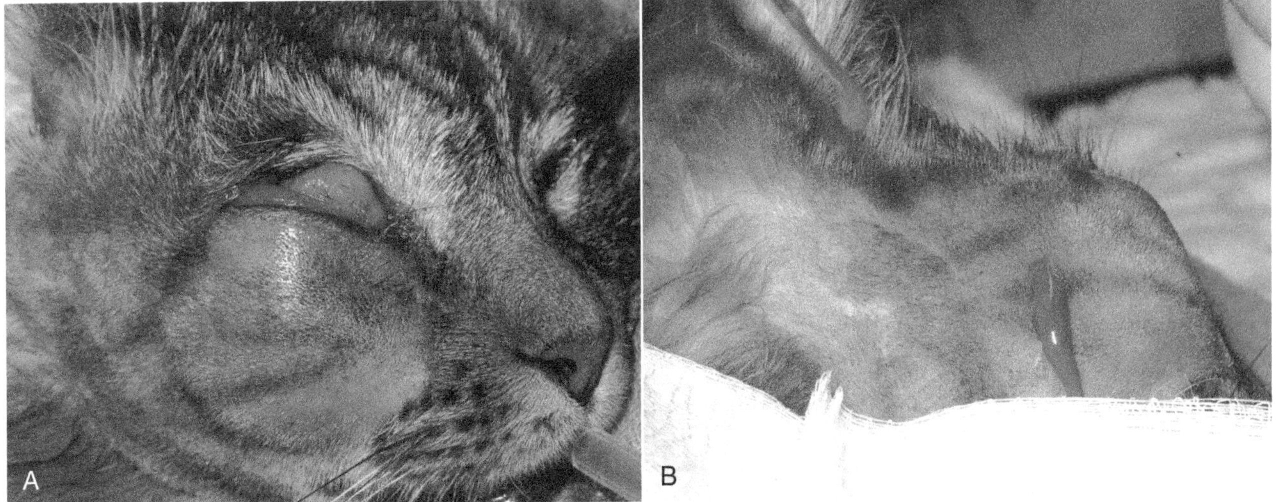

FIGURE 57-4 **A,** Six-year-old female spayed domestic shorthair cat with a cat bite abscess adjacent to the right eye that was associated with marked chemosis and periocular swelling. **B,** Purulent material discharged from the abscess when it was drained surgically. (Images courtesy University of California, Davis Veterinary Ophthalmology service.)

absent menace responses, and seizures.[9] Penetration of the caudal vertebral column and spinal cord can lead to vertebral fractures, osteomyelitis, bacterial meningitis, and signs of pelvic limb paralysis (Figure 57-5). As in dogs, progression to severe sepsis or septic shock can occur, but most cat bite abscesses rupture and resolve spontaneously.

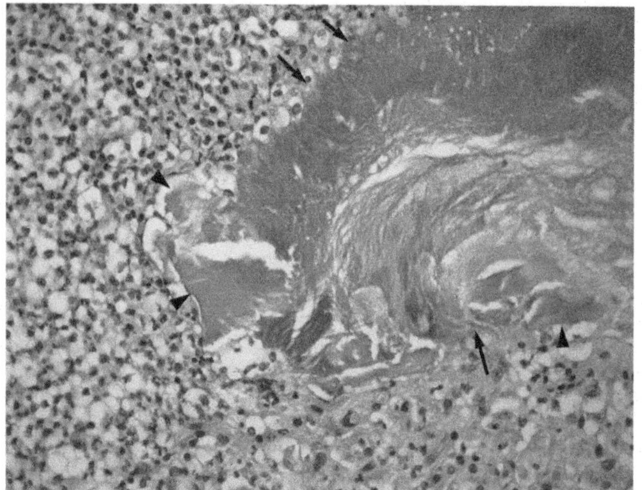

FIGURE 57-5 Histopathology of the vertebral column of a young adult, male domestic shorthair that was found with a bite wound to the base of the tail that drained purulent material and pelvic limb paralysis with absent deep pain sensation. Multiple fractures of caudal vertebrae 4 and 5 were present in association with suppurative osteomyelitis *(arrowheads)*, cellulitis, ascending meningitis, and masses of intralesional bacteria *(arrows)*. Multiple anaerobes were cultured from the lesion. H&E stain.

Cats with dog bite wounds often have life-threatening injuries. Fractures, severe hemorrhage, and hypovolemic shock can dominate the clinical picture. Penetrating injury of cervical structures, the thorax, abdominal organs, brain, or spinal cord can occur (Figure 57-6). Death most often results from trauma rather than infection, but occasionally deep-seated infections or bacteremia develops if the cat survives the initial traumatic episode.

Diagnosis

A diagnosis of bite wound infections is based on history of a fight or bite and physical examination findings that suggest that infection has developed. Cytologic examination of a wound may also assist in diagnosis of infection. The veterinarian should record whether the wound was provoked or unprovoked and note time and location that the wound occurred and the biting animal species involved. Depending on the extent and location of bite wounds, radiographs of the affected region should be considered to assess for underlying damage to bone or body cavities. All cats with cat fight wounds should be tested for FeLV and FIV infection, and the test should be repeated 2 months later because transmission may have occurred at the time of the fight wound (see Chapters 21 and 22).

Laboratory Abnormalities

Laboratory abnormalities in cats or dogs with wound infections are variable and depend on the degree of tissue trauma, the underlying organs involved (if any), and the severity and type of infection. The CBC may show nonregenerative or regenerative anemia, neutrophilia with bandemia, toxic neutrophils,

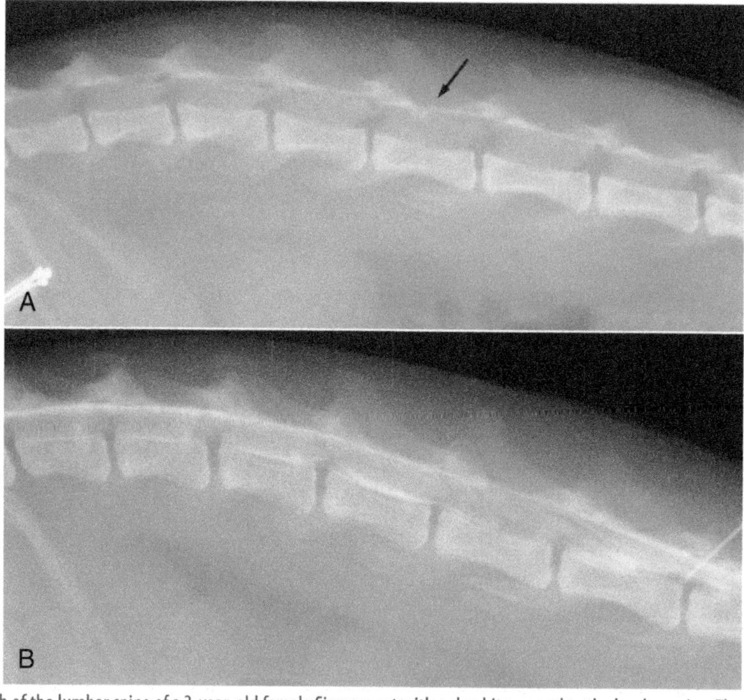

FIGURE 57-6 **A,** Lateral radiograph of the lumbar spine of a 3-year-old female Siamese cat with a dog bite wound to the lumbar spine. The cat was unable to stand and had absent placing reactions in the pelvic limbs. Patellar reflexes were also absent. Two osseous densities are superimposed at the level of the dorsal spinal canal at the level of the fourth lumbar vertebra (L4) *(arrow)*. The dorsoventral view showed deviation of the spinous process of L4 (not shown). CSF analysis revealed mild suppurative inflammation. **B,** Myelogram. A spinal needle is inserted at L5-6 for injection of contrast agent. Spinal cord widening with associated thinning of the contrast column circumferentially is identified over the body of L4. Dorsal deviation and splitting of the ventral contrast column is present over L2-3 as a result of disc protrusion in this region. A decompressive hemilaminectomy over L4 to L6 was performed and a bone fragment was removed; the cat ultimately recovered.

monocytosis, and lymphopenia or lymphocytosis. Animals with severe sepsis or septic shock may be thrombocytopenic. Findings on the chemistry panel include hypoalbuminemia and evidence of muscle damage (increased activities of CK, AST, and sometimes mild increases in serum ALT activity). Increased muscle enzyme activities may be a clue to an underlying cat bite wound in cats with fever of unknown origin. Prolongations of the PT and/or APTT may be present in animals with septic shock and disseminated intravascular coagulation.

Diagnostic Imaging

Plain Radiography

Radiographs of the thorax in dogs or cats with bite wounds may show fractured ribs, pneumothorax, evidence of pulmonary contusions, mediastinal emphysema, diaphragmatic herniation, or pleural effusion due to hemothorax or pyothorax. Abdominal radiographs may show a lack of serosal detail due to hemoabdomen or bacterial peritonitis. Radiographs of the axial or appendicular skeleton may reveal fractures or tooth foreign bodies. In more chronic bite wound infections, evidence of osteomyelitis or septic arthritis may be present, with soft tissue swelling and bony lysis (see also Chapter 85).

Sonographic Findings

Ultrasound of soft tissues can be useful to assess the extent of bite wound infections. Abdominal ultrasound is indicated for animals with bite wounds to the abdomen to assess for evidence of peritonitis or trauma to abdominal organs. Findings in dogs or cats with peritonitis include a hyperechoic mesentery with an irregular outline and free peritoneal fluid, which is typically echogenic (see Chapter 88).

Advanced Imaging

Findings on MRI in cats with brain abscesses secondary to cat bite wounds include space-occupying lesions with well-defined margins that are hyperintense on T2-weighted images, and hypointense T1-weighted images.[9] Marked ring enhancement is usually present. Evidence of brain herniation may be detected.[9]

Cytologic Examination

Cytologic examination of swab or fluid specimens collected from infected wounds typically reveals large numbers of degenerate neutrophils with intracellular bacteria, which may include cocci, rods, or long, filamentous organisms (which are usually anaerobes).

Microbiologic Tests

Isolation and Identification: Dogs

Aerobic bacterial culture and susceptibility and anaerobic bacterial culture are indicated whenever possible from dogs that are suspected to have infected bite wounds. Culture lacks sensitivity for detection of anaerobes, and anaerobic bacterial infections respond predictably to treatment, so anaerobic culture could be considered optional if client finances are limited (see Chapter 37).

The skin around the wound should be clipped and cleaned with chlorhexidine solution, and an aspirate, swab, or devitalized tissue specimen should be collected from as deep within the wound as possible while the animal is sedated or anesthetized. When pockets of purulent material extend subcutaneously away from an open wound, collection of aspirates percutaneously with a needle and syringe can avoid contamination by surface bacteria. Because a positive culture from a wound does not imply infection, results must be interpreted in light of the physical examination and laboratory findings. Susceptibility test results for isolated bacteria can then be used to guide antimicrobial drug treatment. Blood cultures should be considered for dogs with evidence of severe sepsis or septic shock.

Isolation and Identification: Cats

In general, culture of cat bite abscesses in cats is not routinely performed because they almost always respond to drainage with or without systemic antibacterial drug treatment. Cytologic examination and culture are indicated for cat bite abscesses/cellulitis if clinical signs of infection are persistent or recurrent in the face of treatment, or if severe infections that involve underlying bones, joints, or body cavities occur. Culture is also recommended for draining skin lesions in the inguinal region, which may result from infection with rapidly growing mycobacteria (see Chapter 44). Blood cultures are indicated for cats with signs of severe sepsis or septic shock.

Treatment and Prognosis

Surgical Management: Dogs

Dogs with dog bite wounds should be muzzled and the wound(s) covered with a clean, dry bandage immediately after the injury occurs to prevent further contamination of the wound until the animal's condition can be stabilized if necessary. If possible, the dog should then be sedated or anesthetized and a wide area of skin around the wound clipped in order to determine the extent of injury and prepare for surgery. Frequently, this leads to detection of additional full-thickness puncture wounds or lacerations. The skin around the wound should be scrubbed with chlorhexidine or povidone-iodine solution. Full-thickness punctures and lacerations should then be explored, debris and devitalized tissue removed, and specimens collected for culture if infection is suspected. If the abdominal or thoracic cavity has been penetrated, surgical exploration of these cavities is typically required to identify and treat damaged viscera. Wounds should be lavaged extensively with copious quantities of sterile saline or lactated Ringer's solution under moderate pressure (such as using a 60-mL syringe attached to an 18-gauge needle). The use of antibiotics or antiseptics to lavage the wound is not generally recommended, as they can be toxic to tissue and provide minimal benefit for treatment of established wound infections. If used, 0.05% chlorhexidine diacetate (1 part 2% chlorhexidine to 39 parts water) is preferred because it has antibacterial activity in the presence of organic debris, residual antibacterial activity, and minimal systemic absorption and toxicity.

In general, infected wounds that are limited to the subcutaneous tissues and muscle are subsequently managed as open wounds in order to optimize drainage and debridement. Closure of infected wounds can lead to dehiscence and persistence of infection. Whenever possible, the wound is covered with bandages that absorb fluid, reduce dead space, prevent movement and contamination of the wound, and assist in debridement. Hydrophilic bandages are often used for the first 3 to 5 days. Wound closure may be possible for noninfected wounds that are in the "golden period" (first 6 to 8 hours after injury). The reader is referred to small animal surgical texts for additional information on surgical management of bite wound infections and bandaging.[10]

TABLE 57-2

Suitable Antimicrobial Drugs for the Treatment of Bite Wound Infections in Dogs and Cats*

Drug	Species	Dose (mg/kg)	Interval (hours)	Route
Amoxicillin-clavulanic acid	D, C	12.5-20	8-12	PO
Ampicillin-sulbactam	D, C	10-20†	8	IV, IM
Pradofloxacin‡	D	3	24	PO
	C	5-7.5	24	PO
Enrofloxacin	D	5-20	24	IV, IM, PO
Marbofloxacin	D	2.75-5.5	24	PO
Gentamicin	D	9-14	24	IV, IM
Amikacin	D	15-30	24	IV, IM
Metronidazole	D, C	10	8	PO, IV

C, Cat; D, dog.
*Doses of antimicrobial drugs that have activity primarily against gram-negative aerobes are listed for dogs, because isolation of gram-negative aerobes from cat bite abscesses is very rare.
†Dose according to ampicillin component.
‡The pradofloxacin dose for dogs is for the tablet formulation available in Europe. The dose for cats is for the oral suspension. The use of pradofloxacin in dogs may be associated with myelosuppression and is off-label in some countries.

Surgical Management: Cats

As for open dog bite wounds, a wide area of skin around cat bite abscesses should be clipped and scrubbed. The abscess should then be lanced and specimens collected for culture if desired. The abscess cavity should then be lavaged, necrotic tissue debrided, and a placement of a drain should be considered to optimize drainage and prevent early wound closure. Whenever possible, the wound and drain should then be covered with a bandage. The drain is removed in 3 to 5 days. For cats with pyothorax, placement of chest tubes with or without surgical exploration may be required (see Chapter 87). Cats with abscesses that involve the central nervous system have the potential to recover with craniectomy, drainage of purulent material within the abscess, removal of any tooth fragments present, and closure of subcutaneous tissue and the skin.[9]

Antimicrobial Treatment

Contaminated Wounds (First 8 Hours after Injury)

The need for antimicrobial treatment in contaminated, noninfected wounds is controversial, because there is no evidence that it prevents infection of the wound and it may select for infection with bacteria that are resistant to the antimicrobial drug used. Proper wound cleaning and debridement are likely to have the greatest impact on whether infection subsequently develops. Antimicrobial treatment could be considered for deep punctures or large, dirty wounds that require extensive debridement. If deemed necessary, the drug of choice for contaminated wounds is amoxicillin–clavulanic acid, because it has efficacy against most oral cavity commensals of the dog and cat mouth such as *Pasteurella* spp. and a variety of anaerobes, including those that produce β-lactamase enzymes.

Infected Wounds

For severely infected dog bite wounds, initial treatment should consist of parenteral antimicrobial drugs that have activity against gram-negative and gram-positive aerobic and anaerobic bacteria, which includes methicillin-resistant staphylococci (in regions where methicillin-resistant *S. pseudintermedius* is prevalent). Appropriate combinations include ampicillin-sulbactam and an aminoglycoside, or a combination of ampicillin, metronidazole, and an aminoglycoside (Table 57-2). Where methicillin-resistant *S. pseudintermedius* is not prevalent, a fluoroquinolone could be substituted for the aminoglycoside. Subsequent treatment should be based on the results of culture and susceptibility. Amoxicillin-clavulanic acid is the drug of choice for treatment of cat bite abscesses once drainage has been established (although many cat bite abscesses will likely heal with drainage alone). Because *Pasteurella* spp. are not susceptible to clindamycin or first-generation cephalosporins, monotherapy with these drugs should be avoided. Pradofloxacin is also a suitable choice, because it has activity against anaerobes as well as a variety of aerobic bacterial species.

Antimicrobial drug treatment of infected bite wounds that are localized to the skin, subcutaneous tissue, and muscle should continue for 3 to 5 days after signs of infection are no longer evident. The reader is referred to Chapters 85, 87, and 88 for information on the management of osteomyelitis, septic arthritis, pyothorax, and peritonitis.

Rabies Prophylaxis

In regions where rabies occurs, bite wounds may need to be reported to local public health authorities. If the biting animal has an unknown vaccination history, or the bite was from a wild animal that was unavailable for testing, a rabies booster should be administered and the animal monitored for 45 days. If the bitten animal is unvaccinated or has a lapsed vaccination status, additional quarantine or euthanasia may be required (see Chapter 13).

Prognosis

The prognosis for bite wound infections depends on the severity and extent of injury, the immune status of the host, and the organisms involved. Recurrent infections may result from underlying osteomyelitis, foreign bodies, immunodeficiency, or the presence of atypical organisms such as *Mycobacterium* spp., *Nocardia* spp., or *Mycoplasma* spp. (which do not respond to β-lactam drugs). Failure to respond to appropriate treatment should prompt a thorough physical examination; testing for retroviruses in cats; imaging of the affected area; and culture for aerobic and anaerobic bacteria and mycoplasmas. If the clinical picture is suggestive, culture for mycobacteria may also be indicated.

Prevention

Prevention of bite wounds involves education of pet owners in regard to housing cats indoors and use of secure collars and leashes for walking dogs. Intact male dogs should be neutered if they are not to be used for breeding. Proper handling and socialization of puppies as well as behavior training should be encouraged. Pet owners should be instructed to avoid or closely supervise interactions between their dogs and unfamiliar dogs that are breeds of known aggressive tendency, such as American pit bull terriers, Rottweilers, German shepherds, blue heelers, chow chows, and Jack Russell terriers. Special caution is warranted for small-breed dogs, which may provoke larger breed dogs and are more likely to develop life-threatening injuries. Dogs that are unfamiliar with one another or dogs with a history of fighting with one another should never be left together without proper supervision.

Public Health Aspects

Epidemiology of Dog and Cat Bite Wounds

In 2012, the American Pet Products Association estimated that there are 78.2 million owned dogs and 86.4 million owned cats in the United States, and that 39% of households own at least one dog and 33% own at least one cat.[11] In the United Kingdom, around 22% of households own a dog and 18% own a cat.[12] German shepherds, Rottweilers, and Jack Russell terriers are among the top 10 dog breeds owned. Dog and cat bite wounds account for approximately 1% of emergency department visits by humans in the United States, and similar numbers are reported in Europe. Dog bites accounted for more than 70% and cat bites accounted for 13% of animal bite visits to emergency rooms in New York City.[13] The median age of bitten people in one study was 15 years, and in another study it was 28 years.[14,15] Many bites occur in children, especially boys aged 5 to 9 years.[16] Children often have dog bites to the face, neck, and head. Women and the elderly are at risk for cat bite injuries. Patients who seek medical attention more than 8 hours after injury usually have infected wounds.

Dog Bite Infections

Between 3% and 20% of dog bite wounds in humans become infected.[17,18] The infecting organisms generally reflect the flora of the canine oral cavity, but may also derive from the environment or the bitten person's skin or oral cavity. Many infections are polymicrobial, but the organism that most often contributes to dog bite wound infections is *Pasteurella* spp., which is found in 50% of wounds (Table 57-3).[14,19-27] The most common species is *P. canis,* but *P. multocida* (subspecies *multocida, septica,* and *gallicida*), *P. stomatis,* and *P. dagmatis* may also be present. Other common isolates from dog bite wounds include streptococci (especially the α-streptococcus *S. mitis* and *S. pyogenes; S. canis* is rarely isolated), staphylococci, *Corynebacterium* spp., *Neisseria* spp., and anaerobes.[19] Of the staphylococci, *S. aureus* is isolated most often (20% of infections). Infections with *S. pseudintermedius* occur rarely. Anaerobes are present in approximately 70% of infections and are almost always present in combination with other anaerobes and aerobic bacteria.

Cat Bite Infections

Although cat bite wounds are less traumatic to tissue, they are more likely to become infected and progress to infection more rapidly than dog bite wounds.[14] The upper extremities are often affected. As in dog bite wounds, *Pasteurella* spp. are the most common organisms isolated and are present in 75% of wounds.[14,19] The predominant species are *P. multocida* subsp. *multocida* and *P. multocida* subsp. *septica*. Streptococci (including *S. pyogenes*) and staphylococci are also often present, but *S. aureus* is isolated less frequently from cat bite wounds than dog bite wounds. *Neisseria* and *Moraxella* are also often isolated from cat bite wounds (see Table 57-3). The prevalence of infection with anaerobes in cat bite wounds is similar to that in dog bite wounds.[14]

Clinical Manifestations

Infection of bite wounds in humans most often results in localized cellulitis, pain, purulent discharge, a black to gray appearance, and, less often, fever and local lymphadenopathy. Extension to underlying bones or joints can lead to osteomyelitis or septic arthritis, which is especially likely to occur after penetrating cat bite wounds to the hand (Figure 57-7). Rarely, necrotizing fasciitis, bacteremia, meningitis, endocarditis, peritonitis, or brain abscesses develop.[19,28]

Most of the serious consequences of dog or cat bite wound infections occur in immunocompromised humans and involve *P. multocida* or *Capnocytophaga canimorsus.* Severe disease manifestations have also occurred after exposure of wounds to dog or cat saliva through licking, or after invasive medical supplies (such as dialysis tubing) were chewed or licked by a pet.[29] In a few cases, patients have had a history of contact with animals but no known bite or scratch wound.[30-32] Life-threatening infections with *P. multocida* tend to occur in infants, pregnant women with animal contact, patients on chronic glucocorticoid therapy, HIV-infected people, organ-transplant recipients, and patients with chronic liver disease.[28]

Capnocytophaga canimorsus is a capnophilic (carbon dioxide–loving), facultatively anaerobic, filamentous gram-negative bacterial rod that is commonly found in the oral cavity of dogs and cats.[33] Although rarely reported as a cause of illness in dogs or cats, this organism can cause cellulitis, gangrene, bacteremia, meningitis, and endocarditis in humans.[28,33] *C. canimorsus* bacteremia is rare, but humans who are immunocompromised, especially those with chronic alcoholism, cirrhosis, or a history of splenectomy, are at risk for life-threatening *C. canimorsus* infections that progress rapidly, with a mortality of 31%. The virulence factors that contribute to these severe infections are not well understood. The organism does not cause endotoxemia but appears to evade recognition by the immune system and resist phagocytosis.[28] In one series of humans with *C. canimorsus* sepsis, 56% of cases followed a dog bite and 10% of cases followed exposure of a wound to dog saliva by licking.[34] Veterinarians have also developed corneal infections with *C. canimorsus* when dog tooth fragments have struck them in the eye during dental extractions.[35,36] Most affected humans are older than 40 years of age. Clinical manifestations of *C. canimorsus* sepsis include fever, myalgia, and a petechial rash that involves the skin and mucous membranes, which may progress from purpura *(purpura fulminans)* to gangrene over a period of several days. Because *C. canimorsus* is very difficult to grow, early diagnosis and successful treatment require clinical suspicion and early treatment with effective antimicrobial drugs, such as β-lactam/β-lactamase inhibitor combinations, which are also active against *Pasteurella* spp.

TABLE 57-3

Pathogens That Can Infect Humans after a Bite from a Dog or Cat[14,19-27]

	Dog	Cat
Viruses	Rabies	Rabies
Aerobic Gram-positive bacteria	*Streptococcus* (*S. mitis*)* *Staphylococcus* (*S. aureus*) *Corynebacterium* (group G) *Enterococcus* *Bacillus* *Gemella morbillorum* *Actinomyces viscosus* *Lactobacillus* *Dermabacter hominis* *Oerskovia* *Micrococcus lylae* *Pediococcus* *Stomatococcus mucilaginosus*	*Streptococcus* (*S. mitis*) *Staphylococcus* (*S. epidermidis*) *Corynebacterium* (*C. aquaticum*) *Enterococcus* (*E. durans*) *Bacillus* (*B. firmus*) *Actinomyces* *Gemella morbillorum* *Erysipelothrix* *Rothia dentocariosa* *Lactobacillus* *Rhodococcus* spp. *Streptomyces* spp.
Aerobic Gram-negative bacteria	*Pasteurella* (*P. canis*) *Neisseria* (*N. weaveri*) *Moraxella* *Bergeyella zoohelcum* *Capnocytophaga* *Escherichia coli* *Brevibacterium* *Stenotrophomonas maltophilia* *Pseudomonas* *Klebsiella* *Citrobacter* *Flavobacterium* *Eikenella corrodens* *Bartonella*?	*Pasteurella* (*P. multocida*) *Neisseria* (*N. weaveri*) *Moraxella* (*M. catarrhalis*) *Bergeyella zoohelcum* *Capnocytophaga* *Acinetobacter* *Pseudomonas* *Brevibacterium* *Gemella morbillorum* *Actinobacillus* *Alcaligenes* *Enterobacter* *Riemerella anatipestifer* *Klebsiella oxytoca* *Eikenella corrodens* *Flavimonas oryzihabitans* *Aeromonas hydrophila* *Pantoea agglomerans* *Bartonella* *Francisella tularensis* *Yersinia pestis*
Anaerobic bacteria	*Fusobacterium* (*F. nucleatum*) *Bacteroides* (*B. tectum*) *Prevotella* (*P. heparinolytica*) *Porphyromonas* (*P. macacae*) *Propionibacterium* (*P. acnes*) *Peptostreptococcus* *Tannerella forsythia* *Eubacterium* spp. *Campylobacter* spp.	*Fusobacterium* (*F. nucleatum*) *Bacteroides* (*B. tectum*) *Prevotella* (*P. heparinolytica*) *Porphyromonas* (*P. gulae*) *Propionibacterium* (*P. acnes*) *Peptostreptococcus* *Filifactor villosus* *Eubacterium* spp. *Clostridium sordellii* *Veillonella* spp.
Mycoplasmas		*Mycoplasma* spp.
Mycobacteria	*Mycobacterium fortuitum* *Mycobacterium kansasii*	*Mycobacterium fortuitum*
Fungi	*Blastomyces dermatitidis* *Paecilomyces lilacinus*	*Sporothrix schenckii*

*For organisms that are present in >10% of cases, the most common species isolated is listed in parentheses.

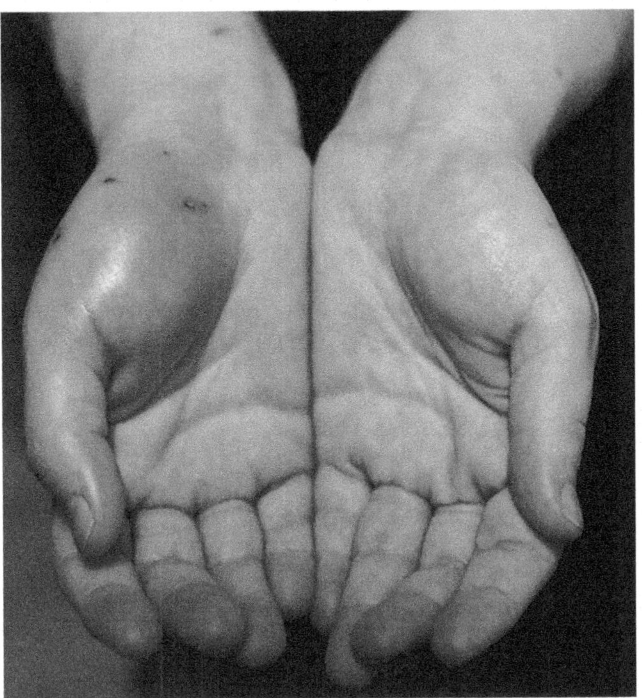

FIGURE 57-7 Cat bite wounds to the base of the thumb of a veterinarian with associated cellulitis. Penetrating cat bite wounds of the hand have a tendency to extend to underlying bones and joints.

Prevention

Veterinarians play an important role in educating the public about prevention of cat and dog bite wounds. Provision of information to clients who intend to purchase a new dog about dog breeds, puppy socialization, dog behavior training, and how to prevent and manage aggression and avoid bites or scratches (to themselves and to others) is encouraged. Veterinarians can also engage in community activities (especially in schools) where young children can be educated about pet ownership and how to avoid wounds and wound infections from their own or someone else's dog or cat. Immunocompromised individuals should be educated about the potential benefits and risks of pet ownership and precautions that can be taken to minimize infections. Finally, care should be taken in the veterinary practice situation to avoid bites or scratches to veterinary staff. Veterinary staff should be educated about the types of infections that can occur in the workplace; likelihood of these infections; risk factors for infection; appropriate preventative measures; and protocols to follow should a bite or scratch wound occur (see General Animal Handling Precautions, Chapter 11). Routine hand-washing practices should be enforced, and licking by dogs or cats should be discouraged. Face protection should be worn by veterinary staff when dental procedures are performed. Bites and scratches may need to be reported to public health authorities, and all staff should be educated about the need to ensure that tetanus and rabies immunizations are not overdue.

CASE EXAMPLE

Signalment: "Murphy", a 5-year-old intact male boxer dog from Vacaville in northern California

History: Murphy was evaluated by the University of California, Davis, veterinary emergency service for dog bite injuries after a fight with another dog in the household. The owner had returned home a few hours earlier to find Murphy bleeding from the neck. The other dog, a 5-year-old male neutered boxer mix, was found hiding and unable to stand with several "scratches" on his body. Murphy had a history of fights with other dogs. Both dogs in the household were fully vaccinated for canine distemper virus, parvovirus, adenovirus, and rabies. There was no other pertinent medical history.

Initial Physical Examination:

Body Weight: 46.2 kg.

General: Quiet, alert, responsive and hydrated. T = 102.1°F (38.9°C), HR = 110, panting, pink and moist mucous membranes, CRT = 1 s.

Integument: The haircoat was full, thick, and dirty. There was a 1-cm superficial laceration on the ventral aspect of the pinna, and approximately 10 puncture wounds on the left ventral cervical region. A 2-cm superficial laceration was present at the cranial aspect of the dorsal midline, and a 5-cm superficial laceration was present on the left flank. No ectoparasites were seen.

Eyes, Ears, Nose, and Throat: Bilateral conjunctival hyperemia and a mucoid ocular discharge were present. No other significant abnormalities were noted.

Musculoskeletal: BCS 6/9, ambulatory.

Cardiovascular, Respiratory, Gastrointestinal, Genitourinary, Lymph Nodes, and Neurologic: No clinically significant abnormalities were detected. Cranial nerve examination was unremarkable. A full neurologic examination was not performed.

Initial Treatment: Murphy was sedated with hydromorphone and dexmedetomidine. The left neck was clipped with a no. 40 clipper blade from the midpoint of the dorsal aspect of the head to the ventral aspect of the left ear and the thorax. The skin was cleaned with 0.05% chlorhexidine solution, and all puncture sites were probed and flushed with sterile saline. The sites were found to be relatively superficial. Drain sites were created with a no. 11 scalpel blade for three wounds, and a 3 × 0.75 inch Penrose drain was placed across a wound site that had the greatest amount of dead space and secured with a single interrupted suture. The dog was sent home with instructions for the owner to administer amoxicillin-clavulanic acid (16 mg/kg PO q12h) and tramadol (2.4 mg/kg PO q8-12h), to monitor the wound for development of excessive discharge, bleeding, swelling, or redness, and to keep the area clean with a washcloth soaked in warm water. Instructions were provided to return in 3 days to have the wound reevaluated and the drain removed.

The owners returned 7 days later for drain removal. At that time, they reported that Murphy had been eating normally, but had been drinking more than usual. His activity level had been normal, but they believed his neck was had become swollen and tender. They had been administering the medications as directed.

Continued

Physical Examination (Day 7):

Body Weight: 46.2 kg.

General: Quiet, alert, responsive, and hydrated but anxious. T = 103.1°F (39.5°C), HR = 114, RR = 36, pink and moist mucous membranes, CRT 1 s.

Integument: There were marked crusts and scabs on the left lateral and ventral aspect of the neck. The Penrose drain was present with minimal amounts of discharge. Serous to purulent discharge was draining from the ventral puncture wounds. There was moderate crusting of the dorsal aspect of the left pinna.

Other Systems: No change from the previous examination.

Treatment (Day 7): The dog was again sedated and purulent material was collected for culture and susceptibility. The eschars were gently removed with forceps and the skin scrubbed with 0.05% chlorhexidine and water. Ultrasound of the neck region revealed pockets of hypoechoic material beneath the skin, and surgical debridement of the area under general anesthesia was recommended. Subsequently Murphy was anesthetized and the wound was explored. No abscesses were found. The devitalized tissue was excised, the wounds flushed vigorously, and two Penrose drains were placed. The neck was bandaged initially, but this interfered with the dog's ability to breathe comfortably, so the bandage was removed. The dog was hospitalized overnight and treated with hydromorphone (0.05 mg/kg, IV, q4h) and warm compresses to the neck (q6h for 5 minutes). He was then sent home with instructions to administer tramadol as previously prescribed, clindamycin (20 mg/kg PO q12h), and enrofloxacin (10 mg/kg PO q24h), and to warm compress the neck every 4 to 6 hours for the next 3 days. They were also instructed to return in 3 to 5 days for reevaluation and drain removal.

Microbiologic Testing:

Direct Smear and Gram Stain: Rare numbers of gram-positive cocci.

Aerobic and Anaerobic Culture and Susceptibility (Swab from Wound): Isolate 1: Methicillin-resistant *Staphylococcus aureus,* resistant to all β-lactams and clindamycin; susceptible to amikacin (≤4 μg/mL), chloramphenicol (8 μg/mL), doxycycline (≤2 μg/mL), enrofloxacin (≤0.25 μg/mL), gentamicin (≤1 μg/mL), marbofloxacin (≤0.25 μg/mL), rifampin (≤1 μg/mL), and trimethoprim-sulfamethoxazole (≤0.50 μg/mL).

Isolate 2: *Enterococcus faecium* (intrinsic resistance to low-level aminoglycosides, cephalosporins, clindamycin, fluoroquinolones, trimethoprim-sulfamethoxazole), resistant to chloramphenicol and rifampin. Intermediate susceptibility to doxycycline (8 μg/mL), erythromycin (1 μg/mL), ticarcillin (64 μg/mL), and ticarcillin-clavulanate (64 μg/mL). Susceptible to ampicillin (1 μg/mL), clavulanic acid–amoxicillin (≤4 μg/mL), penicillin (4 μg/mL), and imipenem (≤1 μg/mL).

Isolate 3: *Pseudomonas aeruginosa,* resistant to ampicillin, amoxicillin-clavulanic acid, all cephalosporins tested, chloramphenicol, and doxycycline. Susceptibility to clindamycin was not reported because this species is usually resistant. Susceptible only to amikacin (≤4 μg/mL), gentamicin (2 μg/mL), enrofloxacin (0.50 μg/mL), imipenem (≤1 μg/mL), ticarcillin (16 μg/mL), ticarcillin–clavulanic acid (16 μg/mL). The MICs for trimethoprim-sulfamethoxazole and marbofloxacin were 2 μg/mL and ≤0.25 μg/mL, respectively.

Anaerobic culture: Moderate numbers of mixed growth that included *Bacteroides ureolyticus* group (β-lactamase negative), *Peptostreptococcus anaerobius,* and *Bacteroides* spp./*Prevotella* spp. (β-lactamase negative).

Diagnosis: Polymicrobial bite wound infection with anaerobes and multiple drug-resistant aerobic gram-positive and gram-negative bacteria.

Outcome: On receipt of the culture and susceptibility test results, the clindamycin was substituted with amoxicillin-clavulanic acid (16 mg/kg PO q12h). Treatment with enrofloxacin was continued and the owners were educated in regard to the public health significance of the infection and the need to wear gloves when handling the wound and for scrupulous hand-washing practices. The dog returned 4 days after surgery for drain removal. The owners reported that the drains had been producing considerable amounts of purulent material and that Murphy was doing well. He was afebrile and the wound was unchanged in appearance. He was again sedated, the area was scrubbed, and crusts were removed. The drains were removed. Murphy recovered uneventfully and the sutures were removed 10 days later at a local veterinary clinic. Five months later he was seen again for multiple bite wounds to the thoracic limbs and right thorax.

Comments: In this dog, bite wound injuries were complicated by infection with multiple gram-negative and gram-positive drug-resistant aerobic bacteria as well as anaerobes. The *S. aureus* and *P. aeruginosa* were resistant to amoxicillin-clavulanic acid, which had been used to prevent infection when the dog was first seen. In contrast, the anaerobes and the *E. faecium* were susceptible to amoxicillin-clavulanic acid, but presumably were able to proliferate and persist in the face of antimicrobial drug treatment as a result of the presence of the other drug-resistant bacteria, purulent material, and dead space. Bite wounds to the neck can be a challenge to manage because of the mobility of this area, which contributes to the maintenance of the dead space. The use of a bandage can reduce dead space, avoid further contamination, and reduce exposure to multidrug-resistant bacteria, but attempts to bandage the wound were not tolerated by this dog. Client education was an important part of management. The owners were instructed to separate the dogs when unattended to avoid further fights. Neutering may also have been of benefit.

SUGGESTED READINGS

Gaastra W, Lipman LJ. *Capnocytophaga canimorsus*. Vet Microbiol. 2010;140:339-346.

Love DN, Malik R, Norris JM. Bacteriological warfare amongst cats: what have we learned about cat bite infections? Vet Microbiol. 2000;74:179-193.

Malik R, Norris J, White J, et al. Wound cat. J Feline Med Surg. 2006;8:135-140.

Oehler RL, Velez AP, Mizrachi M, et al. Bite-related and septic syndromes caused by cats and dogs. Lancet Infect Dis. 2009;9:439-447.

REFERENCES

1. Griffin GM, Holt DE. Dog-bite wounds: bacteriology and treatment outcome in 37 cases. J Am Anim Hosp Assoc. 2001;37:453-460.
2. Meyers B, Schoeman JP, Goddard A, et al. The bacteriology and antimicrobial susceptibility of infected and non-infected dog bite wounds: fifty cases. Vet Microbiol. 2008;127:360-368.
3. Mouro S, Vilela CL, Niza MM. Clinical and bacteriological assessment of dog-to-dog bite wounds. Vet Microbiol. 2010;144:127-132.
4. Love DN, Jones RF, Bailey M, et al. Isolation and characterisation of bacteria from abscesses in the subcutis of cats. J Med Microbiol. 1979;12:207-212.
5. Love DN, Malik R, Norris JM. Bacteriological warfare amongst cats: what have we learned about cat bite infections? Vet Microbiol. 2000;74:179-193.
6. Love DN, Jones RF, Bailey M, et al. Bacteria isolated from subcutaneous abscesses in cats. Aust Vet Practit. 1978;8:87-90.
7. Norris JM, Love DN. The isolation and enumeration of three feline oral *Porphyromonas* species from subcutaneous abscesses in cats. Vet Microbiol. 1999;65:115-122.
8. Malik R, Norris J, White J, et al. Wound cat. J Feline Med Surg. 2006;8:135-140.
9. Costanzo C, Garosi LS, Glass EN, et al. Brain abscess in seven cats due to a bite wound: MRI findings, surgical management and outcome. J Feline Med Surg. 2011;13:672-680.
10. Fossum TW, Hedlund CS, Johnson AL, et al. Surgery of the integumentary system. In: Fossum TW, ed. Small Animal Surgery. 3rd ed. St. Louis, MO: Mosby; 2007:159-259.
11. The Humane Society of the United States. 2012. http://www.humanesociety.org/issues/pet_overpopulation/facts/pet_ownership_statistics.html. Last accessed January 1, 2013.
12. Pet Population 2011. 2011. http://www.pfma.org.uk. Last accessed January 1, 2013.
13. Bregman B, Slavinski S. Using emergency department data to conduct dog and animal bite surveillance in New York City, 2003-2006. Public Health Rep. 2012;127:195-201.
14. Talan DA, Citron DM, Abrahamian FM, et al. Bacteriologic analysis of infected dog and cat bites. Emergency Medicine Animal Bite Infection Study Group. N Engl J Med. 1999;340:85-92.
15. Weiss HB, Friedman DI, Coben JH. Incidence of dog bite injuries treated in emergency departments. JAMA. 1998;279:51-53.
16. Nonfatal dog bite-related injuries treated in hospital emergency departments—United States, 2001. MMWR Morb Mortal Wkly Rep. 2003;52:605-610.
17. Goldstein EJ. Bite wounds and infection. Clin Infect Dis. 1992;14:633-638.
18. Underman AE. Bite wounds inflicted by dogs and cats. Vet Clin North Am Small Anim Pract. 1987;17:195-207.
19. Abrahamian FM, Goldstein EJ. Microbiology of animal bite wound infections. Clin Microbiol Rev. 2011;24:231-246.
20. Zendri E, Martignoni G, Benecchi M, et al. *Paecilomyces lilacinus* cutaneous infection associated with a dog bite. J Am Acad Dermatol. 2006;55:S63-S64.
21. Ngan N, Morris A, de Chalain T. *Mycobacterium fortuitum* infection caused by a cat bite. N Z Med J. 2005;118:U1354.
22. Southern Jr PM. Tenosynovitis caused by *Mycobacterium kansasii* associated with a dog bite. Am J Med Sci. 2004;327:258-261.
23. Ariel I, Haas H, Weinberg H, et al. *Mycobacterium fortuitum* granulomatous synovitis caused by a dog bite. J Hand Surg Am. 1983;8:342-343.
24. Gnann Jr JW, Bressler GS, Bodet 3rd CA, et al. Human blastomycosis after a dog bite. Ann Intern Med. 1983;98:48-49.
25. Thornton DJ, Tustin RC, Pienaar BJ, et al. Cat bite transmission of *Yersinia pestis* infection to man. J S Afr Vet Assoc. 1975;46:165-169.
26. Yuen JC, Malotky MV. *Francisella tularensis* osteomyelitis of the hand following a cat bite: a case of clinical suspicion. Plast Reconstr Surg. 2011;128:37e-39e.
27. McCabe SJ, Murray JF, Ruhnke HL, et al. *Mycoplasma* infection of the hand acquired from a cat. J Hand Surg Am. 1987;12:1085-1088.
28. Oehler RL, Velez AP, Mizrachi M, et al. Bite-related and septic syndromes caused by cats and dogs. Lancet Infect Dis. 2009;9:439-447.
29. Boinett C, Gonzalez A. *Pasteurella multocida* septicaemia in a patient on haemodialysis. BMJ Case Rep. 2009.
30. Bryant BJ, Conry-Cantilena C, Ahlgren A, et al. *Pasteurella multocida* bacteremia in asymptomatic plateletpheresis donors: a tale of two cats. Transfusion. 2007;47:1984-1989.
31. Waghorn DJ, Robson M. Occupational risk of *Pasteurella multocida* septicaemia and premature labour in a pregnant vet. BJOG. 2003;110:780-781.
32. Wade T, Booy R, Teare EL, et al. *Pasteurella multocida* meningitis in infancy-(a lick may be as bad as a bite). Eur J Pediatr. 1999;158:875-878.
33. Gaastra W, Lipman LJ. *Capnocytophaga canimorsus*. Vet Microbiol. 2010;140:339-346.
34. Pers C, Gahrn-Hansen B, Frederiksen W. *Capnocytophaga canimorsus* septicemia in Denmark, 1982-1995: review of 39 cases. Clin Infect Dis. 1996;23:71-75.
35. de Smet MD, Chan CC, Nussenblatt RB, et al. *Capnocytophaga canimorsus* as the cause of a chronic corneal infection. Am J Ophthalmol. 1990;109:240-242.
36. Chodosh J. Cat's tooth keratitis: human corneal infection with *Capnocytophaga canimorsus*. Cornea. 2001;20:661-663.

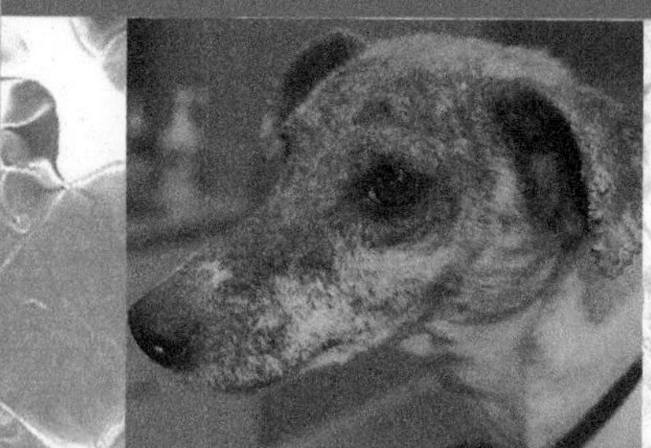

SECTION 3
Fungal and Algal Diseases

CHAPTER 58

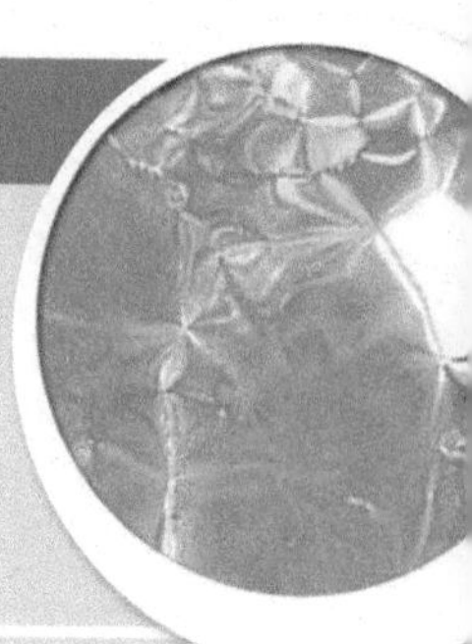

Dermatophytosis

Jane E. Sykes and Catherine A. Outerbridge

Overview of Dermatophytosis

First Described: Dermatophytosis was described independently by several scientists in the 1830s and 1840s,[1] but probable descriptions of ringworm date back to ancient Greek times. Dermatophytes were more fully characterized in the early 1900s by Sabouraud.[2]

Causes: *Microsporum* and *Trichophyton* species (especially *Microsporum canis, Microsporum gypseum,* and *Trichophyton mentagrophytes*) (teleomorph name, *Arthroderma* spp.)

Geographic Distribution: Worldwide, especially warm and humid climates

Mode of Transmission: Direct contact with other infected hosts, fomite transmission

Major Clinical Signs: Cutaneous lesions include alopecia, erythema, crusting and scaling, and sometimes nodular or draining lesions (kerions and dermatophytic mycetomas).

Differential Diagnoses: Alopecic lesions must be differentiated from self-traumatic alopecia secondary to allergic dermatitis, sarcoptic mange, or demodicosis. If scale and crusting are also present, bacterial folliculitis, superficial pyoderma, and pemphigus foliaceus are differential diagnoses. Nodular lesions must be differentiated from eosinophilic granuloma, feline acne (cats), and mast cell tumors (dogs).

Human Health Significance: Dermatophytosis is a zoonosis. Young children and the immunocompromised can develop extensive cutaneous lesions.

Etiology and Epidemiology

Dermatophytosis (ringworm or tinea) is a superficial cutaneous infection with one or more of the keratinophilic fungi that belong to the genera *Microsporum, Trichophyton,* or *Epidermophyton.* Transmission of dermatophytes occurs by close contact with other infected animals or through contact with contaminated fomites (which includes the haircoats of animals and arthropods such as fleas or houseflies). Dermatophyte spores survive more than a year in the environment under optimal conditions of temperature and humidity, and they resist most routinely used hospital disinfectants, which facilitates transmission. Dermatophytes are somewhat host species specific and are classified as *geophilic, zoophilic,* or *anthropophilic* (Table 58-1).[3-8] Geophilic dermatophytes are soil saprophytes. The most common geophilic dermatophyte that infects dogs or cats is *Microsporum gypseum,* which is most prevalent in warm, humid tropical and subtropical environments. Zoophilic dermatophytes are adapted to animal hosts and are rarely found in soil. The most common zoophilic dermatophyte that infects dogs and especially cats is *Microsporum canis*; this organism accounts for more than 90% of dermatophyte isolates from cats worldwide and more than 60% of isolates from dogs.[3,9,10] Sylvatic dermatophytes are zoophilic dermatophytes that are adapted to rodents or hedgehogs. The most common sylvatic dermatophyte that infects dogs and cats is *Trichophyton mentagrophytes.* Anthropophilic dermatophytes are adapted to human hosts and do not survive in the soil; they include *Microsporum audouinii, Trichophyton tonsurans, Trichophyton rubrum,* and *Epidermophyton floccosum.* Rarely, these species infect or contaminate dogs or cats that have a history of close contact with infected humans.[4,11-16] Mixed infections with multiple dermatophyte species occur rarely in dogs.[10]

Risk factors for dermatophytosis in dogs and cats include young age and concurrent immunosuppressive disorders, especially endogenous or iatrogenic hyperadrenocorticism. Dermatophytosis is more common in cats than in dogs, but the prevalence varies with geographic location. Positive dermatophyte cultures occurred in 6% of submissions from dogs or cats in the southern United States (3.8% for dogs and 14.9% for cats),[17] and in the United Kingdom, 16% were positive (10% for dogs and 16% for cats).[9] Higher prevalences of detection (19% to 43%) have been reported in some studies

TABLE 58-1

Zoophilic and Geophilic Dermatophyte Species Reported to Infect Dogs and/or Cats[3-8]

Dermatophyte Species	Classification	Primary Reservoir	Species Affected	Geographic Distribution
Microsporum canis	Zoophilic	Cats, dogs, horses	All mammals	Temperate and tropical locations worldwide
Microsporum gypseum	Geophilic	Soil	All mammals	Worldwide
*Microsporum persicolor**	Zoophilic	Voles, field mice	Dogs, cats	Europe
Trichophyton mentagrophytes	Zoophilic	Rodents	All mammals	Worldwide
Trichophyton erinacei	Zoophilic	Hedgehogs	Dogs	Europe and New Zealand
Trichophyton simii	Zoophilic	Primates	Dogs, cats	India and the Far East
*Trichophyton terrestre**	Geophilic	Soil	All mammals	Worldwide

*Do not invade hair; the role of *T. terrestre* in disease causation is controversial.

of cats and dogs, with and without skin lesions, from parts of continental Europe.[3,5,10] Dermatophytosis (especially geophilic dermatophytosis) is more prevalent in regions with high warmth and humidity. Shelter cats, the vast majority of which lack skin lesions, are more likely to carry dermatophytes on their haircoats than healthy pet cats. Dermatophytes were cultured from 5.5% and 19% of all shelter cats depending on geographical region,[18,19] whereas the prevalence of *M. canis* isolation from healthy pet cats is generally less than 2.5%.[18] Animals admitted to breeding or boarding facilities that have a history of dermatophytosis are also at risk of infection, whereas dermatophytes are generally not detectable on the haircoats of animals in facilities without a history of infection.[20] Retrovirus-infected cats are no more likely to carry dermatophytes than retrovirus-negative cats,[21] but retrovirus-infected cats carry a greater range of species and may be more likely to develop skin lesions (dermatophytosis). Genetic factors may also be important. Persian and Himalayan cats and Yorkshire and Jack Russell terriers appear to be predisposed to dermatophytosis.[3,9,17] In particular, Persian cats are thought to be at greater risk for development of dermatophytic mycetomas (see Clinical Features). Dogs that hunt and burrow in soil may be at increased risk for infection by geophilic or sylvatic dermatophytes, which may explain the common distribution of lesions on the face and distal thoracic limbs for these dermatophyte species (Figure 58-1).

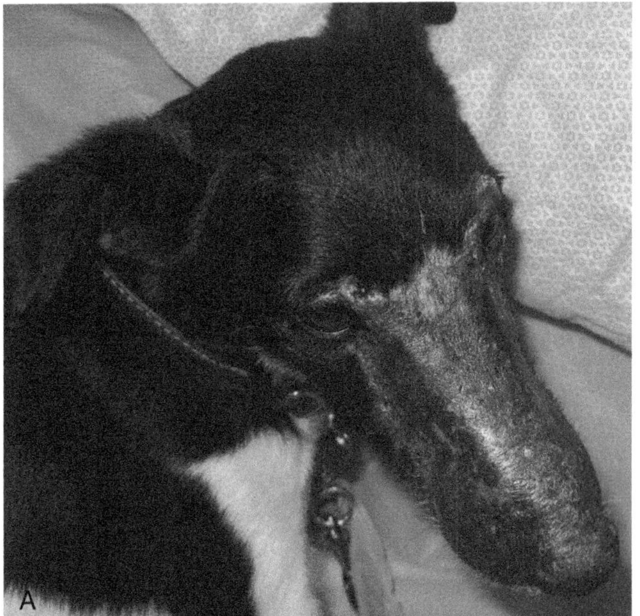

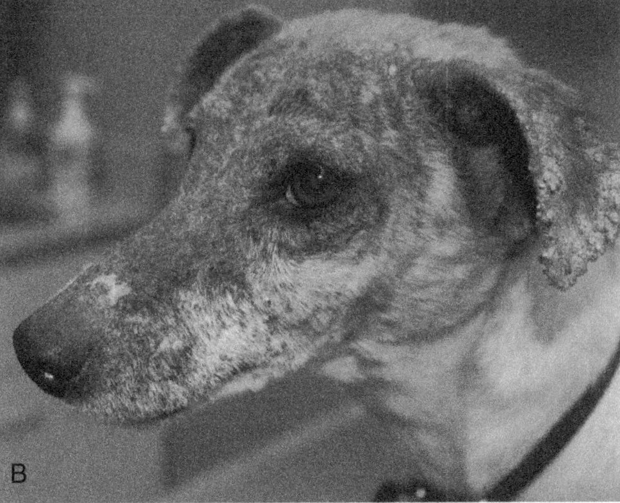

FIGURE 58-1 Chronic *Trichophyton mentagrophytes* infections. There is alopecia, crusting, hyperpigmentation, and ulceration of the muzzle and periocular skin. **A,** Four-and-a-half-year-old male neutered fox terrier. **B,** Six-year-old female spayed Jack Russell terrier. (Courtesy University of California, Davis, Veterinary Dermatology Service.)

Clinical Features

Signs and Their Pathogenesis

Pathogenic dermatophytes invade keratinized tissue that has been macerated or traumatized. Infections are localized to the stratum corneum, hair shafts, and claws. The clinical expression of the disease is affected by the fungal species and strain involved and the host response to infection.[22] Infectious arthrospores, which are formed by the segmentation and fragmentation of fungal hyphae, adhere to the surfaces of skin and nails, germinate, and secrete proteases. These proteases, such as subtilisins, fungalysins, and a variety of acidic proteases,[22,23] digest keratin into short peptides or amino acids, which are then used by the fungus as a source of nutrition. The pattern of proteases secreted by different dermatophyte strains may influence the clinical expression of disease. On the host, dermatophytes reproduce asexually through production of conidia.

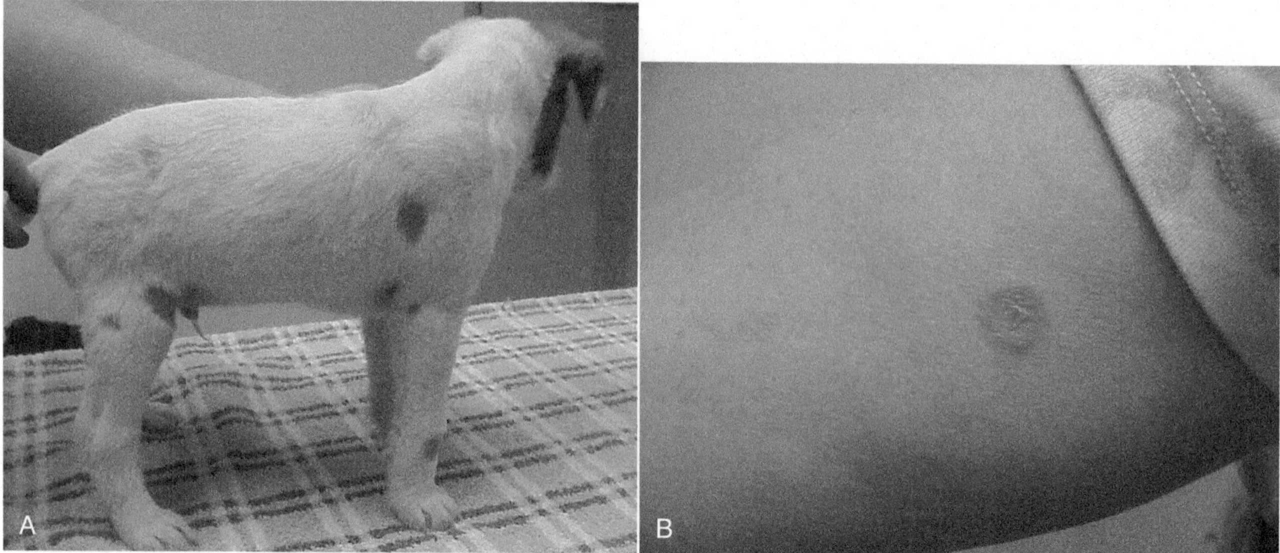

FIGURE 58-2 **A,** Jack Russell terrier puppy with multifocal classic well-circumscribed lesions caused by infection by *Microsporum canis.* **B,** On questioning, the owner of the affected litter of puppies revealed that she also had a lesion on her arm. (Courtesy Dr. Terry Nagle.)

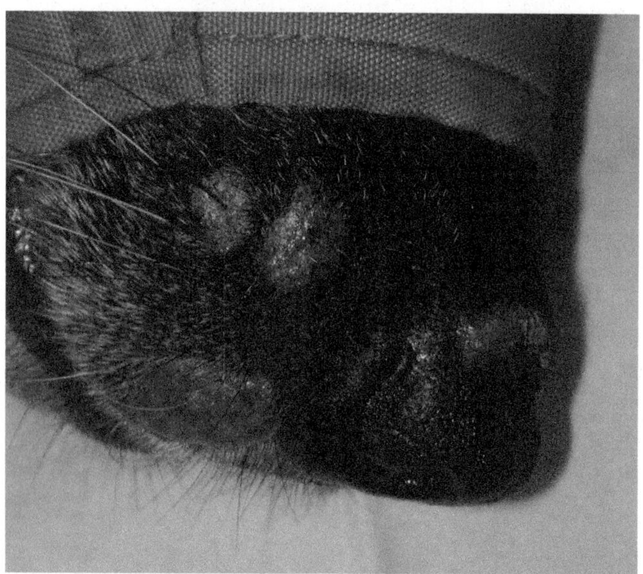

FIGURE 58-3 Nine-year-old female spayed labrador retriever with multiple kerions on the muzzle due to *Microsporum canis* infection. Another dog in the household had similar lesions that were less severe. (Courtesy University of California, Davis, Veterinary Dermatology Service.)

Dermatophyte lesions form after an incubation period of 1 to 3 weeks. Classically, lesions are single or multiple and consist of circular regions of alopecia with an erythematous margin, superficial scale and crust, and follicular papules and pustules (Figure 58-2). Central healing may occur, sometimes with hyperpigmentation or hair regrowth in the center of the lesion. Pruritis is variable. Infection by *T. mentagrophytes* in dogs can result in progressive alopecia, with dramatic scaling and/or crusting and inflammation and in some cases scarring (see Figure 58-1). A *kerion* or *kerion reaction* (also known as nodular dermatophytosis) is a localized, nodular inflammatory lesion that results from dermatophyte infection and may be associated with infection by *M. gypseum, T. mentagrophytes,* or *M. canis* (Figure 58-3).[10,24,25]

Longhaired cats may develop a poor haircoat, shed excessively, and vomit hairballs more frequently, because infected hair shafts are friable and prone to breakage. Persian and Himalayan cats (and very rarely, domestic longhair cats and dogs) with *M. canis* infections can develop dermatophytic mycetomas, which are coalescing subcutaneous nodular lesions that often drain purulent fluid (Figure 58-4).[26-31] These develop when dermatophytes invade the dermis and subcutaneous tissues, presumably after traumatic implantation of fungal organisms from the haircoat of an already colonized or infected animal. These lesions have also been referred to as granulomatous dermatitis, Majocchi's granuloma, or "pseudomycetomas," although use of the last term was not recommended by the International Society for Human and Animal Mycology (ISHAM) committee for nomenclature of fungal diseases.[32] In contrast to true mycetomas (eumycetomas), dermatophytic mycetomas are not caused by soil saprophytes, and lesions are often multiple and coalescing, rather than single and localized.[10]

Physical Examination Findings

In dogs, dermatophytosis can occur anywhere on the body but most often occurs on the face, distal limbs, and tail. Dogs are more likely than cats to present with classical, localized, well-circumscribed lesions. Claw infection is manifested by erythema and thickening of the ungual fold, deformity and friability of the claw, and sometimes footpad involvement (Figure 58-5). Kerions most commonly develop on the muzzle or distal limbs, and with digital pressure they typically have a boggy or exudative appearance (see Figure 58-4).

Lesions in cats are extremely pleomorphic and can consist of one or more areas of partial alopecia with scale and crusts, especially on the pinnae and pinnal margins, nasal bridge, distal limbs, or tail (Figure 58-6). Some lesions resemble miliary dermatitis or are focal, pruritic lesions that resemble eosinophilic plaques. Cats with dermatophytic mycetomas have focal (and rarely disseminated) nodular, sometimes ulcerated cutaneous lesions, usually on the dorsum or neck, which may drain serous or purulent fluid (see Figure 58-4).

Diagnosis

Diagnosis of dermatophytosis is based on clinical suspicion together with the results of Wood's lamp examination, skin and hair cytology, skin scrapings (to evaluate for demodicosis), and/or fungal culture (Table 58-2). In both dogs and cats, lesions are rarely symmetric. This asymmetry can help differentiate dermatophytosis from other diagnoses that more commonly cause symmetrical lesions. However, diagnosis that is solely based on the appearance of lesions and/or Wood's lamp examination is not recommended, because it can lead to misdiagnosis and unnecessary treatment that may be expensive and even harmful. In addition, mixed processes can occur, such as co-infections with dermatophytes and staphylococci or dermatophytes and *Demodex* mites. Because dermatophytosis can take on a wide range of appearances in cats, it should be considered a possible differential diagnosis in cats with *any* skin disease.[33]

Laboratory Abnormalities

Complete Blood Count, Serum Biochemical Tests, and Urinalysis

The results of routine laboratory testing in dogs and cats with dermatophytosis are typically unremarkable or show abnormalities associated with predisposing disease conditions (such as hyperadrenocorticism).

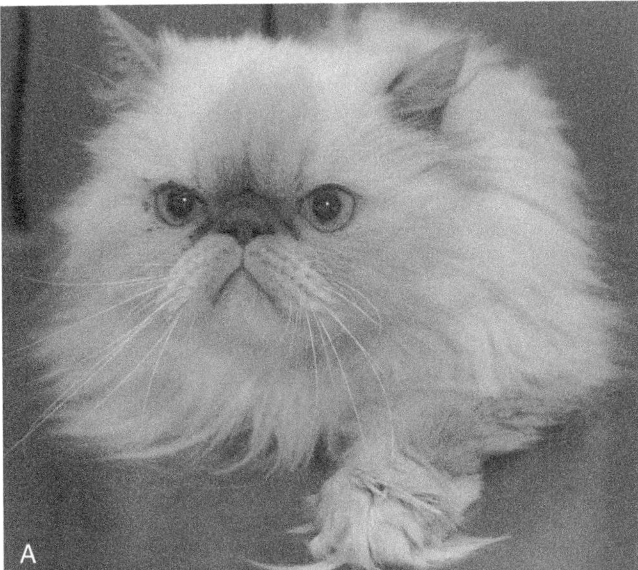

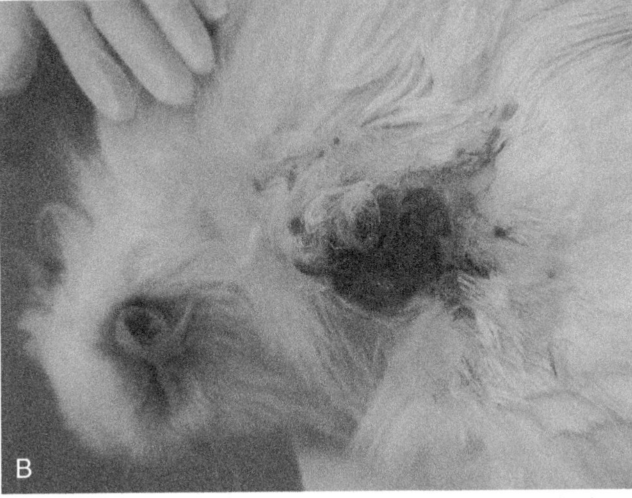

FIGURE 58-4 **A** and **B,** Twelve-year-old female spayed Himalayan with a dermatophytic mycetoma. Ulceration and fistulation are present. Ultimately, surgical excision of the mycetoma was required. (Courtesy University of California, Davis, Veterinary Dermatology Service.)

Microbiologic Tests

Wood's Lamp Examination

A positive Wood's lamp examination is characterized by the presence of apple-green fluorescence along the length of a hair shaft (Figure 58-7). The fluorescence results from tryptophan metabolites produced by some *M. canis* strains when they grow within the hair shaft; the metabolite is not produced when the organism grows on scale or the claw. A significant proportion of *M. canis* infections do not fluoresce,[3,9] and other dermatophyte species of veterinary significance do not produce fluorescent metabolites, so the sensitivity of Wood's lamp examination is low. The lamp should be allowed to warm up for several minutes before it is used, and the lights should be turned off during the examination. False-positive results can occur if topical ointments, scale, lint, keratinized debris, or sebum are present and incorrectly interpreted as dermatophyte fluorescence. Hairs that fluoresce can be plucked and submitted for cytologic examination and fungal culture.

Cytologic Examination

Cytologic examination of hairs plucked from lesions or the circumference of lesions may reveal fungal hyphae or chains of arthroconidia (ectothrix spores) in some affected animals; macroconidia, which form in culture, are not seen (Figure 58-8). Addition of a clearing agent such as 10% or 20% potassium hydroxide (KOH) or chlorphenolac is recommended, which removes scale and debris that can interfere with organism identification. Potassium hydroxide solutions must be gently heated with the hair for 10 minutes for clearing to occur, or incubated

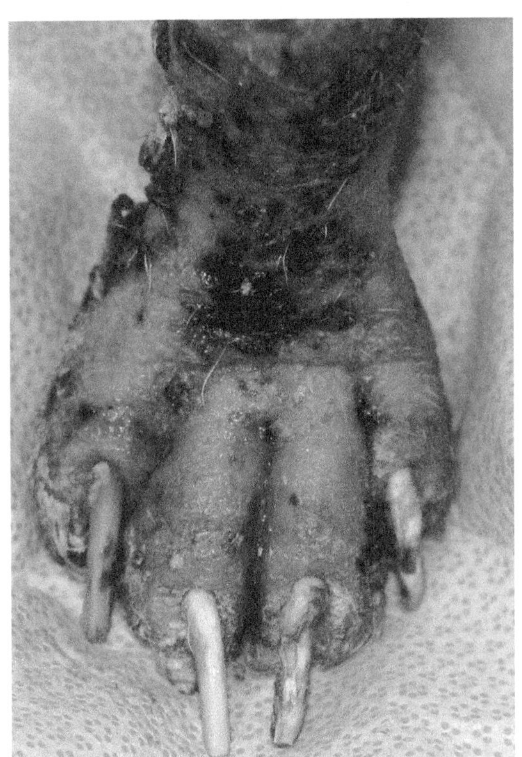

FIGURE 58-5 Foot of a 9-year-old intact male terrier mix with dermatophytosis caused by *Microsporum gypseum*. The dog competed in rodent hunting events that occurred in underground tunnels. Severe, chronic dermatitis with ulceration and alopecia that involved multiple distal limbs and claws was present. The claws were irregular and discolored. (Courtesy University of California, Davis, Veterinary Dermatology Service.)

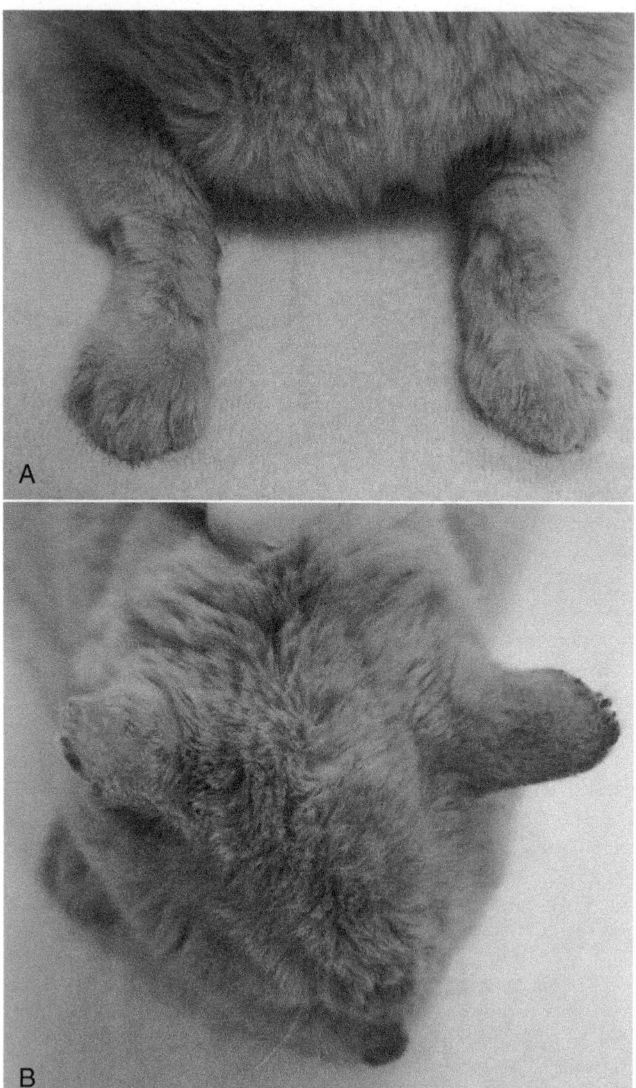

FIGURE 58-6 Eighteen-year-old male neutered domestic shorthair cat with dermatophytosis caused by *Trichophyton mentagrophytes*. The paws **(A)**, pinnae **(B)**, and nasal bridge were involved. (Courtesy University of California, Davis, Veterinary Dermatology Service.)

overnight at room temperature. Chlorphenolac, which is composed of chloral hydrate, phenol, and lactic acid, is not readily available and is toxic, but it does not require heating or prolonged incubation. Examination of hairs mounted in mineral oil can still yield positive results in the absence of a clearing agent.[25] Cytologic examination has low sensitivity when compared with culture, and experience is required for proper organism identification.

Fungal Culture

Culture is the gold standard for diagnosis of dermatophytosis. Ten to 12 hairs (ideally those that appear damaged or broken) should be plucked from the edge of lesions with sterile forceps and placed in a clean, dry paper envelope (preferably) or a sterile tube or container at room temperature. Scrapings of crusts from the edge of lesions or nail clippings (after cleaning the nail with 70% alcohol) can also be submitted (see also Chapter 4 for specimen collection methods for dermatophytes). Alternatively, a brand-new toothbrush (out of the package) can be used to collect specimens from lesions or the entire coat of a suspect animal by vigorous brushing for several minutes. The toothbrush is then submitted to the laboratory. Macerated tissue cultures can be performed on biopsy specimens from animals that have nodular dermatophytosis or dermatophytic mycetomas.

The most commonly used media for culture are Dermatophyte Test Medium (DTM) or Sabouraud's dextrose agar. In-house DTM cultures, if performed, should be interpreted with caution. Flat Petri plates (as opposed to vials) should be used in order to facilitate inoculation and species identification. Inoculated media should be incubated at 24°C to 30°C; incubation at room temperature is more likely to result in false negatives.[34] Growth occurs within 14 days, and often within 5 to 7 days, but may take up to 21 days (particularly for treated animals). Dermatophyte colonies, which are white or cream and powdery (Figure 58-9), should not be confused with those of saprophytic molds, which may be brown, green, black, gray, or mixed in color. The DTM turns red when the first dermatophyte colony is visible. Color changes that occur after the first colony appears may result from growth of saprophytic fungi. All suspicious colonies must be confirmed as dermatophytes and speciated based

TABLE 58-2

Diagnostic Assays Available for Dermatophytosis

Assay	Specimen Type	Target	Performance
Wood's lamp examination	Haircoat	Fluorescent *Microsporum canis* strains in hair	Low sensitivity (around 50%) for detection of *M. canis* when performed properly. Other dermatophyte species do not fluoresce. The presence of scale, sebum, debris, and topical ointments may lead to false positive results. When positive, allows identification of suitable specimens for cytology and/or culture.
Cytology	Hair pluck specimens	Dermatophyte hyphae and arthrospores	When positive, allows early institution of treatment. Low sensitivity. Incubation with clearing agents may increase sensitivity, but these may not be readily available. Other fungal conidia that contaminate the haircoat or debris may be mistaken for dermatophyte elements.
Culture	Plucked hair specimens, scale and nail clippings	All dermatophyte species	Gold standard for diagnosis of dermatophytosis. Prolonged incubation times may be required.
Histopathology	Skin biopsies	Dermatophytes	Organisms may be visualized with silver stains, periodic acid–Schiff stain, or immunohistochemistry.

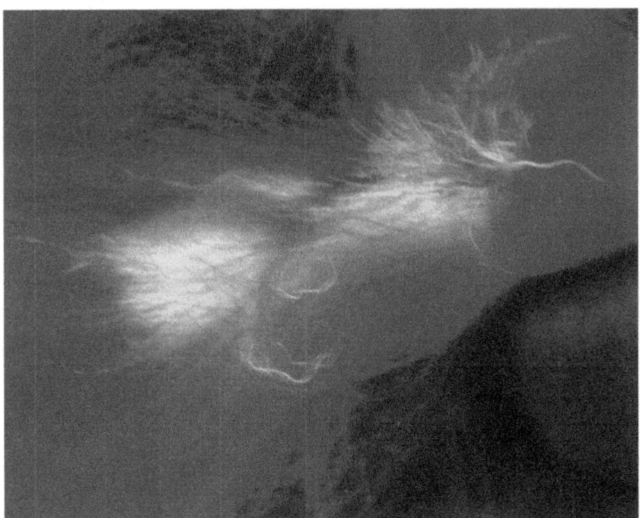

FIGURE 58-7 Positive Wood's lamp examination in a 2-year-old male neutered Persian that was seen for pruritis and hair loss. (Courtesy University of California, Davis, Veterinary Dermatology Service.)

on spore morphology through the use of microscopy (see Figure 58-9). Spores form after 7 to 10 days of growth. The individual performing the identification should wear gloves. Tape is placed over the colony and transferred to a slide, on which a drop of stain is applied. A coverslip is then applied. Lactophenol cotton blue or new methylene blue are suitable stains. Dysgonic strains of *M. canis* have been described that have atypical morphology in culture, but these are rare.[27,35] Whenever possible, submission to a veterinary diagnostic laboratory that follows Clinical and Laboratory Standards Institute (CLSI) guidelines is recommended to ensure proper quality assurance for culture and identification of dermatophytes. This also minimizes the risk of laboratory-acquired infections and contamination of the practice environment. Matrix-assisted laser desorption/ionization–time of flight mass spectrometry (MALDI-TOF) offers promise for rapid identification of dermatophytes in veterinary diagnostic microbiology laboratories in the future.[36]

Molecular Diagnosis Using the Polymerase Chain Reaction

PCR assays have been developed that detect and differentiate between dermatophytes that infect dogs and cats.[37,38] Sensitive real-time PCR assays have been described for use in humans,[39,40] but their use has not been reported for the diagnosis of dermatophytosis in dogs or cats. PCR assays have the potential to be

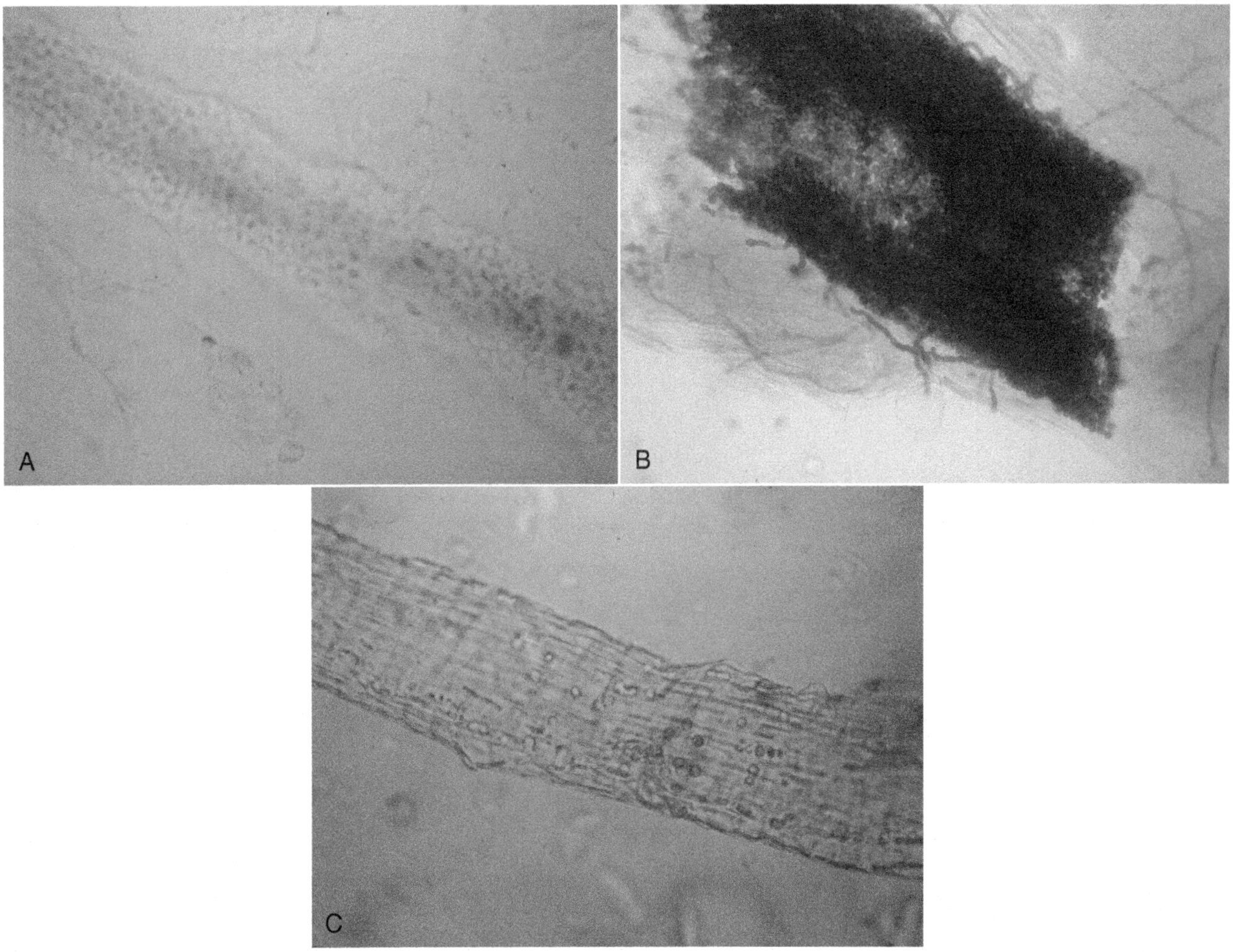

FIGURE 58-8 Cytology images of hairs infected with dermatophytes. **A,** Unstained preparation. Large numbers of *Microsporum canis* spores are seen that surround the hair shaft. **B,** Parker ink-KOH stain. Arthrospores and hyphae can be seen. **C,** Unstained preparation of a hair infected by *Microsporum gypseum*.

more sensitive than culture, with a more rapid turnaround time, and have the potential to facilitate assessment of treatment efficacy and control of disease in group-housed animals.

Pathologic Findings

Histopathology of biopsy specimens from dogs or cats with dermatophytosis may reveal spores and hyphae within intrafollicular hair shafts, in association with a variable pyogranulomatous inflammatory response (Figure 58-10). Special stains such as periodic acid–Schiff (PAS) or Gomori's methenamine silver can increase the sensitivity for detection of fungal elements.[41] Immunohistochemical stains have also been used to detect *M. canis* within lesions.[26] Occasionally, dermatophytes produce a superficial pustular histologic lesion. Acantholytic keratinocytes can be seen in biopsies from some dogs, which may lead to misdiagnosis of pemphigus foliaceus.[41] Histopathology of representative skin biopsies is especially useful for diagnosis of dermatophytic mycetomas, kerions, and fungal paronychia, because organisms are typically present in low numbers in these lesions and culture may be negative. Histopathology of dermatophytic mycetomas reveals pyogranulomatous inflammation and PAS-positive fungal elements that are embedded in an eosinophilic amorphous material within the dermis.

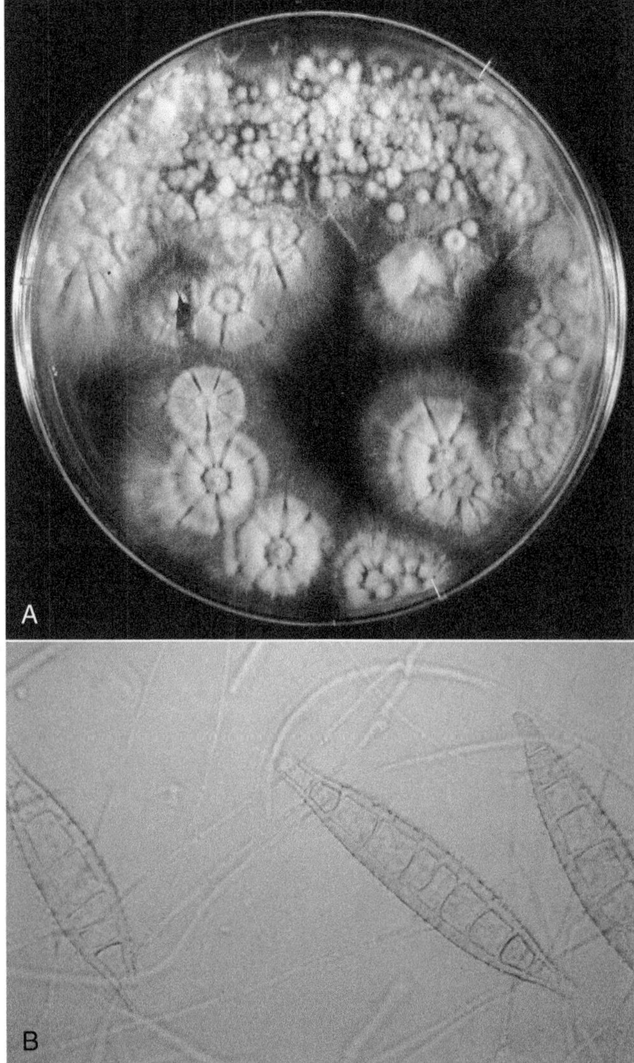

FIGURE 58-9 Selected cultural characteristics of dermatophytes. **A,** *Microsporum canis* from a cat with a dermatophytic mycetoma growing on inhibitory mold agar. **B,** Macroconidia of *M. gypseum* after growth in culture.

Treatment and Prognosis

Most otherwise healthy animals with dermatophytosis clear the infection without specific antifungal treatment within 3 months of diagnosis. Nevertheless, treatment is strongly recommended for animals that reside in multianimal households and those that live with immunocompromised humans (which includes children and older people, e.g., 60+ years of age) because of the highly contagious nature of the infection. The general approach to treatment includes the use of systemic antifungal drugs, with or without topical treatment, together with environmental decontamination. Lesions should be mapped and photographed before treatment is initiated so that progress can be monitored over time.

Management of dermatophytosis in multicat households can be frustrating, because (1) all in-contact cats must be treated; (2) some cats are colonized and have no visible lesions; and (3) testing and treatment require considerable energy, time, monitoring, and expense. For group-housed animals, all in-contact animals should be examined and cultured using the toothbrush technique. Ideally all animals with positive cultures (and definitely those with clinical signs) should be treated with both systemic and topical antifungal therapy, whereas all unaffected, culture-negative animals should be monitored for development of lesions and treated with topical antifungal drugs (ideally lime sulfur).

Topical Antifungal Drug Treatment

Topical antifungal drug treatment is not as effective as systemic treatment, but inactivates fungal spores on the haircoat and reduces environmental contamination. Spot treatments are not recommended, because spores are distributed all over the haircoat even when skin lesions are localized. The two most effective topical treatments are lime sulfur (1:16 dilution, or 237 mL in 3.6 L of water) or 0.2% enilconazole, both of which should be applied twice weekly.[42-44] Miconazole-chlorhexidine shampoos are also an option but may not be as effective as lime sulfur.[45,46] Lime sulfur shampoos, sprays, or dips have a foul odor and can

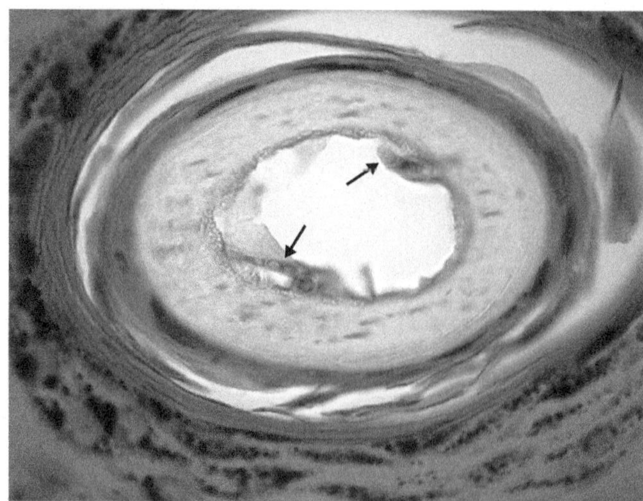

FIGURE 58-10 Histopathology that shows a cross-sectional view of a hair shaft from a 3-year-old female spayed Boston terrier. Fungal hyphae are visible within the hair shaft *(arrows)*.

TABLE 58-3

Antimicrobial Drugs That Can Be Used for Systemic Treatment of Dermatophytosis*

Drug	Dose (mg/kg)	Route	Interval (hours)
Itraconazole†	5	PO	12-24
Fluconazole	5-10	PO	12-24
Ketoconazole	10	PO	12
Terbinafine†	30-40	PO	24
Griseofulvin† (microsized)	25	PO	12
Griseofulvin (ultramicrosized)	15	PO	12

*See also Chapter 9 for more information on adverse reactions and drug administration before use.
†Administer itraconazole capsules, terbinafine, and griseofulvin with food. Reduce dose of itraconazole to 3 mg/kg q24h if using the suspension in cats.

stain light-colored haircoats but are safe for all age groups. A reformulated lime sulfur product with an odor-masking agent was not as effective in one clinical trial as a traditional lime sulfur preparation.[46] Lime sulfur products are most commonly used in the United States but may not be readily available in other parts of the world. Anecdotally, lime sulfur solutions have been reported to cause oral ulcerations in cats, but these were not detected in studies that evaluated cats that were allowed to lick their coats after treatment.[46,47] Ingestion of enilconazole can cause hypersalivation, anorexia, and vomiting, and there are rare anecdotal reports of severe adverse effects that include death.[11] Use of an Elizabethan collar is recommended to prevent cats from licking topical solutions from the haircoat until the treatment has dried. Chlorhexidine alone or povidone-iodine are not sufficiently active against spores and are not recommended. Whether or not the haircoat should be clipped before application of these treatments is controversial. Clipping removes contaminated hair and facilitates penetration of topical treatments, but may also serve to contaminate the environment and may create or exacerbate skin lesions if clipping disrupts the skin. It is recommended that clipping be used for longhaired cats and all cats in an affected Persian or Himalayan cattery. Clippers must be thoroughly disinfected with 10% bleach or concentrated accelerated hydrogen peroxide solutions afterward.

Systemic Antifungal Drug Treatment

Systemic antifungal drug treatment decreases the duration and severity of feline dermatophytosis (Table 58-3).[42] However, it should be used in conjunction with topical treatment and environmental decontamination when groups of animals are affected. Antifungal drugs with activity against dermatophytes are griseofulvin, ketoconazole, fluconazole, itraconazole, and terbinafine (see Chapter 9 for additional information on these drugs). Itraconazole is the drug of choice for treatment of dermatophytosis, because adverse reactions are uncommon and it has equal or greater efficacy when compared with griseofulvin.[48] Fluconazole is less active than other azole antifungal drugs against dermatophytes in vitro (as is the case for other fungi),[49,50] but controlled clinical trials that compare the efficacy of fluconazole to that of itraconazole for treatment of dermatophytosis are needed. The chitin inhibitor lufenuron (traditionally administered orally to prevent flea infestations) has been evaluated for treatment of dermatophytosis,[51,52] but its efficacy has been questioned and its use is no longer recommended.[10,11,24]

Environmental Decontamination

In some situations, environmental decontamination is extremely difficult or impossible because of the hardiness of dermatophyte spores and their widespread dispersal on surfaces that cannot be adequately disinfected. Even concentrated (1:10) bleach solutions are not 100% active against dermatophyte spores; complete disinfection requires undiluted household bleach or 1% formalin. Both are too toxic and caustic for routine use.

All potentially contaminated beds and blankets should be either discarded or washed with bleach through the use of a hot cycle and a hot dryer. Leashes, collars, and grooming equipment should be discarded, and carpets and furniture should be vacuumed to remove all visible hair and then steam cleaned. Because vacuum cleaners are a source of recontamination, they may need to be replaced after initial cleaning efforts; at the very least the vacuum bag should be discarded. Disinfection of hard surfaces should be performed with 1:10 to 1:100 bleach solution, 0.2% enilconazole solution, or (where available) an enilconazole fogger. Vehicles and carriers used to transport animals must also be appropriately cleaned. According to label information, concentrated (1:16) accelerated hydrogen peroxide solutions may also inactivate dermatophytes and reduce environmental contamination, but this requires further evaluation (see Chapter 11).

Duration of Treatment

The duration of treatment of dogs and cats with dermatophytosis is based on serial physical examinations and importantly, follow-up culture results. Usually, several months of treatment are required. In general, animals should be examined and a culture performed at least monthly (and no more frequently than weekly) during treatment. Treatment should be continued until two successive cultures are negative and active lesions have resolved. For group-housed animals, at least three successive negative cultures are suggested. Some authors advocate once-weekly cultures because this may permit earlier discontinuation of treatment.[11] If serial cultures are not possible because of financial limitations, treatment should be continued for 2 to 4 weeks after complete resolution of clinical signs. Typically, treatment is continued for at least 10 to 12 weeks.

Prognosis

The prognosis is good for resolution of dermatophytosis in young animals, especially in households with only a single animal or very low numbers of animals. Complicated disease such as dermatophytic mycetomas are difficult to resolve and require very long treatment durations; in some cats with mycetomas, surgery may ultimately be required for complete lesion resolution. The prognosis for rapid resolution of dermatophytosis may also be worse for animals with irreversible underlying immunocompromise. Hair regrowth may not occur in regions of scarring.

Immunity and Vaccination

Resolution of dermatophytosis depends on a delayed type-hypersensitivity immune response, which involves the activity of macrophages and IFN-γ.[22] Less invasive dermatophytes may evade the host immune response by limiting their presence to the superficial corneal epithelial cells and hair shafts. A vaccine for prevention of feline *M. canis* infections was licensed in the United States in the mid-1990s but was not sufficiently efficacious and is no longer available.

Prevention

Prevention of dermatophytosis relies on avoidance of contact with infected or carrier animals or fomites, but this may be impossible in some situations. For scenarios that involve group-housed animals, clean (culture-negative) animals, incoming animals, and animals undergoing treatment (culture-positive) must be kept in separate rooms, and ideally in individual cages. Once animals in the contaminated room are culture negative, they are moved to the clean room, and the contaminated room is thoroughly disinfected. Culture and topical treatment should be considered for any incoming animals to a clean facility.

In veterinary hospitals, animals with known dermatophytosis should be scheduled for examination late in the day and should be carried directly from the parking lot to an appropriate examination room that can subsequently be easily cleaned (the animal should not wait in the reception area). Strict attention to barrier precautions is required (see Chapter 11). If hospitalization is necessary, animals with suspected or documented *M. canis* infections should be housed in isolation.

Public Health Aspects

Forms of human dermatophytosis include tinea capitis (scalp), tinea pedis ("athlete's foot"), tinea barbae (bearded area), tinea cruris ("jock itch"), tinea corporis (body), tinea imbricata (a variant of tinea corporis), tinea manuum (hand), tinea faciei (face), and tinea unguium (nails).[1] Dermatophyte species that cause disease in dogs and cats have the potential to cause human disease. *Microsporum canis* is the most common zoophilic dermatophyte implicated. Zoophilic dermatophytes are most often associated with tinea capitis or tinea corporis. A high prevalence of infection with *M. canis* has been reported in children that have tinea capitis (scalp infection) from continental Europe and Asia.[53-55] *M. canis* is now a rare cause of tinea capitis in the United States, with most cases caused by anthropophilic dermatophytes such as *T. tonsurans*.[56]

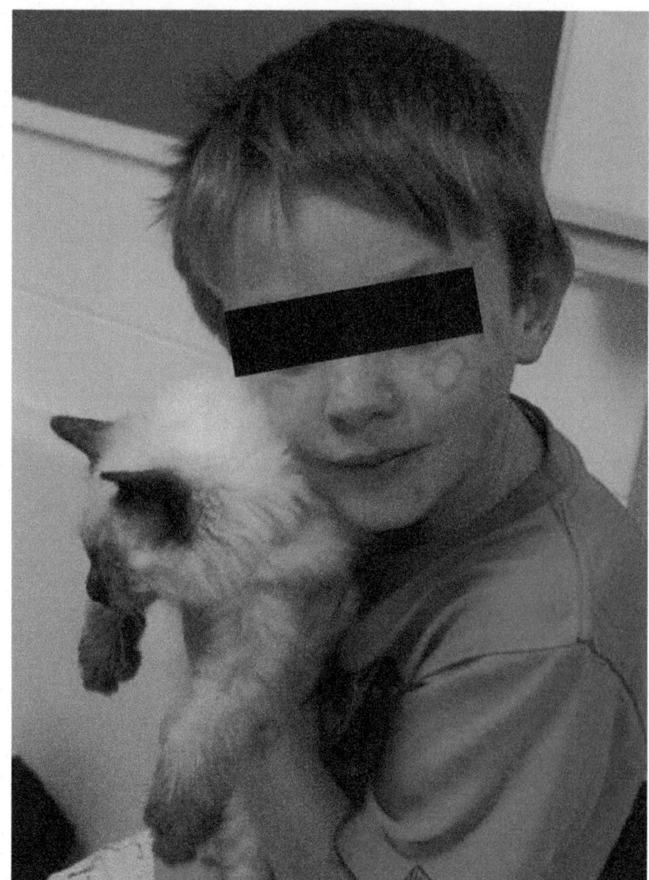

FIGURE 58-11 Boy with multiple lesions of dermatophytosis on the face and body. The boy had juvenile rheumatoid arthritis. The boy's cat had a lesion on the right side of its face. (Courtesy Dr. Richard Malik.)

Young children and the immunocompromised (e.g., transplant recipients) are most susceptible to dermatophytosis and may develop deep, recalcitrant, and/or disseminated lesions as a result of contact with infected pets.[57,58] Disease has been described in veterinarians and veterinary students.[11,35] In general, zoophilic and geophilic species evoke a more profound inflammatory response than anthropophilic dermatophytes; the latter tend to cause more chronic infections in people.[1] Typical "ringworm" lesions in humans are erythematous, circular lesions with a raised margin (Figure 58-11), but atypical forms that mimic other skin diseases such as atopic dermatitis and lupus have been described.[59] Humans who handle infected animals should wear protective clothing and gloves. Young children or the immunocompromised should avoid any contact with these animals. Toothbrush cultures should be considered for cats that are adopted from shelters or multicat households before they are introduced to households where immunocompromised individuals reside.

CASE EXAMPLE

Signalment: "Jack", a 4.5-year-old male neutered smooth-coated fox terrier from northern California

History: Jack was evaluated for chronic diarrhea, a distended abdomen, and loss of hair on the face. Jack's owners adopted him when he was 14 months old, at which time he had no clinical signs of illness. At 2 years of age, the owners noted that Jack began to rub his muzzle on objects. The intensity of this behavior at times resulted in excoriations that would bleed. Jack had been seen at another veterinary clinic where he was treated with a diet that was "hypoallergenic." The owners then continued to try to feed a variety of different diets for the skin problem, with a change to a new diet approximately every 3 months. The most recently fed diets were a prescription intestinal diet and a prescription venison and potato diet. Diet trials were never strict elimination trials, because the dog was fed the same treats throughout the diet trial process. There was no improvement in the skin lesions, which progressed to cause alopecia that involved the entire aspect of his face (see Figure 58-1, *A*). Approximately 18 months before Jack was evaluated, intermittent diarrhea had developed. The diarrhea was brown, occurred once or twice a day, and was sometimes accompanied by tenesmus. It occasionally contained mucus but never blood, and varied from soft to watery in consistency. In addition to this history, over the preceding 2 years, Jack had been treated intermittently with prednisone (0.5 to 0.75 mg/kg PO q12h) for the pruritus. The prednisone never improved the skin condition but was occasionally associated with resolution of the diarrhea. Other medications used at various time points over the previous 2 years included hydroxyzine, metronidazole, tylosin, cephalexin, and a topical otic preparation that contained thiabendazole, neomycin, and dexamethasone. Although Jack's appetite was generally good, he was described as a picky eater and had intermittent lethargy when his diarrhea was severe. The owners reported that over the most recent few weeks he had lost weight and muscle mass and had developed a distended abdomen. Jack lived on a ranch with multiple other dogs (the owner bred poodles and shelties), cats, and horses, none of which were unwell or had skin lesions. He spent most of his time outdoors on the farm and loved to dig in rodent holes.

Current medications: Prednisone, 1.4 mg/kg PO q12h

Physical Examination:

Body Weight: 7.1 kg.

General: Bright, alert, responsive, hydrated. T = 100.3°F (37.9°C), HR = 120 beats/min, RR = 40 breaths/min, mucous membranes pink/pigmented, CRT <2 s.

Integument: A dull, unkempt haircoat was noted. An area of partial alopecia with crusts was present over the right caudal tarsus. Diffuse, complete alopecia with serocellular and hemorrhagic crusting and multifocal, discrete ulcerations was present over the entire dorsal muzzle (see Figure 58-1, *A*). The skin within the alopecic area was hyperpigmented and had a shiny appearance compatible with scarring. Periocular alopecia with crusts was also present bilaterally and was confluent with the erythematous, advancing edge of the facial lesion. The skin on the ventral abdomen was thin with prominent subcutaneous vessels.

Eyes, Ears, and Throat: No clinically significant abnormalities of the eyes or ears were noted. On oral examination, the dentition was severely worn, and there was mild to moderate periodontal disease.

Musculoskeletal: Normal ambulation. Body condition score was 3/9.

Cardiovascular and Respiratory Systems: No clinically significant abnormalities were noted.

Gastrointestinal and Genitourinary: The abdomen was moderately distended with a palpable fluid wave. Rectal examination revealed only a moderate amount of formed but soft feces.

Lymph Nodes: No peripheral lymphadenopathy was detected.

Laboratory Findings:

CBC:

HCT 39.8% (40%-55%)
MCV 69.7 fL (65-75 fL)
MCHC 34.2 g/dL (33-36 g/dL)
WBC 18,810 cells/μL (6000-13,000 cells/μL)
Neutrophils 16,177 cells/μL (3000-10,500 cells/μL)
Band neutrophils 188 cells/μL
Lymphocytes 376 cells/μL (1000-4000 cells/μL)
Monocytes 1693 cells/μL (150-1200 cells/μL)
Eosinophils 376 cells/μL (0-1500 cells/μL)
Platelets clumped, rare nucleated RBC/100 WBC.

Serum Chemistry Profile:

Sodium 144 mmol/L (145-154 mmol/L)
Potassium 4.1 mmol/L (3.6-5.3 mmol/L)
Chloride 115 mmol/L (108-118 mmol/L)
Bicarbonate 24 mmol/L (16-26 mmol/L)
Phosphorus 1.9 mg/dL (3.0-6.2 mg/dL)
Calcium 6.6 mg/dL (9.7-11.5 mg/dL)
BUN 10 mg/dL (5-21 mg/dL)
Creatinine 0.5 mg/dL (0.3-1.2 mg/dL)
Glucose 108 mg/dL (64-123 mg/dL)
Total protein 2.9 g/dL (5.4-7.6 g/dL)
Albumin 1.5 g/dL (3.0-4.4 g/dL)
Globulin 1.4 g/dL (1.8-3.9 g/dL)
ALT 85 U/L (19-67 U/L)
AST 109 U/L (19-42 U/L)
ALP 23 U/L (21-170 U/L)
Creatine kinase 309 U/L (51-399 U/L)
GGT < 3 U/L (0-6 U/L)
Cholesterol 88 mg/dL (135-361 mg/dL)
Total bilirubin < 0.1 mg/dL (0-0.2 mg/dL)
Magnesium 1.8 mg/dL (1.5-2.6 mg/dL).

Serum Vitamin B_{12} and Folate: Vitamin B_{12} 314 ng/L (272-875 ng/L), folate 9.1 ng/mL (6.5-18.6 ng/mL).

Serum Ionized Magnesium Concentration: 0.44 mmol/L (0.40-0.52 mmol/L).

Urinalysis (Cystocentesis): SGr 1.018; pH 6.5, no protein, bilirubin, hemoprotein, or glucose, 0-2 WBC/HPF, no RBC/HPF, no crystals or bacteria, rare granular casts, few lipid droplets.

Imaging Findings:

Thoracic Radiographs: No abnormalities were detected in the thorax. In the portion of visible abdomen, there was decreased serosal detail.

Abdominal Ultrasound: There was marked thickening of the mucosal layer of the small intestine diffusely, with hyperechoic striations. A moderate volume of anechoic peritoneal effusion was present.

Cytologic Findings: Abdominal effusion: the fluid was colorless with a total protein of 0.3 g/dL, low numbers of erythrocytes, and 380 nucleated cells/μL (38% neutrophils, 2% small mononuclear cells, and 60% large mononuclear cells). Nucleated cells were a mixture of nondegenerate neutrophils and mononuclear cells of normal morphology. One large cluster of reactive mesothelial cells was observed. The fluid was interpreted as a transudate.

Microbiologic Testing: Skin scrapings and hair pluck cytology (trichogram) (from face and tarsus): Large numbers of dermatophyte hyphae and spores were present. No mites were seen.

Fungal culture (hair specimens from periphery of lesions on face and tarsus): Small numbers of *Trichophyton mentagrophytes* grew after 4 days.

Diagnosis: Protein-losing enteropathy (suspect lymphangiectasia), likely iatrogenic hyperadrenocorticism, and dermatophytosis due to *T. mentagrophytes* infection.

Treatment: Before the results of the fungal culture became available, fluconazole (7 mg/kg PO q24h) was prescribed based on the high index of suspicion from cytologic identification of fungal elements, together with an oatmeal shampoo to be used twice weekly. The dose of prednisone was reduced to 0.5 mg/kg PO q12h and strict instructions were given to feed a prescription low-fat diet and no other foods (including treats). At a recheck 3 weeks later, the owners reported that Jack was doing very well. His diarrhea, abdominal distention, and facial pruritus had resolved; he was more energetic; and his appetite had improved. Physical examination revealed resolution of crusts and evidence of new hair growth. Body weight had reduced to 6.2 kg and no evidence of abdominal distention was present. The only abnormalities on the chemistry panel were mild hypoproteinemia (5.1 g/dL) and hypocholesterolemia (110 mg/dL). Albumin was 3.1 g/dL and globulin was 2.2 g/dL. Abdominal ultrasound examination showed resolution of ascites. The prednisone dose was decreased to 0.4 mg/kg PO q24h, but diarrhea returned, so the dose was increased again to 0.4 mg/kg PO q12h. A repeat fungal culture (hair pluck specimen) 3 months after starting treatment was negative; culture was not performed earlier because lesions still appeared active, even though they had improved. Additional follow-up showed complete resolution of abnormalities on the serum chemistry panel and serum B_{12} and folate concentrations in the middle of the reference range. Ultimately management of the diarrhea required a cottage cheese and rice–based diet (balanced by a veterinary nutritionist) and a low dose of prednisone (0.4 mg/kg PO every 4 days). However, despite resolution of crusts and pruritis, hair cultures continued to periodically grow small numbers of *T. mentagrophytes* 1 year later, and fluconazole was never discontinued.

Comments: Persistent dermatophytosis in this dog was likely due to underlying immunosuppressive disease/drug treatment that could not be completely reversed, and possibly reinfection. The dog was likely exposed as a result of digging in rodent holes, based on the history and the dermatophyte species isolated. Poor client compliance and client financial limitations were factors that may also have contributed to an inability to control the infection.

SUGGESTED READINGS

Chermette R, Ferreiro L, Guillot J. Dermatophytoses in animals. Mycopathologia. 2008;166:385-405.

Moriello KA. Treatment of dermatophytosis in dogs and cats: review of published studies. Vet Dermatol. 2004;15:99-107.

Vermout S, Tabart J, Baldo A, et al. Pathogenesis of dermatophytosis. Mycopathologia. 2008;166:267-275.

REFERENCES

1. Weitzman I, Summerbell RC. The dermatophytes. Clin Microbiol Rev. 1995;8:240-259.
2. Sabouraud R. Les teignes. Paris: Masson et Cie; 1910.
3. Cafarchia C, Romito D, Sasanelli M, et al. The epidemiology of canine and feline dermatophytoses in southern Italy. Mycoses. 2004;47:508-513.
4. Ranganathan S, Arun Mozhi Balajee S, Mahendra Raja S. A survey of dermatophytosis in animals in Madras, India. Mycopathologia. 1997;140:137-140.
5. Seker E, Dogan N. Isolation of dermatophytes from dogs and cats with suspected dermatophytosis in Western Turkey. Prev Vet Med. 2011;98:46-51.
6. Muller A, Guaguere E, Degorce-Rubiales F, et al. Dermatophytosis due to *Microsporum persicolor*: a retrospective study of 16 cases. Can Vet J. 2011;52:385-388.
7. Fairley RA. The histological lesions of *Trichophyton mentagrophytes* var erinacei infection in dogs. Vet Dermatol. 2001;12:119-122.
8. Pierard-Franchimont C, Hermanns JF, Collette C, et al. Hedgehog ringworm in humans and a dog. Acta Clin Belg. 2008;63:322-324.
9. Sparkes AH, Gruffydd-Jones TJ, Shaw SE, et al. Epidemiological and diagnostic features of canine and feline dermatophytosis in the United Kingdom from 1956 to 1991. Vet Rec. 1993;133:57-61.
10. Chermette R, Ferreiro L, Guillot J. Dermatophytoses in animals. Mycopathologia. 2008;166:385-405.
11. Moriello K, DeBoer DJ. Cutaneous fungal infections. In: Greene CE, ed. Infectious Diseases of the Dog and Cat. 4th ed. St Louis, MO: Elsevier; 2012:588-606.
12. Kushida T, Watanabe S. Canine ringworm caused by *Trichophyton rubrum*; probable transmission from man to animal. Sabouraudia. 1975;13(Pt 1):30-32.
13. Kano R, Hirai A, Yoshiike M, et al. Molecular identification of *Trichophyton rubrum* isolate from a dog by chitin synthase 1 (CHS1) gene analysis. Med Mycol. 2002;40:439-442.
14. Brilhante RS, Cordeiro RA, Gomes JM, et al. Canine dermatophytosis caused by an anthropophilic species: molecular and phenotypical characterization of *Trichophyton tonsurans*. J Med Microbiol. 2006;55:1583-1586.
15. Terreni AA, Gregg Jr WB, Morris PR, et al. *Epidermophyton floccosum* infection in a dog from the United States. Sabouraudia. 1985;23:141-142.
16. Stenwig H, Taksdal T. Isolation of *Epidermophyton floccosum* from a dog in Norway. Sabouraudia. 1984;22:171-172.
17. Lewis DT, Foil CS, Hosgood G. Epidemiology and clinical features of dermatophytosis in dogs and cats at Louisiana State University: 1981-1990. Vet Dermatol. 1991;2:53-58.
18. Mignon BR, Losson BJ. Prevalence and characterization of *Microsporum canis* carriage in cats. J Med Vet Mycol. 1997;35:249-256.

19. Moriello KA, Kunkle G, DeBoer DJ. Isolation of dermatophytes from the hair coats of stray cats from selected animal shelters in two different geographic regions of the United States. Vet Dermatol. 1994;5:57-62.
20. Moriello KA, Deboer DJ. Fungal flora of the haircoat of cats with and without dermatophytosis. J Med Vet Mycol. 1991;29:285-292.
21. Reche Jr A, Daniel AG, Lazaro Strauss TC, et al. Cutaneous mycoflora and CD4:CD8 ratio of cats infected with feline immunodeficiency virus. J Feline Med Surg. 2010;12:355-358.
22. Vermout S, Tabart J, Baldo A, et al. Pathogenesis of dermatophytosis. Mycopathologia. 2008;166:267-275.
23. Sriranganadane D, Waridel P, Salamin K, et al. Identification of novel secreted proteases during extracellular proteolysis by dermatophytes at acidic pH. Proteomics. 2011;11:4422-4433.
24. Outerbridge CA. Mycologic disorders of the skin. Clin Tech Small Anim Pract. 2006;21:128-134.
25. Cornegliani L, Persico P, Colombo S. Canine nodular dermatophytosis (kerion): 23 cases. Vet Dermatol. 2009;20:185-190.
26. Abramo F, Vercelli A, Mancianti F. Two cases of dermatophytic pseudomycetoma in the dog: an immunohistochemical study. Vet Dermatol. 2001;12:203-207.
27. Thian A, Woodgyer AJ, Holloway SA. Dysgonic strain of *Microsporum canis* pseudomycetoma in a domestic long-hair cat. Aust Vet J. 2008;86:324-328.
28. Nobre Mde O, Negri Mueller E, Teixeira Tillmann M, et al. Disease progression of dermatophytic pseudomycetoma in a Persian cat. Rev Iberoam Micol. 2010;27:98-100.
29. Bergman RL, Medleau L, Hnilica K, et al. Dermatophyte granulomas caused by *Trichophyton mentagrophytes* in a dog. Vet Dermatol. 2002;13:49-52.
30. Chang SC, Liao JW, Shyu CL, et al. Dermatophytic pseudomycetomas in four cats. Vet Dermatol. 2011;22:181-187.
31. Bond R, Pocknell AM, Tozet CE. Pseudomycetoma caused by *Microsporum canis* in a Persian cat: lack of response to oral terbinafine. J Small Anim Pract. 2001;42:557-560.
32. Odds FC, Arai T, Disalvo AF, et al. Nomenclature of fungal diseases: a report and recommendations from a Sub-Committee of the International Society for Human and Animal Mycology (ISHAM). J Med Vet Mycol. 1992;30:1-10.
33. Chermette R, Bussieras S, Jeanmonod P, et al. Dermatophytie à *Trichophyton rubrum* chez un chien et son propriétaire. Première description en France. Bull Soc Fr Mycol Med. 1990;19:219-223.
34. Guillot J, Latie L, Deville M, et al. Evaluation of the dermatophyte test medium RapidVet-D. Vet Dermatol. 2001;12:123-127.
35. Hermoso de Mendoza M, Hermoso de Mendoza J, Alonso JM, et al. A zoonotic ringworm outbreak caused by a dysgonic strain of *Microsporum canis* from stray cats. Rev Iberoam Micol. 2010;27:62-65.
36. Nenoff P, Erhard M, Simon JC, et al. MALDI-TOF mass spectrometry—a rapid method for the identification of dermatophyte species. Med Mycol. 2013;51:17-24.
37. Cafarchia C, Gasser RB, Figueredo LA, et al. An improved molecular diagnostic assay for canine and feline dermatophytosis. Med Mycol. 2013;51:136-143.
38. Nardoni S, Franceschi A, Mancianti F. Identification of *Microsporum canis* from dermatophytic pseudomycetoma in paraffin-embedded veterinary specimens using a common PCR protocol. Mycoses. 2007;50:215-217.
39. Yuksel T, Ilkit M. Identification of rare macroconidia-producing dermatophytic fungi by real-time PCR. Med Mycol. 2012;50:346-352.
40. Jensen RH, Arendrup MC. Molecular diagnosis of dermatophyte infections. Curr Opin Infect Dis. 2012;25:126-134.
41. Peters J, Scott DW, Erb HN, et al. Comparative analysis of canine dermatophytosis and superficial pemphigus for the prevalence of dermatophytes and acantholytic keratinocytes: a histopathological and clinical retrospective study. Vet Dermatol. 2007;18:234-240.
42. Moriello KA. Treatment of dermatophytosis in dogs and cats: review of published studies. Vet Dermatol. 2004;15:99-107.
43. Diesel A, Verbrugge M, Moriello KA. Efficacy of eight commercial formulations of lime sulphur on in vitro growth inhibition of *Microsporum canis*. Vet Dermatol. 2011;22:197-201.
44. Hnilica KA, Medleau L. Evaluation of topically applied enilconazole for the treatment of dermatophytosis in a Persian cattery. Vet Dermatol. 2002;13:23-28.
45. Moriello KA, Verbrugge M. Use of isolated infected spores to determine the sporocidal efficacy of two commercial antifungal rinses against *Microsporum canis*. Vet Dermatol. 2007;18:55-58.
46. Newbury S, Moriello KA, Kwochka KW, et al. Use of itraconazole and either lime sulphur or Malaseb Concentrate Rinse (R) to treat shelter cats naturally infected with *Microsporum canis*: an open field trial. Vet Dermatol. 2011;22:75-79.
47. Newbury S, Moriello K, Verbrugge M, et al. Use of lime sulphur and itraconazole to treat shelter cats naturally infected with *Microsporum canis* in an annex facility: an open field trial. Vet Dermatol. 2007;18:324-331.
48. Moriello KA, DeBoer DJ. Efficacy of griseofulvin and itraconazole in the treatment of experimentally induced dermatophytosis in cats. J Am Vet Med Assoc. 1995;207:439-444.
49. Perea S, Fothergill AW, Sutton DA, et al. Comparison of in vitro activities of voriconazole and five established antifungal agents against different species of dermatophytes using a broth macrodilution method. J Clin Microbiol. 2001;39:385-388.
50. Mota CR, Miranda KC, Lemos Jde A, et al. Comparison of in vitro activity of five antifungal agents against dermatophytes, using the agar dilution and broth microdilution methods. Rev Soc Bras Med Trop. 2009;42:250-254.
51. Guillot J, Malandain E, Jankowski F, et al. Evaluation of the efficacy of oral lufenuron combined with topical enilconazole for the management of dermatophytosis in catteries. Vet Rec. 2002;150:714-718.
52. Ben-Ziony Y, Arzi B. Use of lufenuron for treating fungal infections of dogs and cats: 297 cases (1997-1999). J Am Vet Med Assoc. 2000;217:1510-1513.
53. Tsoumani M, Jelastopulu E, Bartzavali C, et al. Changes of dermatophytoses in southwestern Greece: an 18-year survey. Mycopathologia. 2011;172:63-67.
54. del Boz J, Crespo V, Rivas-Ruiz F, et al. A 30-year survey of paediatric tinea capitis in southern Spain. J Eur Acad Dermatol Venereol. 2011;25:170-174.
55. Zhu M, Li L, Wang J, et al. Tinea capitis in Southeastern China: a 16-year survey. Mycopathologia. 2010;169:235-239.
56. Coloe JR, Diab M, Moennich J, et al. Tinea capitis among children in the Columbus area, Ohio, USA. Mycoses. 2010;53:158-162.
57. Trabelsi S, Aouinet A, Abderrahim E, et al. First case of subcutaneous dermatomycoses in a Tunisian renal transplant patient. Tunis Med. 2012;90:196-199.
58. Chiapello LS, Dib MD, Nuncira CT, et al. Mycetoma of the scalp due to *Microsporum canis*: hystopathologic, mycologic, and immunogenetic features in a 6-year-old girl. Diagn Microbiol Infect Dis. 2011;70:145-149.
59. Atzori L, Aste N, Pau M. Tinea faciei due to *Microsporum canis* in children: a survey of 46 cases in the district of Cagliari (Italy). Pediatr Dermatol. 2012;29:409-413.

CHAPTER 59

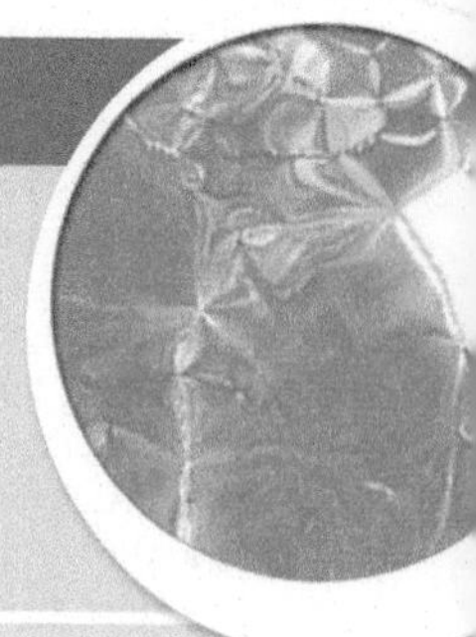

Malassezia Infections

Jane E. Sykes, Terry M. Nagle, and Stephen D. White

Overview of *Malassezia* Dermatitis

First Described: 1874, in France, by Louis-Charles Malassez (the fungus was initially named *Pityrosporum ovale*)[1]

Cause: *Malassezia pachydermatis*; less commonly, lipid-dependent species such as *Malassezia globosa, Malassezia sympodialis, Malassezia nana, Malassezia slooffiae,* and *Malassezia furfur* are involved.

Affected Hosts: Dogs and to a lesser extent cats

Geographic Distribution: Worldwide

Mode of Transmission: Direct contact and opportunistic proliferation of commensal organisms

Major Clinical Signs: Cutaneous erythema, pruritus, alopecia, scaling, greasy exudation, hyperpigmentation, lichenification, malodor

Differential Diagnoses: Dermatophytosis, demodicosis, allergic dermatitis, drug eruptions, pyoderma

Human Health Significance: *M. pachydermatis* does not normally colonize human skin but can rarely infect immunosuppressed adults and cause catheter-related infections in neonatal intensive care units.

Etiology and Epidemiology

Malassezia spp. (formerly *Pityrosporum* spp.) are lipophilic yeasts that normally colonize animal and human skin in low numbers. At least 13 species of *Malassezia* exist. The vast majority of species are classified as lipid dependent: when grown in the laboratory, these species have an absolute requirement for long-chain fatty acids, which are used as a source of carbon. In contrast, *Malassezia pachydermatis,* the most commonly isolated yeast species from the skin and ears of healthy dogs and cats, is non–lipid dependent when grown in the laboratory. Lipid-dependent species, including *Malassezia globosa, Malassezia sympodialis, Malassezia nana, Malassezia slooffiae,* and *Malassezia furfur,* can colonize the skin of healthy cats.[2-5]

In healthy dogs, *Malassezia* spp. are most commonly found in the ear canals, on the lips, axillae, interdigital spaces, anal sacs, and occasionally the nose and vagina. It has been suggested that a symbiotic relationship exists between *Malassezia* spp. and commensal staphylococci; each maintains a local microenvironment that benefits the other.

Malassezia spp. are common opportunistic contributors to chronic dermatitis and otitis externa in dogs, and to a lesser extent in cats. They are isolated more frequently from the ears of dogs and cats with otitis externa than from the ears of healthy dogs and cats.[6,7] Dogs with skin disease can have 100- to 10,000-fold increases in skin population densities of *Malassezia* spp. compared with healthy dogs.[8] Species and strains of *Malassezia* vary in virulence and tropism for different anatomic sites and host species.[9,10] A variety of lipid-dependent *Malassezia* spp. occasionally have been isolated from dogs and cats with otitis externa.[6,7,11-14]

Malassezia spp. infection can occur in dogs and cats of any age, breed, and sex, but some dog breeds are thought to be predisposed, including American cocker spaniels, West Highland white terriers, basset hounds, poodles, and Australian silky terriers.[15] Sphynx and Devon Rex cats have high rates of *Malassezia* spp. colonization when compared with domestic shorthair cats.[16]

Clinical Features

Signs and Their Pathogenesis

Malassezia spp. proliferate opportunistically, becoming pathogenic with alterations in host defenses or the skin surface microclimate. Examples of underlying diseases include allergic dermatitis, endocrinopathies, intertrigo, primary keratinization/cornification disorders, and, in cats, underlying neoplasia or retrovirus infections.[17,18] A history of treatment with antibiotics was a predisposing factor in one study.[19] Prolonged glucocorticoid treatment can also lead to yeast proliferation. The yeasts adhere to the cells of the stratum corneum and secrete lipases, proteinases, phospholipases, and acid sphingomyelinases.[20] The resulting skin lesions may be localized or generalized, are thought to result from inflammation, and, in some animals, hypersensitivity reactions to yeast antigens.[21,22] The more erythematous the interdigital region is in an atopic dog, the more likely a *Malassezia* spp. infection is present.[23]

The most commonly affected anatomic sites are the ear canals, skin folds (including the periocular and perioral skin, ventral neck, axillae, inguinal regions, and perineum), and interdigital skin (Figure 59-1). Clinical signs include erythema, pruritus, alopecia, scaling, and a greasy exudate. The claw beds may develop a reddish-brown stain. Chronicity results in hyperpigmentation, lichenification, and stenosis of the ear canal, and a pungent, offensive odor develops. Pruritus may result in excoriations. Devon Rex and Sphynx cats can develop a greasy dermatitis associated with increased numbers of *Malassezia* spp., which can respond dramatically to antifungal drug treatment.[8]

Physical Examination

A thorough physical and dermatologic examination aids diagnosis of *Malassezia* spp. infection and provides important clues

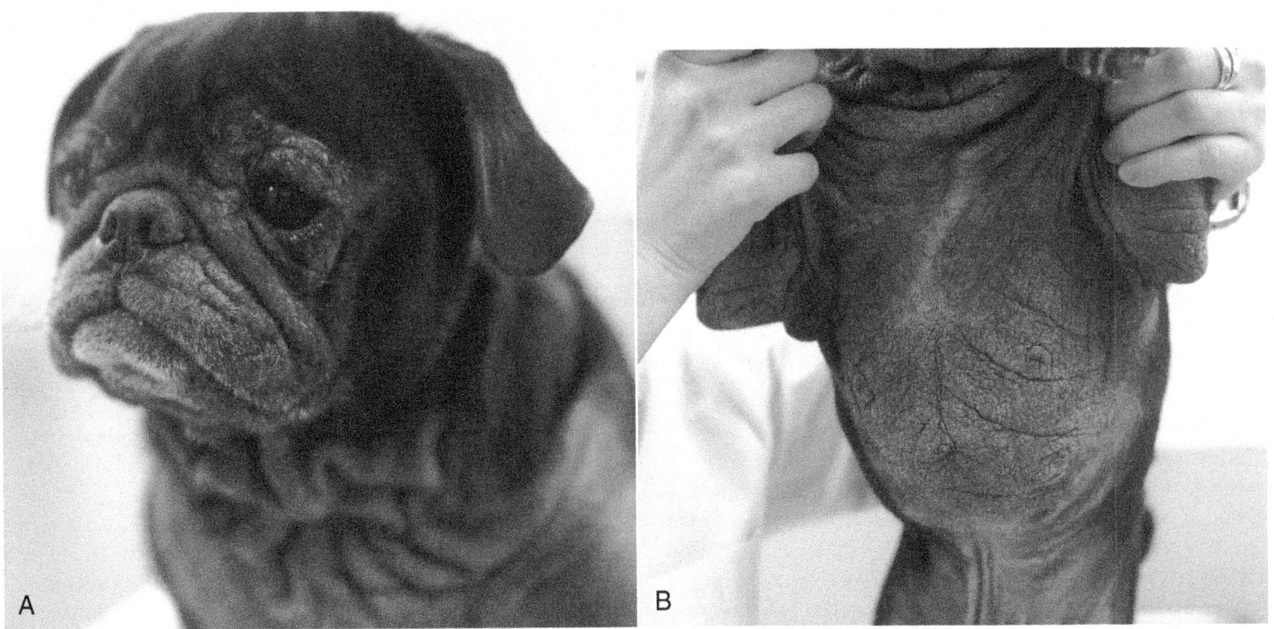

FIGURE 59-1 Five-year-old male neutered pug with a 1 year history of otitis externa and generalized pruritus. *Malassezia* dermatitis and bacterial pyoderma secondary to underlying atopic dermatitis was diagnosed. Note the distribution of lesions, which affect the facial folds and ventral neck **(A)** and axillae **(B)**.

as to the underlying disorder leading to opportunistic proliferation of *Malassezia* spp. It also allows identification of lesions consistent with concurrent pyoderma (see Chapter 84).

Diagnosis

Diagnosis of *Malassezia* spp. dermatitis is based on clinical signs, findings on cytologic examination, and a positive response to antifungal drug treatment.

Microbiologic Testing

Skin Scrapings

Skin scrapings are important in animals suspected to have *Malassezia* spp. dermatitis in order to rule out demodicosis, which can mimic *Malassezia* spp. dermatitis.

Cytologic Examination

Cytology is an important tool for diagnosis and is generally performed using clear (not frosted) acetate (Scotch) tape preparations of the skin. The tape is pressed to the skin, dipped in the final step basophilic (blue) Diff-Quik solution, rinsed, and applied to a slide on which a drop of immersion oil has been placed. Alternatively, the tape is pressed against the affected skin several times and then placed on a dry glass slide, and a small amount of the basophilic Diff-Quik solution is injected under the tape. The tape is then examined using a light microscope, with an additional drop of immersion oil to allow identification of bacteria and *Malassezia* spp. using the 100× objective. The yeasts stain deeply basophilic and exhibit wide-based budding, resembling "footprints," "peanuts," or "snowmen" (Figure 59-2). An inflammatory cellular response is often not present, even when *Malassezia* spp. contribute to disease progression.

Estimation of yeast counts, although only semiquantitative, may help to determine the role of *Malassezia* in otitis and dermatitis, but there are no clear guidelines as to what constitutes a normal yeast population size. In addition, yeast counts do not take into account other factors, such as strain variation in virulence or host hypersensitivity.[10,24] For *Malassezia* spp. dermatitis, mean counts of 1 or more yeast per oil immersion field (1000× magnification) are considered abnormal in dogs.[25] For ears, a mean yeast count of approximately 5 or more organisms per oil immersion field has been suggested as abnormal.[25] Cats may be colonized with higher numbers of yeasts, and 12 or more organisms per high dry field has been suggested as abnormal in feline ear canals in another study.[26] The ear canals of healthy dogs and cats have mean counts of 2 or fewer yeasts per high dry field (400× magnification), and intermediate counts represent a gray zone.[26]

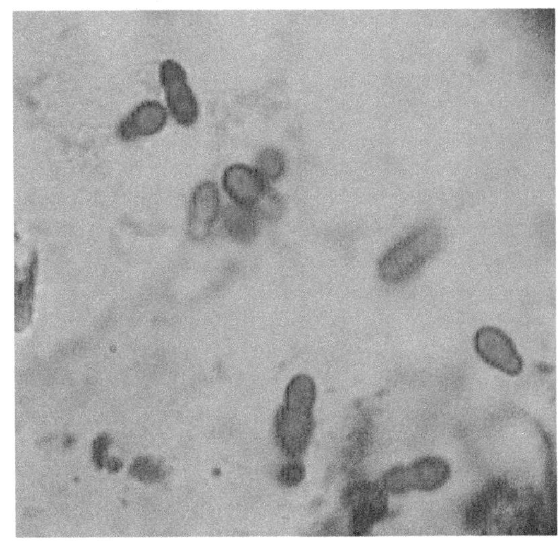

FIGURE 59-2 Tape preparation from the skin of a dog with *Malassezia* dermatitis. Note broad-based budding yeasts, which have the appearance of a footprint. Modified Wright's stain, 1000× oil magnification.

Fungal Culture

Fungal culture and susceptibility testing for *Malassezia* spp. is not routinely performed for clinical diagnostic purposes,

TABLE 59-1

Systemic Antifungal Drugs Used for Treatment of *Malassezia* Dermatitis and Otitis Externa in Dogs

Drug	Dose (mg/kg)	Route	Interval (hours)	Duration (days)
Ketoconazole	5 to 10	PO	12	3 to 4 weeks or until cytologic resolution
Itraconazole	5*	PO	24	
Fluconazole	5	PO	24	
Terbinafine	30	PO	24	

*Dose applies to the capsules. Reduce dose to 3 mg/kg if using the suspension.

although methods that use broth dilution or E-testing for susceptibility testing have been described. The organism can be cultured from a tape preparation, which in the laboratory is mounted on a drop of olive oil that has been placed on fungal isolation media.[25] Growth occurs within 7 days of incubation. Currently, most *Malassezia* spp. infections are broadly susceptible and respond well to treatment of the yeast infection and any underlying disorders present. One azole-resistant isolate of *M. pachydermatis* was identified in a dog with dermatitis, but this was not associated with resistance in vivo.[27]

Treatment and Prognosis

Treatment of *Malassezia* spp. dermatitis and otitis requires identification and, if possible, treatment of the underlying cause, in addition to antifungal drug treatment. Because *Malassezia* spp. infection is superficial, topical treatments may be adequate to resolve infection. A variety of topical otic preparations are available for treatment of *Malassezia* otitis. These contain antifungals such as clotrimazole, miconazole, or posaconazole, which are generally combined with a glucocorticoid and an antibacterial (see Chapter 84). There is good evidence that *Malassezia* dermatitis can be successfully treated with twice-weekly shampooing with a 2% miconazole/2% chlorhexidine shampoo (e.g., Malaseb, DVM Pharmaceuticals) for 3 weeks,[24] and this can also prevent recurrence. A 3% chlorhexidine shampoo may be equally efficacious.[28] Systemic antifungals that have been shown to have efficacy for treatment of *Malassezia* infections include ketoconazole, itraconazole, fluconazole, and terbinafine, which are generally administered for 3 weeks (Table 59-1).[29,30] Longer periods of treatment may be required for severe infections or infections of the claw bed.[8] Administration of terbinafine on two consecutive days each week (i.e., in a pulsatile fashion) may be as effective as daily administration, but more studies are required.[31] Treatment should be monitored through serial dermatologic examinations and cytologic evaluation of tape preparations. The prognosis for resolution depends on the ability to identify and address the underlying cause for proliferation of *Malassezia* spp.

Public Health Aspects

In human beings, *Malassezia* infections most commonly result from infection by *M. furfur*. This organism belongs to the normal human cutaneous flora and proliferates opportunistically following immunocompromise. Yeast proliferation can lead to *Malassezia* folliculitis, seborrheic dermatitis, catheter-related fungemia, and a variety of other invasive infections.[32] Administration of lipid-containing total parenteral nutrition solutions is a risk factor for disseminated infections in humans, which often occur in neonates.[33,34]

M. pachydermatis is not part of the normal human cutaneous microflora. Human disease associated with *M. pachydermatis* infection occurs rarely. Nosocomial infections with *M. pachydermatis* have been reported in neonates in intensive care units.[35] One epidemic was associated with colonization of health care workers' pet dogs with a strain identical to that causing disease, as determined by molecular typing with pulsed-field gel electrophoresis.[36] Cutaneous infections have also been reported in adults with underlying immunosuppressive disease.[30] Owners of dogs with atopic skin disease were 11 times more likely to carry *M. pachydermatis* on their hands than owners of healthy dogs, as determined using culture (39% vs. 6%).[25] The owners of both groups of dogs were equally likely to carry the yeast on their hands as determined by PCR testing (93% and 94%). It was concluded that mechanical carriage of the organism by dog owners appears to be of low risk to human health, given how rarely disease due to *M. pachydermatis* occurs. Hand washing is likely to reduce the rate of carriage of *M. pachydermatis*, but this has not been well studied.

CASE EXAMPLE

See case example in Chapter 84.

SUGGESTED READING

Tragiannidis A, Bisping G, Koehler G, et al. Minireview: *Malassezia* infections in immunocompromised patients. Mycoses. 2010;53(3):187-195.

REFERENCES

1. Malassez L. Note sur la champignon de la pelade. Arch Physiol Norm et Pathol. 1874;1:203-212.
2. Bond R, Anthony RM, Dodd M, et al. Isolation of *Malassezia sympodialis* from feline skin. J Med Vet Mycol. 1996;34(2):145-147.
3. Bond R, Howell SA, Haywood PJ, et al. Isolation of *Malassezia sympodialis* and *Malassezia globosa* from healthy pet cats. Vet Rec. 1997;141(8):200-201.
4. Crespo MJ, Abarca ML, Cabañes FJ. Isolation of *Malassezia furfur* from a cat. J Clin Microbiol. 1999;37(5):1573-1574.
5. Volk AV, Belyavin CE, Varjonen K, et al. *Malassezia pachydermatis* and *M. nana* predominate amongst the cutaneous mycobiota of Sphynx cats. J Fel Med Surg. 2010;12(12):917-922.

6. Cafarchia C, Gallo S, Capelli G, et al. Occurrence and population size of *Malassezia* spp. in the external ear canal of dogs and cats both healthy and with otitis. Mycopathologica. 2005;160(2):143-149.
7. Dizotti CE, Coutinho SD. Isolation of *Malassezia pachydermatis* and *M. sympodialis* from the external ear canal of cats with and without otitis externa. Acta Vet Hung. 2007;55(4):471-477.
8. Bond R. Superficial veterinary mycoses. Clin Dermatol. 2010;28(2): 226-236.
9. Duarte ER, Hamdan JS. RAPD differentiation of *Malassezia* spp. from cattle, dogs and humans. Mycoses. 2010;53(1):48-56.
10. Machado ML, Cafarchia C, Otranto D, et al. Genetic variability and phospholipase production of *Malassezia pachydermatis* isolated from dogs with diverse grades of skin lesions. Med Mycol. 2010;48(6):889-892.
11. Cafarchia C, Latrofa MS, Figueredo LA, et al. Physiological and molecular characterization of atypical lipid-dependent *Malassezia* yeasts from a dog with skin lesions: adaptation to a new host? Med Mycol. 2011;49:365-374.
12. Crespo MJ, Abarca ML, Cabaûes FJ. Otitis externa associated with *Malassezia sympodialis* in two cats. J Clin Microbiol. 2000;38(3):1263-1266.
13. Crespo MJ, Abarca ML, Cabaûes FJ. Atypical lipid-dependent *Malassezia* species isolated from dogs with otitis externa. J Clin Microbiol. 2000;38(6):2383-2385.
14. Shokri H, Khosravi A, Rad M, et al. Occurrence of *Malassezia* species in Persian and domestic short hair cats with and without otitis externa. J Vet Med Sci. 2010;72(3):293-296.
15. Scott DW, Miller WH, Griffin CE. Bacterial skin diseases. In: Muller and Kirk's Small Animal Dermatology. 6th ed. Philadelphia, PA: WB Saunders; 2001:274-335.
16. Volk AV, Belyavin CE, Varjonen K, et al. *Malassezia pachydermatis* and *M. nana* predominate amongst the cutaneous mycobiota of Sphynx cats. J Fel Med Surg. 2010;2(12):917-922.
17. Sierra P, Guillot J, Jacob H, et al. Fungal flora on cutaneous and mucosal surfaces of cats infected with feline immunodeficiency virus or feline leukemia virus. Am J Vet Res. 2000;61(2):158-161.
18. Perrins N, Gaudiano F, Bond R. Carriage of *Malassezia* spp. yeasts in cats with diabetes mellitus, hyperthyroidism and neoplasia. Med Mycol. 2007;45(6):541-546.
19. Plant JD, Rosenkrantz WS, Griffin CE. Factors associated with and prevalence of high *Malassezia pachydermatis* numbers on dog skin. J Am Vet Med Assoc. 1992;201(6):879-882.
20. Coutinho SD, Paula CR. Proteinase, phospholipase, hyaluronidase and chondroitin-sulphatase production by *Malassezia pachydermatis*. Med Mycol. 2000;38(1):73-76.
21. Bond R, Curtis CF, Hendricks A, et al. Intradermal test reactivity to *Malassezia pachydermatis* in atopic dogs. Vet Rec. 2002;150(14):448-449.
22. Kim HJ, Kim ET, Lim CY, et al. The immunoglobulin G response to *Malassezia pachydermatis* extracts in atopic and non-atopic dogs. Can Vet J. 2010;51(8):869-872.
23. White SD, Bourdeau P, Blumstein P, et al. Comparison via cytology and culture of carriage of *Malassezia pachydermatis* in atopic and healthy dogs. In: Kwochka KW, Willemse T, von Tscharner C, eds. Advances in Veterinary Dermatology. vol. 3. Oxford, UK: Butterworth Heinemann; 1998:292-298.
24. Negre A, Bensignor E, Guillot J. Evidence-based veterinary dermatology: a systematic review of interventions for *Malassezia* dermatitis in dogs. Vet Dermatol. 2009;20(1):1-12.
25. Morris DO. *Malassezia pachydermatis* carriage in dog owners. Emerg Infect Dis. 2005;11(1):83-88.
26. Ginel PJ, Lucena R, Rodriguez JC, et al. A semiquantitative cytological evaluation of normal and pathological samples from the external ear canal of dogs and cats. Vet Dermatol. 2002;13(3):151-156.
27. Nijima M, Kano R, Nagata M, et al. An azole-resistant isolate of *Malassezia pachydermatis*. Vet Microbiol. 2011;149:288-290.
28. Maynard L, Rème CA, Viaud S. Comparison of two shampoos for the treatment of *Malassezia* dermatitis: a randomised controlled trial. J Small Anim Pract. 2011;52:566-572.
29. Rosales MS, Marsella R, Kunkle G, et al. Comparison of the clinical efficacy of oral terbinafine and ketoconazole combined with cephalexin in the treatment of *Malassezia* dermatitis in dogs—a pilot study. Vet Dermatol. 2005;16(3):171-176.
30. Sickafoose L, Hosgood G, Snook T, et al. A noninferiority clinical trial comparing fluconazole and ketoconazole in combination with cephalexin for the treatment of dogs with *Malassezia* dermatitis. Vet Ther. 2010;11(2):E1-E13.
31. Berger DJ, Lewis TP, Schick AE, et al. Comparison of once-daily versus twice-weekly terbinafine administration for the treatment of canine *Malassezia* dermatitis – a pilot study. Vet Dermatol. 2012;23:418–e79.
32. Tragiannidis A, Bisping G, Koehler G, et al. Minireview: *Malassezia* infections in immunocompromised patients. Mycoses. 2010;53(3):187-195.
33. Dankner WM, Spector SA, Fierer J, et al. *Malassezia* fungemia in neonates and adults: complication of hyperalimentation. Rev Infect Dis. 1987;9(4):743-753.
34. Chryssanthou E, Broberger U, Petrini B. *Malassezia pachydermatis* fungaemia in a neonatal intensive care unit. Acta Paediatr. 2001;90(3):323-327.
35. Larocco M, Dorenbaum A, Robinson A, et al. Recovery of *Malassezia pachydermatis* from eight infants in a neonatal intensive care nursery: clinical and laboratory features. Pediatr Infect Dis J. 1988;7(6):398-401.
36. Chang HJ, Miller HL, Watkins N, et al. An epidemic of *Malassezia pachydermatis* in an intensive care nursery associated with colonization of health care workers' pet dogs. N Engl J Med. 1998;338(11):706-711.

CHAPTER 60

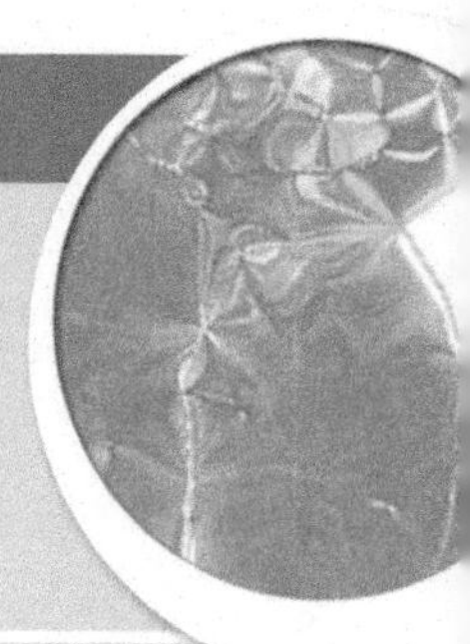

Blastomycosis

Jane E. Sykes and Lindsay K. Merkel

Overview of Blastomycosis

First Described: 1894, in the United States by Thomas Casper Gilchrist.[1] The organism was initially mistaken for a protozoan parasite.

Cause: *Blastomyces dermatitidis* (an ascomycete, teleomorph *Ajellomyces dermatitidis*)

Affected Hosts: Primarily humans and dogs, but also other mammalian species that include cats, horses, ferrets, and sea lions

Geographic Distribution: Primarily North America, especially the south-central and upper midwestern states of the United States; Canadian provinces that border the Great Lakes; and a small area of the northeastern United States and southeastern Canada near the St. Lawrence river

Mode of Transmission: Inhalation of conidia from the environment; rarely cutaneous inoculation

Major Clinical Signs: Fever, inappetence, weight loss, cough, tachypnea, respiratory difficulty, nodular or ulcerative cutaneous lesions, ocular lesions (uveitis, chorioretinitis, panophthalmitis), lameness, neurologic signs

Differential Diagnoses: Neoplasia, other deep mycoses, protothecosis, mycobacterial infections, systemic protozoal infections (leishmaniasis, toxoplasmosis, neosporosis), aspiration or foreign body pneumonia

Human Health Significance: *B. dermatitidis* causes disease in humans, but direct transmission from animals to humans does not occur (with the exception of rare bite wound transmission from infected dogs). Dogs are a sentinel for human exposure.

Etiology and Epidemiology

Blastomyces dermatitidis is a dimorphic fungus that grows as a mycelial form in the environment and as a thick-walled budding yeast in tissues (at 37°C). Hyphae within soil produce conidia that are 2 to 10 μm in diameter. The conidia are thought to be aerosolized and inhaled by the host, where they transform into yeasts and produce a localized pulmonary or disseminated disease known as blastomycosis (Figure 60-1). The organism's name *(dermatitidis)* stems from the fact that the skin is a common site to which the organism disseminates.

B. dermatitidis is primarily found in the eastern parts of the United States, especially around the Great Lakes, along the Ohio and Mississippi river valleys, and in the southeastern states (Figure 60-2). A smaller focus of endemicity exists in the St. Lawrence river region in the northeast, which extends up into Ontario, Canada. Disease may also be seen in parts of Canada around the Great Lakes and has also been reported from Saskatchewan.[2,3] Occasionally disease appears in nontraveled dogs that reside in non-endemic parts of the United States, such as in Wyoming and South Dakota. Canine blastomycosis has also been reported from India.[4] Human blastomycosis occurs in Africa, but a different serotype is involved. Interestingly, reports of canine disease from Africa are absent from the literature. Blastomycosis was described in Europe in a dog with a travel history to the United States.[5]

The ecologic niche of *B. dermatitidis* appears to be warm, moist, sandy soil that is rich in organic debris such as decaying vegetation. However, this has not been thoroughly defined because the fungus is difficult to isolate from the environment. No consistent seasonality has been linked to disease. Genetic differences have been reported among isolates of *B. dermatitidis* within the United States. Using PCR-based typing methods, several different genotypes have been described (A, B, C, D, and E).[6] Analysis by microsatellite typing suggests the existence of at least two genetically distinct groups, group 1 and group 2, the geographic distributions of which overlap.[7] In human patients, group 2 isolates may be more likely to be associated with disease in older patients with comorbid conditions, and group 2 isolates are also more likely to be associated with dissemination than group 1 isolates.[8]

Young adult, large-breed (>15 kg) dogs are predisposed to blastomycosis, and a slight male predisposition has been

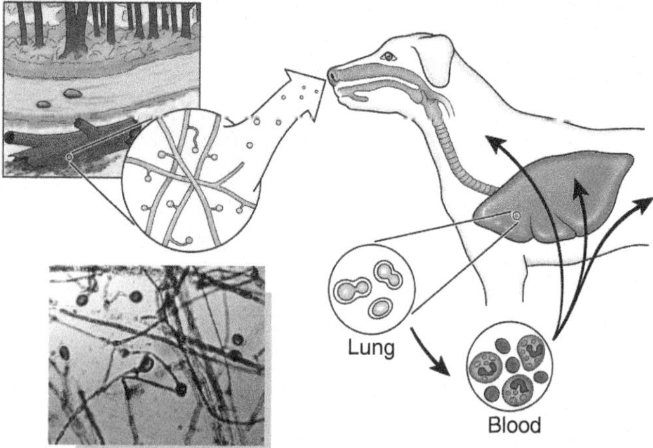

FIGURE 60-1 Life cycle of *Blastomyces dermatitidis*. From the lung, the organism can disseminate to a variety of tissues, but especially the eye, lymph nodes, skin, and bones.

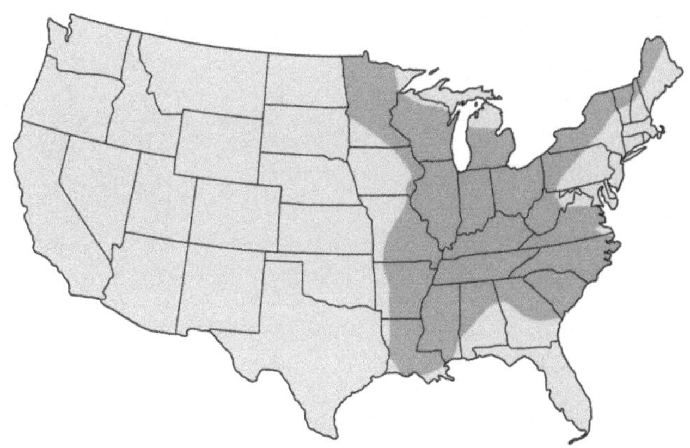

FIGURE 60-2 Approximate geographic distribution of *Blastomyces dermatitidis* in the United States.

identified in some studies.[9] Overrepresented breeds include coonhounds, pointers, Weimaraners, Labrador retrievers, golden retrievers, and Doberman pinschers.[9,10] This may reflect the increased likelihood of exposure of these dog types to organisms in the environment, because they are more likely to be used in outdoor activities such as hunting. Dogs younger than 6 months of age and as old as 17 years may be affected, but dogs in the 2- to 4-year age group have the highest risk of infection with the 4- to 6-year age group a close second.[9,10] Residence less than 400 m from a body of water increased the risk of blastomycosis by a factor of 10 in one study from Louisiana,[10] and exposure to sites of soil disturbance or excavation may also increase the risk of infection. In one report, *B. dermatitidis* was isolated from a woodpile near the Wisconsin River; over 14 years, 4 of 9 dogs housed in a kennel close to the woodpile developed blastomycosis.[11] Most affected dogs are immunocompetent. Blastomycosis is rarely reported in cats from endemic regions of the United States and, as with other soil-borne mycoses such as histoplasmosis and cryptococcosis, blastomycosis can occur in cats that have been housed entirely indoors.[12,13] In one study, 10% of 41 affected cats tested positive for FeLV antigen.[14]

Clinical Features

Signs and Their Pathogenesis

Infection most often results from inhalation of conidia in the environment. Direct inoculation of organisms followed by localized cutaneous disease and/or osteomyelitis *(inoculation blastomycosis)* occurs rarely in dogs and human patients.[15,16] Once within the host, the conidia transform into yeasts that can resist destruction by neutrophils. The yeasts trigger a pyogranulomatous inflammatory response. Important virulence factors include a cell surface glycoprotein known as BAD-1 (previously known as WI-1), and other cell wall components such as α-1,3-glucan and possibly melanin.[17,18] BAD-1 is an adhesin that binds to host cell receptors on macrophages. It may also contribute to the yeast's ability to evade the host immune response by influencing cytokine secretion and impairing complement activation.[17,19] In some animals, the organism spreads hematogenously from the lungs to associated lymph nodes and other extrapulmonary sites. Extrapulmonary sites of predilection include the skin, eye, bone, reproductive tissues (prostate and testes), and the central nervous system (CNS). However,

TABLE 60-1

Physical Examination Findings in 115 Dogs with Blastomycosis[9]

Clinical Sign	Percent of Dogs
Fever	62
Lymphadenopathy	56
Harsh lung sounds	50
Skin lesions	49
Chorioretinitis	43
Anterior uveitis	42
Cough	32
Emaciation	25
Retinal detachment	23
Cutaneous mass	16
Glaucoma	16
Tachypnea	16
Dehydration	15
Bony mass/swelling	14
Nasal discharge	8
Neurologic signs	6
Prostatomegaly	5
Mammary mass	3
Orchitis	2
Synovial effusion	2

virtually any tissue in the body may be affected, and infection has been reported in the mammary glands, nasal or oral cavities, cardiac tissues (myocardium, endocardium, and pericardium), and very rarely in the kidneys, liver, spleen, peritoneum, gastrointestinal tract, and urinary bladder.[20]

Clinical signs are variable. Dogs may develop subclinical infections, acute or chronic disease that is localized to the lungs and associated lymph nodes, or severe and progressive signs that result from dissemination of the organism to multiple extrapulmonary sites. The incubation period is variable and not precisely known, but is estimated to range from 5 to 12 weeks. Nonspecific signs of illness such as lethargy, weakness, fever, inappetence, and weight loss are common (Table 60-1). Other common clinical manifestations (between 20% and 50% of affected dogs) include signs of respiratory involvement (such as cough and increased respiratory rate), lymphadenopathy, ocular manifestations, cutaneous lesions, and lameness.[10,21] Lameness may result from fungal osteomyelitis, arthritis, or rarely, hypertrophic osteopathy.[22] Gastrointestinal signs (vomiting, diarrhea, hematemesis, and melena); polyuria or polydipsia; mammary gland masses; laryngeal masses; nasal discharge, sneezing and/or epistaxis; testicular masses; dysuria or hematuria secondary to prostatic involvement; cardiac arrhythmias; and neurologic signs due to meningoencephalitis or ependymitis occur less frequently.[10,23-29] Neurologic involvement secondary to extension of intranasal or retrobulbar *Blastomyces* granulomas through the calvarium can also occur.[25,29] Rarely, thromboembolic disease has been reported.[30]

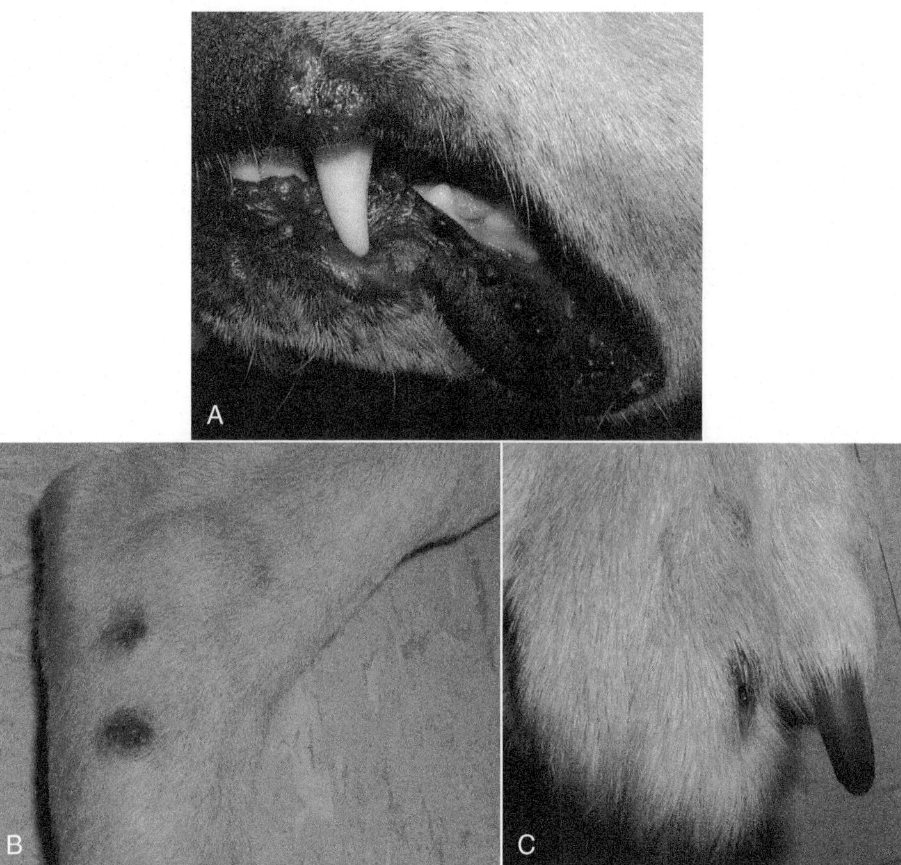

FIGURE 60-3 Disseminated blastomycosis in a labrador retriever. Nodular cutaneous lesions are present on the muzzle (**A**). There are also multiple, ulcerated, and draining skin lesions on the distal limbs (**B**) and digit (**C**). (Courtesy Dr. Sheila Torres, University of Minnesota.)

In cats, clinical signs of blastomycosis are similar to those in dogs, although neurologic and gastrointestinal involvement may be more prevalent.[31]

Physical Examination Findings

Physical examination abnormalities in dogs with blastomycosis commonly include fever, thin body condition, dehydration, and signs of respiratory involvement. Fever is present in approximately 50% of affected dogs and is usually low grade (103°F to 104°F or 39.4°C to 40.0°C) but occasionally exceeds 106°F (41.1°C).[20,27] Respiratory signs include cough, tachypnea, increased respiratory effort, and increased lung sounds on thoracic auscultation. Other common findings on physical examination are firm cutaneous or subcutaneous masses, draining or ulcerated skin lesions, and peripheral lymphadenopathy. Careful palpation of the entire skin surface can reveal small skin lesions. Cutaneous and subcutaneous lesions are frequently found on the trunk, limbs, and digits and can also involve the muzzle (Figure 60-3). Lesions of the tongue, gingiva, or mucocutaneous junctions may also be present (Figure 60-4). Facial swelling, exophthalmos, or facial deformity has been described in some affected dogs.[25,32] Dogs with nasal cavity involvement can have stertorous respiration, decreased nasal airflow, or nasal discharge. Ocular signs may be unilateral or bilateral and include chorioretinitis (sometimes with retinal detachment); lesions consistent with optic neuritis; endophthalmitis or panophthalmitis; uveitis with aqueous flare, iris bombé, synechia, and miosis; cataract formation; conjunctivitis; keratitis;

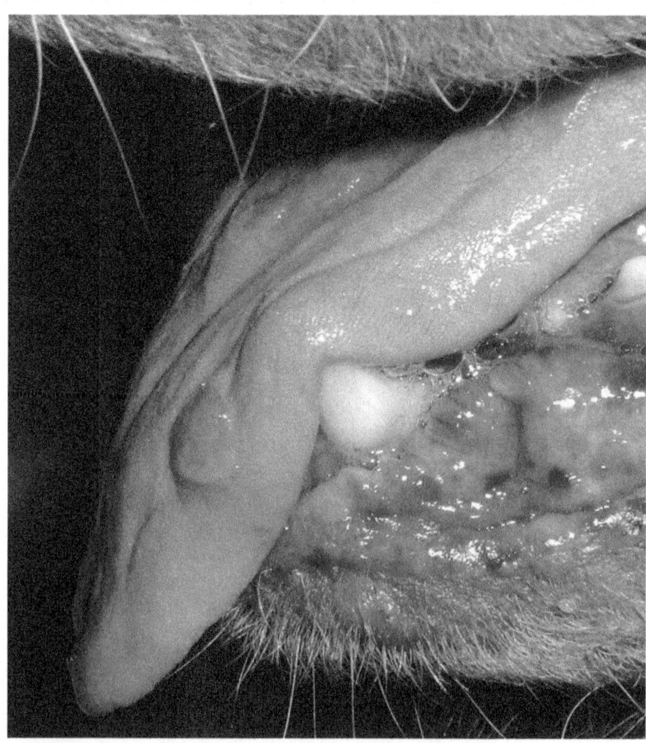

FIGURE 60-4 Nodular and ulcerated lesions of the tongue in a dog with disseminated blastomycosis. (Courtesy Dr. Sheila Torres, University of Minnesota.)

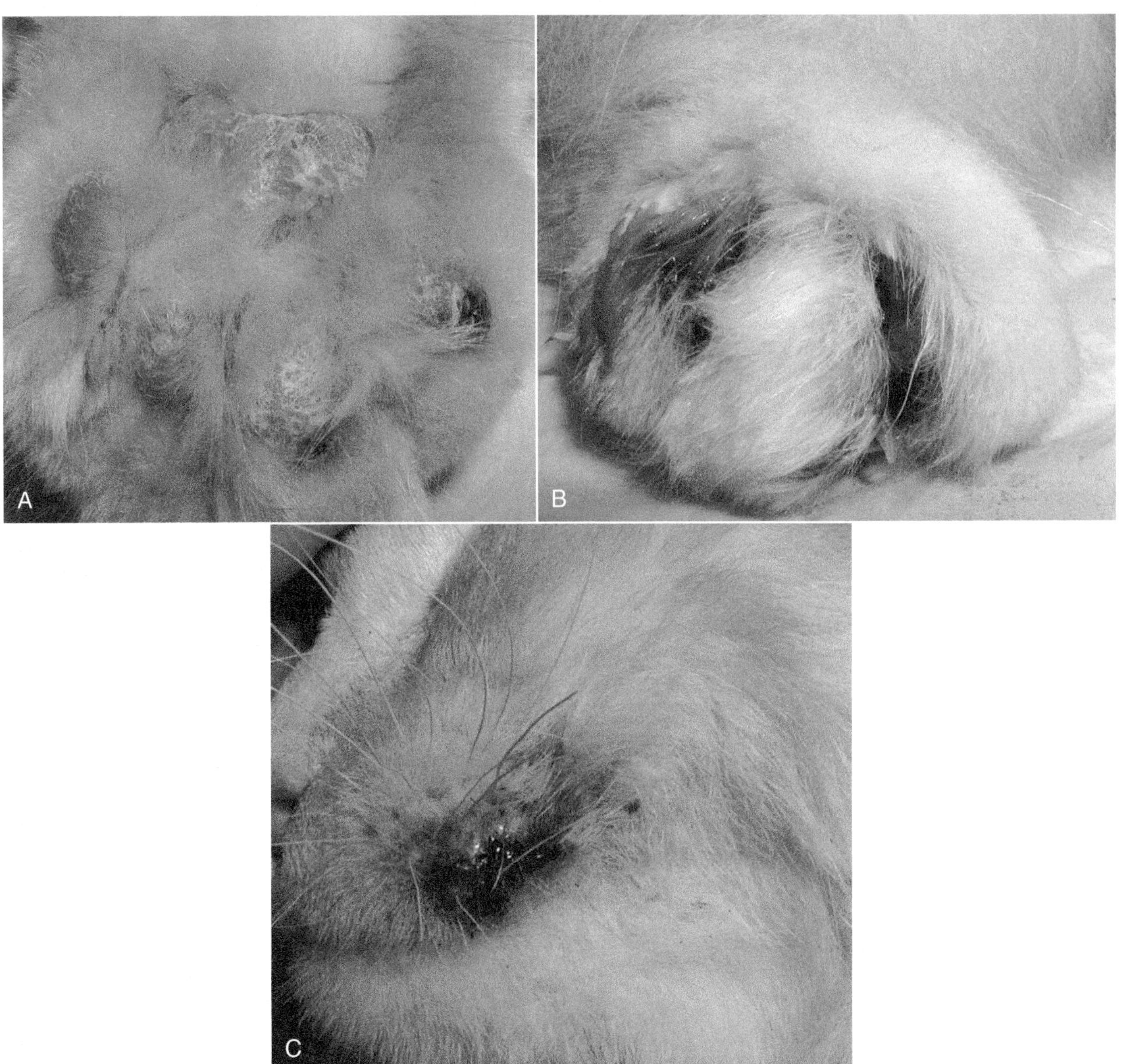

FIGURE 60-5 Cutaneous lesions in a cat with disseminated blastomycosis that involved the footpads **(A)**, interdigital folds **(B)**, and lips **(C)**. (Courtesy Dr. Sheila Torres, University of Minnesota.)

and photophobia.[33,34] Severe ocular involvement may result in increased intraocular pressures and/or loss of vision. Dogs with musculoskeletal involvement may be lame, have firm swellings associated with long bones, or exhibit joint swelling, warmth, and/or pain. Dogs with testicular blastomycosis may have scrotal swelling or palpable testicular masses. Neurologic signs are present in fewer than 5% of affected dogs and can include seizures, hypermetria, decreased placing reactions, tetraparesis, circling, ataxia, blindness, decreased or absent menace and/or pupillary light reflexes, nystagmus, and decreased facial sensation.

Physical examination findings in cats with blastomycosis are similar to those described in dogs. These include fever, thin body condition, peripheral lymphadenopathy, tachypnea, increased or decreased lung sounds, ocular abnormalities (chorioretinitis with retinal detachment, uveitis, panophthalmitis, and secondary glaucoma), nodular or draining skin lesions (Figure 60-5), and a variety of neurologic signs that include obtundation, ataxia, pelvic limb paresis, circling, hyperesthesia, decreased placing reactions, and blindness.[13,31,35-37]

Diagnosis

A diagnosis of blastomycosis is usually suspected based on the presence of suspicious clinicopathologic abnormalities in a dog or cat from an endemic area. The diagnosis is usually confirmed through cytologic examination of fine needle aspirates of affected tissues (especially skin lesions and lymph nodes), impression smears of draining skin lesions, respiratory lavage specimens (transtracheal washes or bronchoalveolar lavage), or body fluids (especially CSF or ocular fluid, but also synovial fluid or urine sediment). Other methods of diagnosis include histopathology (e.g., of bone or tissue biopsies), fungal culture, and PCR-based assays (Table 60-2). Serologic assays that detect antigen and antibody are also available, but when used alone, these do not confirm a diagnosis of blastomycosis.

TABLE 60-2

Diagnostic Assays Currently Available for Blastomycosis in Dogs and Cats

Assay	Specimen Type	Target	Performance
Cytologic examination	Aspirates of affected tissues, body fluids, impression smears of skin lesions	*Blastomyces dermatitidis* yeasts	Organisms are usually present in variable numbers but occasionally may not be visualized. Organisms may appear disrupted after treatment with antifungal drugs.
Fungal culture	Aspirates or biopsies of affected tissues, body fluids	*B. dermatitidis*	Rarely indicated. Sensitive and specific and may be required for animals when cytologic examination is negative. Risk of laboratory-acquired infections. Slow turnaround time (may require several weeks of incubation).
Antibody serology (gel ID)	Serum	Antibodies to *B. dermatitidis*	When present in conjunction with consistent clinical signs, positive test results usually indicate active infection, but the potential for false positives exists. Negative test results occur commonly in dogs and cats with blastomycosis (low sensitivity).
Antigen assay (ELISA)	Urine, serum	*B. dermatitidis* antigen	Highly sensitive (>90%) when urine is used as the test specimen. False positives are extremely rare in dogs that lack fungal disease, but cross-reactivity with other fungal pathogens may occur (especially *Histoplasma*), so positive results are not diagnostic for blastomycosis.
Real-time PCR assays	Whole blood	*B. dermatitidis* DNA	Not yet validated in adequate numbers of dogs or cats with blastomycosis; usefulness requires further evaluation.
Histopathology	Biopsy specimens from affected tissues	*B. dermatitidis* yeasts	Sensitive, but yeasts may be difficult to find in some infections. Special stains may assist organism detection.

Laboratory Abnormalities

Complete Blood Count

The hemogram of dogs or cats with blastomycosis can be unremarkable. However, a mild, normocytic, normochromic nonregenerative anemia is present in many affected animals. Mild to moderate neutrophilia is also present in many dogs and may be accompanied by a mild to moderate bandemia.[10,38] Mild monocytosis, lymphocytosis, or lymphopenia may be detected.

Serum Biochemical Tests

Serum biochemistry findings in animals with blastomycosis include mild to moderate hyperglobulinemia due to a polyclonal gammopathy, hypoalbuminemia, and, uncommonly, mild hypercalcemia.[10,38] Hypoalbuminemia was present in 70 of 91 (77%) of dogs in one study, hyperglobulinemia in 58%, and hypercalcemia in 14% of dogs.[10]

Urinalysis

The urinalysis is usually unremarkable in animals with blastomycosis, but occasionally proteinuria, pyuria, hematuria, or cylindruria are present. Rarely, *B. dermatitidis* yeasts are identified in the sediment.

Cerebrospinal Fluid Analysis

CSF analysis in dogs with CNS blastomycosis can reveal increased total nucleated cell counts and increased CSF protein concentration.[39] Nucleated cells typically consist of a mixture of small and large mononuclear cells and neutrophils.

Diagnostic Imaging

Plain Radiography

Radiographic patterns in dogs with blastomycosis vary considerably and include unstructured, miliary, or nodular interstitial patterns; a bronchointerstitial pattern; alveolar or mixed alveolar-interstitial patterns; pulmonary mass lesions (>3 cm in diameter); or single or multiple large (0.5 to 2.9 cm) pulmonary nodules that can resemble metastatic pulmonary neoplasia (Figure 60-6).[10,40,41] Tracheobronchial lymphadenopathy is present in approximately 25% of dogs.[40] Pleural thickening and mild pleural effusion are uncommonly identified (≤10% of

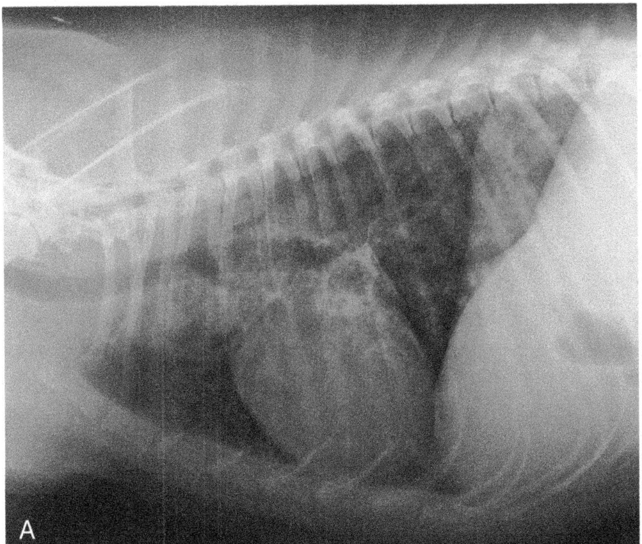

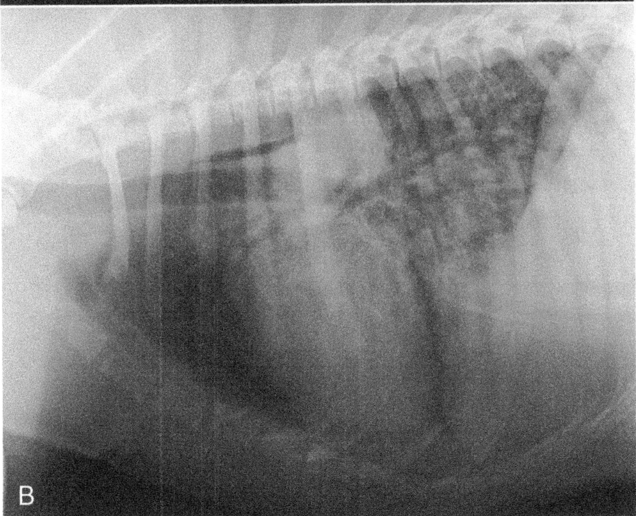

FIGURE 60-6 Radiographic patterns in pulmonary blastomycosis. **A**, Lateral thoracic radiograph from a 2-year-old female spayed Labrador retriever with a 1-week history of cough and inappetence. A diffuse miliary nodular interstitial pattern is present. **B**, Lateral thoracic radiograph from a 5-year-old female spayed German shepherd dog with lethargy and inappetence. An alveolar pattern is present in the caudal lung lobes, along with marked hilar lymphadenopathy. There is also a nodular lesion in the cranial lung lobes just ventral to the trachea. (Courtesy Daniel Cronk, University of Minnesota.)

affected dogs). Focal bronchiectasis has also been described. In one study, only 2 of 125 dogs with blastomycosis had no visible abnormalities on thoracic radiography. Findings in affected cats include diffuse miliary or nodular interstitial patterns, lobar consolidation, and/or pleural effusion.[13,31]

Radiographs of affected bone typically show osteolysis, often accompanied by periosteal proliferation and soft tissue swelling. Pathologic fractures may be identified (Figure 60-7). Evidence of hypertrophic osteopathy was present bilaterally along the humerus, radius, ulna, metacarpi, and phalanges of a dog with a mass lesion in the right middle lung lobe.[22]

Advanced Imaging

Computed tomographic findings in dogs with CNS blastomycosis include intra-axial, intranasal, or retrobulbar mass lesions that are uniformly or heterogeneously contrast enhancing.[25] An intra-axial contrast-enhancing mass lesion was also described in a cat.[42] Intranasal or retrobulbar mass lesions can invade the cribriform plate or other parts of the skull, with associated osteolysis. Meningeal or periventricular contrast enhancement may also be present.[25,26] MRI findings have not been extensively described. One dog had a retrobulbar mass lesion that extended through the calvarium; the lesion was iso- to hypointense on T2-weighted images, slightly hypointense on T1-weighted images, and showed strong homogenous contrast enhancement.[29]

Microbiologic Tests

Cytologic Examination

Cytologic examination of fine-needle aspirates, respiratory wash specimens, or body fluids frequently reveals large numbers of *B. dermatitidis* yeasts. The yeasts are 8 to 15 μm in diameter, have a thick, refractile cell wall, and exhibit broad-based budding (Figure 60-8). Daughter cells are nearly as large as the parent cell when they detach. A pyogranulomatous inflammatory response is usually present. Occasionally, organisms are not seen; the sensitivity of transtracheal lavage for diagnosis of pulmonary blastomycosis in two studies of 17 and 39 dogs was 76% and 69%,[38,41] whereas the sensitivity of fine-needle aspiration of the lung was 46 of 57 (81%).[38]

Serologic Diagnosis

Serologic assays that detect antibody and those that detect *B. dermatitidis* antigen are available on a commercial basis in North America. The most widely available antibody assay uses gel immunodiffusion (ID) (see Chapter 2), which detects antibodies to the *B. dermatitidis* A antigen. Unfortunately, gel ID assays have variable and generally unacceptable sensitivity for diagnosis of blastomycosis in dogs and cats, which has ranged from 17% to 91%.[10,31,38,43-45] An enzyme immunoassay that used crude mold-phase *B. dermatitidis* as the antigen had a sensitivity of 76.1%,[43] and a radioimmunoassay designed to detect antibody responses to the BAD-1 antigen had a sensitivity of 92%.[45] The specificity of the gel ID assay exceeds 95% based on limited studies of healthy dogs or dogs with diagnoses other than blastomycosis.[44,45] However, because false-positive test results have the potential to occur as a result of exposure and recovery in endemic areas or as a result of cross-reactivity to other infectious agents, diagnosis based on positive antibody serology alone is not recommended.

An assay that detects *Blastomyces* cell wall galactomannan antigen (MiraVista Diagnostics, Indianapolis, IN) has largely replaced antibody assays for serologic diagnosis of canine blastomycosis. The performance of this assay was evaluated in 46 dogs with confirmed blastomycosis.[43] When urine was used, the sensitivity was 93.5%, whereas when serum was assayed, sensitivity was 87%. Only 1 of 43 control dogs without blastomycosis had a positive test result. In human patients, the sensitivity of urine galactomannan antigen testing was 90%, and specificity was 99% in patients without fungal infections. However, 96% of humans with histoplasmosis tested positive as a result of cross-reactivity.[46] Positive test results can also occur in dogs and cats that have histoplasmosis, although the extent to which this occurs requires further study. It is possible that cross-reactivity may also occur when other mycoses are present.

Fungal Culture

B. dermatitidis can be isolated from clinical specimens on routine fungal media in the laboratory. Growth of a white mold

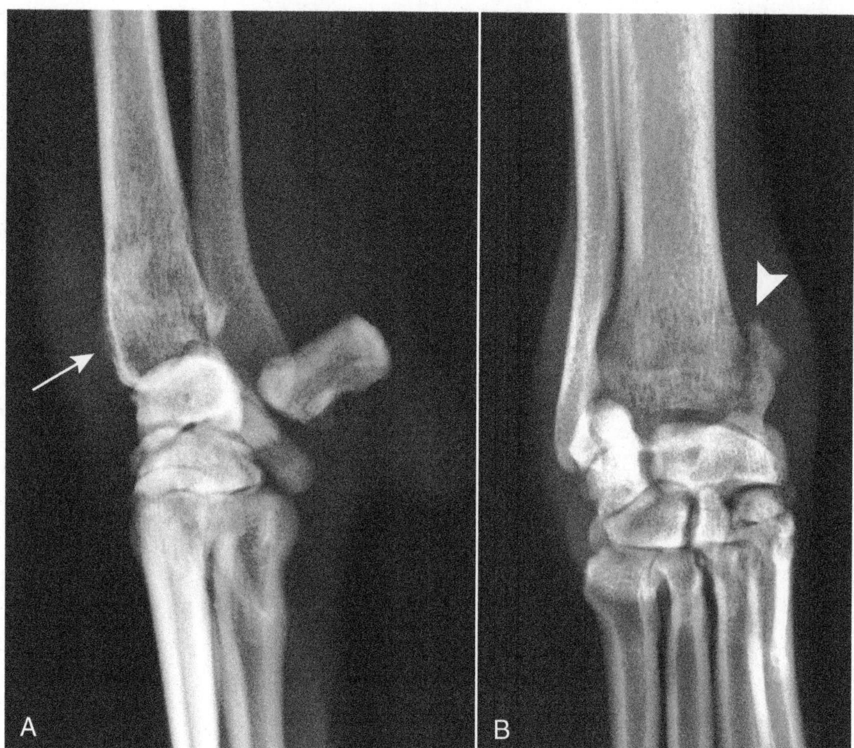

FIGURE 60-7 Lateral **(A)** and anteropalmar **(B)** radiograph of the right carpus showing an osteolytic and osteoproductive *(small arrow)* lesion with a pathologic fracture *(arrowhead)* and associated soft tissue swelling in the distal radius of a 6-year-old male neutered Labrador retriever with disseminated blastomycosis. (Image courtesy Daniel Cronk, University of Minnesota.)

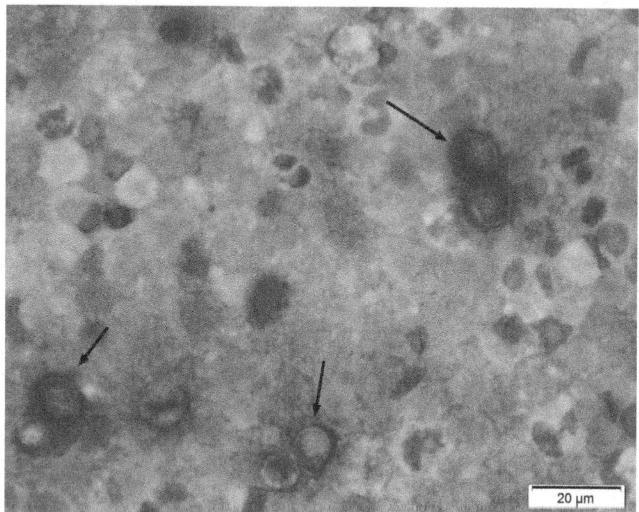

FIGURE 60-8 Cytology of a fine-needle aspirate of a skin lesion from a dog with blastomycosis. *Blastomyces* yeasts *(arrows)* have a thick wall and exhibit broad-based budding. A pyogranulomatous inflammatory response is also present. (Image courtesy Dr. Jed Overmann, University of Minnesota.)

typically appears after incubation for 1 to 3 weeks, but occasionally incubation periods of up to 5 weeks are required. The organism is identified based on the morphology of its conidia, which are round to oval and attached to hyphae (see Figure 60-1). Because *B. dermatitidis* grows as a mycelium in the laboratory, culture is a laboratory health hazard and should be performed only if necessary. The laboratory should be warned of the possibility of a dimorphic fungal infection, so that appropriate precautions are taken.

Molecular Diagnosis Using the Polymerase Chain Reaction

Real-time PCR assays have been developed that rapidly detect *B. dermatitidis* in clinical specimens from humans,[47,48] but are not currently used routinely for diagnosis in dogs and cats. The sensitivity of one assay was 86% when compared with culture of clinical specimens.[48] PCR assays have not been widely applied to the diagnosis of blastomycosis in dogs and cats.

Pathologic Findings

Gross pathologic findings in dogs with blastomycosis include thin body condition; characteristic skin lesions; bony proliferations that may be accompanied by pathologic fracture; enlargement of the peripheral and/or tracheobronchial lymph nodes; ocular lesions; lung consolidation; and firm, pale, pulmonary nodules or masses that range in size from 1 mm to several centimeters in diameter. Masses may be caseous on cut surface. Animals with CNS involvement may have masses within the brain, secondary hydrocephalus, or retrobulbar or caudal nasal cavity granulomas that may invade the cribriform plate and extend along optic nerves.[27,39] Rarely, pleural and/or peritoneal effusion and nodular lesions within abdominal viscera have been reported.[20] Testicular and prostatic masses can also be found.[27] Histopathology reveals granulomatous or pyogranulomatous inflammatory infiltrates in a variety of organs, often with intralesional budding yeasts (Figure 60-9). Multinucleated giant cells, fibroblasts, and large numbers of lymphocytes may also be present. Ocular lesions include uveitis, choroiditis, retinal detachment, retinal degeneration, lens rupture, cataracts, optic

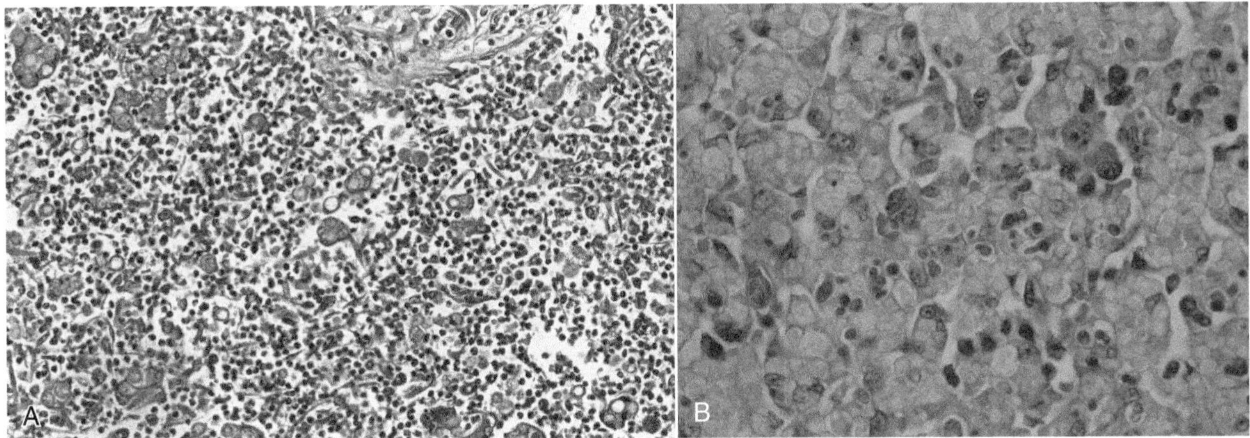

FIGURE 60-9 Histopathologic findings in dogs with blastomycosis. **A,** Histopathology of the lymph node from a 10-year-old female spayed Australian shepherd dog with blastomycosis. Severe pyogranulomatous lymphadenitis is present with moderate numbers of large yeast organisms. (Image courtesy Dr. Catherine Benson, University of Minnesota.) **B,** Histopathology of the lung of another Australian shepherd dog that had a pulmonary and a mediastinal abscess due to *Blastomyces dermatitidis*. Abundant yeast organisms are present. 1000x oil magnification. (Image courtesy Dr. Patricia Pesavento, University of California, Davis.)

neuritis, and vitritis.[27,34] Secondary hepatic and renal amyloidosis was described in one dog.[49]

Organisms are not always detected in lesions, even in untreated dogs. Special stains such as silver stains, periodic acid–Schiff, and immunohistochemical stains can assist in the identification of *B. dermatitidis* yeasts within sections,[34,49,50] but failure to detect yeasts does not rule out blastomycosis.

Treatment and Prognosis

Antimicrobial Treatment

The most widely used treatment for blastomycosis in dogs is itraconazole, which is effective as a single agent in many dogs.[38,51] Itraconazole has largely replaced the use of ketoconazole for treatment of blastomycosis. The recommended dose of itraconazole for dogs is 5 mg/kg PO q24h. This dose has an equivalent efficacy as a dose of 5 mg/kg PO q12h and a lower rate of adverse effects such as anorexia.[51] The duration of azole treatment should be based on serial monitoring of clinical signs and radiographic lesions (e.g., every 4 to 8 weeks). Most dogs require at least 3 to 6 months of treatment, and some dogs require treatment for more than 1 year, especially those with osteoarticular infections or widespread dissemination. Because fluconazole is less active, its use is not recommended for treatment of human blastomycosis, unless itraconazole is not tolerated.[52] Treatment with deoxycholate amphotericin B or lipid-complexed amphotericin B is also effective and could be considered for dogs with severe disease with widespread dissemination, for animals that do not respond to azole mono therapy, or for those that do not tolerate itraconazole (see Box 9-1).[38,53] Cats with blastomycosis have also been treated with variable success with combinations of amphotericin B and azoles or amphotericin B alone.[13,31] In human patients, the use of deoxycholate or lipid-complexed amphotericin B is recommended for severe pulmonary or disseminated disease, followed by step-down itraconazole therapy after there has been a satisfactory clinical response.[52] Whether protocols that include amphotericin B offer a survival advantage over azole monotherapy for dogs or cats has not been well studied in a prospective fashion. Other drugs that have been used successfully to treat human blastomycosis include voriconazole and posaconazole.[54,55] Because of its ability to penetrate the CNS and eye, voriconazole has been recommended for treatment of human CNS blastomycosis after initial treatment with lipid-complexed amphotericin B.[55]

Urine *Blastomyces* galactomannan antigen concentration declines with effective antifungal drug treatment.[43] It is not yet clear whether treatment should be continued until antigenuria is undetectable when radiographic lesions resolve earlier. It is possible that the immune system of some dogs may continue to clear antigen even after treatment is discontinued.

Supportive Care

Other treatments that may be required for treatment of dogs or cats with severe pulmonary blastomycosis are supplemental oxygen, nebulization and coupage, intravenous fluid therapy, and, in some cases, mechanical ventilation.[38] Mechanical ventilation was used to treat 5 (4%) of 125 dogs with pulmonary blastomycosis in one report, none of which survived.[38] Dogs with CNS involvement may require treatment with anticonvulsants in order to control seizure activity. The concurrent use of systemic glucocorticoids should also be considered to control brain inflammation and edema, although whether this ultimately improves outcome is not known. For animals that lack CNS involvement, NSAIDs can be used to control pyrexia. Topical anti-inflammatory and antiglaucoma agents may be indicated if ocular involvement is present. Enucleation may ultimately be required if endophthalmitis is present to control ocular pain and eliminate infection. Treatment of osteomyelitis or large pulmonary granulomas that are refractory to antifungal chemotherapy may require surgical treatment by amputation or lung lobectomy, respectively.

Prognosis

Cure rates of 50% to 75% have been reported in dogs with blastomycosis.[51,56] An additional 20% of dogs experience relapse of disease after treatment is discontinued.[51] Clinical signs and radiographic lesions can worsen in the first few days of treatment in some affected dogs,[40] possibly as a result of the inflammatory response to dying organisms. The median time for resolution of primary radiographic patterns in dogs with

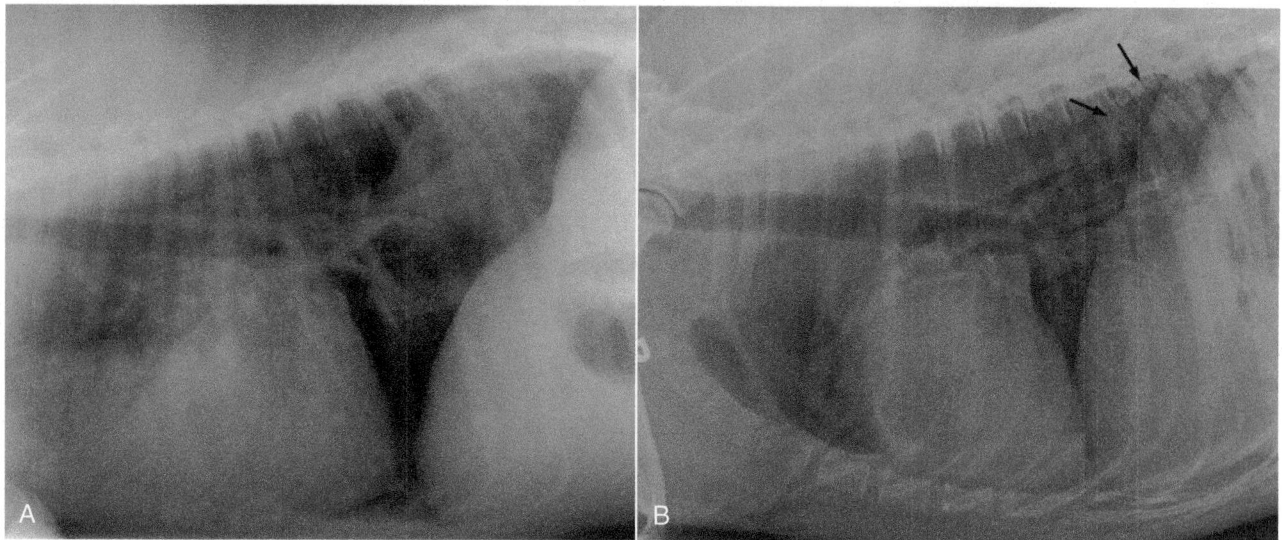

FIGURE 60-10 Lateral thoracic radiographs from a young adult male neutered golden retriever with blastomycosis. **A,** A nodular soft tissue pattern is present diffusely throughout all lung lobes, which coalesces to alveolar infiltrates in the left caudal lung lobe and right cranial lung lobe. **B,** Residual pulmonary infiltrates are present in the right cranial lung lobe after 14 months of itraconazole treatment. There is also a large bulla in the left caudal lung lobe *(arrows)*.

pulmonary blastomycosis in one study was 186 days (range, 4 to >355 days).[40] Significantly longer mean treatment durations were required for radiographic improvement of large pulmonary masses when compared with alveolar and interstitial patterns. The most common radiographic sequela to pulmonary blastomycosis is development of one or more pulmonary bullae. Unstructured interstitial patterns may also persist, presumably as a result of pulmonary fibrosis (Figure 60-10).[40]

Involvement of the CNS, severe lung disease, and a high band neutrophil count are negative prognostic factors.[38,51,56] In one study, the median band neutrophil count in dogs that did not survive was 1200 cells/μL (range, 0 to 3980 cells/μL), whereas that in survivors was 0 cells/μL (range, 0 to 2380 cells/μL).[38] In that study, 63% of 125 dogs with blastomycosis survived. The prognosis for survival in animals with neurologic involvement is particularly poor. The prognosis for resolution of endophthalmitis is also poor; only 20% of eyes with endophthalmitis respond favorably to antifungal drug treatment.[33] Nevertheless, eyes that do not undergo enucleation can ultimately progress to phthisis bulbi after completion of treatment, without recurrence of systemic infection.[33]

Immunity and Vaccination

Immunity to blastomycosis is initially dependent on phagocyte function, especially neutrophils and alveolar macrophages, which can clear conidia. However, once the organisms have transitioned to the yeast form, control of infection also depends on T lymphocytes, which stimulate macrophages to kill the yeasts.[52] Humoral immunity is not essential for resolution of infection. An experimental vaccine that includes a genetically engineered, live-attenuated BAD-1 deletion mutant *B. dermatitidis* strain protected mice from experimental infection, was safe in 25 beagles and 78 foxhounds in a field trial, and induced specific immune responses to *B. dermatitidis* antigens.[57,58] Although further study is required, this vaccine holds promise for prevention of blastomycosis in dogs that reside in hyperendemic regions of the United States.

Prevention

Avoidance of specific foci of hyperendemicity where other dogs or humans have contracted blastomycosis may prevent blastomycosis, but this is not always possible.

Public Health Aspects

Like dogs, humans acquire *B. dermatitidis* infection from the environment. Dogs are considered sentinels for human exposure and infection,[59] although whether strains that infect dogs also infect humans requires further study. The incidence of blastomycosis in dogs is approximately 8 times that in humans, and disease has been reported in humans and dogs that reside in the same household.[59,60] Approximately 50% of human infections are asymptomatic.[52] When illness develops, it typically occurs 30 to 45 days after exposure and is often a mild, self-limiting influenza-like illness with fever and cough. Blastomycosis is suspected in endemic areas when respiratory signs persist and fail to respond to treatment with antibacterial drugs. Radiographic abnormalities resemble those in dogs, although hilar lymphadenopathy is not often seen. Chronic pulmonary blastomycosis can resemble pulmonary neoplasia or tuberculosis. Rarely, blastomycosis-associated acute respiratory distress syndrome (ARDS) develops, which is associated with mortality rates that exceed 50%.[52] Dissemination to extrapulmonary sites similar to those involved in dogs occurs in 20% to 25% of affected humans. Serious infections can occur in immunocompromised patients such as those with AIDS, solid organ transplant recipients, and humans treated with TNF-α blockers (used to treat inflammatory diseases such as Crohn's disease, psoriasis, and rheumatoid arthritis).[52,61,62]

Inoculation blastomycosis that involves the skin and underlying bone has been described in veterinary personnel after sharps injuries or bite wounds from dogs with blastomycosis. One involved a needle-stick injury after a lung aspirate in a dog with suspected blastomycosis, and another was an accident that occurred during a necropsy.[63,64] Bite wounds from dogs with blastomycosis can result in localized disease; disseminated disease occurred in a renal transplant recipient.[65-67] A veterinary technician developed pulmonary blastomycosis after *B. dermatitidis* was cultured unexpectedly in a veterinary clinic in-house laboratory.[68] Although these routes of transmission are rare, prevention of sharps injuries, avoidance and proper management of bite wounds, and use of accredited veterinary laboratories for isolation of microorganisms from dogs and cats may reduce the risk of inoculation or laboratory-acquired blastomycosis in veterinary staff. The bandaging of skin lesions has been discouraged because it has the potential to promote transition of the organism to the mold form, but this has not been documented to occur. The body of deceased pets with blastomycosis should be disposed of promptly and by cremation.

CASE EXAMPLE

Signalment: "Sam," a 3-year-old male neutered golden retriever from Burlingame in northern California

History: Sam was evaluated by the Veterinary Emergency and Critical Care Service at the University of California, Davis, for pulmonary blastomycosis, which had been diagnosed at a local veterinary clinic. Sam had a 1-week history of lethargy and inappetence. The day after illness was noted, Sam was taken to a local veterinary clinic. Routine blood work showed only anemia (hematocrit 34%), thrombocytosis (554,000 platelets/μL), and a mildly increased serum alkaline phosphatase activity (199 U/L). Thoracic radiographs showed hilar lymphadenopathy, a mild diffuse miliary interstitial pattern, and focal alveolar infiltrates in the right cranial and left caudal lung lobe. Cytologic examination of a transtracheal lavage specimen showed pyogranulomatous inflammation with moderate numbers of yeasts that had morphology consistent with *Blastomyces dermatitidis*. Serology (gel immunodiffusion) for detection of antibodies to *B. dermatitidis* was negative. Treatment with itraconazole (5 mg/kg PO q24h) was commenced, and after 2 days the dose was increased to 10 mg/kg PO q24h because of lack of clinical improvement. Subsequently the dog's rectal temperature increased to 105°F (40.6°C) and a day later, radiographs showed an increase in the severity of the alveolar infiltrates. Treatment with carprofen (2.4 mg/kg PO q12h) was initiated, and subcutaneous fluids were administered. This was associated with resolution of pyrexia, but the dog remained lethargic and exercise intolerant and the owners noted right pelvic limb lameness. The dog was referred for further evaluation.

Approximately 6 weeks before he became ill, Sam had been taken to Georgian Bay in Ontario, Canada, for 1 week. He had also been in the Vermont region for 2 months before that time. Other travel had been limited to various bayside and mountainous parts of northern California. The owner's brother's dog, which had traveled with Sam to Ontario and Vermont, had also been diagnosed with blastomycosis 3 weeks earlier.

Physical Examination:

Body Weight: 41.5 kg.

General: Quiet, alert and responsive. T = 103.5°F (39.7°C), HR = 120 beats/min, panting, CRT <2 s, mucous membranes were moist and slightly cyanotic.

Eyes, Ears, Nose, and Throat: No clinically significant abnormalities were detected. A fundoscopic examination with dilated pupils was unremarkable.

Musculoskeletal: BCS 4/9; no obvious lameness or pain on palpation was appreciated.

Respiratory: Increased respiratory effort was present. Lung sounds were increased diffusely on thoracic auscultation and partially obscured the heart sounds. Markedly increased respiratory effort was evident when the dog's gait was assessed as part of an orthopedic examination. An intermittent nonproductive cough was also appreciated.

All Other Systems: No clinically significant abnormalities were detected. No obvious neurologic deficits were noted, but a full neurologic examination was not performed.

Laboratory Findings: Blood oxygen saturation (pulse oximetry) = 91%, improved to 95% with flow-by supplemental oxygen

CBC:

HCT 37.3% (40%-55%)
MCV 71.2 fL (65-75 fL)
MCHC 35.1 g/dL (33-36 g/dL)
WBC 14,640 cells/μL (6000-13,000 cells/μL)
Neutrophils 11,273 cells/μL (3000-10,500 cells/μL)
Band neutrophils 586 cells/μL
Lymphocytes 1318 cells/μL (1000-4000 cells/μL)
Monocytes 1318 cells/μL (150-1200 cells/μL)
Eosinophils 146 cells/μL (0-1500 cells/μL)
Platelets 387,000 platelets/μL (150,000-400,000 platelets/μL)
Rare slight toxicity of band neutrophils was reported.

Serum Chemistry Profile:

Sodium 148 mmol/L (145-154 mmol/L)
Potassium 5.0 mmol/L (4.1-5.3 mmol/L)
Chloride 116 mmol/L (105-116 mmol/L)
Bicarbonate 15 mmol/L (16-26 mmol/L)
Phosphorus 6.6 mg/dL (3.0-6.2 mg/dL)
Calcium 9.9 mg/dL (9.9-11.4 mg/dL)
BUN 11 mg/dL (8-21 mg/dL)
Creatinine 0.5 mg/dL (0.5-1.6 mg/dL)
Glucose 81 mg/dL (60-104 mg/dL)
Total protein 5.6 g/dL (5.4-7.4 g/dL)
Albumin 1.8 g/dL (2.9-4.2 g/dL)
Globulin 3.8 g/dL (2.3-4.4 g/dL)
ALT 15 U/L (19-67 U/L)
AST 32 U/L (21-54 U/L)
ALP 148 U/L (15-127 U/L)
GGT 0 U/L (0-6 U/L)
Cholesterol 318 mg/dL (135-345 mg/dL)
Total bilirubin 0.4 mg/dL (0-0.4 mg/dL).

Urinalysis: SGr 1.015; pH 5.0, no protein (SSA), 1+ bilirubin, no hemoprotein, no glucose, no WBC, rare RBC/HPF, rare transitional epithelial cells, and a few amorphous crystals were seen.

Continued

Imaging Findings:

Thoracic Radiographs: A nodular soft tissue pattern was present diffusely throughout all lung lobes, which coalesced to alveolar infiltrates in the left caudal lung lobe and right cranial lung lobe (see Figure 60-10). The cardiac silhouette was mildly enlarged. Increased soft tissue opacity was noted in the perihilar region.

Abdominal Ultrasound: The spleen was mildly enlarged, and there was mild mesenteric lymphadenopathy.

Diagnosis: Acute, severe pulmonary blastomycosis.

Treatment: Sam was placed in an oxygen cage with an inspired oxygen concentration (FiO_2) of 40% to 60%. An arterial blood gas revealed a pH of 7.301, pCO_2 of 36.6 mm Hg, pO_2 of 79.1 mm Hg, HCO_3 of 16.8 mmol/L, base deficit of 7.8 mmol/L, and measured O_2 saturation of 92.8%. The dog was also treated with crystalloid fluids (lactated Ringer's solution with 20 mEq/L KCl; 80 mL/hr, IV) and nebulization and coupage (q6h). For the first 24 hours, respiratory rate ranged from 90 to 105 breaths/min and a nonproductive cough occurred every few hours. The dog drank water, but was inappetent. Treatment with lipid-complexed amphotericin B was initiated (1 mg/kg IV on a Monday-Wednesday-Friday basis) and carprofen administration continued. By day 4, Sam was afebrile, eating, and oxygen saturation was 96% with an FiO_2 of 46%. However, increased respiratory effort developed when oxygen supplementation was discontinued, and arterial blood gas analysis showed a pH of 7.335, pCO_2 of 27.2 mm Hg, pO_2 of 65.8 mm Hg, HCO_3 of 13.9 mmol/L, and base deficit of 10.6 mmol/L (room air). By day 5, Sam was playing with toys in the oxygen cage, and his appetite was excellent. Treatment with itraconazole (5 mg/kg PO q24h) was resumed in addition to the amphotericin B. By day 8, oxygen saturation was 95% with an FiO_2 of 30%. Thoracic radiographs showed persistent radiographic abnormalities, organization of the alveolar infiltrates, and apparent bronchiectasis. Survey radiographs of the appendicular skeleton showed no evidence of osteomyelitis. The dog was discharged after 11 days of hospitalization (cumulative amphotericin B dose of 6 mg/kg). An additional seven treatments of amphotericin B were then administered at the local veterinary clinic. Serial renal panels showed no evidence of nephrotoxicity.

At a recheck 1 month after the date of first evaluation, Sam remained somewhat lethargic and exercise intolerant, but had gained 3 kg. The frequency of cough had decreased from approximately 8 times a day to once or twice daily over the previous 2 weeks. An arterial blood gas showed a pO_2 of 93.5 mm Hg, hematocrit was 27.8% with 39,400 reticulocytes/μL, and there was persistent hypoalbuminemia (2.0 mg/dL) and hyperglobulinemia (4.8 mg/dL). There was mild radiographic improvement in the pulmonary lesions. Treatment with itraconazole was continued for an additional 14 months, with serial monitoring of thoracic radiographs at 1, 2, 3, 8, and 14 months. At the 14-month time point, Sam had returned to his normal energetic self, weighed 45 kg, but had persistent mild infiltrates in the right cranial lung lobe on thoracic radiographs and a bulla in the left cranial lung lobe. There was also a mild to moderate generalized interstitial pattern with multiple small soft tissue opaque nodules that had not changed from the previous evaluation. One month after the itraconazole was discontinued, thoracic radiographs remained unchanged. Relapse did not occur. Sam was ultimately euthanized at 8 years of age as a result of an unrelated neoplastic disease.

Comments: This case is an example of acute pulmonary blastomycosis that followed travel to an endemic area. Another dog that traveled to the same area also developed disease. Sam appeared to require more aggressive therapy than itraconazole alone, so amphotericin B was instituted, which was followed by gradual recovery from the infection. Although lipid-complexed amphotericin B was used, treatment with deoxycholate amphotericin B may also have led to cure. No evidence of dissemination was clearly identified. The lameness observed by the client may have represented weakness or exercise intolerance, but it is possible that bone involvement was present but not evident radiographically. The case also illustrates the residual pulmonary lesions that can develop in dogs with pulmonary blastomycosis, and the need for serial radiographic evaluations to assess these lesions. Although not performed in this dog, serial monitoring of antigenuria may also ultimately help determine the most appropriate time to discontinue therapy.

SUGGESTED READINGS

Arceneaux KA, Taboada J, Hosgood G. Blastomycosis in dogs: 115 cases (1980-1995). J Am Vet Med Assoc. 1998;213:658-664.

Crews LJ, Feeney DA, Jessen CR, et al. Radiographic findings in dogs with pulmonary blastomycosis: 125 cases (1989-2006). J Am Vet Med Assoc. 2008;232:215-221.

Smith JA, Kauffman CA. Blastomycosis. Proc Am Thorac Soc. 2010; 7:173-180.

Spector D, Legendre AM, Wheat J, et al. Antigen and antibody testing for the diagnosis of blastomycosis in dogs. J Vet Intern Med. 2008;22:839-843.

REFERENCES

1. Gilchrist TC. Protozoan dermatitis. J Cutan Gen Dis. 1894; 12:496-499.
2. Harasen GL, Randall JW. Canine blastomycosis in southern Saskatchewan. Can Vet J. 1986;27:375-378.
3. Hoff B. North American blastomycosis in two dogs in Saskatchewan. Can Vet J. 1973;14:122-123.
4. Iyer PKR. Pulmonary blastomycosis in a dog in India. Indian J Vet Pathol. 1983;7:60-62.
5. Kucher I, Christiansen E, Schneider-Haiss M. Blastomykose bei einer Rottweiler-Hündin. Kleintierpraxis. 1998;43:627-631.
6. Meece JK, Anderson JL, Klein BS, et al. Genetic diversity in *Blastomyces dermatitidis*: implications for PCR detection in clinical and environmental samples. Med Mycol. 2010;48:285-290.
7. Meece JK, Anderson JL, Fisher MC, et al. Population genetic structure of clinical and environmental isolates of *Blastomyces dermatitidis*, based on 27 polymorphic microsatellite markers. Appl Environ Microbiol. 2011;77:5123-5131.
8. Meece JK, Anderson JL, Gruszka S, et al. Variation in clinical phenotype of human infection among genetic groups of *Blastomyces dermatitidis*. J Infect Dis. 2013;207:814-822.
9. Rudmann DG, Coolman BR, Perez CM, et al. Evaluation of risk factors for blastomycosis in dogs: 857 cases (1980-1990). J Am Vet Med Assoc. 1992;201:1754-1759.
10. Arceneaux KA, Taboada J, Hosgood G. Blastomycosis in dogs: 115 cases (1980-1995). J Am Vet Med Assoc. 1998;213:658-664.

11. Baumgardner DJ, Paretsky DP. The in vitro isolation of *Blastomyces dermatitidis* from a woodpile in north central Wisconsin, USA. Med Mycol. 1999;37:163-168.
12. Blondin N, Baumgardner DJ, Moore GE, et al. Blastomycosis in indoor cats: suburban Chicago, Illinois, USA. Mycopathologia. 2007;163:59-66.
13. Breider MA, Walker TL, Legendre AM, et al. Blastomycosis in cats: five cases (1979-1986). J Am Vet Med Assoc. 1988;193:570-572.
14. Davies C, Troy GC. Deep mycotic infections in cats. J Am Anim Hosp Assoc. 1996;32:380-391.
15. Gray NA, Baddour LM. Cutaneous inoculation blastomycosis. Clin Infect Dis. 2002;34:E44-E49.
16. Marcellin-Little DJ, Sellon RK, Kyles AE, et al. Chronic localized osteomyelitis caused by atypical infection with *Blastomyces dermatitidis* in a dog. J Am Vet Med Assoc. 1996;209:1877-1879.
17. Finkel-Jimenez B, Wuthrich M, Klein BS. BAD1, an essential virulence factor of *Blastomyces dermatitidis*, suppresses host TNF-alpha production through TGF-beta-dependent and -independent mechanisms. J Immunol. 2002;168:5746-5755.
18. Nosanchuk JD, van Duin D, Mandal P, et al. *Blastomyces dermatitidis* produces melanin in vitro and during infection. FEMS Microbiol Lett. 2004;239:187-193.
19. Wuthrich M, Finkel-Jimenez B, Brandhorst TT, et al. Analysis of non-adhesive pathogenic mechanisms of BAD1 on *Blastomyces dermatitidis*. Med Mycol. 2006;44:41-49.
20. Nielsen C, Olver CS, Schutten MM, et al. Diagnostic peritoneal lavage for identification of blastomycosis in a dog with peritoneal involvement. J Am Vet Med Assoc. 2003;223:1623-1627:1600.
21. Menges RW, Furcolow ML, Selby LA, et al. Clinical and epidemiologic studies on seventy-nine canine blastomycosis cases in Arkansas. Am J Epidemiol. 1965;81:164-179.
22. Brockus CW, Hathcock JT. Hypertrophic osteopathy associated with pulmonary blastomycosis in a dog. Vet Radiol Ultrasound. 1988;29:184-188.
23. Totten AK, Ridgway MD, Sauberli DS. *Blastomyces dermatitidis* prostatic and testicular infection in eight dogs (1992-2005). J Am Anim Hosp Assoc. 2011;47:413-418.
24. Ditmyer H, Craig L. Mycotic mastitis in three dogs due to *Blastomyces dermatitidis*. J Am Anim Hosp Assoc. 2011;47:356-358.
25. Hecht S, Adams WH, Smith JR, et al. Clinical and imaging findings in five dogs with intracranial blastomycosis (*Blastomyces dermatitidis*). J Am Anim Hosp Assoc. 2011;47:241-249.
26. Saito M, Sharp NJ, Munana K, et al. CT findings of intracranial blastomycosis in a dog. Vet Rad Ultrasound. 2002;43:16-21.
27. Wilson RW, van Dreumel AA, Henry JN. Urogenital and ocular lesions in canine blastomycosis. Vet Pathol. 1973;10:1-11.
28. Salinardi BJ, Marretta SM, McCullough SM, et al. Pharyngeal-laryngeal blastomycosis in a dog. J Vet Dent. 2003;20:146-147.
29. Baron ML, Hecht S, Westermeyer HD, et al. Intracranial extension of retrobulbar blastomycosis (*Blastomyces dermatitidis*) in a dog. Vet Ophthalmol. 2011;14:137-141.
30. McGuire NC, Vitsky A, Daly CM, et al. Pulmonary thromboembolism associated with *Blastomyces dermatitidis* in a dog. J Am Anim Hosp Assoc. 2002;38:425-430.
31. Miller PE, Miller LM, Schoster JV. Feline blastomycosis: a report of three cases and literature review (1961 to 1988). J Am Anim Hosp Assoc. 1990;26:417-424.
32. Bromel C, Sykes JE. Epidemiology, diagnosis, and treatment of blastomycosis in dogs and cats. Clin Tech Small Anim Pract. 2005;20:233-239.
33. Bloom JD, Hamor RE, Gerding Jr PA. Ocular blastomycosis in dogs: 73 cases, 108 eyes (1985-1993). J Am Vet Med Assoc. 1996;209:1271-1274.
34. Hendrix DV, Rohrbach BW, Bochsler PN, et al. Comparison of histologic lesions of endophthalmitis induced by *Blastomyces dermatitidis* in untreated and treated dogs: 36 cases (1986-2001). J Am Vet Med Assoc. 2004;224:1317-1322.
35. Meschter C, Heiber K. Blastomycosis in a cat in lower New York State. Cornell Vet. 1989;79:259-262.
36. McEwen SA, Hulland TJ. Cerebral blastomycosis in a cat. Can Vet J. 1984;25:411-413.
37. Nasisse MP, van Ee RT, Wright B. Ocular changes in a cat with disseminated blastomycosis. J Am Vet Med Assoc. 1985;187:629-631.
38. Crews LJ, Feeney DA, Jessen CR, et al. Utility of diagnostic tests for and medical treatment of pulmonary blastomycosis in dogs: 125 cases (1989-2006). J Am Vet Med Assoc. 2008;232:222-227.
39. Nafe LA, Turk JR, Carter JD. Central nervous system involvement of blastomycosis in the dog. J Am Anim Hosp Assoc. 1983;19:933-936.
40. Crews LJ, Feeney DA, Jessen CR, et al. Radiographic findings in dogs with pulmonary blastomycosis: 125 cases (1989-2006). J Am Vet Med Assoc. 2008;232:215-221.
41. McMillan CJ, Taylor SM. Transtracheal aspiration in the diagnosis of pulmonary blastomycosis (17 cases: 2000-2005). Can Vet J. 2008;49:53-55.
42. Smith JR, Legendre AM, Thomas WB, et al. Cerebral *Blastomyces dermatitidis* infection in a cat. J Am Vet Med Assoc. 2007;231:1210-1214.
43. Spector D, Legendre AM, Wheat J, et al. Antigen and antibody testing for the diagnosis of blastomycosis in dogs. J Vet Intern Med. 2008;22:839-843.
44. Legendre AM, Becker PU. Evaluation of the agar-gel immunodiffusion test in the diagnosis of canine blastomycosis. Am J Vet Res. 1980;41:2109-2111.
45. Klein BS, Squires RA, Lloyd JK, et al. Canine antibody response to *Blastomyces dermatitidis* WI-1 antigen. Am J Vet Res. 2000;61:554-558.
46. Connolly P, Hage CA, Bariola JR, et al. *Blastomyces dermatitidis* antigen detection by quantitative enzyme immunoassay. Clin Vaccine Immunol. 2012;19:53-56.
47. Sidamonidze K, Peck MK, Perez M, et al. Real-time PCR assay for identification of *Blastomyces dermatitidis* in culture and in tissue. J Clin Microbiol. 2012;50:1783-1786.
48. Babady NE, Buckwalter SP, Hall L, et al. Detection of *Blastomyces dermatitidis* and *Histoplasma capsulatum* from culture isolates and clinical specimens by use of real-time PCR. J Clin Microbiol. 2011;49:3204-3208.
49. Sherwood BF, LeMay JC, Castellanos RA. Blastomycosis with secondary amyloidosis in the dog. J Am Vet Med Assoc. 1967;150:1377-1381.
50. Sekhon AS, Marien GR, Easton B, et al. A canine case of North American blastomycosis in Alberta, Canada. Mycoses. 1988;31:454-458.
51. Legendre AM, Rohrbach BW, Toal RL, et al. Treatment of blastomycosis with itraconazole in 112 dogs. J Vet Intern Med. 1996;10:365-371.
52. Smith JA, Kauffman CA. Blastomycosis. Proc Am Thorac Soc. 2010;7:173-180.
53. Krawiec DR, McKiernan BC, Twardock AR, et al. Use of an amphotericin B lipid complex for treatment of blastomycosis in dogs. J Am Vet Med Assoc. 1996;209:2073-2075.
54. Proia LA, Harnisch DO. Successful use of posaconazole for treatment of blastomycosis. Antimicrob Agents Chemother. 2012;56:4029.
55. Bariola JR, Perry P, Pappas PG, et al. Blastomycosis of the central nervous system: a multicenter review of diagnosis and treatment in the modern era. Clin Infect Dis. 2010;50:797-804.
56. Legendre AM, Selcer BA, Edwards DF, et al. Treatment of canine blastomycosis with amphotericin B and ketoconazole. J Am Vet Med Assoc. 1984;184:1249-1254.
57. Wuthrich M, Krajaejun T, Shearn-Bochsler V, et al. Safety, tolerability, and immunogenicity of a recombinant, genetically engineered, live-attenuated vaccine against canine blastomycosis. Clin Vaccine Immunol. 2011;18:783-789.
58. Wuthrich M, Filutowicz HI, Klein BS. Mutation of the WI-1 gene yields an attenuated *Blastomyces dermatitidis* strain that induces host resistance. J Clin Invest. 2000;106:1381-1389.
59. Sarosi GA, Eckman MR, Davies SF, et al. Canine blastomycosis as a harbinger of human disease. Ann Intern Med. 1979;91:733-735.

60. Baumgardner DJ, Paretsky DP. Blastomycosis: more evidence for exposure near one's domicile. WMJ. 2001;100:43-45.
61. Pappas PG. Blastomycosis in the immunocompromised patient. Semin Respir Infect. 1997;12:243-251.
62. Gauthier GM, Safdar N, Klein BS, et al. Blastomycosis in solid organ transplant recipients. Transpl Infect Dis. 2007;9:310-317.
63. Ramsey DT. Blastomycosis in a veterinarian. J Am Vet Med Assoc. 1994;205:968.
64. Graham Jr WR, Callaway JL. Primary inoculation blastomycosis in a veterinarian. J Am Acad Dermatol. 1982;7:785-786.
65. Gnann Jr JW, Bressler GS, Bodet 3rd CA, et al. Human blastomycosis after a dog bite. Ann Intern Med. 1983;98:48-49.
66. Butka BJ, Bennett SR, Johnson AC. Disseminated inoculation blastomycosis in a renal transplant recipient. Am Rev Respir Dis. 1984;130:1180-1183.
67. Jaspers RH. Letter: Transmission of *Blastomyces* from animals to man. J Am Vet Med Assoc. 1974;164:8.
68. Cote E, Barr SC, Allen C. Possible transmission of *Blastomyces dermatitidis* via culture specimen. J Am Vet Med Assoc. 1997;210:479-480.

CHAPTER 61

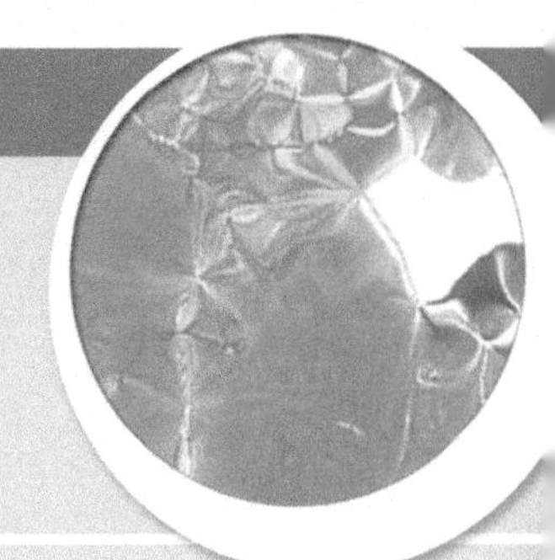

Histoplasmosis

Jane E. Sykes and Joseph Taboada

> **Overview of Histoplasmosis**
>
> First Described: 1905, Panama (by Samuel Darling), in a person from Martinique, where it was initially mistaken for a protozoal pathogen.[1]
>
> Cause: *Histoplasma capsulatum* (an ascomycete)
>
> Affected Hosts: Many mammalian species including dogs, cats, and humans
>
> Geographic Distribution: Worldwide; but especially the Ohio, Missouri, Tennessee, and Mississippi river valleys of the United States; and Latin America
>
> Mode of Transmission: Inhalation of microconidia from the environment
>
> Major Clinical Signs: Cough, tachypnea, organomegaly, gastrointestinal signs, pallor; signs are often non-specific in cats.
>
> Differential Diagnoses: Other deep mycoses, protothecosis, mycobacterial infections, hemic neoplasia, leishmaniosis, histiocytic colitis
>
> Human Health Significance: *H. capsulatum* also causes disease in humans but direct transmission from animals to humans does not occur

Etiology and Epidemiology

Histoplasma capsulatum is a dimorphic, soil-borne fungus that is found worldwide, but especially along the Mississippi, Missouri, Tennessee, and Ohio river valleys of the United States, as well as in Latin America (Figure 61-1). Endemic areas within the United States span the central portion of the United States from western Virginia to central Texas. Disease has also been reported in cats or dogs from northern California[2]; Brazil[3]; Italy[4]; Queensland in Australia[5]; Japan[6]; and western Canada.[7,8] Eight clades of the organism have been identified by genetic analysis: North American (class 1 and class 2), Latin American (group A and group B), and one each of Australian, Indonesian, Eurasian, and African. These may vary in virulence. All except the Eurasian clade, which is derived from the Latin American group A clade, may be distinct phylogenetic species.[9] A possible ninth clade, which is related to, but distinct from, North American class 1 also appears to infect cats in North America outside the accepted endemic range.[10] Three variants have also been described based on pathogenicity and morphology—*H. capsulatum* var. *capsulatum*, *H. capsulatum* var. *duboisii*, and *H. capsulatum* var. *farciminosum*—although the phylogenetic value of these variants has been debated.[6,9] *H. capsulatum* var. *duboisii* occurs primarily in Africa and Japan. *H. capsulatum* var. *farciminosum* infections occur primarily in horses, but have also been reported in humans and dogs.

H. capsulatum grows best in soil where temperatures are between 22°C and 29°C, where annual rainfall is 35 to 50 inches, and where relative humidity is 67% to 87%. These conditions are typically found between latitudes of 45 degrees north to 30 degrees south.[11] *H. capsulatum* can be found in the intestinal tracts and guano of bats, which are the primary reservoir of the organism and serve to disseminate it geographically.[12] Bat caves can maintain perfect growth conditions for *H. capsulatum*. Although *H. capsulatum* can be found in high concentrations in decaying avian guano (especially around blackbird or starling roosts and chicken coops), it is not found in fresh feces or shed in the feces of birds.

Cats are as susceptible, or slightly more susceptible, to histoplasmosis than dogs. Affected cats can be as young as 2 months and, in some cases, older than 15 years.[13] The mean age of affected cats has varied from around 4 years to 9 years.[14] For dogs, a mean age of 4.3 years was reported (range, 5 months to 10 years).[15] Dogs in the 2- to 4-year and 4- to 7-year age groups were more likely to develop histoplasmosis than dogs less than 2 years of age.[16] Sporting or working dogs may be at greater risk of infection because of increased exposure; in a study using the Veterinary Medical Database, pointers were strongly overrepresented.[16] Weimaraners and Brittany spaniels were also at increased risk. Among cats, Persian cats may be slightly overrepresented. A sex predisposition has not been clearly identified in dogs or cats, but more female than male dogs were affected in some case series.[14,15,17-19] This contrasts to human histoplasmosis and other systemic mycoses in dogs, which affect males more often than females.[20] The overwhelming majority of cats with histoplasmosis are retrovirus negative, but a significant percentage of cats in two studies (16% and 28%, respectively) were co-infected with FeLV.[13,14] A small percentage of cats have underlying comorbidities such as lymphoma, feline infectious peritonitis, or a history of glucocorticoid treatment.[13] Comorbidities described in dogs include dirofilariasis[15] and metastatic carcinoma.[6] Disease can occur in cats that are housed exclusively indoors.

Clinical Features

Signs and Their Pathogenesis

In the soil, the mycelial phase of *H. capsulatum* forms macroconidia and microconidia (Figure 61-2). The microconidia are thought to be the form inhaled by mammalian hosts, because they are small enough (2 to 5 μm) to enter the terminal bronchioles and alveoli. Within the lungs (i.e., at a temperature of 37°C), the microconidia transition to a unicellular yeast, which replicates by budding. The fungus binds to CD11-CD18 integrins on alveolar macrophages and is phagocytized. It then replicates within these cells through control of the phagolysosomal environment and ultimately destroys them, with subsequent replication in other resident alveolar macrophages and inflammatory phagocytes that are recruited to the lung.[21] Acquisition of iron by the fungus is essential for growth in vivo.[22] Some animals control the initial infection but remain latently infected with small numbers of yeasts. Subsequent immune suppression can lead to reactivation of infection years later. Thus, the incubation period can range from 2 to 3 weeks to as long as several years.

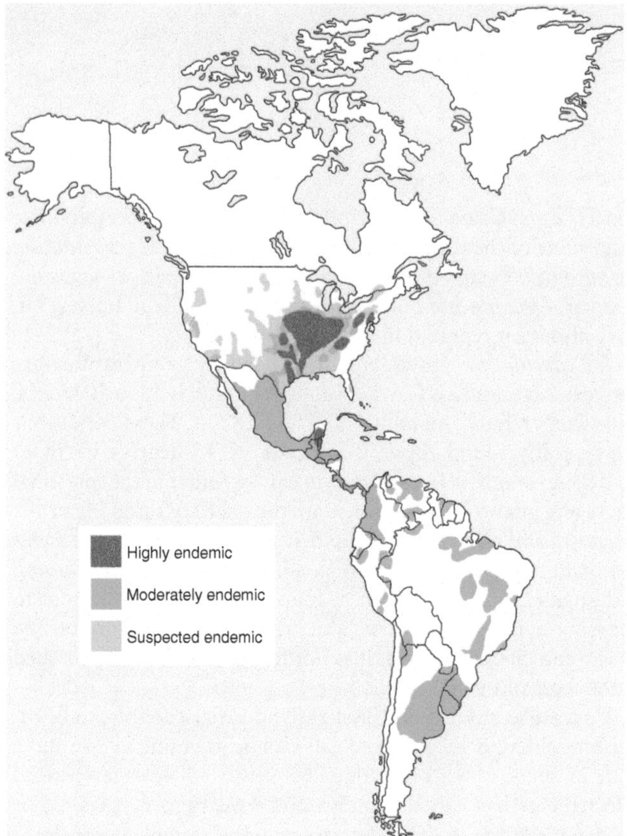

FIGURE 61-1 Approximate geographic distribution of histoplasmosis in the Americas.

The clinical manifestations and rate of disease progression depend on the host immune response to infection, the infectious dose, and the *Histoplasma* strain, which can vary geographically. The vast majority of infections are probably subclinical.[23] Replication of the organism leads to a granulomatous inflammatory response in the lungs. Occasionally, the inflammatory response is followed by fibrosis and scarring. The yeasts migrate to local lymph nodes (such as the hilar lymph node) and other tissues that contain mononuclear cells, such as the liver and spleen. When the cell-mediated immune response is defective or absent, disseminated disease occurs (referred to in human patients as *progressive disseminated histoplasmosis* [PDH][20]), which may be acute or chronic. In addition to lymph nodes, liver, and spleen, other common sites of dissemination are the bone marrow, small and/or large intestinal tract, pancreas, skin, bones, central nervous system (CNS), and eyes. Dogs with histoplasmosis in the United States appear to be particularly susceptible to intestinal involvement. Severe infiltration of the small and large intestines leads to malabsorption, diarrhea, severe weight loss, and hematochezia, often without evidence of respiratory involvement.

Clinical signs in cats are commonly vague and nonspecific, such as weight loss, inappetence, weakness, dehydration, and fever.[13,14] Approximately 40% of cats show respiratory signs such as dyspnea and tachypnea, and to a lesser extent, cough and nasal discharge. However, respiratory signs may be absent

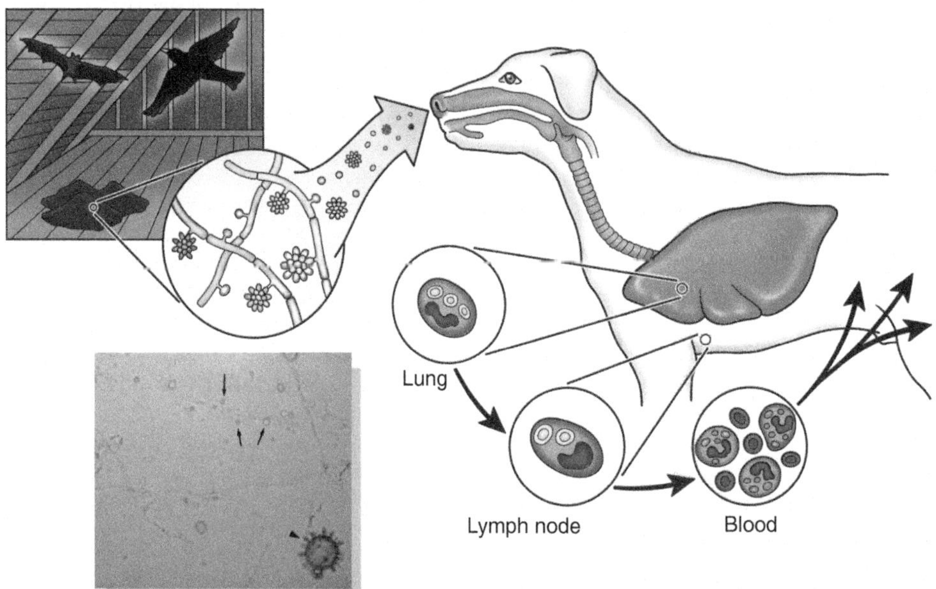

FIGURE 61-2 Life cycle of *Histoplasma capsulatum*. In the environment, the organism forms macroconidia (*arrowhead*, inset) and microconidia (*arrows*, inset). The microconidia are thought to be inhaled into the lungs of mammalian hosts. Within the lung, the organisms transform into yeasts that infect alveolar macrophages and then disseminate to local lymph nodes and the systemic circulation.

in some cats with dissemination of infection to nonpulmonary sites. Ocular signs such as chorioretinitis and/or posterior or anterior uveitis occur in approximately one quarter of cats with histoplasmosis, and around 20% of cats have signs of skeletal involvement.[13,14,17] Nodular or ulcerated and draining skin lesions, peripheral lymphadenopathy, vomiting, diarrhea, oral ulceration, myelopathy, and/or hematuria due to bladder wall involvement have also been reported.[4,14,17,24-29] Clinical signs associated with gastrointestinal involvement are much less likely to occur in cats than in dogs. A high proportion of affected cats that were necropsied had severe disseminated disease.[13]

In dogs, diarrhea, decreased appetite, weight loss, lethargy, fever (up to 40°C or 104°F), and mucosal pallor are the most common clinical signs.[7,8,15,18] In addition to inappetence, weight loss, and diarrhea, other clinical signs referable to the gastrointestinal tract include melena, tenesmus, hematochezia, dyschezia, and/or increased frequency of defecation.[8,15,18] Profuse diarrhea may be chronic and persist for several months. Hilar lymphadenopathy is common, and may be an incidental finding on thoracic radiographs, or it may be severe and contribute to signs of cough. Other signs include respiratory difficulty, icterus, vomiting, hepatomegaly, lymphadenomegaly, nasal discharge, ocular signs, polyuria and polydipsia, lameness due to osteomyelitis, and neurologic signs such as seizures or paralysis/paresis.[8,15,30-32] Affected dogs in Japan have had chronic cutaneous or gingival lesions in the absence of pulmonary or gastrointestinal involvement,[33-36] although disseminated disease has also been described.[6] Skin nodules were also reported in an Australian dog with histoplasmosis.[5] Varied clinical manifestations of histoplasmosis in different parts of the world as a result of strain variation in *H. capsulatum* also occur in humans.[20]

Physical Examination Findings

Physical examination findings in cats with histoplasmosis can be minimal or can include thin body condition or emaciation; fever; pale and/or rarely icteric mucous membranes; peripheral lymphadenopathy; respiratory signs such as dyspnea, tachypnea, and increased or decreased lung sounds; single or multiple cutaneous nodules, ulcerations, and/or draining tracts (Figure 61-3); lameness; and detection of organomegaly, abdominal masses, and/or pain on palpation of the abdomen. Ocular signs include chorioretinitis, optic neuritis, anterior uveitis, retinal detachment, panophthalmitis, and glaucoma (Figure 61-4).

In dogs, lethargy, fever, thin body condition, and pale mucous membranes are most often found on physical examination. Other physical examination abnormalities include dehydration, hepatomegaly, icterus, and/or ascites; tachypnea, increased respiratory effort, and increased lung sounds; lymphadenomegaly that involves one or more peripheral lymph nodes; abnormal stool quality on rectal examination (diarrhea, hematochezia, or melena); nasal and ocular discharge; tachycardia; tongue lesions; and cutaneous nodules, ulceration, or draining tracts.[5,8,15,18,30,37,38] Ocular examination can reveal uveitis, evidence of optic neuritis, or chorioretinitis with retinal detachment.[18,39,40] One dog was seen for lameness, hyperemia, and edema of the left pelvic limb because of a sclerosing pyogranulomatous inflammatory mass in the inguinal region that resulted in venous occlusion.[37] Rarely, neurologic signs such as ataxia, obtundation, head tilt,

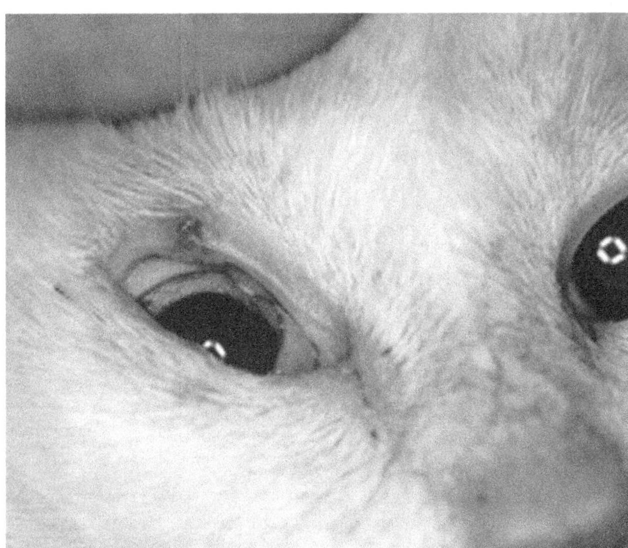

FIGURE 61-3 Cutaneous lesion on the eyelid of a cat with histoplasmosis. (Courtesy Dr. Amy Grooters, Louisiana State University.)

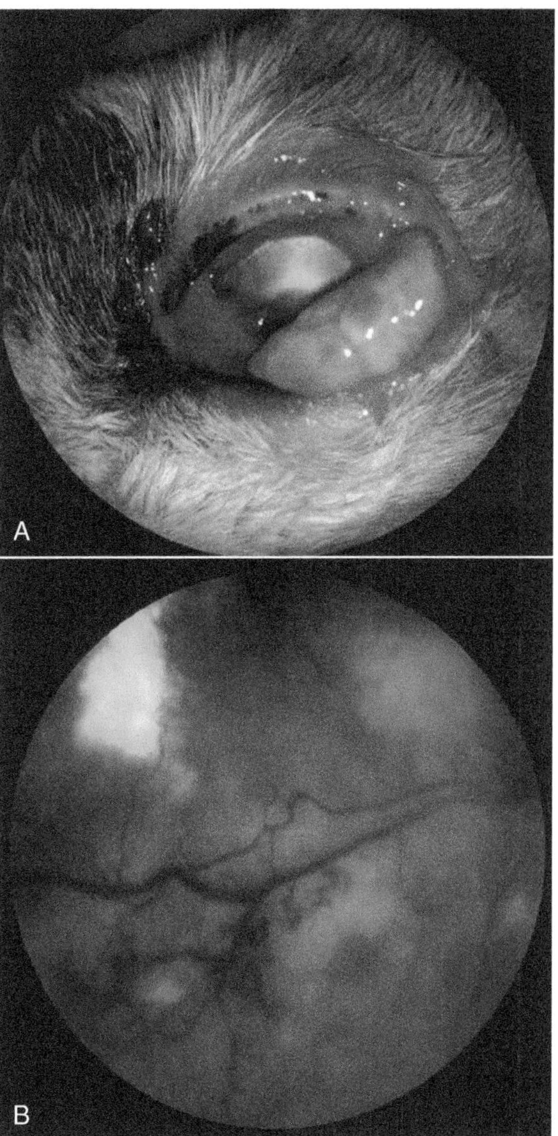

FIGURE 61-4 Ocular changes in cats with histoplasmosis. **A,** Blepharitis. **B,** Granulomatous chorioretinitis with multifocal pigmented lesions. (A, From Ketring KL, Glaze MB. Atlas of Feline Ophthalmology. 2nd ed. Hoboken, NJ: Wiley-Blackwell; 2012. B, Courtesy of Dr. Mary Belle Glaze, Gulf Coast Animal Eye Clinic, Houston, TX.)

nystagmus, strabismus, seizures, facial paralysis, and tetraparesis may be present on physical examination as a result of hepatic encephalopathy or meningoencephalitis.[40-42]

Diagnosis

Laboratory Abnormalities

Complete Blood Count

The CBC in dogs and cats with histoplasmosis reflects the presence of systemic inflammation, gastrointestinal hemorrhage, and/or bone marrow infiltration by fungal organisms. In both dogs and cats, anemia is a common abnormality, may be mild to severe, and is usually normocytic, normochromic, and nonregenerative.[14,15,17,18,43,44] Increased numbers of nucleated erythrocytes occur in some affected dogs.[8,44] The total white cell count or neutrophil count may be normal, increased, or decreased.[15,17,18,43] Most affected cats have a normal or decreased white cell count,[14,43] but leukocytosis due to neutrophilia and monocytosis may be more common in affected dogs.[15,44] Increased numbers of band neutrophils with toxic neutrophils, lymphopenia, monocytopenia, and thrombocytopenia can be present in some severely affected animals.[14,17,18,43,45] Thrombocytopenia can be a result of platelet consumption, sequestration, and/or myelophthisis. Rarely, eosinophilia is present.[46]

Serum Biochemical Tests

Mild to severe hypoalbuminemia is present in most (>75%) affected dogs and cats. Cats with liver involvement may have increased activities of serum ALT and AST.[17,43] Hyperbilirubinemia and increased serum ALP activity are rarely reported.[17] Hypercalcemia and hyperglobulinemia have been described in a few affected cats.[17] Hyperglobulinemia; mild to moderate increases in the activity of serum ALT, AST, ALP, and GGT; and hyperbilirubinemia can be found in dogs.

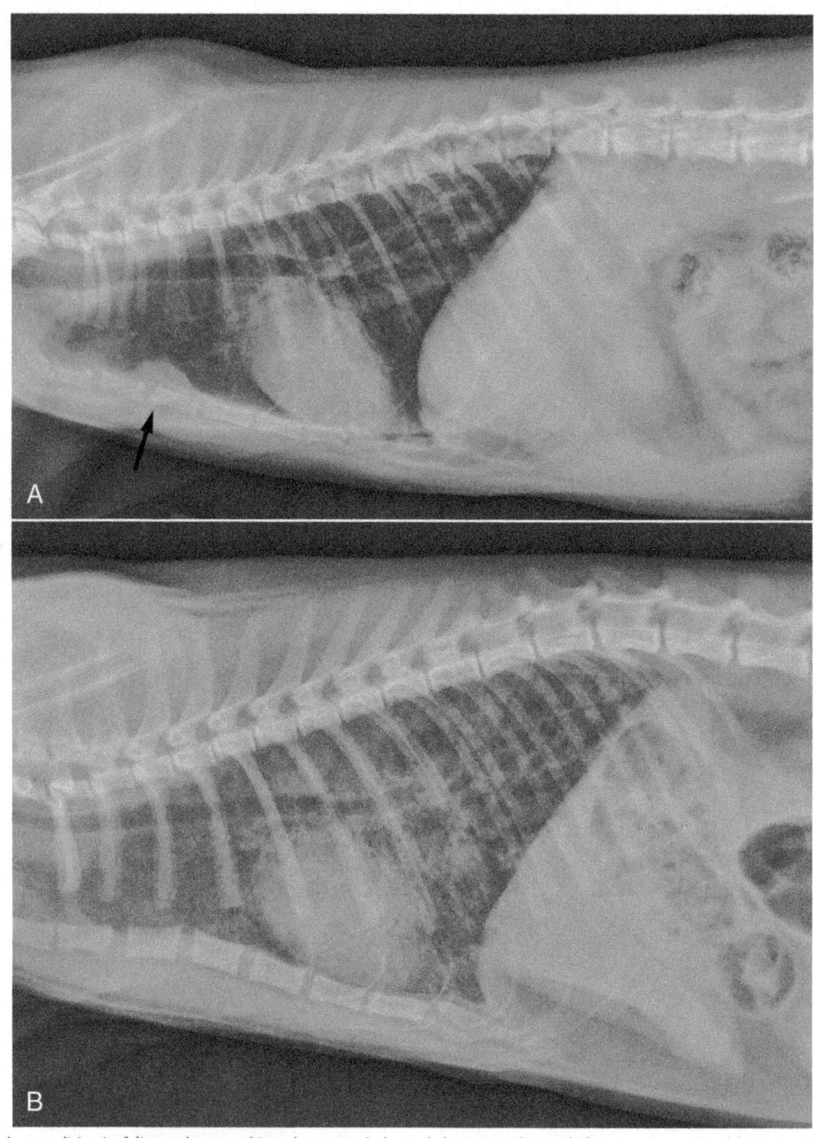

FIGURE 61-5 Radiographic abnormalities in feline pulmonary histoplasmosis. **A,** Lateral thoracic radiograph from an 8-month-old intact male domestic shorthair cat with disseminated histoplasmosis. There is a diffuse bronchointerstitial pulmonary pattern and evidence of sternal lymphadenopathy *(arrow)*. In the viewable abdomen, marked splenomegaly can be appreciated. **B,** Lateral thoracic radiograph from a 7-month-old male neutered domestic shorthair cat with histoplasmosis that was evaluated for tachypnea and dyspnea of 10 days duration. There is a diffuse, severe, interstitial-to-coalescing and patchy pulmonary pattern that obscures visualization of the pulmonary vasculature and cardiac contours. (Courtesy of Lorrie Gaschen, Louisiana State University.)

Urinalysis

Results of urinalysis are usually within normal limits, but low urine specific gravity and bilirubinuria may be present in dogs with hepatic involvement.

Coagulation Testing

A few dogs with acute PDH have had coagulation abnormalities characterized by increased PT and PTT and fibrin degradation product or D-dimer concentrations.[31,44] Coagulation abnormalities in dogs with histoplasmosis may result from disseminated intravascular coagulation and possibly severe hepatic involvement (see also Canine Case Example).

Diagnostic Imaging

Plain Radiography

In cats, thoracic radiographic findings in histoplasmosis usually consist of diffuse, linear, nodular, or miliary interstitial patterns, but mixed interstitial-alveolar-bronchial patterns, pleural effusion, or an absence of abnormal findings can also occur (Figure 61-5).[14,19,43,47] Plain thoracic radiographs in dogs may show alveolar, interstitial, and/or bronchial patterns, tracheobronchial lymphadenopathy, lung lobe consolidation, and/or rarely pleural effusion.[31,45,47,48] Lesions in dogs sometimes mineralize, which does not seem to occur in cats. Abdominal radiographs may show hepatomegaly, splenomegaly, or decreased serosal detail due to ascites. Radiographic evidence of osteomyelitis may be present in cats, with associated soft tissue swelling and sometimes pathologic fractures. Osteomyelitis is rarely described in dogs.[30,32]

Sonographic Findings

Findings on abdominal sonographic examination of dogs with histoplasmosis include hepatic enlargement and hypoechogenicity, abdominal lymphadenopathy, splenomegaly, and ascites. A thickened intestinal wall may be present with disruption of bowel wall architecture. Adrenomegaly, abdominal lymphadenopathy, and occasionally renomegaly have been described in cats.[14]

Endoscopy

Colonoscopic findings in dogs with colonic histoplasmosis include irregularity, ulceration, and increased granularity and friability of the colonic wall (Figure 61-6).

Microbiologic Tests

Diagnostic assays currently available for histoplasmosis in dogs and cats are described in Table 61-1.

Cytologic Examination

Cytologic examination of aspirates or impression smears of affected tissues (e.g., fine-needle aspirates of liver, spleen, lymph nodes, lung, bone marrow), rectal scrapings, or Cytospin preparations of lung wash specimens or body fluids (e.g., CSF, synovial fluid, ascites, or pleural effusion) usually reveals pyogranulomatous or granulomatous inflammation. *H. capsulatum* yeasts can be seen extracellularly and intracellularly (usually within mononuclear phagocytes). Most extracellular organisms are probably an artifact of smear preparation. Occasionally one or more organisms are seen in circulating monocytes, neutrophils, or eosinophils in severely ill animals with disseminated disease (Figure 61-7). Cytologic evidence of fungemia was detected in nearly 20% of affected cats in one study.[13] The bone marrow is a common site to yield organisms in cats, even when hematologic abnormalities are minimal.

Cytologically, the yeasts are 2 to 4 μm in diameter, oval, have a basophilic center, and are surrounded by a clear halo, which results from shrinkage artifact (see Figure 61-7). They are similar in size to *Sporothrix* spp., although different in shape. A variety of stains can be used, such as Diff-Quik and Wright stains. The organism is not encapsulated, despite its name. Organisms may not be identified within chronic, fibrosing lesions.[37,49]

Serologic Testing

Both antibody and antigen (ELISA) assays are available for serodiagnosis of histoplasmosis. Antibody assays for *Histoplasma capsulatum* are based on gel immunodiffusion or complement fixation and have had poor diagnostic sensitivity.[13,15,17] False positives reportedly occur in recovered animals, although the specificity of antibody assays in dogs and cats is not well documented. In human patients, acute and convalescent antibody testing is useful for diagnosis of acute pulmonary histoplasmosis, and a single positive antibody titer is used as an aid for diagnosis of chronic histoplasmosis. In particular, a positive CSF antibody titer can be useful for diagnosis of culture-negative chronic *H. capsulatum* meningitis. An ELISA assay for *H. capsulatum* antigen (MiraVista Diagnostics, Indianapolis, IN) is widely used in human patients for diagnosis of histoplasmosis, and urine is the preferred specimen for testing because it results in a higher sensitivity than when serum is assayed.[49] In human patients with AIDS and severe PDH, the sensitivity of the assay is 95% when urine is used, and 86% when serum is used.[49] The sensitivity is lower in human patients with pulmonary histoplasmosis, but use of a combination of urine antigen and serum antigen increases sensitivity to 83%.[50] False positives occur in people with other disseminated mycoses, including blastomycosis, penicilliosis, and coccidioidomycosis,[51,52] so the

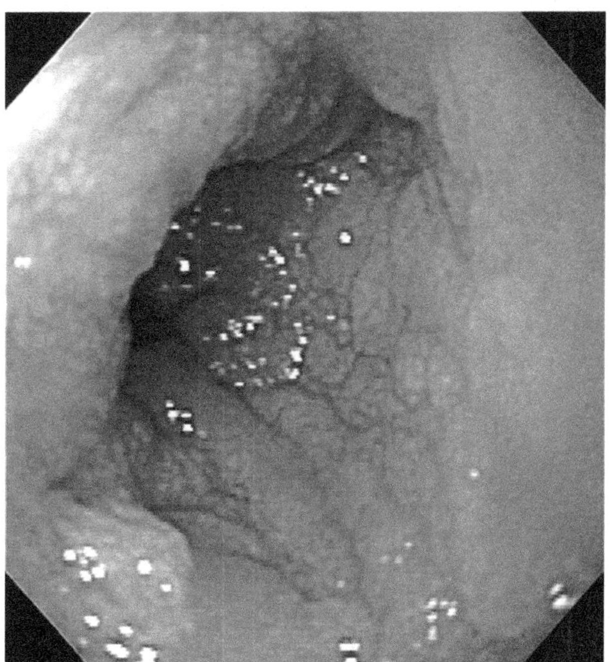

FIGURE 61-6 Colonoscopy image from a dog with disseminated histoplasmosis with large intestinal involvement. The mucosa is thickened and granular. (Courtesy Dr. Michael Willard, Texas A&M University.)

TABLE 61-1

Diagnostic Assays Currently Available for Histoplasmosis in Dogs and Cats

Assay	Specimen Type	Target	Performance
Cytologic examination	Aspirates of affected tissues, bone marrow aspirates, sometimes blood smears or buffy coat preparations, body fluids	*Histoplasma capsulatum* organisms (usually in large numbers) within mononuclear phagocytes and granulocytes	Organisms are usually present but, in the absence of experience, may be confused with protozoa such as *Leishmania* or other fungi such as *Sporothrix schenckii*. False negatives can occur in animals with very chronic clinical manifestations.
Fungal culture	Aspirates or biopsies of affected tissues, body fluids, whole blood	*H. capsulatum*	Rarely indicated. Sensitive and specific and may be required for animals with chronic histoplasmosis when cytologic examination is negative. Risk of laboratory-acquired infections. Slow turnaround time (several weeks of incubation may be required).
Antibody serology (complement fixation or gel immunodiffusion)	Serum	Antibodies to *H. capsulatum*	Positive test results indicate exposure but do not indicate active infection or correlate with clinical disease. Negative test results occur commonly in animals with histoplasmosis (low sensitivity).
Antigen assay (ELISA)	Urine, serum	*H. capsulatum* antigen	Sensitivity and specificity require further evaluation in dogs and cats, although the assay appears to be sensitive and specific in cats when urine is tested. Cross-reactivity with other fungal pathogens may occur, so positive results are not diagnostic for histoplasmosis. Cross-reactivity is seen with blastomycosis, a systemic fungal infection with an overlapping geographic range.
Real-time PCR assays	See fungal culture	*H. capsulatum* DNA	Not yet validated in adequate numbers of dogs or cats with histoplasmosis; usefulness requires further evaluation.
Histopathology	Biopsy specimens from affected tissues	*H. capsulatum* yeasts	Yeasts can be difficult to find in chronic infections. Special stains may assist organism detection.

assay must always be used in conjunction with other diagnostic assays in order to determine the identity of the infecting fungal pathogen. Antigen levels become undetectable with successful treatment.[53] The antigen assay has also been used for the diagnosis of histoplasmosis in cats and dogs.[37,54] In one study, the urine of 17 of 18 cats with confirmed histoplasmosis was positive, whereas none of 26 cats with other diagnoses were positive.[54] Additional studies that evaluate larger numbers of cats and dogs with and without confirmed histoplasmosis, as well as those with other fungal infections, are required to further establish the sensitivity and specificity of this assay.

Fungal Culture

H. capsulatum can be isolated from clinical specimens on routine fungal media. There is a risk of laboratory-acquired infection when the organism grows in the mycelial form on artificial media, so culture should be performed only if necessary, and the laboratory should be warned of the possibility of a dimorphic fungal infection, so that appropriate precautions are taken. Although most cultures are positive within 2 or 3 weeks, growth may require up to 6 weeks of incubation. The organism is identified based on morphology (see Figure 61-2).

Molecular Diagnosis Using the Polymerase Chain Reaction

Real-time PCR assays have been developed for rapid detection of *H. capsulatum* in clinical specimens from affected humans[55,56] but currently are not used routinely for diagnosis. The sensitivity of one assay was 73% when compared with culture of clinical specimens.[55] PCR assays have not been widely applied to the diagnosis of histoplasmosis in dogs and cats; further studies are required to determine their usefulness.

Pathologic Findings

Gross pathologic findings in dogs and cats with histoplasmosis consist of miliary nodules or larger focal lesions in the lungs and other organs, and enlarged lymph nodes, which may be mineralized in dogs with chronic disease. In dogs, the intestinal tract may be thickened and focal or diffuse mucosal hemorrhage may be present. The liver and spleen may be enlarged with rounded borders, and the liver may be mottled with a reticulated appearance. Pleural and peritoneal effusions are occasionally described.[45] Histopathology yields pyogranulomatous or granulomatous inflammation with intralesional yeasts in a variety of organs (Figure 61-8). Lymphocytes and plasma cells may be present, and in some animals with chronic histoplasmosis, histologic evidence of fibrosis or (in dogs) mineralization is apparent.[37,45] Special stains such as Gomori's methenamine silver or periodic acid–Schiff can aid detection of the yeasts in tissues.

Treatment and Prognosis

Antimicrobial Treatment

Antifungal drugs with activity against *H. capsulatum* include the azole antifungal drugs ketoconazole, itraconazole, and fluconazole

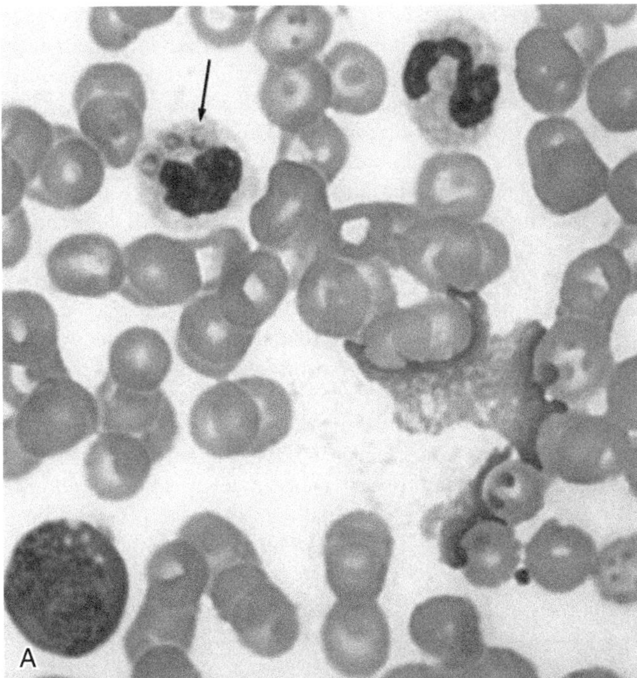

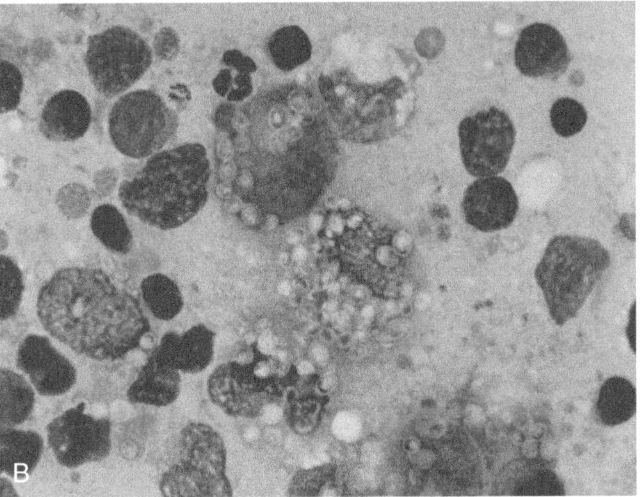

FIGURE 61-7 **A,** Blood smear from a dog with *Histoplasma capsulatum* fungemia. Three organisms can be seen in a circulating neutrophil *(arrow)*. Wright's stain, 1000× magnification. **B,** Fine-needle aspirate cytology from the right popliteal lymph node of the cat in Figure 61-5, *A*. There is pyogranulomatous inflammation with large numbers of intracellular yeast organisms with morphology consistent with that of *H. capsulatum*. Wright's stain, 1000× magnification. (Courtesy Angela Royal, Louisiana State University.)

(see Chapter 9 for more information and dosing for antifungal drugs). Itraconazole and fluconazole are preferred to ketoconazole since they are more effective and less likely to cause toxicity.[17] In human patients, itraconazole has consistently been more effective than fluconazole. An increased efficacy of itraconazole when compared with fluconazole is likely in dogs and cats as well, although in the authors' experiences, some animals may be cured with fluconazole monotherapy. Limited data suggest that posaconazole may be an effective salvage treatment in human patients with histoplasmosis that fail to respond to treatment with other antifungal drugs, including fluconazole, itraconazole, amphotericin B, and voriconazole.[57] Development of resistance to fluconazole and voriconazole has been documented during treatment of human patients with fluconazole, but not with posaconazole.[58]

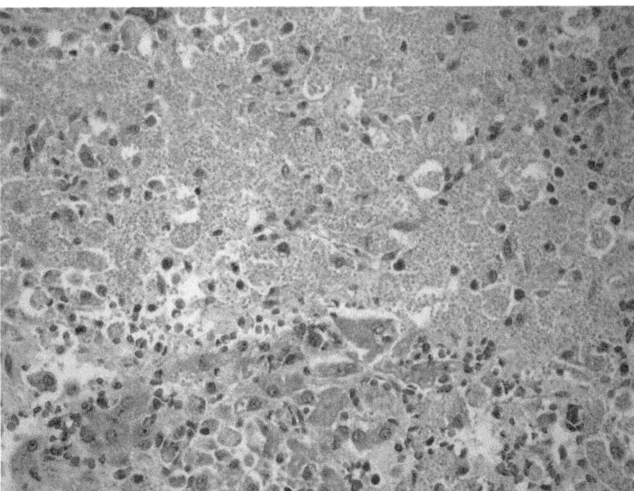

FIGURE 61-8 Histopathology of the liver of a 5-month-old intact male redbone coonhound with disseminated histoplasmosis. There is severe granulomatous inflammation with massive numbers of intrahistiocytic yeast organisms.

Deoxycholate or lipid-complexed amphotericin B should be used initially to treat dogs or cats with severe acute pulmonary, acute disseminated, or CNS disease, after which treatment should be continued with itraconazole. If funds or patient factors do not permit itraconazole treatment, fluconazole can be used as a second-line agent.

The length of treatment and prognosis depend on the severity and chronicity of disease and the immune status of the host. At least 6 months of treatment is generally required. Many animals require treatment for 12 months or longer, and those with chronic disease may require treatment for more than 2 years. The decision to discontinue treatment should be based on lesion resolution (which may require serial imaging studies). Resolution of positive urine antigen titers might also be used to decide when to discontinue treatment, but further study is required to determine whether serial monitoring of *H. capsulatum* antigenuria is useful in making treatment decisions.

Supportive Treatment

Other supportive treatments that may be required depend on the extent of infection and include intravenous crystalloid fluids, supplemental oxygen, blood transfusions for severely anemic animals, nutritional support, antiemetics, and medications to manage consequences of hepatic failure such as hepatic encephalopathy. Topical glucocorticoids and atropine may be required for animals with uveitis, and enucleation may be required to manage persistent ocular infection and pain. The role of systemic glucocorticoids for treatment of chronic manifestations of histoplasmosis is controversial, and they are not recommended for treatment of active or disseminated histoplasmosis.

Immunity and Vaccination

Immunity to *H. capsulatum* is dependent on a Th1 immune response. Production of IFN-γ activates macrophages to destroy the fungus.[59] There is currently no vaccine for prevention of histoplasmosis, but there is interest in development of a vaccine for at-risk human patients because of increasing incidence of the disease.

Prevention

Prevention of histoplasmosis involves avoidance of bat caves and areas previously inhabited by avian species in endemic areas. Nevertheless, histoplasmosis has occurred in animals housed exclusively indoors, and widespread exposure and recovery likely occurs in endemic areas.

Public Health Aspects

As many as 80% of young adults in endemic areas have been previously infected by *H. capsulatum*, but only 1% develop symptoms.[49] Risk factors identified for human histoplasmosis include exposure to soil disrupted as a result of excavation, exploration of caves inhabited by bats, or renovation of buildings inhabited by birds or bats. Males are predisposed in a 4:1 ratio.[20] Several forms of the disease have been described, which include acute pulmonary histoplasmosis, chronic pulmonary histoplasmosis (which may be cavitary or noncavitary), and acute or chronic PDH.[20] Complications of pulmonary histoplasmosis include granulomatous mediastinitis (characterized by enlargement and sometimes calcification of mediastinal lymph nodes, with compression of adjacent structures) or mediastinal fibrosis (characterized by fibrosis of caseous mediastinal lymph nodes). The clinical picture of PDH in humans is similar to that described in dogs; rare clinical manifestations include meningitis, endocarditis, and vascular infections.[20,49] Humans with AIDS or those treated with immunosuppressive drugs (such as tumor necrosis factor antagonists) are at risk for severe PDH, and smokers are predisposed to chronic pulmonary histoplasmosis. Itraconazole prophylaxis is considered for immunosuppressed patients who are at risk for development of the disease.[20]

Transmission of *H. capsulatum* from dogs or cats to humans has not been reported, but disease in dogs and cats may signal the potential for human infection as a result of exposure to the same source of infection; outbreaks have been described that involved both humans and dogs.[60] The bodies of deceased pets with histoplasmosis should be disposed of promptly and by cremation.

CANINE CASE EXAMPLE

Signalment: "Murphy," a 5-month-old intact male redbone coonhound from northern California.

History: Murphy was evaluated at the University of California, Davis, Veterinary Medical Teaching Hospital for a 1-week history of increased respiratory effort, hypersalivation, a single episode of vomiting, and lethargy. After the first day of illness he was taken to a local veterinary clinic where fever (103.2°F or 39.6°C), pale mucous membranes, and a cranial abdominal mass were noted on physical examination. Abdominal radiographs revealed moderate hepatomegaly and mild splenomegaly. He was treated with vitamin K, a single dose of prednisone (2 mg/kg SC), and cephalexin (20 mg/kg PO q8h). Considerable improvement in his mentation was noted. However, after 5 days, anorexia, hypersalivation, vomiting, and liquid diarrhea occurred, and he returned to the local veterinary clinic, where he was hospitalized and treated with intravenous fluids. The following day, obtundation and facial twitching developed, and Murphy was referred for further diagnostics and treatment.

Other Medical History: Murphy had been coughing a week before he became systemically ill, but this subsequently resolved. He was treated for a roundworm infection at that time, which was diagnosed by fecal flotation. Murphy was obtained from a breeder in Oklahoma at 4 months of age. He had always appeared "slow" to the owner, his appetite had never been very good, and he seemed unthrifty. The other puppies in the litter were apparently healthy. There was no known exposure to toxins. The breeder administered his first vaccines, and he was revaccinated for distemper, parvovirus, adenovirus, parainfluenza virus, and *Leptospira* by the local veterinarian when he was acquired.

Physical Examination:

Body Weight: 12.2 kg.

General: Obtundation was noted; the dog was in lateral recumbency and apparently unaware of his surroundings. Facial twitching occurred throughout the examination. T = 102.2°F (39.0°C), HR = 140 beats/min, RR = 50 breaths/min, mucous membranes were moist and pink.

Eyes, Ears, Nose, and Throat: Moderate conjunctivitis was present. There was a mild bilateral serous nasal discharge. No other abnormalities were detected.

Musculoskeletal: Appeared small in stature, BCS 3/9.

Cardiovascular, Respiratory and Lymph Nodes: No clinically significant abnormalities were detected.

Abdominal Palpation: Cranial organomegaly was present.

Laboratory Findings:

Blood Glucose: 70 mg/dL.

Plasma Fasting Ammonia Concentration: 509 µg/dL (0-92 µg/dL).

Canine Distemper Virus Direct Immunofluorescent Antibody (Urine Sediment): Negative.

CBC:

HCT 30.2% (40%-55%)
MCV 61 fL (65-75 fL)
MCHC 36.1 g/dL (33-36 g/dL)
Reticulocytes 49,200/µL (7000-65,000/µL)
WBC 22,000 cells/µL (6000-13,000 cells/µL)
Neutrophils 10,340 cells/µL (3000-10,500 cells/µL)
Band neutrophils 7040 cells/µL
Metamyelocytes 880 cells/µL
Lymphocytes 1100 cells/µL (1000-4000 cells/µL)
Monocytes 1100 cells/µL (150-1200 cells/µL)
Eosinophils 880 cells/µL (0-1500 cells/µL)
Platelets 28,000/µL (150,000-400,000 platelets/µL).

Moderately toxic neutrophils and markedly toxic band neutrophils and metamyelocytes were present. Occasional organisms with morphology consistent with *Histoplasma capsulatum* were seen within both neutrophils and monocytes. The myeloid series was shifted to the myelocyte stage with rare progranulocytes noted. Rare nucleated erythrocytes (metarubricytes) were also present. Many lymphocytes were reactive. Numerous macroplatelets were noted.

Serum Chemistry Profile:

Sodium 143 mmol/L (145-154 mmol/L)
Potassium 4.7 mmol/L (4.1-5.3 mmol/L)

Chloride 108 mmol/L (105-116 mmol/L)
Bicarbonate 18 mmol/L (16-26 mmol/L)
Phosphorus 7.7 mg/dL (3.0-6.2 mg/dL)
Calcium 10.3 mg/dL (9.9-11.4 mg/dL)
BUN 18 mg/dL (8-31 mg/dL)
Creatinine 0.4 mg/dL (0.8-1.6 mg/dL)
Glucose 117 mg/dL (70-118 mg/dL)
Total protein 5.8 g/dL (5.4-7.4 g/dL)
Albumin 2.1 g/dL (2.9-4.2 g/dL)
Globulin 3.7 g/dL (2.3-4.4 g/dL)
ALT 31 U/L (19-70 U/L)
AST 217 U/L (15-43 U/L)
ALP 195 U/L (15-127 U/L)
GGT 24 U/L (0-6 U/L)
Cholesterol 363 mg/dL (135-345 mg/dL)
Total bilirubin 1.1 mg/dL (0-0.4 mg/dL).

Urinalysis (Cystocentesis): SGr 1.044; pH 5.0, 1+ bilirubin, no hemoprotein, no glucose, no protein, 0-1 RBC/HPF, rare WBC/HPF; no crystals, casts, or bacteria seen.

Coagulation Panel: PT 10.7 s (7.5-10.5 s), PTT 24.4 s (9-12 s), fibrin degradation products > 40 μg/mL (<10 μg/mL).

Imaging Findings:

Thoracic Radiographs: There was a diffuse bronchointerstitial pulmonary pattern, especially in the region of the cranial right middle lung lobe. The heart and pulmonary vasculature were slightly small. In the viewable abdomen, the liver was moderately enlarged.

Abdominal Ultrasound: Severe hepatomegaly was present with normal hepatic echogenicity. A large, folded spleen and sublumbar and mesenteric lymphadenomegaly were present.

Microbiologic Testing:

Fecal Flotation: Positive for *Ancylostoma* ova.

Aspiration Cytology (Ultrasound-guided Liver Aspirate): The specimen was bloody and moderately cellular with numerous clusters of platelets and inflammatory cells. Occasional small clusters of hepatocytes were noted, which showed mild to moderate vacuolar degeneration. A few hepatocytes contained intracytoplasmic blue-green pigment consistent with bile. Inflammatory cells consisted primarily of activated macrophages that contained abundant intracellular yeast organisms consistent with *Histoplasma* spp. Lower numbers of nondegenerate neutrophils, mixed lymphocytes, and occasional eosinophils and basophils were also found. Interpretation: *Histoplasma* infection with marked pyogranulomatous inflammation. Mild to moderate hepatic vacuolar degeneration and cholestasis.

CSF Analysis (Cisternal): The fluid was clear and colorless. The protein concentration was 17 mg/dL (reference range, <25 mg/dL). There was fewer than 1 RBC/μL (reference range, <1200 RBC/μL) and 25 nucleated cells/μL (reference range, <2 cells/μL). The differential cell count consisted of 1% neutrophils, 6% lymphocytes, and 93% large mononuclear cells. The cytofuge specimen was cellular, and large, foamy macrophage-like cells predominated. Vacuoles within the cytoplasm contained digested debris, but no organisms could be discerned. Low numbers of small lymphocytes were also noted. Interpretation: Mononuclear pleocytosis.

Diagnosis: Acute progressive disseminated histoplasmosis with suspected *Histoplasma* meningitis; hookworm infestation.

Treatment: Murphy was hospitalized in the intensive care unit and treated with intravenous crystalloids (lactated Ringer's solution with 25 mEq/L KCl and 2.5% dextrose, 75 mL/h), plasma, vitamin K, and heparin (100 units/kg SC q8h). The hookworm infection was treated with fenbendazole (50 mg/kg PO q24h for 3 days). Seizures were controlled with diazepam as needed and phenobarbital (2 mg/kg IM q12h). Hepatic encephalopathy was treated with a warm water enema followed by a 3 mL/kg lactulose enema, then oral lactulose (1 mL/kg PO q8h). Profuse watery diarrhea ensued. Treatment with lipid-complexed amphotericin B was then initiated (2 mg/kg IV over 2 hours, every other day). Initially, clinical signs improved, and Murphy appeared brighter and began eating small amounts of a reduced protein diet. A CBC showed a hematocrit of 30%, 19,988 neutrophils/μL, 263 band neutrophils/μL with slight toxicity, 2367 lymphocytes/μL, 2367 monocytes/μL, 1315 eosinophils/μL, and 65,000 platelets/μL. No *Histoplasma* organisms were seen. The results of a biochemistry profile were similar to those reported at hospitalization, but electrolytes and glucose had normalized and total bilirubin was 2.6 mg/dL.

On day 4 of hospitalization, Murphy developed increased respiratory effort, weakness, and a head tremor. Thoracic radiographs showed a diffuse miliary interstitial infiltrate in the perihilar region and in the region of the right cranial lung lobe, which was slightly more severe than that seen at the time of hospitalization. By day 7 of hospitalization, he remained extremely weak and inappetent, and the owners elected euthanasia because of financial limitations. At necropsy, there was severe hepatomegaly and splenomegaly; the lungs were firm and mottled dark red to pink, and cut surfaces oozed white froth and blood. Histopathology revealed severe, diffuse, granulomatous inflammation with intrahistiocytic yeasts in the lungs, liver, spleen, bone marrow, sublumbar lymph nodes, and tracheobronchial lymph nodes (see Figure 61-8). In the kidneys there was severe, multifocal, granulomatous interstitial nephritis with intrahistiocytic yeasts. Multifocal granulomatous inflammatory lesions with intrahistiocytic yeasts were present in the pancreas, duodenum, jejunum, thyroid glands, and peritoneal fat. Within the brain there was minimal, focal, granulomatous meningitis.

Comments: In this dog, the diagnosis of disseminated histoplasmosis with fungemia was straightforward because organisms were seen in a peripheral blood smear. The dog likely acquired infection in Oklahoma where the fungus is endemic. Overwhelming infection suggested a possible underlying immunodeficiency, although severe disease is common without obvious immunodeficiency in dogs. The dog had evidence of disseminated intravascular coagulation, hepatic encephalopathy, and granulomatous meningitis. Had treatment with amphotericin B, azole antifungal drugs, and additional supportive care continued, recovery might have occurred, but the costs of this treatment without guaranteed success led the owners to elect euthanasia. Clearly the burden of intact fungal organisms at necropsy was still massive despite several treatments with amphotericin B. Even in human patients, overall cure rates for *H. capsulatum* meningitis are no better than 50%.

FELINE CASE EXAMPLE

Signalment: "Shaq," an 8-month-old intact male domestic shorthair cat from east central Louisiana.

History: Shaq was evaluated at the Louisiana State University (LSU) Veterinary Medical Teaching Hospital for a 3-week history of lethargy and intermittent anorexia. Occasional right pelvic limb lameness had been noted. He was taken to a local veterinary clinic, where fever and an enlarged right popliteal lymph node were noted on physical examination. A bite wound was suspected at the local veterinarian's clinic, and Shaq was treated with an injectable long-acting cephalosporin and oral amoxicillin. After 2 weeks of continued waxing and waning lethargy, Shaq was brought to the emergency service at LSU.

Current Medications: Amoxicillin.

Other Medical History: Shaq was an indoor/outdoor cat who has always lived in Louisiana. He ate a commercial kitten food and was vaccinated at 3 to 4 months of age, which included an FIV vaccination. FeLV and FIV infection status was unknown.

Physical Examination:

Body Weight: 3.2 kg.

General: The cat was quiet but alert and responsive. His mucous membranes were pink and moist, and his CRT was less than 2 s. Rectal temperature was 104.9°F (40.5°C), and heart rate was 216 beats/min.

Eyes, Ears, Nose, and Throat: Normal; no fundic examination abnormalities were noted.

Musculoskeletal: Normal; no pain was noted on palpation of the right pelvic limb. The right popliteal lymph node was moderately enlarged, movable, and nonpainful.

Cardiovascular: No murmurs or arrhythmias were auscultated, and a strong pulse quality was present.

Respiratory: Tachypnea was present but no significant abnormalities were detected on auscultation.

Abdominal Palpation: Cranial organomegaly (splenomegaly) was present.

Lymph Nodes: Other than the right popliteal lymph node, lymph nodes were palpably normal.

Laboratory Findings:

CBC:

HCT 28.6% (30%-48%)
MCV 33 fL (41-57 fL)
MCHC 30.0 g/dL (30-35 g/dL)
Reticulocytes 22,100/μL
WBC 10,300 cells/μL (6000-10,000 cells/μL)
Neutrophils 6500 cells/μL (2500-12,500 cells/μL)
Lymphocytes 3700 cells/μL (1500-7000 cells/μL)
Monocytes 100 cells/μL (0-800 cells/μL)
Eosinophils 0 cells/μL (0-1500 cells/μL)
Platelets 515,000/μL (190,000-368,000 platelets/μL)
WBC and RBC morphology were considered normal.
Plasma protein 8.2 g/dL (6-7.5 g/dL).

Serum Chemistry Profile:

Sodium 164 mmol/L (150-165 mmol/L)
Potassium 3.7 mmol/L (4.0-5.0 mmol/L)
Chloride 126 mmol/L (121-126 mmol/L)
Phosphorus 6.5 mg/dL (3.1-7.5 mg/dL)
Calcium 10.3 mg/dL (8.8-9.3 mg/dL)
BUN 28 mg/dL (16-22 mg/dL)
Creatinine 1.1 mg/dL (1.7-1.9 mg/dL)
Glucose 125 mg/dL (77-96 mg/dL)
Total protein 7.8 g/dL (6.5-7.1 g/dL)
Albumin 3.0 g/dL (2.8-3.1 g/dL)
Globulin 4.8 g/dL (37.-4.1 g/dL)
ALT 77 U/L (24-44 U/L)
AST 16 U/L (0-36 U/L)
ALP 41 U/L (33-72 U/L)
Total bilirubin 0.2 mg/dL (0-0.4 mg/dL).

Urinalysis: Not performed.

Imaging Findings:

Thoracic Radiographs: There was a diffuse mild bronchointerstitial pulmonary pattern that was somewhat patchy in the caudodorsal lung fields. A smooth, broad-based soft tissue opaque structure that was sharply marginated by the surrounding lung was evident dorsal to sternebrae 3 to 4; this was consistent with sternal lymphadenopathy. In the visible abdomen, the spleen was moderately enlarged (see Figure 61-5, *A*).

Abdominal Ultrasound: A large spleen was present with diffusely heterogenous echogenicity.

Microbiologic Testing:

Fecal Flotation: Negative.

FeLV/FIV ELISA Serology: Negative for FeLV antigen, positive for FIV antibody.

Aspiration Cytology (Popliteal Lymph Node Aspirate): Smears contained large numbers of adequately preserved nucleated cells with a low number of erythrocytes. The nucleated cell population consisted of high numbers of small lymphocytes (75%), low numbers of neutrophils (20%), and highly vacuolated macrophages (5%). The macrophages contained large numbers of oval, 2- to 3-μm–diameter yeast that were surrounded by a thin clear halo and had small, eccentric, crescent-shaped purple nuclei. Interpretation: Pyogranulomatous inflammation with intracellular *Histoplasma* spp. yeasts (see Figure 61-7, *B*).

Histoplasma *Quantitative Antigen EIA (Urine):* 9.3 ng/mL (positive).

Diagnosis: Disseminated histoplasmosis.

Treatment: Shaq was hospitalized in the intensive care unit and treated with intravenous crystalloids (Normosol-R with 25 mEq/L KCl, 8 mL/h) and his temperature was monitored. The fungal infection was treated with itraconazole oral solution (10 mg/kg PO q24h). His temperature fluctuated between 103.6°F and 105.3°F (39.8°C and 40.7°C) over the next 48 hours, but he maintained a good appetite and was bright and alert. On day 3, Shaq was discharged from the hospital with instructions to continue the itraconazole treatment. He was still febrile but was bright and alert and eating well. Recommendations were to recheck monthly at the local veterinary clinic for exam and chemistry panel. A urinary *Histoplasma* Quantitative Antigen EIA was repeated after 2 months of treatment and was 2.0 ng/mL, which was still positive but indicated a probable treatment response. Recheck at 6 months revealed a normal physical examination, thoracic radiograph, CBC, and chemistry panel with the exception of an increased serum ALT activity at 221 U/L (0-90 U/L). It was recommended that the local veterinarian repeat the *Histoplasma* antigen assay and discontinue itraconazole if negative.

Comments: In this cat, a diagnosis of disseminated histoplasmosis was straightforward because organisms were seen in a lymph node aspirate. If they had not been present on cytologic examination of the lymph node aspirate, cytologic examination of a splenic or a bone marrow aspirate would have been most likely to reveal organisms. The vague presentation with mild respiratory signs is typical of infection in cats. The positive result for FIV antibody was likely due to the previous vaccination. Treatment is probably best continued until the result of the urine antigen assay is negative, but if the titer remains low and clinical signs have resolved, discontinuation of itraconazole treatment may be appropriate with retesting for antigenuria. An increase in urine antigen concentration may indicate relapse and need for further therapy. The increased ALT (221 U/L) was likely due to itraconazole therapy and did not necessitate alteration in treatment as long as the cat otherwise appeared normal.

SUGGESTED READINGS

Aulakh HK, Aulakh KS, Troy GC. Feline histoplasmosis: a retrospective study of 22 cases (1986-2009). J Am Anim Hosp Assoc. 2012;48:182-187.

Cook AK, Cunningham LY, Cowell AK, et al. Clinical evaluation of urine *Histoplasma capsulatum* antigen measurement in cats with suspected disseminated histoplasmosis. J Feline Med Surg. 2012;14:512-515.

Kroetz DN, Deepe GS. The role of cytokines and chemokines in *Histoplasma capsulatum* infection. Cytokine. 2012;58:112-117.

Lin Blache J, Ryan K, Arceneaux K. Histoplasmosis. Compend Contin Educ Vet. 2011;33:E1-E11.

REFERENCES

1. Darling ST. A protozoal general infection producing pseudotubercles in the lungs and focal necrosis in the liver, spleen, and lymph nodes. JAMA. 1906;46:1283-1285.
2. Johnson LR, Fry MM, Anez KL, et al. Histoplasmosis infection in two cats from California. J Am Anim Hosp Assoc. 2004;40:165-169.
3. Brilhante RS, Coelho CG, Sidrim JJ, et al. Feline histoplasmosis in Brazil: clinical and laboratory aspects and a comparative approach of published reports. Mycopathologia. 2012;173:193-197.
4. Mavropoulou A, Grandi G, Calvi L, et al. Disseminated histoplasmosis in a cat in Europe. J Small Anim Pract. 2010;51:176-180.
5. Mackie JT, Kaufman L, Ellis D. Confirmed histoplasmosis in an Australian dog. Aust Vet J. 1997;75:362-363.
6. Murata Y, Sano A, Ueda Y, et al. Molecular epidemiology of canine histoplasmosis in Japan. Med Mycol. 2007;45:233-247.
7. Sanford SE, Straube U. Ontario. Disseminated histoplasmosis in a young dog. Can Vet J. 1991;32:692.
8. Tyre E, Eisenbart D, Foley P, et al. Histoplasmosis in a dog from New Brunswick. Can Vet J. 2007;48:734-736.
9. Kasuga T, White TJ, Koenig G, et al. Phylogeography of the fungal pathogen *Histoplasma capsulatum*. Mol Ecol. 2003;12:3383-3401.
10. Arunmozhi Balajee S, Hurst SF, Chang L, et al. Multilocus sequence typing of *Histoplasma capsulatum* in formalin-fixed paraffin-embedded tissues from cats living in non-endemic regions reveals a new phylogenetic clade. Med Mycol. 2012:Oct 17 [Epub].
11. Zeidberg LD, Ajello L, Webster RH. Physical and chemical factors in relation to *Histoplasma capsulatum* in soil. Science. 1955;122:33-34.
12. Taylor ML, Hernandez-Garcia L, Estrada-Barcenas D, et al. Genetic diversity of *Histoplasma capsulatum* isolated from infected bats randomly captured in Mexico, Brazil, and Argentina, using the polymorphism of (GA)(n) microsatellite and its flanking regions. Fungal Biol. 2012;116:308-317.
13. Davies C, Troy GC. Deep mycotic infections in cats. J Am Anim Hosp Assoc. 1996;32:380-391.
14. Aulakh HK, Aulakh KS, Troy GC. Feline histoplasmosis: a retrospective study of 22 cases (1986-2009). J Am Anim Hosp Assoc. 2012;48:182-187.
15. Mitchell M, Stark DR. Disseminated canine histoplasmosis: a clinical survey of 24 cases in Texas. Can Vet J. 1980;21:95-100.
16. Selby LA, Becker SV, Hayes Jr HW. Epidemiologic risk factors associated with canine systemic mycoses. Am J Epidemiol. 1981;113:133-139.
17. Hodges RD, Legendre AM, Adams LG, et al. Itraconazole for the treatment of histoplasmosis in cats. J Vet Intern Med. 1994;8:409-413.
18. Clinkenbeard KD, Cowell RL, Tyler RD. Disseminated histoplasmosis in dogs: 12 cases (1981-1986). J Am Vet Med Assoc. 1988;193:1443-1447.
19. Wolf AM, Green RW. The radiographic appearance of pulmonary histoplasmosis in the cat. Vet Radiol. 1987;28:34-37.
20. Deepe GS. *Histoplasma capsulatum*. In: Mandell GL, Bennett JE, Dolin R, eds. Principles and Practice of Infectious Diseases. 7th ed. Philadelphia, PA: Elsevier; 2010:3305-3318.
21. Newman SL, Gootee L, Hilty J, et al. Human macrophages do not require phagosome acidification to mediate fungistatic/fungicidal activity against *Histoplasma capsulatum*. J Immunol. 2006;176:1806-1813.
22. Hilty J, George Smulian A, Newman SL. *Histoplasma capsulatum* utilizes siderophores for intracellular iron acquisition in macrophages. Med Mycol. 2011;49:633-642.
23. Emmons CW, Rowley DA, Olson BJ, et al. Histoplasmosis; proved occurrence of inapparent infection in dogs, cats and other animals. Am J Hyg. 1955;61:40-44.
24. Goad MEP, Roenick WJ. Osseous histoplasmosis in a cat. Fel Pract. 1983;13:32-36.
25. Tamulevicus AM, Harkin K, Janardhan K, et al. Disseminated histoplasmosis accompanied by cutaneous fragility in a cat. J Am Anim Hosp Assoc. 2011;47:e36-e41.
26. Lamm CG, Rizzi TE, Campbell GA, et al. Pathology in practice. *Histoplasma capsulatum* infections. J Am Vet Med Assoc. 2009;235:155-157.
27. Vinayak A, Kerwin SC, Pool RR. Treatment of thoracolumbar spinal cord compression associated with *Histoplasma capsulatum* infection in a cat. J Am Vet Med Assoc. 2007;230:1018-1023.
28. Taylor AR, Barr JW, Hokamp JA, et al. Cytologic diagnosis of disseminated histoplasmosis in the wall of the urinary bladder of a cat. J Am Anim Hosp Assoc. 2012;48:203-208.
29. Kobayashi R, Tanaka F, Asai A, et al. First case report of histoplasmosis in a cat in Japan. J Vet Med Sci. 2009;71:1669-1672.
30. Burk RL, Jones BD. Disseminated histoplasmosis with osseous involvement in a dog. J Am Vet Med Assoc. 1978;172:1416-1417.
31. Gilor C, Ridgway MD, Singh K. DIC and granulomatous vasculitis in a dog with disseminated histoplasmosis. J Am Anim Hosp Assoc. 2011;47:e26-e30.
32. Lau RE, Kim SN, Pirozok RP. *Histoplasma capsulatum* infection in a metatarsal of a dog. J Am Vet Med Assoc. 1978;172:1414-1416.
33. Nishifuji K, Ueda Y, Sano A, et al. Interdigital involvement in a case of primary cutaneous canine histoplasmosis in Japan. J Vet Med A Physiol Pathol Clin Med. 2005;52:478-480.

34. Kagawa Y, Aoki S, Iwatomi T, et al. Histoplasmosis in the skin and gingiva in a dog. J Vet Med Sci. 1998;60:863-865.
35. Ueda Y, Sano A, Tamura M, et al. Diagnosis of histoplasmosis by detection of the internal transcribed spacer region of fungal rRNA gene from a paraffin-embedded skin sample from a dog in Japan. Vet Microbiol. 2003;94:219-224.
36. Sano A, Miyaji M. Canine histoplasmosis in Japan. Nihon Ishinkin Gakkai Zasshi. 2003;44:239-243.
37. Clemans JM, Deitz KL, Riedesel EA, et al. Retroperitoneal pyogranulomatous and fibrosing inflammation secondary to fungal infections in two dogs. J Am Vet Med Assoc. 2011;238:213-219.
38. Olson GA, Wowk BJ. Oral lesions of histoplasmosis in a dog. Vet Med Small Anim Clin. 1981;76:1449-1451.
39. Huss BT, Collier LL, Collins BK, et al. Polyarthropathy and chorioretinitis with retinal detachment in a dog with systemic histoplasmosis. J Am Anim Hosp Assoc. 1994;30:217-224.
40. Gwin RM, Makley Jr TA, Wyman M, et al. Multifocal ocular histoplasmosis in a dog and cat. J Am Vet Med Assoc. 1980;176:638-642.
41. Meadows RL, MacWilliams PS, Dzata G, et al. Diagnosis of histoplasmosis in a dog by cytologic examination of CSF. Vet Clin Pathol. 1992;21:122-125.
42. Schaer M, Johnson KE, Nicholson AC. Central nervous system disease due to histoplasmosis in a dog: a case report. J Am Anim Hosp Assoc. 1983;19:311-316.
43. Clinkenbeard KD, Cowell RL, Tyler RD. Disseminated histoplasmosis in cats: 12 cases (1981-1986). J Am Vet Med Assoc. 1987;190:1445-1448.
44. Carakostas MC, Miller RI, Gossett KA. Clinical laboratory evaluation of deep mycotic diseases in dogs. J Small Anim Pract. 1984;25:687-693.
45. Kowalewich N, Hawkins EC, Skowronek AJ, et al. Identification of *Histoplasma capsulatum* organisms in the pleural and peritoneal effusions of a dog. J Am Vet Med Assoc. 1993;202:423-426.
46. Clinkenbeard KD, Cowell RL, Tyler RD. Identification of *Histoplasma* organisms in circulating eosinophils of a dog. J Am Vet Med Assoc. 1988;192:217-218.
47. Burk RL, Corley EA, Corwin LA. The radiographic appearance of pulmonary histoplasmosis in the dog and cat: a review of 37 case histories. J Am Vet Radiol Soc. 1978;19:2-7.
48. Miller BM, Waterhouse G, Alford RH, et al. *Histoplasma* infection of abdominal aortic aneurysms. Ann Surg. 1983;197:57-62.
49. Kauffman CA. Histoplasmosis: a clinical and laboratory update. Clin Microbiol Rev. 2007;20:115-132.
50. Swartzentruber S, Rhodes L, Kurkjian K, et al. Diagnosis of acute pulmonary histoplasmosis by antigen detection. Clin Infect Dis. 2009;49:1878-1882.
51. Wheat J, Wheat H, Connolly P, et al. Cross-reactivity in *Histoplasma capsulatum* variety *capsulatum* antigen assays of urine samples from patients with endemic mycoses. Clin Infect Dis. 1997;24:1169-1171.
52. Kuberski T, Myers R, Wheat LJ, et al. Diagnosis of coccidioidomycosis by antigen detection using cross-reaction with a *Histoplasma* antigen. Clin Infect Dis. 2007;44:e50-e54.
53. Hage CA, Kirsch EJ, Stump TE, et al. *Histoplasma* antigen clearance during treatment of histoplasmosis in patients with AIDS determined by a quantitative antigen enzyme immunoassay. Clin Vaccine Immunol. 2011;18:661-666.
54. Cook AK, Cunningham LY, Cowell AK, et al. Clinical evaluation of urine *Histoplasma capsulatum* antigen measurement in cats with suspected disseminated histoplasmosis. J Feline Med Surg. 2012;14:512-515.
55. Martagon-Villamil J, Shrestha N, Sholtis M, et al. Identification of *Histoplasma capsulatum* from culture extracts by real-time PCR. J Clin Microbiol. 2003;41:1295-1298.
56. Babady NE, Buckwalter SP, Hall L, et al. Detection of *Blastomyces dermatitidis* and *Histoplasma capsulatum* from culture isolates and clinical specimens by use of real-time PCR. J Clin Microbiol. 2011;49:3204-3208.
57. Restrepo A, Tobon A, Clark B, et al. Salvage treatment of histoplasmosis with posaconazole. J Infect. 2007;54:319-327.
58. Wheat LJ, Connolly P, Smedema M, et al. Activity of newer triazoles against *Histoplasma capsulatum* from patients with AIDS who failed fluconazole. J Antimicrob Chemother. 2006;57:1235-1239.
59. Kroetz DN, Deepe GS. The role of cytokines and chemokines in *Histoplasma capsulatum* infection. Cytokine. 2012;58:112-117.
60. Davies SF, Colbert RL. Concurrent human and canine histoplasmosis from cutting decayed wood. Ann Intern Med. 1990;113:252-253.

CHAPTER 62

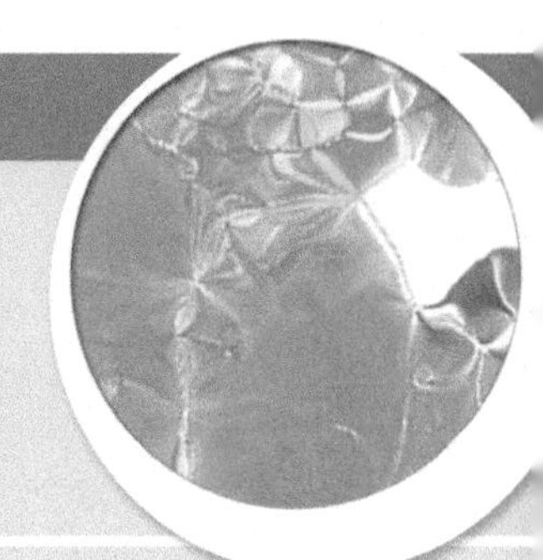

Cryptococcosis

Jane E. Sykes and Richard Malik

Overview of Cryptococcosis

First Described: 1894, in a human patient in Germany (independently by Busse and Buschke)[1]

Causes: *Cryptococcus gattii, Cryptococcus neoformans,* rarely other cryptococcal species (a basidiomycete, teleomorph *Filobasidiella* spp.)

Affected Hosts: Cats, dogs, humans, and a variety of other domestic and wild animal species

Geographic Distribution: Worldwide

Major Mode of Transmission: Inhalation of basidiospores from the environment

Major Clinical Signs: Nodular or ulcerative cutaneous lesions, upper respiratory tract signs, chorioretinitis, neurologic signs secondary to meningoencephalitis. In dogs, *Cryptococcus* can also disseminate to abdominal organs and cause gastrointestinal signs such as vomiting, diarrhea, and inappetence.

Differential Diagnoses: For cats, differential diagnoses for cutaneous lesions include other deep mycoses (especially sporotrichosis), mycobacteriosis, nocardiosis, neoplasia (especially squamous cell carcinoma), herpetic dermatitis and eosinophilic granuloma complex. Differential diagnoses for suspected cryptococcal rhinitis include nasal lymphoma, foreign bodies, sinonasal/sino-orbital aspergillosis, oronasal fistulae and neutrophilic rhinitis. For ocular and central nervous system lesions, differential diagnoses include neoplasia (especially lymphoma), toxoplasmosis, feline infectious peritonitis, and otogenic bacterial meningitis. For dogs, differential diagnoses include other disseminated mycoses (especially histoplasmosis and blastomycosis), mycobacteriosis, actinomycosis and nocardiosis, other causes of rhinitis (such as foreign bodies, nasal aspergillosis, oronasal fistulas, lymphoplasmacytic rhinitis, rhinosporidiosis), neoplasia (especially round cell neoplasia), toxoplasmosis, neosporosis, severe inflammatory bowel disease, and pancreatitis.

Human Health Significance: Human infections occur as a result of exposure to organisms in the environment and are often associated with underlying immune compromise.

Etiology and Epidemiology

Cryptococcosis is an important fungal infection of people and animals worldwide and the most common systemic mycosis of cats. The infection is acquired from the environment, and disease transmission from one animal to another has not been reported. Occasional outbreaks of cryptococcosis in people and animals may result from exposure to common environmental sources.[2,3] Various domestic and native mammals may be infected, which include cats, dogs, ferrets, horses, camelids, goats, sheep, cattle, dolphins, birds, koalas, and other marsupials.[4-10] The incidence of cryptococcosis in cats is eightfold higher than that in dogs.[11]

The genus *Cryptococcus* contains at least 19 encapsulated yeast species. *Cryptococcus neoformans* and *Cryptococcus gattii* (formerly *C. neoformans* var. *gattii*) cause the vast majority of infections in dogs, cats, and humans. *C. gattii* has emerged as a pathogen of immunocompetent humans in temperate regions of North America, in particular on the west coast of the United States and in British Columbia, Canada. Other species, particularly *Cryptococcus laurentii* and *Cryptococcus albidus,* rarely cause disease in people and animals, but may be emerging as a result of immunocompromise.[12-14] *Cryptococcus magnus* was isolated from the external ear canal of a cat with otitis externa,[15] and *C. laurentii* has been isolated from the external ear canal of dogs.[16]

Cryptococcus spp. are dimorphic, basidiomycetous fungi. The life cycle of the fungus is thought to involve growth in host tissues as an encapsulated haploid budding yeast, combined with the ability to undergo a transition to a filamentous form (or teleomorph) in the environment. Two mating types of *Cryptococcus* spp. exist, α and **a**. The α-type is vastly more prevalent in environmental and clinical samples. Under appropriate laboratory conditions, the two mating types fuse and adopt a dikaryotic filamentous state, also known as the *perfect state.* This is followed by production of basidia, which are small, club-shaped structures on which basidiospores form (Figure 62-1).[17] Cells of the α mating type can also undergo asexual reproduction via a process known as monokaryotic fruiting, which also involves filamentation and spore formation.[17-19] Although they have never been observed in nature, basidiospores (or possibly desiccated yeasts) are thought to be the main form that, when inhaled, gives rise to mammalian disease.[20] In animal tissues, basidiospores convert to the yeast form, which is round to oval with a variably sized capsule. The capsule is primarily (90% to 95%) composed of a polysaccharide known as glucuronoxylomannan (GXM), with smaller amounts of galactoxylomannan. The capsule enlarges after infection of mammalian hosts and protects the fungus from phagocytosis and environmental insults such as desiccation. Within tissues, *Cryptococcus* reproduces by forming one or two daughter cells (buds) that are connected to the parent cell by a narrow base (Figure 62-2).

Historically, five serotypes of *Cryptococcus* (A, B, C, D, and AD) were recognized on the basis of antigenic differences in the capsular polysaccharide. Based on the results of molecular

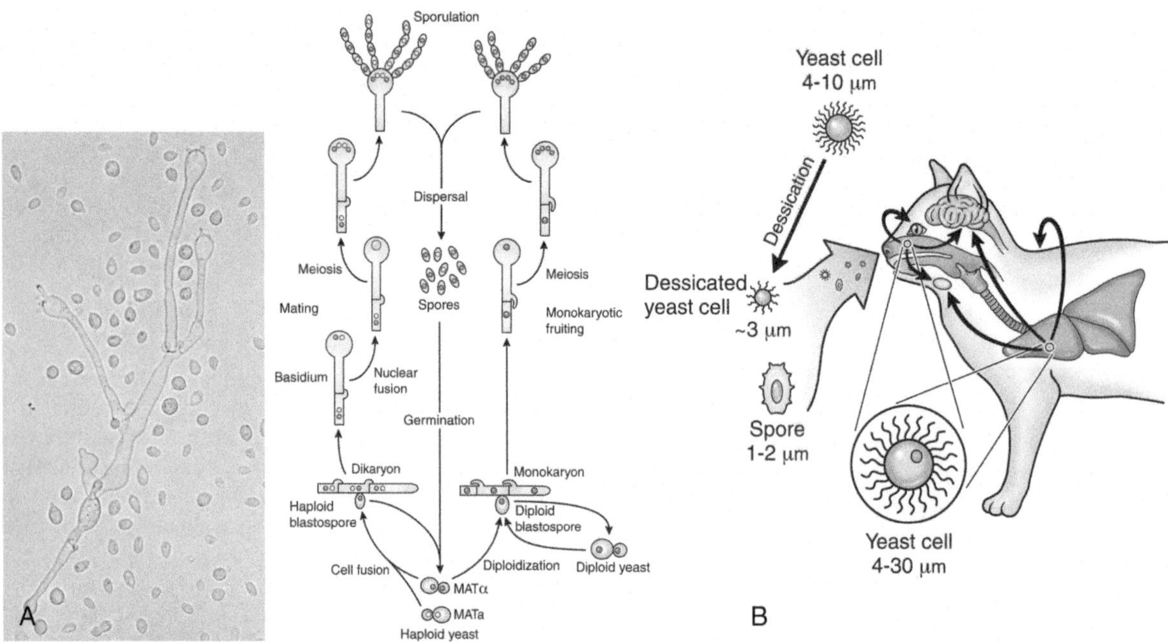

FIGURE 62-1 Life cycle of *Cryptococcus* spp. **A,** Spores result from either mating between cells of opposite mating types (MATa or MATα) and subsequent formation of dikaryotic hyphae or unisexual mating of MATα cells (monokaryotic fruiting). In both cases, sexual development within the filamentous form results in meiosis and basidiospore formation. The spores germinate to produce haploid, yeast-like cells that divide by budding. **B,** Spores, and potentially desiccated yeast cells, are inhaled. Germination of spores or vegetative growth of yeast cells in the upper or lower respiratory tract results in the proliferation of budding yeasts. Dissemination to a variety of tissues can then occur, but especially to the lymph nodes, nasal cavity, skin, and CNS. (Modified from Kronstad JW, Attarian R, Cadieux B, et al. Expanding fungal pathogenesis: *Cryptococcus* breaks out of the opportunistic box. Nat Rev Microbiol 2011;9:193-203. Basidiospore image courtesy Patrik Inderbitzen, University of California, Davis.)

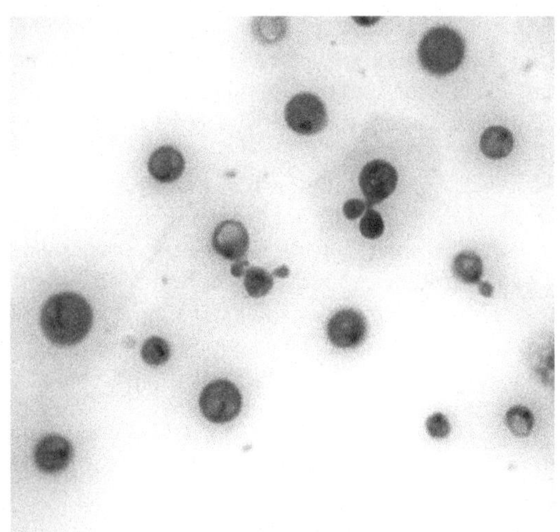

FIGURE 62-2 CSF cytology from an 8-year-old male neutered domestic shorthair cat with cryptococcal meningitis. Large numbers of budding cryptococcal yeasts are present.

typing methods such as PCR fingerprinting and multilocus sequence typing, cryptococcal strains from around the world are divided into eight major molecular types: VNI and VNII (*C. neoformans* serotype A); VNIII (*C. neoformans* serotype AD); VNIV (*C. neoformans* serotype D), and VGI, VGII, VGIII, and VGIV (*C. gattii*, serotypes B and C).[21] Hybrid strains also exist. Differences in epidemiology, pathogenicity, clinical features, and drug susceptibility have been associated with each species and molecular type.

Cats of all ages may be affected,[22] but young adult cats appear to be at increased risk. In dogs, cryptococcosis is diagnosed predominantly in young adult dogs. In one study, the median age of cats and dogs was 6 and 4 years, respectively.[11] No clear sex predisposition exists. Siamese, birman, and ragdoll cats have been predisposed in Australian studies but were not found to be at risk in the United States.[11,23] Similarly, German shepherd dogs, Doberman pinschers, and great Danes appear to be predisposed in Australia, whereas in the United States, American cocker spaniel dogs are strongly predisposed.[5,11,22,24,25]

Most cats and dogs with cryptococcosis do not have identifiable underlying immunosuppressive illness. The prevalence of retrovirus infection in cat populations with cryptococcosis does not differ from that in cat populations without cryptococcosis.[11,22] However, some cats with cryptococcosis that are co-infected with FeLV appear to respond more slowly to treatment and may be more likely to have relapses.[26] Cryptococcosis is occasionally reported in cats treated with immunosuppressive therapy or chemotherapy for malignancy.[11,27] Concurrent opportunistic infections have been reported in other cats (e.g., toxoplasmosis), as well as in dogs (e.g., neosporosis or papillomatosis), suggesting underlying immunodeficiency.[11,28]

Cryptococcus neoformans

C. neoformans has a worldwide distribution. It primarily infects human patients who are immunocompromised, especially AIDS patients. The realized environmental niche for *C. neoformans* is weathered bird (especially pigeon) guano, in which it mates prolifically.[29] It can also be found in decaying plant matter in hollows of certain trees.[30] The organism can remain viable for at least 2 years in environments such as pigeon lofts. The majority of human cryptococcal infections result from infection with *C. neoformans* var. *grubii* (VNI). *C. neoformans* var. *grubii* is the most common *Cryptococcus* species isolated from dogs and cats in southeastern Australia and accounts for more than 70% of infections.[22,23,25] Across the United States, most dogs with cryptococcosis are infected with *C. neoformans*, but infection of cats with this species is rare.[11,31]

Cryptococcus gattii

C. gattii is endemic in Australia, New Zealand, Papua New Guinea, Southeast Asia, parts of Latin America, California, Mexico, Hawaii, Central and South Africa, and, to a lesser extent, certain parts of Europe (Austria, Germany, France, Italy, Greece, and Spain).[32,33] Since 1999, an epidemic of infections with *C. gattii* has occurred in humans and domestic and wild animals in British Columbia in Canada, especially Vancouver Island, and the Pacific Northwest of the United States.[34-36] The main molecular types identified in this epidemic have been molecular types VGIIa and, to a much lesser extent, VGIIb and, in Oregon, also VGIIc. *C. gattii* molecular type VGII can be found on living tree bark (Garry oak, maple, cedar, and pine) and in air, and has also been found in freshwater and seawater. Proximity to areas with soil disturbance was a risk factor for dogs and cats.[37] In California, almost all cats are infected with *C. gattii* VGIII, with occasional VGII infections.[11,31] The ecologic niche of this molecular type in the United States remains unclear. Approximately 25% of affected cats are housed exclusively indoors.[11]

In eastern Australia, 20% to 30% of human, feline, and canine cryptococcosis is caused by C. *gattii*,[23,38] whereas in western Australia, approximately 50% of cats and dogs are infected with *C. gattii*.[5] Most *C. gattii* isolates from eastern Australia belong to VGI; VGII predominates in southwestern and northern Australia.[5,39] *C. gattii* VGI in Australia is exclusively associated with dead plant material in eucalyptus tree hollows. Cats in rural environments are at risk of infection.

In contrast to *C. neoformans*, *C. gattii* isolates from the Pacific northwest and British Columbia can infect apparently immunocompetent humans.[40] *C. gattii* molecular type VGIII infections have been reported in immunosuppressed humans in southern California.[41] When disease occurs in immunocompetent hosts, it is often characterized by the presence of pulmonary mass lesions (cryptococcomas) and sometimes intracranial cryptococcomas.[42] As a result, pulmonary cryptococcomas are more commonly described in human patients infected with *C. gattii* compared with those infected with *C. neoformans*.[43]

Clinical Features

Signs and Their Pathogenesis

Based on the small size of basidiospores, the lung is thought to be the primary site of infection in humans. In cats, dogs, and koalas, the nasal cavity may be the primary site of infection (see Figure 62-1); significant pulmonary parenchymal involvement in these species is rare. Colonization of the nasal cavity may be followed by development of cryptococcal rhinitis in some (but not all) dogs and cats. However, some nasal cavity involvement may result from hematogenous dissemination, because injection of *Cryptococcus* spp. into the carotid artery of cats can lead to development of lesions on the bridge of the nose. Some localized cutaneous lesions may result from direct cutaneous inoculation (e.g., after a cat scratch), but skin lesions are usually interpreted as the result of dissemination or extension from the nasal cavity.

The pathogenesis of cryptococcosis depends on the size of the inoculum, virulence of the cryptococcal strain, and host immunity. *Cryptococcus* has been aptly described as "a sugar-coated killer with designer genes."[44] *Cryptococcus* has several important virulence factors, including its polysaccharide capsule, laccase (which makes melanin), and other enzymes such as

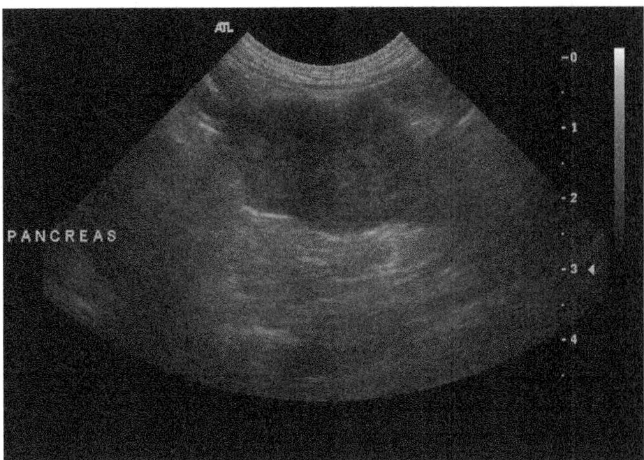

FIGURE 62-3 Ultrasound image that shows an enlarged and hypoechoic pancreas in a 7-year-old female spayed basset mixed-breed dog with systemic cryptococcosis caused by *Cryptococcus neoformans* var. *grubii* (molecular type VNI). The dog was evaluated for gastrointestinal signs that were associated with severe cryptococcal pancreatitis and enteritis. The dog's lungs, heart, kidneys, liver, mesenteric lymph nodes, peritoneum, brain, and meninges were also involved at necropsy.

phospholipase, urease, and superoxide dismutase.[17,42] Capsular polysaccharide is continuously shed into the host's extracellular fluid, which includes blood, urine, and CSF. The capsule inhibits phagocytosis, depletes complement, and is well known for its ability to inhibit effective T cell responses. The ability of *C. neoformans* and *C. gattii* to grow at mammalian body temperature is also an important virulence factor and is lacking in other species of *Cryptococcus*.

The incubation period can range from 2 to 13 months.[45,46] Exposure and self-limiting infection may occur in some individuals, with reactivation of viable cryptococci in residual granulomatous foci months or years later with immunosuppressive drug therapy or illness.[42] Because of this delay, a travel history to areas where *Cryptococcus* is highly endemic (such as British Columbia or the west coast of the United States) may be present in animals and humans residing in non-endemic regions. After infection is established within the lung or nasal cavity, the organism can spread hematogenously to other sites, particularly the lymph nodes, eye, skin, and central nervous system (CNS) (see Figure 62-1). *Cryptococcus* spp. has a strong tendency to invade the meninges and typically causes meningitis or meningoencephalitis. In humans, cerebral cryptococcosis is often associated with increased intracranial pressure, and this probably also occurs in cats and dogs. Spread of infection to the eye, either along the optic nerves from the brain or as a result of hematogenous spread, may result in concurrent cryptococcal optic neuritis and chorioretinitis. In animals with nasal cavity involvement, extension of infection into the brain may also follow osteomyelitis of the cribriform plate or of the ventral wall of the frontal sinus. Middle ear involvement can also occur.[47] Infection also often spreads from the nasal cavity to the mandibular lymph nodes.

Multifocal cutaneous involvement in cats and dogs reflects hematogenous dissemination from the primary site of infection, as do lesions in bone (e.g., digits) or periarticular soft tissues. Dogs infected with *C. neoformans* often develop widely disseminated disease, with involvement of sites such as the gastrointestinal system, pancreas, mesenteric lymph nodes, kidneys, myocardium, and thyroid gland (Figure 62-3).[11,24,48,49] In contrast, dogs infected with *C. gattii* molecular type VGII in the

United States tend to have isolated caudal nasal cavity cryptococcomas, which can extend through the cribriform plate into the brain (Figure 62-4).

Clinical Features in Cats

Cryptococcosis is often a chronic infection in cats, and affected cats are usually otherwise well but occasionally have mild lethargy and inappetence. Fever is rare, and when it occurs, it tends to be low-grade. Upper respiratory tract signs due to nasal cavity involvement are common, sometimes with associated mandibular lymphadenopathy. Single or multifocal ulcerated or nonulcerated cutaneous masses may also be present (Figure 62-5).

Lower respiratory tract signs such as tachypnea are uncommon but can occur as a result of pleural effusion or severe mediastinal lymphadenomegaly. Neurologic signs vary depending on the location of lesions in and around the CNS (see Physical Examination Findings), and, rarely, cats with CNS involvement lack obvious neurologic signs. Optic neuritis and chorioretinitis develop in as many as one third of affected cats and almost always indicate CNS involvement.

Other signs include peripheral lymphadenomegaly (which may be unassociated with skin lesions and is often asymmetric), lameness due to osteomyelitis or cryptococcal arthritis, and swollen digits. Rarely, involvement of the abdominal lymph nodes, kidneys, spleen, liver, thyroid, and salivary glands occur.

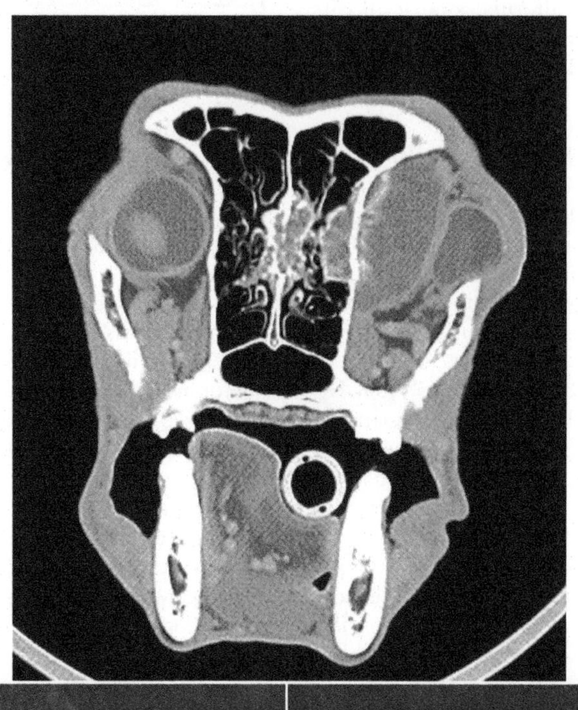

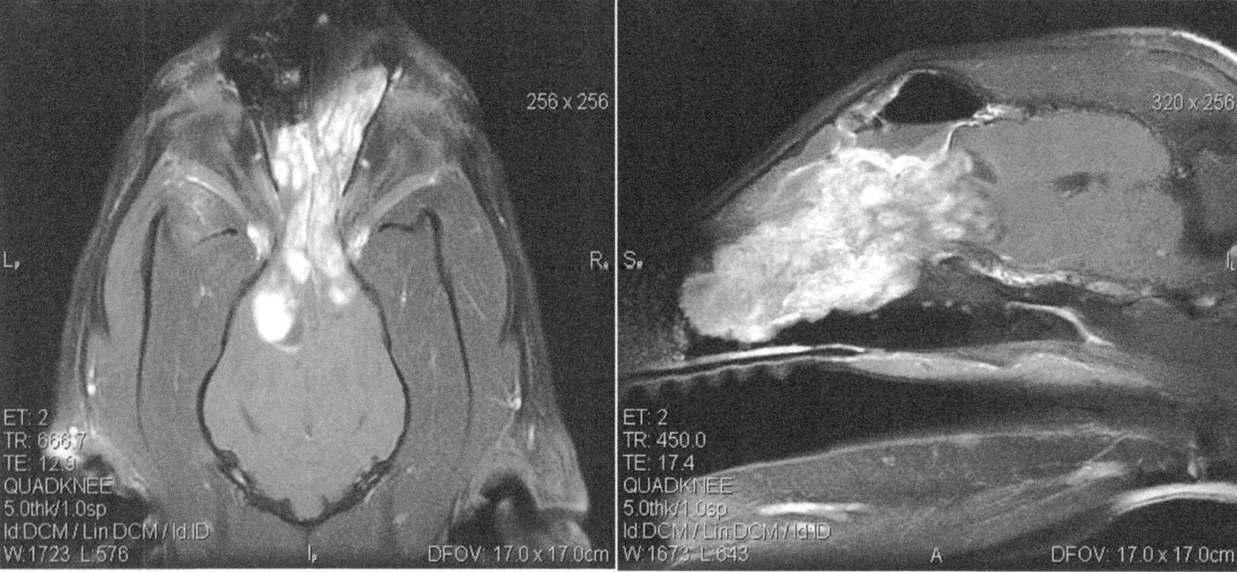

FIGURE 62-4 Caudal nasal cryptococcosis in dogs infected with *Cryptococcus gattii*. **A,** CT scan showing a large caudal nasal cavity cryptococcoma at necropsy that invaded the cribriform plate and retrobulbar space in a 5-year-old Doberman pinscher infected with *C. gattii* molecular type VGIIa. There is a palisading periosteal response along the lateral margin of the right frontal and lacrimal bones. **B** and **C,** Postcontrast magnetic resonance images of the head of a 2-year-old intact male malamute with a 1-week history of abnormal behavior and seizures. *Cryptococcus gattii* was isolated from the nasal cavity. A large, contrast-enhancing mass is present in the caudal nasal cavity that invades the cribriform plate and extends into the brain. (Courtesy Dr. Stacey Hoffman.)

Clinical Features in Dogs

In contrast to cats, dogs frequently develop severe disseminated disease. In one study, 80% of dogs had involvement of multiple anatomic sites, and 50% of dogs had involvement of sites other than the nasal cavity, skin, lungs, lymph nodes, kidney, eye, and CNS.[11] Weight loss, lethargy, and inappetence are common nonspecific findings. Rhinosinusitis from cryptococcosis may be subclinical in dogs, so its incidence may be underestimated.[11,25] However, sneezing and mucopurulent nasal discharge can also occur. Neurologic signs were present in two thirds of affected dogs from California.[11] Dogs can also primarily show signs of gastrointestinal or pancreatic involvement, such as vomiting, diarrhea, and abdominal pain.

Cutaneous involvement is uncommon in dogs but, as in cats, may be a marker for disseminated disease. Although rarely detected antemortem, more than half of dogs have lower respiratory involvement at necropsy.[11] Other clinical signs that are infrequently present in dogs include peripheral lymphadenomegaly or lameness (due to osteomyelitis or arthritis).

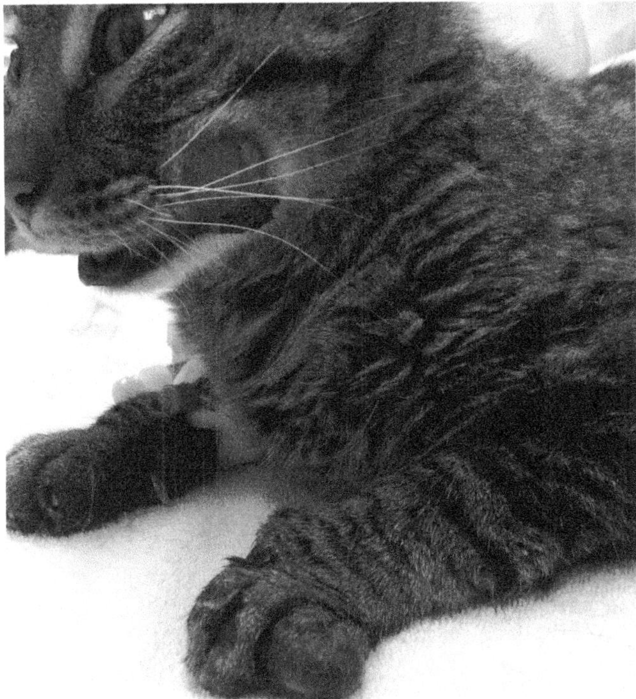

FIGURE 62-5 Multiple ulcerated skin lesions in a cat from northern California with disseminated cryptococcosis caused by *Cryptococcus gattii* molecular type VGIII.

Physical Examination Findings

Cats

Upper respiratory tract signs are common physical examination findings in cats with cryptococcosis. These include sneezing; snuffling; and mucopurulent, serous, or hemorrhagic nasal discharge that is unilateral or bilateral. In some cats, a fleshy mass protrudes from the nostril. Other cats have one or more firm to fluctuant, ulcerated or nonulcerated, subcutaneous swellings over the bridge of the nose. These swellings may communicate with the frontal sinus or nasal cavity, and palpation of the lesions may reveal crepitus due to subcutaneous emphysema. Cats with nasopharyngeal cryptococcosis develop stertor, stridor, and, occasionally, otitis media. Mandibular lymphadenopathy is often present. Ulcerated or proliferative lesions of the buccal mucosa can also be found. Multifocal skin lesions consist of nodules or masses that are fluctuant to firm, up to several centimeters in diameter, and may ulcerate (see Figure 62-5).

Neurologic examination abnormalities in cats with CNS involvement include obtundation; atypical behavior; slow menace, palpebral, or pupillary light responses; mydriasis or anisocoria (Figure 62-6, *A*); twitching or tremors; and seizures, circling, head pressing, ataxia, paresis, abnormal placing reactions, head tilt, nystagmus, and spinal pain.[9] Fundoscopic examination may reveal granulomatous chorioretinitis, exudative retinal detachment, papilledema, evidence of optic neuritis, and/or retinal hemorrhage (Figure 62-6, *B*). Severe ocular

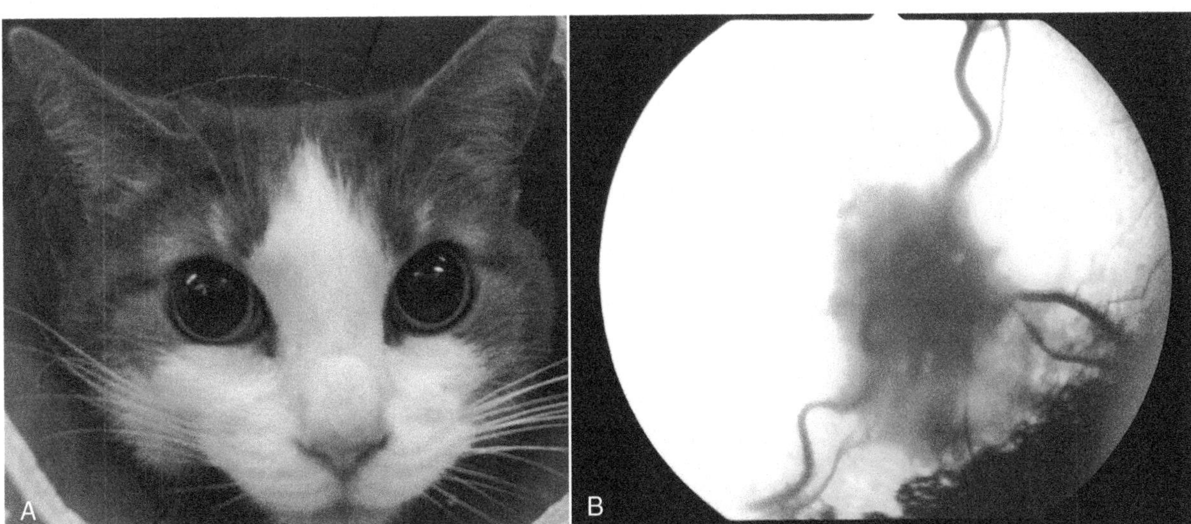

FIGURE 62-6 Ocular abnormalities in cats with disseminated cryptococcosis. **A,** Bilateral mydriasis in an 8-year-old male neutered domestic shorthair with cryptococcal meningoencephalitis. Fundoscopic examination was within normal limits. **B,** Granulomatous chorioretinitis and retinal detachment in another cat with cryptococcosis. (Courtesy University of California, Davis, Veterinary Ophthalmology Service.)

TABLE 62-1

Diagnostic Assays Currently Available for Cryptococcosis in Dogs and Cats

Assay	Specimen Type	Target	Performance
Cytologic examination	Aspirates of affected tissues, body fluids, impression smears of skin lesions or biopsies	*Cryptococcus* organisms	High sensitivity, but occasionally organisms are not visualized (such as in the CSF of some animals with CNS cryptococcosis).
Fungal culture	Aspirates or biopsies of affected tissues, body fluids such as CSF and urine	*Cryptococcus* spp.	Generally sensitive and specific, but false negatives are possible if specimen size is low. Requires several days' incubation. Allows species identification and antifungal drug susceptibility testing.
Antigen assay (latex agglutination)	Serum, CSF	*Cryptococcus* polysaccharide antigen	Sensitivity and specificity exceed 90%. False negatives can occur in dogs and with localized infections in cats. False positives are generally of low magnitude (<1:200 and usually <1:16). Titers vary between kits.
Real-time PCR assays	Biopsies, body fluids, aspirates	*Cryptococcus* DNA	Not yet validated in adequate numbers of dogs or cats with cryptococcosis; usefulness requires further evaluation.
Histopathology	Biopsy specimens from affected tissues	*Cryptococcus* spp. yeasts	High sensitivity, with rare false negatives. Special stains such as Mayer's mucicarmine and immunohistochemical stains facilitate organism detection and identification.

lesions or optic neuritis may result in blindness with dilated and unresponsive pupils.

Dogs

Many dogs with cryptococcosis are lethargic or obtunded because of disseminated disease and/or CNS involvement. When fever occurs, it is typically low grade. Other CNS signs in dogs include absent or slow menace, gag, pupillary light responses, nystagmus, mydriasis, head tilt, strabismus, anisocoria, facial paralysis, paraparesis, abnormal placing reactions, ataxia, circling, seizures, twitching or tremors, reluctance to open the mouth, absent or decreased segmental reflexes, and, commonly, cervical hyperesthesia.[9,24] Some dogs show signs that resemble those of cervical disc herniation. The most common ocular abnormalities are chorioretinitis, papilledema, evidence of optic neuritis, and retinal detachment. Decreased nasal airflow may be present in dogs with nasal cavity cryptococcomas. Nodules, masses, or ulcers may involve any portion of the integument, and the nose, tongue, buccal mucosa, hard palate, lips, or nail beds.

Diagnosis

Definitive diagnosis of cryptococcosis is usually straightforward and based on evaluation of representative tissue specimens with cytology, culture, and occasionally histopathology, with or without serologic detection of cryptococcal antigen in body fluids (Table 62-1). Suitable specimens include nasal swabs, nasal washings, needle aspirates from mass lesions or enlarged lymph nodes, bronchoalveolar lavage specimens, pleural fluid, CSF, and urine.

Laboratory Abnormalities

Complete Blood Count, Serum Chemistry Profile, and Urinalysis

Changes in the CBC, chemistry panel, and urinalysis in animals with cryptococcosis are generally mild and nonspecific. Mild to moderate nonregenerative anemia; leukocytosis, often with monocytosis; and eosinophilia are the most common findings. Dogs with disseminated disease may have a neutrophilia with a left shift. The serum biochemical profile reflects specific organ involvement in animals with disseminated disease. Occasionally, cryptococcal yeasts are found on examination of the urine sediment.

Cerebrospinal Fluid Examination

The CSF in cats and dogs with neurologic signs due to cryptococcosis may have an increased protein concentration (usually between 10 and 140 mg/dL in cats, but may be several hundred or rarely more than 1000 mg/dL in dogs).[9] Leukocyte counts can range from 2 to more than 1000 cells/μL in both dogs and cats. A mixed cellular pleocytosis is generally present, with neutrophils or large mononuclear cells generally outnumbering other cell types. Some dogs have a marked eosinophilic pleocytosis. Cryptococcal yeasts are visible in most but not all animals with cryptococcal meningitis (see Figure 62-2).[9] Marked deterioration in neurologic status occasionally occurs in animals with CNS cryptococcosis immediately after CSF collection. Many animals have intracranial mass lesions or increased CSF pressure, which can increase the risk of cerebellar herniation following a cisternal tap. Wherever possible, attempts to make a diagnosis with serum antigen testing or collection of specimens from other anatomic sites should be considered as an alternative to diagnosis by CSF analysis.

Diagnostic Imaging

Plain Radiography

Thoracic radiographs in dogs and cats are often normal. In some animals, interstitial to alveolar infiltrates or small nodular lesions are present. Occasionally, large pulmonary nodules, hilar lymphadenopathy, a mediastinal granuloma, or pleural effusion are found.[41]

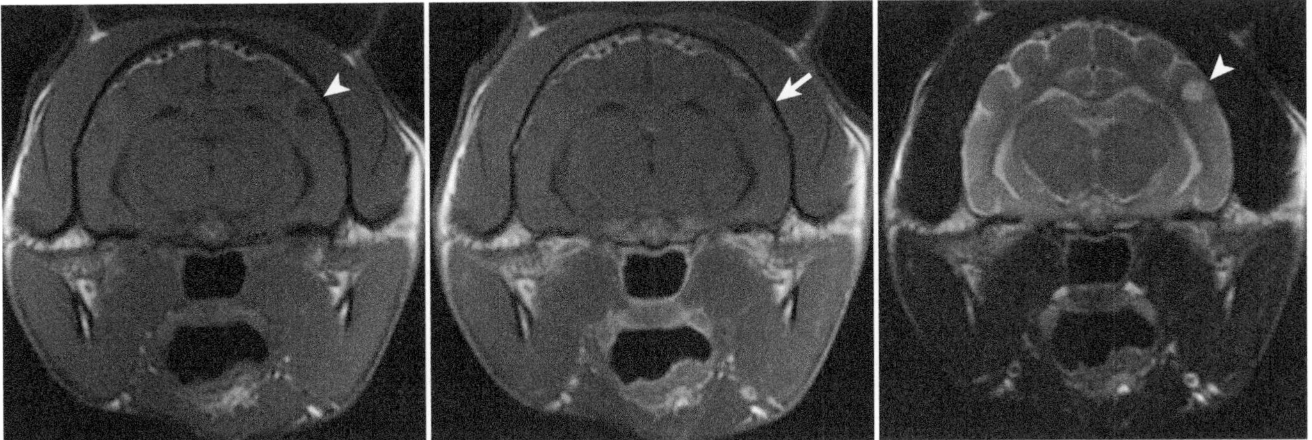

FIGURE 62-7 Transverse T1-weighted pre-contrast *(left)*, T1-weighted post-contrast *(center)*, and T2-weighted *(right)* MRI of the brain of an 8-year-old male neutered domestic shorthair with cryptococcosis. There is a focal lesion in the gray matter of the right cerebral cortex at the junction of the parietal and occipital lobes *(arrowhead)*. The lesion is T2 hyperintense, T1 hypointense, and rim-enhancing *(arrow)*. These signal characteristics were consistent with a pseudocyst lesion.

Computed Tomography

In cats with nasal cryptococcosis, computed tomography (CT) of the nasal cavity can reveal soft tissue and fluid opacification of the nasal cavity or frontal sinus, peripherally contrast-enhancing mass lesions of the nasal planum, and lysis of the nasal bones or of the cribriform plate.[11] In dogs, CT findings in the nasal cavity include peripherally contrast-enhancing mass lesions within the frontal sinuses, caudal nasal cavity, nasopharynx, or the retrobulbar space and associated osteomyelitis (see Figure 62-4, *A*). CNS abnormalities such as ventricular dilation and intra-axial contrast-enhancing mass lesions have been described in dogs using CT.[9] However, MRI is more sensitive for detection of CNS lesions in human patients,[42] and the same is probably true for dogs and cats.

Magnetic Resonance Imaging

MRI abnormalities in cats with CNS cryptococcosis consist of single or multifocal contrast-enhancing mass lesions that tend to be hyperintense on T2-weighted images and hypointense on T1-weighted images, as well as mild to moderate, diffuse or focal meningeal enhancement.[9] Some cats have lesions that appear fluid-filled on T2-weighted images but have a greater T1-weighted intensity than expected for acellular fluid ("high T2, low T1 lesions") (Figure 62-7).[9] MRI in dogs may show contrast-enhancing mass lesions that are hyperintense on T2-weighted images and of variable intensity on T1-weighted images, as well as meningeal enhancement (see Figure 62-4, *B*). Ventriculomegaly and/or cribriform plate osteomyelitis may also be evident.

Sonographic Findings

Over 80% of cats with cryptococcosis have normal abdominal ultrasound examinations. Cats with kidney involvement can have iso- to hypoechoic intraparenchymal mass lesions on ultrasound, with or without associated renal failure. These sometimes involve the renal pelvis. However, cats with renal involvement can also have normal abdominal ultrasound examinations.[11]

Ultrasonographic findings in dogs include intra-abdominal lymphadenomegaly, multifocal gastric and small intestinal thickening, changes suggestive of pancreatitis, renal mass lesions, and/or ascites (see Figure 62-3).[11,48]

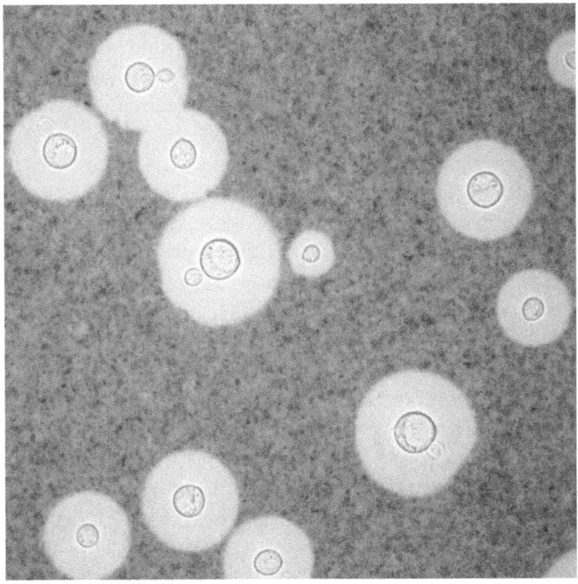

FIGURE 62-8 India ink stained preparation of *Cryptococcus gattii* yeasts that had been grown in culture. 1000× oil magnification. (Courtesy Greg Hodges and George Thompson III, University of California, Davis.)

Microbiologic Tests

Cytologic Examination

Cytologic examination can be performed on aspirates, body fluids, or impression smears of biopsy specimens. Romanowsky-type stains, new methylene blue, and Gram stain are all satisfactory for making a cytologic diagnosis. India ink can be used to examine CSF for cryptococcal yeasts, which appear unstained and silhouetted against a black background. India ink staining of CSF is still used routinely in the diagnosis of human cryptococcal infections (Figure 62-8).[42] However, lymphocytes and fat droplets can sometimes be confused with the organism.

Although cytologic examination of nasal or cutaneous exudates, aspirates, or body fluids for organisms is a rapid and sensitive test for cryptococcosis, negative test results do not eliminate the possibility of cryptococcosis. Generally, organisms are found only by cytologic examination of CSF in 60% to 80% of dogs and cats.[11] If a sufficient index of suspicion exists, additional diagnostic tests such as histopathology, antigen testing, and/or fungal culture are indicated.

Fungal Culture

Cryptococcus spp. are readily cultured from aspirates, exudate, CSF, urine, and tissue specimens. Attempts to culture the organism are recommended whenever possible before treatment is initiated, because isolation confirms the diagnosis, can be used to differentiate *C. gattii* from *C. neoformans*, and permits antifungal susceptibility testing for cases that subsequently fail to respond adequately to antifungal drug treatment. Some veterinary diagnostic laboratories still report all *Cryptococcus* isolates as *C. neoformans* in the absence of tests to discriminate between *C. neoformans* and *C. gattii*. If the report lists *C. neoformans* as the isolate, the laboratory must therefore be consulted to determine whether *C. neoformans* was differentiated from *C. gattii*. However, whether the clinician needs to know whether the isolate is *C. neoformans* or *C. gattii* is debatable because at this time, species identification does not clearly influence treatment recommendations or prognosis. If *Cryptococcus* is isolated from a contaminated site such as the nasal cavity, a diagnosis of cryptococcosis should be supported with cytologic or histopathologic evidence of active infection. This is because subclinical colonization occurs in some animals.

C. neoformans and *C. gattii* grow on almost all laboratory media, but fungal isolation media (such as Sabouraud's dextrose agar) and incubation temperatures of 25°C or 30°C in addition to incubation at 37°C are preferred when fungi are being considered in the differential diagnosis. Antibiotics are added to the medium for isolation of *Cryptococcus* spp. from contaminated sites, such as the nasal cavity. Colonies usually are visible in 2 to 3 days, but sometimes incubation for up to 10 days is required. Unlike other dimorphic fungi, *Cryptococcus* grows as a yeast, rather than a mold, on routine fungal media and so is less likely to represent a laboratory hazard than organisms that grow as molds. The organisms form white, creamy colonies. Often *C. gattii* colonies are more mucoid than *C. neoformans* colonies. The organism is identified based on its microscopic morphology and response to biochemical tests in commercial yeast identification kits (see Chapter 4). Canavanine-glycine-bromothymol blue (CGB) agar is used to differentiate between *C. neoformans* and *C. gattii*.[50] Unlike *C. neoformans*, *C. gattii* grows on CGB agar and turns the media a brilliant deep blue (Figure 62-9). Fungal culture of the CSF is frequently positive in patients with CNS cryptococcosis and should be performed even if the organism cannot be demonstrated cytologically or serologically. Culture of urine specimens collected using cystocentesis is also indicated when cryptococcosis is suspected, even when obvious renal involvement is not present and cytologic abnormalities are not present. Identification of molecular types for epidemiologic purposes requires specialized techniques such as multilocus sequence typing or PCR fingerprinting. However, matrix-assisted laser desorption/ionization–time of flight mass spectrometry (MALDI-TOF) can also rapidly differentiate between *Cryptococcus* species as well as molecular types, and may be used in veterinary clinical microbiology laboratories in the future.[51]

Most cryptococcal isolates from dogs or cats are susceptible to amphotericin B, 5-flucytosine, and azoles. Rarely, resistance to 5-flucytosine and azole antifungal drugs (especially fluconazole) is detected. In general, minimum inhibitory concentrations (MICs) for fluconazole are higher than those for other azole drugs, and this does not imply resistance in vivo. In the human literature it has been suggested that when the MIC rises during treatment, or if the initial MIC is at least 16 μg/mL for fluconazole, or at least 128 μg/mL for flucytosine, failure of antifungal drug treatment may result from drug resistance.[42]

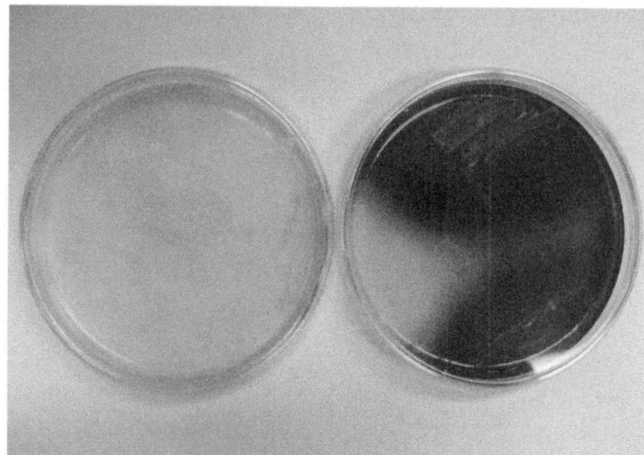

FIGURE 62-9 Growth of *C. neoformans (left)* and *C. gattii (right)* on canavanine-glycine-bromothymol blue agar. *Cryptococcus neoformans* does not grow well in the presence of canavanine and does not utilize glycine, so the medium color remains unchanged. *Cryptococcus gattii* grows in the presence of L-canavanine and utilizes glycine as the sole carbon and nitrogen source, which raises the pH of the medium and causes the bromothymol blue indicator in the medium to turn the agar a vivid cobalt blue color.

Serologic Testing

Latex agglutination assays for detection of cryptococcal polysaccharide capsular antigen are widely used for diagnosis of cryptococcosis in veterinary patients and are sensitive and specific.[11,52,53] ELISA assays are also available, and the performance of a rapid lateral-flow assay (CrAg, IMMY Diagnostics, Norman, OK) is under investigation in the authors' laboratories. Serologic assays detect the antigen of all *C. gattii* and *C. neoformans* molecular types and can be used on serum or CSF. These can provide a rapid diagnosis when organisms cannot be visualized or cultured. When positive, serum cryptococcal antigen assays can be advantageous in animals with neurologic signs when CSF collection is unacceptably risky or if a diagnosis of cryptococcosis is unlikely but requires additional evidence for exclusion.

In human patients, commercial kits typically have at least 90% sensitivity and specificity.[42] Results have been similar for small animal patients,[11,52,53] although false negative results may be more common in dogs than in cats.[11] False positive test results are reduced when test specimens are pretreated in the laboratory with pronase (a proteinase).[42] In human patients, titers below 1:8 can represent false-positive results, although false-positive titers of up to 1:200 have rarely been detected in cats.[11] These cats had other causative etiologies identified that explained their clinical signs. In some cats these low positive titers may represent subclinical colonization. Attempts to obtain cytologic or histopathologic confirmation of infection in animals with titers of 1:200 or less are recommended.

Antigen titers are frequently extremely high (>1:65,536) in cats and dogs with cryptococcosis, but even a titer of 1:2 can indicate cryptococcal infection.[52] Titer results from different kits vary considerably; therefore, the methodology should not be altered when monitoring the response to treatment. A good prognosis is indicated by a decrease in antigen titer, whereas

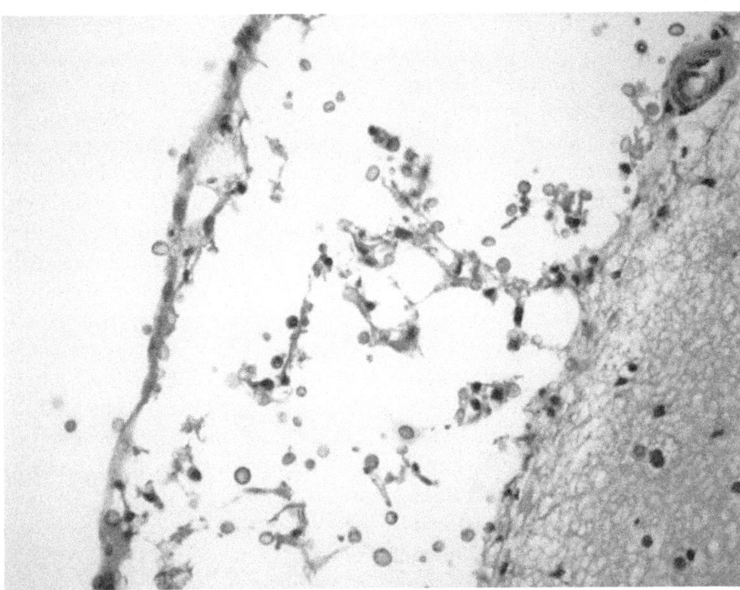

FIGURE 62-10 Histopathology showing the meninges of a cat with cryptococcosis. Numerous round yeast organisms occupy the meningeal spaces. H&E stain.

a persistent titer after treatment suggests continued infection. Reductions in the titer typically lag behind clinical improvement. No correlation has been found between pretreatment antigen titer and outcome.

Because the sensitivity of cryptococcal antigen testing is not 100%, cryptococcosis should not be ruled out on the basis of a negative antigen titer alone. This is especially important in dogs, because false negatives are more common in dogs than in cats.[11] False negatives are most common in animals with localized ocular, CNS, or solitary cutaneous lesions. For dogs and cats suspected to have cryptococcal meningoencephalomyelitis that have negative serum antigen titers, CSF should be submitted for cytologic examination, antigen titers, and fungal culture.

Molecular Diagnosis Using the Polymerase Chain Reaction

Real-time PCR assays for *Cryptococcus* spp. are offered on a commercial basis by some veterinary diagnostic laboratories. These assays can confirm the presence of *Cryptococcus* DNA in tissues or body fluids when other means fail. However, because a diagnosis of cryptococcosis is usually apparent based on the methods described earlier, PCR is currently not regarded as a routinely useful clinical tool. Because *Cryptococcus* DNA has been detected using PCR assays in small intestinal contents from healthy dogs and dogs with chronic enteropathies,[54] positive results on intestinal biopsies may not reflect cryptococcosis. Similarly, because subclinical nasal cavity colonization can occur, positive results on nasal biopsies may not represent invasive disease. Because false positives also have the potential to occur as a result of contamination in the PCR laboratory, a PCR diagnosis of cryptococcosis should always be supported by cytologic or histopathologic evidence of infection and/or culture of *Cryptococcus* spp. from a normally sterile site.

Pathologic Findings

Lesions associated with cryptococcosis vary from gelatinous masses that consist almost exclusively of organisms to well-ordered granulomas or pyogranulomas that typically occur in patients with improved cell-mediated immune (CMI) responses. The gelatinous appearance is a reflection of the large amount of capsular polysaccharide present in lesions. In sections stained with hematoxylin-eosin, *Cryptococcus* yeasts are faint, eosinophilic, round to oval bodies that are surrounded by a clear halo (the unstained capsule). The organism is more easily visualized with periodic acid–Schiff, methenamine silver, or Fontana-Masson stain, although the capsule still does not stain well with these methods. With Mayer's mucicarmine stain, the cryptococcal capsule takes on a rose-red color, and the organism appears pink against a blue background. Other fungi with similar morphologic features do not stain with Mayer's mucicarmine. Some *Cryptococcus* strains have poorly developed capsules. If necessary, immunohistochemistry can be used to differentiate *Cryptococcus* from other fungi and some reagents can provide information on the identity of the species and serotype present.[55]

Cats

In cats that die or are euthanized as a result of cryptococcosis, histopathology of lesions within the nasal cavity may reveal granulomatous rhinitis. CNS cryptococcosis consists of either meningitis[41] or meningoencephalomyelitis, with single or multiple cerebral granulomas (Figure 62-10). Extension of infection from the meninges along perforating arteries into the Virchow-Robin spaces can result in cystic collections of yeast organisms known as gelatinous pseudocysts.[9] Ocular lesions include pyogranulomatous to granulomatous chorioretinitis, optic neuritis, uveitis, endophthalmitis, panophthalmitis, and retinal separation. Other affected organs include skin and subcutaneous tissues, kidneys, and lymph nodes. Renal granulomas have been found in some cats with disseminated disease. Granulomas can also occasionally be found in the spleen, adrenal glands, thyroid glands, and liver.

Dogs

Dogs that die or are euthanized because of cryptococcosis often have CNS infection, ocular involvement, or widely disseminated disease. The lesions consist of granulomatous or pyogranulomatous meningoencephalitis, sometimes with pseudocyst formation; neuritis of the optic, facial, or vestibular nerves; and pyogranulomatous or granulomatous chorioretinitis. Inflammatory lesions that contain *Cryptococcus* yeasts may also be present in the lungs, nasal cavity, kidneys, pancreas, liver, myocardium, gastrointestinal tract, and spleen. Less commonly, involvement of the peritoneum, thyroid, tongue, prostate, pleura, joints, mediastinum, urinary bladder, and adrenal gland has been detected at necropsy.

Treatment and Prognosis

Treatment recommendations for dogs and cats with cryptococcosis have been based on evidence-based studies performed in human patients and clinical experiences; evidence-based studies are lacking for veterinary patients. The most common problems encountered are the high cost of therapy, requirement for multiple hospital visits, and the need for regular medication of pets for a protracted period. Immunocompromised animals (which may include purebred dogs with no obvious underlying immunodeficiency) are especially likely to have persistent or progressive infection in the face of treatment. In many affected animals, treatment must be continued for years or the life of the animal. Surgical debulking could be considered before treatment for large cryptococcomas to improve drug penetration. However, even large cryptococcomas can resolve with medical treatment alone, and surgery should only be performed if lesions can be easily and safely resected. The reader is referred to Chapter 9 for detailed information on antifungal drugs.

Cats

Cats with localized cutaneous disease can sometimes be treated successfully with azole monotherapy. The initial drug of choice is fluconazole (10 mg/kg PO q12h), because of its good penetration of the brain, eye, and urinary tract; low cost; and minimal adverse effects.

Treatment should be continued until there is complete lesion resolution and the cryptococcal antigen titer becomes negative. A four- to fivefold reduction in the antigen titer suggests an adequate response. In cats with *C. gattii* molecular type VGI or *C. neoformans* infections, this typically takes 2 to 12 months (median, 4 months),[56] although longer periods of therapy may be required for some cats. For recovered animals that achieve an antigen titer of 0, the titer can be monitored every 3 to 6 months, so that any recurrence is diagnosed early. However, in the authors' experience, many cats with *C. gattii* molecular type VGII and VGIII infections in North America fail to respond completely to fluconazole treatment, antigen titers persist at high levels, and relapse occurs after an initial treatment response. In some of these cats, treatment with itraconazole (5-10 mg/kg PO q24h [capsules] or 3-5 mg/kg PO q24h [solution]) or ketoconazole can lead to clinical remission. Liver enzyme activities should be monitored monthly during treatment with azole antifungal drugs to monitor for hepatotoxicity (see Chapter 9).

Amphotericin B is the most effective anticryptococcal agent. Penetration of the CNS and vitreous is poor, but clinical responses still occur in cats and dogs with CNS and ocular cryptococcosis, presumably because the blood-brain barrier is compromised. A combination of amphotericin B and 5-flucytosine (250 mg PO q8h) is considered the optimal therapy for cats (and humans, but not dogs) with CNS cryptococcosis, or for those that fail to respond to azole drugs. Fluconazole can be substituted for 5-flucytosine if 5-flucytosine is unaffordable. However, 5-flucytosine shows synergy when combined with amphotericin B and effectively penetrates the blood-brain barrier. Because resistance can develop rapidly when 5-flucytosine is used alone, it is used chiefly to improve the efficacy of other antifungal drugs. Lipid-complexed amphotericin B preparations are not necessarily more effective but are less nephrotoxic, which may translate into greater efficacy because higher doses can be used, although at a substantially increased cost. In human patients, higher doses of amphotericin B more effectively sterilize the CSF. The reader is referred to Chapter 9 for dosing protocols for various formulations of amphotericin B. Treatment with 5-flucytosine (or fluconazole) and amphotericin B is continued for 2 to 4 weeks (ideally 4 weeks) or until azotemia develops, after which treatment is continued with azole monotherapy. Additional courses of amphotericin B may be required to maintain clinical remission in some cats. Although controlled trials have not been performed, some cats with CNS cryptococcosis have shown apparent response to addition of terbinafine to the treatment regimen, when other drugs failed to resolve clinical signs.[57]

Dogs

If affordable to the owner, dogs with disseminated disease or CNS involvement should be treated initially with deoxycholate or lipid-complexed amphotericin B and fluconazole. Dogs treated with flucytosine frequently develop toxic epidermal necrolysis, typically 10 to 14 days after starting therapy, which precludes treatment with flucytosine in this species.[58] Some dogs with CNS involvement respond to azole monotherapy, although residual neurologic signs may persist.[9] Other potential outcomes include incomplete recovery, with persistent active infection despite therapy, or relapse after prolonged clinical remission. In one dog, surgical debridement of an extradural spinal cord granuloma combined with fluconazole treatment controlled spinal cord infection.[59] Again, azoles are fungistatic and rely on a CMI response and phagocytosis to remove cryptococcal yeasts from the host, which may be lacking in some dogs with cryptococcosis. Treatment of a dog with intestinal cryptococcosis with terbinafine was associated with long-term disease resolution when treatment with azoles, surgical debulking, and amphotericin B failed.[48]

Other Antifungal Drugs

Other antifungal drugs that are effective for treatment of cryptococcosis include voriconazole and posaconazole, although these can be unaffordable for many clients. Voriconazole penetrates the CNS and so is potentially advantageous for treatment of cryptococcal meningoencephalitis. However, virtually all cats and some dogs do not tolerate voriconazole treatment because of gastrointestinal, neurologic, and cardiac adverse effects. In humans, posaconazole is well tolerated, and it has been used to treat other fungal infections without complication in cats (see Chapter 9), so it could be an option for cats with refractory disease. Unpredictable serum levels have led to increased interest in therapeutic serum level determination in humans.

Supportive Care

Because many cats and dogs with CNS involvement deteriorate clinically during initial treatment with antifungal drugs as a result of the inflammatory response to dying yeasts, anti-inflammatory doses of short-acting glucocorticoids may be necessary to support animals with CNS cryptococcosis for the first few days to weeks of treatment and may increase survival rate at 10 days after initiation of treatment.[9] Deterioration of neurologic status in the first few days of treatment is not a negative prognostic indicator if the animal can be supported through this phase. Supportive care with IV fluid therapy, tube feeding, and antiseizure medications may be necessary. Rarely, dogs or cats require supplemental oxygen because of respiratory involvement.

Prognosis

In general, cats show significant clinical improvement within 1 to 2 weeks of starting therapy. In studies from Australia, around 75% of cats were treated successfully.[5,56] As many as 60% of cats may be cured after an initial course of therapy, although some cats that show an initial favorable response to therapy can relapse, sometimes as long as 10 years after therapy is discontinued.[56] In one study, the median survival time of cats with CNS cryptococcosis was only 13 days (range, 0 to 4050 days), but a median survival time was never reached if cats survived at least 3 days after diagnosis, so supportive care during this phase may be critical.[9]

The prognosis is more guarded for dogs. Six of 11 dogs with cryptococcosis in Australia were treated successfully.[56] In a study from the western United States[9] and another from southwestern Australia,[5] the success rate was lower, around 30%. The median survival time for dogs with CNS cryptococcosis was 7 days (range, 0 to 3680 days).[9]

In human patients with cryptococcosis, negative prognostic indicators include underlying immunosuppressive disease or drugs, abnormal mental state, high organism burden at presentation (as defined by large numbers of yeasts in the CSF and/or high antigen titers), and a poor anti-inflammatory response in the CSF (<20 cells/μL).[60] The presence of CNS disease appears to negatively affect outcome in both cats and dogs.[56,61] In dogs and cats with CNS involvement, the presence of altered mental status at first evaluation was associated with increased mortality ($P = 0.03$).[9]

Immunity and Vaccination

Cryptococcosis can occur in apparently immunocompetent or in immunodeficient individuals, although those with deficiencies of cell-mediated immunity are most commonly infected. Production of Th1 type cytokines such as Il-2, TNF-α, and IFN-γ and a granulomatous inflammatory response are important for elimination of infection, and decline in the CD4+ T cell count to less than 50 to 100 cells/μL correlates well with the risk of infection in HIV-infected humans.[42] No vaccines are available.

Prevention

Prevention of cryptococcosis may be possible through avoidance of exposure to ecologic niches of the organism, such as pigeon feces. Nevertheless, cryptococcosis occurs in animals housed exclusively indoors, and widespread exposure and recovery likely occurs in endemic areas.

Public Health Aspects

Cryptococcosis is an important opportunistic fungal infection of people with AIDS, in particular those who are not treated with highly active antiretroviral therapy. Human infection is acquired from the environment and not by direct contact with infected animals, although intense exposure to avian excrement has been associated with some cryptococcosis cases in HIV-infected humans.[62] Malignancy, chemotherapy, immunosuppressive drug therapy, diabetes mellitus, splenectomy, cirrhosis, or sarcoidosis can also predispose to the disease. Severe meningitis and disseminated infections can develop in immunodeficient patients.

The organism does not aerosolize from sites of tissue infection, so the disease cannot spread among people or animals. The major public health significance of infected pets is that cats may act as a sentinel for infection of human beings, because of their susceptibility to infection. In the diagnostic laboratory, culture of *Cryptococcus* is not a significant health hazard, because only the yeast form is grown routinely, and this form does not aerosolize from media. During handling of infected tissues or cultures, precautions should be taken to prevent inadvertent cutaneous inoculation of the organism. Veterinarians should consider patient sedation for procedures that involve fine-needle aspiration in order to avoid inadvertent needle-stick injuries, which have caused localized cutaneous infection in the human health care setting.[63] Because sporotrichosis is a major differential diagnosis for cats with cutaneous lesions, gloves should always be worn and hand hygiene performed when handling cats with suspicious lesions (see Chapter 64).

CASE EXAMPLE

Signalment: "Simon," an 8-year-old male neutered domestic shorthair cat from northern California

History: Simon was evaluated by the University of California, Davis, Veterinary Medical Teaching Hospital (VMTH) for a 5-week history of progressive weakness, inappetence, and weight loss. Initially the owners noted that he was reluctant to jump and had a low tail carriage, and intermittent episodes of head shaking and sneezing were also noted. He also had episodes of clenching the furniture with his claws. Three weeks before he was brought to the VMTH, Simon was seen at a local veterinary clinic where a physical examination was unremarkable. Broad-spectrum antimicrobial drugs were prescribed (amoxicillin-clavulanic acid and enrofloxacin for 7 days), and he was treated with subcutaneous fluids (lactated Ringer's solution, 150 mL, once). Over the following 5 days his clinical signs lessened, but then anorexia developed. Physical examination 2 days after the onset of anorexia revealed a rectal temperature of 102.5°F (39.2°C) and weight loss (3.7 kg at the previous visit to 3.2 kg). A CBC and biochemistry panel showed mild lymphopenia (1157 cells/μL, reference range 1500-7000 cells/μL). Treatment with metronidazole (39 mg/kg PO q24h) and prednisone (3 mg/kg PO q24h) was instituted. Three days before he was brought to the VMTH, he began panting and vocalizing. The metronidazole was discontinued and the prednisone dose was reduced to 1.5 mg/kg PO q24h. The following day, the owners noted that Simon's eyelids were twitching, and he urinated and defecated on himself in the litter box. Clindamycin (6 mg/kg PO q12h) was prescribed

Continued

for suspected toxoplasmosis, and Simon was referred for further evaluation.

Simon had no other previous medical or surgical history apart from being neutered as a kitten. He had access to the outdoors and there were no other cats in the household. There had been no changes in his thirst or urination, no vomiting or diarrhea, and he was last vaccinated at 5 years of age. He had killed a large rat approximately 5 weeks earlier and had not been himself since.

Physical Examination:

Body Weight: 2.9 kg.

General: Obtunded but responsive, estimated as 5% dehydrated. T = 100.2°F (37.9°C), HR = 200 beats/min, RR = 60 breaths/min, CRT <2 s.

Eyes, Ears, Nose, and Throat: Bilateral mydriasis and absent pupillary light reflexes were noted. There was no evidence of nasal discharge and nasal airflow was normal. Mucous membranes were pink and slightly tacky. Fundic examination was within normal limits.

Musculoskeletal: Body condition score 4/9, ambulatory. The cat had a slow gait with a short stride.

Respiratory: Tachypnea was present with a normal respiratory effort. Normal breath sounds were present on auscultation.

Cardiovascular, Gastrointestinal, Genitourinary and Lymph Nodes: No clinically significant abnormalities were detected. The urinary bladder was small.

Neurologic Examination: The cat was mildly obtunded, walked with a crouched stance and behaved as if nonvisual. Bilateral mydriasis and absent menace and pupillary light reflexes were confirmed. Intermittent horizontal nystagmus with the fast phase to the left was present. Cranial nerve examination was otherwise normal. Placing and hopping reactions were delayed in the left pelvic limb. There was a decreased left patellar reflex, but other segmental reflexes were intact. There was no apparent pain on spinal palpation, but the cat appeared painful when the tail was raised. Neuroanatomic location: Multifocal CNS disease.

Laboratory Findings:

CBC:

HCT 27.2% (30%-50%)
MCV 48.3 fL (42-53 fL)
MCHC 29.8 g/dL (30-33.5 g/dL)
Reticulocytes 8400 cells/μL (7000-60,000 cells/μL)
WBC 12,360 cells/μL (4500-14,000 cells/μL)
Neutrophils 11,000 cells/μL (2000-9000 cells/μL)
Lymphocytes 828 cells/μL (1000-7000 cells/μL)
Monocytes 445 cells/μL (50-600 cells/μL)
Eosinophils 87 cells/μL (150-1100 cells/μL)
Basophils 0 cells/μL (0-50 cells/μL)
Platelets 357,000/μL (180,000-500,000 platelets/μL).

Serum Chemistry Profile:

Sodium 150 mmol/L (151-158 mmol/L)
Potassium 4.3 mmol/L (3.6-4.9 mmol/L)
Chloride 115 mmol/L (117-126 mmol/L)
Bicarbonate 19 mmol/L (15-21 mmol/L)
Phosphorus 5.4 mg/dL (3.2-6.3 mg/dL)
Calcium 10 mg/dL (9.0-10.9 mg/dl)
BUN 21 mg/dL (18-33 mg/dL)
Creatinine 1.2 mg/dL (1.1-2.2 mg/dL)
Glucose 136 mg/dL (63-118 mg/dL)
Total protein 7.5 g/dL (6.6-8.4 g/dL)
Albumin 3.8 g/dL (2.2-4.6 g/dL)
Globulin 3.7 g/dL (2.8-5.4 g/dL)
ALT 37 U/L (27-101 U/L)
AST 28 U/L (17-58 U/L)
ALP 8 U/L (14-71 U/L)
GGT < 3 U/L (0-4 U/L)
Cholesterol 177 mg/dL (89-258 mg/dL)
Total bilirubin < 0.1 mg/dL (0-0.2 mg/dL).

Urinalysis: SGr 1.018; pH 7.0; 25 mg/dL protein; no bilirubin, hemoprotein, glucose; rare WBC/HPF, 0 RBC/HPF, few amorphous crystals, few lipid droplets.

ELISA for FeLV Antigen and FIV Antibody: Negative.

Latex Agglutination for Cryptococcus Antigen: Positive at 1:32,768.

Imaging Findings:

Plain Thoracic and Abdominal Radiographs: The only abnormality present was mild lateral spondylosis of the caudal lumbar spine.

Abdominal Ultrasonography: The liver was mildly enlarged and contained multiple small hyperechoic foci. In the kidneys, mild cortical hyperechogenicity and decreased corticomedullary distinction were present.

Magnetic Resonance Imaging (Brain): Precontrast images showed a well-defined, round T2-hyperintense, T1-hypointense lesion in the gray matter of the right cerebral cortex at the junction of the parietal and occipital lobes (see Figure 62-7). Postcontrast images showed moderate contrast enhancement of this lesion. There was mild contrast enhancement of the meninges ventral to the right preoptic area. There was moderate, focal contrast enhancement of the gray matter at the lateral aspect of the right pyriform lobe. There was contrast enhancement of the medial aspect of both pyriform lobes adjacent to the hypophysis. Impressions: Multifocal contrast-enhancing lesions with T2 hyperintensity and a cystic lesion in the right cerebral cortex.

Cytologic Findings: CSF analysis (cisternal): Protein concentration 29 mg/dL (reference range, <25 mg/dL). The specimen had a moderate increase in cellularity with a low number of erythrocytes. Numerous thick-capsuled yeast organisms with frequent narrow budding forms were noted, consistent with *Cryptococcus* spp. Nucleated cells consisted of nondegenerate neutrophils admixed with low numbers of variably vacuolated macrophages and small lymphocytes. The differential cell count was 83% neutrophils, 7% small mononuclear cells, and 10% large mononuclear cells.

Microbiologic Testing: Fungal culture (CSF): *Cryptococcus gattii*. Multilocus sequence typing revealed the organism belonged to *C. gattii* molecular type VGIIa.

Diagnosis: *Cryptococcus gattii* meningoencephalitis.

Treatment: Simon was treated with deoxycholate amphotericin B (0.25 mg/kg in 30 mL 5% dextrose IV over 30 minutes on Monday, Wednesday, and Friday for five treatments). Before and after this treatment, 0.9% NaCl was administered at twice maintenance rate and kidney analytes were monitored. Flucytosine (62.5 mg PO q8h) and prednisone (2.5 mg PO q24h) were also administered. An esophagostomy tube was placed for enteral nutrition because of persistent inappetence. By day 7, Simon appeared more alert, pupillary light reflexes and menace responses were present but weak, and nystagmus had resolved. He was discharged from the hospital on day 12, with instructions to continue treatment with fluconazole (50 mg PO q12h) and prednisone (2.5 mg PO q48h), in addition to esophagostomy tube feeding. On day 24, he was reevaluated for lethargy of several days' duration. Physical examination showed resolution of cranial nerve abnormalities, but delayed hopping reactions in all limbs were present. He was treated with six additional amphotericin B treatments over 2 weeks. He began eating, and the esophageal feeding tube was removed on day 40. Three months after diagnosis, his neurologic signs had almost completely resolved with the exception of occasional tremors, persistent mild placing reaction deficits, and lumbosacral pain. A cryptococcal antigen titer was positive at 1:65,536. The fluconazole was replaced with itraconazole solution (3 mg/kg PO q12h). After an additional month, the antigen titer was 1:1024, a serum chemistry profile was unremarkable, and the owners felt that Simon was a normal cat. The prednisone treatment was discontinued thereafter. A year later, the antigen titer was 1:20. At a recheck examination 2 years later the cat was neurologically normal. The owner declined further antigen testing and chose to continue treatment with itraconazole.

Comments: This cat had CNS cryptococcosis caused by *Cryptococcus gattii* molecular type VGIIa, a hypervirulent molecular type that emerged in British Columbia and the Pacific Northwest. The treatment plan was limited by client financial concerns, which meant that the initial course of amphotericin B and flucytosine treatment was short, and a second course of amphotericin B was required. Subsequently, treatment with fluconazole was associated with limited improvement, but a change to itraconazole was followed by dramatic clinical improvement and reduction in antigen titers.

SUGGESTED READINGS

Datta K, Bartlett KH, Baer R, et al. Spread of *Cryptococcus gattii* into Pacific Northwest region of the United States. Emerg Infect Dis. 2009;15:1185-1191.

Kronstad JW, Attarian R, Cadieux B, et al. Expanding fungal pathogenesis: *Cryptococcus* breaks out of the opportunistic box. Nat Rev Microbiol. 2011;9:193-203.

Trivedi SR, Malik R, Meyer W, et al. Feline cryptococcosis: impact of current research on clinical management. J Feline Med Surg. 2011;13:163-172.

REFERENCES

1. Knoke M, Schwesinger G. One hundred years ago: the history of cryptococcosis in Greifswald. Medical mycology in the nineteenth century. Mycoses. 1994;37:229-233.
2. Stephen C, Lester S, Black W, et al. Multispecies outbreak of cryptococcosis on southern Vancouver Island, British Columbia. Can Vet J. 2002;43:792-794.
3. Lester SJ, Kowalewich NJ, Bartlett KH, et al. Clinicopathologic features of an unusual outbreak of cryptococcosis in dogs, cats, ferrets, and a bird: 38 cases (January to July 2003). J Am Vet Med Assoc. 2004;225:1716-1722.
4. Rotstein DS, West K, Levine G, et al. *Cryptococcus gattii* VGI in a spinner dolphin (*Stenella longirostris*) from Hawaii. J Zoo Wildl Med. 2010;41:181-183.
5. McGill S, Malik R, Saul N, et al. Cryptococcosis in domestic animals in Western Australia: a retrospective study from 1995-2006. Med Mycol. 2009;47:625-639.
6. Datta K, Bartlett KH, Baer R, et al. Spread of *Cryptococcus gattii* into Pacific Northwest region of the United States. Emerg Infect Dis. 2009;15:1185-1191.
7. Krockenberger MB, Canfield PJ, Barnes J, et al. *Cryptococcus neoformans* var. *gattii* in the koala (*Phascolarctos cinereus*): serological evidence for subclinical cryptococcosis. Med Mycol. 2002;40:273-282.
8. Malik R, Alderton B, Finlaison D, et al. Cryptococcosis in ferrets: a diverse spectrum of clinical disease. Aust Vet J. 2002;80:749-755.
9. Sykes JE, Sturges BK, Cannon MS, et al. Clinical signs, imaging features, neuropathology, and outcome in cats and dogs with central nervous system cryptococcosis from California. J Vet Intern Med. 2010;24:1427-1438.
10. Malik R, Krockenberger MB, Cross G, et al. Avian cryptococcosis. Med Mycol. 2003;41:115-124.
11. Trivedi SR, Sykes JE, Cannon MS, et al. Clinical features and epidemiology of cryptococcosis in cats and dogs in California: 93 cases (1988-2010). J Am Vet Med Assoc. 2011;239:357-369.
12. Kano R, Kitagawat M, Oota S, et al. First case of feline systemic *Cryptococcus albidus* infection. Med Mycol. 2008;46:75-77.
13. Labrecque O, Sylvestre D, Messier S. Systemic *Cryptococcus albidus* infection in a Doberman Pinscher. J Vet Diagn Invest. 2005;17:598-600.
14. Johnson LB, Bradley SF, Kauffman CA. Fungaemia due to *Cryptococcus laurentii* and a review of non-*neoformans* cryptococcaemia. Mycoses. 1998;41:277-280.
15. Kano R, Hosaka S, Hasegawa A. First isolation of *Cryptococcus magnus* from a cat. Mycopathologia. 2004;157:263-264.
16. Bernardo FM, Martins HM, Martins ML. A survey of mycotic otitis externa of dogs in Lisbon. Rev Iberoam Micol. 1998;15:163-165.
17. Kronstad JW, Attarian R, Cadieux B, et al. Expanding fungal pathogenesis: *Cryptococcus* breaks out of the opportunistic box. Nat Rev Microbiol. 2011;9:193-203.
18. Wickes BL, Mayorga ME, Edman U, et al. Dimorphism and haploid fruiting in *Cryptococcus neoformans*: association with the alpha-mating type. Proc Natl Acad Sci U S A. 1996;93:7327-7331.
19. Hull CM, Heitman J. Genetics of *Cryptococcus neoformans*. Annu Rev Genet. 2002;36:557-615.
20. Velagapudi R, Hsueh YP, Geunes-Boyer S, et al. Spores as infectious propagules of *Cryptococcus neoformans*. Infect Immun. 2009;77:4345-4355.
21. Ngamskulrungroj P, Gilgado F, Faganello J, et al. Genetic diversity of the *Cryptococcus* species complex suggests that *Cryptococcus gattii* deserves to have varieties. PLoS One. 2009;4:e5862.
22. Malik R, Wigney DI, Muir DB, et al. Cryptococcosis in cats: clinical and mycological assessment of 29 cases and evaluation of treatment using orally administered fluconazole. J Med Vet Mycol. 1992;30:133-144.
23. O'Brien CR, Krockenberger MB, Wigney DI, et al. Retrospective study of feline and canine cryptococcosis in Australia from 1981 to 2001: 195 cases. Med Mycol. 2004;42:449-460.
24. Berthelin CF, Bailey CS, Kass PH, et al. Cryptococcosis of the nervous system in dogs: part 1. Epidemiologic, clinical, and neuropathologic features. Prog Vet Neurol. 1994;5:88-97.
25. Malik R, Dill-Macky E, Martin P, et al. Cryptococcosis in dogs: a retrospective study of 20 consecutive cases. J Med Vet Mycol. 1995;33:291-297.

26. Jacobs GJ, Medleau L, Calvert C, et al. Cryptococcal infection in cats: factors influencing treatment outcome, and results of sequential serum antigen titers in 35 cats. J Vet Intern Med. 1997;11:1-4.
27. Kano R, Fujino Y, Takamoto N, et al. PCR detection of the *Cryptococcus neoformans* CAPS9 gene from a biopsy specimen from a case of feline cryptococcosis. J Vet Diagn Invest. 2001;13:439-442.
28. Barrs VR, Martin P, Nicoll RG, et al. Pulmonary cryptococcosis and *Capillaria aerophila* infection in an FIV-positive cat. Aust Vet J. 2000;78:154-158.
29. Nielsen K, De Obaldia AL, Heitman J. *Cryptococcus neoformans* mates on pigeon guano: implications for the realized ecological niche and globalization. Eukaryot Cell. 2007;6:949-959.
30. Lazera MS, Pires FD, Camillo-Coura L, et al. Natural habitat of *Cryptococcus neoformans* var. *neoformans* in decaying wood forming hollows in living trees. J Med Vet Mycol. 1996;34:127-131.
31. Trivedi SR, Malik R, Meyer W, et al. Feline cryptococcosis: impact of current research on clinical management. J Feline Med Surg. 2011;13:163-172.
32. Viviani MA, Cogliati M, Esposto MC, et al. Molecular analysis of 311 *Cryptococcus neoformans* isolates from a 30-month ECMM survey of cryptococcosis in Europe. FEMS Yeast Res. 2006;6:614-619.
33. Sorrell TC. *Cryptococcus neoformans* variety *gattii*. Med Mycol. 2001;39:155-168.
34. Marr KA. *Cryptococcus gattii* as an important fungal pathogen of western North America. Expert Rev Anti Infect Ther. 2012;10:637-643.
35. Bartlett KH, Cheng PY, Duncan C, et al. A decade of experience: *Cryptococcus gattii* in British Columbia. Mycopathologia. 2012;173:311-319.
36. MacDougall L, Kidd SE, Galanis E, et al. Spread of *Cryptococcus gattii* in British Columbia, Canada, and detection in the Pacific Northwest. USA. Emerg Infect Dis. 2007;13:42-50.
37. Duncan CG, Stephen C, Campbell J. Evaluation of risk factors for *Cryptococcus gattii* infection in dogs and cats. J Am Vet Med Assoc. 2006;228:377-382.
38. Mitchell DH, Sorrell TC, Allworth AM, et al. Cryptococcal disease of the CNS in immunocompetent hosts: influence of cryptococcal variety on clinical manifestations and outcome. Clin Infect Dis. 1995;20:611-616.
39. Campbell LT, Currie BJ, Krockenberger M, et al. Clonality and recombination in genetically differentiated subgroups of *Cryptococcus gattii*. Eukaryot Cell. 2005;4:1403-1409.
40. Speed B, Dunt D. Clinical and host differences between infections with the two varieties of *Cryptococcus neoformans*. Clin Infect Dis. 1995;21:28-34: discussion 35–26.
41. Chaturvedi S, Dyavaiah M, Larsen RA, et al. *Cryptococcus gattii* in AIDS patients, southern California. Emerg Infect Dis. 2005;11:1686-1692.
42. Perfect JR. *Cryptococcus neoformans*. In: Mandell GL, Bennett JE, Dolin R, eds. Principles and Practice of Infectious Diseases. 7th ed. Philadelphia, PA: Elsevier; 2010:3287-3303.
43. Perfect JR. The triple threat of cryptococcosis: it's the body site, the strain, and/or the host. MBio. 2012;3.
44. Perfect JR. *Cryptococcus neoformans*: a sugar-coated killer with designer genes. FEMS Immunol Med Microbiol. 2005;45: 395-404.
45. Georgi A, Schneemann M, Tintelnot K, et al. *Cryptococcus gattii* meningoencephalitis in an immunocompetent person 13 months after exposure. Infection. 2009;37:370-373.
46. MacDougall L, Fyfe M. Emergence of *Cryptococcus gattii* in a novel environment provides clues to its incubation period. J Clin Microbiol. 2006;44:1851-1852.
47. Beatty JA, Barrs VR, Swinney GR, et al. Peripheral vestibular disease associated with cryptococcosis in three cats. J Feline Med Surg. 2000;2:29-34.
48. Olsen GL, Deitz KL, Flaherty HA, et al. Use of terbinafine in the treatment protocol of intestinal *Cryptococcus neoformans* in a dog. J Am Anim Hosp Assoc. 2012;48:216-220.
49. Malik R, Hunt GB, Bellenger CR, et al. Intra-abdominal cryptococcosis in two dogs. J Small Anim Pract. 1999;40:387-391.
50. Kwon-Chung KJ, Polacheck I, Bennett JE. Improved diagnostic medium for separation of *Cryptococcus neoformans* var. *neoformans* (serotypes A and D) and *Cryptococcus neoformans* var. *gattii* (serotypes B and C). J Clin Microbiol. 1982;15: 535-537.
51. Firacative C, Trilles L, Meyer W. MALDI-TOF MS enables the rapid identification of the major molecular types within the *Cryptococcus neoformans/Cryptococcus gattii* species complex. PLoS One. 2012;7:e37566.
52. Malik R, McPetrie R, Wigney DI, et al. A latex cryptococcal antigen agglutination test for diagnosis and monitoring of therapy for cryptococcosis. Aust Vet J. 1996;74:358-364.
53. Medleau L, Marks MA, Brown J, et al. Clinical evaluation of a cryptococcal antigen latex agglutination test for diagnosis of cryptococcosis in cats. J Am Vet Med Assoc. 1990;196:1470-1473.
54. Suchodolski JS, Morris EK, Allenspach K, et al. Prevalence and identification of fungal DNA in the small intestine of healthy dogs and dogs with chronic enteropathies. Vet Microbiol. 2008;132:379-388.
55. Krockenberger MB, Canfield PJ, Kozel TR, et al. An immunohistochemical method that differentiates *Cryptococcus neoformans* varieties and serotypes in formalin-fixed paraffin-embedded tissues. Med Mycol. 2001;39:523-533.
56. O'Brien CR, Krockenberger MB, Martin P, et al. Long-term outcome of therapy for 59 cats and 11 dogs with cryptococcosis. Aust Vet J. 2006;84:384-392.
57. Sykes JE. Unpublished observations, 2012.
58. Malik R, Medeiros C, Wigney DI, et al. Suspected drug eruption in seven dogs during administration of flucytosine. Aust Vet J. 1996;74:285-288.
59. Kerwin SC, McCarthy RJ, VanSteenhouse JL, et al. Cervical spinal cord compression caused by cryptococcosis in a dog: successful treatment with surgery and fluconazole. J Am Anim Hosp Assoc. 1998;34:523-526.
60. Bicanic T, Harrison TS. Cryptococcal meningitis. Br Med Bull. 2004;72:99-118.
61. Duncan C, Stephen C, Campbell J. Clinical characteristics and predictors of mortality for *Cryptococcus gattii* infection in dogs and cats of southwestern British Columbia. Can Vet J. 2006;47:993-998.
62. Fessel WJ. Cryptococcal meningitis after unusual exposures to birds. N Engl J Med. 1993;328:1354-1355.
63. Casadevall A, Mukherjee J, Yuan R, et al. Management of injuries caused by *Cryptococcus neoformans*–contaminated needles. Clin Infect Dis. 1994;19:951-953.

CHAPTER 63

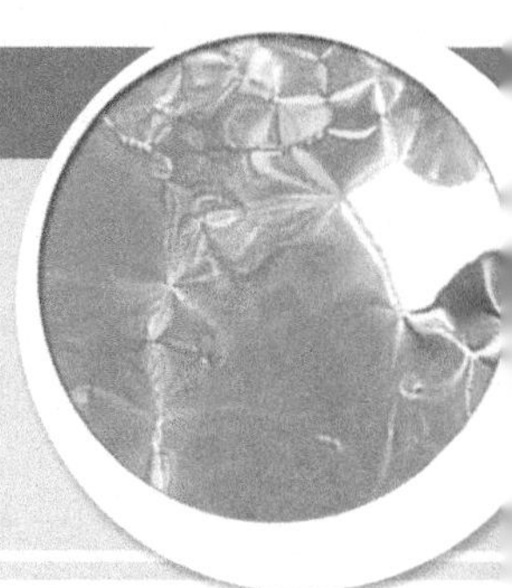

Coccidioidomycosis

Jane E. Sykes

Overview of Coccidioidomycosis

First Described: 1892 (by the medical student Alejandro Posadas), in a person from Buenos Aires, Argentina, where it was initially mistaken for a protozoan (*Coccidia*)[1]

Cause: *Coccidioides immitis* and *Coccidioides posadasii* (ascomycetes, no known teleomorph)

Affected Hosts: Primarily humans and dogs, but also a variety of other animals that include cats, domestic farm animal species, and a variety of wildlife hosts

Geographic Distribution: Southwestern United States, Mexico, and parts of Central and South America (northeastern Brazil, Argentina, Paraguay, and Bolivia)

Mode of Transmission: Inhalation of arthroconidia from the environment; rarely cutaneous inoculation

Major Clinical Signs: Cough, fever, inappetence, weight loss, tachypnea, increased respiratory effort, lameness, subcutaneous masses or draining skin lesions, lymphadenopathy, neurologic signs, ascites due to right-sided heart failure (pericarditis), ocular lesions (uveitis, chorioretinitis, endophthalmitis)

Differential Diagnoses: Neoplasia, other deep mycoses, mycobacteriosis, actinomycosis or nocardiosis, toxoplasmosis or neosporosis, systemic immune-mediated disease

Human Health Significance: Direct transmission from animals to humans does not usually occur, although sharps injuries or bite wounds from affected animals may be a source of human infection. Dogs are a sentinel for human exposure.

Etiology and Epidemiology

Coccidioides spp. are dimorphic, soil-borne fungi that exist in the environment as a mycelium and in tissues (at 37°C) as peculiar structures known as *spherules*. The mycelium consists of chains of haploid, multinucleated, barrel-shaped arthroconidia (or arthrospores) that alternate with smaller, thin-walled, nonviable cells. The arthroconidia remain viable in the soil for long periods. They ultimately fragment from each other and are subsequently aerosolized and inhaled by animal hosts (Figure 63-1). This can be followed by the development of coccidioidomycosis, a localized pulmonary disease or a serious multisystemic disease if dissemination occurs in the face of inadequate immune responses.

In the environment, *Coccidioides* spp. are distributed in the lower Sonoran life zone, regions characterized by semiarid to arid soils, low elevations above sea level, and hot summers. Worldwide, *Coccidioides* spp. are found in the southwestern United States, Mexico, and parts of Central and South America, specifically Colombia, Guatemala, Honduras, Venezuela, northeastern Brazil, Argentina, Paraguay, and Bolivia (Figure 63-2). In the southwestern United States, highly endemic regions are the south-central valley of California, especially Bakersfield ("valley fever") and Arizona, especially Tucson and Phoenix.[2] Infections also occur in non-endemic regions in dogs and humans that have a travel history to endemic regions.

Two species of *Coccidioides* have been identified, *C. posadasii* and *C. immitis*. These appear to cause similar clinical manifestations and have similar antifungal drug susceptibilities, but further studies are required.[3] The geographic range of *C. immitis* is largely limited to the central valley of California, whereas *C. posadasii* is found elsewhere.[4] However, there may be some overlap in the distribution of these organisms.

Infection of animals and humans with *Coccidioides* spp. often follows a cycle of moist conditions (required for growth of the organism in the soil), a dry period, then soil disruption, such as may occur with heavy rainfall, earthquakes, dust storms, prolonged droughts, or construction.[5-7] Dogs of any breed, age, or sex may be affected, although large-breed, young adult dogs predominate in case series.[8,9] In dogs seen at the University of California Veterinary Medical Teaching Hospital, boxers, poodles, pointers, Labrador and golden retrievers, German shepherds, Australian shepherds, Dalmatians, Scottish terriers, dachshunds, and beagles are overrepresented when compared with the hospital patient population.[10] Risk factors for infection in dogs from Arizona include being housed outdoors during the day rather than indoors, roaming areas more than 1 acre, and walking in the desert.[11] Latent infections may also occur in dogs, and these can reactivate after treatment with immunosuppressive drugs, such as corticosteroids and chemotherapeutic agents, including after previous recovery from coccidioidomycosis.

Although not as prevalent as in dogs, coccidioidomycosis also occurs in cats.[12] In a study of 48 cats from Arizona, cats ranged in age from 1 to 15 years (median, 5 years) and there was no obvious sex or breed predisposition.[12] One cat was infected with FIV, and all cats tested were FeLV negative. Interestingly, a search of the author's hospital and pathology database from 1990 to 2012 revealed not a single cat with coccidioidomycosis, which might suggest cats are less susceptible to *C. immitis* infection than to *C. posadasii* infection.

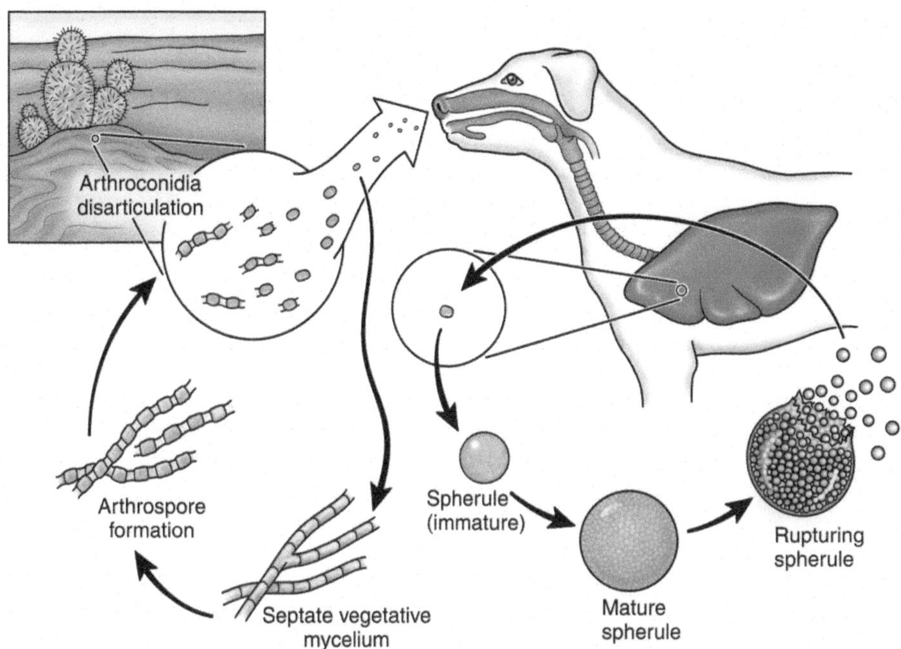

FIGURE 63-1 Life cycle of *Coccidioides* spp. Hyphae fragment into arthroconidia, which are inhaled and form spherules in tissues. The spherules rupture and release endospores, which form new spherules. In some dogs, the organism disseminates from the lungs to a variety of other tissues, but especially local lymph nodes, bone, skin, the pericardium, the eye, and the central nervous system.

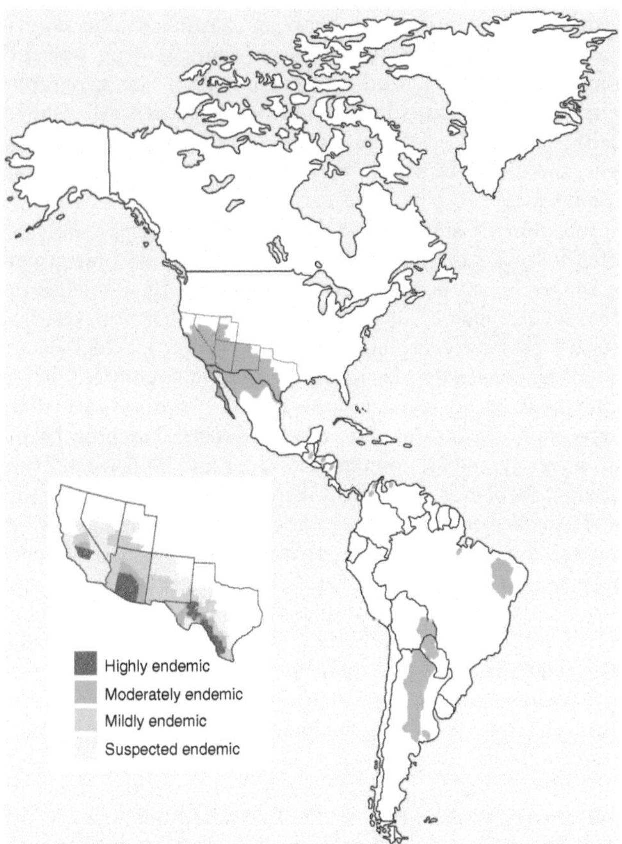

FIGURE 63-2 Geographic distribution of *Coccidioides* spp. worldwide. The inset shows the distribution of *Coccidioides* species in the southwestern United States.

Clinical Features

Signs and Their Pathogenesis

The clinical signs of coccidioidomycosis depend on factors such as the infectious dose and the immune status of the host. Arthroconidia are inhaled and are phagocytosed by alveolar macrophages. They then enlarge into a spherule, which measures 8 to 100 μm in diameter. Hundreds of endospores then develop within the spherule, which are released when the mature spherule ruptures. These attract neutrophils, which leads to a pyogranulomatous inflammatory response. Each released endospore that escapes immune destruction then enlarges into a new spherule, and the cycle continues. Endospores can revert to mycelial growth when removed from the site of infection. In hosts that are unable to mount an effective immune response, endospores disseminate by lymphatics to tracheobronchial lymph nodes and hematogenously to a variety of body sites. Inoculation coccidioidomycosis can rarely occur, and generally results in lesions that are localized to the site of the wound. In one report, it followed removal of a foxtail from a wound.[13]

Most infections in endemic areas are subclinical.[14] Development of clinical signs often follows a subacute to chronic course, with variable and often mild systemic signs such as intermittent fever, lethargy, inappetence, and weight loss.[8,15] Many dogs otherwise appear healthy, with occasional periods of inappetence.[8] Clinical signs may be present for days to years before veterinary attention is sought.[9] Signs of respiratory tract involvement include a harsh cough, increased respiratory effort, tachypnea and/or exercise intolerance.[9,15] Cough may be chronic and is sometimes associated with gagging or retching; occasionally it results from bronchial compression by enlarged tracheobronchial lymph nodes. Rarely, diffuse pneumonia follows a fulminant course, with signs that resemble acute bacterial pneumonia or septic shock, as reported in immunocompromised human patients.[2]

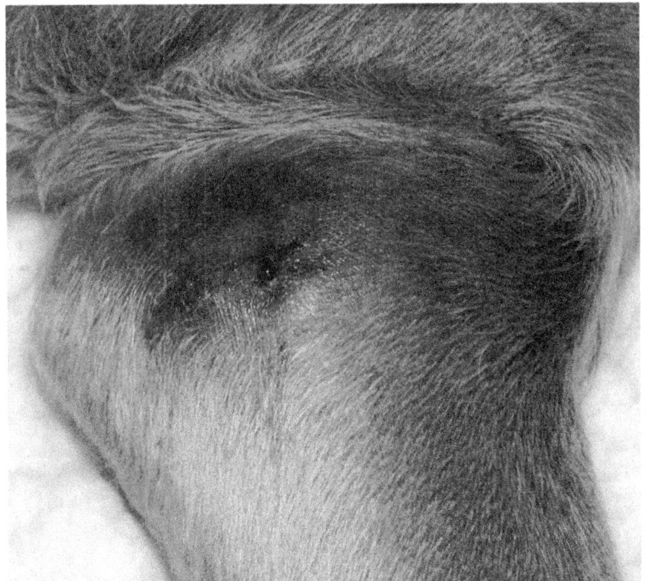

FIGURE 63-3 Draining skin lesion on the left elbow of a 5-year-old shepherd mix with disseminated coccidioidomycosis. Radiography revealed a mixed productive and destructive lesion of the distal humerus and proximal ulna. Productive lesions of the sixth and seventh ribs were also present. Arthrocentesis revealed suppurative inflammation with no growth on culture. Diagnosis was ultimately made by biopsy of the synovium and serology. The *Coccidioides* titer was 1:64.

A smaller percentage of infected dogs develop disseminated infections. Sites of dissemination often include osteoarticular sites, the central nervous system (CNS), skin, peripheral lymph nodes, eyes, testes, prostate, and the pericardium.[9,10] Rarely, sites such as the liver, spleen, gastrointestinal tract, or urinary system are affected.[8] Sometimes dissemination to only one anatomic site is evident; in other dogs multiple sites are involved. A history of respiratory signs may be absent.[8] Bone involvement may manifest as lameness and/or one or more firm swellings associated with the appendicular or axial skeleton. Dogs with skin involvement may have subcutaneous masses ulcerated skin lesions that drain serosanguineous fluid (Figure 63-3).[8] Skin lesions may overlie sites of osteomyelitis. Neurologic signs result from meningoencephalitis and include obtundation, blindness, nystagmus, absent menace reflexes, diminished gag responses, ataxia, abnormal placing reactions, pacing, circling, cervical pain, tetraparesis, and seizures.[9,16,17] Ocular manifestations of coccidioidomycosis include chorioretinitis, uveitis, optic neuritis, and endophthalmitis.[9,18,19] Involvement of abdominal organs such as the liver and gastrointestinal tract can lead to inappetence, vomiting, and/or diarrhea.[8] Pericarditis may lead to signs of right-sided cardiac failure, with ascites and pleural effusion.[8]

Physical Examination Findings

Fever is present in up to two thirds of dogs with coccidioidomycosis (range, 103°F to 106°F) on physical examination. Other common findings in dogs are lethargy, weakness, thin body condition or profound muscle atrophy, tachypnea, increased respiratory effort, inducible or spontaneous cough, and/or increased lung sounds.[9] Lameness and firm, often painful bony swellings with associated muscle atrophy may be present in dogs with osteomyelitis. Less often, focal or (very rarely) generalized peripheral lymphadenomegaly, subcutaneous masses or draining skin lesions, or swollen joints are present. Dogs with pericardial coccidioidomycosis may have abdominal distention with a palpable fluid wave, tachycardia, tachypnea, jugular pulses, muffled breath and heart sounds due to pleural effusion, mucosal pallor, prolonged capillary refill time, and weak pulses.[20] Neurologic signs, when present, include obtundation, apparent blindness, ataxia, nystagmus, spinal pain, circling, and tetraparesis. The most common ocular abnormality is uveitis, but keratitis, conjunctivitis, granulomatous chorioretinitis, optic neuritis, retinal detachment, and endophthalmitis with secondary glaucoma have also been described.[9,18,19]

Of 48 cats with coccidioidomycosis, fever was present in 31%. Skin lesions were present in more than 50% of 48 affected cats and included draining skin lesions, subcutaneous granulomas, and abscesses.[12] Tachypnea or increased respiratory effort was present in 25% of affected cats, and lameness in fewer than 20% of cats. Ocular abnormalities were present in 13% of cats. Conjunctival masses, periorbital swellings, chorioretinitis, retinal detachment, endophthalmitis, and/or anterior uveitis have been described.[21,22] A small percentage of cats have neurologic signs such as hyperesthesia, posterior paresis, seizures, and ataxia. Dissemination to abdominal organs such as the spleen can occur.[23]

Diagnosis

Coccidioidomycosis is usually suspected based on a history of travel to or residence in an endemic region, and consistent clinical signs and radiographic findings. Because the disease is not prevalent in some endemic regions (such as coastal southern California), early diagnosis requires a high index of suspicion in these regions. The diagnosis can be confirmed with cytologic examination of aspirates or body fluids, serologic assays that detect antibodies to *Coccidioides* spp., histopathology, and/or fungal culture (Table 63-1).

Laboratory Abnormalities

Complete Blood Count

CBC findings in dogs with coccidioidomycosis are nonspecific and resemble those of other deep mycoses. Most affected dogs have mild, normocytic, normochromic, nonregenerative anemia and mild leukocytosis. Leukocytosis results from a neutrophilia, occasionally with a left shift and evidence of neutrophil toxicity.[9,20] A monocytosis and lymphopenia may also be present, but in contrast to human infections, eosinophilia is not typically present.

Serum Biochemical Tests

Almost all dogs with coccidioidomycosis have hypoalbuminemia, and approximately half of affected dogs and cats have hyperglobulinemia (up to 7.8 mg/dL in one study).[9,12] Hypoalbuminemia is usually mild to moderate, but rarely may be more severe (<1.5 g/dL). Uncommonly, mild hypercalcemia is present. Increased activity of serum ALP may be present in some dogs, possibly as a result of bone involvement.

Urinalysis

The urinalysis is often normal, but significant proteinuria (urine protein-to-creatinine ratios as high as 9.5, reference range <1) has been reported in some dogs with coccidioidomycosis.[9] It is not clear whether proteinuria of this magnitude results from glomerulonephritis secondary to chronic immune stimulation or another comorbidity.

TABLE 63-1

Diagnostic Assays Currently Available for Coccidioidomycosis in Dogs and Cats

Assay	Specimen Type	Target	Performance
Cytologic examination	Aspirates of affected tissues, body fluids, impression smears of skin lesions	*Coccidioides* spherules and/or endospores	Low sensitivity and organisms may be difficult to accurately identify in some specimens. Immature spherules may be mistaken for other fungi or cellular aggregates or debris.
Fungal culture	Aspirates or biopsies of affected tissues, body fluids such as CSF or pleural effusion, transtracheal or bronchoalveolar lavage specimens	*Coccidioides* spp.	Generally sensitive and specific, but false negatives are possible if specimen size is low. Can require several weeks' incubation. A significant laboratory health hazard.
Antibody serology (gel immunodiffusion)	Serum, CSF	IgG or IgM antibodies to *Coccidioides* spp.	Sensitivity is close to 100%. Quantification of an IgG antibody titer is possible. Titers decline with successful treatment. In hyperendemic areas, titers as high as 1:16 have the potential to exist in subclinically infected or recovered dogs, so positive serology should be supported with other diagnostic tests for coccidioidomycosis.
Serology for *Coccidioides* antigen	Serum, urine	*Coccidioides* spp. galactomannan antigen	Low sensitivity (≤20%); false positives can occur in dogs with histoplasmosis or blastomycosis. Not recommended.
Real-time PCR assays	Biopsies, body fluids, respiratory lavage specimens, aspirates	*Coccidioides* DNA	Not yet validated in adequate numbers of dogs or cats with coccidioidomycosis; usefulness requires further evaluation.
Histopathology	Biopsy specimens from affected tissues, such as bone biopsies	*Coccidioides* spp. spherules	Limited sensitivity in dogs; submission of multiple biopsies is recommended when possible. Often only one or two spherules are visualized. Special stains such as periodic acid–Schiff and silver stains facilitate organism detection.

Cerebrospinal Fluid Analysis

CSF analysis in dogs with CNS coccidioidomycosis usually reveals an increase in protein concentration (generally <300 mg/dL, reference range <25 mg/dL) and a mild to moderate increase in the nucleated cell count (usually <50 cells/μL, reference range <2 cells/μL).[9] The differential cell count may show mixed, predominantly lymphocytic, mixed mononuclear, or neutrophilic pleocytosis. Organisms are generally not observed.

Diagnostic Imaging

Plain Radiography

Thoracic radiographs in dogs with disseminated coccidioidomycosis are often unremarkable. The most common radiographic finding in dogs with pulmonary coccidioidomycosis is mild to severe hilar lymphadenomegaly (Figure 63-4, *A*), which was present in 10 of 19 dogs with coccidioidomycosis from California.[9] Hilar lymphadenopathy can also be present in affected cats.[12] Although hilar lymphadenopathy can be the only finding, most dogs with hilar lymphadenopathy also have pulmonary infiltrates, which are usually mild to moderate and interstitial. Nodular interstitial, interstitial-alveolar, bronchointerstitial infiltrates, and/or sternal lymphadenomegaly can also be present (Figure 63-4, *B* and *C*).[9,15] Dogs with pericarditis can have cardiomegaly and pleural effusion, with hepatomegaly and decreased abdominal detail.[20]

Radiographs of affected bones in both dogs and cats with *Coccidioides* osteomyelitis reveal local periosteal proliferation as well as osteolysis and soft tissue swelling. Lesions can resemble osteosarcomas (Figure 63-5).[8,12]

Sonographic Findings

Abdominal ultrasound examination of dogs with coccidioidomycosis is typically unremarkable. Mild hepatosplenomegaly and abdominal lymphadenomegaly have been described in a small proportion of dogs.[9] Ascites, hepatomegaly, and distended hepatic veins may be evident in dogs with pericarditis.[20]

Echocardiography in dogs with *Coccidioides* spp. pericarditis can reveal thickening and mass lesions of the pericardium, adherence of the pericardium to the epicardium, pericardial and pleural effusion, and evidence of cardiac tamponade (see Figure 86-3).[20]

Advanced Imaging

Advanced imaging findings in dogs with coccidioidomycosis have not been extensively reported in the literature. Focal, contrast-enhancing intra-parenchymal mass lesions in the brain or osteomyelitis of the skull may be identified on computed tomography (CT) of the head.[24] Thoracic CT findings include contrast-enhancing miliary nodular pulmonary lesions; single or multifocal larger nodules or masses; tracheobronchial, sternal,

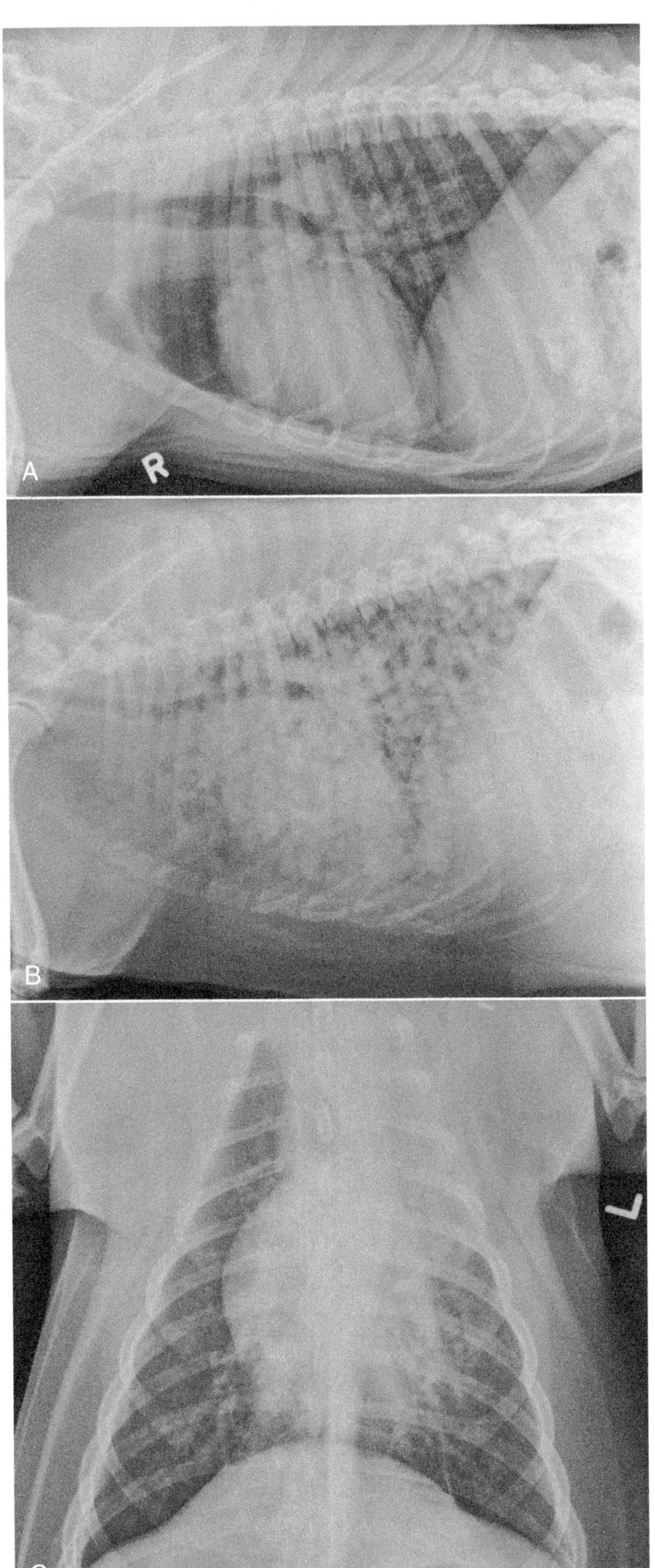

FIGURE 63-4 Thoracic radiographic patterns in coccidioidomycosis. **A,** Lateral thoracic radiograph from a 7-year-old intact male English pointer that shows several tracheobronchial lymphadenomegaly and focal pulmonary infiltrates. **B,** Lateral thoracic radiograph from a 3-year-old intact female Rottweiler with cough, anorexia, and respiratory distress. There are diffuse nodular and peribronchial infiltrates throughout the pulmonary parenchyma and possible hilar lymphadenopathy. Necropsy revealed necrogranulomatous interstitial pneumonia with intralesional spherules. The spleen, liver, and kidney were also involved. **C,** Dorsoventral thoracic radiograph from a 2-year-old female spayed Labrador retriever with cough and inappetence. There is an alveolar pattern in the left cranial lung lobe.

or mediastinal lymphadenopathy; focal regions of alveolar or peribronchial infiltrates; lobar consolidation; pleural or mediastinal thickening; and, rarely, pleural effusion (Figure 63-6).

MRI of the brain in dogs with CNS coccidioidomycosis may show focal hyperintense lesions within the brain on T2-weighted images (Figure 63-7). These are typically isointense on T1-weighted images and enhance with contrast. Other findings include ventricular dilation and/or meningeal enhancement.

Microbiologic Tests

Cytologic Examination

Cytologic examination of aspirates of affected tissues, pleural effusion, or respiratory lavage specimens typically reveals granulomatous or pyogranulomatous inflammation, sometimes with rare multinucleated giant cells, scattered eosinophils, and/or a reactive lymphocyte population. However, occasionally a suppurative inflammatory response predominates. Spherules may be visualized as round, deeply basophilic, double-walled, slightly crinkled structures that range in diameter from 8 to 70 μm. Spherules are generally low in number, frequently associated with cellular aggregates, but often they are not evident or easily identified. Usually their internal structure is not easily discernible, but occasionally endospores are seen in association with ruptured spherules (Figure 63-8). The endospores are 2 to 5 μm in diameter, are surrounded by a thin, nonstaining halo, and have small, round to oval, densely aggregated, eccentric nuclei. Endospores may be found extracellularly or within phagocytes. In one report, only endospores were visualized in a fine-needle aspirate from a bone lesion; intact spherules were not seen.[13]

Because cytology is relatively insensitive for diagnosis of coccidioidomycosis when compared with other deep mycoses, serologic testing for coccidioidomycosis should always be considered when cytology of tissue aspirates, body fluids, or lung washes reveals pyogranulomatous, suppurative, or granulomatous inflammation but organisms are not seen, and exposure to *Coccidioides* is possible based on the history.

Serologic Diagnosis

Serologic assays that detect antibodies to *Coccidioides* spp. are important diagnostic tests for coccidioidomycosis because organism detection assays have low sensitivity. Most diagnostic laboratories screen serum specimens with qualitative gel immunodiffusion (ID) assays for IgG or IgM antibodies (see Chapter 2). Detection of IgM (tube precipitin) or IgG (complement fixating) antibodies is reported, depending on the antigen preparation used in the assay. In dogs, IgM is detectable within 2 to 5 weeks of infection, and IgG appears after 8 to 12 weeks.[10] Quantification of an IgG antibody response can then be performed by quantitative ID, whereby serial dilutions of patient serum are subjected to gel ID.[14] In human patients, the complement fixation test is often used to quantify IgG antibody, but frequent false-positive results have been described with this method in dogs as a result of anticomplementary properties of canine serum.[25] The complement fixation test is positive in most cats with coccidioidomycosis; titers have ranged from 1:2 to 1:128.[12]

False-negative serologic test results are extremely rare in dogs with coccidioidomycosis tested at the author's institution,[9,20] but they have been described in dogs from Arizona.[26,27] Antibody titers usually range from 1:2 to 1:256; the median titer was 1:32 in one study.[9] There is no clear correlation between the magnitude of the IgG titer and the severity of illness in dogs.

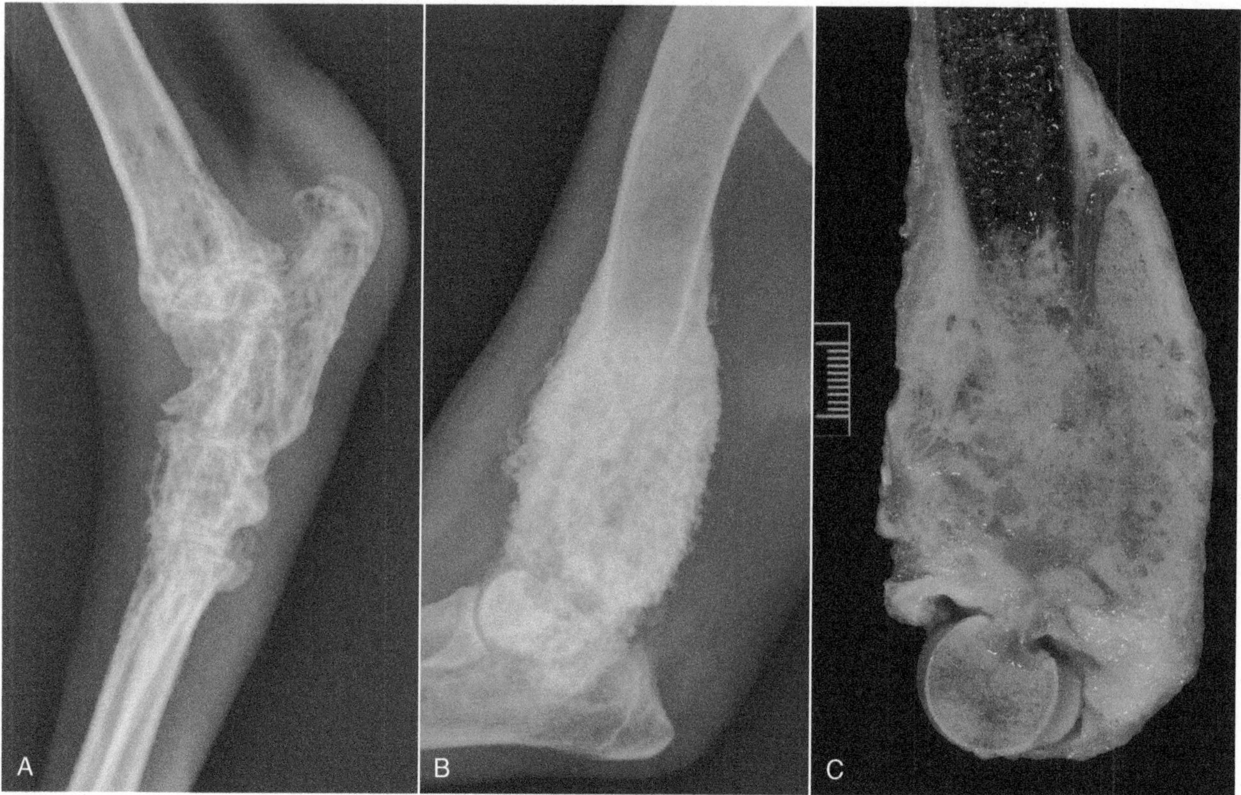

FIGURE 63-5 Osteomyelitis caused by *Coccidioides* spp. **A,** Left tarsus of a 4-year-old female spayed Dalmatian that was evaluated for signs of right-sided congestive heart failure due to pericarditis. Severe osteolysis is present. **B,** Right humerus of a 4-year-old female spayed shepherd mix. There is a mixed productive and lytic lesion of the distal diaphysis of the right humerus. **C,** Lesion in **(B)** at necropsy. (Courtesy University of California, Davis, Veterinary Anatomic Pathology Service.)

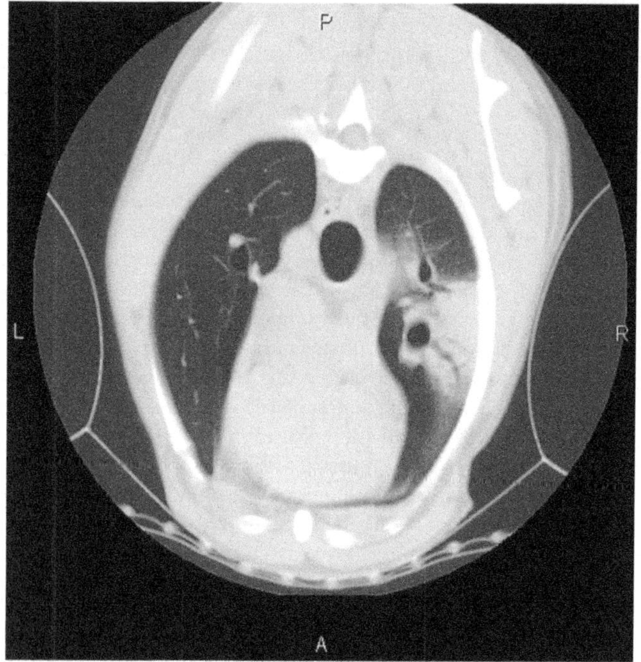

FIGURE 63-6 Computed tomography scan of the thorax of a 2-year-old intact male Labrador retriever with coccidioidomycosis. There are infiltrates in the caudal aspect of the right cranial lung lobe that extend from the mediastinum to the pleural surface. The walls of the right cranial bronchus and associated airways are thickened. Bronchial lymphadenomegaly was also identified.

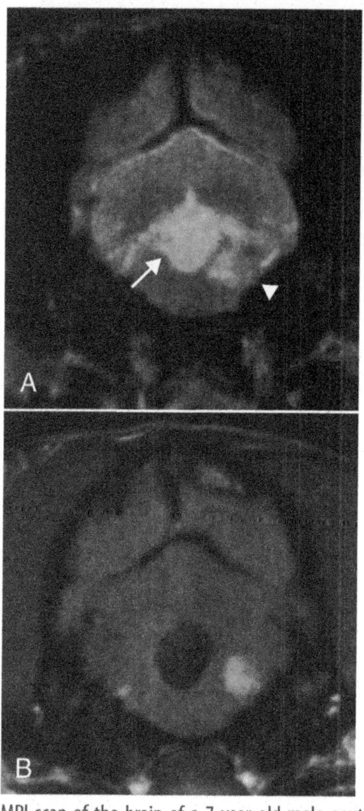

FIGURE 63-7 MRI scan of the brain of a 7-year-old male neutered shih tzu with disseminated coccidioidomycosis. **A,** A small focus of increased signal intensity on T2-weighting is present in the left lateral aspect of the brainstem *(arrowhead)*. Ventricular dilation is also present *(arrow)*. **B,** T1-weighted image after administration of gadolinium. The lesion in the brainstem is contrast enhancing.

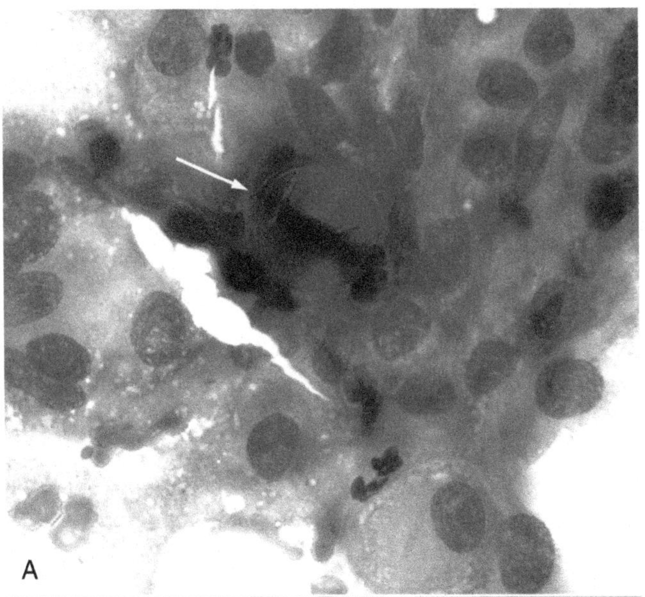

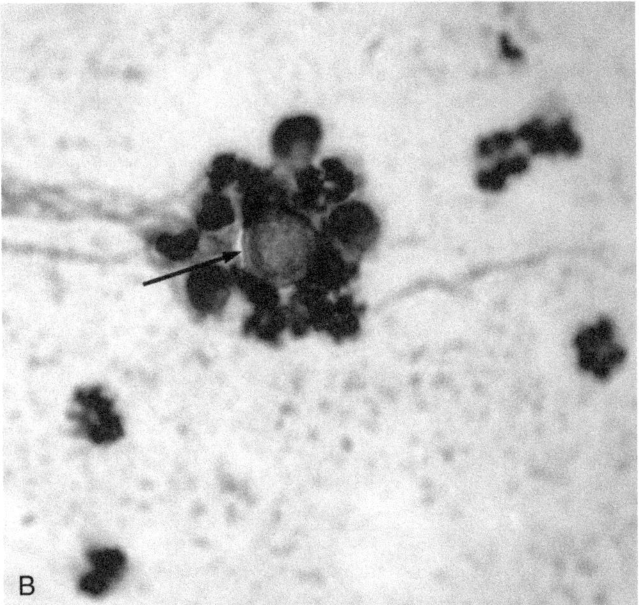

FIGURE 63-8 Cytologic appearance of *Coccidioides* spp. spherules. **A,** Spherules often appear as deeply basophilic, crinkled, intact, or ruptured ball-like structures *(white arrow)*. **B,** Sometimes, a refractile spherule wall is appreciated *(arrow)* and endospores are visualized as granular material within the spherule.

Dogs with active infection can have titers as low as 1:2, and healthy dogs in hyperendemic areas in Arizona can have titers as high as 1:16.[14] As a result, positive titers of 1:16 or lower must be interpreted in light of clinicopathologic abnormalities, and in hyperendemic areas, other diagnostic tests (such as culture, cytology or histopathology) should be used to confirm the diagnosis if possible. Latex agglutination and ELISA (EIA) assays for detection of anti-*Coccidioides* antibody have also been developed, but these are not widely used in veterinary medicine, and their use has been associated with a significant number of false-positive reactions in humans.[2,25,28]

A serologic assay that detects *Coccidioides* antigen in urine is available for diagnosis of coccidioidomycosis in human patients, such as in immunocompromised patients who lack the ability to produce significant quantities of antibody. However, preliminary data suggest that this assay has unacceptable sensitivity (≤20%) for diagnosis of coccidioidomycosis in dogs when serum, urine, or both specimens are tested, and false-positive reactions occur in a small proportion of dogs with blastomycosis or histoplasmosis.[29]

Fungal Culture

Coccidioides spp. can be isolated from clinical specimens on routine fungal media in the laboratory, but a negative culture result does not rule out coccidioidomycosis. Growth of a gray-white, downy mold that is tan to brown when visualized through the bottom of the plate usually appears after incubation for several days. Isolates can be identified based on their light microscopic appearance, with or without molecular methods. Culture of *Coccidioides* spp. is a serious laboratory health hazard and should only be performed if necessary and by suitably equipped laboratories. The clinician should warn the laboratory of the possibility of dimorphic fungal infection if suspected.

Molecular Diagnosis Using the Polymerase Chain Reaction

Real-time PCR assays have been used for rapid detection of *Coccidioides* spp. in respiratory specimens or CSF from affected humans, although sensitivity has been limited.[2,30] PCR assays have also been used in epidemiologic studies to identify major growth sites of *Coccidioides* spp. in soil.[31] PCR assays have not yet been widely applied to the diagnosis of coccidioidomycosis in dogs and cats.

Pathologic Findings

Gross pathologic findings in dogs with coccidioidomycosis include mottling and consolidation of the pulmonary parenchyma; single or multiple pale masses, nodular lesions, or emphysematous bullae within the lungs (Figure 63-9); enlarged and firm tracheobronchial, mediastinal, or sternal lymph nodes; plaque-like lesions on the pleura; and pleural and pericardial effusion. The interior of masses or nodules may be firm, caseous, or liquefied. The pericardium and epicardium may be thickened with mass lesions and adhesions between the pericardium and epicardium.[20] Ascites may also be present in dogs with pericarditis. Dogs with disseminated disease may have diffuse muscle atrophy, one or more enlarged peripheral lymph nodes, irregular bony swellings with associated draining skin lesions, and/or evidence of arthritis and synovitis. Meningoencephalitis may be evident as mass lesions within the brain parenchyma, ventricular dilation secondary to obstruction of CSF flow by inflammatory lesions, regional discoloration within the brain, and/or discoloration and thickening of the meninges. Rarely, prostatic enlargement, hepatic congestion and friability, multifocal nodular lesions within the myocardium or other parenchymal organs, and ocular lesions are present (see Physical Examination Findings for a description of ocular lesions).

Histopathology of affected tissues reveals large numbers of neutrophils and macrophages and sometimes marked fibrosis, with occasional endosporulating or non-endosporulating spherules. Multinucleated giant cells may be present and can contain spherules.[26] Spherules have a thick wall, and endospores may be visualized in mature spherules (Figure 63-10). Often only one or two spherules are visualized, and in some cases they are not found at all. Use of special stains such as periodic acid–Schiff and Gomori's methenamine silver can enhance organism identification within lesions. The presence of large numbers of spherules has been described in some affected cats.[23,32] Chronic, diffuse glomerulonephritis was present in 3 of 13 dogs with

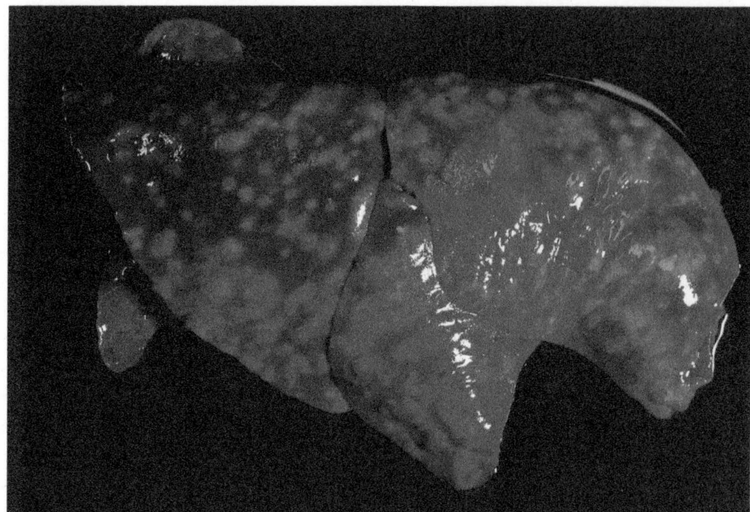

FIGURE 63-9 Lungs of the dog in Figure 63-4, *B*. Multiple pale nodules are present throughout the lung parenchyma.

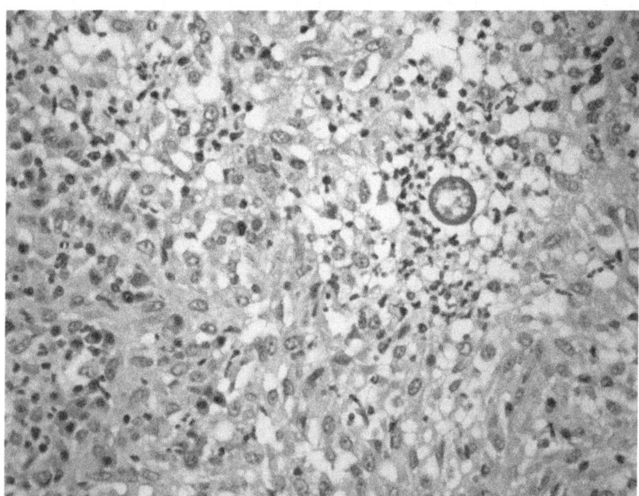

FIGURE 63-10 Histopathology of the tarsus of the dog in Figure 63-5, *A*. A single mature spherule is surrounded by a pyogranulomatous inflammatory response. The spherule contains many endospores.

coccidioidomycosis that had full necropsy examinations at the author's hospital; an additional dog with renal lesions had multiple renal pyogranulomas with intralesional spherules.[24]

Treatment and Prognosis

Successful treatment of coccidioidomycosis is limited by the high cost of treatment and the often advanced nature of the disease by the time it is diagnosed in some dogs. Treatment consists of a combination of antifungal drug therapy and supportive care; in some cases, surgery is required. Usually a minimum of 6 months of treatment is required.

Antimicrobial Treatment

Animals with coccidioidomycosis can respond well to azole monotherapy with fluconazole or itraconazole. Ketoconazole has been used successfully to treat dogs and cats in the past but is no longer the drug of first choice owing to its lower activity and increased rate of adverse effects. Fluconazole is the least expensive azole and may be a better choice than itraconazole for dogs with CNS involvement, because of its superior penetration of the CNS. The dose of fluconazole used by the author is 5 mg/kg PO q12h. Itraconazole (5 mg/kg PO q24h) is preferred for animals with bone involvement and may be effective in dogs that fail to respond to treatment with fluconazole. In human patients, itraconazole demonstrated a greater response rate in a blinded comparison with fluconazole.[33] Compounded formulations of itraconazole should be avoided. Small dogs are best treated with itraconazole solution (10 mg/mL), which has higher bioavailability than the capsules (see Chapter 9). If capsules are used, they should be administered with food. If clinical signs do not improve with azole treatment, therapeutic drug monitoring could be considered to ensure that serum drug concentrations are adequate. Periodic monitoring of liver enzymes is recommended for animals treated with azole antifungals.

Treatment with deoxycholate or lipid-complexed amphotericin B is recommended either alone or in combination with an azole for dogs with refractory or severe disease (see Chapter 9 for dosing protocols). However, studies that compare amphotericin B to azole monotherapy in dogs have not been performed. Voriconazole and posaconazole have been used to treat refractory coccidioidomycosis in human patients, but they are not considered first-line drugs.[2] Their use for treatment of affected dogs or cats is limited by expense. Voriconazole could be considered for treatment of refractory meningoencephalitis if client finances permit its use, because it has excellent penetration of the CNS.

Surgical Management

Ultimately, some dogs with severe and persistent osteomyelitis require amputation to control the infection, and enucleation may be required for dogs with endophthalmitis. Successful treatment of *Coccidioides* pericarditis has been reported after subtotal pericardiectomy and epicardial excision, which should be performed in conjunction with antifungal drug therapy. Referral to a specialist surgeon with experience with the technique is strongly recommended. The perioperative mortality rate in one study was reported as 24%, and the 2-year survival rate after discharge was 82%.[20]

Supportive Care

Other treatments that may be required for dogs with severe pulmonary coccidioidomycosis are similar to those described for blastomycosis and include oxygen supplementation, nebulization and coupage, drainage of thoracic effusions, nutritional support, anti-inflammatory drugs, and intravenous fluid therapy. Concurrent treatment with glucocorticoids and antiseizure medications may be necessary to reduce the severity of neurologic signs in dogs with CNS coccidioidomycosis. Topical prednisolone acetate solution and antiglaucoma agents may be required for dogs with ocular lesions.

Prognosis

The prognosis for resolution for coccidioidomycosis depends on the severity of infection and the extent of dissemination. The duration of treatment ranges from 6 months to many years, and in some cases, lifelong treatment is needed. IgG antibody titers decrease with successful treatment, which in general should be continued until lesions resolve and the titer is 1:2 or lower. Residual radiographic opacities may be present in some dogs as a result of scar tissue formation. Dogs with localized pulmonary infection have the best prognosis; the prognosis appears to be poor for dogs with CNS involvement. Dogs with *Coccidioides* osteomyelitis may require lifelong treatment with itraconazole.

Immunity and Vaccination

Immunity to *Coccidioides* spp. depends primarily on cell-mediated immunity, specifically T lymphocytes. No vaccine is currently available commercially for prevention of the disease.

Prevention

Prevention of coccidioidomycosis requires avoidance of hyperendemic areas (especially parts of Arizona and south-central California), which may not be possible. In endemic areas, dogs should be kept away from sites of soil disturbance (such as construction sites) and housed indoors during dust storms; digging should be discouraged. Housing dogs indoors during the day in endemic regions may reduce the chance of infection. Nevertheless, it should be remembered that clinical infections develop in only a minority of exposed dogs.

Public Health Aspects

Coccidioidomycosis is a serious infection in human patients and has similar clinical manifestations to those described in dogs. The incidence of human coccidioidomycosis has increased in Arizona in the last decade, possibly as a result of population growth, immigration of immunologically naïve people, and construction. Construction and agricultural workers, archeologists, and excavators are at high risk for coccidioidomycosis.[2] African American and Filipino patients, as well as patients with AIDS and women in the third trimester of pregnancy, are at highest risk for disseminated disease, which occurs in approximately 0.5% of infected humans.

Because of their susceptibility to infection, dogs have been used as a sentinel for human exposure to environmental sources of *Coccidioides* spp. in seroprevalence studies.[34] Direct transmission between infected veterinary patients and humans has not been reported. However, fatal coccidioidomycosis occurred in a veterinary resident after necropsy of a horse with disseminated disease.[35] Inoculation coccidioidomycosis was reported in a veterinary technician from Arizona after a bite from a cat that was later diagnosed with disseminated disease.[23] Inoculation coccidioidomycosis also has the potential to occur if sharps injuries occur during aspiration of affected tissues, surgical procedures, or necropsy examinations. Proper sedation or anesthesia should always be used if coccidioidomycosis is suspected in dogs or cats seen at veterinary clinics and the potential for a sharps injury exists. If accidental inoculation occurs, immediate attention should be sought from a physician. Prolonged fluconazole prophylaxis is generally recommended with monitoring of *Coccidioides* serology and liver function tests. Bandaging of skin lesions should be avoided. Necropsies should be performed without delay with suitable protective clothing, and the carcasses of animals that die from coccidioidomycosis should immediately be incinerated, because conversion of the organism to a mycelial form can occur after death of an animal. For the same reason, burial is not recommended because of the potential for contamination of the environment. Fluconazole prophylaxis is also indicated after accidental laboratory exposure to inocula.[36]

CASE EXAMPLE

Signalment: "Jenny", a 2-year-old female spayed Labrador retriever from Oxnard in southwestern California

History: Jenny was evaluated for a 2-month history of cough, inappetence, and lethargy. For the first 3 days of illness, the owner noted only an intermittent harsh, nonproductive cough. On day 4, the dog became lethargic and inappetent, so she was taken to a local veterinary clinic. Thoracic radiographs revealed alveolar infiltrates in the left cranial lung lobe. A diagnosis of bacterial pneumonia was suspected, so Jenny was treated with enrofloxacin (6 mg/kg PO q24h), amoxicillin-clavulanic acid (12.5 mg/kg PO q12h), and metronidazole (8 mg/kg PO q12h) for 2 weeks. After the first week of treatment, there was no improvement, so a long-acting cephalosporin was administered (cefovecin, 8 mg/kg SC once). Two days later, treatment with prednisone (0.3 mg/kg PO q12h) was initiated, which was followed by mild improvement in the clinical signs. Jenny's owner then sought a second opinion on day 20 after onset of clinical signs, and *Coccidioides* serology was performed. The titer was positive for IgG at 1:64. The prednisone was discontinued, and treatment was initiated with fluconazole (6.7 mg/kg PO q12h). However, after 1 month of treatment, thoracic radiographic abnormalities were unchanged. The fluconazole was substituted with a compounded itraconazole formulation (5 mg/kg PO q12h). However, after an additional 2 weeks of treatment, there had been no further improvement in the cough, so the owner was referred to the University of California, Davis.

Continued

According to the owner, Jenny had a poor appetite for dog food but was eating home-cooked chicken, rice, and vegetables. Her activity level had been low. The cough occurred many times throughout the day and was unrelated to exercise and eating. Occasionally she had paroxysms of cough with a terminal retch. Other medical history included canine parvovirus infection when she was 8 weeks old and "kennel cough" when she was 9 months old, which resolved after 10 days. The owners lived in a semirural area just north of Los Angeles. The only travel had been to Atascadero, further north on the California coast. She was the only animal in the household. There had been ongoing construction around the house to replace a septic system with a sewer, which began 4 to 6 weeks before the onset of clinical signs.

Physical Examination:

General: Quiet but alert and responsive, hydrated. T = 102.6°F (39.2°C), HR = 100 beats/min, RR = 24 breaths/min, CRT = 1 s.

Eyes, Ears, Nose, and Throat: No abnormalities were noted. A dilated fundoscopic examination was unremarkable.

Musculoskeletal: Body condition score was 4/9. The dog was ambulatory with no lameness or muscle atrophy.

Respiratory: Harsh breath sounds were present in all lung fields. A harsh cough with a terminal retch was readily elicited on tracheal palpation.

Cardiovascular, Gastrointestinal, Genitourinary, and Lymph Nodes: No clinically significant abnormalities were detected.

Imaging Findings: Thoracic radiographs were compared to the two-view thoracic study performed 2 weeks previously, which was available for review. The initial radiographs showed a dense alveolar pattern throughout the left cranial lung lobe and increased opacity in the region of the hilar lymph nodes with splaying of the mainstem bronchi (see Figure 63-4, *C*). These abnormalities had improved slightly in the 10-day recheck interim, but alveolar infiltrates were still present throughout the left cranial lung lobe. There was a persistent, mild, diffuse pulmonary interstitial pattern in the remaining pulmonary parenchyma, which was most severe in the caudodorsal lung fields. This was considered excessive for the age of the patient. The cardiovascular structures were within normal limits.

Microbiologic Testing: *Coccidioides* serology: positive by qualitative gel immunodiffusion for complement-fixing antibody (IgG), negative for IgM. Quantitative immunodiffusion revealed an IgG titer of 1:128.

Serum itraconazole concentration: <0.31 μg/mL (undetectable).

Diagnosis: Pulmonary coccidioidomycosis.

Treatment: The itraconazole capsules prescribed at the previous veterinary clinic were examined and found to contain a white powder rather than granules. Treatment was changed to brand-name itraconazole (Sporanox), because compounded formulations can be unstable. Instructions were given to administer the itraconazole (5 mg/kg PO q24h) with food to improve absorption. Aspirin was also prescribed (12 mg/kg PO q12h). One month later Jenny's cough and activity level had improved considerably. A CBC was within normal limits, and a biochemistry panel showed hypoalbuminemia (3.3 g/dL, reference range 3.4-4.3 g/dL) and hyperglobulinemia (3.4 g/dL, reference range 1.7-3.1 g/dL). Liver enzyme activities were within reference ranges. Thoracic radiographs showed resolution of hilar lymphadenopathy with persistence of the alveolar infiltrates in the left cranial lung lobe. The IgG antibody titer to *Coccidioides* was 1:64. Three months later, the cough had resolved completely, and after 6 months of treatment, there was complete resolution of thoracic radiographic abnormalities and the titer was 1:32. At this point, the owner switched to a generic formulation of itraconazole because of financial concerns. After an additional 3 and 6 months of treatment, the IgG titer was 1:16 and 1:8, respectively, with no further clinical signs. Treatment was continued for an additional 3 months (i.e., total of 15 months of treatment), and the dog remains alive and apparently healthy at the time of writing.

Comments: This is an interesting case of pulmonary coccidioidomycosis that occurred outside the hyperendemic central valley region in California. Exposure may have resulted from soil disturbance as a result of sewer work. Because of the low suspicion for the disease, the disease was mistaken for bacterial pneumonia. The owner had limited financial resources, so an extensive respiratory work-up (including respiratory lavage with cytology and culture) was declined. When *Coccidioides* serology was positive, fluconazole was prescribed, but there was no improvement. The decision to treat with compounded itraconazole was made because of client financial limitations, but serum drug levels with this treatment were undetectable. Fortunately, disease ultimately resolved with a change to a noncompounded formulation, and there was progressive decline in serial IgG titers (which were always performed by the same laboratory). Whether treatment beyond complete resolution of the radiographic abnormalities was necessary is unknown.

SUGGESTED READINGS

Greene RT, Troy GC. Coccidioidomycosis in 48 cats: a retrospective study (1984-1993). J Vet Intern Med. 1995;9:86-91.

Johnson LR, Herrgesell EJ, Davidson AP, et al. Clinical, clinicopathologic, and radiographic findings in dogs with coccidioidomycosis: 24 cases (1995-2000). J Am Vet Med Assoc. 2003;222:461-466.

Shubitz LE, Butkiewicz CD, Dial SM, et al. Incidence of *Coccidioides* infection among dogs residing in a region in which the organism is endemic. J Am Vet Med Assoc. 2005;226:1846-1850.

REFERENCES

1. Hirschmann JV. The early history of coccidioidomycosis: 1892-1945. Clin Infect Dis. 2007;44:1202-1207.
2. Thompson 3rd GR. Pulmonary coccidioidomycosis. Semin Respir Crit Care Med. 2011;32:754-763.
3. Ramani R, Chaturvedi V. Antifungal susceptibility profiles of *Coccidioides immitis* and *Coccidioides posadasii* from endemic and non-endemic areas. Mycopathologia. 2007;163:315-319.
4. Fisher MC, Koenig GL, White TJ, et al. Molecular and phenotypic description of *Coccidioides posadasii* sp. nov., previously recognized as the non-California population of *Coccidioides immitis*. Mycologia. 2002;94:73-84.

5. Flynn NM, Hoeprich PD, Kawachi MM, et al. An unusual outbreak of windborne coccidioidomycosis. N Engl J Med. 1979;301:358-361.
6. Schneider E, Hajjeh RA, Spiegel RA, et al. A coccidioidomycosis outbreak following the Northridge, Calif, earthquake. JAMA. 1997;277:904-908.
7. Park BJ, Sigel K, Vaz V, et al. An epidemic of coccidioidomycosis in Arizona associated with climatic changes, 1998-2001. J Infect Dis. 2005;191:1981-1987.
8. Maddy KT. Disseminated coccidioidomycosis of the dog. J Am Vet Med Assoc. 1958;132:483-489.
9. Johnson LR, Herrgesell EJ, Davidson AP, et al. Clinical, clinicopathologic, and radiographic findings in dogs with coccidioidomycosis: 24 cases (1995-2000). J Am Vet Med Assoc. 2003;222:461-466.
10. Davidson AP, Pappagianis D. Canine coccidioidomycosis: 1970 to 1993. Stanford University, CA: 5th International Conference on Coccidioidomycosis; 1994:155-162.
11. Butkiewicz CD, Shubitz LE, Dial SM. Risk factors associated with *Coccidioides* infection in dogs. J Am Vet Med Assoc. 2005;226:1851-1854.
12. Greene RT, Troy GC. Coccidioidomycosis in 48 cats: a retrospective study (1984-1993). J Vet Intern Med. 1995;9:86-91.
13. Beaudin S, Rich LJ, Meinkoth JH, et al. Draining skin lesion from a desert poodle. Vet Clin Pathol. 2005;34:65-68.
14. Shubitz LE, Butkiewicz CD, Dial SM, et al. Incidence of *Coccidioides* infection among dogs residing in a region in which the organism is endemic. J Am Vet Med Assoc. 2005;226:1846-1850.
15. Millman TM, O'Brien TR, Suter PF, et al. Coccidioidomycosis in the dog: its radiographic diagnosis. J Am Vet Radiol Soc. 1979;20:50-65.
16. Burtch M. Granulomatous meningitis caused by *Coccidioides immitis* in a dog. J Am Vet Med Assoc. 1998;212:827-829.
17. Pryor Jr WH, Huizenga CG, Splitter GA, et al. *Coccidioides immitis* encephalitis in two dogs. J Am Vet Med Assoc. 1972;161:1108-1112.
18. Angell JA, Merideth RE, Shively JN, et al. Ocular lesions associated with coccidioidomycosis in dogs: 35 cases (1980-1985). J Am Vet Med Assoc. 1987;190:1319-1322.
19. Shively JN, Whiteman CE. Ocular lesions in disseminated coccidioidomycosis in 2 dogs. Pathol Vet. 1970;7:1-6.
20. Heinritz CK, Gilson SD, Soderstrom MJ, et al. Subtotal pericardectomy and epicardial excision for treatment of coccidioidomycosis-induced effusive-constrictive pericarditis in dogs: 17 cases (1999-2003). J Am Vet Med Assoc. 2005;227:435-440.
21. Angell JA, Shively JN, Merideth RE, et al. Ocular coccidioidomycosis in a cat. J Am Vet Med Assoc. 1985;187:167-169.
22. Tofflemire K, Betbeze C. Three cases of feline ocular coccidioidomycosis: presentation, clinical features, diagnosis, and treatment. Vet Ophthalmol. 2010;13:166-172.
23. Gaidici A, Saubolle MA. Transmission of coccidioidomycosis to a human via a cat bite. J Clin Microbiol. 2009;47:505-506.
24. Sykes JE. Unpublished observations, 2012.
25. Gershman N, Villaba W, Neel K. Detection of canine IgG and IgM antibodies to *Coccidioides immitis* using a novel enzyme-linked immunosorbent assay (EIA) method. Stanford University, CA: 5th International Conference on Coccidioidomycosis; 1994:137-146.
26. Graupmann-Kuzma A, Valentine BA, Shubitz LF, et al. Coccidioidomycosis in dogs and cats: a review. J Am Anim Hosp Assoc. 2008;44:226-235.
27. Greene RT. Coccidioidomycosis and paracoccidioidomycosis. In: Greene CE, ed. *Infectious Diseases of the Dog and Cat*. 4th ed. St. Louis, MO: Elsevier Saunders; 2012:634-645.
28. Yturraspe DJ. Clinical evaluation of a latex particle agglutination test and a gel diffusion precipitin test in the diagnosis of canine coccidioidomycosis. J Am Vet Med Assoc. 1971;158:1249-1256.
29. Kirsch EJ, Greene RT, Prahl A, et al. Evaluation of *Coccidioides* antigen detection in dogs with coccidioidomycosis. Clin Vaccine Immunol. 2012;19:343-345.
30. Vucicevic D, Blair JE, Binnicker MJ, et al. The utility of *Coccidioides* polymerase chain reaction testing in the clinical setting. Mycopathologia. 2010;170:345-351.
31. Lauer A, Baal JD, Baal JC, et al. Detection of *Coccidioides immitis* in Kern County, California, by multiplex PCR. Mycologia. 2012;104:62-69.
32. Reed RE, Hoge RS, Trautman RJ. Coccidioidomycosis in two cats. J Am Vet Med Assoc. 1963;143:953-956.
33. Galgiani JN, Catanzaro A, Cloud GA, et al. Comparison of oral fluconazole and itraconazole for progressive, nonmeningeal coccidioidomycosis. A randomized, double-blind trial. Mycoses Study Group. Ann Intern Med. 2000;133:676-686.
34. Gautam R, Srinath I, Clavijo A, et al. Identifying areas of high risk of human exposure to coccidioidomycosis in Texas using serology data from dogs. Zoonoses Public Health, 2012.
35. Kohn GJ, Linne SR, Smith CM, et al. Acquisition of coccidioidomycosis at necropsy by inhalation of coccidioidal endospores. Diagn Microbiol Infect Dis. 1992;15:527-530.
36. Stevens DA, Clemons KV, Levine HB, et al. Expert opinion: what to do when there is *Coccidioides* exposure in a laboratory. Clin Infect Dis. 2009;49:919-923.

CHAPTER 64

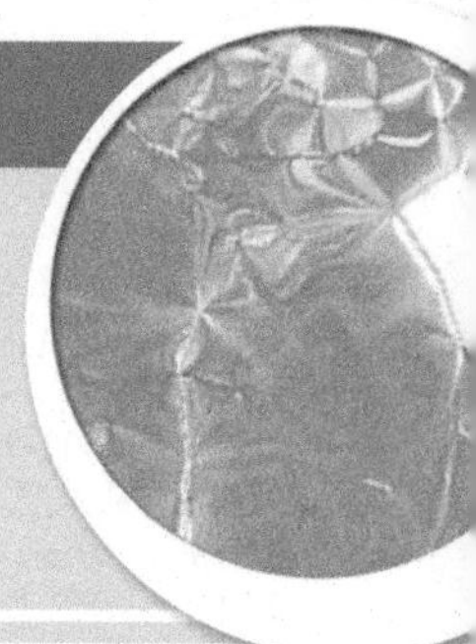

Sporotrichosis

Jane E. Sykes

> **Overview of Sporotrichosis**
>
> First Described: 1896, in Maryland, USA, by Benjamin Schenk[1]
>
> Cause: *Sporothrix schenckii* complex fungi (ascomycetes, teleomorph *Ophiostoma stenoceras*)
>
> Affected Hosts: Cats, dogs, humans, and a variety of other mammalian and avian species
>
> Geographic Distribution: Tropical and temperate zones worldwide
>
> Mode of Transmission: Cutaneous inoculation or inhalation of conidia
>
> Major Clinical Signs: Cutaneous nodules or draining skin lesions, lymphadenopathy
>
> Differential Diagnoses: Other deep mycoses (especially cryptococcosis in cats), mycobacterial infections, nocardiosis or actinomycosis, leishmaniosis, squamous cell carcinoma, feline eosinophilic granuloma complex, feline herpesviral dermatitis, foreign body granulomas
>
> Human Health Significance: Many human infections are acquired from the environment, but direct transmission can follow contact between infected cats and humans, and especially cat bites or scratches.

Etiology and Epidemiology

Organisms that belong to the *Sporothrix schenckii* species complex are dimorphic, saprophytic fungi that cause sporotrichosis, a subacute to chronic disease that most often results from cutaneous or subcutaneous inoculation of the organism through a puncture wound, but can also follow inhalation of the fungus. Sporotrichosis has been described in cats, dogs, humans, and a variety of other domestic and wild animal hosts that include equine species, ruminants, swine, rats, mice, hamsters, armadillos, domestic fowl, chimpanzees, and dolphins.

Sporothrix species thrive in humid conditions (92% to 100%) and at mean temperatures between 25°C and 30°C. They prefer moist soil that is rich in decaying vegetation, as well as sphagnum moss, wood, thorns, or hay, where they grow as mycelia. The fungus is distributed worldwide in tropical and temperate zones but is most prevalent in tropical or subtropical regions of the Americas. Regions of endemicity include Mexico, Brazil, Uruguay, Peru, Japan, India, and South Africa; sporotrichosis is uncommon in Europe. Although all *Sporothrix* isolates have in the past been grouped into one species, multiple genotypes exist that vary in virulence and geographic distribution.[2-4] As a result, an *S. schenckii* species complex has been identified, which includes at least six species: *S. schenckii* sensu stricto, *Sporothrix brasiliensis, Sporothrix globosa, Sporothrix mexicana, Sporothrix albicans,* and *Sporothrix luriei.*[5-7] The epidemiology of the various members of the complex is as yet incompletely understood. *S. globosa* has a worldwide distribution, whereas *S. brasiliensis* appears to be limited to Brazil. *S. schenckii, S. brasiliensis,* and *S. albicans* have been isolated from cats, and *S. schenckii* and *S. luriei* have been isolated from dogs.[8]

Cats are more susceptible to sporotrichosis than dogs and are thought to facilitate spread of organisms in the environment.[9] Contaminated claw or bite wounds, as well as autoinoculation during grooming, are thought to be important modes of transmission.[10] Male cats are overrepresented in most studies (60% to 70% of affected cats), which may reflect the tendency of male cats to roam outdoors and be involved in aggressive interactions.[10-13] In Rio de Janeiro, a large outbreak of sporotrichosis has occurred over the past decade, which has involved more than 1000 humans, 60 dogs, and 1500 cats.[1] Of affected cats in this outbreak, *Sporothrix* spp. were isolated from 100% of 76 cutaneous lesions, 66% of 71 swab specimens from the nasal cavity, 41% of 79 oral swab specimens, and 40% of 38 nail fragments.[14] The fungus was also isolated from 3 of 84 apparently healthy cats that were in contact with affected animals. Twenty percent of cats were positive for antibodies to FIV, 1% of cats were positive for FeLV antigen, and 1% of cats were positive for both FIV antibodies and FeLV antigen.[10] More than 85% of affected cats were less than 4 years of age. Of isolates from affected humans in the outbreak, most were *S. brasiliensis,* but *S. schenckii* sensu stricto and *S. globosa* were also isolated.[7]

In dogs, sporotrichosis is relatively rare. Cutaneous introduction of the organism with plant foreign bodies has been suggested in some cases. In one dog, the portal of entry was thought to be an alligator bite wound.[15] In the Brazilian outbreak, contact with cats appeared to be an important mode of transmission to dogs.[16] No clear breed or sex predisposition has been identified, and dogs in the Brazilian outbreak ranged in age from 6 months to 12 years (median, 4 years). Mixed sporotrichosis and cryptococcosis was reported in a dog from Ontario.[17]

Clinical Features

Signs and Their Pathogenesis

Transmission of *Sporothrix* primarily results from cutaneous inoculation of organisms in the environment, but can also result from inhalation of conidia. Direct contact with cats that have sporotrichosis (without an apparent break in the skin) can also result in transmission.[10] Once within tissues, the organism

TABLE 64-1

Proposed Classification Scheme for Clinical Forms of Sporotrichosis in Human Patients[1]

Group	Subcategory	Relevance to Cats and Dogs
Cutaneous	Fixed (or localized) Lymphocutaneous Multifocal (or disseminated)	All forms described in cats and dogs, but fixed or multifocal disease most common
Mucosal	Ocular Nasal Other	Occurs in cats and dogs
Extracutaneous	Pulmonary Osteoarticular Meningeal Generalized (or disseminated)	Pulmonary and generalized disease is primarily described in cats. Pulmonary, generalized, and osteoarticular disease occur rarely in dogs.
Special forms	Spontaneous regression Hypersensitivity (erythema nodosum, erythema multiforme)	Spontaneous regression has been described in cats and especially dogs

converts into a yeast form. The yeast form has a cell wall that contains glucans, a glycoprotein fraction known as peptidorhamnomannan, and galactose-containing polysaccharides. The cell wall also contains melanin, which may protect the yeast from oxidative damage.[1,9] Adhesins on the surface of the organism bind fibronectin, which appears to be important for virulence.[18] Organisms that are thermotolerant (able to survive at temperatures closer to body temperature, or 37°C) may be more likely to cause invasive disease.[9]

Several clinical forms of sporotrichosis are recognized in human patients. The clinical form of disease that develops depends on host factors and the virulence of the infecting *Sporothrix* strain. A suggested classification system for human sporotrichosis categorizes the distribution of lesions into cutaneous, mucosal, or extracutaneous (Table 64-1). Cutaneous lesions are crusted, plaque-like, or nodular lesions that often ulcerate or drain serosanguineous fluid. They may be fixed (localized), track along the course of lymphatics (lymphocutaneous), or be multifocal (sometimes referred to as disseminated cutaneous disease) (Figures 64-1 and 64-2). More than 50% of human patients develop the lymphocutaneous form and the infection spreads proximally along lymphatics, with formation of multiple secondary nodules (also known as gummata) that may ulcerate. This form has not been clearly recognized in cats and appears to be uncommon to rare in dogs.[16] Up to 80% of cats with sporotrichosis have multiple, widely distributed cutaneous lesions.[10,13] These may develop as a result of autoinoculation during grooming, or they can be a manifestation of a disseminated (or generalized) systemic infection.

Extracutaneous disease follows inhalation of conidia or hematogenous spread of *Sporothrix* from sites of cutaneous

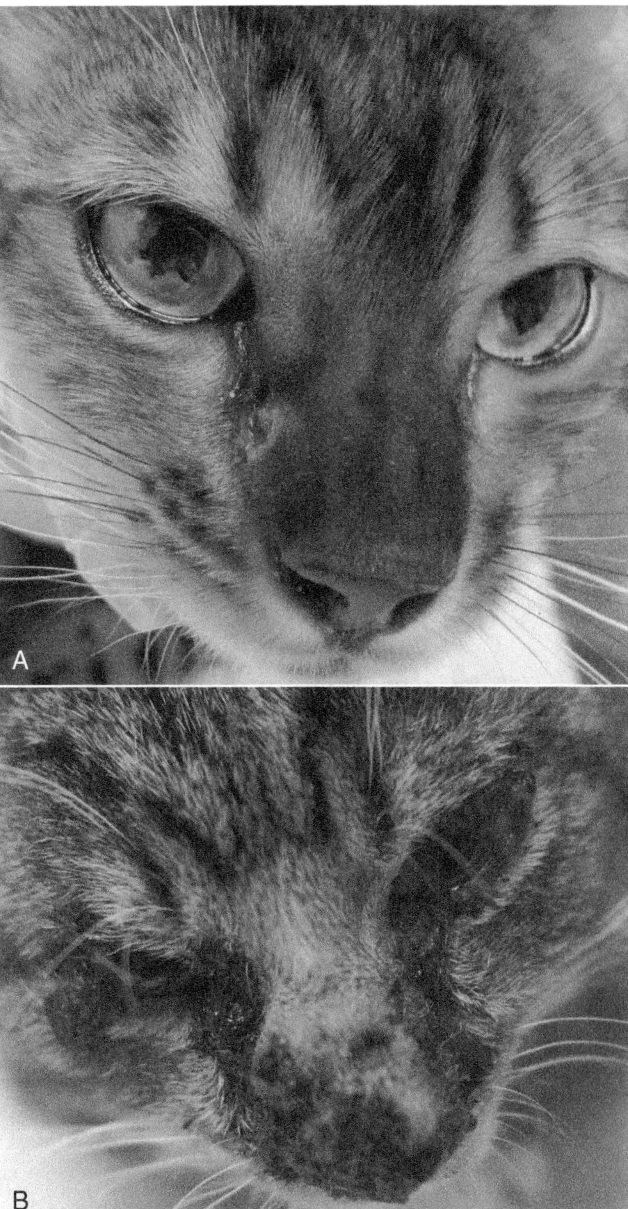

FIGURE 64-1 Cutaneous and mucosal sporotrichosis. **A,** 2-year-old female spayed Bengal that had ulcerated lesions of the face, thoracic limb, and tail. **B,** Cutaneous and conjunctival sporotrichosis in a 1-year-old male neutered domestic shorthair. (Courtesy University of California, Davis, Veterinary Dermatology Service.)

inoculation. Transmission by inhalation is thought to occur in some cats, because pulmonary and nasal cavity disease with associated respiratory signs are common in cats.[10-13,19] Respiratory signs include sneezing, cough, tachypnea, increased respiratory effort, stertor, and/or nasal discharge. Respiratory signs were present in 44% of 347 cats in the Brazilian outbreak[10] and can also occur in dogs.[13,16] Sneezing may occur before the onset of cutaneous lesions in cats, and some cats or dogs show only respiratory signs. Cats also can develop generalized disease, with involvement of multiple organ systems, which include the lungs, liver, spleen, kidneys, lymph nodes, and testicles.[13,20] Co-infection with FIV does not appear to be a risk factor for dissemination.[21] Isolation of *Sporothrix* species from the blood of 35% of 49 cats with focal or multifocal cutaneous involvement was reported.[21] Clinical signs of systemic involvement include fever, generalized

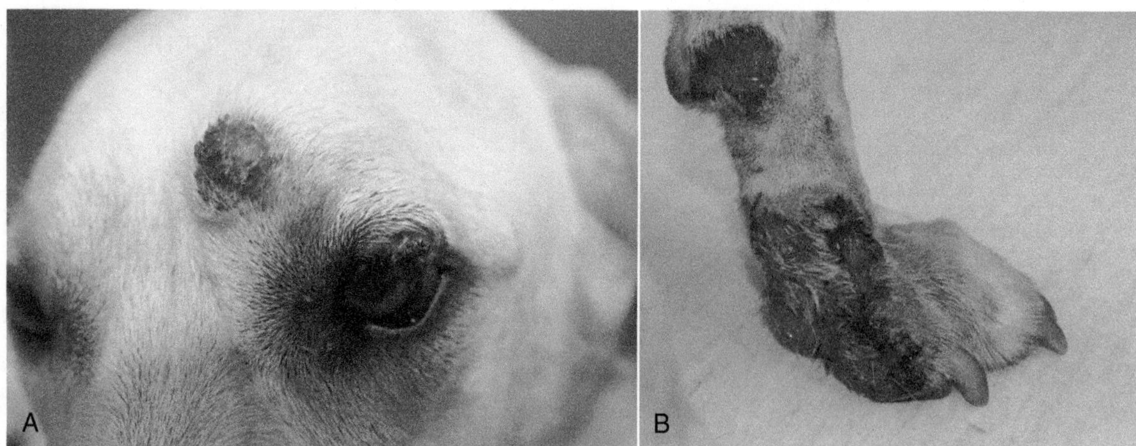

FIGURE 64-2 Multifocal ulcerated cutaneous lesions on the head **(A)** and left thoracic limb **(B)** caused by *Sporothrix* spp. in a 2-year-old male neutered Labrador retriever. (Courtesy University of California, Davis, Veterinary Dermatology Service.)

TABLE 64-2

Diagnostic Assays Currently Available for Sporotrichosis in Dogs and Cats

Assay	Specimen Type	Target	Performance
Cytologic examination	Aspirates of cutaneous nodules, impression smears of skin lesions or biopsies	*Sporothrix* yeasts	High sensitivity (approximately 80%) in cats. Sensitivity is lower in dogs.
Fungal culture	Aspirates, swabs, or biopsies of affected tissues	*Sporothrix* spp.	Generally sensitive (around 75%), but false negatives can occur if specimen size is low. Most specific method. Requires several weeks' incubation. Allows species identification via molecular methods and antifungal drug susceptibility testing.
Histopathology	Biopsy specimens from affected tissues	*Sporothrix* spp. yeasts	Sensitivity is higher (>60%) in cats when compared with dogs (<20%). Special stains such as Gomori's methenamine silver and immunohistochemical stains facilitate organism detection and identification.

lymphadenomegaly, anorexia, dehydration, vomiting, and weight loss. These signs were each reported in fewer than 20% of cats with sporotrichosis; vomiting occurred in fewer than 5% of the cats.[10] Weight loss, vomiting, or anorexia can also occur in dogs.[13,16] Other rare forms of extracutaneous sporotrichosis described in humans include osteoarticular and meningeal sporotrichosis. Osteoarticular sporotrichosis occurs rarely in dogs and may manifest clinically as lameness and synovial effusion.[12,22]

Physical Examination Findings

In cats, cutaneous lesions are most often found on the head (especially the bridge of the nose and the nasal planum, eyelids, and/or pinnae) and have a similar appearance to those caused by *Cryptococcus* spp. (see Figure 64-1).[10,12,23] Other common sites for skin lesions are the distal limbs, digits, and tail, but lesions can also be found elsewhere on the body. Swelling of the conjunctiva or lesions in the oral cavity or nasal cavity can be present in some affected cats (see Figure 64-1). Cutaneous or subcutaneous lesions are often firm nodules that sometimes enlarge to form soft cutaneous masses. Nodules can ulcerate and drain serosanguineous to purulent fluid, but are usually not painful or pruritic.[12] In some cases, ulcerations and draining skin lesions are not associated with the formation of discrete nodules. Lesions range in diameter from a few millimeters to several centimeters. Extensive zones of necrosis with exposure of underlying muscle and bone have also been described.[10] Regional lymphadenomegaly may be detected. Other less frequent physical examination findings in cats are fever, nasal discharge, decreased nasal airflow, tachypnea, increased respiratory effort, dehydration, and thin body condition.

In dogs, lesions consist of single or multiple ulcers or nodules on the head, trunk, forelimbs, and/or digits (see Figure 64-2). Rarely, they course along lymphatics.[12,13,16,24] The nasal planum was affected in 59% of 44 dogs in one study, and 21% of dogs had nasal mucosal involvement.[16] Regional lymphadenomegaly is common.

Diagnosis

Diagnosis of sporotrichosis rests on identification of the organism by cytologic or histopathologic evaluation, or by fungal culture of lesions (Table 64-2). A high degree of suspicion is required for the disease in non-endemic regions. Sporotrichosis should be considered in any dog or cat with cutaneous lesions suggestive of cryptococcosis or other deep mycoses, and especially any cat with ulcerative or nodular lesions of the face.

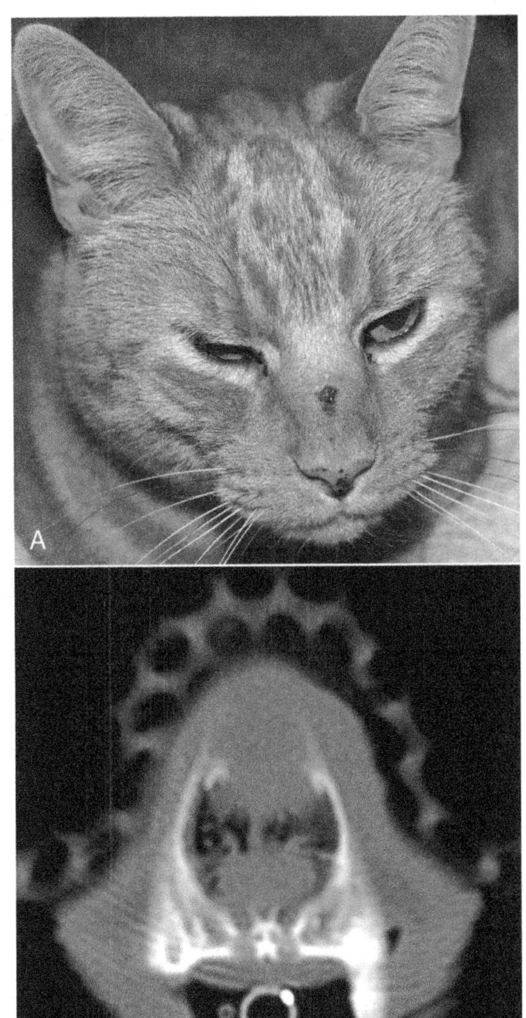

FIGURE 64-3 Nasal sporotrichosis with communication to the overlying skin in a 14-year-old male neutered domestic shorthair. **A,** The cat had a 1-year history of sneezing and a 2-month history of a mass on the bridge of the nose. **B,** Computed tomography revealed a nasal cavity mass with nasal bone destruction and involvement of the subcutaneous tissues.

Laboratory Abnormalities

Complete Blood Count

In many dogs and cats with sporotrichosis, the CBC is unremarkable. The most common abnormalities are mild anemia and leukocytosis due to a neutrophilia, sometimes with a mild left shift.[10,24] Monocytosis, eosinophilia, lymphocytosis, or lymphopenia may also be present. Approximately 50% of dogs in the Brazilian outbreak were anemic, and around 20% had eosinophilia or neutrophilia.[16]

Serum Biochemical Tests

The most frequent serum biochemistry findings in cats and dogs with sporotrichosis are hyperglobulinemia and hypoalbuminemia.[10,16] Rarely, increased liver enzyme activities are present in affected dogs.[16]

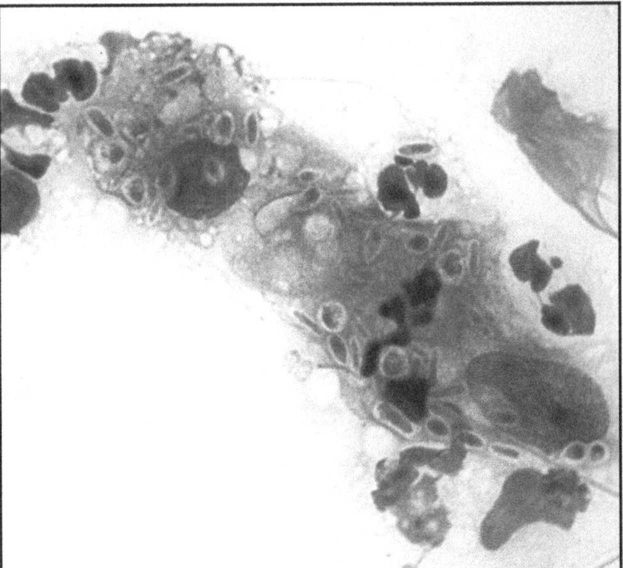

FIGURE 64-4 Cytology of an impression smear from a skin lesion of the cat in Figure 64-1, *A*. There are large numbers of extracellular and intracellular pleomorphic yeasts, with morphology consistent with *Sporothrix* spp.

Urinalysis

Urinalysis in animals with sporotrichosis usually reveals no clinically significant abnormalities.

Diagnostic Imaging

Plain Radiography

Findings on plain thoracic radiographs in cats with pulmonary sporotrichosis have not been described in detail. An interstitial infiltrate was described in one affected cat.[20] Thoracic radiographs were performed on one dog and five cats seen at the author's teaching hospital, but no radiographic abnormalities were present. Radiographs of bones that underlie skin lesions typically reveal only soft tissue swelling; rarely is underlying osteomyelitis detected.

Advanced Imaging

In the author's hospital, computed tomography (CT) of the nasal cavity in a cat with a lesion on the bridge of the nose revealed an irregular rim-enhancing mass within the nasal cavity that invaded through the nasal bones to involve the subcutaneous tissues (Figure 64-3). Severely thickened turbinate mucosa, an intranasal soft tissue density mass, and focal osteolysis were reported on nasal CT in a dog with signs of nasal cavity disease due to sporotrichosis.[25]

Microbiologic Tests

Cytologic Examination

Cytologic examination of impression smears or aspirates of skin lesions typically reveals pyogranulomatous inflammation. In cats, large numbers of round to cigar-shaped yeasts can be found intracellularly within neutrophils or macrophages and extracellularly (Figure 64-4). The yeasts are 4 to 6 μm in diameter and can exhibit a single bud with a narrow base. The sensitivity of cytologic examination of impression smears from skin lesions of 806 cats with sporotrichosis from Brazil was 79%.[26] Yeasts are usually not found in bronchoalveolar lavage fluid from cats with respiratory signs.[19] In general, dogs have very low numbers of

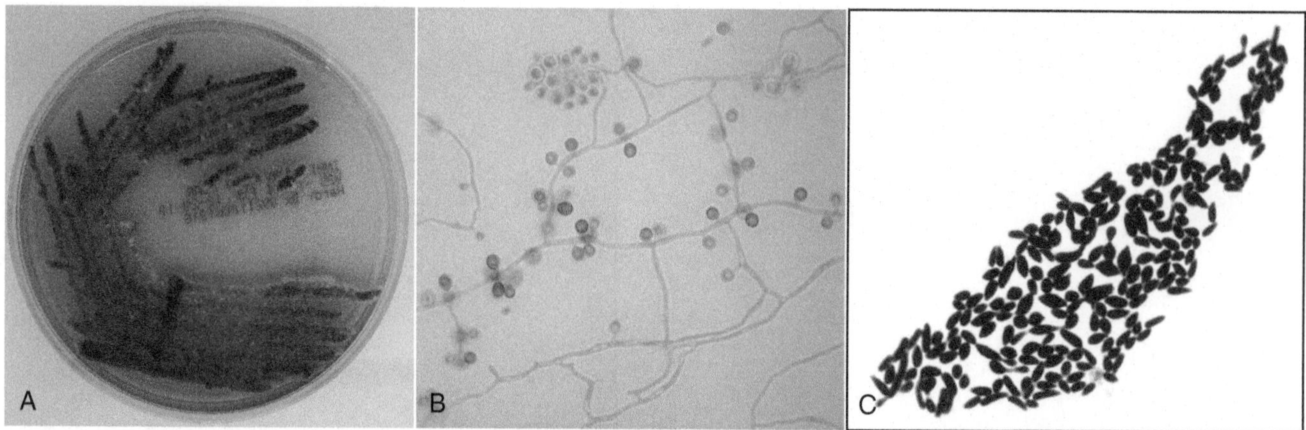

FIGURE 64-5 *Sporothrix schenckii* growing on laboratory media. **A,** The fungus grows on fungal isolation media as a white mold at 30°C with production of pigmented conidia. **B,** Using light microscopy, the mold form is characterized by the production of conidia in a flower-like arrangement. Lactophenol cotton blue stain, 1000× oil magnification. **C,** At 37°C, the organism converts to the yeast form. Gram stain, 1000× oil magnification.

organisms in skin lesions, which leads to a high proportion of false-negative results.[12,16] *Sporothrix* spp. may be confused with *Histoplasma capsulatum, Cryptococcus* spp., *Candida* spp., *Leishmania infantum,* and potentially other protozoan parasites such as *Toxoplasma gondii* and *Neospora caninum.*

Fungal Culture

Definitive diagnosis of sporotrichosis can be made by isolation and identification of the organism from clinical specimens (such as skin biopsies, blood, nasal swabs, or respiratory lavage specimens), preferably in both mycelial and yeast forms. The sensitivity of isolation from skin biopsies exceeds 75% in both dogs and cats.[10,13,16] The chance of successful culture is reduced if swab specimens of exudate instead of biopsies are submitted. The organism grows in culture as a white mold, which becomes brown to black as a result of production of pigmented conidia, which are arranged in florets on a stem (conidiophore) (Figure 64-5). Although growth can occur in 5 to 7 days, sometimes several weeks of incubation may be required.[9] When the organism is incubated on rich media such as brain-heart infusion at 37°C, it converts to oval to cigar-shaped yeasts. The organism can then be identified based on light microscopic appearance of the mold and yeast forms (see Figure 64-5, *B* and *C*). Determination of the *Sporothrix* species present requires subsequent molecular analysis by specialized laboratories.[27] Antifungal susceptibility testing can be performed, but established breakpoints are not available. Nevertheless, it may be of help for treatment of refractory cases (see Case Example).

Serologic Diagnosis

ELISA assays that detect antibody to *Sporothrix* cell wall antigens have been developed for diagnosis of human and feline sporotrichosis.[28,29] These assays are not widely available for diagnosis of sporotrichosis in cats or dogs. Currently, no antigen assays are available, but cross-reactivity with the *H. capsulatum* antigen assay occurs in human patients.[30]

Molecular Diagnosis Using the Polymerase Chain Reaction

PCR assays have been described for detection of *Sporothrix* spp. in lesions.[31,32] These have not been widely applied to the diagnosis of sporotrichosis in cats or dogs.

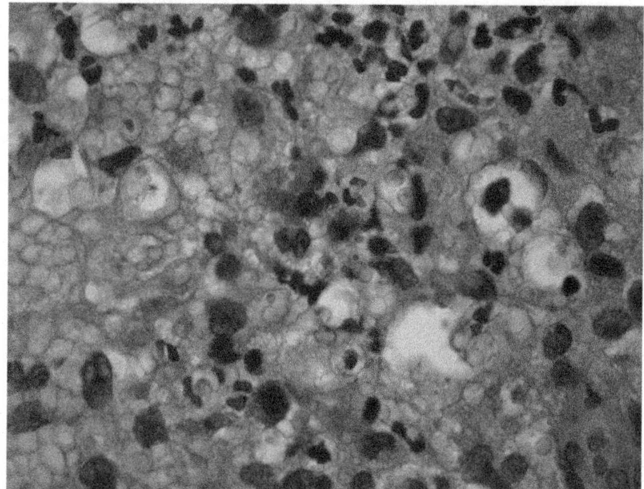

FIGURE 64-6 Histopathology of a biopsy from the skin of an 11-year-old female spayed domestic shorthair cat. Granulomatous inflammation is present with abundant intracytoplasmic fungal organisms consistent with *Sporothrix* spp.

Pathologic Findings

Gross pathologic findings at necropsy in cats with generalized sporotrichosis include multifocal, pinpoint (1 mm) white nodular lesions within the lungs and lymphadenomegaly.[20] Histopathology of lesions from cats usually reveals pyogranulomatous inflammation with a variable number of neutrophils, histiocytes, multinucleated giant cells, and lymphocytes, with fewer plasma cells, eosinophils, and mast cells (Figure 64-6).[12,13] Organized granuloma formation, with focal accumulations of macrophages and sometimes an outer layer of plasma cells, is found in a minority (<15%) of skin biopsies from affected cats[10] and in more than 30% of skin biopsies from affected dogs.[16,33] Intracellular and extracellular yeasts are seen on histopathology in more than 60% of skin biopsies from affected cats.[10,13] In contrast, organisms were found in biopsy specimens from fewer than 20% of dogs with sporotrichosis.[16,33] The presence of the Splendore-Hoeppli phenomenon ("asteroid bodies") around yeasts is commonly described in human infections, but this is not typically observed in dogs or cats.[9] Application of stains such as periodic acid–Schiff (PAS) and especially Gomori's methenamine silver (GMS) increase the chance that organisms are detected.[12,34] However, despite the use of such stains, diagnosis of canine sporotrichosis can be frustrating because of the scarcity of organisms in tissues. The use of immunohistochemistry (IHC) to aid histologic diagnosis has been reported, although this is not readily available.[34] In one study, the sensitivity of PAS, GMS, and IHC for detection of *Sporothrix* spp. in dogs with sporotrichosis was 20%, 44%, and 66%, respectively.[34] The use of the stains in combination increased the sensitivity to over 80%.

Treatment and Prognosis

Antimicrobial Treatment

The treatment of choice for sporotrichosis in dogs, cats, and humans is itraconazole (see Chapter 9 for recommended doses). In human patients, use of itraconazole results in cure rates for cutaneous sporotrichosis that exceed 90%.[35] Itraconazole resistance has been documented in some *Sporothrix* isolates from animals.[8] Fluconazole is considered less active than itraconazole for treatment of human sporotrichosis but was used successfully to treat disseminated disease in a cat.[12] Treatment of human, canine, and feline sporotrichosis with ketoconazole is more likely to result in relapses, and development of drug toxicity may limit therapy.[10,12,22] In affected cats from Brazil, clinical cure was 1.3 times more likely in cats treated with itraconazole than in cats treated with ketoconazole.[11]

Alternative antifungal drugs for animals with refractory disease include supersaturated potassium or sodium iodide, terbinafine, or amphotericin B. Oral administration of supersaturated potassium iodide (SSKI) for 30 days beyond complete resolution of clinical signs was used to treat sporotrichosis in cats, dogs, or humans before the widespread availability of itraconazole. However, treatment failures and toxic side effects that include anorexia, vomiting, diarrhea, and lethargy are common (41% of cats in one recent report).[10,22,36,37] It has been recommended that the use of SSKI be reserved for fixed cutaneous, lymphocutaneous, or mucosal forms of the disease in human patients. Because of its extremely bitter taste, potassium iodide (KI) capsules have also been used to treat affected cats, with a cure rate of 48% after 4 to 5 months.[23] Inappetence occurred in 52% of cats, and a smaller percentage of cats developed weight loss, diarrhea, or vomiting. Increased liver enzyme activities can also occur. The dose range used was 2.5 to 20 mg/kg PO q24h (median, 15 mg/kg). The dose was increased in 2.5 mg/kg increments every 5 days from an initial dose of 5 mg/kg PO q24h. Alterations in thyroid function can be an adverse effect of KI treatment in humans.[35] Treatment with terbinafine was successful in a human with nasal sporotrichosis that failed treatment with KI and itraconazole.[38]

Although amphotericin B is effective, nephrotoxicity and the need for parenteral administration have limited its use. The primary indication for amphotericin B is for treatment of sporotrichosis that is refractory to itraconazole. Intralesional amphotericin B administration in combination with itraconazole was used successfully to treat fixed or multifocal cutaneous lesions in cats that were refractory to itraconazole alone.[39] The solution was prepared by addition of 5 mL of 2% lidocaine and 5 mL of distilled water to a 50 mg vial of amphotericin B (final concentration, 5 mg/mL). A total of 0.5 to 1.5 mL (median 0.7 mL) was administered intralesionally once a week to once every other week, and 73% of the cats were cured. The number of treatments administered ranged from 1 to 5 (median, 2 treatments per cat). Sterile abscess formation at the site of administration occurred in 15% of cats.

Lastly, localized hyperthermia has been used as a safe and inexpensive method to treat fixed cutaneous and lymphocutaneous sporotrichosis in human patients and was used as the sole treatment in a cat with localized cutaneous disease.[40] In that case, a thermal bag that reached a temperature of 40°C to 42°C was applied twice daily for 15 minutes. When used alone, this method is not likely to be effective in animals with disseminated disease. Surgery or cryotherapy are other alternatives suggested for treatment of localized sporotrichosis in human patients.[35]

Prognosis

Treatment durations of 4 to 6 months are usually required for successful treatment of sporotrichosis. A median time to clinical cure of 26 weeks (range, 8 to 131 weeks) was reported for 175 cats treated with itraconazole.[11] Treatment should be continued for a month after lesions resolve. Some cats may require more than a year of antifungal drug treatment.[10] In general, the prognosis for cure of sporotrichosis is good, with more than 70% of cats in some studies cured of the disease, regardless of the number of skin lesions present.[10,12] Lower cure rates of 38% for itraconazole and 29% for ketoconazole were reported in another study.[11] Co-infection with FIV does not seem to alter the likelihood of treatment success,[10] but the presence of respiratory signs was associated with a twofold increase in death rate.[11] Relapse (or re-infection) may occur between 3 and 18 months after discontinuation of antifungal drug therapy. Spontaneous regression of a persistent cutaneous lesion was also described in a cat.[10] Euthanasia may result from expense related to antifungal drug therapy or concerns for zoonotic transmission.

Spontaneous regression of cutaneous lesions has been described in 15% of 33 dogs.[16] Nearly 80% of dogs were cured after itraconazole or ketoconazole treatment for 2 to 15 months (median, 2.5 months for itraconazole and 3.5 months for ketoconazole).

Immunity and Vaccination

Immunity imparted by T cells appears to be important in limiting the extent of sporotrichosis.[9,41] There is no vaccine.

Prevention

Indoor housing and neutering may reduce sporotrichosis in cats. Isolation of affected cats from other cats and dogs while they are properly treated may also reduce transmission.

Public Health Aspects

Many human sporotrichosis cases result from cutaneous inoculation of organisms in soil or on plant material. Activities associated with human sporotrichosis include rose gardening, topiary production, armadillo hunting, mining, carpentry, forestry work, Christmas tree farming, and hay baling, and outbreaks have been reported after common exposure of multiple individuals to a source of contaminated plant material. Laboratory-acquired infections have also been described.[42,43] Zoonotic transmission has followed bites or scratches from squirrels, horses, dogs, pigs, mules, insects, and especially cats.

In one study from Malaysia, slightly more human sporotrichosis cases resulted from cat bites or scratches than from exposure to plant foreign bodies.[44] Direct transmission can occur from infected cats to humans without an apparent break in the skin. In the epidemic in Rio de Janeiro, disease in cats preceded that in humans and dogs. Nearly 85% of affected humans reported contact with sick cats, and more than half of these individuals reported a history of a scratch or a bite. Women were more likely than men to be affected, especially those involved in domestic activities and animal care.[45] Five percent of the cases were veterinarians or veterinary technicians. Of cats with sporotrichosis from 225 residences in this outbreak, 91 people who had contact with infected cats acquired the infection.[10] In contrast, no human cases were associated with a series of 23 veterinary cases from northern California.[12] Generalized extracutaneous sporotrichosis with involvement of multiple organs has been described in immunocompromised humans, such as those with AIDS.[46,47]

In contrast to feline sporotrichosis, canine sporotrichosis is of minimal zoonotic importance. As occurs in humans, dogs have a paucity of organisms within tissues. There were no reports of transmission to humans as a result of contact with affected dogs in the Rio de Janeiro outbreak.[16]

Owners of dogs and cats with sporotrichosis should be told to minimize contact with affected animals. If contact is necessary, gloves should be worn and proper hand washing performed. Owners should also be informed of the potential for exposure to organisms in the environment.[6]

CASE EXAMPLE

Signalment: "Bingo," a 2-year-old male neutered domestic longhair cat from Fairfield in northern California

History: Bingo was referred to the University of California, Davis, Veterinary Medical Teaching Hospital for evaluation of refractory cryptococcosis. Initially Bingo's owners noted signs of snuffling, sneezing, and nasal discharge, which they attributed to a "cold." One month later a lump appeared on Bingo's nose. Bingo was taken to a local veterinary clinic where cytologic examination of an impression smear of the mass revealed organisms that were suspected to be *Cryptococcus* spp. A CBC showed no abnormalities. The owners declined treatment with itraconazole because of financial limitations, so fluconazole was prescribed (10 mg/kg PO q12h). Despite this treatment, the respiratory signs persisted, nodular skin lesions appeared on the face, and mandibular lymphadenopathy developed. Bingo had been an indoor-outdoor cat but had been housed exclusively indoors for the previous few months. He lived with five other indoor cats and a dog, all of which were well. His appetite and activity level had been normal and he was fed a commercial dry cat food. According to the owners, Bingo had tested negative for FeLV and FIV approximately 1 year previously.

Physical Examination:

Body Weight: 5.7 kg.

General: Bright, alert, responsive, and hydrated. T = 102.2°F (39.0°C), HR = 140 beats/min, RR = 40 breaths/min, CRT 1 s.

Integument, Ears, Eyes, Nose, and Throat: Ulcerated, firm cutaneous nodules (1 cm) were present on the left pinna and first digit of the left thoracic limb (0.25 cm). An ulceration (0.5 cm) was present on the bridge of the nose, which was markedly swollen (Figure 64-7, *A*). There was decreased nasal airflow bilaterally that was more severe on the left side, and mild left-sided mucoid nasal discharge. Marked soft tissue swelling occluded the left nares. There was moderate, left-sided serous ocular discharge. No lesions were detected on fundoscopic examination.

Musculoskeletal: Body condition score was 6/9, ambulatory.

Cardiovascular: No clinically significant abnormalities were detected.

Respiratory: There was a mild increase in respiratory effort with stertor. Thoracic auscultation revealed referred upper airway sounds.

Gastrointestinal and Genitourinary: Abdominal palpation was unremarkable. A small amount of dried feces and a tapeworm proglottid protruded from the anus.

Lymph Nodes: Only the left mandibular lymph node was enlarged (2 cm in diameter).

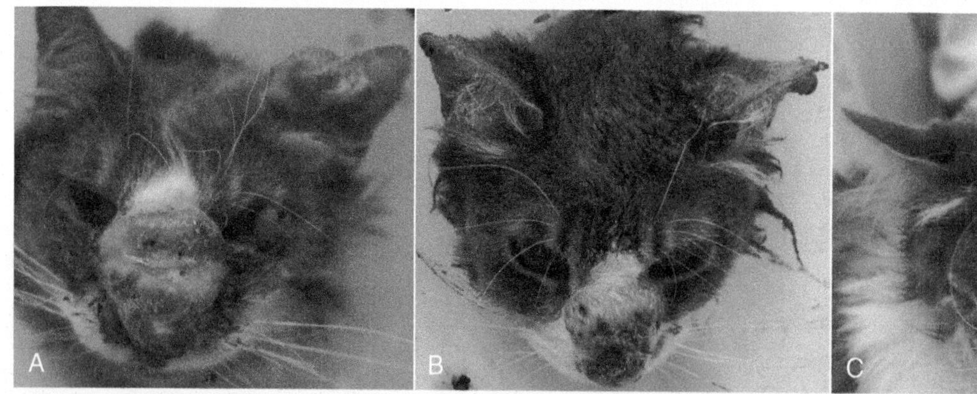

FIGURE 64-7 Effect of treatment with itraconazole and amphotericin B in a 2-year-old male neutered domestic longhair cat with multifocal cutaneous and mucosal sporotrichosis. **A,** Before institution of treatment. **B,** After itraconazole and eight treatments with amphotericin B. **C,** After an additional 7 months of itraconazole treatment.

Microbiologic Testing: Latex agglutination for *Cryptococcus* antigen: Negative.

Cytologic examination of impression smears from the nares: Erythrocytes, neutrophils, and occasional epithelial cells were present. No fungal elements were identified.

Histopathology of a biopsy from the nasal cavity: Pyogranulomatous inflammation with intralesional fungi with morphology consistent with *Sporothrix* spp.

Diagnosis: Sporotrichosis with nasal and multifocal cutaneous involvement.

Treatment: Bingo was treated with a compounded form of itraconazole (5 mg/kg PO q12h). Clinical improvement did not occur after 2 weeks, so terbinafine was added (30 mg/kg PO q24h). One month later, two nodules appeared on the conjunctiva of the left eye, and the lesions on the left pinna, left thoracic limb, and nasal bridge had enlarged. Mild subcutaneous emphysema of the face was also apparent during respiration. The cat was bright and appetent, but body weight had decreased to 5.1 kg. No abnormalities were detected on the CBC and serum biochemistry panel. Large numbers of *Sporothrix* yeasts were seen on impression smears of the thoracic limb lesion. Fungal culture yielded *S. schenckii* sensu stricto (identified at the University of Texas Health Science Center at San Antonio based on ITS, D1/D2, and calmodulin gene sequencing). Antifungal drug susceptibility testing revealed minimum inhibitory concentrations of 1, 2, 0.06, greater than 64, 1, 1, and 16 μg/mL for amphotericin B, 5-flucytosine, terbinafine, fluconazole, itraconazole, posaconazole, and voriconazole, respectively. A serum itraconazole concentration was less than 0.31 μg/mL. Subsequently the cat was hospitalized and treated with itraconazole (Sporanox) solution (3 mg/kg PO q12h) and deoxycholate amphotericin B (0.25 mg/kg IV). Terbinafine treatment was discontinued. Cutaneous lesions were also treated with local hyperthermia (15 minutes q8h). After eight amphotericin B treatments, the lesions had halved in size (Figure 64-7, *B*). An additional three treatments were administered, after which a mild increase in BUN concentration developed (43 mg/dL, reference range 18-33 mg/dL). Serum creatinine was within the reference range (1.4 mg/dL, reference range 1.1-2.2 mg/dL). The serum itraconazole concentration was 4.03 μg/mL. A new lesion appeared on the right distal thoracic limb, and impression smears of the lesion revealed large numbers of *Sporothrix* yeasts. The itraconazole dose was increased to 5 mg/kg PO q12h, but was reduced by the owner to 5 mg/kg PO q48h after 5 months because Bingo's appetite was slightly decreased. When the cat was reevaluated 7 months after completion of amphotericin treatment, lesions had improved dramatically (Figure 64-7, *C*). The owner was encouraged to increase the dose of itraconazole to 5 mg/kg PO q24h, but the cat was subsequently lost to follow-up.

Comments: This cat had nasal and multifocal cutaneous sporotrichosis that was somewhat refractory to treatment with antifungal drugs. The disease was initially mistaken for cryptococcosis. Limited client financial resources and compliance may have influenced treatment outcome in this case; costs of fungal culture, identification, and antifungal susceptibility testing were not charged to the client. Fluconazole was ineffective, and the antifungal susceptibility panel suggested resistance to this azole. The use of compounded itraconazole resulted in suboptimal serum drug concentrations. However, once treatment with amphotericin B, a brand name itraconazole formulation, and heat compression of lesions was instituted, gradual clinical improvement occurred. The change in itraconazole formulation alone might have been sufficient to cause disease resolution. The owners were told to wear gloves when handling the cat and to wash their hands afterward. No disease was reported in the owners or any other animals in the household.

SUGGESTED READINGS

Barros MB, de Almeida Paes R, Schubach AO. *Sporothrix schenckii* and sporotrichosis. Clin Microbiol Rev. 2011;24:633-654.

Crothers SL, White SD, Ihrke PJ, et al. Sporotrichosis: a retrospective evaluation of 23 cases seen in northern California (1987-2007). Vet Dermatol. 2009;20:249-259.

Vasquez-del-Mercado E, Arenas R, Padilla-Desgarenes C. Sporotrichosis. Clin Dermatol. 2012;30:437-443.

REFERENCES

1. Lopes-Bezerra LM, Schubach A, Costa RO. *Sporothrix schenckii* and sporotrichosis. An Acad Bras Cienc. 2006;78:293-308.
2. Brito MM, Conceicao-Silva F, Morgado FN, et al. Comparison of virulence of different *Sporothrix schenckii* clinical isolates using experimental murine model. Med Mycol. 2007;45:721-729.
3. Kong X, Xiao T, Lin J, et al. Relationships among genotypes, virulence and clinical forms of *Sporothrix schenckii* infection. Clin Microbiol Infect. 2006;12:1077-1081.
4. Zhang Z, Liu X, Lv X, et al. Variation in genotype and higher virulence of a strain of *Sporothrix schenckii* causing disseminated cutaneous sporotrichosis. Mycopathologia. 2011;172:439-446.
5. Romeo O, Scordino F, Criseo G. New insight into molecular phylogeny and epidemiology of *Sporothrix schenckii* species complex based on calmodulin-encoding gene analysis of Italian isolates. Mycopathologia. 2011;172:179-186.
6. Marimon R, Serena C, Gene J, et al. In vitro antifungal susceptibilities of five species of *Sporothrix*. Antimicrob Agents Chemother. 2008;52:732-734.
7. Oliveira MM, Almeida-Paes R, Muniz MM, et al. Phenotypic and molecular identification of *Sporothrix* isolates from an epidemic area of sporotrichosis in Brazil. Mycopathologia. 2011;172:257-267.
8. Oliveira DC, Lopes PG, Spader TB, et al. Antifungal susceptibilities of *Sporothrix albicans*, *S. brasiliensis*, and *S. luriei* of the *S. schenckii* complex identified in Brazil. J Clin Microbiol. 2011;49:3047-3049.
9. Barros MB, de Almeida Paes R, Schubach AO. *Sporothrix schenckii* and sporotrichosis. Clin Microbiol Rev. 2011;24:633-654.
10. Schubach TM, Schubach A, Okamoto T, et al. Evaluation of an epidemic of sporotrichosis in cats: 347 cases (1998-2001). J Am Vet Med Assoc. 2004;224:1623-1629.
11. Pereira SA, Passos SR, Silva JN, et al. Response to azolic antifungal agents for treating feline sporotrichosis. Vet Rec. 2010;166:290-294.

12. Crothers SL, White SD, Ihrke PJ, et al. Sporotrichosis: a retrospective evaluation of 23 cases seen in northern California (1987-2007). Vet Dermatol. 2009;20:249-259.
13. Madrid IM, Mattei AS, Fernandes CG, et al. Epidemiological findings and laboratory evaluation of sporotrichosis: a description of 103 cases in cats and dogs in southern Brazil. Mycopathologia. 2012;173:265-273.
14. Schubach TM, de Oliveira Schubach A, dos Reis RS, et al. *Sporothrix schenckii* isolated from domestic cats with and without sporotrichosis in Rio de Janeiro, Brazil. Mycopathologia. 2002;153:83-86.
15. Moriello KA, Franks P, Delany-Lewis D, et al. Cutaneous-lymphatic and nasal sporotrichosis in a dog. J Am Anim Hosp Assoc. 1987;24:621-626.
16. Schubach TM, Schubach A, Okamoto T, et al. Canine sporotrichosis in Rio de Janeiro, Brazil: clinical presentation, laboratory diagnosis and therapeutic response in 44 cases (1998-2003). Med Mycol. 2006;44:87-92.
17. Shany M. A mixed fungal infection in a dog: sporotrichosis and cryptococcosis. Can Vet J. 2000;41:799-800.
18. Teixeira PA, de Castro RA, Nascimento RC, et al. Cell surface expression of adhesins for fibronectin correlates with virulence in *Sporothrix schenckii*. Microbiology. 2009;155:3730-3738.
19. Leme LR, Schubach TM, Santos IB, et al. Mycological evaluation of bronchoalveolar lavage in cats with respiratory signs from Rio de Janeiro, Brazil. Mycoses. 2007;50:210-214.
20. Schubach TM, Schubach Ade O, Cuzzi-Maya T, et al. Pathology of sporotrichosis in 10 cats in Rio de Janeiro. Vet Rec. 2003;152:172-175.
21. Schubach TM, Schubach A, Okamoto T, et al. Haematogenous spread of *Sporothrix schenckii* in cats with naturally acquired sporotrichosis. J Small Anim Pract. 2003;44:395-398.
22. Goad DL, Goad ME. Osteoarticular sporotrichosis in a dog. J Am Vet Med Assoc. 1986;189:1326-1328.
23. Reis EG, Gremiao ID, Kitada AA, et al. Potassium iodide capsule treatment of feline sporotrichosis. J Feline Med Surg. 2012;14:399-404.
24. Sykes JE, Torres SM, Armstrong PJ, et al. Itraconazole for treatment of sporotrichosis in a dog residing on a Christmas tree farm. J Am Vet Med Assoc. 2001;218:1440-1443:1421.
25. Whittemore JC, Webb CB. Successful treatment of nasal sporotrichosis in a dog. Can Vet J. 2007;48:411-414.
26. Pereira SA, Menezes RC, Gremiao ID, et al. Sensitivity of cytopathological examination in the diagnosis of feline sporotrichosis. J Feline Med Surg. 2011;13:220-223.
27. de Oliveira MM, Sampaio P, Almeida-Paes R, et al. Rapid identification of *Sporothrix* species by T3B fingerprinting. J Clin Microbiol. 2012;50:2159-2162.
28. Fernandes GF, Lopes-Bezerra LM, Bernardes-Engemann AR, et al. Serodiagnosis of sporotrichosis infection in cats by enzyme-linked immunosorbent assay using a specific antigen, SsCBF, and crude exoantigens. Vet Microbiol. 2011;147:445-449.
29. Bernardes-Engemann AR, Costa RC, Miguens BR, et al. Development of an enzyme-linked immunosorbent assay for the serodiagnosis of several clinical forms of sporotrichosis. Med Mycol. 2005;43:487-493.
30. Assi M, Lakkis IE, Wheat LJ. Cross-reactivity in the *Histoplasma* antigen enzyme immunoassay caused by sporotrichosis. Clin Vaccine Immunol. 2011;18:1781-1782.
31. Hu S, Chung WH, Hung SI, et al. Detection of *Sporothrix schenckii* in clinical samples by a nested PCR assay. J Clin Microbiol. 2003;41:1414-1418.
32. Kano R, Watanabe K, Murakami M, et al. Molecular diagnosis of feline sporotrichosis. Vet Rec. 2005;156:484-485.
33. de Miranda LH, Quintella LP, dos Santos IB, et al. Histopathology of canine sporotrichosis: a morphological study of 86 cases from Rio de Janeiro (2001-2007). Mycopathologia. 2009;168:79-87.
34. Miranda LH, Quintella LP, Menezes RC, et al. Evaluation of immunohistochemistry for the diagnosis of sporotrichosis in dogs. Vet J. 2011;190:408-411.
35. Vasquez-del-Mercado E, Arenas R, Padilla-Desgarenes C. Sporotrichosis. Clin Dermatol. 2012;30:437-443.
36. Burke MJ, Grauer GF, Macy DW. Successful treatment of cutaneolymphatic sporotrichosis in a cat with ketoconazole and sodium iodide. J Am Anim Hosp Assoc. 1983;19:542-547.
37. Anderson NV, Ivoghli D, Moore WS, et al. Cutaneous sporotrichosis in a cat: a case report. J Am Anim Hosp Assoc. 1973;9:526-529.
38. Heidrich D, Stopiglia CD, Senter L, et al. Successful treatment of terbinafine in a case of sporotrichosis. An Bras Dermatol. 2011;86:S182-S185.
39. Gremião I, Schubach T, Pereira S, et al. Treatment of refractory feline sporotrichosis with a combination of intralesional amphotericin B and oral itraconazole. Aust Vet J. 2011;89:346-351.
40. Honse CO, Rodrigues AM, Gremiao ID, et al. Use of local hyperthermia to treat sporotrichosis in a cat. Vet Rec. 2010;166:208-209.
41. Carlos IZ, Sassa MF, da Graca Sgarbi DB, et al. Current research on the immune response to experimental sporotrichosis. Mycopathologia. 2009;168:1-10.
42. Cooper CR, Dixon DM, Salkin IF. Laboratory-acquired sporotrichosis. J Med Vet Mycol. 1992;30:169-171.
43. Thompson DW, Kaplan W. Laboratory-acquired sporotrichosis. Sabouraudia. 1977;15:167-170.
44. Tang MM, Tang JJ, Gill P, et al. Cutaneous sporotrichosis: a six-year review of 19 cases in a tertiary referral center in Malaysia. Int J Dermatol. 2012;51:702-708.
45. Barros MB, Schubach AO, Schubach TM, et al. An epidemic of sporotrichosis in Rio de Janeiro, Brazil: epidemiological aspects of a series of cases. Epidemiol Infect. 2008;136:1192-1196.
46. Freitas DF, de Siqueira Hoagland B, do Valle AC, et al. Sporotrichosis in HIV-infected patients: report of 21 cases of endemic sporotrichosis in Rio de Janeiro, Brazil. Med Mycol. 2012;50:170-178.
47. Hardman S, Stephenson I, Jenkins DR, et al. Disseminated *Sporothrix schenckii* in a patient with AIDS. J Infect. 2005;51:e73-e77.

CHAPTER 65

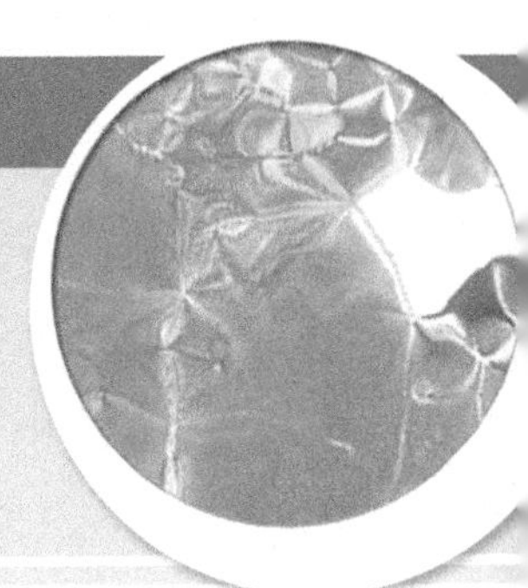

Aspergillosis

Jane E. Sykes

Overview of Aspergillosis

First Described: Invasive aspergillosis was first described in 1815 in a jackdaw bird (Mayer)[1]

Cause: *Aspergillus* spp. (an ascomycete, teleomorphs *Neosartorya, Emericella, Eurotium*)

Affected Hosts: Dogs, cats, humans, and a variety of other animal species

Geographic Distribution: Worldwide

Mode of Transmission: Inhalation of conidia from the environment

Major Clinical Signs: Sinonasal aspergillosis: nasal discharge, sneezing, epistaxis, depigmentation of the nares in dogs. Sino-orbital aspergillosis (especially cats): exophthalmos, mass lesions or ulcers in the pterygopalatine fossa. Disseminated aspergillosis: inappetence, weight loss, spinal pain, lameness, pelvic limb paresis or paralysis, cough, vomiting.

Differential Diagnoses: Sinonasal aspergillosis: neoplasia, inflammatory rhinitis, oronasal fistulas, cryptococcosis, nasal mites (dogs), foreign bodies, and polyps (cats). Disseminated aspergillosis: bacterial discospondylitis, bacterial pyelonephritis, and other systemic fungal infections, especially paecilomycosis and penicilliosis.

Human Health Significance: Human *Aspergillus* infections are acquired from the environment. Direct transmission from affected dogs and cats to humans does not occur.

Aspergillosis is the disease caused by pathogenic fungi that belong to the genus *Aspergillus*. *Aspergillus* species are ubiquitous, saprophytic, hyaline molds, the spores of which can be found in soil, water, air, and decaying vegetation. It is estimated that an individual person inhales several hundred *Aspergillus* spores each day.[2] *Aspergillus* species cause a variety of noninvasive, semi-invasive, and invasive forms of disease in dogs and cats that include keratomycosis, fungal otitis externa, sinonasal aspergillosis (SNA), sino-orbital aspergillosis (SOA), bronchopulmonary aspergillosis, and disseminated aspergillosis. *Aspergillus* species that can cause disease in dogs and cats are shown in Table 65-1.[3-14] Teleomorphs (sexual forms) of the fungus have been identified for some *Aspergillus* species. Currently, these are named differently and include fungi that belong to the genera *Neosartorya, Emericella,* and *Eurotium*. The name *Aspergillus* may be retained even when teleomorphs are isolated from lesions, to avoid confusion through the use of unfamiliar names.[12] Because accurate identification of *Aspergillus* species (especially rare species) requires advanced molecular techniques, organisms can be misidentified based on their morphology in culture alone. As a result, use of the term "species complex" is recommended when molecular techniques are not used for identification purposes.[15]

Because the etiology, epidemiology, clinical signs, diagnosis, and treatment of upper respiratory tract (URT) aspergillosis, systemic aspergillosis, and keratomycosis/otomycosis differ, they are considered separately in this chapter.

Upper Respiratory Tract Aspergillosis

Etiology and Epidemiology

In dogs, SNA is a subacute to chronic, noninvasive disease of the nasal cavity and sinuses. It is most often caused by *Aspergillus fumigatus*. Rarely, infection by other species, such as *Aspergillus niger* complex organisms (such as *Aspergillus tubingensis*) or *Aspergillus flavus* and the closely related fungus *Penicillium*, occurs. SNA occurs worldwide. Any breed of dog can be affected, but disease is most common in large, nonbrachycephalic breeds, especially German shepherd dogs, Rottweilers, Border collies, Rhodesian ridgebacks, and retrievers. Dogs of any age can be affected (median age around 6 years).[16] No clear sex predisposition exists. SNA is thought to occur when local immune mechanisms fail as a result of uncharacterized genetic or acquired immunodeficiency syndromes, and occasionally as a result of implantation of a foreign body or other preexisting nasal disease, such as nasal neoplasia. Rarely, it occurs in conjunction with other systemic diseases such as hyperadrenocorticism, diabetes mellitus, or systemic autoimmune disorders. However, in most cases, affected dogs are otherwise systemically well and have no evidence of immune compromise. Impaired cell-mediated immune responses have been detected in dogs with SNA, but it is unclear whether this is a cause or consequence of *Aspergillus* infection.[17]

Upper respiratory tract aspergillosis is relatively uncommon in cats, and includes SNA and SOA. Approximately 50 cases of URT aspergillosis have been reported in cats to date.[3] Fungi that belong to the *A. fumigatus* complex and, rarely, other *Aspergillus* species may also be involved (see Table 65-1). A novel organism with a proposed name of *Aspergillus felis* sp. nov. appears to cause SOA in cats,[12] whereas SNA is caused predominantly by *A. fumigatus* sensu stricto.[3] Brachycephalic breeds such as Persians and Himalayan Persians appear to be predisposed to SNA and especially to SOA, but both conditions occur in any breed of cat. Affected cats range in age from 1 to 13 years (median, 5 years). No clear sex predisposition exists.[3] Most cats with URT aspergillosis test negative for retrovirus infection; only one cat with SNA in the

TABLE 65-1

Aspergillus Species Associated with Disease in Dogs and Cats[3-14]

Clinical Form	Host Species	*Aspergillus* species*
Keratomycosis	Cats	*A. fumigatus* *A. flavus*
	Dogs	Not reported
Otomycosis	Cats	*A. fumigatus*
	Dogs (very rare)	*A. ochraceus* *A. versicolor* *A. niger*
Sinonasal aspergillosis	Dogs	*A. fumigatus* *A. niger* *A. nidulans* *A. flavus* *A. tubingensis*
	Cats	*A. fumigatus* *A. niger* *A. udagawae* *A. flavus* *Neosartorya* spp.
Sino-orbital aspergillosis	Cats	*A. felis* sp. nov.
Bronchopulmonary aspergillosis	Dogs and cats	*A. fumigatus* *A. flavus* (dog)
Disseminated aspergillosis	Dogs	*A. terreus* *A. deflectus* *A. fumigatus* *A. niger* *A. flavipes* *A. lentulus* *A. carneus* *A. versicolor* *A. alabamensis* *A. felis* sp. nov.
	Cats	*A. fumigatus*

*Some isolates have not been identified beyond the species complex level (including some *A. flavus*, *A. fumigatus*, and *A. niger*).

literature was co-infected with FeLV.[18] Five of 8 cats with SNA evaluated at the author's teaching hospital had diabetes mellitus.[4]

Clinical Features

Signs and Their Pathogenesis

Aspergillus conidia (or spores), which are 2 to 3 μm in diameter, are inhaled and deposit in the nasal cavity and/or sinuses, where they adhere to epithelial cells. In the absence of adequate immune defenses, the conidia enlarge and germinate to form hyphae. SNA is a noninvasive disease, and the fungus does not extend beyond the mucosal epithelium.[19] Production of toxins by the fungus and a profound host inflammatory response is thought to explain the extensive turbinate and bony destruction that follows fungal colonization. Toxins produced by *A. fumigatus* include aflatoxin, hemolysin, fumagillin, and gliotoxin,[2] but the role that these toxins play in canine SNA has not been determined. Gliotoxin induces ciliostasis and apoptosis and can suppress the host immune response.[2] The fungus also produces proteases and phospholipases. Chemokines such as Il-8 and monocyte chemoattractant protein-1 (MCP-1/CCL2) are secreted by host inflammatory cells in response to the fungus, which may recruit neutrophils and macrophages to the site of infection.[20] Severe disease is associated with destruction of nasal bones, the cribriform plate, and/or the orbit.

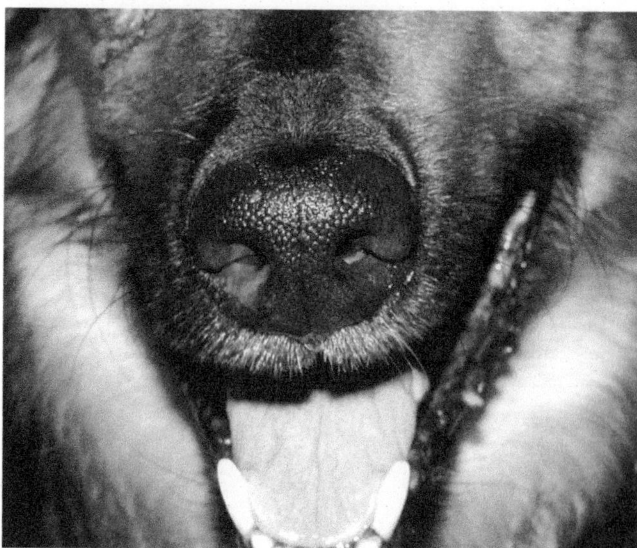

FIGURE 65-1 Unilateral depigmentation and ulceration of the nares of a 7-year-old shepherd mix with sinonasal aspergillosis. (Courtesy Dr. Lynelle Johnson, Small Animal Internal Medicine Service, University of California, Davis.)

Clinical signs of SNA in dogs and cats consist of sneezing, reverse sneezing, serous to mucopurulent nasal discharge, depigmentation of the nasal planum, and, less commonly, epistaxis. Nasal discharge is initially unilateral but can become bilateral as disease progresses. Animals with advanced disease can be lethargic and inappetent and may lose weight. Nasal pain can manifest in dogs as pawing at the face, hiding, or withdrawal when approached. Destruction of the nasolacrimal duct or invasion of the orbit can lead to epiphora. Osteolysis of the cribriform plate is often subclinical, but occasionally leads to meningitis with neurologic signs such as obtundation or seizures.

In cats with SOA, *Aspergillus* invades the submucosal tissue of the nasal cavity and sinus and extends through the orbital bone and into the retrobulbar space. A profound granulomatous inflammatory response to the fungus results in the formation of a retrobulbar mass, with clinical signs that include exophthalmos, protrusion of the third eyelid, mass lesions in or ulceration of the pterygopalatine fossa, and, rarely, blindness due to invasion of the optic nerve or optic chiasm.[3,21-23] Inappetence and dysphagia can also develop.[22] Occasionally, the clinical signs of SOA develop after initial signs of SNA, such as sneezing and nasal discharge.[3,21]

Physical Examination Findings

Physical examination findings in dogs with SNA include unilateral or bilateral serous or mucopurulent nasal discharge, epistaxis, pain on palpation of the face, mild mandibular lymphadenomegaly, and sometimes depigmentation and ulceration of the nares (Figure 65-1).[24,25] Nasal airflow is usually normal or increased because of turbinate lysis. Serous ocular discharge occurs uncommonly as a result of destruction of the bones of the orbit. Rarely, palpation of the nasal bones or the hard palate can reveal defects

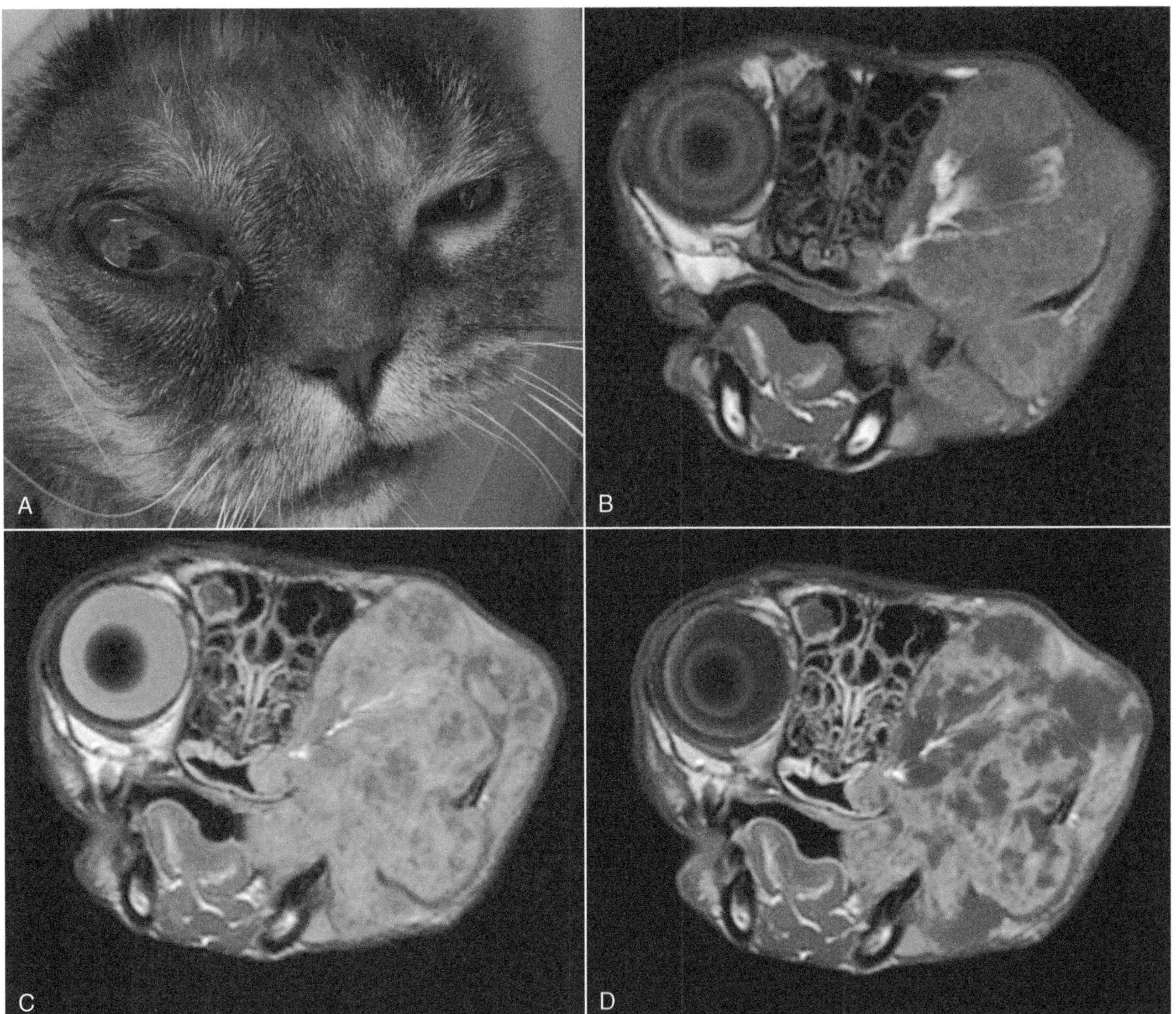

FIGURE 65-2 **A,** Seven-year-old male neutered Scottish fold cat with exophthalmos, conjunctivitis, and blindness of the right eye secondary to sino-orbital aspergillosis. A 1- to 2-cm mass was also identified in the pterygopalatine fossa on oral examination. **B-D,** MRI image of the head of the same cat. The right eye was displaced rostrally by a large retrobulbar mass that is mildly, heterogeneously hyperintense on T1-weighted images **(B)**, hyperintense on T2-weighted images **(C)**, and enhanced with contrast **(D)**. The mass extends medial to the ramus of the mandible and enters the nasopharynx as well as the oropharynx. A small T1-hyperintense structure is noted in the left frontal sinus.

in the underlying bone. Dogs with cribriform plate involvement and meningitis may be obtunded or dehydrated. Dogs with severe epistaxis can have evidence of melena on rectal examination secondary to swallowed blood. Most affected dogs are afebrile.

Physical examination findings in cats with SNA consist of serous or mucopurulent nasal discharge, sneezing, stertor, epistaxis, and, in some cases, facial distortion.[3] Cats with SOA usually have unilateral exophthalmos and deviation of the globe; bilateral involvement has also been described (Figure 65-2).[3,22,23] There may be resistance to ocular retropulsion and protrusion of the third eyelid. Miosis, an absent pupillary light response, and an absent menace response may be present. On examination of the oral cavity, most affected cats also have a mass or ulcer in the pterygopalatine fossa ipsilateral to the affected eye. Other less common findings are exposure keratitis and corneal ulceration, mandibular lymphadenomegaly, pain on opening the mouth, and/or ulceration of the hard palate.[3,22]

Diagnosis

Early diagnosis of URT aspergillosis relies on a high degree of suspicion for the disease and availability of client financial resources, because there is a lack of sensitive, noninvasive diagnostic tests for the disease. Definitive diagnosis requires a combination of imaging, visualization of fungal plaques by rhinoscopy/sinuscopy, and identification of fungal structures on cytology or histopathology. Imaging should be performed before rhinoscopy to avoid the influence of iatrogenic hemorrhage on the results.

Laboratory Abnormalities

Dogs with SNA often have no abnormalities on the CBC, serum chemistry profile, or urinalysis. Occasionally, mild nonregenerative anemia; mild neutrophilia, rarely with a left shift; mild eosinophilia; and/or mild hypoalbuminemia are present.[4] Cats

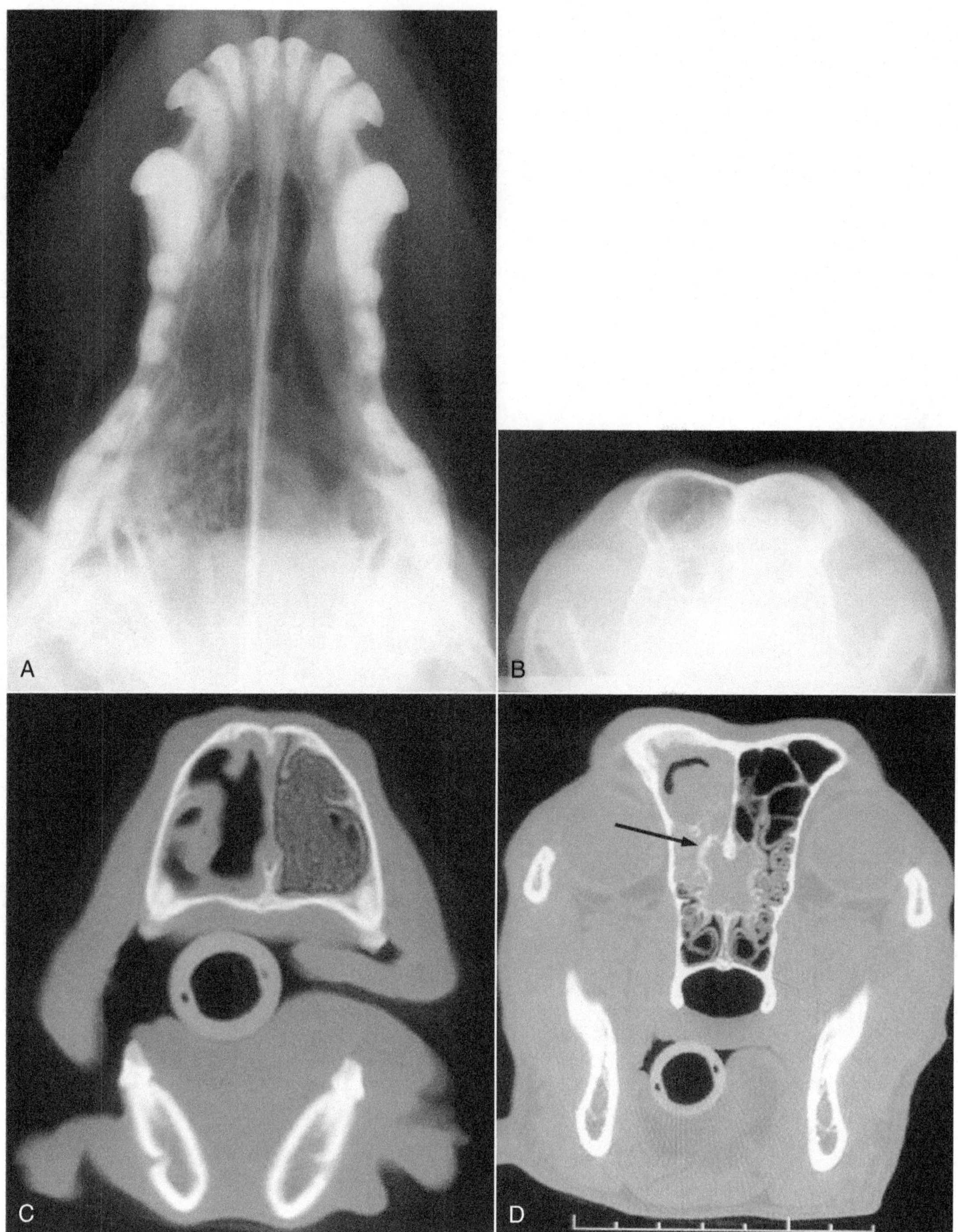

FIGURE 65-3 Plain radiographs (**A** and **B**) and CT scan images (**C** and **D**) of the nasal cavity of a 6-year old female spayed golden retriever with sinonasal aspergillosis. **A,** Open-mouth view. There is marked loss of detail in the left nasal cavity. **B,** Skyline projection of the frontal sinuses. There is increased opacity in the left frontal sinus. **C,** A transverse image through the nasal cavity shows marked turbinate loss on the left side. **D,** Transverse image through the frontal sinuses and region of the cribriform plate. There is moderate fluid accumulation and irregular soft tissue structures in the left frontal sinus, and the frontal bone that overlies the sinus is thickened and irregular. Bony destruction at the level of the cribriform plate is present (*arrow*).

with SOA may have a mild mature neutrophilia and sometimes mild to severe hyperglobulinemia.[3,21]

Diagnostic Imaging

Advanced Imaging

Whenever possible, computed tomography (CT) or MRI are preferred imaging modalities for the nasal cavity because of their increased sensitivity over plain radiography for evaluation of the nasal cavity, sinuses, and cribriform plate.[26] Bony changes are best appreciated on CT. Findings on CT or MRI in canine and feline SNA include loss of nasal turbinates and defects in the nasal septum; increased soft tissue opacity within the nasal cavity and/or sinuses due to mucosal inflammation, fluid accumulation, or fungal plaques; hyperostosis of the frontal bones; and mandibular or retropharyngeal lymph node enlargement.[3,26-29] Osteolysis of the cribriform plate, orbit, frontal bones, and, rarely, the maxillary or palatine bones may be present (Figure 65-3, C). Meningeal enhancement is sometimes evident on contrast

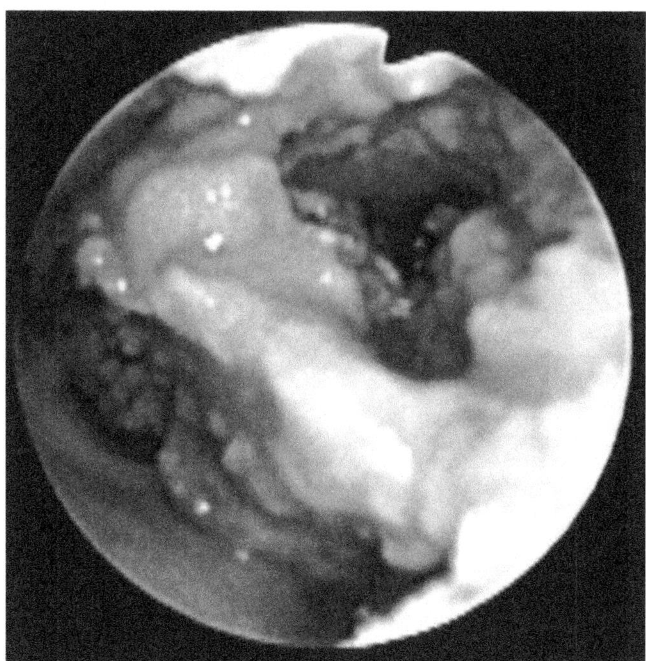

FIGURE 65-4 Rhinoscopic view of a large gray fungal plaque in the nasal cavity of an 8-year-old female pit bull terrier with sinonasal aspergillosis.

administration in dogs with cribriform plate destruction.[25] Fungal plaques and mucosal secretions fail to enhance with contrast and cannot be readily distinguished from each other. In some dogs, lesions are limited to the frontal sinus.[27]

Advanced imaging of the head in cats with SOA reveals a retrobulbar mass that enhances diffusely or heterogeneously with contrast. Displacement of the globe, osteolysis of the orbit, mandibular lymphadenomegaly, and changes consistent with SNA can also be present. With MRI, retrobulbar masses are T2-hyperintense. Invasion of temporal and masseter muscles by the mass may also be apparent on MRI (see Figure 65-2).[30]

Plain Radiography

Plain skull radiographs in dogs with SNA may show unilateral or bilateral loss of turbinate detail, destruction of the nasal septum, and/or increased soft tissue opacity within the nasal cavity. The open-mouth view provides optimum evaluation of the turbinates (see Figure 65-3, *A*). A "skyline" view of the nasal sinuses may show opacification of one or both sinuses and frontal bone hyperostosis (see Figure 65-3, *B*).[26]

Rhinoscopy and Sinuscopy

Visualization of fungal plaques by rhinoscopy and sinuscopy confirms a diagnosis of SNA. Plaques are white, gray, yellow, black, greenish, or a mixture of these colors and are adhered to the nasal mucosa or mucosa of the frontal sinus (Figure 65-4). Caudal rhinoscopy is performed with a flexible endoscope, after which a rigid telescope or flexible endoscope is used to examine the rostral portions of the nasal cavity. In some cases, extensive turbinate destruction allows a flexible endoscope to be passed directly into the frontal sinuses through the nasofrontal opening. If this is not possible, but CT or MRI findings suggest the possibility of frontal sinus lesions, trephination or surgical exploration of the frontal sinuses is necessary to visualize (and treat) this region. After trephination, a rigid endoscope can be used to examine the frontal sinus through the trephination site.

Microbiologic Tests

Cytologic Examination

Cytologic examination of blind or rhinoscopy-directed mucosal swabs, brush specimens of the nasal cavity, or nasal biopsies from dogs or cats with SNA can reveal *Aspergillus* hyphae and sometimes also conidia. Hyphae stain well with Wright's stains. They are septate and branch at 45-degree angles (see Figure 4-3). Large numbers of degenerate neutrophils, ciliated epithelial cells, and/or bacteria are also usually present. In one study, the sensitivity of cytologic examination was 93% when cytology brush specimens were examined and 100% when squash preparations of biopsies were examined, but it was 20% or less when nasal discharge or smears made from blind swab specimens were examined.[31]

Cytologic examination of ultrasound- or CT-guided aspirates of retrobulbar masses from cats with SOA reveals a mixed inflammatory response and sometimes fungal hyphae.

Fungal Culture

Aspergillus fumigatus can be readily grown on routine laboratory media. Colonies of mold generally appear within 96 hours, but occasionally longer incubation times are required.[32] In the absence of supportive rhinoscopic, cytologic, or histopathologic findings, positive cultures from the nasal cavity (or other nonsterile sites) require cautious interpretation because *Aspergillus* may be found within the URT of healthy animals. Nevertheless, in two separate studies, no dogs with nonfungal nasal disorders had positive culture results for *Aspergillus*.[16,32] In one of these studies (which included 21 dogs with SNA and 37 dogs with nonfungal nasal disease), the sensitivity of fungal culture of nasal biopsies for diagnosis of canine SNA was 81%.[16] In the other study, fungal culture of biopsy specimens or plaque specimens collected by rhinoscopic guidance (≥75%) was more sensitive than culture of blindly collected nasal swab specimens (<20%).[32]

Growth of an *A. fumigatus* complex organism from guided aspirates or biopsy specimens collected from a retrobulbar mass in a cat strongly suggests a diagnosis of SOA. In one study, fungal culture of nasal biopsies or aspirates from cats with SOA and SNA had a sensitivity greater than 95%.[3]

Serologic Diagnosis

Both serum antibody and antigen assays have been evaluated for diagnosis of URT aspergillosis. Assays for detection of serum antibodies to *Aspergillus* include ELISA and gel immunodiffusion (ID) assays (see Figure 2-7). Assay types vary in their sensitivity and specificity for diagnosis of SNA, and clinical performance data for some assays used in commercial veterinary diagnostic laboratories may not be available. The sensitivity of one gel ID assay (Meridian Bioscience) for diagnosis of canine SNA was 57% to 77%,[16,25,33] and the specificity was at least 98%.[16,33] The sensitivity and specificity of another gel ID assay (Immuno-Mycologics, OK) was 31% and 97%, respectively.[34] The sensitivity and specificity of an ELISA that detects antibodies against a purified *Aspergillus* antigen extract was 88% and 97%, respectively.[33] Thus, negative results with these antibody assays do not rule out SNA, but positive results strongly suggest the disease is present. The sensitivity and specificity of serum antibody assays for diagnosis of feline URT aspergillosis has not been evaluated in a large number of cats, but both positive and negative assay results have been reported in affected cats.[3,28,35]

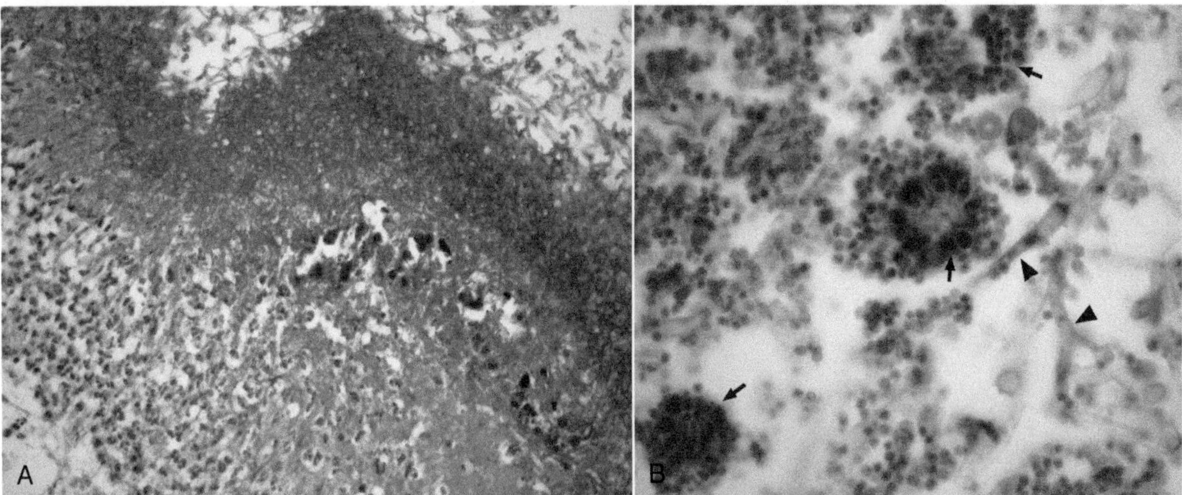

FIGURE 65-5 Histopathology of a nasal biopsy from a 4-year-old intact male Border collie with sinonasal aspergillosis. **A,** There is a profound neutrophilic inflammatory response beneath a thick mat of fungal hyphae, which stain magenta. Periodic acid–Schiff stain, 400× magnification. **B,** *Aspergillus* hyphae *(arrowheads),* conidiophores *(small arrows)* and conidia (spores) can be seen on the surface of the lesion. H&E stain, 1000× oil magnification.

A serum *Aspergillus* galactomannan antigen ELISA assay (Platelia), originally developed for diagnosis of invasive aspergillosis in humans, has been studied for the diagnosis of SNA and SOA in dogs and cats, but its sensitivity and specificity have been low.[5,33,36,37] Only 4 of 17 dogs with SNA were positive in one study, and only weak positive results were obtained (galactomannan indices 0.5-0.8, reference range <0.5).[33] False positive results occurred in 11 of 62 dogs without SNA (galactomannan indices of 0.5-1.5). Only 3 of 13 cats with URT aspergillosis tested positive, and false-positive results were obtained in a number of cats without URT aspergillosis (specificity 78%).[38]

Molecular Detection Using the Polymerase Chain Reaction

The use of real-time PCR assays that detect *Aspergillus* DNA in nasal biopsy specimens has been evaluated for diagnosis of SNA in dogs, but assays evaluated had either unacceptably high rates of false-positive test results (PenAsp assay) or a low sensitivity (*Aspergillus* genus-specific PCR).[34] For both assays, dogs with SNA had higher DNA copy numbers than control dogs or dogs with lymphoplasmacytic rhinitis or neoplasia, but there was considerable overlap in copy numbers between dogs with SNA and those without SNA.

Pathologic Findings

Histopathology of nasal biopsies from dogs with SNA usually reveals branching, septate fungal hyphae in a background of lymphoplasmacytic and neutrophilic inflammation; occasionally the neutrophilic component predominates. Variable numbers of macrophages and eosinophils may also be present, as well as necrotic debris. Other findings include osteolysis, turbinate remodeling, and intralesional bacteria. Occasionally, intralesional plant material is detected. Mats of fungal hyphae may be present if a plaque is submitted for examination. Conidiophores and conidia can be found because the fungus is exposed to air within the nasal cavity (Figure 65-5). The sensitivity of rhinoscopically guided nasal biopsy for diagnosis of canine SNA in one study was 82% (18 of 22 dogs).[25] In that study, three to five biopsy specimens were collected from each side of the nasal cavity.

Histopathology of biopsies of retrobulbar mass lesions in cats with SOA reveals granulomatous inflammation with necrosis and intralesional branching hyphae. A mixed inflammatory reaction (epithelioid macrophages, eosinophils, neutrophils, lymphocytes, and plasma cells) and a peripheral zone of fibrosis surround the granulomas. Inflammatory lesions may efface muscle and bone.

Treatment and Prognosis

Successful treatment of SNA is challenging. Because of the large size of the nasal cavity and sinuses, clinical signs are often not apparent until disease is advanced. Delays in diagnosis can occur because of the costly and invasive nature of diagnosis and treatment and the need for specialized imaging techniques and endoscopic expertise. Owners of adult dogs that develop persistent nasal discharge (e.g., present for at least 1 week) should be encouraged to pursue advanced imaging and rhinoscopy as soon as possible so that the disease can be recognized and treated early. Treatment with antibacterial drugs alone is discouraged, because primary bacterial infections of the nasal cavity in adult dogs are rare.

In general, treatment of SNA requires thorough mechanical debridement of plaques with endoscopic biopsy forceps until no visible fungus remains, which may necessitate extended anesthesia. In some cases, treatment is performed immediately after imaging and rhinoscopy, which further prolongs the period of anesthesia. If plaques within the frontal sinuses cannot be accessed by antegrade rhinoscopy through the nasofrontal opening, frontal sinus trephination and curettage or open surgical debridement of the frontal sinus may be required. Provided the cribriform plate is intact, debridement is followed by repeated lavage with 0.9% saline and suction, followed by topical antifungal drug therapy with clotrimazole or enilconazole. Additional systemic antifungal drug treatment could also be considered, but whether this improves outcome over topical therapy alone is unknown.

Topical Antifungal Drug Treatment

A variety of noninvasive and invasive protocols for topical antifungal drug treatment of canine SNA have been described with varied rates of success. Currently, there is a lack of masked, randomized clinical trials with consistent and long-term follow-up evaluation that indicate clear benefit of one treatment over another. The protocol described here is used at the author's institution. A similar protocol has been used successfully to treat SNA in cats.[38]

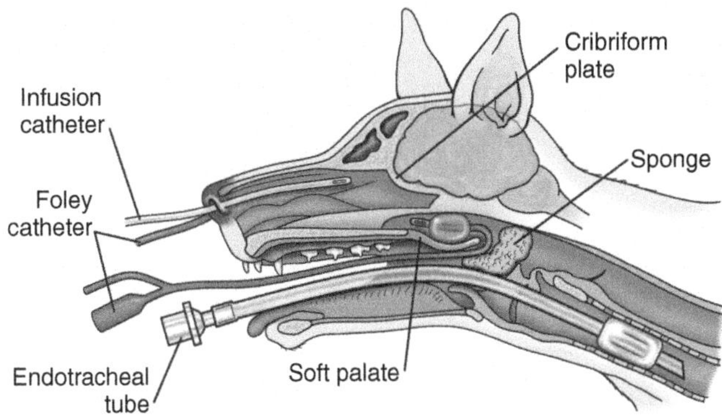

FIGURE 65-6 Diagram illustrating placement of catheters for topical treatment of canine sinonasal aspergillosis with clotrimazole or enilconazole.

A 24F Foley catheter is retroflexed over the soft palate and the balloon inflated until it can be palpated above the soft palate (Figure 65-6). Placement of the catheter is facilitated by insertion of a stiff guidewire into the catheter. The tip of the catheter can then be bent into a U shape and hooked over the soft palate, after which the balloon is inflated. The nasopharynx is packed with moistened laparotomy pads, a gauze pad is placed over the incisive papilla, and the proximal end of the catheter is clamped across the guidewire to prevent leakage of antifungal drug from the nasal cavity. A 10F polypropylene catheter is inserted into each nostril to the level of the medial canthus, or alternatively these two catheters can be placed directly into the frontal sinus with endoscopic guidance.[24,39] The tip of an additional 12F Foley catheter is inserted into each of the nares, the balloon inflated, and the catheters clamped so the nares are occluded. Cotton-tipped swabs can also be inserted into the nares to prevent outflow of antifungal drug. Clotrimazole (1%) or enilconazole (1% or 2%) solution is then administered through the polypropylene catheters. For large-breed dogs, 50 to 60 mL of solution is administered per side, and if frontal sinus trephination was performed, half of the solution can be administered into a catheter placed in the trephination site. The patient is rotated 45 degrees every 15 minutes over an hour to distribute the drug into the nasal cavity and sinuses. The catheters and sponges are then removed with the dog's head tilted downward at an angle of 30 degrees, and the material is allowed to drain from the nasal cavity for 10 minutes. Debridement and a second treatment are then routinely performed 1 month later; sometimes, a third treatment may be necessary. Clotrimazole can be irritating to tissues, and solutions that contain propylene glycol can cause pharyngeal irritation and edema.[40] Enilconazole solutions may be less irritating, but there is no evidence that they are more effective than clotrimazole.

When cribriform plate destruction is present, topical treatment can lead to the development of life-threatening neurologic signs or failure to recover from anesthesia. Nevertheless, treatment has also been performed without complication in some dogs with minor defects in the cribriform plate.[25] Systemic azole antifungal drug therapy could be considered as an alternative in this situation.

Use of topical antifungal creams has been studied in order to improve retention in the sinonasal cavities and reduce procedure time.[24,41] In one study, 1% clotrimazole solution (25 or 60 mL based on patient size) was administered through a catheter placed through a trephination site in each frontal sinus, followed by a 1% clotrimazole cream (10 or 20 g).[41] Debridement was not performed, so the mean treatment time was only 32 minutes. Of 14 dogs treated, 10 had resolution of clinical signs, but outcome was based only on telephone follow-up at 6 to 24 months, and not endoscopic reevaluation. In another study, 15 g of 1% bifonazole cream was administered into the frontal sinus using endoscopic guidance either alone or after topical treatment with enilconazole.[24] Dogs were also treated with ketoconazole or itraconazole. All 12 dogs treated with a combined enilconazole-bifonazole treatment were considered cured after a second treatment, but 2 of 5 dogs treated with bifonazole alone had persistent disease. Bifonazole has limited availability in the United States.

Systemic Antifungal Drug Treatment

Although their efficacy for treatment of SNA has been debated, azole antifungals with activity against molds (i.e., ketoconazole, itraconazole, posaconazole, or voriconazole) have been used either as monotherapy for dogs with cribriform plate involvement or in combination with topical antifungal drugs. Debridement before commencing systemic antifungal drug treatment is recommended if client finances permit, because effective drug concentrations are not likely to be obtained within fungal plaques.

Cats with SOA must be treated with systemic antifungal drugs such as an azole (itraconazole or posaconazole) and/or amphotericin B; the use of terbinafine in combination with these drugs has also been reported.[3] One cat was successfully treated with caspofungin followed by posaconazole monotherapy. More than 50% of treated cats failed treatment in one study.[3] The optimum treatment for SOA requires further study.

Prognosis

The prognosis for SNA depends on the extent of disease at the time of diagnosis. Success rates vary from less than 30% to 100%, but methods to assess treatment success and follow-up times have not been consistent. Serial serologic testing by gel ID is not useful to monitor treatment success.[25] Even if infection is eliminated based on endoscopic reevaluation and biopsy, dogs with extensive turbinate loss are predisposed to recurrent bacterial infections of the nasal cavity, which result in persistent nasal discharge and sneezing. One study showed no difference in the prevalence of sneezing and nasal discharge between dogs that responded to initial treatment and dogs that failed to respond.[25] Recurrence of SNA due to persistent infection or re-infection by *Aspergillus* spp. can also occur. The prognosis for complete remission of SOA in cats is guarded to poor.

Public Health Aspects

There are no reports of transmission of SNA from affected dogs to humans. Whether the handling of affected dogs by immunosuppressed humans poses a risk to their health is unknown, but such individuals should probably minimize contact with affected animals. If contact is necessary, they should be encouraged to discuss the problem with their medical practitioner. At the least, gloves should be worn and proper hand washing practiced.

Systemic Aspergillosis

Etiology and Epidemiology

Systemic aspergillosis may involve the respiratory tract (bronchopulmonary aspergillosis) or may be a disseminated disease of multiple organ systems. Localized bronchopulmonary aspergillosis is rare in dogs and cats, and often follows underlying local or systemic immunodeficiency.[6,42-44] German shepherds appear to be predisposed to a form of bronchopulmonary aspergillosis characterized by the development of cavitary lung lesions.[6,45-47] Bronchopulmonary aspergillosis is typically associated with infection by *A. fumigatus* complex fungi, whereas disseminated aspergillosis in dogs is most often caused by *Aspergillus terreus* or *Aspergillus deflectus*. Other *Aspergillus* species have also been isolated from dogs with disseminated disease (see Table 65-1).

In dogs, disseminated aspergillosis may occur as a result of an uncharacterized genetic immunodeficiency, because female German shepherds are strongly predisposed to the disease, and immunosuppressive drug treatment is rarely present in the history of affected dogs.[7] Two thirds of affected dogs seen at the author's institution were German shepherds, and German shepherds were 43-fold more likely to develop the disease than other dog breeds.[7] Rhodesian ridgebacks were also predisposed. Females are 3 times as likely to develop disseminated aspergillosis as males, and the median age of affected dogs is 4.5 years (range, 2 to 8 years). Concurrent or sequential infections with other opportunistic pathogens have been described in some dogs.[4,48]

Disseminated and bronchopulmonary aspergillosis are rare in cats.[42,49,50] Affected cats often have recognizable underlying immunosuppressive conditions such as diabetes mellitus, cancer chemotherapy, or severe viral infections. The remainder of this chapter focuses on systemic aspergillosis in dogs.

Clinical Features

Signs and Their Pathogenesis

Pulmonary or disseminated aspergillosis is thought to develop after inhalation of *Aspergillus* conidia, which lodge in the alveoli and adhere to epithelial cells. In the absence of adequate local immune defenses, the conidia enlarge and germinate to form hyphae. Invasion of the bloodstream and dissemination to distant sites may occur as a result of systemic immunosuppression. Fungal virulence factors are also likely to be important, although why *A. terreus* and *A. deflectus* are more likely than *A. fumigatus* to cause disseminated disease in dogs is unclear. Human disseminated aspergillosis is most often caused by *A. fumigatus*–complex fungi.[51]

Anatomic sites of predilection in dogs with disseminated aspergillosis are the vertebral endplates and discs, renal pelvis, spleen, long bones, and lymph nodes. However, any organ may be affected, including the liver, heart, cardiac valves, pancreas, eyes, lungs, brain, bone marrow, meninges, small intestine, skin, spinal cord, thyroid, adrenal glands, prostate, and trachea. Nasal cavity involvement is not generally a feature of the bronchopulmonary or disseminated forms, and dogs with disseminated disease often lack evidence of pulmonary involvement. The median duration of illness before admission in one study was 1 month (range, 2 days to 9 months).[7] The most frequent clinical signs are lethargy, inappetence, pain, lameness, and neurologic signs secondary to discospondylitis (especially ataxia and paresis) (Table 65-2). Other signs include apparent blindness, circling, head tilt, seizures, respiratory distress, and vomiting. Cough, increased respiratory effort, and rarely hemoptysis may occur in dogs with bronchopulmonary aspergillosis.[6,47]

Physical Examination Findings

Physical examination findings in dogs with disseminated aspergillosis are listed in Table 65-3. On physical examination, dogs with disseminated aspergillosis often have muscle wasting and/or a thin body condition. Fever (up to 104.2°F or 40.1°C) is present in one quarter of affected dogs.[7] Musculoskeletal abnormalities include spinal pain, lameness, and, rarely, inability to stand. Neurologic signs include vestibular abnormalities, ataxia, mental dullness, paraparesis, vision impairment, hemiparesis, circling, and seizures. Dogs with respiratory involvement may cough and have harsh lung sounds and/or increased respiratory effort. Peripheral lymphadenomegaly may be detected. Ocular abnormalities include chorioretinitis, hyphema, and panophthalmitis.[7] Rarely, arrhythmias are detected secondary to myocardial involvement, but myocardial involvement is often subclinical.

TABLE 65-2

Historical Signs in 30 Dogs with Disseminated Aspergillosis

Sign	Percent of Dogs
Inappetence or anorexia	20
Pain	27
Lameness	13
Neurologic signs (especially pelvic limb ataxia and paresis)	20
Respiratory signs (especially cough)	13
Vomiting	7

From Schultz RM, Johnson EG, Wisner ER, et al. Clinicopathologic and diagnostic imaging characteristics of systemic aspergillosis in 30 dogs. J Vet Intern Med. 2008;22:851-859.

TABLE 65-3

Physical Examination Findings in 30 Dogs with Disseminated Aspergillosis

Finding	Percent of Dogs
Muscle wasting/thin body condition	40
Fever	27
Spinal pain	17
Vestibular signs	17
Peripheral lymphadenomegaly	17
Ocular abnormalities	13
Lameness	13
Ataxia	10
Paraparesis	10
Cough, increased breath sounds	10
Mental dullness	7
Vision impairment	7
Hemiparesis	7
Circling, seizures, arrhythmia	3

From Schultz RM, Johnson EG, Wisner ER, et al. Clinicopathologic and diagnostic imaging characteristics of systemic aspergillosis in 30 dogs. J Vet Intern Med. 2008;22:851-859.

TABLE 65-4

Selected Hematologic and Serum Biochemistry Analysis Results in 30 Dogs with Disseminated Aspergillosis

Variable	Median (Range)	No. (%) with Low Values	No. (%) with High Values	Reference Range
Hematocrit (%)	42% (14%-46%)	8 (31%)	0	40%-55%
Neutrophils (cells/μL)	12,643 (7584-28,321)	0	21 (81%)	3000-10,500
Band neutrophils (cells/μL)	0 (0-3051)	0	10 (38%)	Rare
Monocytes (cells/μL)	1608 (499-3760)	0	16 (62%)	150-1200
Lymphocytes (cells/μL)	1566 (115-3998)	4 (15%)	0	1000-4000
Platelets (cells/μL)	262,000 (86,000-400,000)	1 (4%)	0	150,000-400,000
Albumin (g/dL)	2.7 (1.3-3.6)	6 (24%)	0	2.9-4.2
Globulin (g/dL)	4.4 (2.3-5.8)	0	12 (48%)	2.3-4.4
Creatinine (g/dL)	1.1 (0.5-7.8)	0	9 (36%)	0.5-1.6
BUN (mg/dL)	19 (8-196)	0	9 (36%)	8-31
Calcium (mg/dL)	10.8 (9.9-13.9)	0	8 (32%)	9.9-11.4
ALT (IU/L)	37 (19-609)	0	3 (12%)	19-67
ALP (IU/L)	78 (21-1920)	0	3 (12%)	15-127

Diagnosis

Laboratory Abnormalities

Complete Blood Count

Most dogs with disseminated aspergillosis have leukocytosis due to a neutrophilia (Table 65-4).[7] A left shift and toxic neutrophils may also be present. Normocytic, normochromic nonregenerative anemia occurs in approximately one third of affected dogs and may be secondary to inflammatory disease or renal failure.

Serum Biochemical Tests

Common abnormalities in the serum biochemical profiles of dogs with systemic aspergillosis include hyperglobulinemia, azotemia, hypercalcemia, and hypoalbuminemia (see Table 65-4).

Urinalysis

The urine specific gravity of azotemic dogs with disseminated aspergillosis is usually in the isosthenuric range because of renal failure. Hematuria, proteinuria, and pyuria may also be detected. Fungal hyphae were identified in the urine sediment of 2 (8%) of 25 dogs with disseminated aspergillosis in one study.[7]

Cerebrospinal Fluid Analysis

Analysis of the CSF in dogs with neurologic signs or spinal pain due to disseminated aspergillosis can show no abnormalities, or an increased nucleated cell count and CSF protein concentration. The differential cell count reveals mixed or primarily mononuclear or neutrophilic pleocytosis. Abnormalities of the CSF were identified in 8 of 10 dogs with disseminated aspergillosis at the author's teaching hospital.[4]

Diagnostic Imaging

Plain Radiography

Plain thoracic radiographs in dogs with bronchopulmonary aspergillosis may show a bronchial pattern or lung lobe consolidation.[44] Consolidation and cavitary lesions may be seen in the lungs of German shepherd dogs (Figure 65-7).[45-47] Abnormalities in dogs with disseminated aspergillosis include enlarged tracheobronchial and/or sternal lymph nodes, cranial mediastinal masses, pleural effusion, and/or pulmonary alveolar infiltrates.[7]

Spinal radiographs reveals evidence of discospondylitis in approximately half of dogs with disseminated aspergillosis, with a median of 2 sites affected (range, 1 to 9 sites).[7] Productive and destructive bony changes consistent with osteomyelitis may be present in other parts of the skeleton (Figure 65-8). Most dogs

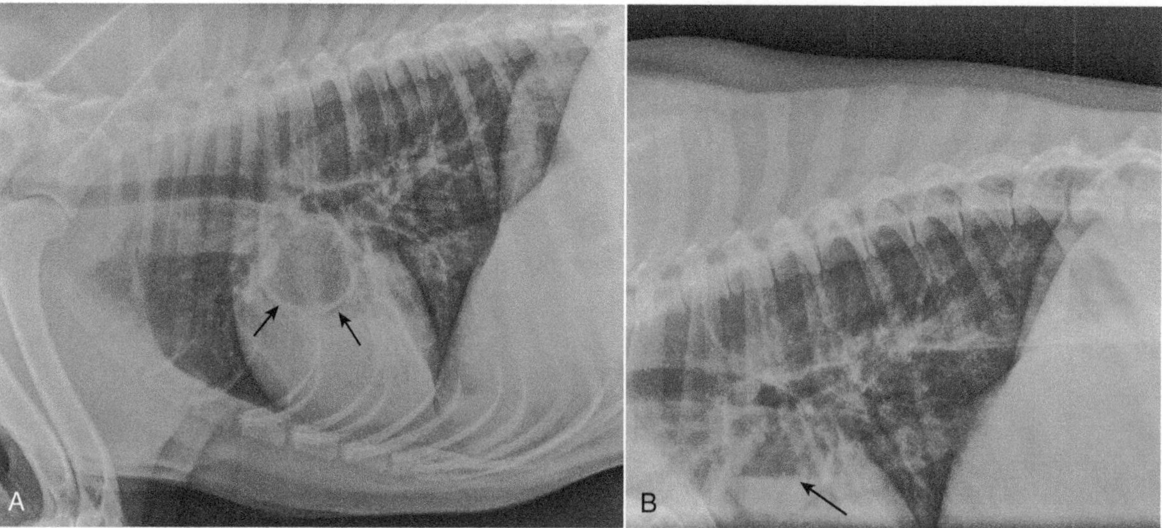

FIGURE 65-7 Lateral thoracic radiograph of a 2-year-old male neutered German shepherd that had a 4-month history of cough and exercise intolerance. **A,** A cavitary lesion *(arrows)* and alveolar infiltrates in the right middle lung lobe are present. **B,** On a horizontal beam projection, a fluid line is present *(arrow)* within the dependent aspect of the lesion.

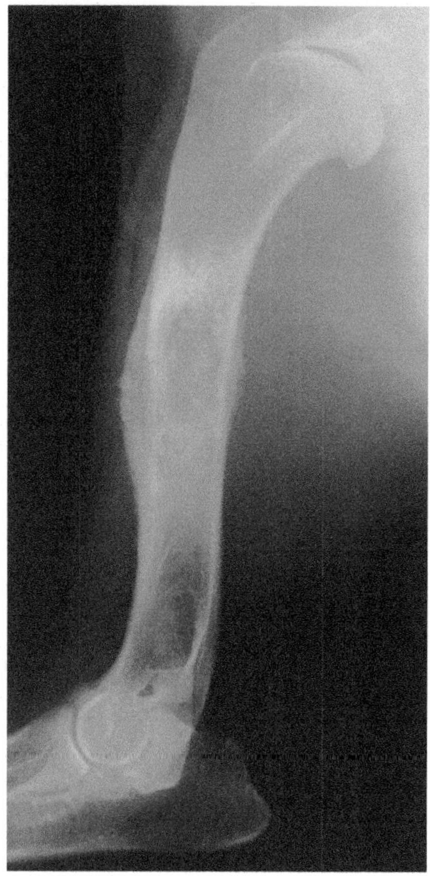

FIGURE 65-8 Lateral radiograph of the left humerus of a 2-year-old male neutered German shepherd with disseminated aspergillosis. A primarily osteoproductive lesion is present in the mid-diaphysis.

have multiple affected sites, which include the vertebral bodies, sternebrae, ribs, scapula, humerus, and tibia.[7]

Sonographic Findings

Abdominal ultrasound abnormalities in dogs with disseminated aspergillosis are most often in the kidneys, spleen, and

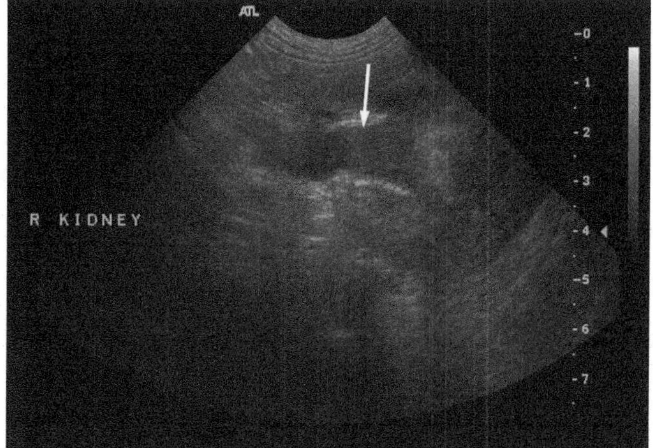

FIGURE 65-9 Ultrasound image of the right kidney of a 6-year-old female spayed German shepherd dog with disseminated aspergillosis. There is dilation of the renal pelvis, which contains echogenic material *(arrow)*.

abdominal lymph nodes.[7] Renal abnormalities include pyelectasia, a distorted and mottled architecture, decreased corticomedullary distinction, echogenic debris within the renal pelvis and proximal ureter, nodules or masses within the renal cortex, and papillary blunting (Figure 65-9). Occasionally, hydronephrosis is detected. Splenic abnormalities include hypoechoic nodules or masses, splenomegaly, changes consistent with infarction, or a mottled echotexture. Abdominal lymph nodes may be enlarged and/or hypoechoic. Other findings include diffuse hepatic or pancreatic hypoechogenicity, ascites, or evidence of venous thrombosis.

Advanced Imaging

MRI of the head in dogs with *Aspergillus* infections that have disseminated to the central nervous system (CNS) may reveal multifocal lesions that are hypo- to isointense and enhance with contrast on T1-weighted images. These lesions are hyperintense or heterogenous on T2-weighted and fluid attenuated inversion recovery (FLAIR) images. Mild or severe meningeal enhancement may also be present.

TABLE 65-5

Diagnostic Assays Available for Aspergillosis in Dogs or Cats

Assay	Specimen Type	Target	Performance
Cytologic examination	Aspirates of affected tissues, body fluids, impression smears of biopsies	Fungal hyphae (with or without conidia in tissues exposed to air)	False negatives can occur when specimen size is small or low numbers of fungi are present. Cytology of brush specimens optimizes sensitivity for dogs with SNA. Identification to species level requires culture and molecular testing.
Fungal culture	Aspirates or biopsies of affected tissues, body fluids	*Aspergillus* species	Sensitivity for diagnosis of canine SNA is at least 75% when endoscopically guided nasal biopsies are cultured. Specificity is >95%. Culture of a typical species (*A. terreus* or *A. deflectus*) from a dog with signs consistent with disseminated disease strongly suggests disseminated aspergillosis. Molecular testing by PCR may be required to identify beyond the species complex level.
Antibody serology (gel ID or ELISA)	Serum	Antibodies to *Aspergillus* species	Assays vary in sensitivity and specificity. In general, positive results support a diagnosis of canine SNA, but negative results do not rule out the disease. Insensitive for diagnosis of disseminated aspergillosis.
Galactomannan antigen assay (ELISA)	Urine, serum	*Aspergillus* spp. galactomannan cell wall antigen	Insensitive for diagnosis of SNA, SOA, and probably bronchopulmonary disease. Very sensitive for diagnosis of disseminated aspergillosis. Cross-reactivity with other fungal pathogens may occur (especially other molds). False positives also occur with Plasmalyte administration.
Real-time PCR assays	Whole blood	*Aspergillus* spp. DNA	Assays studied lack sensitivity or specificity for diagnosis of canine SNA. Usefulness for diagnosis of disseminated aspergillosis requires further study.
Histopathology	Biopsy specimens from affected tissues	Fungal hyphae (with or without conidia in tissues exposed to air)	Sensitivity for diagnosis of canine SNA in rhinoscopically guided biopsies was 82%. Hyphae are usually visualized in biopsies from animals with disseminated aspergillosis, but lesions may be difficult to access for biopsy. Special stains assist organism detection.

Microbiologic Tests

Diagnostic assays available for aspergillosis in dogs or cats are described in Table 65-5.

Cytologic Examination

Hyphae with morphology consistent with *Aspergillus* spp. may be present in aspirates of lymph nodes, kidney, lung tissue, or bone from dogs with systemic aspergillosis (see Figure 4-3).[7] Cytologic examination of pleural effusion, airway lavage specimens, or urine may also reveal hyphae. False-negative results occur when organism numbers are low or specimen size is small. Accurate identification of the organism present requires fungal culture.

Fungal Culture

Aspergillus spp. are readily isolated on routine laboratory media. Isolation of *Aspergillus* spp. (especially *A. terreus* or *A. deflectus*) from normally sterile sites such as urine, blood, or aspirates of lymph node, bone, intervertebral disc, liver, or splenic tissue supports a diagnosis of disseminated aspergillosis. Approximately 50% of dogs with disseminated aspergillosis have positive urine cultures for *Aspergillus* spp., and around one third of dogs have positive blood or CSF cultures.[7] Isolation of *A. fumigatus* from airway washes should be interpreted more cautiously as it may represent contamination. Concurrent cytologic evidence of fungal hyphae is required for definitive diagnosis in this situation.

Once growth of mold occurs in culture, *Aspergillus* species can be identified to the complex level based on conidiophore morphology (Figure 65-10). Accurate identification to the species level requires molecular techniques such as PCR, then sequencing, which are performed by laboratories with special expertise (e.g., the Fungus Testing Laboratory at the University of Texas Health Science Center at San Antonio). Such laboratories can also perform antifungal drug susceptibility testing. However, because clinical breakpoints have not been established for dogs or cats, the relevance of minimum inhibitory concentrations for molds remains unclear.

Serologic Diagnosis

An *Aspergillus* galactomannan antigen ELISA assay (Platelia) has high sensitivity for diagnosis of disseminated aspergillosis in dogs when serum or urine specimens are tested.[36] In the author's hospital, all of 12 dogs with disseminated aspergillosis had positive test results, with galactomannan indices (GMIs) that ranged from 6.4 to 12.2 (reference range, <0.5). Two dogs with localized pulmonary disease had serum GMIs of 0.14 and 0.77, which suggests that, as for SNA, the sensitivity of this assay for diagnosis of bronchopulmonary aspergillosis may be low. High-level

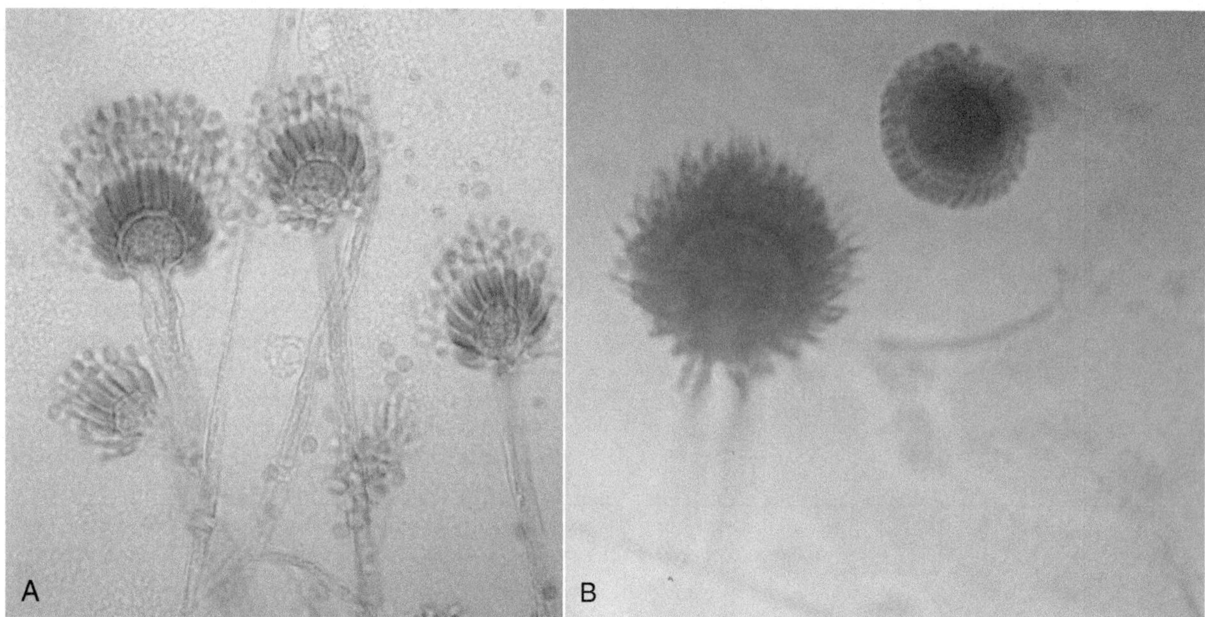

FIGURE 65-10 **A,** Morphology of *Aspergillus fumigatus*. **B,** Morphology of *Aspergillus terreus*, which has an "upswept" appearance. The conidiophore is the specialized hyphal branch that bears the conidia (spores). The vesicle is the dilated top part of the conidiophore. Phialides are flask-shaped projections from the vesicle from which the conidia arise.

false positive test results (GMIs >1.5) appear to only occur in dogs with other fungal infections, especially those caused by *Penicillium* or *Paecilomyces*, and dogs treated with Plasmalyte intravenous fluid therapy. Plasmalyte contains sodium gluconate, which is produced by fermentation by *Aspergillus niger*; carry-over of small amounts of galactomannan during production of the fermentation product is thought to occur.[52] Low-level false positives (0.5-1.5) can occur in dogs infected with other fungi (such as *Cryptococcus* spp.), some dogs with nonfungal disease such as neoplasia, or some dogs treated with penicillin derivatives. In summary, a strong positive assay result in a dog with clinical abnormalities consistent with disseminated aspergillosis and no history of Plasmalyte administration within the last 72 hours supports a diagnosis of a mold infection, but fungal culture is required to confirm that *Aspergillus* is the causative agent. A negative result in a dog with disseminated disease suggests that *Aspergillus* is not the cause, but it does not rule out the possibility of infection with another mold species.

Assays that detect antibodies to *Aspergillus* species are insensitive for diagnosis of systemic aspergillosis.[7] This may reflect underlying host immunodeficiency (and hence inability to produce antibodies), or antibodies in affected dogs may not cross-react with the antigens used in the test kits. For example, one widely used gel ID assay (Meridian Bioscience) contains a purified carbohydrate preparation from mycelial phase cultures of *A. fumigatus, A. niger,* and *A. flavus,* but not *A. terreus* or *A. deflectus.*

Molecular Diagnosis Using the Polymerase Chain Reaction

Several real-time PCR assays have been developed and applied for the diagnosis of invasive aspergillosis in humans.[53,54] The sensitivity and specificity of these assays has varied.[54] To date, they have not been widely applied to diagnosis of disseminated aspergillosis in dogs.

Pathologic Findings

Gross pathologic findings in dogs with disseminated aspergillosis include enlarged and/or congested lymph nodes; multifocal, pale, tan to white masses or nodules within a variety of parenchymal organs or the pleura (Figure 65-11, *A*); evidence of discospondylitis and/or osteomyelitis; serosanguineous pleural effusion; and/or mottled and congested lung lobes. Splenic infarction is also a common finding. The renal pelvis may be dilated and contain soft, granular material. Histopathology reveals granulomatous or pyogranulomatous inflammation with abundant intralesional fungal hyphae in a variety of tissues. Some species, such as *A. terreus,* also produce accessory conidia (aleuriospores) in tissues, which may be free or extend from hyphae. Fibrinoid necrosis of blood vessels and associated hemorrhage may be present. Special stains such as Gomori's methenamine silver or periodic acid–Schiff can delineate fungal hyphae in tissues (Figure 65-11, *B*). Immunohistochemistry has also been used to identify *Aspergillus.*[55,56]

Treatment and Prognosis

Many dogs with disseminated aspergillosis have advanced disease at the time of evaluation, sometimes with respiratory distress, pathologic fractures, and vertebral subluxations and cord compression. The prognosis for these dogs is poor. In one study, 57% of 30 dogs were euthanized within a week of examination (median, 3 days).[7] However, dogs that lack severe CNS signs, pain, or respiratory distress may enter remission for months and occasionally years when treated with antifungal drugs. These dogs maintain high antigen titers or persistently positive urine cultures, and they ultimately relapse and die from the disease. Sometimes, euthanasia is performed earlier because continued treatment is unaffordable.

The relative efficacy of different antifungal drug treatment regimens for disseminated aspergillosis in dogs has not been studied prospectively. The most widely used treatments have been itraconazole, voriconazole, posaconazole, and/or amphotericin B. Terbinafine has been used in addition to azole therapy with limited success in the author's experience.[7] *Aspergillus* species are intrinsically resistant to fluconazole, so the use of fluconazole is not recommended. Although expensive, treatment with

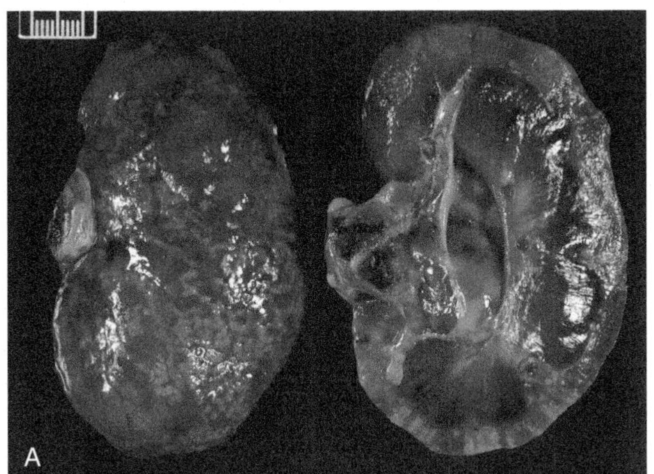

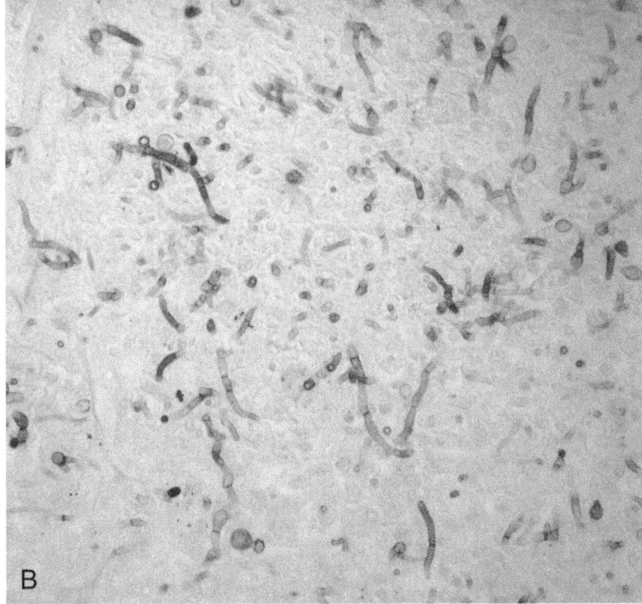

FIGURE 65-11 **A,** Kidney at necropsy from a 5-year-old female English setter with disseminated aspergillosis caused by *Aspergillus terreus*. Numerous small coalescing tan nodules are present throughout the cortex, and the capsular surface is irregular. There is a blood clot adjacent to the renal pelvis. (Image courtesy University of California, Davis, Veterinary Anatomic Pathology Service.) **B,** Histopathology from a 5-year-old male neutered German shepherd dog with disseminated *A. terreus* infection that involved multiple parenchymal organs. Large numbers of septate, branching hyphae are seen. Gomori's methenamine silver stain, 1000× oil magnification.

voriconazole or posaconazole can result in remissions of many months' duration in some dogs.[7,57] Posaconazole in particular has shown promising activity in human patient and mouse models of invasive *A. terreus* infection.[58,59] Many dogs require treatment with multiple antifungal drugs to maintain remission, either in combination or in series. *A. terreus* strains from humans with invasive aspergillosis can become resistant to azoles during treatment.[60] *A. terreus* strains isolated from human patients are also relatively resistant to amphotericin B,[59,61] but clinical improvement can still occur after treatment of infected dogs with amphotericin B (see Chapter 9).[7] Echinocandins (such as caspofungin) are also active against *Aspergillus*, but expense and the need for intravenous administration has limited their use in dogs.

Dogs with localized bronchopulmonary aspergillosis have the best prognosis. These dogs are sometimes cured after treatment with itraconazole alone. Lung lobectomy may be required for successful treatment of German shepherds with cavitary lung lesions.[7,45,46]

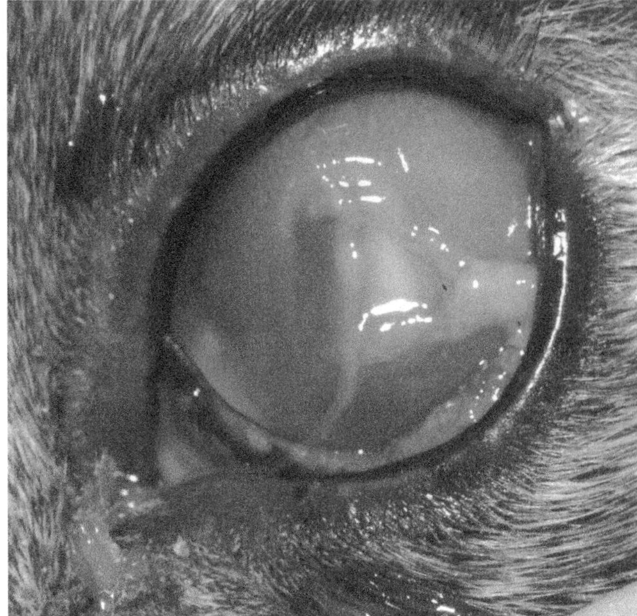

FIGURE 65-12 Severe ulcerative keratitis in a 12-year-old female spayed domestic shorthair caused by an *Aspergillus fumigatus* complex organism. The condition was successfully treated using topical voriconazole and a conjunctival island graft. (Courtesy the University of California, Davis, Veterinary Ophthalmology Service.)

Immunity and Vaccination

Immunity to disseminated aspergillosis is critically dependent on the function of neutrophils and dendritic cells, as well as effective T cell function.[62] A vaccine to prevent the disease is not available.

Public Health Aspects

In human patients, invasive aspergillosis primarily occurs in immunosuppressed humans with hematologic malignancy, or after solid organ transplantation or hematopoietic stem cell transplantation.[51] Infections are acquired from the environment. Transmission from affected dogs has not been described. Most cases (>70%) are caused by *A. fumigatus*. Infection with *A. terreus* is rare, and *A. deflectus* is not a recognized human pathogen.

KERATOMYCOSIS AND OTOMYCOSIS CAUSED BY *ASPERGILLUS* SPECIES

Infection of the cornea[8,63] and ear canal[9,10] by *Aspergillus* species occur rarely in dogs and cats (see Table 65-1; Figure 65-12). Diagnosis of these conditions requires visualization of hyphae on cytologic examination or histopathology of biopsy specimens in addition to fungal culture to rule out the possibility of contamination or colonization. One cat with *A. flavus* keratomycosis had a history of feline herpesvirus-1–associated conjunctivitis and keratitis[8] and was successfully treated with 1% topical voriconazole (q2h to q4h). Cats with *Aspergillus* otomycosis often have a history of diabetes mellitus.[4] Dogs with otomycosis may have a history of underlying allergic dermatitis and otitis externa that has been extensively treated with topical and oral antibiotics.[10]

CASE EXAMPLE

Signalment: "Zach," a 2-year-old male neutered German shepherd from Roseville in northern California

History: Zach was evaluated at the University of California, Davis, Veterinary Oncology Service for possible bone cancer. Two months previously, the owners noted that Zach vocalized when he stood up from rest. He was taken to a local veterinary clinic where he was diagnosed with lumbosacral pain and treated with carprofen (1.5 mg/kg PO q12h). Two weeks later, right pelvic limb lameness developed. Pelvic radiographs showed evidence of moderate osteoarthrosis of the left coxofemoral joint. Carprofen treatment was continued. After an additional 2 weeks, lethargy, inappetence, increased thirst and urination, and left thoracic limb lameness developed, and Zach began vomiting once daily. Radiographs of the left thoracic limb revealed an osteoproductive lesion in the mid-diaphysis of the left humerus, which was interpreted as a primary or metastatic bone tumor (see Figure 65-8). Zach was one of two dogs in the household, was normally fed a dry commercial dog food diet, and was up to date on vaccinations, which included those for distemper, adenovirus, parvovirus, rabies, *Borrelia,* and *Bordetella.*

Physical Examination:

Body Weight: 33.5 kg.

General: Quiet, alert, and responsive. T = 103.4°F (39.7°C), HR = 120 beats/min, panting, CRT <2 s, mucous membranes moist and pink.

Eyes, Ears, Nose, and Throat: No clinically significant abnormalities were detected. Fundoscopic examination revealed multiple hyporeflective regions, consistent with chorioretinitis, in the right fundus.

Musculoskeletal: BCS was 4/9, and generalized muscle wasting was present. There was no evidence of lameness or bone pain on orthopedic examination.

Cardiovascular, Respiratory, Gastrointestinal, Genitourinary, and Lymph Nodes: No clinically significant abnormalities were present.

Laboratory Findings:

CBC:

HCT 32.8% (40%-55%)
MCV 65.2 fL (65-75 fL)
MCHC 35.7 g/dL (33-36 g/dL)
WBC 18,530 cells/μL (6000-13,000 cells/μL)
Neutrophils 13,768 cells/μL (3000-10,500 cells/μL)
Lymphocytes 2687 cells/μL (1000-4000 cells/μL)
Monocytes 1334 cells/μL (150-1200 cells/μL)
Eosinophils 741 cells/μL (0-1500 cells/μL)
Platelets 262,000 platelets/μL (150,000-400,000 platelets/μL).

Serum Chemistry Profile:

Sodium 152 mmol/L (145-154 mmol/L)
Potassium 3.8 mmol/L (4.1-5.3 mmol/L)
Chloride 113 mmol/L (105-116 mmol/L)
Bicarbonate 24 mmol/L (16-26 mmol/L)
Phosphorus 5.7 mg/dL (3.0-6.2 mg/dL)
Calcium 11.8 mg/dL (9.9-11.4 mg/dL)
BUN 31 mg/dL (8-21 mg/dL)
Creatinine 1.9 mg/dL (0.5-1.6 mg/dL)
Glucose 107 mg/dL (60-104 mg/dL)
Total protein 6.8 g/dL (5.4-7.4 g/dL)
Albumin 2.8 g/dL (2.9-4.2 g/dL)
Globulin 4.0 g/dL (2.3-4.4 g/dL)
ALT 15 U/L (19-67 U/L)
AST 27 U/L (21-54 U/L)
ALP 28 U/L (15-127 U/L)
GGT 2 U/L (0-6 U/L)
Cholesterol 205 mg/dL (135-345 mg/dL)
Total bilirubin 0.1 mg/dL (0-0.4 mg/dL).

Urinalysis: SGr 1.010; pH 7.0, 1+ protein (SSA), no bilirubin, 3+ hemoprotein, no glucose, 10-15 WBC/HPF, 50-60 RBC/HPF, 0-2 transitional epithelial cells, a few amorphous crystals, and a few budding organisms were seen.

Imaging Findings:

Thoracic Radiographs: The cardiopulmonary structures were unremarkable.

Bone Survey Radiographs: Single lateral radiographs of the distal left antebrachium, distal right antebrachium, and distal left and right pelvic limbs were performed. An additional lateral radiograph of the left humerus was also obtained and compared with referral radiographs taken 1 month previously. This showed progression of a primarily osteoproductive lesion in the mid-diaphysis of the left humerus. An additional site of chronic active periosteal reaction was noted along the distal caudal aspect of the left femur. Patchy increases in medullary density were identified in the distal diaphysis of both humeri.

Abdominal Ultrasound: Hypoechoic mottling of the splenic hilus was identified. There was bilateral renal pyelectasia with echogenic material within the renal pelves bilaterally (see Figure 65-9). There was marked blunting of the renal pelves bilaterally with mild hydroureter.

Microbiologic Findings: Cytologic examination of a fine needle aspirate of lesion in left humerus: Smears were moderately cellular with a dense, proteinaceous background and moderate amounts of cellular debris. Nucleated cells consisted of a population of numerous activated macrophages and variably degenerate neutrophils that were evenly distributed throughout the smear as well as in variably sized aggregates. Numerous multinucleated giant cells were noted. Throughout the specimen were moderate numbers of small, round, yeast organisms as well as numerous fungal hyphae, which were found intracellularly and extracellularly. The fungal hyphae were negative staining, branching, and septate, often with bulging ends.

Fungal culture and susceptibility (left humerus fine needle aspirate, sent to University of Texas for molecular identification): Moderate numbers of *Aspergillus terreus.* MICs for amphotericin B, itraconazole, and voriconazole were 2, 0.125, and 0.25 μg/mL, respectively.

Aerobic urine bacterial culture: Six colonies of *A. terreus.*

Aspergillus antibody serology (gel immunodiffusion, Meridian Bioscience, Ltd.): Negative.

Diagnosis: Disseminated *Aspergillus terreus* infection.

Treatment: Zach was treated with intravenous fluids (lactated Ringer's solution with 20 mEq/L KCl at 75 mL/hr), lipid-complexed amphotericin B (1 mg/kg IV on a Monday-Wednesday-Friday basis for 4 weeks), and itraconazole (5 mg/kg PO q12h). Over the course of amphotericin B treatment, Zach's inappetence, lethargy, and lameness resolved and his serum creatinine and BUN concentrations remained stable with values of 2.1 mg/dL and 49 mg/dL, respectively, by the end of treatment. At a recheck 2 months after treatment was initiated, fungal culture of the urine revealed a single colony of *A. terreus*, and the creatinine was 1.7 mg/dL. After an additional month, bone survey radiographs showed significant remodeling of the left humeral and left femoral lesions. A serum biochemistry panel showed mildly increased creatinine concentration (1.8 mg/dL) and a serum ALT activity of 364 U/L; the increased serum ALT activity was thought to be secondary to itraconazole administration. Ultrasound of the abdomen showed mild pelvic dilatation, and the echogenic material within the renal pelves had disappeared. Fungal culture of the urine was negative. Four months after treatment was initiated, intermittent vocalization and right pelvic limb lameness developed. Pain was detected only on lumbosacral palpation. Radiographs of this region revealed focal osteolysis of the ventral caudal aspect of the sixth lumbar vertebra. Clinical improvement did not occur after treatment with carprofen and tramadol.

Two weeks later, Zach developed respiratory distress and was seen by the Veterinary Emergency and Critical Care Service. Mild dehydration, pyrexia (105.8°F or 41.0°C), gagging, and ptyalism were detected on physical examination. Thoracic radiographs were unremarkable, but a soft tissue density was seen in the pharyngeal region on cervical radiographs. Blood cultures were negative. Zach was sedated, and on oral examination, multiple large soft tissue masses were observed within the pharynx and around the rim of the epiglottis. Aspiration of the masses revealed suppurative inflammation and possible occasional fungal hyphae. Bronchoscopy was performed, and numerous yellow plaque-like lesions were visualized on the tracheal mucosa. Cytologic examination of biopsies of these lesions revealed fungal hyphae. The owner elected euthanasia. Necropsy findings included severe, locally extensive mural granulomas of the tracheal mucosa with intralesional fungal hyphae and suppurative and eosinophilic pharyngitis with necrosis and edema. There was evidence of healed pyelonephritis and granulomatous nephritis with intralesional fungal hyphae. Granulomatous osteomyelitis with intralesional hyphae was present in the left femur and humerus. There were multiple granulomas in the pancreas and spleen.

Comments: Disseminated aspergillosis in this dog was initially confused with bone neoplasia. An *Aspergillus* antibody titer was negative, which illustrates the lack of sensitivity of this assay for diagnosis of disseminated disease. Galactomannan antigen testing was not performed, but bone lesions were readily accessible for aspiration and culture. The small, round yeast organisms visualized together with the hyphae were likely accessory conidia, which can be found in *A. terreus* infections. Treatment with lipid-complexed amphotericin B and itraconazole was initially associated with clinical remission, but infection was not eliminated. Based on necropsy examination, the cause of the suppurative pharyngeal masses that impaired respiration was not clear. Fungal cultures of the masses were negative.

SUGGESTED READINGS

Barrs VR, Halliday C, Martin P, et al. Sinonasal and sino-orbital aspergillosis in 23 cats: aetiology, clinicopathological features and treatment outcomes. Vet J. 2012;191:58-64.

Day MJ. Canine sino-nasal aspergillosis: parallels with human disease. Med Mycol. 2009;47(suppl 1):S315-S323.

Schultz RM, Johnson EG, Wisner ER, et al. Clinicopathologic and diagnostic imaging characteristics of systemic aspergillosis in 30 dogs. J Vet Intern Med. 2008;22:851-859.

REFERENCES

1. Denning DW. Invasive aspergillosis. Clin Infect Dis. 1998;26:781-803:quiz 804-785.
2. Abad A, Fernandez-Molina JV, Bikandi J, et al. What makes *Aspergillus fumigatus* a successful pathogen? Genes and molecules involved in invasive aspergillosis. Rev Iberoam Micol. 2010;27:155-182.
3. Barrs VR, Halliday C, Martin P, et al. Sinonasal and sino-orbital aspergillosis in 23 cats: aetiology, clinicopathological features and treatment outcomes. Vet J. 2012;191:58-64.
4. Sykes JE. Unpublished observations, 2012.
5. Kano R, Itamoto K, Okuda M, et al. Isolation of *Aspergillus udagawae* from a fatal case of feline orbital aspergillosis. Mycoses. 2008;51:360-361.
6. Southard C. Bronchopulmonary aspergillosis in a dog. J Am Vet Med Assoc. 1987;190:875-877.
7. Schultz RM, Johnson EG, Wisner ER, et al. Clinicopathologic and diagnostic imaging characteristics of systemic aspergillosis in 30 dogs. J Vet Intern Med. 2008;22:851-859.
8. Labelle AL, Hamor RE, Barger AM, et al. *Aspergillus flavus* keratomycosis in a cat treated with topical 1% voriconazole solution. Vet Ophthalmol. 2009;12:48-52.
9. Ghibaudo G, Peano A. Chronic monolateral otomycosis in a dog caused by *Aspergillus ochraceus*. Vet Dermatol. 2010;21:522-526.
10. Coyner K. Otomycosis due to *Aspergillus* spp. in a dog: case report and literature review. Vet Dermatol. 2010;21:613-618.
11. Zhang S, Corapi W, Quist E, et al. *Aspergillus versicolor*, a new causative agent of canine disseminated aspergillosis. J Clin Microbiol. 2012;50:187-191.
12. Barrs VR, van Doorn T, Houbraken J, et al. *Aspergillus felis* sp. nov. – an emerging pathogen of cats, dogs and humans. Proceedings of the International Society for Companion Animal Infectious Diseases. 2012: Abstract 017.
13. Talbot JJ, Martin P, Johnson LR, et al. What causes sinonasal aspergillosis in dogs? A molecular approach to species identification. Proceedings of the International Society for Companion Animal Infectious Diseases. 2012: Abstract 018.
14. Burrough E, Deitz K, Kinyon J, et al. Disseminated aspergillosis in a dog due to *Aspergillus alabamensis*. Med Mycol Case Reports. 2012;1:1-4.
15. Pitt JI, Samson RA. Nomenclatural considerations in naming species of *Aspergillus* and its teleomorphs. Stud Mycol. 2007;59:67-70.
16. Pomrantz JS, Johnson LR, Nelson RW, et al. Comparison of serologic evaluation via agar gel immunodiffusion and fungal culture of tissue for diagnosis of nasal aspergillosis in dogs. J Am Vet Med Assoc. 2007;230:1319-1323.
17. Day MJ. Canine sino-nasal aspergillosis: parallels with human disease. Med Mycol. 2009;47(suppl 1):S315-S323.
18. Goodall SA, Lane JG, Warnock DW. The diagnosis and treatment of a case of nasal aspergillosis in a cat. J Small Anim Pract. 1984;25:627-633.
19. Peeters D, Day MJ, Clercx C. An immunohistochemical study of canine nasal aspergillosis. J Comp Pathol. 2005;132:283-288.
20. Peeters D, Peters IR, Clercx C, et al. Quantification of mRNA encoding cytokines and chemokines in nasal biopsies from dogs with sino-nasal aspergillosis. Vet Microbiol. 2006;114:318-326.
21. Hamilton HL, Whitley RD, McLaughlin SA. Exophthalmos secondary to aspergillosis in a cat. J Am Anim Hosp Assoc. 2000;36:343-347.

22. Giordano C, Gianella P, Bo S, et al. Invasive mould infections of the naso-orbital region of cats: a case involving *Aspergillus fumigatus* and an aetiological review. J Feline Med Surg. 2010;12:714-723.
23. Barachetti L, Mortellaro CM, Di Giancamillo M, et al. Bilateral orbital and nasal aspergillosis in a cat. Vet Ophthalmol. 2009;12:176-182.
24. Billen F, Guieu LV, Bernaerts F, et al. Efficacy of intrasinusal administration of bifonazole cream alone or in combination with enilconazole irrigation in canine sino-nasal aspergillosis: 17 cases. Can Vet J. 2010;51:164-168.
25. Pomrantz JS, Johnson LR. Repeated rhinoscopic and serologic assessment of the effectiveness of intranasally administered clotrimazole for the treatment of nasal aspergillosis in dogs. J Am Vet Med Assoc. 2010;236:757-762.
26. Saunders JH, Clercx C, Snaps FR, et al. Radiographic, magnetic resonance imaging, computed tomographic, and rhinoscopic features of nasal aspergillosis in dogs. J Am Vet Med Assoc. 2004;225:1703-1712.
27. Johnson LR, Drazenovich TL, Herrera MA, et al. Results of rhinoscopy alone or in conjunction with sinuscopy in dogs with aspergillosis: 46 cases (2001-2004). J Am Vet Med Assoc. 2006;228:738-742.
28. Whitney BL, Broussard J, Stefanacci JD. Four cats with fungal rhinitis. J Feline Med Surg. 2005;7:53-58.
29. Peeters D, Clercx C. Update on canine sinonasal aspergillosis. Vet Clin North Am Small Anim Pract. 2007;37:901-916, vi.
30. Smith LN, Hoffman SB. A case series of unilateral orbital aspergillosis in three cats and treatment with voriconazole. Vet Ophthalmol. 2010;13:190-203.
31. De Lorenzi D, Bonfanti U, Masserdotti C, et al. Diagnosis of canine nasal aspergillosis by cytological examination: a comparison of four different collection techniques. J Small Anim Pract. 2006;47:316-319.
32. Billen F, Clercx C, Le Garerres A, et al. Effect of sampling method and incubation temperature on fungal culture in canine sinonasal aspergillosis. J Small Anim Pract. 2009;50:67-72.
33. Billen F, Peeters D, Peters IR, et al. Comparison of the value of measurement of serum galactomannan and *Aspergillus*-specific antibodies in the diagnosis of canine sino-nasal aspergillosis. Vet Microbiol. 2009;133:358-365.
34. Peeters D, Peters IR, Helps CR, et al. Whole blood and tissue fungal DNA quantification in the diagnosis of canine sino-nasal aspergillosis. Vet Microbiol. 2008;128:194-203.
35. Tomsa K, Glaus TM, Zimmer C, et al. Fungal rhinitis and sinusitis in three cats. J Am Vet Med Assoc. 2003;222:1380-1384, 1365.
36. Garcia RS, Wheat LJ, Cook AK, et al. Sensitivity and specificity of a blood and urine galactomannan antigen assay for diagnosis of systemic aspergillosis in dogs. J Vet Intern Med. 2012;26:911-919.
37. Whitney J, Beatty JA, Martin P, et al. Evaluation of serum galactomannan detection for diagnosis of feline upper respiratory tract aspergillosis. Vet Microbiol. 2013;162:180-185.
38. Furrow E, Groman RP. Intranasal infusion of clotrimazole for the treatment of nasal aspergillosis in two cats. J Am Vet Med Assoc. 2009;235:1188-1193.
39. McCullough SM, McKiernan BC, Grodsky BS. Endoscopically placed tubes for administration of enilconazole for treatment of nasal aspergillosis in dogs. J Am Vet Med Assoc. 1998;212:67-69.
40. Caulkett N, Lew L, Fries C. Upper-airway obstruction and prolonged recovery from anesthesia following intranasal clotrimazole administration. J Am Anim Hosp Assoc. 1997;33:264-267.
41. Sissener TR, Bacon NJ, Friend E, et al. Combined clotrimazole irrigation and depot therapy for canine nasal aspergillosis. J Small Anim Pract. 2006;47:312-315.
42. Hazell KL, Swift IM, Sullivan N. Successful treatment of pulmonary aspergillosis in a cat. Aust Vet J. 2011;89:101-104.
43. Sykes JE, Mapes S, Lindsay LL, et al. *Corynebacterium ulcerans* bronchopneumonia in a dog. J Vet Intern Med. 2010;24:973-976.
44. Adamama-Moraitou KK, Pardali D, Day MJ, et al. *Aspergillus fumigatus* bronchopneumonia in a Hellenic shepherd dog. J Am Anim Hosp Assoc. 2011;47:e13-e18.
45. Kulendra E, Halfacree Z, Goggs R, et al. Cavitary pulmonary lesion associated with *Aspergillus fumigatus* infection in a German shepherd dog. J Small Anim Pract. 2010;51:271-274.
46. Whitley NT, Cauvin A, Burton C, et al. Long term survival in two German shepherd dogs with *Aspergillus*-associated cavitary pulmonary lesions. J Small Anim Pract. 2010;51:561.
47. Guerin SR, Walker MC, Kelly DF. Cavitating mycotic pneumonia in a German shepherd dog. J Small Anim Pract. 1993;34:36-39.
48. Krockenberger MB, Swinney G, Martin P, et al. Sequential opportunistic infections in two German Shepherd dogs. Aust Vet J. 2011;89:9-14.
49. Fox JG, Murphy JC, Shalev M. Systemic fungal infections in cats. J Am Vet Med Assoc. 1978;173:1191-1195.
50. Ossent P. Systemic aspergillosis and mucormycosis in 23 cats. Vet Rec. 1987;120:330-333.
51. Steinbach WJ, Marr KA, Anaissie EJ, et al. Clinical epidemiology of 960 patients with invasive aspergillosis from the PATH alliance registry. J Infect. 2012;65:453-464.
52. Hage CA, Reynolds JM, Durkin M, et al. Plasmalyte as a cause of false-positive results for *Aspergillus* galactomannan in bronchoalveolar lavage fluid. J Clin Microbiol. 2007;45:676-677.
53. White PL, Linton CJ, Perry MD, et al. The evolution and evaluation of a whole blood polymerase chain reaction assay for the detection of invasive aspergillosis in hematology patients in a routine clinical setting. Clin Infect Dis. 2006;42:479-486.
54. Johnson GL, Bibby DF, Wong S, et al. A MIQE-compliant real-time PCR assay for *Aspergillus* detection. PLoS One. 2012;7:e40022.
55. Butterworth SJ, Barr FJ, Pearson GR, et al. Multiple discospondylitis associated with *Aspergillus* species infection in a dog. Vet Rec. 1995;136:38-41.
56. Perez J, Mozos E, de Lara FC, et al. Disseminated aspergillosis in a dog: an immunohistochemical study. J Comp Pathol. 1996;115:191-196.
57. Legendre AM. Unpublished observations, 2012.
58. Salas V, Pastor FJ, Rodriguez MM, et al. In vitro activity and in vivo efficacy of posaconazole in treatment of murine infections by different isolates of the *Aspergillus terreus* complex. Antimicrob Agents Chemother. 2011;55:676-679.
59. Hachem RY, Kontoyiannis DP, Boktour MR, et al. *Aspergillus terreus*: an emerging amphotericin B–resistant opportunistic mold in patients with hematologic malignancies. Cancer. 2004;101:1594-1600.
60. Arendrup MC, Jensen RH, Grif K, et al. In vivo emergence of *Aspergillus terreus* with reduced azole susceptibility and a Cyp51a M217I alteration. J Infect Dis. 2012;206:981-985.
61. Escribano P, Pelaez T, Recio S, et al. Characterization of clinical strains of *Aspergillus terreus* complex: molecular identification and antifungal susceptibility to azoles and amphotericin B. Clin Microbiol Infect. 2012;18:E24-E26.
62. Park SJ, Burdick MD, Mehrad B. Neutrophils mediate maturation and efflux of lung dendritic cells in response to *Aspergillus fumigatus* germ tubes. Infect Immun. 2012;80:1759-1765.
63. Qualls Jr CW, Chandler FW, Kaplan W, et al. Mycotic keratitis in a dog: concurrent *Aspergillus* sp. and *Curvularia* sp. infections. J Am Vet Med Assoc. 1985;186:975-976.

CHAPTER 66

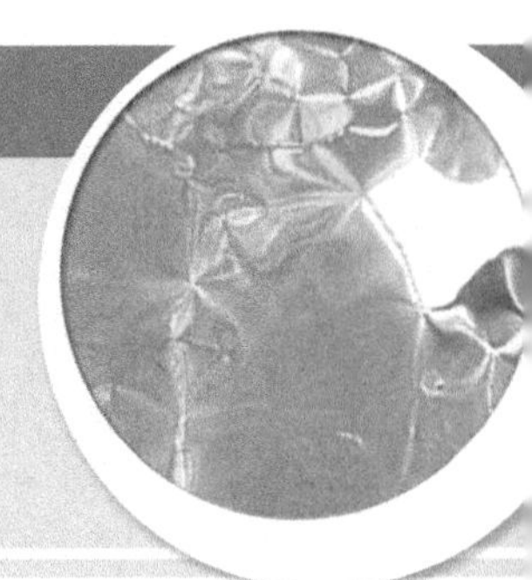

Rhinosporidiosis

Jane E. Sykes

> **Overview of Rhinosporidiosis**
>
> First Described: In the 1890s, in Argentina (by Malbran and then by Seeber)[1]
>
> Cause: *Rhinosporidium seeberi* (kingdom Protista, class Mesomycetozoea)
>
> Affected Hosts: Dogs, humans, horses, rarely cats and other domestic animals
>
> Geographic Distribution: Worldwide but especially in warm, wet environments such as the south-eastern and south-central United States
>
> Mode of Transmission: Unclear; possibly exposure to contaminated water sources in association with trauma
>
> Major Clinical Signs: Sneezing, epistaxis, mass protruding from nares
>
> Differential Diagnoses: Nasal neoplasia, cryptococcosis, sinonasal aspergillosis, nasal mites *(Pneumonyssoides caninum)*, foreign bodies
>
> Human Health Significance: Human infections by *R. seeberi* are likely acquired from the environment, and direct transmission from affected animals to humans has not been described.

Etiology and Epidemiology

Rhinosporidiosis is caused by *Rhinosporidium seeberi,* which causes slow-growing tumor-like masses in the nasal cavity. Although once thought to be a fungus, molecular methods have identified this organism as an aquatic protistan parasite (class Mesomycetozoea). The organism is taxonomically located where animals and fungi diverge and is closely related to pathogens of fish.[2] The organism is difficult or impossible to culture. Rhinosporidiosis has been most widely reported in humans and dogs, but cats, horses, and other mammalian and avian species may also be affected. There is some evidence that host-specific strains of *R. seeberi* exist.[3]

In humans, rhinosporidiosis is most prevalent in southern India, Sri Lanka, and Argentina but also occurs in North America, Africa, Europe, and Asia. In dogs and cats, rhinosporidiosis has been reported from many regions of the United States, Ontario in Canada,[4] Argentina,[5] Italy in continental Europe,[6] and the United Kingdom.[7] Within the United States, the disease is most often reported in dogs and cats from the south-central and southeastern states (Figure 66-1). The overwhelming majority of affected dogs are young-adult to middle-aged (with a range of 1 to 13 years of age), otherwise-healthy, large-breed hunting dogs such as Labrador and golden retrievers, Doberman pinschers, Siberian huskies, German shepherds, and Rhodesian ridgebacks. However, small-breed dogs can also be affected.[7] No clear sex predisposition has been identified, but of cases in the literature, males have outnumbered females. Affected cats have been outdoor cats. One affected cat had concurrent nasal adenocarcinoma,[8] but other cats have had no reported comorbidities.

Although the mode of transmission of *R. seeberi* is not precisely understood, disease often occurs in association with contact with aquatic or marshy environments. It is thought that spores are released into the environment, where they contact susceptible human and animal hosts.[2] Spores may be introduced into tissues after trauma to the mucous membranes, where they form sporangia that produce new spores. Because disease in humans also occurs in arid regions, airborne spore transmission has also been suggested.

Clinical Features

Signs and Their Pathogenesis

In dogs and cats, infection by *R. seeberi* leads to formation of pedunculate or sessile masses within the nasal cavity, usually in the rostral third.[6] The polyps range in size from a few millimeters to several centimeters. Clinical signs consist of subacute (weeks) to chronic (>1 year) sneezing with or without epistaxis, snuffling, and sometimes a serous, mucoid, or serosanguineous unilateral nasal discharge. Sneezing may be frequent and severe and associated with excitement or increased

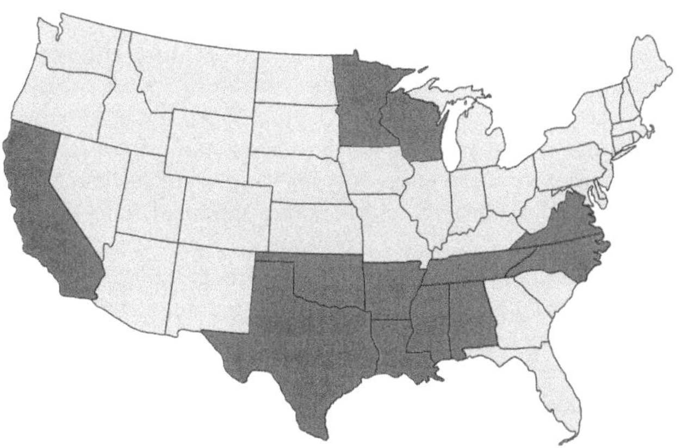

FIGURE 66-1 States within the United States in which rhinosporidiosis has been reported in dogs and cats.

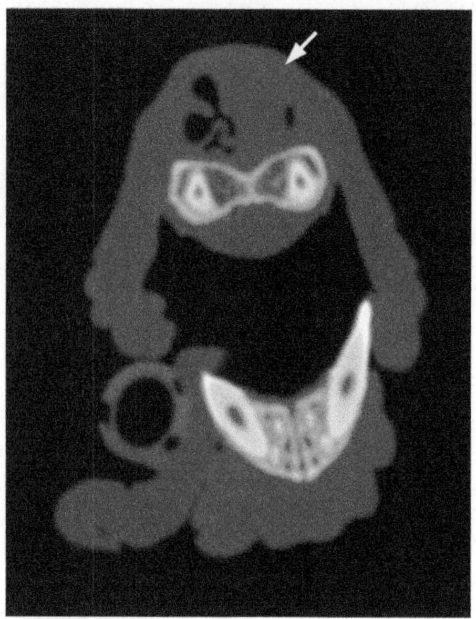

FIGURE 66-2 CT scan of the nasal cavity of a 16-month-old female Labrador retriever with rhinosporidiosis. A soft tissue mass that enhanced with contrast is present in the rostral nasal cavity *(arrow)*.

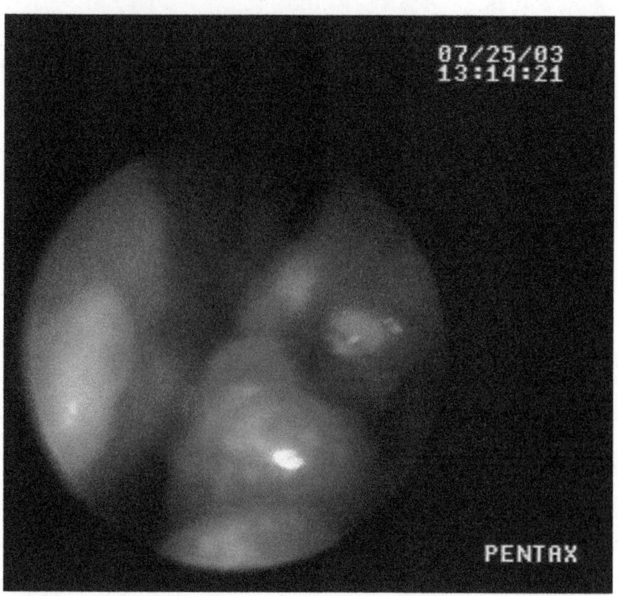

FIGURE 66-3 Rhinoscopic image of a polypoid mass caused by *Rhinosporidium seeberi* in the nasal cavity of a 10-year-old intact female yellow Labrador retriever.

activity. In some dogs, a polypoid pink mass protrudes from the nasal cavity. The masses are often stippled with white-yellowish granules less than 1 mm in diameter, which represent mature sporangia.[6]

Diagnosis

Most animals with rhinosporidiosis have no significant abnormalities on blood work. Plain radiography is insensitive for detection of nasal masses caused by *R. seeberi*.[6] Computed tomography (CT) reveals soft tissue masses in the rostral third of the nasal cavity that can enhance with contrast (Figure 66-2). In some cases evidence of turbinate loss is present. The masses, which can be visualized directly using rostral rhinoscopy, are pink to gray and may be covered with miliary white to yellow foci, but these are not always clearly visible (Figure 66-3).

Definitive diagnosis requires cytology or histopathology of the masses. Cytologic examination of smears from nasal swabs, cytology brush specimens, or impression smears made from biopsies of the polyps reveals suppurative to pyogranulomatous inflammation with dysplastic epithelial cells and numerous immature to mature *R. seeberi* endospores, which occur singly or in clusters.[9] Sometimes sporangia that contain hundreds of endospores are visualized. Mature endospores stain intensely, are round to oval and 10 to 15 µm in diameter, and have a thick cell wall (Figure 66-4). Immature endospores are 2 to 4 µm in diameter and contain a paracentral, light pink-purple structure that may represent nuclear material, as well as one to two smaller, spherical, dark purple structures.[9]

Histopathology reveals abundant sporangia in various stages of development and a mild to severe pyogranulomatous inflammatory response (Figure 66-5). Lymphocytes, plasma cells, and, in some cases, multinucleate giant cells and evidence of turbinate remodeling with activated osteoclasts and osteoblasts may be present. Juvenile sporangia are small (<100 µm in diameter) and have a single nucleus that is surrounded by fibrillar material. Mature sporangia are up to 500 µm in diameter and may

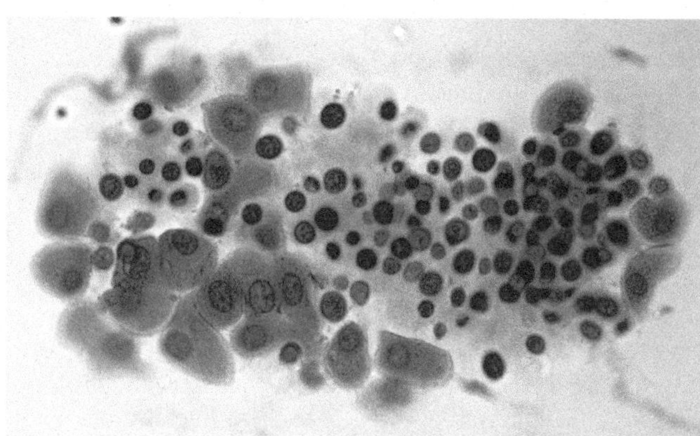

FIGURE 66-4 Impression smear of a biopsy taken from the nasal cavity of a 6-year-old female spayed Labrador retriever with rhinosporidiosis. A large cluster of endospores is present together with several epithelial cells.

be seen releasing endospores at the polyp surface through a pore in the sporangial wall. Although the organisms stain well with special stains such as periodic acid–Schiff, Gomori's methenamine silver, and Mayer's mucicarmine, these stains are usually not required for diagnosis.[6]

Treatment and Prognosis

The treatment of choice for dogs and cats is surgical removal of polyps, which generally requires rhinotomy. Because the polyps are often rostrally located, excisions can often be extended caudally from the nares. Many dogs have no recurrence of clinical signs thereafter, but some dogs develop relapse within months of surgery.[5,10,11] Treatment of these dogs can be frustrating and costly. Povidone-iodine is active against *R. seeberi* in vitro and could be applied in the form of gauze packs topically after surgery in an attempt to minimize the chance of recurrence (see Case Example).[12] In some dogs, apparent transient or long-term responses to treatment with ketoconazole[7,13] or dapsone (1.1 mg/kg PO q8-12h)[11]

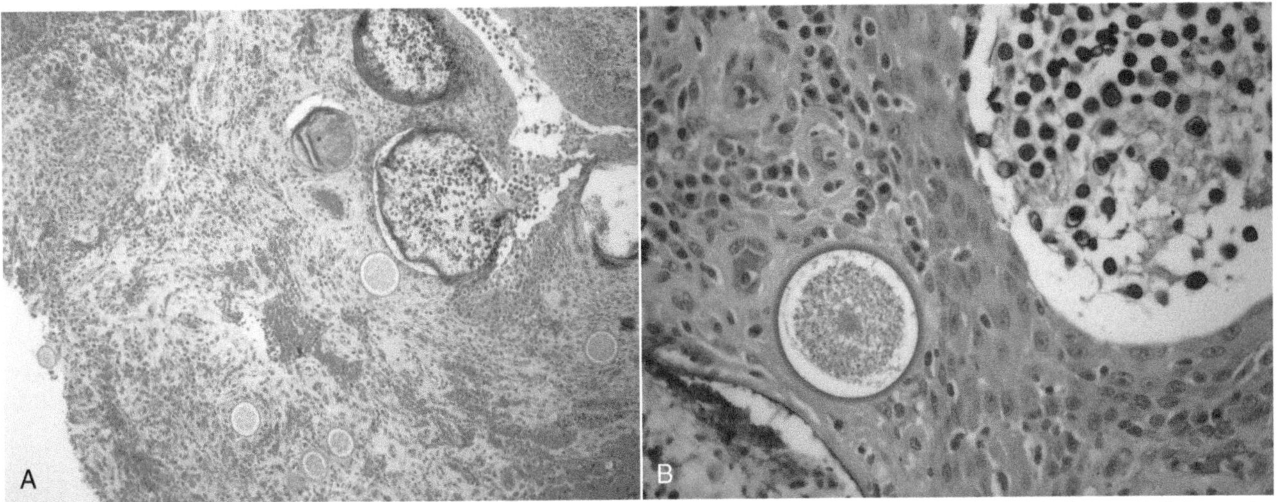

FIGURE 66-5 Histopathology of a polyp caused by *Rhinosporidium seeberi*. **A,** Low-power image that shows sporangia in various stages of development. **B,** High-power image (1000× oil magnification) that shows a juvenile sporangium adjacent to a mature sporangium, which contains endospores *(right)*. H&E stain.

have been described. Responses to dapsone have also been described in human patients. Dapsone could be used to treat dogs with refractory disease, but because both dapsone and ketoconazole can have significant adverse effects, careful monitoring is required. Dapsone is a sulfur drug (diaminophenyl sulfone) that can cause bone marrow suppression in dogs[14] and has the potential to cause hepatotoxicity and cutaneous drug reactions. Treatment of cats with dapsone is not recommended because of a high prevalence of adverse effects in this species, specifically neurotoxicosis and anemia.

Public Health Aspects

In humans, rhinosporidiosis usually involves the nasal cavity or nasopharynx, but involvement of the conjunctiva, genitalia, or skin can occur.[15] Rarely, cutaneous disease is disseminated. Disease is most often reported in males. Infection is likely acquired from the environment, and transmission from animals to humans has not been described. It is possible that strains of *R. seeberi* that infect humans may differ from those that infect dogs.

CASE EXAMPLE

Signalment: "Sarah," a 16-month-old intact female Labrador retriever from the central valley of northern California

History: Sarah was evaluated by her local veterinary clinic for a 1-month history of sneezing, which occurred throughout the day and was more frequent and severe during periods of excitement. The owners had not observed nasal discharge, and they were concerned about the possibility of a foreign body. A limited rhinoscopic examination with an otoscope cone at the local veterinary clinic revealed a large, fleshy, irregular mass in the dorsal meatus near the nares. Histopathology on a biopsy of the mass yielded a diagnosis of rhinosporidiosis, and Sarah was referred to the University of California, Davis, Veterinary Medical Teaching Hospital for further evaluation and treatment.

Sarah had been obtained from a breeder in Oregon as a puppy and since then had been a duck hunting dog in California. During the hunting season, she waded and swam in stagnant and fresh water sources. The owners also had ponds in their backyard. She was otherwise healthy and was fed a dry commercial dog food diet.

Physical Examination:

Body Weight: 32.2 kg.

General: Excited, alert, responsive, and hydrated. T = 101.6°F (38.7°C), HR = 140 beats/min, panting, CRT <2 s, mucous membranes moist and pink.

Eyes, Ears, Nose, and Throat: The dog's face was symmetrical with no pain on palpation, and normal ocular retropulsion. There was no evidence of nasal discharge. Nasal airflow was absent on the right side. Minimal dental calculus was present. There were no other clinically significant findings.

Musculoskeletal: BCS 4/9. Adequate musculature, normal gait.

Cardiovascular, Respiratory, Gastrointestinal, Genitourinary, and Lymph Nodes: No clinically significant abnormalities were detected.

Laboratory Findings: Preanesthetic laboratory assessment: PCV 44%, total solids 6.6 g/dL. Serum urea nitrogen was estimated at 15-26 mg/dL with a reagent strip.

Imaging Findings: Computed tomography of the head: A round, 0.9 × 1.7 × 2.3 cm, soft tissue mass was present in the rostral, dorsal right nasal cavity extending from the level of the incisors to the root of the right maxillary canine tooth. The mass was moderately and heterogeneously contrast enhancing. The superficial soft tissues overlying the mass

Continued

were thickened and contrast enhancing. The remainder of the nasal cavities and sinuses appeared within normal limits. The mandibular and medial retropharyngeal lymph nodes appeared within normal limits.

Diagnosis: Nasal rhinosporidiosis.

Treatment: A rhinotomy was performed using an anterolateral approach, and a single 1.5 cm × 0.5 cm pedunculated mass was identified attached to the mucosal layer of the nasal septum. The mass was resected with sharp dissection and diathermy. A povidone-iodine–soaked gauze pad was placed on the site of resection for 7 minutes, and the nasal vestibule was packed with an iodine-soaked gauze pad for 1 hour after surgical closure. Histopathology of the resected mass confirmed the diagnosis of nasal rhinosporidiosis. The dog was discharged with instructions to administer tramadol (3 mg/kg PO q12h) for pain relief and dapsone (0.8 mg/kg PO q8h for 2 weeks, then 0.8 mg/kg PO q12h for 3 months). At a recheck 2 weeks later, the sneezing had reduced in frequency, but vomiting was reported every 2 days approximately 2 hours after the morning dose of dapsone. A CBC and biochemistry panel were unremarkable. The frequency of dapsone administration was reduced to twice daily. Subsequently Sarah did well with no recurrence of disease or adverse effects of medication.

Comments: In this dog, topical povidone-iodine and dapsone were used after rhinotomy in an attempt to prevent recurrence. The owners were warned about the possibility of reinfection if Sarah continued her hunting activities.

SUGGESTED READING

Caniatti M, Roccabianca P, Scanziani E, et al. Nasal rhinosporidiosis in dogs: four cases from Europe and a review of the literature. Vet Rec. 1998;142:334-338.

REFERENCES

1. Fredricks DN, Jolley JA, Lepp PW, et al. *Rhinosporidium seeberi*: a human pathogen from a novel group of aquatic protistan parasites. Emerg Infect Dis. 2000;6:273-282.
2. Mendoza L, Vilela R, Rosa PS, et al. *Lacazia loboi* and *Rhinosporidium seeberi*: a genomic perspective. Rev Iberoam Micol. 2005;22:213-216.
3. Silva V, Pereira CN, Ajello L, et al. Molecular evidence for multiple host-specific strains in the genus *Rhinosporidium*. J Clin Microbiol. 2005;43:1865-1868.
4. Hoff B, Hall DA. Rhinosporidiosis in a dog. Can Vet J. 1986;27:231-232.
5. Castellano MC, Idiart JR, Martin AA. Rhinosporidiosis in a dog. Vet Med Small Anim Clinician. 1984;79:45.
6. Caniatti M, Roccabianca P, Scanziani E, et al. Nasal rhinosporidiosis in dogs: four cases from Europe and a review of the literature. Vet Rec. 1998;142:334-338.
7. Miller RI, Baylis R. Rhinosporidiosis in a dog native to the UK. Vet Rec. 2009;164:210.
8. Brenseke BM, Saunders GK. Concurrent nasal adenocarcinoma and rhinosporidiosis in a cat. J Vet Diagn Invest. 2010;22:155-157.
9. Meier WA, Meinkoth JH, Brunker J, et al. Cytologic identification of immature endospores in a dog with rhinosporidiosis. Vet Clin Pathol. 2006;35:348-352.
10. Mosier DA, Creed JE. Rhinosporidiosis in a dog. J Am Vet Med Assoc. 1984;185:1009-1010.
11. Allison N, Willard MD, Bentinck-Smith J, et al. Nasal rhinosporidiosis in two dogs. J Am Vet Med Assoc. 1986;188:869-871.
12. Arseculeratne SN, Atapattu DN, Balasooriya P, et al. The effects of biocides (antiseptics and disinfectants) on the endospores of *Rhinosporidium seeberi*. Indian J Med Microbiol. 2006;24:85-91.
13. Easley JR, Meuten DJ, Levy MG, et al. Nasal rhinosporidiosis in the dog. Vet Pathol. 1986;23:50-56.
14. Lees GE, McKeever PJ, Ruth GR. Fatal thrombocytopenic hemorrhagic diathesis associated with dapsone administration to a dog. J Am Vet Med Assoc. 1979;175:49-52.
15. Prasad K, Veena S, Permi HS, et al. Disseminated cutaneous rhinosporidiosis. J Lab Physicians. 2010;2:44-46.

CHAPTER 67

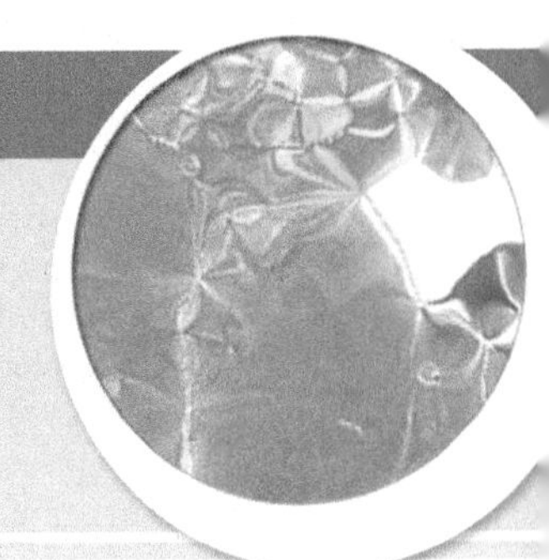

Candidiasis

Jane E. Sykes

Overview of Candidiasis

First Described: The etiology of candidiasis as a fungus was recognized in Stockholm around 1840 (Fredrik Berg),[1] but the disease was described as far back as around 400 BC by Hippocrates.

Cause: *Candida* spp. (an ascomycete)

Affected Hosts: Dogs, cats, humans, and a variety of other animal species

Geographic Distribution: Worldwide

Mode of Transmission: Usually invasion of commensal yeasts secondary to immune suppression

Major Clinical Signs: Local dermatitis; otitis externa; keratitis; lower urinary tract signs; abdominal pain, icterus, and/or ascites due to peritonitis; or severe systemic infections with fever, inappetence, ocular inflammation, lameness due to osteomyelitis, respiratory distress, vomiting

Differential Diagnoses: Other systemic fungal or bacterial infections

Human Health Significance: Human infections by *Candida* species result from invasion by normal flora, but human-to-human transmission of *Candida* strains can also occur. Whether resistant *Candida* species can be transferred from animals to colonize humans or vice versa is not known.

Etiology and Epidemiology

Candida species are yeasts that are typically benign counterparts of the normal gastrointestinal, urogenital, and cutaneous flora but can invade tissues and cause disease as a result of disruption of normal host defenses. *Candida* species can also be isolated from soil, inanimate objects, and hospital environments. The yeasts are small (3 to 6 μm) and ovoid (blastospores) and reproduce by budding. Budding results in the formation of new yeast cells, pseudohyphae (chains of elongated yeast cells), and true septate hyphae. Disease syndromes caused by *Candida* species that occur in dogs and cats are listed in Box 67-1. More than 200 species of *Candida* exist, but only a few species have been identified as pathogens in dogs and cats (Table 67-1[2-10]). The most commonly isolated species is *Candida albicans,* and only *C. albicans* appears to cause disseminated disease in dogs and cats. Local or disseminated infections where *Candida* is present with a mixture of bacterial species can occur. Local infections (such as UTIs) with two different *Candida* species have also been reported.[2,11]

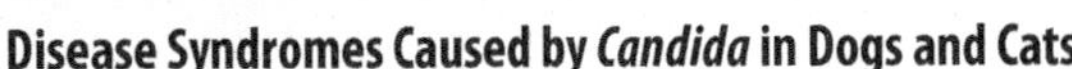

BOX 67-1

Disease Syndromes Caused by *Candida* in Dogs and Cats

Keratitis
Cutaneous candidiasis
Otitis externa and otitis media
Urinary tract infections
Gastrointestinal candidiasis
Peritonitis
Disseminated infections

When compared with human patients, candidiasis is uncommonly described in dogs and cats. Predisposing factors in dogs or cats with local or disseminated candidiasis have included diabetes mellitus,[2,3,12] treatment with immunosuppressive drugs or broad-spectrum antibacterial drugs,[2,13] a history of gastrointestinal surgery,[4,5] parvoviral infections,[14-16] and/or underlying malignancy.[2,17] Often more than one of these factors is in the history. Disseminated candidiasis has most often been described in dogs, but also occurs in cats.[5,18] Although most animals have underlying immunocompromising conditions, disseminated candidiasis has been described in apparently immunocompetent animals,[19,20] which may reflect an unidentified underlying genetic immunodeficiency. Cats with candidiasis usually test negative for FeLV or FIV infection.

Analysis of the author's hospital population suggests that cats are at least as likely as dogs to develop *Candida* UTIs.[11] In other studies, *Candida* species were isolated from the urine of 0.2% of more than 8000 dogs with UTIs[21] and 0.2% of more than 2000 dogs with persistent or recurrent UTIs.[22] Urethrostomy or indwelling cystostomy tube placement may be in the history of some cats and dogs with *Candida* UTIs, respectively.[2,6] Local mucocutaneous infections can occur at the site of long-term placement of feeding tubes.[7]

Clinical Features

Signs and Their Pathogenesis

Disruption of normal barriers is necessary to allow *Candida* spp. to invade the host. Concurrent use of broad-spectrum antibiotics suppresses the normal bacterial flora and allows *Candida* to proliferate, which increases the risk that organisms will be introduced into tissues. *Candida* can adhere to a variety of tissue components such as epithelial and endothelial cells, fibronectin, and thrombi, as well as other bacteria and inanimate objects such as catheters.[23] The yeasts can also form biofilms on medical devices and produce a huge variety of hydrolytic enzymes. Within tissues, neutrophils are a key defense against *Candida*.[24] *Candida* blastospores are phagocytized and destroyed by neutrophils. Mononuclear cells play a less important role. Reactive oxygen species, hydrolytic enzymes, and antimicrobial peptides contribute to the intracellular destruction of blastospores by neutrophils. Thus, any condition that impairs neutrophil numbers or function, such as neutropenia or diabetes mellitus, predisposes dogs and cats to candidiasis. A large number of other cytokines, complement, dendritic cells, and lymphocytes are also involved in the immune response to *Candida*.[24] The formation of hyphae by *Candida* promotes tissue invasion, which may be followed by life-threatening fungemia and dissemination to multiple organs. This ability of *Candida* to change its morphology ("morphologic dimorphism") is thought to be an important virulence factor.

Lower urinary tract candidiasis may be subclinical or associated with dysuria, stranguria, and/or hematuria. Systemic signs of pyrexia, lethargy, inappetence, and weight loss have also been described in affected dogs and cats,[6] but these signs may result from the presence of other predisposing diseases. Ascending infections may lead to development of *Candida* pyelonephritis.

Cutaneous candidiasis may manifest as erythema, scaling, alopecia, erosions, and crusting, often where disruption of cutaneous or mucocutaneous regions has occurred (such as a previous surgical site or a feeding tube or cystotomy stoma). Persistent disease in the face of systemic or topical treatment with broad-spectrum antibiotics should raise suspicion for candidiasis. Dogs with *Candida* otitis externa often have a history of chronic bacterial otitis externa that has been treated aggressively with systemic or topical antibacterials.

Overgrowth of *Candida* in the gastrointestinal tract may occur in animals that are immunosuppressed or treated with glucocorticoids and/or broad-spectrum antibacterial drugs. In some cases, invasion of the mucosa into the lamina propria or deeper tissues occurs (e.g., intestinal candidiasis). Intestinal candidiasis is occasionally identified at necropsy in puppies that die after treatment for parvoviral enteritis and may be a reason for persistent vomiting, diarrhea, and death despite aggressive fluid and antibacterial drug therapy.[14] *Candida* spp. may also contribute to ulcerative glossitis in puppies with parvovirus infection (Figure 67-1).

TABLE 67-1

***Candida* Species Associated with Disease in Dogs and/or Cats [2-10]**

Species	Clinical Manifestations
Candida albicans	Dermatitis, UTI, otitis externa, keratitis, disseminated infections
Candida glabrata (formerly *Torulopsis glabrata*)	UTI, feeding-tube site infections
Candida krusei	UTI, feeding tube site infections
Candida guilliermondii	UTI, dermatitis
Candida parapsilosis	UTI, otitis, dermatitis
Candida tropicalis	UTI
Candida rugosa	UTI

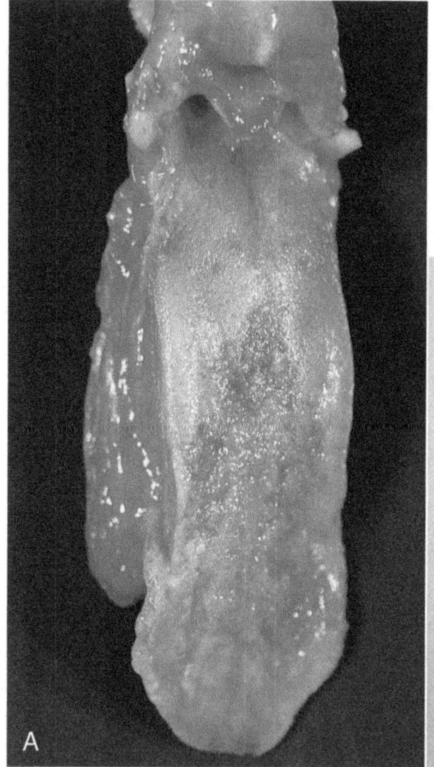

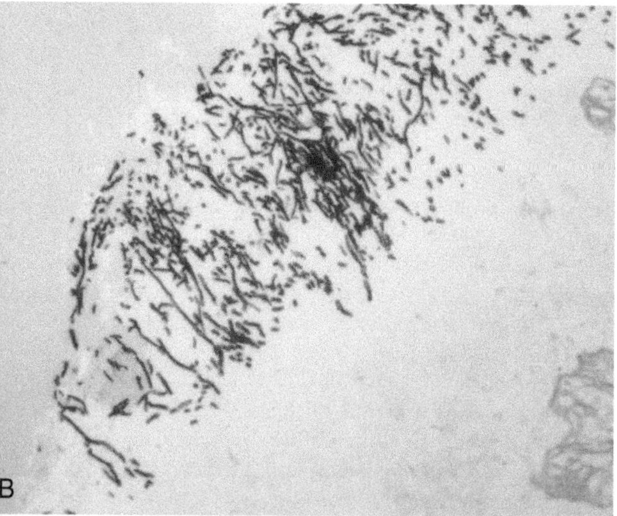

FIGURE 67-1 **A,** Tongue ulcerations at necropsy in a 2-month-old mixed-breed puppy that was euthanized because of canine parvoviral infection. **B,** Histopathology revealed multifocal ulcerative glossitis, pharyngitis, and esophagitis with intralesional yeasts and pseudohyphae. Gomori's methenamine silver stain. (Image courtesy University of California Davis Anatomic Pathology Service.)

Candida peritonitis can follow intestinal surgery, treatment with broad-spectrum antibacterial drugs, and subsequent enterotomy site dehiscence.[4,5] Mixed infections with *Candida* and intestinal flora may develop. Affected dogs are febrile, have abdominal pain, and may have other gastrointestinal signs such as vomiting and diarrhea.

Disseminated candidiasis results from hematogenous spread of *Candida* from intestinal, urinary, or possibly corneal or cutaneous sites.[12,15,25] A diagnosis of disseminated candidiasis should be considered whenever *Candida* infections are identified in the eye, skin, or urinary tract of an animal that has (or subsequently develops) severe systemic illness. Clinical signs of disseminated candidiasis in dogs include fever, inappetence, anorexia, weight loss, and a variety of other clinical signs that reflect underlying immunosuppressive disease processes and specific organs involved. The latter can include the pancreas, liver, mesentery, spleen, kidneys, heart, lungs, lymph nodes, and, less often, the bone, intestinal tract, eyes, meninges, thyroid, and/or prostate gland.[3,12,15,17,20,25-28] Ocular signs in animals with disseminated disease include keratitis and corneal ulceration, uveitis, chorioretinitis, and endophthalmitis.[11,12,28] *Candida* keratitis may also occur as a localized process, sometimes secondary to aggressive treatment of corneal ulceration secondary to other disease processes with topical broad-spectrum antibacterial drugs. Thromboembolic disease may complicate disseminated infections. Pulmonary thromboembolism may result in respiratory distress and death.[3,11]

Diagnosis

Laboratory Abnormalities

Laboratory abnormalities in dogs and cats with candidiasis result from the underlying disease process (such as diabetes mellitus or systemic neoplastic disease) as well as the location and severity of the fungal infection. Laboratory abnormalities in dogs or cats with *Candida* UTIs may be absent, or there may be evidence of renal failure with azotemia and isosthenuria. Grossly, urine may contain flocculent white debris. Urinalysis may reveal proteinuria, pyuria, and, in some cases, hematuria and/or *Candida* fungal elements (see Case Example). Dogs and cats with disseminated candidiasis or *Candida* peritonitis frequently have had nonregenerative anemia and mild to marked neutrophilia with bandemia and toxic neutrophil changes (in contrast to other deep mycoses, where hematologic abnormalities are often mild or absent). Lymphopenia may be present as a result of underlying immunosuppressive illness or drug therapy. Some dogs are thrombocytopenic and have coagulation abnormalities consistent with disseminated intravascular coagulation.[3] Findings on the serum biochemistry panel in dogs with disseminated candidiasis are variable and nonspecific but may include metabolic acidosis, moderate to severe hypoalbuminemia, and increased liver enzyme activities.

Diagnostic Imaging

Plain thoracic radiographs in dogs with disseminated candidiasis may be unremarkable or show increased pulmonary interstitial opacity, thoracic lymphadenomegaly, and/or pleural or pericardial effusion.[13,5,20] Abdominal ultrasound examination in dogs with *Candida* peritonitis or disseminated disease may reveal echogenic ascites fluid, mesenteric hyperechogenicity, changes consistent with pancreatitis, abdominal lymphadenomegaly, or increased echogenicity of the renal cortices or hepatic parenchyma.

Microbiologic Tests

Definitive diagnosis of candidiasis requires visualization of the organism within lesions by cytologic or histopathologic examination and confirmation of its identity using culture.

Cytologic Examination

Candida blastospores, pseudohyphae, and true hyphae can be visualized in swab specimens from the ear canal (ear cytology); tape preparations from the skin; urine sediment or other body fluids (Figure 67-2); or ultrasound-guided aspirates of abdominal lesions.

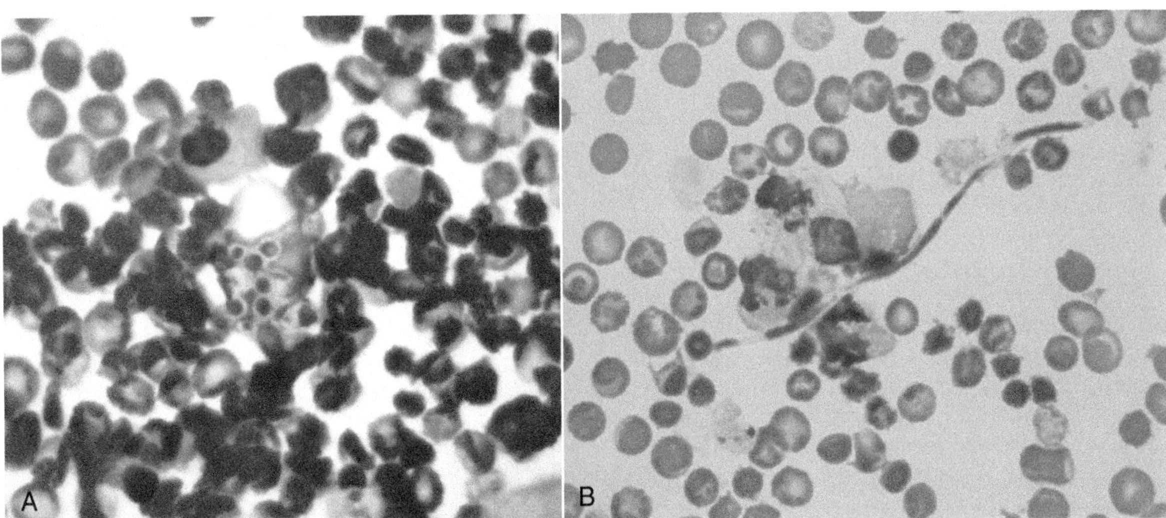

FIGURE 67-2 *Candida albicans* within urine sediment from a 5-year-old female spayed Labrador retriever being treated for multicentric lymphoma and acute-onset hematuria. Both budding **(A)** and filamentous **(B)** fungal elements are visible. (Image courtesy Dr. Barrak Pressler, The Ohio State University. From Bartges J, Polzin D. Nephrology and Urology of Small Animals. John Wiley and Sons, 2011.)

Fungal Culture

Candida grows on routine bacteriologic media as well as fungal media such as Sabouraud dextrose agar. Creamy white colonies appear within 2 to 3 days, and so isolation of the yeast may be reported when it is present in specimens submitted for aerobic bacterial culture, which are typically incubated only for this period of time. If *Candida* is suspected based on the history, fungal culture (rather than bacterial culture alone) should be requested because *Candida* grows best on fungal isolation media. Because *Candida* can be isolated from the skin and mucous membranes of healthy dogs and cats, infection must be confirmed with cytology or histopathology when *Candida* is isolated from these sites.

Identification of *Candida* isolates is based on morphology and biochemical reactions. Preliminary differentiation of *C. albicans* from other *Candida* species can be made based on the ability of *C. albicans* to produce germ tubes when exposed to serum. Matrix-assisted laser desorption/ionization–time of flight (MALDI-TOF) mass spectrometry (see Chapter 3) accurately and rapidly identifies *Candida* species[29] and may replace these methods in the future. Isolation of *Candida* allows not only definitive identification but also antifungal susceptibility testing (see Figure 4-8). This is important for *Candida* because some isolates (especially *C. glabrata* and *C. krusei*) can exhibit antifungal drug resistance.

Pathologic Findings

Gross pathologic findings at necropsy in animals with disseminated candidiasis include peritoneal or pleural effusion, enlarged and edematous lymph nodes, congestion and necrotic whitish foci within affected organs, evidence of tissue thrombosis, and formation of a gray-white or yellow-green fibrinonecrotic layer on affected mucosal surfaces.[3,5,14,15,20,26] Concurrent underlying disease processes are also often identified.

Histopathology of affected tissues reveals yeasts, pseudohyphae, and septate hyphae with an associated inflammatory response that is composed primarily of neutrophils, macrophages, and lymphocytes. Multinucleated giant cells may also be present.[15,20,26] Pseudohyphae and hyphae predominate in invasive infections (see Figure 4-1). Evidence of blood vessel invasion, thrombosing vasculitis, and infarction may be seen, with multifocal mycotic granulomas in affected organs.[15] The organism is most readily visualized with special stains such as periodic acid–Schiff and Gomori's methenamine silver. Immunohistochemistry has also been used to identify *Candida* within lesions.[15,20] When mixed infections with *Candida* and other bacteria are present, tissue gram stains may reveal bacterial rods and/or cocci in addition to gram-positive fungal elements.

Treatment and Prognosis

Treatment of candidiasis should involve management of underlying immunosuppressive disorders, if possible, and specific antifungal drug treatment. Systemic antibacterial drugs should be discontinued if not clearly indicated, or the spectrum of activity should be narrowed as much as possible. Cutaneous and corneal infections are usually treated with a combination of topical antiseptics or antifungal medications and systemic antifungal drugs until lesions resolve.[8]

Dogs and cats with *Candida* UTIs should initially be treated with antifungal drugs that achieve high concentrations in the urine, such as fluconazole with or without 5-flucytosine. Systemic antifungals alone may be adequate to resolve *Candida* UTIs in some animals, although resolution has been reported in some animals in the absence of antifungal drug therapy.[2] Persistent infection may result from drug resistance, adverse effects of treatment that necessitate treatment discontinuation, or inadequate drug penetration into balls of fungus that line the bladder wall (see Case Example). Intravesicular treatment with 1% clotrimazole may be effective in these cases.[30,31] Under anesthesia, the bladder is catheterized with a Foley catheter, emptied, then lavaged with sterile saline. The bladder is then filled with 1% clotrimazole solution (e.g., 30 to 50 mL for a cat). The animal is rotated to promote contact of the solution with the uroepithelium, and after the solution has been in the bladder for an hour, the catheter is removed and the animal is allowed to recover. Treatment is continued weekly until *Candida* can no longer be isolated from the urine. Typically one to four treatments are required.[11,30] Ultrasound-guided administration of clotrimazole via cystocentesis to a dog with *Candida* cystitis was described in one report.[31]

Successful treatment of systemic candidiasis in dogs or cats is rarely described. One dog with *Candida* peritonitis was treated successfully by surgical exploration and lavage of the abdomen, placement of an abdominal drain, and intravenous fluconazole.[4] In addition, aggressive supportive measures were required that included intravenous fluid therapy, fresh frozen plasma, antiemetics, gastroprotectants, total parenteral nutrition, and antibacterial drugs for a suspected catheter-related infection. Antifungal drugs other than fluconazole used to treat invasive candidiasis in human patients include amphotericin B or an echinocandin such as caspofungin,[32] both of which must be administered parenterally.

Prevention

Prevention of candidiasis involves avoidance of excessive immunosuppression as well as discriminate use of antibacterial drugs, which should be tailored to the results of culture and susceptibility whenever possible. Whether *Candida* species carried on the hands of humans can colonize dogs and cats is not known, but routine hand washing and the wearing of gloves when immunosuppressed animals are handled or intravascular devices are placed should minimize the chance of health care–associated infections. Although prophylactic antifungal drug treatment has been used to prevent invasive candidiasis in human high-risk groups, the low incidence of candidiasis in immunosuppressed dogs and cats does not warrant the use of prophylactic antifungal drugs in this group.

Public Health Aspects

Candida species (especially *C. albicans*) are common causes of mucosal disease in humans. Since 2000, *Candida* has also emerged as an extremely important cause of invasive infections owing to the more widespread use of invasive medical devices and immunosuppressive drugs. In hospitalized human patients, *Candida* is reportedly the fourth most common organism isolated from the bloodstream.[33] Although many human infections result from invasion of tissues by commensal yeasts in the face of immune suppression, horizontal transmission of *Candida* and hospital-acquired infections have been described.[34] Whether *Candida* isolates from dogs or cats colonize humans is not known.

CASE EXAMPLE

Signalment: "Lizzie", an 18-year-old female spayed domestic shorthair from the San Francisco Bay area (Figure 67-3, *A*)

History: Lizzie was evaluated by the University of California, Davis, Veterinary Medical Teaching Hospital for a 12-hour history of dysuria and hematuria. The owner described multiple episodes of urination and defecation outside the litter box with stranguria, hematuria, and tenesmus. Lizzie was also observed repeatedly grooming her perineum. The cat had been diagnosed with diabetes mellitus 10 years previously, and more recently with feline bronchial disease, a thoracolumbar (T3 to L3) myelopathy, generalized osteoarthritis, chronic constipation, bilateral cataracts, chronic kidney disease, and recurrent bacterial UTIs (*Streptococcus bovis* group, *Escherichia coli, Enterococcus faecalis,* then *Aerococcus viridans*). She also had a cardiac murmur secondary to dynamic right ventricular outflow tract obstruction. The historical UTIs had been treated with a variety of antimicrobial drugs selected based on the results of aerobic bacterial urine culture and susceptibility (most recently doxycycline, but also amoxicillin-clavulanic acid or marbofloxacin in the past). Her current medications consisted of prozinc insulin (3.5 units SC q12h), lactulose (2 mL PO q12h), a soluble fiber supplement (1 teaspoon with food twice daily), inhaled fluticasone (110-μg puff q12h), theophylline (12 mg/kg PO q24h), and doxycycline (5 mg/kg PO q12h). Her most recent blood work (collected 1 month previously) showed a creatinine of 1.8 mg/dL (reference range, 1.1-2.2 mg/dL) and a BUN of 34 (reference range, 18-33 mg/dL), which were similar to values obtained over the course of the previous 5 years. She was an indoor-only cat and was fed a commercial cat food with occasional turkey meat from the delicatessen. Her appetite was good, there had been no weight loss noted, her water consumption was unchanged, and there had been no vomiting or diarrhea. She had not been vaccinated for the past 4 years but was on regular flea preventative medication (nitenpyram as well as fipronil).

Physical Examination:

Body Weight: 4.1 kg.

General: Quiet, alert and responsive, T = 100.5°F (38.1°C), HR = 170 beats/min, RR = 28 breaths/min, CRT <1 s, pale pink mucous membranes.

Integument: A dull, slightly unkempt haircoat with mild scale was noted.

Eyes, Ears, Nose, and Throat: Immature cataracts were present bilaterally, and all teeth were absent on examination of the oral cavity. No other clinically significant abnormalities were detected.

Musculoskeletal: BCS was 4/9, and there was mild generalized muscle atrophy. The cat was reluctant to ambulate, and appeared painful on manipulation of the elbows, stifles, and coxofemoral joints bilaterally. Crepitus was detected on manipulation of the tarsus.

Cardiovascular and Respiratory Systems: A grade II/VI left parasternal heart murmur was auscultated. Pulses were strong and synchronous. No other abnormalities were detected.

Abdominal Palpation: The abdomen was soft and nonpainful. Both kidneys were small (approximately 2 cm in diameter) and irregular. The urinary bladder was approximately 5 cm in diameter and soft. Severe erythema was noted around the vulva.

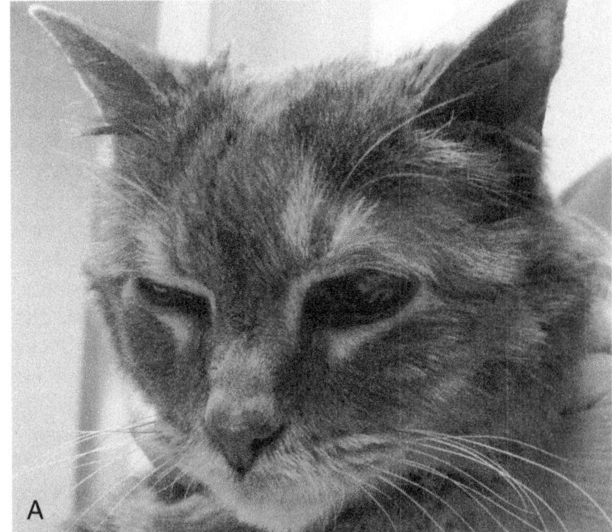

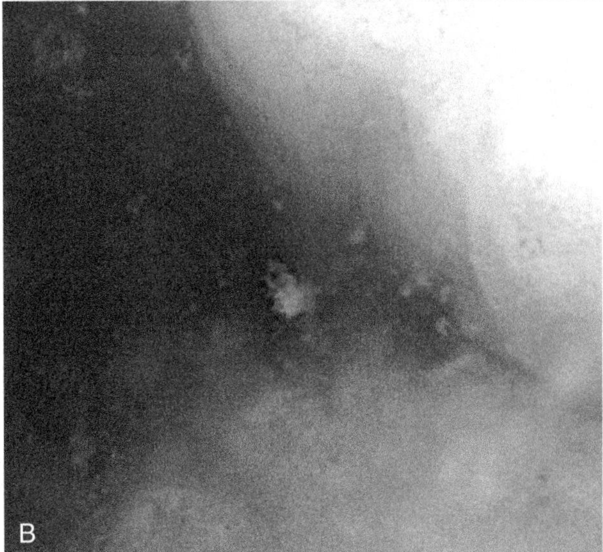

FIGURE 67-3 **A,** 18-year-old female spayed domestic shorthair with a *Candida albicans* urinary tract infection, as well as diabetes mellitus, feline bronchial disease, a myelopathy, and generalized osteoarthritis. **B,** Bladder lumen as viewed by cystoscopy. The urine contains large amounts of fluffy white debris that was loosely adherent to the bladder wall.

Lymph Nodes: All were <1 cm in diameter.

Laboratory Findings: Urinalysis: SGr 1.030; pH 6.0, 75 mg/dL protein, 1000 mg/dL glucose, no ketones or bilirubin, 250 erythrocytes/μL hemoprotein, >100 WBC/HPF, >100 RBC/HPF, few transitional and squamous epithelial cells, many budding yeast organisms

Microbiologic Testing: Aerobic bacterial urine culture: 10^5 organisms/mL *Candida albicans* were cultured.

Yeast antifungal drug susceptibility panel: Susceptible to 5-flucytosine (0.5 μg/mL), caspofungin (0.25 μg/mL), fluconazole (0.25 μg/mL), itraconazole (0.06 μg/mL), voriconazole (0.015 μg/mL). Minimum inhibitory concentrations for amphotericin B and posaconazole were 0.5 μg/mL

Continued

and 0.03 μg/mL, respectively (no interpretative criteria available).

Diagnosis: Susceptible *C. albicans* UTI.

Treatment: Lizzie was treated with fluconazole (50 mg PO q12h). At a recheck examination 10 days later, the owner reported ongoing pollakiuria and incontinence. A fungal urine culture again revealed 10^5 *C. albicans*/mL with a similar susceptibility profile. Addition of flucytosine was recommended (250 mg PO q8h) but was considered unaffordable to the owners. Treatment was continued for another month with little clinical improvement and persistence of infection. A blood glucose curve revealed two-hourly blood glucose concentrations that were "high", 470, 368, 300, 383, and 423 mg/dL, respectively, so the insulin dose was increased to 4 U q12h. Two weeks later the owner described some improvement in the urinary incontinence and reduction in stranguria, but again 10^5 *C. albicans*/mL was cultured from the urine, and persistent urine scalding was noted around the perineum and on the pelvic limbs on physical examination. Body weight was 3.8 kg, and a blood glucose curve revealed two-hourly blood glucose concentrations that were 457, 301, 209, 227, 300, and 296 mg/dL, respectively.

Topical treatment with clotrimazole was elected. Before the procedure was performed, a preanesthetic evaluation was done. A CBC showed a normocytic, normochromic, nonregenerative anemia (HCT 28.3%; RR, 30%-50%), mature neutrophilia (15,206 cells/μL; RR, 2000-9000 cells/μL), lymphopenia (919 cells/μL; 1000-7000 cells/μL), and monocytopenia (33 cells/μL; 50-600 cells/μL). A serum biochemistry profile was unremarkable with the exceptions of a BUN concentration of 49 mg/dL (18-33 mg/dL) and a glucose concentration of 314 mg/dL (63-118 mg/dL). Urinalysis showed a specific gravity of 1.022; pH 6.0, 25 mg/dL protein, 1000 mg/dL glucose, 0-2 WBC/HPF, 0-2 RBC/HPF, and moderate numbers of budding yeast organisms and fungal structures. Thoracic radiographs revealed mild cardiomegaly and a diffuse, static bronchial pattern consistent with the previous diagnosis of feline bronchial disease. Abdominal ultrasound findings included an enlarged and hyperechoic liver, mild diffuse thickening of the gastrointestinal mucosa and submucosa, decreased renal corticomedullary distinction bilaterally with thickening of the renal cortices, a markedly thickened and irregular urinary bladder wall that contained hypoechoic, ill-defined nodules, and thick sediment within the urinary bladder lumen. Cystoscopy revealed a large amount of white, fluffy debris adherent to an edematous bladder wall as well as in the lumen (Figure 67-3, *B*). A 10F Foley catheter was placed over a 0.025-inch guidewire. The bladder was flushed and the majority of the debris removed. A total of 47 mL of 1% clotrimazole solution was infused into the bladder, and the solution was allowed to remain in place for 1 hour. The solution was removed and Lizzie was allowed to recover from anesthesia. Treatment with fluconazole was continued, although the dose was lowered (25 mg PO q12h). At a recheck 2 weeks later, the owners reported that Lizzie was more active and was no longer pollakiuric, although she still urinated outside the litter box and intermittent vomiting had been noted. A CBC, biochemistry panel, and urinalysis revealed nonregenerative anemia (HCT 21.2%); lymphopenia (349 cells/μL); monocytopenia (70 cells/μL); increased activities of serum ALT (1028 U/L; RR, 27-101 U/L), AST (226 U/L; RR, 17-58 U/L), and ALP (223 U/L; RR, 14-17 U/L); hypercholesterolemia (324 U/L; RR, 89-258 U/L); and hyperbilirubinemia (0.7 mg/dL; RR, 0-0.2 mg/dL). Aerobic bacterial urine culture revealed more than 10^5 CFU/mL of hemolytic *E. coli*, and fungal culture of the urine was negative. The fluconazole was discontinued, after which the vomiting ceased and liver enzyme activities returned to reference ranges. Multiple bacterial UTIs were diagnosed over the following 6 months, but *Candida* was never again isolated from the urine.

Comments: In this cat, the *C. albicans* UTI may have occurred secondary to a combination of factors that likely included poorly controlled diabetes mellitus, chronic kidney disease, neurologic disease, and repeated treatment with broad-spectrum antimicrobial drugs. Systemic antifungal drug treatment and improved control of diabetes mellitus were initially used as treatment strategies but failed, probably because of the large mats of fungus that were adherent to the bladder wall. Fortunately, a single topical clotrimazole treatment resulted in resolution of the yeast infection. The hepatopathy that developed was thought to be secondary to fluconazole toxicity, since it resolved when the drug was discontinued.

SUGGESTED READINGS

Cheng SC, Joosten LA, Kullberg BJ, et al. Interplay between *Candida albicans* and the mammalian innate host defense. Infect Immun. 2012;80:1304-1313.

Ong RK, Raisis AL, Swindells KL. *Candida albicans* peritonitis in a dog. J Vet Emerg Crit Care (San Antonio). 2010;20:143-147.

Pressler BM, Vaden SL, Lane IF, et al. *Candida* spp. urinary tract infections in 13 dogs and seven cats: predisposing factors, treatment, and outcome. J Am Anim Hosp Assoc. 2003;39:263-270.

REFERENCES

1. Barnett JA. A history of research on yeasts 12: medical yeasts part 1, *Candida albicans*. Yeast. 2008;25:385-417.
2. Pressler BM, Vaden SL, Lane IF, et al. *Candida* spp. urinary tract infections in 13 dogs and seven cats: predisposing factors, treatment, and outcome. J Am Anim Hosp Assoc. 2003;39:263-270.
3. Heseltine JC, Panciera DL, Saunders GK. Systemic candidiasis in a dog. J Am Vet Med Assoc. 2003;223:821-824:810.
4. Ong RK, Raisis AL, Swindells KL. *Candida albicans* peritonitis in a dog. J Vet Emerg Crit Care (San Antonio). 2010;20:143-147.
5. Rogers CL, Gibson C, Mitchell SL, et al. Disseminated candidiasis secondary to fungal and bacterial peritonitis in a young dog. J Vet Emerg Crit Care (San Antonio). 2009;19:193-198.
6. Jin Y, Lin D. Fungal urinary tract infections in the dog and cat: a retrospective study (2001-2004). J Am Anim Hosp Assoc. 2005;41:373-381.
7. Boutilier P, Carr A. Fungal colonization and failure of a long-term gastrostomy tube in a cat. Can Vet J. 2005;46:709-710.
8. Mueller RS, Bettenay SV, Shipstone M. Cutaneous candidiasis in a dog caused by *Candida guilliermondii*. Vet Rec. 2002;150:728-730.
9. Dale JE. Canine dermatosis caused by *Candida parapsilosis*. Vet Med Small Anim Clin. 1972;67:548-549.

10. Ozawa H, Okabayashi K, Kano R, et al. Rapid identification of *Candida tropicalis* from canine cystitis. Mycopathologia. 2005;160:159-162.
11. Sykes JE. Unpublished observations, 2012.
12. Gerding Jr PA, Morton LD, Dye JA. Ocular and disseminated candidiasis in an immunosuppressed cat. J Am Vet Med Assoc. 1994;204:1635-1638.
13. Mohri T, Takashima K, Yamane T, et al. Purulent pericarditis in a dog administered immune-suppressing drugs. J Vet Med Sci. 2009;71:669-672.
14. Ochiai K, Valentine BA, Altschul M. Intestinal candidiasis in a dog. Vet Rec. 2000;146:228-229.
15. Rodriguez F, Fernandez A, Espinosa de los Monteros A, et al. Acute disseminated candidiasis in a puppy associated with parvoviral infection. Vet Rec. 1998;142:434-436.
16. Langheinrich KA, Nielsen SW. Histopathology of feline panleukopenia: a report of 65 cases. J Am Vet Med Assoc. 1971;158:suppl 2:863+.
17. Matsuda K, Sakaguchi K, Kobayashi S, et al. Systemic candidiasis and mesenteric mast cell tumor with multiple metastases in a dog. J Vet Med Sci. 2009;71:229-232.
18. Miller WW, Albert RA. Ocular and systemic candidiasis in a cat. J Am Anim Hosp Assoc. 1988;24:521-524.
19. Lorenzini R, De Bernardis F. Antemortem diagnosis of an apparent case of feline candidiasis. Mycopathologia. 1986;93:13-14.
20. Brown MR, Thompson CA, Mohamed FM. Systemic candidiasis in an apparently immunocompetent dog. J Vet Diagn Invest. 2005;17:272-276.
21. Ling GV, Norris CR, Franti CE, et al. Interrelations of organism prevalence, specimen collection method, and host age, sex, and breed among 8,354 canine urinary tract infections (1969-1995). J Vet Intern Med. 2001;15:341-347.
22. Norris CR, Williams BJ, Ling GV, et al. Recurrent and persistent urinary tract infections in dogs: 383 cases (1969-1995). J Am Anim Hosp Assoc. 2000;36:484-492.
23. Karkowska-Kuleta J, Rapala-Kozik M, Kozik A. Fungi pathogenic to humans: molecular bases of virulence of *Candida albicans, Cryptococcus neoformans* and *Aspergillus fumigatus*. Acta Biochim Pol. 2009;56:211-224.
24. Cheng SC, Joosten LA, Kullberg BJ, et al. Interplay between *Candida albicans* and the mammalian innate host defense. Infect Immun. 2012;80:1304-1313.
25. Holoymoen JI, Bjerkas I, Olberg IH, et al. Disseminated candidiasis (moniliasis) in a dog. A case report. Nord Vet Med. 1982;34:362-367.
26. Skoric M, Fictum P, Slana I, et al. A case of systemic mycosis in a Hovawart dog due to *Candida albicans*. Veterinarni Medicina. 2011;56:260-264.
27. Kuwamura M, Ide M, Yamate J, et al. Systemic candidiasis in a dog, developing spondylitis. J Vet Med Sci. 2006;68:1117-1119.
28. Linek J. Mycotic endophthalmitis in a dog caused by *Candida albicans*. Vet Ophthalmol. 2004;7:159-162.
29. Rosenvinge FS, Dzajic E, Knudsen E, et al. Performance of matrix-assisted laser desorption-time of flight mass spectrometry for identification of clinical yeast isolates. Mycoses. 2012.
30. Toll J, Ashe CM, Trepanier LA. Intravesicular administration of clotrimazole for treatment of candiduria in a cat with diabetes mellitus. J Am Vet Med Assoc. 2003;223:1156-1158:1129.
31. Forward ZA, Legendre AM, Khalsa HD. Use of intermittent bladder infusion with clotrimazole for treatment of candiduria in a dog. J Am Vet Med Assoc. 2002;220:1496-1498:1474-1495.
32. Azie N, Neofytos D, Pfaller M, et al. The PATH (Prospective Antifungal Therapy) Alliance registry and invasive fungal infections: update 2012. Diagn Microbiol Infect Dis. 2012;73:293-300.
33. Pappas PG. Invasive candidiasis. Infect Dis Clin North Am. 2006;20:485-506.
34. Ben Abdeljelil J, Saghrouni F, Emira N, et al. Molecular typing of *Candida albicans* isolates from patients and health care workers in a neonatal intensive care unit. J Appl Microbiol. 2011;111:1235-1249.

CHAPTER 68

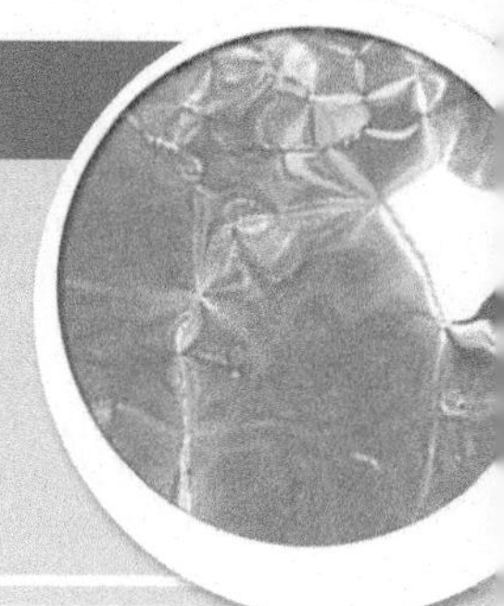

Miscellaneous Fungal Diseases

Amy M. Grooters

In contrast to the well-recognized fungal pathogens that cause endemic mycoses (such as *Blastomyces, Histoplasma,* and *Cryptococcus*), miscellaneous fungal pathogens comprise large groups of fungi with unfamiliar names that traditionally have caused disease only sporadically. These opportunistic fungi have low inherent virulence and typically cause infection only when normal host resistance mechanisms are compromised. Over the past 30 years, these opportunists have become increasingly important in human patients because immunocompromise associated with chemotherapy, organ transplantation, and HIV infection has become more prevalent. Similarly, over the past 5 to 10 years, the frequency with which opportunistic fungal infections are encountered in small animal patients has increased significantly in association with the use of multiagent immunosuppressive therapy (especially with cyclosporine) to treat immune-mediated disease in dogs. Thus, veterinarians are increasingly likely to encounter patients infected by an opportunistic fungal pathogen with which they are unfamiliar.

Unlike the common endemic fungal pathogens (for which a definitive diagnosis can often be made simply by visualizing the unique morphologic features of the organism in cytologic or histologic samples), opportunistic fungi can only be identified to genus and species level by culture or molecular methods. However, they can be assigned to categories based on their morphologic features in tissue, such as pigmentation, hyphal diameter, and frequency of septation. These categories include *phaeohyphomycosis* (pigmented hyphal or yeast forms), *hyalohyphomycosis* (nonpigmented hyphal forms), *eumycotic mycetoma* (fibrosing granuloma with black or white tissue grains consisting of aggregates of pigmented or nonpigmented fungi, respectively), and *zygomycosis* (wide, infrequently septate, nonpigmented hyphae associated with pyogranulomatous and eosinophilic inflammation). Because of its similarities to pythiosis and lagenidiosis, zygomycosis is discussed in Chapter 69. Although identification of a specific pathogen after culture is ideal, classification of opportunistic mycoses based on the categories just listed is usually sufficient to allow the clinician to make a reasonable prediction about clinical course and prognosis and to make appropriate treatment decisions. Because many opportunistic fungi are common contaminants and can normally be found on skin, nasal mucosa, and other nonsterile sites, culture- or PCR-based identification of a potential opportunistic fungal pathogen from a skin specimen, nasal swab, or exudate should not be considered evidence of fungal infection unless there is supportive histologic or cytologic evidence of tissue invasion by a morphologically compatible organism.

Overview of Phaeohyphomycoses

Causes: *Alternaria, Bipolaris, Cladophialophora, Curvularia, Exophiala, Fonsecaea, Moniliella, Phialophora, Ramichloridium, Ulocladium,* and *Scolecobasidium,* among many others

Affected Hosts: A variety of animal hosts that include dogs, cats, horses, and humans

Geographic Distribution: Worldwide

Mode of Transmission: Cutaneous inoculation of organisms from the environment

Major Clinical Signs: Localized cutaneous nodules that may appear pigmented, often on the nose or digits; occasionally meningoencephalitis, with associated neurologic signs

Differential Diagnosis: Neoplasia, cryptococcosis, blastomycosis, sporotrichosis, hyalohyphomycosis, zygomycosis, mycobacterial infections, actinomycosis, nocardiosis

Human Health Significance: Direct transmission from animals to humans has not been described; humans develop infections from environmental sources.

Phaeohyphomycosis

Etiology and Epidemiology

The term "phaeohyphomycosis" refers to cutaneous, subcutaneous, cerebral, or disseminated infections caused by pigmented (also known as dematiaceous) fungi that contain melanin in their cell walls.[1] Infection usually results from cutaneous inoculation. Fungal genera that have been identified as agents of phaeohyphomycosis in veterinary patients include *Alternaria, Bipolaris, Cladophialophora, Curvularia, Exophiala, Fonsecaea, Moniliella, Phialophora, Ramichloridium, Ulocladium,* and *Scolecobasidium,* among others (Table 68-1).

Clinical Features

The most common clinical manifestations of phaeohyphomycosis in immunocompetent small animals are lesions associated with the digits, pinnae, nasal planum, or nasal cavity in cats (Figure 68-1).[2-8] Cutaneous lesions occur less often in dogs.[9] In addition, granulomatous meningoencephalitis caused by pigmented fungi

TABLE 68-1

Causative Agents and Histologic/Cytologic Characteristics Associated with Miscellaneous Fungal and Pseudofungal Pathogens

Disease	Causative Agents	Histologic and Cytologic Characteristics
Phaeohyphomycosis	*Alternaria, Bipolaris, Phialophora, Cladophialophora (Cladosporium), Curvularia, Exophiala, Fonsecaea, Moniliella, Ochroconis, Ramichloridium,* others	Pyogranulomatous inflammation associated with pigmented, irregularly septate hyphae or yeast-like cells that may be solitary or may cluster in small groups or chains
Hyalohyphomycosis	*Acremonium, Fusarium, Geotrichum, Geosmithia, Paecilomyces, Phialosimplex, Pseudallescheria, Sagenomella, Scedosporium, Schizophyllum,* others	Pyogranulomatous inflammation associated with hyphal elements that have nonpigmented (transparent, hyaline) walls; *Phialosimplex* may cause yeast-like forms in tissue
Mycetoma (black-grain)	*Curvularia*	Pyogranulomatous inflammation associated with aggregates of pigmented fungal organisms (which appear grossly as pigmented tissue grains)
Mycetoma (white-grain)	*Pseudallescheria boydii, Acremonium*	Pyogranulomatous inflammation associated with aggregates of nonpigmented fungal organisms (which appear grossly as nonpigmented tissue grains)
Pythiosis	*Pythium insidiosum*	Pyogranulomatous and eosinophilic inflammation associated with broad (2-7 µm), infrequently septate hyphae (see Chapter 69)
Lagenidiosis	*Lagenidium*	Pyogranulomatous and eosinophilic inflammation associated with broad (4-25 µm), infrequently septate hyphae (see Chapter 69)
Zygomycosis	*Conidiobolus* spp., *Basidiobolus ranarum* in dogs; *Rhizomucor, Mucor,* and *Cokeromyces* in cats	Pyogranulomatous and eosinophilic inflammation associated with broad (5-20 µm), infrequently septate hyphae with thick prominent eosinophilic sleeve (see Chapter 69)
Aspergillosis	*Aspergillus terreus, A. deflectus, A. flavipes, A. fumigatus,* others	Suppurative to granulomatous inflammation associated with multiple, nonpigmented, 3- to 6-µm, septate hyphae with parallel walls and 45-degree angle branching (see Chapter 65)
Candidiasis	*Candida albicans,* other *Candida* spp.	Suppurative inflammation with numerous 2- to 6-µm oval yeasts, pseudohyphae (chains of oval yeast cells), and true hyphae (see Chapter 67)

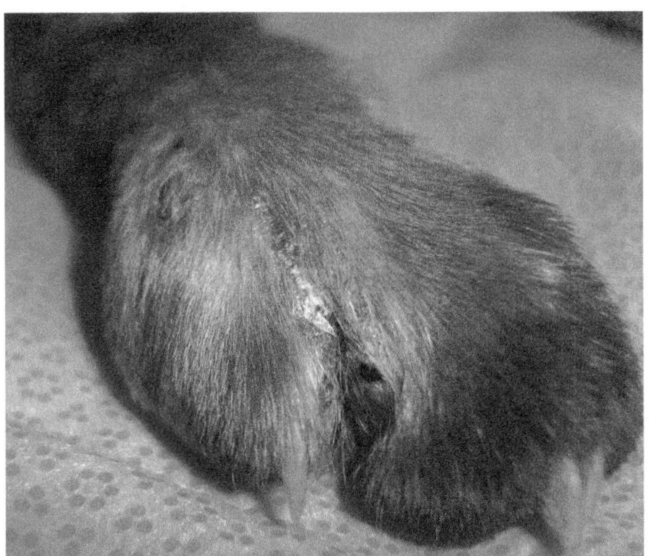

FIGURE 68-1 Left distal thoracic limb of an 8-year-old male neutered Burmese cat with digital phaeohyphomycosis. (Courtesy University of California, Davis, Veterinary Dermatology Service.)

(especially *Cladophialophora bantiana*) have been described both in dogs and cats.[10-14] In immunocompromised patients, the most common presentation appears to be multifocal cutaneous lesions in dogs treated with multiagent immunosuppressive therapy, especially that which includes cyclosporine.[15-17]

Animals with phaeohyphomycosis typically have cutaneous nodules or a visible nasal mass. Infected tissues may appear grossly pigmented, and thus masses may be confused with melanomas. Phaeohyphomycoses tend to be locally invasive and may extend to involve regional lymph nodes (Figure 68-2). Systemic dissemination more often occurs in animals treated with immunosuppressive drugs, but disseminated infections have also been described in apparently immunocompetent patients.[18,19] Animals with central nervous system (CNS) phaeohyphomycosis may have neurologic signs such as obtundation, seizures, abnormal placing reactions, circling, tremors, ataxia, and abnormal cranial nerve function.

Diagnosis

Laboratory and Imaging Abnormalities

Results of a CBC, biochemistry panel, and urinalysis in animals with cutaneous phaeohyphomycoses are typically unremarkable. Animals with disseminated disease can have abnormalities

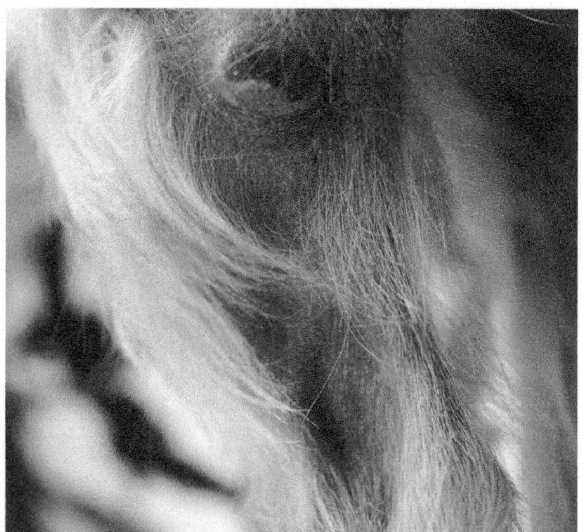

FIGURE 68-2 Popliteal lymphadenopathy and abscessation caused by *Curvularia* spp. infection in a 1-year-old female Yorkshire terrier with cutaneous phaeohyphomycosis. (Courtesy Amy Grooters, Louisiana State University, Baton Rouge, LA.)

associated with underlying immunosuppressive illness or drug treatment. Imaging with computed tomography (CT) or MRI in animals with CNS involvement may reveal focal or multifocal contrast-enhancing lesions that may be associated with hydrocephalus (Figure 68-3).

Cytologic and Histologic Findings

On histologic or cytologic examination, fungi that cause phaeohyphomycosis appear as dark-walled, irregularly septate hyphae or as yeast-like cells, solitary or in small groups or chains (Figure 68-4). Pigmentation may not always be apparent on cytologic examination (Figure 68-5). The presence of melanin in the walls of lightly-pigmented hyphae can be confirmed by the examination of unstained sections, by lowering the microscope condenser during examination, or by utilization of a Fontana-Masson stain for melanin.

Culture

Organisms that cause phaeohyphomycosis are readily isolated on routine fungal culture of infected tissue biopsies as well as from fine-needle aspirate specimens from infected lymph nodes. Further identification is based on colony and conidial morphology (see also Figure 4-7, *B*) and PCR and sequencing of ribosomal RNA genes. Because pigmented fungi are common laboratory contaminants and can sometimes be isolated from nonsterile sites on healthy animals (such as skin), positive cultures from potentially contaminated sites should only be considered significant if accompanied by cytologic or histologic evidence of fungal infection with a morphologically compatible organism.

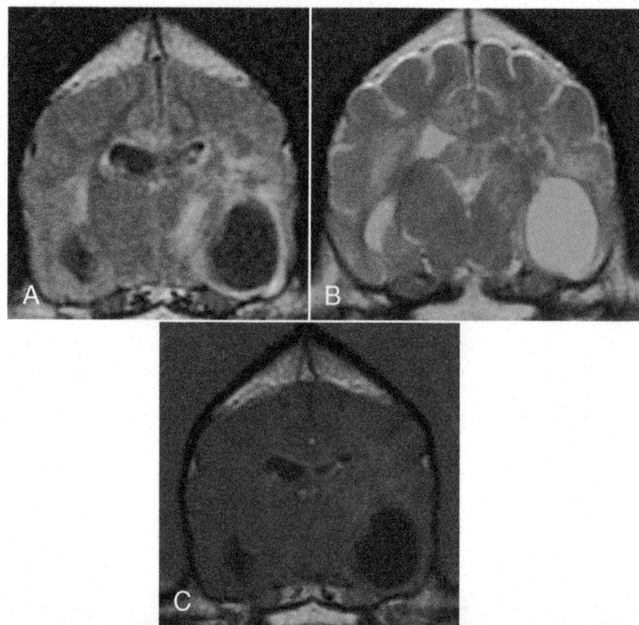

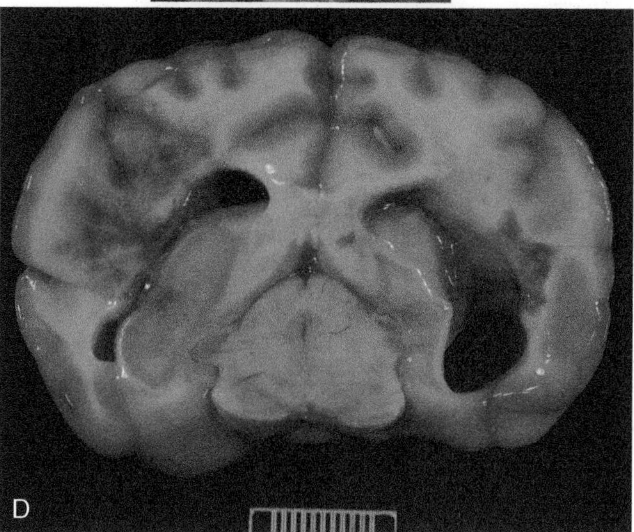

FIGURE 68-3 Axial T1 postcontrast, T2, and FLAIR magnetic resonance images (**A, B,** and **C**, respectively) of the brain of a 6-year-old male neutered Border collie mix that was evaluated for neurologic signs including seizures and progressive obtundation. In the images shown, there is bilateral but asymmetric ventricular dilation that is severe on the right and mild to moderate on the left (asymmetric hydrocephalus). Multifocal regions of contrast enhancement are also present (**A**). Some of these regions appeared nodular; others had a ring-like appearance. There is also marked contrast enhancement of the ventricular ependymal lining. The regions of contrast enhancement correlate with regions of T2 and FLAIR hyperintensity (**B** and **C**) and were isointense on precontrast T1-weighted sequences (not shown). Meningoencephalitis caused by *Cladophialophora bantiana* and secondary hydrocephalus was diagnosed on brain biopsy and at necropsy (**D**). Olive-green pigmented masses can be seen on both the left and right sides of the brain. Interestingly, the dog also had cutaneous protothecosis. (Courtesy University of California, Davis, Veterinary Neurology and Anatomic Pathology Services.)

Treatment and Prognosis

Pigmented fungi are often poorly responsive to medical therapy, in part because melanin is a virulence factor. Aggressive surgical resection is the treatment of choice for solitary cutaneous phaeohyphomycosis lesions. The surgeon should attempt to obtain wide margins at the time of the initial surgery. Digit amputation is usually indicated for lesions of the distal phalanx. Medical therapy with itraconazole or posaconazole is recommended for 3 to 6 months after surgery, because recurrence of disease at the surgical site is common.

For nonresectable lesions, treatment with itraconazole (10 mg/kg/day) often results in partial or complete resolution of cutaneous lesions, but recurrence is very common, so prolonged courses (6 to 12 months) should be recommended. Voriconazole or posaconazole may be more effective than itraconazole for the treatment of phaeohyphomycosis but are significantly

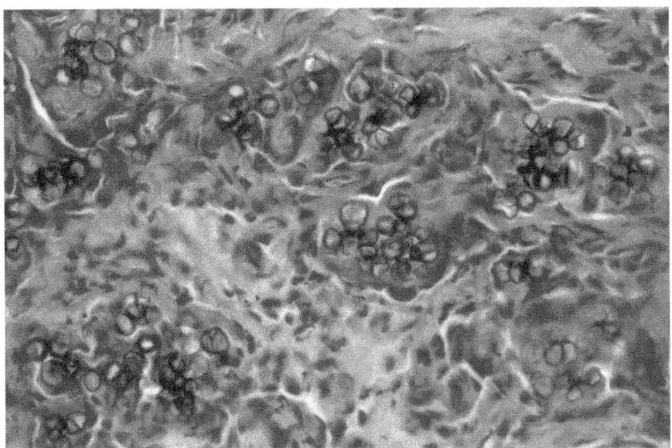

FIGURE 68-4 Histopathology showing small groups of pigmented, yeast-like fungal organisms in tissue from a nasal mass in a cat with phaeohyphomycosis; H&E stain. (Courtesy Amy Grooters, Louisiana State University, Baton Rouge, LA.)

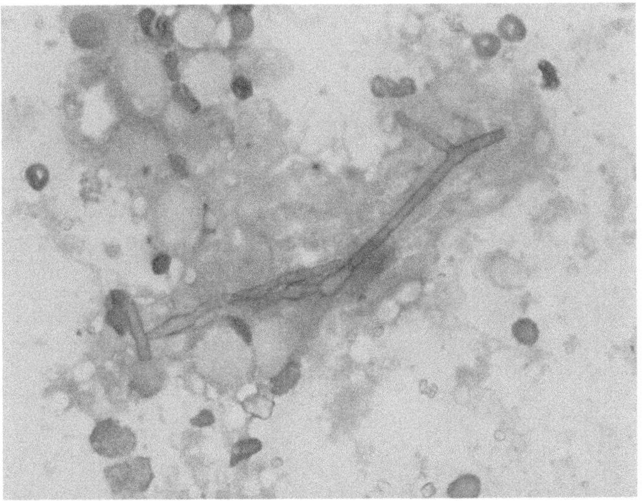

FIGURE 68-5 Impression smear from the brain of the dog in Figure 68-3. Septate, branching hyphae are present, but pigmentation is not clearly apparent. Wright's stain, 1000× magnification. (Courtesy University of California, Davis, Veterinary Pathology Service.)

more expensive. In addition, voriconazole administration is not recommended in cats because of significant adverse effects (see Chapter 9). Recently, long-term voriconazole therapy (7 to 10 mg/kg/day for 10 to 12 months) was used successfully to treat intracranial phaeohyphomycosis in one dog[10] and mycotic peritonitis caused by *Exophiala* in another.[20] Early combination therapy with amphotericin B, flucytosine, and extended-spectrum azoles has been recommended for treatment of human patients with CNS infections,[21] but flucytosine can be prohibitively expensive and is generally not tolerated by dogs (see Chapter 9).

In the author's experience, cutaneous phaeohyphomycosis that occurs in dogs receiving immunosuppressive drug therapy can be resolved in many cases with itraconazole (10 mg/kg/day) administered for at least 6 months if the immunosuppressive drug therapy can be tapered quickly. However, dissemination of disease can also occur, sometimes despite appropriate antifungal therapy. Discontinuation of cyclosporine treatment in these animals appears to be important for achieving a good outcome.

Public Health Aspects

Phaeohyphomycosis in humans clinically resembles that in dogs and cats and may include localized cutaneous lesions in immunocompetent hosts; life-threatening CNS infections in immunocompromised or apparently immunocompetent hosts (especially brain abscesses caused by *C. bantiana*); and, rarely, disseminated phaeohyphomycosis, primarily in immunocompromised hosts.[21] Infections caused by pigmented fungi are acquired from the environment. Although there is no evidence of transmission between mammalian hosts, routine precautions (such as wearing gloves when handling infected tissues or exudate) should be followed. Precautions should also be taken to prevent needlestick injuries if phaeohyphomycosis is suspected.

Overview of Hyalohyphomycoses

Causes: *Acremonium, Fusarium, Geotrichum, Paecilomyces, Pseudallescheria, Sagenomella, Scedosporium,* others

Affected Hosts: A variety of animal hosts that include dogs, cats, and humans

Geographic Distribution: Worldwide

Mode of Transmission: Inhalation or cutaneous inoculation of organisms in the environment

Major Clinical Signs: Keratitis; cutaneous lesions; osteomyelitis; pneumonia; disseminated disease with involvement of lymph nodes, kidneys, liver, spleen, bone, intervertebral discs, and/or CNS

Differential Diagnosis: Neoplasia, aspergillosis, penicilliosis, phaeohyphomycoses, sporotrichosis, cryptococcosis, blastomycosis, candidiasis, endemic mycoses, nocardiosis, actinomycosis, mycobacteriosis, zygomycosis

Human Health Significance: Direct transmission from animals to humans has not been described; humans develop infections from environmental sources.

Hyalohyphomycosis

Etiology and Epidemiology

The term "hyalohyphomycosis" refers to infections caused by fungi that are nonpigmented (hyaline or transparent) in tissue. Genera that have been described as agents of hyalohyphomycosis in veterinary patients include *Fusarium, Acremonium, Paecilomyces* (especially *Paecilomyces variotii* and *Paecilomyces lilacinus*), *Pseudallescheria boydii* (anamorph *Scedosporium apiospermum*), *Sagenomella, Phialosimplex, Geosmithia,* and *Geomyces,* among others (see Table 68-1). By convention, infections caused by *Aspergillus* and *Penicillium* species are not included in the term "hyalohyphomycosis," because aspergillosis and penicilliosis can usually be identified as such based on their clinicopathologic features. In general, hyalohyphomycosis occurs more often in dogs than in cats.

Clinical Features

Hyalohyphomycosis ranges from a local disease confined to the skin (Figure 68-6), nasal mucosa, or cornea to osteomyelitis,

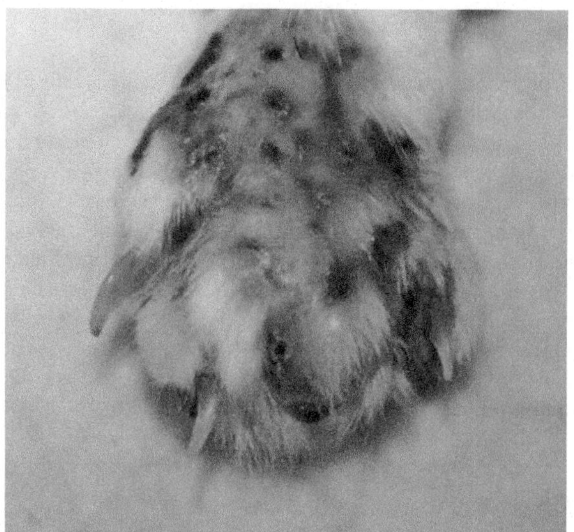

FIGURE 68-6 *Scedosporium prolificans* infection in a domestic shorthair cat. There are multiple draining skin lesions and soft tissue swelling. (Courtesy Spencer Jang, University of California, Davis.)

pneumonia, and disseminated disease that can involve one or more organs including the kidneys, bone marrow, lymph nodes, liver, spleen, bones, intervertebral discs, and CNS, sometimes with associated fungemia.[22-30]

Traditionally, the disseminated and corneal forms of hyalohyphomycosis have been most commonly identified. Therefore, animals with no overt signs of systemic disease that present with cutaneous or bone lesions that contain nonpigmented hyphae should still be evaluated for occult lesions in the chest and abdomen. Like phaeohyphomycosis, hyalohyphomycosis is an increasingly common cause of multifocal skin lesions in dogs receiving multiagent immunosuppressive therapy. These dogs may or may not have accompanying extracutaneous lesions.

Diagnosis

Cytologic and Histologic Findings

Cytologically and histologically, fungi that cause hyalohyphomycosis are nonpigmented, frequently septate, branching hyphae that are often pleomorphic (Figures 68-7 and Figure 4-6). Special stains such as periodic acid–Schiff and Gomori's methenamine silver may be used to identify organisms more readily.

Culture

The fungi that cause hyalohyphomycosis are readily isolated by routine fungal culture methods from infected tissues as well as from fine-needle aspirate specimens from infected lymph nodes, bones, or abdominal organs. Because these fungi are common laboratory contaminants and can sometimes be isolated from the skin or hair of healthy animals, positive cultures from nonsterile sites should be considered significant only if accompanied by cytologic or histologic evidence of fungal infection with a morphologically compatible organism. Species identification is based on conidial morphology (Figure 68-8) and may require PCR and sequencing of ribosomal RNA genes. Species identification may assist in selection of antifungal drug treatments, because some species are predictably less susceptible to conventional antifungal drugs (see Treatment and Prognosis). Proper identification and antifungal drug susceptibility testing are best performed by laboratories that specialize in mycoses (e.g., the

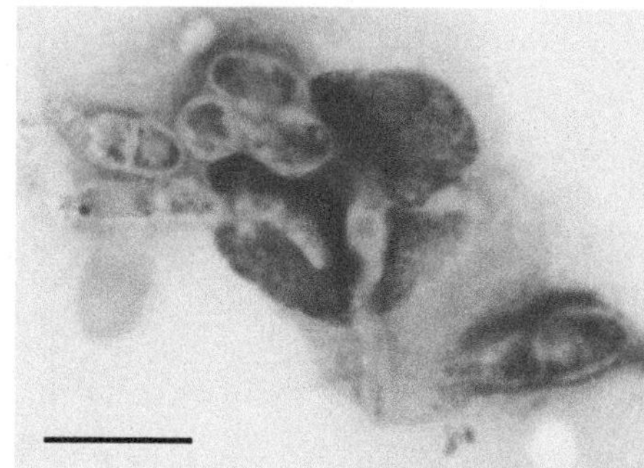

FIGURE 68-7 Fine needle aspirate cytology from a lytic bone lesion in a 4-year-old female spayed mixed breed dog with hyalohyphomycosis. Note the septate, nonpigmented fungal hyphae present within the macrophage; Wright-Giemsa stain, bar = 10 µm. (Courtesy Kaikhushroo Banajee, Louisiana State University, Baton Rouge, LA.)

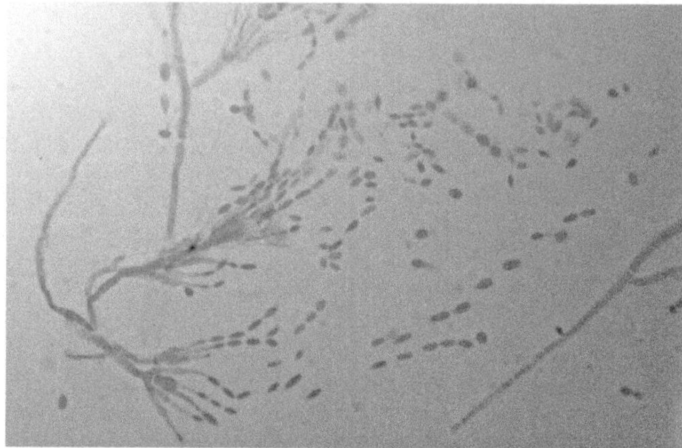

FIGURE 68-8 Cytologic appearance of *Paecilomyces variotii* growing in culture in the laboratory. Lactophenol cotton blue, 1000× magnification. (Courtesy Spencer Jang, University of California, Davis.)

University of Texas Health Science Center at San Antonio) and may be useful for selection of treatments for difficult cases. Nevertheless, evidence that supports a correlation between in vitro susceptibility data and clinical response to treatment is lacking.

Antigen Testing

The Platelia *Aspergillus* galactomannan antigen ELISA assay is positive in some, but not all, animals with hyalohyphomycoses such as paecilomycosis. This results from antigenic cross-reactivity (see Chapter 65).[31] In most dogs with disseminated paecilomycosis that test positive, the magnitude of positive results is somewhat lower than those in dogs with disseminated aspergillosis, but occasionally results are strongly positive (galactomannan indices >6).

Treatment and Prognosis

Treatment of hyalohyphomycosis has traditionally been challenging because many animals have disseminated disease. Drugs used most often to treat hyalohyphomycosis in small animals include itraconazole and amphotericin B, but different fungal species vary in their susceptibility to antifungal drugs, and some species, such as *Pseudallescheria boydii* and *Paecilomyces lilacinus,* are relatively resistant to conventional antifungal drugs in vitro.[32,33] The newer triazoles, voriconazole and posaconazole, and the echinocandins, such as caspofungin, may be more active against these fungi than itraconazole but are significantly more expensive. In contrast, *Paecilomyces variotii* is usually susceptible to amphotericin B but is less susceptible to voriconazole. Although treatment of disseminated hyalohyphomycosis with antifungal drugs can prolong survival, clinical signs often recur even if signs initially resolve. Therefore, disseminated hyalohyphomycosis generally carries a guarded to poor prognosis.

Cutaneous hyalohyphomycosis that develops in an animal receiving immunosuppressive drug therapy may respond well to oral azole antifungal drugs or may rapidly disseminate. Therefore, fungal skin lesions that develop in immunocompromised patients should be treated aggressively, and a guarded prognosis should be offered. This author most often uses itraconazole (10 mg/kg/day) administered orally for at least 6 months. Other options include amphotericin B, voriconazole, or posaconazole. Combination therapies have been recommended for difficult cases in human patients.[21] Discontinuation of cyclosporine and rapid tapering of other immunosuppressive medications in these patients appears to be important for achievement of a good outcome.

Public Health Aspects

Hyalohyphomycosis in humans is acquired as a result of infection by fungi in the environment. Keratitis and nailbed infections (onychomycosis) can occur in immunocompetent humans. Invasive infections occur in immunocompromised patients such as transplant recipients, patients with AIDS, and leukemic or neutropenic patients. Although there is no evidence to suggest that transmission between mammalian hosts is possible, routine precautions (such as wearing gloves when handling infected tissues or exudate) should be followed. Precautions should especially be taken to prevent needle-stick injuries if hyalohyphomycosis is suspected.

Eumycotic Mycetoma

The term "mycetoma" refers to localized mycotic or actinomycotic infections of the skin, subcutaneous tissue, muscle, or bone that are characterized by the presence of colonies or aggregates of organisms that form "grains" in tissue. Actinomycotic mycetomas are caused by bacteria such as *Actinomyces* spp. or *Nocardia* spp. (see Chapters 42 and 43), dermatophytic mycetomas are caused by dermatophytes (see Chapter 58), and eumycotic mycetomas are caused by nondermatophyte fungi. Lesions result from traumatic implantation of soil organisms into tissue. The grains or granules of eumycotic mycetomas are pigmented (for black-grain mycetoma, caused by dematiaceous fungi) or hyaline (for white-grain mycetoma, caused by nonpigmented fungi), depending on the type of fungal pathogen involved (see Table 68-1).

Black-grain mycetomas are most often caused by *Curvularia* species and typically are associated with chronic nonhealing wounds and cutaneous nodules on the extremities. Lesions often develop weeks to months after a traumatic incident in the same area. Draining tracts are often present, and black grains may be observed in the exudate. White-grain mycetomas, usually caused by *Pseudallescheria boydii* or *Acremonium* spp., most often occur as body-wall and/or intra-abdominal granulomas that develop subsequent to surgical wound contamination or dehiscence. Interestingly, the lesions associated with white-grain mycetoma may not be evident until months or even a year or more after the surgical event. Affected dogs may be evaluated for a draining mass on the body wall or clinical signs of peritonitis.

The treatment of choice for eumycotic mycetoma is aggressive surgical excision of infected tissues, including amputation if clinically indicated. Response to medical therapy is generally poor, but administration of itraconazole, voriconazole, or posaconazole may be considered as adjunctive therapy following surgical excision when wide margins cannot be achieved. Dissemination of eumycotic mycetoma beyond local tissues is rare, but disease within the abdomen or other local tissues may be extensive. The prognosis is guarded if complete surgical resection is not possible.

CASE EXAMPLE

Signalment: "CJ", a 1-year-old male intact boxer dog from central Louisiana

History: CJ was initially evaluated for acute ataxia and abnormal limb placement. Based on results of CSF analysis as well as MRI of the brain and spinal cord, inflammatory central nervous system disease was diagnosed, and treatment with prednisone (1 mg/kg PO q12h) was initiated. Despite a good initial response, neurologic signs recurred 2 weeks later, at which time cytosine arabinoside (50 mg/m² SC q12h, for four doses, repeated every 3 weeks) and azathioprine (1.6 mg/kg PO q48h) were added to the treatment protocol. Neurologic signs again improved, but 7 weeks later, the dog was evaluated for ulcerative lesions on the distal extremities that had been present for 1 week and lethargy that had been present for 3 days.

Physical Examination:

Body Weight: 29 kg.

General: Alert and responsive, but painful on ambulation because of ulcerative lesions on all four feet. Vital parameters were within normal limits. Peripheral lymph nodes were palpably normal.

Dermatologic Examination: Pitting edema and multifocal ulcerative lesions were present on all four distal extremities, with sloughing of multiple footpads (Figure 68-9, *A* and *B*). Some of the pad lesions were proliferative and extended into the interdigital area (Figure 68-9, *C*). Multiple light brown colored areas could be visualized within the fibrinonecrotic material that covered the area of the left metacarpal pad (see Figure 68-9, *B*). In addition, a 1-cm ulcerated lesion was present on the left pinna, a crusted lesion was present on the tip of the tail, and a small subcutaneous mass was present in the right saphenous area. Larger (3 cm) ulcerated lesions partially covered with eschar were present on the medial aspect of the right tarsus and the dorsal aspect of the left antebrachium. Major differential diagnoses considered were opportunistic fungal infection and drug eruption.

Cytology and Histology Findings: Cytologic evaluation of the left pinnal lesion, subcutaneous right saphenous mass, and right popliteal lymph node revealed septic neutrophilic to pyogranulomatous inflammation with septate, branching, 3- to 7-μm fungal hyphae, both extracellularly and within neutrophils. Pigmentation of hyphae was not observed.

Continued

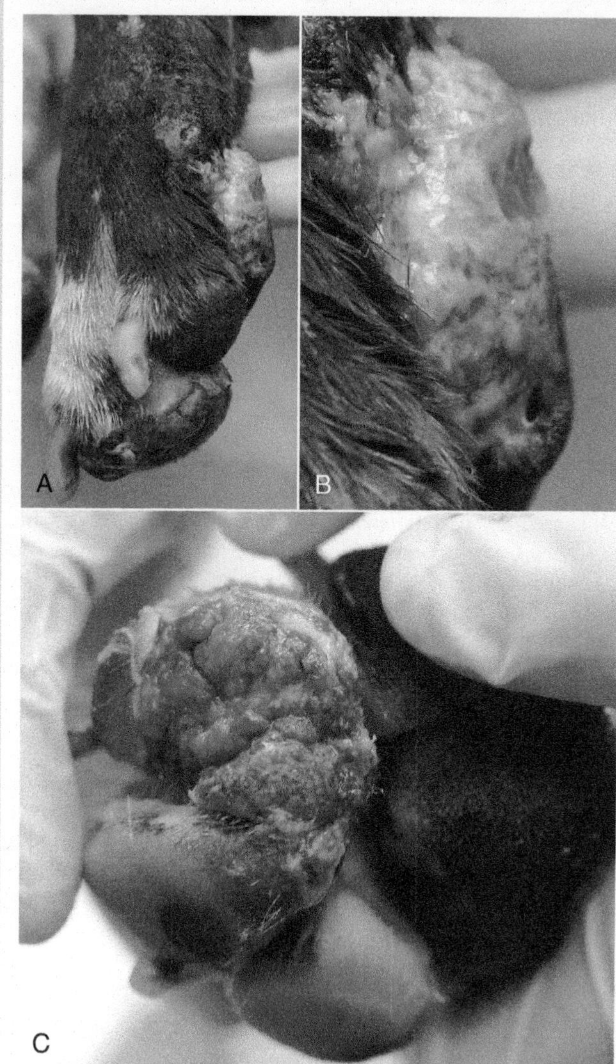

FIGURE 68-9 **A-C,** Phaeohyphomycosis of the left thoracic limb that developed after multiagent immunosuppressive therapy in 1-year-old boxer with inflammatory central nervous system disease. (Courtesy Amy Grooters, Louisiana State University, Baton Rouge, LA.)

Histologic evaluation of punch biopsies obtained from cutaneous lesions on the left front foot, right hind foot, and right forelimb revealed severe pyogranulomatous dermatitis with intralesional septate, pigmented hyphae.

Diagnosis: Disseminated cutaneous phaeohyphomycosis extending to regional lymphadenitis.

Treatment and Outcome: Pentoxifylline (30 mg/kg PO q24h) was administered because of suspected vasculitis associated with the cutaneous lesions. Antifungal therapy with itraconazole (10 mg/kg PO q24h) was initiated, but lesion progression was observed over the next several days, so lipid-complexed amphotericin B treatment (2 mg/kg diluted in 5% dextrose, IV, over several hours three times weekly) was initiated. Unfortunately, 2 days later lesions had progressed rapidly with appearance of new draining tracts and abscess formation. Because of the poor prognosis and pain associated with the lesions, the dog was euthanized.

Comments: As was noted here, pigmentation of hyphae may not always be visible on cytologic examination of lesions caused by phaeohyphomycosis, in part because hyphae and the cells that phagocytize them often take up enough color with the Wright-Giemsa stain to mask the pigmentation. Therefore, in this case, evaluation of histologic samples was important for differentiating phaeohyphomycosis from hyalohyphomycosis. Culture would have been ideal for definitive identification of the opportunistic fungal organism that caused the infection in this dog, but was not performed.

SUGGESTED READINGS

Grooters AM, Foil CS. Miscellaneous fungal infections. In: Greene CE, ed. Infectious Diseases of the Dog and Cat. 4th ed. Philadelphia, PA: WB Saunders; 2012:675-688.

Naggie S, Perfect JR. Molds: hyalohyphomycosis, phaeohyphomycosis and zygomycosis. Clin Chest Med. 2009;30:337-353.

REFERENCES

1. Revankar SG, Sutton DA. Melanized fungi in human disease. Clin Microbiol Rev. 2010;23:884-928.
2. Dye C, Johnson EM, Gruffydd-Jones TJ. *Alternaria* species infection in nine domestic cats. J Feline Med Surg. 2009;11:332-336.
3. Maeda H, Shibuya H, Yamaguchi Y, et al. Feline digital phaeohyphomycosis due to *Exophiala jeanselmei*. J Vet Med Sci. 2008;70:1395-1397.
4. Knights CB, Lee K, Rycroft AN, et al. Phaeohyphomycosis caused by *Ulocladium* species in a cat. Vet Rec. 2008;162:415-416.
5. Beccati M, Vercelli A, Peano A, et al. Phaeohyphomycosis by *Phialophora verrucosa*: first European case in a cat. Vet Rec. 2005;157:93-94.
6. Fondati A, Gallo MG, Romano E, et al. A case of feline phaeohyphomycosis due to *Fonsecaea pedrosoi*. Vet Dermatol. 2001;12:297-301.
7. Abramo F, Bastelli F, Nardoni S, et al. Feline cutaneous phaeohyphomycosis due to *Cladophialophora bantiana*. J Feline Med Surg. 2002;4:157-163.
8. Tennant K, Patterson-Kane J, Boag AK, et al. Nasal mycosis in two cats caused by *Alternaria* species. Vet Rec. 2004;155:368-370.
9. Rajeev S, Clifton G, Watson C, et al. *Fonsecaea pedrosoi* skin infection in a dog. J Vet Diagn Invest. 2008;20:379-381.
10. Bentley RT, Faissler D, Sutherland-Smith J. Successful management of an intracranial phaeohyphomycotic fungal granuloma in a dog. J Am Vet Med Assoc. 2011;239:480-485.
11. Giri DK, Sims WP, Sura R, et al. Cerebral and renal phaeohyphomycosis in a dog infected with *Bipolaris* species. Vet Pathol. 2011;48:754-757.

12. Anor S, Sturges BK, Lafranco L, et al. Systemic phaeohyphomycosis (*Cladophialophora bantiana*) in a dog—clinical diagnosis with stereotactic computed tomographic-guided brain biopsy. J Vet Intern Med. 2001;15:257-261.
13. Bouljihad M, Lindeman CJ, Hayden DW. Pyogranulomatous meningoencephalitis associated with dematiaceous fungal (*Cladophialophora bantiana*) infection in a domestic cat. J Vet Diagn Invest. 2002;14:70-72.
14. Simmons JK, McManamon R, Rech RR, et al. Pathology in Practice. Necrotizing pyogranulomatous meningoencephalitis with intralesional fungal hyphae, consistent with *Cladophialophora bantiana*. J Am Vet Med Assoc. 2010;236(3):295-297.
15. Dedola C, Stuart AP, Ridyard AE, et al. Cutaneous *Alternaria infectoria* infection in a dog in association with therapeutic immunosuppression for the management of immune-mediated haemolytic anaemia. Vet Dermatol. 2010;21:626-634.
16. Swift IM, Griffin A, Shipstone MA. Successful treatment of disseminated cutaneous phaeohyphomycosis in a dog. Aust Vet J. 2006;84:431-435.
17. Herraez P, Rees C, Dunstan R. Invasive phaeohyphomycosis caused by *Curvularia* species in a dog. Vet Pathol. 2001;38:456-459.
18. Coldrick O, Brannon CL, Kydd DM, et al. Fungal pyelonephritis due to *Cladophialophora bantiana* in a cat. Vet Rec. 2007;161:724-728.
19. Elies L, Balandraud V, Boulouha L, et al. Fatal systemic phaeohyphomycosis in a cat due to *Cladophialophora bantiana*. J Vet Med A Physiol Pathol Clin Med. 2003;50(10):50-53.
20. Murphy KF, Malik R, Barnes A, et al. Successful treatment of intraabdominal *Exophiala dermatitidis* infection in a dog. Vet Rec. 2011;168:217.
21. Naggie S, Perfect JR. Molds: hyalohyphomycosis, phaeohyphomycosis and zygomycosis. Clin Chest Med. 2009;30:337-353.
22. Foley JE, Norris CR, Jang SS. Paecilomycosis in dogs and horses and a review of the literature. J Vet Intern Med. 2002;16:238-243.
23. Holahan ML, Loft KE, Swenson CL, et al. Generalized calcinosis cutis associated with disseminated paecilomycosis in a dog. Vet Dermatol. 2008;19:368-372.
24. Caro-Vadillo A, Garcia-Real I, Paya-Vicens MJ, et al. Fungal rhinitis caused by *Scedosporium apiospermum* in a Labrador retriever. Vet Rec. 2005;157:175-177.
25. Erne JB, Walker MC, Strik N, et al. Systemic infection with *Geomyces* organisms in a dog with lytic bone lesions. J Am Vet Med Assoc. 2007;230:537-540.
26. Tanaka H, Takizawa K, Baba O, et al. Basidiomycosis: *Schizophyllum commune* osteomyelitis in a dog. J Vet Med Sci. 2008;70:1257-1259.
27. Grant DC, Sutton DA, Sandberg CA, et al. Disseminated *Geosmithia argillacea* infection in a German shepherd dog. Med Mycol. 2009;47:221-226.
28. Armstrong PF, Sigler L, Sutton DA, et al. Fungal myelitis caused by *Phialosimplex caninus* in an immunosuppressed dog. Med Mycol. 2012;50:509-512.
29. Marlar AB, Miller PE, Canton DD, et al. Canine keratomycosis: a report of eight cases and literature review. J Am Anim Hosp Assoc. 1994;30:331-340.
30. Rampazzo A, Kuhnert P, Howard J, et al. *Hormographiella aspergillata* keratomycosis in a dog. Vet Ophthalmol. 2009;12:43-47.
31. Garcia RS, Wheat LJ, Cook AK, et al. Sensitivity and specificity of a blood and urine galactomannan antigen assay for diagnosis of systemic aspergillosis in dogs. J Vet Intern Med. 2012;26:911-919.
32. Lackner M, de Hoog GS, Verweij PE, et al. Species-specific antifungal susceptibility patterns of *Scedosporium* and *Pseudallescheria* species. Antimicrob Agents Chemother. 2012;56(5):2635-2642.
33. Pastor FJ, Guarro J. Clinical manifestations, treatment and outcome of *Paecilomyces lilacinus* infections. Clin Microbiol Infect. 2006;12(10):948-960.

CHAPTER 69

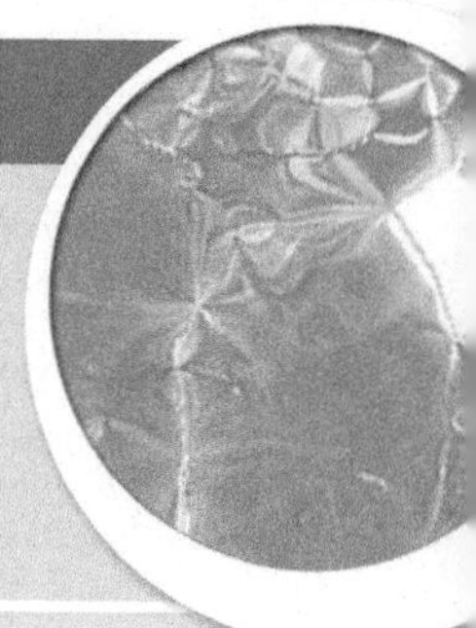

Pythiosis, Lagenidiosis, and Zygomycosis

Amy M. Grooters

Pythiosis, lagenidiosis, and zygomycosis are often grouped together because of similarities in their clinical presentations and histologic characteristics (all three cause pyogranulomatous and eosinophilic inflammation associated with large, infrequently septate hyphae with nonparallel walls). Despite their clinicopathologic similarities, however, the pathogens that cause these infections are taxonomically diverse. *Pythium insidiosum* and *Lagenidium* species are water molds in the class Oomycetes and as such are more closely related to red algae and *Prototheca* spp. than to true fungi, including the zygomycetes.[1] Important traits that distinguish oomycetes from fungi include the production of motile, flagellate zoospores that act as infective elements in wet environments, and the fact that the oomycete cell membrane generally lacks ergosterol.[2] In addition, there are clinically relevant differences in prognosis, recommended treatment, and epidemiology that make it important to distinguish among pythiosis, lagenidiosis, and zygomycosis. Although *P. insidiosum* has been recognized as a pathogen in dogs and horses for more than 25 years, *Lagenidium* species have only been recognized as mammalian pathogens since 1999. In comparison to pythiosis and lagenidiosis, infections caused by the zygomycetes are rare.

> **Overview of Pythiosis**
>
> First Described: 1884, India (Smith)[3], in horses
>
> Cause: *Pythium insidiosum* (kingdom Stramenopila, class Oomycota), related to algae and *Prototheca* spp.
>
> Affected Hosts: Horses and dogs; less commonly cats, sheep, cattle, exotic species, and humans
>
> Geographic Distribution: Tropical, subtropical, and some temperate regions worldwide, especially the Gulf Coast region of the United States
>
> Mode of Transmission: Likely penetration of damaged skin or mucosa by motile zoospores, usually after exposure to standing freshwater sources
>
> Major Clinical Signs: Ulcerative, nodular, and mass-like cutaneous lesions with draining tracts (cutaneous form); weight loss, anorexia, vomiting, diarrhea, hematochezia (gastrointestinal form)
>
> Differential Diagnosis: For suspected gastrointestinal pythiosis, differential diagnoses include neoplasia, zygomycosis, histoplasmosis, eosinophilic gastroenteritis, or chronic intestinal foreign bodies; for suspected cutaneous pythiosis, they include lagenidiosis, zygomycosis, mycobacterial infections, actinomycosis, or furunculosis.
>
> Human Health Significance: *P. insidiosum* is a rare cause of disease in human patients; infection is not transmitted directly from affected animals to people.

PYTHIOSIS

Etiology and Epidemiology

Pythium insidiosum is an aquatic oomycete that causes severe, progressive gastrointestinal or cutaneous disease that is often fatal. The infective form of *P. insidiosum* is thought to be the motile flagellate zoospore, which is an asexual reproductive structure produced in wet environments in association with plant material.[4] Zoospores of *P. insidiosum* are attracted to damaged tissue, and likely cause infection by encystation on and invasion of damaged skin or gastrointestinal mucosa.[5] In support of this mechanism of infection, clinical reports have long suggested an association between pythiosis and frequent exposure to warm freshwater habitats. However, some infections occur in dogs with no history of access to lakes or ponds.

Globally, pythiosis occurs in tropical and subtropical climates, including Southeast Asia, eastern coastal Australia, and South America (Figure 69-1). In the United States, the disease occurs most often in the Gulf Coast states, but it has also been recognized throughout the South; along the East Coast as far north as Maryland and New Jersey; in the Midwest including Missouri, Kansas, southern Illinois, and Indiana; and in the West in Arizona and California.[6]

Pythiosis is most common in young, large-breed dogs, especially Labrador retrievers and other outdoor working breeds. Infected dogs are typically evaluated by veterinarians in the fall, winter, and early spring.[7] Pythiosis is uncommon in cats compared to dogs, and specific breed and sex predilections have not been observed in the cases described to date. However, the development of cutaneous pythiosis in very young animals (less than 1 year of age) appears to occur more often in cats than in dogs. For both species, affected animals are typically immunocompetent.

Clinical Features

The clinical signs associated with pythiosis are caused by gastrointestinal or cutaneous lesions, or by extension of disease into regional lymph nodes or adjacent tissues. Generally, gastrointestinal and cutaneous lesions do not occur together in the same animal. Disseminated pythiosis has only been described in one dog.[8]

Gastrointestinal Pythiosis

Gastrointestinal pythiosis in dogs is characterized by severe, segmental, transmural thickening of the stomach wall (Figure 69-2), small intestine, colon, rectum, or, rarely, the

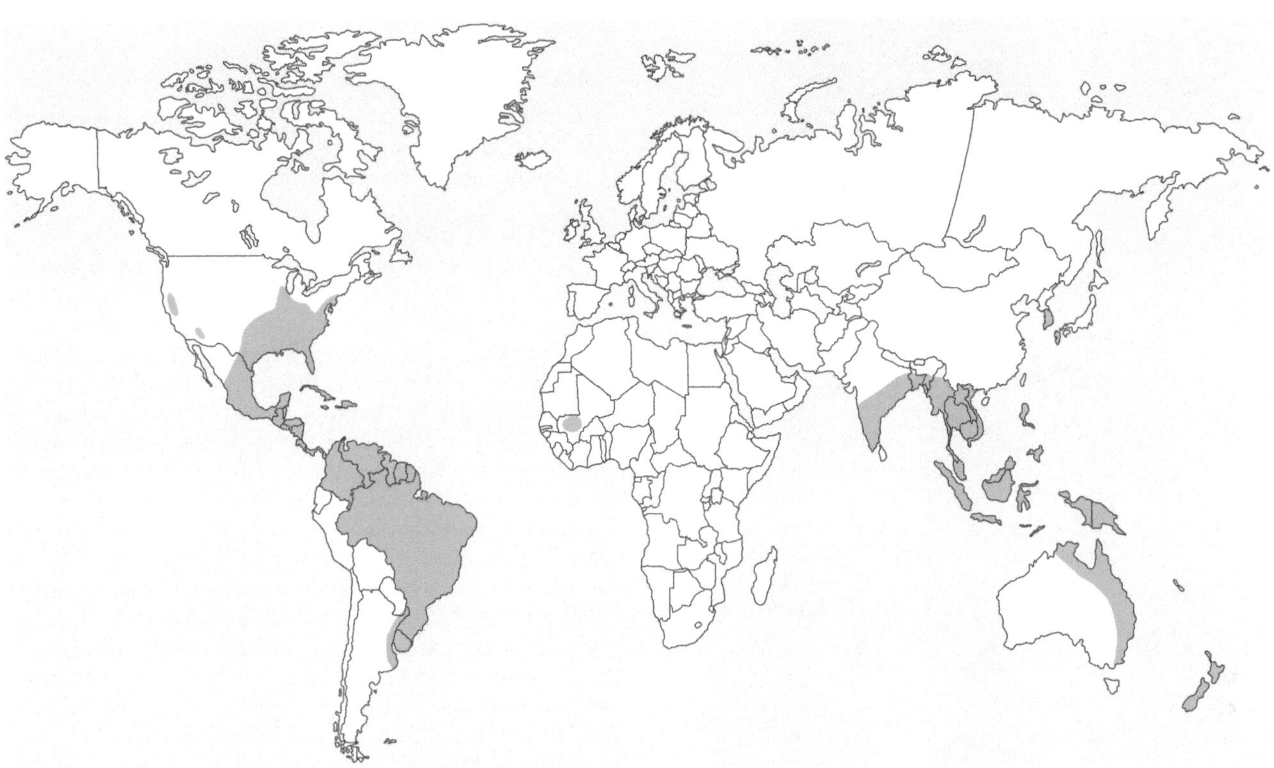

FIGURE 69-1 Worldwide geographic distribution of pythiosis.

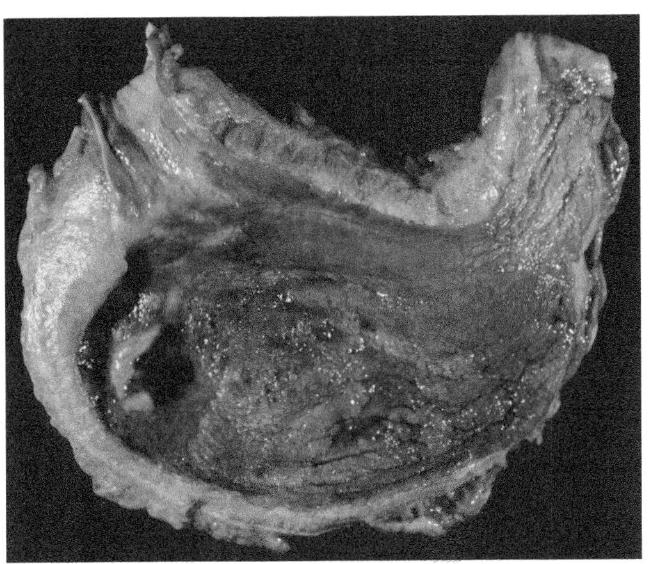

FIGURE 69-2 Gastric pythiosis in a 1-year-old male neutered mixed breed dog. Note extreme thickening of the gastric wall. (Courtesy Amy Grooters, Louisiana State University, Baton Rouge, LA.)

esophagus, and it is not uncommon to find multiple segmental lesions in the same patient.[7,9,10] The most commonly affected regions of the gastrointestinal tract are the gastric outflow area, proximal duodenum, and ileocolic junction. Mesenteric lymphadenopathy is common but is usually caused by reactive hyperplasia rather than infection. Extension of disease into the mesenteric root often causes severe mesenteric lymphadenopathy, with the lymph nodes embedded in a single large, firm mass that is palpable in the cranial to mid abdomen. Invasion of mesenteric vessels may result in bowel ischemia, infarction, perforation, or acute hemoabdomen. In addition, infection may extend into adjacent tissues such as the pancreas or the uterus. Gastrointestinal pythiosis is rare in cats but has been described in two young adult male cats with focal intestinal lesions that were amenable to surgical resection.[11]

Dogs with gastrointestinal pythiosis typically have a history of chronic progressive weight loss, vomiting, diarrhea, anorexia, and sometimes hematochezia, depending on the location of the lesions. Regurgitation may be present in dogs with esophageal involvement. Physical examination usually reveals a poor body condition and sometimes a palpable abdominal mass. Signs of systemic illness such as lethargy or depression are absent unless intestinal obstruction, infarction, or perforation occurs.

Cutaneous Pythiosis

Cutaneous pythiosis in dogs occurs most often at the base of the tail, or on the extremities, ventral neck, or perineum,[8,12] and is characterized by nonhealing wounds and invasive masses that contain ulcerated nodules and draining tracts (Figure 69-3). In contrast to gastrointestinal pythiosis, regional lymphadenopathy associated with cutaneous pythiosis often reflects extension of infection rather than just reactive hyperplasia. Extension of cutaneous disease to tissues other than regional lymph nodes is rare, but the author has observed a single, focal pulmonary lesion caused by *P. insidiosum* in one dog with cutaneous pythiosis on a distal extremity.

In cats, lesions associated with cutaneous pythiosis include cervical, inguinal, or truncal subcutaneous masses; draining nodular lesions or ulcerated plaque-like lesions on the tailhead or extremities[12]; and periorbital and nasopharyngeal lesions.[13]

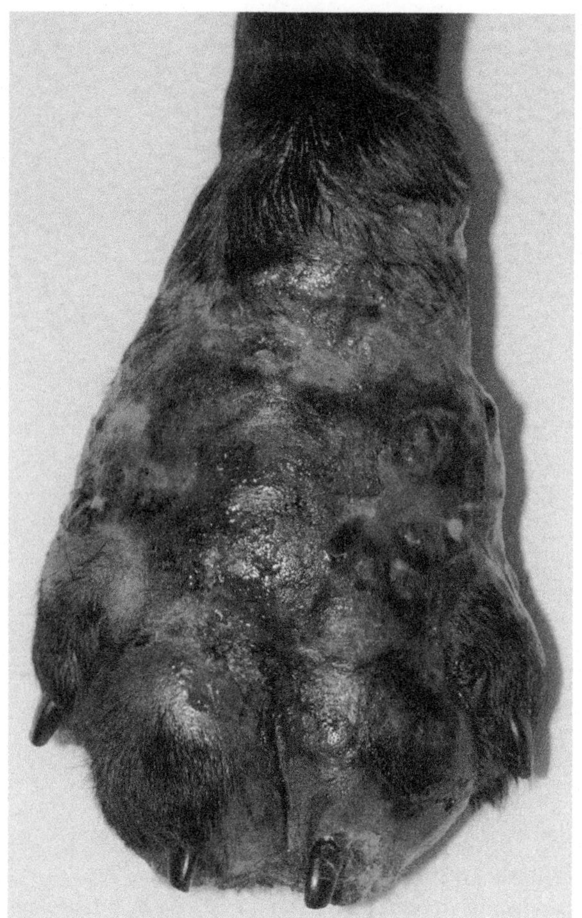

FIGURE 69-3 Cutaneous pythiosis in a 6-month-old female Labrador retriever. (Courtesy Amy Grooters, Louisiana State University, Baton Rouge, LA.)

Diagnosis

Laboratory Abnormalities

The most common laboratory abnormalities associated with pythiosis are eosinophilia, anemia, hyperglobulinemia, and hypoalbuminemia. Hypercalcemia has been described once.[14]

Imaging Findings

In dogs with gastrointestinal pythiosis, common radiographic findings include poor abdominal detail and the presence of an abdominal mass. Evidence of small bowel obstruction may also be observed. In rare cases of esophageal pythiosis, thoracic radiographs reveals increased soft tissue opacity in the region of the esophagus and deviation of the trachea. Abdominal ultrasonography is the tool of choice for imaging animals suspected to have gastrointestinal pythiosis and usually reveals severe segmental thickening of the gastrointestinal tract and mesenteric lymphadenopathy. In addition, Doppler ultrasonography may identify the presence of vascular pathology (such as an aneurysm) that can result from invasion of mesenteric vessels. In the author's practice, abdominal ultrasonography is a critical tool for determining the location and extent of disease in dogs with gastrointestinal pythiosis to determine the likelihood that surgical resection could be performed successfully and to assess prognosis. In addition, ultrasonography facilitates the acquisition of fine-needle aspirate specimens from affected segments of the gastrointestinal tract and enlarged lymph nodes. In animals with cutaneous pythiosis, computed tomography may provide information about the extent of disease and may assist with surgical planning when lesions are not located on an extremity.[15]

Microbiologic Tests

Diagnostic assays currently available for pythiosis, lagenidiosis, and zygomycosis in dogs and cats are described in Table 69-1.

TABLE 69-1

Diagnostic Assays Currently Available for Pythiosis, Lagenidiosis, and Zygomycosis in Dogs and Cats

Assay	Specimen Type	Target	Performance
Cytologic examination	Aspirates of affected tissues	Broad, rarely septate fungal hyphae with tapered, rounded ends	Does not reliably differentiate among pythiosis, lagenidiosis, and zygomycosis.
Culture	Biopsies of affected tissues	*Pythium insidiosum*, *Lagenidium* spp., or zygomycetes	Special tissue handling and expertise required for *P. insidiosum* culture (see text). The use of swab specimens or aspirates may result in false negatives. Species identification requires the use of molecular techniques.
Antibody serology	Serum	Antibodies to *P. insidiosum* or *Lagenidium* spp.	Assays that detect anti-*Pythium* antibodies allow early, noninvasive diagnosis of pythiosis in dogs. Positive test results correlate with active disease, and titers fall with successful treatment. Assays that detect *Lagenidium* antibodies in dogs are less specific and may be positive in animals with other diseases.
Histopathology	Biopsies of affected tissues	Broad, rarely septate fungal hyphae with tapered, rounded ends	Does not reliably differentiate among pythiosis, lagenidiosis, and zygomycosis. Use of special stains may facilitate detection.
PCR assays	Biopsies of affected tissues	*P. insidiosum* DNA	Not widely available.

Cytologic Examination

Cytologically, pythiosis is characterized by pyogranulomatous and eosinophilic inflammation that can be visualized on impression smears made from draining skin lesions or fine-needle aspirates of a thickened gastrointestinal wall or enlarged lymph nodes. Hyphae are observed occasionally in cytologic samples, and their morphologic appearance (broad, rarely septate with tapered, rounded ends) in conjunction with a typical inflammatory response can provide a tentative diagnosis of pythiosis, lagenidiosis, or zygomycosis.[14]

Culture

Isolation of *P. insidiosum* from infected tissues is not difficult but does require specific specimen handling and culture techniques. For best results, unrefrigerated tissue specimens should be wrapped in a saline-moistened gauze sponge and shipped at ambient temperature to arrive within 24 hours at a laboratory that has experience with culture of pathogenic oomycetes. Small pieces of fresh, nonmacerated tissue are placed directly on the surface of vegetable extract agar supplemented with streptomycin and ampicillin (or an alternative selective medium) and incubated at 37°C.[16] Mycelial growth is typically observed within 12 to 24 hours. Isolation of *P. insidiosum* from swabs of exudate collected from draining skin lesions is generally unsuccessful. Because generation of the sexual reproductive structures that are necessary for definitive morphologic classification of pathogenic oomycetes rarely occurs in the laboratory, identification of *P. insidiosum* isolates is based on species-specific PCR amplification[17] or rRNA gene sequencing. Although production of zoospores is an important supporting feature for the identification of pathogenic oomycetes, it is not specific for *P. insidiosum.*

Molecular Diagnosis using the Polymerase Chain Reaction

A species-specific PCR assay has been used to identify *P. insidiosum* DNA in fresh, frozen, or paraffin-embedded tissues, as well as DNA extracted directly from cultured isolates.[18] However, such assays are not widely available on a commercial basis.

Serologic Testing

A highly sensitive and specific ELISA for the detection of anti–*P. insidiosum* antibodies in dogs is currently available through the author's laboratory at Louisiana State University.[19] This assay provides a means for early, noninvasive diagnosis and also allows response to therapy to be monitored. Following complete surgical resection of infected tissues, a dramatic decrease in antibody levels is typically detected within 2 to 3 months. In contrast, antibody levels remain high in animals that go on to develop clinical recurrence following surgical treatment. This same ELISA has been adapted for detection of anti–*P. insidiosum* antibodies in domestic and exotic cats, and although case numbers are too small to generate strong estimates of sensitivity and specificity, in the author's experience they appear to be high.

Pathologic Findings

Histologically, pythiosis is characterized by eosinophilic pyogranulomatous inflammation, with multiple foci of necrosis that are surrounded and infiltrated by neutrophils, eosinophils, and macrophages. In addition, discrete granulomas composed of epithelioid macrophages, plasma cells, multinucleate giant cells, and fewer neutrophils and eosinophils are often observed. Organisms are typically found within areas of necrosis or at the center of granulomas. Vasculitis is occasionally present. In gastrointestinal pythiosis, inflammation centers on the submucosal and muscular layers rather than the mucosa and lamina propria. Therefore, the diagnosis of pythiosis may be missed if endoscopic biopsies that fail to reach deeper tissues are submitted. Similarly, disease in animals with cutaneous pythiosis is typically found in the deep dermis and subcutis, necessitating deep wedge biopsies rather than punch biopsies for optimal evaluation. *Pythium insidiosum* hyphae are not routinely visualized on H&E-stained sections but may be identified as clear spaces surrounded by a narrow band of eosinophilic material. Hyphae are readily visualized in sections stained with Gomori's methenamine silver (GMS) but usually do not stain well with periodic acid–Schiff (PAS). They are wide (mean, 4 µm; range, 2 to 7 µm), have nonparallel walls, are infrequently septate, and occasionally branch at right angles.[7,8]

Treatment and Prognosis

Aggressive surgical resection of all infected tissues with wide margins is the treatment of choice for pythiosis. In animals with cutaneous lesions that are confined to a single distal extremity, amputation should be recommended unless there is evidence of regional lymph node infection. In patients with gastrointestinal pythiosis, segmental lesions should be resected with 5-cm margins whenever possible. Because mesenteric lymph nodes are usually reactive rather than infected, the presence of nonresectable mesenteric lymphadenopathy should not dissuade the surgeon from pursuing resection of a segmental bowel lesion. Enlarged regional lymph nodes should, however, always be biopsied for prognostic information. In animals with cutaneous pythiosis, the surgeon should attempt to obtain skin margins of 5 cm and deep margins of two fascial planes.[15] Enlarged regional lymph nodes in dogs with cutaneous pythiosis are often infected rather than reactive; therefore, they should be evaluated cytologically or histologically before amputation or other aggressive resection is attempted.

Unfortunately, many dogs with pythiosis are not brought to a veterinarian until late in the course of disease, when complete excision is not possible. In addition, the anatomic location of the lesion may prevent complete surgical excision when gastrointestinal pythiosis involves the esophagus, gastric outflow tract, rectum, or mesenteric root, or when cutaneous pythiosis involves the ventral thorax, base of the tail, or trunk. Still, very aggressive surgery such as a partial gastrectomy[14] or massive resection of cutaneous lesions combined with reconstructive techniques[15] can sometimes result in a successful outcome.

Local postoperative recurrence of pythiosis is common (especially when wide surgical margins cannot be achieved) and can occur either at the site of resection or in regional lymph nodes. For this reason, postoperative medical therapy is often recommended when the surgeon is not confident that margins of at least 5 cm were achieved. In the author's practice, dogs with focal midjejunal lesions that are resected with wide margins and dogs without regional lymphadenopathy that undergo amputation for distal extremity lesions are not routinely treated with postoperative antifungal medication. All other patients with pythiosis typically are treated with itraconazole (10 mg/kg PO q24h) and terbinafine (5 to 10 mg/kg PO q24h) for at least 2 to 3 months after surgical resection. Unfortunately, if resection is incomplete, lesions often progress despite medical therapy, and clinical signs recur within weeks to months.

To monitor for recurrence, ELISA serology should be performed at the time of surgery and 2 to 3 months later. In animals that have had a complete surgical resection and subsequently show no recurrence of disease, serum antibody levels usually drop 50% or more within 3 months. If this occurs, medical therapy can be discontinued. In the author's experience, surgery is curative in a majority of animals with a distal limb lesion treated with amputation, or with a midjejunal lesion that the surgeon believes was completely resected with good margins.

Medical therapy for nonresectable pythiosis is typically unrewarding, likely because ergosterol (the target for most currently available antifungal drugs) is generally lacking in the oomycete cell membrane. Despite this fact, clinical and serologic cures occur in some patients treated with a combination of itraconazole (10 mg/kg PO q24h) and terbinafine (5 to 10 mg/kg PO q24h).[20] Although the percentage of animals that respond to this treatment is still low, the combination protocol anecdotally appears to be superior to itraconazole or amphotericin B alone.

Dogs with nonresectable gastrointestinal pythiosis are often treated with anti-inflammatory doses of glucocorticoids in an effort to palliate clinical signs and to decrease vomiting so that oral antifungal drugs can be administered. Prednisone (1 mg/kg/day) routinely causes improvement in clinical signs in the short term. Surprisingly, the author has observed complete and long-term resolution of gastrointestinal lesions (based on serial ultrasonographic examinations and serologic testing) in a small number of dogs treated with prednisone alone. Although this is certainly not recommended as a primary treatment for animals with resectable lesions, it is a reasonable option in animals with nonresectable gastrointestinal lesions, especially when financial concerns preclude the use of antifungal medication. The author has not observed this effect of prednisone in dogs with cutaneous pythiosis.

An immunotherapy product derived from antigens of *P. insidiosum* has been used successfully to treat pythiosis in horses and people.[21,22] Unfortunately, although controlled trials have not been completed, the efficacy of this product in dogs appears to be poor, and clinical improvement has not been observed in any of the author's patients.

Public Health Aspects

Human infections caused by *P. insidiosum* are rare. Infections are acquired from the environment and have resulted in keratitis, periorbital cellulitis, and arteritis of the lower extremities. Most cases have been reported from Thailand, and almost all patients have thalassemia. Extremely rare reports of the disease exist from humans in North, South, and Central America, Australia, and other parts of Asia, many of whom are apparently healthy. Although there is no evidence to suggest that transmission between mammalian hosts is possible, routine precautions (such as wearing gloves when handling infected tissues or exudate) should be followed.

Overview of Lagenidiosis

First Described: 2003, Louisiana, USA, in dogs (Grooters and others)[23]

Cause: *Lagenidium* spp.

Affected Hosts: Dogs

Geographic Distribution: Southeastern United States

Mode of Transmission: Likely penetration of damaged skin or mucosa by motile zoospores

Major Clinical Signs: Ulcerative, nodular, and mass-like cutaneous lesions with draining tracts (cutaneous form); pelvic limb edema; local, thoracic, or abdominal lymphadenopathy; rupture of infected great vessels in the abdomen may result in hemoabdomen

Differential Diagnosis: Neoplasia, pythiosis, zygomycosis, mycobacterial infections, actinomycosis, snake bite

Human Health Significance: *Lagenidium* spp. infection is acquired from the environment; infection is not transmitted from affected animals to people.

LAGENIDIOSIS

Etiology and Epidemiology

Most species in the genus *Lagenidium* are pathogens of insects, crustaceans, algae, and nematodes. The most well studied species, *Lagenidium giganteum*, is a mosquito larval pathogen that was previously used as a biologic pesticide for control of mosquito populations. Within the past 15 years, two novel oomycetes that appear to belong to the genus *Lagenidium* have been isolated from dogs with cutaneous lesions. The first of these species causes uniformly fatal dermatologic and disseminated disease in dogs in the southeastern United States.[23] The second pathogenic *Lagenidium* species is less common than the first and causes a chronic ulcerative nodular dermatopathy that has a prolonged course and does not appear to extend beyond local tissues. Although strong antigenic and molecular similarities suggest that the first canine pathogen is closely related to *L. giganteum*, differences in their molecular and in vitro growth characteristics suggest that they are likely distinct species. Sporulation and infectivity for these pathogens is thought to be similar to that associated with *P. insidiosum* and *L. giganteum*, causing infection through production of motile aquatic zoospores that adhere to and encyst in damaged tissues.

The epidemiologic features of lagenidiosis are similar in many respects to those associated with cutaneous pythiosis. Affected animals are typically young to middle-aged dogs that live in the southeastern United States. Although most affected dogs have lived in Florida or Louisiana, cases in Texas, Tennessee, Alabama, Georgia, South Carolina, Maryland, Virginia, Indiana, and Illinois have also been identified. A number of infected dogs have had frequent exposure to lakes or ponds. None have had historical evidence of immunocompromise or were treated with immunosuppressive therapy before development of the infection.

Clinical Features

Dogs with *Lagenidium* infection are typically evaluated for progressive, multifocal or focal, cutaneous or subcutaneous lesions

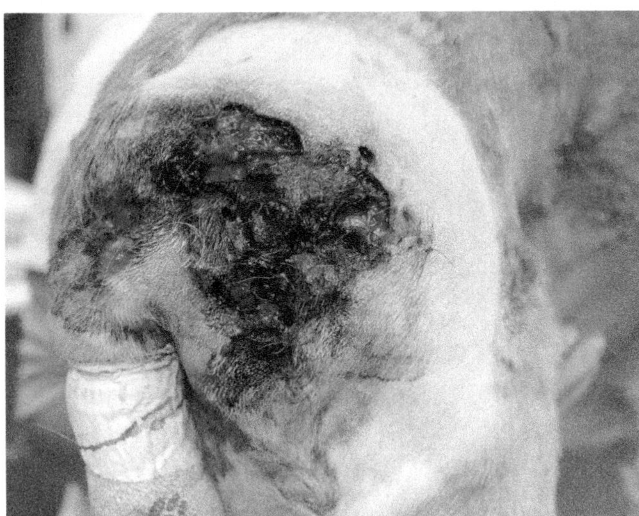

FIGURE 69-4 Tailhead mass caused by lagenidiosis in a 9-year-old female spayed mixed breed dog. Note the extensive tissue necrosis. (Courtesy Amy Grooters, Louisiana State University, Baton Rouge, LA.)

that involve the extremities, mammary region, perineum, or trunk.[23] These lesions may appear as firm dermal or subcutaneous nodules, or as ulcerated, thickened, edematous areas of deep cellulitis with regions of necrosis and numerous draining tracts (Figure 69-4). As with cutaneous pythiosis, skin lesions in dogs with lagenidiosis tend to be progressive, locally invasive, and poorly responsive to medical therapy.

In dogs infected with the more aggressive species of *Lagenidium*, regional lymphadenopathy is often noted and may occur in the absence of obvious cutaneous lesions. Unlike dogs with cutaneous pythiosis, these dogs typically have occult lesions in the thorax or abdomen, which may involve the great vessels, sublumbar and/or inguinal lymph nodes, lung, pulmonary hilus, and cranial mediastinum. Animals with great vessel or sublumbar lymph node involvement usually have cutaneous or subcutaneous lesions on the pelvic limbs and often develop pelvic limb edema. Sudden death caused by great vessel rupture and associated hemoabdomen may occur in these animals.

In dogs infected with the less aggressive species of *Lagenidium*, lesions tend to be locally invasive but rarely extend beyond cutaneous and subcutaneous tissues. Distant lesions in the thorax and abdomen have not been identified, and the clinical course appears to be chronic and slowly progressive; some dogs have lesions that are somewhat stable for several years.

Diagnosis

Because of its clinical, epidemiologic, and histologic similarities to pythiosis, lagenidiosis is often misdiagnosed as pythiosis during routine histologic evaluation. In addition, because many pathologists are more familiar with the zygomycetes than the oomycetes, lagenidiosis may also be misdiagnosed as zygomycosis. Although there are subtle differences in hyphal size, morphology, and distribution among these three infections, histologic lesions associated with lagenidiosis are still often labeled as "suspected pythiosis" or "suspected zygomycosis" during routine evaluation. For this reason, clinicians should always attempt to confirm a suspected histologic diagnosis with serology, culture, or molecular diagnostic assays.

Laboratory Abnormalities

Laboratory abnormalities are often absent in dogs with lagenidiosis; when present, they most often include hyperglobulinemia and eosinophilia. Hypercalcemia has been associated with *Lagenidium* infection in one dog with cutaneous lesions on all four limbs and severe infection and enlargement of popliteal, inguinal, and superficial cervical lymph nodes.

Imaging Findings

Radiographic imaging of the thorax and sonographic imaging of the abdomen are essential parts of the diagnostic evaluation in dogs suspected to have lagenidiosis because of the potential for occult lesions in the thorax or abdomen. These may include solitary pulmonary nodules; sublumbar, inguinal, and medial iliac lymphadenopathy; thickening and invasion of the wall of the aorta or caudal vena cava (sometimes with associated aneurysm); and retroperitoneal or epaxial masses. Thoracic and abdominal lesions have not been observed in dogs infected with the less aggressive *Lagenidium* species.

Microbiologic Tests

Cytologic Examination

Cytologic examination of lymph node aspirates or impression smears made from draining lesions in dogs with lagenidiosis reveal pyogranulomatous to eosinophilic inflammation with or without broad, poorly septate hyphae.

Culture

The diagnosis of lagenidiosis is best made by culture followed by PCR and rRNA gene sequencing, which not only provides a definitive diagnosis but is also the only tool currently available that differentiates between the two pathogenic species. Isolation techniques for *Lagenidium* spp. are similar to those described for *P. insidiosum*, but with peptone-yeast-glucose (PYG) agar. For best results, small pieces of fresh, nonmacerated tissue are placed directly on the surface of the agar and incubated at 37°C. Growth is typically observed within 24 to 48 hours. Because production of the sexual reproductive structures necessary for morphologic classification has not yet been possible, definitive identification of *Lagenidium* species is currently based on rRNA gene sequencing. Although genus-specific PCR assays have been used to identify *Lagenidium* DNA extracted from cultured isolates or from infected tissue specimens,[18] the clinical importance of differentiating between the two pathogenic species in regard to prognosis and treatment makes culture and rRNA gene sequencing the preferred technique.

Serologic Testing

In dogs with supportive clinical signs and histologic findings, immunoblot serology for the detection of anti-*Lagenidium* antibodies in canine serum can suggest lagenidiosis but must be interpreted in conjunction with results of serologic testing for *P. insidiosum* infection because of the potential for cross-reactivity in serum from dogs with pythiosis. In addition, the author has observed nonspecific anti-*Lagenidium* seroreactivity in dogs with other fungal or nonfungal infections. Therefore, based on currently available data, serology alone should not be used as a basis for the diagnosis of lagenidiosis. Serology is not helpful for differentiating between infection by the two canine pathogenic species of *Lagenidium*.

Pathologic Findings

Histologically, lagenidiosis shares many characteristics with pythiosis and zygomycosis, including pyogranulomatous and

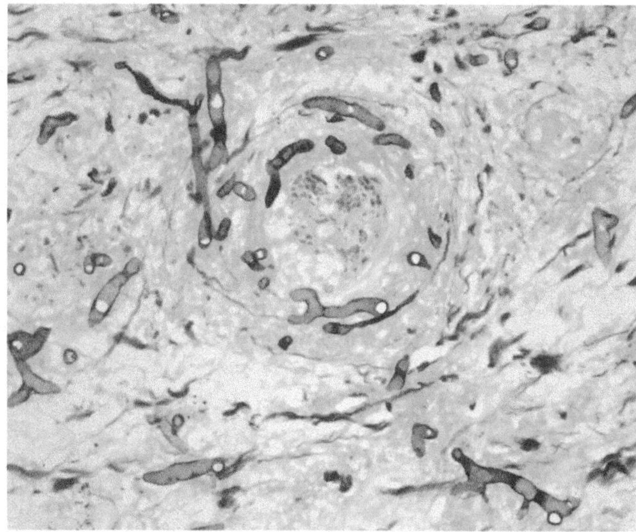

FIGURE 69-5 Broad, thick-walled infrequently septate hyphae associated with granulomatous vasculitis in a lymph node from a dog infected with the more aggressive species of *Lagenidium*. (Courtesy Amy Grooters, Louisiana State University, Baton Rouge, LA.)

eosinophilic inflammation associated with broad, irregularly branching, infrequently septate hyphae with nonparallel walls. Multinucleated giant cells and plasma cells are commonly present. In contrast to *P. insidiosum*, *Lagenidium* spp. hyphae are often visible on H&E-stained sections. On GMS-stained sections, numerous broad, thick-walled, irregularly septate hyphae are easily recognized (Figure 69-5). *Lagenidium* hyphae typically demonstrate a great deal of variability in size, but in general are larger than *P. insidiosum* hyphae, ranging from 7 to 25 μm in diameter, with an average of 12 μm for the more aggressive pathogen and 7.5 μm for the less aggressive pathogen. In some sections, hyphae appear as round or bulbous structures, and right-angle branching is occasionally observed. A scant to thin eosinophilic sleeve may be noted around the hyphae.

Treatment and Prognosis

As with pythiosis, aggressive surgical resection of infected tissues is the treatment of choice for lagenidiosis when disease is confined to a resectable cutaneous lesion. Unfortunately, the vast majority of dogs infected with the more common (and more aggressive) *Lagenidium* pathogen have nonresectable disease in the thorax, abdomen, or regional lymph nodes by the time the initial diagnosis is made, and in the author's experience, the disease is routinely fatal. In dogs infected with the less aggressive species, surgery that achieves 3- to 5-cm margins is often curative. Because the species of *Lagenidium* present is often not known early in the course of diagnostic evaluation, any dog suspected of having lagenidiosis should be evaluated with thoracic radiography and abdominal ultrasonography before surgical resection of cutaneous lesions is attempted. As with pythiosis, medical therapy for lagenidiosis is usually ineffective. However, treatment with a combination of itraconazole (10 mg/kg PO q24h) and terbinafine (5 to 10 mg/kg PO q24h) along with repeated aggressive surgical resection was curative in one dog with recurrent multifocal cutaneous lesions caused by the less aggressive pathogen.

Public Health Aspects

Infections caused by *Lagenidium* species are acquired from the environment. Although there is no evidence to suggest that transmission between mammalian hosts is possible, routine precautions (such as wearing gloves when handling infected tissues or exudate) should be followed.

Overview of Zygomycosis (Entomophthoramycosis and Mucormycosis)

First Described: Reports of zygomycosis in humans date back to the 1800s.

Causes: *Basidiobolus* and *Conidiobolus* spp. (kingdom Fungi, order Entomophthorales); *Rhizopus, Absidia, Mucor* spp., and others (kingdom Fungi, order Mucorales)

Affected Hosts: Dogs, cats, humans, horses, sheep, other mammalian species

Geographic Distribution: Worldwide

Mode of Transmission: Inhalation, ingestion, or cutaneous exposure to organisms in soil and decaying organic matter

Major Clinical Signs: Entomophthoramycoses are associated with chronic, slowly progressive subcutaneous, retrobulbar, or nasal infections in immunocompetent animals; mucormycoses are associated with systemic (respiratory or gastrointestinal) or cutaneous-subcutaneous infections in immunocompromised animals.

Differential Diagnosis: Neoplasia, pythiosis, lagenidiosis, other deep mycoses (especially blastomycosis), mycobacterial infections, actinomycosis

Human Health Significance: Disease in humans results from exposure to organisms in the environment, and direct transmission between animals has not been reported.

ZYGOMYCOSIS

Etiology and Epidemiology

The term "zygomycosis" refers to infections caused by fungi in the class Zygomycetes, which includes pathogenic fungi of the genera *Basidiobolus* and *Conidiobolus* (order *Entomophthorales*) and the genera *Rhizopus, Absidia, Mucor*, and others (order *Mucorales*). In human and veterinary patients, the *Entomophthorales* typically cause chronic localized infections in subcutaneous tissue or nasal submucosa of immunocompetent patients that usually reside in tropical or subtropical locations (entomophthoramycoses), whereas the *Mucorales* tend to cause acute, rapidly progressive disease in debilitated or immunocompromised individuals worldwide (mucormycoses). *Basidiobolus* spp. and *Conidiobolus* spp. cause cutaneous lesions in dogs that are grossly and histologically similar to those caused by *P. insidiosum* and *Lagenidium* spp. Culture-confirmed infections caused by pathogens in the order *Mucorales* have not been well documented in dogs but have been described in a small number of cats. Unfortunately, clinical and pathologic information about zygomycosis in small

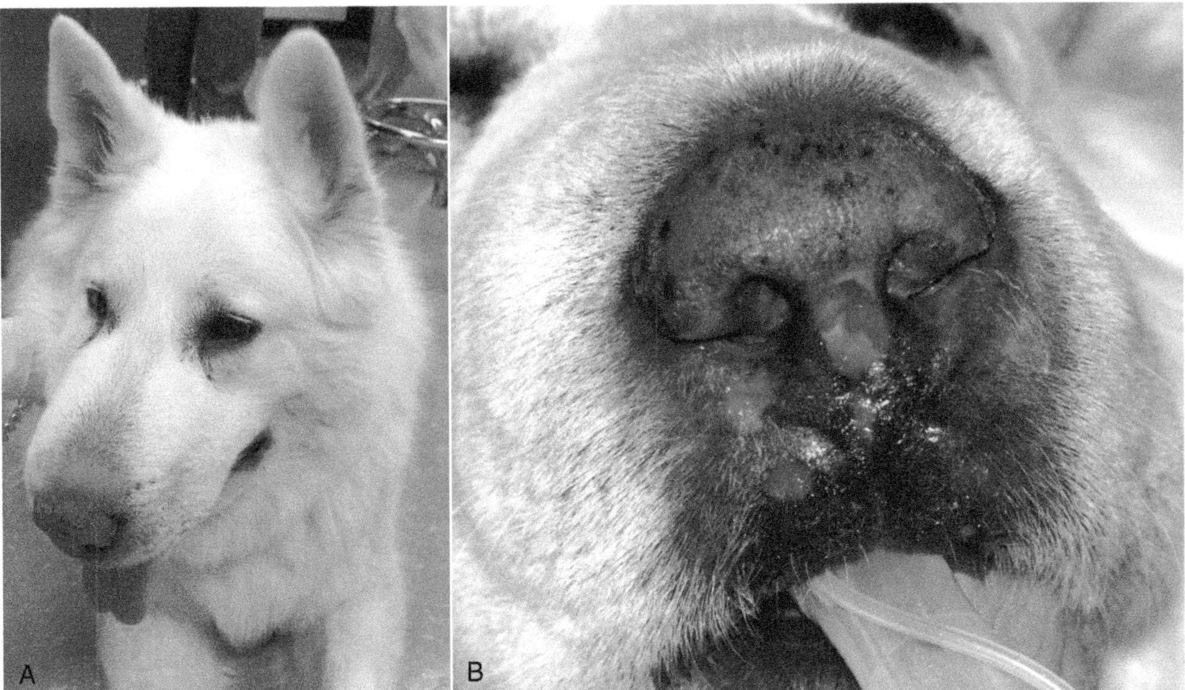

FIGURE 69-6 **A,** Nasopharyngeal *Conidiobolus* spp. infection in a 4-year-old male neutered German shepherd dog. **B,** Note the severe swelling of the nose and muzzle and ulceration of the nasal planum. (Courtesy Amy Grooters, Louisiana State University, Baton Rouge, LA.)

animal patients is lacking because disease is uncommon to rare, and establishment of a definitive diagnosis has historically required tissue biopsy and culture. As a result, small animal patients with zygomycosis often go undifferentiated from those with pythiosis.

Basidiobolus and *Conidiobolus* species are saprophytes commonly found in soil and decaying plant matter. Cutaneous infection with *Basidiobolus* or *Conidiobolus* likely occurs by percutaneous inoculation of spores via minor trauma or insect bites. Infection may also result from inhalation or ingestion of spores.

Clinical Features

In dogs, humans, horses, sheep, and other mammalian species, conidiobolomycosis occurs most often as a nasopharyngeal infection with or without local dissemination into tissues of the face, retropharyngeal region, and retrobulbar space. Manifestations of infection in dogs may include nasal or facial swelling or deformity, nasal discharge, ulceration of the nasal planum or hard palate, exophthalmos, chemosis, ocular discharge, and sometimes skin lesions near the eye (Figure 69-6). In animals with retrobulbar disease that extends into the brain, neurologic signs may occur. *Conidiobolus* infection has been described in a single dog as a cause of multifocal nodular draining subcutaneous lesions and regional lymphadenopathy[24] and as a cause of pneumonia in a dog that was receiving chemotherapy.[25] Basidiobolomycosis is a rare cause of ulcerative skin lesions in dogs and has also been reported as a cause of respiratory disease in a dog.[26] Disseminated *Basidiobolus* infection involving the gastrointestinal tract and other abdominal organs has been described in two dogs.[7,27]

In cats, culture-confirmed cases of zygomycosis are sparse and have been limited to single reports of cats infected with fungi in the order *Mucorales. Rhizomucor* was identified as the cause of duodenal perforation in a 7-month-old cat,[28] and *Cokeromyces recurvatus* was isolated from abdominal fluid in a 16-year-old cat following jejunal perforation caused by lymphosarcoma.[29] In addition, a subcutaneous mass caused by a *Mucor* species on the dorsum of the nose of a 14-year-old cat was treated successfully with posaconazole.[30]

Diagnosis

Because of their histologic similarities, zygomycosis is often confused with pythiosis (which is much more common) when tissue biopsies are evaluated. Unfortunately, there are no serologic, immunohistochemical, or molecular techniques that are routinely available for the diagnosis of zygomycosis, making identification of infected animals reliant on fungal culture of fresh tissues. As a result, a definitive diagnosis of zygomycosis is often elusive.

Laboratory and Imaging Abnormalities

Laboratory abnormalities are not well described in animals with zygomycosis. Diagnostic imaging in the form of computed tomography often provides important information about the location and extent of disease in animals with nasopharyngeal and retrobulbar lesions caused by *Conidiobolus* spp. In addition, ocular ultrasonography may help to characterize the extent of disease in dogs with retrobulbar lesions.

Cytologic and Histologic Findings

The cytologic and histologic features of zygomycosis are similar to those associated with pythiosis and lagenidiosis. On

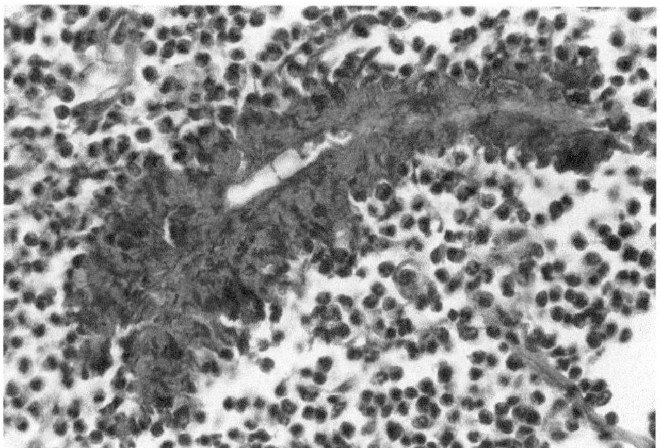

FIGURE 69-7 *Conidiobolus* spp. hyphae in a tissue biopsy from an ulcerated palate lesion in a 3-year-old female boxer. Note the large amount of amorphous eosinophilic material (sleeve) surrounding the hyphal segment; H&E stain. (Courtesy Amy Grooters, Louisiana State University, Baton Rouge, LA.)

GMS-stained sections, hyphae are broad, thin-walled, and occasionally septate. The histologic hallmark of zygomycosis is the presence of a wide (2.5 to 25 µm) eosinophilic sleeve that surrounds the hyphae and makes them easily located on H&E-stained sections (Figure 69-7). This finding helps to differentiate zygomycosis from pythiosis and lagenidiosis, in which eosinophilic sleeves tend to be thin or absent. The hyphal diameter is also significantly larger for *Basidiobolus* spp. (mean 9 µm; range, 5-20 µm) and *Conidiobolus* spp. (mean 8 µm; range, 5-13 µm) than for *P. insidiosum* (mean, 4 µm; range, 2-7 µm).[31]

Treatment and Prognosis

Recommendations for the treatment of zygomycosis are not straightforward because attempted therapy has only been described in a few patients with culture-confirmed diagnoses. Although anecdotal information as well as a small number of cases in the literature suggest that cutaneous zygomycosis may be less aggressive than cutaneous pythiosis or lagenidiosis, progression of lesions and sometimes even dissemination despite treatment have also been observed in zygomycete-infected dogs. The author's current recommendation for dogs with nasopharyngeal conidiobolomycosis is treatment with itraconazole (10 mg/kg PO q24h) for at least 6 months. Recurrence is common after medication is discontinued, so a prolonged course is usually prescribed. Newer oral azoles such as posaconazole would also be reasonable choices but are significantly more expensive. Cutaneous zygomycosis in small animal patients should be treated with aggressive surgical resection of infected tissues whenever possible, followed by itraconazole therapy for 2 to 3 months. If resection is not possible, treatment with itraconazole, posaconazole, or lipid-complexed amphotericin B should be recommended.

Public Health Aspects

Zygomycosis in human patients is rare. Infections are acquired from the environment. Although there is no evidence to suggest that transmission between mammalian hosts occurs, routine precautions (such as wearing gloves when handling infected tissues or exudate) should be followed.

CASE EXAMPLE

Signalment: "Jasper," an 18-month-old intact male Labrador retriever from central Louisiana

History: Jasper was evaluated for a 1-month history of frequent vomiting and persistent diarrhea and a 2-week history of intermittent anorexia. In addition, the owner reported that the dog had lost approximately 6 kg. The diarrhea was watery and yellowish-brown and was produced in large quantity; hematochezia had not been noted. A fecal flotation and heartworm antigen test performed by the referring veterinarian 1 week before the dog was evaluated at the author's institution had been negative. Treatment with metronidazole (17 mg/kg PO q12h) and a change to an easily digestible prescription diet had failed to improve the vomiting and diarrhea. The patient was a field trial dog used for duck and dove hunting in central Louisiana. He frequently worked in rice fields and occasionally in bodies of fresh water and was generally housed in an outdoor kennel.

Physical Examination:

Body Weight: 30 kg.

General: Bright, alert, and responsive. Body temperature = 102.7°F (39.2°C), HR = 110 beats/min, RR = 20 breaths/min, mucous membranes pink, CRT ~ 2 s.

Eyes, ears, nose, and throat: No significant abnormalities were noted.

Musculoskeletal: The dog was underweight with a body condition score of 3/9.

Cardiovascular and Respiratory: Strong femoral pulses. No murmurs or arrhythmias were auscultated. Respiratory rate and effort were normal.

Gastrointestinal and Genitourinary: The patient showed signs of discomfort during abdominal palpation; a large, firm, tubular mass was palpated in the midabdomen. Mild prostatomegaly was detected on rectal examination.

Lymph nodes: All palpable peripheral lymph nodes were normal in size and shape.

Laboratory Findings:

CBC:

HCT 33.7% (37%-55%)
MCV 61.7 fL (62-77 fL)
MCHC 20.8 g/dL (32-37 g/dL)
WBC 10,600 cells/µL (8000-14,500 cells/µL)
Neutrophils 6200 cells/µL (3000-11,500 cells/µL)
Lymphocytes 1700 cells/µL (1000-4800 cells/µL)
Monocytes 1100 cells/µL (100-1400 cells/µL)
Platelets 254,000/µL (220,000-600,000 platelets/µL).

Serum Chemistry Profile:

Sodium 142 mmol/L (140-153 mmol/L)
Potassium 4.4 mmol/L (3.8-5.5 mmol/L)
Chloride 110 mmol/L (107-115 mmol/L)
Bicarbonate 20 mmol/L (17-27 mmol/L)
Phosphorus 4.6 mg/dL (3.4-6.3 mg/dL)
Calcium 9.1 mg/dL (9.4-11.4 mg/dL)

BUN 11 mg/dL (8-22 mg/dL)
Creatinine 0.7 mg/dL (0.5-1.7 mg/dL)
Glucose 96 mg/dL (80-115 mg/dL)
Total protein 5.7 g/dL (5.8-7.5 g/dL)
Albumin 2.0 g/dL (2.6-4.2 g/dL)
Globulin 3.7 g/dL (2.5-4.0 g/dL)
ALT 34 U/L (0-60 U/L)
AST 22 U/L (0-50 U/L)
ALP 13 U/L (0-100 U/L)
Creatine kinase 134 U/L (0-200 U/L)
Cholesterol 158 mg/dL (150-240 mg/dL)
Total bilirubin 0.2 mg/dL (0-0.4 mg/dL).

Urinalysis: SGr 1.041, pH 7.5, 3+ protein, 3+ bilirubin, negative hemoglobin, negative glucose, negative ketones, 0-5 WBC/HPF, 0 RBC/HPF, many lipid droplets.

Imaging Findings:

Plain Abdominal Radiographs: There was a generalized loss of serosal detail in the abdomen. Gas was present in the gastrointestinal tract, but there was no evidence of abnormal intestinal tract dilation.

Abdominal Ultrasound: A severely thickened segment of small bowel could be visualized extending from the cranial to the caudal abdomen. The wall of this bowel segment measured 1.1 cm in thickness and lacked normal layering (Figure 69-8, *A*). Mesenteric lymph nodes were enlarged and heterogenous (Figure 69-8, *B*). There was a small amount of free abdominal fluid.

Cytology Findings: Cytologic evaluation of ultrasound-guided mesenteric lymph node aspirates revealed reactive lymphoid hyperplasia. Examination of ultrasound-guided aspirates of the thickened segment of bowel showed that the cellularity was too low for cytologic evaluation.

Serology Findings: ELISA serology for anti–*Pythium insidiosum* antibodies: Positive at 69%. Results of this assay are expressed as percent positivity in comparison with a strong positive control sample, with values > 40% positivity having been shown to be 100% specific for pythiosis in dogs. Values in healthy dogs range from 3% to 15%.[19]

Diagnosis: Jejunal pythiosis.

Treatment: Abdominal exploratory revealed a 50-cm segment of the mid-jejunum that was severely thickened and firm. This segment was resected with 5-cm margins. After an uneventful postoperative recovery, the dog's vomiting, diarrhea, and anorexia resolved quickly. He was treated with itraconazole (10 mg/kg PO q24h) and terbinafine (8.3 mg/kg PO q24h) for 2 months in an effort to decrease the chance of recurrence of disease at the site of resection. Liver enzyme activities and serum bilirubin concentration were monitored during this time and remained within reference intervals.

Histopathologic Findings: Both the resected segment of jejunum as well as jejunal and ileocolic lymph nodes were submitted for histologic examination. Results revealed severe transmural eosinophilic pyogranulomatous enteritis and lymphoid hyperplasia. In the jejunal lesion, wide (3- to 8-μm), poorly septate hyphae with nonparallel walls were visualized on GMS-stained sections. No organisms were observed in the lymph node sections.

Follow-up: At reevaluation 2 months after resection of the jejunal lesion, the dog remained free of clinical signs and had gained 3 kg body weight. Reevaluation of anti–*Pythium insidiosum* antibody serology at that time yielded a percent positivity of 20%. Because the rapid decrease in antibody levels from 69% to 20% was strongly suggestive of a surgical cure of gastrointestinal pythiosis, oral antifungal medications were discontinued. Reevaluation of anti–*Pythium insidiosum* antibody serology 2 years later yielded results within the range observed in healthy dogs (6%).

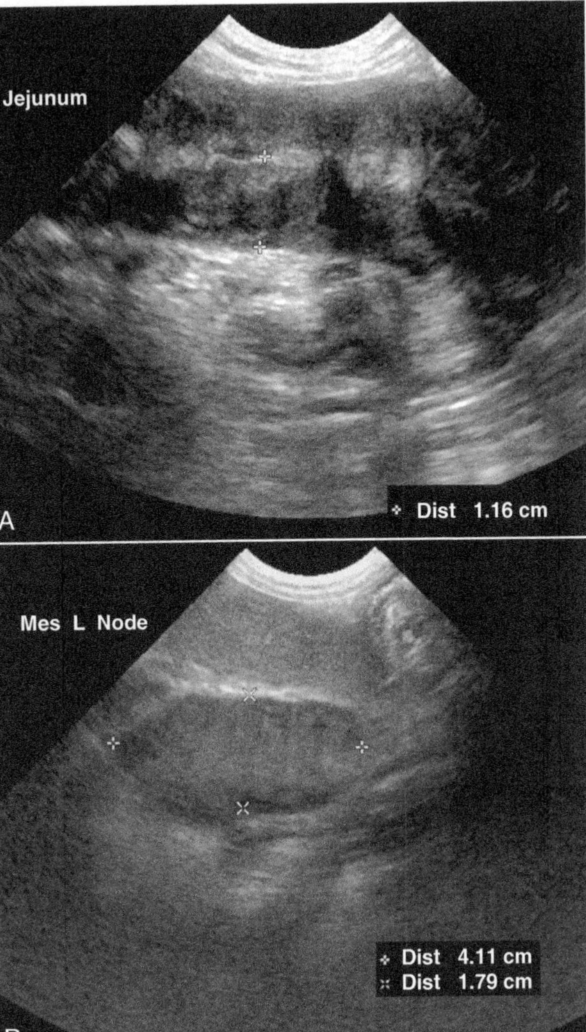

FIGURE 69-8 Sonographic images of the abdomen of the dog described in the case example. Note the severe thickening and loss of layering in the wall of the jejunum **(A)** and the enlarged, heterogenous appearance of the mesenteric lymph node **(B)**.

Comments: Although most dogs with gastrointestinal pythiosis have nonresectable lesions, those with mid-jejunal lesions can often be surgically cured. Preoperative abdominal ultrasound is essential since it helps to determine whether or not a gastrointestinal lesion might be surgically resectable. Because medical therapy alone is often unsuccessful for the treatment of gastrointestinal pythiosis, surgery should be pursued unless there is clear evidence that lesions are nonresectable. Postoperative medical therapy was probably not necessary in the case described

Continued

here, since the postoperative clinical course and follow-up serology results strongly supported a surgical cure. In the author's experience, most dogs with a midjejunal lesion are surgically cured when the surgeon is confident that greater than 5-cm margins of healthy tissue were obtained with the resection and lymph node histology shows hyperplasia rather than infection. In such cases, medical treatment with itraconazole and terbinafine can be offered as optional but likely unnecessary therapy for 2 months until follow-up serology is performed.

SUGGESTED READINGS

Chayakulkeeree M, Ghannoum MA, Perfect JR. Zygomycosis: the re-emerging fungal infection. Eur J Clin Microbiol Infect Dis. 2006;25(4):215-229.

Grooters AM. Pythiosis and lagenidiosis. In: Bonagura JD, ed. Kirk's Current Veterinary Therapy XIV. St. Louis, MO: Saunders; 2008.

Grooters AM. Pythiosis, lagenidiosis, and zygomycosis in small animals. Vet Clin North Am Small Anim Pract. 2003;33:695-720.

REFERENCES

1. Kwon-Chung KJ. Phylogenetic spectrum of fungi that are pathogenic to humans. Clin Infect Dis. 1994;19(suppl 1):S1-S7.
2. Grooters AM. Pythiosis, lagenidiosis, and zygomycosis in small animals. Vet Clin North Am Small Anim Pract. 2003;33:695-720.
3. Smith F. The pathology of bursattee. Vet J. 1884;19:16-17.
4. Gaastra W, Lipman LJ, De Cock AW, et al. *Pythium insidiosum:* an overview. Vet Microbiol. 2010;146:1-16.
5. Mendoza L, Hernandez F, Ajello L. Life cycle of the human and animal oomycete pathogen *Pythium insidiosum*. J Clin Microbiol. 1993;31:2967-2973.
6. Berryessa NA, Marks SL, Pesavento PA, et al. Gastrointestinal pythiosis in 10 dogs from California. J Vet Intern Med. 2008;22:1065-1069.
7. Miller RI. Gastrointestinal phycomycosis in 63 dogs. J Am Vet Med Assoc. 1985;186:473-478.
8. Foil CSO, Short BG, Fadok VA, et al. A report of subcutaneous pythiosis in five dogs and a review of the etiologic agent *Pythium* spp. J Am Anim Hosp Assoc. 1984;20:959-966.
9. Fischer JR, Pace LW, Turk JR, et al. Gastrointestinal pythiosis in Missouri dogs: eleven cases. J Vet Diagn Invest. 1994;6:380-382.
10. Patton CS, Hake R, Newton J, et al. Esophagitis due to *Pythium insidiosum* infection in two dogs. J Vet Intern Med. 1996;10:139-142.
11. Rakich PM, Grooters AM, Tang KN. Gastrointestinal pythiosis in two cats. J Vet Diagn Invest. 2005;17:262-269.
12. Thomas RC, Lewis DT. Pythiosis in dogs and cats. Compend Contin Ed Pract Vet. 1998;20:63-74.
13. Bissonnette KW, Sharp NJ, Dykstra MH, et al. Nasal and retrobulbar mass in a cat caused by *Pythium insidiosum*. J Med Vet Mycol. 1991;29:39-44.
14. LeBlanc CJ, Echandi RL, Moore RR, et al. Hypercalcemia associated with gastric pythiosis in a dog. Vet Clin Pathol. 2008;37:115-120.
15. Thieman KM, Kirkby KA, Flynn-Lurie A, et al. Diagnosis and treatment of truncal cutaneous pythiosis in a dog. J Am Vet Med Assoc. 2011;239:1232-1235.
16. Grooters AM, Whittington A, Lopez MK, et al. Evaluation of microbial culture techniques for the isolation of *Pythium insidiosum* from equine tissues. J Vet Diagn Invest. 2002;14:288-294.
17. Grooters AM, Gee MK. Development of a nested PCR assay for the detection and identification of *Pythium insidiosum*. J Vet Intern Med. 2002;16:147-152.
18. Znajda NR, Grooters AM, Marsella R. PCR-based detection of *Pythium* and *Lagenidium* DNA in frozen and ethanol-fixed animal tissues. Vet Dermatol. 2002;13:187-194.
19. Grooters AM, Leise BS, Lopez MK, et al. Development and evaluation of an enzyme-linked immunosorbent assay for the serodiagnosis of pythiosis in dogs. J Vet Intern Med. 2002;16:142-146.
20. Hummel J, Grooters A, Davidson G, et al. Successful management of gastrointestinal pythiosis in a dog using itraconazole, terbinafine, and mefenoxam. Med Mycol. 2011;49:539-542.
21. Hubert JD, Grooters AM. Treatment of equine pythiosis. Compend Contin Ed Pract Vet. 2002;13:187-194.
22. Wanachiwanawin W, Mendoza L, Visuthisakchai S, et al. Efficacy of immunotherapy using antigens of *Pythium insidiosum* in the treatment of vascular pythiosis in humans. Vaccine. 2004;22:3613-3621.
23. Grooters AM, Hodgin EC, Bauer RW, et al. Clinicopathologic findings associated with *Lagenidium* sp. infection in six dogs: initial description of an emerging oomycosis. J Vet Intern Med. 2003;17:637-646.
24. Hillier A, Kunkle GA, Ginn PE, et al. Canine subcutaneous zygomycosis caused by *Conidiobolus* sp.: a case report and review of *Conidiobolus* infections in other species. Vet Dermatol. 1994;5:205-213.
25. Hawkins EC, Grooters AM, Cowgill ES, et al. Treatment of *Conidiobolus* sp. pneumonia with itraconazole in a dog receiving immunosuppressive therapy. J Vet Intern Med. 2006;20:1479-1482.
26. Greene CE, Brockus CW, Currin MP, et al. Infection with *Basidiobolus ranarum* in two dogs. J Am Vet Med Assoc. 2002;221:528-532:500.
27. Miller RI, Turnwald GH. Disseminated basidiobolomycosis in a dog. Vet Pathol. 1984;21:117-119.
28. Cunha SC, Aguero C, Damico CB, et al. Duodenal perforation caused by *Rhizomucor* species in a cat. J Feline Med Surg. 2011;13:205-207.
29. Nielsen C, Sutton DA, Matise I, et al. Isolation of *Cokeromyces recurvatus*, initially misidentified as *Coccidioides immitis*, from peritoneal fluid in a cat with jejunal perforation. J Vet Diagn Invest. 2005;17:372-378.
30. Wray JD, Sparkes AH, Johnson EM. Infection of the subcutis of the nose in a cat caused by *Mucor* species: successful treatment using posaconazole. J Feline Med Surg. 2008;10:523-527.
31. Miller RI, Campbell RS. The comparative pathology of equine cutaneous phycomycosis. Vet Pathol. 1984;21:325-332.

CHAPTER 70

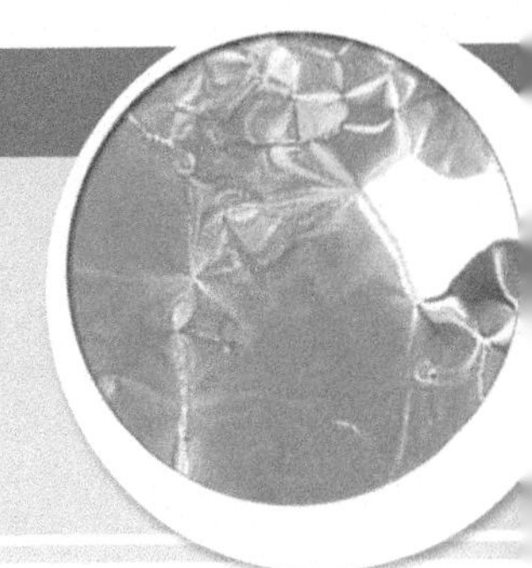

Protothecosis

Jane E. Sykes

Overview of Protothecosis

First Described: *Prototheca* spp. was first isolated from tree slime in the 1880s. Naturally occurring protothecosis was not described until 1952, in cattle (mastitis). Canine disease was reported in 1969, 5 years after the first description of human protothecosis (Van Kruiningen and othes).[1]

Cause: *Prototheca* spp. (lower algae, Chlorophyceae)

Affected Hosts: Dogs, cats, cattle, humans, other domestic and wild animal species

Geographic Distribution: Worldwide except Antarctica, but especially in warm, humid climates and where there is organic matter with a high water content

Mode of Transmission: Cutaneous inoculation of organisms into tissues, or possibly systemic invasion in the face of immunosuppression by organisms that have been ingested or colonize the intestinal tract

Major Clinical Signs: Cutaneous nodules or masses or systemic illness with weight loss, blindness due to ocular involvement, polyuria and polydipsia, hematochezia, vomiting, lameness, neurologic signs

Differential Diagnoses: Chlorellosis (a rare algal disease), a variety of fungal diseases (e.g., histoplasmosis, cryptococcosis, sporotrichosis), intestinal pythiosis, neoplasia (especially round cell neoplasia), toxoplasmosis, neosporosis, granulomatous colitis of boxer dogs, inflammatory bowel disease

Human Health Significance: Human infections occur as a result of exposure to organisms in the environment and are often associated with underlying immune compromise.

Etiology and Epidemiology

Protothecosis is an uncommon cutaneous or systemic disease caused by *Prototheca* species, which are unicellular algae. *Prototheca* spp. lack chlorophyll, and as a result they are dependent on a saprophytic lifestyle. Although ubiquitous in nature, they are especially prevalent in warm, humid climates (e.g., southern and southeastern United States, northeastern Australia, southern continental Europe, Japan) in aqueous environments where decaying organic matter is present. They have been isolated from tree slime, sewage, fresh and saltwater sources, fish tanks, soil, animal excrement, and foodstuffs. Routine water chlorination may not inactivate *Prototheca*.[2] *Prototheca* spp. also colonize the skin and gastrointestinal and respiratory tracts of humans.[3]

The algae are round to oval, 5 to 30 μm in diameter, have a thick cell wall, and reproduce asexually by endosporulation (internal division), which results in a sporangium that contains up to multiple sporangiospores. Rupture of the sporangium releases sporangia into tissues, and the cycle continues. Although the classification of *Prototheca* species is still in flux, six species are currently recognized: *Prototheca zopfii, Prototheca wickerhamii, Prototheca blaschkeae, Prototheca stagnora, Prototheca ulmea,* and *Prototheca cutis* (Table 70-1).[4] Only *P. zopfii* and *P. wickerhamii* have been identified as causes of disease in dogs and cats. Two genotypes of *P. zopfii* are recognized. *P. zopfii* genotype 1 is a weakly pathogenic variant and has been isolated from a minority of protothecal mastitis cases in dairy cows.[4,5] In contrast, *P. zopfii* genotype 2 may be the most virulent *Prototheca* variant. It causes the vast majority of bovine *Prototheca* mastitis cases worldwide and most protothecosis in dogs.[4] *P. wickerhamii* is often associated with cutaneous disease and has to date been isolated from all affected cats, some dogs, and almost all human patients (see Table 70-1). In dogs, disease caused by *P. wickerhamii* may follow a less aggressive clinical course than that caused by *P. zopfii* genotype 2.[6]

Protothecosis is an uncommon and sporadic disease of dogs and is rare in cats. In dogs, protothecosis is usually a serious

TABLE 70-1

Major Species (and Genotypes) of *Prototheca* and Their Clinical Relevance

Species	Host Species Infected	Clinical Manifestations
P. zopfii genotype 1	Cattle	Mastitis (low pathogenicity)
P. zopfii genotype 2	Dogs, humans, cattle, other	Mastitis (cattle), disseminated infections (dogs)
P. wickerhamii	Dogs, cats	Cutaneous disease
P. blaschkeae	Cattle, humans	Mastitis (cattle), cutaneous disease (humans)
P. stagnora	Nonpathogenic	NA
P. ulmea	Nonpathogenic	NA
P. cutis	Humans	Cutaneous disease

NA, Not applicable.

disseminated disease, but localized cutaneous disease occurs occasionally. Most affected dogs do not have a history of immunosuppressive drug therapy or illness. Boxer dogs and collies may be predisposed,[6] possibly secondary to an underlying genetic immunodeficiency, although a variety of other small- and large-breed dogs also can be affected. Occasionally protothecosis occurs in dogs in conjunction with infection by other opportunistic pathogens such as *Neospora*,[7] which supports the likelihood that underlying immune deficiency is present. At the author's hospital, disseminated protothecosis was diagnosed in a canine renal transplant recipient that was treated with cyclosporine, and lymphocutaneous *P. wickerhamii* infection was diagnosed in a dog treated with chemotherapy for lymphoma.[7] The median age of affected dogs in one series of 17 dogs was 4 years (range, 18 months to 11 years), and approximately 70% of the affected dogs were female.[6] Cats with protothecosis have single or multiple nodular skin lesions; disseminated disease has not been reported. Affected cats are typically FIV and FeLV negative, are otherwise in good health, and have ranged in age from 3 to 16 years.[8-13]

Clinical Features

Signs and Their Pathogenesis

The pathogenesis of protothecosis is not fully understood. Infection may occur secondary to cutaneous inoculation of organisms, which may be followed by development of localized cutaneous nodules or dissemination through lymphatic or hematogenous spread. It is also possible that systemic invasion by organisms that are ingested or colonize the gastrointestinal tract occurs. An incubation period of 10 days to several weeks has been suggested for human protothecosis, based on recollection of penetrating injuries before onset of disease.[2]

In dogs, *Prototheca* can disseminate to a variety of tissues, but especially the colon, eyes, brain and meninges, kidneys, and long bones. This results in clinical signs of inappetence and weight loss; acute or chronic large bowel diarrhea (often with hematochezia and tenesmus); blindness; neurologic signs such as obtundation, seizures, or ataxia; polyuria and polydipsia; and sometimes lameness due to osteomyelitis.[6,13-16] Deafness is often reported in association with disseminated protothecosis and may occur as a result of central nervous system (CNS) or inner ear involvement.[13,16,17] Ocular lesions include granulomatous chorioretinitis, uveitis, and panophthalmitis. Other affected organs include the liver, skeletal muscle, thyroid gland, lymph nodes, spleen, pancreas, stomach, small intestine, omentum, myocardium, aorta, spinal cord, and/or lungs.[16-19] Involvement of these organs may lead to other signs such as vomiting, small bowel diarrhea, and/or melena. Sudden death has also been reported, possibly secondary to myocardial involvement.[6,20,21]

Physical Examination Findings

Cutaneous lesions in dogs are nodular and may ulcerate. They often involve the footpads or distal limbs and associated draining lymph nodes, but involvement of other sites such as the trunk and planum nasale can also occur. In cats, single or multiple firm and sometimes ulcerated cutaneous nodules may be present. Lesions may be located on the head, footpads, and distal limbs and tailbase[8-10] and can resemble those caused by *Cryptococcus* or *Sporothrix*.

Dogs with disseminated disease may be obtunded and/or dehydrated and can have a thin body condition. Some dogs are febrile, but rectal temperature may also be normal. Ocular involvement may be manifested by blindness or evidence of conjunctivitis, hyphema, uveitis, cataract formation, panophthalmitis, or granulomatous chorioretinitis, often with retinal detachment. Arrhythmias with pulse deficits may be present in dogs with protothecal myocarditis.[7] Neurologic signs include obtundation, blindness, deafness, ataxia, abnormal placing reactions, circling, head tilt, nystagmus, strabismus, and abnormalities of cranial nerve function such as absent or decreased facial sensation, palpebral, menace, or gag reflexes.[6,14,22-25] Dried fecal material or blood may be present around the anus, and rectal examination may reveal the presence of hematochezia, increased fecal mucus, or melena.

Diagnosis

Laboratory Abnormalities

Complete Blood Count and Serum Biochemical Tests

The CBC in dogs with disseminated protothecosis is often normal. Occasionally it reveals nonregenerative anemia and/or leukocytosis due to a neutrophilia and sometimes monocytosis.[15,16,18] Mild bandemia and/or eosinophilia may be present in some dogs. The serum biochemistry panel may also be normal or reveal hyperglobulinemia due to a polyclonal gammopathy. Mild to moderate azotemia may be evident in dogs with renal involvement.[15,18] Hypoalbuminemia and hypocholesterolemia may occur with severe bowel involvement.[6]

Urinalysis

The urinalysis in dogs with disseminated protothecosis may be unremarkable or reveal isosthenuria, hematuria, pyuria, proteinuria, and the presence of *Prototheca* organisms in the sediment.[15] Urinalysis and urine culture should be performed in all dogs suspected to have protothecosis, because more than half of affected dogs shed algae into the urine.

Cerebrospinal Fluid Cytology

CSF analysis in dogs with CNS protothecosis may be normal or reveal markedly increased total nucleated cell count (sometimes >1000 cells/μL) and increased CSF protein concentration (often >500 mg/dL).[18,22,23] Eosinophilic pleocytosis has been described in some dogs,[22,25] but eosinophils are not always present.[23] *Prototheca* algae may also be found in the CSF.[22,23]

Diagnostic Imaging

Plain Radiography

Thoracic radiographs in dogs with disseminated protothecosis are usually unremarkable.[15,18,19,21] Radiographs of affected long bones may reveal periosteal proliferative and/or osteolytic lesions due to osteomyelitis.[6]

Sonographic Findings

Findings on abdominal ultrasound examination in dogs with disseminated protothecosis include hyperechogenicity of the renal cortices,[15] a thickened colonic wall with loss of normal bowel wall layering,[6] and abdominal lymphadenopathy. Some dogs have no abdominal sonographic abnormalities despite the presence of disseminated disease with colonic and renal involvement.[7]

Other Imaging

Colonoscopy in dogs with protothecosis that has disseminated to the large intestine may reveal a hyperemic, friable, thickened, irregular, and ulcerated mucosa.[6]

Magnetic resonance imaging of the brain of one dog with CNS involvement revealed mild to moderate ventriculomegaly, mild protrusion of the cerebellar vermis through the foramen magnum, syringomyelia, meningeal contrast enhancement, and a focus of increased signal intensity in the brain on T2-weighted and fluid attenuated inversion recovery (FLAIR) sequences.[23] As it enlarged, the focus developed contrast enhancement and caused deformation of a lateral ventricle.

Microbiologic Tests

Specific diagnostic assays for protothecosis are described in Table 70-2.

Cytologic Examination

Prototheca organisms may be seen using cytologic examination of rectal scrapings; fine-needle aspirates of lymph nodes or bone or skin lesions; CSF or vitreal or aqueous humor; and urine sediment. The organisms are spheroid, ovoid, bean-shaped or elliptical, and range in diameter from 1.5 to 30 μm (*P. zopfii*) or up to 10 μm (*P. wickerhamii*). They have a thick, hyaline cell wall that does not take up stain, and a basophilic, granular cytoplasm. Multiple daughter cells (2 to usually <10) may be seen inside the cell (Figure 70-1). In the case of *P. wickerhamii*, the endospores are arranged symmetrically like a daisy or soccer ball, whereas the endospores of *P. zopfii* are

TABLE 70-2

Diagnostic Assays Available for Protothecosis

Assay	Specimen Type	Target	Performance
Cytologic examination	Aspirates of affected tissues, urine sediment, vitreous or aqueous humor, CSF	*Prototheca* algae	Usually large numbers of organisms are present, so sensitivity is high, but false negatives can still occur (such as when urine sediment or CSF are examined). Organisms may be confused with other fungi or *Chlorella* species, so confirmation of the diagnosis requires culture.
Culture	Urine, blood, CSF, vitreous or aqueous humor, aspirates or biopsies of affected tissues	*Prototheca* species	*Prototheca* spp. grow rapidly (usually within 3 days) on routine media such as blood agar and Sabouraud dextrose agar. Allows species identification and subsequent genotyping.
Histopathology	Skin or colonic biopsies, enucleated eyes, tissues collected at necropsy	*Prototheca* algae	Usually large numbers of organisms are present, so sensitivity is high. Organisms are highlighted with PAS or silver stains. Organisms may be confused with other fungi or *Chlorella* species, so confirmation of protothecosis requires culture.

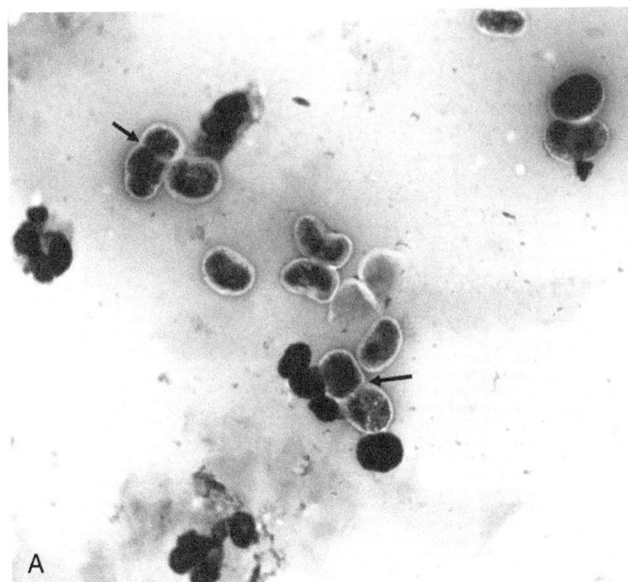

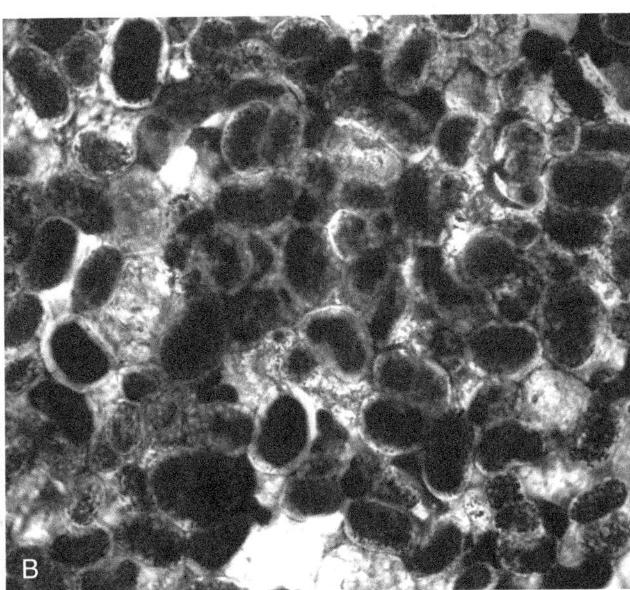

FIGURE 70-1 **A,** Cytology of a subretinal aspirate from an 8-year-old intact male mixed breed dog with panophthalmitis due to *Prototheca* spp. infection. Moderate numbers of oval to bean-shaped organisms are present in a proteinaceous background that contained variably degenerate and ruptured neutrophils. The organisms have a thin clear capsule with deep purple cytoplasmic granulation. Sometimes endosporulation is evident *(arrows)*. Wright's stain, 1000× oil magnification. **B,** Cytology of a bone aspirate from a 2-year-old female mixed breed dog that developed acute vision loss. Physical examination revealed bilateral retinal detachment and a nonpainful swelling of the right distal medial humerus. Abundant numbers of *Prototheca* algae are present. (Courtesy Dr. Emily Pieczarka.)

distributed randomly.[2] The algae may be mistaken for fungi such as *Blastomyces, Coccidioides,* or *Cryptococcus.* Because large numbers of organisms are typically present, the sensitivity of cytologic examination for diagnosis of algal infection is high. However, failure to find organisms does not rule out protothecosis.

Culture

Prototheca species can be readily cultured in the microbiology laboratory on standard media (such as blood agar and Sabouraud dextrose agar), and yeast-like colonies are usually visible within 7 days. Suitable specimens for culture include aspirates or biopsies of affected tissue and body fluids such as urine, CSF, and vitreous or aqueous humor. *Prototheca zopfii* was also cultured from the blood of a dog with disseminated disease.[21] Biochemical testing of isolates allows identification of the *Prototheca* species present and excludes other possible causes such as the green alga *Chlorella,* a very rare cause of disseminated disease in dogs that can closely resemble *Prototheca* in its microscopic appearance.[2,26] Differentiation of *P. zopfii* genotypes requires PCR and ribosomal RNA gene sequencing. Matrix-assisted laser desorption/ionization–time of flight (MALDI-TOF) mass spectrometry offers promise for rapid identification to the species and genotype level in the clinical microbiology laboratory in the future.[4,27]

Antifungal susceptibility testing has been performed for *Prototheca* but has not been standardized, and the clinical relevance of the results is not clear.[2]

Molecular Diagnosis Using the Polymerase Chain Reaction

Real-time PCR assays have been developed that detect and differentiate *Prototheca* species,[28] but these are not available on a commercial basis for diagnosis of protothecosis in animals.

Pathologic Findings

Gross pathologic findings in dogs with disseminated protothecosis include enlarged lymph nodes and gray, tan, or white nodular lesions or streaks in affected organs.[13,16,18,25] The colonic wall may be thickened and contain bloody fluid. Malacic foci may be present in the brain, or the brain may appear normal grossly, even when meningoencephalitis is present.[7,24] Histopathologic examination of affected tissues typically reveals large numbers of sporulating and nonsporulating algae accompanied by a mixed inflammatory response and foci of necrosis (Figure 70-2, *A*). In some tissues the inflammatory response can be minimal to absent.[16,18] Organisms may be seen free and

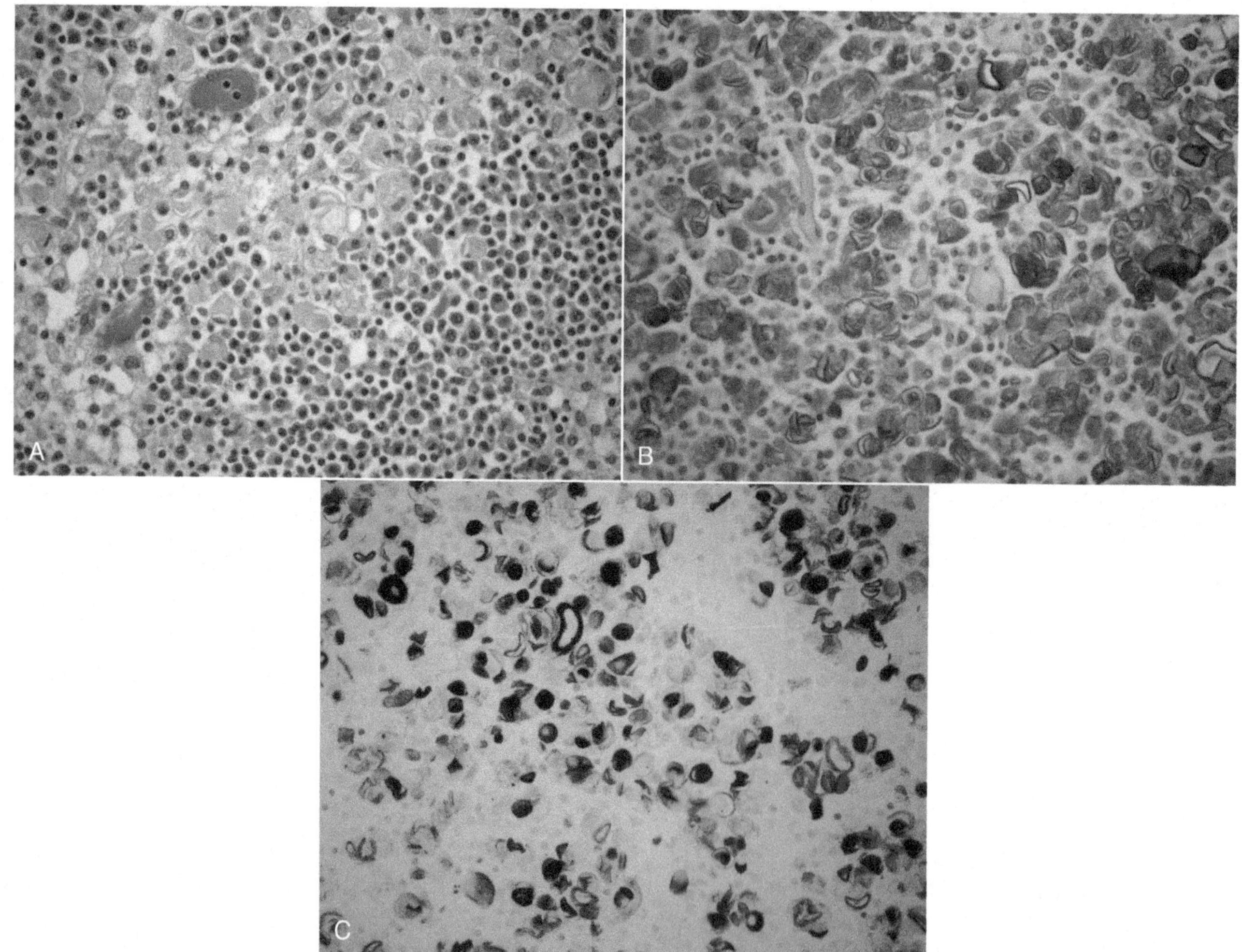

FIGURE 70-2 Histopathology of the renal lymph node of a 6-year-old spayed female shih tzu with protothecosis that was being treated with cyclosporine after renal transplantation. Numerous *Prototheca* organisms are present. The organisms range in diameter from 5 to 15 μm and have several morphologic forms. Sporulating forms are up to 15 μm in diameter and contain two to four wedge-shaped endospores (daughter cells). Many of the organisms present as clear, refractile, oval to polyhedral bodies composed of a thick wall and devoid of cytoplasm and nuclei. **A,** H&E stain. **B,** Periodic acid–Schiff stain. **C,** Gomori's methenamine silver.

within macrophages. The cell wall stains well with Gomori's methenamine silver and periodic acid–Schiff (PAS) stain, but in contrast to *Chlorella*, cytoplasmic granules of *Prototheca* are PAS negative. Cutaneous lesions in cats have been associated with a granulomatous inflammatory response with multinucleated giant cells and, in some cases, necrosis and neutrophilic inflammation.[9,11]

Treatment and Prognosis

Surgical excision can be curative for localized cutaneous protothecosis and should be performed whenever possible.[9] Medical treatment of protothecosis is challenging. In human patients, treatment is generally with amphotericin B, which in some cases results in complete cure. Addition of a tetracycline has also been recommended.[2] Outcomes with azole antifungals alone are often poor, although clinical responses occur in some dogs with itraconazole alone.[7] In one human patient, a combination of amikacin and tetracycline led to cure.[29] Treatment of canine disseminated protothecosis with amphotericin B leads to remission in some cases, but relapse typically occurs when the drug is discontinued, or dogs fail to respond to treatment and ultimately die or are euthanized as a result of the disease.[6,21] One dog with protothecal meningoencephalitis appeared to improve clinically after treatment with oral itraconazole and intrathecal amphotericin B, but was euthanized 4 weeks later because of progressive disease.[23]

Other treatments that may be required for protothecosis include intravenous fluid therapy, antiemetics, topical prednisolone acetate ophthalmic drops for uveitis, or ocular enucleation to control pain and/or remove a focus of infection that fails to respond to chemotherapy (see Case Example). Other treatments such as metronidazole, sulfasalazine, or dietary manipulation may help to control signs of protothecal colitis.

Public Health Aspects

Protothecosis is an uncommon disease of humans and most often caused by *P. wickerhamii*. Infection is acquired from environmental sources, and direct transmission of other animals or humans does not appear to be important. Mortality is low (<5%), and two thirds of infections are chronic and localized to the skin.[2] Joint infections and tendonitis have been described after surgical or accidental wounds; some have been traced back to cleaning an aquarium.[30] Disseminated infections and a syndrome called olecranon bursitis (which follows elbow trauma) account for the remaining third of cases. Underlying local or systemic immune defects can be identified in many patients; topical, local, or systemic glucocorticoid treatment is the most frequently identified risk factor. Other immunosuppressive disorders that may predispose humans to protothecosis include diabetes mellitus and malignancy. Severe disseminated disease has been described in bone marrow and kidney transplant recipients,[31,32] in those with long-standing indwelling catheters or endotracheal tubes, and rarely in AIDS patients.[30,33]

CASE EXAMPLE

Signalment: "Merlot," a 3-year-old female spayed Siberian husky dog from San Francisco, CA

History: Merlot was evaluated at the University of California, Davis, Veterinary Medical Teaching Hospital for a 1-month history of hemorrhagic diarrhea, inappetence, and weight loss. Initially the diarrhea contained fresh blood and mucus but more recently contained only blood. The diarrhea occurred frequently and in small quantities. The owner reported that Merlot had lost approximately 5 kg over the past month and had increased thirst and urination. There had been no history of vomiting, and Merlot's activity level was normal. Her diet consisted of a commercial dry dog food.

At a local veterinary clinic, multiple fecal flotations had been negative, and Merlot had been treated with metronidazole, aminopentamide, bismuth subsalicylate, enrofloxacin, loperamide, tetracycline, metoclopramide, and a highly digestible diet without clinical response. A barium series had recently been performed, and findings were consistent with gastroenteritis.

Merlot had moved to San Francisco from Massachusetts 4 months before the clinical signs began. On the way over the owner stopped in Texas, where Merlot became lost in a field for 30 minutes. The owner reported that Merlot was taken to a dog park in San Francisco several times a week. No other history of illness existed.

Physical Examination:

Body Weight: 18.2 kg.

General: Bright, alert, responsive, and hydrated. T = 102.3°F (39.1°C), HR = 80 beats/min, panting, mucous membranes pink, CRT = 1 s.

Integument, Eyes, Ears, Nose, and Throat: Dried barium was present on the dog's lips, and there were no other clinically significant findings. Fundoscopic examination revealed a region of retinal separation in the left ocular fundus that was adjacent to, dorsomedial to, and approximately the size of the optic disc. The lesion appeared to contain yellowish fluid.

Musculoskeletal: Thin but well-muscled. Body condition score was 3/9.

Cardiorespiratory: No clinically significant findings.

Gastrointestinal/Genitourinary: No masses were palpated in the abdomen. The dog vocalized and appeared painful on caudal abdominal palpation. Frank blood was present on the glove after rectal examination.

Peripheral Lymph Nodes: All peripheral lymph nodes were normal in size.

Laboratory Findings:

CBC:

HCT 48.6% (40%-55%)
MCV 70.9 fL (65-75 fL)
MCHC 34.6 g/dL (33-36 g/dL)
WBC 12,100 cells/μL (6000-13,000 cells/μL)
Neutrophils 9438 cells/μL (3000-10,500 cells/μL)
Lymphocytes 2057 cells/μL (1000-4000 cells/μL)

Monocytes 363 cells/μL (150-1200 cells/μL)
Eosinophils 242 cells/μL (0-1500 cells/μL)
Platelets 259,000/μL (150,000-400,000 platelets/μL).

Serum Chemistry Profile:
Sodium 150 mmol/L (145-154 mmol/L)
Potassium 4.3 mmol/L (3.6-5.3 mmol/L)
Chloride 114 mmol/L (108-118 mmol/L)
Bicarbonate 28 mmol/L (16-26 mmol/L)
Phosphorus 4.2 mg/dL (3.0-6.2 mg/dL)
Calcium 9.8 mg/dL (9.7-11.5 mg/dl)
BUN 21 mg/dL (5-21 mg/dL)
Creatinine 1.2 mg/dL (0.3-1.2 mg/dL)
Glucose 99 mg/dL (64-123 mg/dL)
Total protein 6.4 g/dL (5.4-7.6 g/dL)
Albumin 2.9 g/dL (3.0-4.4 g/dL)
Globulin 3.5 g/dL (1.8-3.9 g/dL)
ALT 61 U/L (19-67 U/L)
AST 42 U/L (19-42 U/L)
ALP 126 U/L (21-170 U/L)
Cholesterol 145 mg/dL (135-361 mg/dL)
Total bilirubin 0 mg/dL (0-0.2 mg/dL).

Urinalysis: SGr 1.005; pH 6.0; no protein (SSA), bilirubin, hemoprotein, or glucose; 0-1 WBC/HPF, rare RBC/HPF, rare transitional epithelial cells; no crystals, casts or bacteria. Moderate numbers of encapsulated organisms were present that measured 10 × 17 μm.

Imaging Findings: Abdominal ultrasound examination: No abnormalities were identified.

Microbiologic Testing: Centrifugal zinc sulfate fecal flotation: Negative, but yeast-like bodies were observed.

Giardia and *Cryptosporidium* fluorescent antibody testing (fecal specimen): Negative.

Cytologic examination of rectal scrapings: Moderate numbers of neutrophils, small numbers of gram-positive coccobacilli, and small numbers of what appeared to be algae were present.

Aerobic bacterial urine culture: Small numbers of *Prototheca zopfii*.

Algal susceptibility testing: MICs for amphotericin B, fluconazole, and itraconazole were 0.5 μg/mL, >64 μg/mL, and 1 μg/mL, respectively.

Histopathology (rectal biopsy obtained by proctoscopy): erosive and hemorrhagic colitis, eosinophilic and lymphoplasmacytic, moderate, with marked expansion of the lamina propria by intralesional spherical organisms (protothecal colitis).

Aerobic bacterial and fungal culture of a rectal biopsy: Small numbers of mixed enteric species and *P. zopfii*.

Diagnosis: Disseminated *P. zopfii* infection with ocular and colonic involvement.

Treatment: Merlot was initially treated with lipid-complexed amphotericin B (3 mg/kg IV) on a Monday, Wednesday, and Friday basis for five doses, after which increased serum creatinine concentration was noted (1.7 mg/dL). She was also treated with oxytetracycline (21 mg/kg PO q8h). She was discharged after 11 days with instructions to administer itraconazole (5 mg/kg PO q12h) and lufenuron (5 mg/kg PO q24h). At a recheck examination 2 weeks later, the owners reported Merlot's appetite had improved slightly and that she was defecating once to twice a day. Each bowel movement was followed by a small amount of diarrhea at the end of defecation, with bloody mucoid material occasionally present. In the 2 weeks since her previous visit, a foxtail had been removed from her right pelvic limb and she had been sprayed in the face by a skunk. Physical examination revealed a body weight of 19.2 kg (1 kg weight gain), but aqueous flare and multifocal retinal separations were present in both eyes. Urinalysis was unremarkable, and rectal scrapings showed no evidence of algal organisms. A biochemistry panel showed normalization of the creatinine and mildly increased activity of ALT, likely secondary to itraconazole administration. Topical prednisolone acetate ophthalmic drops and two additional amphotericin B treatments were administered, but bilateral retinal detachment, blindness, then bilateral hyphema and apparent ocular pain developed despite this treatment. Bilateral enucleation was performed. Histopathology of the globes showed bilateral granulomatous uveitis and retinitis with intralesional *Prototheca* organisms. In the left eye, posterior synechiae, intraocular hemorrhage, and cataract formation were identified.

At a recheck examination 3 months after enucleation, Merlot was eating well and had no signs of large bowel diarrhea. Her body weight was stable and physical examination, a CBC, a biochemistry panel, and cytologic examination of a rectal scraping were unremarkable. Itraconazole treatment was continued at a lower dose (5 mg/kg PO q24h), and the lufenuron was discontinued. Two months later, and shortly after a new puppy was introduced, Merlot developed vomiting and diarrhea with small amounts of hematochezia, and her body weight dropped to 17.5 kg. A serum biochemistry panel showed mild hypoalbuminemia (2.6 g/dL). Cytologic examination of a rectal scraping again revealed *Prototheca* organisms, and a fecal flotation was negative. Merlot was treated with fenbendazole and the dose of itraconazole was increased to 7.5 mg/kg PO daily, after which diarrhea resolved. Four months later (14 months after initial diagnosis), the dog remained in remission but was subsequently lost to follow-up.

Comments: Diagnosis of protothecosis in this dog was straightforward and initially based on routine urine sediment examination. Culture was then used to identify the causative agent as *P. zopfii*. Colonic involvement was confirmed using proctoscopy and biopsy. The most likely place that *Prototheca* infection was acquired was in Texas, but it is possible that infection was acquired elsewhere. Partial clinical remission was observed after treatment with lipid-complexed amphotericin B and itraconazole, but enucleation was required to control pain. Remission was prolonged (>1 year) even though only seven amphotericin B treatments were administered in the first 2 months after diagnosis. Lufenuron is a chitin synthetase inhibitor. Chitin is present in the cell walls of some algae (including *Chlorella*), but whether *Prototheca* possess chitin in their cell walls is not clear.

SUGGESTED READINGS

Lass-Florl C, Mayr A. Human protothecosis. Clin Microbiol Rev. 2007;20:230-242.

Quigley RR, Knowles KE, Johnson GC. Disseminated chlorellosis in a dog. Vet Pathol. 2009;46:439-443.

Stenner VJ, Mackay B, King T, et al. Protothecosis in 17 Australian dogs and a review of the canine literature. Med Mycol. 2007;45:249-266.

REFERENCES

1. Van Kruiningen HJ, Garner FM, Schiefer B. Protothecosis in a dog. Pathol Vet. 1969;6:348-354.
2. Lass-Florl C, Mayr A. Human protothecosis. Clin Microbiol Rev. 2007;20:230-242.
3. Sonck CE, Koch Y. *Prototheca* as parasites of skin. Mykosen. 1971;14:475-482.
4. Ahrholdt J, Murugaiyan J, Straubinger RK, et al. Epidemiological analysis of worldwide bovine, canine and human clinical *Prototheca* isolates by PCR genotyping and MALDI-TOF mass spectrometry proteomic phenotyping. Med Mycol. 2012;50:234-243.
5. Ricchi M, Goretti M, Branda E, et al. Molecular characterization of *Prototheca* strains isolated from Italian dairy herds. J Dairy Sci. 2010;93:4625-4631.
6. Stenner VJ, Mackay B, King T, et al. Protothecosis in 17 Australian dogs and a review of the canine literature. Med Mycol. 2007;45:249-266.
7. Sykes JE. Unpublished observations, 2012.
8. Coloe PJ, Allison JF. Protothecosis in a cat. J Am Vet Med Assoc. 1982;180:78-79.
9. Dillberger JE, Homer B, Daubert D, et al. Protothecosis in two cats. J Am Vet Med Assoc. 1988;192:1557-1559.
10. Endo S, Sekiguchi M, Kishimoto Y, et al. The first case of feline *Prototheca wickerhamii* infection in Japan. J Vet Med Sci. 2010;72:1351-1353.
11. Finnie JW, Coloe PJ. Cutaneous protothecosis in a cat. Aust Vet J. 1981;57:307-308.
12. Kaplan W, Chandler FW, Holzinger EA, et al. Protothecosis in a cat: first recorded case. Sabouraudia. 1976;14:281-286.
13. Migaki G, Font RL, Sauer RM, et al. Canine protothecosis: review of the literature and report of an additional case. J Am Vet Med Assoc. 1982;181:794-797.
14. Lane LV, Meinkoth JH, Brunker J, et al. Disseminated protothecosis diagnosed by evaluation of CSF in a dog. Vet Clin Pathol. 2012;41:147-152.
15. Pressler BM, Gookin JL, Sykes JE, et al. Urinary tract manifestations of protothecosis in dogs. J Vet Intern Med. 2005;19:115-119.
16. Gaunt SD, McGrath RK, Cox HU. Disseminated protothecosis in a dog. J Am Vet Med Assoc. 1984;185:906-907.
17. Cook Jr JR, Tyler DE, Coulter DB, et al. Disseminated protothecosis causing acute blindness and deafness in a dog. J Am Vet Med Assoc. 1984;184:1266-1272.
18. Rakich PM, Latimer KS. Altered immune function in a dog with disseminated protothecosis. J Am Vet Med Assoc. 1984;185:681-683.
19. Buyukmihci N, Rubin LF, DePaoli A. Protothecosis with ocular involvement in a dog. J Am Vet Med Assoc. 1975;167:158-161.
20. Blogg JR, Sykes JE. Sudden blindness associated with protothecosis in a dog. Aust Vet J. 1995;72:147-149.
21. Moore FM, Schmidt GM, Desai D, et al. Unsuccessful treatment of disseminated protothecosis in a dog. J Am Vet Med Assoc. 1985;186:705-708.
22. Gupta A, Gumber S, Bauer RW, et al. What is your diagnosis? Cerebrospinal fluid from a dog. Eosinophilic pleocytosis due to protothecosis. Vet Clin Pathol. 2011;40:105-106.
23. Young M, Bush W, Sanchez M, et al. Serial MRI and CSF analysis in a dog treated with intrathecal amphotericin B for protothecosis. J Am Anim Hosp Assoc. 2012;48:125-131.
24. Salvadori C, Gandini G, Ballarini A, et al. Protothecal granulomatous meningoencephalitis in a dog. J Small Anim Pract. 2008;49:531-535.
25. Tyler DE, Lorenz MD, Blue JL, et al. Disseminated protothecosis with central nervous system involvement in a dog. J Am Vet Med Assoc. 1980;176:987-993.
26. Quigley RR, Knowles KE, Johnson GC. Disseminated chlorellosis in a dog. Vet Pathol. 2009;46:439-443.
27. von Bergen M, Eidner A, Schmidt F, et al. Identification of harmless and pathogenic algae of the genus *Prototheca* by MALDI-MS. Proteomics Clin Appl. 2009;3:774-784.
28. Ricchi M, Cammi G, Garbarino CA, et al. A rapid real-time PCR/DNA resolution melting method to identify *Prototheca* species. J Appl Microbiol. 2011;110:27-34.
29. Zhao J, Liu W, Lv G, et al. Protothecosis successfully treated with amikacin combined with tetracyclines. Mycoses. 2004;47:156-158.
30. Pascual JS, Balos LL, Baer AN. Disseminated *Prototheca wickerhamii* infection with arthritis and tenosynovitis. J Rheumatol. 2004;31:1861-1865.
31. Lass-Florl C, Fille M, Gunsilius E, et al. Disseminated infection with *Prototheca zopfii* after unrelated stem cell transplantation for leukemia. J Clin Microbiol. 2004;42:4907-4908.
32. Mohd Tap R, Sabaratnam P, Salleh MA, et al. Characterization of *Prototheca wickerhamii* isolated from disseminated algaemia of kidney transplant patient from Malaysia. Mycopathologia. 2012;173:173-178.
33. Kaminski ZC, Kapila R, Sharer LR, et al. Meningitis due to *Prototheca wickerhamii* in a patient with AIDS. Clin Infect Dis. 1992;15:704-706.

CHAPTER 71

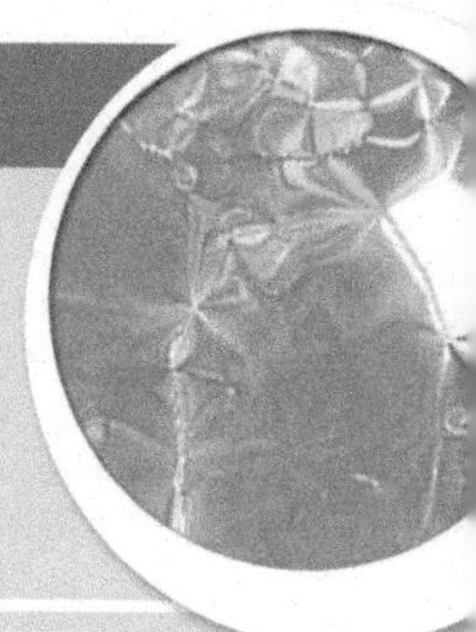

Pneumocystosis

Remo Lobetti

> **Overview of Pneumocystosis**
>
> First Described: *Pneumocystis* was first discovered in Brazil in 1909 (Chagas), when it was initially mistaken for a trypanosome.[1] It was first reported in dogs in the 1950s.[2]
>
> Causes: *Pneumocystis* spp. (an ascomycete)
>
> Affected Hosts: Dogs, humans, pigs, horses, goats, nonhuman primates; *Pneumocystis* species appear to have host specificity.
>
> Geographic Distribution: Worldwide
>
> Mode of Transmission: Opportunistic invasion of immunosuppressed hosts after transmission by aerosol
>
> Major Clinical Signs: Weight loss, respiratory distress, exercise intolerance, variable cough
>
> Differential Diagnoses: Canine distemper virus infection, bacterial pneumonia, mycobacterial infections, other fungal causes of pneumonia, pulmonary neoplasia (especially lymphoma), parasitic lung disease, acute respiratory distress syndrome, pulmonary fibrosis
>
> Human Health Significance: Severely immunocompromised humans are at risk for pneumocystosis, but only *P. jirovecii* infects humans. Whether humans can become colonized with *Pneumocystis* strains that infect dogs is not known.

Etiologic Agent and Epidemiology

Pneumocystis is a saprophyte of low virulence with a worldwide distribution. Its primary habitat is the mammalian lung, where it causes opportunistic pneumonia. *Pneumocystis* pneumonia has been reported in dogs, pigs, horses, goats, primates, and humans. Subclinical or latent infections are common in rats, mice, guinea pigs, rabbits, cats, sheep, and various wildlife species. Most reports of pneumonia due to *Pneumocystis* spp. infection are linked with documented or suspected immunodeficiency syndromes in the host.[3]

The taxonomy of *Pneumocystis* is uncertain. Previously it was classified as a unicellular protozoan in the phylum Sarcomastigophora. However, ultrastructurally the reproductive behavior of *Pneumocystis* is similar to the ascospore formation by yeasts, and its organelles and staining properties by light microscopy resemble those of pathogenic fungi. Phylogenetic classification based on 16S-like rRNA sequences indicates that *Pneumocystis* is most closely related to the fungi of the class Ascomycetes, especially *Saccharomyces cerevisiae*, and so it has been reclassified as fungus, "albeit an odd one."[4] Biologically, it behaves similarly to a protozoan, because it is susceptible to drugs used to treat protozoal infections but resistant to most antifungal drugs. The morphology of *Pneumocystis* organisms and the histopathology of the lesions they produce in humans and animals throughout the world are similar. Although controversial, five species of *Pneumocystis* have been described, which appear to be highly host specific: two species that infect rats, *Pneumocystis carinii* and *Pneumocystis wakefieldiae*; one species that infects mice, *Pneumocystis murina*; a species that infects rabbits, *Pneumocystis oryctolagi*; and *Pneumocystis jirovecii* (pronounced "yee row vet zee"), which infects humans.[5-7] Species designations for the organisms isolated from dogs and other animals require further genetic and biologic study, although DNA analysis of *Pneumocystis* that infected a Cavalier King Charles spaniel suggested that dogs are infected with a unique species, with the proposed name of *Pneumocystis canis*.[8] Biologic differences between isolates from different hosts are supported by the relative difficulty of experimental cross-host species transmission. Because historically *P. carinii* was thought to cause *Pneumocystis* pneumonia in humans, *Pneumocystis* pneumonia has long been referred to as "PCP." Despite the name change to *P. jirovecii* in the 1970s, the term PCP has been retained for convenience. For purposes of this chapter, the organism will be referred to simply as *Pneumocystis*. Strain differences may also exist within species of *Pneumocystis*.

Pneumocystis appears to be maintained in nature by transmission from infected to susceptible hosts. The primary mode of spread is thought to be airborne droplet transmission.[9] Sporadic disease may occur as a result of activation of latent infection by stress, crowding, and immunosuppressive therapy during hospitalization. Clinical disease can also be experimentally activated by treatment with glucocorticoids or cytotoxic chemotherapy. A higher prevalence of infection was found in dogs with distemper compared with a corresponding control population.[10] Genetic analysis of isolates from humans suggests that recent acquisition of infection from another person, rather than reactivation of infection, may be responsible for clinical illness.[11,12]

Most affected dogs have been young miniature dachshunds (less than 1 year of age) or Cavalier King Charles spaniels.[8,13-17] Affected miniature dachshunds and Cavalier King Charles spaniels may possess an underlying primary immune deficiency.[17,18]

Clinical Features

Signs and Their Pathogenesis

Pneumocystis is inhaled and can colonize the lower respiratory tracts of clinically healthy mammals; however, it rarely multiplies to large numbers in the lungs of healthy hosts. Transmission of infection to neonates can occur via aspiration of contaminated amniotic fluid when the placenta is infected. When impaired host resistance (especially reduced CD4 T-lymphocyte counts) or preexisting pulmonary disease is present, rapid proliferation of organisms can occur.[19] The entire life cycle of *Pneumocystis* is completed within alveolar spaces (Figure 71-1). In this location, two main forms, the trophozoite (1 to 4 μm in diameter) and cyst (8 μm), are found. Trophozoites adhere closely to alveolar epithelial cells and are thought to undergo sexual reproduction by conjugation, with formation of a diploid zygote. The zygote becomes a sporocyte (or precyst) and undergoes meiosis followed by mitosis. This leads to formation of a mature, thick-walled cyst or spore case, which contains eight haploid ascospores. The cyst ruptures, and the spores transform into trophozoites, which replicate asexually to form more trophozoites, or sexually to form more cyst forms. The transmissible form has not been identified.[7]

The overgrowth and clustering of *Pneumocystis* within alveolar spaces leads to blockage of capillaries and decreased gas exchange. Intra-alveolar organisms are often accompanied by thickening of alveolar septa, but they seldom invade the pulmonary interstitium and are rarely phagocytosed by alveolar macrophages. With an adequate immune response, the body eliminates the infection, but the removal of large numbers of organisms and cellular debris may take up to 8 weeks. Both the presence of the organisms and the mild inflammatory response they provoke contribute to pulmonary damage.

Although *Pneumocystis* infections are usually confined to the lungs, organisms are rarely reported in extrapulmonary sites. In humans, extrapulmonary pneumocystosis occurs primarily when there is overwhelming pulmonary infection, profound underlying immunodeficiency, and after long-term use of aerosolized pentamidine for prophylaxis against *P. jirovecii* pneumonia in HIV-infected patients.[20] Sites of extrapulmonary infection include lymph nodes, spleen, liver, bone marrow, gastrointestinal tract, eyes, thyroid gland, adrenal glands, kidneys, heart, pancreas, and external auditory canal. Extrapulmonary pneumocystosis has been described in one dog.

The typical clinical history in dogs with pneumocystosis is that of gradual weight loss and respiratory difficulty that progresses over 1 to 4 weeks. The weight loss, which occurs in spite of a good appetite in most dogs, may be associated with diarrhea and occasional vomiting. Cough is not always reported, but reduced exercise tolerance is uniform. Infected animals often show a minimal or temporary response to antibiotic and glucocorticoid therapy.

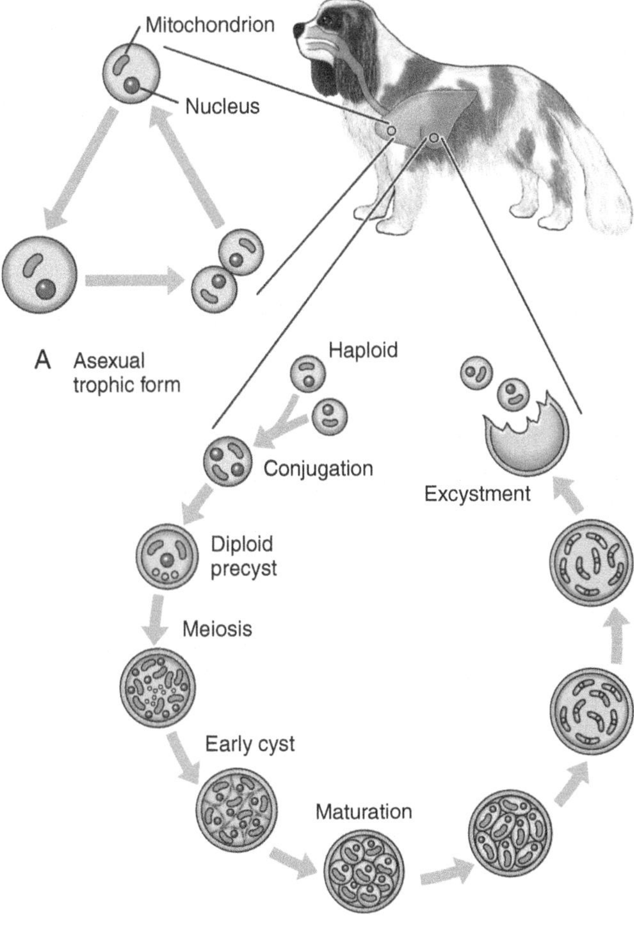

FIGURE 71-1 Life cycle of *Pneumocystis* species. Trophozoites adhere to alveolar epithelial cells in the lungs and undergo both asexual **(A)** and sexual **(B)** reproduction. Sexual reproduction is initiated by conjugation, which results in formation of a zygote. Meiosis occurs followed by mitosis, which leads to the formation of 8 ascospores within a mature cyst. The cyst ruptures, releasing spores that become trophozoites. (Modified from Walzer PD, Smulian AG. Pneumocystis species. In: Mandell GL, Bennett JE, Dolin R, eds. Principles and Practice of Infectious Diseases, 7 ed. Philadelphia, PA: Elsevier; 2010:3377-3390.)

Physical Examination Findings

Abnormalities on physical examination of dogs with pneumocystosis include dyspnea, tachycardia, and increased dry respiratory sounds on thoracic auscultation. Animals are often in poor condition and cachectic and can show dermatologic changes, such as superficial bacterial pyoderma and demodicosis (Figure 71-2). Although the mucous membranes are generally of normal color, they may be cyanotic in severely affected animals. Affected dogs remain relatively alert and afebrile, although mild pyrexia may be present.

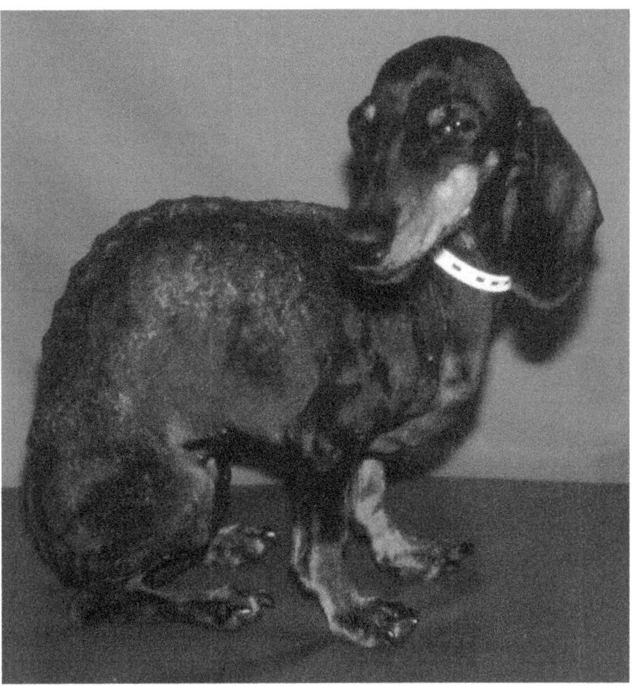

FIGURE 71-2 One-year-old dachshund with pneumocystosis. Note the thin body condition and alopecia secondary to generalized demodectic mange.

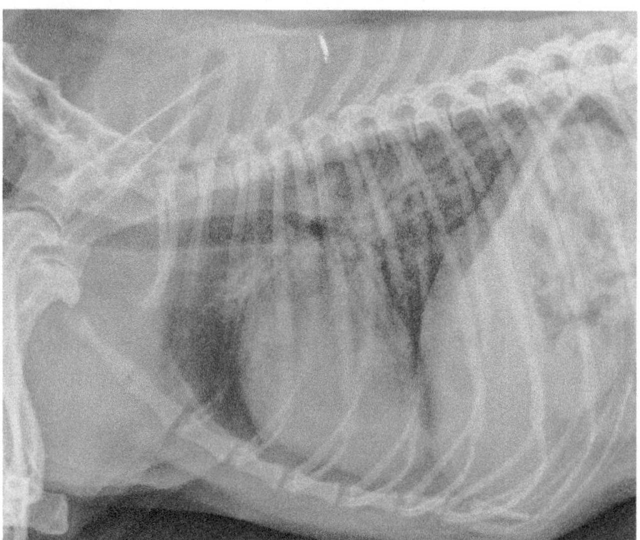

FIGURE 71-3 Lateral thoracic radiographs from a 1-year-old male neutered Cavalier King Charles spaniel with pneumocystosis. A diffuse marked interstitial pattern is present. Mild right-sided cardiomegaly was also identified.

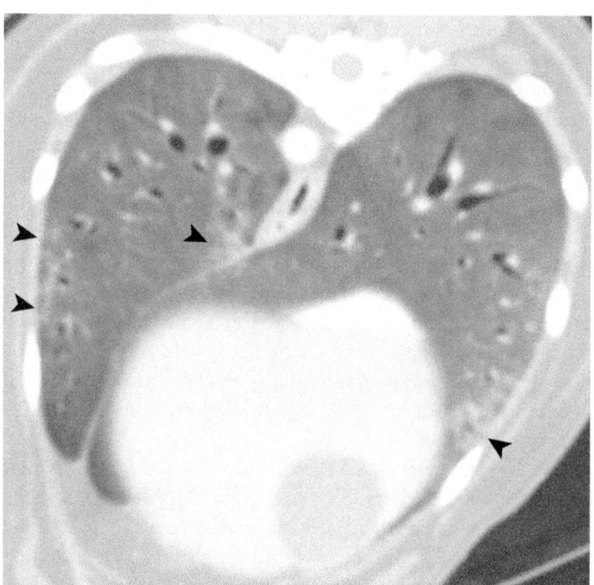

FIGURE 71-4 Thoracic CT scan from a 4-year-old female spayed Cavalier King Charles spaniel with pneumocystosis that was evaluated for lethargy, inappetence, and respiratory distress. There is a diffuse interstitial pattern and focal peripheral alveolar infiltrates *(arrowheads)*.

Diagnosis

Laboratory Abnormalities

Complete Blood Count

Hematologic abnormalities in dogs with pneumocystosis are nonspecific. Neutrophilic leukocytosis is the most consistent finding. Less frequently, eosinophilia or monocytosis are found. Lymphocyte counts can be elevated, normal, or low. Polycythemia may occur secondary to arterial hypoxemia from impaired gaseous exchange. Thrombocytosis is often present in miniature dachshunds. Artifactual thrombocytopenia and megathrombocytosis have been observed in Cavalier King Charles spaniels, which may have a hereditary basis that is likely unrelated to the suspected immunodeficiency.

Serum Chemistry Profile

Total serum proteins are usually within reference limits in dogs with pneumocystosis, with a low to borderline-low globulin level, which correlates with low γ-globulin levels on serum protein electrophoresis.[17] In some dogs, mild hyperglobulinemia is present.[21] Mild hypoalbuminemia may also be detected. Arterial hypoxemia, hypocapnia, and increased arterial blood pH indicate an uncompensated respiratory alkalosis. The arterial pO_2 is often lower than expected based on the clinical signs and thoracic radiographs.

Diagnostic Imaging

Findings on thoracic radiography include diffuse, bilaterally symmetric, miliary-interstitial to alveolar lung disease, with compensatory emphysema in severely infected animals.[22] Interstitial patterns are most common (Figure 71-3). Solitary lesions, unilateral involvement, cavitary lesions, spontaneous pneumothorax, and lobar infiltrates have also been described. Tracheal elevation, right-sided heart enlargement, and pulmonary arterial enlargement reflect cor pulmonale secondary to diffuse pulmonary disease. Computed tomography (CT) scans may show diffuse pulmonary interstitial infiltrates and small focal regions of increased opacity (Figure 71-4), but CT findings in dogs with pneumocystosis have not been extensively described.

Microbiologic Tests

Diagnostic assays available for pneumocystosis in dogs or cats are described in Table 71-1. Identification of pneumonia in a Cavalier King Charles spaniel or miniature dachshund should always raise suspicion for pneumocystosis.

Cytologic Diagnosis

The diagnosis of pneumocystosis requires direct demonstration of *Pneumocystis* cysts in biopsy specimens, respiratory fluids, or occasional extrapulmonary sites. Transtracheal, endotracheal, or bronchoalveolar lavage specimens, lung aspirates, and oropharyngeal secretions may contain organisms. Transtracheal lavage specimens have been useful for detection of organisms in dogs.[17] No cytologic technique is as reliable or as definitive as histopathologic examination of lung biopsy specimens for documentation of active *Pneumocystis* infection. However, lung biopsy is more invasive, has potential complications of hemorrhage or pneumothorax, and is associated with additional costs and hospitalization. *Pneumocystis* organisms are difficult to detect in respiratory secretions or lavage specimens, and success in finding them usually depends on the experience of the examiner and the collection and processing of specimens. Polychrome stains, such as Wright's, Giemsa, and methylene blue, will demonstrate nuclei of trophozoites and intracystic sporozoites in cytologic specimens, but the walls of cysts and trophozoites will not be apparent (Figure 71-5). Diff Quik stain may be useful to rapidly identify organisms.[23]

Serologic Diagnosis

Serologic assays are available for detection of human infections with *P. jirovecii*; however, their diagnostic value is uncertain, since many immunodeficient humans who develop pneumocystosis fail to produce antibody titers, and healthy individuals frequently have high titers. Increased antibody titers to *Pneumocystis* persist for long periods, offering a valuable

TABLE 71-1

Diagnostic Assays Available for Pneumocystosis in Dogs or Cats

Assay	Specimen Type	Target	Performance
Cytologic examination	Lung aspirates; transtracheal, endotracheal, or bronchoalveolar lavage specimens	*Pneumocystis* trophozoites and cysts	False negatives can occur when specimen size is small or low numbers of organisms are present. Identification to the genus level requires immunostaining or PCR assay.
PCR assays	Lung aspirates; transtracheal, endotracheal, or bronchoalveolar lavage specimens	*Pneumocystis* spp. DNA	The sensitivity and specificity of assays may vary depending on assay design. Assays designed to detect *P. jirovecii* may not detect organisms that infect dogs. In the absence of cytologic evidence of *Pneumocystis* infection, the significance of a positive PCR result must be interpreted in light of clinical findings, because of the potential for subclinical colonization.
Histopathology	Lung biopsy or necropsy specimens	*Pneumocystis* trophozoites and cysts	Large numbers of organisms are usually found filling alveolar spaces. Cyst forms are best demonstrated with silver stains or periodic acid–Schiff. The identity of the organisms can be confirmed with immunohistochemistry or PCR assay.

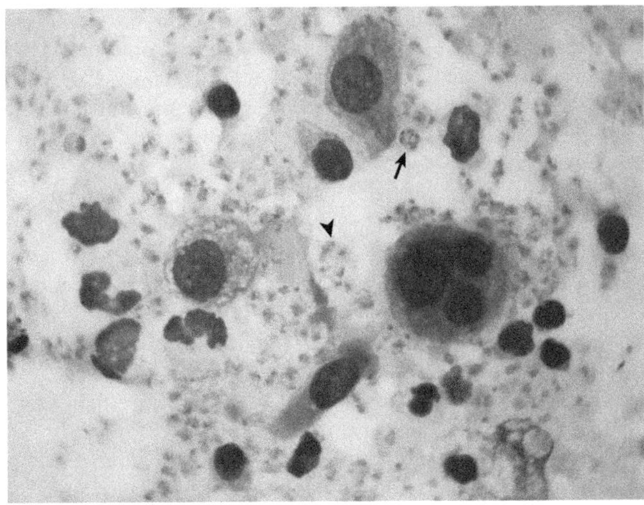

FIGURE 71-5 Impression smear of lung tissue from a 1-year-old male neutered Cavalier King Charles spaniel with pneumocystosis. Large foamy and activated macrophages are present, as well as fewer neutrophils and lymphocytes. Abundant trophozoites are present and range in size from 1 to 2 μm *(arrowhead)*. Organisms can also be seen within a cyst *(arrow)*. Wright's stain.

index of infection in epidemiologic studies. However, they are of limited use for an immediate diagnosis.[24] Circulating *Pneumocystis* antigen has been detected in human serum by counter-immunoelectrophoresis and ELISA methods. However, antigenemia also is found in up to 15% of clinically healthy humans. Direct fluorescent antibody assays can specifically detect organisms in sputum, tracheal aspirates, or pulmonary tissue.[25] Immunoperoxidase techniques also can be used to identify *Pneumocystis* in impression smears or formalin-fixed, paraffin-embedded lung sections.[26]

Fungal Culture

Pneumocystis cannot be cultured in the laboratory from clinical specimens.

Molecular Diagnosis Using the Polymerase Chain Reaction

PCR assays have been used to detect *Pneumocystis* in bronchoalveolar lavage specimens from humans[12,27-29] and in lung tissue from dogs.[16,30] The sensitivity of PCR assays on bronchoalveolar lavage fluids from infected humans is greater than that of conventional staining.[31] DNA analysis of PCR products has been used to type isolates from humans and animals.[8] Some PCR assays (especially specific real-time PCR assays) that detect *P. jirovecii* may not detect *Pneumocystis* organisms that infect dogs because of sequence differences.

Immunologic Findings

The majority of the immunologic studies of pneumocystosis in dogs have been done in the miniature dachshund.[17,32] Lymphocyte stimulation assay results, using phytohemagglutinin and pokeweed mitogen, show severe immunosuppression, especially when compared to controls, even though a normal lymphocyte count can be present. Immunoglobulin fraction quantification consistently reveals deficiencies of IgA, IgM, and IgG. Low globulin levels, immunoglobulin deficiencies, and decreased lymphocyte function have been reported in the Cavalier King Charles spaniel.[18,30] The absence of immunoglobulins in the presence of pathologic changes is a significant finding, since affected dogs have chronic infections, which should result in an immunoglobulin response. Immunoglobulin deficiencies are still present after the *Pneumocystis* and skin infections have resolved, which supports the presence of a primary defect. Lymphocyte transformation studies and the results of immunoglobulin quantification suggest that both T- and B-cell abnormalities exist in affected dogs. Serum complement activity in affected miniature dachshunds has been normal. CD3 and CD79a lymphocyte staining of lymph nodes and spleen shows marked absence of B cells with the presence of T cells. Immunologic abnormalities in the miniature dachshund are similar to those described in human patients that have common variable immunodeficiency syndrome (also known as acquired or adult-onset hypogammaglobulinemia). Common variable immunodeficiency syndrome is a primary immunodeficiency disease characterized by little or no antibody production by B lymphocytes, normal or decreased numbers of B lymphocytes, and abnormal T-lymphocyte function.[33]

Pathologic Findings

Gross Pathologic Findings

Pathologic findings in pneumocystosis are primarily confined to the lungs, although dissemination to regional lymph nodes, spleen, liver, bone marrow, and other organs has been reported. On gross examination, the lungs are firm, consolidated, and pale brown or gray. They do not collapse when the chest cavity is opened. Unlike many pneumonic processes, fluid is not expressed from cut surfaces of the lung. The pulmonary and mediastinal lymph nodes are often enlarged. Small amounts of fluid may be found in the pleural cavity. Cardiac enlargement, when present, has been right sided in all cases.

Histopathologic Findings

On histologic examination, alveolar spaces are filled with aggregates of amorphous, foamy, eosinophilic material that has a frothy, honeycomb-like pattern (Figure 71-6). A few macrophages and detached alveolar lining cells may be present, but polymorphonuclear leukocytes are absent. Special stains are needed to identify cyst forms. Little or no phagocytosis of intact *Pneumocystis* organisms is present. However, nonviable organisms (such as those seen after treatment) are often phagocytosed, and macrophages may contain Gomori's methenamine silver (GMS)-positive granular material that represents the residuum of cyst wall degradation. In some instances, alveolar septa are markedly thickened by dense accumulations of plasma cells, lymphocytes, and macrophages (lymphoplasmacytic pneumonia). The septa may be widened by fibrosis in chronic infections. With GMS stain, cyst forms are spherical, ovoid, or crescent-shaped structures that range from 4 to 7 μm in diameter and have dot-like, argyrophilic (stain with silver), focal cyst wall thickenings. Cyst walls also can be demonstrated with other stains such as toluidine blue, and they fluoresce when stained with orange G of a Papanicolaou stain. The internal structure of trophozoites in tissue sections and smears are best demonstrated with Giemsa stain. On ultrastructural examination, intact alveoli are filled with compact aggregates of trophozoite and cyst forms. Trophozoites commonly line alveoli.

Appropriate histologic staining is essential to ensure detection of *Pneumocystis* organisms. Routine hematoxylin and eosin stain does not readily demonstrate the developmental forms of *Pneumocystis*. Only the nuclei of intracystic sporozoites and trophozoites are stained. Various modifications of methenamine silver staining can be employed to stain the cyst walls brownish-black; trophozoites will not be detected. The cyst wall also stains with periodic acid–Schiff stain (see Figure 71-6).

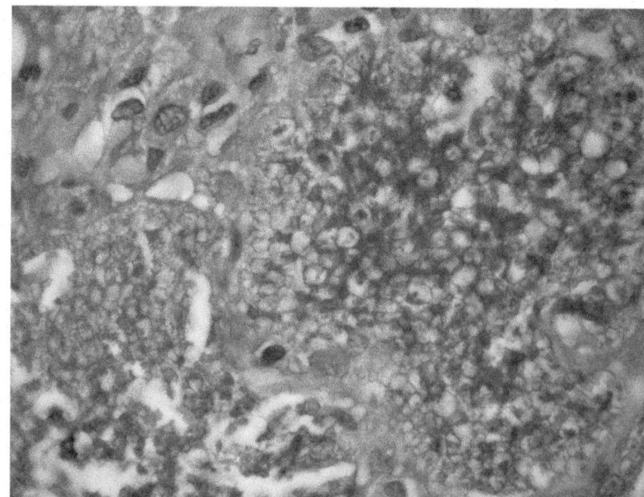

FIGURE 71-6 Histopathology of the lung of an 18-month-old male neutered Cavalier King Charles spaniel with pneumocystosis. Foamy, honeycomb-like material fills the alveoli. Periodic acid–Schiff stain.

Treatment and Prognosis

Specific antimicrobial chemotherapy is most beneficial when pneumocystosis is suspected (usually based on the affected dog breed) or diagnosed during its early stages. The treatment of choice is trimethoprim and a sulfonamide (TMS). Pentamidine isethionate (an aromatic diamidine) has also been effective in humans, but TMS is more effective and less toxic. TMS has also been used as prophylaxis in immunodeficient humans.

Treatment with TMS has been reported in 8 dogs;[16,17,22] 4 were dachshunds that subsequently recovered.[22] A TMS dose of 15 mg/kg, every 8 hours, or 30 mg/kg, every 12 hours, for 3 weeks was used; the longest reported follow-up in these studies was for 4 months. Folic acid supplementation should be given if adverse effects such as leukopenia and anemia are observed or if long-term therapy is required. In human infections, resistance to sulfonamides has been noted among some strains of *P. jirovecii*.[34]

Other treatment options include atovaquone, clindamycin and primaquine, and dapsone-trimethoprim combinations. Atovaquone is licensed for the treatment of human pneumocystosis.[35] This drug, which also has been used to treat canine babesiosis (see Chapter 10), is not as effective against *Pneumocystis* infections in humans as pentamidine or TMS but has lower toxicity. In humans, pentamidine or atovaquone has also been administered by aerosol, but this is less effective than oral administration and is not recommended.[36,37]

Combination therapy with clindamycin and primaquine is now the preferred alternative to treatment with TMS in humans (e.g., for patients intolerant of TMS)[37] but has not been reported for treatment of dogs. Dapsone and trimethoprim or pyrimethamine, in combination, have been effective in experimental animals and in clinical trials in immunosuppressed humans with pneumocystosis.[38] *Pneumocystis* is resistant to azole antifungal drugs and amphotericin B (because it lacks ergosterol in its cell wall), but the anthelmintics benzimidazole and albendazole have been effective in experimental infections.[39,40]

Nonspecific immunostimulants such as cimetidine and levamisole have been given adjunctively to treat affected miniature dachshunds,[41] without much success. Supportive care is essential for any patient with *Pneumocystis* pneumonia because of disturbed alveolar gaseous exchange. Supplemental oxygen therapy may be needed, and ventilatory assistance may also be required. Immunosuppressive agents should be discontinued if possible. Antimicrobial chemotherapy of pulmonary pneumocystosis results in a decline in arterial oxygen related to the inflammatory reaction to dying organisms. Administration of anti-inflammatory doses of glucocorticoids during specific treatment for *P. jirovecii* infection improves pulmonary function and survival in humans.[37,42-44]

Public Health Aspects

Pneumocystis organisms are ubiquitous in the environment. However, molecular and epidemiologic evidence suggests that spread may occur between humans because of localized outbreaks. Humans and animals are exposed to the same environmental sources of *Pneumocystis*. *Pneumocystis* species that infect dogs are likely different from those that infect humans, but further studies are required to verify this. The primary risk factor for clinical pneumocystosis in humans is immunodeficiency (especially HIV infection, hematologic malignancies and solid tumors, transplant recipients, and collagen vascular disorders).[37] Thus, the greatest risk for acquisition of infection from a pet would be if the animal was clinically ill from *Pneumocystis* pneumonia and the person in close contact was immunocompromised.

CASE EXAMPLE

Signalment: "Tessa", a 1-year-old intact female miniature dachshund (see Figure 71-2)

History: Tessa was evaluated for a history of chronic tachypnea and weight loss. The clinical signs had been nonresponsive to various treatments that had included multiple antibiotics, bronchodilators, mucolytics, multivitamins, and glucocorticoids. From 2 months of age, she had a history of recurrent infections including otitis externa, hemorrhagic enteritis, tonsillitis, folliculitis, and pyogranulomatous dermatitis. These conditions had responded each time to supportive care.

Physical Examination:

Body Weight: 4.5 kg.

General: Quiet, alert, and responsive. Ambulatory on all four limbs. Rectal temperature = 101.8°F (38.8°C), HR = 138 beats/min, RR = 129 breaths/min, mucous membranes pink, CRT = 1 s.

Integument: A poor coat was present with focal alopecia on the head and back.

Musculoskeletal: Body condition score was 3/9 with diffuse and symmetrical muscle atrophy.

Respiratory: An increased respiratory rate with increased abdominal effort was noted; tracheal palpation elicited a dry cough.

All Other Systems: No clinically significant abnormalities were noted.

Laboratory Findings:

CBC:

HCT 54% (40-55%)
MCV 68 fL (65-75 fL)
MCHC 35.7 g/dL (33-36 g/dL)
WBC 34,600 cells/μL (6000-15,000 cells/μL)
Neutrophils 23,200 cells/μL (3000-11,000 cells/μL)
Band neutrophils 700 cells/μL (0-300 cells/μL)
Lymphocytes 5500 cells/μL (1000-4800 cells/μL)
Monocytes 4800 cells/μL (100-2000 cells/μL)
Basophils 350 cells/μL (100 cells/μL)
Platelets 730,000 platelets/μL (200,000-500,000 platelets/μL).

Serum Chemistry Profile:

Sodium 147 mmol/L (145-154 mmol/L)
Potassium 4.6 mmol/L (3.6-5.3 mmol/L)
Phosphorus 4.8 mg/dL (3.0-6.2 mg/dL)
Calcium 10.9 mg/dL (9.7-11.5 mg/dL)
BUN 17 mg/dL (5-21 mg/dL)
Creatinine 0.5 mg/dL (0.3-1.2 mg/dL)
Glucose 132 mg/dL (64-123 mg/dL)
Total protein 5.1 g/dL (5.3-7.5 g/dL)
Albumin 3.5 g/dL (2.3-3.5 g/dL)
Globulin 1.6 g/dL (2-3.7 g/dL)
ALT 65 U/L (10-60 U/L)
ALP 210 U/L (100-250 U/L)
Cholesterol 196 mg/dL (135-361 mg/dL)
Total bilirubin 0.1 mg/dL (0-0.2 mg/dL)
α-globulins 0.8 g/dL (0.8-1.6 g/dL)
β-globulins 0.6 g/dL (0.7-1.3 g/dL)
γ-globulins 0.3 g/dL (0.4-1.1 g/dL).

Urinalysis: SGr 1.045; pH 6.0, negative for protein, bilirubin, blood, and glucose. Inactive sediment.

Imaging Findings: On thoracic radiographs the cardiovascular structures appeared within normal limits. A diffuse interstitial pulmonary pattern was present.

Cytology Findings: Transtracheal wash cytology demonstrated active, blastic alveolar macrophages with phagocytic vacuolization, large numbers of neutrophils, and many free and phagocytosed *Pneumocystis* organisms.

Aerobic Bacterial Culture: Culture of the transtracheal wash fluid yielded no growth after 48 hours' incubation.

Fecal Examination: Fecal flotation: Negative for parasites.

Diagnosis: *Pneumocystis* spp. pneumonia.

Treatment: The dog was treated with a potentiated sulfonamide at 15 mg/kg PO q8h for 3 weeks, which resulted in a complete recovery.

Comments: This dog was diagnosed with pneumocystosis as a result of a primary immune deficiency disease, most likely common variable immunodeficiency syndrome. The latter would also explain the history of chronic skin infections and gastroenteritis. CD3 and CD79a lymphocyte staining of a peripheral lymph node biopsy showed a marked absence of B cells.

SUGGESTED READINGS

Chabe M, Aliouat-Denis CM, Delhaes L, et al. *Pneumocystis*: from a doubtful unique entity to a group of highly diversified fungal species. FEMS Yeast Res. 2011;11:2-17.

Watson PJ, Wotton P, Eastwood J, et al. Immunoglobulin deficiency in Cavalier King Charles Spaniels with *Pneumocystis* pneumonia. J Vet Intern Med. 2006;20:523-527.

REFERENCES

1. Miller R, Huang L. *Pneumocystis jirovecii* infection. Thorax. 2004;59:731-733.
2. Sedlmeier H, Dahme E. *Pneumocystis carinii* infection in dog. Zentralbl Allg Pathol. 1955;93:150-155.
3. Lobetti R. *Pneumocystis carinii* infection in miniature dachshunds. Compend Cont Educ Pract Vet. 2001;23:320-327.

4. Stringer JR. *Pneumocystis*. Int J Med Microbiol. 2002;292:391-404.
5. Stringer JR, Beard CB, Miller RF, et al. A new name (*Pneumocystis jiroveci*) for *Pneumocystis* from humans. Emerg Infect Dis. 2002;8:891-896.
6. Hughes WT. *Pneumocystis carinii* vs. *Pneumocystis jiroveci*: another misnomer (response to Stringer et al.). Emerg Infect Dis. 2003;9:276-277:author reply 277–279.
7. Chabe M, Aliouat-Denis CM, Delhaes L, et al. *Pneumocystis*: from a doubtful unique entity to a group of highly diversified fungal species. FEMS Yeast Res. 2011;11:2-17.
8. English K, Peters SE, Maskell DJ, et al. DNA analysis of *Pneumocystis* infecting a Cavalier King Charles spaniel. J Eukaryot Microbiol. 2001(suppl):106S.
9. Bartlett MS, Smith JW. *Pneumocystis carinii*, an opportunist in immunocompromised patients. Clin Microbiol Rev. 1991;4:137-149.
10. Sukura A, Laakkonen J, Rudback E. Occurrence of *Pneumocystis carinii* in canine distemper. Acta Vet Scand. 1997;38:201-205.
11. Beard CB, Carter JL, Keely SP, et al. Genetic variation in *Pneumocystis carinii* isolates from different geographic regions: implications for transmission. Emerg Infect Dis. 2000;6:265-272.
12. Kovacs JA, Gill VJ, Meshnick S, et al. New insights into transmission, diagnosis, and drug treatment of *Pneumocystis carinii* pneumonia. JAMA. 2001;286:2450-2460.
13. Brownlie SE. A retrospective study of diagnosis in 109 cases of canine lower respiratory disease. J Small Anim Pract. 1990;31:371-376.
14. Canfield PJ, Church DB, Malik R. *Pneumocystis* pneumonia in a dog. Aust Vet Practit. 1993;23:150-154.
15. Ramsey IK, Foster A, McKay J, et al. *Pneumocystis carinii* pneumonia in two Cavalier King Charles spaniels. Vet Rec. 1997;140:372-373.
16. Sukura A, Saari S, Jarvinen AK, et al. *Pneumocystis carinii* pneumonia in dogs—a diagnostic challenge. J Vet Diagn Invest. 1996;8:124-130.
17. Lobetti RG, Leisewitz AL, Spencer JA. *Pneumocystis carinii* in the miniature dachshund: case report and literature review. J Small Anim Pract. 1996;37:280-285.
18. Watson PJ, Wotton P, Eastwood J, et al. Immunoglobulin deficiency in Cavalier King Charles Spaniels with *Pneumocystis* pneumonia. J Vet Intern Med. 2006;20:523-527.
19. Kelly MN, Shellito JE. Current understanding of *Pneumocystis* immunology. Future Microbiol. 2010;5:43-65.
20. Watts JC, Chandler FW. Evolving concepts of infection by *Pneumocystis carinii*. Pathol Annu. 1991(26 Pt 1):93-138.
21. Sykes JE. Unpublished observations, 2012.
22. Kirberger RM, Lobetti RG. Radiographic aspects of *Pneumocystis carinii* pneumonia in the miniature Dachshund. Vet Radiol Ultrasound. 1998;39:313-317.
23. Cregan P, Yamamoto A, Lum A, et al. Comparison of four methods for rapid detection of *Pneumocystis carinii* in respiratory specimens. J Clin Microbiol. 1990;28:2432-2436.
24. Daly KR, Huang L, Morris A, et al. Antibody response to *Pneumocystis jirovecii* major surface glycoprotein. Emerg Infect Dis. 2006;12:1231-1237.
25. Ng VL, Virani NA, Chaisson RE, et al. Rapid detection of *Pneumocystis carinii* using a direct fluorescent monoclonal antibody stain. J Clin Microbiol. 1990;28:2228-2233.
26. Kondo H, Hikita M, Ito M, et al. Immunohistochemical study of *Pneumocystis carinii* infection in pigs: evaluation of *Pneumocystis* pneumonia and a retrospective investigation. Vet Rec. 2000;147:544-549.
27. Kitada K, Oka S, Kimura S, et al. Detection of *Pneumocystis carinii* sequences by polymerase chain reaction: animal models and clinical application to noninvasive specimens. J Clin Microbiol. 1991;29:1985-1990.
28. Lu JJ, Chen CH, Bartlett MS, et al. Comparison of six different PCR methods for detection of *Pneumocystis carinii*. J Clin Microbiol. 1995;33:2785-2788.
29. Roux P, Lavrard I, Poirot JL, et al. Usefulness of PCR for detection of *Pneumocystis carinii* DNA. J Clin Microbiol. 1994;32:2324-2326.
30. Hagiwara Y, Fujiwara S, Takai H, et al. *Pneumocystis carinii* pneumonia in a Cavalier King Charles Spaniel. J Vet Med Sci. 2001;63:349-351.
31. Flori P, Bellete B, Durand F, et al. Comparison between real-time PCR, conventional PCR and different staining techniques for diagnosing *Pneumocystis jiroveci* pneumonia from bronchoalveolar lavage specimens. J Med Microbiol. 2004;53:603-607.
32. Lobetti R. Common variable immunodeficiency in miniature dachshunds affected with *Pneumocystis carinii* pneumonia. J Vet Diagn Invest. 2000;12:39-45.
33. Cunningham-Rundles C, Knight AK. Common variable immune deficiency: reviews, continued puzzles, and a new registry. Immunol Res. 2007;38:78-86.
34. Calderon E, de la Horra C, Montes-Cano MA, et al. [Genotypic resistance to sulfamide drugs among patients with *Pneumocystis jiroveci* pneumonia]. Med Clin (Barc). 2004;122:617-619.
35. Stoeckle M, Tennenberg A. Atovaquone for *Pneumocystis carinii* pneumonia. Ann Intern Med. 1995;122:314:author reply 314–315.
36. Chan C, Montaner J, Lefebvre EA, et al. Atovaquone suspension compared with aerosolized pentamidine for prevention of *Pneumocystis carinii* pneumonia in human immunodeficiency virus–infected subjects intolerant of trimethoprim or sulfonamides. J Infect Dis. 1999;180:369-376.
37. Walzer PD, Smulian AG. *Pneumocystis* species. In: Mandell GL, Bennett JE, Dolin R, eds. Principles and Practice of Infectious Diseases. 7th ed. Philadelphia, PA: Elsevier; 2010:3377-3390.
38. Hughes WT. Use of dapsone in the prevention and treatment of *Pneumocystis carinii* pneumonia: a review. Clin Infect Dis. 1998;27:191-204.
39. Bartlett MS, Queener SF, Shaw MM, et al. *Pneumocystis carinii* is resistant to imidazole antifungal agents. Antimicrob Agents Chemother. 1994;38:1859-1861.
40. Bartlett MS, Edlind TD, Lee CH, et al. Albendazole inhibits *Pneumocystis carinii* proliferation in inoculated immunosuppressed mice. Antimicrob Agents Chemother. 1994;38:1834-1837.
41. Farrow BR, Watson AD, Hartley WJ, et al. *Pneumocystis* pneumonia in the dog. J Comp Pathol. 1972;82:447-453.
42. Consensus statement on the use of corticosteroids as adjunctive therapy for *Pneumocystis* pneumonia in the acquired immunodeficiency syndrome. The National Institutes of Health–University of California Expert Panel for Corticosteroids as Adjunctive Therapy for *Pneumocystis* Pneumonia. N Engl J Med. 1990;323:1500-1504.
43. Bozzette SA, Finkelstein DM, Spector SA, et al. A randomized trial of three anti-*Pneumocystis* agents in patients with advanced human immunodeficiency virus infection. NIAID AIDS Clinical Trials Group N Engl J Med. 1995;332:693-699.
44. Masur H. Prevention and treatment of *Pneumocystis* pneumonia. N Engl J Med. 1992;327:1853-1860.

SECTION 4
Protozoal Diseases

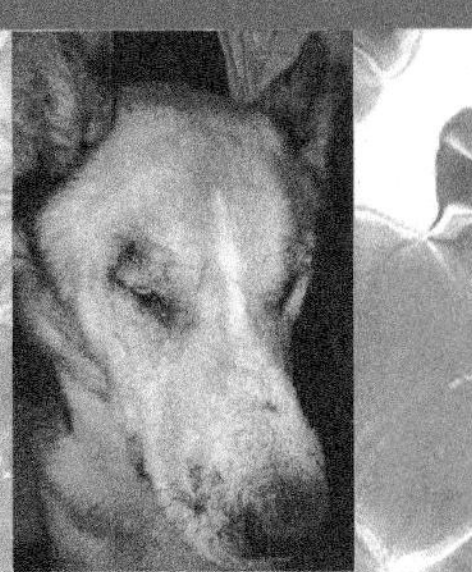

CHAPTER 72

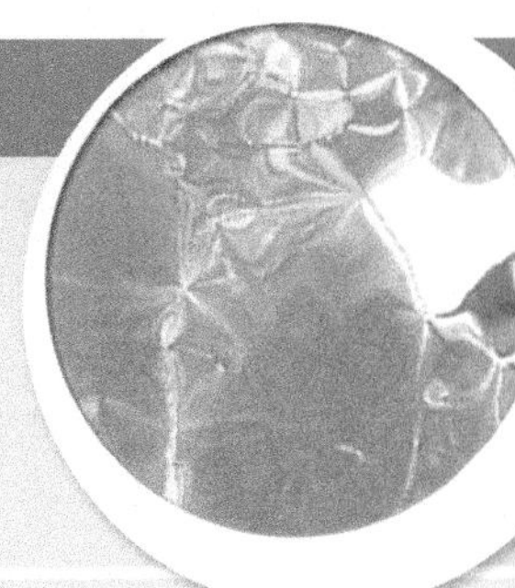

Toxoplasmosis

Michael R. Lappin

> **Overview of Toxoplasmosis**
>
> First Described: The organism that was ultimately named *Toxoplasma gondii* was first described in France in 1908 (Nicolle and Manceaux)[1]
>
> Cause: *Toxoplasma gondii,* a coccidial protozoan parasite (phylum Apicomplexa)
>
> Affected Host Species: Cats are the definitive host and are the only species known to complete the sexual phase of *T. gondii* culminating in the passage of oocysts in feces. Cats and most other vertebrates can serve as intermediate hosts; invertebrates can serve as transport hosts by mechanical carriage of *T. gondii* oocysts.
>
> Geographic Distribution: *T. gondii* has a worldwide distribution except in the absence of cats
>
> Major Clinical Signs: Fever, ocular inflammation, ataxia, seizures, muscle pain, and respiratory distress are the most common clinical signs in cats; dogs have similar signs but develop illness less frequently than cats.
>
> Differential Diagnoses: In the dog, *Neospora caninum* induces the most similar clinical signs; many other chronic intracellular bacterial infections and fungal infections in dogs and cats need to be considered a differential diagnoses for many of the clinical and laboratory abnormities induced by *T. gondii.*
>
> Human Health Significance: There is significant risk to the fetus after transplacental infection and to any immunocompromised person.

Etiologic Agent and Epidemiology

Toxoplasma gondii is a coccidian that is one of the most prevalent parasites infecting warm-blooded vertebrates around the world.[2-4] Only cats complete the sexual phase in the gastrointestinal tract (also known as the enteroepithelial cycle) and pass environmentally resistant oocysts in feces (Figure 72-1). Sporozoites develop within shed oocysts after 1 to 5 days of exposure to oxygen and appropriate environmental temperature and humidity (Figure 72-2). This process is known as sporulation. After oocyst ingestion, released sporozoites can penetrate the intestinal tracts of cats or intermediate hosts and disseminate in blood or lymph as tachyzoites during active infection. *T. gondii* can penetrate most mammalian cells and replicates asexually within infected cells until the cell is destroyed. If an appropriate immune response occurs, replication of tachyzoites is attenuated and slowly dividing bradyzoites develop that persist within cysts in extraintestinal tissues. These tissue cysts form readily in the central nervous system (CNS), muscles, and visceral organs. Live bradyzoites may persist in tissue cysts for the life of the host.

It is likely that most *T. gondii*–infected cats and dogs harbor tissue cysts for life. Thus, the presence of serum antibodies is likely to indicate current infection. *T. gondii* seroprevalence rates vary by the lifestyle of the cat or dog. In general, increased seroprevalence correlates with increased age as a result of increased risk of exposure over time. It also correlates with outdoor exposure, since animals with access to the outdoors are most likely to contact infected intermediate hosts. In a recent study of clinically ill cats, *T. gondii* antibodies were detected in 31.6% of the 12,628 cats tested.[5] The seroprevalence was lowest in regions with low humidity (Figure 72-3). In another study of feral cats in Florida, *T. gondii* antibodies were detected in 12.1% of the cats.[6] Although *T. gondii* infection is common among cats, the oocyst shedding period is generally less than 21 days. Thus, detection of *T. gondii* oocysts in feline feces is uncommon. For example, in two studies in the United States, *T. gondii* oocysts were detected in feces of fewer than 1% of cats.[7,8]

Dogs do not produce *T. gondii* oocysts, but they can mechanically transmit oocysts after they ingest feline feces.[9] The tissue phases of *T. gondii* infection occur in dogs and may be associated with clinical disease. Approximately 20% of dogs in the United States are seropositive for *T. gondii* antibodies.[10] Before 1988, many dogs diagnosed with toxoplasmosis based

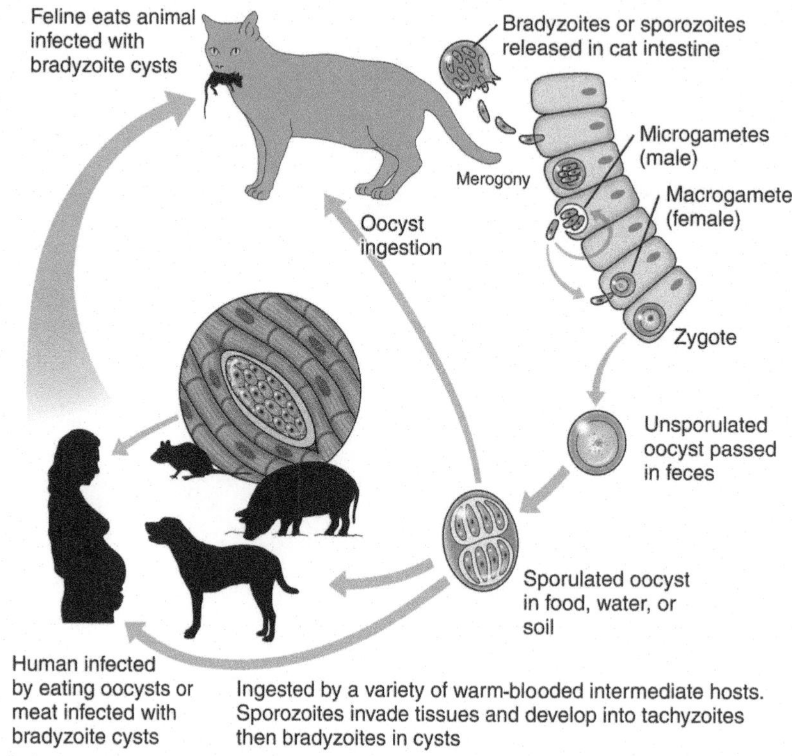

FIGURE 72-1 Life cycle of *Toxoplasma gondii*. Cats are most often infected when they ingest bradyzoite cysts in tissues of prey. The bradyzoites transform into merozoites and undergo repeated cycles of schizogony in the cat's intestinal tract. The merozoites then transform into microgametes (male) and macrogametes (female). When a microgamete penetrates a macrogamete, a zygote forms. The zygote is shed as an unsporulated oocyst in the feces, which is not infectious. Sporulation occurs after 1 to 5 days. The extraintestinal cycle occurs in cats or other intermediate hosts after they ingest sporulated oocysts or tissue cysts. Sporozoites penetrate intestinal cells and transform into tachyzoites, which rapidly multiply in nucleated cells throughout the body in the face of immunosuppression. This can result in severe disease in the developing fetus. Ultimately organisms are contained by the immune system within bradyzoite cysts in muscle, brain, and visceral organs (latent infection).

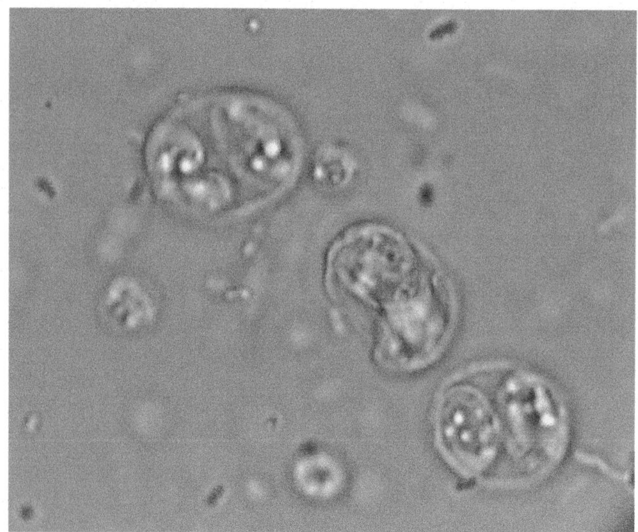

FIGURE 72-2 Sporulated oocysts of *Toxoplasma gondii*. The oocysts are 10 × 12 μm in diameter.

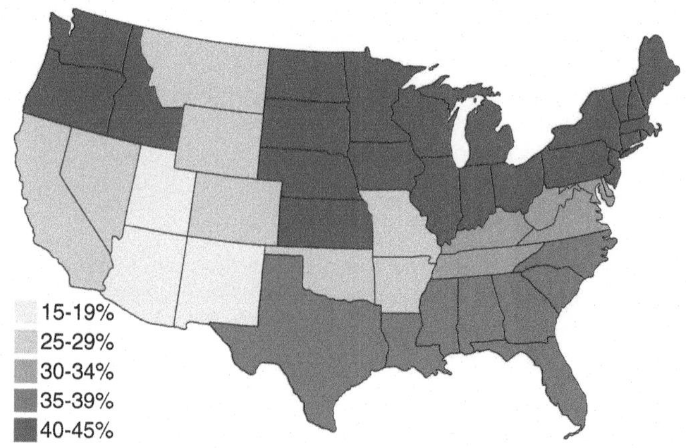

FIGURE 72-3 Continental United States regional seroprevalence in clinically ill cats. Results were based on the presence of *Toxoplasma gondii*-specific IgG or IgM in serum. Information was available from 3,640 serum specimens. (From Vollaire MR, Radecki SV, Lappin MR. Seroprevalence of *Toxoplasma gondii* antibodies in clinically ill cats in the United States. Am J Vet Res 2005;66:874-877.)

on histologic evaluation were in fact infected with *Neospora caninum* (see Chapter 73).

Clinical Features

Signs and Their Pathogenesis

Infection of warm-blooded vertebrates occurs after ingestion of any of the three life stages of *T. gondii* (sporozoite, tachyzoites, bradyzoites) or it can occur by transplacental transmission. Cats can also be infected through the transmammary route.[11] In dogs, evidence for venereal transmission also exists, and repeated transplacental infection has been documented.[12,13]

Most cats are not coprophagic, so most are infected when they ingest *T. gondii* bradyzoites in tissue cysts during carnivorous feeding. After ingestion, the bradyzoites transform into merozoites, which replicate in the epithelial cells of the intestinal tract, then transform into microgametes and macrogametes.

When a microgamete penetrates a macrogamete, a zygote forms. The zygote then transforms into an unsporulated oocyst, which is shed in feces for 3 to 21 days. After sporulation (formation of sporozoites within the oocyst), oocysts can survive in the environment for months to years and are resistant to most disinfectants. The *T. gondii* oocyst shedding prepatent period is stage dependent (ingestion of bradyzoites has a shorter prepatent period than ingestion of sporozoites) but is not dose dependent.[14] In addition, transmission of *T. gondii* is most efficient when cats consume tissue cysts (carnivorism) and when intermediate hosts consume oocysts (fecal-oral transmission). Infection of rodents with *T. gondii* leads to clinical signs of altered behavior, so that the rodent becomes less fearful of cats.[15] This may increase the likelihood that the definitive host (cat) will become infected and potentiate the sexual phase of the organism.

Whether clinical toxoplasmosis develops is dependent on both host and parasite effects. Some strains of *T. gondii* may be more pathogenic than others, and some strains may have specific tissue affinities, such as a tendency to cause ocular disease in cats.[16,17] If a poor immune response is mounted after primary infection, overwhelming tachyzoite replication that results in tissue necrosis is the major cause of disease.[2-4] This mechanism is also likely in cats or dogs with chronic (latent) toxoplasmosis that then become immune suppressed. One example is activation of *T. gondii* infection in cats or dogs after administration of immunosuppressive drugs such as cyclosporine.[18-21] Other immunosuppressive conditions such as FIV infection can also result in activation of toxoplasmosis.[22] The mechanisms for chronic clinical toxoplasmosis have not been fully determined.[2] *T. gondii* antigens and antigen-containing immune complexes have been documented in the serum of affected cats. Persistent infection was not associated with chronic kidney failure in cats of one study.[23-25]

The large majority of cats infected with *T. gondii* never develop detectable clinical abnormalities. In general, the enteroepithelial cycle in the cat rarely leads to clinical signs. Only 10% to 20% of experimentally inoculated cats develop self-limiting, small bowel diarrhea for 1 to 2 weeks following primary oral inoculation with *T. gondii* tissue cysts; this is presumed to be from the enteroepithelial replication of the organism. *T. gondii* enteroepithelial stages were found in intestinal tissues from two cats with inflammatory bowel disease that had positive response to administration of anti-*Toxoplasma* drugs.[26] Eosinophilic fibrosing gastritis was recently described in a *T. gondii*–infected cat.[27]

Fatal extraintestinal toxoplasmosis in cats can develop from overwhelming intracellular replication of tachyzoites following primary infection; hepatic, pulmonary, CNS, and pancreatic tissues are commonly involved.[2-4,28-30] Kittens infected by the transplacental or transmammary routes develop the most severe signs of extraintestinal toxoplasmosis and generally die of pulmonary or hepatic disease. Common clinical signs in cats with disseminated toxoplasmosis include lethargy, anorexia, and respiratory distress. Disseminated toxoplasmosis has been documented in cats concurrently infected with FeLV, FIV, or feline infectious peritonitis virus, as well as following cyclosporine administration for allergic dermatitis, immune-mediated disorders, or after renal transplantation.[18,19,31]

Chronic toxoplasmosis occurs in some cats and should be on the differential diagnosis list for cats with uveitis, chorioretinitis (Figure 72-4), cutaneous lesions, fever, muscle hyperesthesia, myocarditis with arrhythmias, weight loss, anorexia, seizures, ataxia, icterus, diarrhea, respiratory distress, or pancreatitis.[2-4,32-42] Toxoplasmosis appears to be a common infectious cause of uveitis in cats; anterior uveitis or posterior uveitis can occur, and the manifestations can be either unilateral or bilateral.[2,41,42] Kittens infected transplacentally or through the transmammary route commonly develop ocular disease.[16]

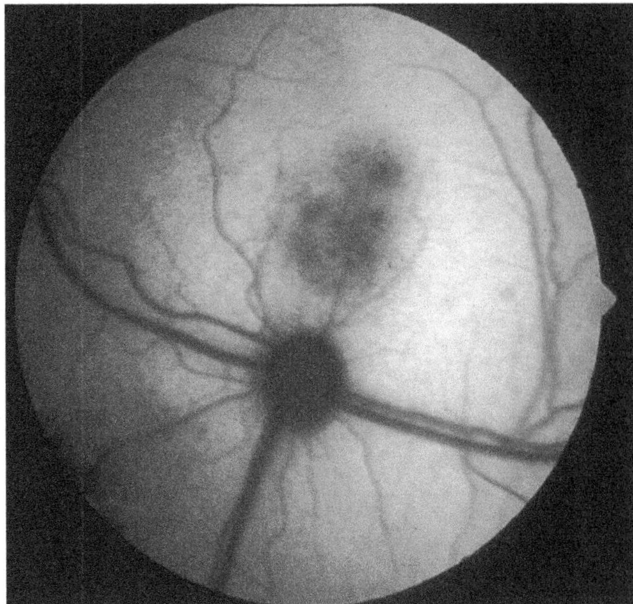

FIGURE 72-4 *Toxoplasma gondii*–associated chorioretinitis in an experimentally inoculated cat.

In dogs, respiratory, gastrointestinal, or neuromuscular infection with associated signs of fever, vomiting, diarrhea, respiratory distress, ataxia, seizures, and icterus occurs most commonly with generalized toxoplasmosis.[2,43-50] Generalized toxoplasmosis is most common in immunosuppressed dogs, such as those with canine distemper virus infection or those treated with cyclosporine to prevent renal transplant rejection. Neurologic signs depend on the location of the primary lesions and include ataxia, seizures, tremors, cranial nerve deficits, paresis, and paralysis. Dogs with myositis present with weakness, stiff gait, or muscle atrophy. Rapid progression to tetraparesis and paralysis with lower motor neuron dysfunction can occur. One study associated *T. gondii* antibodies with polyradiculoneuritis in dogs.[49] Some dogs with suspected neuromuscular toxoplasmosis probably have neosporosis. Myocardial infection with ventricular arrhythmias occurs in some infected dogs. Retinitis, anterior uveitis, iridocyclitis, nodular conjunctivitis, and optic neuritis occur in some dogs with toxoplasmosis, but they are less common than in cats.[50] Cutaneous disease also has been reported, which can manifest as pustules, pruritus, subcutaneous nodules, and/or alopecia.[21,51]

Diagnosis

Diagnosis of toxoplasmosis requires interpretation of specific microbiologic tests (Table 72-1) in light of the presence of consistent clinical abnormalities. No clinical abnormalities are specific for the disease.[2-4]

Laboratory Abnormalities

Complete Blood Count

T. gondii should be on the differential diagnosis list for cats or dogs with appropriate clinical findings and nonregenerative anemia, neutrophilic leukocytosis or neutropenia, lymphocytosis or lymphopenia, monocytosis, and/or eosinophilia.

TABLE 72-1

Microbiologic Assays for Diagnosis of *Toxoplasma gondii* Infection

Assay	Specimen Type	Assay Target	Comments
Fecal flotation	Feces	*T. gondii* oocysts	The negative predictive value of this assay is poor for clinical toxoplasmosis, since most cats cease shedding by the time illness occurs.
Fecal PCR assay	Feces	*T. gondii* DNA	As for fecal flotation.
Cytologic examination	Effusions, skin lesions, tissue aspirates	*T. gondii* tachyzoites and occasionally bradyzoites	Confirms current infection and is generally associated with disease. Organisms cannot be readily distinguished from *Neospora caninum.*
Histopathology	Multiple tissues	*T. gondii* tachyzoites and bradyzoites	If the organisms are detected in the presence of inflammation and necrosis, clinical toxoplasmosis is likely. Can be difficult to differentiate *T. gondii* from tissue protozoans such as *N. caninum* in dogs. Immunohistochemistry can be used to differentiate the two species.
PCR assay	Effusions, blood, multiple tissues	*T. gondii* DNA	*T. gondii* DNA can be amplified from the blood of normal dogs and cats and so PCR on blood has a low positive predictive value. Amplification of specific DNA confirms infection, and if appropriate clinical signs and inflammation are present, positive results document clinical toxoplasmosis.
Serology for *T. gondii* IgM	Serum	*T. gondii* IgM antibodies	Most consistent with recent infection but can be induced during reinfection and by other immune drugs such as glucocorticoids. Positive results do not correlate with active disease.*
T. gondii IgG	Serum	*T. gondii* IgG antibodies	Most consistent with infection of > 10 days duration. Positive results do not correlate with active disease.*
Agglutination assays	Serum	*T. gondii* antibodies	Hypothetically detects all antibody classes but can be falsely negative in animals that only possess anti-*Toxoplasma* IgM antibody. Positive results do not correlate with active disease.*

*Results of serum antibody assays are combined with clinical findings to aid in making a diagnosis of clinical toxoplasmosis.

Serum Chemistry Profile

Depending on the organ system involved, cats with clinical toxoplasmosis may have increases in serum protein and bilirubin concentrations, as well as increased activities of creatine kinase, ALT, ALP, and lipase.[2-4] Findings are similar for dogs; dogs with chronic toxoplasmosis may develop hyperglobulinemia that is generally polyclonal.[52]

Urinalysis

Proteinuria and bilirubinuria have been detected in some dogs or cats with clinical toxoplasmosis.

Cerebrospinal Fluid Analysis

CSF protein concentrations and cell counts are often higher than normal, with the predominant white blood cells in CSF being small mononuclear cells. However, increased neutrophils also are commonly found in cats with acute CNS toxoplasmosis. Increased CSF protein concentrations and mixed inflammatory cell infiltrates occur in dogs with CNS toxoplasmosis.

Diagnostic Imaging

Radiographs

Pulmonary toxoplasmosis most commonly causes diffuse interstitial to alveolar patterns (Figure 72-5); pleural effusion has rarely been documented as well.

Sonography

Ultrasound findings consistent with pancreatitis or diffuse hepatitis could be noted in dogs or cats with involvement of these tissues due to *T. gondii* infection. Intra-abdominal lymphadenomegaly may be noted in dogs or cats with polysystemic disease.

Advanced Imaging

MRI findings in dogs and cats with toxoplasmosis may be unremarkable, or focal or mass lesions may be identified in the brain and/or spinal cord. On MRI, lesions are often isointense on T1-weighted imaging and hyperintense on T2-weighted imaging, and they may enhance peripherally or uniformly with contrast (Figure 72-6).[53-55]

Microbiologic Testing

Cytologic Diagnosis

Using cytologic examination, *T. gondii* bradyzoites or tachyzoites can be detected in tissues, effusions, bronchoalveolar lavage fluids, aqueous humor, or CSF (Figure 72-7).[32,35,36,38] A definitive antemortem diagnosis of toxoplasmosis can be made if the organism is identified; however, this is uncommon, particularly in association with sublethal disease. In the dog, *N. caninum* tachyzoites cannot be distinguished from those of *T. gondii* on cytologic examination, and so further diagnostics are needed to make a definitive diagnosis.[2]

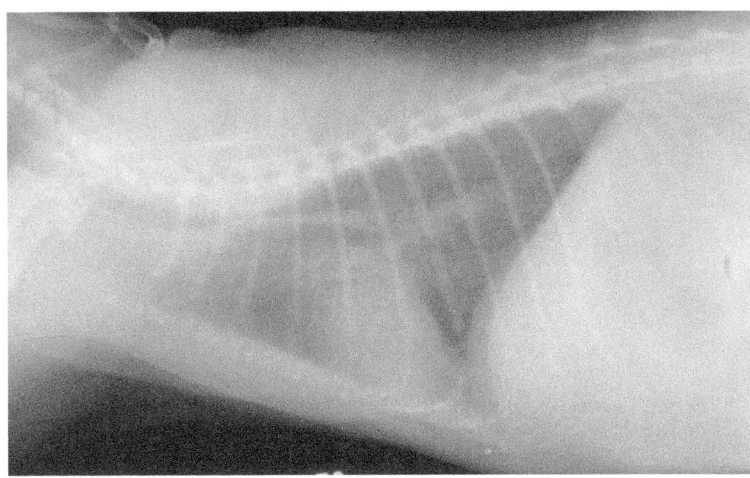

FIGURE 72-5 Thoracic radiographs of a 7-year-old female spayed domestic shorthair cat with pulmonic toxoplasmosis that developed one month after renal transplantation. There is a diffuse interstitial pattern. The cat subsequently developed respiratory arrest and tachyzoites were seen in fluid that was suctioned from the endotracheal tube used for resuscitation. Necropsy revealed severe, diffuse, necrotizing pneumonia with intralesional tachyzoites. Histiocytic, lymphoplasmacytic, and necrotizing lesions with intralesional tachyzoites were also seen in the renal allograft, ureter, bladder, liver, pancreas, peritoneum, muscularis mucosa of the stomach, and myocardium. Tachyzoites were not seen in the brain, but there was perivascular inflammation that suggested the possibility of infection. Immunohistochemistry confirmed that the tachyzoites were *T. gondii*.

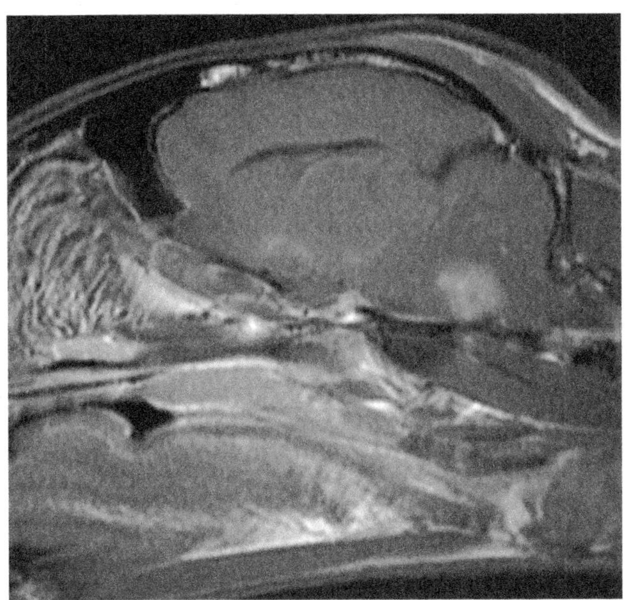

FIGURE 72-6 T1-weighted postcontrast sagittal magnetic resonance image from an 11-year-old female spayed domestic longhair that was evaluated for a 5-day history of inappetence, ataxia, abnormal vocalization, and circling. The cat was FIV and FeLV negative and had no other immunosuppressive conditions. A contrast-enhancing lesion is present in the right brainstem. CSF analysis revealed a mixed monocytic (primarily lymphocytic) pleocytosis with a total nuclear cell count of 36 cells/μL and a total protein concentration of 78 mg/dL. Meningoencephalitis secondary to *T. gondii* infection was confirmed at necropsy.

Fecal Flotation

T. gondii oocysts measure 10 × 12 μm. When identified in feces of cats with diarrhea, this suggests infection by *T. gondii*.[2-4,56] However, *Besnoitia* and *Hammondia* infections of cats produce morphologically similar oocysts. If oocysts of this size are detected in feces of dogs, *N. caninum* infection is most likely if clinical disease is present.[2] However, *T. gondii* oocysts can be present if the dog has ingested infected feline feces. PCR assays are available to differentiate *T. gondii* and *N. caninum*. Alternately, serum antibody responses can be followed sequentially to attempt to determine the infecting genus. Overall, detection of oocysts in cats has a poor negative predictive value for clinical toxoplasmosis, because most clinical toxoplasmosis results from disseminated infections that occur after oocyst shedding has been completed.

Serologic Diagnosis in Cats

Detection of *T. gondii* antibodies in serum is used most frequently for the diagnosis of clinical toxoplasmosis. A multitude of different techniques have been assessed, including ELISA, immunofluorescent antibody (IFA), Western blot immunoassay, and a variety of agglutination tests.[57-67] A latex agglutination assay and an indirect hemagglutination assay are available commercially. These assays can be applied to serum from either dogs or cats and theoretically detect all classes of immunoglobulin directed against *T. gondii*. However, they rarely detect antibody in feline serum samples when only IgM is present.[60] ELISA, IFA, and Western blot immunoassays have been adapted to detect IgM, IgG, and IgA antibody responses by using heavy-chain–specific secondary antibodies.[57,63,64] *T. gondii*–specific serum IgA antibody responses are similar to IgG antibody responses, and this antibody class is usually measured only in research studies. Several commercial laboratories in the United States offer *T. gondii* IgM and IgG testing by ELISA.[68] The following are common findings concerning *T. gondii* IgM and IgG antibody test results in cats.

***Toxoplasma gondii* IgM antibody titers.**

- Using ELISA, approximately 80% of healthy, experimentally infected cats have detectable *T. gondii*–specific IgM in serum within 2 to 4 weeks after inoculation with *T. gondii*; these titers generally are negative within 16 weeks after infection.[57,58]
- As occurs in some healthy women, persistent IgM titers (>16 weeks) have been documented commonly in cats co-infected with FIV and in cats with ocular toxoplasmosis.[41,65] Because of these findings and the fact that some cats never have a detectable IgM response, IgM titers cannot accurately be used to predict when a cat is shedding oocysts. If a clinician is concerned that an individual cat is shedding *T. gondii* oocysts, fecal flotation or a fecal PCR assay should be performed.

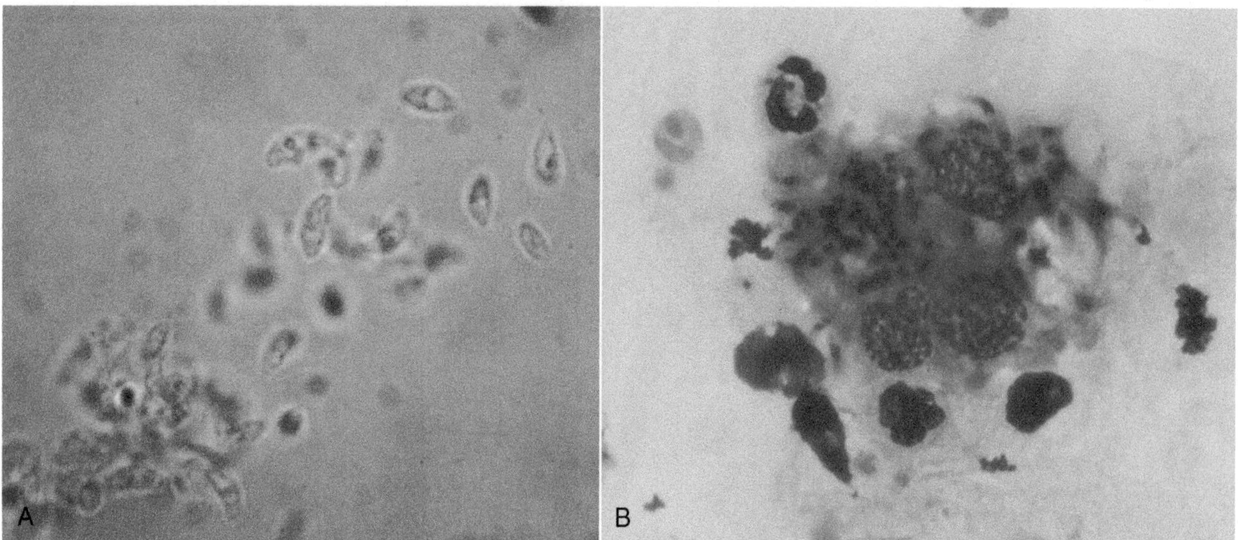

FIGURE 72-7 **A,** Tachyzoites of *Toxoplasma gondii* from the peritoneal cavity of a cat with fulminant toxoplasmosis. Unstained specimen. **B,** Cluster of tachyzoites in a tracheobronchial lavage specimen from a 12-year-old male neutered cat that developed respiratory distress 3 weeks after renal transplantation. Wright's stain, 1000× oil magnification.

- In one study of cats with clinical toxoplasmosis, *T. gondii* IgM titers were detected in the serum of 93% of the cats, whereas *T. gondii* IgG titers were detected in only 60% of the cats. Thus, IgM antibodies have a higher positive predictive value than IgG for clinical feline toxoplasmosis.[57,65]
- Some cats with chronic *T. gondii* infections that are initially IgM positive, but then become IgM negative, again became IgM positive after repeat inoculation with *T. gondii* and immunosuppression through inoculation with FIV and administration of glucocorticoids.[57,67] However, clinical signs of toxoplasmosis do not develop in these cats. Thus, presence of IgM antibodies in feline serum does not always mean that clinical toxoplasmosis is present.

***Toxoplasma gondii* IgG titers.**

- *T. gondii*–specific IgG can be detected by ELISA in serum in the majority of healthy experimentally inoculated cats within 3 to 4 weeks after infection.[57,58]
- By the time IgG antibodies are detected, the oocyst shedding period has usually been completed. Thus, IgG-seropositive cats are of minimal public health risk.
- *T. gondii* IgG antibody titers can be detected for at least 6 years after infection in experimentally inoculated cats; because the organism probably persists in tissues for life, IgG antibodies probably do as well.[62]
- Single, high IgG titers do not necessarily suggest recent or active *T. gondii* infection; healthy cats can have titers that exceed 1:10,000 as long as 6 years after experimental induction of toxoplasmosis.[62]
- Some cats with low *T. gondii* antibody titers can become seronegative based on the cutoff value used in an individual assay even though *T. gondii* is still within tissues. Based on an approximate 10% interassay variation in the ELISA technique, some cats with low positive IgG titers (1:64) can be positive for IgG antibodies on one analysis and negative on a subsequent analysis or vice versa.
- An increasing *T. gondii* IgG titer documents recent or active infection, but in experimentally infected cats, the time span from the first detectable positive IgG titer to the maximal IgG titer is approximately 2 to 3 weeks. Thus, some cats with clinical toxoplasmosis will have reached their maximal IgG titer by the time they are evaluated serologically.
- Rising *T. gondii* IgG antibody titers occur in healthy infected cats as well as cats with clinical toxoplasmosis and so, when assessed alone, do not prove clinical toxoplasmosis.
- In humans and cats that reactivate chronic *T. gondii* infection after immune suppression, IgG titers only rarely increase.

In dogs, assays that detect IgM and IgG titers are available in some commercial laboratories.[68] There have been very few research studies that assess canine serologic responses to *T. gondii* in different situations. However, most of the findings documented in cats appear to be true in dogs, based on the author's clinical experience.

For the reasons just discussed, antibody test results alone cannot be used to make a diagnosis of feline or canine toxoplasmosis. However, the following combination can be used to make a presumptive antemortem diagnosis:

- Demonstration of antibodies in serum that suggest exposure to *T. gondii*
- Demonstration of an IgM titer higher than 1:64, or a fourfold or greater rise in IgG titer, which suggests recent or active infection
- Clinical signs of disease consistent with toxoplasmosis
- Exclusion of other common causes of the clinical syndrome
- Positive response to appropriate treatment

Because *T. gondii* infection cannot be eliminated, most cats and dogs will be antibody positive for life, so there is little reason to repeat serum antibody titers after the clinical disease has resolved or to administer drugs with *T. gondii* activity to cats or dogs without clinical signs of toxoplasmosis.

Other serologic assays. Assays that measure *T. gondii* antigens or immune complexes have been evaluated in some cats. However, as for antibody tests, antigen or immune complexes can be detected in cats with or without clinical illness. These assays are not offered commercially.[23,24,57]

Molecular Diagnosis Using Nucleic Acid–Based Testing

Recently, PCR assays have been used to document *T. gondii* DNA in feces and can be used to differentiate *T. gondii* from other organisms.[56] *T. gondii* DNA can be amplified from the blood of

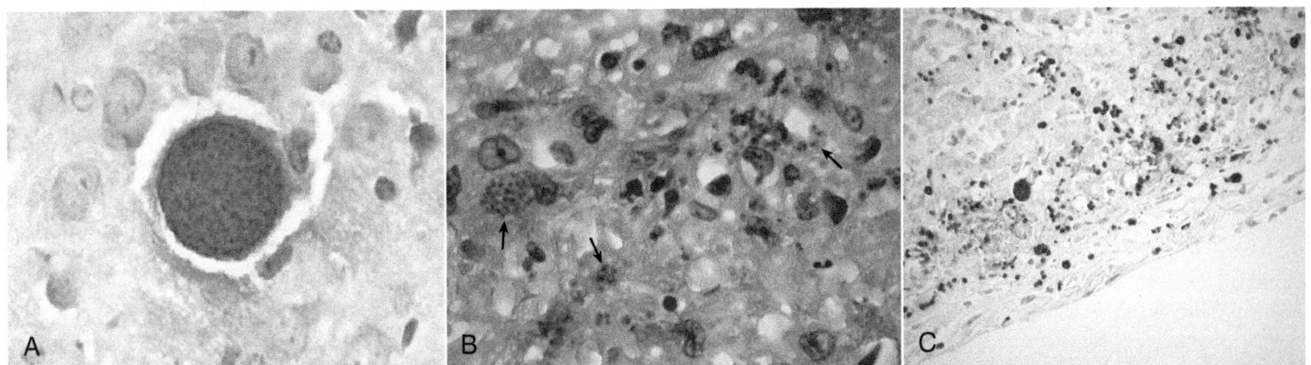

FIGURE 72-8 Histopathologic findings in *Toxoplasma gondii* infections. **A,** A tissue cyst filled with *Toxoplasma gondii* bradyzoites in the brain tissues of an experimentally infected mouse. **B,** Pancreas of the cat in Figure 72-5. There is pyogranulomatous inflammation with intralesional tachyzoites *(arrows)*. H&E stain. **C,** Immunohistochemistry clearly demonstrates the presence of *T. gondii* tachyzoites in the pancreas (brown staining).

TABLE 72-2

Antimicrobial Drugs That May Be Used to Treat Clinical Toxoplasmosis in Dogs and Cats

Drug	Dose	Route	Interval	Duration
Azithromycin	10 mg/kg	PO	q24h	4 weeks
Clindamycin	10-12 mg/kg	PO	q12h	4 weeks
Ponazuril	20 mg/kg	PO	q24h	4 weeks
Trimethoprim-sulfa	15 mg/kg	PO	q12h	4 weeks

If a positive response to treatment is achieved by week 4 but the animal is still improving slowly, continue treatment for 1 week past clinical resolution or when maximal response is recognized.

healthy cats and dogs, and so positive PCR assay results do not correlate with clinical disease.[69,70] Thus, PCR assays are used most frequently with cytologic examination or histopathology to document that the organisms seen were *T. gondii*, or to detect *T. gondii* in aqueous humor or CSF in conjunction with serology.[42,44-46,70]

The combination of detection of *T. gondii*–specific antibody in serum, blood, aqueous humor, or CSF and amplification of *T. gondii* DNA by PCR assay is the most accurate way to diagnose ocular or CNS toxoplasmosis. Whereas *T. gondii*–specific IgA, IgG, and DNA can be detected in aqueous humor and CSF of both normal and clinically ill cats, *T. gondii*–specific IgM has only been detected in the aqueous humor or CSF of clinically ill cats and so may be the best indicator of clinical disease. Whether this is true for dogs has not been assessed to date.

Pathologic Findings

Gross Pathologic Findings

T. gondii infection generally induces pyogranulomatous reactions and necrosis. The pyogranulomas may be visualized grossly depending on the organ involved. Effusions that are characteristic of modified transudates or exudates may be found on necropsy.

Histopathologic Findings

Histopathology in animals with toxoplasmosis usually reveals pyogranulomatous inflammation with necrosis. *T. gondii* tachyzoites or bradyzoites are commonly detected (Figure 72-8, *A* and *B*). However, if necrosis is severe, the organism may be obscured. In these cases, DNA can often be amplified from the tissues, or the agent can be visualized after immunohistochemical staining (Figure 72-8, C). Because *T. gondii* and *N. caninum* induce similar syndromes in dogs, performance of PCR assays for both organisms in dogs is indicated in order to differentiate between them.

Treatment and Prognosis

Cats or dogs with suspected clinical toxoplasmosis should be administered supportive care as needed. Clindamycin hydrochloride or a trimethoprim-sulfonamide combination has been prescribed most frequently for the specific treatment of clinical toxoplasmosis (Table 72-2).[2-4,66] One of the drugs should be prescribed for 1 week, since most clinical signs of toxoplasmosis will begin to resolve within that time period. If a positive response is recognized, treatment should be continued for a total of 4 weeks if possible. If there is a poor response to therapy after the first 7 days, an alternative drug should be considered. Recurrence of clinical signs may be more common in cats or dogs treated for less than 4 weeks.[72]

Azithromycin has been used successfully in a limited number of cats, but the optimal duration of therapy is unknown. Pyrimethamine combined with sulfa drugs is effective for the treatment of human toxoplasmosis but commonly results in toxicity in cats. Pyrimethamine has been administered successfully with other drugs for the treatment of neosporosis in dogs and so may be effective for treatment of clinical toxoplasmosis in this species. Ponazuril has been used experimentally in *T. gondii*–infected rodents and should be studied for the treatment of feline toxoplasmosis.[71,73] Currently, an optimal treatment regimen for the use of this drug for this purpose in cats is unknown. However, ponazuril (20 mg/kg PO q24h for 28 days) was apparently successful in the treatment of a dog with suppurative keratitis and necrotizing conjunctivitis due to *T. gondii* infection.[50] Addition of fluconazole to pyrimethamine and trimethoprim was also effective in rodent models of toxoplasmosis and requires further study.[74] Cats or dogs with suspected *Toxoplasma* uveitis should be treated with anti-*Toxoplasma* drugs in combination with topical or systemic glucocorticoids to avoid secondary lens luxations and glaucoma. Enucleation may be required if lens luxations and glaucoma develop from persistent uveitis.

The prognosis is poor for cats or dogs with hepatic, CNS, or pulmonary disease caused by tachyzoite replication, particularly in those that are immunocompromised by anti-inflammatory drugs or retrovirus co-infection. If they survive, cats or dogs with CNS involvement may not experience complete resolution of neurologic signs after treatment.

Immunity and Vaccination

There is no evidence to suggest that any drug can eliminate *T. gondii* infection in dogs or cats. Thus, recurrence of disease is always possible, and infected dogs and cats often remain seropositive. In cats, if repeat oocyst shedding occurs, the number of oocysts shed is small and shedding is of short duration. Systemic reactivation of *T. gondii* infection after administration of immunosuppressive drugs can occur in both dogs and cats.

Several types of vaccines have been studied to block oocyst shedding in cats, but there is no vaccine for prevention of clinical toxoplasmosis in dogs or cats.

Prevention

To avoid exposure to *T. gondii,* cats and dogs should not be allowed to hunt or be fed undercooked meats. Care should be taken to control transport hosts such as cockroaches that have been shown to carry *T. gondii* oocysts.

Public Health Aspects

Primary *T. gondii* infection in immunocompetent humans results in self-limiting fever, malaise, and lymphadenopathy that may not be recognized or is misdiagnosed. Primary infection of mothers by *T. gondii* during gestation can lead to clinical toxoplasmosis in the fetus; stillbirth, CNS disease, and ocular disease are common clinical manifestations (Figure 72-9). As T-helper cell counts decline, approximately 10% of people with AIDS develop toxoplasmic encephalitis from reactivation of bradyzoites in tissue cysts.

People most commonly acquire toxoplasmosis by ingestion of sporulated oocysts or tissue cysts, or transplacentally. To prevent toxoplasmosis, humans should avoid consumption of undercooked meats or ingestion of sporulated oocysts. In a study of 6282 meat samples from 698 retail meat stores, using a feline bioassay, *T. gondii* was detected in none of the beef or chicken specimens tested and only a small number of pork specimens.[75] However, *T. gondii* has been detected in the tissues of free-ranging chickens.[76] Although exposure to cats is epidemiologically associated with acquiring toxoplasmosis in some studies, touching individual cats is probably not a common way to acquire toxoplasmosis for the following reasons[2-4,77-81]:

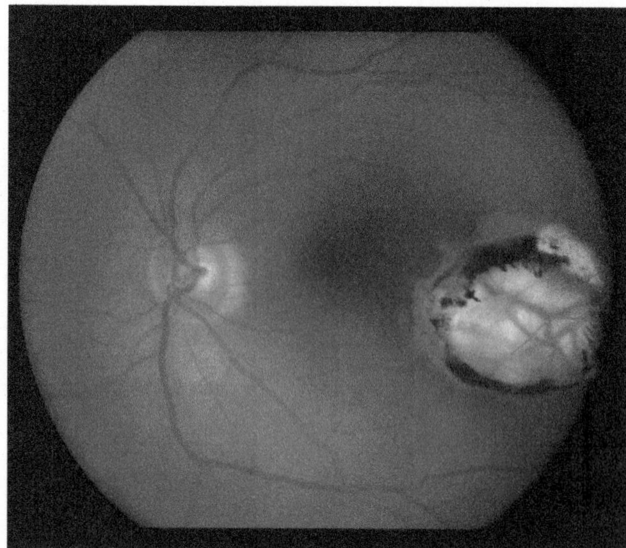

FIGURE 72-9 Healed chorioretinitis in a 60-year-old woman who had recovered from congenital toxoplasmosis. The infection resulted in a permanent visual deficit. (Image courtesy Mrs. Susan Sykes.)

- Cats generally only shed oocysts for days to several weeks after primary inoculation.
- Repeat oocyst shedding is rare, even in cats receiving glucocorticoids or cyclosporine, or in those infected with FIV or FeLV.
- Cats inoculated with tissue cysts 16 months after primary inoculation do not shed oocysts.
- Cats are very fastidious and usually do not allow feces to remain on their skin for time periods long enough to lead to oocyst sporulation; the organism was not isolated from the fur of cats that had been shedding millions of oocysts 7 days previously.

However, because some cats will repeat oocyst shedding when exposed a second time, cat feces should always be handled carefully. If a fecal specimen from a cat contains oocysts that measure 10 × 12 μm, it should be assumed that the organism present is *T. gondii.* The feces should be collected and removed daily until the oocyst shedding period is complete; administration of clindamycin (20 mg/kg PO daily) may shorten the oocyst shedding period if started after infection is documented.[2,82]

Because humans are not commonly infected with *T. gondii* through contact with individual cats, testing healthy cats for evidence of *T. gondii* infection is not recommended.[79] Fecal examination is an adequate procedure to determine when cats are actively shedding oocysts but cannot indicate when a cat has shed oocysts in the past. There is no serologic assay that accurately indicates this, and most cats that are shedding oocysts are seronegative. Most seropositive cats have completed the oocyst shedding period and are unlikely to repeat shedding; most seronegative cats would shed the organism if infected. If owners are concerned that they may have toxoplasmosis, they should see their physicians for testing.

Dogs do not complete the enteroepithelial phase of *T. gondii* but can mechanically transmit oocysts after ingesting feline feces.[9]

CASE EXAMPLE

Signalment: "Fluffy," a 3-year-old male neutered Siamese mix from Evans in northern Colorado

History: Fluffy was referred after being treated for anterior uveitis and recurrent fever at another clinic. The clinical signs had been noted for approximately 1 month. Fluffy was entirely indoors in a suburban environment, but adopted from a humane society at around 6 months of age. His last vaccines (rabies, feline herpesvirus-1, feline calicivirus, and panleukopenia virus) were administered 6 months before the uveitis was first noted. He was fed a commercial processed food. There were no other animals at the house. He was treated with selamectin monthly but had not received his dose this month because of the fever. The fever seemed intermittent, and when normal, Fluffy had normal appetite and attitude. The uveitis persisted in spite of treatment with amoxicillin-clavulanic acid administered daily for 10 days and topical 1% prednisolone acetate applied three times daily.

Physical Examination:

Body Weight: 4.2 kg

General: Quiet, alert, and responsive. Ambulatory on all four limbs. T = 104.3°F (40.2°C), HR = 180 beats/min, RR = 30 breaths/min, mucous membranes pink, CRT = 1 s.

Integument: A dull haircoat was present. There was no evidence of ectoparasites.

Eyes: Bilateral anterior uveitis was present; fundoscopic examination was difficult due to aqueous flare.

Musculoskeletal: Body condition score was 4/9; possible discomfort was detected on muscle palpation.

Gastrointestinal: The cranial abdomen was tense with abdominal splinting noted on palpation.

All Other Systems: No significant abnormalities were noted.

Laboratory Findings:

Complete Blood Count: All values were within reference ranges.

Serum Biochemistry Profile: All values were within reference ranges except for the activity of serum AST (190 U/L; reference range, 19-42 U/L) and the activity of serum CK (2000 U/L; reference range, 50-125 U/L).

Urinalysis: No significant abnormalities; SGr = 1.041.

Imaging Findings: Thoracic and abdominal radiographs and abdominal ultrasound were offered but declined by the owner.

Microbiologic Testing: Serologic testing: FeLV antigen negative; FIV antibody negative; serum *Bartonella* IgG negative; *Bartonella* PCR assay negative on whole blood; *T. gondii* serum IgM 1:256; *T. gondii* serum IgG 1:1024.

Diagnosis: Suspected chronic, and possibly recurrent, toxoplasmosis.

Treatment: Clindamycin (12 mg/kg PO q12h) was administered for 28 days; fever resolved on day 3 of treatment. Prednisolone acetate was continued every 6 hours topically bilaterally for the first 14 days and was discontinued after anterior uveitis resolved. Subsequently, chorioretinal scars were noted on fundoscopic examination.

Comments: The findings were suggestive of chronic recurrent toxoplasmosis, which does not respond to treatment with β-lactam antibiotics. Myositis or pancreatitis may have contributed to some of the clinical and laboratory findings. These tissues commonly contain tissue cysts with *T. gondii* bradyzoites that can repeatedly replicate as tachyzoites, which in turn results in acute disease. *T. gondii* IgM can be detected in some cats with recurrent disease. Fluffy may have been infected with *T. gondii* when he was a stray and had an exacerbation or alternatively may have been infected more recently in the home environment by ingestion of a transport host (cockroach, etc.) or intermediate host (rodent).

SUGGESTED READINGS

Jones JL, Dubey JP. Foodborne toxoplasmosis. Clin Infect Dis. 2012;55:845-851.

Robert-Gangneux F, Dardé M-L. Epidemiology and diagnostic strategies for toxoplasmosis. Clin Microbiol Rev. 2012;25:264-296.

REFERENCES

1. Nicolle C, Manceaux L. Sur une infection à corps de Leishman (ou organismes voisins) du gondii. C R Seances Acad Sci. 1908;147:763-766.
2. Dubey JP, Lindsay DS, Lappin MR. Toxoplasmosis and other intestinal coccidial infections in cats and dogs. Vet Clin North Am Small Anim Pract. 2009;39:1009-1034.
3. Lappin MR. Update on the diagnosis and management of *Toxoplasma gondii* infection in cats. Top Companion Anim Med. 2010;25:136-141.
4. Lappin MR. Toxoplasmosis. In: Couto G, Nelson R, eds. Small Animal Internal Medicine. St Louis, MO: Mosby Elsevier; 2010:1366-1373.
5. Vollaire MR, Radecki SV, Lappin MR. Seroprevalence of *Toxoplasma gondii* antibodies in clinically ill cats in the United States. Am J Vet Res. 2005;66:874-877.
6. Luria BJ, Levy JK, Lappin MR, et al. Prevalence of infectious diseases in feral cats in Northern Florida. J Feline Med Surg. 2004;6:287-296.
7. Spain CV, Scarlett JM, Wade SE, et al. Prevalence of enteric zoonotic agents in cats less than 1 year old in central New York State. J Vet Intern Med. 2001;15:33-38.
8. Dabritz HA, Miller MA, Atwill ER. Detection of *Toxoplasma gondii*–like oocysts in cat feces and estimates of the environmental oocyst burden. J Am Vet Med Assoc. 2007;231:1676-1684.
9. Lindsay DS, et al. Mechanical transmission of *Toxoplasma gondii* oocysts by dogs. Vet Parasitol. 1997;73:27-33.
10. Levy JK, Lappin MR, Glaser AL, et al. Prevalence of infectious diseases in cats and dogs rescued following Hurricane Katrina. J Am Vet Med Assoc. 2011;238:311-317.
11. Powell CC, Brewer M, Lappin MR. Detection of *Toxoplasma gondii* in the milk of experimentally infected lactating cats. J Vet Parasitol. 2001;102:29-33.
12. Arantes TP, Lopes WD, Ferreira RM, et al. *Toxoplasma gondii*: evidence for the transmission by semen in dogs. Exp Parasitol. 2009;123:190-194.
13. Bresciani KD, Costa AJ, Toniollo GH, et al. Transplacental transmission of *Toxoplasma gondii* in reinfected pregnant female canines. Parasitol Res. 2009;104:1213-1217.

14. Dubey JP. Comparative infectivity of oocysts and bradyzoites of *Toxoplasma gondii* for intermediate (mice) and definitive (cats) hosts. Vet Parasitol. 2006;140:69-75.
15. Vyas A, Kim SK, Giacomini N, et al. Behavioral changes induced by *Toxoplasma* infection of rodents are highly specific to aversion of cat odors. Proc Natl Acad Sci U S A. 2007;104:6442-6447.
16. Powell CC, Lappin MR. Clinical ocular toxoplasmosis in neonatal kittens. Vet Ophthalmol. 2001;4:87-92.
17. Spycher A, Geigy C, Howard J, et al. Isolation and genotyping of *Toxoplasma gondii* causing fatal systemic toxoplasmosis in an immunocompetent 10-year-old cat. J Vet Diagn Invest. 2011;23:104-108.
18. Beatty J, Barrs V. Acute toxoplasmosis in two cats on cyclosporin therapy. Aust Vet J. 2003;81:339.
19. Bernsteen L, Gregory CR, Aronson LR, et al. Acute toxoplasmosis following renal transplantation in three cats and a dog. J Am Vet Med Assoc. 1999;215:1123-1126.
20. Lappin MR, Scorza V. *Toxoplasma gondii* oocyst shedding in normal cats and cats treated with cyclosporine [Abstract]. Proceedings of the American College of Veterinary Internal Medicine Annual Forum, Denver CO, June 16, 2011.
21. Webb JA, et al. Cutaneous manifestations of disseminated toxoplasmosis in an immunosuppressed dog. J Am Anim Hosp Assoc. 2005;41:198-202.
22. Davidson MG, Rottman JB, English RV, et al. Feline immunodeficiency virus predisposes cats to acute generalized toxoplasmosis. Am J Pathol. 1993;143:1486-1497.
23. Lappin MR, Cayatte S, Powell CC, et al. Detection of *Toxoplasma gondii* antigen containing immune complexes in the serum of cats. Am J Vet Res. 1993;54:415-419.
24. Lappin MR, Greene CE, Prestwood AK, et al. Enzyme-linked immunosorbent assay for the detection of circulating antigens of *Toxoplasma gondii* in the serum of cats. Am J Vet Res. 1989;50:1586-1590.
25. Hsu V, Grant DC, Zajac AM, et al. Prevalence of IgG antibodies to *Encephalitozoon cuniculi* and *Toxoplasma gondii* in cats with and without chronic kidney disease from Virginia. Vet Parasitol. 2011;176:23-26.
26. Peterson JL, Willard MD, Lees GE, et al. Toxoplasmosis in two cats with inflammatory intestinal disease. J Am Vet Med Assoc. 1991;99:473-476.
27. McConnell JF, Sparkes AH, Blunden AS, et al. Eosinophilic fibrosing gastritis and toxoplasmosis in a cat. J Feline Med Surg. 2007;9:82-86.
28. Dubey JP, Carpenter JL. Histologically confirmed clinical toxoplasmosis in cats: 100 cases (1952-1990). J Am Vet Med Assoc. 1993;203:1556-1566.
29. Dubey JP, Johnstone I. Fatal neonatal toxoplasmosis in cats. J Am Anim Hosp Assoc. 1982;18:461-467.
30. Dubey JP, Carpenter JL. Neonatal toxoplasmosis in littermate cats. J Am Vet Med Assoc. 1993;203:1546-1549.
31. Nordquist BC, Aronson LR. Pyogranulomatous cystitis associated with *Toxoplasma gondii* infection in a cat after renal transplantation. J Am Vet Med Assoc. 2008;232:1010-1012.
32. Park CH, Ikadai H, Yoshida E, et al. Cutaneous toxoplasmosis in a female Japanese cat. Vet Pathol. 2007;44:683-687.
33. Pfohl JC, Dewey CW. Intracranial *Toxoplasma gondii* granuloma in a cat. J Feline Med Surg. 2005;7:369-374.
34. Simpson KE, Devine BC, Gunn-Moore D. Suspected *Toxoplasma*-associated myocarditis in a cat. J Feline Med Surg. 2005;7:203-208.
35. Hawkins EC, Davidson MG, Meuten DJ, et al. Cytologic identification of *Toxoplasma gondii* in bronchoalveolar lavage fluid of experimentally infected cats. J Am Vet Med Assoc. 1997;210:648-650.
36. Brownlee L, Sellon RK. Diagnosis of naturally occurring toxoplasmosis by bronchoalveolar lavage in a cat. J Am Anim Hosp Assoc. 2001;37:251-255.
37. Alves L, Gorgas D, Vandevelde M, et al. Segmental meningomyelitis in 2 cats caused by *Toxoplasma gondii.* J Vet Intern Med. 2011;25:148-152.
38. Falzone C, Baroni M, De Lorenzi D, et al. *Toxoplasma gondii* brain granuloma in a cat: diagnosis using cytology from an intraoperative sample and sequential magnetic resonance imaging. J Small Anim Pract. 2008;49:95-99.
39. Kul O, Atmaca HT, Deniz A, et al. Clinicopathologic diagnosis of cutaneous toxoplasmosis in an Angora cat. Berl Munch Tierarztl Wochenschr. 2011;124:386-389.
40. Lindsay SA, Barrs VR, Child G, et al. Myelitis due to reactivated spinal toxoplasmosis in a cat. J Feline Med Surg. 2010;12:818-821.
41. Lappin MR, Roberts SM, Davidson MG, et al. Enzyme-linked immunosorbent assays for the detection of *Toxoplasma gondii*–specific antibodies and antigens in the aqueous humor of cats. J Am Vet Med Assoc. 1992;201:1010-1016.
42. Powell CC, McInnis CL, Fontenelle JP, et al. *Bartonella* species, feline herpesvirus-1, and *Toxoplasma gondii* PCR assay results from blood and aqueous humor samples from 104 cats with naturally occurring endogenous uveitis. J Feline Med Surg. 2010;12:923-938.
43. Dubey JP, Carpenter JL, Topper MJ, et al. Fatal toxoplasmosis in dogs. J Am Anim Hosp Assoc. 1989;25:659-664.
44. Al-Qassab S, Reichel MP, Su C, et al. Isolation of *Toxoplasma gondii* from the brain of a dog in Australia and its biological and molecular characterization. Vet Parasitol. 2009;164:335-339.
45. da Silva AV, Pezerico SB, de Lima VY, et al. Genotyping of *Toxoplasma gondii* strains isolated from dogs with neurological signs. Vet Parasitol. 2005;127:23-27.
46. Langoni H, Matteucci G, Medici B, et al. Detection and molecular analysis of *Toxoplasma gondii* and *Neospora caninum* from dogs with neurological disorders. Rev Soc Bras Med Trop. 2012;45:365-368.
47. Plugge NF, Ferreira FM, Richartz RR, et al. Occurrence of antibodies against *Neospora caninum* and/or *Toxoplasma gondii* in dogs with neurological signs. Rev Bras Parasitol Vet. 2011;20:202-206.
48. Dubey JP, Chapman JL, Rosenthal BM, et al. Clinical *Sarcocystis neurona, Sarcocystis canis, Toxoplasma gondii*, and *Neospora caninum* infections in dogs. Vet Parasitol. 2006;137:36-49.
49. Holt N, Murray M, Cuddon PA, et al. Seroprevalence of various infectious agents in dogs with suspected acute canine polyradiculoneuritis. J Vet Intern Med. 2011;25:261-266.
50. Swinger RL, Schmidt Jr KA, Dubielzig RR. Keratoconjunctivitis associated with *Toxoplasma gondii* in a dog. Vet Ophthalmol. 2009;12:56-60.
51. Hoffmann AR, Cadieu J, Kiupel M, et al. Cutaneous toxoplasmosis in two dogs. J Vet Diagn Invest. 2012;24:636-640.
52. Yarim GF, Nisbet C, Oncel T, et al. Serum protein alterations in dogs naturally infected with *Toxoplasma gondii*. Parasitol Res. 2007;101:1197-1202.
53. Pfohl JC, Dewey CW. Intracranial *Toxoplasma gondii* granuloma in a cat. J Feline Med Surg. 2005;7(6):369-374.
54. Falzone C, Baroni M, De Lorenzi D, et al. *Toxoplasma gondii* brain granuloma in a cat: diagnosis using cytology from an intraoperative sample and sequential magnetic resonance imaging. J Small Anim Pract. 2008;49(2):95-99.
55. Alves L, Gorgas D, Vandevelde M, et al. Segmental meningomyelitis in 2 cats caused by *Toxoplasma gondii*. J Vet Intern Med. 2011;25:148-152.
56. Salant H, Spira DT, Hamburger J. A comparative analysis of coprologic diagnostic methods for detection of *Toxoplasma gondii* in cats. Am J Trop Med Hyg. 2010;82:865-870.
57. Lappin MR. Feline toxoplasmosis: interpretation of diagnostic test results. Semin Vet Med Surg. 1996;11:154-160.
58. Lappin MR, Greene CE, Prestwood AK, et al. Diagnosis of recent *Toxoplasma gondii* infection in cats by use of an enzyme-linked immunosorbent assay for immunoglobulin M. Am J Vet Res. 1989;50:1580-1585.
59. Lappin MR, Bush DJ, Reduker DW. Feline serum antibody responses to *Toxoplasma gondii* and characterization of target antigens. J Parasitol. 1994;80:73-80.

60. Lappin MR, Powell CC. Comparison of latex agglutination, indirect hemagglutination, and ELISA techniques for the detection of *Toxoplasma gondii*-specific antibodies in the serum of cats. J Vet Intern Med. 1991;5:299-301.
61. Dabritz HA, Gardner IA, Miller MA, et al. Evaluation of two *Toxoplasma gondii* serologic tests used in a serosurvey of domestic cats in California. J Parasitol. 2007;93:806-816.
62. Dubey JP. Duration of immunity to shedding *Toxoplasma gondii* oocysts by cats. J Parasitol. 1995;81:410-415.
63. Cannizzo KP, Lappin MR, Cooper CM, et al. *Toxoplasma gondii* antigen recognition by serum IgM, IgG, and IgA of queens and their neonatally infected kittens. Am J Vet Res. 1996;57:1327-1330.
64. Burney DP, Lappin MR, Cooper CM, et al. Detection of *Toxoplasma gondii*-specific IgA in the serum of cats. Am J Vet Res. 1995;56:769-773.
65. Lappin MR, George JW, Pedersen NC, et al. Primary and secondary *Toxoplasma gondii* infection in normal and feline immunodeficiency virus-infected cats. J Parasitol. 1996;82:733-742.
66. Lappin MR, Greene CE, Dawe DL. Clinical feline toxoplasmosis: serologic diagnosis and therapeutic management of 15 cases. J Vet Intern Med. 1989;3:139-143.
67. Lappin MR, Dawe DL, Lindl PA, et al. The effect of glucocorticoid administration on oocyst shedding, serology, and cell-mediated immune responses of cats with recent or chronic toxoplasmosis. J Am Anim Hosp Assoc. 1992;27:625-632.
68. Colorado State University Veterinary Diagnostic Laboratories. http://www.dlab.colostate.edu. Last accessed January 13, 2013.
69. Burney DP, Spilker M, McReynolds L, et al. Detection of *Toxoplasma gondii* parasitemia in experimentally inoculated cats. J Parasitol. 1999;5:947-951.
70. Lee JY, Lee SE, Lee EG, et al. Nested PCR-based detection of *Toxoplasma gondii* in German shepherd dogs and stray cats in South Korea. Res Vet Sci. 2008;85:125-127.
71. Mitchell SM, Zajac AM, Kennedy T, et al. Prevention of recrudescent toxoplasmic encephalitis using ponazuril in an immunodeficient mouse model. J Eukaryot Microbiol. 2006;53:S164-S165.
72. Lappin M. Unpublished observations, 2012.
73. Mitchell SM, Zajac AM, Davis WL, et al. Efficacy of ponazuril in vitro and in preventing and treating *Toxoplasma gondii* infections in mice. J Parasitol. 2004;90:639-642.
74. Martins-Duarte ES, de Souza W, Vommaro RC. *Toxoplasma gondii:* the effect of fluconazole combined with sulfadiazine and pyrimethamine against acute toxoplasmosis in a murine model. Exp Parasitol. 2012.
75. Dubey JP, Hill DE, Jones JL, et al. Prevalence of viable *Toxoplasma gondii* in beef, chicken, and pork from retail meat stores in the United States: risk assessment to consumers. J Parasitol. 2005;91:1082-1093.
76. Gonçalves IN, Uzêda RS, Lacerda GA, et al. Molecular frequency and isolation of cyst-forming coccidia from free ranging chickens in Bahia State, Brazil. Vet Parasitol. 2012;190:74-79.
77. Angulo FJ, Glaser CA, Juranek DD, et al. Caring for pets of immunocompromised persons. J Am Vet Med Assoc. 1994;205:1711-1722.
78. Dabritz HA, Conrad PA. Cats and *Toxoplasma*: implications for public health. Zoonoses Public Health. 2010;57:34-52.
79. Jones JL, Dargelas V, Roberts J, et al. Risk factors for *Toxoplasma gondii* infection in the United States. Clin Infect Dis. 2009;49:878-884.
80. Kaplan JE, Benson C, Holmes KK, et al. Guidelines for prevention and treatment of opportunistic infections in HIV-infected adults and adolescents. Recommendations from CDC, the National Institutes of Health, and the HIV Medicine Association of the Infectious Diseases Society of America. MMWR Recomm Rep. 2009;58(RR04):1-198.
81. Wallace MR, Rossetti RJ, Olson PE, et al. Cats and toxoplasmosis risk in HIV-infected adults. JAMA. 1993;269:76-77.
82. Malmasi A, Mosallanejad B, Mohebali M, et al. Prevention of shedding and re-shedding of *Toxoplasma gondii* oocysts in experimentally infected cats treated with oral clindamycin: a preliminary study. Zoonoses Public Health. 2009;56:102-104.

CHAPTER 73

Neosporosis

Jane E. Sykes

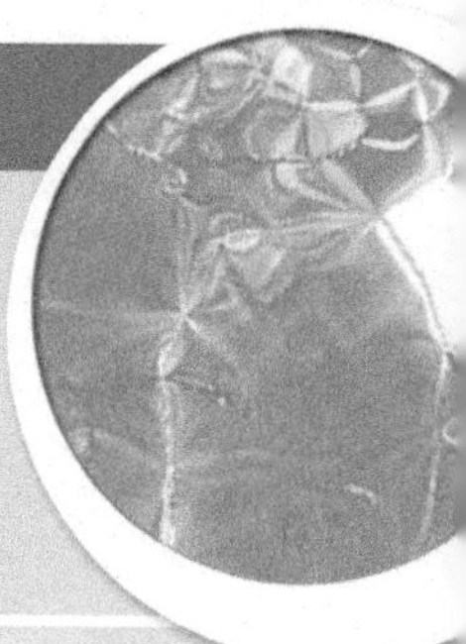

Overview of Neosporosis

First Described: 1984, in boxer dogs in Norway (Bjerkas and others)[1]

Cause: *Neospora caninum,* a coccidial protozoan parasite (phylum Apicomplexa)

Affected Hosts: Dogs are the definitive hosts and are the only species known to complete the sexual phase of *N. caninum* replication with passage of oocysts in the feces. Clinical illness primarily occurs in dogs and cattle, but sheep, deer, and water buffalo may also act as intermediate hosts.

Geographic Distribution: Worldwide

Mode of Transmission: Dogs can be infected transplacentally or through the transmammary route. Postnatally, dogs may be infected after they ingest infected tissues of intermediate hosts or bovine fetal membranes

Major Clinical Signs: Ascending paralysis, muscle atrophy, neurologic (especially cerebellar) signs, nodular dermatitis, respiratory distress

Differential Diagnoses: Toxoplasmosis, sarcocystosis, hepatozoonosis, deep mycoses, protothecosis, rabies, canine distemper virus infection, West Nile virus infection, canine monocytic ehrlichiosis, migrating ascarid infections, neuronal storage diseases, granulomatous meningoencephalitis, immune-mediated neuromuscular disease, primary or metastatic neoplasia

Human Health Significance: There is no clear evidence that *N. caninum* infects humans.

Etiology and Epidemiology

Neospora caninum is an obligately intracellular protozoan pathogen that closely resembles *Toxoplasma gondii*; before its description in 1984, it was misidentified as *T. gondii.* In contrast to *T. gondii,* domestic dogs and wild canids (coyotes, dingos, and probably wolves), and not cats, act as definitive hosts of *N. caninum* and shed oocysts after ingestion of *N. caninum* tissue cysts (enteroepithelial cycle) (Figure 73-1). Clinical neosporosis results from systemic replication of *N. caninum* tachyzoites (which divide by a process known as endodyogeny) and has been described in dogs and certain domestic and wild herbivores such as cattle, sheep, goats, deer, and marsupials. A related parasite, *Neospora hughesi,* sporadically causes myeloencephalitis in horses.[2] This organism has an unknown definitive host that is unlikely to be the dog, based on experimental infection studies.[3]

N. caninum is one of the most important causes of infertility, abortion, and neonatal mortality in cattle worldwide. Sheep can also develop reproductive and neonatal disease, but the economic importance of *N. caninum* in sheep is less clear when compared with cattle.[4] Herbivores likely become infected when they ingest oocysts shed in canine feces or through subclinical transplacental transmission. Oocysts sporulate and become infective 24 to 72 hours after they are shed in canine feces and can survive in the environment for prolonged periods. After oocysts are ingested, sporozoites are released in the intestinal tract and penetrate intestinal epithelial cells. Organisms can then disseminate to a variety of tissues, where they ultimately encyst as bradyzoite cysts. In dogs, pregnancy is associated with reactivation of bradyzoite cysts, with replication of tachyzoites and subsequent abortion or transplacental transmission. In breeding dogs, repeated reactivation of *N. caninum* replication occurs in late gestation with successive pregnancies, so that multiple litters of puppies can be affected. Transmission may also occur via the transmammary route. Infection of immunologically naïve cattle late in pregnancy is most likely to lead to transplacental spread with abortion (also known as *exogenous* transplacental transmission).[5] However, transplacental transmission as a result of reactivation of latent infection during pregnancy (*endogenous* transplacental transmission) can also occur.[6] The pregnant cow typically shows no other overt clinical signs of infection. Although antibodies to *N. caninum* have been found in cats and humans, naturally occurring neosporosis has not been described in these species.

Aside from transplacental transmission, dogs can become infected and shed oocysts when they ingest bovine placental material as well as other bovine tissues, such as muscle, liver, brain, and heart muscle.[7] This horizontal transmission is important and is thought to maintain infection in the dog population.[8] The DNA of *N. caninum* has been found in birds, small rodents, and lagomorphs, but whether predation of these species leads to oocyst shedding by dogs is not clear.[4] Experimental evidence suggests that ingestion of infected chicken eggs by dogs may lead to oocyst shedding.[9] However, ingestion of *oocysts* by dogs does not lead to oocyst shedding or development of tissue cysts.[10] When dogs do shed oocysts, the shedding begins 5 to 13 days after infection, and only low numbers of oocysts are shed for a short period (several days); seroconversion does not always occur. Rarely, protracted oocyst shedding (several months) by dogs has been described.[11] Puppies shed more oocysts than adult dogs,[12] and the number of oocysts shed decreases with repeated exposures to bradyzoite cysts.

In dogs, seroprevalence increases with age (because of an increased likelihood of exposure through horizontal transmission over time) and is higher in free-roaming dogs than in pet

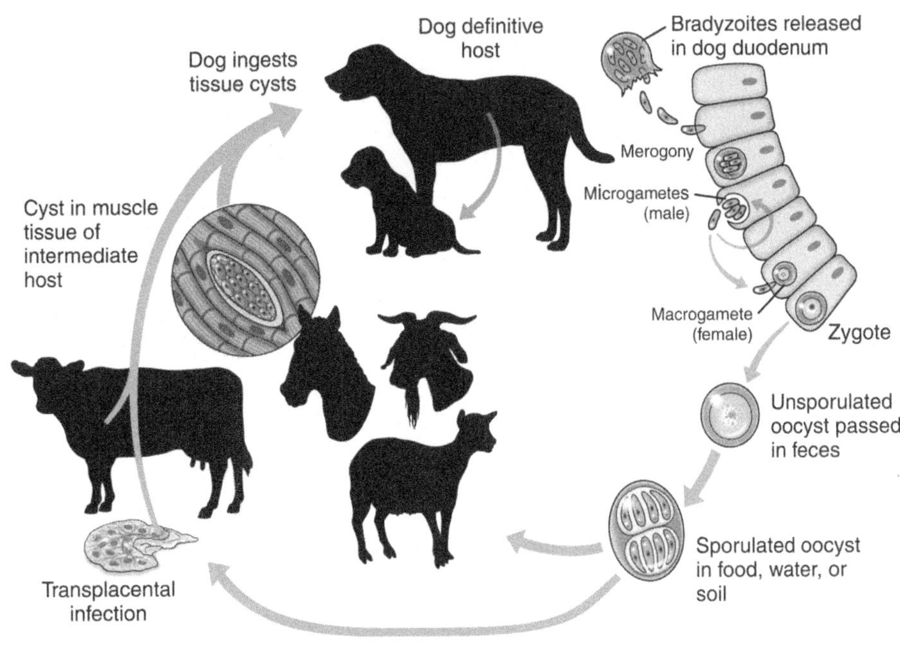

FIGURE 73-1 Life cycle of *Neospora caninum*. Dogs become infected when they ingest tissue cysts in bovine placental material and other bovine tissues. Bradyzoites are released in the intestine and transform into merozoites, where they undergo merogony. A zygote forms and is shed in the feces as an unsporulated oocyst. In addition, organisms can penetrate the dog's intestinal tract and form tissue cysts. Reactivation of these cysts in pregnancy can result in repeated transplacental transmission to the fetus. Herbivores are infected when they ingest sporulated oocysts. Infection of cattle can lead to transplacental spread of tachyzoites and abortion.

dogs. Dogs that reside on cattle farms or dogs in rural areas are also more likely to be seropositive than dogs that reside in urban areas.[13-16] Introduction of infected dogs to a farm can lead to outbreaks of abortion in cattle on the farm,[17] and the more dogs present on a farm, the greater the chance that cattle will be exposed. Although mixed breed dogs are more likely to be seropositive (exposed) than purebred dogs, purebred dogs often develop clinical neosporosis,[18] possibly because of genetic defects in cell-mediated immune function. Commonly affected breeds in the literature and/or in the author's practice include boxers, Rhodesian ridgebacks, bull mastiffs, greyhounds, basset hounds, Labrador retrievers, Rottweilers, and West Highland white terriers.

Clinical Features

Signs and Their Pathogenesis

Although exposure to *N. caninum* is common, clinical disease is uncommon in dogs. The development of clinical neosporosis, the signs that develop, and their rate of progression may depend on the virulence of the infecting *N. caninum* strain and the age and immunocompetence of the host.[4,19] Many affected dogs are infected transplacentally, after which clinical signs usually become apparent from 4 weeks to 6 months of age. Up to 50% of puppies in a litter can be infected, but not all puppies develop signs simultaneously, and sometimes only one puppy in the litter develops clinical illness.[20] Stillbirths and neonatal deaths may also be reported.[18] Reactivation of subclinical infection can occur in older dogs after treatment with immunosuppressive drugs or chemotherapy.[21-23] Horizontal acquisition of infection by adult dogs may occur through consumption of raw meat; one dog that developed neosporosis had a history of being fed raw elk meat.[22]

Transplacental infection of puppies usually leads to myositis and polyradiculoneuritis that initially involves the lumbosacral spinal nerve roots. This is manifested as ascending paralysis, muscle atrophy, and fibrous muscle contracture with arthrogryposis (joint contracture), hyperextension of the pelvic limbs, and loss of patellar reflexes.[18] Early signs of disease include exercise intolerance, ataxia, a high-stepping gait, splaying of the pelvic limbs, a "bunny hopping" gait, urinary incontinence, and/or muscle pain.[18,24-26] Clinical signs progress in some dogs to lethargy, tetraplegia, inability to fully open the mouth, dysphagia, and respiratory difficulty. Involvement of esophageal muscle may lead to megaesophagus.[27,28] Mandibular paralysis, vomiting, and lethargy were described as the only clinical signs in one affected dog.[28] Although ocular lesions are not a major clinical feature of neosporosis, focal chorioretinitis has been reported in some puppies.[29] Less often, young dogs develop signs of hepatitis; pneumonia; meningoencephalomyelitis; or myocarditis with arrhythmias, acute onset of respiratory distress, or sudden death.[26,27,30,31] Puppies with neuromuscular signs may have subclinical infection of other organ systems.[27]

In contrast to puppies, adult dogs typically develop polymyositis and/or meningoencephalomyelitis, with a variety of neurologic signs.[19,27,32] Although lesions can occur throughout the central nervous system (CNS),[27] *N. caninum* has a predilection for the cerebellum.[19] Some dogs can develop cerebellar atrophy.[19,33] Disseminated infections that involve the myocardium, liver, pancreas, lungs, skin, and/or eyes can also occur in adult dogs but are less common than encephalitis. In one unusual case, *N. caninum* tachyzoites were found in the peritoneal fluid of a dog with bacterial peritonitis.[34]

Physical Examination Findings

Physical examination findings in puppies with polyradiculoneuritis-myositis vary from mild ataxia and muscle atrophy to

TABLE 73-1

Diagnostic Assays Available for Neosporosis in Dogs

Assay	Specimen Type	Target	Performance
Fecal flotation	Feces	*N. caninum* oocysts	Dogs with clinical neosporosis typically do not shed oocysts so this has a very low sensitivity and is not used routinely for diagnosis. Oocysts cannot be readily distinguished from those of *Hammondia heydorni*.
Fecal PCR assay	Feces	*N. caninum* DNA	As for fecal flotation.
Cytologic examination	CSF, aspirates of skin lesions, rarely specimens from the respiratory tract	*N. caninum* tachyzoites	Insensitive except in the case of skin lesions. Confirms active infection and is generally associated with disease. Organisms cannot be readily distinguished from *Toxoplasma gondii*.
Serology (IFA or ELISA)	Serum or CSF	Antibodies to *N. caninum*	Assays can vary in performance between laboratories. A fourfold increase in titer is associated with recent infection. Dogs with chronic neosporosis may not show a rise in titer, but titers >1:800 in conjunction with consistent clinical signs suggest neosporosis.
Histopathology	Muscle biopsies, multiple tissues collected at necropsy	*N. caninum* bradyzoites and tachyzoites	If organisms are detected in the presence of inflammation and necrosis, clinical neosporosis is likely. May be difficult to differentiate *N. caninum* and *T. gondii*. Immunohistochemistry can aid in the differentiation of the two species.
PCR assay	Muscle or skin biopsies, body fluids (especially CSF), tissues collected at necropsy	*N. caninum* DNA	Assay performance may vary between laboratories. Because positive PCR results can occur in healthy dogs, they must be interpreted in light of clinical signs and other findings in the specimens tested.

tetraparesis with rigid extension of one or both pelvic limbs and arthrogryposis. Reduced patellar and sometimes other segmental reflexes (including the perianal reflex) are often present.[18,24,35,36] Severely affected dogs may be lethargic and exhibit respiratory difficulty, and it may only be possible to open the mouth a few centimeters. Fever is rare.[18]

Adult dogs with *N. caninum* meningoencephalitis may be obtunded and exhibit signs that include ataxia, circling, head tilt, nystagmus, hypermetria, head tremors, delayed placing reactions, abnormal cranial nerve function, anisocoria, depressed segmental reflexes, tetraparesis, cervical hyperesthesia, and seizures.

Dogs with myocardial involvement may develop acute onset of respiratory difficulty and cyanosis.[18,27] Cutaneous involvement is manifested as dermatitis with single or multifocal firm nodules, crusting, and/or ulceration, which can appear at additional sites over time and may or may not be accompanied by other systemic signs of infection.[21,37-40] Rarely, dogs with pulmonary involvement are evaluated for cough or respiratory difficulty.[41]

Diagnosis

Neosporosis should be suspected in young dogs (<1 year of age) that develop ascending paralysis and muscle atrophy. It should also be suspected in dogs that develop neurologic (and especially cerebellar) signs or nodular dermatitis, especially in predisposed breeds or dogs treated with immunosuppressive drugs. Diagnosis most often relies on serology or detection of protozoal organisms in body fluids, aspirates, or tissues using light microscopy and/or PCR assays (Table 73-1). Often, antemortem diagnosis is based only on serologic testing because organisms are not easily found.

Laboratory Abnormalities

Complete Blood Count, Serum Biochemistry Panel, and Urinalysis

As for toxoplasmosis, there are no specific hematologic or biochemical abnormalities that suggest neosporosis. The CBC is often normal, but occasionally mild nonregenerative anemia, mild eosinophilia, or monocytosis is evident.[18,32] The serum biochemistry panel reveals increased creatine kinase activity in dogs with myositis.[19,23,24,26] Occasionally, increased activity of serum ALT (due to hepatitis or severe myositis) or hyperglobulinemia is evident.[23,32] The urinalysis is generally unremarkable.

Cerebrospinal Fluid Analysis

The CSF of dogs with *N. caninum* meningoencephalitis may be normal or show mild to markedly increased total nuclear cell count (TNCC) (sometimes >1000 cells/μL) and mild to markedly increased CSF protein concentration.[19,32] Usually, a mononuclear pleocytosis is present, but occasionally the response is mixed or primarily composed of neutrophils or eosinophils.[19,24,32,35] *N. caninum* tachyzoites are rarely seen in CSF.[22,32]

Diagnostic Imaging

Plain Radiography

Thoracic radiographs in dogs with neosporosis are usually unremarkable but may show a diffuse interstitial pattern in dogs with pneumonia, or evidence of megaesophagus in dogs with neuromuscular signs.[18]

Sonographic Findings

Abnormalities are rarely detected on abdominal ultrasound examination of dogs with neosporosis.

Advanced Imaging

MRI of adult dogs with cerebellar signs associated with *N. caninum* infection may show moderate to marked bilateral cerebellar atrophy.[19] Meningeal contrast enhancement may be present.[19,32] Single or multifocal T2-weighted and FLAIR hyperintensities that enhance with contrast on T1-weighted images may be present within the cerebellum or other parts of the brain (Figure 73-2). Mild to moderate heterogenous T2-weighted and FLAIR hyperintensities can also be seen in the masseter and temporalis muscles, which may appear atrophied.

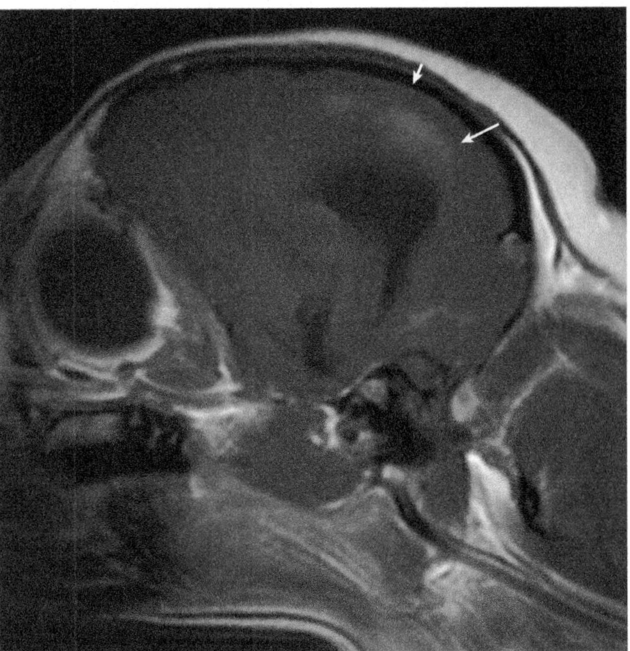

FIGURE 73-2 Sagittal T1-weighted postcontrast MRI image from a 4-year-old female spayed Chihuahua with suspected *Neospora caninum* meningoencephalitis. Multiple poorly defined regions of contrast enhancement were identified in the cerebral cortices *(large arrow)*, and mild meningeal enhancement was evident *(small arrow)*. CSF analysis revealed a mononuclear pleocytosis, and *Neospora* DNA was detected using PCR in the cerebrospinal fluid.

Electrodiagnostic Testing

Electromyography in dogs with neosporosis may reveal spontaneous fibrillation potentials, positive sharp waves, and repetitive discharges.[24,26] In some dogs, nerve conduction studies have revealed reduced conduction velocities and compound muscle action potentials.[24]

Microbiologic Tests

Cytologic Examination

The tachyzoites of *N. caninum* may be visualized within aspirates of skin lesions (which often contain many organisms) and rarely in CSF or other body fluids. They are approximately 6 × 1 μm and oval to crescent-shaped.[22,32,34,37] They may be seen singly, in pairs, or in larger groups, extracellularly and intracellularly, and are often associated with a pyogranulomatous inflammatory response (Figure 73-3). In the dog, *N. caninum* tachyzoites cannot be distinguished from those of *T. gondii* on cytologic examination. Because some cross-reactivity between *N. caninum* and *T. gondii* can occur with immunocytochemistry depending on the antibodies used, the use of PCR assays is recommended to definitively identify organisms as *N. caninum*. For unknown reasons, such cross-reactivity may be most likely to occur in dermal neosporosis.[8]

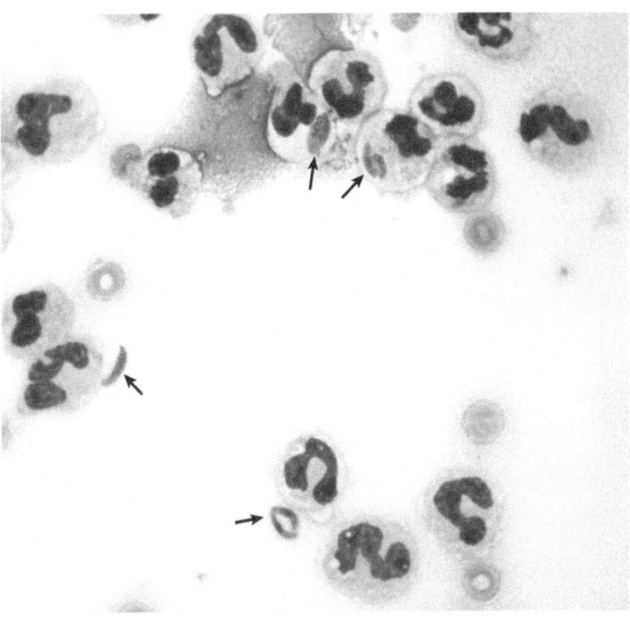

FIGURE 73-3 Cytology of abdominal fluid sediment in a 7-year old male neutered Rhodesian ridgeback showing intracellular and extracellular *Neospora caninum* tachyzoites *(arrows)*. Nucleated cells are predominantly nondegenerate to mildly degenerate neutrophils.

Fecal Flotation

Fecal flotation with sugar or zinc sulfate solutions can be used to detect the oocysts of *N. caninum* in feces. However, clinically affected dogs do not typically shed oocysts. When oocysts are seen, they are indistinguishable from those of *Hammondia heydorni* or *Toxoplasma gondii*.

Serologic Diagnosis

Serologic assays are available commercially that detect antibody to *N. caninum* in serum and/or in CSF. Titers are often higher in serum than in the CSF of affected dogs. Indirect IFA assays are widely used, but ELISA assays have also been developed and may be used to detect IgM and IgG antibody. Seroconversion usually occurs within 2 to 3 weeks of infection, and a rising serum titer can be identified in acutely infected dogs.[26] This rise may not occur in chronically infected dogs, so in this case a single high titer in a dog with consistent clinical signs is suggestive of the diagnosis. Some dogs with neosporosis have extremely

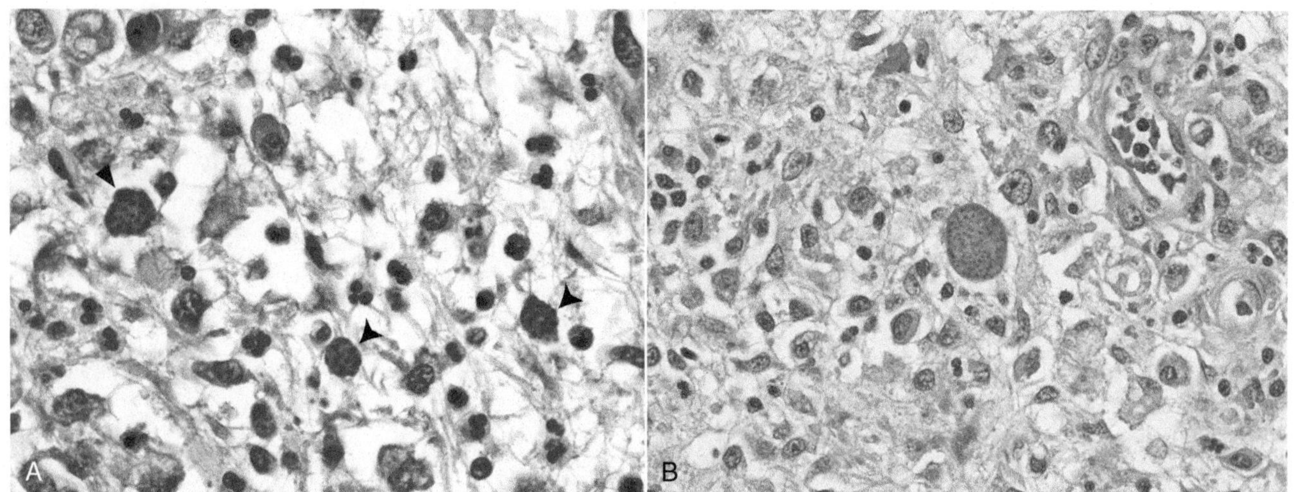

FIGURE 73-4 Histopathology of the cerebellum from a 6-year-old intact male Rhodesian ridgeback with neosporosis. **A,** Large areas of malacia were present admixed with a marked granulomatous inflammatory infiltrate and abundant protozoal cysts *(arrowheads)*. **B,** The protozoal cysts had a thick wall and stained positive with anti-*Neospora* antibodies (not shown). (Courtesy Dr. Robert Higgins, University of California, Davis Veterinary Anatomic Pathology Service.)

high serum titers (e.g., in the tens of thousands), but others have only low antibody titers. The latter situation might reflect the presence of underlying immunodeficiency and inability to produce antibodies. Because interassay variation may cause results to differ between laboratories,[42] the same laboratory should always be used when paired titers are performed or when titers are monitored over time.

Some weak serologic cross-reactivity may occur between the antigens of *T. gondii* and *N. caninum*, so low titers to *T. gondii* may be present in dogs infected with *N. caninum*. Cross-reactivity appears to be less common when IFA assays are used.[42] Serologic cross-reactivity can also occur to *N. hughesi*, again at a slightly lower titer,[43] but the extent to which this organism infects dogs is not clear.

Molecular Diagnosis Using the Polymerase Chain Reaction

Both conventional and real-time PCR assays have been developed for diagnosis of neosporosis.[44-46] Some are available for diagnosis on a commercial basis from veterinary diagnostic laboratories. Suitable specimens for testing include CSF, tissue biopsies (e.g., muscle), or tissues collected at necropsy. The sensitivity and specificity of these assays has the potential to vary considerably between laboratories, and more information is required on how these assays perform for antemortem diagnosis of clinical neosporosis in dogs. Because *N. caninum* DNA can be detected in tissues from healthy dogs, PCR results must always be interpreted in light of the clinicopathologic findings and serologic test results. In one study, *N. caninum* DNA was detected in the liver and/or spleen of one third of shelter dogs that had been euthanized, and PCR assay results did not always correlate with the results of serology.[44] PCR assays can be used to confirm that organisms seen in tissues or body fluids are truly *N. caninum* and not another protozoan parasite such as *Sarcocystis* or *T. gondii*.[23]

Pathologic Findings

Gross pathologic findings may be absent in dogs with neosporosis, or foci of discoloration may be present in the brain and spinal cord, and/or there may be evidence of meningitis (e.g., meningeal thickening or adherence of the meninges to the brain or cranial vault). White streaks within muscle may be found in affected puppies.[24] Histopathology in these puppies reveals polyradiculoneuritis with myelin loss and axonal degeneration, and there may be evidence of muscle fiber degeneration and fibrosis.

Examination of the brain and spinal cord of dogs with CNS involvement usually reveals multifocal nonsuppurative meningoencephalitis and/or myelitis with neuronal degeneration and necrosis, perivascular cuffing, and gliosis. Both gray and white matter can be affected, and the cerebellum may be primarily involved. A mixed inflammatory response with myonecrosis and sometimes dystrophic mineralization may be seen in affected skeletal or cardiac muscle. Bradyzoite cysts and/or tachyzoites may be evident (Figure 73-4). Bradyzoite cysts are up to 100 μm in diameter and have a wall that is 4 μm in diameter, which is thicker than that for *T. gondii*. Skin biopsies from dogs with dermal neosporosis contain tachyzoites and pyogranulomatous inflammation. Occasionally (such as in acute, fulminant infections in immunosuppressed dogs), tachyzoites are found in other tissues, including the peripheral nerves, the eye, reproductive tissues, adrenal glands, lung, liver, kidney, spleen, and esophageal muscle.[27] If intralesional protozoa are identified, immunohistochemistry and PCR assays can be used to distinguish *N. caninum* from other protozoal species.[40] Although serologic cross-reactivity between *N. caninum* and *T. gondii* is uncommon, it can occur with some antibodies, so immunohistochemistry is best performed with a panel of antibodies to each protozoan parasite.

In healthy dogs or dogs that die of other diseases, rare bradyzoite cysts in the absence of an inflammatory response may be found at necropsy in skeletal muscle and the CNS.

Treatment and Prognosis

The primary antimicrobial drug that has been used to treat neosporosis in dogs is clindamycin (Table 73-2). Treatment is usually only temporarily, partially, or completely ineffective, and long periods (>8 weeks) of treatment may be required.[18,19,39] Bradyzoite cysts persist despite treatment with clindamycin.[47] Treatment appears to be most effective for cutaneous neosporosis, although one dog developed neurologic signs when treatment was discontinued, such that reinstitution of long-term treatment was needed.[39] Other treatments that have been successful (or partially successful)

TABLE 73-2

Antimicrobials Used to Treat Neosporosis in Dogs

Drug	Dose (mg/kg)	Route	Interval (hours)	Duration (days)
Clindamycin	10-12 mg/kg	PO	q8h	At least 4 weeks
Trimethoprim-sulfa	15 mg/kg	PO	q12h	At least 4 weeks
Pyrimethamine	1 mg/kg	PO	q24h	At least 4 weeks
Ponazuril	20 mg/kg	PO	q24h	At least 4 weeks

are trimethoprim-sulfadiazine-pyrimethamine, combinations of clindamycin and trimethoprim-sulfadiazine, or combinations of clindamycin and pyrimethamine. The efficacy of ponazuril for treatment of canine neosporosis requires further study but shows promise based on studies in mice and cattle.[8] Treatment should be continued so long as clinical improvement is occurring. The prognosis for puppies once muscle contracture has developed is poor. It has been suggested that once neosporosis has been diagnosed in a puppy, all dogs in a litter should be treated, because the later treatment is initiated after the onset of clinical signs, the worse the prognosis.[48] At the minimum, puppies whose littermates have succumbed to neosporosis should have their serum antibody titer to *N. caninum* checked, and treatment should be considered for those with positive titers. The use of immunosuppressive drugs should be avoided in seropositive puppies.

A low dose of glucocorticoids (e.g., prednisone, 0.5 mg/kg PO q12h) in addition to antiprotozoals is often used to treat *N. caninum* meningoencephalomyelitis, but no prospective controlled trials have been performed to determine if this alters outcome. Very high doses of methylprednisolone acetate reactivate experimental *N. caninum* infections in dogs.[49] Physiotherapy may also be beneficial for young dogs with polyradiculoneuritis-myositis.

Immunity and Vaccination

Immunity to *N. caninum* is dependent on cell mediated immune responses. No vaccines for canine neosporosis exist.

Prevention

Neosporosis on farms can be prevented by not allowing dogs to access bovine placental materials, dead calves, or raw or undercooked meat and by preventing dogs from defecating around livestock. Predation should also be discouraged. The use of a muzzle for dogs that work on farms has been suggested to prevent *Neospora* abortions in cattle.[8] It may be necessary to stop the breeding of bitches that have puppies that develop neosporosis, and the owners of puppies that are diagnosed with neosporosis should be advised to inform the breeder of the diagnosis. No drugs are known to prevent transplacental transmission. Where possible, avoidance of excessive pharmacologic immunosuppression (e.g., with glucocorticoids, cyclosporine, azathioprine, or other immunosuppressive drugs) may help to prevent the disease in adult dogs. However, the relative rarity of reactivated neosporosis in adult dogs does not justify routine serologic screening of dogs for infection before commencing immunosuppressive drug treatment.

Public Health Aspects

Although antibodies to *N. caninum* have been detected in the serum of humans, the DNA of *N. caninum* has never been found in humans, and currently *N. caninum* is not thought to be a zoonotic risk.

CASE EXAMPLE

Signalment: "Lenny," a 6-year-old intact male Rhodesian ridgeback from coastal northern California

History: Lenny was evaluated on a referral basis for a 1-week history of an abnormal gait. The owner first noticed that Lenny was not paying attention during an obedience show. Over the next few days Lenny was observed to stumble on stairs, and he also fell from a bed. For the 3 days before evaluation the owner had noted that Lenny appeared uncoordinated and off balance. There had been no changes in his mentation and no evidence of inappetence, vomiting, diarrhea, or changes in thirst or urination. A soft, intermittent nonproductive cough had been noted since the onset of the other clinical signs. Bloodwork at a local veterinary clinic showed a normal CBC, increased activity of serum creatine kinase (2922 U/L, reference range [RR] 10-200 U/L), ALT (155 U/L, RR 5-60 U/L), and AST (135 U/L, RR 5-55 U/L). Serum thyroxine concentration was within the reference range. A urinalysis was unremarkable and aerobic bacterial urine culture was negative. Serology for antibodies to *Borrelia burgdorferi*, *Anaplasma* spp., *Ehrlichia canis*, and antigen of *Dirofilaria immitis* (4Dx SNAP test, IDEXX Laboratories) was negative. A *T. gondii* titer was pending. Lenny was treated with clindamycin (7.5 mg/kg PO q12h) and doxycycline (5 mg/kg PO q12h) with no signs of improvement.

Lenny had traveled extensively to Iowa, Colorado, and Kentucky but had no history of toxin exposure or trauma. He was fed a raw diet that consisted of turkey necks, chicken meat, lamb, and vegetables. He was up to date on routine vaccinations (distemper, adenovirus, parvovirus, and rabies) and on heartworm prophylaxis, but did not receive flea or tick prophylaxis and had been exposed to ticks in the past. He had been bred once and only one of three puppies survived. There was no other significant medical history.

Physical Examination:

Body Weight: 40.2 kg.

General: Bright and alert, hydrated. T = 100.5°F (38.1°C), HR = 80 beats/min, panting, mucous membranes pink and moist, CRT 1 s.

Musculoskeletal: Body condition score was 4/9. Truncal ataxia was present with a wide-based stance (see Neurologic Examination). There was no evidence of lameness or muscle atrophy.

All Other Systems: With the exception of the neurologic examination, no other clinically significant abnormalities were detected.

Neurologic Examination: The dog was alert and responsive. Truncal ataxia was present with hypermetria that was most pronounced on the left side. Head tremors were also noted. A slight left-sided head tilt was present, together with a decreased to absent menace response on the left side. There was normal physiologic nystagmus and no evidence of spontaneous nystagmus. Delayed placing reactions were detected in all four limbs but were most pronounced on the right side. Spinal reflexes were within normal limits. Neuroanatomic location: cerebellar/vestibular disease.

Laboratory Findings: Muscle biochemistry panel: AST 85 U/L (21-54 U/L), creatine kinase 1683 U/L (46-320 U/L).

Imaging Findings:

Thoracic Radiographs and Abdominal Ultrasound Examination: No abnormalities were detected.

Magnetic Resonance Imaging (Brain): On T2-weighted images, there was increased intensity of the vermis and left cerebellar hemisphere. The cerebellum appeared normal on T1-weighted images. Subtle regions of contrast enhancement were suspected in the left cerebellum on sagittal T1-weighted postcontrast images.

Other Testing: CSF analysis: Total nucleated cell count was 62 cells/μL (normal <2 cells/μL); total protein was 75 mg/dL (normal <25 mg/dL). There were 86% eosinophils, 8% small mononuclear cells, 5% large mononuclear cells, and 1% nondegenerate neutrophils. The large mononuclear cells were mostly of unremarkable morphology but occasionally had mildly increased cytoplasmic vacuolation. No infectious agents were seen.

Microbiologic Testing: Serologic testing (IFA): *Neospora caninum* serum antibody titer positive at 1:20,480; the CSF titer was 1:640.

Zinc sulfate fecal flotation: Negative for parasite ova.

Fecal Baermann examination: Negative for parasite larvae.

Treatment: Before the *Neospora* titers were available, a diagnosis of eosinophilic meningoencephalitis was made, and the dog was treated with prednisone (0.5 mg/kg PO q12h) but showed no clinical improvement over the subsequent 3 days. A second CSF specimen collected at that time had a cell count of 37 cells/μL and a total protein concentration of 59 mg/dL, with no change in the differential cell count. Lenny was discharged from the hospital, and once the *N. caninum* serology results became available (1 week later), treatment with trimethoprim-sulfamethoxazole (15 mg/kg PO q12h) and ponazuril (10 mg/kg, or 2.5 mL of 15% ponazuril paste PO q24h) was added. A baseline Schirmer tear test (performed to monitor for keratoconjunctivitis sicca secondary to sulfamethoxazole) was negative. At a recheck examination 3 weeks later, all neurologic signs were persistent but mildly improved. A CBC showed mild, nonregenerative anemia (34.9%) and mild bandemia (198 cells/μL). Serum CK activity was 88 U/L. CSF analysis showed a total protein concentration of 33 mg/dL and a TNCC of 2 cells/μL, with 0% eosinophils, 51% small mononuclear cells, and 49% mildly reactive large mononuclear cells. The serum and CSF antibody titers to *N. caninum* were both 1:5120. A Schirmer tear test was normal. Two weeks later, the trimethoprim-sulfamethoxazole was discontinued. Neurologic signs persisted but continued to show mild but slow improvement over the next 3 weeks. The ponazuril was discontinued, but after an additional 3 weeks, the head tremors worsened slightly. Blood work was unchanged, CSF analysis (cisternal and lumbar) was within normal limits, and serum and CSF *N. caninum* antibody titers were 1:1280 and 1:640, respectively. The prednisone was also discontinued. Two months later (4 months after initial diagnosis), severe ataxia and falling returned over a 2-week period. The owner declined reinstitution of antiprotozoal treatment and elected euthanasia. A complete necropsy revealed severe, locally extensive, necrotizing granulomatous encephalitis that was localized to the cerebellum. Abundant protozoal cysts were present within the cerebellar lesions, which were identified using immunohistochemical stains as *N. caninum*. Protozoa were not visualized in any other tissues.

Diagnosis: Granulomatous cerebellitis secondary to *N. caninum* infection.

Comments: Neosporosis in this dog resulted from cerebellar encephalitis, which illustrated the suggested predilection of *N. caninum* for the cerebellum. Development of encephalitis rather than polyradiculoneuritis-myositis is typical of neosporosis in adult dogs. It is possible this dog contracted neosporosis as a result of consumption of a raw food diet; tissue cysts have been identified in CNS tissues of a lamb,[50] and chickens are suspected as intermediate hosts based on seropositivity and positive PCR assay results on brain tissue.[51] The inflammatory response in the CSF was profoundly eosinophilic, as previously reported in other dogs with neosporosis. Fecal flotation was negative for *N. caninum* oocysts, which is expected given the life cycle of the parasite and the short shedding period with low numbers of oocysts shed. The fecal examinations were performed to evaluate for the possibility of visceral larva migrans, given the CSF eosinophilia. Although treatment with trimethoprim-sulfamethoxazole and then ponazuril led to resolution of CSF abnormalities, clinical signs showed only mild improvement. Treatment of neosporosis with glucocorticoids remains controversial, but attempts to reduce the prednisone dose were associated with worsening of clinical signs. Ultimately, all treatment was discontinued because of minimal improvement in clinical signs but resolution of laboratory abnormalities. Relapse subsequently ensued, and the diagnosis was confirmed at necropsy.

SUGGESTED READINGS

Dubey JP, Lappin MR. Toxoplasmosis and neosporosis. In: Greene CE, ed. Infectious Diseases of the Dog and Cat, 4th ed. St. Louis, MO: Elsevier Saunders; 2012.

Dubey JP, Schares G. Neosporosis in animals—the last five years. Vet Parasitol. 2011;180:90-108.

Garosi L, Dawson A, Couturier J, et al. Necrotizing cerebellitis and cerebellar atrophy caused by *Neospora caninum* infection: magnetic resonance imaging and clinicopathologic findings in seven dogs. J Vet Intern Med. 2010;24:571-578.

REFERENCES

1. Bjerkas I, Mohn SF, Presthus J. Unidentified cyst-forming sporozoon causing encephalomyelitis and myositis in dogs. Z Parasitenkd. 1984;70:271-274.
2. Pusterla N, Conrad PA, Packham AE, et al. Endogenous transplacental transmission of *Neospora hughesi* in naturally infected horses. J Parasitol. 2011;97:281-285.
3. Walsh CP, Duncan RB, Zajac AM, et al. *Neospora hughesi*: experimental infections in mice, gerbils, and dogs. Vet Parasitol. 2000;92:119-128.
4. Dubey JP, Schares G. Neosporosis in animals—the last five years. Vet Parasitol. 2011;180:90-108.
5. McCann CM, McAllister MM, Gondim LF, et al. *Neospora caninum* in cattle: experimental infection with oocysts can result in exogenous transplacental infection, but not endogenous transplacental infection in the subsequent pregnancy. Int J Parasitol. 2007;37:1631-1639.
6. Williams DJ, Hartley CS, Bjorkman C, et al. Endogenous and exogenous transplacental transmission of *Neospora caninum*—how the route of transmission impacts on epidemiology and control of disease. Parasitology. 2009;136:1895-1900.
7. Cavalcante GT, Monteiro RM, Soares RM, et al. Shedding of *Neospora caninum* oocysts by dogs fed different tissues from naturally infected cattle. Vet Parasitol. 2011;179:220-223.
8. Reichel MP, Ellis JT, Dubey JP. Neosporosis and hammondiosis in dogs. J Small Anim Pract. 2007;48:308-312.
9. Furuta PI, Mineo TW, Carrasco AO, et al. *Neospora caninum* infection in birds: experimental infections in chicken and embryonated eggs. Parasitology. 2007;134:1931-1939.
10. Bandini LA, Neto AF, Pena HF, et al. Experimental infection of dogs (*Canis familiaris*) with sporulated oocysts of *Neospora caninum*. Vet Parasitol. 2011;176:151-156.
11. McGarry JW, Stockton CM, Williams DJ, et al. Protracted shedding of oocysts of *Neospora caninum* by a naturally infected foxhound. J Parasitol. 2003;89:628-630.
12. Gondim LF, McAllister MM, Gao L. Effects of host maturity and prior exposure history on the production of *Neospora caninum* oocysts by dogs. Vet Parasitol. 2005;134:33-39.
13. Antony A, Williamson NB. Prevalence of antibodies to *Neospora caninum* in dogs of rural or urban origin in central New Zealand. N Z Vet J. 2003;51:232-237.
14. Basso W, Venturini L, Venturini MC, et al. Prevalence of *Neospora caninum* infection in dogs from beef-cattle farms, dairy farms, and from urban areas of Argentina. J Parasitol. 2001;87:906-907.
15. Sicupira PM, de Magalhaes VC, Galvao Gda S, et al. Factors associated with infection by *Neospora caninum* in dogs in Brazil. Vet Parasitol. 2012;185:305-308.
16. Bruhn FR, Figueiredo VC, Andrade Gda S, et al. Occurrence of anti-*Neospora caninum* antibodies in dogs in rural areas in Minas Gerais, Brazil. Rev Bras Parasitol Vet. 2012;21:161-164.
17. Dijkstra T, Barkema HW, Hesselink JW, et al. Point source exposure of cattle to *Neospora caninum* consistent with periods of common housing and feeding and related to the introduction of a dog. Vet Parasitol. 2002;105:89-98.
18. Barber JS, Trees AJ. Clinical aspects of 27 cases of neosporosis in dogs. Vet Rec. 1996;139:439-443.
19. Garosi L, Dawson A, Couturier J, et al. Necrotizing cerebellitis and cerebellar atrophy caused by *Neospora caninum* infection: magnetic resonance imaging and clinicopathologic findings in seven dogs. J Vet Intern Med. 2010;24:571-578.
20. Heckeroth AR, Tenter AM. Immunoanalysis of three litters born to a Doberman bitch infected with *Neospora caninum*. Parasitol Res. 2007;100:837-846.
21. Ordeix L, Lloret A, Fondevila D, et al. Cutaneous neosporosis during treatment of pemphigus foliaceus in a dog. J Am Anim Hosp Assoc. 2002;38:415-419.
22. Galgut BI, Janardhan KS, Grondin TM, et al. Detection of *Neospora caninum* tachyzoites in cerebrospinal fluid of a dog following prednisone and cyclosporine therapy. Vet Clin Pathol. 2010;39:386-390.
23. Fry DR, McSporran KD, Ellis JT, et al. Protozoal hepatitis associated with immunosuppressive therapy in a dog. J Vet Intern Med. 2009;23:366-368.
24. Cuddon P, Lin DS, Bowman DD, et al. *Neospora caninum* infection in English Springer Spaniel littermates. Diagnostic evaluation and organism isolation. J Vet Intern Med. 1992;6:325-332.
25. Ishigaki K, Noya M, Kagawa Y, et al. Detection of *Neospora caninum*-specific DNA from cerebrospinal fluid by polymerase chain reaction in a dog with confirmed neosporosis. J Vet Med Sci. 2012;74:1051-1055.
26. Hay WH, Shell LG, Lindsay DS, et al. Diagnosis and treatment of *Neospora caninum* infection in a dog. J Am Vet Med Assoc. 1990;197:87-89.
27. Barber JS, Payne-Johnson CE, Trees AJ. Distribution of *Neospora caninum* within the central nervous system and other tissues of six dogs with clinical neosporosis. J Small Anim Pract. 1996;37:568-574.
28. Mayhew PD, Bush WW, Glass EN. Trigeminal neuropathy in dogs: a retrospective study of 29 cases (1991-2000). J Am Anim Hosp Assoc. 2002:262-270.
29. Dubey JP, Koestner A, Piper RC. Repeated transplacental transmission of *Neospora caninum* in dogs. J Am Vet Med Assoc. 1990;197:857-860.
30. Pumarola M, Anor S, Ramis AJ, et al. *Neospora caninum* infection in a Napolitan mastiff dog from Spain. Vet Parasitol. 1996;64:315-317.
31. Meseck EK, Njaa BL, Haley NJ, et al. Use of a multiplex polymerase chain reaction to rapidly differentiate *Neospora caninum* from *Toxoplasma gondii* in an adult dog with necrotizing myocarditis and myocardial infarct. J Vet Diagn Invest. 2005;17:565-568.
32. Gaitero L, Anor S, Montoliu P, et al. Detection of *Neospora caninum* tachyzoites in canine cerebrospinal fluid. J Vet Intern Med. 2006;20:410-414.
33. Lorenzo V, Pumarola M, Siso S. Neosporosis with cerebellar involvement in an adult dog. J Small Anim Pract. 2002;43:76-79.
34. Holmberg TA, Vernau W, Melli AC, et al. *Neospora caninum* associated with septic peritonitis in an adult dog. Vet Clin Pathol. 2006;35:235-238.
35. Peters M, Wagner F, Schares G. Canine neosporosis: clinical and pathological findings and first isolation of *Neospora caninum* in Germany. Parasitol Res. 2000;86:1-7.
36. Ruehlmann D, Podell M, Oglesbee M, et al. Canine neosporosis: a case report and literature review. J Am Anim Hosp Assoc. 1995;31:174-183.
37. Boyd SP, Barr PA, Brooks HW, et al. Neosporosis in a young dog presenting with dermatitis and neuromuscular signs. J Small Anim Pract. 2005;46:85-88.
38. Poli A, Mancianti F, Carli MA, et al. *Neospora caninum* infection in a Bernese cattle dog from Italy. Vet Parasitol. 1998;78:79-85.
39. McInnes LM, Irwin P, Palmer DG, et al. In vitro isolation and characterisation of the first canine *Neospora caninum* isolate in Australia. Vet Parasitol. 2006;137:355-363.
40. Perl S, Harrus S, Satuchne C, et al. Cutaneous neosporosis in a dog in Israel. Vet Parasitol. 1998;79:257-261.
41. Greig B, Rossow KD, Collins JE, et al. *Neospora caninum* pneumonia in an adult dog. J Am Vet Med Assoc. 1995;206:1000-1001.

42. Silva DA, Lobato J, Mineo TW, et al. Evaluation of serological tests for the diagnosis of *Neospora caninum* infection in dogs: optimization of cut off titers and inhibition studies of cross-reactivity with *Toxoplasma gondii*. Vet Parasitol. 2007;143:234-244.
43. Gondim LF, Lindsay DS, McAllister MM. Canine and bovine *Neospora caninum* control sera examined for cross-reactivity using *Neospora caninum* and *Neospora hughesi* indirect fluorescent antibody tests. J Parasitol. 2009;95:86-88.
44. Ghalmi F, China B, Kaidi R, et al. Detection of *Neospora caninum* in dog organs using real time PCR systems. Vet Parasitol. 2008;155:161-167.
45. Langoni H, Matteucci G, Medici B, et al. Detection and molecular analysis of *Toxoplasma gondii* and *Neospora caninum* from dogs with neurological disorders. Rev Soc Bras Med Trop. 2012;45:365-368.
46. Schatzberg SJ, Haley NJ, Barr SC, et al. Use of a multiplex polymerase chain reaction assay in the antemortem diagnosis of toxoplasmosis and neosporosis in the central nervous system of cats and dogs. Am J Vet Res. 2003;64:1507-1513.
47. Dubey JP, Vianna MC, Kwok OC, et al. Neosporosis in Beagle dogs: clinical signs, diagnosis, treatment, isolation and genetic characterization of *Neospora caninum*. Vet Parasitol. 2007;149:158-166.
48. Dubey JP, Lappin MR. Toxoplasmosis and neosporosis. In: Greene CE, ed. Infectious Diseases of the Dog and Cat, 4th ed. St. Louis, MO: Elsevier Saunders; 2012.
49. Dubey JP, Lindsay DS. Neosporosis in dogs. Vet Parasitol. 1990;36:147-151.
50. Dubey JP, Hartley WJ, Lindsay DS, et al. Fatal congenital *Neospora caninum* infection in a lamb. J Parasitol. 1990;76:127-130.
51. Costa KS, Santos SL, Uzeda RS, et al. Chickens (*Gallus domesticus*) are natural intermediate hosts of *Neospora caninum*. Int J Parasitol. 2008;38:157-159.

CHAPTER 74

Leishmaniosis

Jane E. Sykes, Gad Baneth, and Christine A. Petersen

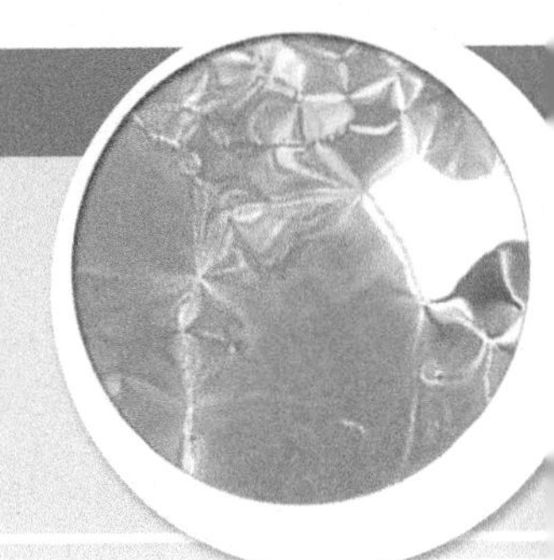

Overview of Leishmaniosis

First Described: The cause of visceral leishmaniosis was first described in India in 1903 (separately by William Leishman and Charles Donovan)[1]

Causes: Canine and feline visceral leishmaniosis is caused by *Leishmania infantum* (syn. *L. chagasi*) (phylum Euglenozoa, class Kinetoplasta, family Trypanosomatidae). Other species such as *L. braziliensis* cause localized cutaneous lesions in South America (American tegumentary leishmaniosis).

Affected Hosts: Dogs and less commonly cats; also humans, rodents, wild canids, and marsupial species

Geographic Distribution: Primarily southern Europe and the Middle East, central and South America; also some parts of the United States. Travel-related disease can occur in non-endemic regions worldwide.

Mode of Transmission: *Phlebotomus* and *Lutzomyia* sandflies. Transmission through blood transfusion as well as vertical transmission can occur.

Major Clinical Signs: Weight loss, inappetence, scaling and/or ulcerative cutaneous lesions, onychogryphosis, fever, keratoconjunctivitis, uveitis, lymphadenopathy, hepatosplenomegaly, pallor, lameness, signs of renal failure

Differential Diagnoses: Differential diagnoses in dogs with visceral disease include canine monocytic ehrlichiosis, babesiosis, histoplasmosis, brucellosis, hemic neoplasia, and primary autoimmune diseases such as systemic lupus erythematosus. Differential diagnoses for cutaneous lesions in dogs include demodectic or sarcoptic mange, pyoderma, *Malassezia* dermatitis, cutaneous vasculitis, and pemphigus foliaceus. Differential diagnoses for cutaneous lesions in cats include squamous cell carcinoma, cutaneous vasculitis, herpesviral dermatitis, and dermatophytosis. The primary differential for American tegumentary leishmaniasis is sporotrichosis.

Human Health Significance: Human infections are primarily transmitted by sandflies and involve a large number of different *Leishmania* species. Dogs are considered the major reservoir for *L. infantum* infections. Precautions should be taken when handling potentially infected tissue and blood specimens.

CANINE LEISHMANIOSIS

Etiology and Epidemiology

The leishmaniases are a group of zoonotic vector-borne diseases caused by various species of the protozoa *Leishmania,* which are primarily transmitted by sandflies. Around 30 species of *Leishmania* exist worldwide, and at least 20 species cause disease in humans, although the taxonomy of *Leishmania* spp. has been highly debated.[2,3] There are two subgenera of *Leishmania, Leishmania* and *Vianna,* which develop in the foregut or the hindgut/midgut of the sandfly vector, respectively. Human and animal disease due to *Leishmania* spp. is distributed across five continents (Africa, Asia, Europe, and the Americas) and nearly 100 countries (Figure 74-1). Disease syndromes in humans are divided into cutaneous leishmaniasis (CL), mucosal leishmaniasis (ML), and visceral leishmaniasis (VL). Disease syndromes in dogs are divided into visceral leishmaniosis and American tegumentary leishmaniosis, a localized cutaneous form that occurs in parts of South America. The term 'leishmaniosis' as opposed to 'leishmaniasis' is preferred to distinguish the disease in animals from that in humans.

Leishmania species are transmitted by female sandflies of the genus *Phlebotomus* in the Old World (Africa, Asia, and Europe) and *Lutzomyia* in the New World (i.e., the Americas). The regional prevalence of leishmaniasis, and the type of disease syndrome that develops, varies with the infecting *Leishmania* species present, sandfly species in the region, and host responses to infection. Some sandfly species transmit certain *Leishmania* species primarily to humans (anthroponotic leishmaniasis), whereas other sandfly species transmit *Leishmania* species to mammalian host species, such as dogs, cats, and rodents. Dogs and rodents are important reservoirs for *Leishmania* infection of humans (zoonotic leishmaniasis). Thus, the major mammalian reservoirs for the disease in a region depend on the *Leishmania* species and the sandfly species present.

The life cycle of *Leishmania* alternates between two major forms: the *promastigote* and the *amastigote* (Figure 74-2). The promastigote resides in the gut of the sandfly vector and is an elongated, flagellated form. Promastigotes are inoculated into tissues when the sandfly feeds, where they are phagocytized by macrophages in the dermis and transform into intracellular, nonmotile, ovoid, or round amastigotes. The amastigotes survive and replicate within macrophage phagolysosomes, and eventually the infected macrophages rupture. Released amastigotes then infect other macrophages that have been attracted to the site of infection. If the infected host fails to control the infection, amastigotes disseminate via regional lymphatics and the blood to infect the entire reticuloendothelial system. Intracellular amastigotes that are ingested by a female sandfly during

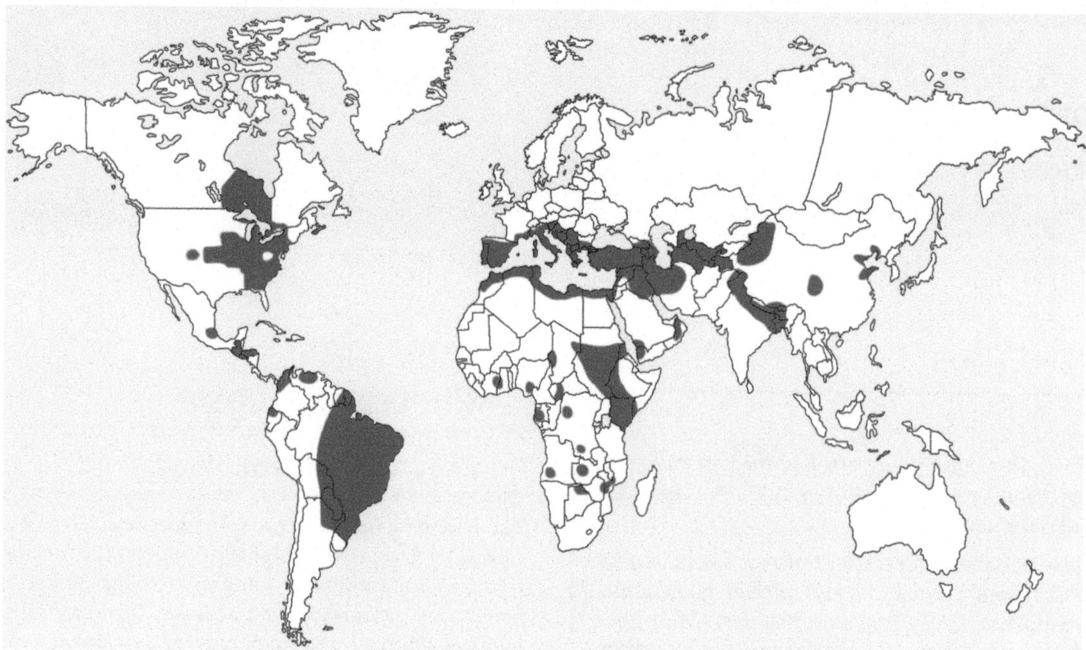

FIGURE 74-1 Geographic distribution of visceral leishmaniases in humans and dogs.

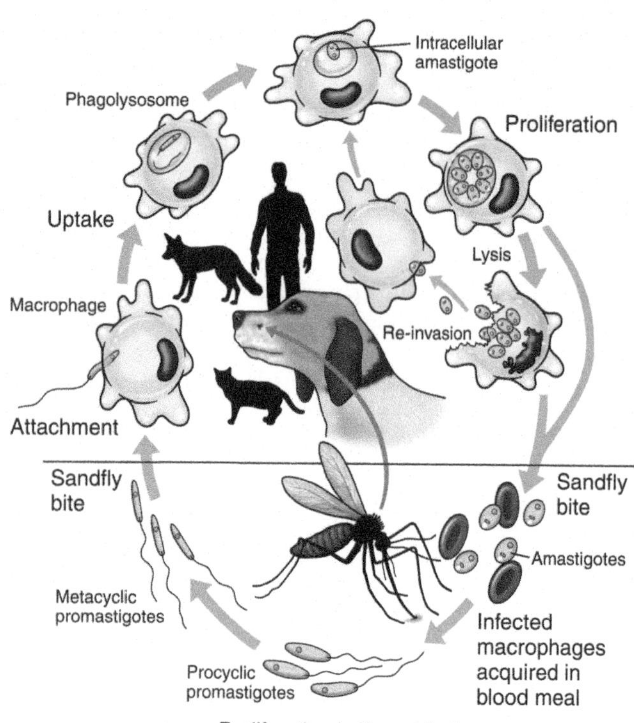

FIGURE 74-2 Life cycle of *Leishmania infantum*. Dogs, cats, and humans become infected when they are bitten by a sandfly. Promastigotes are inoculated into the dermis and penetrate macrophages. Within the macrophage, they transform into amastigotes and replicate within a phagolysosome. The macrophage ruptures and new macrophages are infected. If the host fails to control the infection in the skin, amastigotes disseminate via regional lymphatics and the blood to infect the entire reticuloendothelial system. Amastigotes that are ingested by a female sandfly during feeding convert back into promastigotes, and replication of promastigotes within the sandfly completes the life cycle.

feeding convert back into promastigotes over a period of about 1 week, and replication of promastigotes within the sandfly completes the life cycle. Sandflies breed in cracks in the walls of dwellings, rubble, and in rodent burrows, feed primarily at night, and fly a maximum of 2.5 km from their breeding sites. As a result, the prevalence of infection in dogs can vary considerably between adjacent regions. Lesser modes of transmission of *Leishmania* spp. include vertical transmission from bitches to puppies, venereal transmission, and blood transfusion.[4-7] These modes of transmission become more obvious in regions where suitable sandfly vectors do not exist. Aggressive interactions between dogs also have the potential to transmit infection, but this route has not been proven.

Canine visceral leishmaniosis in dogs and cats is caused by *Leishmania infantum* (also referred to as *Leishmania chagasi* in Central and South America). *L. infantum* is endemic in the Mediterranean basin, the Middle East, and Asia and may have been introduced to Latin America by early explorers and their domestic dogs.[8] Because leishmaniosis has a long incubation period and prolonged disease course, travel-related leishmaniosis in dogs and cats is diagnosed sporadically in regions where sandfly transmission does not occur, such as parts of Scandinavia, Switzerland, Japan, the United Kingdom, and the western United States (most often in dogs imported from southern Europe).[9-13] In highly endemic regions of the Mediterranean and Brazil, infection rates among dogs vary widely but may reach 80%.[14-17] At least 2.5 million dogs are infected in southwestern Europe alone.[14] The disease may be spreading northward in Europe, and has recently appeared in nontraveled dogs in countries such as Germany and Hungary.[5,18,19] Spread of *Leishmania* spp. into new areas can occur when humans bring infected dogs into regions where competent insect vectors exist, or when sandfly populations expand as a result of factors such as climate change.

Risk factors for infection in dogs include age at least 2 years, prolonged exposure to the outdoors, lack of topical insecticide use, and, in some studies, a short haircoat.[20-23] Some authors have described a bimodal age distribution that peaks at 3 years and at greater than 8 years of age.[24] Sex is not an important risk factor for infection. Factors that promote proliferation of sandfly populations, such as poor sanitation and limited garbage collection, as well as the occurrence of stray dogs around homes, also put dogs at risk of infection.[25] In Europe, German shepherd dogs, boxers, Rottweilers, cocker spaniels, and Dobermans may be at increased risk for leishmaniosis; the Ibizan hound in Spain appears to be resistant to clinical disease.[24,26-29] Concurrent diseases are common in dogs with leishmaniosis in endemic regions and include transmissible venereal tumor,[30] demodicosis,[31] sarcoptic mange,[32] and a variety of other vector-borne diseases such as canine monocytic ehrlichiosis, babesiosis, hepatozoonosis, and dirofilariasis.[32-36] Concurrent lymphoma has also been described.[32]

Uncommonly, dogs worldwide are infected by other species of *Leishmania*, which include *Leishmania donovani, Leishmania tropica, Leishmania braziliensis, Leishmania peruviana, Leishmania mexicana, Leishmania panamensis, Leishmania guyanensis, Leishmania amazonensis,* and other as-yet-uncharacterized species.[37-45] *L. braziliensis, L. guyanensis,* and *L. panamensis* have been isolated from dogs with American tegumentary leishmaniosis. Outbreaks of American tegumentary leishmaniosis have occurred in humans and dogs.[43]

Canine Leishmaniosis in North America

Most sporadic cases of visceral leishmaniosis in dogs in North America are diagnosed in dogs with a travel history to other continents. Infected dogs continue to be introduced every year as a result of travel from endemic regions in Europe and Latin America. In addition, over the past 30 years, visceral disease has been described in dogs in the United States that have had no apparent travel history. These have included a basenji dog from a kennel in Texas and dogs of foxhound breed from Ohio, Oklahoma, and Colorado.[46-49] Involvement of multiple dogs in a foxhound kennel was reported in Oklahoma,[47] and outbreaks in foxhounds have also been described in New York, Alabama, and Michigan.[50] Spread to other dogs has occurred as a result of transplacental transmission and, in rare cases, transfusion of infected blood.[4,6] A competent arthropod vector for *Leishmania* spp. has not yet been identified in the United States, and infection has not been detected in surveys of non-foxhound dogs in the United States.[51]

Clinical Features

Signs and Their Pathogenesis

The outcome of *Leishmania* spp. infection is variable. Some dogs completely eliminate the infection, and a small percentage of dogs develop severe, life-threatening disease. Some dogs remain persistently but subclinically infected, with the possibility of reactivation later in life with immunosuppression; these dogs also act as reservoir hosts and can infect sandflies.[52] In general, dogs that mount strong T-cell–mediated immune responses eliminate the infection, whereas those that mount weak cell-mediated immune responses and marked, nonprotective humoral (IgG) immune responses develop clinical disease.[53] Host genetic factors are important in determining progression to clinical disease, and several candidate genes have been identified in dogs that may influence susceptibility.[28,54-56] When clinical disease appears, it occurs after a long incubation period (up to 7 years) and varies from mild papular or exfoliative dermatitis to severe disseminated disease due to massive proliferation of histiocytes, B lymphocytes, and plasma cells in reticuloendothelial tissues and immune-mediated consequences of chronic, persistent infection.

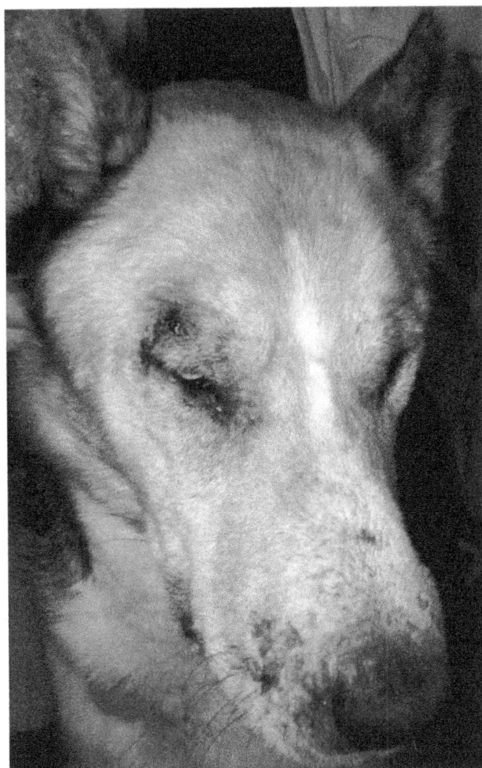

FIGURE 74-3 Periocular alopecia and crusting in an 8-year-old male neutered husky mix with visceral leishmaniosis. The dog was evaluated in northern California but had a travel history to Spain. Lesions are also present on the muzzle and the pinnae.

Cutaneous lesions most commonly manifest as alopecia, scaling, and/or ulceration but can be nodular or papular (Figure 74-3). They are often noticed before signs of systemic infection develop, despite the fact that they occur as a consequence of parasite dissemination. Many dogs also develop onychogryphosis (abnormally long or brittle claws).

Systemic signs of visceral leishmaniosis include fever, weight loss, muscle atrophy, inappetence, and lethargy; oral ulceration; progressive splenomegaly and lymphadenomegaly; mucosal pallor due to anemia; and rarely, hepatomegaly (Table 74-1). Development of autoantibodies and circulating immune complexes is thought to lead to immune-mediated thrombocytopenia and/or thrombocytopathia and signs such as epistaxis or melena, lameness and joint swelling due to immune-mediated polyarthritis, myositis, uveitis, vasculitis, and glomerulonephritis.[57-62] Positive antinuclear antibody tests are found in up to 50% of dogs tested.[32,61,63] Many dogs also have positive Coombs' tests.[32,63]

Glomerular injury ultimately culminates in nephrotic syndrome and/or failure of tubular function for many dogs, with polyuria and polydipsia, vomiting, diarrhea, and dehydration. Renal failure may occur in the absence of other lesions.[32] Anemia may be due to a combination of factors that include blood loss, inflammation, renal failure, immune-mediated destruction, and marrow aplasia or hypoplasia. In addition to uveitis, other ocular lesions include blepharitis, conjunctivitis, panophthalmitis, and keratoconjunctivitis. Keratoconjunctivitis results from direct infection of the lacrimal gland by *Leishmania*.[64]

Atypical presentations of canine visceral leishmaniosis have also been reported. Almost any organ can be affected, with reports of *Leishmania* prostatitis and infertility[65]; nodular lesions

TABLE 74-1

Clinical Signs in Dogs with Visceral Leishmaniosis

Clinical Sign	Prevalence (%)
Lymphadenomegaly	65-90
Cutaneous lesions	51-89
Weight loss	25-64
Lethargy	11-60
Pallor	58
Splenomegaly	10-53
Polydipsia	4-40
Abnormal locomotion or polyarthritis	3-38
Pyrexia	4-36
Onychodystrophy	20-31
Diarrhea	30
Vomiting	26
Ocular lesions (keratoconjunctivitis, uveitis, panophthalmitis, blepharitis)	7-24
Inappetence	17
Polyphagia	15
Epistaxis	6-15
Melena	13

Data from Ciaramella P, Oliva G, Luna RD, et al. A retrospective clinical study of canine leishmaniasis in 150 dogs naturally infected by *Leishmania infantum*. Vet Rec 1997;141:539-543; Slappendel RJ. Canine leishmaniasis. A review based on 95 cases in The Netherlands. Vet Q 1988;10:1-16; Koutinas AF, Carlotti DN, Koutinas C, et al. Claw histopathology and parasitic load in natural cases of canine leishmaniosis associated with *Leishmania infantum*. Vet Dermatol 2010;21:572-577.

of the tongue and other mucosal surfaces[66,67]; pancreatitis[68]; gastrointestinal tract, myocardial, or pulmonary involvement[69-71]; osteomyelitis[72,73]; meningitis[74]; and granuloma formation within the spinal cord.[75]

American Tegumentary Leishmaniosis

American tegumentary leishmaniosis in dogs is characterized by development of a nodular skin lesion at the site of a sandfly bite that enlarges and eventually may ulcerate. Lesions most often occur on regions of the body that have less hair, such as the nose, perineal region, scrotum, and pinnae.[43,76]

Physical Examination Findings

Physical examination findings in dogs with visceral disease include lethargy, muscle atrophy or cachexia, variable and typically low-grade fever, focal or generalized peripheral lymphadenomegaly, and hepatosplenomegaly on abdominal palpation (Figure 74-4). Lymphadenomegaly can be severe and be suggestive of lymphoma. Although not always detected, skin lesions consist of scaling and crusting, hyperkeratosis, alopecia, erythema, and cutaneous ulceration and may be nonpruritic or pruritic. They most often occur on the limbs, pinnae, muzzle, and periocular regions. Mucocutaneous lesions can also occur. Ocular involvement may be associated with mucopurulent ocular discharge, blepharitis, and anterior uveitis.

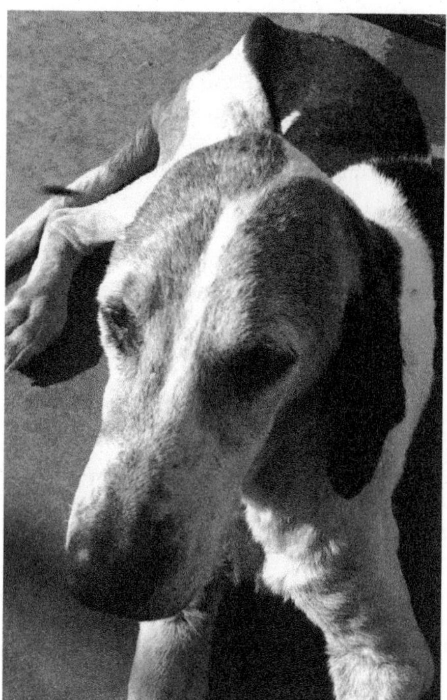

FIGURE 74-4 Poor body condition of 8-year-old male intact foxhound that was seropositive and PCR positive for *Leishmania infantum*. (Courtesy Dr. Christine Petersen, Iowa State University.)

Onychogryphosis may be present. Lameness or reluctance to move may be associated with joint swelling, crepitus, and pain.[72] Epistaxis may also be noted.

Diagnosis

Diagnosis of leishmaniosis may be straightforward, such as when organisms are seen cytologically in impression smears of typical skin lesions, or it may require assessment of the results of a combination of diagnostic assays in light of clinicopathologic findings (Table 74-2). Specific diagnostic assays include cytologic or histopathologic examination of affected tissues, serology, culture of the organism, or the results of PCR assays on affected tissues or blood. In endemic areas, diagnosis may be challenging (1) because dogs may be infected with the parasite for long periods of time in the absence of clinical signs, so the significance of positive test results may be unclear, and (2) because co-infections with other vector-borne pathogens may complicate the clinical picture and cause signs that resemble those of leishmaniosis.

Laboratory Abnormalities

Complete Blood Count

The most common CBC abnormality in dogs with leishmaniosis is a mild to moderate, normocytic, normochromic, nonregenerative anemia. Mild thrombocytopenia is present in up to 50% of affected dogs.[32,63,77] Total leukocyte, neutrophil, lymphocyte, monocyte, and eosinophil counts may be decreased, within the reference range, or increased. Pancytopenia may be present. Although most dogs are lymphopenic, some have moderate to severe lymphocytosis.[77]

Serum Biochemical Tests

Changes on serum biochemistry analysis in dogs with leishmaniosis include hyperglobulinemia, hypoalbuminemia, and

TABLE 74-2

Diagnostic Assays Currently Available for Leishmaniosis in Dogs and Cats

Assay	Specimen Type	Target	Performance
Cytologic examination	Aspirates of lymph nodes, spleen, or bone marrow; impression smears of skin lesions; rarely blood smears or buffy-coat preparations	*Leishmania infantum* amastigotes within mononuclear phagocytes	In the absence of experience, organisms may be confused with fungi such as *Histoplasma capsulatum* or *Sporothrix schenckii*. Organisms may be few in number and in some cases are absent.
Leishmania culture	Aspirates or biopsies of affected tissues	*L. infantum*	Sensitive and specific but requires special techniques and expertise that are not widely available.
Antibody serology (IFA or ELISA)	Serum	Antibodies to *L. infantum*	Most infected dogs test positive (sensitivity > 90%), but positive test results occur in healthy animals, so results must be interpreted in light of clinical signs. Sensitivity may be lower in cats. False positives can occur in dogs exposed to *Trypanosoma* spp. (IFA) and dogs vaccinated with *Leishmania* vaccines.
Real-time PCR assays	Conjunctival swabs, aspirates of affected tissues, lymph node, bone marrow, whole blood, skin biopsies	*L. infantum* DNA	May be useful in dogs with suggestive lesions in which organisms cannot be found cytologically. Sensitivity and specificity depends on assay design. Quantitative PCR may be useful for evaluation of treatment efficacy.
Histopathology	Biopsy specimens from affected tissues (e.g., skin lesions)	*L. infantum* amastigotes	Use of immunohistochemistry may increase sensitivity and can be used to confirm the presence of *Leishmania* spp. in tissues.

IFA, Immunofluorescent antibody.

mild to moderate azotemia.[32,63,77] Hyperglobulinemia and hypoalbuminemia are present in more than 75% of affected dogs. Serum globulin concentration ranges from mild to severe (up to 8 g/dL) and reflects a polyclonal gammopathy; monoclonal gammopathy is rare.[78] Azotemia has been reported in 16% to 38% of dogs. Some studies have shown mild to moderate increases in liver enzyme activities.

Urinalysis

Dogs with leishmaniosis may have proteinuria or isosthenuria, secondary to glomerular and tubulointerstitial renal function impairment, respectively. Cylindruria may be detected.

Synovial Fluid Examination

Cytologic examination of synovial fluid from dogs with *Leishmania* polyarthritis reveals increased numbers of neutrophils and/or lymphocytes.[72] In some cases, *Leishmania* amastigotes are visible within macrophages in the synovial fluid.

Bone Marrow Examination

Bone marrow cytologic alterations described in canine leishmaniosis include erythrophagocytosis, erythroid hypoplasia and dysplasia, eosinophilic hypoplasia, granulocytic hyperplasia, and increased numbers of lymphocytes and plasma cells.[79,80] Amastigotes may also be visible.

Diagnostic Imaging

Abdominal radiography or ultrasonography in dogs or cats with visceral leishmaniosis can reveal abdominal lymphadenomegaly, splenomegaly, and hepatomegaly. Radiographic lesions of long bones in dogs with bone involvement consist of soft periosteal proliferation, increased or decreased intramedullary opacity, and/or cortical and medullary destruction.[63,72] Lesions tend to be bilateral and symmetrical. Joint radiographs in dogs with signs of arthritis may reveal erosive changes, or arthritis may be non-erosive.

Microbiologic Tests

Cytologic Examination

Identification of *Leishmania* spp. amastigotes in lesions with cytology is diagnostic for leishmaniosis (Figure 74-5). Organism densities are particularly high in skin lesions, bone marrow, and the spleen, but specimens collected from other tissues, such as lymph node and hepatic aspirates, may also contain organisms. Organisms are not found in some lesions, and inexperienced microscopists may fail to identify organisms when present or confuse them with other parasites, such as *Trypanosoma,*

Histoplasma, or *Sporothrix schenckii*. Rarely, organisms are seen in circulating white blood cells.[81]

Serologic Diagnosis

Serologic assays based on immunofluorescent antibody (IFA), ELISA, Western immunoblot, and agglutination techniques have all been used for serodiagnosis of canine leishmaniosis, or for screening apparently healthy dogs in endemic areas for evidence of infection. IFA is commonly used by veterinary practitioners in Europe[82] and has a diagnostic sensitivity that ranges from 90% to 100% and a specificity of 80% to 100% in dogs that have not received a *Leishmania* vaccine. Dogs with *Trypanosoma* spp. infections may have false-positive test results due to serologic cross-reactivity between *Trypanosoma* and *Leishmania* antigens. ELISA assays based on recombinant antigens often have higher specificity and are technically less difficult to perform than IFA.[42,83] A rapid lateral flow assay is available commercially (SNAP Canine *Leishmania* Antibody Test Kit, IDEXX Laboratories) that had an overall sensitivity of 95% and a specificity of 91% in one study of 400 dogs from Brazil.[83] Other immunochromatographic assays are available that vary in their sensitivity.

Negative serologic test results may reflect delayed seroconversion in some animals, which can take several months to occur. However, many dogs with clinical signs have already seroconverted because of the long incubation period. Importantly, in endemic areas, positive serologic test results do not imply that disease is due to *Leishmania* spp. infection, because subclinical infections are widespread. Thus, for diagnosis of clinical leishmaniosis, results must be interpreted in conjunction with clinical findings and cytologic and histopathologic evaluation of affected tissues. Because seroconversion occurs in dogs that have received the *Leishmania* vaccine, current serologic assays cannot be used to efficiently differentiate between infected and vaccinated animals.[84]

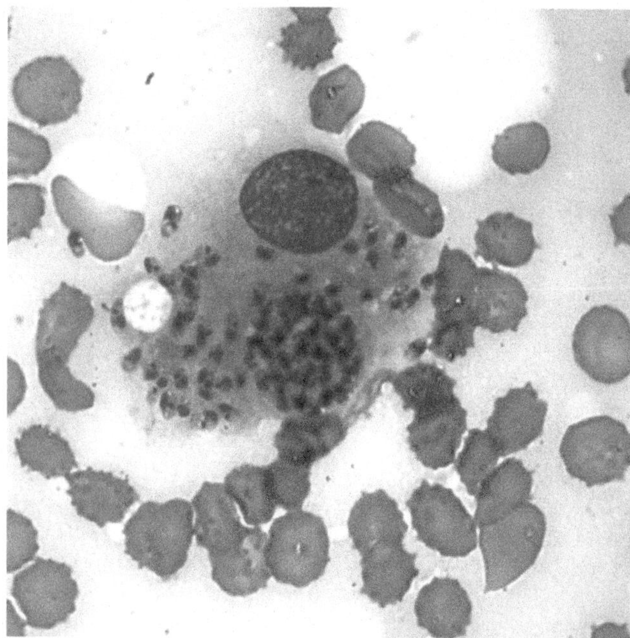

FIGURE 74-5 Bone marrow aspirate cytology findings in a dog with visceral leishmaniosis. Numerous *Leishmania* amastigotes can be seen within a histiocyte. (Courtesy Dr. Sheri Ross, University of California, Davis – San Diego.)

Molecular Diagnosis Using the Polymerase Chain Reaction

Several different conventional and real-time PCR assays have been developed and evaluated for detection of *Leishmania* spp. in dogs and cats. Real-time PCR assays that detect *Leishmania* spp. are now offered on a commercial basis by some veterinary diagnostic laboratories worldwide. Suitable specimens for testing include splenic, hepatic, lymph node, or bone marrow aspirates; whole blood; skin biopsies; conjunctival swabs; and even oral swabs. Conjunctival swabs; aspirates of spleen, bone marrow, or lymph nodes; and skin biopsies are most likely to yield positive results.[85,86] Positive PCR assay results in endemic areas do not confirm that disease is caused by *Leishmania* spp., because dogs without clinical signs can test positive.[87] However, in one study, clinical disease subsequently appeared in 71% of ELISA-positive dogs that lacked clinical signs but had medium to high parasite loads (more than 10 parasites/mL of blood) as determined with a quantitative PCR assay.[86] PCR assays may also be useful in order to monitor the efficacy of treatment.

Culture

Leishmania spp. can be isolated in culture from specimens such as lymph nodes, skin biopsies, spleen, or bone marrow, although special media and expertise are required, and incubation times of up to 30 days may be needed.

Pathologic Findings

Gross Pathologic Findings

Gross pathologic findings in dogs with visceral leishmaniosis include cachexia; generalized enlargement of the spleen, lymph nodes, and sometimes the liver; focal pale nodular lesions in a variety of organs; bone and joint lesions; and gastrointestinal ulcerations.

Histopathologic Findings

Histopathology of most affected tissues in dogs with leishmaniosis typically reveals granulomatous to pyogranulomatous and lymphoplasmacytic inflammation, with variable numbers of intrahistiocytic amastigotes (Figure 74-6). Skin lesions are accompanied by orthokeratotic to parakeratotic

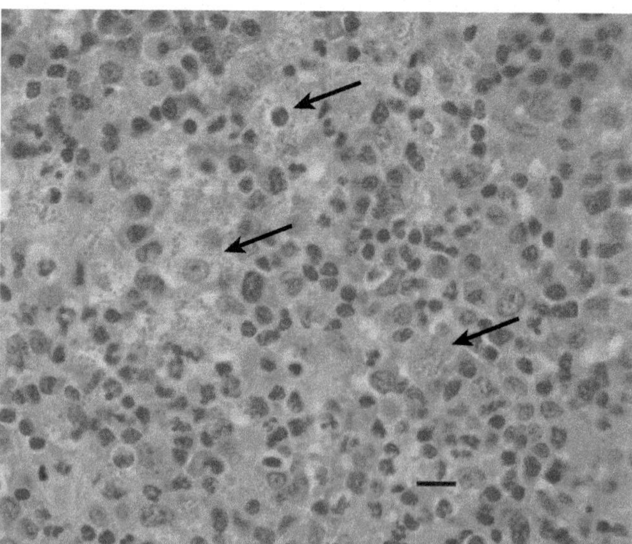

FIGURE 74-6 Histopathology of the spleen in a dog with visceral leishmaniosis. Multiple amastigotes (which have a granular appearance, *arrows*) are present within macrophages. H&E stain; bar = 20 μm. (Courtesy Dr. Christine Petersen, Iowa State University.)

hyperkeratosis, acanthosis, and ulceration. Claw histopathology in dogs with onychogryphosis reveals lichenoid mononuclear cell infiltration, with or without basal keratinocyte vacuolation and dermo-epidermal clefting; organisms are generally not visible.[88] Renal lesions consist of membranoproliferative glomerulonephritis, lymphoplasmacytic tubulointerstitial nephritis, and rarely amyloidosis (Figure 74-7).[46,89-91] Immunohistochemistry can be used to unambiguously detect *Leishmania* amastigotes in tissue sections. Immunohistochemistry may permit detection of *Leishmania* spp. when organisms are not seen with routine histopathology.[70,92] In situ hybridization has also been used to identify *Leishmania* amastigotes in paraffin-embedded specimens.[92]

Treatment and Prognosis

Antiprotozoal Therapy

Drugs with activity against *Leishmania* spp. include the pentavalent antimonials meglumine antimoniate (Glucantime) and sodium stibogluconate; allopurinol; amphotericin B; and miltefosine (Table 74-3). Ketoconazole has also been used. Unfortunately, regardless of the treatment used, complete parasitologic cure is rare, and relapses are frequent.[93,94] In endemic areas, reinfections occur and contribute to apparent treatment failures. Staging systems and consensus treatment guidelines have been published (Table 74-4).[29,95]

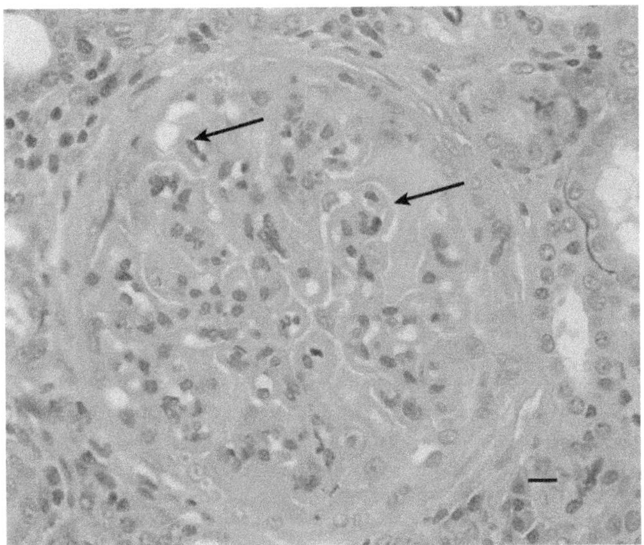

FIGURE 74-7 Histopathology of the kidney in a dog with visceral leishmaniosis. There is marked thickening of glomerular capillary loops *(arrows)* indicative of glomerulonephritis. H&E stain. Bar = 50 μm. (Courtesy Dr. Christine Petersen, Iowa State University.)

Pentavalent antimonials are thought to inhibit protozoal enzymes and damage protozoal DNA, whereas allopurinol interferes with protein synthesis by *Leishmania* spp. (see Chapter 10 for more information on these drugs). In general, a combination of meglumine antimoniate (100 mg/kg SC q24h for 4 weeks) and allopurinol (10 mg/kg PO q12h until clinical signs have resolved and quantitative serology becomes negative) is the treatment of choice for dogs with leishmaniosis.[96] Clinical improvement generally occurs within 1 to 2 months of treatment initiation if no overt renal disease is present. Complete or near-complete clinical remission rates of 65% to 100% have been reported with combination therapy, with relapse rates of around 10%.[93,97] Dogs that relapse can be retreated with one or more cycles of meglumine. Relapses can occur years after treatment is initiated, even in the face of allopurinol treatment. Rarely, xanthine urolithiasis complicates long-term allopurinol treatment.[97] A liposomal form of meglumine antimoniate (LMA) (6.5 mg/kg of stibogluconate every 4 days), when used together with allopurinol (20 mg/kg PO q24h) and administered for 140 days, significantly reduced clinical signs and parasite load and blocked transmission of the parasite to sandflies, but was associated with apparent cure in only 50% of treated dogs.[98] Unfortunately, resistance to antimonials has emerged among some *Leishmania* isolates in highly endemic areas such as southern Europe. Antimonials are also not readily available for treatment of dogs in the United States.

Miltefosine activates proteases in *Leishmania* spp. and causes apoptotic death of the parasite (see Chapter 10). Miltefosine can be used as an alternative to meglumine antimoniate in conjunction with allopurinol for 1 month, after which monotherapy with allopurinol is continued.[99] Unfortunately this combination protocol does not result in parasitologic cure, and relapse is common. Even a second cycle of miltefosine treatment failed to eliminate the parasite in one study.[99]

TABLE 74-3

Suggested Drug Doses for Treatment of Canine Visceral Leishmaniosis

Drug	Dose (mg/kg)	Route	Interval (hours)	Duration and Comments
Allopurinol	10	PO	12	At least 6 to 12 months or until both clinical signs disappear and quantitative serology becomes negative
Meglumine antimoniate	75-100 50	SC	24 12	30 days. Use with allopurinol. Meglumine antimoniate is the first-line treatment where available.
Miltefosine	2	PO	24	28 days. Use with allopurinol where miltefosine is available.
Lipid-complexed amphotericin B	3	IV	Every 48 hours on Monday, Wednesday, and Friday	Dilute to 1 mg/mL in D5W and administer over 1 to 2 hours until a cumulative dose of 21 mg/kg is reached. Monitor kidney values (see Chapter 9). Optimal dosing schedule for dogs is unknown.

TABLE 74-4

Clinical Staging of Canine Visceral Leishmaniosis Based on Serologic Status, Clinical Signs, Laboratory Findings, Type of Treatment, and Prognosis for Each Stage

Clinical Stage	Antibody Titer	Clinical Signs	Laboratory Findings	Therapy	Prognosis
Stage I	Negative or low positive (<3- to 4-fold increase above the laboratory cutoff)	Mild signs such as peripheral lymphadenopathy or papular dermatitis	Usually none, creatinine <1.4 mg/dL, UPC <0.5	None, allopurinol monotherapy, or combination therapy	Good
Stage II	Positive (low or high)	Diffuse or symmetrical cutaneous lesions, ulcerations, anorexia, weight loss, fever, and/or epistaxis	Anemia, hyperglobulinemia, and/or hypoalbuminemia present. Substage a: nonazotemic, nonproteinuric Substage b: nonazotemic, UPC 0.5-1	Combination therapy	Good to guarded
Stage III	Medium to high	Stage II abnormalities plus signs of immune-complex disease (vasculitis, arthritis, glomerulonephritis)	Stage II abnormalities plus IRIS* stage I with UPC >1, or IRIS stage II	Combination therapy	Guarded to poor
Stage IV	Medium to high	Stage III abnormalities plus nephrotic syndrome, pulmonary thromboembolism, or end-stage renal disease	Stage II abnormalities plus IRIS stage III or IV; marked proteinuria (UPC >5)	Consider monotherapy with allopurinol. Follow IRIS guidelines for treatment of chronic kidney disease.	Poor

Data from Solano-Gallego L, Koutinas A, Miro G, et al. Directions for the diagnosis, clinical staging, treatment and prevention of canine leishmaniosis. Vet Parasitol 2009;165:1-18.

*International Renal Interest Society, http://www.iris-kidney.com/guidelines/en

Lipid-complexed amphotericin B is the treatment of choice for human visceral leishmaniasis. Limited reports of the use of both deoxycholate and lipid-complexed forms of amphotericin B to treat dogs with leishmaniosis exist.[100,101] The need for intravenous administration of amphotericin B and its nephrotoxicity has limited its use for treatment of disease in dogs. In one study, use of liposomal amphotericin B (Ambisome) to treat canine leishmaniosis was associated with rapid resolution of clinical signs, but cytologic evidence of parasites persisted in lymph node aspirates.[100] However, treatment was administered for less than 2 weeks (and for some groups of dogs in the study, only 3 days). The FDA-approved regimen for liposomal amphotericin B treatment of immunocompetent human patients consists of seven infusions over 21 days (days 1 through 5, 10, and 21), for a total dose of 21 mg/kg.[102]

Because of the likelihood of relapse in dogs after treatment, the World Health Organization does not advocate treatment of pet dogs with anti-*Leishmania* chemotherapy protocols used to treat humans and instead suggests monotherapy with allopurinol.[103]

Supportive Care

Dogs with renal failure secondary to *Leishmania* infection may require supplemental fluid therapy and medications that address complications of uremia and/or protein-losing nephropathy, such as antacids, antiemetics, phosphate binders, low-protein diets, and antihypertensive drugs.

Immunity and Vaccination

Although immunity to leishmaniosis is complex and not well understood, it is clear that it is strongly dependent on the development of a robust Th1-cell–mediated immune response. Production of cytokines such as IFN-γ and TNF-α activates macrophages to destroy amastigotes, which occurs through nitric oxide–mediated mechanisms. Dogs that resist leishmaniosis exhibit strong delayed type hypersensitivity responses to leishmanial antigen when it is administered intradermally. A balance between Th1 and Th2 immune responses appears to be important in determining the clinical outcome of infection.

Several vaccines against leishmaniosis have been evaluated in dogs under field conditions. One of these vaccines, Leishmune, became licensed for prevention of leishmaniasis in dogs in Brazil in 2011.[53] Leishmune is composed of a promastigote antigen (fucose-mannose ligand) and the adjuvant saponin.[104,105] The vaccine has not been approved in Europe because of adverse effects induced by the saponin adjuvant. Efficacy in initial field trials was approximately 80% and has correlated with a reduction in human leishmaniasis in the area.[53] The vaccine is also licensed in Brazil for immunotherapy, and reduces clinical signs in infected dogs,[106] but when used without antiprotozoal drugs did not reduce 4.5-year mortality when compared with infected control dogs.[107] Another vaccine (CaniLeish, Virbac) composed of purified excreted-secreted proteins of *Leishmania infantum* (LiESP) is licensed in Europe for prevention of canine leishmaniosis. This vaccine stimulates a Th1-dominated anti–*L. infantum* response within 3 weeks of administration.[108]

Prevention

In addition to vaccination, use of ectoparasiticides such as deltamethrin-impregnated dog collars or spot-on repellants that contain permethrin can prevent canine leishmaniosis.[111-114] Indoor housing or use of fine-mesh netting around dogs and humans when sandflies feed at night (from dusk to dawn) is also recommended. Because of transplacental transmission, neutering may also reduce the spread of *Leishmania*.[6] Potential blood donors should be screened with serology and PCR assays and should only be used if both assays are negative.[29]

A dopamine-based oral suspension Leisguard is available in some parts of Europe for prevention of leishmaniosis in dogs that travel to regions where the disease is endemic. This contains the dopamine D2 receptor antagonist domperidone, which activates phagocytic cells and enhances intracellular killing of the parasite.[109] A prospective, randomized controlled trial showed that Leisguard prevented transmission of leishmaniosis to naïve dogs in a kennel.[115] The drug was administered q24h for two 30-day periods at the estimated beginning and end of the vector activity period. Leisguard may also hasten recovery when used for treatment of affected dogs in combination with meglumine antimoniate and allopurinol,[110] but additional studies are required.

Public Health Aspects

An estimated 12 million people worldwide have leishmaniasis, and at least 350 million people are estimated to be at risk. Approximately 0.2 to 0.4 million new cases of VL and 0.7 to 1.2 million cases of CL are believed to occur in humans annually, and it has been estimated that 20,000 to 40,000 leishmaniasis deaths occur per year.[116]

VL in humans is also known as kala-azar. It is caused mostly by *L. donovani* and *L. infantum* (referred to as *L. chagasi* in Central and South America), but also by *L. tropica*. More than 90% of VL cases globally occur in India, Bangladesh, Sudan, South Sudan, Brazil, and Ethiopia. Many cases are due to *L. donovani*, for which humans are the primary reservoir.[116] *L. infantum* causes VL in central Asia, China, the Mediterranean basin, the Middle East, and Latin America. Most disease associated with *L. infantum* infection occurs in children (infantile leishmaniasis) and immunocompromised adults, such as those with AIDS. *L. infantum* is also responsible for some CL in humans. Dogs are considered the primary reservoirs for *L. infantum*, and control of disease in dogs has been associated with reduction in human cases in the area. Nevertheless, other canine species, such as foxes, may also play a role as reservoirs.

Human CL occurs in the Americas, the Mediterranean basin, and western Asia from the Middle East to Central Asia, and especially in Afghanistan, Algeria, Colombia, Brazil, Iran, Syria, Ethiopia, North Sudan, Costa Rica, and Peru. In Africa and western Asia, CL is caused by *L. major, L. tropica,* and *L. aethiopica,* whereas in the Americas, the most common causes are *L. mexicana* and *L. braziliensis*. Mucocutaneous disease occurs primarily in South America and is caused by *L. braziliensis*, for which rodents and other small mammals are the primary reservoirs.[117]

Recommendations of the World Health organization for the control of leishmaniasis in humans consist of treatment of human disease; culling of wild and feral seropositive dogs; and insecticidal treatment of human homes, such as with pyrethroid sprays.[103] The effectiveness of the culling of seropositive or infected dogs is controversial.[42,118] At present this is only undertaken systematically in Brazil. Concerns raised include the ethics of destruction of pet dogs, delays between detection of seropositive dogs and culling, and the persistence of other subclinically or clinically infected canine and wildlife reservoirs. Vaccination of dogs may be more effective than the culling of seropositive dogs and could overcome the ethical concerns that relate to culling.[53]

FELINE LEISHMANIOSIS

Cats are relatively resistant to leishmaniosis, but cases have been described from southern Europe, the Middle East, Latin America, and Texas.[119,120] The cat from Texas was infected with *L. mexicana*. *L. infantum* and a variety of other *Leishmania* species such as *L. braziliensis* and *L. venezuelensis* have also been isolated from cats. Serologic studies of cats in endemic areas have generally revealed seroprevalences of less than 10%, although 34 (36%) of 95 stray cats from the Yucatán peninsula in Mexico had antibodies to *L. infantum, L. braziliensis,* or *L. mexicana*.[119] Disease in cats may be associated with concurrent FIV infection.[121,122] The extent to which cats are a reservoir for infection of humans is unclear.

Clinical signs of leishmaniosis in cats include cutaneous lesions, weight loss, lymphadenopathy, oral ulceration, mucopurulent ocular and nasal discharge, keratitis, altered mentation, diarrhea, and/or tachypnea. Cutaneous lesions consist of nodules, scaling and crusting, erythema, ulceration, and alopecia. Cutaneous lesions can occur anywhere and may be localized or generalized, but are often on the pinnae, bridge of the nose, limbs, or dorsal trunk. In one study, 50% of cats with skin lesions had evidence of visceral spread.[121]

Diagnosis of leishmaniosis in cats is similar to that in dogs, although cats often have low antibody titers.[121] Limited information exists in regard to treatment of feline leishmaniosis. Treatment with allopurinol monotherapy may result in clinical improvement or disease resolution in some cats.[123] Surgery may be curative for localized cutaneous lesions.[12]

CASE EXAMPLE

Signalment: "Fausto," an 8-year-old male neutered husky mix from northern California

History: Fausto was referred to the University of California, Davis, Veterinary Medical Teaching Hospital (VMTH) for evaluation of suspected autoimmune disease. The dog had a 6-month history of progressive skin lesions that began as crusting and ulceration around the elbow and stifle joints. This was followed by development of similar lesions above both eyes and on the dog's ears and dorsal muzzle. Three months after the skin lesions appeared, Fausto became stiff and lethargic and was lame and reluctant to walk. At that time, Fausto was taken to a local veterinary clinic where an injection of triamcinolone acetonide (Vetalog) was administered, and he was prescribed carprofen and trimethoprim-sulfamethoxazole. There was no improvement in the clinical signs. The day before he was brought to the VMTH, the owner had taken Fausto to a local emergency clinic because he was reluctant to move. Blood work and arthrocentesis (left and right tarsal joints) were performed. The blood work showed a normocytic, normochromic nonregenerative anemia (HCT 31%); mild hypoalbuminemia (2.4 g/dL); and moderate hyperglobulinemia (7.7 g/dL). Cytologic examination of the synovial fluid revealed large numbers of nondegenerate neutrophils, which was considered consistent with immune-mediated polyarthritis. Cephalexin and carprofen were prescribed, and the dog was referred for further evaluation.

The owner had not noticed any coughing, sneezing, vomiting, diarrhea, or changes in thirst or urination. Fausto was fed 3 cups of a commercial dry chicken and rice–based dog food once a day, and his appetite was good. He was fully vaccinated for rabies, canine distemper virus, canine adenovirus, and canine parvovirus. The dog did not receive heartworm prophylaxis medication but was treated with fipronil once a month for flea control. There was one other healthy dog in the household. The owner and his dogs had moved to California from Barcelona, Spain, a few weeks earlier, around the time that the skin lesions appeared. In Spain, Fausto had worn a collar to prevent insect bites.

Physical Examination:

Body Weight: 34.4 kg.

General: Quiet, alert, and responsive, but reluctant to ambulate. T = 102.7°F (39.3°C), HR = 132 beats/min, panting but eupneic, mucous membranes moist and pink.

Integument: Multiple focal regions of crusting, erythema, hyperpigmentation, thickening, and sometimes ulceration were present over the elbows and stifles, prepuce, ventral aspect of the mandible, above both eyes, and on both pinnae. Moderate pruritis was present.

Musculoskeletal: BCS 5/9. The dog was able to walk but had a shifting lameness. Pain was detected on extension of the joints, but there was no palpable effusion present.

Abdominal Palpation: Splenomegaly was detected.

Lymph Nodes: Superficial cervical and popliteal lymph nodes were all enlarged (approximately 3 cm in diameter).

All Other Systems: No significant abnormalities were detected.

Laboratory Findings:

CBC:

HCT 32.4% (40%-55%)
MCV 62.7 fL (65-75 fL)
MCHC 35.2 g/dL (33-36 g/dL)
Reticulocyte count 54,500 cells/μL
WBC 9300 cells/μL (6000-13,000 cells/μL)
Neutrophils 7533 cells/μL (3000-10,500 cells/μL)
Lymphocytes 930 cells/μL (1000-4000 cells/μL)
Monocytes 651 cells/μL (150-1200 cells/μL)
Eosinophils 186 cells/μL (0-1500 cells/μL)
Platelets 338,000 platelets/μL (150,000-400,000 platelets/μL).

Serum Chemistry Profile:

Sodium 140 mmol/L (145-154 mmol/L)
Potassium 4.4 mmol/L (4.1-5.3 mmol/L)
Chloride 107 mmol/L (105-116 mmol/L)
Bicarbonate 15 mmol/L (16-26 mmol/L)
Phosphorus 3.8 mg/dL (3.0-6.2 mg/dL)
Calcium 10.4 mg/dL (9.9-11.4 mg/dL)
BUN 16 mg/dL (8-31 mg/dL)
Creatinine 0.9 mg/dL (0.3-1.2 mg/dL)
Glucose 109 mg/dL (70-118 mg/dL)
Total protein 10.7 g/dL (5.4-7.4 g/dL)
Albumin 2.1 g/dL (2.9-4.2 g/dL)
Globulin 8.6 g/dL (2.3-4.4 g/dL)
ALT 12 U/L (19-67 U/L)
AST 39 U/L (21-54 U/L)
ALP 43 U/L (15-127 U/L)
GGT 3 U/L (0-6 U/L)
Cholesterol 191 mg/dL (135-345 mg/dL)
Total bilirubin 0.1 mg/dL (0-0.4 mg/dL).

Serum Protein Electrophoresis: There was a marked increase in gamma-globulin with mild hypoalbuminemia. The gammopathy was polyclonal.

Urinalysis (Cystocentesis): SGr 1.037; pH 7.0, 4+ protein, 1+ bilirubin, 1+ hemoprotein, no glucose or ketones, rare WBC/HPF, 1-3 RBC/HPF, rare hyaline casts, few lipid droplets.

Urine Protein-to-Creatinine Ratio: 2.99 (normal, <0.5).

Microbiologic Testing: IFA serology for antibodies for *Ehrlichia* spp., *Anaplasma* spp., *Rickettsia* spp., *Bartonella clarridgeiae, Bartonella vinsonii* subsp. *berkhoffii*, and *Bartonella henselae*: Negative.

Western immunoblot for antibodies to *Borrelia burgdorferi*: Negative.

Knott's and ELISA antigen test for *Dirofilaria immitis* infection: Negative.

Aerobic bacterial, anaerobic bacterial, and *Mycoplasma* culture of synovial fluid: Negative.

Aspiration cytology (right and left superficial cervical and popliteal lymph nodes): A heterogeneous population of lymphocytes was present, which consisted primarily of small mature lymphocytes and slightly increased numbers of intermediate-sized lymphocytes and lymphoblasts. Large numbers of plasma cells were noted. A few macrophages, nondegenerate neutrophils, and eosinophils were scattered throughout the specimen.

Bone marrow aspiration cytology: Many unit particles were present. Unit particles were normocellular, and a small amount of storage iron was noted. There were normal numbers of megakaryocytes. The myeloid-to-erythroid ratio was mildly increased; both series were synchronous and complete. Increased numbers of plasma cells were noted throughout the specimen, with few small lymphocytes. Macrophages occasionally contained intracytoplasmic organisms consistent with *Leishmania* spp. amastigotes. Interpretation: Mild erythroid hypoplasia, *Leishmania* spp., and mild plasma cell hyperplasia.

Skin biopsy: There was a thick band of inflammatory cells that extended from the superficial to the mid-dermis. The inflammatory infiltrate was composed of dense sheets of large foamy macrophages admixed with smaller numbers of lymphocytes and plasma cells and few neutrophils. Many of the large macrophages contained multiple, round to oval, intracytoplasmic basophilic organisms that were 1 to 2 μm in diameter. The epidermis was hyperplastic and hyperkeratotic and was covered by exudate admixed with keratin, degenerate neutrophils, and cellular debris.

Diagnosis: Canine visceral leishmaniosis.

Treatment and Outcome: Fausto was initially treated with a combination of allopurinol (10 mg/kg PO q8h), ketoconazole (9 mg/kg PO q12h), cephalexin (30 mg/kg PO q12h for 4 weeks, for secondary bacterial pyoderma), and carprofen (4.4 mg/kg PO q24h). At a recheck examination 2 weeks later, the dog's owner reported that 1 or 2 days after treatment was started, Fausto became intensely pruritic. Fausto's appetite also decreased and he developed increased thirst and urination, but the lameness resolved. Physical examination showed severe crusting and ulceration of the face, with an associated foul odor. This extended from the dorsal nasal planum to the temporal and supraocular regions, as well as the inner aspect and tips of the pinnae. The lesions on the limbs were static or slightly improved from the last visit. A CBC was unchanged, and a serum chemistry profile showed worsened hyperglobulinemia (9.3 g/dL) and hypoalbuminemia (1.9 g/dL). A drug reaction was suspected, and the cephalexin was replaced with clavulanic acid–amoxicillin. Over the next month, the skin lesions improved. The owner subsequently obtained meglumine antimoniate from Spain, and treatment was changed to allopurinol (10 mg/kg PO q12h) and meglumine antimoniate (88 mg/kg SC q24h for 1 month). However, 6 days later, the dog developed prolapsed third eyelids and was unable to catch treats when they were thrown to him. Physical examination showed healing skin lesions with evidence of hair regrowth, prolapsed third eyelids, risus sardonicus, and erect ears. A presumptive diagnosis of localized tetanus was made. A serum chemistry panel showed an albumin of 2.5 g/dL and a globulin of 6.4 g/dL. The urine protein-to-creatinine ratio was 0.2. Fausto was treated with metronidazole (10 mg/kg PO q8h for 14 days) and tetanus antitoxin (20,000 U in 250 mL saline over 1 hour, IV, once). Clinical signs of tetanus had almost resolved 11 days later when the owner was contacted by telephone. The dog was subsequently lost to follow-up.

Comments: This case is an interesting example of travel-related canine visceral leishmaniosis that was ultimately complicated by what appeared to be a cutaneous drug reaction to cephalexin and then localized tetanus. The diagnosis of leishmaniosis was suspected based on the clinical signs together with the travel history from southern Europe. The bone marrow aspirate and skin biopsies were obtained simultaneously for the sole purpose of diagnosis of leishmaniosis; impression smears of the skin lesions failed to yield organisms, and the lymph node aspirates were also negative. The owner and his dog traveled back to Spain in order to obtain the meglumine antimoniate, which could not be obtained in the United States. The development of tetanus may have followed wound contamination or use of contaminated needles by the owner for subcutaneous injection of the meglumine.

SUGGESTED READINGS

Maroli M, Gradoni L, Oliva G, et al. Guidelines for prevention of leishmaniasis in dogs. J Am Vet Med Assoc. 2010;236:1200-1206.

Oliva G, Roura X, Crotti A, et al. Guidelines for treatment of leishmaniasis in dogs. J Am Vet Med Assoc. 2010;236:1192-1198.

Paltrinieri S, Solano-Gallego L, Fondati A, et al. Guidelines for diagnosis and clinical classification of leishmaniasis in dogs. J Am Vet Med Assoc. 2010;236:1184-1191.

Solano-Gallego L, Koutinas A, Miro G, et al. Directions for the diagnosis, clinical staging, treatment and prevention of canine leishmaniosis. Vet Parasitol. 2009;165:1-18.

Solano-Gallego L, Miro G, Koutinas A, et al. LeishVet guidelines for the practical management of canine leishmaniosis. Parasit Vectors. 2011;4:86.

REFERENCES

1. Dutta AK. Pursuit of medical knowledge: Charles Donovan (1863-1951) on kala-azar in India. J Med Biogr. 2008;16:72-76.
2. Schonian G, Mauricio I, Cupolillo E. Is it time to revise the nomenclature of Leishmania? Trends Parasitol. 2010;26:466-469.
3. Antinori S, Schifanella L, Corbellino M. Leishmaniasis: new insights from an old and neglected disease. Eur J Clin Microbiol Infect Dis. 2012;31:109-118.
4. Owens SD, Oakley DA, Marryott K, et al. Transmission of visceral leishmaniasis through blood transfusions from infected English foxhounds to anemic dogs. J Am Vet Med Assoc. 2001;219:1076-1083.
5. Naucke TJ, Lorentz S. First report of venereal and vertical transmission of canine leishmaniosis from naturally infected dogs in Germany. Parasit Vectors. 2012;5:67.
6. Boggiatto PM, Gibson-Corley KN, Metz K, et al. Transplacental transmission of *Leishmania infantum* as a means for continued disease incidence in North America. PLoS Negl Trop Dis. 2011;5:e1019.
7. Silva FL, Oliveira RG, Silva TM, et al. Venereal transmission of canine visceral leishmaniasis. Vet Parasitol. 2009;160:55-59.
8. Leblois R, Kuhls K, Francois O, et al. Guns, germs and dogs: on the origin of *Leishmania chagasi*. Infect Genet Evol. 2011;11:1091-1095.
9. Sykes JE. Unpublished observations, 2012.
10. Teske E, van Knapen F, Beijer EG, et al. Risk of infection with *Leishmania* spp. in the canine population in the Netherlands. Acta Vet Scand. 2002;43:195-201.
11. Shaw SE, Langton DA, Hillman TJ. Canine leishmaniosis in the United Kingdom: a zoonotic disease waiting for a vector? Vet Parasitol. 2009;163:281-285.
12. Rufenacht S, Sager H, Muller N, et al. Two cases of feline leishmaniosis in Switzerland. Vet Rec. 2005;156:542-545.

13. Kawamura Y, Yoshikawa I, Katakura K. Imported leishmaniasis in dogs, U.S. military bases. Japan. Emerg Infect Dis. 2010;16: 2017-2019.
14. Moreno J, Alvar J. Canine leishmaniasis: epidemiological risk and the experimental model. Trends Parasitol. 2002;18:399-405.
15. Berrahal F, Mary C, Roze M, et al. Canine leishmaniasis: identification of asymptomatic carriers by polymerase chain reaction and immunoblotting. Am J Trop Med Hyg. 1996;55:273-277.
16. Solano-Gallego L, Morell P, Arboix M, et al. Prevalence of *Leishmania infantum* infection in dogs living in an area of canine leishmaniasis endemicity using PCR on several tissues and serology. J Clin Microbiol. 2001;39:560-563.
17. Leontides LS, Saridomichelakis MN, Billinis C, et al. A cross-sectional study of *Leishmania* spp. infection in clinically healthy dogs with polymerase chain reaction and serology in Greece. Vet Parasitol. 2002;109:19-27.
18. Tanczos B, Balogh N, Kiraly L, et al. First record of autochthonous canine leishmaniasis in Hungary. Vector Borne Zoonotic Dis. 2012;12:588-594.
19. Ready PD. Leishmaniasis emergence in Europe. Euro Surveill. 2010;15:19505.
20. Shang LM, Peng WP, Jin HT, et al. The prevalence of canine *Leishmania infantum* infection in Sichuan Province, southwestern China detected by real time PCR. Parasit Vectors. 2011;4: 173.
21. Cortes S, Vaz Y, Neves R, et al. Risk factors for canine leishmaniasis in an endemic Mediterranean region. Vet Parasitol. 2012;189:189-196.
22. Cardoso L, Rodrigues M, Santos H, et al. Sero-epidemiological study of canine *Leishmania* spp. infection in the municipality of Alijo (Alto Douro, Portugal). Vet Parasitol. 2004;121:21-32.
23. Galvez R, Miro G, Descalzo MA, et al. Emerging trends in the seroprevalence of canine leishmaniasis in the Madrid region (central Spain). Vet Parasitol. 2010;169:327-334.
24. Abranches P, Silva-Pereira MC, Conceicao-Silva FM, et al. Canine leishmaniasis: pathological and ecological factors influencing transmission of infection. J Parasitol. 1991;77:557-561.
25. Bigeli JG, Oliveira Jr WP, Teles NM. Diagnosis of *Leishmania* (Leishmania) *chagasi* infection in dogs and the relationship with environmental and sanitary aspects in the municipality of Palmas, State of Tocantins, Brazil. Rev Soc Bras Med Trop. 2012;45:18-23.
26. Solano-Gallego L, Llull J, Ramos G, et al. The Ibizian hound presents a predominantly cellular immune response against natural *Leishmania* infection. Vet Parasitol. 2000;90:37-45.
27. Miranda S, Roura X, Picado A, et al. Characterization of sex, age, and breed for a population of canine leishmaniosis diseased dogs. Res Vet Sci. 2008;85:35-38.
28. Quilez J, Martinez V, Woolliams JA, et al. Genetic control of canine leishmaniasis: genome-wide association study and genomic selection analysis. PLoS One. 2012;7:e35349.
29. Solano-Gallego L, Koutinas A, Miro G, et al. Directions for the diagnosis, clinical staging, treatment and prevention of canine leishmaniosis. Vet Parasitol. 2009;165:1-18.
30. Marino G, Gaglio G, Zanghi A. Clinicopathological study of canine transmissible venereal tumour in leishmaniotic dogs. J Small Anim Pract. 2012;53:323-327.
31. Mozos E, Perez J, Day MJ, et al. Leishmaniosis and generalized demodicosis in three dogs: a clinicopathological and immunohistochemical study. J Comp Pathol. 1999;120:257-268.
32. Ciaramella P, Oliva G, Luna RD, et al. A retrospective clinical study of canine leishmaniasis in 150 dogs naturally infected by *Leishmania infantum*. Vet Rec. 1997;141:539-543.
33. Cardoso L, Mendao C, Madeira de Carvalho L. Prevalence of *Dirofilaria immitis, Ehrlichia canis, Borrelia burgdorferi* sensu lato, *Anaplasma* spp. and *Leishmania infantum* in apparently healthy and CVBD-suspect dogs in Portugal—a national serological study. Parasit Vectors. 2012;5:62.
34. Cardoso L, Yisaschar-Mekuzas Y, Rodrigues FT, et al. Canine babesiosis in northern Portugal and molecular characterization of vector-borne co-infections. Parasit Vectors. 2010;3: 27.
35. Mekuzas Y, Gradoni L, Oliva G, et al. *Ehrlichia canis* and *Leishmania infantum* co-infection: a 3-year longitudinal study in naturally exposed dogs. Clin Microbiol Infect. 2009;15(suppl 2): 30-31.
36. Tabar MD, Francino O, Altet L, et al. PCR survey of vector-borne pathogens in dogs living in and around Barcelona, an area endemic for leishmaniasis. Vet Rec. 2009;164:112-116.
37. Abreu-Silva AL, Calabrese KS, Cupolilo SM, et al. Histopathological studies of visceralized *Leishmania* (Leishmania) *amazonensis* in mice experimentally infected. Vet Parasitol. 2004;121: 179-187.
38. Guessous-Idrissi N, Berrag B, Riyad M, et al. Short report: *Leishmania tropica*: etiologic agent of a case of canine visceral leishmaniasis in northern Morocco. Am J Trop Med Hyg. 1997;57: 172-173.
39. Hassan MM, Osman OF, El-Raba'a FM, et al. Role of the domestic dog as a reservoir host of *Leishmania donovani* in eastern Sudan. Parasit Vectors. 2009;2:26.
40. Reithinger R, Davies CR. American cutaneous leishmaniasis in domestic dogs: an example of the use of the polymerase chain reaction for mass screening in epidemiological studies. Trans R Soc Trop Med Hyg. 2002;96(suppl 1):S123-S126.
41. Marco JD, Barroso PA, Calvopina M, et al. Species assignation of *Leishmania* from human and canine American tegumentary leishmaniasis cases by multilocus enzyme electrophoresis in North Argentina. Am J Trop Med Hyg. 2005;72:606-611.
42. Silva DA, Madeira MF, Teixeira AC, et al. Laboratory tests performed on *Leishmania* seroreactive dogs euthanized by the leishmaniasis control program. Vet Parasitol. 2011;179:257-261.
43. Velez ID, Carrillo LM, Lopez L, et al. An epidemic outbreak of canine cutaneous leishmaniasis in Colombia caused by *Leishmania braziliensis* and *Leishmania panamensis*. Am J Trop Med Hyg. 2012;86:807-811.
44. Tolezano JE, Uliana SR, Taniguchi HH, et al. The first records of *Leishmania* (Leishmania) *amazonensis* in dogs (*Canis familiaris*) diagnosed clinically as having canine visceral leishmaniasis from Aracatuba County, Sao Paulo State, Brazil. Vet Parasitol. 2007;149:280-284.
45. Sun K, Guan W, Zhang JG, et al. Prevalence of canine leishmaniasis in Beichuan County, Sichuan, China and phylogenetic evidence for an undescribed *Leishmania* sp. in China based on 7SL RNA. Parasit Vectors. 2012;5:75.
46. Freeman KS, Miller MD, Breitschwerdt EB, et al. Leishmaniasis in a dog native to Colorado. J Am Vet Med Assoc. 2010;237:1288-1291.
47. Anderson DC, Buckner RG, Glenn BL, et al. Endemic canine leishmaniasis. Vet Pathol. 1980;17:94-96.
48. Sellon RK, Menard MM, Meuten DJ, et al. Endemic visceral leishmaniasis in a dog from Texas. J Vet Intern Med. 1993;7:16-19.
49. Swenson CL, Silverman J, Stromberg PC, et al. Visceral leishmaniasis in an English foxhound from an Ohio research colony. J Am Vet Med Assoc. 1988;193:1089-1092.
50. Gaskin AA, Schantz P, Jackson J, et al. Visceral leishmaniasis in a New York foxhound kennel. J Vet Intern Med. 2002;16:34-44.
51. Freeman K. Update on the diagnosis and management of *Leishmania* spp. infections in dogs in the United States. Top Companion Anim Med. 2010;25:149-154.
52. Molina R, Amela C, Nieto J, et al. Infectivity of dogs naturally infected with *Leishmania infantum* to colonized *Phlebotomus perniciosus*. Trans R Soc Trop Med Hyg. 1994;88:491-493.
53. Palatnik-de-Sousa CB. Vaccines for canine leishmaniasis. Front Immunol. 2012;3:69.
54. Altet L, Francino O, Solano-Gallego L, et al. Mapping and sequencing of the canine NRAMP1 gene and identification of mutations in leishmaniasis-susceptible dogs. Infect Immun. 2002;70:2763-2771.

55. Sanchez-Robert E, Altet L, Sanchez A, et al. Polymorphism of Slc11a1 (Nramp1) gene and canine leishmaniasis in a case-control study. J Hered. 2005;96:755-758.
56. Quinnell RJ, Kennedy LJ, Barnes A, et al. Susceptibility to visceral leishmaniasis in the domestic dog is associated with MHC class II polymorphism. Immunogenetics. 2003;55:23-28.
57. Petanides TA, Koutinas AF, Mylonakis ME, et al. Factors associated with the occurrence of epistaxis in natural canine leishmaniasis (*Leishmania infantum*). J Vet Intern Med. 2008;22: 866-872.
58. Paciello O, Oliva G, Gradoni L, et al. Canine inflammatory myopathy associated with *Leishmania infantum* infection. Neuromuscul Disord. 2009;19:124-130.
59. Lopez R, Lucena R, Novales M, et al. Circulating immune complexes and renal function in canine leishmaniasis. Zentralbl Veterinarmed B. 1996;43:469-474.
60. Terrazzano G, Cortese L, Piantedosi D, et al. Presence of anti-platelet IgM and IgG antibodies in dogs naturally infected by *Leishmania infantum*. Vet Immunol Immunopathol. 2006;110:331-337.
61. Smith BE, Tompkins MB, Breitschwerdt EB. Antinuclear antibodies can be detected in dog sera reactive to *Bartonella vinsonii* subsp. *berkhoffii*, *Ehrlichia canis*, or *Leishmania infantum* antigens. J Vet Intern Med. 2004;18:47-51.
62. Ginel PJ, Camacho S, Lucena R. Anti-histone antibodies in dogs with leishmaniasis and glomerulonephritis. Res Vet Sci. 2008;85: 510-514.
63. Slappendel RJ. Canine leishmaniasis. A review based on 95 cases in The Netherlands. Vet Q. 1988;10:1-16.
64. Naranjo C, Fondevila D, Altet L, et al. Evaluation of the presence of *Leishmania* spp. by real-time PCR in the lacrimal glands of dogs with leishmaniosis. Vet J. 2012;193:168-173.
65. Mir F, Fontaine E, Reyes-Gomez E, et al. Subclinical leishmaniasis associated with infertility and chronic prostatitis in a dog. J Small Anim Pract. 2012;53:419-422.
66. Font A, Roura X, Fondevila D, et al. Canine mucosal leishmaniasis. J Am Anim Hosp Assoc. 1996;32:131-137.
67. Viegas C, Requicha J, Albuquerque C, et al. Tongue nodules in canine leishmaniosis—a case report. Parasit Vectors. 2012;5:120.
68. Carrasco L, de Lara FC, Martin E, et al. Acute haemorrhagic pancreatitis associated with canine visceral leishmaniasis. Vet Rec. 1997;141:519-521.
69. Pinto AJ, Figueiredo MM, Silva FL, et al. Histopathological and parasitological study of the gastrointestinal tract of dogs naturally infected with *Leishmania infantum*. Acta Vet Scand. 2011;53:67.
70. Toplu N, Aydogan A. An immunohistochemical study in cases with usual and unusual clinicopathological findings of canine visceral leishmaniosis. Parasitol Res. 2011;109:1051-1057.
71. Lopez-Pena M, Aleman N, Munoz F, et al. Visceral leishmaniasis with cardiac involvement in a dog: a case report. Acta Vet Scand. 2009;51:20.
72. Agut A, Corzo N, Murciano J, et al. Clinical and radiographic study of bone and joint lesions in 26 dogs with leishmaniasis. Vet Rec. 2003;153:648-652.
73. de Souza AI, Juliano RS, Gomes TS, et al. Osteolytic osteomyelitis associated with visceral leishmaniasis in a dog. Vet Parasitol. 2005;129:51-54.
74. Vinuelas J, Garcia-Alonso M, Ferrando L, et al. Meningeal leishmaniosis induced by *Leishmania infantum* in naturally infected dogs. Vet Parasitol. 2001;101:23-27.
75. Cauduro A, Favole P, Lorenzo V, et al. Paraparesis caused by vertebral canal leishmaniotic granuloma in a dog. J Vet Intern Med. 2011;25:398-399.
76. Cavalcanti A, Lobo R, Cupolillo E, et al. Canine cutaneous leishmaniasis caused by neotropical *Leishmania infantum* despite of systemic disease: a case report. Parasitol Int. 2012;61:738-740.
77. Freitas JC, Nunes-Pinheiro DC, Lopes Neto BE, et al. Clinical and laboratory alterations in dogs naturally infected by *Leishmania chagasi*. Rev Soc Bras Med Trop. 2012;45:24-29.
78. Font A, Closa JM, Mascort J. Monoclonal gammopathy in a dog with visceral leishmaniasis. J Vet Intern Med. 1994;8:233-235.
79. Foglia Manzillo V, Restucci B, Pagano A, et al. Pathological changes in the bone marrow of dogs with leishmaniosis. Vet Rec. 2006;158:690-694.
80. Tropia de Abreu R, Carvalho MG, Carneiro CM, et al. Influence of clinical status and parasite load on erythropoiesis and leucopoiesis in dogs naturally infected with *Leishmania* (Leishmania) *chagasi*. PLoS One. 2011;6:e18873.
81. Giudice E, Passantino A. Detection of *Leishmania* amastigotes in peripheral blood from four dogs—short communication. Acta Vet Hung. 2011;59:205-213.
82. Galvez R, Miro G, Descalzo MA, et al. Questionnaire-based survey on the clinical management of canine leishmaniosis in the Madrid region (central Spain). Prev Vet Med. 2011;102:59-65.
83. Marcondes M, Biondo AW, Gomes AA, et al. Validation of a *Leishmania infantum* ELISA rapid test for serological diagnosis of *Leishmania chagasi* in dogs. Vet Parasitol. 2011;175:15-19.
84. de Amorim IF, Freitas E, Alves CF, et al. Humoral immunological profile and parasitological statuses of Leishmune vaccinated and visceral leishmaniasis infected dogs from an endemic area. Vet Parasitol. 2010;173:55-63.
85. Lombardo G, Pennisi MG, Lupo T, et al. Detection of *Leishmania infantum* DNA by real-time PCR in canine oral and conjunctival swabs and comparison with other diagnostic techniques. Vet Parasitol. 2012;184:10-17.
86. Martinez V, Quilez J, Sanchez A, et al. Canine leishmaniasis: the key points for qPCR result interpretation. Parasit Vectors. 2011;4:57.
87. de Queiroz NM, da Silveira RC, de Noronha Jr AC, et al. Detection of *Leishmania* (L.) *chagasi* in canine skin. Vet Parasitol. 2011;178:1-8.
88. Koutinas AF, Carlotti DN, Koutinas C, et al. Claw histopathology and parasitic load in natural cases of canine leishmaniosis associated with *Leishmania infantum*. Vet Dermatol. 2010;21:572-577.
89. Costa FA, Goto H, Saldanha LC, et al. Histopathologic patterns of nephropathy in naturally acquired canine visceral leishmaniasis. Vet Pathol. 2003;40:677-684.
90. Nieto CG, Navarrete I, Habela MA, et al. Pathological changes in kidneys of dogs with natural *Leishmania* infection. Vet Parasitol. 1992;45:33-47.
91. Zatelli A, Borgarelli M, Santilli R, et al. Glomerular lesions in dogs infected with *Leishmania* organisms. Am J Vet Res. 2003;64:558-561.
92. Dinhopl N, Mostegl MM, Richter B, et al. In situ hybridisation for the detection of *Leishmania* species in paraffin wax-embedded canine tissues using a digoxigenin-labelled oligonucleotide probe. Vet Rec. 2011;169:525.
93. Noli C, Auxilia ST. Treatment of canine Old World visceral leishmaniasis: a systematic review. Vet Dermatol. 2005;16:213-232.
94. Andrade HM, Toledo VP, Pinheiro MB, et al. Evaluation of miltefosine for the treatment of dogs naturally infected with *L. infantum* (= *L. chagasi*) in Brazil. Vet Parasitol. 2011;181:83-90.
95. Oliva G, Roura X, Crotti A, et al. Guidelines for treatment of leishmaniasis in dogs. J Am Vet Med Assoc. 2010;236:1192-1198.
96. Paradies P, Sasanelli M, Amato ME, et al. Monitoring the reverse to normal of clinico-pathological findings and the disease free interval time using four different treatment protocols for canine leishmaniosis in an endemic area. Res Vet Sci. 2012;93: 843-847.
97. Torres M, Bardagi M, Roura X, et al. Long term follow-up of dogs diagnosed with leishmaniosis (clinical stage II) and treated with meglumine antimoniate and allopurinol. Vet J. 2011;188:346-351.
98. da Silva SM, Amorim IF, Ribeiro RR, et al. Efficacy of combined therapy with liposome-encapsulated meglumine antimoniate and allopurinol in treatment of canine visceral leishmaniasis. Antimicrob Agents Chemother. 2012;56:2858-2867.
99. Manna L, Vitale F, Reale S, et al. Study of efficacy of miltefosine and allopurinol in dogs with leishmaniosis. Vet J. 2009;182:441-445.

100. Oliva G, Gradoni L, Ciaramella P, et al. Activity of liposomal amphotericin B (AmBisome) in dogs naturally infected with *Leishmania infantum*. J Antimicrob Chemother. 1995;36:1013-1019.
101. Cortadellas O. Initial and long-term efficacy of a lipid emulsion of amphotericin B desoxycholate in the management of canine leishmaniasis. J Vet Intern Med. 2003;17:808-812.
102. Murray HW. Leishmaniasis in the United States: treatment in 2012. Am J Trop Med Hyg. 2012;86:434-440.
103. Control of the leishmaniasis. Report of a meeting of the WHO Expert Committee on the Control of Leishmaniases. Geneva, 22–26 March 2010. http://www.who.int/leishmaniasis/surveillance/en/. Last accessed January 13, 2013.
104. Parra LE, Borja-Cabrera GP, Santos FN, et al. Safety trial using the Leishmune vaccine against canine visceral leishmaniasis in Brazil. Vaccine. 2007;25:2180-2186.
105. Nogueira FS, Moreira MA, Borja-Cabrera GP, et al. Leishmune vaccine blocks the transmission of canine visceral leishmaniasis: absence of *Leishmania* parasites in blood, skin and lymph nodes of vaccinated exposed dogs. Vaccine. 2005;23:4805-4810.
106. Santos FN, Borja-Cabrera GP, Miyashiro LM, et al. Immunotherapy against experimental canine visceral leishmaniasis with the saponin enriched-Leishmune vaccine. Vaccine. 2007;25:6176-6190.
107. Borja-Cabrera GP, Santos FN, Santos FB, et al. Immunotherapy with the saponin enriched-Leishmune vaccine versus immunochemotherapy in dogs with natural canine visceral leishmaniasis. Vaccine. 2010;28:597-603.
108. Moreno J, Vouldoukis I, Martin V, et al. Use of a LiESP/QA-21 vaccine (CaniLeish) stimulates an appropriate Th1-dominated cell-mediated immune response in dogs. PLoS Negl Trop Dis. 2012;6:e1683.
109. Gomez-Ochoa P, Sabate D, Homedes J, et al. Use of the nitroblue tetrazolium reduction test for the evaluation of Domperidone effects on the neutrophilic function of healthy dogs. Vet Immunol Immunopathol. 2012;146:97-99.
110. Lanaro E. Efficacy of a combined therapy with meglumine antimoniate and domperidone for treatment of canine leishmaniosis. In: 73rd Congresso Internazionale Multisala SCIVAC. 2012:531.
111. Gavgani AS, Hodjati MH, Mohite H, et al. Effect of insecticide-impregnated dog collars on incidence of zoonotic visceral leishmaniasis in Iranian children: a matched-cluster randomised trial. Lancet. 2002;360:374-379.
112. Giffoni JH, de Almeida CE, dos Santos SO, et al. Evaluation of 65% permethrin spot-on for prevention of canine visceral leishmaniasis: effect on disease prevalence and the vectors (Diptera: Psychodidae) in a hyperendemic area. Vet Ther. 2002;3:485-492.
113. Reithinger R, Coleman PG, Alexander B, et al. Are insecticide-impregnated dog collars a feasible alternative to dog culling as a strategy for controlling canine visceral leishmaniasis in Brazil? Int J Parasitol. 2004;34:55-62.
114. Otranto D, Paradies P, Lia RP, et al. Efficacy of a combination of 10% imidacloprid/50% permethrin for the prevention of leishmaniasis in kennelled dogs in an endemic area. Vet Parasitol. 2007;144:270-278.
115. Gomez-Ochoa P, Sabate D, Homedes J, et al. Clinical efficacy of a Leisguard-based program strategically established for the prevention of canine leishmaniosis in endemic areas with low prevalence [Abstract]. In: 73rd Congresso Internazionale Multisala SCIVAC. 2012:545.
116. Alvar J, Velez ID, Bern C, et al. Leishmaniasis worldwide and global estimates of its incidence. PLoS One. 2012;7:e35671.
117. Dantas-Torres F. Dogs as reservoirs for *Leishmania braziliensis*. Emerg Infect Dis. 2011;17:326-327:author reply 327.
118. Costa CH. How effective is dog culling in controlling zoonotic visceral leishmaniasis? A critical evaluation of the science, politics and ethics behind this public health policy. Rev Soc Bras Med Trop. 2011;44:232-242.
119. Longoni SS, Lopez-Cespedes A, Sanchez-Moreno M, et al. Detection of different *Leishmania* spp. and Trypanosoma cruzi antibodies in cats from the Yucatan Peninsula (Mexico) using an iron superoxide dismutase excreted as antigen. Comp Immunol Microbiol Infect Dis. 2012;35:469-476.
120. Craig TM, Barton CL, Mercer SH, et al. Dermal leishmaniasis in a Texas cat. Am J Trop Med Hyg. 1986;35:1100-1102.
121. Vides JP, Schwardt TF, Sobrinho LS, et al. *Leishmania chagasi* infection in cats with dermatologic lesions from an endemic area of visceral leishmaniosis in Brazil. Vet Parasitol. 2011;178:22-28.
122. Sobrinho LS, Rossi CN, Vides JP, et al. Coinfection of *Leishmania chagasi* with *Toxoplasma gondii*, feline immunodeficiency virus (FIV) and feline leukemia virus (FeLV) in cats from an endemic area of zoonotic visceral leishmaniasis. Vet Parasitol. 2012;187:302-306.
123. Leiva M, Lloret A, Pena T, et al. Therapy of ocular and visceral leishmaniasis in a cat. Vet Ophthalmol. 2005;8:71-75.

CHAPTER 75

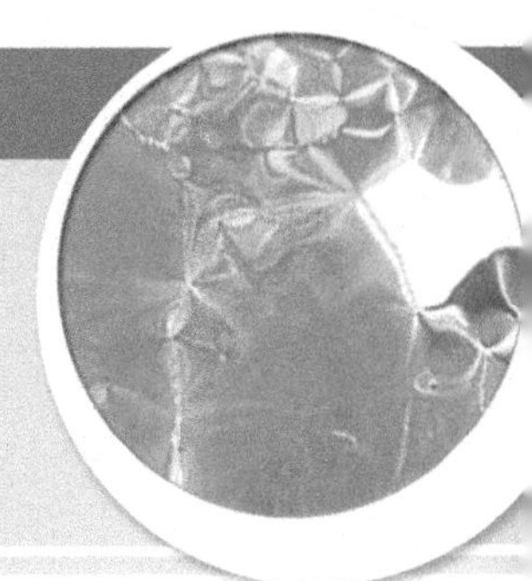

Babesiosis

Adam J. Birkenheuer

> **Overview of Babesiosis in Dogs and Cats**
>
> First Described: Early descriptions of intraerythrocytic parasites in dogs with signs of babesiosis were made in Africa in 1893 (Hutcheon).[1] The first documented case of canine babesiosis in the United States was in 1934 (Eaton).[2]
>
> Cause: *Babesia canis, Babesia gibsoni, Babesia conradae* (dogs); *Babesia felis, Babesia cati* (cats), several other unnamed species (phylum Apicomplexa)
>
> Affected Hosts: Domestic dogs and cats
>
> Geographic Distribution: Worldwide, but different *Babesia* species vary in their geographic distribution
>
> Mode of Transmission: A variety of tick vector species; fighting or biting interactions; vertical transmission; blood transfusion
>
> Major Clinical Signs: Lethargy, pallor, splenomegaly. Dogs with severe babesiosis caused by *B. canis rossi* may show neurologic signs, anuria, tachypnea, and poor perfusion parameters.
>
> Differential Diagnoses: Hemoplasmosis, primary immune-mediated hemolytic anemia and/or thrombocytopenia, other causes of hemolysis such as oxidative toxins or microangiopathic hemolysis (e.g., with splenic hemangiosarcoma). Canine monocytic ehrlichiosis, Rocky Mountain Spotted Fever, and bacterial endocarditis should also be considered.
>
> Human Health Significance: *Babesia* species that infect dogs and cats are not known to infect humans.

Etiology and Epidemiology

Babesiosis, caused by infection with organisms from the genus *Babesia*, is characterized by hemolytic anemia, fever, and splenomegaly. *Babesia* infections can also be subclinical or cause severe life-threatening illness. *Babesia* spp. are intraerythrocytic protozoan parasites of the phylum Apicomplexa. Altogether, more than 100 species of *Babesia* have been described, and with the advent of molecular techniques such as PCR assays, new species and genotypes are identified each year. Historically, species have been named and identified based on the vertebrate host and the size of the parasite (large or small *Babesia* species). Large *Babesia* spp. are 3 to 7 μm in length, whereas small *Babesia* spp. are 1 to 3 μm in length. In most parts of the world, tick vectors are the most important means of transmission of *Babesia* species. However, for some *Babesia* species, such as *Babesia gibsoni* in North America and Europe, direct transmission between dogs, through fighting (and exchange of blood), or congenital transplacental transmission, is believed to be the most common route of transmission when competent tick vectors are absent.[3-5]

When ticks are involved in transmission, sporozoites are released from the tick salivary glands as the tick feeds and they enter the bloodstream of the vertebrate host (Figure 75-1). They then attach to, and are endocytosed by, erythrocytes. Within erythrocytes, they undergo asexual reproduction (merogony), and the daughter cells infect new erythrocytes. A naïve tick then ingests infected erythrocytes. It is unclear whether transformation from merozoite to gametocyte begins in the vertebrate host or in the tick. In the tick midgut, the sexual phase of reproduction occurs when the gametocytes fuse to form a zygote. The zygote invades epithelial cells of the tick gut. The resultant forms, ookinetes, leave the epithelial cell and invade either the salivary gland or the ovary, where they participate in transstadial and transovarial transmission, respectively. Prior to transmission, another asexual form of reproduction occurs in the salivary gland, sporogony.

Babesiosis in Dogs

Canine babesiosis is a disease of worldwide importance. Initially, two species of *Babesia* were recognized in dogs (*Babesia canis* and *B. gibsoni*); however, now at least nine genetically distinct canine piroplasms have been described. *Babesia* species that infect dogs vary in their geographic distribution, which in turn has been subject to change due to movement of infected animals, movement of tick vectors, and reclassification with improved diagnostic techniques. As new species have been recognized, it has become more important for the clinician to understand the differences in diagnosis, prognosis, and treatment for infection with each species.

Babesia canis

Babesia canis is the most common large *Babesia* species and has three distinct subspecies: *B. canis vogeli, B. canis canis,* and *B. canis rossi.* It has been proposed that these are in fact three distinct species (*B. vogeli, B. canis,* and *B. rossi*).[6] *B. canis vogeli* is transmitted by the brown dog tick (*Rhipicephalus sanguineus*). Infection is most commonly diagnosed in warm, humid regions of the world, and the disease occurs throughout the year in endemic regions. *B. canis vogeli* can be found in Africa, Asia, Australia, Europe, and the Americas. In the United States, disease is most often diagnosed in the southern regions. *B. canis vogeli* reported seroprevalence in dogs has ranged from 3.8% to 59%.[7] The prevalence of seroreactivity is higher in adult dogs than in dogs younger than 1 year.[8] In an antibody serosurvey of dogs in Florida, 46% of 393 greyhounds were seroreactive.[7] The prevalence of seroreactive dogs within these kennels ranged from 17% to 100%; the lower prevalence was noted in kennels

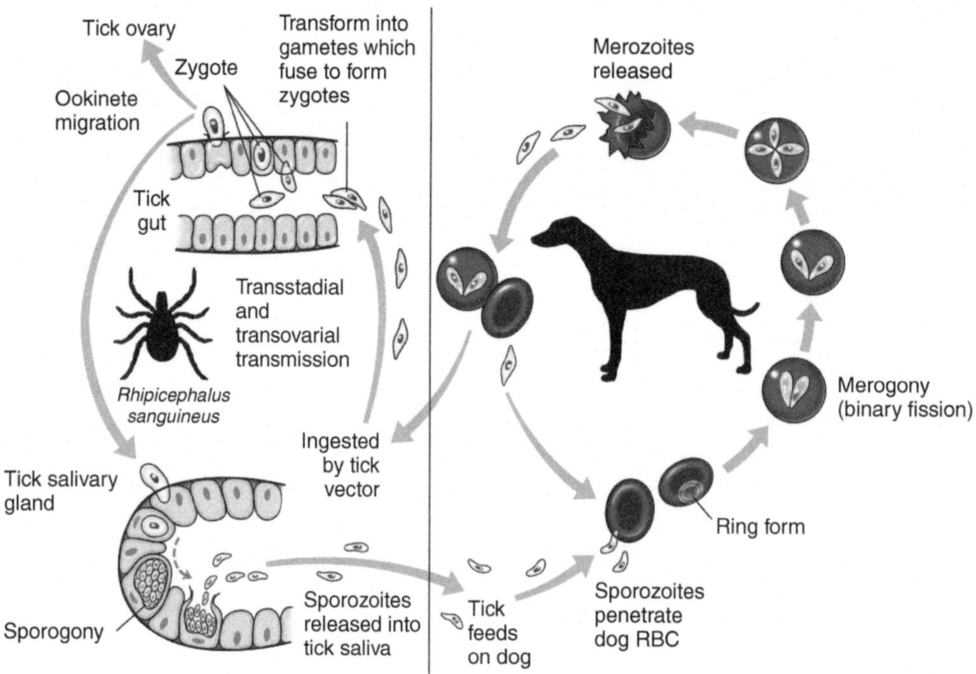

FIGURE 75-1 Life cycle of *Babesia canis*.

with more intensive tick control. None of 50 non-greyhound, individually housed adult pet dogs within the same geographic area were seroreactive, which implicated environment and breed susceptibility as possible risk factors in endemic areas.[7] Transplacental transmission of *B. canis vogeli* infections is strongly suspected but unproven in an experimental setting.[9]

B. canis canis is found in Europe and Africa. It is transmitted by the ornate cow tick, *Dermacentor reticulatus,* but *R. sanguineus* may also be a vector.[10] The incidence of infection is highest in the fall and spring. Higher prevalence rates are most commonly found in rural or suburban areas that are adjacent to prairies or woodlands that provide suitable habitat for *D. reticulatus.*[11] *B. canis canis* infection is most often diagnosed in France. Infections are being reported more frequently from other European countries such as Croatia, Poland, and Germany, possibly due to changes in the distribution of *D. reticulatus.*[12] Outbreaks of disease due to *B. canis canis* infection in Polish sled dogs share many similarities with those due to *B. canis vogeli* infection in North American greyhounds.[13]

B. canis rossi is transmitted by the yellow dog tick, *Haemaphysalis elliptica* (formerly *Haemaphysalis leachi*).[14] Reports of *B. canis rossi* infection have been limited to Africa, with the vast majority of reports coming from South Africa, where more than 10% of the dogs evaluated in some veterinary hospitals may be affected.[15,16] The incidence of infection is highest during the summer months. Breed predispositions for infection have not been well studied, but the traditional fighting breeds (American pit bull terriers, Staffordshire bull terriers, and bull terriers) are more likely to die when they are diagnosed with severe babesiosis.[17]

Unnamed Large *Babesia* Species

A large *Babesia* sp. has been isolated from dogs in North America that had been splenectomized or were undergoing chemotherapy for cancer. Infected dogs have been identified in North Carolina, New Jersey, New York, and Texas.[18-20] A tick vector has not been identified. A different novel large *Babesia* sp. was reported in a dog from Great Britain that never traveled outside of that country.[21] The dog died as a result of infection.

Babesia gibsoni

Infections with *B. gibsoni* occur throughout the world, and the insidious nature of this infection has allowed the inadvertent transport of infected dogs from Asia to other areas. *B. gibsoni* can be found in Africa, Asia, Australia, North and South America, and Europe. Depending on the availability of suitable vectors, two distinct epidemiologic scenarios exist for *B. gibsoni*: tick transmission and direct transmission between dogs.[22,23] *B. gibsoni* is transmitted primarily by the tick vectors *Haemaphysalis bispinosa* and *Haemaphysalis longicornis,* and possibly by *R. sanguineus.*[24-28] In its original endemic area of Asia, the geographic range of *B. gibsoni* correlates with that of *H. bispinosa,* and tick infestation is a risk factor for infection in nonfighting breeds. In the United States where competent tick vectors are not endemic, *B. gibsoni* infections occur in dogs engaged in fighting activities.[23,29] Most dogs with *B. gibsoni* infection in the United States have been American pit bull terriers.[29,30] However, an increased prevalence of infection has even been noted in fighting breeds in areas such as Japan, where *Haemaphysalis* spp. are endemic. In fighting breeds, transmission has been associated with a fight or bite by an infected dog or having been born to an infected bitch. Perinatal transmission is believed to occur.[3-5]

Babesia conradae

B. conradae (previously referred to as "the California isolate" and the "western piroplasm" and historically misidentified as *B. gibsoni*)[31] has been detected primarily in dogs from southern California.[31,32] Tick vectors have not been identified. Transmission studies that attempted to prove vector competence for *R. sanguineus* and *Dermacentor variabilis* were unsuccessful or inconclusive.[33] The author has identified *R. sanguineus* as well as soft-bodied ticks, *Ornithodoros coriaceus,* on *B. conradae*–infected dogs. A high prevalence of *B. conradae* infection was noted in a kennel of greyhound mixed-breed dogs that were used to hunt coyotes.[34] A history of coyote fights was a risk factor for infection. *B. conradae* DNA was detected in the spleen of 1 of 50 coyotes, so fighting may be one mode of transmission for this *Babesia* species.

Babesia microti–Like Organism

A *B. microti*–like parasite (also referred to as *Babesia annae* or *Theileria annae*) has been identified in dogs, the majority of which have lived in, or traveled to, northwestern Spain.[35-38] A single American pit bull terrier confiscated from a suspected dog-fighting operation in North America was also infected.[39] A high percentage of European and North American foxes are infected with a genetically identical parasite.[40,41] A tick vector has not been definitively identified, but in Spain an association between *Ixodes hexagonus* infestation and *B. microti*–like infection has been observed.[42]

Feline Babesiosis

Feline babesiosis has not been studied as extensively as canine babesiosis. Several small *Babesia* species have been identified in cats, which include *Babesia felis, Babesia cati,* and *Babesia leo. Babesia felis* is a highly pathogenic *Babesia* species that infects domestic cats in southern Africa and the Sudan.[43] Infection of domestic cats has primarily been identified along the coast of South Africa.[44,45] Affected cats are usually younger than 3 years, and there is no recognized breed or sex predilection. *Babesia cati* is less pathogenic and found primarily in India. *Babesia leo* has been detected in lions *(Panthera leo)* in Kruger National Park, as well as a single domestic cat in a molecular survey.[46] A small piroplasm was visualized in blood smears from feral cats in Rio de Janeiro, Brazil, but no molecular data were available to confirm the identity of these organisms.[47]

Large *Babesia* species also appear to infect cats. DNA sequences, most similar to those of *B. canis canis* and a *B. microti*–like parasite, have been amplified from the blood of three cats with retroviral infections from Spain and Portugal, but no organisms were visualized.[48] *B. canis presentii* was identified in two cats in Israel.[49] Another *B. canis*–like parasite has been identified in a naturally infected cat from Poland.[50] Feline babesiosis has not been reported in the United States.

Clinical Features

Clinical Signs and Their Pathogenesis

Canine Babesiosis

The pathogenicity of *Babesia* organisms is determined primarily by the species and strain involved. Host factors, such as the age of the host and the immunologic response generated against the parasite or vector tick, are also important. Although most often subclinically infected, dogs infected with "avirulent" species such as *B. canis vogeli* may have severe clinical disease. Similarly, dogs infected with "virulent" species such as *B. canis rossi* may be subclinically infected without overt clinical or laboratory findings. However, features that should raise clinical suspicion for babesiosis include fever, thrombocytopenia, hemolytic anemia, and splenomegaly. Dogs often have nonspecific signs such as lethargy, anorexia, and weakness (Box 75-1). Occasionally owners note jaundice, mucosal pallor, or discoloration of the urine caused by bilirubinuria or hemoglobinuria. Dogs infected with *B. canis vogeli* may have fever of unknown origin only without overt hematologic abnormalities.[51] Co-infections with other tick- or bloodborne pathogens may also influence the clinical signs of disease.

Box 75-1

Clinical Findings in Dogs with Babesiosis

Prevalence	Duration
Common signs	**Hyperacute signs (primarily *B. canis rossi*)**
Anorexia	Hypothermia
Lethargy	Shock
Weakness	Coma
Pyrexia	Disseminated intravascular coagulation
Weight loss	Metabolic acidosis
Uncommon/atypical signs (predominantly *B. canis rossi*)	Death
Ascites	**Acute signs**
Edema	Hemolytic anemia
Constipation	Icterus
Diarrhea	Splenomegaly
Ulcerative stomatitis	Lymphadenopathy
Hemorrhage	Vomiting
Congested mucous membranes	**Chronic signs**
Polycythemia	Intermittent pyrexia
Ocular and nasal discharge	Partial anorexia
Respiratory distress	Loss of body condition
Masticatory myositis	Lymphadenomegaly
Temporomandibular joint pain	Splenomegaly
Back pain	No signs
Central nervous system signs (seizures, ataxia, paresis)	

Parasite antigens are incorporated on the erythrocyte surface and induce host-opsonizing antibodies, which in turn leads to removal of infected erythrocytes by the mononuclear-phagocyte system. Soluble parasite antigens can also adhere to the surface of noninfected erythrocytes and platelets. This may lead to their opsonization by antibodies, with or without complement, and account for hemolytic anemia and thrombocytopenia that is often not correlated with the level of parasitemia. Parasitemia and anemia are more severe in splenectomized dogs, and splenectomy may precipitate disease in dogs with chronic subclinical infections. Mechanisms other than immune-mediated destruction that contribute to erythrocyte damage include increased erythrocyte osmotic fragility, direct injury of erythrocytes by *Babesia* parasites, accumulation of cyclic nucleotides, and oxidative injury.[52-56] Lipid peroxidation increases erythrocyte rigidity and slows the passage of erythrocytes through capillary beds. Soluble parasite proteases activate the kallikrein system and induce fibrinogen-like protein formation. These proteins make erythrocytes more "sticky," and they sludge in capillary beds, which contributes to anemia and many of the other potential clinical signs. The most severe sludging occurs in the central nervous system (CNS) and muscles.

Thrombocytopenia may result from immune-mediated or coagulatory consumption of platelets. Despite severely decreased platelet counts, bleeding is rarely observed in dogs infected with most *Babesia* strains, and other abnormal coagulation test results are uncommon (with the exceptions of *B. conradae* and also *B. canis rossi*). Dogs with *B. conradae* infection have experienced life-threatening hemorrhages, the pathogenesis of which requires further study.[57]

Other possible complications include membranoproliferative glomerulonephritis, which may have an immune-mediated pathogenesis.[58-60] Renal failure occurs in up to 40% of dogs infected with *B. microti*–like parasites, and their presence has been associated with increased mortality.[35,36,38,61,62] Nonregenerative anemia, azotemia, and proteinuria with high urine protein/creatinine ratios were found in these dogs.[35]

Severe Babesiosis

Virulent *B. canis canis* and especially *B. canis rossi* strains induce a profound systemic inflammatory response, which can result in a severe sepsis-like syndrome with multiple organ dysfunction (see Chapter 86). The majority of dogs infected with *B. canis rossi* have uncomplicated babesiosis and can be treated as outpatients. However, up to 31% of the dogs examined at a university clinic required hospitalization, and 10% of hospitalized dogs did not survive.[17] Severe clinical illness in dogs infected with *B. canis rossi* results from hypotension, acute renal failure (ARF), neurologic complications, disseminated intravascular coagulation (DIC), a hepatopathy, and acute respiratory distress syndrome (ARDS). Tissue hypoxia results from anemia, shock, vascular stasis, excessive endogenous production of carbon monoxide, parasitic damage to hemoglobin, and decreased ability of hemoglobin to off-load oxygen.[53,63] Lactic acid generation from tissue hypoxia can result in severe metabolic acidosis.[64]

"Red biliary syndrome" is a paradoxical phenomenon of severe intravascular hemolysis (manifested as hemoglobinemia and hemoglobinuria) in combination with hemoconcentration (high-reference-range or elevated hematocrit).[63] The hemoconcentration is thought to occur when plasma shifts from the vascular to the extravascular compartment as a result of increased capillary permeability, with a resultant decrease in blood volume. Hemoconcentration has been associated with cerebral babesiosis, DIC, ARF, and ARDS.

Neurologic complications result from sludging of parasitized erythrocytes in CNS capillary beds, with congestion and macroscopic and microscopic hemorrhages. Severe hypoglycemia can also result in neurologic signs. Other complications of severe babesiosis include pancreatitis, rhabdomyolysis, ocular involvement, upper respiratory signs, cardiac arrhythmias, necrosis of the extremities, and fluid accumulation. Pulmonary, CNS, and renal complications are associated with a higher rate of mortality. Persistent lactate concentrations above 40 mg/dL are a poor prognostic indicator for survival.[65]

Feline Babesiosis

Cats with babesiosis from southern Africa generally show lethargy, anorexia, weakness, an unkempt haircoat, and/or diarrhea.[45] Fever and icterus are less common. Anemia can be severe and is the underlying reason for the clinical signs. The disease is chronic, and signs may not be apparent until a later stage of illness. Cats usually adapt to the anemia and may have only mild clinical signs until they are stressed by handling. Complications of the hemolytic anemia have included hepatopathy, pulmonary edema, renal failure, CNS signs, and concurrent infections.

Physical Examination Findings

Physical examination abnormalities in most dogs with babesiosis consist of fever, mucosal pallor, lethargy, splenomegaly, and bounding pulses. Fever is not consistently identified, because it often waxes and wanes. Tachycardia and tachypnea may be present in severely anemic dogs. Mucosal hemorrhages and/or epistaxis may be present in dogs with *B. conradae* infection (Figure 75-2), and excessive bleeding from venipuncture sites may be noted.

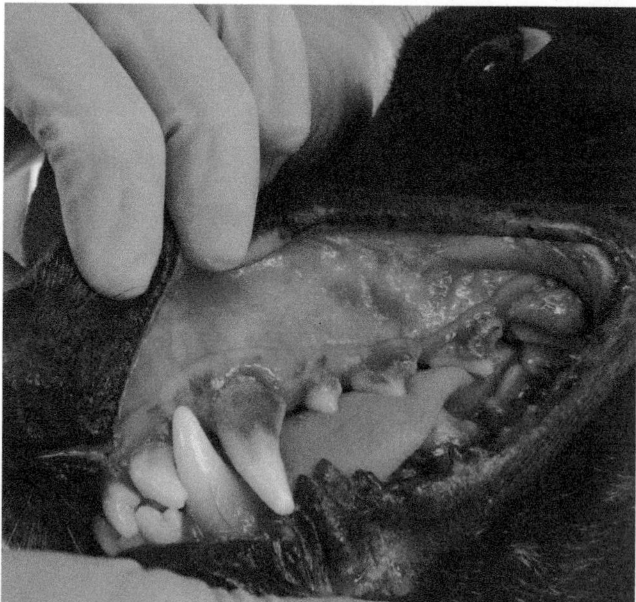

FIGURE 75-2 Greyhound infected with *Babesia conradae*. Mucosal hemorrhages are apparent. These resolved after treatment with atovaquone and azithromycin. (Courtesy Dr. Jane Sykes, University of California, Davis.)

Dogs with severe babesiosis may show CNS signs such as incoordination, pelvic limb paresis, muscle tremors, nystagmus, anisocoria, intermittent loss of consciousness, seizures, stupor, coma, aggression, or vocalization.[63] Dogs with red biliary syndrome may have congested mucous membranes or icterus. Other clinical abnormalities in dogs with severe babesiosis include tachypnea, increased lung sounds, and cardiac arrhythmias.

Affected cats may be lethargic, pale, tachycardic, and tachypneic, and in some cases, icteric.

Diagnosis

Laboratory Abnormalities

Complete Blood Count

In dogs with babesiosis, the primary hematologic abnormalities are anemia and thrombocytopenia. Thrombocytopenia is often present, even when anemia is absent. A mild, normocytic, normochromic anemia is generally noted in the first few days after infection, which becomes macrocytic, hypochromic, and regenerative as the disease progresses. Uncommonly with *B. canis rossi* infections, a relative polycythemia may be noted.[63] Leukocyte abnormalities are inconsistently observed but may include leukocytosis (with or without a left shift), leukopenia, neutrophilia, neutropenia, lymphocytosis, and/or eosinophilia.[34,66-68] Leukopenia or a low-normal leukocyte count due to relative neutropenia has been frequently observed in dogs from Europe with *B. canis* infections and dogs from the United States with *B. conradae* infections.[34,68] Autoagglutination, positive direct antiglobulin (Coombs') tests, and spherocytosis may also be present.

TABLE 75-1

Diagnostic Assays Available for Babesiosis in Dogs and Cats

Assay	Specimen Type	Target	Performance
Cell culture	Whole blood	*Babesia* spp.	Not widely offered or utilized for routine diagnostic purposes. Requires several weeks' incubation.
Cytology	Whole blood, buffy-coat smears (the area just below the buffy coat), tissue aspirates	*Babesia* spp.	Rapid and specific (i.e., when merozoites are identified by experienced cytologists, the sample is likely to be infected with *Babesia* spp.; however, *Babesia* spp. cannot be accurately differentiated based on morphology alone). Less sensitive than PCR.
Immunofluorescent antibody serology	Serum	Antibodies to *Babesia* spp.	Acute and convalescent serology may be required for diagnosis of acute infection, because initial results may be negative in dogs with acute disease and positive results may reflect previous exposure rather than active infection. Cross-reactivity can occur between *Babesia* spp. Some dogs do not develop detectable antibody titers despite chronic infection.
PCR	Whole blood, splenic aspirates	*Babesia spp*. DNA	Confirms active infection. Sensitivity and specificity varies depending on assay design and specimen type. Both false-positive and false-negative results are possible; PCR results must be interpreted in light of the clinical signs. Serial sampling (i.e., two or more tests on specimens obtained 2-4 weeks apart) will increase sensitivity, especially in chronically infected animals.

In cats, anemia associated with *B. felis* infection is typically macrocytic, hypochromic, and regenerative.[69] Thrombocytopenia is an inconsistent finding.

Serum Chemistry Profile

There are no pathognomonic biochemical findings in dogs with babesiosis. Common findings in North American dogs include hyperglobulinemia (which may be present in the absence of other laboratory abnormalities), mildly increased liver enzyme activities, and, less commonly, hyperbilirubinemia. A study of dual infections with *B. canis* and *Ehrlichia canis* showed that the prevalence of hyperglobulinemia was higher in dogs with dual infections than in dogs with a single infection caused by either organism.[70] Hyperbilirubinemia is a consistent finding during acute disease caused by *B. canis canis* and *B. canis rossi* but not by *B. gibsoni* or *B. conradae*.[34,67] Dogs with severe *B. canis rossi* infections may have hemoglobinemia, moderately increased liver enzyme activities, increased BUN and serum creatinine concentrations, hypoalbuminemia, hypoglycemia, and metabolic acidosis.

Cats infected with *B. felis* typically have elevated serum ALT activity and total bilirubin concentrations. Serum protein values are usually within reference limits, but hyperglobulinemia can occur. Renal parameters are unaffected.[69]

Urinalysis

Urinalysis abnormalities in dogs with babesiosis are variable but include bilirubinuria, hemoglobinuria, proteinuria, and, in rare cases, granular casts. Some dogs have pigmenturia consisting most commonly of bilirubin, and occasionally hemoglobin.

Coagulation Testing

The most consistent hemostatic abnormality in complicated and uncomplicated babesiosis is thrombocytopenia. DIC has been reported; however, complete confirmation of DIC in animals with babesiosis may be difficult because of the nature of the underlying disease process and the reported unreliability of the human fibrin degradation product test for evaluating canine specimens. Dogs with *B. conradae* infection appear to have altered platelet function tests.[57]

Microbiologic Testing

There are three basic methods available for specific diagnosis of *Babesia* infections: microscopic identification, serologic testing, and nucleic acid–based detection methods (Table 75-1). The true clinical sensitivity and specificity of most of the available tests is unknown, but all modalities can have either false-positive or false-negative results. Therefore, there is no "perfect" test for *Babesia* infection, and in some cases, multiple diagnostic tests are indicated.

Cytologic Diagnosis

Light microscopic examination is highly specific for the identification of *Babesia* organisms, but because of its limit of detection (0.001% parasitemia), it has relatively poor sensitivity and is not a suitable screening test. Several species/genotypes are virtually indistinguishable by light microscopy, making accurate identification to the species level impossible. However, when cytologic detection is used in combination with the history, signalment, physical examination, clinicopathologic data, and geographic location, the clinician may be able to predict the most likely species present.

Babesia canis are large, pyriform organisms and usually exist singly or in pairs (Figure 75-3, *A*). Smaller single intracellular organisms are likely to be *B. gibsoni* or *B. conradae* (see Figure 75-3, *B* and C). However, when the parasites are rapidly replicating, the classic intraerythrocytic forms may not predominate and some more atypical irregular, amoeboid parasite forms with a wide range of sizes can be detected. During these phases of infection, some small *Babesia* spp. have large forms and some large *Babesia* spp. have small forms. In chronic infection, the level of parasitemia is often low, especially in *B. canis*–infected dogs, and thorough examination of thin blood smears is necessary. Evaluation of stained slides requires experience and a significant time commitment on the part of the laboratory technician. For *B. canis* infections, blood collected from the peripheral capillary beds of the ear tip or nailbed may yield higher numbers of parasitized cells.[71] Rarely, phagocytized organisms and erythrocyte fragments are seen in neutrophils. Methods that concentrate and stain buffy-coat specimens may improve the sensitivity of parasite detection.[72,73]

Serologic Diagnosis

Because *Babesia* parasites are difficult to detect, especially in chronic carriers, immunodiagnostics may be used to screen for exposure. Immunofluorescent antibody (IFA) assays are used most commonly to detect antibodies to *Babesia* species. Laboratory methods differ, and each laboratory should be consulted for cutoff antibody titers. As a general guideline, titers to *B. canis* or *B. gibsoni* of 1:64 or greater on a single specimen are supportive of exposure. Serologic assays for *B. conradae* are not widely available at the time of writing.

Titers to multiple *Babesia* species must be measured if antibody testing is performed in geographic areas where more than one species of *Babesia* exists. Cross-reactivity between *Babesia* spp. makes parasite identification by PCR necessary to definitively identify a given species. There are also many documented instances in which parasites or parasite DNA have been detected but anti-*Babesia* antibodies could not be detected. Very young dogs or dogs tested early in the disease course may have negative antibody test results, so convalescent serology is required in some cases. Antibodies were not detected in 36% of dogs with *B. canis* parasitemia in one study.[8] ELISAs that target several different antigens have been developed for use in antibody or antigen detection tests and offer promise for serodiagnosis of canine babesiosis in the future. However, there are no

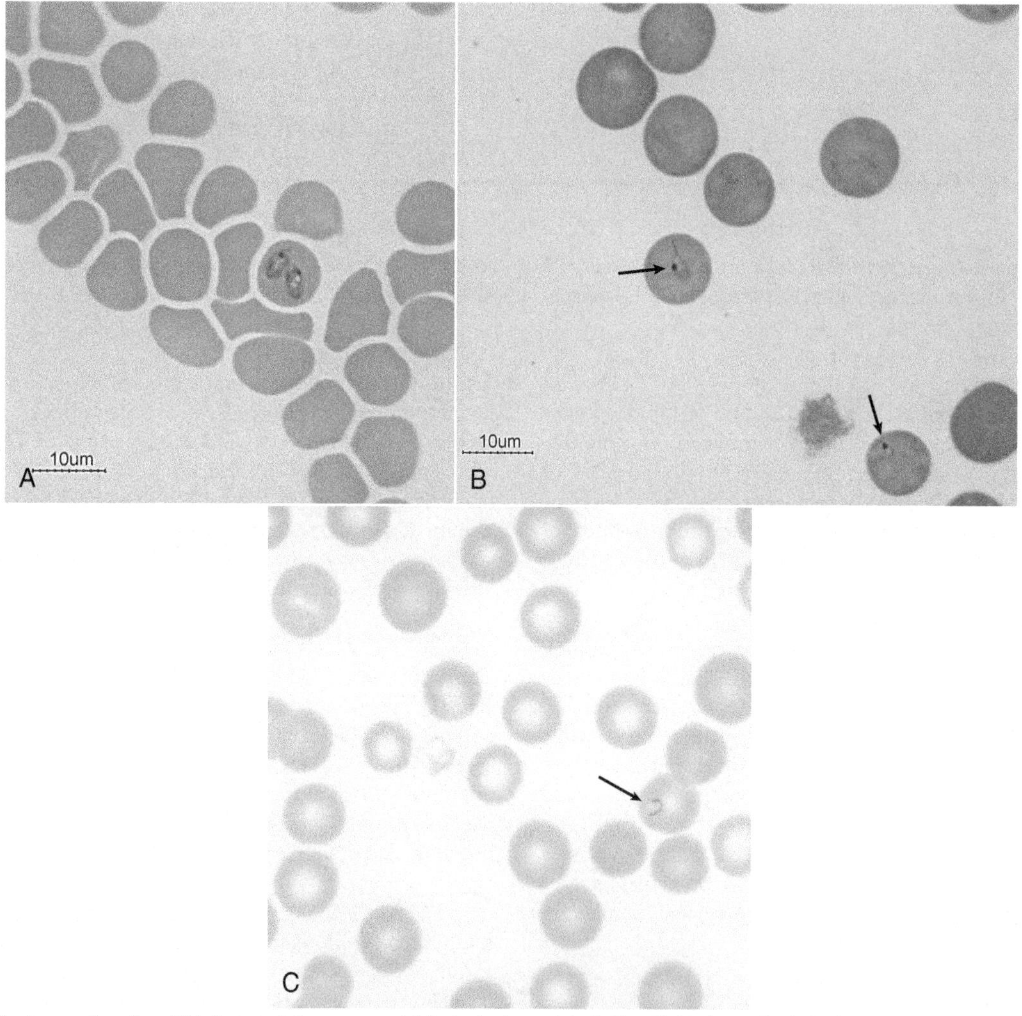

FIGURE 75-3 Blood smears from dog with babesiosis. **A,** Large unnamed *Babesia* piroplasm originally identified in dogs in North Carolina. A pair of large, piriform-shape merozoites are present within an erythrocyte. **B,** Individual merozoites of *Babesia gibsoni* in erythrocytes *(arrows)*. **C,** *Babesia conradae* merozoite within an erythrocyte *(arrow)*. Polychromasia and anisocytosis are also present. Although considered a small *Babesia* species, in this image, the organism is relatively large. Wright's stain, 1000×.

commercially available ELISA assays for the detection of anti-*Babesia* antibodies in the United States.

Molecular Diagnosis Using the Polymerase Chain Reaction

Genetic methods such as PCR assays are the most sensitive and specific means of detecting active infection with *Babesia*. Some assays have a lower limit of detection that is more than 1300-fold more sensitive than the level (0.001% parasitized erythrocytes) of light microscopy.[74] Many different PCR assays have been published for the identification and differentiation of *Babesia* infections, and several commercial diagnostic laboratories offer real-time PCR assays for detection of *Babesia* infection. Species identification can then be accomplished by DNA sequencing or by the use of species-specific PCR assays. PCR assays that are designed to detect multiple *Babesia* spp. (i.e., a broad-range *Babesia* PCR) can facilitate screening. A well-designed species-specific assay will only detect one species, and a negative test may lead clinicians to falsely conclude that the patient is not infected with *Babesia* because the wrong species was targeted for testing. In addition, broad-range PCR assays have been helpful for identification of novel *Babesia* species.

Pathologic Findings

The most striking pathologic findings occur in dogs that die from severe babesiosis (usually associated with *B. canis rossi*). These include staining of tissues with hemoglobin or bilirubin, hepatosplenomegaly, lymphadenomegaly, and kidneys that are a dark-reddish color. Edema and hemorrhage, which may indicate vascular injury and poor tissue oxygenation in severely affected dogs, are often most severe in the lungs. Nonparasitized cells often line the endothelial surface with parasitized cells sludged in the lumen. Pathologic changes in the brain of these dogs include congestion, macroscopic and microscopic hemorrhages, sequestration of parasitized erythrocytes in capillary beds, and pavementing of parasitized cells against the endothelium. Cardiac histologic changes include hemorrhage, necrosis, inflammatory infiltrate, and fibrosis. Microthrombi of many tissues may be evident in animals exhibiting signs of DIC. Impression smears of the spleen may substantiate the diagnosis of babesiosis at necropsy. Nonspecific findings in dogs with all forms of babesiosis include erythroid hyperplasia in the bone marrow, extramedullary hematopoiesis of the liver and spleen, mononuclear phagocyte system hyperplasia, and centrilobular necrosis of the liver. Vasculitis has been observed in *B. conradae* infections and is associated with hepatitis and lymphadenitis with multifocal deposits of IgM in inflamed arteries and renal glomeruli.[60] In chronic canine babesiosis and feline babesiosis, the only gross finding may be splenomegaly.

Treatment and Prognosis

Antiprotozoal Treatment

Dogs

Dogs generally show clinical improvement within 24 to 72 hours of treatment with antibabesial drugs, but some animals take as long as 7 days to respond (Table 75-2). Imidocarb

TABLE 75-2

Selected Antibabesial Compounds Used in the Treatment of Dogs and Cats

					Organism			
Generic Name*	Dose (mg/kg)	Route	Interval (hours)	Duration (days)	*Babesia canis*	*Babesia gibsoni*	*Babesia conradae*	*Babesia felis*
Imidocarb dipropionate†	5-6.6 7.5	IM IM	Once Once	Repeat in 14 NA	+++	+	+	—
Diminazene aceturate	3.5-5	IM	Once‡	NA	+++	++	?	+
Azithromycin§ *and* Atovaquone§	10 13.3	PO PO	24 8	10 10	+++	+++	+++	?
Clindamycin‖ *and* Doxycycline *and* Metronidazole	25 5 15	PO PO PO	12 12 12	90 90 90	+	+	?	?
Primaquine phosphate	0.5 1 mg *per cat*#	PO IM	24 36	1-3 6	? —	— —	? ?	+++ +++

+++, Very good; ++, good; +, fair to poor; —, not effective; ?, unknown.
*For specific information on each drug, see Chapter 10.
†For combination therapy, a dose of 3.5 mg/kg diminazene has been followed by a dose of 6.0 mg/kg imidocarb.
‡Not available in the United States, except by compassionate use. For *B. canis*, this dose is sufficient; for *B. gibsoni*, repeat dose in 24 hours. Total dosages of 7 mg/kg or higher are associated with an increased risk of neural and parasympathomimetic toxicity.
§These two drugs should be used in combination. Atovaquone must be given with a fatty meal to facilitate absorption. The suspension causes minimal gastrointestinal side effects.
‖Anecdotal evidence for activity against *B. canis*. Not effective in clearing the infection. Not recommended as sole therapy because of the potential to develop resistance. Further documentation needed to establish efficacy of this combination (see text).
#Note that 1 mg/kg is a lethal dose.

dipropionate is active against *B. canis*.[75] Imidocarb can eliminate *B. canis*, eliminates infection in ticks that engorge on treated animals for up to 4 weeks after treatment, and prevents infection for up to 6 weeks after a single injection.[76] A single dose of 7.5 mg/kg or a single dose of 6 mg/kg given the day after a dose of diminazene (3.5 mg/kg) also clears infection.[77] In areas where reinfection is likely, some practitioners use a lower dose, 2 mg/kg SC once, that does completely clear infection. This approach is an attempt to induce a state of premunition. Premunition is the immunity of existing infection in which chronic subclinically affected carriers may be resistant to reinfection or at least have reduced morbidity with new infections. In contrast, animals that have been cleared of infection are more susceptible to reinfection with recurrent clinical disease. The risk of this approach is that clinical babesiosis may relapse in some chronic carriers. Therefore, this approach is not recommended for the treatment of canine babesiosis in many parts of the United States, where vector transmission and risk for reinfection are thought to be low. Imidocarb does not clear *B. gibsoni* infections, but reduces morbidity and mortality. Therefore, this is a reasonable alternative treatment for *B. gibsoni* if the owner cannot immediately afford more effective treatments. The same may be true for *B. conradae* infections. Pretreatment with atropine (0.5 mg/kg SC 30 minutes before injection) reduces the adverse effects of imidocarb (see Chapter 10).

Other related aromatic diamidines include diminazene aceturate, phenamidine isethionate, and pentamidine isethionate (see Chapter 10). Although these are not available for treatment of dogs in the United States, the first two of these drugs have been used in many other countries and are highly active against *B. canis*. They do not clear *B. gibsoni* infections, but can reduce morbidity and mortality.

Atovaquone and azithromycin combination therapy is the most effective treatment for *B. gibsoni* and *B. conradae* infections (see Table 75-2).[78,79] Atovaquone and azithromycin are given for 10 days. Atovaquone must be administered with a fatty meal to maximize drug absorption. The treatment appeared to sterilize *B. gibsoni* infections or reduce the parasitemia below detectable limits in approximately 80% of dogs in a randomized double-blind placebo-controlled trial.[79] However, in another study, this combination only eliminated *B. gibsoni* infection (or reduced parasitemia below detectable limits of PCR assay), in 2 of 7 dogs.[80] It also did not clear experimental infection with two Australian isolates of *B. gibsoni*.[81] When atovaquone is used alone to treat *B. gibsoni* infection, recrudescence of infection develops more than 30 days after treatment.[81] Drug resistance has been identified in vitro, so atovaquone should always be used in combination with other drugs. Mutations in the genes that encode the putative molecular target of atovaquone have been identified in *B. gibsoni* isolated from dogs that failed to clear infection after atovaquone treatment.[80,82]

In this author's experience, dogs that fail to clear *B. gibsoni* infections after initial treatment with atovaquone and azithromycin will not clear their infection after a follow-up treatment with the same drugs, although clinical disease may resolve. There are also two commercially available formulations of atovaquone: a single-drug liquid suspension that is very well tolerated, and a combination tablet product (atovaquone and proguanil hydrochloride). Although the combination product is less expensive, it causes severe vomiting in some patients. Because drug absorption is critical and resistance to atovaquone can develop or be selected, this author recommends *only* use of the suspension. Dogs that have been splenectomized before treatment do not appear to clear infections with treatment.[83] Likewise, immunosuppressive therapy may reduce the ability of antibabesial treatment to clear dogs of *B. gibsoni* infection. The recommended follow-up after treatment with atovaquone and azithromycin is a minimum of two PCR tests approximately 60 and 90 days after completing treatment.

An alternative treatment strategy can be used to treat *B. gibsoni* infections that fail to respond to atovaquone and azithromycin.[84] This regimen involves a combination of clindamycin, metronidazole, and doxycycline for a minimum of 3 months (see Table 75-2). In an uncontrolled study, 3 of 4 experimentally infected dogs had negative PCR assay results after treatment, whereas 1 dog remained persistently infected and experienced clinical relapses during treatment.[84] Clearance of the infection as determined by PCR was not detected until 30 and 72 days after completing a 90-day treatment course in 2 dogs. The PCR test result became negative in the third dog 12 days into treatment. Three of the dogs were initially treated with three doses of diminazene aceturate. In another study, 3 naturally infected dogs that had clinical relapse after or during atovaquone and azithromycin treatment had clinical recoveries after treatment with the clindamycin, metronidazole, and doxycycline combination.[80] The small number of cases reported and the high degree of variability in the PCR results after treatment make the efficacy of this combination uncertain. However, as with the atovaquone-azithromycin combination, PCR testing should be performed 60 and 90 days after completing therapy.

Aggressive supportive care and monotherapy with clindamycin (25 mg/kg PO q12h for 7 to 21 days) has been recommended if specific antibabesial drugs are not available. At this dosage, clinical abnormalities resolve even if organism clearance does not occur. This author *does not* recommend this practice for *B. gibsoni*–infected dogs, because it has the potential to select for macrolide resistance and interfere with subsequent atovaquone and azithromycin treatment.

Other treatments that have been used to treat *B. canis* infections are quinuronium sulfate and 1% trypan blue solution. Trypan blue does not clear infections and results in bluish discoloration of tissues and plasma.

Cats

Treatment of feline babesiosis has not been as critically evaluated, but most antibabesial drugs appear ineffective. Primaquine phosphate, an antimalarial compound, administered orally or as an intramuscular injection, is currently the drug of choice (see Table 75-2). However, the effective dose, 0.5 mg/kg, is very close to the lethal dose (1 mg/kg). In experimental studies, rifampin and trimethoprim-sulfadiazine were not as effective as primaquine.[85]

Supportive Care

Other supportive care measures that may be required to treat animals with babesiosis are packed red blood cell transfusions and intravenous crystalloid fluid therapy. The administration of the plasma component of whole blood is unnecessary in the majority of dogs with babesiosis and can place the patient at risk of volume overload. If rehydration is required, crystalloid replacement solutions are preferable. Whether glucocorticoids are indicated to counteract the immune-mediated complications of babesiosis is controversial. In one study, 21% of

134 dogs with *B. canis rossi* infection had hemolytic anemias that did not respond to antibabesial therapy alone.[63] This seems less common with *B. canis vogeli* or *B. gibsoni* infections, because these often respond completely to antibabesial treatment alone. In most dogs that require glucocorticoids, the glucocorticoid dosage can be tapered and discontinued within a 2- to 3-week period. Continued glucocorticoid therapy may predispose the animals to other infections and has the potential to induce babesial relapse.[86]

Immunity and Vaccination

The duration of protective immunity against *B. canis* infection is limited. Antibody titers may gradually decline between 3 and 5 months after infection.[76] Recovered dogs are protected against homologous infection within 5 to 8 months after infection.[76] Cross-protection between strains does not occur, and seropositivity does not guarantee protection against heterologous challenge.

A vaccine produced from cell-culture–derived exoantigens of *B. canis canis* is available in Europe.[87] An efficacy of 70% to 100% has been reported, with the disease occasionally seen in the vaccinates generally being mild. Other field studies have been less impressive. Vaccination does not prevent infection but appears to block initiation of many of the pathologic processes involved in disease pathogenesis.[88,89] Vaccines may limit parasitemia and reduce development of anemia and splenomegaly. A bivalent vaccine derived from soluble parasite antigens from *B. canis canis* and *B. canis rossi* (Nobivac Piro, MSD Animal Health South Africa) reduces clinical signs after challenge with both species.[90,91] Differences in strain antigenicity limit the usefulness of the commercial vaccine in other areas. Because *B. canis* vaccines do not cross protect against all *B. canis* subspecies, they are highly unlikely to protect against other *Babesia* species.

Prevention

Treatment of babesiosis is expensive and may be ineffective, so prevention is of paramount importance. Preventive measures alone may be sufficient to control *B. canis* outbreaks in kennels in the southeastern United States. The primary means of prevention is tick control (see Prevention section in Chapter 28). Early tick identification and removal is important because it likely takes a minimum of 2 to 3 days of feeding for transmission of the parasite to occur. Dogs should be tested, treated if necessary, and quarantined before being introduced into a colony. The use of amitraz-impregnated collars significantly reduced new infections in a *B. canis rossi*–endemic area. In this study none of 20 dogs treated with the collars acquired infections, compared to 27% of 30 control dogs that received no tick prevention.[92] Prevention of aggressive interactions with other dogs (especially fighting breeds such as American pit bull terriers) may also prevent infection. All prospective canine blood donors should be tested for babesiosis with serology and PCR assays, and animals positive by either or both methods should not be used for blood donation.

Of 16,000 greyhounds adopted through rescue leagues in 1995, 20% to 60% were seropositive for *B. canis*. Much of this screening was done before the availability of PCR assays, and serologic testing results likely overestimate the true prevalence of infection. The likelihood that an adopted greyhound will develop clinical babesiosis or directly transmit infection to other dogs is low. However, the risk to other dogs is great if the infected animal is placed in a breeding kennel in which dogs are housed together and tick control is not adequate, or if the animal is used as a blood donor. Treatment with imidocarb dipropionate may eliminate the *B. canis* carrier status. This approach should be considered in situations in which risk of spread is likely. In other situations, the owner should be made aware of the seropositive status so that should clinical signs consistent with babesiosis arise, the attending veterinarian can be alerted to the possibility of the disease. Splenectomy should be avoided if possible in these dogs should it become indicated.

Public Health Aspects

Canine and feline *Babesia* spp. do not appear to pose a zoonotic risk to immunocompetent humans. Their risks to immunocompromised individuals are unknown, but as with many infectious diseases, people who are undergoing chemotherapy, are infected with HIV, or have been splenectomized should exercise special caution when handling blood samples from dogs. Babesiosis is a rare tick-borne zoonosis of people in Europe and in the United States, and isolated uncharacterized *Babesia* infections have been reported in Africa and Mexico.[93] The majority of infections are mild or asymptomatic; however, some result in severe illness and death. Splenectomized people or those older than 55 years are especially at risk.[94,95] No *Babesia* species has been identified that is host specific for people. Sylvan cycles with wild animal reservoirs occur in nature. People serve as accidental hosts for *Babesia* of animals when they are bitten by infected ticks. Transmission through blood transfusion has also been described. *B. microti* is the primary parasite that infects people in the northeast and upper Midwest of the United States. The vector tick is *Ixodes scapularis*, which can co-transmit anaplasmosis and Lyme borreliosis. The hemolytic disease with flu-like symptoms is usually mild and self-limiting or easily treated with clindamycin and quinine. Both asymptomatic infections and clinical babesiosis with severe anemia have been reported in people in California and Washington and is caused by the more recently described parasite *Babesia duncani*.[96-98]

Babesia divergens causes a severe form of human babesiosis in Europe, which usually occurs in people who have had a splenectomy and is often fatal. Babesiosis was also identified in splenectomized people from Italy and Austria with a new strain (EU1) that was more closely related to *Babesia odocoilei*.[98] Identical isolates of *Babesia* have been found in *Ixodes ricinus* ticks from Slovenia, suggesting a more widespread distribution of this organism in Europe.

CASE EXAMPLE

Signalment: "Dora," a 4-year-old female spayed American Staffordshire terrier from North Carolina

History: Dora was evaluated for a 3- to 4-day history of anorexia and lethargy. Before referral, an ELISA that detects heartworm antigen and antibodies to *E. canis* or *B. burgdorferi* antigens was performed and the results were negative. The dog had mild anemia (HCT 28.4%) and moderate thrombocytopenia (59,000 platelets/μL) on an automated hematology analyzer. Amoxicillin–clavulanic acid, doxycycline, and famotidine were prescribed. The patient began showing signs of increased energy and appetite as well as an increase in the HCT (38%) and platelet count (147,000 platelets/μL) after 4 weeks of treatment. However, because the values did not return to within reference range, the case was referred.

Physical Examination:

Body Weight: 24.2 kg.

General: Bright, alert, responsive, hydrated. T = 101.6°C (38.7°F), HR = 100 beats/min, RR = 24 breaths/min, mucous membranes pink, CRT <2 s. Physical examination was otherwise unremarkable.

Selected Laboratory Findings:

	Pretreatment	Posttreatment	Reference Range
PCV (%)	41	52	39-58
Platelet count (× 10^3/μL)	80	361	190-468
TP (g/dL)	6.3	6.5	5.2-7.3
Albumin (g/dL)	2.7	3.8	3-3.9
Globulin (g/dL)	3.5	2.7	1.7-3.8
Albumin/globulin ratio	0.78	1.38	0.9-1.8
Visualization of *Babesia* on microscopic examination of blood smear	Negative	Negative	
Babesia canis IFA	1:256	ND	
Ehrlichia canis IFA	<1:16	ND	
Bartonella vinsonii IFA	<1:16	ND	
Bartonella henselae IFA	<1:16	ND	
Rickettsia rickettsii IFA	1:64	ND	
SNAP 4Dx ELISA	Negative for all agents	ND	
Babesia spp. PCR	Positive (*B. gibsoni*)	Negative	

Diagnosis: *Babesia gibsoni* infection.

Treatment: Atovaquone and azithromycin.

Comments: Dogs with babesiosis often have a positive clinical response to doxycycline, which leads clinicians to suspect rickettsial infection. Although fever is considered a classic sign of babesiosis, most dogs are afebrile during initial examination, and waxing and waning fever is often documented with serial rectal temperatures. Thrombocytopenia is often a more prominent hematologic finding than anemia and may be the only finding in some cases. Babesiosis may be associated with changes in both albumin and globulin concentrations. Hypoalbuminemia can be secondary to proteinuria (not documented in this case). Globulins are often increased, although they may not be above the high end of the reference range. Organisms are frequently not observed on routine examination of stained blood smears, and PCR assay is required to document infection. Panels that detect antibodies to tick-borne pathogens typically either do not include *Babesia* spp. at all or only detect antibodies against *B. canis*. Serologic cross-reactivity between species can occur, leading to inappropriate diagnosis and treatment recommendations. The positive titer to *Rickettsia* spp. was interesting, but in this geographic location, approximately 20% to 25% of healthy dogs are seropositive to *Rickettsia* spp., so its significance was unclear. Although acute phase serology for *B. gibsoni* was not done, a convalescent titer to *B. gibsoni* at a follow up examination was 1:64.

SUGGESTED READINGS

Birkenheuer AJ, Correa MT, Levy MG, et al. Geographic distribution of babesiosis among dogs in the United States and association with dog bites: 150 cases (2000-2003). J Am Vet Med Assoc. 2005;227:942-947.

Di Cicco MF, Downey ME, Beeler E, et al. Re-emergence of *Babesia conradae* and effective treatment of infected dogs with atovaquone and azithromycin. Vet Parasitol. 2012;187:23-27.

Jefferies R, Ryan UM, Jardine J, et al. *Babesia gibsoni*: detection during experimental infections and after combined atovaquone and azithromycin therapy. Exp Parasitol. 2007;117:115-123.

REFERENCES

1. Hutcheon D. Diseases amongst dogs. Malignant jaundice or bilious fever of the dog. Agric J Cape Good Hope. 1893;6:476-477.
2. Eaton P. *Piroplasma canis* in Florida. J Parasitol. 1934;20:312-313.
3. Abu MIH, Naito I, et al. *Babesia* infections in puppies: probably due to transplacental transmission. J Vet Med B Infect Dis Immunol Food Hyg Vet Public Health. 1973;609:203-206.
4. Fukumoto S, Suzuki H, Igarashi I, et al. Fatal experimental transplacental *Babesia gibsoni* infections in dogs. Int J Parasitol. 2005;35:1031-1035.
5. Itoh N, Itoh S. A case of canine babesiosis possibly developed by transplacental infection. J Jpn Vet Med Assoc. 1990;43:275-276.
6. Uilenberg G, Franssen FF, Perie NM, et al. Three groups of *Babesia canis* distinguished and a proposal for nomenclature. Vet Q. 1989;11:33-40.
7. Taboada J, Harvey JW, Levy MG, et al. Seroprevalence of babesiosis in Greyhounds in Florida. J Am Vet Med Assoc. 1992;200:47-50.
8. Bobade PA, Oduye OO, Aghomo HO. Prevalence of antibodies against *Babesia canis* in dogs in an endemic area. Rev Elev Med Vet Pays Trop. 1989;42:211-217.

9. Harvey JW, Taboada J, Lewis JC. Babesiosis in a litter of pups. J Am Vet Med Assoc. 1988;192:1751-1752.
10. Cassini R, Zanutto S, Frangipane di Regalbono A, et al. Canine piroplasmosis in Italy: epidemiological aspects in vertebrate and invertebrate hosts. Vet Parasitol. 2009;165:30-35.
11. Bourdoiseau G. Canine babesiosis in France. Vet Parasitol. 2006;138:118-125.
12. Zygner W, Gorski P, Wedrychowicz H. New localities of *Dermacentor reticulatus* tick (vector of *Babesia canis canis*) in central and eastern Poland. Pol J Vet Sci. 2009;12:549-555.
13. Welc-Faleciak R, Rodo A, Sinski E, et al. *Babesia canis* and other tick-borne infections in dogs in Central Poland. Vet Parasitol. 2009;166:191-198.
14. Apanaskevich DA, Horak IG, Camicas JL. Redescription of *Haemaphysalis (Rhipistoma) elliptica* (Koch, 1844), an old taxon of the *Haemaphysalis (Rhipistoma) leachi* group from East and southern Africa, and of *Haemaphysalis (Rhipistoma) leachi* (Audouin, 1826) (Ixodida, Ixodidae). Onderstepoort J Vet Res. 2007;74:181-208.
15. Collett MG. Survey of canine babesiosis in South Africa. J S Afr Vet Assoc. 2000;71:180-186.
16. Shakespeare AS. The incidence of canine babesiosis amongst sick dogs presented to the Onderstepoort Veterinary Academic Hospital. J S Afr Vet Assoc. 1995;66:247-250.
17. Reyers F, Leisewitz AL, Lobetti RG, et al. Canine babesiosis in South Africa: more than one disease. Does this serve as a model for falciparum malaria? Ann Trop Med Parasitol. 1998;92:503-511.
18. Birkenheuer AJ, Neel J, Ruslander D, et al. Detection and molecular characterization of a novel large *Babesia* species in a dog. Vet Parasitol. 2004;124:151-160.
19. Holman PJ, Backlund BB, Wilcox AL, et al. Detection of a large unnamed *Babesia* piroplasm originally identified in dogs in North Carolina in a dog with no history of travel to that state. J Am Vet Med Assoc. 2009;235:851-854.
20. Sikorski LE, Birkenheuer AJ, Holowaychuk MK, et al. Babesiosis caused by a large *Babesia* species in 7 immunocompromised dogs. J Vet Intern Med. 2010;24:127-131.
21. Holm LP, Kerr MG, Trees AJ, et al. Fatal babesiosis in an untravelled British dog. Vet Rec. 2006;159:179-180.
22. Konishi K, Sakata Y, Miyazaki N, et al. Epidemiological survey of *Babesia gibsoni* infection in dogs in Japan by enzyme-linked immunosorbent assay using B. *gibsoni* thrombospondin-related adhesive protein antigen. Vet Parasitol. 2008;155:204-208.
23. Matsuu A, Kawabe A, Koshida Y, et al. Incidence of canine *Babesia gibsoni* infection and subclinical infection among Tosa dogs in Aomori Prefecture. Japan. J Vet Med Sci. 2004;66:893-897.
24. Swaminath CS, Shortt HE. The arthropod vector of *Babesia gibsoni*. Indian J Med Res. 1937;25:499-503.
25. Higuchi S, Fujimori M, Hoshi F, et al. Development of *Babesia gibsoni* in the salivary glands of the larval tick, *Rhipicephalus sanguineus*. J Vet Med Sci. 1995;57:117-119.
26. Higuchi S, Izumitani M, Hoshi H, et al. Development of *Babesia gibsoni* in the midgut of larval tick, *Rhipicephalus sanguineus*. J Vet Med Sci. 1999;61:689-691.
27. Higuchi S, Fujimori M, Hoshi F, et al. Observations on the development of *Babesia gibsoni* in the midgut of adult female *Rhipicephalus sanguineus* ticks. Jpn J Parasitol. 1994;43:308-311.
28. Sen SK. The vector of canine piroplasmosis due to *Piroplasma gibsoni*. Indian J Vet Sci Anim Husb. 1933;3:356-363.
29. Birkenheuer AJ, Correa MT, Levy MG, et al. Geographic distribution of babesiosis among dogs in the United States and association with dog bites: 150 cases (2000-2003). J Am Vet Med Assoc. 2005;227:942-947.
30. Wang C, Ahluwalia SK, Li Y, et al. Frequency and therapy monitoring of canine *Babesia* spp. infection by high-resolution melting curve quantitative FRET-PCR. Vet Parasitol. 2010;168:11-18.
31. Kjemtrup AM, Conrad PA. A review of the small canine piroplasms from California: *Babesia conradae* in the literature. Vet Parasitol. 2006;138:112-117.
32. Kjemtrup AM, Wainwright K, Miller M, et al. *Babesia conradae*, sp. nov., a small canine *Babesia* identified in California. Vet Parasitol. 2006;138:103-111.
33. Yamane I, Gardner SR, Telford T, et al. Vector competence of *Rhipicephalus sanguineus* and *Dermacentor variabilis* for American isolates of *Babesia gibsoni*. Exp Appl Acarol. 1993;17:913-919.
34. Dear JD, Owens SD, Biondo A, et al. *Babesia conradae* infection in coyote hunting dogs infected with multiple blood-borne pathogens. In: American College of Veterinary Internal Medicine Forum, New Orleans, LA, 2012.
35. Camacho AT, Guitian EJ, Pallas E, et al. Azotemia and mortality among *Babesia microti*–like infected dogs. J Vet Intern Med. 2004;18:141-146.
36. Camacho AT, Pallas E, Gestal JJ, et al. Infection of dogs in north-west Spain with a *Babesia microti*–like agent. Vet Rec. 2001;149:552-555.
37. Garcia AT. Piroplasma infection in dogs in northern Spain. Vet Parasitol. 2006;138:97-102.
38. Zahler M, Rinder H, Schein E, et al. Detection of a new pathogenic *Babesia microti*–like species in dogs. Vet Parasitol. 2000;89:241-248.
39. Yeagley TJ, Reichard MV, Hempstead JE, et al. Detection of *Babesia gibsoni* and the canine small *Babesia* "Spanish isolate" in blood samples obtained from dogs confiscated from dogfighting operations. J Am Vet Med Assoc. 2009;235:535-539.
40. Birkenheuer AJ, Horney B, Bailey M, et al. *Babesia microti*–like infections are prevalent in North American foxes. Vet Parasitol. 2010;172:179-182.
41. Criado-Fornelio A, Martinez-Marcos A, Buling-Sarana A, et al. Molecular studies on *Babesia, Theileria* and *Hepatozoon* in southern Europe. Part I. Epizootiological aspects. Vet Parasitol. 2003;113:189-201.
42. Camacho AT, Pallas E, Gestal JJ, et al. *Ixodes hexagonus* is the main candidate as vector of *Theileria annae* in northwest Spain. Vet Parasitol. 2003;112:157-163.
43. Penzhorn BL, Schoeman T, Jacobson LS. Feline babesiosis in South Africa: a review. Ann N Y Acad Sci. 2004;1026:183-186.
44. Penzhorn BL, Stylianides E, Coetzee MA, et al. A focus of feline babesiosis at Kaapschehoop on the Mpumalanga escarpment. J S Afr Vet Assoc. 1999;70:60.
45. Jacobson LS, Schoeman T, Lobetti RG. A survey of feline babesiosis in South Africa. J S Afr Vet Assoc. 2000;71:222-228.
46. Bosman AM, Venter EH, Penzhorn BL. Occurrence of *Babesia felis* and *Babesia leo* in various wild felid species and domestic cats in Southern Africa, based on reverse line blot analysis. Vet Parasitol. 2007;144:33-38.
47. Mendes-de-Almeida F, Faria MC, Branco AS, et al. Sanitary conditions of a colony of urban feral cats (*Felis catus* Linnaeus, 1758) in a zoological garden of Rio de Janeiro, Brazil. Rev Inst Med Trop Sao Paulo. 2004;46:269-274.
48. Criado-Fornelio A, Martinez-Marcos A, Buling-Sarana A, et al. Presence of *Mycoplasma haemofelis, Mycoplasma haemominutum* and piroplasmids in cats from southern Europe: a molecular study. Vet Microbiol. 2003;93:307-317.
49. Baneth G, Kenny MJ, Tasker S, et al. Infection with a proposed new subspecies of *Babesia canis, Babesia canis* subsp. *presentii*, in domestic cats. J Clin Microbiol. 2004;42:99-105.
50. Adaszek L, Ukaszewska J, Winiarczyk S, et al. The first case of feline babesiosis in Poland. Zycie Weterynaryjne. 2008;83:668-670.
51. Birkenheuer AJ. Unpublished observations, 2012.
52. Hossain MA, Yamato O, Yamasaki M, et al. Serum from dogs infected with *Babesia gibsoni* inhibits maturation of reticulocytes and erythrocyte 5′-nucleotidase activity in vitro. J Vet Med Sci. 2003;65:1281-1286.
53. Lobetti RG, Reyers F. Met-haemoglobinuria in naturally occurring *Babesia canis* infection. J S Afr Vet Assoc. 1996;67:88-90.
54. Makinde MO, Bobade PA. Osmotic fragility of erythrocytes in clinically normal dogs and dogs infected with parasites. Res Vet Sci. 1994;57:343-348.

55. Murase T, Ueda T, Yamato O, et al. Oxidative damage and enhanced erythrophagocytosis in canine erythrocytes infected with *Babesia gibsoni*. J Vet Med Sci. 1996;58:259-261.
56. Otsuka Y, Yamasaki M, Yamato O, et al. Increased generation of superoxide in erythrocytes infected with *Babesia gibsoni*. J Vet Med Sci. 2001;63:1077-1081.
57. Sykes JE. Unpublished observations, 2012.
58. Pomianowski A, Lew S, Kuleta Z, et al. Peritoneal dialysis in a dog with acute renal failure caused by the infection with *Babesia canis*. Pol J Natural Sci. 2008;23:257-267.
59. Suh M, Chung M. Pathogenicity in experimentally infected dogs with *Babesia gibsoni*. Kor J Vet Res. 2000;40:587-599.
60. Wozniak EJ, Barr BC, Thomford JW, et al. Clinical, anatomic, and immunopathologic characterization of *Babesia gibsoni* infection in the domestic dog (*Canis familiaris*). J Parasitol. 1997;83:692-699.
61. Camacho AT, Pallas E, Gestal JJ, et al. Natural infection by a *Babesia microti*–like piroplasm in a splenectomised dog. Vet Rec. 2002;150:381-382.
62. Guitian FJ, Camacho AT, Telford SR, 3rd. Case-control study of canine infection by a newly recognised *Babesia microti*–like piroplasm. Prev Vet Med. 2003;61:137-145.
63. Jacobson LS, Clark IA. The pathophysiology of canine babesiosis: new approaches to an old puzzle. J S Afr Vet Assoc. 1994;65:134-145.
64. Leisewitz AL, Jacobson LS, de Morais HS, et al. The mixed acid-base disturbances of severe canine babesiosis. J Vet Intern Med. 2001;15:445-452.
65. Nel M, Lobetti RG, Keller N, et al. Prognostic value of blood lactate, blood glucose, and hematocrit in canine babesiosis. J Vet Intern Med. 2004;18:471-476.
66. Omamegbe JO, Uche UE. Haemogram studies in Nigerian local dogs suffering from ancylostomiasis, babesiosis, and trypanosomiasis. Bull Anim Health Prod Afr. 1985;33:335-338.
67. Irwin PJ, Hutchinson GW. Clinical and pathological findings of *Babesia* infection in dogs. Aust Vet J. 1991;68:204-209.
68. Zygner W, Gojska O, Rapacka G, et al. Hematological changes during the course of canine babesiosis caused by large *Babesia* in domestic dogs in Warsaw (Poland). Vet Parasitol. 2007;145:146-151.
69. Schoeman T, Lobetti RG, Jacobson LS, et al. Feline babesiosis: signalment, clinical pathology and concurrent infections. J S Afr Vet Assoc. 2001;72:4-11.
70. Matthewman LA, Kelly PJ, Bobade PA, et al. Infections with *Babesia canis* and *Ehrlichia canis* in dogs in Zimbabwe. Vet Rec. 1993;133:344-346.
71. Bohm M, Leisewitz AL, Thompson PN, et al. Capillary and venous *Babesia canis rossi* parasitaemias and their association with outcome of infection and circulatory compromise. Vet Parasitol. 2006;141:18-29.
72. Mattia AR, Waldron MA, Sierra LS. Use of the Quantitative Buffy Coat system for detection of parasitemia in patients with babesiosis. J Clin Microbiol. 1993;31:2816-2818.
73. Comazzi S, Paltrinieri S, Manfredi MT, et al. Diagnosis of canine babesiosis by Percoll gradient separation of parasitized erythrocytes. J Vet Diagn Invest. 1999;11:102-104.
74. Birkenheuer AJ, Levy MG, Breitschwerdt EB. Development and evaluation of a seminested PCR for detection and differentiation of *Babesia gibsoni* (Asian genotype) and *B. canis* DNA in canine blood samples. J Clin Microbiol. 2003;41:4172-4177.
75. Adeyanju BJ, Aliu YO. Chemotherapy of canine ehrlichiosis and babesiosis with imidocarb dipropionate. J Am Anim Hosp Assoc. 1982;18:827-830.
76. Vercammen F, De Deken R, Maes L. Duration of protective immunity in experimental canine babesiosis after homologous and heterologous challenge. Vet Parasitol. 1997;68:51-55.
77. Penzhorn BL, Lewis BD, de Waal DT, et al. Sterilisation of *Babesia canis* infections by imidocarb alone or in combination with diminazene. J S Afr Vet Assoc. 1995;66:157-159.
78. Di Cicco MF, Downey ME, Beeler E, et al. Re-emergence of *Babesia conradae* and effective treatment of infected dogs with atovaquone and azithromycin. Vet Parasitol. 2012;187:23-27.
79. Birkenheuer AJ, Levy MG, Breitschwerdt EB. Efficacy of combined atovaquone and azithromycin for therapy of chronic *Babesia gibsoni* (Asian genotype) infections in dogs. J Vet Intern Med. 2004;18:494-498.
80. Sakuma M, Setoguchi A, Endo Y. Possible emergence of drug-resistant variants of *Babesia gibsoni* in clinical cases treated with atovaquone and azithromycin. J Vet Intern Med. 2009;23:493-498.
81. Jefferies R, Ryan UM, Jardine J, et al. *Babesia gibsoni*: detection during experimental infections and after combined atovaquone and azithromycin therapy. Exp Parasitol. 2007;117:115-123.
82. Matsuu A, Miyamoto K, Ikadai H, et al. Short report: cloning of the *Babesia gibsoni* cytochrome B gene and isolation of three single nucleotide polymorphisms from parasites present after atovaquone treatment. Am J Trop Med Hyg. 2006;74:593-597.
83. Stegeman JR, Birkenheuer AJ, Kruger JM, et al. Transfusion-associated *Babesia gibsoni* infection in a dog. J Am Vet Med Assoc. 2003;222:959-963:952.
84. Suzuki K, Wakabayashi H, Takahashi M, et al. A possible treatment strategy and clinical factors to estimate the treatment response in *Babesia gibsoni* infection. J Vet Med Sci. 2007;69:563-568.
85. Penzhorn BL, Lewis BD, Lopez-Rebollar LM, et al. Screening of five drugs for efficacy against *Babesia felis* in experimentally infected cats. J S Afr Vet Assoc. 2000;71:53-57.
86. Masuda T, Baba E, Arakawa A. Relapse of canine babesiosis after prednisolone treatment. Mod Vet Pract. 1983;64:931-932.
87. Moreau Y, Vidor E, Bissuel G, et al. Vaccination against canine babesiosis: an overview of field observations. Trans R Soc Trop Med Hyg. 1989;83(suppl):95-96.
88. Schetters TH, Kleuskens J, Scholtes N, et al. Strain variation limits protective activity of vaccines based on soluble *Babesia canis* antigens. Parasite Immunol. 1995;17:215-218.
89. Schetters TP, Kleuskens JA, Scholtes NC, et al. Vaccination of dogs against *Babesia canis* infection. Vet Parasitol. 1997;73:35-41.
90. MSD Animal Health South Africa. 2009. http://www.msd-animal-health.co.za/whats_new/informative_articles/995.aspx. Last accessed October 20, 2012.
91. Schetters TP, Kleuskens J, Carcy B, et al. Vaccination against large *Babesia* species from dogs. Parassitologia. 2007;49(suppl 1):13-17.
92. Last RD, Hill JM, Matjila PT, et al. A field trial evaluation of the prophylactic efficacy of amitraz-impregnated collars against canine babesiosis (*Babesia canis rossi*) in South Africa. J S Afr Vet Assoc. 2007;78:63-65.
93. Kjemtrup AM, Conrad PA. Human babesiosis: an emerging tick-borne disease. Int J Parasitol. 2000;30:1323-1337.
94. Persing DH, Herwaldt BL, Glaser C, et al. Infection with a *Babesia*-like organism in northern California. N Engl J Med. 1995;332:298-303.
95. Falagas ME, Klempner MS. Babesiosis in patients with AIDS: a chronic infection presenting as fever of unknown origin. Clin Infect Dis. 1996;22:809-812.
96. Quick RE, Herwaldt BL, Thomford JW, et al. Babesiosis in Washington State: a new species of *Babesia*? Ann Intern Med. 1993;119:284-290.
97. Conrad PA, Kjemtrup AM, Carreno RA, et al. Description of *Babesia duncani* n.sp. (Apicomplexa: Babesiidae) from humans and its differentiation from other piroplasms. J Parasitol. 2006;36:779-789.
98. Herwaldt BL, de Bruyn G, Pieniazek NJ, et al. *Babesia divergens*–like infection, Washington State. Emerg Infect Dis. 2004;10:622-629.

CHAPTER 76

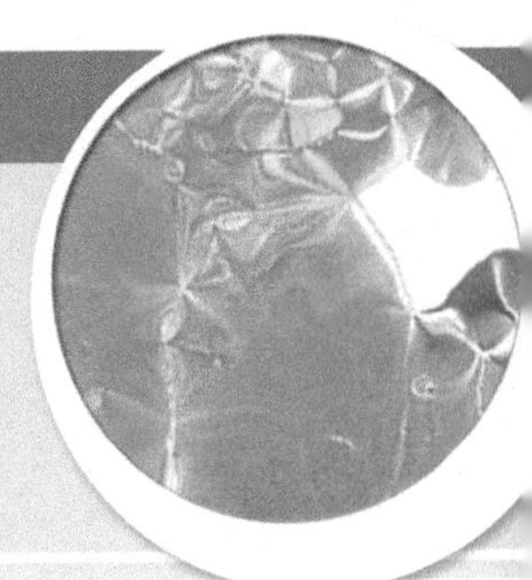

Cytauxzoonosis

Leah A. Cohn

> **Overview of Cytauxzoonosis**
>
> First Described: *Cytauxzoon felis* was first described in domestic cats from Missouri in 1976[1]
>
> Cause: *Cytauxzoon felis,* a hemoprotozoan parasite (phylum Apicomplexa)
>
> Affected Hosts: Any felid; bobcats are the major reservoir host.
>
> Mode of Transmission: *Amblyomma americanum* (Lone Star tick), possibly *Dermacentor variabilis* (American dog tick)
>
> Geographic Distribution: South central, southeastern, and mid-Atlantic United States, and South America
>
> Major Clinical Signs: Lethargy, anorexia, dyspnea, fever, icterus, anemia
>
> Differential Diagnosis: Hemotropic mycoplasmosis, tularemia, cholangiohepatitis, sepsis, primary immune-mediated hemolytic anemia, oxidative toxicities, toxoplasmosis, feline infectious peritonitis
>
> Human Health Significance: *Cytauxzoon felis* is not known to infect humans.

Etiology and Epidemiology

Cytauxzoonosis, a life-threatening acute febrile illness of cats, is caused by the hemoprotozoan parasite *Cytauxzoon felis,* an apicomplexan parasite within the order Piroplasmida and family Theileriidae.[2] The parasite infects both domestic and wild Felidae, but not other mammals.[3] Both *Amblyomma americanum* (Lone Star ticks) and *Dermacentor variabilis* (American dog ticks) harbor the pathogen and are competent transmission vectors, although it is likely that *Amblyomma* ticks are the more important natural disease vectors.[4-6]

As for other apicomplexan parasites, the parasite life cycle involves sexual reproduction in the vector tick and asexual reproduction in the mammalian host. The parasite is inoculated into the host as a sporozoite when an infected tick vector feeds. As for other members of the *Theileriidae* family, the pathogen exists within the mammalian host in both a non-erythrocytic (schizont) and an erythrocytic (piroplasm) form. Approximately 2 weeks after inoculation, schizogony occurs, whereby mononuclear cells become distended with parasites.[7,8] When these cells rupture, merozoites are released and endocytosed by RBCs, where they are known as piroplasms.[8] The piroplasms are ingested by naïve ticks during feeding (Figure 76-1). The acute illness, known as cytauxzoonosis, occurs during the schizogenous phase of infection, whereas piroplasms can be found both during illness and in healthy carrier cats.

There is no breed, sex, or age predisposition for infection, and retroviral infection has not been proven to predispose cats to infection or disease.[9] Often, infected cats are young adults and previously quite healthy. They are typically outdoor or indoor/outdoor cats from wooded suburban or rural areas, where they are more likely to encounter a tick that has recently fed on an infected bobcat *(Lynx rufus),* the predominant reservoir host.[9,10] Often, multiple cats in a neighborhood are affected nearly simultaneously, which likely reflects the presence of infected ticks. Infection occurs most commonly in spring and summer when the tick vector is most active.[9] Originally identified in only the south-central United States, the geographic range of *C. felis* has expanded simultaneously with expansion in the range of the vector Lone Star ticks. Infections in domestic cats are now recognized throughout the south-central, southeastern, and mid-Atlantic states, and the pathogen has been identified in bobcats as far north as Pennsylvania and North Dakota (Figure 76-2).[10,11]

Clinical Features

Signs and Their Pathogenesis

Owners of cats with cytauxzoonosis usually notice an acute onset of profound lethargy and anorexia in a previously healthy cat. Less consistently, owners report vocalization, elevation of the nictitans, tachypnea and/or dyspnea, or icterus, or that the cat feels warm to the touch.[12] The vast majority of the considerable pathologic damage that occurs during acute illness is due to the schizogenous phase of parasitemia.[8] The degree of schizogony appears to be correlated with severity of disease; bobcats (the natural host) undergo a brief and milder schizogenous phase as compared to domestic cats, and correspondingly illness is less pronounced in bobcats than in domestic cats.[13] Schizont-distended mononuclear cells occlude small veins and capillaries, most notably in the liver, lung, spleen, and lymph nodes.[8,14] Obstruction fuels hypoxic tissue damage and release of inflammatory cytokines, which can lead to systemic inflammatory response syndrome, sepsis, disseminated intravascular coagulation (DIC), and multisystem organ failure. The presence of piroplasms may trigger hemolysis in the later stages of the acute illness; however, hemolysis abates in surviving cats, and hemolytic anemia has not been noted in chronic carriers.[15-18]

Physical Examination Findings

Physical examination findings associated with acute cytauxzoonosis are nonspecific.[8,12,19] The most consistent single finding is fever. Although temperatures greater than 104°F (40°C) are

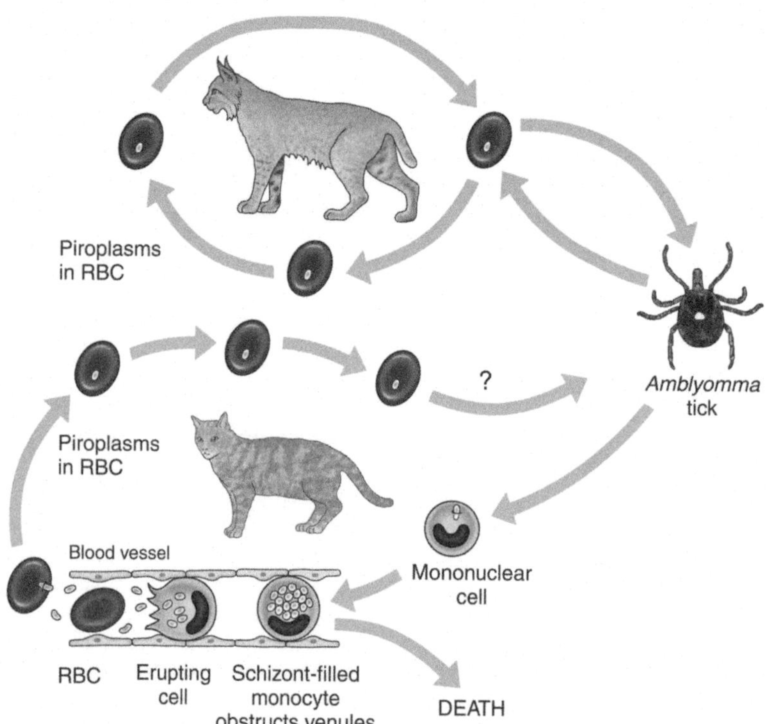

FIGURE 76-1 Life cycle of *Cytauxzoon felis*. The parasite is maintained in bobcats (top) which are subclinically infected. The sexual cycle of the organism occurs in *Amblyomma americanum* hard ticks, which then transmit sporozoites to domestic cats. Sporozoites invade mononuclear cells, where they undergo schizogony. Schizont-filled monocytes obstruct venules and capillaries and cause multiorgan failure and death. In cats that survive the schizogony phase, the organism infects erythrocytes and forms piroplasms. The importance of domestic cats as a reservoir for infection of ticks is unknown. The schizogony stage in the bobcat is relatively mild and brief.

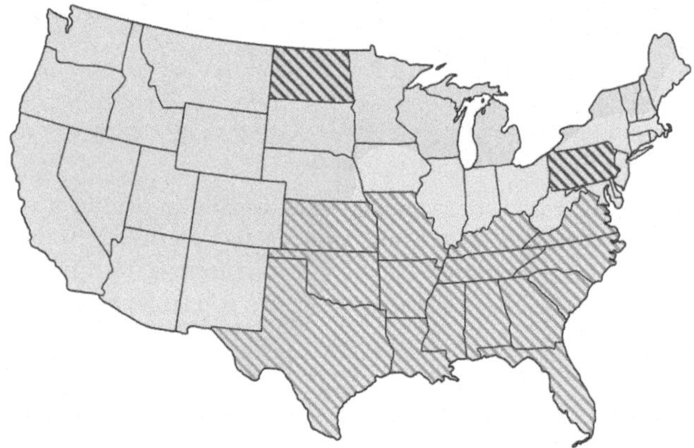

FIGURE 76-2 Geographic distribution of *Cytauxzoon felis* infections. Shaded areas show confirmed cases in either domestic cats *(blue)*, or bobcats only (ND and PA). The yellow region represents the distribution of *Amblyomma americanum* ticks.

common, body temperature drops in moribund animals, and many cats are hypothermic for several hours before death.[8,12] Cats are almost always lethargic. Icterus and pallor are common findings but may not be present initially. The nictitating membrane is commonly elevated (Figure 76-3). Both tachycardia and tachypnea, with or without increased respiratory effort, are also common. Cardiac murmurs are sometimes auscultated, especially in anemic cats. Splenomegaly, hepatomegaly, and lymphadenomegaly may be appreciable. Cats may have seizures or become obtunded shortly before death. Because the onset of illness occurs as long as 2 weeks after the cat is bitten by a tick, ectoparasites are not consistently found on examination.

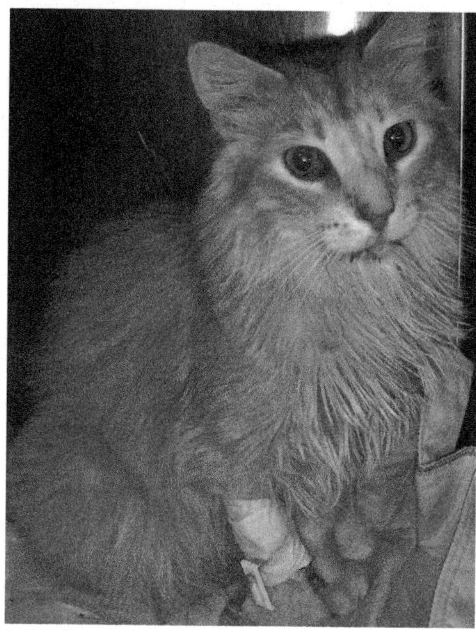

FIGURE 76-3 Cat with *Cytauxzoon felis* infection. There is elevation and hyperemia of the nictitating membranes.

Diagnosis

Laboratory Abnormalities

Complete Blood Count

Abnormalities on the CBC in cats with cytauxzoonosis commonly include pancytopenia or bicytopenia and characteristic signet ring

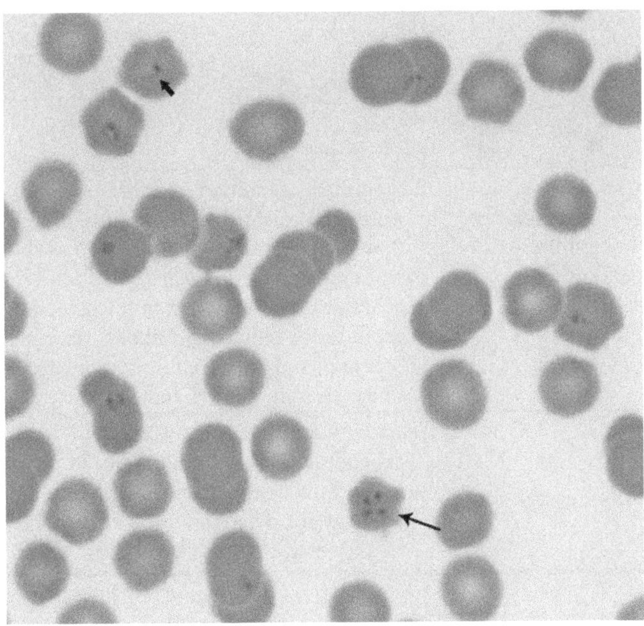

FIGURE 76-4 Wright-Giemsa–stained peripheral blood smear from a cat with cytauxzoonosis at 1000× magnification. Multiple RBC contain signet ring–shaped piroplasms *(short arrow)*; a single RBC demonstrates a tetrad form *(long arrow)*. (Courtesy Dr. Marlyn Whitney, University of Missouri Veterinary Medical Diagnostic Laboratory.)

intraerythrocytic inclusions (see Cytologic Examination) (Figure 76-4). Various combinations of neutropenia, lymphopenia, thrombocytopenia, and nonregenerative anemia are observed.[12,19,20] Occasionally, neutrophilia or bandemia are observed. Although thrombocytopenia is usually identified and may be related to DIC or vasculitis, platelet clumping is common even in healthy cats and can result in false thrombocytopenia. Anemia may be absent at the onset of illness but usually develops about the same time piroplasms become identifiable. Because of the acute nature of the disease, anemia is initially nonregenerative. In recovered carrier cats, cell counts rebound to values within reference ranges, and chronic anemia is not a feature of the carrier state.[15,17,18,21]

Serum Chemistry Profile

Although there are no specific findings on serum chemistry analysis, a number of abnormalities are commonly identified in cats with cytauxzoonosis. Hyperbilirubinemia is common and may result from hepatic vascular occlusion and/or hemolysis. The activities of serum ALP and ALT increase in a minority of sick cats, and increases are usually mild to moderate.[12] Mild to moderate hyperglycemia is common in stressed, sick cats. Mild hypoproteinemia, hypocalcemia, hyponatremia, and hypokalemia can occur during acute illness.[12,19] No consistent abnormalities have been reported on serum chemistry analysis for recovered carrier cats.[17,21]

Urinalysis

Urinalysis results are rarely reported for cats with cytauxzoonosis.[19] Certainly, hyperbilirubinemia may be reflected by bilirubinuria, and hyperglycemia that surpasses the renal threshold may cause mild glucosuria. In the author's experience, the urinalysis is otherwise unremarkable.

Clotting Function

Acute cytauxzoonosis is a form of sepsis and, as such, is expected to be associated with altered coagulability. Thrombocytopenia is common in affected cats, but because platelet clumping occurs readily in cats, the frequency of true thrombocytopenia may be overestimated.[12,19,20] Although not often assayed, prolongation of APTT and PT in several affected cats suggests that DIC is a common complication.[22,23]

Diagnostic Imaging

Imaging studies do not contribute directly to the diagnosis of cytauxzoonosis, and results are seldom reported in the literature. Splenomegaly, hepatomegaly, or both may be identified either on plain radiographs or on abdominal ultrasound examination. Although thoracic radiographic findings are seldom documented in the literature, the author has commonly identified diffuse interstitial pulmonary patterns on radiographs from cats with respiratory signs. Less commonly, alveolar lung patterns or pleural effusion are recognized.

Microbiologic Testing

Diagnostic assays currently available for cytauxzoonosis in cats are described in Table 76-1.

Cytologic Examination of Aspirates or Blood Smears

Careful microscopic examination for intracellular parasites is the most commonly used method for diagnosis of infection. A well-made thin blood smear stained with Wright's stain or Diff Quik should be carefully scanned for either RBC piroplasms or schizont-laden mononuclear cells. Schizont-distended mononuclear cells are sometimes, but not usually, found on careful examination of the entire feathered edge of the blood smear during acute illness (Figure 76-5). If these cells are identified, a diagnosis of acute cytauxzoonosis is confirmed. More commonly, microscopic review allows identification of piroplasms within RBCs. Unfortunately, because illness is most associated with schizogenous replication, illness precedes development of piroplasms in up to half of cats examined. When cytauxzoonosis is suspected but piroplasms are not identified, reexamination of another blood smear the following day may yield positive results. Piroplasms are most often 1 to 1.5 μm, signet ring–shaped inclusions, but tetrad, "safety pin," and coccoid organisms are seen on occasion (see Figures 76-4 and 76-5).[8] Stain precipitate, Howell-Jolly bodies, or other RBC pathogens such as *Mycoplasma haemofelis* have features that distinguish them from *C. felis* piroplasms, but a less experienced microscopist may misidentify them as *C. felis*. Importantly, recovered cats may harbor piroplasms for months to years after initial infection. It is important to realize that piroplasms might be discovered incidentally in chronic carrier cats that survived infection in the distant past. Thus, although identification of piroplasms confirms infection, piroplasms alone (especially in low numbers) cannot confirm that current illness is due to cytauxzoonosis.

When compared with peripheral blood, mononuclear cells distended with merozoites are more commonly identified on fine-needle aspiration (FNA) from spleen, liver, lymph nodes, or lungs of affected cats. Because schizogony precedes piroplasm development, FNA of these organs can rapidly confirm a diagnosis when piroplasms are absent (Figure 76-6).

Molecular Diagnosis using the Polymerase Chain Reaction

PCR assays are the most sensitive diagnostic test for cytauxzoonosis.[18,24] Several commercial veterinary diagnostic laboratories that perform molecular diagnostics offer PCR analysis of whole blood samples for *Cytauxzoon felis* DNA. As with any PCR test, only

TABLE 76-1

Diagnostic Assays Currently Available for Cytauxzoonosis in Cats

Assay	Specimen Type	Target	Performance
Cytologic examination	Whole blood smears, aspirates of lymph nodes, spleen, liver, lung	*Cytauxzoon felis* piroplasms in erythrocytes, or merozoites/schizonts in mononuclear cells or reticuloendothelial tissues	Piroplasms may initially not be visible in acutely ill cats or may be confused with other erythrocyte inclusions such as hemoplasmas or Howell-Jolly bodies. Schizonts may be found in fine-needle aspirates of reticuloendothelial tissues before piroplasms are found on blood smear examination in some cats.
PCR assays	Whole blood	*C. felis* DNA	Sensitivity and specificity may vary depending on assay design, but PCR assays may be more sensitive than cytology for detection of piroplasms, especially in chronic carrier cats.

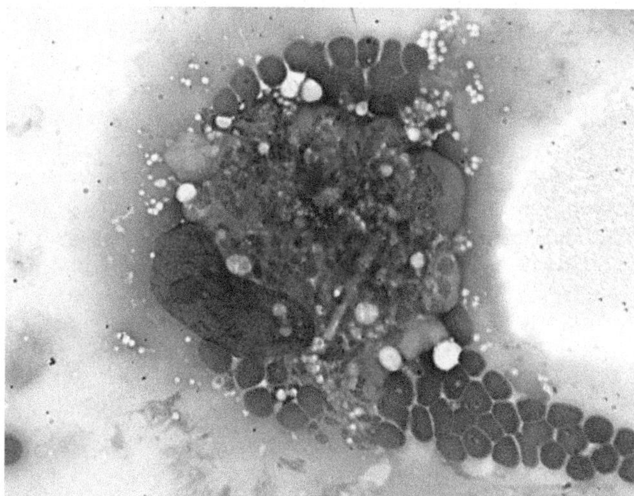

FIGURE 76-5 Wright-Giemsa–stained peripheral blood smear from a cat with cytauxzoonosis at 1000× magnification. A mononuclear cell massively distended with a schizont is surrounded by multiple RBCs, a few of which contain *Cytauxzoon felis* piroplasms.

reputable laboratories should be used; quality control is crucial. Because of the delay inherent in any mail-out PCR test, presumptive disease treatment needs to precede the results of PCR testing.

Healthy, chronic carrier cats have been identified by PCR assays applied to peripheral blood samples.[18,25,26] Although the importance of such carrier cats in propagation of infection is not known, they are competent hosts for transmission of infection to other cats via the bite of a tick vector.[27] Some cat owners may request screening of healthy cats that reside in the same neighborhood as a cat with cytauxzoonosis; such screening is best accomplished with PCR assays. Unfortunately, no method has been confirmed to completely eliminate parasitemia from chronic carrier cats.[21,28,29]

Other Diagnostic Assays

To date, *C. felis* has not been successfully cultured in vitro. Although serologic tests have been developed for detection of antibodies to *C. felis,* they are not practical for disease diagnosis, because illness likely precedes antibody formation.[30]

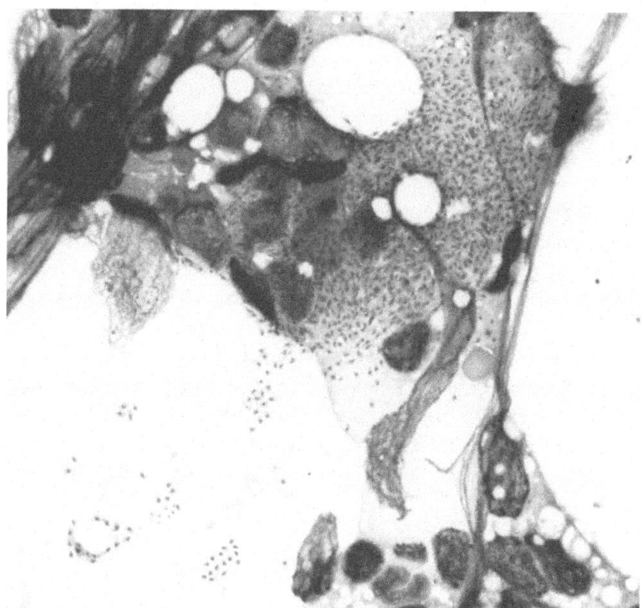

FIGURE 76-6 Fine-needle aspirate of a lymph node from a cat with cytauxzoonosis. Large numbers of merozoites (which have a granular appearance) erupt from a mononuclear cell.

Pathologic Findings

Gross Pathologic Findings

Icterus and pallor are common gross pathologic findings in cats that die from cytauxzoonosis.[8,19,31] The spleen and liver are often enlarged, and mesenteric lymph nodes may be enlarged and edematous.[8,19,31] The lungs are often wet and fail to collapse. Pleural effusion is sometimes identified, as is pericardial effusion.[32] Petechial hemorrhages are occasionally found on the serosal surface of organs.[8,33]

Although histopathology is not a commonly performed antemortem diagnostic test, a diagnosis of cytauxzoonosis is easily confirmed at necropsy by histopathology.[19,31,33] Numerous venules and capillaries, especially in the spleen, liver, and lungs, are occluded with markedly enlarged merozoite-distended mononuclear cells (Figure 76-7).[19,33,34] The germinal centers of

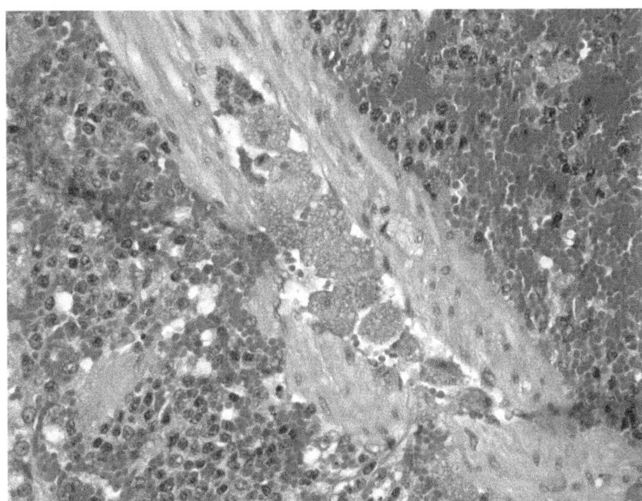

FIGURE 76-7 Histopathologic image of a section of spleen from a cat that died of cytauxzoonosis. Schizont-distended mononuclear cells obstruct blood vessels. H&E stain, 400× magnification. (Courtesy Dr. Linda Berent, University of Missouri Veterinary Medical Diagnostic Laboratory.)

lymphoid tissues contain many parasitized mononuclear cells as well, but organisms are not found in lymphocytes themselves.[8] Pulmonary lesions, which are common, are typified by moderate to severe vascular occlusion of medium-caliber vessels and interstitial pneumonia with edema and neutrophil accumulation.[35]

Treatment and Prognosis

Antiprotozoal Drugs

Currently, the treatment of choice for feline cytauxzoonosis is a combination of atovaquone suspension (Mepron, GlaxoSmithKline, Research Triangle Park, NC) and azithromycin (see also Chapter 10) (Table 76-2). Both drugs are administered orally for 10 days.[12] Although atovaquone is expensive, a single bottle will treat many cats. Compounding pharmacies may supply reasonably priced atovaquone in smaller quantities. In recovered carrier cats, the combination of atovaquone and azithromycin does not consistently eliminate parasitemia, but in most treated cats, pathogen burden drops to levels below PCR detection and piroplasms are no longer visible on peripheral blood smears.[19]

Other antiprotozoal therapies have been investigated for the treatment of cytauxzoonosis. Parvaquone and buparvaquone, both used to treat related *Theileria* infections, were ineffective for treatment of experimental cytauxzoonosis.[36] Imidocarb dipropionate has not proved to be an effective treatment for cytauxzoonosis; only 25% of cats treated with the drug survived.[12] Additionally, imidocarb does not reduce the parasite burden in carrier cats.[29] Diminazene aceturate is a drug used extensively in Africa, South America, and the far East for treatment of protozoal diseases. In a retrospective report, 5 of 6 cats treated with diminazene aceturate at 2 mg/kg IM, plus supportive care, survived acute cytauxzoonosis.[22] The author has used diminazene to treat four additional cats with cytauxzoonosis, and only one survived. Studies in naturally infected cats are difficult to conduct because this drug is not approved for use in the United States. As with imidocarb, diminazene aceturate was unable to eliminate or reduce parasitemia from healthy carrier cats.[21,30]

TABLE 76-2

Antimicrobial Drugs Indicated for Treatment of Feline Cytauxzoonosis

Drug	Dose (mg/kg)	Route	Interval (hours)	Duration (days)
Atovaquone/azithromycin combination:				
Atovaquone *and*	15	PO	8	10
Azithromycin	10	PO	24	10

Supportive Care

Cats with cytauxzoonosis are critically ill and require supportive care. Crystalloid fluids address dehydration, correct prerenal azotemia, and may improve organ perfusion but should be used judiciously in cats with evidence of pulmonary damage or pleural effusion. Whole blood or packed RBC transfusion is often necessary during the hemolytic stage of acute illness. Plasma administration may be useful in cats with DIC, and although the recommendation is controversial, some clinicians advocate treatment with heparin at 200 units/kg SC q8h.[12] Because affected cats may be severely febrile and apparently in pain, antipyretic, anti-inflammatory, and analgesic drugs are often used. Unfortunately, no controlled studies have examined whether these therapies improve or worsen clinical outcome. The author does not usually administer either glucocorticoids or nonsteroidal anti-inflammatory drugs but has treated cats with buprenorphine as an analgesic. There are numerous reports of antibacterial drugs used in the therapy of cats with cytauxzoonosis, but the drugs utilized (enrofloxacin, doxycycline, and/or sodium ampicillin) seem unlikely to have contributed substantially to any improved outcome.[19,37] Cats typically have a poor appetite during recovery from cytauxzoonosis. Early placement of a nasoesophageal or esophagostomy feeding tube not only allows for provision of enteral nutrition and hydration, but facilitates administration of oral medications (i.e., atovaquone and azithromycin) with minimal stress to the patient.

Prognosis

In the early history of the disease, treatment options for cytauxzoonosis were considered ineffective and the disease was regarded as uniformly fatal. However, it is now recognized that some cats become infected without recognized clinical illness, and others survive illness with supportive or specific medical care.[12,15,18,26,38] Either differences in the individual cat's immune response to infection or reduced pathogenicity of the infecting organism are possible explanations for chronic infection in cats with no history of prior illness. The latter theory is supported by finding many cats with chronic infection but no history of illness in a limited geographic region around northwestern Arkansas.[15,27,39]

Despite occasional recognition of subclinically infected cats, most infected cats become extremely ill and die in the absence of aggressive treatment.[19,39] Even when treated with atovaquone and azithromycin, only 60% of infected cats survive.[12] Because most cats that die despite therapy do so within a day of presentation, even the most active antiprotozoal compound may not prevent death in a proportion of infected cats once clinical illness is recognized.

Immunity and Vaccination

Cats that survive experimentally induced schizogenous infection appear to be immune to illness on re-infection, although experimental inoculation with piroplasms alone does not provide protection.[36,40,41] Resistance to re-infection with *C. felis* offers hope that successful vaccine development may be possible, but safe and effective vaccines against apicomplexan parasites are notoriously difficult to develop.[42] Inoculation of cats with a less pathogenic *Cytauxzoon* species *(C. manul)* failed to reduce mortality associated with *C. felis* challenge.[43] Many veterinarians in endemic regions have observed clinical illness indistinguishable from cytauxzoonosis in cats known to have survived cytauxzoonosis in previous years. Because no attempt has been made to look for schizonts in the cats experiencing a second illness, it is unclear if these cats have recrudescent cytauxzoonosis, re-infection, or some other illness altogether.

Prevention

For now, prevention relies on avoidance of tick exposure. Given the sensitivity of domestic cats to many commonly used ectoparasiticides, the arsenal of acaricides available for cats is limited to flumethrin-impregnated collars, fipronil, and possibly selamectin, although the latter does not make a label claim of efficacy against ticks in cats.[44,45] Given their potent activity against ticks and their safety in cats, flumethrin-impregnated collars offer the greatest potential for prevention of cytauxzoonosis in cats that reside in endemic areas. However, no ectoparasiticide prevents tick bites entirely.[12,46] Where possible, cats in endemic areas should be kept indoors to minimize tick exposure.

Recovered cats may remain carriers, and may serve as reservoirs for infection of naïve ticks.[6] For this reason, recovered cats should also be kept indoors and ectoparasite control practices instituted in order to minimize the risk of transmission to other cats via tick bite. Treatment of recovered cats with imidocarb dipropionate or diminazene aceturate does not reduce piroplasm parasitemia, but treatment with atovaquone and azithromycin may reduce the parasite burden and potentially reduce the risk of transmission to feeding ticks.[29,30]

Public Health Aspects

Cytauxzoon felis is not known to infect humans. However, infected cats have the potential to be infected with other vector-borne pathogens, so precautions should be taken to avoid needlestick injuries or direct skin contact with blood from infected cats.

CASE EXAMPLE

Signalment and History: "Ginger," a 2-year-old female spayed domestic longhaired cat that lived near Springfield, Missouri, was evaluated for a 1-day history of anorexia and lethargy in April of the year. The cat was an indoor/outdoor cat with no known history of tick exposure. There were no other cats in the household.

Physical Examination: On examination, the cat's rectal temperature was 105.6°F (40.9°C), with a heart rate of 200 beats/min and a respiratory rate of 28 breaths/min. The spleen was prominent on abdominal palpation and the nictitans was elevated (see Figure 76-3), but examination was otherwise unremarkable.

Laboratory Findings: Blood was obtained for a CBC and retrovirus testing. The cat tested negative for FeLV antigen and FIV antibody. The cat had a mild, nonregenerative anemia (PCV 27%) and leukopenia (4200 cells/μL, reference range 5500-19,500 cells/μL). Although the platelet count was low, platelet clumps were present. Plasma in the spun hematocrit tube was icteric. No parasites were observed on microscopic slide review.

Because of a high degree of suspicion for cytauxzoonosis, a fine-needle aspirate was obtained from the spleen. Multiple markedly enlarged mononuclear cells containing numerous merozoites were observed.

Diagnosis: Cytauxzoonosis.

Treatment and Outcome: A nasoesophageal tube was placed to facilitate administration of atovaquone suspension (15 mg/kg PO q8h) and azithromycin (10 mg/kg PO q24h). A cephalic vein catheter was placed and intravenous crystalloid fluids administered at a maintenance rate. Heparin (200 units/kg SC q8h) and buprenorphine (0.01 mg/kg SC q8h) were administered.

The following day, the cat's PCV was 20% and icterus was evident on physical examination. Additionally, many piroplasms were visible on cytologic analysis of a smear of peripheral blood. A serum chemistry profile confirmed hyperbilirubinemia and a mild increase in the activity of serum ALT but was otherwise unremarkable.

By day 3, the PCV was 12%, and both respiratory and heart rate were increased. The cat was administered a single unit of whole blood, after which the PCV increased to 19%. Nutritional support was administered via the nasoesophageal tube, but otherwise treatment remained unchanged.

On day 5, the PCV dropped to 11%, which necessitated another whole blood transfusion. The cat remained tachypneic after transfusion. Thoracic radiographs revealed pleural effusion and a marked diffuse interstitial lung pattern. The cat was treated with supplemental oxygen, and 25 mL of a clear, yellow, modified transudate was removed using thoracocentesis.

By day 7, the cat no longer required supplemental oxygen to maintain respiratory function, and the anemia was regenerative. The cat was discharged from the hospital on day 8 with continued administration of atovaquone and azithromycin at home, but all other treatments were discontinued.

On recheck examination 1 week later, the cat was seemingly normal to the owners, and no abnormalities were detected on physical examination. The PCV was 29%, platelet and WBC counts had normalized, and a single piroplasm was observed on careful review of the entire feathered edge of the blood smear. The cat's owners were advised to keep the cat entirely indoors and to use an ectoparasiticide regularly to minimize any risk that the cat could serve as a reservoir for infection of ticks. The cat remained healthy 1 year later.

SUGGESTED READINGS

Brown HM, Lockhart JM, Latimer KS, et al. Identification and genetic characterization of *Cytauxzoon felis* in asymptomatic domestic cats and bobcats. Vet Parasitol. 2010;(172):311-316.

Cohn LA, Birkenheuer AJ, Brunker JD, et al. Efficacy of atovaquone and azithromycin or imidocarb dipropionate in cats with acute cytauxzoonosis. J Vet Intern Med. 2011;25:55-60.

Reichard MV, Baum KA, Cadenhead SC, et al. Temporal occurrence and environmental risk factors associated with cytauxzoonosis in domestic cats. Vet Parasit. 2008;152:314-320.

REFERENCES

1. Wagner JE. A fatal cytauxzoonosis-like disease in cats. J Am Vet Med Assoc. 1976;168(7):585-588.
2. Lack JB, Reichard MV, Van Den Bussche RA. Phylogeny and evolution of the piroplasmida as inferred from 18S rRNA sequences. Int J Parasitol. 2012;42:353-363.
3. Kier AB, Wightman SR, Wagner JE. Interspecies transmission of *Cytauxzoon felis*. Am J Vet Res. 1982;43:102-105.
4. Blouin EF, Kocan AA, Glenn BL, et al. Transmission of *Cytauxzoon felis* Kier, 1979 from bobcats, *Felis rufus* (Schreber), to domestic cats by *Dermacentor variabilis* (Say). J Wildl Dis. 1984;20:241-242.
5. Bondy Jr PJ, Cohn LA, Tyler JW, et al. Polymerase chain reaction detection of *Cytauxzoon felis* from field-collected ticks and sequence analysis of the small subunit and internal transcribed spacer 1 region of the ribosomal RNA gene. J Parasitol. 2005;91:458-461.
6. Reichard MV, Edwards AC, Meinkoth JH, et al. Confirmation of *Amblyomma americanum* (Acari: Ixodidae) as a vector for *Cytauxzoon felis* (Piroplasmorida: Theileriidae) to domestic cats. J Med Entomol. 2010;47:890-896.
7. Simpson CF, Harvey JW, Lawman MJ, et al. Ultrastructure of schizonts in the liver of cats with experimentally induced cytauxzoonosis. Am J Vet Res. 1985;46:384-390.
8. Kier AB, Wagner JE, Kinden DA. The pathology of experimental cytauxzoonosis. J Comp Pathol. 1987;97:415-432.
9. Reichard MV, Baum KA, Cadenhead SC, et al. Temporal occurrence and environmental risk factors associated with cytauxzoonosis in domestic cats. Vet Parasitol. 2008;152:314-320.
10. Shock BC, Murphy SM, Patton LL, et al. Distribution and prevalence of *Cytauxzoon felis* in bobcats (*Lynx rufus*), the natural reservoir, and other wild felids in thirteen states. Vet Parasitol. 2011;175:325-330.
11. Birkenheuer AJ, Marr HS, Warren C, et al. *Cytauxzoon felis* infections are present in bobcats (*Lynx rufus*) in a region where cytauxzoonosis is not recognized in domestic cats. Vet Parasitol. 2008;153:126-130.
12. Cohn LA, Birkenheuer AJ, Brunker JD, et al. Efficacy of atovaquone and azithromycin or imidocarb dipropionate in cats with acute cytauxzoonosis. J Vet Intern Med. 2011;25:55-60.
13. Blouin EF, Kocan AA, Kocan KM, et al. Evidence of a limited schizogenous cycle for *Cytauxzoon felis* in bobcats following exposure to infected ticks. J Wildl Dis. 1987;23:499-501.
14. Wagner JE. A fatal cytauxzoonosis-like disease in cats. J Am Vet Med Assoc. 1976;168:585-588.
15. Meinkoth J, Kocan AA, Whitworth L, et al. Cats surviving natural infection with *Cytauxzoon felis*: 18 cases (1997-1998). J Vet Intern Med. 2000;14:521-525.
16. Kocan AA, Blouin EF, Glenn BL. Hematologic and serum chemical values for free-ranging bobcats, *Felis rufus* (Schreber), with reference to animals with natural infections of *Cytauxzoon felis* Kier, 1979. J Wildl Dis. 1985(21):190-192.
17. Lewis KM, Cohn LA, Birkenheuer AJ. Lack of evidence for perinatal transmission of *Cytauxzoon felis* in domestic cats. Vet Parasitol. 2012;188:172-174.
18. Brown HM, Latimer KS, Erikson LE, et al. Detection of persistent *Cytauxzoon felis* infection by polymerase chain reaction in three asymptomatic domestic cats. J Vet Diagn Invest. 2008;20:485-488.
19. Hoover JP, Walker DB, Hedges JD. Cytauxzoonosis in cats: eight cases (1985-1992). J Am Vet Med Assoc. 1994;(205):455-460.
20. Franks PT, Harvey JW, Shields RP, et al. Hematological findings in experimental feline cytauxzoonosis. J Am Anim Hosp Assoc. 1988;24:395-401.
21. Lewis KM, Cohn LA, Marr H, et al. Diminazene diaceturate for the treatment of chronic *Cytauxzoon felis* parasitemia in naturally infected cats. J Vet Intern Med. 2012;26:1490-1493.
22. Greene CE, Latimer K, Hopper E, et al. Administration of diminazene aceturate or imidocarb dipropionate for treatment of cytauxzoonosis in cats. J Am Vet Med Assoc. 1999;215:497-500.
23. Garner MM, Lung NP, Citino S, et al. Fatal cytauxzoonosis in a captive-reared white tiger (*Panthera tigris*). Vet Pathol. 1996;33:82-86.
24. Birkenheuer AJ, Marr H, Alleman AR, et al. Development and evaluation of a PCR assay for the detection of *Cytauxzoon felis* DNA in feline blood samples. Vet Parasitol. 2006;137:144-149.
25. Haber MD, Tucker MD, Marr HS, et al. The detection of *Cytauxzoon felis* in apparently healthy free-roaming cats in the USA. Vet Parasitol. 2007;146:316-320.
26. Lewis KM, Cohn LA, Downey M, et al. Evaluation of *Cytauxzoon felis* infection status in captive-born wild felids housed in areas endemic for this pathogen. J Am Vet Med Assoc. 2012;241:1088-1092.
27. Reichard MV, Meinkoth JH, Edwards AC, et al. Transmission of *Cytauxzoon felis* to a domestic cat by *Amblyomma americanum*. Vet Parasitol. 2009;161:110-115.
28. Cohn LA, Birkenheuer AJ, Ratcliff E. Comparison of two drug protocols for clearance of *Cytauxzoon felis* infections [Abstract]. J Vet Intern Med. 2008;22:704.
29. Lewis KM, Cohn LA, Marr H, et al. High dose diminazene diaceturate does not eliminate parasitemia in cats with chronic *Cytauxzoon felis* infection. Proceedings of the American College of Veterinary Internal Medicine Forum. New Orleans: LA; 2012.
30. Cowell RL, Fox JC, Panciera RJ, et al. Detection of anticytauxzoon antibodies in cats infected with a *Cytauxzoon* organism from bobcats. Vet Parasitol. 1988;28:43-52.
31. Aschenbroich SA, Rech RR, Sousa RS, et al. Pathology in practice. *Cytauxzoon felis* infection. J Am Vet Med Assoc. 2012;240:159-161.
32. Butt MT, Bowman D, Barr MC, et al. Iatrogenic transmission of *Cytauxzoon felis* from a Florida panther (*Felix concolor coryi*) to a domestic cat. J Wildl Dis. 1991;27:342-347.
33. Wagner JE, Ferris DH, Kier AB, et al. Experimentally induced cytauxzoonosis-like disease in domestic cats. Vet Parasitol. 1980;6:305-311.
34. Susta L, Torres-Velez F, Zhang J, et al. An in situ hybridization and immunohistochemical study of cytauxzoonosis in domestic cats. Vet Pathol. 2009;46:1197-1204.
35. Snider TA, Confer AW, Payton ME. Pulmonary histopathology of *Cytauxzoon felis* infections in the cat. Vet Pathol. 2010;47:698-702.
36. Motzel SL, Wagner JE. Treatment of experimentally induced cytauxzoonosis in cats with parvaquone and buparvaquone. Vet Parasitol. 1990;35:131-138.
37. Walker DB, Cowell RL. Survival of a domestic cat with naturally acquired cytauxzoonosis. J Am Vet Med Assoc. 1995;206:1363-1365.
38. Brown HM, Lockhart JM, Latimer KS, et al. Identification and genetic characterization of *Cytauxzoon felis* in asymptomatic domestic cats and bobcats. Vet Parasitol. 2010;172:311-316.
39. Brown HM, Berghaus RD, Latimer KS, et al. Genetic variability of *Cytauxzoon felis* from 88 infected domestic cats in Arkansas and Georgia. J Vet Diagn Invest. 2009;21:59-63.
40. Glenn BL, Kocan AA, Blouin EF. Cytauxzoonosis in bobcats. J Am Vet Med Assoc. 1983;183:1155-1158.
41. Ferris DH. A progress report on the status of a new disease of American cats: cytauxzoonosis. Comp Immun Microbiol Infect Dis. 1979;1:269-276.
42. Sharma S, Pathak S. Malaria vaccine: a current perspective. J Vector Borne Dis. 2008;45:1-20.

43. Joyner PH, Reichard MV, Meinkoth JH, et al. Experimental infection of domestic cats (*Felis domesticus*) with *Cytauxzoon manul* from Pallas' cats (*Otocolobus manul*). Vet Parasitol. 2007;146:302-306.
44. Bishop BF, Bruce CI, Evans NA, et al. Selamectin: a novel broad-spectrum endectocide for dogs and cats. Vet Parasitol. 2000;91:163-176.
45. Stanneck D, Kruedewagen EM, Fourie JJ, et al. Efficacy of an imidocloprid/flumethrin collar against fleas and ticks on cats. Parasit Vectors. 2012;5:82.
46. Dryden MW. Flea and tick control in the 21st century: challenges and opportunities. Vet Dermatol. 2009;20:435-440.

CHAPTER 77

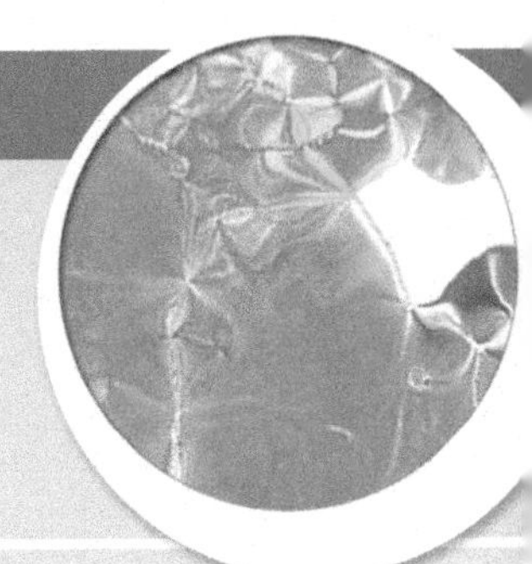

Canine and Feline Hepatozoonosis

Nancy Vincent-Johnson

Overview of Canine Hepatozoonosis

First Described: *Hepatozoon canis*, India, 1905 (James)[1]; *Hepatozoon americanum*, USA, 1978 (Craig and others)[2]

Cause: *Hepatozoon canis, Hepatozoon americanum* (phylum Apicomplexa)

Affected Hosts: Domestic dogs, possibly some wild carnivores

Geographic Distribution: *H. americanum*, southeastern and south-central United States; *H. canis*, Asia, Africa, southern Europe, the Middle East, the Americas.

Mode of Transmission: Primarily by ingestion of tick vectors. For *H. americanum*, the vector is *Amblyomma maculatum;* for *H. canis*, the vector is *Rhipicephalus sanguineus*. Other tick species (*Amblyomma, Rhipicephalus*, and *Haemaphysalis* spp.) may also be involved.

Major Clinical Signs: Dogs with *H. americanum* infections most often show lethargy, fever, weight loss, locomotory abnormalities, hyperesthesia, mucopurulent ocular discharge, signs related to protein-losing nephropathy such as polyuria and polydipsia. Dogs with severe *H. canis* infections may show fever and lethargy.

Differential Diagnoses: Sterile or infectious meningitis, bacterial discospondylitis, Lyme borreliosis, canine monocytic ehrlichiosis, toxoplasmosis, sarcocystosis, systemic immune-mediated diseases such as systemic lupus erythematosus

Human Health Significance: Canine *Hepatozoon* species are not known to infect humans.

Etiology and Epidemiology

Apicomplexan protozoal parasites from the genus *Hepatozoon* include more than 300 species that infect a wide variety of amphibians, reptiles, birds, and mammals.[3] Despite its name, canine hepatozoonosis is not a zoonotic disease and rarely affects the liver. Canine hepatozoonosis is caused by one of two species of *Hepatozoon* currently known to cause disease in dogs, *Hepatozoon canis* and *Hepatozoon americanum* (compared in Table 77-1). First described in India in 1905, *H. canis* has long been known as the agent that infects dogs in many regions of the Old World, including Asia, Africa, southern Europe, and the Middle East, and more recently has been identified in the New World in both North and South America (Figure 77-1).[1,3-20] *Hepatozoon americanum* causes American canine hepatozoonosis, which occurs in dogs primarily in the southeastern and south-central United States. It was first confused with *H. canis* in 1978 in dogs from the Gulf Coast region of Texas and has subsequently been detected in dogs from Louisiana, Oklahoma, Alabama, Georgia, Florida, and Tennesee.[2,21-25] In 1997, it was identified as a distinct species, *H. americanum*.[26,27] Occasional cases have been identified in diverse locations across the United States, including Washington, California, Nebraska, Vermont, and Virginia.[17] Because infection is chronic, the infection may be diagnosed in dogs with a history of travel to endemic areas. The DNA of a *Hepatozoon felis*–like organism was detected in a dog from southern California, but the clinical significance and epidemiology of this organism are unknown.[28]

Recent reports indicate that *H. canis* also exists in the United States, although infection with *H. americanum* is diagnosed much more frequently. *H. canis* has been identified in dogs from Mississippi, Louisiana, Alabama, Georgia, Oklahoma, and Virginia and in a dog that lived in New Jersey but was born in a Texas shelter.[16,17,29] A few dogs have mixed infections with both *H. americanum* and *H. canis*. Domestic cats can also be infected by *Hepatozoon* spp., which include *H. felis* and possibly *H. canis* or closely related species (see later section on feline infections and Table 77-1).[30,31]

Because dogs or other vertebrates serve as intermediate hosts, a vector is needed to complete the sexual phase of the life cycle of *Hepatozoon* species. In the case of *H. americanum*, the definitive host is the Gulf Coast tick, *Amblyomma maculatum,* whereas the definitive host of *H. canis* is the brown dog tick, *Rhipicephalus sanguineus*.[32,33] In Japan, *Haemaphysalis* spp. ticks have been implicated as vectors of *H. canis*, and in Brazil, *Amblyomma ovale* and *Rhipicephalus (Boophilus) microplus* are suspected vectors.[34-36]

As it feeds on an infected dog, the nymphal tick ingests circulating leukocytes that contain gamonts. Within the tick's gut, the gamonts are freed from the cells and undergo further development before fertilization occurs. The resulting zygote divides through sporogony and develops into an oocyst within the hemocoel of the tick (Figure 77-2). Oocysts mature while the tick molts to the adult stage. In the case of *H. americanum,* the larval stage of the tick can also become infected, resulting in a nymph that contains viable oocysts capable of transmitting the disease.[37] Each mature oocyst contains hundreds of sporocysts, with each sporocyst containing 10 to 26 infective sporozoites. Unlike most tick-borne diseases, hepatozoonosis is not transmitted through the bite of an infected tick but rather by *ingestion* of an infected tick. This typically occurs when the dog grooms itself but can also occur if the dog feeds on tick-infested prey. Once ingested, exposure to bile in the dog's intestinal tract results in release of the sporozoites, which penetrate the intestinal epithelial wall and are transported to the target organs and tissues, likely within mononuclear cells.

TABLE 77-1

Comparison of *Hepatozoon canis* Infection, American Canine Hepatozoonosis, and Feline Hepatozoonosis

	H. canis Infection	American Canine Hepatozoonosis	Feline Hepatozoonosis
First described	India, 1905	Texas Gulf Coast, 1978	India, 1908
Etiologic agent	*Hepatozoon canis*	*Hepatozoon americanum*	Multiple poorly defined *Hepatozoon* sp.
Primary vector	*Rhipicephalus sanguineus* (brown dog tick)	*Amblyomma maculatum* (Gulf Coast tick)	Unknown
Route of transmission	Ingestion of tick (not a tick bite)	Ingestion of tick (not a tick bite)	Probably ingestion of tick (not a tick bite)
Additional routes of transmission	Transplacental from dam to puppy	Ingestion of cystozoites in transport hosts; transplacental is likely	Unknown
Affected mammalian hosts	Dogs, foxes, jackals, hyenas, other carnivores	Dogs, coyotes, possibly bobcats, ocelots, and other wildlife	Domestic cats, wild felids
Geographic distribution	Africa, Middle East, Asia, southern Europe, South America, United States	Primarily southern and southeastern United States	India, Africa, Israel, Brazil, Spain, France, Thailand, United States (Hawaii)
Severity of disease	Subclinical to mild; occasionally severe, esp. if immunosuppressed	Usually severe, even in absence of immunosuppression	Typically subclinical unless immunosuppressed
Major clinical signs	Lethargy, fever, weight loss	Fever, pain, lameness, ocular discharge	Nonspecific
Common laboratory abnormalities	Anemia Extreme leukocytosis is rare but may occur with high parasitemia	Marked leukocytosis (20,000-200,000 cells/μL), anemia, elevated ALP activity, low glucose concentration	Elevated CK activity
Radiographic lesions	Nonspecific; rare periostitis	Common; periosteal bone proliferation	Not reported
Histopathology findings	No muscle lesions "wheel-spoked" meronts in spleen, bone marrow, lymph nodes	Myositis, onion-skin cysts, pyogranulomas, and meronts in skeletal muscle	Meronts in myocardium and skeletal muscle
Blood smear findings	Gamonts common; parasitemia of 1%-5% is typical; rarely see parasitemia of 5%-100%	Rarely observed gamonts; parasitemia is usually <0.1%	Parasitemia is rare; when present usually <1% of neutrophils
Human health significance	None known	None known	None known

In *H. americanum* infections, infected cells preferentially travel to skeletal muscle, where each organism develops within its host cell, which becomes lodged between myocytes (Figure 77-3). Concentric layers of mucopolysaccharide are laid down by the host cell to form an "onion-skin cyst," which may protect the organism from the immune response (Figure 77-4). Merogony occurs within the cyst, and on maturation of the meront, the cyst ruptures, and merozoites are released. This elicits a severe inflammatory response, with recruitment of neutrophils and monocytes to the area. A pyogranuloma develops in the space where the cyst existed (Figure 77-5). Many of these inflammatory cells become infected with a single zoite. Angiogenesis within the pyogranuloma results in a highly vascular structure from which the infected cells can reenter circulation. The intracellular parasites can travel to other target sites, where they continue the asexual reproductive cycle, or they may become gamonts. The gamonts are then ingested by feeding ticks, which completes the life cycle. Some of the onion-skin cysts lie dormant for varying lengths of time; their activation is responsible for the waxing and waning nature of the disease as well as the relapse of clinical signs that can occur months after perceived clinical cure.

In *H. canis* infections, infected cells are carried by lymph or blood to the spleen, bone marrow, lymph nodes, and other organs such as the liver, kidney, and lungs where the organisms divide asexually through merogony (Figure 77-6). Two types of meronts form: the "wheel spoke" meront, which contains 20 to 30 micromerozoites which form around a central round structure (Figure 77-7), and a meront that contains up to four macromerozoites.[38] Once released from the mature meront, micromerozoites invade neutrophils and monocytes and become

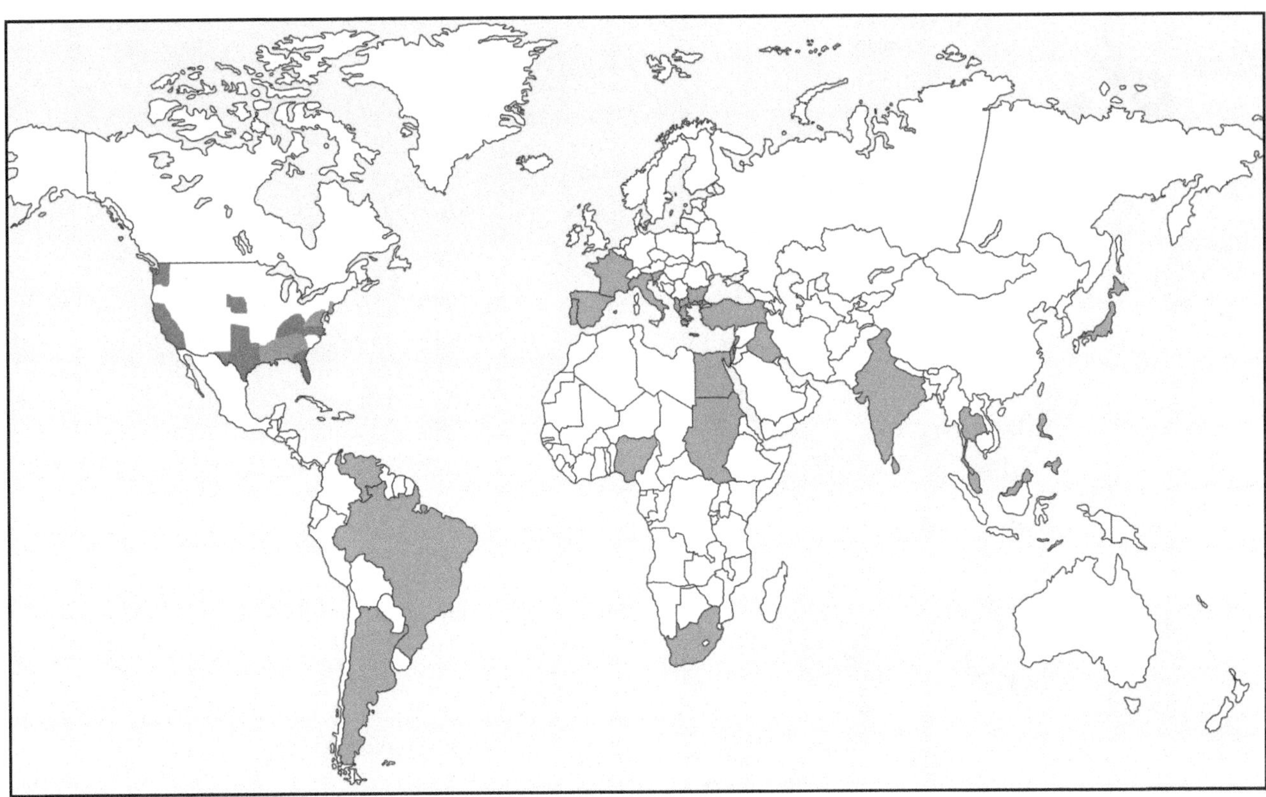

FIGURE 77-1 Geographic distribution of reported *Hepatozoon canis* and *Hepatozoon americanum* infections. Both species exist in the United States. (Blue, *Hepatozoon canis;* red, *Hepatozoon americanum;* purple both species.)

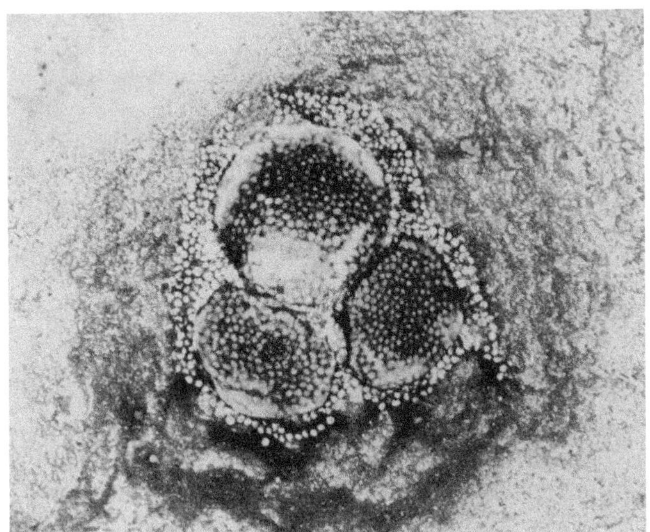

FIGURE 77-2 *Hepatozoon americanum* oocysts from the hemocoel of an *Amblyomma maculatum* tick. Hundreds of small, round sporocysts are present within each oocyst. Each sporocyst contains 10 to 26 infective sporozoites.

gamonts, which can then be ingested by feeding ticks (Figure 77-8). The larger macromerozoites are believed to be responsible for the production of secondary meronts in the target tissues, which continue the asexual cycle of merogony. Another tissue stage found in dogs with *H. canis* but not *H. americanum* infections is a small monozoic cyst that resembles the cystozoite found in transport hosts of other *Hepatozoon* species.[39]

Other modes of transmission also occur in hepatozoonosis. Transplacental transmission from dam to puppies has been documented for *H. canis* infections and likely occurs in *H. americanum* infections as well.[40] Ingestion of tissue from wild animals or prey may transmit *H. americanum*.[41-43] Laboratory rodents fed *H. americanum* oocysts developed cystozoites, but they did not develop gamonts or meronts or become ill. Cystozoite-laden rodent tissue fed to naïve dogs resulted in *H. americanum* infection along with its classical clinical signs. Investigation of a natural outbreak in a pack of hunting beagles revealed that clinical signs of American canine hepatozoonosis arose 4 to 6 weeks after some of the dogs were allowed to consume a wild rabbit carcass, whereas dogs not allowed to consume the rabbit did not develop clinical signs. The predation route of transmission has not yet been proven to occur with *H. canis*.

The geographic distribution of American canine hepatozoonosis aligns closely with the range of the Gulf Coast tick. Although this tick is endemic in the states that surround the Gulf of Mexico, its range is expanding and it has been found as far north as Kansas and Kentucky.[44] Larval and nymphal stages of *A. maculatum* preferentially feed on birds and small rodents. Surveys of wildlife have revealed the presence of *Hepatozoon* spp. that are related but not identical to *H. americanum* in small rodents and rabbits.[45] Although a reservoir species has not yet been identified, dogs are likely an aberrant, rather than natural, host of *H. americanum*. *H. americanum* or closely related species have been identified in coyotes, bobcats, and ocelots.[46-49] Because these wild animals were in good physical condition at the time of capture, they may represent a reservoir host in nature. In contrast to adult animals, coyote puppies developed classic signs of *H. americanum* infection after experimental transmission.[50]

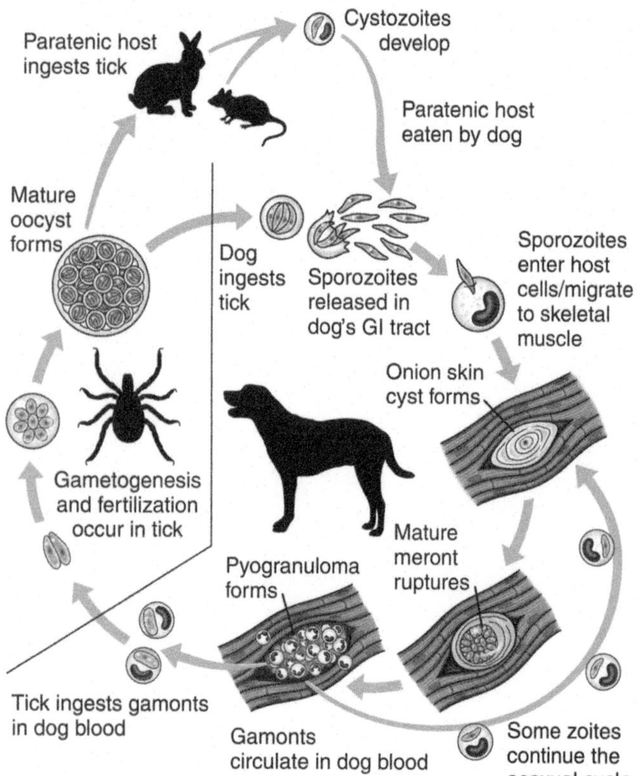

FIGURE 77-3 Life cycle of *Hepatozoon americanum*.

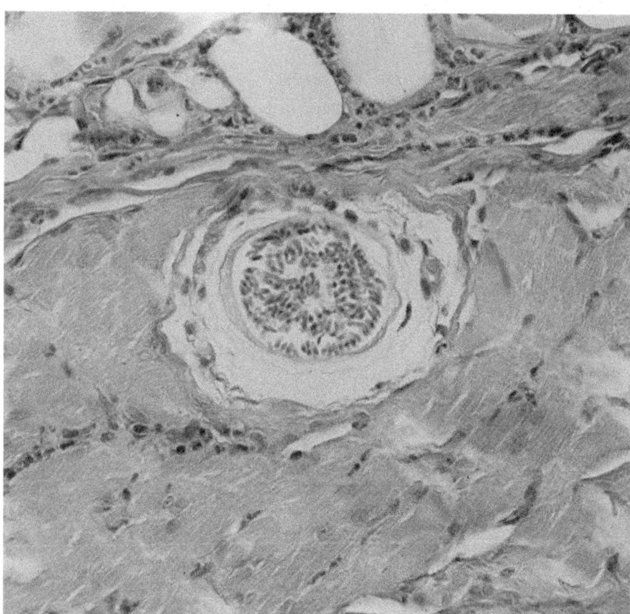

FIGURE 77-4 Skeletal muscle containing a developing meront of *H. americanum*. The mucopolysaccharide layers produced by the host cell protect the developing organisms from the host's immune system.

Dogs are believed to be the natural host reservoir of *H. canis*. The brown dog tick, which serves as the definitive host of *H. canis*, is found worldwide, and all three stages preferentially feed on dogs. Life stages of *H. canis* or morphologically indistinguishable *Hepatozoon* spp. have been reported in numerous carnivore species around the world, including several species of fox, jackal, African wild dog, hyena, palm civet, cheetah, leopard, lion, and Pallas cat.[30]

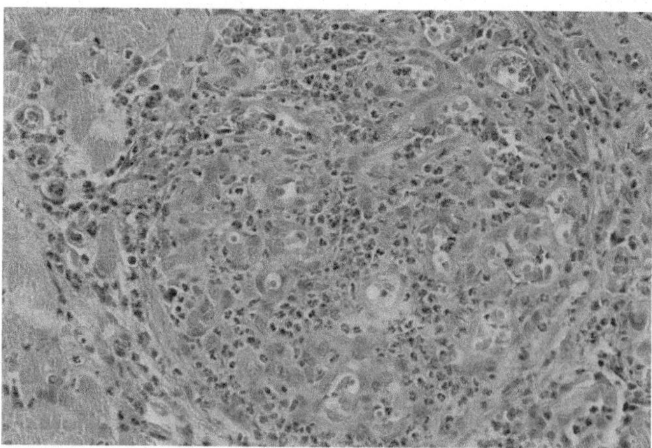

FIGURE 77-5 Pyogranuloma in skeletal muscle of a dog infected with *Hepatozoon americanum*. Zoites displace the nucleus in several of the inflammatory cells.

There is no sex or breed predilection for hepatozoonosis, but hunting dogs, rural dogs, and dogs allowed to roam are most at risk.

Clinical Features

Signs and Their Pathogenesis

Dogs with *H. americanum* infection exhibit a moderate to severe illness, whereas most dogs infected with *H. canis* have no or only mild signs of illness. Immunosuppression or concurrent disease is an important factor in expression of illness in *H. canis* but not in *H. americanum* infections. Co-infections with other pathogens such as *Ehrlichia, Babesia, Anaplasma, Leishmania,* parvovirus, or canine distemper virus can allow establishment of a new *H. canis* infection as well as progression or reactivation of an existing infection.

Clinical signs of *H. americanum* infection are associated with the strong inflammatory response that occurs when meronts rupture, leukocytes are recruited, and pyogranulomas form in skeletal muscle. The earliest lesions occur 3 weeks after infection.[51] As the organisms multiply, the infection disseminates, which results in more severe inflammation that waxes and wanes over time. The inflammation causes fever and myositis, which is associated with locomotor abnormalities and hyperesthesia (Table 77-2). The clinical signs can mimic those of meningitis or discospondylitis. Many affected dogs also develop bone lesions that are evident radiographically and resemble lesions seen in hypertrophic osteopathy, except they are proximal rather than distal in distribution (Figure 77-9). It is unknown whether the bone lesions result from nearby localized muscle inflammation or from humoral factors. Dogs usually have a mucopurulent ocular discharge that may be caused by pyogranulomatous inflammation of the extraocular muscles or of the lacrimal gland (Figure 77-10). Return of ocular discharge is frequently the first indication of a relapse following treatment. Dogs with American canine hepatozoonosis frequently maintain a fairly normal appetite; however, weight loss, cachexia, and muscle atrophy occur over time. There may be a history of polyuria and polydipsia that is due to glomerulonephritis or amyloidosis, which can occur secondary to long-standing inflammation. Nephrotic syndrome and thromboembolic complications may ensue. Less common clinical signs include

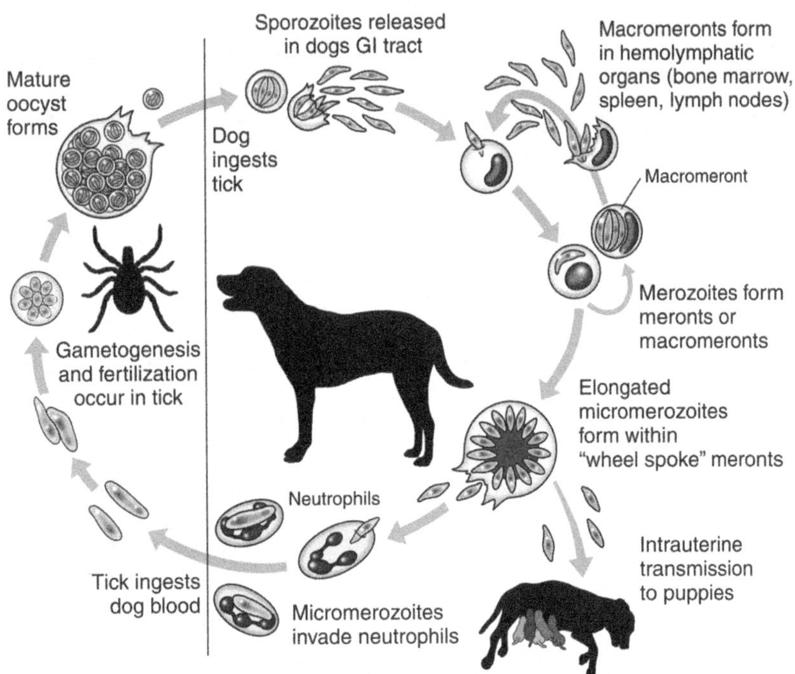

FIGURE 77-6 Life cycle of *Hepatozoon canis.*

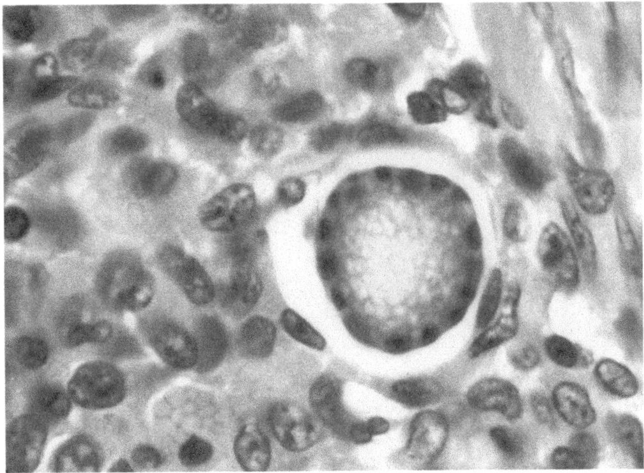

FIGURE 77-7 *Hepatozoon canis* meront in splenic tissue of a dog from Israel demonstrating the typical "wheel spoke" pattern. (Courtesy of Dr. Gad Baneth, Koret School of Veterinary Medicine, Israel.)

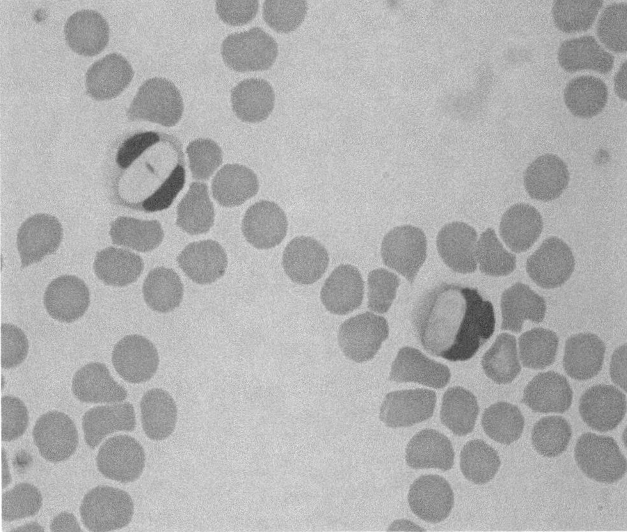

FIGURE 77-8 Two *Hepatozoon canis* gamonts in neutrophils on a blood smear. The gamonts of *Hepatozoon americanum* are nearly identical in appearance to those of *H. canis,* although they are rarely seen. 1000x magnification. (Courtesy of Dr. Gad Baneth, Koret School of Veterinary Medicine, Israel.)

diarrhea, mucosal pallor, cough, abnormal lung sounds, and lymphadenomegaly.

Most dogs infected with *H. canis* have a low level of parasitemia, with less than 5% of circulating leukocytes infected with gamonts.[52] These dogs have a limited inflammatory reaction. About 15% of parasitemic dogs have a high level of parasitemia (>800 gamonts/μL). The degree of parasitemia correlates with the severity of clinical signs; the sickest dogs have a level of parasitemia that approaches 100% of infected circulating leukocytes. These dogs may have hepatitis, glomerulonephritis, or pneumonitis in addition to severe anemia, fever, and cachexia.

Physical Examination Findings

With *H. americanum* infection, fever (up to 105.6°F or 40.9°C) is common, although because of the waxing and waning nature of the disease, body temperature may be normal at any given time.[23] Because of the myositis, dogs are typically evaluated for gait abnormalities, which range from lameness or stiffness to recumbency and an inability to rise. Hyperesthesia is common and may appear as cervical, back, joint, or generalized pain. Lethargy is common, and cachexia and generalized muscle atrophy may be apparent. Mucopurulent ocular discharge is often present. Other ocular lesions seen on occasion include focal retinal scars or hyper-reflectivity, increased retinal pigmentation, papilledema, and uveitis with active inflammatory fundic lesions. Mucosal pallor and lymphadenomegaly may also be present.

TABLE 77-2

Frequency of Clinical Signs in 22 Dogs with American Canine Hepatozoonosis

Clinical Sign	Number of Dogs (%)
Fever	19 (86)
Weight loss	18 (82)
Mucopurulent ocular discharge	17 (77)
Low tear production	8 (36)
Muscle atrophy	14 (64)
Pain (all types)	14 (64)
Joints	2 (9)
Lumbar	4 (18)
Cervical	5 (23)
Generalized	3 (14)
Stiffness	12 (55)
Generalized weakness	9 (41)
Pelvic limb paresis and ataxia	5 (23)
Inability to rise	5 (23)
Anorexia	5 (23)

From Vincent-Johnson NA. American canine hepatozoonosis. Vet Clin North Am Small Anim Pract. 2003;33:905-920. Data from Macintire DK, Vincent-Johnson N, Dillon AR, et al. Hepatozoonosis in dogs: 22 cases (1989-1994). J Am Vet Med Assoc. 1997;210:916-922.

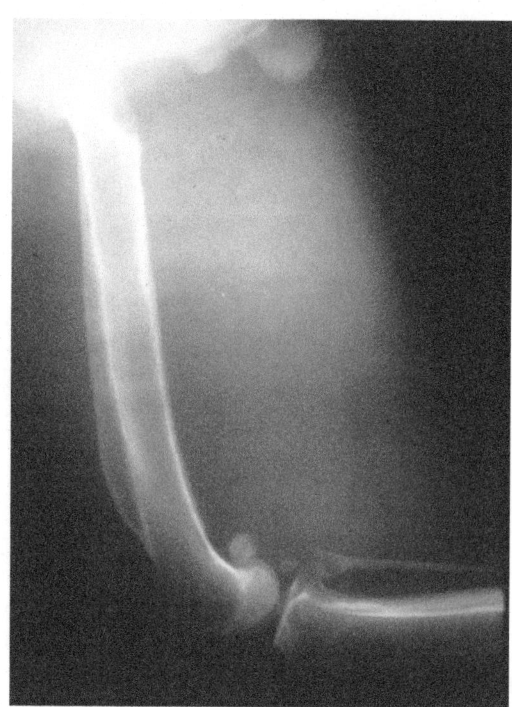

FIGURE 77-9 Radiograph of the pelvic limb of a dog with *Hepatozoon americanum* infection. There is smooth periosteal proliferation on the cranial aspect of the femur. (From Vincent-Johnson NA. American canine hepatozoonosis. Vet Clin North Am Small Anim Pract. 2003;33:905-920.)

Dogs with mild *H. canis* infections may have pale mucous membranes and lethargy. Dogs with high parasitemia often exhibit fever, lethargy, and severe weight loss or cachexia, even if they maintain a good appetite. Splenomegaly and lymphadenomegaly may be detected. Dogs often have physical examination abnormalities that relate to the presence of co-infections or other comorbidities.

Diagnosis

Laboratory Abnormalities

Complete Blood Count

The most common laboratory abnormality in *H. americanum* infection is leukocytosis, which is often extreme (Table 77-3). White cell counts are typically 20,000 to 200,000 cells/μL, with reported means of 76,807 and 85,700 cells/μL.[23,53] The leukocytosis is due to a mature neutrophilia, although sometimes there is a mild to moderate left shift. A mild normocytic, normochromic nonregenerative anemia is typical. Platelets are usually normal to increased, sometimes with thrombocytosis up to 916,000 platelets/μL. When thrombocytopenia is evident, concurrent tick-borne diseases such as ehrlichiosis should be considered.

The most common laboratory finding in *H. canis* infection is anemia, which is usually normocytic, normochromic, and occasionally regenerative.[52] Platelets are decreased about one third of the time, but this may be due to concurrent infection with *Ehrlichia canis* or other disease. The white blood cell count is typically normal in cases with low parasitemia but is elevated in dogs with high parasitemia. Some dogs have neutrophil counts of 50,000 to 150,000/μL with close to 100% of these cells containing gamonts.

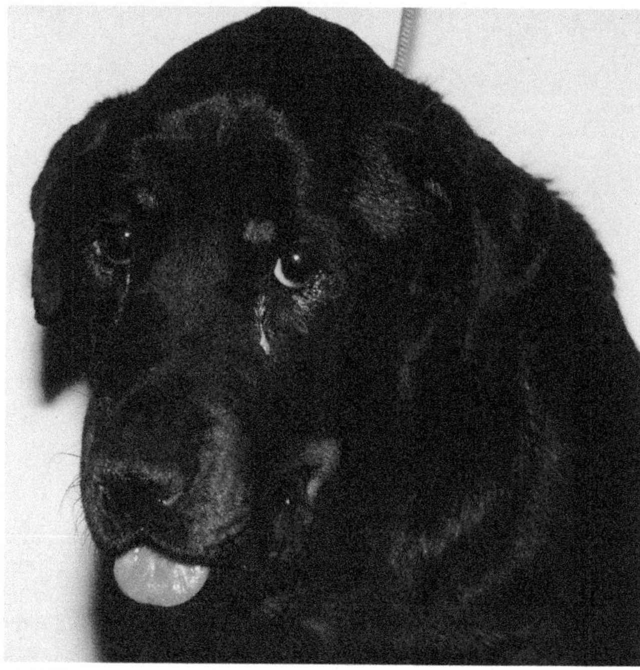

FIGURE 77-10 Rottweiler with *Hepatozoon americanum* infection. Note the hunched appearance, muscle atrophy, and mucopurulent ocular discharge.

Serum Chemistry Profile

In *H. americanum* infection, a mild elevation in the activity of ALP is typical, possibly due to periosteal new bone formation. Serum glucose concentration is often decreased (40 to 60 mg/dL) and occasionally as low as 5 mg/dL. This is not a true hypoglycemia, but rather a laboratory artifact due to

TABLE 77-3

Frequency of Laboratory and Radiographic Findings in 22 Dogs with American Canine Hepatozoonosis

Finding	Number of Dogs (%)
Moderate to marked leukocytosis*	22 (100)
Mature neutrophilia	15 (68)
Mild left shift	7 (31)
Elevated ALP activity	22 (100)
Hypoglycemia	20 (91)
Hypoalbuminemia	19 (86)
Periosteal proliferation on radiography	18 (82)
Anemia (nonregenerative)	14 (64)
Hypocalcemia	14 (64)
Normal platelet count	11 (50)
Thrombocytosis	9 (41)
Hyperphosphatemia	7 (32)
Low BUN concentration	7 (32)
Hyperglobulinemia	4 (11)
Hypercalcemia	2 (9)
Elevated CK activity	1 (5)

From Vincent-Johnson NA. American canine hepatozoonosis. Vet Clin North Am Small Anim Pract. 2003;33:905-920. Data from Macintire DK, Vincent-Johnson N, Dillon AR, et al. Hepatozoonosis in dogs: 22 cases (1989-1994). J Am Vet Med Assoc. 1997;210:916-922.
*Minimum white cell count was 27,800 cells/μL.

utilization of glucose in the specimen by the high number of white blood cells. Hypoalbuminemia is common and may be due to chronic inflammation, decreased protein intake, or renal loss from secondary glomerulonephritis or amyloidosis. Except in dogs with significant renal damage, BUN concentration is often low. The combination of increased activity of serum ALP and low glucose, BUN, and albumin concentrations may mislead the clinician to suspect liver disease. Serum bile acid concentrations are normal or only slightly elevated. Surprisingly, the activity of serum CK is consistently within the normal range even though *H. americanum* infection causes severe myositis.

Common serum chemistry findings in *H. canis* infection include hyperproteinemia, hyperglobulinemia, and hypoalbuminemia. The hyperglobulinemia is due to a polyclonal gammopathy.[52,54] Increases in the activities of ALP and CK are usually present.

Diagnostic Imaging

Plain Radiography

Many dogs with *H. americanum* infection show radiographic abnormalities of the skeletal system; therefore, radiographs of the pelvis or long bones can be useful to support a clinical diagnosis of American canine hepatozoonosis. Young dogs are more likely than older dogs to show bone lesions. In experimental infections, bone lesions are recognizable histologically within 5 weeks postexposure.[55] Disseminated, symmetric periosteal new bone formation occurs most frequently and severely on the diaphysis of long bones but occurs to a lesser degree on flat and irregular bones. The radiographic appearance can vary from subtle irregular periosteal exostoses to thick parallel pseudocortices. *H. americanum* infection typically affects the more proximal bones while sparing the distal bones.[56]

In *H. canis* infections, radiographic bone lesions are rare. Periostitis has only been described in three reports from Japan, India, and Italy, and in an experimental infection in Israel.[4,57]

Microbiologic Testing

Diagnostic assays currently available for hepatozoonosis in dogs are described in Table 77-4.

Cytologic Diagnosis

The sexual stage of *H. americanum* and *H. canis*, the gamont, appears as a light blue to clear oblong structure with a faintly staining nucleus within the cytoplasm of neutrophils or monocytes stained with Diff Quik or Giemsa. The gamonts of the two species look nearly identical, although there is a slight difference in size: *H. canis* gamonts measure approximately 11.0 × 4.3 μm while *H. americanum* gamonts are slightly smaller at 8.8 × 3.9 μm.[26]

In dogs with *H. americanum* infection, gamonts are rarely found within monocytes or neutrophils on peripheral blood smears. When present, infected cells rarely exceed 0.1% of the circulating leukocytes; several thousand cells may have to be examined before an infected cell is found. The chance that gamonts are detected can be increased by examination of buffy-coat smears. Neither bone marrow nor lymph node aspirates are of much value in making a definitive diagnosis of *H. americanum* infection; organisms are not usually seen in these specimens.

In most dogs with *H. canis* infections, gamonts are found on blood smear examination in 0.5% to 5% of neutrophils and monocytes. Parasitemia may approach 100% in heavy infections. Gamonts may also be identified in dogs that are apparently healthy.

Serologic Diagnosis

An ELISA assay for detection of antibodies to *H. americanum* has been developed at Oklahoma State University for research purposes, but this assay is not available commercially to veterinary practitioners.[58] Both an indirect immunofluorescent antibody (IFA) assay and ELISA assays for *H. canis* antibodies have been developed and used for epidemiologic studies in countries outside of the United States.[59-62] Positive serologic test results indicate exposure but do not prove active infection or correlate with clinical disease. Thus, serologic testing is mostly of use for epidemiologic studies and for screening blood donor animals.

Molecular Diagnosis Using the Polymerase Chain Reaction

A real-time PCR assay that detects *Hepatozoon* spp. is available commercially to veterinary practitioners through the Auburn University Molecular Diagnostics Laboratory.[63] Other commercial veterinary diagnostic laboratories also offer real-time PCR assays for detection of *Hepatozoon* species. The assay performed at Auburn University detects as few as seven genomic copies of *Hepatozoon* spp. per mL of blood, and it distinguishes between infection with *H. canis* and *H. americanum*.[16,17] Although highly sensitive and specific, false negatives can occur early in the course of infection or in dogs with chronic disease where the numbers of circulating gamonts are extremely low or absent. Muscle biopsy should be performed in dogs suspected

TABLE 77-4

Diagnostic Assays Currently Available for Hepatozoonosis in Dogs

Assay	Specimen Type	Target	Performance
Cytologic examination	Whole blood smears	*Hepatozoon* spp. gamonts in leukocytes	False negatives are common because of low circulating numbers of gamonts, especially in clinical *H. americanum* infections.
Antibody serology (ELISA or immunofluorescent antibody)	Serum	Antibodies to *H. canis*	Positive test results indicate exposure but do not indicate the presence of the organism in circulating leukocytes and do not correlate with clinical disease.
Real-time PCR assays	Whole blood	*H. americanum* or *H. canis* DNA	Sensitivity and specificity may vary depending on assay design, but in general PCR assays are more sensitive than cytology. False-negative results may occur when organism levels are very low, such as early in disease or in very chronic infections.
Histopathology	Muscle biopsy specimens	*H. americanum* cysts, meronts, and pyogranulomas	Most reliable method of diagnosis of *H. americanum* infection, but requires anesthesia.

to have *H. americanum* infection but that have negative PCR assay results.

Pathologic Findings

Gross Pathologic Findings

In dogs with *H. americanum* infection, muscle atrophy and cachexia are consistent findings on gross necropsy examination. Pyogranulomas may appear as multiple 1- to 2-mm–diameter white-tan foci.[23] These are scattered diffusely throughout skeletal and cardiac muscle but may also be observed in other tissues. Roughening and thickening of bony surfaces are often present. Less common findings include lymphadenomegaly, congestion of the gastric mucosa, splenic coagulative necrosis, and pulmonary congestion.

In dogs with *H. canis* infection, the spectrum of gross pathologic lesions depends on the severity of the infection. In heavy infections, splenomegaly and hepatomegaly are common findings and these organs often exhibit diffuse white necrotic foci that are 1 to 2 mm in diameter.[14] The necrotic areas may be larger and nodular and can also be found in other tissues, such as pancreas and pleura. Lymphadenomegaly is common, and pneumonia may be present.

Histopathologic Findings

For *H. americanum* infections, muscle biopsy has long been considered the most reliable method for diagnosis. Small pieces of muscle (approximately 2 cm × 2 cm) are obtained from the biceps femoris or semitendinosus muscles under general anesthesia.[25] Submission of multiple specimens increases sensitivity, especially in low-level infections. Muscle lesions consist of large onion-skin cysts, pyogranulomas, and myositis. The cysts are round to oval and have mean cross-section dimensions of 186 × 150 μm.[26] At the center of the cyst is a host cell nucleus and protozoa, but depending on the plane of the cut surface, these may or may not be visible. Surrounding the center of the cyst are concentric layers of mucopolysaccharide. Occasionally meronts in various stages of development are observed within these cystic structures. The highly vascular pyogranulomas are packed with neutrophils and macrophages, many of which contain a single zoite. Myositis is characterized by muscle necrosis and atrophy with infiltration of neutrophils, macrophages, and occasional lymphocytes between muscle fibers. Although consistently identified in skeletal and cardiac muscle, *H. americanum* cysts, meronts, and pyogranulomas can sporadically be found in adipose tissue, intestinal smooth muscle, pancreas, liver, lymph node, spleen, skin, salivary gland, lung, and kidney.[64] Renal damage is common and manifests as focal pyogranulomatous inflammation with mild glomerulonephritis, lymphoplasmacytic interstitial nephritis, mesangioproliferative glomerulonephritis, or occasionally amyloidosis. Amyloid deposits have also been found in the spleen, lymph nodes, small intestines, and liver of affected dogs. Various organs can show vascular changes, which include fibrinoid degeneration of vessel walls, mineralization and proliferation of the vascular intima, and pyogranulomatous vasculitis.

In *H. canis* infections, "wheel-spoked" meronts are present in varying numbers and stages of development throughout hemolymphatic target organs, such as bone marrow, spleen, and lymph nodes. The meronts are approximately 30 μm in diameter and on central cross-section appear as a circle of micromerozoite nuclei surrounding a central core. Meronts can be found in small numbers as an incidental finding in dogs from endemic areas.[65] Inflammation associated with meronts can range from none to very severe. In heavy infections, microscopic lesions may include hepatitis with Kupffer's cell hyperplasia and inflammatory infiltrates, interstitial pneumonia and thickening of alveolar septae with inflammatory infiltrates, glomerulonephritis or interstitial nephritis with multifocal necrosis, and focal splenic necrosis.

Treatment and Prognosis

Although no treatment effectively eliminates the tissue stages of *H. americanum*, remission of clinical signs can be achieved using a combination of a trimethoprim-sulfa, clindamycin, and pyrimethamine for 14 days (Table 77-5).[66] Response to therapy is usually dramatic, with resolution of clinical abnormalities within 48 to 72 hours of initiating therapy. Ponazuril

TABLE 77-5

Antimicrobial Drugs Indicated for Treatment of American Canine Hepatozoonosis

Drug	Dose* (mg/kg)	Route	Interval (hours)	Duration (days)
TCP combination:				
Trimethoprim-sulfonamide *and*	15	PO	12	14
Clindamycin *and*	10	PO	8	14
Pyrimethamine *and*	0.25	PO	24	14
Decoquinate†	10-20	PO	12	730

Adapted from Baneth G, Macintire DK, Vincent-Johnson N, et al. Hepatozoonosis. In Greene CE, ed. Infectious Diseases of the Dog and Cat, 3 ed. St. Louis, MO: Saunders; 2006:698-711.
TCP, Trimethoprim-sulfadiazine, clindamycin, and pyrimethamine; *PO*, by mouth.
*Dose per administration at specified interval.
†Use the decoquinate 6% (27.2 g/lb) powder, Deccox (Alpharma Inc., Fort Lee, NJ). One teaspoonful is equivalent to approximately 180 mg decoquinate. Administer at a rate of 1 teaspoon per 10 kg of body weight and feed q12h mixed into moist dog food.

(10 mg/kg PO q12h for 14 days) is an alternative therapeutic option.[67] Either of these protocols must be followed by long-term administration of decoquinate in order to prevent relapse. Without the addition of decoquinate, relapse occurs in most dogs 2 to 6 months following treatment. Although these dogs generally respond well to another round of combination therapy, subsequent relapses occur more frequently, and eventually disease becomes refractory to treatment. Persistent infections and multiple relapses lead to complications such as glomerulonephropathy, amyloidosis, vasculitis, and cachexia, which carry a guarded to poor prognosis. Decoquinate, a livestock anticoccidial agent, apparently breaks the asexual recycling of infection by arresting development of the merozoites after their release from meronts. Two years of daily decoquinate therapy is recommended.[66] Alternatively, a PCR assay can be performed every 3 to 6 months, and when the PCR becomes negative, treatment can be discontinued. Mild relapses can occur even during treatment with decoquinate. If clinical signs are severe, another course of combination therapy is indicated. Long-term administration of decoquinate results in extended survival times and excellent quality of life with a good prognosis. During the initial few days of treatment with either antiprotozoal regimen, administration of a nonsteroidal anti-inflammatory drug at standard dosages can provide relief from fever and pain.

Hepatozoon canis infections are treated with imidocarb dipropionate (5 to 6 mg/kg SC or IM every 14 days) until gamonts are no longer seen on blood smear examination.[52] Although some dogs require only one or two treatments, at least 8 weeks of treatment may be required for dogs with heavy infections. Doxycycline (10 mg/kg/day PO for 21 to 28 days) is frequently given in conjunction with imidocarb dipropionate. It has been recommended that all dogs, even those with only mild disease, be treated, because parasitemia may increase over time. A recent study showed that despite negative blood smears, dogs remained positive by PCR or buffy-coat examination even when treated repeatedly over 8 months.[68] This study also found that buffy-coat examination was twice as sensitive as blood smear examination in detecting gamonts, and PCR was even more sensitive for detection of persistent infection. Addition of toltrazuril does not seem to provide any additional benefit to imidocarb therapy.[69] Despite lack of a parasitologic cure, clinical cure is achieved in many dogs. Dogs with low parasitemia generally have a good long-term prognosis for survival, whereas those with high parasitemia have a guarded prognosis.

Immunity and Vaccination

Current treatments do not cure *H. americanum* or *H. canis* infections, so dogs remain susceptible to relapse of disease, especially if immunosuppressed. In experimental *H. canis* infections, treatment with an immunosuppressive dose of glucocorticoids was followed by the appearance of parasitemia.[33] Vaccines for *H. americanum* or *H. canis* infections are not available.

Prevention

Since both *H. canis* and *H. americanum* are transmitted by ingestion of ticks, the use of topical acaricides, environmental parasiticides, and immediate removal of ticks from dogs are the most important means of prevention. Because *H. americanum*, and possibly *H. canis*, can also be transmitted through ingestion of cystozoites in muscle from other animals, dogs should not be allowed to roam, scavenge, or engage in predatory behavior. Dogs should not be fed uncooked or undercooked game meat. Although *Hepatozoon* spp. have not been shown to be transmitted through blood transfusion, it seems logical that dogs infected with *Hepatozoon* species be avoided as blood donor dogs. To prevent congenital infections of puppies, infected females either should not be bred or should receive treatment before breeding.

Public Health Aspects

Only one case of human infection with a *Hepatozoon* spp. has been reported. Gamonts were identified on blood smears of an adult man from the Philippines who suffered from anemia and icterus, but no parasites were found in liver or bone marrow biopsies.[70] Because hepatozoonosis is transmitted by tick ingestion rather than a tick bite, tick ingestion is an unlikely route of transmission for humans. However, caution should be used when removing ticks from dogs or when handling tick-infested dogs or blood from infected dogs because of the unknown zoonotic potential of organisms that cause canine disease and the possibility that known human pathogens may also be present.

Hepatozoonosis in Domestic Cats

Feline hepatozoonosis occurs primarily in areas where canine hepatozoonosis exists, and it has been reported in a number of countries, including India, South Africa, Nigeria, Brazil, Israel, Spain, France, and Thailand.[30,31] In the United States, there is one report of hepatozoonosis in a domestic cat from Hawaii.[71] A survey of blood specimens from stray cats in Bangkok, Thailand, showed that 32.3% were positive by PCR for a *Hepatozoon* sp. most closely related to *H. canis*, whereas only 0.7% of the cats had gamonts observed on blood smears.[7] In Israel, *Hepatozoon* DNA was amplified from the blood of 36% of 152 cats, and infected cats were significantly more likely to have access to the outdoors.[31] The vast majority of cats were infected with an organism that resembled *H. felis*, although 2 cats were infected with an organism that resembled *H. canis*. Most infections were subclinical. Meronts have also been found in the myocardium and skeletal muscles of cats with no signs of illness. Cats with clinical hepatozoonosis are commonly immunosuppressed because of infection with FIV or FeLV. A range of clinical signs has been reported, including weakness, intermittent anorexia, weight loss, fever, lymphadenomegaly, ulcerative glossitis, hypersalivation, anemia, serous ocular discharge, and icterus. Treatment success has been reported with oral doxycycline at 5 mg/kg PO once a day for 10 days.[72]

CASE EXAMPLE

Signalment: "Pepper," a 1.5-year-old male miniature schnauzer from Opelika, AL (Figure 77-11)

History: Pepper was seen for a 1-month duration of illness characterized by intermittent fever (104.0°F to 105.0°F [40.0°C to 40.6°C]), lethargy, and ocular discharge. His owner reported that Pepper had also been stiff and reluctant to move. Despite a fairly good appetite, he had lost weight and muscle mass. The fever and other clinical signs had been nonresponsive to antibiotics, which included enrofloxacin and doxycycline, prescribed at the onset of illness. Pepper was a house dog but spent time outdoors in a rural environment. No vomiting, coughing, or sneezing had been reported, but he had had mild diarrhea at the onset of illness that resolved after a week. He had also had a mild increase in thirst and urination. He was fed a high-quality commercial dry dog food, received monthly heartworm preventive, and was current on all vaccinations, including canine distemper, hepatitis, parvovirus, and rabies vaccines. He had not traveled outside of the local area. The owner mentioned that she had had another dog that died about 1 year earlier after exhibiting similar clinical signs, but a diagnosis was not made.

Current medications: Aspirin 11 mg/kg PO q12h for pain.

Physical Examination:

Body Weight: 7.6 kg.

General: Quiet, slightly lethargic, but responsive. Reluctant to walk or stand; appeared painful. T = 103.8°F (39.9°C), HR = 96 beats/min, RR = 32 breaths/min, mucous membranes pink, CRT = 1.5 s.

Integument: The skin and haircoat appeared normal with no evidence of ectoparasites.

Eyes, Ears, Nose, and Mouth: A moderate amount of mucopurulent ocular discharge was present bilaterally. No other abnormalities were identified.

Musculoskeletal: Body condition score was 3/9 with moderate generalized muscle atrophy. The dog exhibited hyperesthesia during palpation of trunk, head, neck, and limb muscles. The dog's gait was very stiff and slow.

All Other Systems: Apart from abdominal splinting on palpation of the abdomen, no clinically significant abnormalities were present.

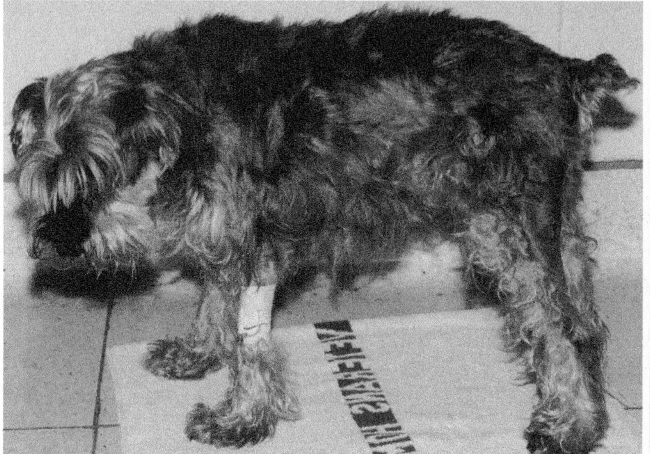

FIGURE 77-11 "Pepper," a 1.5-year-old male miniature schnauzer with *H. americanum* infection.

Ophthalmic Exam: Pupillary light reflex (direct and consensual): Normal.

Conjunctiva: injected bilaterally, mucopurulent discharge bilaterally.

Cornea and lens: Normal.

Schirmer Tear Test: Right eye = 18 mm; left eye = 16 mm (normal > 15 mm).

Fluorescein stain: Negative.

Tonometry: Normal.

Fundoscopic examination: A small grayish, slightly raised focal lesion was identified in the right fundus.

Laboratory Findings:

CBC:

PCV 38.7% (37%-55%)
MCV 68.7 fL (60-77 fL)
MCHC 35.4 g/dL (32-36 g/dL)
WBC 39,200 cells/μL (6000-17,000 cells/μL)
Neutrophils 35,672 cells/μL (3000-11,400 cells/μL)
Lymphocytes 1176 cells/μL (1000-4000 cells/μL)
Monocytes 2352 cells/μL (150-1200 cells/μL)
Eosinophils 0 (100-750 cells/μL)
Platelets 607,000 platelets/μL (200,000-400,000 platelets/μL).
The clinical pathologist's blood smear review showed no evidence of microorganisms.

Serum Chemistry Profile:
BUN 8 mg/dL (10-25 mg/dL)
Creatinine 0.6 mg/dL (0.3-1.0 mg/dL)
ALP 142 U/L (19-50 U/L)
ALT 37 U/L (17-66 U/L)
Creatine kinase 148 U/L (92-357 U/L)
Total bilirubin 0.3 mg/dL (0.1-0.3 mg/dL)
Glucose 52 mg/dL (80-100 mg/dL)
Sodium 153 mmol/L (146-160 mmol/L)
Potassium 4.7 mmol/L (3.5-5.9 mmol/L)
Chloride 118 mmol/L (108-125 mmol/L)
Calcium 10.3 mg/dL (9.5-11.8 mg/dL)
Phosphorus 3.9 mg/dL (3.3-5.8 mg/dL)
Total protein 6.4 g/dL (5.1-7.3 g/dL)
Albumin 2.7 g/dL (2.6-3.5 g/dL)
Globulin 3.7 g/dL (3.6-5.0 g/dL)
Total CO_2 21.8 mmol/L (13.9-31.5 mmol/L).

Urinalysis: SGr 1.035; pH 8.0, protein 1+, bilirubin negative, hemoprotein negative, glucose negative, 0 WBC/HPF, 0 RBC/HPF, no crystals, moderate lipid droplets.

Imaging Findings:

Pelvic Radiographs: Bilateral smooth periosteal bone formation was present on the ilium and femurs.

Abdominal Ultrasound Examination: No abnormalities were detected.

Bone Marrow Aspirate: The bone marrow smears were highly cellular with many particles. Megakaryocytes were adequate. In a 500-cell count, the M:E ratio was 1.7 (reference range 1.3-2.1) with normal maturation sequences in both red and white series. Multiple smears examined showed no evidence of microorganisms.

Muscle Biopsy: Histopathology showed infiltration of neutrophils and monocytes between muscle fibers. There were rare onion-skin cysts and one focal pyogranuloma. Many of the monocytes and neutrophils within the granuloma contained a single zoite. Findings were consistent with *Hepatozoon americanum* infection.

Cytology Findings: Although negative at the initial evaluation, blood smears and buffy-coat smears performed a few days later showed oblong "jellybean" inclusions in the cytoplasm of <0.1% of the leukocytes. These were characteristic of *Hepatozoon* gamonts.

Diagnosis: American canine hepatozoonosis (*Hepatozoon americanum* infection).

Treatment: Triple combination therapy consisting of (1) pyrimethamine 0.5 mg/kg PO q24h for 14 days; (2) sulfadiazine/trimethoprim 15 mg/kg PO q12h for 14 days; and (3) clindamycin 10 mg/kg PO q8h for 14 days. This was associated with resolution of fever within 24 hours. According to his owner, Pepper was back to normal within 7 days. After the 14-day course of triple combination therapy was completed, Pepper was started on decoquinate 15 mg/kg PO q12h with food. At day 74, the owners ran out of decoquinate and Pepper missed 2 days of treatment before a refill was obtained. Eight days later, the owners called to say that Pepper was doing poorly, could not get up, and his eyes were matted shut with a yellow-green discharge. Physical exam and CBC findings were similar to initial findings. Another 14-day course of triple combination therapy with pyrimethamine, sulfadiazine/trimethoprim, and clindamycin was prescribed. Once again, Pepper's clinical signs resolved within a few days. Pepper has continued on the decoquinate twice daily with no further breaks in doses and no more relapses.

Comments: American canine hepatozoonosis was suspected in this dog because of the geographic location in an endemic area of the southeastern United States, a waxing and waning fever, muscle pain, ocular discharge, leukocytosis, and other laboratory findings. As initially occurred in this case, organisms often cannot be seen on blood smear or buffy-coat exam. Muscle biopsy has been considered the most reliable way to diagnose infection, although PCR is also a very sensitive and specific diagnostic tool. This case illustrates the typical relapsing nature of the disease and the need for continuous long-term decoquinate therapy. After missing only a few doses of decoquinate, this dog suffered a relapse days later. He made a quick recovery with a second round of triple combination therapy. Effective treatment requires daily decoquinate therapy with no breaks for at least 2 years or until PCR of whole blood becomes negative.

SUGGESTED READINGS

Baneth G. Perspectives on canine and feline hepatozoonosis. Vet Parasitol. 2011;181:3-11.

Little SE, Allen KE, Johnson EM, et al. New developments in canine hepatozoonosis in North America: a review. 4th International Canine Vector-Borne Disease Symposium, Seville, Spain, 26-28 March 2009. Parasites Vectors. 2009;2(Suppl I):S5.

Vincent-Johnson NA. American canine hepatozoonosis. Vet Clin North Am Small Anim Pract. 2003;33:905-920.

REFERENCES

1. James SP. On a parasite found in the white corpuscles of the blood of dogs. Sci Mem Offrs Med Sanit Deps India. 1905;14:1-12.
2. Craig TM, Smallwood JE, Knauer KW, et al. *Hepatozoon canis* infection in dogs: clinical, radiographic, and hematologic findings. J Am Vet Med Assoc. 1978;173(8):967-972.
3. Smith TG. The genus *Hepatozoon*. J Parasitol. 1996;82:565-585.
4. Murata T, Shiramizu K, Hara Y, et al. First case of *Hepatozoon canis* infection of a dog in Japan. J Vet Med Sci. 1991;53:1097-1099.
5. Rajamanickam C, Wiesenhutter E, Zin FMD, et al. The incidence of canine haematozoa in peninsular Malaysia. Vet Parasitol. 1985;17:151-157.
6. Novilla MN, Kwapien RP, Peneyra RS. Occurrence of canine hepatozoonosis in the Philippines. Proc Helminthol Soc Wash. 1977;44:98-101.
7. Jittapalapong S, Rungphisutthipongse O, Maruyama S, et al. Detection of *Hepatozoon canis* in stray dogs and cats in Bangkok, Thailand. Ann N Y Acad Sci. 2006;1081:479-488.
8. McCully RM, Basson PA, Bigalke RD, et al. Observations on naturally acquired hepatozoonosis of wild carnivores and dogs in the Republic of South Africa. Onderstepoort J Vet Res. 1975;42:117-134.
9. Ezeokoli CD, Ogunkoya AB, Abdullah R, et al. Clinical and epidemiological studies on canine hepatozoonosis in Zaria, Nigeria. J Small Anim Pract. 1983;24:455-460.
10. Oyamada M, Davoust B, Boni M, et al. H. Detection of *Babesia canis rossi*, *B. canis vogeli*, and *Hepatozoon canis* in dogs in a village of eastern Sudan by using a screening PCR and sequencing methodologies. Clin Diagn Lab Immunol. 2005;12:1343-2136.

11. Kontos V, Koutinas A. Canine hepatozoonosis: a review of 11 naturally occurring cases. Bull Hell Vet Med Soc. 1990;41:73-81.
12. Fischer S, Hartmann K, Gothe R. *Hepatozoon canis*: eine importierte parasitare Infektion bei Hunden. Tierarztl Prax. 1994;22: 172-180.
13. Hervas J, Carrasco L, Gomez-Villamanddos JC, et al. Acute fatal hepatozoonosis in a puppy: histopathological and ultrastructural study. Vet Rec. 1995;137:518-519.
14. Baneth G, Harmelin A, Presentey BZ. *Hepatozoon canis* in two dogs. J Am Vet Med Assoc. 1995;206:1891-1894.
15. Elias E, Homans PA. *Hepatozoon canis* infection in dogs: clinical and hematological findings; treatment. J Small Anim Pract. 1988;29:55-62.
16. Allen LE, Li Y, Kaltenboeck B, et al. Diversity of *Hepatozoon* species in naturally infected dogs in the southern United States. Vet Parasitol. 2008;154:220-225.
17. Li Y, Wang C, Allen KE, et al. Diagnosis of canine *Hepatozoon* spp. infection by quantitative PCR. Vet Parasitol. 2008;157:50-58.
18. Gondim LF, Kohayagawa A, Alencar NX, et al. Canine hepatozoonosis in Brazil: description of eight naturally occurring cases. Vet Parasitol. 1998;74:319-323.
19. Eiras DF, Basabe J, Scodellaro CF, et al. First molecular characterization of canine hepatozoonosis in Argentina: evaluation of asymptomatic *Hepatozoon canis* infection in dogs from Buenos Aires. Vet Parasitol. 2007;149:275-279.
20. Criado-Fornelio A, Rey-Valeiron C, Buling A, et al. New advances in molecular epizootiology of canine hematic protozoa from Venezuela, Thailand, and Spain. Vet Parasitol. 2007;144:261-269.
21. Gossett KA, Gaunt SD, Aja DS. Hepatozoonosis and ehrlichiosis in a dog. J Am Anim Hosp Assoc. 1985;21:265-267.
22. Baker JL, Craig TM, Barton CC, et al. *Hepatozoon canis* in a dog with oral pyogranulomas and neurologic disease. Cornell Veterinarian. 1988;78:179-183.
23. Macintire DK, Vincent-Johnson N, Dillon AR, et al. Hepatozoonosis in dogs: 22 cases. J Am Vet Med Assoc. 1989-1994;1997(210):916-922.
24. Panciera RJ, Gatto NT, Crystal MA, et al. Canine hepatozoonosis in Oklahoma. J Am Anim Hosp Assoc. 1997;33:221-225.
25. Macintire DK, Vincent-Johnson NA. Canine hepatozoonosis. In: Bonagura, ed. Kirk's Current Veterinary Therapy XIII Small Animal Practice. Philadelphia, PA: WB Saunders; 2000:310-313.
26. Vincent-Johnson NA, Macintire DK, Lindsay DS, et al. A new *Hepatozoon* species from dogs: description of the causative agent of canine hepatozoonosis in North America. J Parasitol. 1997;83(6):1165-1172.
27. Baneth G, Barta JR, Shkap V, et al. Genetic and antigenic evidence supports the separation of *Hepatozoon canis* and *Hepatozoon americanum* at the species level. J Clin Microbiol. 2000;3: 1298-1301.
28. Dear JD, Owens SD, Biondo A, et al. *Babesia conradae* infection in coyote hunting dogs infected with multiple blood-borne pathogens. Proceedings of the 2012 American College of Veterinary Internal Medicine Forum. New Orleans: LA; June 2012.
29. Little L, Baneth G. Cutaneous *Hepatozoon canis* infection in a dog from New Jersey. J Vet Diagn Invest. 2011;23:585-588.
30. Baneth G, Macintire DK, Vincent-Johnson NA, et al. Hepatozoonosis. In: Greene, ed. Infectious Diseases of the Dog and Cat, 3rd ed. Philadelphia, PA: WB Saunders; 2006:698-711.
31. Baneth G, Sheiner A, Eyal O, et al. *Hepatozoon felis* infection in domestic cats – morphologic description and genetic characterization. Proceedings of the 2nd Symposium of the International Society for Companion Animal Infectious Diseases. San Francisco: CA; 2012; Abstract O16.
32. Mathew JS, Ewing SA, Panciera RJ, et al. Experimental transmission of *Hepatozoon americanum* to dogs by the Gulf Coast tick, *Amblyomma maculatum* Koch. J Parasitol. 1998;80:1-14.
33. Baneth G, Samish M, Alekseev E, et al. Transmission of *Hepatozoon canis* to dogs by naturally fed or percutaneously injected *Rhipicephalus sanguineus* ticks. J Parasitol. 2001;87:606-611.
34. Murata T, Inoue M, Taura Y, et al. Detection of *Hepatozoon canis* oocyst from ticks collected from the infected dogs. J Vet Med Sci. 1995;57:111-112.
35. Forlano M, Scofield A, Elisei C, et al. Diagnosis of *Hepatozoon* spp. in *Amblyomma ovale* and its experimental transmission in domestic dogs in Brazil. Vet Parasitol. 2005;134:1-7.
36. de Miranda RL, de Castro JR, Olegario MM, et al. Oocysts of *Hepatozoon canis* in *Rhipicephalus (Boophilus) microplus* collected from a naturally infected dog. Vet Parasitol. 2011;177:392-396.
37. Ewing SA, DuBois JG, Mathew JS, et al. Larval Gulf Coast ticks (*Amblyomma maculatum*) [Acari: Ixodidae] as host for *Hepatozoon americanum* [Apicomplexa: Adeleorina]. Vet Parasitol. 2002;103:43-51.
38. Baneth G, Samish M, Shkap V. Life cycle of *Hepatozoon canis* (Apicomplexa: Adeleorina: hepatozoidae) in the tick *Rhipicephalus sanguineus* and domestic dog (*Canis familiaris*). J Parasitol. 2007;93:283-299.
39. Baneth G, Shkap V. Monozoic cysts of *Hepatozoon canis*. J Parasitol. 2003;89:379-381.
40. Murata T, Makoto I, Susumu T, et al. Vertical transmission of *Hepatozoon canis* in dogs. J Vet Med Sci. 1993;55:867-868.
41. Johnson EM, Allen KE, Panciera RJ, et al. Infectivity of *Hepatozoon americanum* cystozoites for a dog. Vet Parasitol. 2008;154:148-150.
42. Johnson EM, Allen KE, Panciera RJ, et al. Experimental transmission of *Hepatozoon americanum* to New Zealand White rabbits (*Oryctolagus cuniculus*) and infectivity of cystozoites for a dog. Vet Parasitol. 2009;164:162-166.
43. Johnson EM, Panciera RJ, Allen KE, et al. Alternate pathway of infection with *Hepatozoon americanum* and the epidemiologic importance of predation. J Vet Intern Med. 2009;23:1315-1318.
44. Ewing SA, Mathew JS, Panciera RJ. Transmission of *Hepatozoon americanum* (Apicomplexa: Adeleorina) by ixodids (Acari: Ixodidae). J Med Entomol. 2002;39(4):631-634.
45. Allen K, Yabsley M, Johnson E, et al. Novel *Hepatozoon* in vertebrates from the southern United States. J Parasitol. 2011;97:648-653.
46. Davis DS, Robinson RM, Craig TM. Naturally occurring hepatozoonosis in a coyote. J Wildl Dis. 1978;14:244-246.
47. Lane JR, Kocan AA. *Hepatozoon* sp. infection in bobcats. J Am Vet Med Assoc. 1983;183:1323-1324.
48. Mercer SH, Jones LP, Rappole JH, et al. *Hepatozoon* sp. in wild carnivores in Texas. J Wildl Dis. 1988;24:574-576.
49. Kocan AA, Breshears M, Cummings C, et al. Naturally occurring hepatozoonosis in coyotes from Oklahoma. J Wildl Dis. 1999;35(1):86-89.
50. Kocan AA, Cummings CA, Panciera RJ, et al. Naturally occurring and experimentally transmitted *Hepatozoon americanum* in coyotes from Oklahoma. J Wildl Dis. 2000;36(1):149-153.
51. Panciera RJ, Ewing SA, Mathew JS, et al. Canine hepatozoonosis: comparison of lesions and parasites in skeletal muscle of dogs experimentally or naturally infected with *Hepatozoon americanum*. Vet Parasitol. 1999;82:261-272.
52. Baneth G, Weigler B. Retrospective case-control study of hepatozoonosis in dogs in Israel. J Vet Intern Med. 1997;11:365-370.
53. Barton CL, Russo EA, Craig TM, et al. Canine hepatozoonosis: a retrospective study of 15 natural occurring cases. J Am Anim Hosp Assoc. 1985;21:125-134.
54. Gavazza A, Bizzeti M, Papini R. Observations on dogs found naturally infected with *Hepatozoon canis* in Italy. Revue Med Vet. 2003;154:565-571.
55. Drost WT, Cummings CA, Mathew JS, et al. Determination of time of onset and location of early skeletal lesions in young dogs experimentally infected with *Hepatozoon americanum* using bone scintigraphy. Vet Radiol Ultrasound. 2003;44:86-91.
56. Panciera RJ, Mathew JS, Ewing SA, et al. Skeletal lesions of canine hepatozoonosis caused by *Hepatozoon americanum*. Vet Pathol. 2000;37:225-230.

57. Baneth G. Perspectives on canine and feline hepatozoonosis. Vet Parasitol. 2011;181:3-11.
58. Mathew JS, Saliki JT, Ewing SA, et al. An indirect enzyme-linked immunosorbent assay for diagnosis of American canine hepatozoonosis. J Vet Diagn Invest. 2001;13:17-21.
59. Shkap V, Baneth G, Pipano E. Circulating antibodies to *Hepatozoon canis* demonstrated by immunofluorescence. J Vet Diagn Invest. 1994;6:121-123.
60. Baneth G, Shkap V, Presentey BZ, et al. *Hepatozoon canis*: the prevalence of antibodies and gamonts in dogs in Israel. Vet Res Commun. 1996;20:41-46.
61. Gonen L, Strauss-Ayali D, Shkap V, et al. An enzyme-linked immunosorbent assay for antibodies to *Hepatozoon canis*. Vet Parasitol. 2004;122:131-139.
62. Mylonakis ME, Leontides L, Gonen L, et al. Anti-*Hepatozoon canis* serum antibodies and gamonts in naturally-occurring canine monocytic ehrlichiosis. Vet Parasitol. 2005;129:229-233.
63. Auburn University College of Veterinary Medicine Molecular Diagnostics. http://www.vetmed.auburn.edu/molecular-diagnostics. Last accessed January 21, 2013.
64. Vincent-Johnson NA. American canine hepatozoonosis. Vet Clin North Am Small Anim Pract. 2003;33:905-920.
65. Baneth G, Vincent-Johnson N. Hepatozoonosis. In: Shaw SE, Day MJ, eds. Arthropod-borne Infectious Diseases of the Dog and Cat. London: Manson; 2005:78-88.
66. Macintire DK, Vincent-Johnson NA, Kane CW, et al. Treatment of dogs infected with *Hepatozoon americanum:* 53 cases (1989-1998). J Am Vet Med Assoc. 2001;218:77-82.
67. Companion Animal Parasite Council Current Advice on Parasite Control. Vector-borne Diseases: American Hepatozoonosis. 2012. http://www.capcvet.org/capc-recommendations/american-hepatozoonosis/. Last accessed January 21, 2013.
68. Sasanelli M, Paradies P, Greco B, et al. Failure of imidocarb dipropionate to eliminate *Hepatozoon canis* in naturally infected dogs based on parasitological and molecular evaluation methods. Vet Parasitol. 2010;171:194-199.
69. Pasa S, Voyvoda H, Karagenc T, et al. Failure of combination therapy with imidocarb dipropionate and toltrazuril to clear *Hepatozoon canis* infection in dogs. Parasitol Res. 2011;109:919-926.
70. Carlos ET, Cruz FB, Cabiles CC, et al. *Hepatozoon* sp. in the WBC of a human patient. Univ Philipp Vet. 1971;15:5-7.
71. Ewing GO. Granulomatous cholangiohepatitis in a cat due to a protozoan parasite resembling *Hepatozoon canis*. Feline Pract. 1977;7:37-40.
72. Baneth G, Lavy E, Presentey BZ. *Hepatozoon* sp. parasitemia in a domestic cat. Feline Pract. 1995;23:10-12.

CHAPTER 78

Trypanosomiasis

Stephen C. Barr, Ashley B. Saunders, and Jane E. Sykes

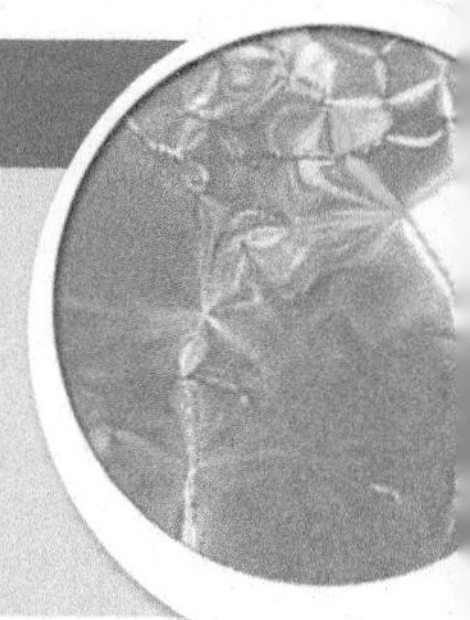

Overview of American Trypanosomiasis

First Described: Chagas' disease (American trypanosomiasis) was first described in humans in 1909 (Carlos Chagas).[1]

Cause: *Trypanosoma cruzi,* a protozoan parasite (phylum Sarcomastigophora, family Trypanosomatidae)

Affected Hosts: Dogs, humans, and more than 150 other domestic or wildlife mammalian species

Geographic Distribution: Central and South America; to a lesser extent southern United States (especially southeastern Texas)

Mode of Transmission: A bite from, or ingestion of, reduviid (kissing bug) vectors, primarily *Triatoma* species. Transmission through blood transfusion and vertical transmission can occur.

Major Clinical Signs: American trypanosomiasis in puppies manifests as lethargy, inappetence, mucosal pallor, lymphadenopathy, splenomegaly, arrhythmias, or sudden death. Neurologic signs such as pelvic limb ataxia and exaggerated spinal reflexes may also occur. Adult dogs may show lethargy, arrhythmias, signs of right- or left-sided congestive heart failure, or sudden death.

Differential Diagnoses: The differential diagnoses for suspected Chagas' myocarditis include dilated cardiomyopathy of large-breed dogs, parvoviral myocarditis in puppies, canine monocytic ehrlichiosis, babesiosis, and leishmaniosis. The primary differential diagnoses for suspected Chagas' meningoencephalitis in puppies are canine distemper virus infection and neosporosis, but other infectious and inflammatory causes of meningoencephalitis should also be considered.

Human Health Significance: Transmission to humans has the potential to occur after needle-stick injuries; caution is advised when handling tissues or clinical specimens from dogs with suspected trypanosomiasis.

AMERICAN TRYPANOSOMIASIS

Etiology and Epidemiology

Chagas' disease, or American trypanosomiasis, is caused by the flagellated protozoan *Trypanosoma cruzi.* In North America, disease in dogs usually manifests as cardiac disease typified by arrhythmias or myocarditis (acute or chronic), and, rarely, neurologic disease.[2-7] However, many infected dogs are subclinically infected for life. Cats can become infected, but disease in cats has not been recognized. *Trypanosoma cruzi* is an important vector-borne zoonosis in the Americas, particularly South and parts of Central America, and is the leading cause of dilated cardiomyopathy in humans.[8] Within the United States, most cases in dogs occur in Texas and especially involve working dogs that reside in southeastern Texas (Figure 78-1).[9-11] A few affected dogs have been reported from other southern states,[5,6,12-14] and as far north as Missouri.[15] The seroprevalence in dogs from Louisiana and Texas has generally been in the range of 12% to 22%, with seroprevalences of <10% in other states where canine disease has been identified.[16] Canine Chagas' disease is of importance to veterinary practitioners because it can be difficult to diagnose, is a potential zoonosis, and there is a lack of therapeutic options.

Trypanosoma cruzi exists in three morphologic forms. The form that circulates freely in the host's peripheral blood is the *trypomastigote.* This form is 15 to 20 μm long, with a flattened spindle-shaped body and a centrally placed vesicular nucleus. A single flagellum originates near a large, subterminal kinetoplast (situated posterior to the nucleus) and passes along the body to project anteriorly (Figure 78-2). The host intracellular or *amastigote* form is approximately 1.5 to 4.0 μm in diameter, is roughly spheroid, and contains both a nucleus and a rod-like kinetoplast. A small flagellum is present, but this is rarely obvious under light microscopy. The third morphologic form, the *epimastigote,* is found in the arthropod vector, a reduviid or "kissing bug" (subfamily Triatomae). Epimastigotes are flagellated and spindle shaped with the kinetoplast situated anterior to the nucleus. When a vector is involved in transmission, infection occurs when trypomastigotes are deposited in the triatomine's feces at the insect bite site. This is the main mode of transmission to humans in South America.

Transmission of *T. cruzi* in endemic countries depends on the confluence of vectors, reservoirs, parasites, and hosts (both people and animals) in a single habitat. Only three Triatomae species (*Triatoma infestans* [the main vector in South America], *Triatoma dimidiata,* and *Rhodnius prolixus*) that feed on man in endemic regions in South America display the appropriate behavior that enables them to transmit *T. cruzi* effectively. These species feed on blood from both people and domestic reservoir mammals (dog, cat, guinea pigs), reproduce prolifically while cohabiting close to people, and defecate soon after taking a blood meal, meaning that they are usually still on the host near the bite wound when they defecate.[17] Infection rates in these vectors can be as high as 100% south of the equator. By contrast, domestic transmission cycles probably do not occur in the United States, except in areas of southeastern

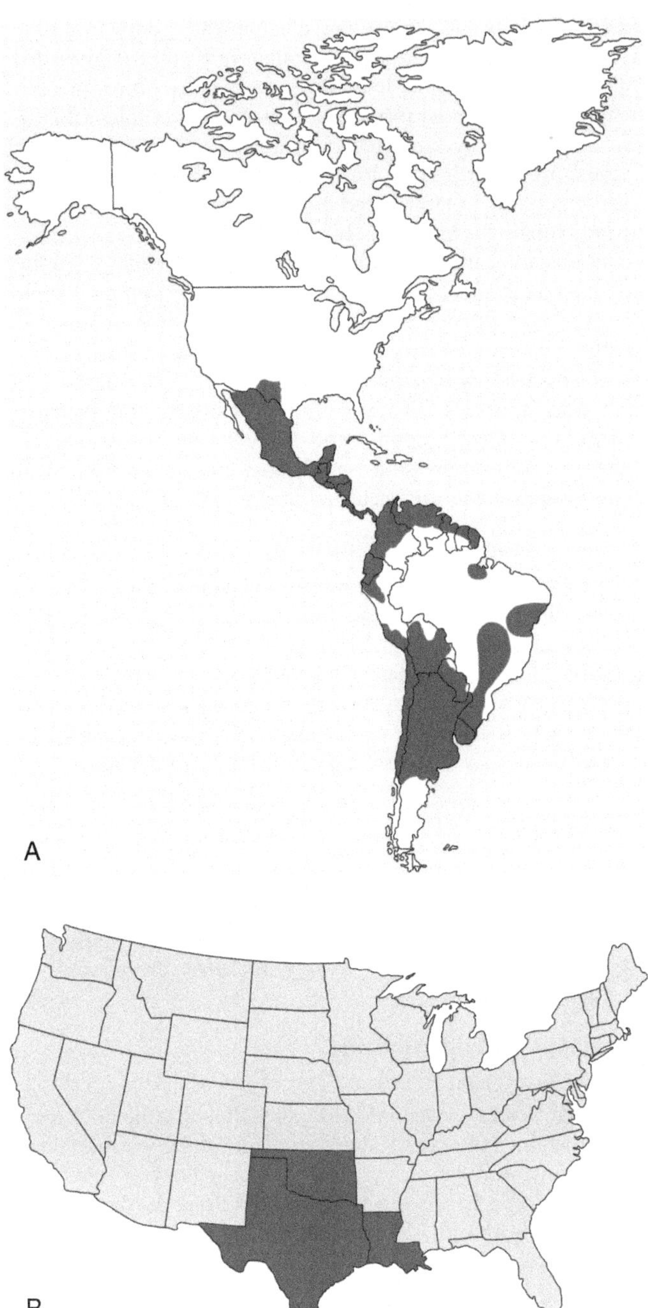

FIGURE 78-1 **A,** Approximate distribution of Chagas' disease in humans in the Americas. Insect-transmitted human Chagas' disease has also been rarely reported in Tennessee, California and Louisiana. **B,** States within the United States where Chagas' disease is most prevalent in dogs. Disease in Texas primarily occurs in the southeast. Occasional cases have been reported in other southern states and as far north as Virginia and Missouri.

Texas where there is evidence to suggest that the dog can be involved in domestic transmission cycles involving vectors and man.[18] Generally, though, the two principal vectors in the United States (*Triatoma protracta* and *Triatoma sanguisuga*) have low infection rates (20%), display different feeding habits, and defecate about 20 minutes after feeding, often when they have long fled the host.[19] As a result, it is more likely that dogs in North America become infected when they eat infected triatomines or their excreta. Certainly, opossums[20] and armadillos[21] become infected by this route, and outbreaks have occurred in humans following ingestion of contaminated food

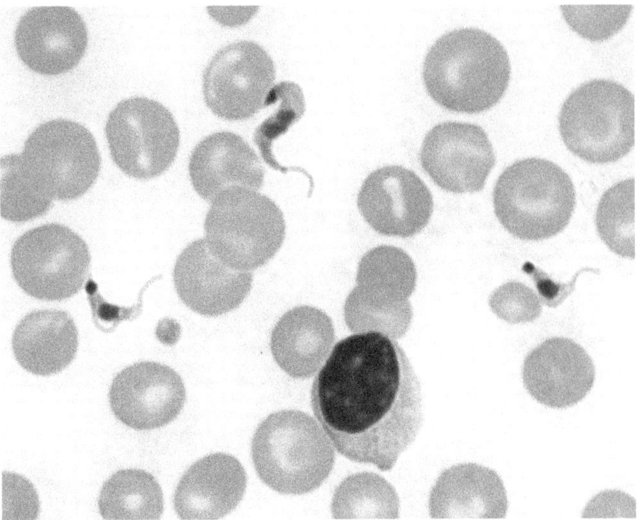

FIGURE 78-2 Trypomastigotes of *Trypanosoma cruzi* in a blood smear of a dog. Wright-Giemsa stain, 1000× oil magnification. (From Barr SC. Canine Chagas' disease (American trypanosomiasis) in North America. Vet Clin North Am. 2009;39:1055-1064.)

or drinks.[22] Blood transfusion and transplacental transmission can also occur, and infection after ingestion of infected milk from lactating bitches has been proposed.[6] Whether ingestion of reservoir hosts leads to transmission is unclear.

Within the United States, the principal wildlife reservoir hosts of *T. cruzi* in the eastern seaboard states south from Maryland and in most other southern states (Texas, Louisiana, and Oklahoma, to name a few) are opossums and raccoons. Armadillos can also be infected.[23] Various mouse, squirrel, and rat species are the main reservoir hosts in New Mexico and California.[24] Isolates of *T. cruzi* from vectors and animal reservoirs in North America are less pathogenic in mice than South American isolates.[23,25] Experimental inoculation of *T. cruzi* isolates from opossums and armadillos into dogs produces a disease consistent with naturally acquired acute and chronic canine trypanosomiasis, so it is likely that dogs in nature are infected with the same isolates as these wildlife hosts.[2-6] Six genotypes of *T. cruzi* have been identified (TcI through TcVI, also known as *discrete typing units* or *DTUs*), which appear to differ in their vector preferences and the extent to which they cause disease.[26]

After infection, trypomastigotes enter macrophages, transform into amastigotes, and multiply by binary fission (Figure 78-3). Alternatively, they spread hematogenously from the site of infection, infect myocardiocytes, transform into amastigotes, multiply, and transform back into trypomastigotes. The host cell then ruptures and trypomastigotes are released back into circulation. Parasitemia in dogs appears as early as 3 days postinfection (DPI), peaks at 17 DPI, and is cytologically undetectable *(subpatent infection)* by 30 DPI.[2] Clinical signs of acute myocarditis, should they occur, develop about 14 DPI with recovery occurring around 28 DPI.[2] Rapid intracellular multiplication ensures a rapid rise in parasitemia before effective immunity develops. Parasitemia steadily rises as more and more intracellular multiplication cycles add to the number of circulating trypomastigotes. The vector becomes infected when it ingests circulating trypomastigotes, which transform into epimastigotes and multiply by binary fission. Transformation of the epimastigotes back into trypomastigotes occurs in the vector's hindgut before the trypomastigotes are passed in the feces.

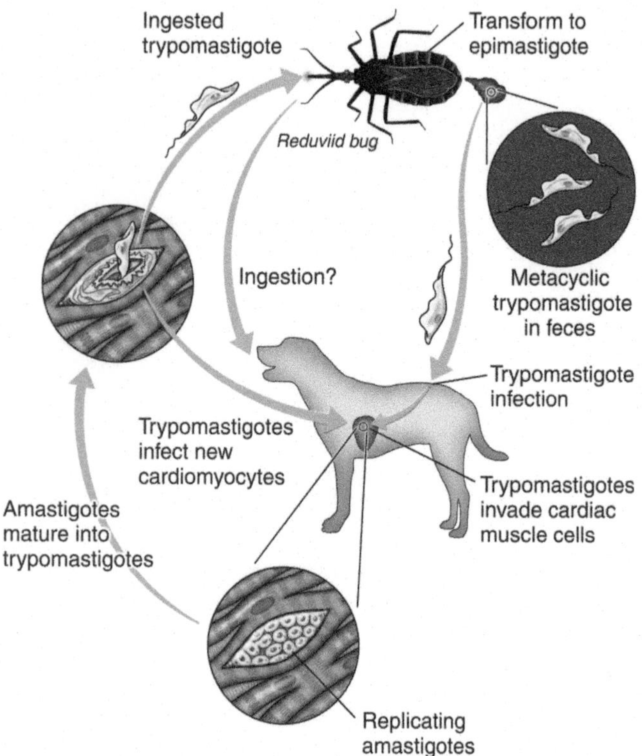

FIGURE 78-3 Life cycle of *Trypanosoma cruzi.* Dogs are infected when a triatome (reduviid bug) defecates at its bite site, and possibly when dogs ingest infected triatomes. Other routes of transmission may also predominate in the United States (see text). Trypomastigotes infect cardiomyocytes (as well as other tissues) and form amastigotes, which replicate locally, leading to myocarditis.

Clinical Features

Signs and Their Pathogenesis

As in humans, there are three phases of Chagas' myocarditis in dogs: acute, indeterminate (or latent), and chronic.[2-6] Acute myocarditis results from cell damage and inflammation as trypomastigotes rupture from myocardiocytes. Lethargy, fever, inappetence, generalized lymphadenopathy, slow capillary refill time with pale mucus membranes, and, in some cases, splenomegaly and hepatomegaly are the main signs in puppies. Diarrhea can also occur. In dogs over 6 months of age, parasitemia develops more slowly and clinical signs are often much less severe or not apparent at all. Sudden death, presumably from cardiac muscle failure or conduction system failures leading to malignant arrhythmias, is not a common occurrence. Although less common than signs referable to cardiac abnormalities, neurologic signs referable to meningoencephalitis (as a direct result of parasitic invasion of the neurologic system) may also occur and include weakness, pelvic limb ataxia, and exaggerated spinal reflexes suggestive of distemper. Humans with Chagas' disease can also develop severe megaesophagus or megacolon due to parasympathetic denervation,[22] but these have not been described in dogs.

Dogs that survive the acute phase enter a prolonged indeterminate phase typified by a lack of clinical signs. Parasitemia becomes cytologically undetectable at about 30 DPI, although it can still be demonstrated by blood culture. The ECG is usually normal during this phase, although ventricular arrhythmias can be induced by exercise.[3] Although not all dogs progress to develop chronic disease, some develop chronic myocarditis with cardiac dilatation over the subsequent 8 to 36 months.[2,3] ECG abnormalities become more prevalent in these dogs and may even result in sudden death. Clinical signs referable to right-sided and eventually, in some, left-sided heart failure occur and can include exercise intolerance, pulse deficits, ascites, pleural effusion, hepatomegaly, and jugular venous congestion.[2] Chronic Chagas' myocarditis is clinically indistinguishable from dilated cardiomyopathy of large breed dogs.[4-6] The pathogenesis of the cardiomyopathy is unknown, but proposed mechanisms include damage to myocardiocytes or the autonomic nervous system by immune-mediated mechanisms or toxic parasitic products, and/or microvascular disease coupled with platelet dysfunction.[27,28] Cardiac dilatation occurs when fibrosis no longer permits efficient compensatory hypertrophy.[27,29] Some *T. cruzi* isolates that infect dogs in the United States are not pathogenic but produce a marked serologic response and a low-level parasitemia following immunosuppression.[2,30] Reactivation of infection with immunosuppression can occur in human patients.[22]

Physical Examination Findings

The most common physical examination findings in puppies with Chagas' disease are lethargy, generalized lymphadenomegaly, splenomegaly, pallor, and arrhythmias. Generalized subcutaneous edema has also been reported.[31] Dogs with chronic Chagas' disease may show signs of right- and/or left-sided congestive heart failure, with tachypnea, ascites, or jugular pulses. Cardiac murmurs and/or arrhythmias may be detected on auscultation of the heart.

Diagnosis

The key to diagnosis of Chagas' disease is a high degree of clinical suspicion. Chagas' disease should be considered in any dog with signs of myocarditis or cardiomyopathy, particularly if it lives or has lived at any time—even years before evaluation—in an endemic region.

Laboratory Abnormalities

Complete Blood Count

During the acute *T. cruzi* infection, the CBC of some dogs may reveal anemia, leukocytosis due to a neutrophilia, eosinophilia, monocytosis, and lymphocytosis.[32,33] Thrombocytopenia, leukopenia, and/or lymphopenia have also been documented.[16] Dogs in the chronic phase of infection may have no hematologic abnormalities.

Serum Biochemical Tests

Serum ALT activity, AST activity, and creatinine and urea nitrogen concentrations can be elevated in dogs with *T. cruzi* infection, especially those that are at risk of death from severe acute myocarditis. Rarely, moderate to severe hypoalbuminemia with or without hyperglobulinemia occurs in acutely affected dogs.[16,31] Serum troponin I levels rise slowly in infected dogs and peak at around 10 to 30 mg/mL by 21 DPI. Serum troponin I levels are elevated in dogs infected after 6 months of age but usually not to such high levels.

Urinalysis

There are no specific findings reported on urinalysis in dogs with Chagas' disease.

Electrocardiography

The ECG of dogs with severe Chagas' myocarditis may show sinus tachycardia, decreased R-wave amplitude, axis shifts, T-wave

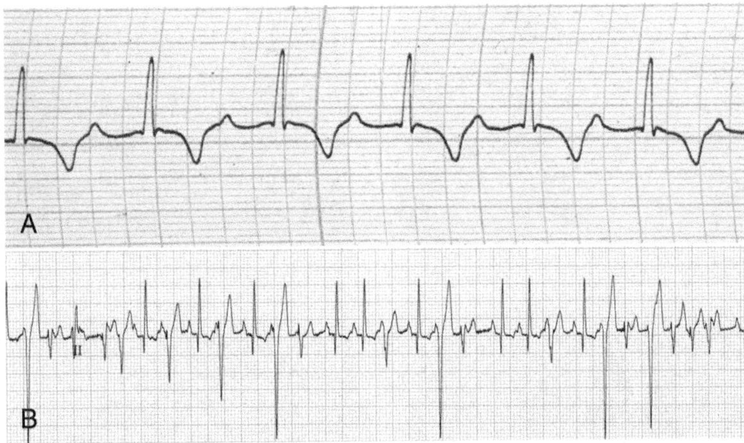

FIGURE 78-4 Electrocardiographic findings in dogs with Chagas' disease. **A,** Second-degree heart block and depressed QRS complexes. (From Barr SC. Canine Chagas' disease (American trypanosomiasis) in North America. Vet Clin North Am. 2009;39:1055-1064.) **B,** Multiform ventricular premature complexes in an 11-year-old, neutered male Labrador retriever presenting for collapse. Recording speed 25 mm/s, sensitivity 10 mm/mV.

inversion, ventricular arrhythmias, and conduction abnormalities, including first-, second-, and third-degree atrioventricular block and right bundle branch block (Figure 78-4).

Diagnostic Imaging

Plain Radiography

Plain thoracic radiographs in dogs with chronic Chagas' myocarditis may reveal cardiomegaly or evidence of congestive heart failure (pulmonary edema or pleural effusion) (Figure 78-5).

Sonographic Findings

Echocardiograms of puppies with acute myocarditis are usually within normal limits. Echocardiographic abnormalities in dogs with chronic Chagas' myocarditis include right ventricular dilation with progression to include a loss of left ventricular function with decreased fractional shortening, reduced ejection fraction, reduced left ventricular free wall thickness, and increased end-systolic volume (Figure 78-6).

Microbiologic Tests

Diagnostic assays for trypanosomiasis in dogs and cats are described in Table 78-1.

Cytologic Examination

During acute disease, trypomastigotes may be detected on blood smear examination (see Figure 78-2). However, only a few parasites may be present on the entire slide, demanding diligent examination, or some form of concentration technique may be used. High-power (400×) examination of the buffy-coat layer from a centrifuged microhematocrit tube may reveal the motile parasites. Examination of a thick-film buffy-coat smear stained with either Wright or Giemsa stains is more sensitive than examination of a blood smear. A highly effective concentration technique involves pelleting trypomastigotes from plasma (obtained by centrifugation of 10 to 50 mL of heparinized blood at 800 × *g* for 10 minutes) by further centrifugation (8000 × *g* for 15 minutes). The pellet from the final centrifugation may be examined microscopically after staining or be submitted for PCR analysis or culture. The larger the volume of the blood specimen collected, the greater the likelihood that organisms will be detected. Trypomastigotes may also be found on cytologic examination of lymph node aspirates and in abdominal effusions. Amastigotes were described in the lymph node of one affected dog that were cytologically indistinguishable from those of *Leishmania*.[31]

Culture

Trypanosoma cruzi can be cultured from blood in liver infusion tryptose (LIT) growth medium. However, several weeks are required before epimastigotes grow in this medium, which is too long to be helpful for making treatment decisions. Although culture is more sensitive than blood smear examination, false-negative results can still occur; in humans the sensitivity of blood culture is estimated to be only 50%.[22] Culture of trypanosomes is a specialized procedure that is not routinely available in veterinary diagnostic laboratories.

Serologic Diagnosis

Serology is extremely useful for the diagnosis of Chagas' disease, especially during the indeterminate and chronic phases when trypomastigotes are very difficult to detect.[34] Indirect fluorescent antibody, ELISA, and radioimmunoprecipitation assays are most commonly used. A rapid immunochromatographic dipstick test has also been developed.[35] Serologic tests confirm the presence of antibodies to *T. cruzi,* but most cross-react with antibodies to *Leishmania*. Further, in rare situations in dogs, the clinical signs of Chagas' disease and leishmaniasis overlap sufficiently that it is necessary to go to considerable lengths to establish a diagnosis.[31] Therefore a detailed history of the likelihood of exposure to *Leishmania* must be known in order to accurately interpret serologic results. A higher antibody titer to *Trypanosoma* than to *Leishmania* may support a diagnosis of trypanosomiasis. Positive serology in association with consistent clinical signs is the most common means of diagnosis of Chagas' disease in dogs. If possible, two different serologic assays should be used to confirm a positive titer, especially in regions of low prevalence. The serum titer usually becomes positive by 21 DPI, when parasitemia is declining, and persists for the life of the animal irrespective of whether clinical signs develop.[30]

Molecular Diagnosis Using the Polymerase Chain Reaction

PCR assays, which detect DNA of *T. cruzi* in various clinical specimens (blood, plasma pellets, lymph node aspirates, or ascites fluid), can be highly specific for *T. cruzi* but can have

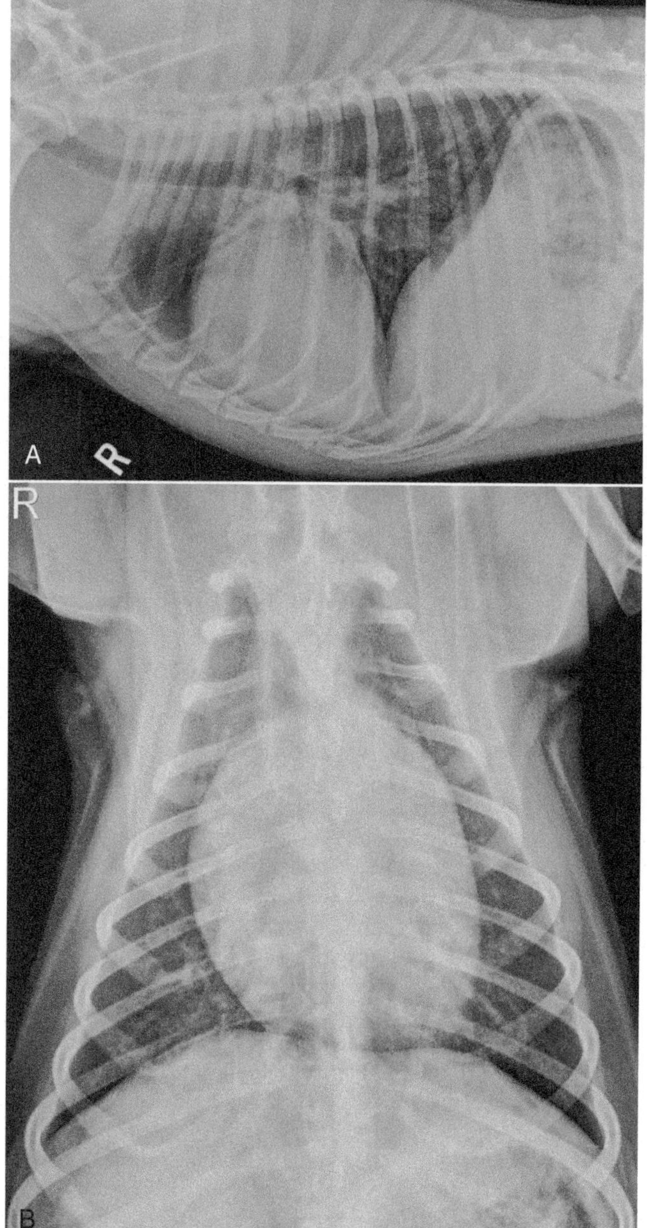

FIGURE 78-5 Right lateral **(A)** and dorsoventral **(B)** thoracic radiographic images of a dog with trypanosomiasis and mild generalized cardiomegaly. The pulmonary veins are slightly larger than the corresponding artery, and a slight interstitial pattern was present throughout the lungs.

variable and sometimes low sensitivity for diagnosis of chronic infections unless multiple specimens are tested.[34] Real-time PCR assays have been developed for diagnosis of human Chagas' disease that detect repetitive sequences found in very high copy number within *T. cruzi*.[36] Because each parasite may have more than 100,000 copies of the sequence, the sensitivity of the assay is increased.[22] The sensitivity of PCR assays varies depending on the *T. cruzi* strain involved.[36,37] PCR may be useful to confirm infection when organisms are not seen on blood smears. Currently, PCR assays for *T. cruzi* are not widely available from veterinary diagnostic laboratories on a commercial basis, but have been used for diagnosis of canine Chagas' disease.[31]

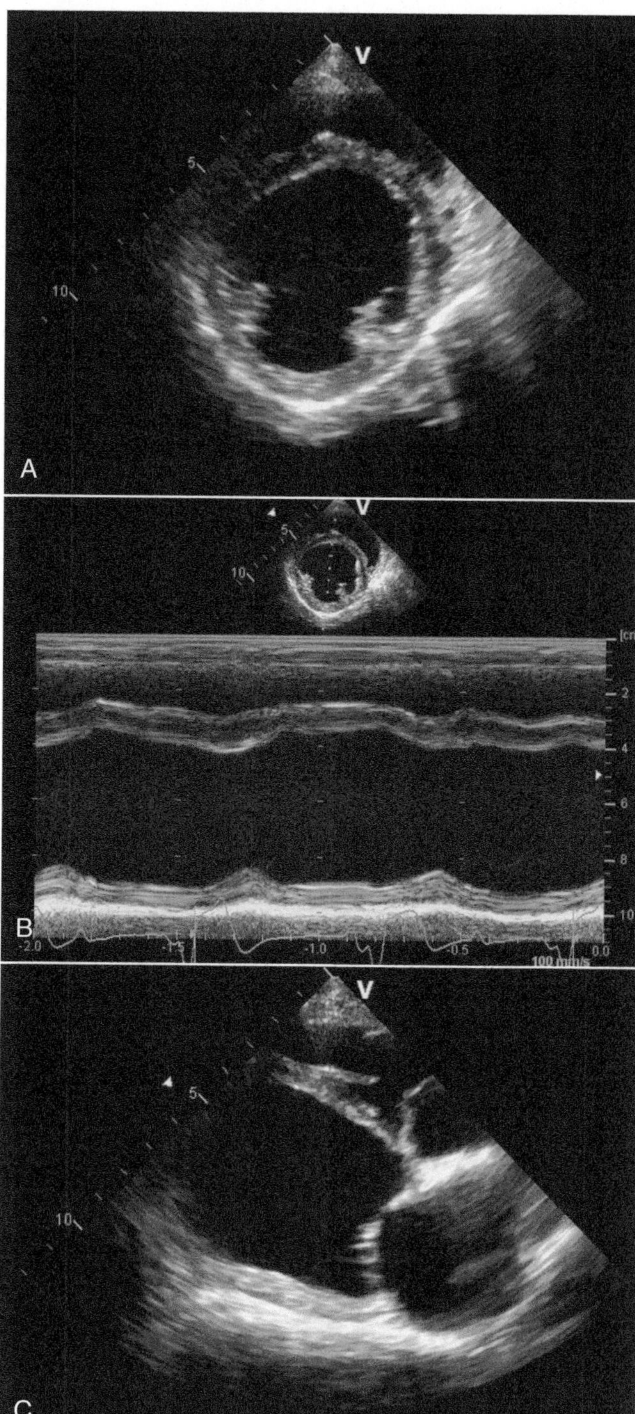

FIGURE 78-6 Two dimensional **(A)** and M-mode **(B)** transthoracic echocardiogram images obtained in a right parasternal short-axis view and long-axis view **(C)** from a dog with Chagas' disease documenting significant left ventricular enlargement and mild right ventricular enlargement.

Pathologic Findings

Gross Pathologic Findings

Gross pathologic findings in dogs with Chagas' disease include lymphadenopathy, evidence of congestive heart failure (ascites, pleural effusion, or congestion of viscera), and biventricular cardiac enlargement with thinning of the ventricular wall. Often the right side of the heart is more enlarged than the left. Hemorrhages and pale foci may be identified in the myocardium.

TABLE 78-1

Diagnostic Assays Currently Available for Trypanosomiasis in Dogs and Cats

Assay	Specimen Type	Target	Performance
Cytologic examination	Aspirates of lymph nodes, spleen, bone marrow, blood smears, or buffy-coat preparations	*Trypanosoma* trypomastigotes or, less commonly, amastigotes	Organisms may be few in number and in chronic trypanosomiasis are often not found.
Trypanosoma culture	Blood or buffy-coat preparations, bone marrow	*Trypanosoma* spp.	Requires special techniques and expertise that are not widely available. Sensitivity may be low in chronic infections.
Antibody serology (immunofluorescent antibody or ELISA)	Serum	Antibodies to *Trypanosoma* spp.	Most infected dogs test positive, but positive test results occur in healthy animals, so results must be interpreted in light of clinical signs. False positives can occur in dogs exposed to *Leishmania* or those vaccinated with *Leishmania* vaccines.
Real-time PCR assays	Whole blood, buffy coats, splenic or lymph node aspirates, CSF	*Trypanosoma* DNA	May be useful in dogs with suggestive clinical signs in which organisms cannot be found cytologically. Sensitivity and specificity depend on assay design. Quantitative PCR may be useful for evaluation of treatment efficacy. Limited availability.

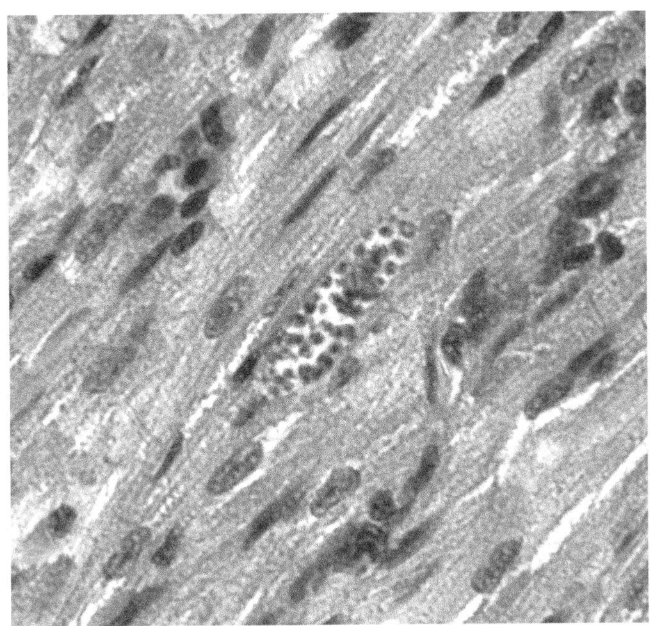

FIGURE 78-7 Pseudocyst of *Trypanosoma cruzi* within a myocardiocyte of an infected dog. H&E stain, 1000× magnification. (From Barr SC. Canine Chagas' disease (American trypanosomiasis) in North America. Vet Clin North Am. 2009;39:1055-1064.)

Histopathologic Findings

Histopathologic findings in Chagas' disease include a severe diffuse granulomatous myocarditis, large numbers of parasitic pseudocysts (intracellular collections of amastigotes), and minimal fibrosis (Figure 78-7). Immunohistochemistry does not distinguish *Leishmania* from *Trypanosoma* amastigotes, because of serologic cross-reactivity.[31] Histopathology of the myocardium in chronic Chagas' myocarditis is characterized by multifocal lymphocytic infiltrates, perivasculitis, and marked fibrosis, and rare, if any, parasitic pseudocysts.[4,27]

TABLE 78-2

Antimicrobials Used to Treat Acute Chagas' Disease in Dogs

Drug*	Dose (mg/kg)	Route	Interval (hours)	Duration (months)
Benznidazole	5-10	PO	24	2
Nifurtimox	2-7	PO	6	3-5
Prednisone	0.5	PO	12	1

*Both benznidazole and nifurtimox are available from the Centers for Disease Control and Prevention, Atlanta, GA.

Treatment and Prognosis

Antimicrobial Treatment

Treatment of dogs with naturally occurring acute Chagas' myocarditis is poorly documented, since this phase is seldom recognized. The use of nifurtimox (usually in association with glucocorticoids)[38] or benznidazole[39] has been reported in the dog (Table 78-2). However, the severe adverse effects of nifurtimox preclude its use, so benznidazole is the drug of choice (see Chapter 10). Benznidazole is available from the Centers for Disease Control and Prevention, Atlanta, GA. After treatment with benznidazole, serum antibody titers usually remain elevated, although they are reported to decline in people. Treatment of experimentally infected dogs with *acute* Chagas' disease with benznidazole reduced or prevented subsequent fibrosis and arrhythmias, even if parasites were not completely eliminated.[40] Benznidazole-resistant strains of *T. cruzi* have been described. Ketoconazole, gossypol, allopurinol, and verapamil have shown promise in other species but are ineffective for the treatment of Chagas' disease in dogs. Ravuconazole and posaconazole also reduce parasite load,[41,42] but to date azole drugs have not been adopted for treatment of humans because they lack significant benefit over benznidazole or nifurtimox.[22] However, the combination of the antiarrhythmic amiodarone and an azole (itraconazole or posaconazole) has synergistic antiprotozoal activity against *T. cruzi* and shows promise as an effective treatment for chronic Chagas' disease in humans.[43,44]

Most dogs are diagnosed with Chagas' disease during the chronic stage. Unfortunately, treatments directed against the parasite at this stage do not significantly alter the outcome of disease.[45] Treatment should be directed toward the myocardial failure and ventricular arrhythmias, although the latter are often refractory to drug therapy. Pacemaker implantation may be required for some dogs with bradyarrhythmias such as third-degree atrioventricular block. In humans with indeterminate and chronic symptomatic Chagas' disease, the benefit of treatment remains controversial and is still under investigation by means of a large, prospective clinical trial (the Benznidazole Evaluation for Interrupting Trypanosomiasis [BENEFIT] trial).[36]

Prognosis

The prognosis for dogs that develop Chagas' disease is poor because of the lack of effective treatments. Dogs diagnosed at an older age (mean of 9 years) survive longer (30 to 60 months) than dogs diagnosed at a younger age (mean of 4.5 years), which survive only up to 5 months postdiagnosis.[11]

Immunity and Vaccination

Recovery from *T. cruzi* infection is not associated with protective immunity. No vaccine is available.

Prevention

The risk of infection by *T. cruzi* can be reduced by limiting contact between dogs and vectors and possible reservoir hosts (raccoons, opossums, armadillos, and skunks). Dogs should not be fed meat from reservoir hosts. Kennels and surrounding structures (chicken houses, wood piles) in endemic areas should be sprayed monthly with a residual insecticide. Dog housing should be upgraded to remove vector nesting sites. Applications of fipronil on the coats of dogs do not appear to prevent infections in dogs or reduce the feeding of vectors,[46] but deltamethrin-treated collars do reduce feeding by *Triatoma infestans*.[47,48] Blood donor dogs should be serologically screened to determine previous exposure to *T. cruzi*. In highly endemic regions (southern Texas), bitches should be screened serologically, and positive animals should not be bred.

Public Health Aspects

American trypanosomiasis is a major human health problem in South and Central America and is increasingly recognized in Mexico.[8,49] It is primarily a problem in impoverished regions where humans live in rural areas. Dogs are considered a reservoir for human infection in these regions because they maintain high levels of parasitemia and are a preferred host for triatomine insects. Cats may also act as a reservoir for human infection in South America.[50] Fewer than one third of infected humans ultimately develop Chagas' disease.[22]

To date, fewer than 10 human cases of Chagas' disease involving transmission by vectors have been reported in the United States (4 in Texas, and 1 each in California, Tennessee, and Louisiana). By far the largest number of people infected with *T. cruzi* in the United States (estimated at approximately 100,000 people) have emigrated from endemic regions such as Mexico and Central America. Consequently, reports of cases associated with transmission by blood transfusion continue to rise.[51,52] Imported cases in tourists who return to the United States have not been described. There are probably several reasons why only a handful of naturally acquired cases have been reported in the United States. First, North American vector species are poorly adapted to living in houses and do not defecate on the host after a blood meal. Higher standards of housing in North America than in parts of Central and South America may also prevent vectors from nesting in human dwellings. Third, some human cases of Chagas' disease in North America may be overlooked because of a low level of suspicion.

Although the risk of a human acquiring infection from an infected dog is extremely low, the severity and difficulty of treating disease in humans makes this disease of considerable public health significance. Veterinarians should be careful when handling blood samples from infected dogs and warn laboratory staff of the potential infectivity of the samples. Accidental needle-stick injuries when administering therapy to or collecting specimens from infected dogs should be reported immediately to the CDC.

Overview of African Trypanosomiasis in Dogs

First Described: Reports of African trypanosomiasis date back to Egyptian times. Trypanosomes were identified as the cause in 1895, when they were detected in cattle by a Scottish microbiologist, David Bruce (after whom *Brucella* was named).[53]

Cause: *Trypanosoma brucei rhodesiense, Trypanosoma congolense, Trypanosoma evansi* (protozoan parasites, family Trypanosomatidae)

Affected Hosts: Dogs and a variety of other mammalian host species. Humans are infected with *T. brucei gambiense* and *T. brucei rhodesiense.*

Geographic Distribution: Central Africa *(T. brucei, T. congolense); T. evansi* is found in Africa as well as in Asia, Latin America, and the Canary Islands in Spain.

Mode of Transmission: A bite from the tsetse fly *(T. brucei or T. congolense)* or mechanical transmission by hematophagous flies *(T. evansi)*

Major Clinical Signs: Lethargy, inappetence, weight loss, pallor, peripheral edema, ascites, hematemesis, hemorrhagic diarrhea, uveitis, corneal edema, neurologic signs due to meningoencephalitis

Differential Diagnoses: These include canine monocytic ehrlichiosis, babesiosis, leishmaniosis, and systemic immune-mediated diseases. Canine distemper virus infection and neosporosis are important differential diagnoses in dogs with meningoencephalitis.

Human Health Significance: Although most *Trypanosoma* species that cause African trypanosomiasis in dogs do not infect humans, *T. brucei rhodesiense* does, so caution is advised when handling tissues or clinical specimens from dogs or cats with suspected trypanosomiasis.

AFRICAN TRYPANOSOMIASIS

African trypanosomiasis is caused by *Trypanosoma brucei* and *Trypanosoma congolense.* These organisms are transmitted by tsetse flies (*Glossina* species), which are only found in Africa. *Trypanosoma brucei* includes *Trypanosoma brucei brucei, T. brucei gambiense,* and *T. brucei rhodesiense,* which are indistinguishable morphologically and are referred to as "*T. brucei* complex" organisms. *T. evansi* also belongs to this group (see later). The epidemiology, host range, and clinical features of disease caused by these *T. brucei* complex organisms differ. *Trypanosoma brucei gambiense* and *T. brucei rhodesiense* cause "sleeping sickness" in humans from Africa (West African and East African trypanosomiasis, respectively) (Figure 78-8). A variety of animal reservoirs of *T. brucei rhodesiense* have been identified, but an animal reservoir for *T. brucei gambiense* has not.[54] Along these lines, only naturally occurring infections with *T. brucei rhodesiense* , and not *T. brucei gambiense*, have been reported in dogs.[55] *Trypanosoma brucei brucei* and *T. congolense* cause trypanosomiasis in a variety of domestic animal species ("nagana") but do not infect humans. Dogs are especially susceptible to *T. congolense* infection. Four types of *T. congolense* have been identified—savannah, forest, Tsavo, and Kilifi—which may vary in pathogenicity. There are several reports of travel-related infections with *T. congolense* in dogs,[56-58] sometimes in association with a long period of latency.[57] It has been suggested that African dogs may exhibit a degree of "trypanotolerance," whereas dogs imported into Africa may be more susceptible to infection and disease.[59]

African trypanosomes exist only as a trypomastigote in the blood of the mammalian host; in contrast to Chagas' disease, there is no amastigote phase. Epimastigotes develop in the salivary glands of the tsetse fly, and the organism is transmitted in saliva when it feeds on the mammalian host. Transmission to the mammalian host results in hemolymphatic spread of the organism over weeks to months with signs that relate to proliferation of mononuclear phagocytes and increased vascular permeability. *T. brucei* complex organisms are well known for their ability to evade the host immune response through extensive variation of their outer surface glycoproteins (known as *variant antigen types*, or *VATs*). The hemolymphatic phase may be followed by the development of meningoencephalitis in some animals. In humans, meningoencephalitis is most apparent with *T. brucei gambiense* infections and results in tremors and progressive daytime somnolescence (hence the term "sleeping sickness"). Pancarditis with arrhythmias and congestive heart failure is a more typical outcome of *T. brucei rhodesiense* infection in humans.

The clinical signs of African trypanosomiasis in dogs include persistent fever, lethargy, anorexia, weight loss, pallor, mucopurulent oculonasal discharge, lymphadenopathy, hepatosplenomegaly, variable peripheral edema, abdominal distention due to ascites, petechial hemorrhages, signs of pancarditis, and ocular signs such as unilateral or bilateral uveitis, corneal edema, and/or keratitis (which can mimic "blue eye" due to canine adenovirus-1). Hemorrhagic vomiting and diarrhea can occur in dogs infected with *T. congolense.*[58,60] Neurologic signs (seizures, tremors, opisthotonos, and hyperreflexia) due to meningoencephalitis have also been described in dogs infected with *T. congolense.*[58]

Laboratory abnormalities in dogs with African trypanosomiasis have been most well described for *T. congolense* infections. The most common findings are regenerative or nonregenerative anemia, leukocytosis or leukopenia, and thrombocytopenia.[57,58,60] Serum biochemistry findings include increased serum liver

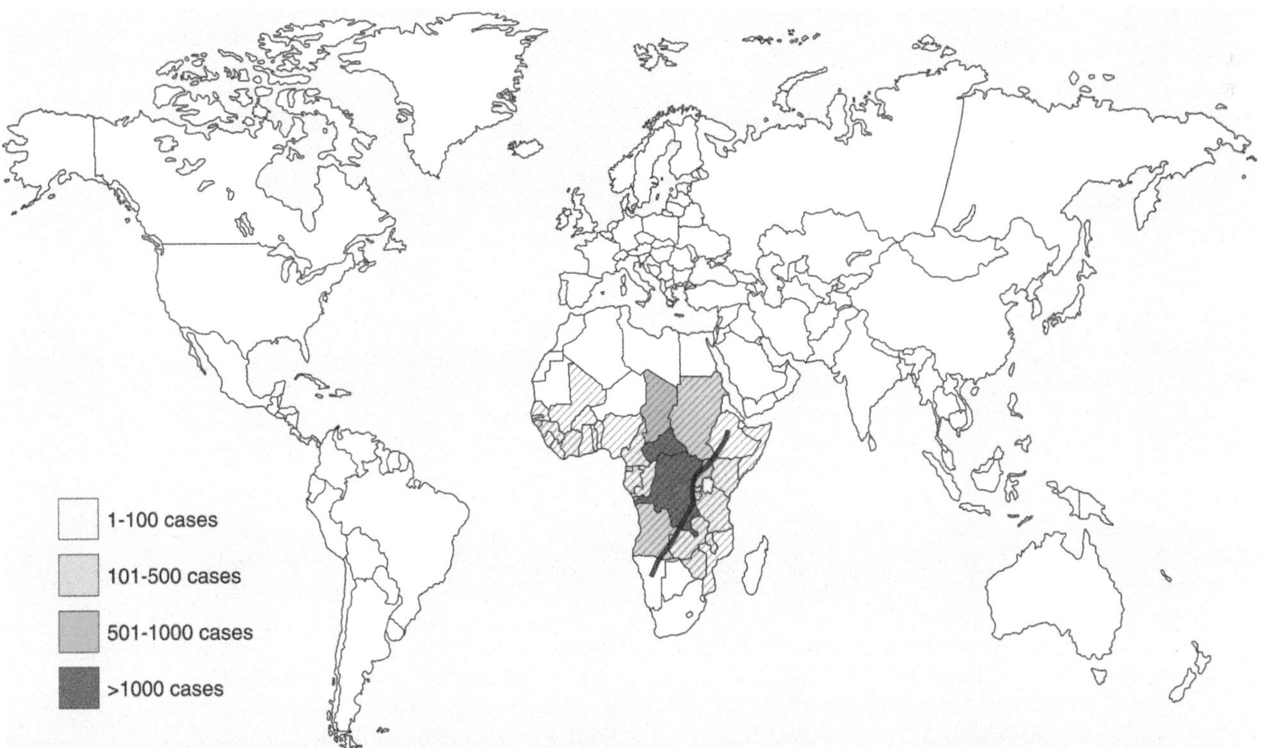

FIGURE 78-8 Map showing geographic distribution of human African trypanosomiasis (green countries) and the number of cases reported in natives in the year 2009. *Trypanosoma brucei gambiense* is found in western Africa and *Trypanosoma brucei rhodesiense* is found in eastern Africa. The line divides the geographic distribution of the two forms of disease. *T. brucei brucei,* which infects dogs, occurs throughout both regions. The hashed lines indicate the countries in which tsetse flies are found. (Modified from Brun R and Blum J. Human African Trypanosomiasis. Inf Dis Clin North Am. 2012;26:261-273.)

enzyme activities, azotemia, hyperglobulinemia, and hypoalbuminemia,[57,58] but one dog had no significant abnormal serum biochemistry findings.[56]

The primary means of diagnosis is cytologic detection of the organism in aspirates, body fluids, or blood smears. Identification of the infecting species requires PCR and sequencing. The treatment of choice for dogs is diminazene aceturate, but this may not always be effective or available. Treatment of the hemolymphatic disease in humans is with pentamidine isethionate *(gambiense)* or suramin *(rhodesiense)*, whereas disease of the central nervous system is treated with the arsenical melarsoprol, but these drugs can have significant adverse effects. Pentamidine was used with apparent success to treat one dog with African trypanosomiasis.[61] Prevention is through the use of insect repellants and indoor housing.

OTHER *TRYPANOSOMA* INFECTIONS

Other *Trypanosoma* species that can infect dogs (and to a lesser extent, cats) include *Trypanosoma evansi* and *Trypanosoma caninum*.

T. evansi causes surra (= "rotten") and is endemic in large parts of Asia, Africa, Latin America, and the Canary Islands of Spain. It causes disease in a variety of mammalian host species that include horses, cattle, dogs, and cats, but not humans. *T. evansi* is very closely related to *T. brucei* and may have derived from *T. brucei* as a result of partial or complete loss of kinetoplast DNA, which stops it from developing within the insect vector. Instead, the organism is transmitted mechanically by biting flies. Ingestion of infected meat may also lead to infection. Because populations of biting flies are greatest during the rainy season, a seasonal incidence of disease has been observed in dogs.[62] Travel-related disease has been described.[63,64] The disease has an acute course; clinical signs and laboratory abnormalities resemble those of African trypanosomiasis, with lethargy, fever, anorexia, weight loss, pallor, lymphadenopathy, vomiting, conjunctivitis, uveitis, corneal edema, and peripheral edema, as well as leukopenia, thrombocytopenia, and anemia on the CBC.[62-65] Hyperglobulinemia and proteinuria have also been reported.[64] Some dogs develop neurologic signs late in the course of disease due to nonsuppurative meningoencephalitis.[64] Definitive diagnosis of infection is based on cytologic examination of blood smears and/or PCR assay. Treatment is usually with diminazene aceturate or suramin, although diminazene aceturate is considered less effective against *T. evansi* than *T. congolense* infection.[64] Untreated infection is usually fatal in dogs.

Trypanosoma caninum is a recently discovered *Trypanosoma* species that has only been identified in dogs from South America, many of which have been apparently healthy.[66,67] The pathogenicity of this organism requires further study. Importantly, infection with *T. caninum* leads to false-positive serologic test results for *Leishmania*, which can confound control methods that rely on culling of dogs that are seropositive for *Leishmania* (see Chapter 74).

CASE EXAMPLE

Signalment: "Duke," a 5-year-old male beagle mix dog from San Antonio, TX

History: Duke's owner reported a 7-day history of inappetence, lethargy, and decreased exercise tolerance. Two months earlier, the dog had been diagnosed with dirofilariasis and was treated with melarsomine dihydrochloride using a split protocol. He had not traveled out of his local area. He was up to date on vaccinations, which included vaccines for distemper, hepatitis, parvovirus, and rabies.

Current medications: Monthly oral ivermectin/pyrantel heartworm preventative.

Physical Examination:

Body weight: 19.9 kg.

General: Lethargic. T = 101.7°F (38.7°C), HR = 142 beats/min, RR = 48 breaths/min, mucous membranes pink, CRT = 1 s.

Integument, Eyes, Ears, Nose, and Throat: Full, shiny haircoat. No evidence of ectoparasites was detected. No other significant abnormalities were noted.

Musculoskeletal: Body condition score was 6/9.

Cardiovascular: An irregular rhythm and a grade 3/6 systolic left apical murmur were detected on thoracic auscultation. Strong femoral pulses were palpated bilaterally.

Respiratory: Mild tachypnea was identified with normal breath sounds and normal respiratory effort.

Gastrointestinal, Genitourinary, and Lymph Nodes: No abnormalities were detected.

Laboratory Findings:

CBC:

PCV 48.3% (31%-56%)
MCV 66.4 fL (60-77 fL)
MCHC 35 g/dL (32-36 g/dL)
WBC 13,100 cells/μL (6000-17,000 cells/μL)
Neutrophils 8777 cells/μL (3000-11,500 cells/μL)
Lymphocytes 2096 cells/μL (1000-4800 cells/μL)
Monocytes 1179 cells/μL (150-1250 cells/μL)
Platelets 238,000 platelets/μL (200,000-500,000 platelets/μL)

Serum Chemistry Profile:

Sodium 144 mmol/L (139-147 mmol/L)
Potassium 3.9 mmol/L (3.3-4.6 mmol/L)
Chloride 118 mmol/L (107-118 mmol/L)
Bicarbonate 22 mmol/L (20-28 mmol/L)
Phosphorus 3.6 mg/dL (2.9-6.2 mg/dL)
Calcium 9.8 mg/dL (9.3-11.8 mg/dL)
BUN 19 mg/dL (5-29 mg/dL)
Creatinine 1.27 mg/dL (0.3-2.0 mg/dL)
Glucose 108 mg/dL (60-135 mg/dL)
Total protein 5.5 g/dL (5.7-7.8 g/dL)
Albumin 2.6 g/dL (2.4-3.6 g/dL)
Globulin 2.9 g/dL (1.7-3.8 g/dL)
ALT 136 U/L (10-130 U/L)
ALP 103 U/L (21-147 U/L)
GGT 11 U/L (0-25 U/L)
Cholesterol 199 mg/dL (120-247 mg/dL)
Total bilirubin 0.2 mg/dL (0-0.8 mg/dL)
Magnesium 2.1 mg/dL (1.7-2.1 mg/dL)

Urinalysis: SGr 1.012; pH 7.5, trace protein (SSA), no bilirubin, no glucose, no WBC/HPF, 0-1 RBC/HPF.

Heartworm Antigen Test: Negative.

Cardiac Troponin I: 0.69 ng/mL (<0.2 ng/mL).

Chagas Immunofluorescent Antibody Titer: Positive at 1:160.

Imaging Findings:

Thoracic Radiographs: The cardiac silhouette was mildly, generally enlarged. The pulmonary veins were mildly larger than the corresponding artery. A mild pulmonary interstitial pattern was present.

Echocardiogram: The left ventricular internal dimensions were enlarged, and systolic function was reduced (fractional shortening 16.1%, area shortening 26.9%; normal is >25% and >50%, respectively). Moderate mitral regurgitation was documented, and the left atrium was enlarged. The right ventricle was mildly dilated. Pulmonic and aortic velocities were within normal limits. No heartworms were visualized.

Additional Testing: Electrocardiogram: Sinus rhythm with frequent, multiform ventricular premature complexes.

Blood pressure: Systolic blood pressure was 115 mm Hg.

Diagnosis: American trypanosomiasis (Chagas' disease).

Treatment: Medication to address cardiac enlargement, dysfunction, and arrhythmias included pimobendan (0.25 mg/kg PO q12h), enalapril (0.5 mg/kg PO q12h), and sotalol (1 mg/kg PO q12h). This was associated with improvement in clinical signs within 1 week of starting treatment.

Comments: This dog was diagnosed with trypanosomiasis based on an index of suspicion in the presence of ventricular enlargement and dysfunction in combination with multiform ventricular arrhythmias. Infection by *Leishmania* could also have caused the positive serologic test result, but this was considered unlikely based on the geographic location and clinical signs. PCR assays or *Trypanosoma* blood culture could have been performed to confirm the diagnosis, but these are not widely available and have low sensitivity when used in chronic infections. Antiprotozoal drugs were not used to treat this dog because they do not appear to alter outcome in chronic Chagas' disease. The dog did very well clinically while being managed with cardiac medications including antiarrhythmics along with routine evaluation. After 2.5 years, ventricular arrhythmias increased in severity and were more difficult to control with antiarrhythmic therapy. He died suddenly at home 5 days after reevaluation.

SUGGESTED READINGS

Museux K, Boulouha L, Majani S, et al. African *Trypanosoma* infection in a dog in France. Vet Rec. 2011;168:590.

Nabity MB, Barnhart K, Logan KS, et al. An atypical case of *Trypanosoma cruzi* infection in a young English Mastiff. Vet Parasitol. 2006;140:356-361.

REFERENCES

1. Chagas C. Nova tripanosomiase humana. Estudos sobre a morfologia e o ciclo evolutivo do *Schizotrypanum cruzi* n. gen., n. sp., agente etiologico de nova entradade morbida do homen. Mem Inst Oswaldo Cruz. 1909;1:1-9.
2. Barr SC, Gossett KA, Klei TR. Clinical, clinicopathologic, and parasitologic observations of trypanosomiasis in dogs infected with North American *Trypanosoma cruzi* isolates. Am J Vet Res. 1991;52:954-960.
3. Barr SC, Holmes RA, Klei TR. Electrocardiographic and echocardiographic features of trypanosomiasis in dogs inoculated with North American *Trypanosoma cruzi* isolates. Am J Vet Res. 1992;53:521-527.
4. Barr SC, Schmidt SP, Brown CC, et al. Pathologic features of dogs inoculated with North American *Trypanosoma cruzi* isolates. Am J Vet Res. 1991;52:2033-2039.
5. Barr SC, Simpson RM, Schmidt SP, et al. Chronic dilatative myocarditis caused by *Trypanosoma cruzi* in two dogs. J Am Vet Med Assoc. 1989;195:1237-1241.
6. Barr SC, Van Beek O, Carlisle-Nowak MS, et al. *Trypanosoma cruzi* infection in Walker hounds from Virginia. Am J Vet Res. 1995;56:1037-1044.
7. Berger SL, Palmer RH, Hodges CC, et al. Neurologic manifestations of trypanosomiasis in a dog. J Am Vet Med Assoc. 1991;198: 132-134.
8. Espinosa R, Carrasco HA, Belandria F, et al. Life expectancy analysis in patients with Chagas' disease: prognosis after one decade (1973-1983). Int J Cardiol. 1985;8:45-56.
9. Barr SC. Canine American trypanosomiasis. Compend Cont Educ Pract Vet. 1991;13:745-755.
10. Kjos SA, Snowden KF, Craig TM, et al. Distribution and characterization of canine Chagas disease in Texas. Vet Parasitol. 2008;152:249-256.
11. Meurs KM, Anthony MA, Slater M, et al. Chronic *Trypanosoma cruzi* infection in dogs: 11 cases (1987-1996). J Am Vet Med Assoc. 1998;213:497-500.
12. Bradley KK, Bergman DK, Woods JP, et al. Prevalence of American trypanosomiasis (Chagas disease) among dogs in Oklahoma. J Am Vet Med Assoc. 2000;217:1853-1857.
13. Snider TG, Yaeger RG, Dellucky J. Myocarditis caused by *Trypanosoma cruzi* in a native Louisiana dog. J Am Vet Med Assoc. 1980;177:247-249.
14. Tippit TS. Canine trypanosomiasis (Chagas' disease). Southwest Vet. 1978;2:97-104.
15. Cohn L. Unpublished observations, 2012.
16. Patel JM, Rosypal AC, Zimmerman KL, et al. Isolation, mouse pathogenicity, and genotyping of *Trypanosoma cruzi* from an English Cocker Spaniel from Virginia, USA. Vet Parasitol. 2012;187:394-398.
17. Carcavallo RU. The subfamily Triatominae (Hemoptera, Reduviidae): systematics and ecological factors. In: Brenner RR, Stoke A, eds. Chagas' Disease Vectors. Boca Raton, FL: CRC Press; 1987:13-18.
18. Beard CB, Pye G, Steurer FJ, et al. Chagas disease in a domestic transmission cycle, southern Texas. USA. Emerg Infect Dis. 2003;9: 103-105.
19. Yaeger RG. The present status of Chagas' disease in the United States. Bull Tulane Univ Med Fac. 1961;21:9-13.
20. Yaeger RG. Transmission of *Trypanosoma cruzi* infection to opossums via the oral route. J Parasitol. 1971;57:1375-1376.
21. Roellig DM, Ellis AE, Yabsley MJ. Oral transmission of *Trypanosoma cruzi* with opposing evidence for the theory of carnivory. J Parasitol. 2009;95:360-364.
22. Kirchhoff LV. *Trypanosoma* species (American Trypanosomiasis, Chagas' disease): biology of trypanosomes. In: Mandell GL, Bennett JE, Dolin R, eds. Principles and Practice of Infectious Diseases. 7th ed. Philadelphia, PA: Elsevier; 2010:3481-3488.
23. Barr SC, Brown CC, Dennis VA, et al. The lesions and prevalence of *Trypanosoma cruzi* in opossums and armadillos from southern Louisiana. J Parasitol. 1991;77:624-627.
24. Woody NC, Woody HB. American trypanosomiasis. I. Clinical and epidemiologic background of Chagas' disease in the United States. J Pediatr. 1961;58:568-580.
25. Barr SC, Dennis VA, Klei TR. Growth characteristics in axenic and cell cultures, protein profiles, and zymodeme typing of three *Trypanosoma cruzi* isolates from Louisiana mammals. J Parasitol. 1990;76:631-638.

26. Zingales B, Miles MA, Campbell DA, et al. The revised *Trypanosoma cruzi* subspecific nomenclature: rationale, epidemiological relevance and research applications. Infect Genet Evol. 2012;12: 240-253.
27. Andrade ZA, Andrade SG, Correa R, et al. Myocardial changes in acute *Trypanosoma cruzi* infection. Ultrastructural evidence of immune damage and the role of microangiopathy. Am J Pathol. 1994;144:1403-1411.
28. Andrade ZA, Andrade SG, Sadigursky M, et al. The indeterminate phase of Chagas' disease: ultrastructural characterization of cardiac changes in the canine model. Am J Trop Med Hyg. 1997;57: 328-336.
29. Tanowitz HB, Kirchhoff LV, Simon D, et al. Chagas' disease. Clin Microbiol Rev. 1992;5:400-419.
30. Barr SC, Dennis VA, Klei TR, et al. Antibody and lymphoblastogenic responses of dogs experimentally infected with *Trypanosoma cruzi* isolates from North American mammals. Vet Immunol Immunopathol. 1991;29:267-283.
31. Nabity MB, Barnhart K, Logan KS, et al. An atypical case of *Trypanosoma cruzi* infection in a young English Mastiff. Vet Parasitol. 2006;140:356-361.
32. Guedes PM, Veloso VM, Mineo TW, et al. Hematological alterations during experimental canine infection by *Trypanosoma cruzi*. Rev Bras Parasitol Vet. 2012;21:151-156.
33. Quijano-Hernandez IA, Castro-Barcena A, Aparicio-Burgos E, et al. Evaluation of clinical and immunopathological features of different infective doses of *Trypanosoma cruzi* in dogs during the acute phase. Scientific World Journal. 2012;2012:635169.
34. Araujo FM, Bahia MT, Magalhaes NM, et al. Follow-up of experimental chronic Chagas' disease in dogs: use of polymerase chain reaction (PCR) compared with parasitological and serological methods. Acta Trop. 2002;81:21-31.
35. Rosypal AC, Hill R, Lewis S, et al. Evaluation of a rapid immunochromatographic dipstick test for detection of antibodies to *Trypanosoma cruzi* in dogs experimentally infected with isolates obtained from opossums (*Didelphis virginiana*), armadillos (*Dasypus novemcinctus*), and dogs (*Canis familiaris*) from the United States. J Parasitol. 2011;97:140-143.
36. Moreira OC, Ramirez JD, Velazquez E, et al. Towards the establishment of a consensus real-time qPCR to monitor *Trypanosoma cruzi* parasitemia in patients with chronic Chagas disease cardiomyopathy: a substudy from the BENEFIT trial. Acta Trop. 2013;125:23-31.
37. Veloso VM, Guedes PM, Andrade IM, et al. *Trypanosoma cruzi*: blood parasitism kinetics and their correlation with heart parasitism intensity during long-term infection of Beagle dogs. Mem Inst Oswaldo Cruz. 2008;103:528-534.
38. Andrade ZA, Andrade SG, Sadigursky M, et al. Experimental Chagas' disease in dogs. A pathologic and ECG study of the chronic indeterminate phase of the infection. Arch Pathol Lab Med. 1981;105: 460-464.
39. Viotti R, Vigliano C, Armenti H, et al. Treatment of chronic Chagas' disease with benznidazole: clinical and serologic evolution of patients with long-term follow-up. Am Heart J. 1994;127:151-162.
40. Caldas IS, da Matta Guedes PM, Dos Santos FM, et al. Myocardial scars correlate with electrocardiographic changes in chronic *Trypanosoma cruzi* infection for dogs treated with benznidazole. Trop Med Int Health. 2013;18:75-84.
41. Diniz Lde F, Caldas IS, Guedes PM, et al. Effects of ravuconazole treatment on parasite load and immune response in dogs experimentally infected with *Trypanosoma cruzi*. Antimicrob Agents Chemother. 2010;54:2979-2986.
42. Veiga-Santos P, Barrias ES, Santos JF, et al. Effects of amiodarone and posaconazole on the growth and ultrastructure of *Trypanosoma cruzi*. Int J Antimicrob Agents. 2012;40:61-71.
43. Paniz-Mondolfi AE, Perez-Alvarez AM, Lanza G, et al. Amiodarone and itraconazole: a rational therapeutic approach for the treatment of chronic Chagas' disease. Chemotherapy. 2009;55:228-233.
44. Benaim G, Sanders JM, Garcia-Marchan Y, et al. Amiodarone has intrinsic anti–*Trypanosoma cruzi* activity and acts synergistically with posaconazole. J Med Chem. 2006;49:892-899.
45. Santos FM, Lima WG, Gravel AS, et al. Cardiomyopathy prognosis after benznidazole treatment in chronic canine Chagas' disease. J Antimicrob Chemother. 2012;67:1987-1995.
46. Gurtler RE, Ceballos LA, Stariolo R, et al. Effects of topical application of fipronil spot-on on dogs against the Chagas disease vector *Triatoma infestans*. Trans R Soc Trop Med Hyg. 2009;103:98-304.
47. Reithinger R, Ceballos L, Stariolo R, et al. Chagas disease control: deltamethrin-treated collars reduce *Triatoma infestans* feeding success on dogs. Trans R Soc Trop Med Hyg. 2005;99:502-508.
48. Reithinger R, Ceballos L, Stariolo R, et al. Extinction of experimental *Triatoma infestans* populations following continuous exposure to dogs wearing deltamethrin-treated collars. Am J Trop Med Hyg. 2006;74:766-771.
49. Estrada-Franco JG, Bhatia V, Diaz-Albiter H, et al. Human *Trypanosoma cruzi* infection and seropositivity in dogs, Mexico. Emerg Infect Dis. 2006;12:624-630.
50. Cardinal MV, Lauricella MA, Ceballos LA, et al. Molecular epidemiology of domestic and sylvatic *Trypanosoma cruzi* infection in rural northwestern Argentina. Int J Parasitol. 2008;38:1533-1543.
51. Kirchhoff LV. American trypanosomiasis (Chagas' disease)—a tropical disease now in the United States. N Engl J Med. 1993;329:639-644.
52. Schmunis GA. *Trypanosoma cruzi*, the etiologic agent of Chagas' disease: status in the blood supply in endemic and nonendemic countries. Transfusion. 1991;31:547-557.
53. Steverding D. The history of African trypanosomiasis. Parasit Vectors. 2008;1:3.
54. Balyeidhusa AS, Kironde FA, Enyaru JC. Apparent lack of a domestic animal reservoir in Gambiense sleeping sickness in northwest Uganda. Vet Parasitol. 2012;187:157-167.
55. Matete GO. Occurrence, clinical manifestation and the epidemiological implications of naturally occurring canine trypanosomosis in western Kenya. Onderstepoort J Vet Res. 2003;70:317-323.
56. Museux K, Boulouha L, Majani S, et al. African *Trypanosoma* infection in a dog in France. Vet Rec. 2011;168:590.
57. Gow AG, Simpson JW, Picozzi K. First report of canine African trypanosomosis in the UK. J Small Anim Pract. 2007;48:658-661.
58. Harrus S, Harmelin A, Presenty B, et al. *Trypanosoma congolense* infection in two dogs. J Small Anim Pract. 1995;36:83-86.
59. Horchner F, Zillmann U, Metzner M, et al. West African dogs as a model for research on trypanotolerance. Trop Med Parasitol. 1985;36:257-258.
60. Ezeokonkwo RC, Ezeh IO, Onunkwo JI, et al. Comparative haematological study of single and mixed infections of mongrel dogs with *Trypanosoma congolense* and *Trypanosoma brucei brucei*. Vet Parasitol. 2010;173:48-54.
61. Hooft EM. Canine African *Trypanosoma*. J Small Anim Pract. 2008;49:487.
62. Singh B, Kalra IS, Gupta MP, et al. *Trypanosoma evansi* infection in dogs: seasonal prevalence and chemotherapy. Vet Parasitol. 1993;50:137-141.
63. Hellebrekers LJ, Slappendel RJ. Trypanosomiasis in a dog imported in The Netherlands. Vet Q. 1982;4:182-186.
64. Defontis M, Richartz J, Engelmann N, et al. Canine *Trypanosoma evansi* infection introduced into Germany. Vet Clin Pathol. 2012;41:369-374.
65. Aquino LP, Machado RZ, Alessi AC, et al. Clinical, parasitological and immunological aspects of experimental infection with *Trypanosoma evansi* in dogs. Mem Inst Oswaldo Cruz. 1999;94:255-260.
66. Madeira MF, Sousa MA, Barros JH, et al. *Trypanosoma caninum* n. sp. (Protozoa: Kinetoplastida) isolated from intact skin of a domestic dog (*Canis familiaris*) captured in Rio de Janeiro, Brazil. Parasitology. 2009;136:411-423.
67. De SPAG, Schubach TM, Figueiredo FB, et al. Isolation of *Trypanosoma caninum* in domestic dogs in Rio de Janeiro, Brazil. Parasitology. 2010;137:1653-1660.

CHAPTER 79

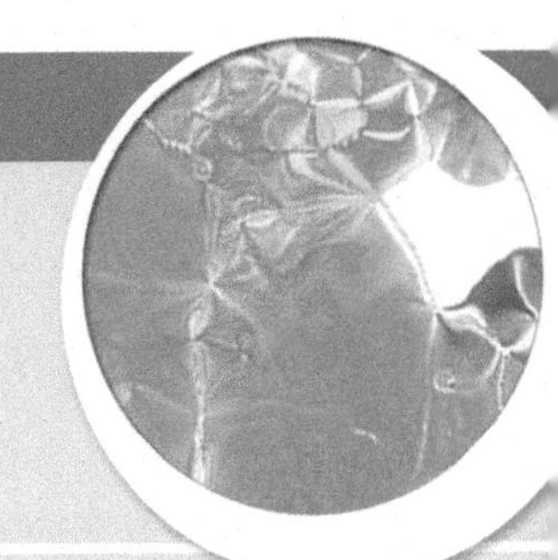

Giardiasis

Michael R. Lappin

Overview of Giardiasis

First Described: Trophozoites that were likely *Giardia* spp. were first described in 1681 by Antonie van Leeuwenhoek (who found the parasite in his own stools[1]) and the genus was established in the early 1900s. Infections of dogs and cats were first described in the 1960s.[2]

Cause: *Giardia duodenalis* (multiple genetic assemblages); a flagellate protozoan (phylum Sarcomastigophora)

Transmission: Fecal-oral

Affected Host Species: Dogs and cats are the definitive hosts for several different *Giardia* assemblages and pass either trophozoites (diarrhea) or cysts (diarrhea or normal stool) in feces.

Intermediate Hosts: Although there are no intermediate hosts, there are multiple potential transport hosts that may carry *Giardia* spp. cysts and indirectly infect dogs or cats.

Geographic Distribution: Worldwide

Major Clinical Signs: Most dogs and cats harbor subclinical infections. Acute watery diarrhea that can contain mucus can occur. Steatorrhea can be observed. Chronic or intermittent diarrhea and weight loss may be noted in animals with concurrent infections or immunocompromise.

Differential Diagnoses: All causes of small bowel diarrhea including *Isospora* spp., *Cryptosporidium* spp., bacterial infections such as salmonellosis, nematode infections, dietary intolerance, exocrine pancreatic insufficiency, and inflammatory bowel disease

Human Health Significance: *Giardia* assemblages that infect dogs (assemblage C and D) or cats (assemblage F) are usually not associated with clinical disease in humans but can be detected in the feces of immunocompromised people. Human assemblages A and B can be found in feces of dogs and cats when animals share human environmental features (such as contaminated water). However, it is unlikely that new human infections with *Giardia* assemblage A or B infections are acquired from the feces of dogs or cats.

Etiologic Agent and Epidemiology

Giardia spp. are protozoans in the flagellate group that have been recognized in the feces of animals and man for many years.[3] *Giardia* spp. occurs in two forms, the trophozoite and the cyst (Figure 79-1). The trophozoite is the active, motile form; it is approximately 15 µm long and 8 µm wide and has a teardrop shape and a ventral adhesive disk (Figure 79-2). Trophozoites are almost never found in normal feces and are susceptible to many environmental conditions; thus, they usually are not associated with transmission among animals. The 12-µm long and 7-µm wide cyst is the environmentally resistant stage primarily responsible for transmission. The cyst contains two incompletely separated but formed trophozoites, the axoneme, fragments of the ventral disks, and as many as four nuclei (Figure 79-3). The cyst can survive several months outside the host in wet and cool conditions but is susceptible to desiccation in dry and hot conditions.

Giardia spp. are transmitted by the direct ingestion of fecal cysts or by indirect ingestion of contaminated water, food, transport hosts, infected prey species, or fomites. The prepatent period (time between ingestion and appearance of cysts in the feces) in cats ranges from 5 to 16 days (mean around 10 days) and in dogs ranges from 4 to 12 days (mean around 8 days). Shedding of *Giardia* cysts by cats may fluctuate from undetectable to concentrations of more than 1 million cysts/g of feces over periods as short as 2 to 7 days.[4] Young dogs shed an average of 2000 cysts per gram of feces; the mean cyst count per gram of feces for all infected dogs (regardless of age) was 706.[5] Most infections are self-limited with cessation of cyst shedding in 27 to 35 days in dogs and cats. However, some infected animals shed cysts for several months.

Although there are many *Giardia* spp., *G. duodenalis* (syn. *G. intestinalis* or *G. lamblia*) is the species that infects people, dogs, and cats.[6] Based on genetic analyses, there are at least seven distinct assemblages (A-G) within *G. duodenalis*. Assemblage A has been amplified from feces of infected humans, dogs, and cats as well as many other mammals. Assemblage B is most commonly amplified from human feces but is occasionally amplified from dog feces. Overall, most dogs are infected with the species-specific assemblages C and D, and cats are infected with assemblage F.[6] It has been proposed that these assemblages be recategorized as separate species of *Giardia* (Table 79-1), but this has not yet been unanimously accepted.[7]

Giardia infections in cats and dogs have been reported in many prevalence studies, case reports, and treatment studies from around the world. Infection rates vary with the assay used and whether or not diarrhea is occurring. However, in general they are approximately 5% to 20% in dogs and cats.[3] In most studies there is no association between the presence of *Giardia* in the feces and clinical signs, because of the high prevalence of subclinical infections.[3,8] Younger or immunosuppressed animals and those living in crowded environments are at the highest risk of showing clinical signs of disease.

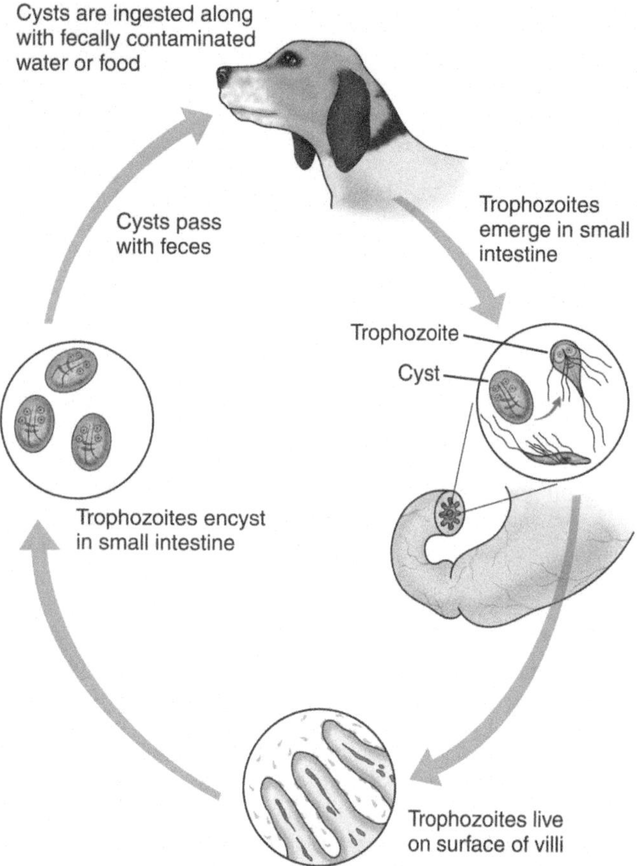

FIGURE 79-1 Life cycle of Giardia duodenalis.

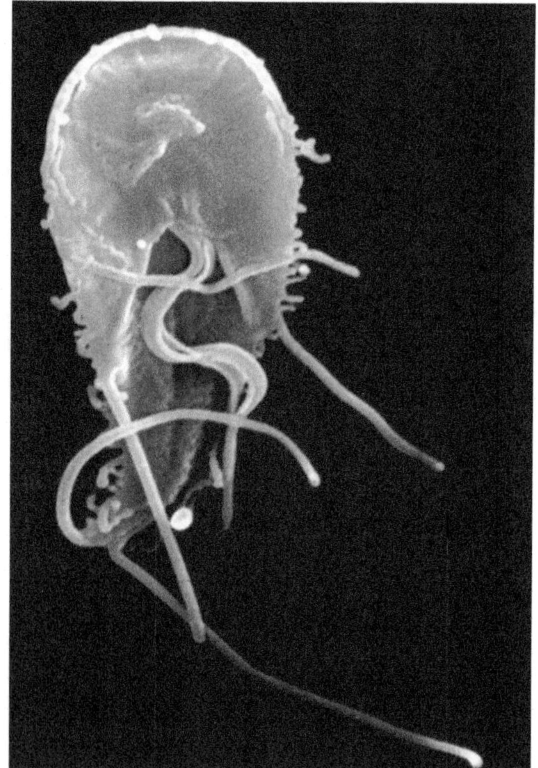

FIGURE 79-2 Electron micrograph of a *Giardia* trophozoite. (Courtesy of Bayer Animal Health. In Tangtrongsup S, Scorza V. Update on the diagnosis and management of *Giardia* spp. infections in dogs and cats. Topics in Companion Animal Medicine. 2010;25:155-162.)

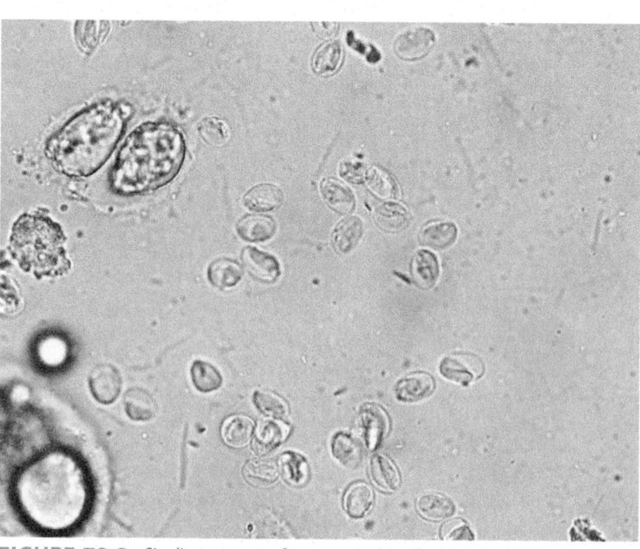

FIGURE 79-3 *Giardia* spp. cysts after concentration by sugar centrifugation (400× magnification). The cysts are approximately 12 μm long and 7 μm wide. (Courtesy of Dr. Lora Ballweber, Colorado State University. In from Tangtrongsup S, Scorza V. Update on the diagnosis and management of *Giardia* spp. infections in dogs and cats. Topics in Companion Animal Medicine. 2010;25:155-162.)

TABLE 79-1

Proposed and Existing Nomenclature in the Genus *Giardia*

Species	Hosts
Giardia duodenalis (assemblage A*)	Wide range of domestic and wild mammals including humans
Giardia enterica (assemblage B)	Humans and other primates, dogs, some species of wild mammals
Giardia canis (assemblage C/D)	Dogs and other canids
Giardia cati (assemblage F)	Cats
Giardia bovis (assemblage E)	Cattle, other hoofed livestock
Giardia simondi (assemblage G)	Rats
Giardia muris	Rodents
Giardia microti	Muskrats and voles
Giardia ardeae	Birds
Giardia psittaci	Birds
Giardia agilis	Amphibians

Modified from Thompson RCA, Smith A. Zoonotic enteric protozoa. Vet Parasitol. 2011;182(1):70-78.

*The *Giardia* assemblages listed currently fall within the single species *Giardia duodenalis*

Clinical Features

Signs and Their Pathogenesis

After *Giardia* spp. cysts are ingested by a susceptible host, gastric acid and pancreatic enzyme exposure in the duodenum induces release of the two trophozoites, which mature quickly and attach to the brush border of the villous epithelium by means of their ventral adhesive disk and a number of parasitic surface molecules, including the giardins (alpha, beta, delta, and gamma giardins) and a network of contractile proteins. In dogs, trophozoites are found from the duodenum to the ileum; in cats, they predominate in the jejunum and ileum. Trophozoites multiply by binary fission and then encyst by an unknown mechanism. Contamination of fomites, which can include arthropods and the coats of animals, or food and especially water sources by *Giardia* cysts is an important mode of transmission, because cysts remain viable for days to weeks in the environment when conditions are cool and moist.

Although the pathogenesis of *Giardia* is not completely understood, in vitro and in vivo studies suggest it is multifactorial with a combination of intestinal malabsorption and hypersecretion as the primary mechanisms associated with development of diarrhea. The host-parasite interaction leads to the upregulation of genes involved in the apoptotic cascade and in the formation of reactive oxygen species.[9] The induction of apoptosis increases gastrointestinal permeability, allowing luminal antigens to activate host immune-dependent pathologic pathways. *Giardia* also alters epithelial claudin proteins that are components of tight junctions.[9] However, *Giardia* can cause clinical signs in the absence of villous atrophy or other signs of mucosal injury.[9] *Giardia* infection stimulates chloride secretion and results in a diffuse loss of brush border microvillus length, which causes epithelial maldigestion and malabsorption of glucose, sodium, and water and reduced disaccharidase activity. Mild to moderate infiltrates of intraepithelial lymphocytes can be recognized and may be associated with the sodium and glucose malabsorption. Loss of epithelial barrier function may have the potential to lead to chronic intestinal disorders, but the mechanisms remain unclear.[9] Mast cell hyperplasia may also contribute to the loss of epithelial barrier function. It is unknown why some people and animals maintain chronic, subclinical infections, but this is likely related to both host and parasite factors.

Although most cats and dogs that shed *Giardia* do not show clinical signs of disease, *Giardia* infection can induce illness in some animals. The primary clinical signs of giardiasis include chronic diarrhea and weight loss. The diarrhea is usually mucoid, pale, and soft and has a strong odor; steatorrhea may be present as well.[3] The presence of blood in the stool is uncommon unless co-infections with other agents such as *Ancylostoma* spp., *Isospora* spp., *Tritrichomonas foetus,* or *Clostridium perfringens* occur. Fever or vomiting is almost never recognized in dogs or cats with giardiasis. Co-infections with other agents such as *Cryptosporidium* spp. or *T. foetus* may potentiate diarrhea in dogs or cats.[10,11] It is currently unknown whether the different assemblages induce different clinical signs in cats and dogs or if there are strains within a given assemblage that are more pathogenic than others.

Diagnosis

Laboratory Abnormalities

Giardia spp. infection alone is rarely associated with CBC or serum biochemical panel abnormalities.

Diagnostic Imaging

Abdominal radiographic abnormalities are uncommon and nonspecific and, when present, are suggestive of diffuse enteritis.

Microbiologic Testing

Because of the small size of *Giardia* cysts and the high subclinical infection rate, giardiasis is commonly misdiagnosed, underdiagnosed, or overdiagnosed.[3,12] Yeasts are easily mistaken for *Giardia*, which leads to false-positive fecal flotation results. *Giardia* cysts are shed intermittently, and repeated fecal analysis may be needed to detect cysts. In addition, cysts can deteriorate in fecal flotation solutions, leading to false-negative results.[12] A variety of different *Giardia* assays have been evaluated for use in cats and dogs (Table 79-2). There is no one test that can be performed on a single fecal specimen that has 100% sensitivity. The following is a discussion of the currently available diagnostic methods.

Cytologic Examination

Feces can be evaluated for the presence of *Giardia* trophozoites by wet mount examination. Approximately 2 mm × 2 mm of fresh diarrheic feces or mucus is mixed with a drop of normal saline solution (warmed to body temperature) on a microscope slide and a coverslip placed. At 100× magnification, trophozoites are recognized by their "falling leaf" motion. Evaluation for structural characteristics is then performed at 400× magnification. Because trophozoites may be associated with mucus, the only visible motility may be the flagella. Although *Giardia* trophozoites can be confused with tritrichomonads that are similar in size, they can be differentiated from tritrichomonads based on their motility and morphology. In contrast to *Giardia* spp., tritrichomonads have an undulating membrane and a rolling form of motility, lack a concave surface, and have only a single nucleus (see Chapter 80).[3] Further testing of feces for *Giardia* antigen, *Giardia* DNA by PCR assay, or fecal culture or PCR assay for *Tritrichomonas foetus* can be used to differentiate the organisms if cytology is inconclusive. Once *Giardia* is detected in a direct smear or wet mount based on motility, further cytologic examination with staining should be performed on a fresh specimen. The application of Lugol's solution, methylene blue, or acid methyl green to the wet mount helps in the visualization of the internal structures of the trophozoites. Trophozoites are rarely found in solid feces.

Concentration Techniques

Giardia cysts are more likely to be detected after fecal concentration techniques. Sheather's sugar centrifugation and zinc sulfate centrifugation are commonly used. In addition to the identification of *Giardia* cysts, ova of other common parasites can easily be identified. *Giardia* cysts can be confused with yeast because of similar size, but *Giardia* cysts have a distinct structure (see Figure 79-3). Because of the intermittent pattern of shedding, at least three specimens should be examined over a period of about 1 week before ruling out *Giardia* spp. infection as a cause of diarrhea. If fecal specimens cannot be examined immediately, storage at 4°C for several days is acceptable, but specimens should not be frozen.

Duodenal Aspirates

Endoscopic sampling of duodenal secretions and then examination of the sediment for trophozoites was once considered the most sensitive technique for detection of *Giardia* spp. infection in dogs, but with the advent of immunologic and molecular techniques, duodenal aspirates are no longer performed. In cats, because of the location of the parasite in the mid to distal small bowel, this technique is unlikely to yield positive results.

Direct Immunofluorescence

A monoclonal antibody–based immunofluorescent antibody (IFA) assay (Merifluor *Cryptosporidium/Giardia,* Meridian

TABLE 79-2

Diagnostic Assays Available for Giardiasis in Dogs or Cats

Assay	Specimen Type	Target	Performance
Cytologic examination	Feces	*Giardia* trophozoites and cysts	False negatives are common and occur when specimen size is small or low numbers of organisms are present, or because of intermittent shedding. False positives can occur when cysts are confused with yeasts.
Centrifugal fecal flotation (concentration techniques)	Feces	*Giardia* cysts	Because of the intermittent pattern of shedding, at least three specimens should be examined over a period of about 1 week before concluding that *Giardia* spp. infection is an unlikely cause of diarrhea. False positives can occur when cysts are confused with yeasts.
Direct immunofluorescence	Feces	*Giardia* cysts	May be more sensitive and specific than centrifugal fecal flotation, but sensitivity for detection of assemblages that infect dogs and cats is not well understood. Sensitivity appears to be similar to that of *Giardia* antigen ELISA assays.
Giardia antigen ELISA assays	Feces	*Giardia* cyst antigen	When used in combination with centrifugal fecal flotation, sensitivity can approach 98%. However, performance varies with the assay used, and the sensitivity of ELISA assays for detection of assemblages from dogs and cats is not well understood. It has been recommended that this assay be used in addition to fecal flotation only during evaluation of dogs and cats with diarrhea and not healthy pets (see text).
PCR assays	Feces	*Giardia* spp. DNA	The sensitivity and specificity of assays may vary depending on assay design. False negatives can occur as a result of PCR inhibitors in feces. The significance of a positive PCR result must be interpreted in light of clinical findings because of subclinical infections.

Diagnostics, Cincinnati, OH) used to detect *Giardia* spp. cysts and *Cryptosporidium* spp. oocysts in human feces has been applied to feces from dogs and cats in multiple studies.[3,13,14] It is believed that *Giardia* cysts from assemblages C, D, and F are detected by this assay, but this hypothesis has not been rigorously assessed using genotyped specimens. The assay gives both immunologic confirmation (fluorescence) and morphologic evaluation (size and shape) to confirm the presence of *Giardia* in feces. In one study, the assay was more sensitive and specific than zinc sulfate flotation but comparable to an antigen-detection technique when used on fecal specimens from shelter dogs.[13] Because *Cryptosporidium* spp. are also associated with small bowel diarrhea, can exist as co-infections with *Giardia,* and are difficult to detect with other techniques, the IFA assay is used frequently by some clinicians (see Chapter 81). A fluorescence microscope is needed to read the IFA slides; therefore, this assay is usually only performed in diagnostic laboratories. If the specimens cannot be examined immediately, they can be stored at 4°C for a maximum of several days but should not be frozen.

Fecal Antigen Detection by Enzyme-Linked Immunosorbent Assays

Several ELISAs are available for detection of *Giardia* antigen in human feces. A veterinary assay is labeled for use with dog and cat feces (SNAP *Giardia,* IDEXX Laboratories, Portland, ME). Results vary with the ELISA assay used, and inconsistent results have been reported with some *Giardia* antigen tests when compared to other techniques. In a study of cats, the SNAP *Giardia* antigen assay had similar sensitivity and specificity when compared to fecal flotation, and when the results of the two techniques were combined, the overall sensitivity was 97.8%.[14] Little information is available as to whether currently available fecal antigen assays detect *Giardia* assemblages C, D, or F (i.e., the canine- and feline-associated assemblages). In one study of 4 assemblage C isolates and 13 assemblage D isolates (which infect dogs), all were positive by the SNAP *Giardia* antigen assay.[15] The Companion Animal Parasite Council currently recommends that fecal antigen tests be used as an addition to fecal flotation only during the evaluation of dogs and cats with diarrhea and not healthy pets, because the clinical and zoonotic impact of an antigen-positive, cyst-negative healthy pet is unknown.[16] It is also unknown how long *Giardia* antigen assays remain positive after resolution of diarrhea. Therefore, if a veterinarian chooses to assess the success of the treatment for giardiasis in cats and dogs, only fecal flotation is recommended for the follow-up evaluation.

Molecular Diagnosis Using the Polymerase Chain Reaction

Giardia spp. DNA can be amplified from feces by PCR assay, and such molecular methods can be used to determine the *Giardia* assemblage present through sequence analysis of the PCR product. However, the assignment of isolates to specific *G. duodenalis* assemblages using PCR assays is not always consistent because different results occur depending on the target sequence amplified.[5,17] Thus, some dog or cat isolates can be genotyped as "potentially zoonotic" using one target gene but as "host specific" with another. It is currently recommended that if the assemblage is to be determined, three genes should be assessed (the assessment of multiple genes using PCR and sequencing is also known as multilocus sequence typing). *Giardia* PCR assays can also be falsely negative because of the presence of PCR inhibitors in feces and so should not be used as the sole *Giardia* spp. assay.

Pathologic Findings

Gross Pathologic Findings

Giardia spp. infection may cause mild intestinal thickening. Because the agent is not enteroinvasive, blood is generally not present within the intestinal lumen unless co-infections are recognized. Animals with chronic clinical signs of disease may be emaciated. Other parasites such as roundworms or hookworms may be found.

Histopathologic Findings

In clinically affected animals with *Giardia* infection, a diffuse loss of brush border microvillus length may be noted on histopathology of the small intestine. Increased numbers of intraepithelial lymphocytes and mast cell hyperplasia may also be present. However, diarrhea has been associated with giardiasis in dogs, cats, and people with normal intestinal biopsy results.

Treatment and Prognosis

Giardia spp. have specific antimicrobial susceptibility patterns, and so it is currently impossible to predict which anti-*Giardia* drug will be effective in individual dogs or cats. Because *Giardia* spp. of dogs and cats can be difficult to culture in the laboratory, there is little in vitro susceptibility test result information available. Although a variety of drugs have been used to treat giardiasis in dogs and cats, there are few studies that have evaluated the efficacy of drugs and varied drug doses in experimentally infected animals. In most studies, fecal specimens were evaluated for only short periods of time after treatment, and immune suppression was not induced to evaluate whether infection was eliminated or merely suppressed. Infection with *Giardia* does not appear to cause permanent immunity, and so re-infection can occur, a finding that also hampers assessment of treatment studies.

Treatment options that are currently available or used historically for dogs or cats with confirmed or suspected giardiasis include albendazole, febantel/pyrantel/praziquantel, fenbendazole, furazolidone, ipronidazole, metronidazole, quinacrine, and tinidazole (Table 79-3). Newer drugs being studied or those with minimal information available for dogs and cats include azithromycin, nitazoxanide, paromomycin, and secnidazole.

Administration of metronidazole is indicated if concurrent infection with *Clostridium* spp. is suspected (see Chapter 48). In cats, metronidazole benzoate is preferred to metronidazole USP because it is better tolerated by most cats.[18] However, metronidazole should not be administered orally for longer than 7 days sequentially or at a total daily dose greater than 50 mg/kg because of the risk for neurotoxicity.[19,20] Ipronidazole, ronidazole, secnidazole, and tinidazole are other drugs with this class that have been used to treat giardiasis in dogs or cats (see Table 79-3). Ipronidazole added to the drinking water could be considered if a large number of dogs are clinically affected.[21] Ronidazole was used

TABLE 79-3

Drugs Used for the Treatment of *Giardia* spp. Infections

Drug	Species	Dose
Febantel, pyrantel, praziquantel	D	Label dose for 3 days
	C	56 mg/kg (based on the febantel component) PO q24h for 5 days
Fenbendazole	D, C	50 mg/kg PO daily for 3-5 days
Ipronidazole	D	126 mg/liter of water PO ad libitum for 7 days
Metronidazole	D, C	15-25 mg/kg PO q12-24h for 5-7 days
Tinidazole	D	44 mg/kg PO q24hr for 3 days
	C	30 mg/kg PO q24hr for 3 days

C, Cat; D, dog.

with hygiene management to control giardiasis in a dog kennel, but the author recommends reserving this drug for the treatment of *T. foetus* infections because of the potential for neurotoxicity and emerging ronidazole-resistant *T. foetus* strains.[22-24] Tinidazole should be considered as a secondary *Giardia* spp. treatment for dogs and cats if metronidazole is not tolerated, but optimal dosing protocols are not known. Secnidazole was evaluated in a small study of cats with minimal recognized toxicity (elevated liver enzyme activity in one cat) and apparent efficacy after one dose.[25] Further research is needed before routine use of this drug can be recommended.

If concurrent nematode infestation is suspected, albendazole, febantel/pyrantel/praziquantel, or fenbendazole may be most effective anti-*Giardia* drugs.[26-35] Albendazole has been associated with bone marrow suppression in some dogs and cats, so some clinicians avoid use of this drug.[35] Febantel/pyrantel/praziquantel is licensed in some countries for treatment of *Giardia* spp. infection in dogs and can be effective when administered daily for 3 days.[26] This combination has also been studied in small numbers of experimentally infected cats.[33] Data from an experimental model suggest that the combination of febantel with pyrantel is synergistic.[34] Many clinicians currently prescribe fenbendazole once daily for 5 days as initial therapy for dogs or cats with diarrhea and *Giardia* infection because of minimal expense and wide safety margin.

If the first drug fails to clear the infection (cyst shedding) or resolve the diarrhea, antimicrobial drug resistance may be present, so a second drug from an alternative class is indicated. Some clinicians currently recommend the concurrent administration of metronidazole and fenbendazole. Other clinicians resort to combination therapy only if there is evidence of a persistent infection that has not been cleared by monotherapy.

Azithromycin was used successfully in the management of giardiasis in one dog.[36] Paromomycin has anti-*Giardia* properties but has been absorbed across the gastrointestinal epithelium and associated with reversible acute renal failure in cats. Nitazoxanide is labeled for the treatment of giardiasis and cryptosporidiosis in humans in some countries and has been studied in some dogs and cats, but optimal protocols for the treatment of giardiasis are unknown. In addition, nitazoxanide is commonly associated with vomiting in dogs and cats.[31] The author currently administers nitazoxanide at 10 mg/kg PO q12h with food for 7 days for the treatment of dogs or cats with small bowel diarrhea and co-infections with *Giardia* spp. and *Cryptosporidium* spp. A longer duration of treatment appears to be required for some dogs and cats, and so treatment should be continued if an initial positive response is noted but clinical resolution is not achieved after the first 7 days.

The addition of fiber to the diet may help control clinical signs of giardiasis in some animals through reduction of bacterial overgrowth or by inhibiting organism attachment to microvilli. Feeding a fat-restricted diet may also be effective. In one study, administration of the probiotic *Enterococcus faecium* SF68 (FortiFlora, Nestle Purina PetCare) lessened *Giardia* spp. shedding in mice when fed before infection and enhanced *Giardia* immune responses.[37] In contrast, administration of this probiotic to dogs with chronic subclinical giardiasis had no measurable effect on cyst shedding.[38] In another study, dogs with acute diarrhea that were housed in shelters responded more rapidly to treatment if the probiotic was administered with metronidazole than if metronidazole was administered alone; many of these dogs were infected with *Giardia* spp.[39]

Bathing all dogs during medical treatment may lessen re-infection rates. In dogs and cats with persistent diarrhea and *Giardia* spp. infection, a more extensive work-up to attempt to diagnose other underlying diseases is indicated if several therapeutic trials fail to control the diarrhea. Potential underlying disorders that should be considered include cryptosporidiosis, tritrichomoniasis (primarily in cats), inflammatory bowel disease, gastrointestinal lymphoma, bacterial overgrowth, exocrine pancreatic insufficiency, and immunodeficiencies.

The primary goal of *Giardia* treatment is to resolve clinical signs of diarrhea. It is controversial whether to treat healthy dogs and cats with *Giardia* spp. cysts in feces, because healthy pets are generally not considered significant human health risks by the Centers for Disease Control and Prevention.[40] This is because infection can recur rapidly or not be cleared, and because all drugs have adverse effects. For example, in one small study of naturally infected dogs, approximately 50% of dogs had adverse events associated with treatment, and more than 60% of treated dogs were still *Giardia* infected when rechecked 34 days after treatment.[31] However, because clinical signs induced by *Giardia* spp. can be intermittent and since some *Giardia* spp. may be of zoonotic concern (especially to the immunocompromised), treatment of healthy infected animals should be discussed with each owner. If treatment is deemed indicated by the clinician and owner, many clinicians currently recommend that a 5-day course of fenbendazole be administered to apparently healthy dogs and cats that test positive for *Giardia* spp. cysts in feces. After treatment, if the animal is healthy and negative for cysts, retesting is not indicated again until the next scheduled wellness examination and fecal flotation. *Giardia*–infected dogs or cats should not be tested for *Giardia* antigen or DNA in feces since it is unknown how long positive assay results persist after treatment.

A common question is how to manage dogs or cats that have normal stool and are *Giardia* antigen positive but *Giardia* cyst negative. These animals may have a low-grade infection, or a low percentage of animals (approximately 2% to 5%) have false-positive antigen test results. To further evaluate for cyst shedding, the veterinarian can perform an IFA test or two additional fecal flotations (three negative centrifugal flotation assays run within 5 days is considered adequate to rule out a *Giardia* infection in both animals and humans). If these other test results are negative, the antigen test was likely falsely positive. If cysts are still identified after fecal centrifugal flotation performed 2 weeks after appropriate administration of a drug with anti-*Giardia* activity, a second course of therapy may be indicated using a drug from a different class. It is recommended that apparently well animals *not* be treated beyond two courses of therapy.[40] No further diagnostics are indicated unless gastrointestinal signs occur or the animal is again due for routine fecal screening (once to twice annually as a minimum for all dogs and cats).

Immunity and Vaccination

Sterilizing immunity to *Giardia* spp. does not occur, and so repeated shedding, clinical signs, and infection may occur. Re-infection occurs even in vaccinated dogs or cats, and so the previously available *Giardia* vaccines have been discontinued.

Prevention

Prevention of *Giardia* infection involves boiling or filtering of water collected from the environment before drinking and disinfection of premises contaminated with infected feces with steam cleaning or quaternary ammonium compounds (1 minute contact time). Transport hosts should be controlled, and treatment and bathing of all animals in the environment could be considered if intermittent diarrhea occurs. Feces from infected animals should be removed from the environment promptly.

Public Health Aspects

In humans, infection with *Giardia* can be asymptomatic or result in acute or chronic gastrointestinal illness. Acute giardiasis is characterized by watery diarrhea, epigastric pain, nausea, vomiting, decreased appetite, and weight loss; these signs occur 6 to 15 days after infection. Young children and immunodeficient individuals are most likely to show clinical signs; chronic infections are also more likely to occur in the immunocompromised. Recent studies suggest that functional gastrointestinal disorders such as irritable bowel syndrome can be associated with a previous *Giardia duodenalis* infection.[41]

Infection with the *Giardia* assemblages of dogs (assemblage C and D) or cats (assemblage F) is usually not associated with clinical disease in humans, but can be detected in the feces of immunocompromised people.[1] Human assemblages A and B can be found in feces of dogs and cats when animals share human environmental features (i.e., contaminated water). However, it is unlikely that new human infections by *Giardia* assemblages A or B are acquired from dogs or cats.[3] Thus, healthy animals that test positive for *Giardia* are probably not significant human health risks if the family members are also healthy. Greater risk is likely to exist for immunocompromised people, and so the potential for contact with infected feces should be minimized.

CASE EXAMPLE

Signalment: "Duke," a 12-week-old intact male Golden retriever from Fort Collins, CO

History: Duke was adopted from a backyard breeder. The puppy was eating well and was in good body condition. Small bowel diarrhea was the only historical complaint. The stool character varied from soft to watery with occasional streaks of white material that was interpreted as mucus. The diarrhea began just after adoption (a week before evaluation). This was also the time that a new commercial puppy food designed for large-breed dogs was introduced by the owner. The puppy's first two vaccines (attenuated live distemper, adenovirus, parvovirus, parainfluenza virus) had been administered at 7 and 10 weeks of age, at which times he also was administered pyrantel pamoate orally for strategic deworming. It was unknown whether or not other littermates had diarrhea or parasitic infections. The resident adult collie was considered normal by the owner, and the adult dog's feces were normal the previous day.

Physical Examination: The dog was bright, alert, and responsive and weighed 11.2 kg. T = 101.3°F (38.5°C), HR = 120 beats/min, RR = 24 breaths/min, mucous membranes pink, and CRT = 1 s. Body condition score was 4/9. The dog's haircoat was normal and there was no evidence of ectoparasites. No clinically significant abnormalities were noted on physical examination.

Results of Microbiologic Testing: Fecal wet mount examination: No motile flagellates were noted.

Zinc sulfate centrifugal fecal flotation: cysts consistent with *Giardia* spp. were noted.

Fecal cytology: no inflammatory cells, spore-forming rods, or spirochetes were detected.

Diagnosis: *Giardia* spp. infection.

Treatment: Fenbendazole (50 mg/kg PO q24h) for 3 days was prescribed together with a commercially available intestinal diet and probiotic (daily for 1 month). The adult housemate was not treated. The feces were normal 2 days later, after which the puppy food was reinstituted by feeding a progressively increasing percentage over 5 days. Clinical signs of diarrhea never developed in the adult dog. A second vaccine was administered at the recheck 1 week later and again with a rabies vaccine at 16 weeks of age, at which time a fecal flotation was negative. The puppy was still clinically healthy at the 16-week vaccine visit.

Comments: The findings were characteristic of *Giardia* spp.–associated diarrhea; however, because *Giardia* spp. cysts are common in both healthy puppies and puppies with diarrhea, it is impossible to definitively make a diagnosis of giardiasis. Since the puppy needed an additional strategic deworming, fenbendazole was chosen rather than metronidazole. Febantel/praziquantel/pyrantel would also have been an appropriate choice. Because the history was also consistent with stress-associated diarrhea (diet change, housing change), the probiotic and diet change were initiated. Both of these adjunct treatments also may aid in the treatment of giardiasis. *Giardia* antigen testing was not performed, because cysts were clearly identified on fecal flotation. *Giardia* assemblage determination was not performed, but could have been considered if immunosuppressed family members lived in the household. If recheck fecal examination is to be performed, only fecal flotation is indicated, not fecal antigen tests or PCR assays. Whether to test or treat in-contact healthy adult dogs is controversial; however, 5% to 10% of healthy dogs are already infected with *Giardia* in most studies, re-infection is common, and drugs are expensive and can be toxic. Thus, many clinicians just treat the animal with clinical signs of disease during the first episode of diarrhea, with the potential to escalate therapies should the problem persist.

SUGGESTED READINGS

Scorza V, Lappin MR. Giardiasis. In: Greene CE, ed. Infectious Diseases of the Dog and Cat. 4th ed. St. Louis, MO: Elsevier; 2012:785-792.

Simpson KW, Rishniw M, Bellosa M, et al. Influence of *Enterococcus faecium* SF68 probiotic on giardiasis in dogs. J Vet Intern Med. 2009;23:476-481.

Thompson RCA, Smith A. Zoonotic enteric protozoa. Vet Parasitol. 2011;182(1):70-78.

REFERENCES

1. Wolfe MS. Giardiasis. Clin Microbiol Rev. 1992;5(1):93-100.
2. Bemrick WJ. Observations on dogs infected with *Giardia*. J Parasitol. 1963;49:1031-1032.
3. Scorza V, Lappin MR. Giardiasis. In: Greene CE, ed. Infectious Diseases of the Dog and Cat. 4th ed. St. Louis, MO: Elsevier; 2012:785-792.
4. Kirkpatrick CE, Farrell JP. Feline giardiasis: Observations on natural and induced infections. Am J Vet Res. 1984;45:2182-2188.
5. Sykes TJ, Fox MT. Patterns of infection with *Giardia* in dogs in London. Trans R Soc Trop Med Hyg. 1989;83:239-240.
6. Scorza AV, Ballweber LR, Tangtrongsup S, et al. Comparisons of mammalian *Giardia duodenalis* assemblages based on the β-giardin, glutamate dehydrogenase and triose phosphate isomerase genes. Vet Parasitol. 2012;189:182-188.
7. Weissenböck H, Ondrovics M, Gurtner S, et al. Development of a chromogenic in situ hybridization for *Giardia duodenalis* and its application in canine, feline, and porcine intestinal tissue samples. J Vet Diagn Invest. 2011;23:486-491.
8. Wang A, Ruch-Gallie R, Scorza V, et al. Prevalence of *Giardia* and *Cryptosporidium* species in dog park attending dogs compared to non-dog park attending dogs in one region of Colorado. Vet Parasitol. 2012;184:335-340.
9. Buret AG. Pathophysiology of enteric infections with *Giardia duodenalis*. Parasite. 2008;15:261-265.
10. Scorza AV. Co-infection of *Cryptosporidium* and *Giardia* in naturally infected cats. Diagnosis and Treatment of Cryptosporidiosis and Giardiasis in Cats and Dogs in the United States. Fort Collins: Colorado State University; 2007.
11. Gookin JL, Stebbins ME, Hunt E, et al. Prevalence of and risk factors for feline *Tritrichomonas foetus* and *Giardia* infection. J Clin Microbiol. 2004;42:2707-2710.

12. Dryden MW, Payne PA, Smith V. Accurate diagnosis of *Giardia* spp. and proper fecal examination procedures. Vet Ther. 2006;7:4-14.
13. Rishniw M, Liotta J, Bellosa M, et al. Comparison of 4 *Giardia* diagnostic tests in diagnosis of naturally acquired canine chronic subclinical giardiasis. J Vet Intern Med. 2010;24:293-297.
14. Mekaru SR, Marks SL, Felley AJ, et al. Comparison of direct immunofluorescence, immunoassays, and fecal flotation for detection of *Cryptosporidium* spp. and *Giardia* spp. in naturally exposed cats in 4 Northern California animal shelters. J Vet Intern Med. 2007;21:959-965.
15. Clark M, Scorza AV, Lappin MR. A commercially available *Giardia* spp. antigen assay detects the assemblages isolated from dogs [Abstract]. Proceedings of the American College of Veterinary Internal Medicine Forum, San Antonio, TX, June 4-7, 2008.
16. Companion Animal Parasite Council. http://www.capcvet.org. Last accessed October 23, 2012.
17. Cacciò SM, Ryan U. Molecular epidemiology of giardiasis. Mol Biochem Parasitol. 2008;160:75-80.
18. Scorza AV, Lappin MR. Metronidazole for the treatment of feline giardiasis. J Feline Med Surg. 2004;6:157-160.
19. Caylor KB, Cassimatis MK. Metronidazole neurotoxicosis in two cats. J Am Anim Hosp Assoc. 2001;37:258-262.
20. Dow SW, LeCouteur RA, Poss ML, et al. Central nervous system toxicosis associated with metronidazole treatment of dogs: five cases (1984-1987). J Am Vet Med Assoc. 1989;195:365-368.
21. Abbitt B, Huey RL, Eugster AK, et al. Treatment of giardiasis in adult Greyhounds, using ipronidazole-medicated water. J Am Vet Med Assoc. 1986;188:67-69.
22. Rosado TW, Specht A, Marks SL. Neurotoxicosis in 4 cats receiving ronidazole. J Vet Intern Med. 2007;21:328-331.
23. Fiechter R, Deplazes P, Schnyder M. Control of *Giardia* infections with ronidazole and intensive hygiene management in a dog kennel. Vet Parasitol. 2012;187:93-98.
24. Gookin JL, Stauffer SH, Dybas D, Cannon DH. Documentation of in vivo and in vitro aerobic resistance of feline *Tritrichomonas foetus* isolates to ronidazole. J Vet Intern Med. 2010;24:1003-1007.
25. Da Silva AS, Castro VS, Tonin AA, et al. Secnidazole for the treatment of giardiasis in naturally infected cats. Parasitol Int. 2011;60:429-432.
26. Montoya A, Dado D, Mateo M, et al. Efficacy of Drontal Flavour Plus (50 mg praziquantel, 144 mg pyrantel embonate, 150 mg febantel per tablet) against *Giardia* sp in naturally infected dogs. Parasitol Res. 2008;103:1141-1144.
27. Barr SC, Bowman DD, Frongillo MF, et al. Efficacy of a drug combination of praziquantel, pyrantel pamoate, and febantel against giardiasis in dogs. Am J Vet Res. 1998;59:1134-1136.
28. Bowman DD, Liotta JL, Ulrich M, et al. Treatment of naturally occurring, asymptomatic *Giardia* sp. in dogs with Drontal Plus flavour tablets. Parasitol Res. 2009;105:S125-S134.
29. Giangaspero A, Traldi G, Paoletti B, et al. Efficacy of pyrantel embonate, febantel and praziquantel against *Giardia* species in naturally infected adult dogs. Vet Rec. 2002;150:184-186.
30. Keith CL, Radecki SV, Lappin MR. Evaluation of fenbendazole for treatment of *Giardia* infection in cats concurrently infected with *Cryptosporidium parvum*. Am J Vet Res. 2003;64:1027-1029.
31. Lappin MR, Clark M, Scorza AV. Treatment of healthy *Giardia* spp. positive dogs with fenbendazole or nitazoxanide. In: Proceedings of the American College of Veterinary Internal Medicine Forum, San Antonio, TX, 2008.
32. Miro G, Mateo M, Montoya A, et al. Survey of intestinal parasites in stray dogs in the Madrid area and comparison of the efficacy of three anthelmintics in naturally infected dogs. Parasitol Res. 2007;100:317-320.
33. Scorza AV, Radecki SV, Lappin MR. Efficacy of a combination of febantel, pyrantel, and praziquantel for the treatment of kittens experimentally infected with *Giardia* species. J Feline Med Surg. 2006;8:7-13.
34. Olson ME, Heine J. Synergistic effect of febantel and pyrantel embonate in elimination of *Giardia* in a gerbil model. Parasitol Res. 2009;105(suppl 1):S135-S140.
35. Stokol T, Randolph JF, Nachbar S, et al. Development of bone marrow toxicosis after albendazole administration in a dog and cat. J Am Vet Med Assoc. 1997;210:1753-1756.
36. Zygner W, Jaros D, Gójska-Zygner O, et al. Azithromycin in the treatment of a dog infected with *Giardia intestinalis*. Pol J Vet Sci. 2008;11:231-234.
37. Benyacoub J, Pérez PF, Rochat F, et al. *Enterococcus faecium* SF68 enhances the immune response to *Giardia intestinalis* in mice. J Nutr. 2005;135:1171-1176.
38. Simpson KW, Rishniw M, Bellosa M, et al. Influence of *Enterococcus faecium* SF68 probiotic on giardiasis in dogs. J Vet Intern Med. 2009;23:476-481.
39. Fenimore A, Groshong L, Scorza V, et al. Evaluation of Enterococcus faecium SF68 supplementation with metronidazole for the treatment of non-specific diarrhea in dogs housed in animal shelters [Poster]. Proceedings of the American College of Veterinary Internal Medicine Forum, New Orleans, LA, 2012.
40. Centers for Disease Control and Prevention. http://www.cdc.gov/hiv/pubs/brochure/oi_pets.htm. Last accessed January 21, 2013.
41. Hanevik K, Dizdar V, Langeland N, et al. Development of functional gastrointestinal disorders after *Giardia lamblia* infection. BMC Gastroenterol. 2009;9:27.

CHAPTER 80

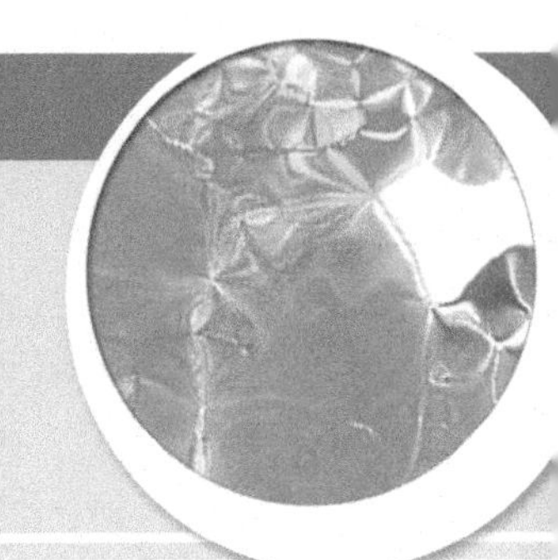

Trichomoniasis

Michael R. Lappin

Overview of Trichomoniasis

First Described: Trophozoites that were likely to be *Tritrichomonas foetus* have been recognized in cat feces for many years, but *T. foetus* was not definitely recognized as the primary cause of trichomonal diarrhea until 2003 (Levy).[1]

Cause: *Tritrichomonas foetus*; flagellate protozoan (phylum Sarcomastigophora, order Trichomonadida)

Affected Host Species: Cats are infected more commonly than dogs. Clinical signs of disease are most common in purebred, young animals that are housed in crowded environments.

Mode of Transmission: Fecal-oral. There are no proven intermediate hosts, but *T. foetus* can survive outside the host for several hours as well as survive transit through slugs, and so transport hosts are possible.

Geographic Distribution: Although infections have not been documented in all countries, *T. foetus* infection of cats is thought to have a worldwide distribution.

Major Clinical Signs: Subclinical infections are common in high-risk cats. Continuous or intermittent large bowel diarrhea is most common in kittens with clinical infections. Swelling of the anus and fecal incontinence can occur.

Differential Diagnoses: All causes of large bowel diarrhea, including *Isospora* spp., *Clostridium perfringens*, dietary intolerance, and inflammatory bowel disease. If motile trophozoites are noted on wet mount examination of feces, *Giardia* spp. and *Pentatrichomonas hominis* are differential diagnoses.

Human Health Significance: There are no known significant human health risks associated with *T. foetus* infections of cats. Nevertheless, cat feces should always be handled as if the possibility of zoonosis exists.

Etiologic Agent and Epidemiology

Members of the order Trichomonadida are flagellates that reproduce by binary fission and do not form cysts (Figure 80-1).[2,3] The trophozoite of *Tritrichomonas foetus* is 10 to 26 µm long and 3 to 5 µm wide and has three anterior flagella (Figure 80-2). In vertebrates, trichomonads are parasites of the gastrointestinal system, the reproductive system, and the upper portions of the respiratory tract. *Tritrichomonas foetus* infects the reproductive tract of both cows and bulls and can cause abortion and other reproductive abnormalities. The organism parasitizes the gastrointestinal system of the cat and can be associated with diarrhea. Genetic characterization of bovine and feline isolates of *T. foetus* has been performed, and minor differences exist.[4-6] Feline isolates of *T. foetus* remained in the reproductive tract of heifers but did not cause the same pathologic changes as a bovine isolate in one study.[7] Similarly, bovine isolates of *T. foetus* may not cause diarrhea in cats as successfully as feline isolates.[8]

T. foetus is transmitted by the direct fecal-oral route. The organism can survive in the environment for hours to days in very moist conditions. Shared litter boxes and mutual grooming likely contribute to transmission from one cat to another.

Cats that harbor *T. foetus* infection have now been documented in multiple countries.[9-27] Cats in crowded environments and purebred catteries are commonly colonized; the organism is uncommon in feral cats. In one of the first large prevalence studies in the United States, 31% of 117 cats owned by 89 different breeders at an international cat show were colonized.[14] In the United Kingdom, 16 (14.4%) of 111 diarrhea specimens were positive for *T. foetus* by PCR assay.[15] *T. foetus*–associated diarrhea is most common in kittens and young cats, but adult cats can also be affected.[14,15] Catteries with a recent history of refractory diarrhea, adult cats with *Isospora* spp. infections, and cats living in a facility with a small number of square feet per cat were

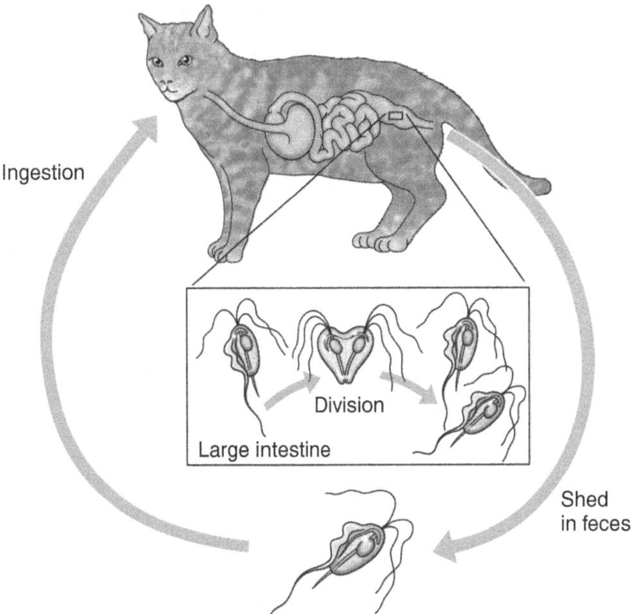

FIGURE 80-1 Life cycle of *Tritrichomonas foetus*. The organism has a direct life cycle, and the parasite replicates by binary fission.

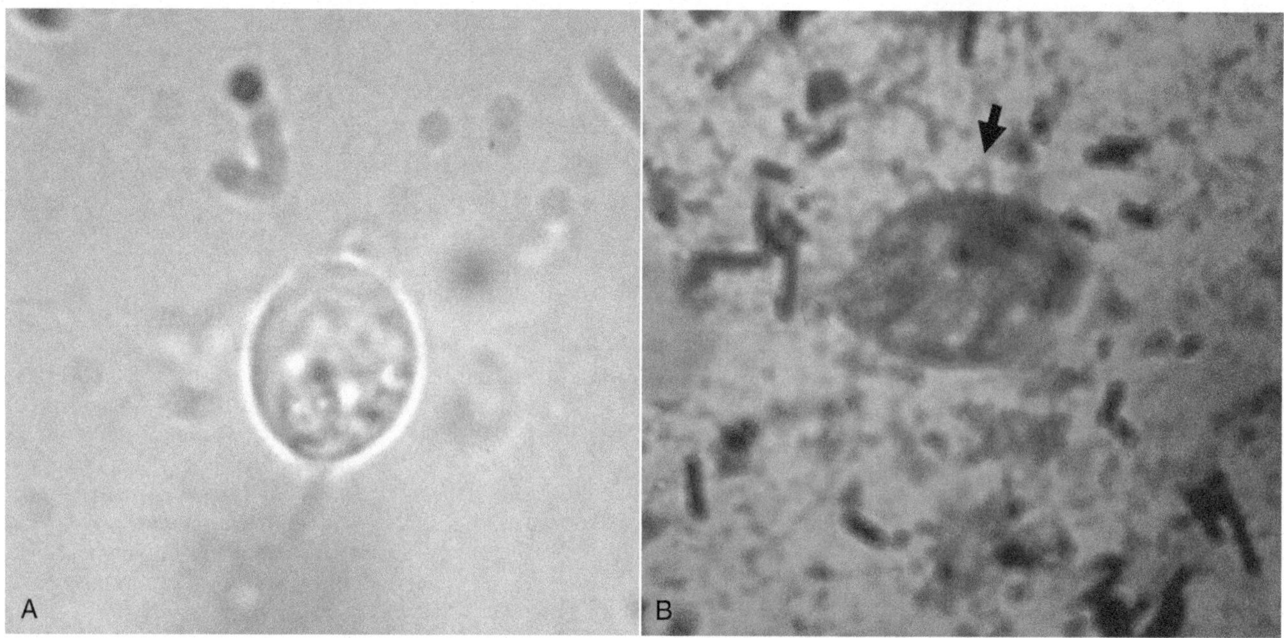

FIGURE 80-2 **A,** *Tritrichomonas foetus* trophozoite seen on a saline wet mount of a fecal specimen. The organism can be recognized by its progressive forward, rolling motility. **B,** Diff Quik stain. The undulating membrane can be clearly visualized coursing along the lateral aspect of the trophozoite *(arrow)*.

more likely to be infected with *T. foetus* in some studies.[14,15] Other co-infections, such as those with *Giardia* spp. and *Cryptosporidium felis,* may also increase the potential for disease.

Clinical Features

Signs and Their Pathogenesis

Tritrichomonas foetus is an obligate parasite that depends on endogenous bacteria and host secretion for nutrients. However, the organism can survive for short periods of time in contaminated water, urine, feces, and cat litter.[28,29] In one study, the organism was shown to survive 30 minutes on dry cat food, several hours in moist cat food, and hours to days in cat feces.[29] The organism also survived transit through the gastrointestinal tract of two types of slugs.[30]

In experimentally infected cats, the location of *T. foetus* is restricted to the ileum, cecum, and colon.[31,32] Fluctuations in the colonic microflora or other factors are necessary to produce the clinical signs of *T. foetus* infection. The organism can persist in cats without diarrhea, and diarrhea can worsen without a change in the organisms present, suggesting that the underlying mechanisms that lead to diarrhea are multifactorial.[31] The organism adheres to the intestinal epithelium and incites a lymphoplasmacytic and neutrophilic inflammatory response.[33] An increased number of *T. foetus* organisms and increased severity of diarrhea was associated with co-infection with *Cryptosporidium* spp. in one study.[31] However, co-infections are not always associated with the presence of *T. foetus*–associated diarrhea.[23] There is little information available as to whether immunosuppression predisposes to chronic infection with *T. foetus*. Administration of prednisolone did not change the fecal consistency or the frequency of positive results on direct fecal exams in one study.[31]

The clinical signs of trichomoniasis are variable and range from subclinical infection to chronic intractable diarrhea. The signs often are intermittent and can resolve with antimicrobial drug treatment, only to recur after treatment is discontinued. The diarrhea is mainly a large bowel diarrhea characterized by increased frequency of defecation and passage of semiformed to liquid, often foul-smelling feces that sometimes are associated with fresh blood and mucus. When the diarrhea is severe, the anus may become edematous and fecal incontinence may develop (Figure 80-3). Although diarrhea may persist, most affected cats maintain a good appetite and body condition score.

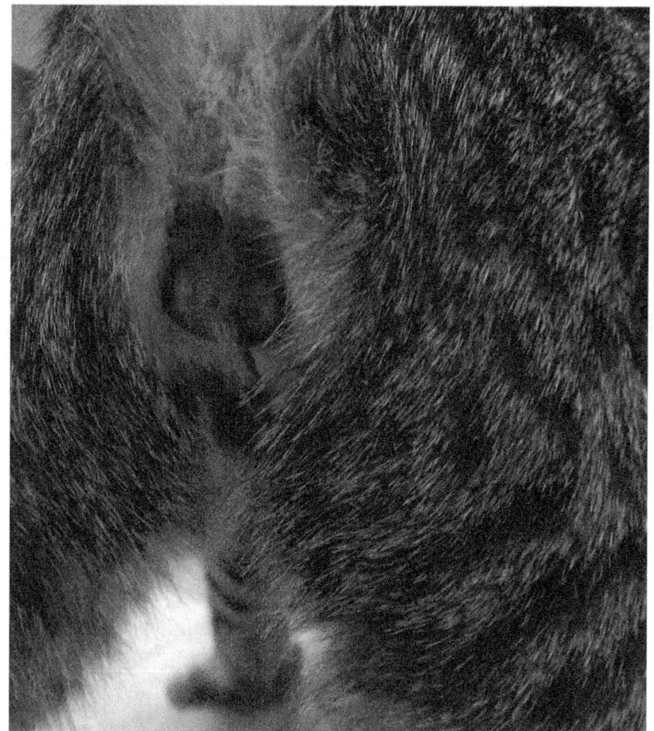

FIGURE 80-3 Anal swelling and evidence of fecal incontinence in a kitten with suspected *Tritrichomonas foetus* infection.

TABLE 80-1

Diagnostic Assays Available for Tritrichomoniasis in Dogs or Cats

Assay	Specimen Type	Target	Performance
Cytologic examination	Feces	*Tritrichomonas* trophozoites	False negatives are common and occur when specimen size is small or low numbers of organisms are present, or because of intermittent shedding. The sensitivity of this method is <20%.
Culture (InPouch test)	Feces	*T. foetus*	Considered the gold standard for diagnosis. May take days for the organism to grow. The sensitivity of this method is approximately 55%. False negatives can occur if feces are dried out, because of intermittent shedding or recent treatment with antiprotozoal drugs, or if the pouch is overgrown by intestinal bacteria.
PCR assays	Feces	*T. foetus* DNA	The sensitivity and specificity of assays may vary depending on assay design. Well designed assays have the highest sensitivity of all diagnostic test methods, but false negatives can occur if specimen size is small or as a result of PCR inhibitors in feces.

Tritrichomonas foetus was detected in the uterine contents of a cat with endometritis and pyometra.[32] However, the organism was not associated with infection or disease of the reproductive tract in a separate study of cats with *T. foetus* infection that were housed in catteries.[34]

Diagnosis

Laboratory Abnormalities

Tritrichomonas foetus infections only rarely lead to systemic laboratory abnormalities. However, if the diarrhea is severe, decreases in potassium, sodium, and chloride concentrations may be present from gastrointestinal losses.

Diagnostic Imaging

Abdominal radiographic or ultrasonographic abnormalities are uncommon, are nonspecific, and, when present, are suggestive of diffuse colitis.

Microbiologic Testing

A direct fecal smear should be performed for all cats with large bowel diarrhea to evaluate for the presence of *T. foetus* trophozoites (Table 80-1), using the technique described for *Giardia* (see Chapter 79). *Tritrichomonas foetus* is similar in size to *Giardia* but can be differentiated by the presence of an undulating membrane, a rapid forward motion, the lack of a concave surface, and a single nucleus. Video clips that demonstrate the classic motility can be found online (http://www.cvm.ncsu.edu/docs/personnel/gookin_jody.html). The trophozoite and its undulating membrane may also be identified on fecal smears stained with Diff Quik stain. The sensitivity of a direct smear using specimens from naturally infected cats was only 14% in one study, so false negatives are common with this method.[31] The sensitivity can be improved by analyzing multiple fecal smears. If *T. foetus* infection is still suspected after the initial work-up, culture can be performed using a commercially available culture system (InPouch TF, BioMed Diagnostics, White City, OR). In this system, a tiny amount of feces is inoculated into the pouch, which can be incubated in the clinic at room temperature and examined daily by microscopy for evidence of protozoal growth. The medium used does not support the growth of *Giardia* spp. or *Pentatrichomonas hominis*, and positive test results suggest infection by *T. foetus*.[35] This assay is considered the gold standard for diagnosis of infection. However, it takes days for positive test results to develop in some cases. Thus, PCR assays are also used by clinicians to document current infection. Several PCR-based assays that are specific for *T. foetus* are also commercially available, and these assays are recommended for assessment of fecal specimens that were found negative by microscopy and fecal culture and to confirm that microscopically observed or cultivated organisms are *T. foetus*.[36] PCR assays are available that are specific for *T. foetus* and do not amplify *Giardia* or *P. hominis* DNA.[37] The DNA of *P. hominis* has been amplified from the feces of cats co-infected with *T. foetus*, but whether this potentiates *T. foetus*–associated clinical disease is currently unknown.[37]

Pathologic Findings

Gross Pathologic Findings

The gross findings associated with *T. foetus* infection in cats are nonspecific and associated primarily with the colon. The colon may be normal or appear mildly thickened with or without hyperemia.

Histopathologic Findings

Lesions associated with *T. foetus* infection in cats are confined to the colon. The organisms are noted in most experimentally infected cats, but not in all sections.[38] Thus, if colonoscopy is performed, multiple specimens should be collected for histopathologic evaluation. The organisms are usually close to the mucosal surface and are associated with mild-to-moderate lymphoplasmacytic and neutrophilic infiltrates; crypt epithelial cell hypertrophy, hyperplasia, and increased mitotic activity; loss of goblet cells; crypt microabscesses; and attenuation of the superficial colonic mucosa.[38] In some cats, *T. foetus* may be detected in the lumen of colonic crypts and can invade the lamina propria. In situ hybridization techniques can be used to identify *T. foetus* and *P. hominis* in biopsy specimens.[39,40]

Treatment and Prognosis

The treatment of choice for *T. foetus* infections is the nitroimidazole drug ronidazole (Table 80-2). Before ronidazole was discovered as an effective treatment, multiple other treatment

TABLE 80-2

Drugs Commonly Used for Treatment of *Tritrichomonas foetus* Infection in Cats

Drug	Dose	Route	Interval (hr)	Minimum duration (days)
Ronidazole	30 mg/kg	PO	24	14
Tinidazole	30 mg/kg	PO	24	14

regimens had been attempted in cats with *T. foetus* infections with generally poor responses.[12,25,41] In some cases, temporary improvement was noted with a variety of drugs, but relapse was invariable. Some of the apparent clinical improvement may have been due to secondary effects of drugs on the intestinal bacterial flora, although treatment may also prolong trophozoite shedding.

A number of drugs have also been tested in vitro to determine *T. foetus* susceptibility patterns.[42] Ronidazole has been the most effective drug used clinically to date and is currently recommended at a dose of 30 mg/kg PO q24h for 14 days.[43] Clinical signs can relapse after administration of ronidazole, but generally resolve again after the treatment regimen is repeated. The pharmacokinetics have been determined for ronidazole in cats.[44,45] Higher doses of ronidazole and twice-daily dose regimens can result in neurologic signs.[46] This likely relates to the high oral bioavailability and slow elimination of the drug by cats.[44] To date, all reported cases of ronidazole-related neurotoxicity have been reversible, but irreversible neurotoxicity can occur in some cats. Not all cats treated with high doses of ronidazole develop toxicity. In one study, a dose of 50 mg/kg PO q12h was used in research cats with no reported adverse effects.[47] Ronidazole is teratogenic and should not be used to treat pregnant or lactating queens or very young kittens. A delayed-release (guar gum) formulation offers promise for targeted delivery of ronidazole to the colon and reduced likelihood of systemic adverse effects in cats.[45]

Some strains of *T. foetus* are resistant to ronidazole.[48] Poor compounding can be another reason for failure of treatment in some situations. Ronidazole also has activity against *Giardia*.[49] However, to lessen potential for selection of resistant strains, ronidazole should be reserved for use for *T. foetus* infections, because multiple other drugs are effective for treatment of giardiasis.

Tinidazole, administered at 30 mg/kg for 14 days, suppressed *T. foetus* shedding to undetectable levels in two of four cats during a 33-week period posttreatment.[50] However, this drug is currently considered inferior to ronidazole because infection was not eliminated in all cats.

Immunity and Vaccination

Immunity to reinfection by *T. foetus* does not occur in the short term after recovery. However, although intestinal infection can be prolonged, the development of effective immune responses as kittens mature is followed by resolution of clinical disease. Vaccines for prevention of *T. foetus* infection in cats are not currently available.

Prevention

Kittens in crowded environments are more susceptible to infection due to stress or immunologic immaturity. Thus, minimizing stress and reduction of population-dense housing conditions will likely reduce the chances of exposure to *T. foetus*. Protocols for eliminating infections or lessening signs of *T. foetus* infection in catteries are available and involve testing, isolation or removal of cats that test positive, and retesting.[51] Treatment with ronidazole does not guarantee cure even if repeated PCR assays are negative, and relapse of infection (or reinfection) can occur months after discontinuation of treatment. For this reason, reintroduction of treated cats to a cattery is not recommended.

Public Health Aspects

Only a single case of an immunosuppressed human infected with *T. foetus* has been reported.[52] The parasite was isolated from a bronchoalveolar lavage specimen in a patient with *Pneumocystis* pneumonia. The authors did not rule out the possibility of a human host-adapted strain of *T. foetus*. However, because of the apparent poor host specificity of *T. foetus* and the close contact between cats and humans, zoonotic transmission should be considered and infected kittens with diarrhea should be handled with care. In addition, the possible presence of other zoonotic pathogens should always be considered in cats with diarrhea.

CASE EXAMPLE

Signalment: "Belle," a 14-week-old, intact female Pixie-bob cat from Seattle, WA

History: Belle was considered a pet quality Pixie-bob and so was sold into a private home at 14 weeks of age. The cattery had three queens and one tom and had bred at least six litters over the previous 2 years. No significant health problems were reported to the adoptive owner, and the cattery was retrovirus free. Belle appeared healthy the day the adoption was completed and was also pronounced healthy by the new attending veterinarian. The breeder had administered one dose of a vaccine for prevention of feline herpesvirus-1, feline calicivirus, and feline panleukopenia virus (FVRCP) and a dose of pyrantel pamoate at 7 and 10 weeks of age. The veterinarian administered an attenuated live FVRCP vaccine subcutaneously, gave one dose of pyrantel pamoate, discharged Belle with selamectin to be applied monthly, and scheduled a recheck at 16 weeks of age for rabies vaccination. Belle was taken to her new home by car for 4 hours and then housed in her private room while attempting to socialize to the two black Labrador retrievers living at the new home. The kitten was not allowed to see the dogs the first 2 days, but the dogs were allowed to sniff under the door of the room Belle was housed in and occasionally barked. On day 3, Belle began having diarrhea that the owner reported to be "pea soup" consistency, with white strands and fresh blood. Tenesmus was also noted.

Physical Examination:

Body Weight: 2.1 kg.

General: Quiet, alert, and responsive. Ambulatory on all four limbs. Body weight was 2.1 kg and body condition score was 4/9. T = 101.3°F (38.5°C), HR = 180 beats/min, RR = 24 breaths/min, mucous membranes pink, CRT = 1 s. The only abnormality detected on physical examination was that the cat postured to defecate, and passed a small volume of diarrhea with streaks of blood and mucus when the caudal abdomen was palpated. Intestinal palpation was unremarkable.

Microbiologic Testing: Fecal wet mount examination: Motile flagellates noted with morphology and motility consistent with that of *Tritrichomonas foetus.*

In-house *Giardia* ELISA assay (SNAP *Giardia*, IDEXX Laboratories): Negative.

Zinc sulfate centrifugal fecal flotation: Negative.

Diagnosis: *Tritrichomonas foetus* infection.

Treatment: FortiFlora (Nestle Purina PetCare) for 1 month and ronidazole at 30 mg/kg PO daily for 14 days were prescribed. The stool normalized 3 days later, and ultimately, Belle learned to tolerate Labrador retrievers. She was clinically healthy at the visit 2 weeks later for rabies vaccination. The breeder was informed of the findings, and it was recommended that the breeder discuss management of this agent in the cattery with a veterinarian.

Comments: The findings were characteristic of a stress-activated *T. foetus* infection associated with moving to the new home and first contact with dogs. Many cats in catteries maintain subclinical infections that may be followed by clinical signs of large bowel diarrhea when the infected cats are subjected to stress. While *T. foetus* can be amplified by PCR assay or grown from feces of dogs, it is unlikely that healthy adult dogs will become clinically ill, and so no tests or treatments were performed on the family dog. In this cat, the clinical scenario was characteristic, so PCR assay or culture were not performed. However, if there had been any doubt that the organisms seen were *T. foetus*, these assays could also have been performed.

SUGGESTED READINGS

Gookin JL. An owners guide to diagnosis and treatment of cats infected with *Tritrichomonas foetus* infection. http://www.cvm.ncsu.edu/docs/personnel/gookin_jody.html. Last accessed January 21, 2013.

Rosado TW, Specht A, Marks SL. Neurotoxicosis in 4 cats receiving ronidazole. J Vet Intern Med. 2007;21:328-331.

REFERENCES

1. Levy MG, Gookin JL, Poore M, et al. *Tritrichomonas foetus* and not *Pentatrichomonas hominis* is the etiologic agent of feline trichomonal diarrhea. J Parasitol. 2003;89:99-104.
2. Scorza V, Lappin MR. Gastrointestinal protozoal infections. In: August J, ed. Consultations in Feline Medicine. 6th ed. Philadelphia: Saunders/Elsevier; 2010:200.
3. Payne PA, Artzer M. The biology and control of *Giardia* spp and *Tritrichomonas foetus*. Vet Clin North Am Small Anim Pract. 2009;39:993-1007.
4. Reinmann K, Müller N, Kuhnert P, et al. *Tritrichomonas foetus* isolates from cats and cattle show minor genetic differences in unrelated loci ITS-2 and EF-1. Vet Parasitol. 2012;185:138-144.
5. Slapeta J, Craig S, McDonell D, et al. *Tritrichomonas foetus* from domestic cats and cattle are genetically distinct. Exp Parasitol. 2010;126:209-213.
6. Sun Z, Stack C, Slapeta J. Sequence differences in the diagnostic region of the cysteine protease 8 gene of *Tritrichomonas foetus* parasites of cats and cattle. Vet Parasitol. 2012;186:445-449.
7. Stockdale H, Rodning S, Givens M, et al. Experimental infection of cattle with a feline isolate of *Tritrichomonas foetus*. J Parasitol. 2007;93:1429-1434.
8. Stockdale HD, Dillon AR, Newton JC, et al. Experimental infection of cats (*Felis catus*) with *Tritrichomonas foetus* isolated from cattle. Vet Parasitol. 2008;154:156-161.
9. Bell ET, Gowan RA, Lingard AE, et al. Naturally occurring *Tritrichomonas foetus* infections in Australian cats: 38 cases. J Feline Med Surg. 2010;12:889-898.
10. Bissett SA, Gowan RA, O'Brien CR, et al. Feline diarrhoea associated with *Tritrichomonas foetus* and *Giardia* co-infection in an Australian cattery. Aust Vet J. 2008;86:440-443.
11. Doi J, Hirota J, Morita A, et al. Intestinal *Tritrichomonas suis* (=*T. foetus*) infection in Japanese cats. J Vet Med Sci. 2012;74:413-417.
12. Foster DM, Gookin JL, Poore MF, et al. Outcome of cats with diarrhea and *Tritrichomonas foetus* infection. J Am Vet Med Assoc. 2004;225:888-892.
13. Frey CF, Schild M, Hemphill A, et al. Intestinal *Tritrichomonas foetus* infection in cats in Switzerland detected by in vitro cultivation and PCR. Parasitol Res. 2009;104:783-788.
14. Gookin JL, Stebbins ME, Hunt E, et al. Prevalence of and risk factors for feline *Tritrichomonas foetus* and *Giardia* infection. J Clin Microbiol. 2004;42:2707-2710.
15. Gunn-Moore DA, McCann TM, Simpson KE. Prevalence of *Tritrichomonas foetus* infection in cats with diarrhoea in the UK. J Feline Med Surg. 2007;9:214-218.
16. Holliday M, Deni D, Gunn-Moore DA. *Tritrichomonas foetus* infection in cats with diarrhoea in a rescue colony in Italy. J Feline Med Surg. 2009;11:131-134.
17. Steiner JM, Xenoulis PG, Read SA, et al. Identification of *Tritrichomonas foetus* DNA in feces from cats with diarrhea from Germany and Austria. J Vet Intern Med. 2007;21:649(abstr).
18. Stockdale HD, Givens MD, Dykstra CC, et al. *Tritrichomonas foetus* infections in surveyed pet cats. Vet Parasitol. 2009;160:13-17.
19. Tysnes K, Gjerde B, Nødtvedt A, et al. A cross-sectional study of *Tritrichomonas foetus* infection among healthy cats at shows in Norway. Acta Vet Scand. 2011;53:39.
20. Xenoulis PG, Saridomichelakis MN, Read SA, et al. Detection of *Tritrichomonas foetus* in cats in Greece. J Feline Med Surg. 2010;12:831-833.
21. Kim YA, Kim HY, Cho SH, et al. PCR detection and molecular characterization of *Pentatrichomonas hominis* from feces of dogs with diarrhea in the Republic of Korea. Kor J Parasitol. 2010;48:9-13.
22. Kingsbury DD, Marks SL, Cave NJ, et al. Identification of *Tritrichomonas foetus* and *Giardia* spp. infection in pedigree show cats in New Zealand. N Z Vet J. 2010;58:6-10.
23. Kuehner KA, Marks SL, Kass PH, et al. *Tritrichomonas foetus* infection in purebred cats in Germany: prevalence of clinical signs and the role of co-infection with other enteroparasites. J Feline Med Surg. 2011;13:251-258.

24. Lim S, Park SI, Ahn KS, et al. First report of feline intestinal trichomoniasis caused by *Tritrichomonas foetus* in Korea. Kor J Parasitol. 2010;48:247-251.
25. Mardell EJ, Sparkes AH. Chronic diarrhoea associated with *Tritrichomonas foetus* infection in a British cat. Vet Rec. 2006;158:765-766.
26. Miró G, Hernández L, Montoya A, et al. First description of naturally acquired *Tritrichomonas foetus* infection in a Persian cattery in Spain. Parasitol Res. 2011;109:1151-1154.
27. Queen EV, Marks SL, Farver TB. Prevalence of selected bacterial and parasitic agents in feces from diarrheic and healthy control cats from Northern California. J Vet Intern Med. 2012;26:54-60.
28. Hale S, Norris JM, Slapeta J. Prolonged resilience of *Tritrichomonas foetus* in cat faeces at ambient temperature. Vet Parasitol. 2009;166:60-65.
29. Rosypal AC, Ripley A, Stockdale Walden HD, et al. Survival of a feline isolate of *Tritrichomonas foetus* in water, cat urine, cat food and cat litter. Vet Parasitol. 2012;185:279-281.
30. Van der Saag M, McDonell D, Slapeta J. Cat genotype *Tritrichomonas foetus* survives passage through the alimentary tract of two common slug species. Vet Parasitol. 2011;177:262-266.
31. Gookin JL, Levy MG, Law JM, et al. Experimental infection of cats with *Tritrichomonas foetus*. Am J Vet Res. 2001;62:1690.
32. Dahlgren SS, Gjerde B, Pettersen HY. First record of natural *Tritrichomonas foetus* infection of the feline uterus. J Small Anim Pract. 2007;48:654-657.
33. Tolbert MK, Stauffer SH, Gookin JL. Feline *Tritrichomonas foetus* adhere to intestinal epithelium by receptor-ligand-dependent mechanisms. Vet Parasitol. 2013;192:75-82.
34. Gray SG, Hunter SA, Stone MR, et al. Assessment of reproductive tract disease in cats at risk for *Tritrichomonas foetus* infection. Am J Vet Res. 2010;71:76-81.
35. Gookin JL, Foster DM, Poore MF, et al. Use of a commercially available culture system for diagnosis of *Tritrichomonas foetus* infection in cats. J Am Vet Med Assoc. 2003;222:1376-1379.
36. Gookin JL, Birkenheuer AJ, St John V, et al. Molecular characterization of trichomonads from feces of dogs with diarrhea. J Parasitol. 2005;91:939-943.
37. Gookin JL, Stauffer SH, Levy MG. Identification of *Pentatrichomonas hominis* in feline fecal samples by polymerase chain reaction assay. Vet Parasitol. 2007;145:11-15.
38. Yaeger MJ, Gookin JL. Histologic features associated with *Tritrichomonas foetus*-induced colitis in domestic cats. Vet Pathol. 2005;42:797-804.
39. Gookin JL, Stone MR, Yaeger MJ, et al. Fluorescence in situ hybridization for identification of *Tritrichomonas foetus* in formalin-fixed and paraffin-embedded histological specimens of intestinal trichomonosis. Vet Parasitol. 2010;172:139-143.
40. Mostegl MM, Wetscher A, Richter B, et al. Detection of *Tritrichomonas foetus* and *Pentatrichomonas hominis* in intestinal tissue specimens of cats by chromogenic in situ hybridization. Vet Parasitol. 2012;183:209-214.
41. Gookin JL, Breitschwerdt EB, Levy MG, et al. Diarrhea associated with trichomonosis in cats. J Am Vet Med Assoc. 1999;215:1450-1454.
42. Kather EJ, Marks SL, Kass PH. Determination of the in vitro susceptibility of feline *Tritrichomonas foetus* to 5 antimicrobial agents. J Vet Intern Med. 2007;21:966-970.
43. Gookin JL, Copple CN, Papich MG, et al. Efficacy of ronidazole for treatment of feline *Tritrichomonas foetus* infection. J Vet Intern Med. 2006;20:536-543.
44. LeVine DN, Papich MG, Gookin JL, et al. Ronidazole pharmacokinetics after intravenous and oral immediate-release capsule administration in healthy cats. J Feline Med Surg. 2011;13:244-250.
45. Papich MG, Levine DN, Gookin JL, et al. Ronidazole pharmacokinetics in cats following delivery of a delayed-release guar gum formulation. J Vet Pharmacol Ther. 2012 Oct 30:[Epub ahead of print].
46. Rosado TW, Specht A, Marks SL. Neurotoxicosis in 4 cats receiving ronidazole. J Vet Intern Med. 2007;21:328-331.
47. Lim S, Park SI, Ahn KS, Oh DS, Shin SS. Efficacy of ronidazole for treatment of cats experimentally infected with a Korean isolate of *Tritrichomonas foetus*. Kor J Parasitol. 2012;50:161-164.
48. Gookin JL, Stauffer SH, Dybas D, et al. Documentation of in vivo and in vitro aerobic resistance of feline *Tritrichomonas foetus* isolates to ronidazole. J Vet Intern Med. 2010;24:1003-1007.
49. Fiechter R, Deplazes P, Schnyder M. Control of *Giardia* infections with ronidazole and intensive hygiene management in a dog kennel. Vet Parasitol. 2012;187:93-98.
50. Gookin JL, Stauffer SH, Coccaro MR, et al. Efficacy of tinidazole for treatment of cats experimentally infected with *Tritrichomonas foetus*. Am J Vet Res. 2007;68:1085-1088.
51. North Carolina State University College of Veterinary Medicine. http://www.cvm.ncsu.edu/docs/personnel/gookin_jody.html. Last accessed January 21, 2013.
52. Duboucher C, Caby S, Dufernez F, et al. Molecular identification of *Tritrichomonas foetus*-like organisms as coinfecting agents of human *Pneumocystis* pneumonia. J Clin Microbiol. 2006;44:1165-1168.

CHAPTER 81

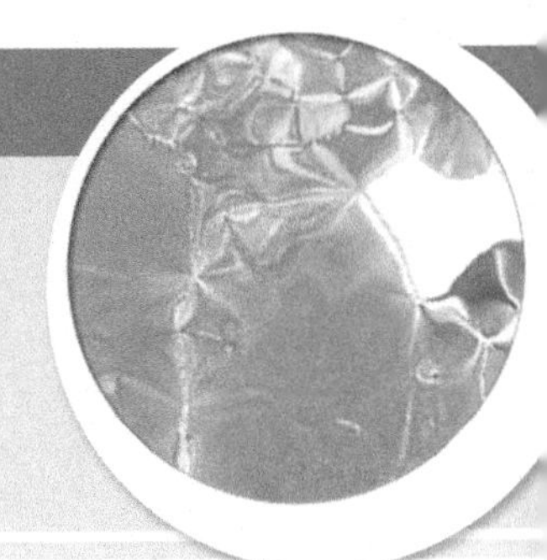

Cryptosporidiosis

Michael R. Lappin

Overview of Cryptosporidiosis

First Described: *Cryptosporidium* was first described in mice in 1907 (Tyzzer).[1] Although *Cryptosporidium* spp. oocysts were reported in feces of cats and dogs in earlier reports, genetic evidence for the existence of host-adapted species was reported in 1998 (cats) and 2000 (dogs).[2,3]

Cause: *Cryptosporidium felis* (cats), *Cryptosporidium canis* (dogs), which are coccidian protozoan parasites (phylum Apicomplexa)

Mode of Transmission: Fecal-oral

Affected Host Species: Dogs and cats are the definitive hosts for the species-adapted *C. canis* or *C. felis*, respectively. Other *Cryptosporidium* spp. such as *Cryptosporidium parvum* may be detected in dog or cat feces, but the potential for disease causation is unclear.

Intermediate Hosts: Although there are no intermediate hosts, there are multiple potential transport hosts that may carry *Cryptosporidium* spp. oocysts and indirectly infect dogs or cats.

Geographic Distribution: Worldwide

Major Clinical Signs: Most dogs and cats harbor subclinical infections. Acute watery diarrhea or chronic or intermittent diarrhea and weight loss may be noted in animals with concurrent infections such as *Giardia* spp. or *Tritrichomonas foetus*, immunocompromise, or coexistent conditions such as inflammatory bowel disease.

Differential Diagnoses: All causes of small bowel diarrhea including *Isospora* spp. infection, *Giardia* spp. infection, dietary intolerance, and inflammatory bowel disease

Human Health Significance: *Cryptosporidium parvum* and *C. hominis* are the species most commonly associated with disease in people; neither of these organisms is common in dogs and cats. Although DNA of *C. felis* and *C. canis* has been amplified from human feces, the disease-inducing potential in humans appears to be minimal. However, immunocompromised people should take extra care to avoid accidental ingestion of dog or cat feces, particularly if diarrhea is present.

Etiologic Agent and Epidemiology

Cryptosporidium spp. are coccidians that reside in the small intestines and are occasionally associated with disease in some infected hosts. There are now 16 accepted species of *Cryptosporidium*, and approximately 50 *Cryptosporidium* genotypes have been described.[4] In the past, most mammalian cryptosporidiosis was attributed to *Cryptosporidium parvum*. However, molecular studies have demonstrated that cats are usually infected with the host-specific *Cryptosporidium felis* and dogs are usually infected with *Cryptosporidium canis*.[4-16] Occasionally, dogs or cats are infected with *C. parvum*.[17] A mixed infection with *Cryptosporidium muris* and *C. felis* was reported in one cat.[18] *Cryptosporidium hominis* is the most common human host–adapted strain and has not been associated with infection in dogs and cats.

Cryptosporidium spp. infections of dogs and cats can be quite common, with prevalence rates generally being 2% to 12% in dogs or cats with or without diarrhea, depending on the method of diagnostic testing.[19-30] In one study of specimens collected from around the United States, *Cryptosporidium* spp. DNA was amplified by PCR assay from feces of 29.4% of cats and 15.1% of dogs with diarrhea.[24] In a study of cats in shelters in upstate New York, fecal flotation identified oocysts in 3.8% of the cats tested.[21]

Clinical Features

Signs and Their Pathogenesis

Cryptosporidium felis and *C. canis* are transmitted among dogs and cats by the ingestion of oocysts in feces from mutual grooming, shared litter boxes, ingestion of contaminated food or water, and possibly ingestion of infected prey species. The oocysts are passed in the feces already sporulated and so are immediately infectious (Figure 81-1). In a study of cats inoculated with *C. parvum*, oocysts were detected by day 7 and *C. parvum* DNA was detected by day 2 after inoculation.[31] In contrast, *C. felis* oocysts are first shed in the feces 3 to 6 days after infection. Approximately 20% of the oocysts produced in the intestine are "thin-walled" oocysts that fail to form an oocyst wall. These oocysts rupture within the intestines, and when the sporozoites are released, auto-infection occurs, which allows for rapid amplification of infection. Thick-walled oocysts are passed in the feces, are environmentally resistant, and are the likely source of new infections. Between 1 and 1000 oocysts of pathogenic species such as *C. parvum* are enough to cause infection in humans.[4]

Although infection of dogs and cats with *Cryptosporidium* spp. is common, most infected animals are clinically normal. In prevalence studies, only rarely is there an association between positive *Cryptosporidium* spp. assay results and the presence of diarrhea.[28] Diarrhea is generally more common in young animals.[32-46] When diarrhea occurs, it is usually watery, without mucus, blood, melena, or straining, and so is classified as small bowel diarrhea (Figure 81-2). Weight loss may also

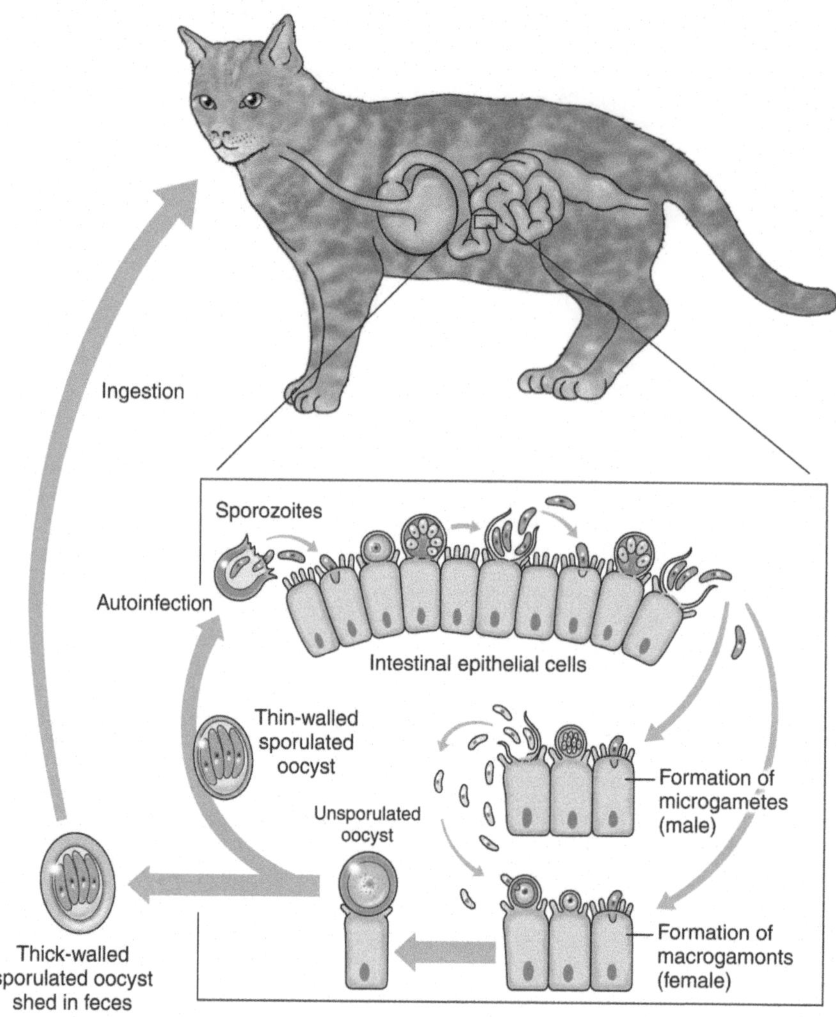

FIGURE 81-1 Life cycle of *Cryptosporidium* spp. Gametogony generates both thin-walled oocysts, which are immediately infective, and thick-walled oocysts, which are shed in the feces already sporulated.

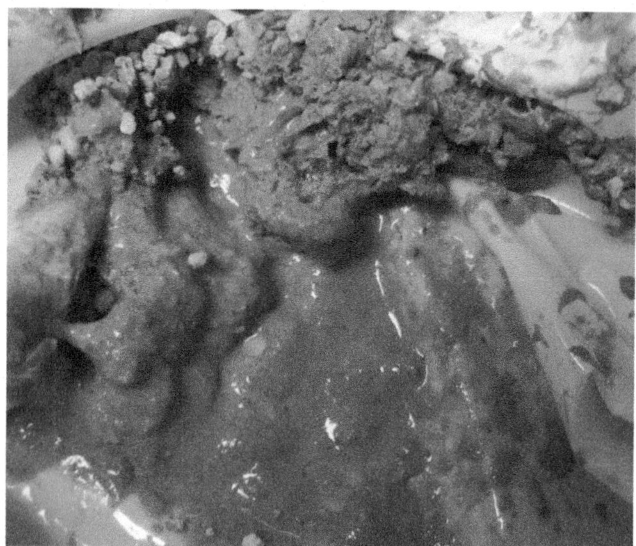

FIGURE 81-2 Characteristic appearance of diarrhea induced by *Cryptosporidium felis* and *Giardia* spp. co-infection. The image is from the case example described at the end of this chapter.

occur. Co-infection with other protozoans such as *Giardia* spp. (dogs and cats) or *Tritrichomonas foetus* (cats) may be associated with more significant illness than infection with just one of the parasites.[47,48] The presence of immunosuppressive diseases such as lymphoma, FeLV infection, canine distemper virus infection, or canine parvovirus infection also can potentiate the development of clinical signs of disease. Clinical signs appear to be more likely in cats infected with *C. felis* than in dogs infected with *C. canis*. In the cat with a mixed *C. muris* and *C. felis* infection, both vomiting and diarrhea were present, and *C. muris* was identified in the stomach in the presence of inflammation.[18]

Little information is available in regard to the pathogenesis of *Cryptosporidium* spp. in cats and dogs; most information is from what is known in humans and mice after infection by *C. parvum*.[49] After ingestion, *Cryptosporidium* spp. sporozoites attach to the intestinal epithelium via interactions among multiple parasite ligands and host receptors. The organism resides between the cell membrane and the cell cytoplasm, which may partially explain its resistance to antiprotozoal chemotherapy. The intestinal epithelial cells act as a physical barrier and produce a variety of cytokines and chemokines in response to the pathogen. Mucosal infiltration with neutrophils, macrophages, and lymphocytes in the lamina propria can result. There is upregulation of both proinflammatory and antiinflammatory

TABLE 81-1

Diagnostic Assays Available for Cryptosporidiosis in Dogs or Cats

Assay	Specimen Type	Target	Performance
Cytologic examination	Feces	*Cryptosporidium* oocysts	Modified acid-fast staining has a sensitivity of approximately 70% and so false negatives are common. However, the technique is more sensitive than fecal flotation.
Fecal flotation	Feces	*Cryptosporidium* oocysts	The small size of the oocysts and small numbers shed by dogs and cats makes this an inadequate screening procedure. The sensitivity is unknown but may be as low as 10%.
Immunofluorescent antibody assay	Feces	*Cryptosporidium* oocysts	IFA assays are available that detect both *Cryptosporidium* spp. oocysts and *Giardia* cysts. Morphology can be evaluated as well as fluorescence, and so this assay is considered by most to be the gold standard. The assay appears to detect *C. felis* and *C. canis*. The sensitivity of the assay is >70%, but false negatives can occur because oocyst numbers fluctuate.
PCR assays	Feces	*Cryptosporidium* DNA	The sensitivity and specificity of assays may vary depending on assay design. Well-designed assays have the highest sensitivity of all diagnostic test methods, but false negatives can occur if low numbers of oocysts are shed, the specimen size is small, or as a result of PCR inhibitors in feces. Use of PCR as a screening assay will result in detection of many subclinical infections.

cytokines, and the ratio of these cytokines likely determines whether diarrhea develops. Cellular immunity mediated by CD4+ and CD8+α/β T cells is an important component for the resolution of *C. parvum* infection. When it occurs, *Cryptosporidium* spp. diarrhea is associated with impaired intestinal absorption and enhanced secretion.[49] It is possible that susceptibility to cryptosporidiosis in animals could have a genetic basis as suggested for humans.[50,51]

Physical Examination Findings

Most dogs or cats colonized with *Cryptosporidium* spp. have a normal physical examination. On abdominal palpation, small intestines may feel slightly thickened. Because some dogs or cats with *Cryptosporidium* spp. infection and diarrhea have had underlying diseases such as inflammatory bowel disease, lymphoma, or infections (especially *T. foetus*, FeLV, canine distemper virus, or canine parvovirus), physical examination findings may reflect the presence of these conditions.

Diagnosis

Laboratory Abnormalities

Cryptosporidium spp. infection alone is rarely associated with CBC or serum biochemistry panel abnormalities. Electrolyte and acid-base changes may be present if diarrhea is severe. If concurrent immunosuppressive conditions such as FeLV infection or FIV infection exist, test results consistent with those conditions may be present.

Diagnostic Imaging

Abdominal radiographic and ultrasonographic abnormalities in dogs and cats with *Cryptosporidium* infection are uncommon, are nonspecific, and, when present, are suggestive of diffuse enteritis.

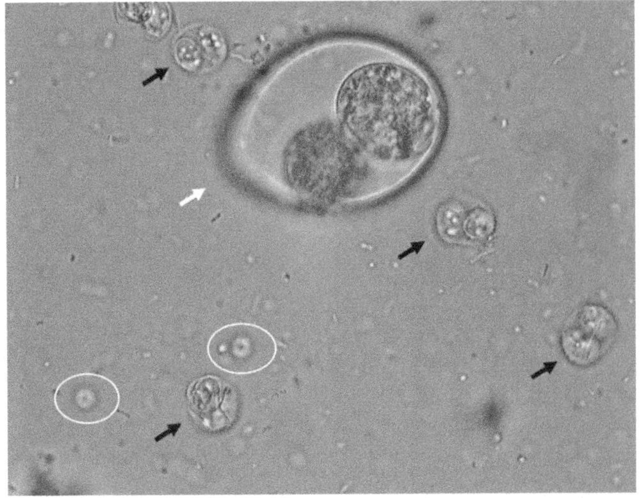

FIGURE 81-3 Fecal flotation from a cat that was co-infected with *Toxoplasma gondii*, *Isospora felis*, and *Cryptosporidium felis*. The image is magnified approximately 2,000×. The black arrows are sporulated *T. gondii oocysts*; the white arrow shows *Isospora felis*; the white circles surround *Cryptosporidium felis* oocysts.

Microbiologic Testing

Specific diagnostic assays for cryptosporidiosis are shown in Table 81-1.

Cytologic Examination

Cryptosporidium felis and *C. canis* oocysts are similar in size; *C. felis* oocysts are 5 μm by 4.5 μm and *C. canis* oocysts are 4.95 μm by 4.71 μm (Figure 81-3). However, their small size means that the oocysts are easy to overlook. Modified acid-fast staining of a thin fecal smear can be performed in the small animal practice to aid in the detection of the organisms

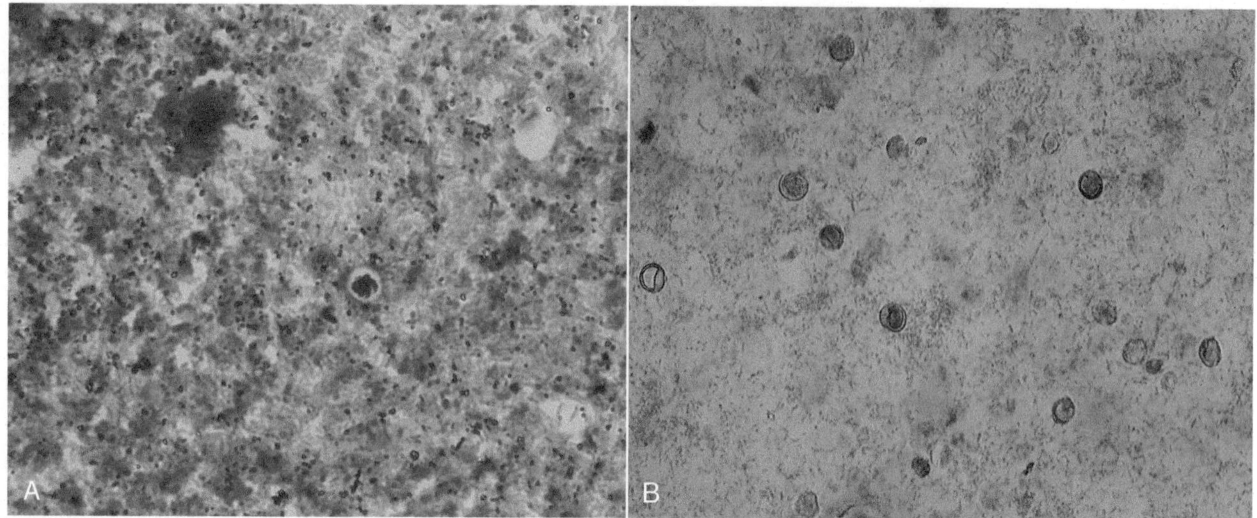

FIGURE 81-4 Acid-fast (Ziehl-Neelsen) stained fecal smears showing *Cryptosporidium felis*. **A,** Smear from a cat with diarrhea that shows a single oocyst of *C. felis*. (From: Marks SL, Willard MD. Diarrhea in kittens. In: August JR, ed. Consultations in Feline Internal Medicine. 5th ed. St. Louis: Saunders; 2006.) **B,** Multiple oocysts of *C. felis* that have a more crinkled appearance. The oocysts are approximately 5 µm in diameter and stain pink to red. (From Ettinger SJ, Feldman EC. Textbook of Veterinary Internal Medicine. 7th ed. St. Louis: Saunders; 2011.)

(Figure 81-4).[23,52] *Cryptosporidium* spp. are generally the only enteric organism of the size just specified that stain pink to red with acid-fast stain. However, in one study, acid-fast staining detected only approximately 70% of *Cryptosporidium* spp.–infected kittens when a single specimen was tested.[52]

Concentration Techniques

Centrifugal fecal flotation is usually performed as part of the initial diagnostic work-up of dogs or cats with small bowel diarrhea.[53] *Cryptosporidium* spp. oocysts are frequently missed because of their small size, and only low numbers of oocysts are passed in infected dog or cat feces (often <500 oocysts/gram of feces).

Direct Immunofluorescent Antibody Testing

A fluorescein-labeled monoclonal antibody system is available that contains monoclonal antibodies that react with *Cryptosporidium* spp. oocysts and *Giardia* spp. cysts (Merifluor IFA, Meridian Biosciences, Cincinnati, OH). In limited studies, this assay appears to detect both *Giardia* spp. and *Cryptosporidium* spp. isolates from dogs and cats.[12,24,31,52] The IFA provides both a morphologic assessment of the oocysts and immunologic identification, which makes false-positive results unlikely.

Fecal Antigen Detection by Enzyme-Linked Immunosorbent Assays

Fecal ELISA antigen tests for *Cryptosporidium* spp. are available for use with human feces, but results of these assays have been variable when applied to feces from infected animals.[12,52,54] The assays use antibodies against *C. parvum* in their design, and so the high false-negative rate in animals may reflect antigenic differences among *C. parvum, C. felis,* and *C. canis*.

Molecular Genetic Techniques

PCR assays are currently available to amplify *Cryptosporidium* spp. DNA from canine or feline feces. These assays appear to be more sensitive than IFA when used with cat feces.[24,31,55] Real-time PCR assays are available commercially through some veterinary diagnostic laboratories. Specific PCR assays are available for each host-adapted species, or PCR products generated with genus-specific assays can be sequenced to identify the *Cryptosporidium* species present. Because *Cryptosporidium* oocysts or DNA can be detected in apparently healthy dogs and cats, positive test results do not prove a disease association.

Pathologic Findings

Gross Pathologic Findings

Cryptosporidium spp. infection can cause mild intestinal thickening. Because the agent is not enteroinvasive, blood is generally not noted in the intestinal lumen unless co-infections are present. Animals with chronic cryptosporidiosis may be emaciated. The concurrent presence of other parasites such as roundworms or hookworms may be noted.

Histopathologic Findings

On histopathology of the gastrointestinal tract, infected cats can exhibit loss of microvilli, degeneration of host epithelial cells, and atrophy of villi and can have lymphocytic-plasmacytic infiltrates.[4,42] Histopathologic findings in infected dogs include severe crypt damage with hyperplasia, dilation, marked villous atrophy, and loss of glands from the mucosa. The lamina propria is generally infiltrated with lymphocytes, plasma cells, and neutrophils.[32,34,35,37] *Cryptosporidium* organisms may be seen in association with the apical membrane of enterocytes. In one puppy with gastrointestinal cryptosporidiosis, *C. canis* were most abundant within the gastric region.[34] This finding was similar to those reported for the cat with *C. felis* and *C. muris* co-infection, whereby *C. muris* was identified in the stomach.

Treatment and Prognosis

There have been no controlled treatment studies in dogs or cats for cryptosporidiosis, and so all protocols discussed should be considered empirical. Because most small animals likely have self-limited disease, feeding highly digestible diets used for small bowel diarrhea may be all that is needed. In addition, administration of probiotics may also have a nonspecific beneficial effect.[56]

More than 100 compounds have been used in an attempt to treat *Cryptosporidium* spp. infections in mammals, and no

TABLE 81-2

Antiprotozoal Drugs Used for the Treatment of Cryptosporidiosis in Cats and Dogs

Drug	Dose	Route	Interval (hours)	Minimum Duration (days)
Azithromycin	10 mg/kg	PO	24	5-7
Nitazoxanide	10-25 mg/kg	PO	12	7
Tylosin	10-15 mg/kg	PO	12	14

compound is consistently effective.[57-60] Paromomycin was initially believed to be effective for treatment of human cryptosporidiosis and was used to treat a cat in one case report.[61] However, this orally administered aminoglycoside can be absorbed across a damaged intestinal epithelium and cause renal and otic toxicity.[62] In addition, in people with AIDS and cryptosporidiosis, the drug has been ineffective.[63] Thus, use of paromomycin in dogs and cats cannot be recommended.

Diarrhea in dogs or cats infected with *Cryptosporidium* spp. sometimes resolves after administration of tylosin (Table 81-2). It is unlikely that tylosin has anti-*Cryptosporidium* effects, and so apparent clinical responses may relate to antibacterial or antiinflammatory effects of the drug. In the one published case report suggesting a tylosin response, clindamycin had been administered before tylosin.[41] However, apparent responses to tylosin have been noted in other cases.[48] Tylosin is very difficult to administer to cats because of its bitter taste and so is usually prescribed in capsules.

Several studies have suggested a beneficial effect of azithromycin for the treatment of cryptosporidiosis in cattle or people.[64,65] Azithromycin (10 mg/kg PO q24h) has been used by the author to treat some cats with suspected cryptosporidiosis, but controlled data are lacking. Vomiting and diarrhea in the cat that was co-infected with *C. felis* and *C. muris* reduced in severity after treatment with azithromycin for 2 weeks. Biopsies were obtained a year later and documented oocysts consistent with *C. muris* in gastric biopsies; *C. felis* was not detected. Azithromycin is believed to have antiinflammatory properties and has effects against other gastrointestinal agents such as *Campylobacter* species. Thus, apparent treatment responses may relate to other drug effects.

Nitazoxanide is labeled for the treatment of cryptosporidiosis in people in some countries and is one of the most widely studied anticryptosporidial drugs.[47,66,67] Nitazoxanide is active against many gastrointestinal pathogens and so may be effective for some co-infections. In a study of research cats infected with both *Tritrichomonas foetus* and *C. felis*, administration of nitazoxanide resulted in temporary resolution of fecal shedding of both organisms and resolution of diarrhea.[47] However, *T. foetus* shedding and diarrhea recurred. The author has administered nitazoxanide (10-25 mg/kg PO q12-24h) in unpublished research studies and to client-owned animals with cryptosporidiosis. The drug is a gastrointestinal irritant and can cause vomiting (see Chapter 10). Thus, it is often administered at 10 mg/kg PO q12h, initially with food. There is no longer a veterinary formulation of nitazoxanide, and so the human product is used (Alinia, Romark Laboratories, Tampa, FL). Because the suspension for children has a low drug concentration, formulation of 500-mg tablets may result in increased ease of administration.

If an apparent clinical response to the first 7 days of therapy with tylosin, azithromycin, or nitazoxanide occurs and toxicity has not been noted, treatment of affected dogs or cats should be continued for 1 week past clinical resolution of diarrhea. Some cats with *Cryptosporidium* spp. infection with or without *Giardia* co-infection have required several weeks of treatment before diarrhea resolves. Whether use of fiber, silymarin, or probiotics in addition to antimicrobial therapy is of benefit is unknown. Some of the cats and dogs with apparently resistant cryptosporidiosis have underlying diseases (i.e., inflammatory bowel disease, *Tritrichomonas foetus*, immunodeficiency syndromes), and so the diagnostic work-up should be continued if therapeutic failures occur. No drug treatment has been shown to consistently eliminate *Cryptosporidium* spp. infections. Thus, the primary goal for the treatment of dogs or cats with cryptosporidiosis is to resolve diarrhea. Since infection is unlikely to be eliminated, following results of *Cryptosporidium* spp. diagnostic tests in normal animals seems to have little clinical utility.

Immunity and Vaccination

Sterilizing immunity to *Cryptosporidium* spp. does not occur, and so repeated shedding, clinical signs, and infection may occur. There are currently no vaccines available for *Cryptosporidium* spp. infection in dogs or cats.

Prevention

Avoidance of contaminated food and water or potential transport hosts is the primary means of prevention. *Cryptosporidium* DNA can be amplified from some raw meat diets.[67] Housing dogs or cats indoors and feeding commercially processed foods may also lessen the chances for exposure. *Cryptosporidium* spp. oocysts are resistant to most frequently used disinfectants, including commercial bleach. Formal saline (10% solution; a formaldehyde solution) and ammonia (5% solution) destroy the viability of the oocysts, but the required contact time is 18 hours. Concentrated ammonia solutions (50%) can inactivate *Cryptosporidium* oocysts after 30 minutes. Moist heat (steam or pasteurization [over 55°C]), freezing and thawing, or thorough drying are more practical means of disinfection. Swimming pools can be disinfected by using high-chlorine concentrations for long periods (3 mg/L of water for 53 hours or 8 mg/L for 20 hours). Exceptional sanitation and use of boiling water for the cleaning of water and food bowls should decrease the possibility of contamination within crowded environments. When a person is infected with cryptosporidiosis, it is advisable to exclude the infected person from the work place, school, or other institutional settings until 48 hours after the last diarrhea episode. This last preventive measure might also be prudent for infected cats or dogs being housed in animal day care environments.

Public Health Aspects

Cryptosporidium is an important cause of water- and food-borne gastrointestinal illness in humans.[68] The organism resists salt water and chlorination and is not readily filtered from water supplies. This, combined with the low dose of organisms required to cause disease has led to significant outbreaks of disease in association with recreational activities that involve water. Young children in day care centers and humans with AIDS are particularly susceptible to disease. Infection may be subclinical or lead to fever, severe abdominal pain, nausea, decreased appetite, weight loss, vomiting, and voluminous watery diarrhea. Life-threatening disseminated infections that involve the respiratory tract, gallbladder, liver, and pancreas in addition to the gastrointestinal tract have been reported in humans with AIDS. The most beneficial treatment for these individuals has been reversal of underlying immunosuppression with highly active antiretroviral therapy (HAART).

The DNA of *C. felis* or *C. canis* have been amplified from the feces of some immunosuppressed people, suggesting that zoonotic transfer of these agents can occur.[69-72] However, *C. felis* or *C. canis* represent the minority of *Cryptosporidium* isolates from people. For example, in one study of 14,469 isolates from humans, 38 were *C. felis* and one was *C. canis*.[70] Overall, it appears unlikely that healthy or immunocompromised people acquire *Cryptosporidium* spp. infection from healthy cats or dogs.[72,73] Thus, the Centers for Disease Control and Prevention does not consider healthy pets to be significant human health risks for HIV-infected people.[74] However, if a dog or cat is known to shed *Cryptosporidium* spp., the family should be informed, and families with immunocompromised individuals or very young children should take particular care to avoid contact with the animal's feces and to practice good hygiene.

CASE EXAMPLE

Signalment: "Ben," a 24-week-old, male neutered, domestic shorthair cat from Denver, CO.

History: Ben and his littermate were adopted into a private home from a large open-admission animal shelter at approximately 18 weeks of age. When adopted, both kittens had diarrhea (see Figure 81-2). The diarrhea had the consistency of toothpaste with no blood or mucus and the kittens were eating well without vomiting. An attenuated live vaccine (feline herpesvirus-1, feline calicivirus, and feline panleukopenia virus) and one dose of pyrantel pamoate had been administered at the shelter on admission. The kittens were taken to a veterinarian immediately after adoption for a general health examination, fecal flotation, FeLV antigen assay, and FIV antibody assay. The kittens were fed a commercial processed food.

Physical Examination: Bright, alert, and responsive. Ambulatory on all four limbs. Body weight was 3.5 kg and body condition score was 4/9. T = 100.3°F (37.9°C), HR = 180 beats/min, RR = 24 breaths/min, mucous membranes pink, CRT = 1 s. No clinically significant abnormalities were noted on the physical examination.

Microbiologic Testing: Centrifugal fecal flotation: *Giardia* spp. cysts were present.

Fecal wet mount examination: No motile flagellates noted.

ELISA assay for FeLV antigen and FIV antibody: Negative.

Initial Diagnosis: *Giardia* spp. infection.

Treatment: Metronidazole benzoate in tuna suspension was administered to both kittens at 20 mg/kg PO twice daily for 7 days. A commercially available intestinal diet was administered to both cats.

Follow-up: The findings were characteristic of *Giardia* spp. infection. However, there was no improvement in stool character after administration of metronidazole and in the week that followed. The rDVM then prescribed a veterinary probiotic to be administered once daily and fenbendazole (50 mg/kg PO q24h) for 5 days with no improvement in stool character. One week after finishing the fenbendazole treatment, the stool character of both cats remained abnormal. At a recheck examination, the physical examination was still normal. A CBC, serum biochemical panel, and abdominal radiographs were normal. Serum B_{12} concentration, folate concentration, feline trypsin-like immunoreactivity, and a commercially available fluorescent antibody assay that detects *Giardia* spp. cysts and *Cryptosporidium* spp. oocysts were performed. The presence of both *Giardia* spp. cysts and *Cryptosporidium* spp. oocysts were the only abnormalities detected. Both cats were treated with nitazoxanide (10 mg/kg PO q12h) for 7 days and the stool consistency improved but was not normal. Treatment was continued for an additional 10 days, and the stool consistency normalized 5 days into treatment.

Comments: Cats with mixed *Giardia* spp. and *Cryptosporidium* spp. infection will fail to respond to drugs with activity against *Giardia* spp. alone. The small size of *Cryptosporidium* spp. oocysts can result in false-negative fecal flotation results, and so the fluorescent antibody assay that detects *Giardia* spp. cysts and *Cryptosporidium* spp. oocysts is indicated for cats with small bowel diarrhea, in particular if there is failure to respond to anti-*Giardia* drugs. Most *Giardia* spp. and *Cryptosporidium* spp. of cats are the host-adapted feline genotypes which are of minimal risk to healthy humans. Genotyping could have been performed if the owner was concerned about zoonotic transfer of infection.

SUGGESTED READING

Fayer R. Cryptosporidium: a water-borne zoonotic parasite. Vet Parasitol. 2004;126:37-56.

REFERENCES

1. Tyzzer EE. A sporozoan found in the peptic glands of the common mouse. Proc Soc Exp Biol Med Assoc. 1907;5:12-13.
2. Sargent KD, Morgan UM, Elliot A, et al. Morphological and genetic characterisation of *Cryptosporidium* oocysts from domestic cats. Vet Parasitol. 1998;77:221-227.
3. Morgan UM, Xiao L, Monis P, et al. *Cryptosporidium* spp. in domestic dogs: the "dog" genotype. Appl Env Microbiol. 2000;66:2220-2223.
4. Scorza V, Lappin MR. Cryptosporidiosis. In: Greene CE, ed. Infectious Diseases of the Dog and Cat. 4th ed. St. Louis: Elsevier; 2012:840.
5. Lappin MR. Small intestinal infections. In: Washabau RJ, Day MJ, eds. Canine and Feline Gastroenterology. 1st ed. Saunders/Elsevier; 2013:683.
6. Fayer R, Trout J, Xiao L, et al. *Cryptosporidium canis* n. sp. from domestic dogs. J Parasitol. 2001;87:1415-1422.
7. Morgan UM, Constantine CC, Forbes DA, et al. Differentiation between human and animal isolates of *Cryptosporidium parvum* using rDNA sequencing and direct PCR analysis. J Parasitol. 1997;83:825-830.
8. Monis PT, Thompson RCA. *Cryptosporidium* and *Giardia*—zoonoses: fact or fiction? Infect Genet Evol. 2003;3:233-244.
9. Bowman DD, Lucio-Forster A. Cryptosporidiosis and giardiasis in dogs and cats: Veterinary and public health importance. Exp Parasitol. 2010;124:121-127.
10. Thompson RCA, Palmer CS, O'Handley R. The public health and clinical significance of *Giardia* and *Cryptosporidium* in domestic animals. Vet J. 2008;177:18-25.
11. Gunn-Moore DA, Scorza V, Wilmot A, et al. *Cryptosporidium felis* in feces from cats in the United Kingdom. Proceedings of the ACVIM Forum, Seattle, WA, June 7, 2007.
12. Rimhanen-Finne R, Enemark HL, Kolehmainen J, et al. Evaluation of immunofluorescence microscopy and enzyme-linked immunosorbent assay in detection of *Cryptosporidium* and *Giardia* infections in asymptomatic dogs. Parasitology. 2007;145:345-348.
13. Wang A, Ruch-Gallie R, Scorza V, et al. Prevalence of *Giardia* and *Cryptosporidium* species in dog park attending dogs compared to non-dog park attending dogs in one region of Colorado. Vet Parasitol. 2012;184:335-340.
14. Sevá Ada P, Funada MR, Souza Sde O, et al. Occurrence and molecular characterization of *Cryptosporidium* spp. isolated from domestic animals in a rural area surrounding Atlantic dry forest fragments in Teodoro Sampaio municipality, State of São Paulo, Brazil. Rev Bras Parasitol Vet. 2010;19:249-253.
15. Scorza V, Tangtrongsup S. Update on the diagnosis and management of *Cryptosporidium* spp infections in dogs and cats. Top Companion Anim Med. 2010;25:163-169.
16. Yoshiuchi R, Matsubayashi M, Kimata I, et al. Survey and molecular characterization of *Cryptosporidium* and *Giardia* spp. in owned companion animal, dogs and cats, in Japan. Vet Parasitol. 2010;174:313-316.
17. Scorza AV, Duncan C, Miles L, et al. Prevalence of selected zoonotic and vector-borne agents in dogs and cats in Costa Rica. Vet Parasitol. 2011;183:178-183.
18. FitzGerald L, Bennett M, Ng J, et al. Morphological and molecular characterisation of a mixed *Cryptosporidium muris/Cryptosporidium felis* infection in a cat. Vet Parasitol. 2011;175:160-164.
19. Spain CV, Scarlett JM, Wade SE, et al. Prevalence of enteric zoonotic agents in cats less than 1 year old in central New York State. J Vet Intern Med. 2001;15:33-38.
20. Nutter FB, Dubey JP, Levine JF, et al. Seroprevalences of antibodies against *Bartonella henselae* and *Toxoplasma gondii* and fecal shedding of *Cryptosporidium* spp, *Giardia* spp, and *Toxocara cati* in feral and pet domestic cats. J Am Vet Med Assoc. 2004;225:1394-1398.
21. Lucio-Forster A, Bowman DD. Prevalence of fecal-borne parasites detected by centrifugal flotation in feline samples from two shelters in upstate New York. J Feline Med Surg. 2011;13:300-303.
22. Hart ML, Suchodolski JS, Steiner JM, Webb CB. Open-label trial of a multi-strain synbiotic in cats with chronic diarrhea. J Feline Med Surg. 2012;14:240-245.
23. de Oliveira Lemos F, Almosny NP, et al. *Cryptosporidium* species screening using Kinyoun technique in domestic cats with diarrhea. J Feline Med Surg. 2012;14:113-117.
24. Scorza V, Lappin MR. Detection of *Cryptosporidium* spp. in feces of dogs and cats in the United States by PCR assay and IFA. [Abstract] J Vet Intern Med. 2005;19:437.
25. Hill S, Lappin MR, Cheney J, et al. Prevalence of enteric zoonotic agents in cats. J Am Vet Med Assoc. 2000;216:687-692.
26. Hackett T, Lappin MR. Prevalence of enteric pathogens in dogs of north-central Colorado. J Am Anim Hosp Assoc. 2003;39(1):52-56.
27. Tzannes S, Batchelor DJ, Graham PA, et al. Prevalence of *Cryptosporidium, Giardia* and *Isospora* species infections in pet cats with clinical signs of gastrointestinal disease. J Feline Med Surg. 2008;10:1-8.
28. Mirzaei M. Epidemiological survey of *Cryptosporidium* spp. in companion and stray dogs in Kerman, Iran. Vet Ital. 2012;48:291-296.
29. Tupler T, Levy JK, Sabshin SJ, et al. Enteropathogens identified in dogs entering a Florida animal shelter with normal feces or diarrhea. J Am Vet Med Assoc. 2012;241:338-343.
30. Queen EV, Marks SL, Farver TB. Prevalence of selected bacterial and parasitic agents in feces from diarrheic and healthy control cats from Northern California. J Vet Intern Med. 2012;26:54-60.
31. Scorza AV, Brewer MM, Lappin MR. Polymerase chain reaction for the detection of *Cryptosporidium* spp. in cat feces. J Parasitol. 2003;89:423-426.
32. Wilson RB, Holscher MA, Lyle SJ. Cryptosporidiosis in a pup. J Am Vet Med Assoc. 1983;183:1005-1006.
33. Sisk DB, Gosser HS, Styer EL, et al. Intestinal cryptosporidiosis in two pups. J Am Vet Med Assoc. 1984;184:835-836.
34. Miller DL, Liggett A, Radi ZA, et al. Gastrointestinal cryptosporidiosis in a puppy. Vet Parasitol. 2003;115:199-204.
35. Turnwald GH, Barta O, Taylor HW, et al. Cryptosporidiosis associated with immunosuppression attributable to distemper in a pup. J Am Vet Med Assoc. 1988;192:79-81.
36. Fukushima K, Helman RG. Cryptosporidiosis in a pup with distemper. Vet Pathol. 1984;21:247-248.
37. Willard MD, Bouly D. Cryptosporidiosis, coccidiosis and total colonic mucosal collapse in an immunosuppressed puppy. J Am Anim Hosp Assoc. 1999;35:405-409.
38. Aydin Y, Guvenc T, Beyaz L, et al. Intestinal cryptosporidiosis associated with distemper in a dog [Abstract]. Ankara Universitesi Veteriner Fakultesi Dergisi. 2004;51:233-235.
39. Greene CE, Jacobs GJ, Prickett D. Intestinal malabsorption and cryptosporidiosis in an adult dog. J Am Vet Med Assoc. 1990;197:365-369.
40. Poonacha KB, Pippin C. Intestinal cryptosporidiosis in a cat. Vet Pathol. 1982;19:708-710.
41. Lappin MR, Dowers K, Edsell D, et al. Cryptosporidiosis and inflammatory bowel disease in a cat. Feline Pract. 1997;25:10-13.
42. Goodwin MA, Barsanti JA. Intractable diarrhea associated with intestinal cryptosporidiosis in a domestic cat also infected with feline leukemia virus. J Am Anim Hosp Assoc. 1990;26:365-368.
43. Brizee-Buxton BL, Crystal MA. Coincident enteric cryptosporidiosis [Correspondence]. J Am Anim Hosp Assoc. 1994;30:307.
44. Monticello TM, Levy MG, Bunch SE, et al. Cryptosporidiosis in a feline leukemia virus-positive cat. J Am Vet Med Assoc. 1987;191:705-706.
45. Lent SF, Burkhardt JE, Bolka D. Coincident enteric cryptosporidiosis and lymphosarcoma in a cat with diarrhea. J Am Anim Hosp Assoc. 1993;29:492-496.
46. Denholm KM, Haitjema H, Gwynne BJ, et al. Concurrent *Cryptosporidium* and parvovirus infections in a puppy. Aust Vet J. 2001;79:98-101.

47. Gookin JL, Levy MG, Law JM, et al. Experimental infection of cats with *Tritrichomonas foetus*. Am J Vet Res. 2001;62:1690-1697.
48. Scorza AV. Diagnosis and Treatment of Cryptosporidiosis and Giardiasis in Cats and Dogs in the United States. PhD Dissertation: Colorado State University; 2007.
49. Buret AG, et al. Pathogenic mechanisms in giardiasis and cryptosporidiosis. In: Ortega Pierres ED, ed. *Giardia* and *Cryptosporidium*: from Molecules to Disease. CAB International; 2009:428-441.
50. Pierce KK, Kirkpatrick BD. Update on human infections caused by intestinal protozoa. Curr Opin Gastroenterol. 2009;25:12-17.
51. Flores J, Okhuysen PC. Genetics of susceptibility to infection with enteric pathogens. Curr Opin Infect Dis. 2009;22:471-476.
52. Marks SL, Hanson TE, Melli AC. Comparison of direct immunofluorescence modified acid-fast staining, and enzyme immunoassay techniques for detection of *Cryptosporidium* spp. in naturally exposed kittens. J Am Vet Med Assoc. 2004;225:1549-1553.
53. Brown RR, Elston TH, Evans L, et al. Feline zoonoses guidelines from the American Association of Feline Practitioners. Comp Cont Ed Pract Vet. 2003;25:936-965.
54. Mekaru SR, Marks SL, Felley AJ, et al. Comparison of direct immunofluorescence, immunoassays, and fecal flotation for detection of *Cryptosporidium* spp. and *Giardia* spp. in naturally exposed cats in 4 Northern California animal shelters. J Vet Intern Med. 2007;21:959-965.
55. Morgan UM. The development of diagnostic PCR primers for *Cryptosporidium* using RAPD-PCR. Mol Biochem Parasitol. 1996;77:103-108.
56. Bybee SN, Scorza AV, Lappin MR. Effect of the probiotic *Enterococcus faecium* SF68 on presence of diarrhea in cats and dogs housed in an animal shelter. J Vet Intern Med. 2011;25:856-860.
57. Smith HV, Corcoran GD. New drugs and treatment for cryptosporidiosis. Curr Opin Infect Dis. 2004;17:667-674.
58. Gargala G. Drug treatment and novel drug target against *Cryptosporidium*. Parasite. 2008;15:275-281.
59. Rossignol JF. *Cryptosporidium* and *Giardia*: treatment options and prospects for new drugs. Exp Parasitol. 2010;124:45-53.
60. Cabada MM, White Jr AC. Treatment of cryptosporidiosis: do we know what we think we know? Curr Opin Infect Dis. 2010;23:494–459.
61. Barr SC, Jamrosz GJ, Hornbuckle WE, et al. Use of paromomycin for treatment of cryptosporidiosis in a cat. J Am Vet Med Assoc. 1994;205:1742-1743.
62. Gookin JL, Riviere JE, Gilger BC, et al. Acute renal failure in four cats treated with paromomycin. J Am Vet Med Assoc. 1999;215:1821-1823.
63. Hewitt RG, Yiannoutsos CT, Higgs ES, et al. Paromomycin: no more effective than placebo for treatment of cryptosporidiosis in patients with advance human immunodeficiency virus infection. Clin Infect Dis. 2000;31:1084-1092.
64. Elitok OM, Pulat H. Efficacy of azithromycin dihydrate in treatment of cryptosporidiosis in naturally infected dairy calves. J Vet Intern Med. 2005;19:590-593.
65. Allam AF, Shehab AY. Efficacy of azithromycin, praziquantel and mirazid in treatment of cryptosporidiosis in school children. J Egypt Soc Parasitol. 2002;32:969-978.
66. Hemphill A, Mueller J, Esposito M. Nitazoxanide, a broad-spectrum thiazolide anti-infective agent for the treatment of gastrointestinal infections. Expert Opin Pharmacother. 2006;7:953-964.
67. Strohmeyer RA, Morley PS, Hyatt DR, et al. Evaluation of bacterial and protozoal contamination of commercially available raw meat diets for dogs. J Am Vet Med Assoc. 2006;228:537-542.
68. Fayer R. Cryptosporidium: a water-borne zoonotic parasite. Vet Parasitol. 2004;126:37-56.
69. Insulander M, Silverlås C, Lebbad M, et al. Molecular epidemiology and clinical manifestations of human cryptosporidiosis in Sweden. Epidemiol Infect. 2012 Aug 9:1-12:[Epub ahead of print].
70. Elwin K, Hadfield SJ, Robinson G, et al. The epidemiology of sporadic human infections with unusual cryptosporidia detected during routine typing in England and Wales, 2000-2008. Epidemiol Infect. 2012;140:673-683.
71. Lim YA, Iqbal A, Surin J, et al. First genetic classification of *Cryptosporidium* and *Giardia* from HIV/AIDS patients in Malaysia. Infect Genet Evol. 2011;11:968-974.
72. Lucio-Forster A, Griffiths JK, Cama VA, et al. Minimal zoonotic risk of cryptosporidiosis from pet dogs and cats. Trends Parasitol. 2010;26:174-179.
73. Glaser CA, Safrin S, Reingold A, et al. Association between *Cryptosporidium* infection and animal exposure in HIV-infected individuals. J Acquir Immune Defic Syndr Hum Retrovirol. 1998;17:79-82.
74. Centers for Disease Control and Prevention. http://www.cdc.gov/hiv/pubs/brochure/oi_pets.htm. Last accessed January 22, 2013.

CHAPTER 82

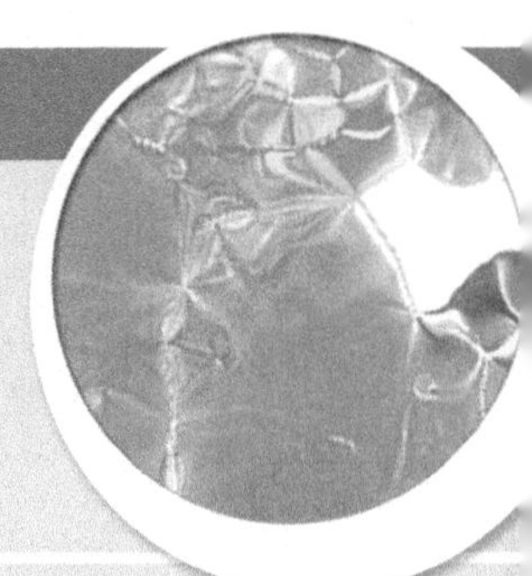

Isosporiasis

Michael R. Lappin

Overview of Isosporiasis

First Described: Coccidian parasites were first described in dogs and cats in the 1800s; the organisms were placed in the genus *Isospora* spp. in 1906.[1]

Cause: *Isospora* spp., a coccidial protozoal parasite (phylum Apicomplexa)

Mode of Transmission: Fecal-oral; ingestion of intermediate hosts

Affected Host Species: Dogs and cats are the definitive host of different *Isospora* spp. The sexual phase of the organism is completed in the gastrointestinal tract, which culminates in the passage of oocysts in feces.

Intermediate Hosts: Most other vertebrates can serve as intermediate hosts; invertebrates can serve as transport hosts by carrying *Isospora* spp. oocysts.

Geographic Distribution: Worldwide

Major Clinical Signs: Most dogs and cats harbor subclinical infections. Watery diarrhea that can contain blood occasionally occurs in puppies and kittens.

Differential Diagnoses: These include other enteropathogenic bacterial (e.g., *Clostridium perfringens, Campylobacter*) and protozoal infections (e.g., *Giardia, Tritrichomonas foetus*), as well as nematode infestations.

Human Health Significance: *Isospora* spp. of dogs and cats do not infect humans.

Etiologic Agent and Epidemiology

Isospora spp. are protozoan coccidian parasites that have been recognized for years as potential pathogens in dogs and cats.[2-4] The sexual phase of reproduction occurs in the gastrointestinal tracts of dogs and cats and culminates in the passage of oocysts in feces. Cats are the definitive hosts for *Isospora felis* and *Isospora rivolta,* and dogs are the definitive hosts for *Isospora canis, Isospora ohioensis, Isospora neorivolta,* and *Isospora burrowsi.*[2] The oocysts vary in microscopic appearance; this can be used to determine which species is present (Table 82-1).[3,4]

Isospora spp. are host specific, have worldwide distribution, and infections are very common, particularly in young animals. In the United States, the Companion Animal Parasite Council reports that prevalence rates for *Isospora* spp. infection in dogs and cats vary from 3% to more than 30%.[5] In a study of more than one million fecal specimens from dogs in the United States, 4.4% contained *Isospora* spp. oocysts.[6] In a study of 1355 cats in the United Kingdom, *I. felis* oocysts were detected in 3%.[7] Gender and breed do not usually influence the *Isospora* spp. shedding rates, but young animals are usually more likely to be shedding oocysts than adults. For example, in one Austrian study, 8.7% of dogs less than 2 years of age were infected; 78% of the positive specimens were in puppies less than 4 months of age.[8] In the study from the United Kingdom, *I. felis* was found in the feces of 9% of cats less than 6 months of age.[7]

Clinical Features

Signs and Their Pathogenesis

Infection by *Isospora* spp. in dogs or cats is initiated by ingestion of sporulated oocysts in the environment or by ingestion of tissues of other infected vertebrate "transport" hosts (Figure 82-1).[9,10] Infection can also occur if the dog or cat ingests sporulated oocysts carried mechanically by flies, cockroaches, or dung beetles.[10] The enteroepithelial phase occurs in the small intestine of infected animals and culminates in the passage of unsporulated oocysts in feces. The prepatent period (time between infection and appearance of oocysts in the feces) and patent period (time that the organism can be detected in the body) vary slightly by the species. In one study of dogs experimentally infected with *I. canis,* the mean prepatent period was 9.8 days (range, 9 to 11 days, n = 22 dogs), the patent period was 8.9 days (range, 7 to 18 days, n = 20 dogs), and all of the puppies developed diarrhea.[9] In contrast, the prepatent period for *I. ohioensis* in one study was 6 to 7 days, and diarrhea was variable.[8] The number of oocysts shed by infected animals can vary dramatically.[8,9] Depending on the environmental conditions, sporulation can occur in as little as 12 hours. Clinical disease is most common in young, debilitated, and immunocompromised animals. All the different *Isospora* spp. replicate in the small intestine, but the regions with the heaviest infection vary by species.

Isospora spp. infections are generally only associated with disease in puppies and kittens. Clinically ill puppies and kittens can exhibit vomiting, abdominal discomfort, inappetence, and watery diarrhea that sometimes contains blood. Depending on the age of the animal and the parasite burden, severe dehydration and death can occur. Puppies and kittens with subclinical infection can repeat shedding and clinical signs of disease during periods of stress.

Diagnosis

Laboratory Abnormalities

Isospora spp. infections only rarely lead to systemic laboratory abnormalities. A regenerative anemia can develop from blood loss in puppies or kittens with heavy parasite loads. Other CBC abnormalities are uncommon. Decreases in serum total protein, albumin, and globulin concentrations can occur concurrently with blood loss. If diarrhea is severe, potassium, sodium, and chloride concentrations may decrease as a result of gastrointestinal losses.

TABLE 82-1

***Isospora* spp. Oocyst Characteristics after Detection by Centrifugal Fecal Flotation**

	Oocyst Dimensions
Cats	
Isospora felis	30 × 40 µm
Isospora rivolta	20 × 25 µm
Dogs	
Isospora burrowsi	17 × 20 µm
Isospora canis	30 × 38 µm
Isospora neorivolta	11 × 13 µm
Isospora ohioensis	19 × 23 µm

Diagnostic Imaging

Abdominal radiographic abnormalities in puppies and kittens with isosporiasis are uncommon and nonspecific and, when present, are suggestive of diffuse enteritis.

Microbiological Testing

The definitive diagnosis of coccidiosis is made by demonstrating oocysts in fecal specimens from affected animals. *Isospora* spp. oocysts are large and often numerous and so are generally easy to identify on microscopic examination of feces after centrifugal fecal flotation (Figure 82-2). However, nondiarrheic animals also can pass *Isospora* spp. oocysts, and so positive test results do not prove a disease association. False-negative fecal flotation results are uncommon in clinically infected animals, but occasionally clinical signs precede oocyst shedding, and so a second fecal flotation may be needed to prove infection in some cases.

Pathologic Findings

Clinically affected puppies and kittens are often emaciated. Other parasites such as roundworms or hookworms may be noted. The small intestines of clinically ill puppies and kittens may be thickened. Microscopic lesions observed in some infected animals include villous atrophy, dilation of lacteals, and hyperplasia of lymph nodes in Peyer's patches.

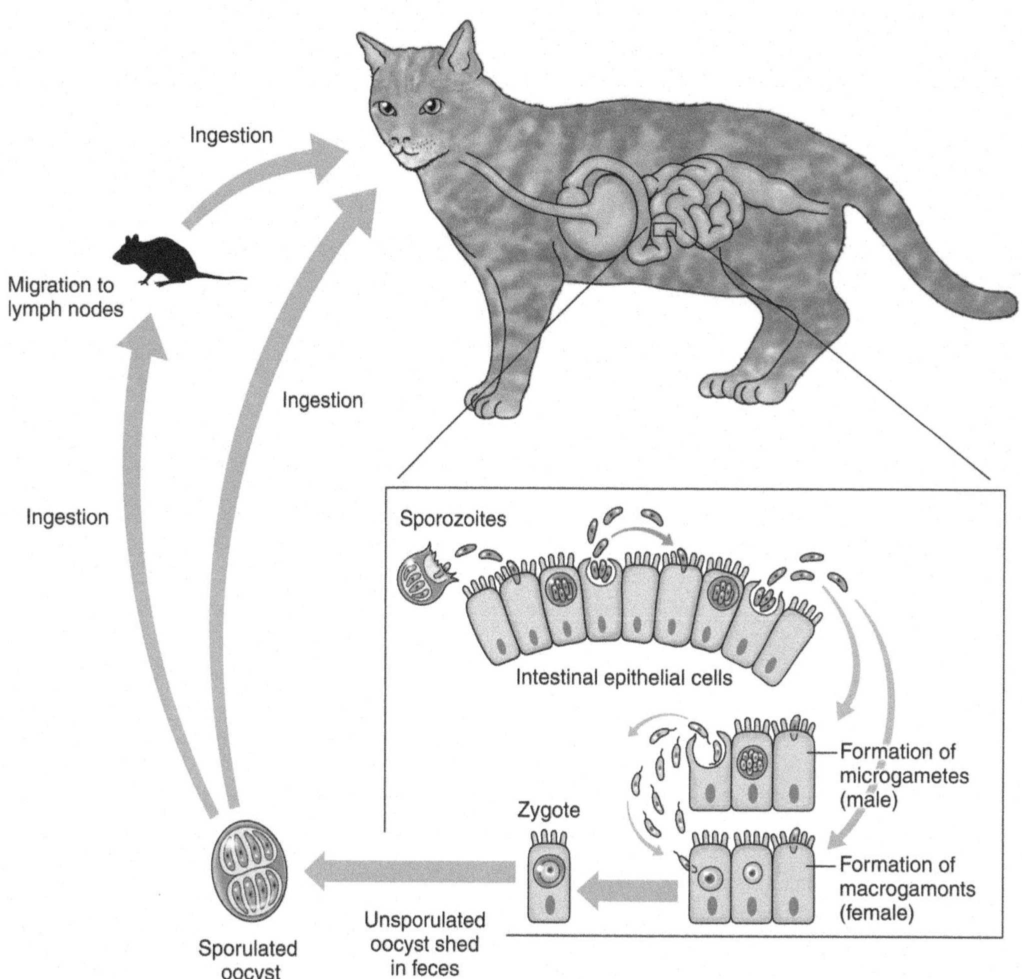

FIGURE 82-1 Life cycle of *Isospora* spp. The host species (in this case, cats) can be infected by ingestion of sporulated oocysts or ingestion of prey that have organisms encysted in their mesenteric lymph nodes. Oocysts shed in the feces can sporulate in as little as 12 hours under optimal environmental conditions.

Treatment and Prognosis

Coccidiosis is generally self-limited, and clinical signs in most puppies and kittens resolve without therapy. However, treatment can speed resolution of clinical disease and may lessen environmental contamination and the potential for infecting other, in-contact animals (Table 82-2). The only approved treatment for coccidiosis in the United States is sulfadimethoxine. Other drug regimens have been used with some success, and these include trimethoprim-sulfa (30 to 60 mg/kg of trimethoprim daily for 6 days in animals >4 kg; or 15 to 30 mg/kg trimethoprim daily for 6 days in animals <4 kg) and a variety of protocols using amprolium alone or in combination with sulfadimethoxine.

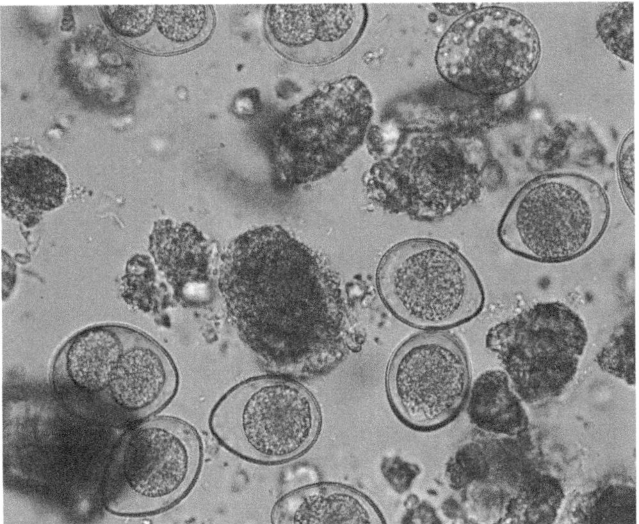

FIGURE 82-2 Oocysts of *Isospora felis* from a kitten with diarrhea (1000× magnification). (From Marks SL, Willard MD. Diarrhea in kittens. In: August JR, ed. Consultations in Feline internal Medicine. 5th ed. St Louis: Saunders Elsevier: 2006; 138.)

Amprolium can cause anorexia, diarrhea, lethargy, and central nervous system disease due to induction of thiamine deficiency.

The use of ponazuril and toltrazuril for the treatment of small animal coccidiosis has recently been studied (see Chapter 10). These drugs are coccidiocidal and so may be superior to other drugs for the treatment for coccidiosis.[11,12] The equine drug ponazuril has been used most frequently in the United States. This drug can be administered off-label at 20 mg/kg PO twice 1 to 7 days apart or at 50 mg/kg PO once, although its efficacy is unclear. Many compounding pharmacies in the United States will appropriately formulate the drug by prescription. In Europe, toltrazuril is available in combination with the anthelmintic emodepside (Procox Oral Suspension for Dogs, Bayer Animal Health) for treatment of isosporiasis and roundworm infections in puppies over 2 weeks of age (see Chapter 10 for additional information). A single 9 mg/kg dose is recommended. Use of prebiotics (food ingredients that stimulate the growth or activity of beneficial bacteria), or probiotics and/or dietary manipulation may speed resolution of diarrhea, but controlled data are lacking.

Most *Isospora* spp.–infected puppies and kittens survive infection, and so the prognosis is considered good to excellent.

Immunity and Vaccination

Immunity to *Isospora* spp. reinfection does not occur, so repeated shedding, clinical signs, and infection may occur. However, although intestinal infection can be prolonged, immune responses usually block the development of clinical disease as puppies and kittens grow older. Vaccines for *Isospora* spp. that infect dogs and cats are not currently available.

Prevention

Isospora spp. oocysts are very resistant to environmental conditions and disinfectants. The key to control is to provide good sanitation, including prompt removal of feces before oocyst sporulation. Steam cleaning can be used to destroy oocysts that

TABLE 82-2

Drugs Used for the Treatment of *Isospora* spp. Infections*

Drug	Species	Dose	Route	Interval and Duration
Amprolium	C D	60-100 mg total 300-400 mg total	PO	q24h for 5 days
Furazolidone	C, D	8-20 mg/kg	PO	q12-24h for 5 days
Ponazuril	C, D	20 mg/kg 50 mg/kg	PO	Twice, 1 to 7 days apart Once
Toltrazuril†	C, D	9 mg/kg	PO	Once
Sulfadimethoxine	C, D	50-60 mg/kg	PO	q24h for 5 to 20 days
Trimethoprim-sulfonamide	C, D	15-30 mg/kg	PO	q12-24h for 5 days
Amprolium-sulfadimethoxine	D	150 mg amprolium and 25 mg/kg sulfadimethoxine	PO	q24h for 14 days

C, Cats; D, dogs.

*Sulfadimethoxine is the only approved drug for the treatment of coccidiosis in the United States. Sulfonamides or trimethoprim-sulfonamide combinations can cause macrocytic anemia, keratoconjunctivitis sicca, type III hypersensitivity reactions (primarily Doberman pinschers), and acute hepatic necrosis. See also Chapter 8.

†In Europe, toltrazuril is available in combination with emodepside (Procox Oral Suspension for Dogs, Bayer Animal Health) for treatment of isosporiasis and roundworm infections in puppies over 2 weeks of age. The suspension contains 18 mg/mL of toltrazuril.

contaminate surfaces. Treatment of dams and queens with anticoccidial agents before parturition can lessen the occurrence of coccidiosis in young animals. In environments with heavy infections, treatment of all in-contact animals, particularly puppies and kittens, could be considered. Ponazuril administered to all at-risk puppies and kittens on intake to shelters may aid in the control of coccidiosis.[12]

Public Health Aspects

Isospora spp. of dogs and cats do not infect people. However, some infected animals are co-infected with other parasites with potential for zoonotic transfer to people, such as *Cryptosporidium* spp. and *Giardia* spp. Thus, a complete diagnostic work-up should be completed for animals with diarrhea.

CASE EXAMPLE

Signalment: "No-name," an 8-week-old, intact male, domestic shorthair cat from a pet store in Fort Collins, CO

History: No-name was housed in a pet store. The kitten appeared small for his age and weighed 25% less than the littermates also housed at the pet store. Although he was eating well, he was thin. Small bowel diarrhea was the other historical complaint, and stool character varied from soft to watery with occasional flecks of what appeared to be fresh blood but no mucus. The source of the kitten was not disclosed. His first vaccine (an attenuated live vaccine for prevention of feline herpesvirus-1, feline calicivirus, and feline panleukopenia virus infections) had been administered subcutaneously 2 weeks previously. He had been fed a commercial processed food followed by a bland diet with no improvement noted in body weight or diarrhea. The other littermates were normal according to the pet store owner. The kitten was administered pyrantel pamoate once on entry to the pet store; no other treatments had been administered.

Physical Examination: Quiet, alert, and responsive. Ambulatory on all four limbs. Body weight was 1.1 kg and body condition score was 3/9. T = 101.3°F (38.5°C), HR = 180 beats/min, RR = 24 breaths/min, mucous membranes pink, CRT = 1 s. The cat's haircoat was dull but there was no evidence of ectoparasites. Abdominal palpation revealed mild diffuse thickening of the small intestinal loops. No other significant abnormalities were detected.

Results of Microbiologic Testing: FeLV antigen ELISA assay: Negative.

FIV antibody ELISA assay: Negative.

Fecal wet mount examination: No motile flagellates were noted.

Fecal flotation: Oocysts that were morphologically consistent with *I. felis* were noted.

Diagnosis: *Isospora felis* infection.

Treatment: Ponazuril at 20 mg/kg PO q24h for 2 days; the littermates were treated as well. A commercially available intestinal diet was administered until the stool normalized 5 days later.

Comments: The findings were characteristic of *Isospora* spp. infection. Although the littermates were clinically normal, ponazuril was administered to try to lessen oocysts shedding into the pet store environment and lessen the potential for reinfection.

SUGGESTED READING

Dubey JP. The evolution of the knowledge of cat and dog coccidia. Parasitology. 2009;136:1469-1475.

REFERENCES

1. Lühe M. Die im Blute schmarotzenden Protozoen und ihre nächsten Verwandten. In: Mese CA, ed. Handbuch der Tropenkrankheiten. Anbang: Coccidia. Leipzig; 1906:69-268.
2. Dubey JP. The evolution of the knowledge of cat and dog coccidia. Parasitology. 2009;136:1469-1475.
3. Lappin MR. Update on the diagnosis and management of *Isospora* spp infections in dogs and cats. Top Companion Anim Med. 2010;25:133-135.
4. Lappin MR. Protozoal diseases. In: Morgan RV, ed. Handbook of Small Animal Practice. New York, NY: Churchill Livingstone; 1997:1169-1186.
5. Companion Animal Parasite Council. http://www.capcvet.org. Last accessed March 8, 2013.
6. Little SE, Johnson EM, Lewis D, et al. Prevalence of intestinal parasites in pet dogs in the United States. Vet Parasitol. 2009;166:144-152.
7. Tzannes S, Batchelor DJ, Graham PA, et al. Prevalence of *Cryptosporidium, Giardia* and *Isospora* species infections in pet cats with clinical signs of gastrointestinal disease. J Feline Med Surg. 2008;10:1-8.
8. Buehl IE, Prosl H, Mundt HC, et al. Canine isosporosis—epidemiology of field and experimental infections. J Vet Med B Infect Dis Vet Public Health. 2006;53:482-487.
9. Mitchell SM, Zajac AM, Charles S, et al. *Cystoisospora canis* Nemeséri, 1959 (syn. *Isospora canis*), infections in dogs: clinical signs, pathogenesis, and reproducible clinical disease in beagle dogs fed oocysts. J Parasitol. 2007;93:345-352.
10. Saitoh Y, Itagaki H. Dung beetles, *Onthophagus* spp., as potential transport hosts of feline coccidia. Nippon Juigaku Zasshi. 1990;52:293-297.
11. Lloyd S. Activity of toltrazuril and diclazuril against *Isospora* species in kittens and puppies. Vet Rec. 2001;148:500-511.
12. Daugschies A, Mundt HC, Letkova V. Toltrazuril treatment of cystoisosporosis in dogs under experimental and field conditions. Parasitol Res. 2000;86:797-799.

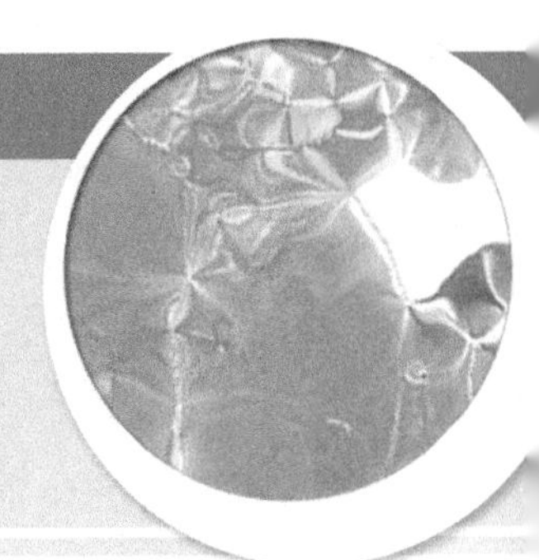

CHAPTER 83

Miscellaneous Protozoal Diseases

Jane E. Sykes

MISCELLANEOUS SYSTEMIC PROTOZOAL INFECTIONS

Besides the systemic protozoal infections described in Chapters 72 to 78, other systemic protozoal infections of dogs and cats include sarcocystosis, amebiasis, rangeliosis, and theileriosis. These are uncommon causes of disease when compared with the other protozoal infections described in this book and are briefly reviewed here. Some have been recognized relatively recently and the life cycle and pathogenesis of these pathogens are not fully understood.

Sarcocystosis

Sarcocystosis is caused by *Sarcocystis* species, which are coccidian parasites that resemble *Toxoplasma* and *Neospora* and have a life cycle that involves intermediate and definitive host species. After ingestion of oocysts, organisms replicate in the intermediate host, forming schizonts, usually in endothelial cells. Merozoites are released from the schizonts and ultimately encyst in tissues as a sarcocyst which contains bradyzoites. On ingestion of tissues from the intermediate host by the definitive host, bradyzoites are released from sarcocysts and replicate in the small intestine, with formation of oocysts. The oocysts are then excreted in feces. Dogs are definitive hosts for numerous species of *Sarcocystis*, but the life cycles of these *Sarcocystis* species are incompletely understood.[1] *Sarcocystis canis* can cause hepatitis, encephalitis, dermatitis, and pneumonia in dogs, with most reports involving puppies.[2-6] *Sarcocystis neurona* is an unusual species with opossums as definitive hosts and several other animal species as intermediate or aberrant hosts, including dogs, cats, marine mammals, and horses.[7,8] There are rare reports of severe *S. neurona*–like infections in dogs and cats, usually with central nervous system signs associated with the schizont stage.[9,10] An unnamed *Sarcocystis* species has been identified as a cause of systemic illness and myositis in dogs.[11] Dogs infected with this *Sarcocystis* species have shown signs of fever, lethargy, anorexia, thrombocytopenia, and increased liver enzyme activities, followed by development of generalized muscle stiffness, muscle atrophy, and increased CK activity. These clinical signs can resemble a systemic immune-mediated disease. Large numbers of sarcocysts are found in muscle biopsies, with an associated inflammatory and necrotizing myopathy (Figure 83-1). Treatment of one dog with decoquinate led to resolution of signs of myositis.

Rangeliosis and Theileriosis

Rangelia vitalii and *Theileria* species are piroplasms that resemble *Babesia* species and are probably transmitted by ticks. *Rangelia vitalii* has been identified only in dogs from southern Brazil. It causes a disease characterized by fever, anemia, thrombocytopenia, icterus, weight loss, lymphadenopathy, hepatosplenomegaly, and cutaneous and mucosal hemorrhages with hematemesis and bloody diarrhea.[12,13] Locally the disease has been referred to as "nambiuvú" ("bloody ear") because of extensive bleeding that can develop on the outer surface of the pinnae.[12] *Rangelia vitalii* replicates in erythrocytes, monocytes, neutrophils, and capillary endothelial cells and can be found in aspirates of reticuloendothelial tissues. Treatment with a single dose of diminazine was effective in the early stages of disease in experimentally infected dogs,[13] but several naturally infected dogs died despite this treatment.[12] Treatment with a combination of doxycycline, imidocarb dipropionate, and prednisone was effective in other studies.[14] A *Babesia microti*–like small piroplasm (also known as the "Spanish isolate" or *Theileria annae*) has been identified in dogs in Europe,[15,16] and a *Theileria* species has also been detected in dogs in South Africa.[17] The extent to which *Theileria* parasites cause clinical disease in dogs and cats requires further study.

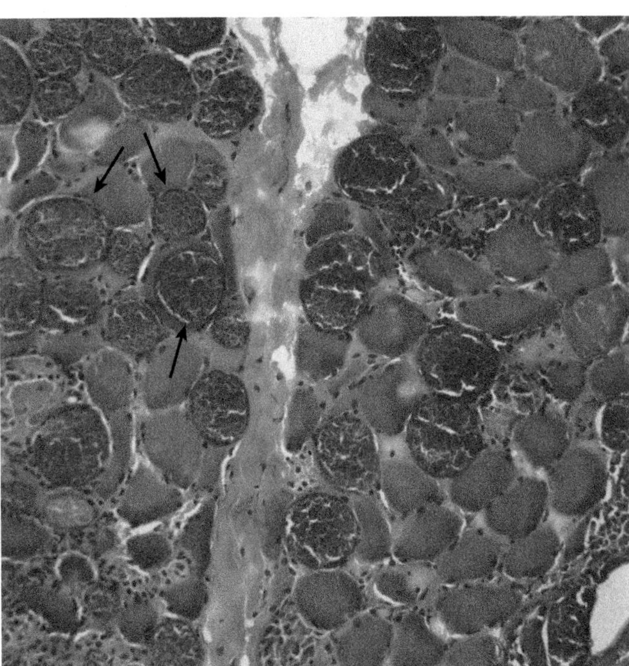

FIGURE 83-1 H&E stained cryosection of a biopsy from the deep digital flexor muscle of an 11-year-old male neutered golden retriever with myositis showing numerous myofibers containing large and encapsulated parasite cysts that were confirmed to be *Sarcocystis* (200× magnification). (From Sykes JE, Dubey JP, Lindsay LL, et al. Severe myositis associated with *Sarcocystis* spp. infection in 2 dogs. J Vet Intern Med. 2011;25:1277-1283.)

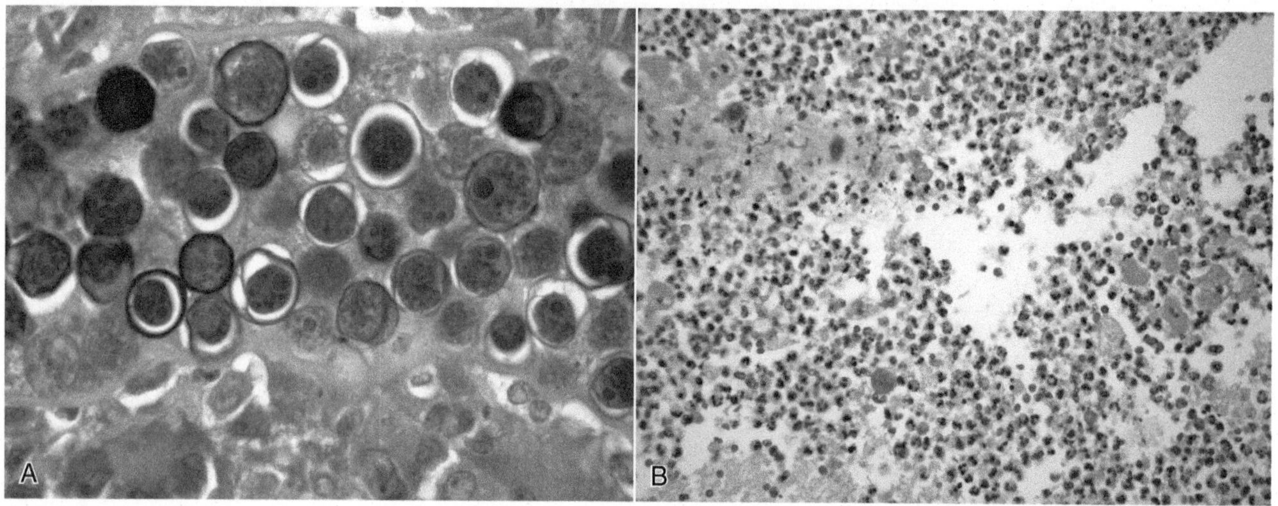

FIGURE 83-2 **A,** Histopathology of the kidney of a 2-year-old male great Dane with disseminated *Balamuthia mandrillaris* infection. Protozoal cysts are present within the renal tubules. Trophozoites were also present within the renal parenchyma (not shown). **B,** Necrotizing encephalitis with intralesional *B. mandrillaris* trophozoites. Cysts were also found in the brain (not shown). 1000x magnification; H&E stain (**A,** From Foreman O, Sykes J, Ball L, et al. Disseminated infection with *Balamuthia mandrillaris* in a dog. Vet Pathol. 2004;41:506-510.)

Systemic Amebiasis

Acanthamoeba spp. and *Balamuthia mandrillaris* are amoebae that can rarely cause granulomatous meningoencephalitis, nephritis, and/or pneumonia in dogs[18-25] as well as humans.[26] Other organs may also be affected, such as the heart, pancreas, and lymph nodes.[21] Affected dogs are febrile and show a variety of neurologic signs, with CSF pleocytosis. Diagnosis is usually based on finding amoebae in tissues with cytology or histopathology (Figure 83-2). Specific PCR assays have been described that can specifically identify the amoeba species involved. Treatment is difficult but in humans is usually with a combination of antiprotozoal and antifungal drugs.

MISCELLANEOUS GASTROINTESTINAL PROTOZOAL INFECTIONS

Several protozoal species can infect the gastrointestinal tracts of dogs and cats in the absence of clinical signs. These include the coccidian species *Hammondia, Besnoitia,* and *Sarcocystis* spp. Cats are definitive hosts for *Hammondia hammondi, Besnoitia* spp., and *Sarcocystis* spp. Dogs are the definitive hosts for *Hammondia heydorni.* In recent years, *H. heydorni* has been associated with diarrhea in puppies that are kept in overcrowded environments.

Amoeba species that can infect the colon include *Balantidium coli* and *Entamoeba histolytica*. Balantidiasis has been reported very rarely in dogs but not in cats. Affected dogs showed signs of large bowel diarrhea with hematochezia and tenesmus, although co-infections with *Trichuris* have been reported.[27,28] *Entamoeba histolytica* infection occurs worldwide and is an important cause of disease in humans and nonhuman primates (Figure 83-3). Infection can occur in both dogs and cats. Most infections are subclinical, but large bowel diarrhea and anorexia can also occur.[29,30] Dogs and cats may acquire infection from humans in the household, so the owners of pets diagnosed with *E. histolytica* infection should be referred to their physicians for medical advice.

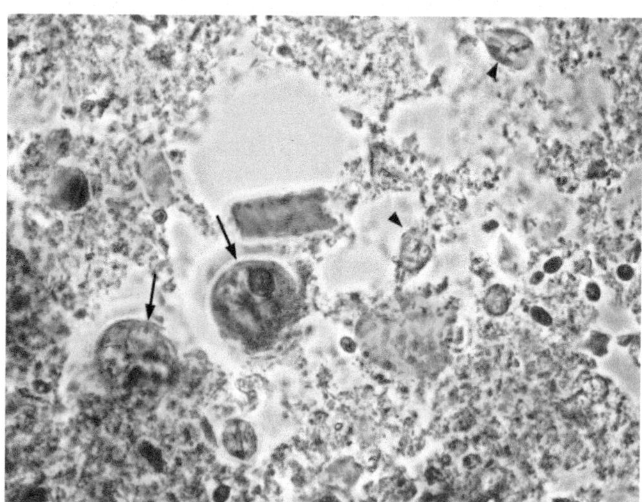

FIGURE 83-3 Fecal smear from a woman who had recently traveled to India and developed severe diarrhea. Trophozoites of *Entamoeba histolytica (arrows)* and *Giardia (arrowheads)* are present. Trichrome stain. (Image courtesy Dr. Patricia Conrad.)

SUGGESTED READINGS

Balamuthia amebic encephalitis—California, 1999-2007. MMWR Morb Mortal Wkly Rep. 2008;57:768-771.

Da Silva AS, Franca RT, Costa MM, et al. Experimental infection with *Rangelia vitalii* in dogs: acute phase, parasitemia, biological cycle, clinical-pathological aspects and treatment. Exp Parasitol. 2011;128:347-352.

Loretti AP, Barros SS. Hemorrhagic disease in dogs infected with an unclassified intraendothelial piroplasm in southern Brazil. Vet Parasitol. 2005;134:193-213.

Sykes JE, Dubey JP, Lindsay LL, et al. Severe myositis associated with *Sarcocystis* spp. infection in 2 dogs. J Vet Intern Med. 2011;25:1277-1283.

REFERENCES

1. Dubey J, Speer CA, Fayer R. Sarcocystosis of Animals and Man. Boca Raton, Florida: CRC Press; 1989.
2. Berrocal A, Lopez A. Pulmonary sarcocystosis in a puppy with canine distemper in Costa Rica. J Vet Diagn Invest. 2003;15:292-294.

3. Trasti SL, Dubey JP, Webb DM, et al. Fatal visceral and neural sarcocystosis in dogs. J Comp Pathol. 1999;121:179-184.
4. Allison R, Williams P, Lansdowne J, et al. Fatal hepatic sarcocystosis in a puppy with eosinophilia and eosinophilic peritoneal effusion. Vet Clin Pathol. 2006;35:353-357.
5. Dubey JP, Speer CA. *Sarcocystis canis* n. sp. (Apicomplexa: Sarcocystidae), the etiologic agent of generalized coccidiosis in dogs. J Parasitol. 1991;77:522-527.
6. Dubey JP, Slife LN, Speer CA, et al. Fatal cutaneous and visceral infection in a Rottweiler dog associated with a *Sarcocystis*-like protozoon. J Vet Diagn Invest. 1991;3:72-75.
7. Dubey JP, Chapman JL, Rosenthal BM, et al. Clinical *Sarcocystis neurona, Sarcocystis canis, Toxoplasma gondii*, and *Neospora caninum* infections in dogs. Vet Parasitol. 2006;137:36-49.
8. Dubey JP, Lindsay DS, Saville WJ, et al. A review of *Sarcocystis neurona* and equine protozoal myeloencephalitis (EPM). Vet Parasitol. 2001;95:89-131.
9. Cooley AJ, Barr B, Rejmanek D. *Sarcocystis neurona* encephalitis in a dog. Vet Pathol. 2007;44:956-961.
10. Bisby TM, Holman PJ, Pitoc GA, et al. *Sarcocystis* sp. encephalomyelitis in a cat. Vet Clin Pathol. 2010;39:105-112.
11. Sykes JE, Dubey JP, Lindsay LL, et al. Severe myositis associated with *Sarcocystis* spp. infection in 2 dogs. J Vet Intern Med. 2011;25:1277-1283.
12. Loretti AP, Barros SS. Hemorrhagic disease in dogs infected with an unclassified intraendothelial piroplasm in southern Brazil. Vet Parasitol. 2005;134:193-213.
13. Da Silva AS, Franca RT, Costa MM, et al. Experimental infection with *Rangelia vitalii* in dogs: acute phase, parasitemia, biological cycle, clinical-pathological aspects and treatment. Exp Parasitol. 2011;128:347-352.
14. Franca RT, Silva AS, Paim FC, et al. *Rangelia vitalii* in dogs in southern Brazil. Comp Clin Pathol. 2010;19:383-387.
15. Simoes PB, Cardoso L, Araujo M, et al. Babesiosis due to the canine *Babesia microti*-like small piroplasm in dogs—first report from Portugal and possible vertical transmission. Parasit Vectors. 2011;4:50.
16. Camacho AT, Pallas E, Gestal JJ, et al. Infection of dogs in north-west Spain with a *Babesia microti*-like agent. Vet Rec. 2001;149:552-555.
17. Matjila PT, Leisewitz AL, Oosthuizen MC, et al. Detection of a *Theileria* species in dogs in South Africa. Vet Parasitol. 2008;157:34-40.
18. Pearce JR, Powell HS, Chandler FW, et al. Amebic meningoencephalitis caused by *Acanthamoeba castellani* in a dog. J Am Vet Med Assoc. 1985;187:951-952.
19. Bauer RW, Harrison LR, Watson CW, et al. Isolation of *Acanthamoeba* sp. from a greyhound with pneumonia and granulomatous amebic encephalitis. J Vet Diagn Invest. 1993;5:386-391.
20. Brofman PJ, Knostman KA, DiBartola SP. Granulomatous amebic meningoencephalitis causing the syndrome of inappropriate secretion of antidiuretic hormone in a dog. J Vet Intern Med. 2003;17:230-234.
21. Dubey JP, Benson JE, Blakeley KT, et al. Disseminated *Acanthamoeba* sp. infection in a dog. Vet Parasitol. 2005;128:183-187.
22. Kent M, Platt SR, Rech RR, et al. Multisystemic infection with an *Acanthamoeba* sp. in a dog. J Am Vet Med Assoc. 2011;238:1476-1481.
23. Foreman O, Sykes J, Ball L, et al. Disseminated infection with *Balamuthia mandrillaris* in a dog. Vet Pathol. 2004;41:506-510.
24. Finnin PJ, Visvesvara GS, Campbell BE, et al. Multifocal *Balamuthia mandrillaris* infection in a dog in Australia. Parasitol Res. 2007;100:423-426.
25. Hodge PJ, Kelers K, Gasser RB, et al. Another case of canine amoebic meningoencephalitis—the challenges of reaching a rapid diagnosis. Parasitol Res. 2011;108:1069-1073.
26. *Balamuthia* amebic encephalitis—California, 1999-2007. MMWR Morb Mortal Wkly Rep. 2008;57:768-771.
27. Bailey WS, Williams AG. *Balantidium* infection in the dog. J Am Vet Med Assoc. 1949;114:238.
28. Ewing SA, Bull RW. Severe chronic canine diarrhea associated with *Balantidium-Trichuris* infection. J Am Vet Med Assoc. 1966;149:519-520.
29. Wittnich C. *Entamoeba histolytica* infection in a German shepherd dog. Can Vet J. 1976;17:259-263.
30. Shimada A, Muraki Y, Awakura T, et al. Necrotic colitis associated with *Entamoeba histolytica* infection in a cat. J Comp Pathol. 1992;106:195-199.

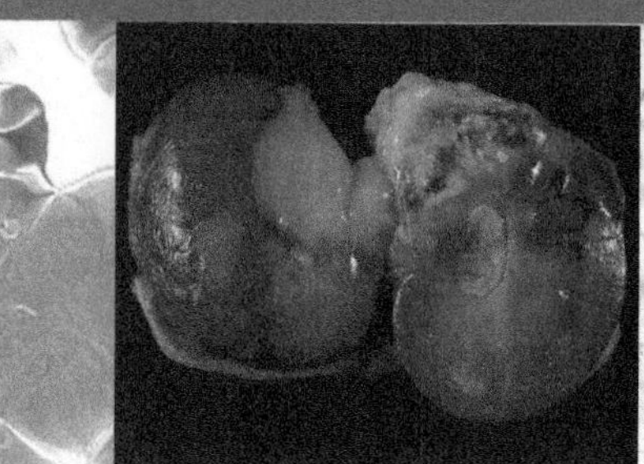

SECTION 5
Infections of Selected Organ Systems

Jane E. Sykes, Terry M. Nagle, and Stephen D. White

CHAPTER 84

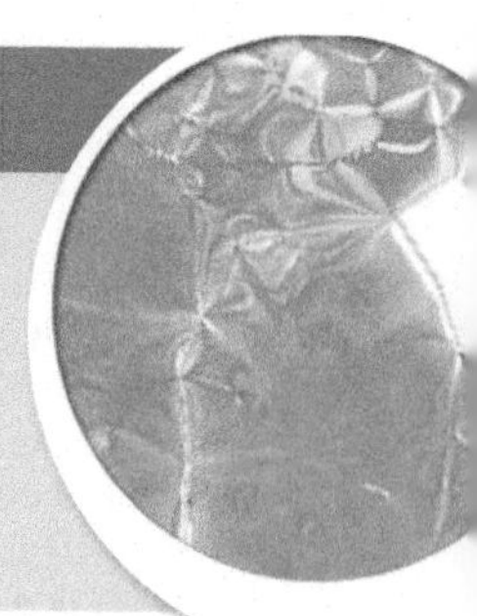

Pyoderma, Otitis Externa, and Otitis Media

Jane E. Sykes, Terry M. Nagle, and Stephen D. White

Overview of Pyoderma

Cause: *Staphylococcus pseudintermedius*; less commonly *Staphylococcus schleiferi* and *Staphylococcus aureus*. Gram-negative bacteria may be involved in dogs with deep pyoderma.

Affected Hosts: Dogs, less commonly cats

Geographic Distribution: Worldwide

Major Clinical Signs: Cutaneous epidermal collarettes, pruritus, erythema, papules, pustules, alopecia. Deep pyoderma is characterized by deep nodules and fistulous tracts. Local lymphadenopathy may be present. Hyperpigmentation and lichenification occur with chronicity.

Differential Diagnoses: Pemphigus foliaceus, dermatophytosis, demodicosis, allergic dermatitis, drug eruptions, erythema multiforme, *Malassezia* dermatitis. For deep pyoderma, sterile pyogranulomatous dermatitis, juvenile cellulitis, neoplasia, foreign body reactions, and deep cutaneous mycoses and pythiosis must be considered.

Human Health Significance: *S. pseudintermedius* prefers not to colonize humans, but zoonotic transmission has been reported. *S. aureus* infections in dogs most likely represent reverse zoonotic transmission from humans to dogs. *S. schleiferi* has also been reported to infect humans.

PYODERMA

Etiology and Epidemiology

Pyoderma is a cutaneous infection with pyogenic (pus-forming) bacteria. Although the term *pyoderma* literally means "pus in the skin," the pus may not always be visible to the naked eye. Pyoderma is the one of the most common disorders of canine skin. It results from impaired local defense mechanisms, which permit secondary bacterial invasion of the skin. The most common underlying skin diseases are allergic dermatitis and endocrine diseases, but a variety of other skin diseases can also predispose to pyoderma. In cats, pyoderma is uncommon to rare, although feline acne can be classified as a pyoderma. Three broad classifications of pyoderma exist, based on the depth of skin and follicle involvement: *surface pyoderma, superficial pyoderma,* and *deep pyoderma.*

Surface pyoderma occurs when bacteria proliferate on the surface of the skin and incite an inflammatory response, without invading the skin. Surface pyodermas include the "fold" pyodermas (also known as *intertrigo*), "hot spots" (also known as *pyotraumatic dermatitis*), and mucocutaneous pyoderma, which commonly affects German shepherd dogs.[1] The last probably has an immunologic as well as a bacterial etiology. Mucocutaneous pyoderma is histologically identical to intertrigo, and differentiation between the two entities must be made clinically.[2] Microbial overgrowth has also been categorized as a surface pyoderma when it involves bacteria (as opposed to just *Malassezia* spp.).

In superficial pyoderma, bacteria infect the superficial epidermal layers that lie immediately under the stratum corneum (the outermost layer of the skin) and the portion of the hair follicle above the sebaceous duct (the infundibulum) (Figure 84-1). This is the most common type of pyoderma. It includes superficial bacterial folliculitis, superficial spreading pyoderma, and "puppy pyoderma" (also known as *impetigo* or *juvenile pustular dermatitis*).

Deep pyoderma is defined by infection deep within the hair follicle, with or without follicular rupture *(furunculosis)* (Figure 84-2) German shepherd dogs seem prone to a more severe and extensive form of deep pyoderma.[3] Other examples include pedal folliculitis and furunculosis, pressure-point pyoderma, pyotraumatic folliculitis and furunculosis, and muzzle folliculitis and furunculosis ("canine acne").

The most common cause of pyoderma in dogs is the coagulase-positive *Staphylococcus pseudintermedius* (previously misidentified as *Staphylococcus intermedius*) (see Chapter 35 for more information on staphylococci).[4] *S. pseudintermedius* is a normal resident of mucosal sites such as the anus and nares and is thought to colonize the skin transiently following grooming and excessive licking in dogs with pruritus.[5] In contrast, the resident flora of the canine skin includes coagulase-negative staphylococci, *Micrococcus* spp., α-hemolytic streptococci, aerobic coryneforms, *Acinetobacter* spp., and some anaerobes. Other organisms implicated in canine pyoderma are *Staphylococcus schleiferi* and, uncommonly, *Staphylococcus aureus*.[6-8] Gram-negative bacteria such as *Pseudomonas aeruginosa*, *Proteus* spp., and *Escherichia coli* may be isolated from dogs with deep pyoderma.[9,10] These organisms are thought to invade secondary to alteration of local environmental conditions by *S. pseudintermedius*. Complete genome sequencing of *S. pseudintermedius* isolated from a dog with pyoderma has shown that *S. pseudintermedius* possesses a number of virulence factors that resemble those produced by *S. aureus*.[11]

Over the past 5 years, clonal spread of methicillin-resistant *S. pseudintermedius* has occurred across Europe and North America.[12] Methicillin resistance has also been described among *S. schleiferi* and *S. aureus* isolates from dogs with pyoderma.[8] These organisms encode an altered penicillin binding protein that incurs resistance to all β-lactam antimicrobials, and many also demonstrate resistance to fluoroquinolone antimicrobials.

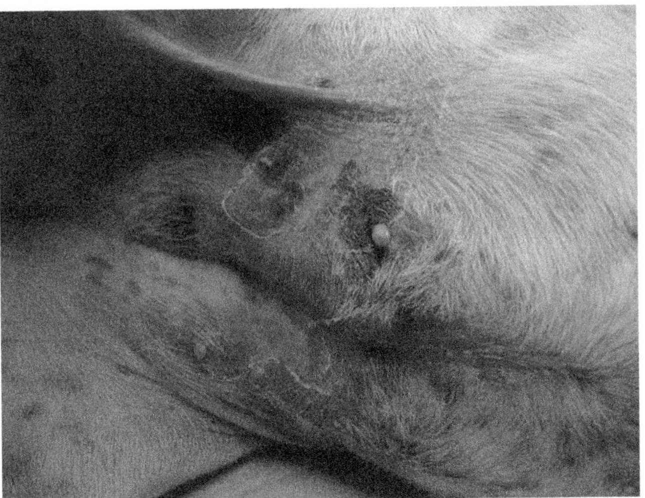

FIGURE 84-1 Superficial bacterial folliculitis manifested by severe erythema, epidermal collarettes, pustules, papules, and plaques in a 10-year-old female spayed pit bull terrier cross dog with underlying atopic dermatitis. Cytologic examination showed numerous cocci and neutrophils. Culture and susceptibility grew a methicillin-susceptible, β-lactamase–producing *Staphylococcus pseudintermedius* that was treated successfully with cephalexin together with management of the underlying atopic skin disease.

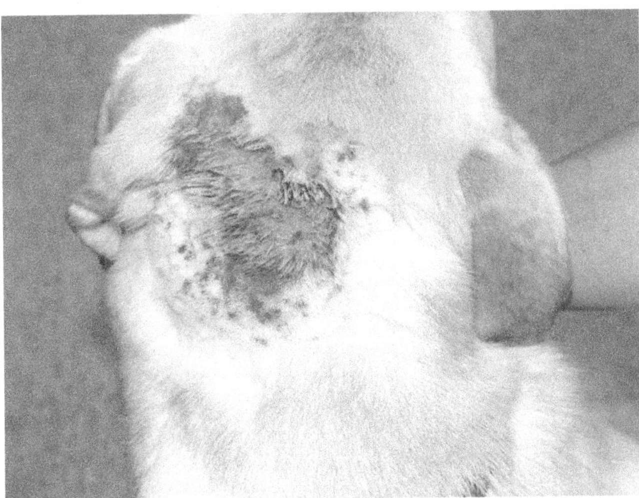

FIGURE 84-2 Deep pyoderma in a 2-year-old male neutered Labrador retriever. Cytology showed numerous cocci and neutrophils. No mites were detected in a skin scraping.

Clinical Features

Signs and Their Pathogenesis

Surface Pyoderma

Surface pyoderma is usually caused by superficial skin trauma, such as the rubbing together of lip, facial, vulvar, and tail folds in dogs with skinfold pyoderma. "Hot spots" occur secondary to self-trauma, such as that secondary to flea allergy dermatitis, and are commonly found in the lumbosacral area. Clinical signs include erythema, variable pruritus, alopecia, moist exudation, and a foul odor. Chronic lesions may be characterized by lichenification and hyperpigmentation. The exact causes of mucocutaneous pyoderma and surface microbial overgrowth have not yet been elucidated. Mucocutaneous pyoderma is characterized by erosions and ulcerations with or without crusting, which involve the lips, nasal planum, nares, perioral skin, and sometimes the anus, vulva, prepuce, and eyelids. It has also been reported in the axillary and inguinal region.[1] Microbial overgrowth syndrome usually involves the ventral aspect of the body and is characterized by erythema, pruritus, a foul odor, erythema, alopecia, hyperpigmentation, lichenification, and excoriations, but no evidence of papules, pustules, epidermal collarettes or crusts.[13]

Superficial Pyoderma

Early lesions of superficial pyoderma are erythematous follicular papules (papules from which a hair shaft protrudes). As pus accumulates within the epidermis and hair follicles, these lesions become pustules. Papules and pustules are *primary skin lesions*. When pustules rupture, crusted papules result. Epidermal collarettes are circles of epidermal scale with a free edge facing toward the center of the circle (see Figure 84-1), and may be remnants of ruptured papules. In thick-coated or shaggy dogs, the scale may become trapped throughout the haircoat as epidermal collarettes exfoliate. Hair fragments are shed from damaged follicles, which results in alopecia. Crusted papules, epidermal collarettes, and alopecia are *secondary lesions*.

Impetigo generally occurs in dogs less than a year of age. In impetigo, pustules are confined to the epidermis, without follicular involvement, and are most commonly found in the poorly haired (glabrous) areas on the ventral abdomen and inguinal region and around the chin. Superficial bacterial folliculitis usually occurs secondary to underlying allergic or atopic dermatitis or endocrinopathies such as hyperadrenocorticism or hypothyroidism. Pruritus is less common in dogs with underlying endocrinopathies. Other conditions that predispose to pyoderma include cornification disorders, genetic skin disorders, and ectoparasitism. In dogs with atopic dermatitis, invasion of the skin by staphylococci can in turn lead to a hypersensitivity response to staphylococcal antigens, which exacerbates the pyoderma.[14]

Deep Pyoderma

Follicular rupture in dogs with deep pyoderma leads to a granulomatous foreign body inflammatory response within the dermis. Deep nodules with fistulation can be seen grossly.

Physical Examination Findings

Because the lesions of bacterial pyoderma are directly visible, in many cases, diagnosis can be made based on a thorough physical examination. Use of a hand lens may be helpful. In some cases, clipping of small areas of the haircoat may be required. This can help to identify epidermal collarettes in dogs with dry scale. Careful attention should be paid to the presence of follicular papules, pustules, crusted papules, epidermal collarettes, alopecia, nodules, fistulous tracts, and the presence or absence of pruritus (Box 84-1). The distribution of lesions should be noted because it can be a clue to underlying disease, such as demodicosis. In dogs with deep pyoderma, the skin may feel warm to the touch, and peripheral lymphadenomegaly may be detected.

BOX 84-1

Physical Examination Findings in Dogs with Pyoderma

Erythema	Epidermal collarettes
Pruritus	Hyperpigmentation
Papules	Hypopigmentation
Crusted papules	Alopecia
Pustules	Peripheral lymphadenopathy

Diagnosis

The diagnostic approach to pyoderma should involve confirmation of the presence of pyoderma and a thorough search for possible underlying causes. The differential diagnosis includes many diseases that predispose to pyoderma, such as demodicosis, dermatophytosis, and pemphigus foliaceus (see Overview). When crusting is present, cornification disorders should be considered, although crusting may also result from self-trauma. The presence or absence of *Malassezia* spp. must also be determined (Chapter 59).

In addition to a thorough physical examination, diagnostic procedures that may be necessary include skin scrapings, cytologic examination, aerobic bacterial culture and susceptibility, and skin biopsy (Table 84-1). Dermatophyte culture is indicated when underlying dermatophytosis is suspected (see Chapter 58). Identification and subsequent treatment of underlying allergic skin disease may require additional testing such as intradermal skin testing, for which referral to a veterinary dermatologist should be considered.

Microbiologic Testing

Skin Scrapings

Skin scrapings should be performed in any dog suspected to have pyoderma to assess for underlying demodicosis. Pustules or papules that are associated with hair follicles should be targeted, because *Demodex* mites have a predilection for this site.

Cytologic Examination

Cytology can be performed on tape preparations of the skin or smears made after swabbing pustules or draining tracts. Cytologic examination is essential in order to identify concurrent

TABLE 84-1

Diagnostic Assays Available for Pyoderma, Otitis Externa, and Otitis Media in Dogs

Assay	Specimen Type	Target	Performance
Cytology	Pyoderma: Swabs or tape preparations of pustules or draining tracts Otitis externa: Swabs from the horizontal ear canal Otitis media: Swabs of the material obtained from the tympanic bulla after myringotomy	Assessment for inflammatory cells, cocci, or rod-shaped bacteria and *Malassezia* spp.	Five to 10 oil immersion fields should be examined. Results of cytology do not address the underlying cause of disease. Neutrophils may be absent in dogs with underlying immunosuppression. Pyoderma: Degenerate neutrophils and intracellular cocci suggest infection. Otitis externa: Any bacteria found with leukocytes are abnormal. In healthy animals, cocci may be found at counts ≤5 (dogs) and ≤4 (cats)/400× magnification.
Histopathology	Pyoderma: Biopsy specimens Otitis externa: Biopsy specimens after total ear canal ablation with bulla osteotomy	Classifies extent and type of pyoderma and aids in identification of other conditions	Useful for refractory pyoderma, deep pyoderma, and when underlying cause not apparent. Occasionally assists diagnosis of underlying cause of otitis externa (such as demodicosis or neoplasia).
Culture	Superficial pyoderma: Swabs from pustules or epidermal collarettes Deep pyoderma: Skin biopsy specimens Otitis externa: Swabs from the horizontal ear canal Otitis media: Swabs or aspirates from the tympanic bulla	Pathogenic bacteria	Allows susceptibility testing in chronic, refractory, or recurrent cases or when gram-negative bacteria are present. Always interpret in light of cytologic findings because of the presence of commensal bacteria and mixed populations of bacteria. False negatives may occur in the face of antimicrobial treatment.

infection with *Malassezia pachydermatis*. Slides should be air-dried and stained with a modified Wright's stain such as Diff Quik. The presence of cocci suggests *S. pseudintermedius* infection (Figure 84-3). Infection is supported by the presence of degenerate neutrophils and intracellular cocci. Inflammatory cells may be absent in dogs with underlying immunosuppressive disorders or those receiving glucocorticoid treatment.

Culture and Susceptibility Testing

Given the rapidly increasing prevalence of methicillin-resistant staphylococci worldwide, aerobic bacterial culture and susceptibility testing is playing a more important role in diagnosis of canine pyoderma. Although probably not necessary for dogs with a first-time diagnosis of pyoderma, culture and susceptibility testing is never contraindicated and should always be offered in dogs with recurrent or refractory pyoderma, or in dogs that have a history of recent treatment with systemic antimicrobial drugs. Refractory pyoderma is pyoderma that fails to respond to treatment within a 3- to 4-week treatment period. Culture also can definitively identify the staphylococcal species involved, which may have public health implications (see Public Health Aspects, later). The results of culture and susceptibility testing must always be interpreted in light of the clinical signs present and any history of antimicrobial drug treatment.

The best lesions for culture in dogs with superficial pyoderma are pustules. A thorough search for pustules is recommended. If pustules cannot be detected, culture can be performed on swab specimens collected from the skin that lies beneath crusts or from epidermal collarettes. No surface antisepsis should be performed. Any hair should be clipped from the lesion using sterile scissors, and crusts should be lifted with sterile forceps. Pustules can be ruptured using a sterile needle, and a swab used to obtain purulent material. Papules can be biopsied using local anesthesia and submitted for culture. In this case, surface antisepsis with a single 70% alcohol wipe is indicated before collection of the biopsy. Culture of biopsy specimens from nodules and furuncles is best for dogs with deep pyoderma. After collection of the biopsy, the epidermis can be removed using a sterile blade and the deeper tissues submitted for macerated tissue culture.

Pathologic Findings

Histopathologic Findings

Findings on histopathology in dogs with uncomplicated pyoderma include a neutrophilic infiltrate and abundant bacterial organisms. Histopathologic evaluation of skin biopsy specimens allows classification of the extent and type of pyoderma and identification of other conditions such as allergic dermatitis, demodicosis, dermatophytosis, pemphigus foliaceus, neoplasia, deep mycoses, and vasculitides. Biopsy should be considered in recurrent or refractory cases, in dogs with deep pyoderma, or when the underlying cause is not apparent. Biopsies can be performed under local anesthesia using a 6-mm punch biopsy. An attempt should be made to include both affected and adjacent healthy tissue when identifying sites for biopsy collection. The biopsy site should be sutured after the specimen has been collected.

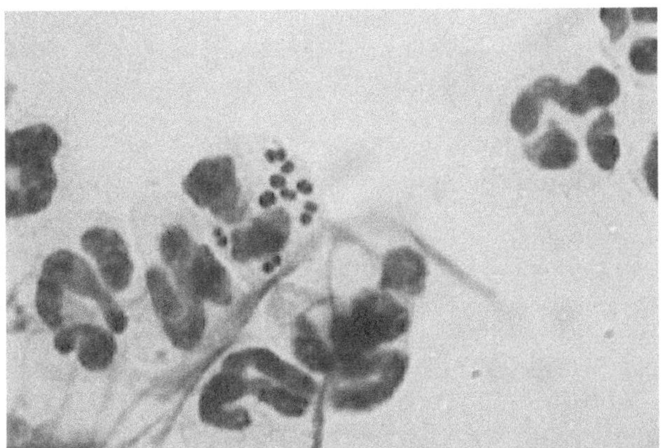

FIGURE 84-3 Cytology showing intracellular cocci (*Staphylococcus pseudintermedius*) and leukocytes in a tape preparation from a dog with pyoderma. Wright's stain, 1000× magnification.

Treatment and Prognosis

Factors to consider when treating dogs for pyoderma include the underlying disease present, the severity and extent of lesions, and the local prevalence of staphylococcal resistance. Veterinarians' reliance on systemic antimicrobial drug treatment has been challenged by the increasing prevalence of multidrug-resistant staphylococci. Topical treatments that help to restore skin structure and function, as well as topical antimicrobial therapy, should be considered as alternatives.[15] In dogs with mild disease, treatment aimed at the underlying disorder may be sufficient to resolve infection (see Prevention).

Topical Treatments

Antibacterial shampoos may be effective alone in some dogs with surface or mild superficial pyoderma and should be used as adjunctive therapy in dogs with deep pyoderma. They aid in debridement, reduce surface bacterial numbers, and decrease pain and pruritus. Options include shampoos that contain benzoyl peroxide, ethyl lactate, chlorhexidine, or triclosan. Initially, they should be used at least twice weekly with a 10-minute contact time. Benzoyl peroxide shampoos can be drying and so are best reserved for dogs with greasy dermatitides. Daily shampooing may be required for dogs with deep pyoderma. If available, treatment with daily whirlpool baths containing chlorhexidine may also be helpful for these dogs.

Topical antimicrobial drugs and antiseptics result in high concentrations of drug at the skin surface that can overwhelm bacterial drug resistance mechanisms, and can be useful when pyoderma is limited to small areas of skin. Aside from having the potential to be messy, these drugs have minimal side effects and result in minimal exposure of bystander organisms (such as gut flora) to antimicrobial drugs. Examples of topical drugs with excellent activity against staphylococci include neomycin, gentamicin, polymyxin B, bacitracin, hydroxyl acids (such as acetic acid), novobiocin, and silver sulfadiazine. Mupirocin and fusidic acid are additional topical antimicrobial drug preparations that may also be useful for treatment of pyoderma that is restricted to small areas. Unfortunately, resistance to mupirocin and fusidic acid has been documented in methicillin-resistant *S. aureus* isolates from humans.[16,17]

Systemic Antimicrobial Drug Therapy

When pyoderma is severe, treatment with systemic antimicrobial drugs may be required. The drug selected for empiric treatment should be based on the local prevalence of resistance, and narrow-spectrum drugs that target staphylococci are preferable. Clindamycin, first-generation cephalosporins (such as cephalexin), and amoxicillin-clavulanic acid are reasonable first choices (Table 84-2). Other acceptable alternatives when the

TABLE 84-2

Suitable First-Tier Drugs for Treatment of Superficial Pyoderma in Dogs

Drug	Dose (mg/kg)	Route	Interval (hours)	Duration (days)
Cephalexin	22 to 30	PO	12	28, and at least 7 days after clinical resolution
Clindamycin	10	PO	12	28
Amoxicillin-clavulanic acid	12.5 to 25	PO	12	28
Lincomycin	15 to 25	PO	12	28
Doxycycline	5	PO	12	28
Trimethoprim-sulfamethoxazole*	15 to 30	PO	12	28

*Concerns exist regarding idiosyncratic and immune-mediated adverse effects in some patients with sulfa drugs, especially with prolonged therapy. Baseline Schirmer's tear testing is recommended, with periodic re-evaluation and owner monitoring for ocular discharge. Avoid in dogs that may be sensitive to potential adverse effects such as keratoconjunctivitis sicca (KCS), hepatopathy, hypersensitivity, and skin eruptions. See also Chapter 8.

local regional susceptibility of *S. pseudintermedius* is known include doxycycline, trimethoprim- or ormetoprim-potentiated sulfonamides, lincomycin, and erythromycin. The use of third-generation cephalosporins for empiric therapy is controversial because their use in particular has been associated with selection for methicillin-resistant staphylococci in humans and they have the potential to select for resistant populations of gram-negative bacteria in the gastrointestinal tract.[18] More research is required to determine whether this is also true in dogs and for all third-generation cephalosporins. When pyoderma is severe, and only when culture and susceptibility indicate the presence of multidrug-resistant staphylococci, the use of chloramphenicol, minocycline, doxycycline, third-generation cephalosporins, rifampin, clarithromycin, azithromycin, amikacin, or fluoroquinolones (such as enrofloxacin, marbofloxacin, orbifloxacin, pradofloxacin, or ciprofloxacin) could be considered as indicated based on culture and susceptibility results. The use of fluoroquinolones in humans and dogs is a risk factor for selection of methicillin-resistant *S. pseudintermedius* and also has the potential for selection of resistant populations of gram-negative bacteria in the gastrointestinal tract.

Treatment should be for a minimum of 4 weeks for superficial pyoderma and 8 weeks for deep pyoderma. A small percentage of dogs with superficial pyoderma require 6 weeks of treatment. For superficial pyodermas, treatment should be continued for at least 7 days beyond clinical resolution of lesions, because inflammation subsides before infection is completely resolved. For deep or recurrent superficial pyoderma, treatment should be continued for 14 days beyond clinical resolution.

Although intermittent administration of antimicrobials on a regular basis ("pulse therapy") has been used to treat some dogs with recurrent pyodermas, there is concern for induction of resistance using these protocols. If this appears to be necessary, referral to a veterinary dermatologist is recommended.

Prevention

Prevention of pyoderma relies on addressing the underlying cause or causes whenever possible. This could include treatment with antihistamines and essential fatty acids, intradermal skin testing and hyposensitization injections, frequent bathing to restore skin condition, dietary management for dogs with food allergies, or breeding practices that aim to select against atopy and dogs with abundant skin folds. Specific prevention of methicillin-resistant staphylococcal infections relies on handwashing and disinfection practices and judicious use of antimicrobial drugs, as outlined earlier, although more data are required in regard to risk factors for development of resistant pyodermas in dogs.

When treatment of the underlying cause or use of topical therapy is unsuccessful in preventing recurrence of pyoderma, subcutaneous administration of autogenous bacterins or commercial bacterial antigens (such as Staphage Lysate, Delmont Laboratories, USA) may be beneficial in some dogs.[19,20] These are generally given once or twice weekly (see Chapter 7).

Public Health Aspects

Although *S. pseudintermedius* prefers not to colonize humans, human infection has been reported occasionally, including among veterinarians.[21-23] A methicillin-susceptible *S. pseudintermedius* was detected as a cause of endocarditis in a human patient,[23] and methicillin-resistant *S. pseudintermedius* has been isolated from human patients with sinusitis.[21] In all cases, pet dog contact was reported and suggested to be the source of infection. In one case, an isolate from the dog matched that isolated from the human as determined using pulsed field gel electrophoresis.

In contrast, contact with human hospitals and children may be risk factors for acquisition of methicillin-resistant *S. aureus* infections by dogs, and *S. aureus* infections appear to be a reverse zoonosis. Colonization is generally transient in dogs and cats, so specific treatment to decolonize dogs and cats is not necessary.[24]

Two subspecies of *S. schleiferi* have been described: *S. schleiferi* subsp. *coagulans,* which is coagulase positive, and *S. schleiferi* subsp. *schleiferi,* which is coagulase negative. Although it may be carried elsewhere on the body, *S. schleiferi* subsp. *coagulans* has been isolated primarily from dogs with otitis externa and was reported as a cause of endocarditis in an immunocompromised human.[25] Coagulase-negative *S. schleiferi* are thought to be a commensal of the skin of both humans and dogs, and although they are common contaminants, they can cause disease in both species.[8,26]

Frequent and *proper* hand washing using soap and water and disinfectant foams or gels is the number one practice that limits spread of these infections in human hospitals. Hands should be washed before and after handling each patient. Clean clothing should be worn and laboratory coats changed regularly. Attention must be paid to regular disinfection of other fomites such as stethoscopes, cell phones, rectal thermometers, computer keyboards and mice, calculators, and bandage scissors. Disinfectant wipes that contain alcohol or accelerated hydrogen peroxide can be used to clean these surfaces.

Overview of Otitis Externa and Otitis Media

Cause: *Staphylococcus pseudintermedius* and *Pseudomonas aeruginosa*; less commonly *S. schleiferi, S. aureus, Proteus mirabilis, Escherichia coli, Corynebacterium* spp., *Klebsiella* spp., enterococci, and β-hemolytic streptococci

Affected Hosts: Dogs, less commonly cats

Geographic Distribution: Worldwide

Major Clinical Signs: Otic erythema, pruritus, head shaking, purulent discharge, swelling, malodor, and pain. Proliferative changes and ulceration occur with chronicity. Vestibular signs, deafness, Horner's syndrome, and facial paralysis occur with middle ear involvement.

Differential Diagnoses: Underlying causes include allergic dermatitis, foreign bodies, neoplasia, hypothyroidism, cornification disorders, pemphigus foliaceus, otoacariasis, dermatophytosis, demodicosis, and drug eruptions. *Malassezia* otitis externa must also be considered.

Human Health Significance: *S. pseudintermedius* prefers not to colonize humans, but zoonotic transmission has been reported.[21] Frequent hand washing is recommended for dogs that are known or suspected to have drug-resistant *Pseudomonas aeruginosa* otitis externa.

OTITIS EXTERNA AND OTITIS MEDIA

Etiology and Epidemiology

Otitis externa, or inflammation of the ear canal, although relatively uncommon in the cat, is one of the most common diseases of dogs, accounting for 10% to 20% of all accessions seen in general veterinary practice.[27] Bacterial and fungal infections of the ear canal are virtually always secondary to an underlying condition, and recognition of the underlying cause or causes of otitis externa is *critical* for effective treatment. Repeated treatment with antimicrobial drugs without regard for the underlying cause leads only to the selection of resistant bacterial populations and treatment failure.

The causative factors for otitis externa have been grouped into predisposing, primary, and perpetuating factors (Box 84-2). Predisposing factors include ear canal conformation, obstructive processes such as tumors within the ear canal, and increased moisture within the ear. Primary causes of otitis externa in dogs are allergic dermatitis, which accounts for as many as 90% of cases,[28] and less commonly endocrinopathies (especially hypothyroidism), foreign bodies, ear mite infestation *(Otodectes cynotis)*, and cornification disorders (such as seborrhea in cocker spaniels). More than 80% of dogs with atopy have otitis externa, and otitis externa may be the only sign of allergic dermatitis.[10] Seasonal occurrence of otitis externa can be a clue to underlying atopic dermatitis. In cats, ear mite infestation accounts for at least 50% of cases, with young cats being predisposed.[29] These factors increase inflammation within the ear, which intensifies bacterial and yeast infections. Chronic inflammation then leads to progressive pathology within the ear canal, tympanic membrane, and middle ear, which prevents resolution of otitis externa. Predisposed breeds include cocker and Brittany spaniels, poodles, and Labrador retrievers.

A variety of bacteria and occasionally yeasts can be isolated from the ear canals of healthy dogs, including *S. pseudintermedius, S. schleiferi, Streptococcus* spp., and *Malassezia pachydermatis*. Gram-negative rods are rarely isolated from normal ears. In dogs with otitis externa, overgrowth of yeast and bacterial organisms occurs within the ear canal. *S. pseudintermedius* is the most common bacterial pathogen isolated from dogs with otitis externa. *Pseudomonas aeruginosa* is frequently isolated from dogs with chronic otitis externa, and this may be challenging to treat effectively because of the development of antimicrobial resistance. Less commonly, *S. schleiferi, S. aureus, Proteus mirabilis, E. coli, Corynebacterium* spp., *Klebsiella* spp., enterococci, and β-hemolytic streptococci are isolated.

Malassezia pachydermatis is the most common fungal cause of otitis externa. In one study, it was isolated from more than 60% of otitic ears.[30] Fungi such as *Candida* spp., *Aspergillus* spp., and dermatophytes are less commonly reported causes. In dogs with bilateral otitis externa, the organisms

BOX 84-2

Major Factors That Predispose to, Cause, and Perpetuate Otitis Externa

Predisposing Factors

Stenotic canals (e.g., shar-pei)
Pendulous pinnae
Excessive moisture (swimming, humidity)
Excessive cerumen production
Trauma from cotton applicators
Topical treatments that irritate the canal
Ear canal neoplasia, polyps, cholesteatomas, or foreign bodies
Immunosuppression

Primary Causes

Parasites, such as *Otodectes cynotis, Demodex canis,* and *Otobius megnini*
Dermatophytosis
Allergic dermatitis (atopy, food and contact hypersensitivities)
Primary idiopathic seborrhea
Hypothyroidism
Foreign bodies (grass awns, sand, inspissated medications)
Cerumen gland hyperplasia

Perpetuating Factors

Aerobic bacterial infection
Malassezia pachydermatis infection
Hyperkeratosis
Hyperplasia
Dermal edema
Fibrosis
Stenosis
Mineralization
Osteomyelitis

present in each ear frequently differ.[31] Unilateral otitis externa may suggest the presence of an underlying foreign body or neoplasia, although bilateral involvement with these causes is possible, and unilateral involvement can occur with symmetric disorders such as allergic dermatitis and ceruminous gland hyperplasia.

Otitis media is inflammation of the middle ear. More than half of dogs with chronic otitis externa have otitis media, although the bacteria present in the external ear canal often differ from those present in the middle ear.[32] The tympanic membrane can rupture and reseal, so it frequently appears intact on examination of the external ear canal. Less commonly, otitis media results from extension of infection from the nasopharynx or hematogenous spread. Evidence of otitis media is sometimes detected during computed tomography (CT) of the skull of cats or dogs with chronic rhinosinusitis.

Clinical Features

Signs and Their Pathogenesis

Early clinical signs of otitis externa are erythema of the pinnae, external meatus, and lining of the ear canal. Progression of disease with proliferation of bacteria and yeasts leads to signs of pruritus, head shaking, ceruminous or purulent discharge from the ear canal, swelling, malodor, lesions resulting from self-trauma (including aural hematomas), and/or pain when the ear is touched or palpated (Figure 84-4). With chronicity, proliferative changes occur that lead to stenosis and occlusion of the ear canal, and the tympanic membrane may rupture. Subsequently, there is fibrosis and mineralization of the ear canal, which uncommonly (but especially with *P. aeruginosa* infections) is accompanied by ulcerations of the canal, sometimes with ongoing pain and debilitation.[28]

Physical, Dermatologic, and Otoscopic Examination Findings

A thorough physical and dermatologic examination may provide clues to the underlying cause of otitis externa. In addition to lesions of the external ear canal (see Signs and their Pathogenesis), examination may reveal signs consistent with underlying endocrine disease, or skin lesions suggestive of underlying allergic dermatitis (atopic, food, or contact dermatitides), parasitic infections, or keratinization disorders.

A complete otoscopic examination of both ears should be performed, starting with the least affected ear. Sedation may be required in animals that are painful or uncooperative, or the animal may need to be reexamined at a later date for otoscopy after treatment has been initiated to reduce pain and inflammation. Usually cytologic examination with or without culture is still possible in these animals.

Either a handheld otoscope or video otoscope can be used for otoscopic examination. Video otoscopy allows a higher degree of magnification and intense illumination of the ear canal (Figure 84-5). The ear canal should be examined for the presence and characteristics of foreign bodies, exudate, erythema, stenosis, proliferation, ulceration, and mass lesions. The tympanic membrane may be visualized in some cases and inspected for rupture, distortion, or discoloration that suggests the presence of hemorrhage or pus within the middle ear. In dogs with chronic otitis externa, ear flushing under general anesthesia may be required in order to properly visualize the tympanic membrane. Proper assessment of the integrity of the tympanum may still not be possible in some dogs. In dogs with severe stenosis or ear canal ulceration, treatment with topical and oral glucocorticoids may be necessary for 4 to 7 days before proper otoscopic examination can be performed. Clients should always be educated regarding the complications of ear canal flushing such as Horner's syndrome, facial nerve paralysis, vestibular signs, and deafness.

Diagnosis

Diagnosis is based on the physical, dermatologic, and otoscopic examination; cytology of the ear canal; culture; and in some cases, advanced imaging. Each ear should be considered as a separate unit, because organisms present in one ear canal may differ from those present in the other.[31]

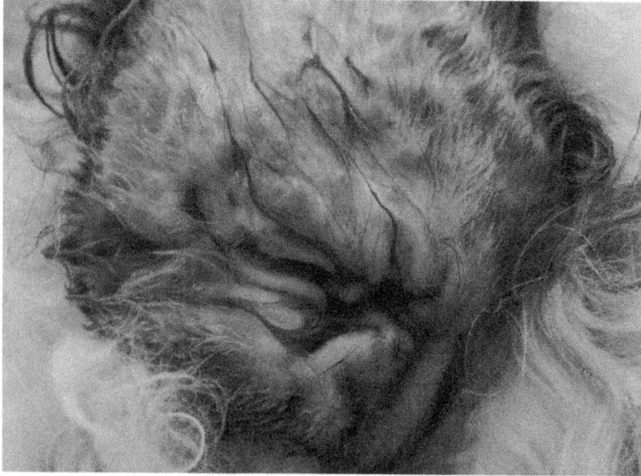

FIGURE 84-4 Chronic, multidrug-resistant *Pseudomonas aeruginosa* otitis externa in a 4-year-old intact male Old English sheepdog showing erythema and multifocal ulcerative lesions on the pinna.

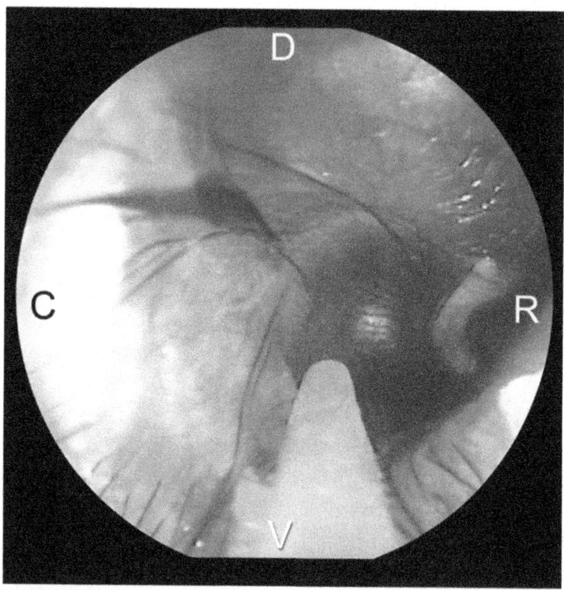

FIGURE 84-5 Proper site for myringotomy, right tympanic membrane. The caudoventral quadrant of the pars tensa is approached with a tomcat catheter. *C*, caudal; *D*, dorsal; *R*, rostral; *V*, ventral. (From Cole LK. Otoscopic evaluation of the ear canal. Vet Clin North Am Small Anim Pract. 2004;34[2]:397-410.)

Microbiologic Testing

Cytologic Examination

Cytologic examination of the ear canal should *always* be performed in dogs and cats seen for otitis externa. The results of otic cytology support culture and susceptibility data, guide initial treatment decisions, and allow the response to treatment to be monitored. In some situations (such as when mites or foreign bodies are found), otoscopy permits diagnosis of the underlying cause. Specimens are collected from the external ear canal with a cotton-tipped applicator before any cleaning or treatment administration. The tip of the swab is directed at the junction of the horizontal and vertical ear canal, being cautious to avoid trauma to the tympanic membrane. For dogs and cats suspected to have otitis media, specimens for cytology and culture should be collected from the middle ear following myringotomy, which is performed in an anesthetized animal by perforating the ventrocaudal quadrant of the tympanum with a small sterile swab, catheter, or spinal needle (see Figure 84-5).

Slides should be labeled according to the ear they are from and briefly heat fixed, because the high lipid content of cerumen causes material to be washed from the slide during staining. After staining with a modified Wright's stain, 10 to 15 oil immersion fields of each slide should be examined for the presence of cocci, rods, fungi (most commonly *Malassezia* spp.), and leukocytes, and the type and number of each should be recorded for each ear. Any bacteria associated with leukocytes are abnormal. Bacterial counts considered abnormal are at least 25/400× magnification (40× objective) for dogs and 15 or more for cats.[33] Normal dogs and cats have 5 or fewer and 4 or fewer organisms/400× magnification, respectively, and intermediate counts represent a gray zone.[33] Rod-shaped bacteria or large numbers of leukocytes are also rarely found in normal ear canals. The presence of leukocytes suggests a true bacterial infection; rarely they can indicate other underlying disease processes, such as pemphigus foliaceus or otocariasis. *Malassezia* spp. are found in the ear canals of healthy dogs and dogs with otitis externa. An inflammatory response is typically not present, even when *Malassezia* spp. are contributing to disease progression. Estimation of yeast counts may be helpful to determine the role of *Malassezia* in otitis. It has been suggested that a mean count of 5 or more yeasts/400× magnification (40× objective) is abnormal in dogs, and 12 or more yeasts/400× magnification is abnormal in cats. Normal dogs and cats have 2 or fewer yeasts/400× magnification.[33] If the presence of mites is suspected, a mineral oil preparation is made on a separate slide, and the slide is examined using low-power magnification.

Bacterial Isolation

Culture allows identification of the species of bacteria present and subsequent documentation of antimicrobial susceptibility. Culture is indicated (1) when bacterial rods (as opposed to cocci) or degenerate neutrophils are present on cytology; (2) when otitis externa is recurrent (within 6 months), or is chronic and refractory to initial treatment; or (3) when otitis media is present. Because culture of the external ear canal does not distinguish among commensal bacteria, overgrowth, and true infection, it must *always* be interpreted in light of cytologic examination findings. As for cytologic examination, each ear canal should be considered as a separate unit. When otitis media is present, the external ear canal and middle ear should be cultured separately.[32]

Diagnostic Imaging

Diagnostic imaging under general anesthesia is indicated for dogs with recurrent otitis externa, those with evidence of chronic disease (such as infection with *P. aeruginosa*), or animals with suspected middle ear involvement. Imaging can be performed using plain radiography or CT. MRI abnormalities in dogs with otitis externa and media have been described, but MRI is less sensitive than CT for evaluation of cartilage and bony detail. MRI is useful for evaluation of the central nervous system (CNS) of dogs and cats that have neurologic signs in conjunction with otitis media and assists in the differentiation between central and peripheral vestibular lesions.

Plain radiography of the tympanic bulla should include lateral, dorsoventral, latero-20 degree ventral-laterodorsal oblique, and rostro-30 degree ventral-caudodorsal open-mouth oblique radiographs. An additional 10-degree ventrodorsal view may assist visualization of the tympanic bulla in cats.[34] Advanced imaging can often be performed more quickly than plain radiography because advanced imaging does not require multiple views and precise positioning. CT also offers advantages of increased sensitivity for detection of changes to the bulla and external ear canal, although false negatives can still occur when otitis media is mild.[35]

Changes found on plain radiography and CT of the ear in dogs and cats with otitis externa include increased soft tissue opacity in association with the lumen or wall of the ear canal, and/or stenosis or mineralization of the wall of the ear canal. In animals with otitis media, increased soft tissue opacity within the tympanic bulla, thickening of the bulla wall, or bony proliferation of the wall of the bulla may be evident (Figure 84-6). Lysis of the bulla may be evident in animals with severe otitis media.

Using MRI, changes suggestive of otitis media include medium-signal intensity material in the bulla on T1-weighted images, with hyperintensity of this material on T2-weighted images.[34,36] After contrast agent administration, meningeal

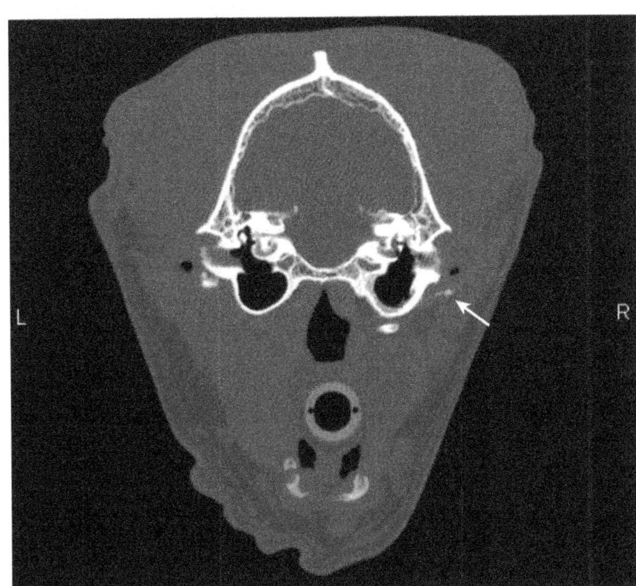

FIGURE 84-6 CT scan showing mineralization of the external ear canals (arrow) and thickening and debris within the right tympanic bulla in a 5-year-old male neutered German shepherd dog with chronic, multidrug-resistant *Pseudomonas aeruginosa* otitis externa and severe, chronic otitis media.

enhancement may be appreciated in animals with otitis interna, or changes suggestive of brain abscessation, such as mass lesions with ring enhancement, may be present (Figure 84-7).[36]

Treatment and Prognosis

Otitis Externa

The decision to treat otitis externa and the specific treatments used depend on assessment of the history, clinical signs, cytologic findings, and, if performed, consideration of culture results as they relate to the most common pathogens present. A plethora of different treatments have been used, because no single treatment is effective for all cases, and many veterinarians and veterinary dermatologists base their choice(s) on familiarity. Regardless of the treatment used to control secondary bacterial infections, attention to identification and treatment of the underlying cause (foreign bodies, allergic dermatitis) is critical for successful long-term resolution of otitis externa. For dogs with chronic or recurrent otitis externa, the importance of regular rechecks at monthly intervals should be emphasized to ensure compliance with medications and an appropriate response to treatment. Clients should be offered referral to a veterinary dermatologist for dogs with recurrent, refractory, or chronic otitis externa, and when *P. aeruginosa* or highly resistant bacterial infections are present.

Treatments for otitis externa may be topical or systemic. The treatment of otitis externa presents challenges because of the difficulty in obtaining adequate drug concentrations in the bacterial exudate that accumulates within the ear canal; difficulties in obtaining owner compliance, especially in dogs that have otic pain; and the potential for ototoxicity with ear cleaners and other topical treatments. Ototoxicity occurs rarely but is unpredictable and may be manifested by vestibular signs, Horner's syndrome, facial paralysis, or deafness. Neurologic signs following ear flushing are especially apt to occur in cats. Usually these signs are transient but occasionally can be permanent. Clients should be taught how to properly lavage the ear canal, administer topical medications, and monitor for and treat ototoxicity. The prognosis for resolution of otitis externa depends strongly on owner compliance in regard to medications and rechecks and the ability to address the underlying cause. Treatment is generally continued until cytologic examination, performed at 2- to 3-week intervals, shows no evidence of bacteria or neutrophils. Infections with *P. aeruginosa* should be treated until *P. aeruginosa* is no longer cultured from the ear canal.

Ear Cleaning

Gentle ear cleaning and flushing removes secretions and some foreign bodies and allows better penetration and activity of antimicrobial drugs. It is essential for resolution of otitis media, provided the tympanic membrane remains open. Some ear cleansers also have antimicrobial properties.[37] Ear cleaners should be warmed to body temperature before use. Ear cleaning in the home may not be possible until several days of oral analgesics and topical antimicrobials have been administered, to counteract pain resulting from infection and inflammation. Once tolerated, cleaning is generally performed on a 12- or 24-hour basis for the first 5 to 7 days, and then every second or third day until clinical signs resolve. Subsequently, weekly maintenance cleaning may be needed to reduce the risk of recurrence while managing the underlying cause of otitis externa. If the tympanum is intact, a routine ear cleanser and dryer can be used. If the integrity of the tympanum is unknown, ceruminolytic agents (such as those containing squalene, dioctyl sodium sulfosuccinate, carbamide peroxide, or triethanolamine polypeptide locate-condensate) should be avoided. Isotonic saline or a tromethamine-ethylenediaminetetraacetate (Tris EDTA) solution can be used twice daily, either before

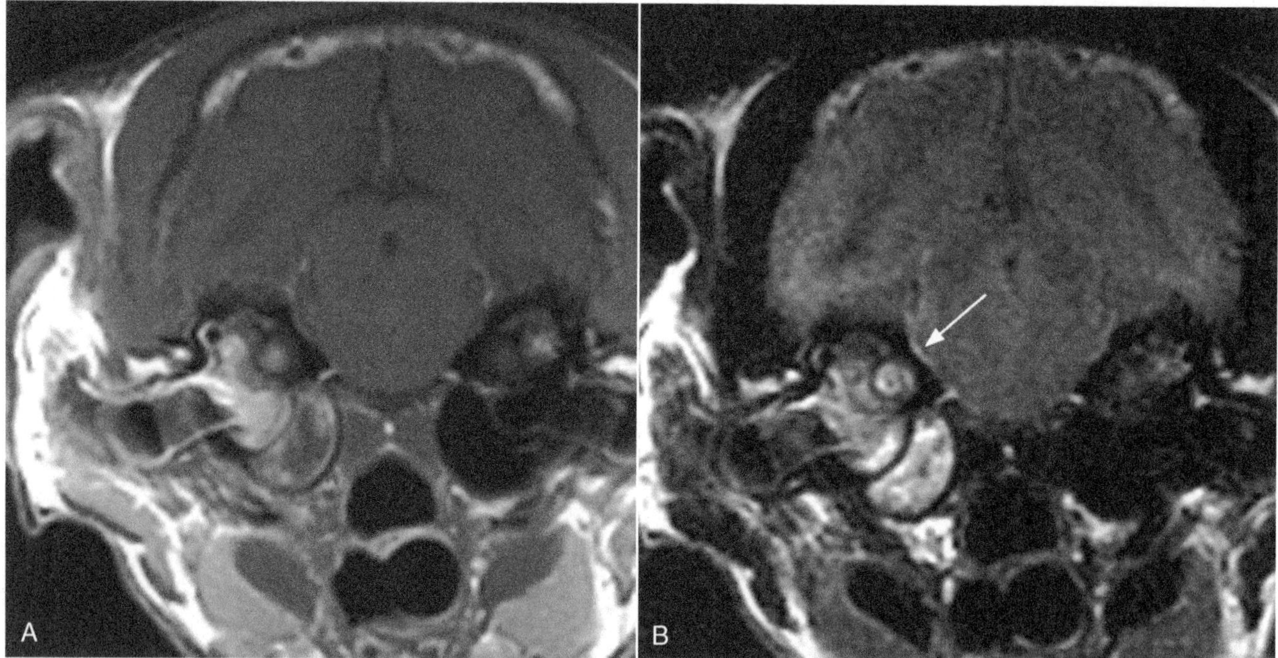

FIGURE 84-7 Post-contrast T1-weighted image **(A)** and FLAIR image **(B)** from an MRI scan of the brain of a 15-year-old female spayed domestic shorthair cat. Precontrast images showed diffuse hyperintensity within the left tympanic bulla. The postcontrast images showed moderate contrast enhancement of the lining of the tympanic bulla and mild enhancement of the lateral meninges of the left cerebellar hemisphere adjacent to the bulla (see arrow on FLAIR image). These findings were consistent with otitis media and edema of the left cerebellar meninges.

topical antimicrobials are instilled or as a solution that contains antimicrobials. Tris EDTA destabilizes the bacterial cell wall and potentiates the effect of topical antimicrobials.[38] Several proprietary solutions are available in the United States (Table 84-3). Preparations that contain acetic or boric acid can also be used once daily, although the potential for these preparations to cause adverse effects in dogs with ruptured tympanums is unknown. If owner-administered treatment fails to remove exudates and otitis persists, flushing and examination of the ear canal and tympanic membrane with warm isotonic saline under anesthesia may be indicated. This may also be necessary for resolution of *P. aeruginosa* infections and for dogs with otitis media.

Glucocorticoids

Systemic and/or topical glucocorticoid treatment may be indicated for dogs with otitis externa if it is accompanied by severe inflammation or proliferative changes in the ear canal, including those with *P. aeruginosa* infections. Treatment with oral prednisolone for 1 to 2 weeks, with subsequent tapering over an additional 4-week period, helps to reduce or resolve inflammation, pain, and proliferative changes (Table 84-4). Treatment with prednisolone is discontinued when these abnormalities have significantly reduced or resolved. Many topical otic preparations also contain glucocorticoids (see next section). These have the disadvantage of making the ear appear healthy to the client, who may then discontinue treatment before bacterial infection has resolved, so client education is important. Dogs with severe proliferative changes may benefit from topical administration of the potent combination of fluocinolone and DMSO. Intralesional triamcinolone acetonide injections have also been used to treat severe proliferative otitis externa,[39] usually with reduction in the dose of concurrently administered systemic glucocorticoids. Referral to a dermatologist is recommended for these cases.

Topical Glucocorticoid/Antibiotic/Antifungal Drugs

Topical preparations that contain glucocorticoids and antimicrobial drugs allow delivery of high concentrations of antimicrobials to the ear canal, with or without local anti-inflammatory effect

TABLE 84-3

Drug Preparations Administered Topically That May Be Used to Treat Canine Otitis Externa

Drug	Dose*	Interval (hours)	Duration	Goal
1:2 solution of enrofloxacin injectable (22.7 mg/mL): dexamethasone sodium phosphate (4 mg/mL)† *or* a 1:2 solution of enrofloxacin:Tris EDTA‡	Fill ear and massage in	12	Until cytologic resolution, 2 to 4 weeks	Antibiotic, anti-inflammatory
Gentamicin/betamethasone/clotrimazole ointment§	4 to 8 drops	12	Until cytologic resolution, 2 to 4 weeks	Antibiotic/anti-inflammatory/antifungal
Gentamicin/mometasone/clotrimazole ointment‖	4 to 8 drops	24	Until cytologic resolution, 2 to 4 weeks	Antibiotic/anti-inflammatory/antifungal
Polymyxin B/prednisolone acetate/miconazole ointment¶	4 to 8 drops	12	Until cytologic resolution, 2 to 4 weeks	Antibiotic/anti-inflammatory/antifungal
Orbifloxacin/mometasone/posaconazole ointment#	4 to 8 drops	24	Until cytologic resolution, 2 to 4 weeks	Antibiotic/anti-inflammatory/antifungal
Enrofloxacin/silver sulfadiazine ointment**	4 to 8 drops	12	Until cytologic resolution, 2 to 4 weeks	Antibiotic with some antifungal properties, promotes reepithelialization. Effect may be potentiated after Tris EDTA flush.
Fluocinolone and DMSO solution††	4 to 8 drops depending on dog size	12	Until significant reduction of pain and inflammation	Anti-inflammatory, antipruritic, and analgesic

*Some clinicians suggest that ointment volumes of up to 1 mL should be used depending on body weight; use a syringe for accurate dosing has been recommended.

†Add 1% miconazole lotion in a 1 (enrofloxacin):1 (dexamethasone sodium phosphate):2 (miconazole) ratio when *Malassezia* spp. is present. If bacteria are absent, a 1:1 solution of miconazole:dexamethasone should be used.

‡Such as TrizEDTA (Dechra Veterinary Products), T8 or T8 Keto (DVM Pharmaceuticals).

§Otomax, Merck Animal Health.

‖Mometamax, Merck Animal Health.

¶Surolan, Vétoquinol.

#Posatex, Merck Animal Health.

**Baytril Otic, Bayer Animal Health Division.

††Synotic, Pfizer Animal Health. Gloves must be worn when handling this medication.

TABLE 84-4

Drug Preparations Administered Orally That May Be Required to Treat Dogs with Otitis Externa

Drug	Dose (mg/kg)	Interval (hours)	Duration	Effect
Tramadol	1 to 4	12	Days to weeks	Analgesic
Prednisolone	0.5	12-24, then taper and discontinue	Days to weeks, until proliferative changes have reduced or resolved	Anti-inflammatory, antipruritic, and analgesic
Cephalexin	30	12	3 to 8 weeks	Antibiotic (initial choice when cocci are seen)
Marbofloxacin	4 to 5.5	24	3 to 8 weeks	Antibiotic (initial choice pending culture when rods are seen)
Ketoconazole, fluconazole, or itraconazole	5	24	Until cytologic resolution	Antifungal (when *Malassezia* spp. are present)

(see Table 84-3). Most acute, first occurrences of otitis externa will respond to topical treatments alone, without the need for systemic treatment. Culture and susceptibility results may not predict the response to treatment with topical antimicrobials, because of the high concentrations that can be achieved safely in the ear canal using such treatments. The choice of topical treatment should be based on the results of cytologic examination and, if possible, an assessment of the integrity of the tympanic membrane. If the integrity of the tympanic membrane is unknown, owners should be warned regarding the potential for ototoxicity, although ototoxicity has the potential to occur with any topical treatment. If the tympanum is intact, all options are acceptable. If the integrity of the tympanum is unknown, and increased numbers of bacteria are present, enrofloxacin solutions appear to be well tolerated. A solution of enrofloxacin and dexamethasone sodium phosphate can be used, or enrofloxacin can be diluted in Tris EDTA (see Table 84-3). Serial cytologic examinations should be used to monitor treatment efficacy and complications such as *Malassezia* overgrowth, which can occur following the use of topical antibiotics alone.

If bacterial rods predominate on cytologic examination, aerobic bacterial culture and susceptibility are indicated; a solution containing an aminoglycoside, polymyxin B, or ticarcillin-clavulanate is a good first empirical choice, although all have the potential to cause ototoxicity. Ototoxicity following topical aminoglycoside administration in dogs appears to be very uncommon,[40] but the risk of ototoxicity may outweigh the benefits of these treatments in service or performance dogs, and proper examination of the tympanum under anesthesia before initiating these treatments is recommended. A variety of other topical treatments have been used by veterinary dermatologists, including those containing antibacterials such as fusidic acid and silver sulfadiazine.[40] Silver sulfadiazine may also promote reepithelialization of ulcerated ears. The presence of *P. aeruginosa* is commonly associated with recurrent otitis externa, poor compliance, and primary causes that have not been addressed. The use of a more potent or expensive topical antimicrobial alone is rarely effective in successfully managing these cases, even in the short term.

Systemic Antimicrobial Drugs

Systemic antimicrobial treatment is not always necessary, even in *P. aeruginosa* otitis. General indications for systemic antibiotic treatment include (1) chronic and recurrent otitis externa; (2) the presence of ulceration; (3) the presence of otitis media; or (4) owner inability to effectively administer topical antimicrobial drugs. The antimicrobial is chosen on the basis of cytologic findings initially, while the results of culture and susceptibility testing are pending. A change in antimicrobial drug may be indicated if the results of susceptibility testing suggest resistance to the initial drug selected. Appropriate initial choices include cephalexin for otitis associated with the presence of cocci, and a fluoroquinolone for otitis associated with the presence of rods (see Table 84-4). Susceptibility panels should include enrofloxacin, marbofloxacin, ciprofloxacin, ticarcillin-clavulanate, and ceftazidime, in addition to those antibiotics routinely tested. Systemic azole antifungal treatment may be required when *Malassezia* spp. are present (see Chapter 59). Treatment is for a minimum of 6 to 8 weeks for dogs with otitis media and should be continued until there is normalization of the ear canals with no evidence of microorganisms on cytologic examination. The tympanic membrane may or may not regenerate. For dogs with highly resistant bacterial infections of the external or middle ear, daily lavage in conjunction with aggressive topical treatment alone may be successful.[40]

Surgery

Surgical treatments are salvage options that are reserved primarily for dogs with irreversible ear canal disease that is not responsive to medical treatment, and include total ear canal ablation (TECA) or total ear canal ablation with bulla osteotomy (TECA-BO). Indications for surgery in dogs with otitis externa include severe proliferative changes that occlude the ear canal, collapse or stenosis of the horizontal canal, or severely calcified periauricular tissues. Lateral wall resections achieve poor control of the disease and are not generally recommended. Addition of the bulla osteotomy to a TECA can help to prevent recurrence of disease due to persistent otitis media, manifested as recurrent infection with draining tracts. Severe intraoperative hemorrhage, postoperative wound infections, recurrent otitis media with draining tract formation, pinna necrosis, permanent or transient facial nerve damage, peripheral vestibular signs, and deafness are potential complications of the procedure, but the overall prognosis for resolution of disease is good. Resected tissue and bulla epithelium should be submitted for histopathology (see Table 84-1), since a previously undiagnosed underlying cause is occasionally detected. Cultures are obtained from the external and middle ear during surgery, and antimicrobials are administered perioperatively and for 4 to 8 weeks postoperatively (depending on the extent of middle ear involvement). Referral to a specialist surgeon is encouraged.

Public Health Aspects

The public health aspects outlined for pyoderma also apply to otitis externa. Hand hygiene should particularly be emphasized to owners of dogs with otitis externa associated with multidrug-resistant gram-negative bacteria, especially *P. aeruginosa*.

CASE EXAMPLE

Signalment: "Carla," a 3-year-old FS cocker spaniel dog from northern California (Figure 84-8)

History: Carla was brought to a veterinary dermatologist for a 1-year history of chronic skin problems that began on her back and progressed to involve her ventral abdomen, paws, lips, and neck. The owner reported she had been licking, scratching, biting, and rubbing the affected areas, and on a scale of 1 to 10 for pruritus, the owner believed she was an 8. She had also been lethargic and her appetite had been decreased. The condition had responded twice to antimicrobial drug treatment in the past (amoxicillin-clavulanic acid, then clindamycin) but returned when they were discontinued, and the third, most recent episode failed to respond to treatment with cephalexin and diphenhydramine. She was obtained as a puppy at 14 weeks of age and had no skin problems for her first 2 years of life. She was treated monthly with spinosad for flea prevention. There was one other healthy dog in the house.

Current medications: Diphenhydramine 2.5 mg/kg PO q12h

Physical Examination:

Body Weight: 10 kg.

General: Quiet, alert, hydrated, responsive. T = 102.5°F (39.2°C), HR = 120 beats/min, eupneic, CRT = 2 s.

Eyes, Ears, Nose, and Throat: Both eyes showed moderate scleral injection, moderate hyperemia with mild chemosis of third eyelid, and moderate tear staining. Both inner pinnae felt greasy with moderate yellow debris in the left ear canal, but no odor was detected. Mild to moderate dental calculus was present.

Integument: There was a full, soft, clean haircoat with moderate scaling but no evidence of ectoparasites. Generalized crusts with erythematous borders were noted. The crusts ranged from small (4-5 mm) round crusts randomly distributed on the dorsum to larger, irregularly shaped consolidated yellow crusts along the ventrum and left cervical region. Marked erythema of the inguinal region was present. There was bilateral erythema and diffuse thickening of the lower lip. Marked bilateral periocular alopecia with marked periocular scaling and crusting and moderate edema and swelling of the lower eyelids was noted. There was also marked erythema and moist skin interdigitally on both palmar and dorsal surfaces of both thoracic limbs, and yellow discoloration was present interdigitally on the dorsal surfaces. Mild to moderate erythema and moist skin was present interdigitally on both plantar and dorsal surfaces of both pelvic limbs.

Musculoskeletal: Body condition score was 8/9, ambulatory.

Genitourinary: There was mild perivulvar alopecia with mild erythema, mild yellow dried vulval discharge.

Other Systems: All other systems examined were within normal limits. All peripheral lymph nodes were <1 cm in diameter.

Cytology Findings:

Tape Preparations: Inguinal skin and dorsal feet: Degenerate neutrophils, cocci (too numerous to count).

Perianal skin: Degenerate neutrophils and 3 to 5 yeasts/oil immersion field.

Interdigital region: Degenerate neutrophils and 1 to 2 yeasts/oil immersion field.

Ear Swab Cytology: Right ear: Degenerate neutrophils and 15 to 20 cocci/oil immersion field.

Left ear: Degenerate neutrophils and cocci (too numerous to count).

Aerobic Bacterial Culture and Susceptibility: Moderate numbers of *Staphylococcus pseudintermedius* and a few *Pseudomonas aeruginosa* were isolated from the skin beneath crusts in the inguinal region.

	Bacteria Isolated	
Drug	***S. pseudintermedius***	***P. aeruginosa***
Amikacin	S ≤ 4.00	S ≤ 4.00
Amoxicillin–clavulanic acid	R	R > 32.00
Ampicillin	R	—
Cefazolin	R	R > 16.00
Cefoxitin	R	R > 16.00
Cefpodoxime	R	R > 16.00
Ceftiofur	R	No Int P > 4.00
Cephalothin	R	R > 16.00
Chloramphenicol	S = 8.00	R > 16.00
Clindamycin	R > 1.00	—
Enrofloxacin	R > 4.00	S ≤ 0.50
Erythromycin	R > 4.00	—
Gentamicin	R > 8.00	S ≤ 1.00
Imipenem	R	S ≤ 1.00
Marbofloxacin	R > 2.00	No Int P ≤ 0.25
Orbifloxacin	R > 4.00	S ≤ 1.00
Oxacillin + 2% NaCl	R	—
Penicillin	R	—
Rifampin	No Int P ≤ 1.00*	—
Tetracycline	S ≤ 2.00	I = 8.00
Ticarcillin-clavulanate	R	S = 16.00
Ticarcillin	R	S = 16.00
Trimethoprim-sulfamethoxazole	R > 2.00	R > 2.00

*No Int P, no interpretative criteria (breakpoint) available.

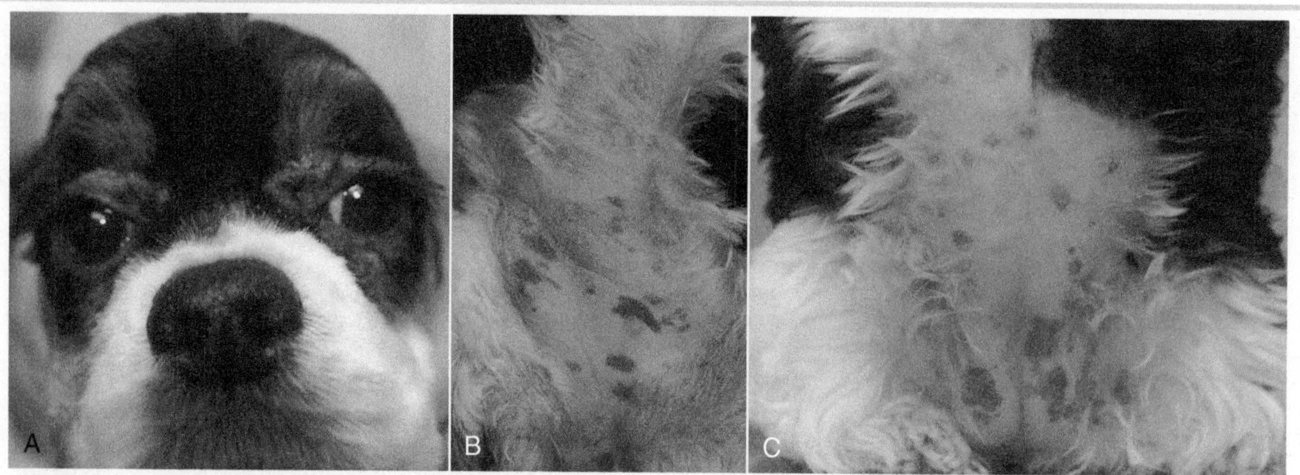

FIGURE 84-8 A 3-year-old FS Cocker spaniel with generalized superficial pyoderma, *Malassezia* spp. dermatitis, and bacterial otitis externa. **A,** Note periocular alopecia, scaling, and crusting. **B,** Consolidated yellow crusting and erythema are present on the ventral abdomen. **C,** Ventral abdomen of the same dog at a recheck 2 months after initiation of treatment.

Diagnosis: Generalized superficial pyoderma (methicillin-resistant *S. pseudintermedius*), *Malassezia* spp. dermatitis, bacterial otitis externa; suspect underlying allergic dermatitis or primary seborrhea of cocker spaniels.

Treatment: Fluconazole, 5 mg/kg PO q24h; prednisolone/trimeprazine 10 mg/4 mg (2 tablets) PO q12h for 2 days, then 10 mg PO q24h for 5 days, 10 mg q48h for 7 days, then one tablet twice weekly; routine ear cleaning twice daily followed 10 minutes later by topical gentamicin/betamethasone/clotrimazole ointment. Treatment with chloramphenicol was also initiated once culture and susceptibility results became available, but because of gastrointestinal adverse effects this was changed to doxycycline, 5 mg/kg PO q12h for 4 weeks. Suspected primary seborrhea was treated with every other day bathing with antiseborrheic shampoo and a spot-on antiseborrhea treatment (Duoxo, Sogeval). At a recheck 6 weeks after the initial visit, lesions and cytologic findings were greatly improved (see Figure 84-8, *C*). Subsequent management of Carla's skin condition required monthly rechecks with adjustment of treatments based on dermatologic examination and cytologic findings, routine ear cleansing with an antiseborrheic micellar ear solution (Duoxo, Sogeval), and a novel single-source protein diet for a suspected underlying food allergy.

Comments: This dog was diagnosed with superficial pyoderma and otitis externa on the basis of the dermatologic examination, cytologic findings, and culture. The *P. aeruginosa* was considered a likely contaminant based on the low numbers of organisms isolated and lack of cytologic evidence of bacterial rods. Failure to identify and address the underlying causes of this dog's pyoderma and otitis externa resulted in inadequate control of the disease, with development of a resistant bacterial infection. Culture and susceptibility testing of a pustule found 7 months after discontinuation of systemic antimicrobial treatment showed an *S. pseudintermedius* isolate with the same susceptibility pattern as the previous isolate, except now with intermediate susceptibility to tetracyclines. Although Carla's skin is much improved, inadequate owner compliance with bathing and medications has been partly responsible for the failure to eliminate the infection.

SUGGESTED READINGS

Matousek JL. Ear Disease. Vet Clin North Am Small Anim Pract. 2004;34(2):XI-XII.

Weese JS, van Duijkeren E. Methicillin-resistant *Staphylococcus aureus* and *Staphylococcus pseudintermedius* in veterinary medicine. Vet Microbiol. 2010;140(3-4):418-429.

REFERENCES

1. Bassett RJ, Burton GG, Robson DC. Antibiotic responsive ulcerative dermatoses in German Shepherd dogs with mucocutaneous pyoderma. Aust Vet J. 2004;82(8):485-489.
2. Gross TL, Ihrke PJ, Waldman EJ, et al. Lichenoid diseases of the dermis. In: Gross TL, Ihrke PJ, Walder EJ, et al, eds. Skin Diseases of the Dog and Cat. Ames, Iowa: Blackwell Science; 2005:261-263.
3. Rosser Jr EJ. German Shepherd dog pyoderma. Vet Clin North Am Small Anim Pract. 2006;36(1):203-211.
4. Sasaki T, Kikuchi K, Tanaka Y, et al. Reclassification of phenotypically identified *Staphylococcus intermedius* strains. J Clin Microbiol. 2007;45(9):2770-2778.
5. Allaker RP, Lloyd DH, Simpson AI. Occurrence of *Staphylococcus intermedius* on the hair and skin of normal dogs. Res Vet Sci. 1992;52(2):174-176.
6. Frank LA, Kania SA, Hnilica KA, et al. Isolation of *Staphylococcus schleiferi* from dogs with pyoderma. J Am Vet Med Assoc. 2003;222(4):451-454.
7. May ER, Hnilica KA, Frank LA, et al. Isolation of *Staphylococcus schleiferi* from healthy dogs and dogs with otitis, pyoderma, or both. J Am Vet Med Assoc. 2005;227(6):928-931.
8. Griffeth GC, Morris DO, Abraham JL, et al. Screening for skin carriage of methicillin-resistant coagulase-positive staphylococci and *Staphylococcus schleiferi* in dogs with healthy and inflamed skin. Vet Dermatol. 2008;19(3):142-149.
9. Hiller A, Alcorn JR, Cole LK, et al. Pyoderma caused by *Pseudomonas aeruginosa* infection in dogs: 20 cases. Vet Dermatol. 2006;17(6):432-439.
10. Scott DW, Miller WH, Griffin CE. Bacterial skin diseases. Muller and Kirk's Small Animal Dermatology. 6th ed. Philadelphia, PA: WB Saunders; 2001:274-335.

11. Tse H, Tsoi HW, Leung SP, et al. Complete genome sequence of the veterinary pathogen *Staphylococcus pseudintermedius* strain HKU10-03 isolated from a case of canine pyoderma. J Bacteriol. 2011;193:1783-1784.
12. Perreten V, Kadlec K, Schwarz S, et al. Clonal spread of methicillin-resistant *Staphylococcus pseudintermedius* in Europe and North America: an international multicentre study. J Antimicrob Chemother. 2010;65(6):1145-1154.
13. Pin D, Carlotti DN, Jasmin P, et al. Prospective study of bacterial overgrowth syndrome in eight dogs. Vet Rec. 2006;158(13):437-441.
14. DeBoer DJ, Marsella R. The ACVD task force on canine atopic dermatitis (XII): the relationship of cutaneous infections to the pathogenesis and clinical course of canine atopic dermatitis. Vet Immunol Immunopathol. 2001;81(3-4):239-249.
15. Hillier A, Lloyd DH, Weese JS, et al. Guidelines for antimicrobial therapy of superficial bacterial folliculitis: Antimicrobial Guidelines Working Group of the International Society for Companion Animal Infectious Diseases. Submitted for publication.
16. Cadilla A, David MZ, Daum RS, et al. Association of high-level mupirocin resistance and multidrug-resistant methicillin-resistant *Staphylococcus aureus* at an academic center in the United States. J Clin Microbiol. 2011;49(1):95-100.
17. Castanheira M, Watters AA, Bell JM, et al. Fusidic acid resistance rates and prevalence of resistance mechanisms among *Staphylococcus* spp. isolated from North America and Australia, 2007-2008. Antimicrob Agents Chemother. 2010;54(9):3614-3617.
18. Tacconelli E, De Angelis G, Cataldo MA, et al. Does antibiotic exposure increase the risk for methicillin-resistant *Staphylococcus aureus* (MRSA) isolation? A systematic review and meta-analysis. J Antimicrob Chemother. 2008;61(1):26-38.
19. Curtis CF, Lamport AI, Lloyd DH. Masked, controlled study to investigate the efficacy of a *Staphylococcus intermedius* autogenous bacterin for the control of canine idiopathic recurrent superficial pyoderma. Vet Dermatol. 2006;17(3):163-168.
20. DeBoer DJ, Moriello KA, Thomas CB, et al. Evaluation of a commercial staphylococcal bacterin for management of idiopathic recurrent superficial pyoderma in dogs. Am J Vet Res. 1990;51(4):636-639.
21. Stegmann R, Burnens A, Maranta C, et al. Human infection associated with methicillin-resistant *Staphylococcus pseudintermedius* ST71. J Antimicrob Chemother. 2010;65(9):2047-2048.
22. Morris DO, Boston RC, O'Shea K, et al. The prevalence of carriage of methicillin-resistant staphylococci by veterinary dermatology practice staff and their respective pets. Vet Dermatol. 2010;21:400-407.
23. Riegel P, Jesel-Morel L, Laventie B, et al. Coagulase-positive *Staphylococcus pseudintermedius* from animals causing human endocarditis. Int J Med Microbiol. 2011;301:237-239.
24. Weese JS, van Duijkeren E. Methicillin-resistant *Staphylococcus aureus* and *Staphylococcus pseudintermedius* in veterinary medicine. Vet Microbiol. 2010;140(3-4):418-429.
25. Kumar D, Cawley JJ, Irizarry-Alvarado JM, et al. Case of *Staphylococcus schleiferi* subspecies *coagulans* endocarditis and metastatic infection in an immune compromised host. Transpl Infect Dis. 2007;9(4):336-338.
26. von Eiff C, Peters G, Heilmann C. Pathogenesis of infections due to coagulase-negative staphylococci. Lancet Infect Dis. 2002;2(11): 677-685.
27. Cole LK. Otoscopic evaluation of the ear canal. Vet Clin North Am Small Anim Pract. 2004;34(2):397-410.
28. Rosser Jr EJ. Causes of otitis externa. Vet Clin North Am Small Anim Pract. 2004;34(2):459-468.
29. Sotiraki ST, Koutinas AF, Leontides LS, et al. Factors affecting the frequency of ear canal and face infestation by *Otodectes cynotis* in the cat. Vet Parasitol. 2001;96(4):309-315.
30. Crespo MJ, Abarca ML, Cabañes FJ. Occurrence of *Malassezia* spp. in the external ear canals of dogs and cats with and without otitis externa. Med Mycol. 2002;40(2):115-121.
31. Oliviera LC, Leite CA, Brilhante RS, et al. Comparative study of the microbial profile from bilateral otitis externa. Can Vet J. 2008;49(8):785-788.
32. Cole LK, Kwochka KW, Kowalski JJ, et al. Microbial flora and antimicrobial susceptibility patterns of isolated pathogens from the horizontal ear canal and middle ear in dogs with otitis media. J Am Vet Med Assoc. 1998;212(4):534-538.
33. Ginel PJ, Lucena R, Rodriguez JC, et al. A semiquantitative cytological evaluation of normal and pathological samples from the external ear canal of dogs and cats. Vet Dermatol. 2002;13(3):151-156.
34. Bischoff MG, Kneller SK. Diagnostic imaging of the canine and feline ear. Vet Clin North Am Small Anim Pract. 2004;34(2): 437-458.
35. Rohleder JJ, Jones JC, Duncan RB, et al. Comparative performance of radiography and computed tomography in the diagnosis of middle ear disease in 31 dogs. Vet Radiol Ultrasound. 2006;47(1):45-52.
36. Sturges BK, Dickinson PJ, Kortz GD, et al. Clinical signs, magnetic resonance imaging features, and outcome after surgical and medical treatment of otogenic intracranial infection in 11 cats and 4 dogs. J Vet Intern Med. 2006;20(3):648-656.
37. Lloyd DH, Bond R, Lamport I. Antimicrobial activity in vitro and in vivo of a canine ear cleanser. Vet Rec. 1998;143(4):111-112.
38. Wooley RE, Jones MS. Action of EDTA-Tris and antimicrobial agent combinations on selected pathogenic bacteria. Vet Microbiol. 1983;8(3):271-280.
39. Griffin CE. Otitis techniques to improve practice. Clin Tech Small Anim Pract. 2006;21(3):96-105.
40. Morris DO. Medical therapy of otitis externa and otitis media. Vet Clin North Am Small Anim Pract. 2004;34(2):541-556.

CHAPTER 85

Osteomyelitis, Discospondylitis, and Infectious Arthritis

Jane E. Sykes and Amy S. Kapatkin

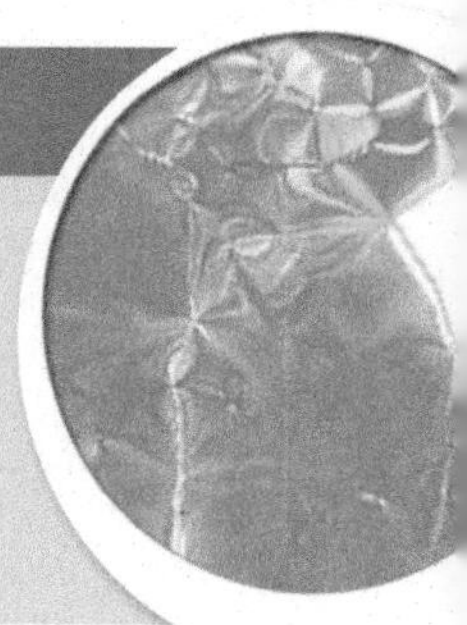

Overview of Musculoskeletal System Infections

Causes: The most common cause of osteomyelitis and infectious monoarthritis in dogs is *Staphylococcus* spp., but streptococci, other gram-negative bacteria, anaerobes, and fungi may be involved. *Bartonella, Nocardia,* and *Mycobacterium* can also cause osteomyelitis. *Brucella* can cause osteomyelitis and discospondylitis. Polyarthritis may be caused by a wide range of gram-positive and gram-negative bacteria; vector-borne bacterial pathogens *(Rickettsia rickettsii, Ehrlichia canis, Anaplasma phagocytophilum, Ehrlichia ewingii, Borrelia burgdorferi);* protozoa *(Leishmania);* and fungi.

Geographic Distribution: Worldwide, although the prevalence of brucellosis and vector-borne and fungal causes varies geographically

Major Clinical Signs: Pain, lameness, fever, inappetence, lethargy, draining skin lesions, and soft tissue swelling may occur with osteomyelitis. Spinal pain, fever, lethargy, inappetence, and pelvic limb paresis or paralysis can occur with discospondylitis. A stiff gait, reluctance to move, lameness, fever, inappetence, lethargy, and swollen joints may occur with polyarthritis.

Differential Diagnoses: Differential diagnoses for suspected osteomyelitis, monoarthritis, and discospondylitis include bone neoplasia, sterile foreign body reactions, and degenerative osteoarthritis. Primary immune-mediated polyarthritis is the major differential diagnosis for suspected infectious polyarthritis.

Human Health Significance: When draining wounds are present, resistant bacteria such as methicillin-resistant *Staphylococcus aureus* associated with osteomyelitis and arthritis in dogs and cats may have the potential to colonize human patients. Discospondylitis and polyarthritis caused by *Brucella* spp. can be transmitted to humans through contact with infected urine. Because vector-borne pathogens and fungi of importance to human health can cause polyarthritis, hospital staff should take special care to avoid sharps injuries when working with animals with polyarthritis.

Infectious osteomyelitis is defined as infection of the cortical bone, periosteum, and myeloid cavity and the associated inflammatory response. The axial and/or appendicular skeleton may be involved. *Discospondylitis* refers to inflammation of the intervertebral discs and adjacent cartilaginous endplates, and almost always results from infection by bacteria or fungi. *Infectious arthritis* refers to inflammation of the synovium, synovial fluid, and associated cartilage secondary to infectious causes.

Osteomyelitis, discospondylitis, and arthritis can result from (1) hematogenous spread of bacteria or fungi to these sites, or (2) from direct introduction of bacteria as a result of penetrating wounds or surgery. When fungi are involved, molds such as *Aspergillus* spp. or *Paecilomyces* spp. are more likely than yeasts to cause discospondylitis; *Candida* has rarely been associated with discospondylitis in dogs.[1] In contrast, osteomyelitis can be caused by opportunistic molds or dimorphic fungi, especially *Coccidioides* spp. or *Blastomyces dermatitidis.* Fungal arthritis is uncommon but has been associated with infection by *Coccidioides* spp., *B. dermatitidis,* and *Cryptococcus* spp.

OSTEOMYELITIS

Etiology, Pathogenesis, and Epidemiology

Bacterial osteomyelitis most often results from direct introduction of bacteria into wounds adjacent to bone. Bacteria can be introduced into the bone as a result of penetrating foreign bodies, surgical wounds (especially orthopedic surgeries with implant placement), traumatic wounds, bite wounds, or extension of soft tissue infections. Tibial plateau leveling osteotomy (TPLO) surgery for cranial cruciate rupture, one of the most common orthopedic surgical procedures performed, has a postoperative infection rate that ranges from 0% to 7%.[2-5] For unknown reasons, the infection rate after TPLO appears to be higher than that after routine "clean" orthopedic surgeries that involve osteotomy (as opposed to fracture repair). In a report that was published before the TPLO procedure was described, the overall infection rate after any orthopedic surgery procedure was 3 of 502 surgeries (<1%).[6] In contrast, radiographically detectable osteomyelitis was reported in 14 (7.3%) of 193 dogs that underwent TPLO surgery and was the single most common complication of the procedure.[3] In another study, the infection rate after fracture repair was 9 (8%) of 110 surgeries.[7] In this study, 20% of the fractures were open. Open fractures were 4 times more likely to be contaminated with bacteria at the time of surgery than the closed fractures, and contaminated wounds were 5 times more likely to develop complications (seroma, drainage, and dehiscence) than those without contamination. Distal radius/ulna and tibial fractures were 10.5 times and 7.5 times more likely to be contaminated than femoral fractures, respectively. Animals with a normal postoperative temperature and a clean surgical wound did not develop postoperative complications.

Although gram-positive aerobes such as staphylococci and, to a lesser extent, streptococci predominate as a cause of osteomyelitis in dogs and cats, the organisms present and the bone(s)

TABLE 85-1

Bacteria Isolated from 31 Dogs with Surgical Site Infections after Tibial Plateau Leveling Operations at the University of California, Davis, Veterinary Medical Teaching Hospital

Bacterial Classification	Bacterial Species	Number of Isolates (%)	Proportion of Staphylococci Methicillin Resistant	Proportion Multidrug Resistant*
Gram-positive aerobes (n = 30)	*Staphylococcus pseudintermedius*	20 (49)	4/20 (20%)	7 (35%)
	Staphylococcus aureus	3 (7)	2/3	1/3
	Coagulase-negative staphylococci	3 (7)	1/3	0
	Staphylococcus schleiferi subsp. *coagulans*	1 (2)	0	0
	Enterococcus spp.	3 (7)	NA	2/3
Gram-negative aerobes (n = 9)	Enterobacteriaceae (*E. coli, Proteus, Klebsiella pneumoniae*)	4 (10)	NA	1/2†
	Pseudomonas aeruginosa	3 (7)	NA	2/3
	Eugonic fermenter-4–like	1 (2)	NA	0
	Pasteurella canis	1 (2)	NA	0
Anaerobes (n = 2)	*Actinomyces*	1 (2)	NA	ND
	Propionibacterium acnes	1 (2)	NA	ND

Mixed infections with 2 or 3 bacterial species or strains were present in 7 (23%) of the dogs (total 41 isolates).
NA, Not applicable; ND, not done.
*Resistant to three or more classes of antimicrobial drugs.
†One of 2 *E. coli* and the *Proteus* isolate did not undergo susceptibility testing because isolation was performed at necropsy.

affected generally reflect the underlying type of injury that led to infection. For example, osteomyelitis that follows surgical site infection is often caused by *Staphylococcus pseudintermedius*, a common commensal of canine skin (Table 85-1). *Staphylococcus aureus* and gram-negative bacterial infections can also cause orthopedic surgical site infections.[5] In contrast, anaerobes and aerobic gram-positive bacteria (staphylococci, enterococci, streptococci) or gram-negative bacteria *(Pseudomonas, E. coli, Klebsiella pneumoniae, Proteus, Pasteurella)* predominate in osteomyelitis that results from bite wound infections, tooth root abscesses, or penetrating foreign bodies.[8,9] Such mixed bacterial infections are also common in dogs with digital osteomyelitis.

Osteomyelitis secondary to bacteremia, also known as *hematogenous osteomyelitis,* is very rare and usually affects young animals. The metaphyseal regions are often involved, sometimes with extension to the epiphyses and joints (Figure 85-1). The pathogenesis remains obscure. It has been suggested that discontinuous endothelium in the primary spongiosa may predispose to extravasation of erythrocytes and bacteria in this region.[10] In humans, blunt trauma appears to contribute to development of focal childhood osteomyelitis, and it has been hypothesized that the periosteum, rather than the metaphysis, may initially be involved.[11] Sternal and vertebral osteomyelitis can also result from hematogenous spread of bacteria. Osteomyelitis occasionally also results from hematogenous spread of fastidious bacteria such as *Brucella, Bartonella, Mycobacterium,* and *Nocardia* spp.

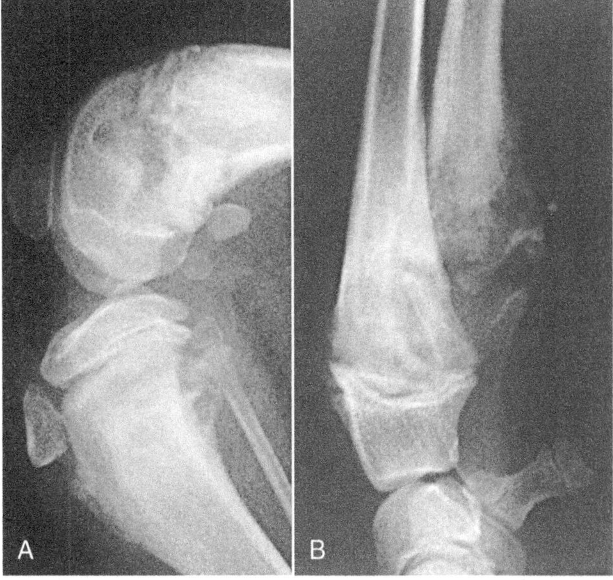

FIGURE 85-1 Polyostotic metaphyseal osteomyelitis in a Border collie puppy that had persistent neutropenia. **A,** Disruption of metaphyseal architecture of distal femur and proximal tibia, with irregular areas of radiolucency and sclerosis and some adjacent periosteal new bone. **B,** Similar changes are evident in the distal radius and ulna. (From Ettinger SJ, Feldman EC, eds. Textbook of Veterinary Internal Medicine. 7th ed. St. Louis, MO: Saunders; 2010.)

Clinical Features

Signs and Their Pathogenesis

The development of bacterial osteomyelitis requires the presence not only of bacteria, but also of compromised bone. Bone necrosis can result from trauma (i.e., fracture), surgery, or underlying bone neoplasia. Bacteria adhere to fibronectin, a connective tissue glycoprotein, through the use of a variety of adhesins. The presence of foreign material promotes persistence of infection in the form of biofilm (Figure 85-2). Within biofilm, bacteria evade opsonization and phagocytosis and are protected from the effects of antimicrobial drugs. Bone sequestra can also

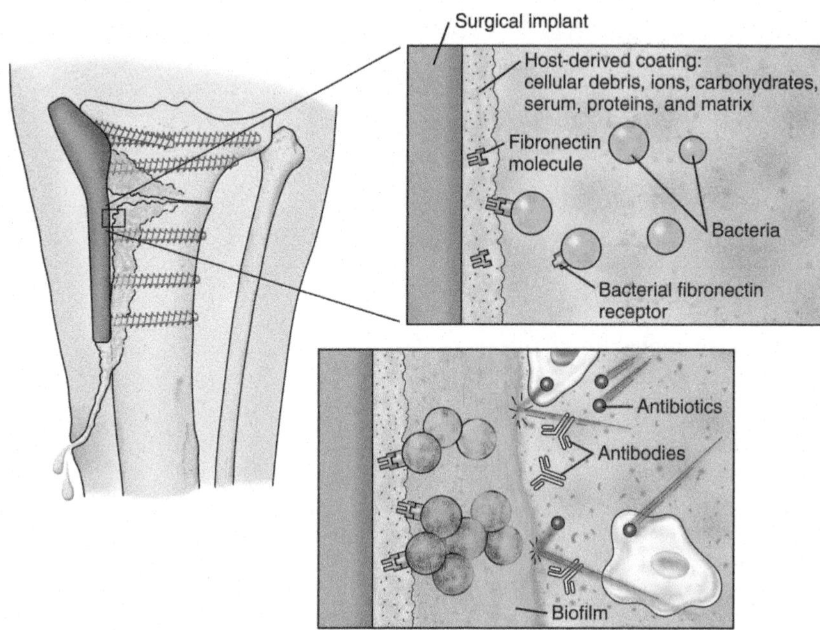

FIGURE 85-2 Pathogenesis of osteomyelitis. Necrotic bone is colonized by bacteria, which adhere to fibronectin and in the presence of foreign material (in this case, an implant) can form biofilm. Biofilm consists of bacterial aggregates embedded in a matrix of exopolysaccharide (bacterial slime). The biofilm protects the bacteria from antibodies, phagocytosis, and antimicrobial drugs.

become colonized by bacteria, which evade host defenses in the absence of adequate blood supply. Loose implants and fracture instability contribute to bone resorption, compromised blood supply, and persistent infection.[10] Some implant types are more apt to be colonized by bacteria. In one study, Slocum TPLO plates were more likely to be removed than other types of TPLO plates because of local bacterial infection and clinical signs of inflammation.[12]

Inflammatory cells recruited to the site of infection release enzymes that cause additional bone necrosis, with destruction of cancellous and cortical bone and abscessation of associated soft tissue. The end result is focal swelling, pain, draining skin lesions, and lameness. Small draining skin lesions often represent the "tip of the iceberg", with extensive bone involvement hidden beneath the skin (Figure 85-2). The presence of anaerobes can be associated with a foul odor or gas production. Fever, inappetence, lethargy, and leukocytosis are occasionally present in animals with acute osteomyelitis but are often absent in chronic osteomyelitis. Occasionally, infection reactivates in dogs years after surgery and implant placement. In human patients, latent periods between infection and development of osteomyelitis can last many decades.[13]

Physical Examination Findings

Physical examination findings in dogs and cats with osteomyelitis include lameness, localized pain, soft tissue swelling, muscle atrophy, and the presence of draining tracts. Fever and lethargy can also be identified in some animals.

Diagnosis

In most cases, osteomyelitis is diagnosed on the basis of history, physical examination, and radiographic findings. Aerobic and anaerobic bacterial culture of affected bone or any implants present is required for definitive diagnosis.

Laboratory Abnormalities

The CBC of animals with osteomyelitis may be unremarkable or reveal mild anemia, neutrophilia with bandemia, and monocytosis. The serum biochemistry panel and urinalysis are usually unremarkable, unless bacteremia or other systemic disease is also present.

Diagnostic Imaging

Radiographic changes in dogs and cats with osteomyelitis vary considerably in extent and character. In some dogs and cats, only soft tissue swelling may be evident. Plain radiography is insensitive and can be poorly specific for diagnosis of osteomyelitis, and interpretation can vary from one board-certified radiologist to another. In one study, plain radiographic findings were interpreted as osteomyelitis by two radiologists in only 5 of 8 dogs with experimentally induced osteomyelitis.[14] One radiologist diagnosed osteomyelitis in only 3 of the 8 dogs, but that radiologist was less likely than the other radiologists to diagnose osteomyelitis when infection was absent.

When radiographic bony changes are evident, they consist of periosteal proliferation, which may be smooth or speculated; focal osteopenia with cortical resorption or thinning; loss of trabecular markings; lucency around implants such as plates or screws; and sequestration (Figure 85-3). Pathologic fractures may be evident in dogs with fungal osteomyelitis. Scintigraphy with technetium-99m ciprofloxacin has also been investigated for diagnosis of osteomyelitis in a rabbit model.[15] False negatives and false positives were common early (4 weeks) in the course of healing, but sensitivity increased to 75% to 100% later in the course of healing, with specificities that approached 100%. Ultrasound imaging, contrast computed tomography (CT), and MRI may be useful for identification of sequestra, foreign material, and abscess formation. Intravenous administration of ultraparamagnetic iron oxide nanoparticles during MRI, which are taken up by macrophages, has shown promise for early detection of vertebral osteomyelitis and differentiation of osteomyelitis from aseptic inflammation.[16]

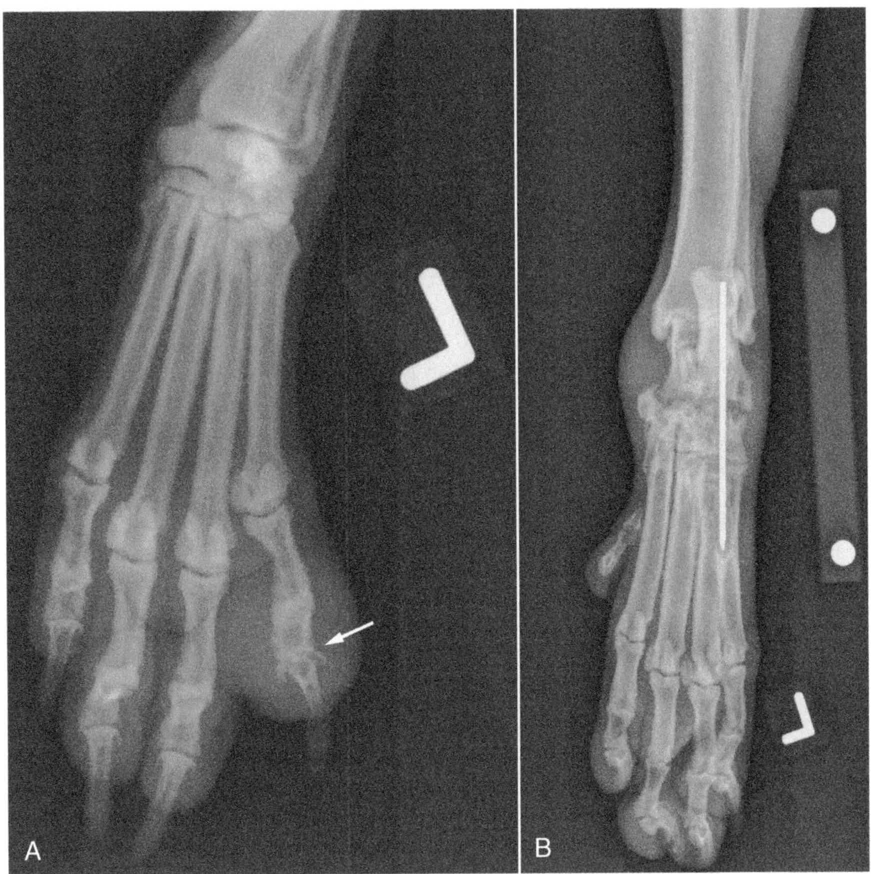

FIGURE 85-3 Radiographic changes in bacterial osteomyelitis. **A,** Osteomyelitis of the third phalanx of the fifth digit in a 7-year-old female spayed fox terrier with systemic lupus erythematosus that had been treated with prednisone and cyclosporine. There is severe soft tissue swelling, moderate lysis of the distal aspect of the third phalanx, and an irregular cortical margin with loss of the normal P2-P3 joint space *(arrow)*. A *Nocardia* sp. was isolated from the draining lymph node. **B,** Radiographs of the left tarsus of a 5-year-old male neutered pit bull terrier with implant-associated osteomyelitis. A partial left tarsal arthrodesis had been performed a year previously after the dog suffered a traumatic injury. Draining tracts then developed in association with the screw heads, and treatment with cephalexin was unsuccessful. There is severe irregular bone lysis on both sides of the proximal intertarsal joint. A surgical pin extends from the proximal calcaneus through the tarsal joint to the level of the mid-diaphysis of the 5th metatarsal bone. There is a region of lucency that surrounds the tip of the surgical pin within the 5th metatarsal bone. The cortex of the 4th metatarsal bone adjacent to the pin is thickened with a slightly irregular periosteal reaction. The first phalanx of the first digit is incomplete (likely congenital). There is marked soft tissue swelling associated with the tarsus. A methicillin-susceptible *Staphylococcus aureus* was cultured from the implant at surgery to remove the pin. Tobramycin-impregnated calcium sulfate beads were used to fill the pin tract.

Microbiologic Tests

Isolation and Identification

Aerobic and anaerobic bacterial culture and susceptibility should be performed on aspirates of pus, bone biopsies, or removed implants from dogs and cats with osteomyelitis. Aspirates should be collected in a sterile manner from the focus of infection to avoid contamination with surface bacteria (e.g., via aspiration of lesions through healthy skin after skin antisepsis, or through collection of biopsies or implants during surgical exploration). Negative culture results may reflect an insufficient specimen size, or the presence of fastidious bacteria such as anaerobes, *Bartonella, Brucella, Nocardia,* or *Mycobacterium* spp. Blood cultures should be performed if hematogenous osteomyelitis is suspected based on the history and clinical findings (young animal, multiple sites affected, sternal or vertebral involvement, other systemic illness or immunosuppression).

Pathologic Findings

Pathologic findings in osteomyelitis depend on the causative agent and chronicity of infection. Inflammatory cell infiltrates may range from suppurative (acute osteomyelitis) to pyogranulomatous or lymphoplasmacytic. The neutrophilic infiltrate in dogs with acute osteomyelitis may be accompanied by the presence of fibrin, free red blood cells, and necrotic debris. There may be evidence of bone resorption with multinucleated osteoclasts and new bone and fibrous tissue formation. In some cases, intralesional bacteria or fragments of foreign material (such as plant material) are observed (Figure 85-4).

Treatment and Prognosis

Treatment recommendations for focal osteomyelitis secondary to trauma, surgery, or foreign body penetration depends on the severity and chronicity of disease, the location of osteomyelitis, the presence or absence of foreign material, and the extent of blood supply to the bone. In animals with fractures, early detection and treatment of osteomyelitis is critical to prevent extensive bone necrosis and nonunion. Antimicrobial drug treatment alone is usually not sufficient to resolve chronic bacterial osteomyelitis, because sequestra and biofilm are avascular and are not effectively penetrated by antimicrobial drugs. In general, treatment requires debridement, removal of sequestra and foreign material (such as implants), dead space removal, extensive lavage with sterile saline, rigid fracture stabilization,

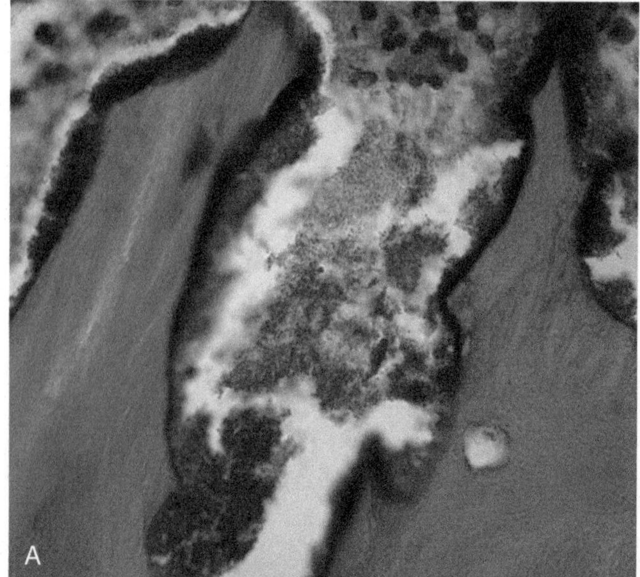

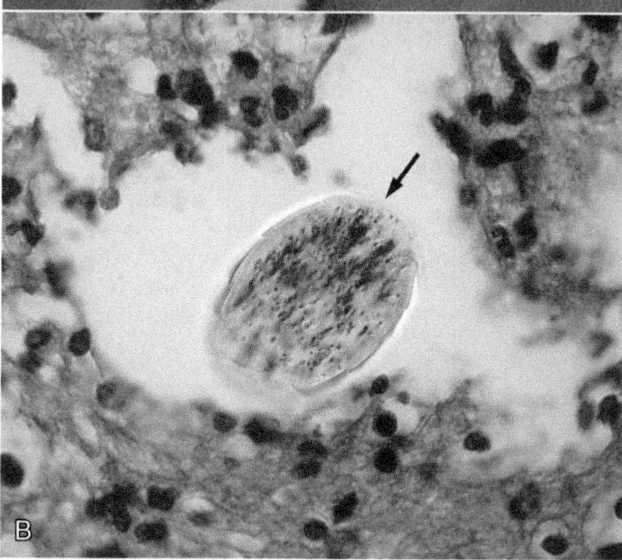

FIGURE 85-4 Histopathology from the right pelvic fourth digit of a 3-year-old intact male Labrador retriever with an open articular fracture and chronic suppurative bacterial osteomyelitis. **A,** Large numbers of bacteria are adhered to bone fragments (eosinophilic material) with an associated neutrophilic inflammatory response. **B,** In other fields, intralesional plant material was visible *(arrow)*.

systemic +/- local administration of appropriate antimicrobial drugs, and grafting of bone deficits. Because implants must ultimately be removed to resolve infection, fractures may need stabilization through alternative means, such as external skeletal fixation. If implants are rigidly stable, they should be left in place until bone healing is complete and then they should be removed in a second surgical procedure. Systemic antimicrobial drug therapy (and often regional antibiotic therapy in the form of antimicrobial drug–impregnated beads) is required while the bone heals. In some cases, foci of osteomyelitis may be removed en bloc without the need for further graft placement or stabilization (e.g., digital osteomyelitis). Resected bone should be submitted for histopathology (to confirm the presence of osteomyelitis and identify other processes such as fungal infection or neoplasia) as well as culture and susceptibility. Wounds are left open after debridement if continued debridement is needed via wet-to-dry bandaging. If all nonviable tissue has been removed, closed irrigation systems or vascularized tissue flaps may be used to manage dead space. A sterile dressing should be used to cover the wounds, with daily bandage changes until exudation resolves. If needed, autogenous cancellous bone graft placement is delayed until infection has been controlled and granulation tissue has begun to fill the wound (usually 1 to 2 weeks after initiation of antimicrobial drug treatment).[17] When graft placement or fracture stabilization is not possible because of financial concerns or uncontrollable infection, amputation may be necessary.

The choice of antimicrobial drugs should be based on the results of aerobic and anaerobic bacterial culture and susceptibility. If the animal is stable, treatment should be withheld until results are available, and medications to manage pain should be administered. If earlier antimicrobial treatment is deemed necessary pending the results of culture and susceptibility, the drug chosen should be based on the history (e.g., postsurgical infection versus bite wound infection) and local prevalence data for the practice (Table 85-2). Clindamycin is a reasonable initial choice for infections that could include susceptible staphylococci and/or anaerobic bacteria and was effective in experimental models of *S. aureus* osteomyelitis in dogs,[18] but a significant proportion of methicillin-resistant staphylococci exhibit clindamycin resistance or inducible clindamycin resistance (see Chapter 35). If gram-negative bacteria or methicillin-resistant staphylococci are suspected, the addition of an aminoglycoside may be necessary if treatment must be instituted before the results of culture and susceptibility become available. However, aminoglycosides penetrate poorly into purulent material, so adequate debridement is essential. Combinations of antibiotics are sometimes required in animals with polymicrobial infections. Systemic antibiotic treatment should be continued for at least 4 to 6 weeks. Longer periods of treatment may be required in some dogs and cats. Antimicrobial drugs should be given parenterally in the hospital for at least the first 3 to 5 days, and for longer if possible.

In addition to systemic treatment, antibiotic-impregnated beads can be used to treat chronic osteomyelitis and septic arthritis in dogs.[19-21] These are prepared in the operating room by mixing an antimicrobial drug with commercially available cement and setting the cement into beads on a suture through the use of a plastic mold or by hand. The beads are counted and strings of beads are placed at the site of infection, where they deliver high concentrations of drug to the site (e.g., initially 500-fold that of normal serum concentrations with systemic treatment), sometimes for several weeks, without systemic adverse effects.[22] The antimicrobial drugs used are generally heat stable, hydrophilic, and have activity against methicillin-resistant staphylococci, such aminoglycosides (gentamicin or tobramycin) or vancomycin. Clindamycin has also been used. Once the antimicrobial drug has diffused from the bead, nonbiodegradable beads such as those composed of polymethylmethacrylate (PMMA) may act as foreign bodies and a nidus for infection, and so a second surgery is usually required for bead removal. Biodegradable materials are also available, and include antibiotic-impregnated collagen, bone graft substitutes such as calcium phosphate or calcium sulfate (plaster of Paris, e.g., Osteoset) beads (Figure 85-5), and a variety of synthetic polymers such as polylactic acid, polylactide-co-glycolides, and cross-linked polydimethylsiloxane.[22] Tobramycin-impregnated calcium phosphate beads have been used successfully to treat osteomyelitis in dogs.[20] Polymers can be engineered to control the duration and concentration of antibiotic treatment at the site.

TABLE 85-2

Suggested Initial Antimicrobial Drug Doses for Stable Animals with Bacterial Orthopedic Infections Pending Culture and Susceptibility Results

Disease	Drug	Dose (mg/kg)	Route	Interval (hours)
Osteomyelitis or monoarthritis	Clindamycin hydrochloride, clindamycin phosphate	11-33 (dogs)	PO	12 (dogs)
		11 (cats)	PO	24 (cats)
		10	IV,* IM	12
	Enrofloxacin†	5-20 (dogs)	IV, IM, PO	24
	Gentamicin sulfate‡	14 (dogs) 8 (cats)	IV, IM, SC	24
	Amikacin‡	15-30 (dogs) 10-14 (cats)	IV, IM, SC	24
Discospondylitis	Ampicillin sodium	20	IV	6
	Ampicillin-sulbactam§	20	IV	8
	Amoxicillin–clavulanic acid	20-25	PO	12
	Cefazolin sodium	20-35	IV, IM	8
	Cephalexin	20-30	PO	6-8

See Chapter 86, Table 86-8, for suggestions for severe sepsis.
*For IV administration, dilute 1:10 in 0.9% saline and administer over 30-60 minutes.
†Addition of fluoroquinolones to clindamycin or a β-lactam is indicated if gram-negative bacteria may be present and methicillin resistance among staphylococci is not prevalent in the region. In cats, other fluoroquinolones such as pradofloxacin or marbofloxacin are preferred because of the risk of retinopathy (see Chapter 8 for doses and contraindications). Use of pradofloxacin has been associated with bone marrow suppression in dogs, especially at high doses.
‡Addition of aminoglycosides to clindamycin or a β-lactam is indicated if gram-negative bacteria and/or methicillin-resistant staphylococci may be present. See Chapter 8 for contraindications.
§Dose based on ampicillin component

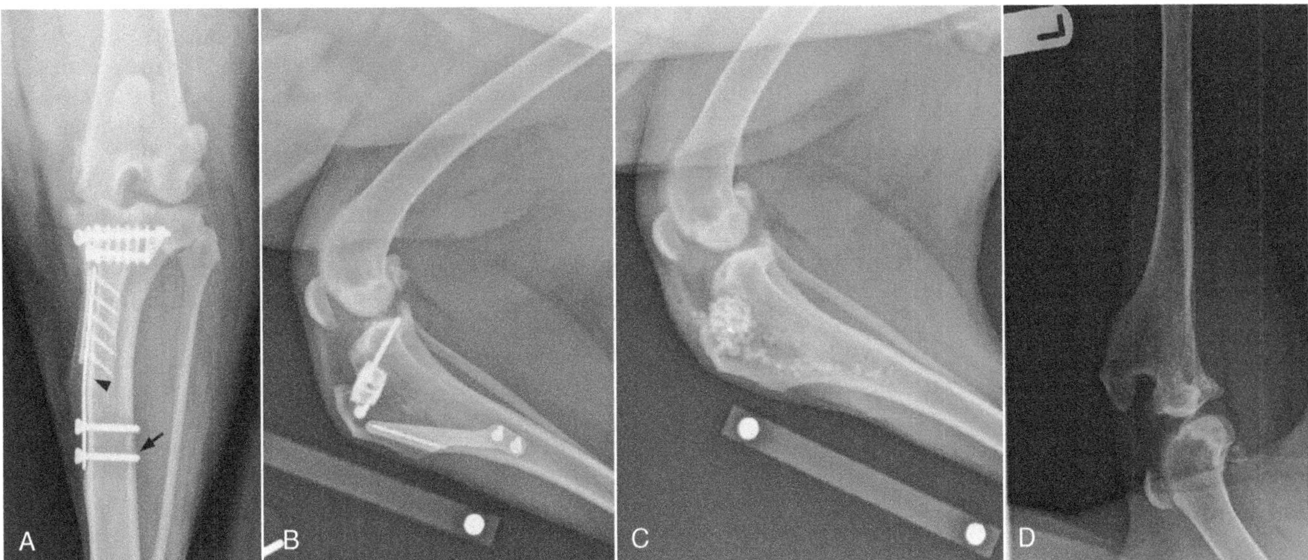

FIGURE 85-5 Lateral radiographs of the left stifle from a 10-year-old female spayed greyhound–pit bull terrier mix that developed osteomyelitis at the site of a left tibial tuberosity advancement surgery (see Case Example). Anteropalmar **(A)** and lateral **(B)** radiographs of the left stifle 13 months after the surgery. The osteotomy site has filled with bone to some extent, but the site is still visible as a result of incomplete union. There was also lucency in the region of the most distal screw *(arrow)* and thinning of the cortical bone adjacent to the plate *(arrowhead)*. **C,** The cage was removed by drilling around it, and calcium sulfate (Osteoset) beads were used to fill the defect. **D,** Radiograph taken 13 months postoperatively showing resolution of osteomyelitis and degradation of the calcium sulfate beads.

Prevention

Although not a substitute for sterile surgical technique and strict hospital infection control measures (see Chapter 11), preoperative antimicrobial drug treatment is an accepted aid for prevention of soft tissue surgical infections and osteomyelitis, especially when orthopedic implants are anticipated. Guidelines published for human medicine state that adequate prophylaxis requires (1) antimicrobial agents with activity against organisms likely to be encountered in the surgical field; (2) timely preoperative antimicrobial drug administration (within 60 minutes of incision); (3) bactericidal concentrations of drug in the serum and tissues during the time that the wound is open; and (4) a duration of 24 hours after surgery.[23] Additional intraoperative doses should be given if the procedure lasts longer than two half-lives of the drug being administered (usually at least 2 hours). In practices where the prevalence of postoperative infections with methicillin-resistant staphylococci is low, preoperative treatment with cefazolin may be effective. Where the regional prevalence of skin colonization with methicillin-resistant staphylococci is high (e.g., >10%), preoperative treatment with cefazolin and an aminoglycoside such as amikacin could be used. Prophylactic treatment should never be continued for longer than 24 hours after surgery because it can select for drug-resistant bacterial infections. In human patients, antibiotic-impregnated implants have been used to prevent attachment of bacteria to their surface.[22] Minimization of surgery time, careful surgical technique, and use of plate types that are associated with a lower risk of postoperative infection (i.e., non–Slocum-type TPLO plates) may also prevent postsurgical osteomyelitis.[12] Metals used in implants should be of the same type (e.g., plate and screws) to minimize the chance of galvanic corrosion. Galvanic corrosion occurs when metals of different electrochemical properties are placed in close proximity in an electrolytic environment. This can predispose to implant loosening, local infection, or sarcoma formation.[24] Currently, it is considered acceptable to leave implants in place after healing unless the animal is very young, there is persistent pain associated with the implant, or radiographic evidence of osteomyelitis or osteopenia is present. This is because the process of implant removal itself can be costly and may be followed by osteomyelitis or fracture. However, owners of pets with implants should be advised that although rare, possible long-term complications of implant placement include reactivation of infection in the future or development of malignancy at the implant site.

Public Health Aspects

Dogs and cats with bacterial osteomyelitis can shed antibiotic-resistant gram-positive and gram-negative bacteria that have the potential to colonize humans and later be a source of human infection. Infections acquired after orthopedic surgeries, especially TPLOs, are problematic. Most dogs are infected with *S. pseudintermedius*, but a smaller percentage of dogs are infected with *S. aureus*, which is more likely to colonize humans (see Table 85-1). However, in some cases, the human in the household may have been the source of *S. aureus* infection. Some hospitals experience a high prevalence (>10%) of postoperative wound infections with methicillin-resistant staphylococci. In a case-control study that included dogs with methicillin-resistant *S. aureus* infection (cases) and dogs with methicillin-susceptible *S. aureus* infection (controls), surgical implant placement was associated with a 33-fold increased risk of methicillin-resistant *S. aureus* infection (P = 0.001).[25] Infected osteomyelitis wounds should be covered with a suitable dressing at all times, and owners should be advised to wear gloves when handling their pets (especially if the wound is infected) and to wash their hands properly afterwards. In the hospital, animals with draining orthopedic surgical wound infections due to methicillin-resistant or multi-drug resistant bacteria should be handled by a limited number of individuals who wear gloves, a gown, and dedicated equipment, and signage should be posted. Hand washing should be performed after protective wear is removed, and all equipment used should be disinfected properly (see Chapter 11).

DISCOSPONDYLITIS

Etiology, Pathogenesis, and Epidemiology

Discospondylitis most often follows hematogenous spread of bacteria or fungi to the cartilaginous vertebral endplates, with extension to the intervertebral discs. Bacteria or fungi are thought to lodge in the endplates because blood flow slows in this region. In most cases, the source of infection cannot be identified, but infection can originate from the urogenital tract, abscesses, skin wounds, respiratory tract infections, or the oral cavity. Occasionally discospondylitis follows extension of infection from an adjacent site, such as following vertebral column surgical site infections, complications of epidural anesthesia, bite wounds, or migrating grass awns.

Risk factors for discospondylitis in dogs include male sex, older age, and breed.[1] Predisposed breeds include great Danes, boxers, Rottweilers, English bulldogs, German shepherd dogs, and Doberman pinschers. German shepherds and Rhodesian ridgebacks are predisposed to systemic mold infections that can target the intervertebral discs.[26] Although discospondylitis is frequently diagnosed in Labrador and golden retrievers, these dogs are popular breeds and were not found to be at risk.[1] Discospondylitis is extremely rare in cats and usually follows trauma such as cat bites, with associated meningomyelitis.[27-31] Concurrent disorders identified in dogs include genitourinary tract infections (prostatitis, orchitis, metritis, and/or urinary tract infection), pyoderma and otitis, immunosuppressive drug treatment, heartworm disease, recent vertebral column surgery, respiratory tract infection, bite wounds and other traumatic injuries, recent nonvertebral surgery, septic arthritis, severe intestinal parasitism, and infective endocarditis.

The incidence of discospondylitis in dogs and prevalence of different causative infectious agents varies geographically. In one study, the incidence of discospondylitis in the southern U.S. states was higher than in northern states.[1] In 123 dogs with discospondylitis from the southern United States, the most common pathogen isolated was *Staphylococcus* (41% of 63 isolates), followed by *Streptococcus* (12%), and *E. coli* (11%).[1] Other bacteria included *Klebsiella, Brucella, Pseudomonas, Proteus,* and *Actinomyces* spp. (<10% each). When the results of *Brucella* serology and culture were combined, 13 of the dogs were diagnosed with brucellosis. Only 2 dogs were infected with fungal organisms, one with *Candida tropicalis* and the other with an unidentified fungal agent. Mixed infections were detected in 11 (9%) of dogs. In 23 dogs with discospondylitis from the Pacific northwest of the United States, 10 of 18 isolates were staphylococci, 3 were streptococci, and 3 were *E. coli; Brucella* infection was not reported and a filamentous fungal species (*Phialemonium* or *Paecilomyces*) was isolated from 2 dogs.[32] In contrast, filamentous fungal species were isolated from nearly one third of dogs diagnosed with discospondylitis at the University of California, Davis (Table 85-3). The most common bacterial isolate was methicillin-susceptible *S. pseudintermedius;* methicillin-resistant staphylococci were not detected. In more than half of dogs with discospondylitis, the causative agent is not identified. Lumbar discospondylitis caused by *Actinomyces* spp. and anaerobic bacteria may occur as a result of migration of inhaled grass awns, which lodge in the retroperitoneal space. Sexually intact male dogs and dogs from the southeastern states are at increased risk for *Brucella canis* discospondylitis,[33] but it can occur in any region and in dogs of any sex.

TABLE 85-3

Infectious Agents Isolated from 31 Dogs with Culture-Positive Discospondylitis Seen at the University of California, Davis, Veterinary Medical Teaching Hospital*

Organism Type	Infectious Agent	Number of Isolates (%)
Gram-positive aerobes (n = 15, 42%)	*Staphylococcus pseudintermedius* (methicillin-susceptible)	12 (33)
	Coagulase-negative staphylococci	2 (6)
	Streptococcus equisimilis	1 (3)
Gram-negative aerobes (n = 5, 14%)	*Klebsiella pneumoniae*	2 (6)
	Escherichia coli	2 (6)
	Brucella canis	1 (3)
Anaerobes (n = 4, 11%)	*Actinomyces* spp., *Prevotella, Fusobacterium, Porphyromonas*	4 (11)
Fungi (n = 11, 31%)	*Aspergillus* spp.	6 (17)
	Paecilomyces spp.	3 (8)
	Other molds	2 (3)

*Based on culture of blood and/or disc material (26 dogs) or urine only (5 dogs; 3 with mold infections, 1 with *E. coli*, and 1 with *K. pneumoniae* infections)

Clinical Features

Signs and Their Pathogenesis

Clinical signs of discospondylitis include fever, lethargy, inappetence, spinal pain, a hunched stance, lameness, reluctance to move, and/or reluctance to jump or climb stairs. The duration of signs is extremely variable, but are usually present for less than one month.[32] Spinal cord compression as a result of vertebral subluxation, abscess formation, disc protrusion or extrusion, and soft tissue proliferation can lead to neurologic deficits such as delayed or absent placing reactions, paresis with ataxia or paralysis, and loss of deep pain sensation. Neurologic deficits were detected in 59 (48%) of 123 dogs in one study,[1]; in another study, paresis or paralysis was detected in 20 of 23 dogs (87%) and 8 of these dogs were nonambulatory.[32] The neurologic signs reflect the severity and location of discospondylitis lesions; in one study the severity of neurologic signs was correlated with the number of compressive lesions and the percentage of spinal cord or cauda equina compression.[32] The majority (50% to 60%) of dogs have lesions in the thoracolumbar spine (especially the lumbosacral junction); cervical lesions are present in fewer than 20% of dogs.[1,32,34,35] Around 30% to 40% of dogs have multiple lesions. Thus, tetraparesis (which reflects the presence of compressive cervical lesions) is less common (<5% of dogs) than pelvic limb paresis or paralysis (33% of dogs). The location of discospondylitis lesions (e.g., L7 to S1 versus C5 to C6) does not seem to affect the likelihood of cord compression.[34]

Physical Examination Findings

Dogs with discospondylitis may have fever (although it is often absent), lethargy, weakness, and pain on palpation or manipulation of the spine. In some dogs, pain is difficult to localize or manifests as apparent abdominal pain when the abdomen is palpated, especially if upward pressure is placed on the spine. Dogs with neurologic deficits can be tetraparetic or have pelvic limb paresis or paralysis. Loss of deep pain sensation can occur in dogs with severe compression lesions. Neurologic examination may reveal delayed or absent placing reactions and exaggerated or reduced segmental reflexes. Evaluation for abnormalities that reflect the presence of concurrent disorders (such as cardiac murmurs in dogs with endocarditis or swollen joints in dogs with polyarthritis) should be carefully performed. Occasionally, discospondylitis is an incidental finding on plain radiography (performed to evaluate concurrent disease such as fever of unknown origin), and clinical signs that suggest discospondylitis are absent.

Diagnosis

Diagnosis of discospondylitis is based on physical examination findings; imaging (plain radiography, CT/MRI); culture of blood, CSF, or aspirates of disc material; and serologic testing for *Brucella* spp. (antibody tests) or fungi (antigen tests). The reader is referred to Chapters 53 (Canine Brucellosis) and Chapter 65 (Aspergillosis) for information on serologic testing for these diseases. Serologic testing for *Aspergillus* galactomannan antigen is inexpensive, and positive results (galactomannan indices >1.5) correlate strongly with an underlying mold infection.[36] Rarely, mixed infections with bacteria and fungi occur, and bacterial contaminants can complicate interpretation of blood and disc aspirates. Thus, all dogs with discospondylitis should ideally be tested for *Aspergillus* antigen before antibiotic treatment is initiated. It is especially important to test predisposed breeds such as German shepherds and Rhodesian ridgebacks. Affected dogs should be evaluated for evidence of disease at other anatomic sites. If possible, this should consist of thoracic radiographs and abdominal ultrasound, echocardiography (for infective endocarditis), and aerobic bacterial culture of the urine.

Laboratory Abnormalities

Often the CBC and biochemistry panel are surprisingly unremarkable in dogs with discospondylitis. There may be mild to moderate neutrophilia with bandemia and/or lymphopenia on the CBC. Mild hypoalbuminemia and mild to moderate hyperglobulinemia are the most common abnormalities on the biochemistry panel. Dogs with fungal discospondylitis may be azotemic

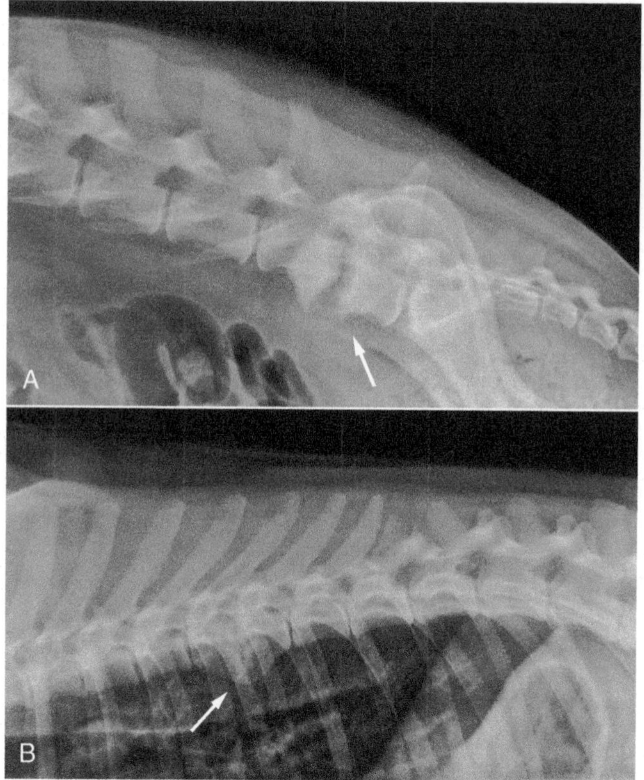

FIGURE 85-6 Radiographic changes in discospondylitis. **A,** Lateral radiograph of the lumbosacral region of a 3-year-old female spayed German shepherd with *Aspergillus* spp. discospondylitis. There is severe destruction of the endplates at L6-L7 *(arrow)* with sclerosis and ventral periosteal proliferation. **B,** Lateral radiograph of the thoracic spine of a 1-year-old female malamute. Resolving discospondylitis is present at T8-T9 *(arrow)*. There is lysis and irregularity to the endplates of these vertebrae. There is bridging spondylosis ventrally.

because of concurrent fungal pyelonephritis.[26] Urinalysis may show pyuria, bacteriuria, funguria, proteinuria, and/or cylindruria in dogs with concurrent urinary tract infections. Analysis of the CSF often reveals mild to markedly increased CSF protein concentration and rarely increased total nucleated cell count.[32]

Diagnostic Imaging

Plain Radiography

Radiographic changes in dogs (and cats) with discospondylitis include narrowing or widening of the intervertebral space, irregularity or lysis of the vertebral body endplates, endplate lucency, sclerosis at the margins of bone loss, proliferative lesions within adjacent vertebral bones and bridging spondylosis, and, in some cases, vertebral subluxation or fracture (Figure 85-6). Because multiple disc spaces are frequently affected, radiographs of the entire spine should be performed to properly assess the extent and severity of disease. Radiographic changes may lag behind clinical signs for as long as 6 weeks in dogs with discospondylitis, so radiographs should be repeated every 1 to 2 weeks if discospondylitis is suspected and plain radiographs are initially normal. Alternatively, advanced imaging with CT or MRI may reveal lesions not seen on plain radiographs. Plain radiography does not allow visualization of the degree of spinal cord compression, so myelography or advanced imaging is required to further evaluate dogs with neurologic signs. Ultrasonography may be useful for detection of retroperitoneal grass awns in dogs with localized lumbar discospondylitis on plain radiography.

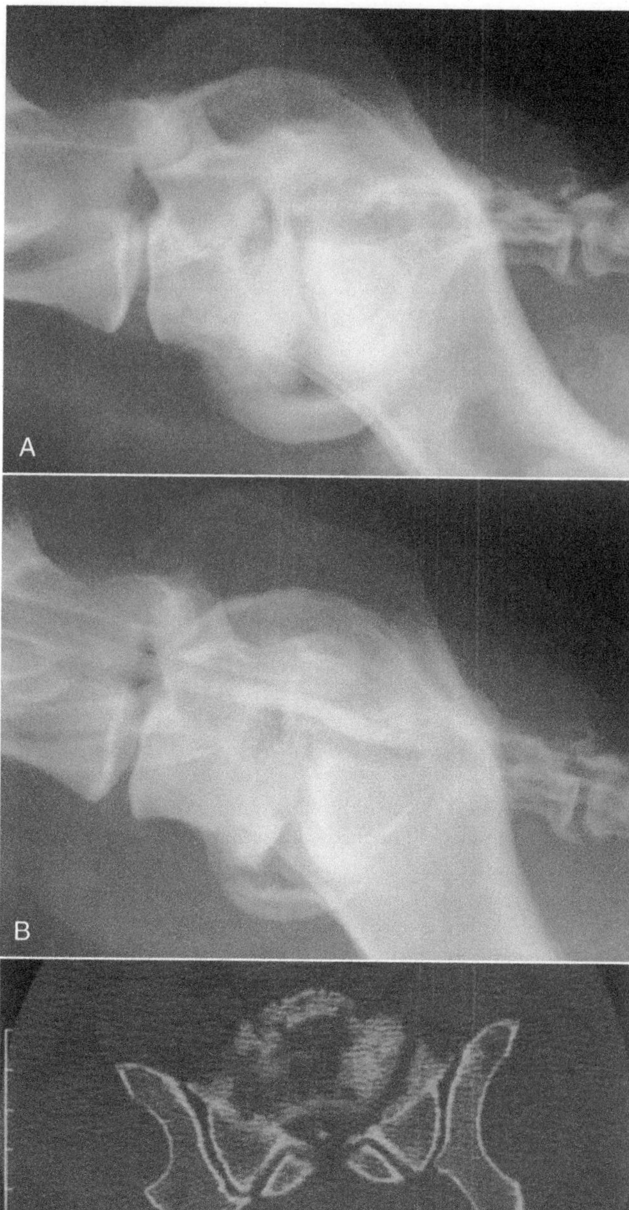

FIGURE 85-7 Images from a 9-year-old intact male Rottweiler with a 3-day history of difficulty standing and decreased appetite. Findings on neurologic examination included lumbosacral spinal pain, left pelvic limb paresis, and right pelvic limb paralysis. Blood and synovial fluid cultures yielded a methicillin-susceptible *Staphylococcus pseudintermedius*. Radiographic findings were consistent with chronic discospondylitis at the lumbosacral disc space and secondary compression of the spinal cord. **A,** Plain lateral radiograph of the pelvis. The lumbosacral joint space is narrowed and there is significant bridging spondylitis, with endplate osteolysis. **B,** Myelogram. Dorsal elevation of the conus is present at the lumbosacral junction. **C,** Contrast tomography of the lumbosacral junction. There is substantial endplate osteolysis. (All images courtesy the University of California, Davis, Veterinary Neurology/Neurosurgery Service.)

Contrast Radiography

Myelography can identify the site(s), type (vertebral subluxation or soft tissue proliferation), and extent of spinal cord compression in dogs with discospondylitis and allow planning for decompressive surgery (Figure 85-7).[34] However, MRI is less

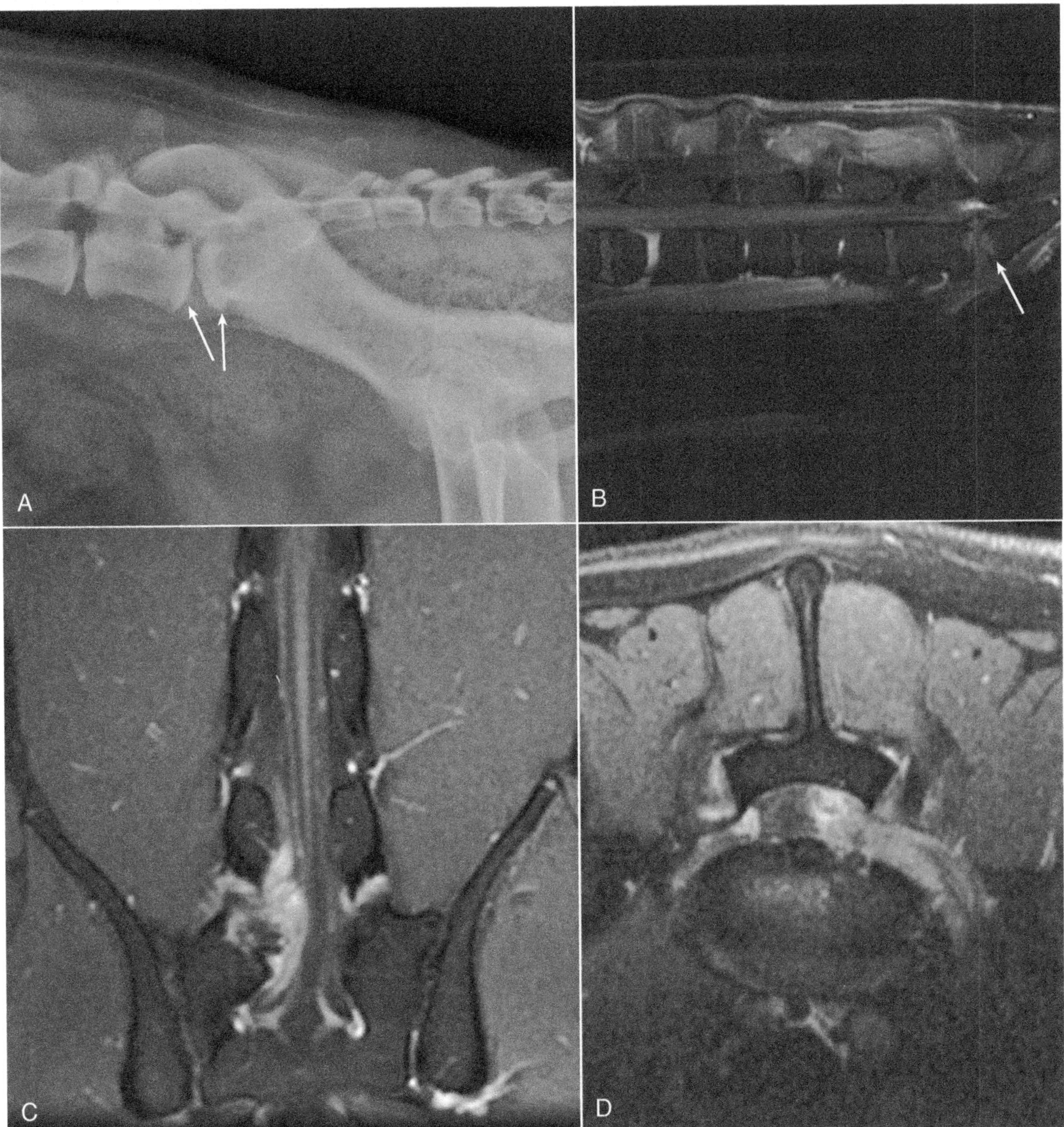

FIGURE 85-8 Images from a 5-year-old intact male German shepherd dog with a history of progressive reluctance to jump over the previous 18 months. Neurologic examination revealed decreased pelvic limb placing reactions and lumbosacral pain. Blood cultures were negative. Clinical signs and radiographic lesions improved dramatically with cephalexin treatment. **A,** Plain right lateral radiograph of the pelvis. The lumbosacral disc space is narrowed and there is vertebral endplate sclerosis *(arrows)*. There is also bony proliferation of the endplates at the level of the vertebral canal. **B,** Sagittal T1-postcontrast MRI with fat saturation, caudal lumbar and lumbosacral vertebral column. There is strong contrast enhancement in the endplates of L7 and S1 *(white arrow)* on either side of the disc space. **C,** Dorsal view. There is diffuse contrast enhancement of the tissues around the 7th lumbar nerve root with displacement of neural structures. **D,** Transverse view. There is marked enlargement and strong uniform enhancement of the right 7th lumbar spinal nerve. The primary differential based on radiologic findings was chronic lumbosacral discospondylitis with regional soft tissue inflammation on the right, and severe neuritis of the right 7th lumbar nerve. The impingement of the right 7th lumbar nerve by contrast-enhancing material was thought to result from granulation tissue formation. (All images courtesy the University of California, Davis, Veterinary Neurology/Neurosurgery Service.)

invasive and is now the preferred method for diagnosis of cord compression due to discospondylitis.

Advanced Imaging

CT and MRI may have increased sensitivity for diagnosis of discospondylitis when compared with plain radiography. MRI is the gold standard for diagnosis of discospondylitis in human patients and is increasingly used for diagnosis and characterization of discospondylitis in dogs.[32,35,37] Affected vertebral bodies are classically hypointense on T1-weighted images and may be hypointense, isointense, or hyperintense on T2-weighted images when compared with normal surrounding structures.[32,35] Hyperintensity of the vertebral bodies in dogs is more commonly observed in short tau inversion recovery (STIR) images, which suppress the signal from fat. Two adjacent vertebrae are consistently involved. Intervertebral discs are hyperintense on T2-weighted and STIR images when discospondylitis is present. Marked uniform or heterogenous contrast enhancement is usually apparent in vertebral endplates, within the disc, and in surrounding soft tissue (Figure 85-8). Paravertebral soft tissues may also be hyperintense on T2-weighted and especially STIR images.[32] With more chronic infection, there is loss of definition and cortical continuity and destruction of cortical margins in T1-weighted images. Distortion and narrowing of the disc space is also apparent, and subluxation and disc protrusion with associated spinal cord compression can be easily identified.

Microbiologic Tests

Isolation and Identification

The optimal specimens for identification of the causative agent of discospondylitis are blood or disc aspirates (or biopsies performed during decompressive surgery), because organisms isolated from these specimens are most likely to reflect those involved in disc destruction. Blood cultures are indicated in all dogs with discospondylitis (see Chapter 3 for blood culture technique and interpretation). Because anaerobes are uncommonly isolated from dogs with discospondylitis and they have predictable susceptibilities, the decision to perform anaerobic blood culture should be considered in light of any underlying disease processes and client financial constraints. Negative blood cultures occur in more than half of dogs with discospondylitis and may reflect low-level bacteremia or fungemia, the presence of fastidious or unculturable organisms such as *Brucella* or anaerobes, or recent antimicrobial drug treatment. Urine cultures may reveal the causative organism when blood cultures are negative, but not uncommonly bacterial species present in the urine differ from the organism present in affected discs. However, isolation of a mold species from the urine suggests a disseminated mycosis. Serologic testing for *Aspergillus* antigen and *Brucella* antibody should be performed in dogs with culture-negative discospondylitis. *Aspergillus* serology should also be considered for dogs that have blood culture-positive discospondylitis, because mixed infections with fungi and bacteria can rarely occur. Dogs with *Paecilomyces* discospondylitis can have positive *Aspergillus* serum and urine antigen tests due to serologic cross-reactions between these fungi.[36]

When blood cultures are negative, disc aspirates can be obtained under anesthesia with fluoroscopic (or other advanced imaging such as CT) guidance after preparation of the skin in a sterile manner.[38] Aspiration is performed with a 22-G, 1.5- to 2.5-inch spinal needle into a syringe that contains a small amount of sterile saline. In one study, 0.3 to 0.5 mL of sterile saline was injected and immediately reaspirated,[38] but dry aspiration can also be performed into the needle. The saline in the syringe can then be used to flush the contents of the needle into a plain sterile tube, which is submitted for bacterial and fungal culture. Only 3 of 11 aspirates or biopsies were positive in one study.[1] However, in another study, positive bacterial cultures were obtained in 9 of 12 disc aspirates.[38] Other specimens that may yield growth include CSF, aspirates of cellulitis or abscesses adjacent to sites of discospondylitis, or synovial fluid. When disease is present at other sites, every effort should be made to perform culture for aerobic and anaerobic bacteria and fungi from these sites in order to identify an infectious etiology.

Pathologic Findings

Gross pathologic findings in dogs with discospondylitis include the presence of pus and necrotic debris in the intervertebral disc spaces, irregularity and collapse of the disc spaces, and discoloration and friability of the vertebral endplates (Figure 85-9). Protrusion of disc material and compression of the spinal cord may be apparent. There may also be evidence of bony callus material (ankylosing spondylosis). The nature of the inflammatory infiltrates on histopathology varies with the chronicity of the lesions and the underlying cause. For example, fungal discospondylitis may be associated with granulomatous or pyogranulomatous inflammation and intralesional fungal hyphae, whereas chronic bacterial discospondylitis may be associated with neutrophilic and lymphoplasmacytic infiltrates, with perilesional fibrosis and granulation tissue. Osteonecrosis may be present, as well as necrosis of compressed spinal tissue.

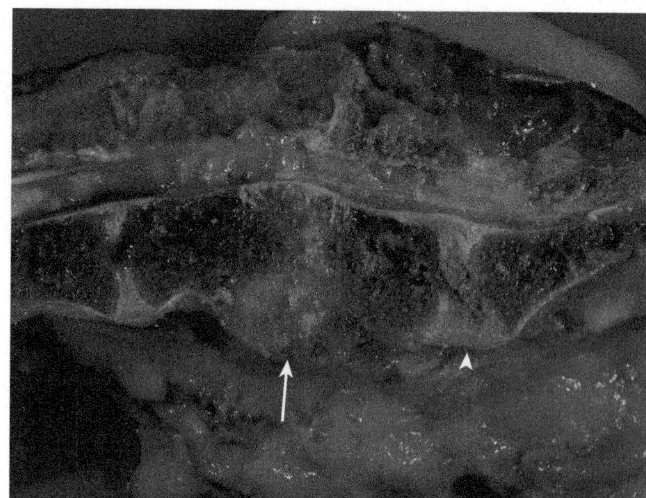

FIGURE 85-9 Vertebral column of a 4-year-old female spayed German shepherd at necropsy that had multifocal discospondylitis caused by *Aspergillus* spp. The L6-L7 disc space *(arrow)* is collapsed with degenerate disc material, sclerotic endplates, and marked ventral proliferation of bone. The lumbosacral disc space *(arrowhead)* has an irregular annulus with friable, pale tan nuclear material that protrudes ventrally. (Courtesy of the University of California, Davis, Veterinary Anatomic Pathology Service.)

Treatment and Prognosis

Treatment of discospondylitis involves prolonged antimicrobial drug treatment and strict restriction of movement for several weeks to prevent herniation of disc material or subluxation, with a gradual increase in movement once lesions have healed. It is important to stress to owners of dogs with discospondylitis that it is a serious, life-threatening condition. Analgesics such as tramadol or fentanyl patches can also be administered provided they do not encourage excessive movement. Non-steroidal anti-inflammatory drugs may also be beneficial.

The antibiotic chosen to treat discospondylitis should ideally be based on the results of culture and susceptibility. Treatment recommendations for dogs with *Brucella* discospondylitis are described in Chapter 53. Dogs with fungal discospondylitis should be treated with antifungal drugs that have activity against molds, such as voriconazole (if finances allow) or itraconazole (*not* fluconazole) with or without amphotericin B; prognosis is guarded, and lifelong treatment may be required (see Chapter 65). Dogs with culture-negative discospondylitis that have negative serum or urine *Aspergillus* galactomannan antigen tests should be treated with high doses of a drug with activity against susceptible staphylococci and *E. coli*, such as amoxicillin-clavulanic acid or cephalexin (see Table 85-2). Amoxicillin-clavulanic acid also has activity against penicillinase-producing anaerobes. However, occasionally gram-negative organisms such as *Klebsiella pneumoniae* cause discospondylitis, and these may not respond to treatment with β-lactam drugs. Addition of a fluoroquinolone or an aminoglycoside should be considered if there is no improvement after 1 week of treatment with a β-lactam drug. For dogs that are systemically unwell or that have neurologic abnormalities, antimicrobials should be administered parenterally in the hospital for as long as possible (ideally at least 10 days) before changing to oral administration. Antimicrobial drugs should be administered for at least 6 to 8 weeks; in some cases treatment may need to be extended for many months. In one study, the mean ± standard deviation for duration of antimicrobial treatment in dogs that were cured of discospondylitis was 54 ± 45 weeks; for dogs with staphylococcal infections, it was 74 ± 62 weeks.[1] Dogs with fungal discospondylitis may require lifelong treatment with antifungal drugs (see Chapter 65). Dogs should be reevaluated clinically and radiographically every 3 to 4 weeks. Improvement is characterized by resolution of bone lysis, sclerosis of bone, and vertebral fusion. Antimicrobial drug treatment should be continued until lysis resolves completely. MRI may be the most sensitive imaging technique to confirm resolution of active infection. Imaging should also be performed 1 to 2 months after antimicrobial drugs are discontinued. If clinical deterioration occurs during treatment, additional imaging (ideally with MRI) should be offered to evaluate for development of new lesions, abscessation, subluxation, fracture, or disc protrusion.

Dogs with severe neurologic deficits (such as paralysis) may require decompressive surgery, debridement of abscesses or vertebral osteomyelitis, and stabilization of the vertebral column. However, return of neurologic function can sometimes occur with antimicrobial drug treatment alone, provided deep pain is present. Decompressive surgery should be performed within 24 hours if deep pain is absent. Referral to a specialist surgeon is recommended in this situation. In one study, 9 of 27 dogs with discospondylitis received some form of decompressive surgery.[34] Physical therapy may also be beneficial in these animals.

Public Health Aspects

The most important public health consideration in dogs with discospondylitis is the possibility of *Brucella* infection. Human disease has occurred as a result of contact with dogs with *Brucella canis* discospondylitis and is typically an influenza-like illness. The possibility of *B. canis* infection should be considered in all dogs with discospondylitis, and precautions such as routine hand washing, minimization of exposure to urine, and the wearing of gloves should be taken until appropriate diagnostic testing has ruled out *Brucella* as a cause.

ARTHRITIS

Etiology, Pathogenesis, and Epidemiology

Infectious arthritis may be classified as *monoarthritis* or *polyarthritis*. Bacterial monoarthritis can follow orthopedic surgeries that involve the joint (such as TPLOs, arthroscopies, or joint arthrodesis), spread from soft tissue or bone infection at adjacent sites, or result from trauma or bite wound infections. Less commonly, monoarthritis follows systemic spread of bacteria to a single joint. Bacterial causes of monoarthritis are similar to those involved in osteomyelitis; the most common cause is *Staphylococcus* spp., especially *S. pseudintermedius* but also *S. aureus* and coagulase-negative staphylococci. Other reported causes are *Streptococcus canis* and *Streptococcus equi* subsp. *zooepidemicus, E. coli,* and *P. aeruginosa*.[39,40]

Systemic spread of bacteria to the joints more often results in polyarthritis. Infection with a variety of bacteria, protozoa, fungi, and, rarely, viruses (West Nile virus) have been associated with polyarthritis in dogs and cats. In areas where tick-borne infections are endemic, the most common bacterial causes are *Anaplasma phagocytophilum, Ehrlichia ewingii, Ehrlichia canis, Borrelia burgdorferi,* and *Rickettsia rickettsii,* but non–vector-borne bacteria such as *Streptococcus canis, Staphylococcus aureus, Erysipelothrix, Salmonella, Brucella,* and mycoplasmas (see Chapter 40) can also be involved. Although its importance as a cause of polyarthritis remains unclear, *Bartonella* should also be considered. Endocarditis is frequently (if not almost always) present in dogs with polyarthritis caused by facultative aerobic gram-positive and gram-negative bacteria, and among dogs with endocarditis, *Streptococcus canis* infections are most likely to be associated with polyarthritis. Worldwide, the most important cause of protozoal polyarthritis in dogs is *Leishmania*. Fungal polyarthritis is uncommon but can result from infection by dimorphic fungi and, rarely, molds such as *Aspergillus*. Infectious polyarthritis is an important differential diagnosis for primary (idiopathic) immune-mediated polyarthritis (IMPA) in dogs. Although infectious polyarthritis is less common than primary IMPA, failure to identify an underlying infection can have disastrous consequences when treatment with immunosuppressive drugs is initiated.

Clinical Features

Clinical signs of monoarthritis may be acute or chronic in onset and include variable fever, lethargy, inappetence, lameness that involves a single limb, and a swollen joint that may be erythematous, warm to the touch, and occasionally drain purulent or blood-tinged fluid (Figure 85-10). The draining lymph node may be enlarged and firm. The most common joints affected in one study were the stifle and elbow joints, followed by the tarsi and coxofemoral joints, and signs developed within 2 to over 8 weeks after articular or periarticular surgery.[40] In polyarthritis, multiple peripheral joints are affected, and dogs (and less commonly cats) show signs of recumbency, reluctance to move, generalized peripheral lymphadenopathy, a stiff gait, and/or shifting leg lameness; drainage of fluid is not usually apparent. Dogs with bacterial polyarthritis can also show signs of severe sepsis (see Chapter 86 as well as the Case Example in Chapter 45).

Diagnosis

Diagnosis of infectious arthritis is based on the history, clinical signs, and cytology and culture of joint fluid; serologic assays for *Brucella canis* and fungal pathogens; and/or molecular diagnostic and/or serologic testing for vector-borne pathogens in endemic regions. Blood cultures may also allow identification of the underlying etiology in dogs with bacterial polyarthritis. As for discospondylitis, dogs with bacterial polyarthritis should ideally be evaluated for evidence of disease at other sites with thoracic

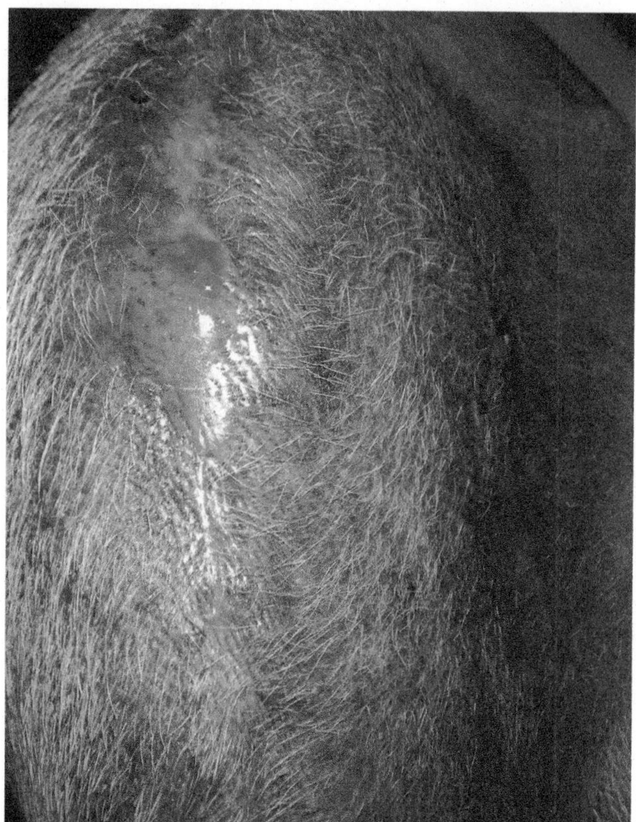

FIGURE 85-10 Surgical site of a 5-year-old male neutered mastiff dog with non–weight-bearing lameness and a draining skin lesion that developed along the incision site approximately 1 month after a tibial plateau leveling operation. The right stifle was swollen and warm. Synovial fluid aspirated from the joint was red and turbid and contained 161,550 nucleated cells/μL (98% nondegenerate neutrophils) and 90,000 red blood cells/μL. Aerobic and anaerobic cultures of the fluid yielded a methicillin-resistant, multidrug-resistant *Staphylococcus pseudintermedius* that was resistant to all β-lactams, macrolides, and clindamycin, fluoroquinolones, and trimethoprim-sulfamethoxazole. The infection was treated successfully with joint exploration, lavage, and oral chloramphenicol for 8 weeks.

radiographs, spinal radiographs (for concurrent discospondylitis) and abdominal ultrasound, echocardiography (for endocarditis), and aerobic bacterial culture of the urine.

Laboratory Abnormalities

Routine laboratory testing in animals with bacterial arthritis typically shows leukocytosis due to a neutrophilia, which can be accompanied by bandemia. Thrombocytopenia may be present in dogs with bacteremia or vector-borne bacterial infections and should prompt diagnostic evaluation for vector-borne infections with PCR assays and serology. Urinalysis may be normal or show pyuria, bacteriuria, proteinuria, and/or cylindruria in dogs with concurrent aerobic bacterial urinary tract infections.

Synovial fluid from affected joints is often yellow or blood-tinged (normal synovial fluid is clear), cloudy, increased in volume, and thin or watery in consistency. Cytologic examination of synovial fluid reveals increased numbers of leukocytes (>5000 cells/μL), with a predominance of nondegenerate and/or degenerate neutrophils. Importantly, in the majority of dogs with septic arthritis, degenerate neutrophils are not visualized,[39,40] so the presence of only nondegenerate neutrophils does not rule out an underlying bacterial infection. Rarely, bacteria or fungal organisms are visualized extracellularly or within leukocytes. Morulae are occasionally seen within neutrophils in synovial fluid of dogs infected with *A. phagocytophilum* or *E. ewingii* (see Figure 29-3C).

Diagnostic Imaging

Radiographs of the joints in dogs and cats with infectious arthritis most often reveal soft tissue swelling and joint effusion. In severe and chronic bacterial monoarthritis, associated osteomyelitis may be present, with subchondral bone lysis, articular erosion, and periarticular new bone formation.

Microbiologic Tests

Isolation and Identification

Confirmation of bacterial arthritis requires culture of synovial fluid or of the synovium itself. Synovial fluid from dogs with neutrophilic polyarthritis should be submitted for aerobic bacterial culture and susceptibility, and anaerobic, fungal, or *Mycoplasma* culture should at least be considered if the history is suggestive. Situations in which anaerobic culture may be indicated include a history of foreign body (such as plant awn) exposure or bite wounds. Although rare, the possibility of *Mycoplasma* arthritis should be considered in cats and dogs with a history of immune compromise, surgery, or bite wounds, and when treatment with β-lactam drugs fails (see Chapter 40). Dogs with fungal polyarthritis may have lesions elsewhere (e.g., chorioretinitis, pulmonary disease) that support a diagnosis of disseminated fungal disease. However, anaerobic and *Mycoplasma* culture may be insensitive (especially when there are delays in specimen transport to the laboratory); *Mycoplasma* and fungal cultures require prolonged incubation; and anaerobes, fungi, and mycoplasmas tend to have predictable susceptibilities. Aerobic blood cultures may assist in identification of bacteria involved in polyarthritis.

If arthroscopy or arthrotomy is performed as part of evaluation and treatment of bacterial monoarthritis, a biopsy of the synovium could also be submitted for culture and susceptibility and may yield growth when synovial fluid culture is negative.[39] In most cases, synovial fluid culture alone is sufficient for diagnosis of bacterial arthritis.

Treatment and Prognosis

Treatment of infectious arthritis depends on whether one joint is involved or whether polyarthritis is present, as well as on the identity of the causative agent. Infectious monoarthritis may require surgical exploration, lavage and drainage, and treatment with appropriate antimicrobial drugs based on the results of culture and susceptibility. Monoarthritis is considered a surgical emergency, and lavage should be performed immediately after diagnosis, either via an ingress-egress approach or with open surgery. For ingress-egress lavage, large-bore (14- to 16-G) needles are inserted percutaneously into two to three fluid pockets around the joint while the animal is heavily sedated or anesthetized. Several liters of sterile saline is then administered through one portal under pressure and allowed to drain from the other portal(s). The sites of ingress and egress are switched until the fluid becomes clear. Arthroscopy can also be used. Arthrotomy may be necessary if there are large accumulations of fibrin or inspissated purulent debris that cannot be effectively flushed from the joint. If implants are present, they should be removed when healing has occurred or if stabilization has failed. If the implant is stable but the bone has not healed, lavage is performed and the implant left in place, because bone can heal if rigidly stable despite infection. Ultimately, the implant must be removed to resolve the infection; removal should be done as soon as possible after healing. Antimicrobial drugs should initially be given parenterally if possible. Treatment should continue until implants can be removed if left in place. Once implants are removed, treatment may need to be continued for another 2 to 4 weeks. If local antibiotic therapy is used in associated osteomyelitis lesions (i.e., impregnated beads), systemic antimicrobial drug treatment should also be used. The prognosis depends on the degree of cartilage and bone destruction, the degree to which progressive osteoarthritis occurs, and the joint affected. Unfortunately, evidence-based clinical studies that document long-term prognosis or prognostic indicators for infectious monoarthritis are not available. In one retrospective study, dogs that fully recovered tended to have a shorter duration of lameness before treatment (median, 11 days compared with 26 days) and lower synovial fluid cell counts (median, 54×10^9 cells/mL compared with 100×10^9 cells/mL) than dogs that never fully recovered, and had significantly lower body weights (median, 29 kg compared with 44 kg).[40]

Polyarthritis caused by vector-borne bacteria usually responds to treatment with doxycycline within 24 to 48 hours. Antimicrobials for treatment of polyarthritis caused by other bacteria should be selected based on the results of cytologic examination of synovial fluid (cocci versus rods) and culture and susceptibility of blood or synovial fluid. Because streptococci, staphylococci, and *Erysipelothrix* are usually involved, a β-lactam drug such as amoxicillin-clavulanic acid (or amoxicillin if streptococci are more likely) could be used. Because bacterial polyarthritis is frequently associated with endocarditis or discospondylitis, the duration of treatment should be based on resolution of these lesions. The reader is referred to Chapter 86 for additional information on treatment of bacteremia and sepsis.

Public Health Aspects

Polyarthritis can be caused by organisms of public health significance, such as *Salmonella, Brucella, S. aureus*, pathogenic fungi, *Leishmania*, and vector-borne bacterial pathogens of importance to human health. This should be kept in mind when handling dogs with polyarthritis. Care should be taken to avoid needle-stick injuries during venipuncture, arthrocentesis, and aspiration of other tissues such as lymph nodes. Deep sedation or anesthesia is recommended for arthrocentesis.

CASE EXAMPLE

Signalment: "Tilly," a 10-year-old female spayed greyhound/pit bull terrier mix from Davis, CA (Figure 85-11).

History: Tilly was brought to the University of California, Davis, VMTH Orthopedic Surgery service for evaluation of a draining tract on her left medial proximal tibia that developed after a tibial tubercle advancement (TTA) surgery for left cranial cruciate ligament tear. The ligament tear had been diagnosed at the VMTH 15 months previously after an acute onset of lameness, and the surgery was performed 2 months after diagnosis at another veterinary hospital after there had been no improvement with conservative management (activity restriction and anti-inflammatory drugs). Immediately after the surgery, the dog was placed on a 10-day course of doxycycline. The tract was first observed 2 weeks after the doxycycline course had finished, and the owner (a veterinary student) noted that the tract subsequently healed over, then drained again. When the wound initially appeared, treatment with doxycycline was reinstituted for a month, with no improvement. A radiograph of the limb was performed at the end of the course of treatment at the VMTH. Soft tissue swelling was identified at the medial aspect of the stifle, but there was no radiographic evidence of implant infection or motion. Regional osteopenia of the left tibial tuberosity and proximal tibia was present, and there was progressive left stifle osteoarthrosis. Culture of the wound yielded very small numbers of *Streptococcus canis* and a coagulase-negative *Staphylococcus*. The wound subsequently closed over again and antibiotic treatment was not initiated, but 11 months later the tract reappeared. Since the surgery, the incision had appeared healthy. Tilly had been bearing progressively more weight on the limb, although some lameness persisted. Other treatments had included activity restriction and carprofen (2 mg/kg PO q12h) for pain relief. Tilly had no other significant medical history apart from multiple lipomas that had been evaluated with fine-needle aspiration cytology, which had not changed in size.

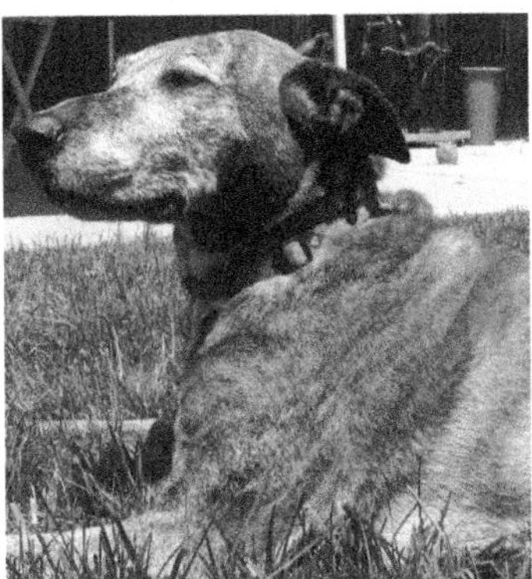

FIGURE 85-11 Tilly, 10-year old female spayed greyhound – pit bull terrier mix that developed osteomyelitis at the site of a left tibial tuberosity advancement surgery.

Physical Examination:

Body Weight: 37.2 kg.

General: Bright, alert, responsive. T = 101.0°F (38.3°C), HR = 80 beats/min, panting.

Eyes, Ears, Nose, and Throat: No abnormalities were identified apart from moderate periodontal disease.

Musculoskeletal: Left pelvic limb lameness was present, but there was intermittent right pelvic limb lameness and muscle atrophy of both pelvic limbs. There was pain on extension of both coxofemoral joints. Examination of the left pelvic limb revealed a 1-cm, open round wound on the medial aspect of the proximal left tibia, which oozed serosanguineous fluid. A positive cranial drawer sign and tibial thrust were present.

All Other Systems: No clinically significant abnormalities were detected.

Imaging Findings:

Plain Radiographs (Pelvis): Bilaterally there was poor coverage of the femoral heads by the acetabulae. The femoral heads and necks were thickened and irregularly margined. There was periarticular osteophytosis of the acetabulae. Atrophy of the pelvic musculature was appreciated bilaterally although somewhat worse on the left than the right. Findings were consistent with bilateral hip dysplasia with severe degenerative change.

Plain Radiographs (Left Stifle): The implants associated with the TTA procedure were in place and intact (see Figure 85-5, *A* and *B*). The osteotomy site had filled in with bone to some extent, although the site was still visible nearly its entire length, and bridging bone was absent at the proximal aspect of the osteotomy and around the basket implant. There was thinning of the cortical bone adjacent to the plate that was associated with the tibial tuberosity and proximal tibial diaphysis, and mild lucency surrounded the medial aspect of the distalmost screw, which suggested implant-associated osteomyelitis. A gap was present between the bone plate and the tibia. Distal to the bone plates, there was smooth periosteal proliferation. The patella was displaced distally. There was moderate intracapsular soft tissue swelling of the stifle. There was also persistent, moderate periarticular osteophytosis of the distal femur and proximal tibia.

Diagnosis: TTA implant-associated osteomyelitis with incomplete union of osteotomy; severe canine hip dysplasia.

Treatment: Surgical exploration of the left stifle joint was performed. The draining tract was followed to the plate and screws. The TTA plate and screws were removed. The cage was removed by drilling around it, which left a 2-cm round defect in the tibia. During the procedure, it was discovered that a titanium plate had been used together with 316L steel screws, which led to concerns that osteomyelitis may have developed secondary to a galvanic reaction. The area was extensively flushed, and the defect was filled with calcium sulfate beads. Beads were also placed in the area previously occupied by the plate (see Figure 85-5, *C*). The fascia, subcutaneous tissue, and skin were closed, and a modified Robert-Jones bandage was placed. Aerobic and anaerobic bacterial cultures of the implant yielded small numbers of methicillin-susceptible *Staphylococcus pseudintermedius*. The organism was resistant to ampicillin, penicillin, ticarcillin, and doxycycline. Tilly was therefore treated with amoxicillin-clavulanic acid (10 mg/kg PO q12h). At the time of suture removal 2 weeks later, Tilly was weight bearing on the left pelvic limb, and the draining tract had resolved. A small draining tract reappeared 2 weeks later, and a swab from the tract again grew *S. pseudintermedius* with the same antibiogram, but only from the enrichment broth. Treatment was continued for an additional month, all lesions resolved, and lameness was reduced. A year later (at the time of writing) the dog was doing well and there had been no recurrence of draining tracts (see Figure 85-5, *D*).

Comments: Diagnosis and treatment of osteomyelitis in this case was delayed because of the lag in radiographic changes and the appearance and disappearance of the draining tract. This illustrates the difficulties associated with diagnosis of osteomyelitis. Although unconfirmed, use of two different metals may have contributed to development of osteomyelitis in this dog, which required costly and difficult surgical intervention with implant removal. The defects were closed with biodegradable beads and infection resolved after 2 months of systemic antimicrobial drug treatment, based on the results of culture and susceptibility.

SUGGESTED READINGS

Burkert BA, Kerwin SC, Hosgood GL, et al. Signalment and clinical features of discospondylitis in dogs: 513 cases (1980-2001). J Am Vet Med Assoc. 2005;227:268-275.

Clements DN, Owen MR, Mosley JR, et al. Retrospective study of bacterial infective arthritis in 31 dogs. J Small Anim Pract. 2005;46:171-176.

Fischer A, Mahaffey MB, Oliver JE. Fluoroscopically guided percutaneous disk aspiration in 10 dogs with discospondylitis. J Vet Intern Med. 1997;11:284-287.

Thompson AM, Bergh MS, Wang C, et al. Tibial plateau levelling osteotomy implant removal: a retrospective analysis of 129 cases. Vet Comp Orthop Traumatol. 2011;24:450-456.

REFERENCES

1. Burkert BA, Kerwin SC, Hosgood GL, et al. Signalment and clinical features of discospondylitis in dogs: 513 cases (1980-2001). J Am Vet Med Assoc. 2005;227:268-275.
2. Pacchiana PD, Morris E, Gillings SL, et al. Surgical and postoperative complications associated with tibial plateau leveling osteotomy in dogs with cranial cruciate ligament rupture: 397 cases (1998-2001). J Am Vet Med Assoc. 2003;222:184-193.
3. Priddy 2nd NH, Tomlinson JL, Dodam JR, et al. Complications with and owner assessment of the outcome of tibial plateau leveling osteotomy for treatment of cranial cruciate ligament rupture in dogs: 193 cases (1997-2001). J Am Vet Med Assoc. 2003;222:1726-1732.
4. Stauffer KD, Tuttle TA, Elkins AD, et al. Complications associated with 696 tibial plateau leveling osteotomies (2001-2003). J Am Anim Hosp Assoc. 2006;42:44-50.
5. Fitzpatrick N, Solano MA. Predictive variables for complications after TPLO with stifle inspection by arthrotomy in 1000 consecutive dogs. Vet Surg. 2010;39:460-474.
6. Griffiths GL, Bellenger CR. A retrospective study of osteomyelitis in dogs and cats. Aust Vet J. 1979;55:587-591.
7. Stevenson S, Olmstead ML, Kowalski J. Bacterial culturing for prediction of postoperative complications following open fracture repair in small animals. Vet Surg. 1986;15:99-102.
8. Johnson KA, Lomas GR, Wood AK. Osteomyelitis in dogs and cats caused by anaerobic bacteria. Aust Vet J. 1984;61:57-61.
9. Muir P, Johnson KA. Anaerobic bacteria isolated from osteomyelitis in dogs and cats. Vet Surg. 1992;21:463-466.
10. Johnson KA. Osteomyelitis in dogs and cats. J Am Vet Med Assoc. 1994;204:1882-1887.

11. Labbe JL, Peres O, Leclair O, et al. Acute osteomyelitis in children: the pathogenesis revisited? Orthop Traumatol Surg Res. 2010;96:268-275.
12. Thompson AM, Bergh MS, Wang C, et al. Tibial plateau levelling osteotomy implant removal: a retrospective analysis of 129 cases. Vet Comp Orthop Traumatol. 2011;24:450-456.
13. Gallie WE. First recurrence of osteomyelitis eighty years after infection. J Bone Joint Surg Br. 1951:110-111:33-B.
14. Braden TD, Tvedten HW, Mostosky UV. The sensitivity and specificity of radiology and histopathology in the diagnosis of post-traumatic osteomyelitis. Vet Comp Orthop Traumatol. 1989;3:98-103.
15. Southwood LL, Kawcak CE, McIlwraith CW, et al. Use of scintigraphy for assessment of fracture healing and early diagnosis of osteomyelitis following fracture repair in rabbits. Am J Vet Res. 2003;64:736-745.
16. Kruskal JB. Can USPIO-enhanced spinal MR imaging help distinguish acute infectious osteomyelitis from chronic infectious and inflammatory processes? Radiology. 2008;248:1-3.
17. Bardet JF, Hohn RB, Basinger R. Open drainage and delayed autogenous cancellous bone grafting for treatment of chronic osteomyelitis in dogs and cats. J Am Vet Med Assoc. 1983;183:312-317.
18. Braden TD, Johnson CA, Wakenell P, et al. Efficacy of clindamycin in the treatment of *Staphylococcus aureus* osteomyelitis in dogs. J Am Vet Med Assoc. 1988;192:1721-1725.
19. Brown A, Bennett D. Gentamicin-impregnated polymethylmethacrylate beads for the treatment of septic arthritis. Vet Rec. 1988;123:625-626.
20. Ham K, Griffon D, Seddighi M, et al. Clinical application of tobramycin-impregnated calcium sulfate beads in six dogs (2002-2004). J Am Anim Hosp Assoc. 2008;44:320-326.
21. Dernell WS, Withrow SJ, Straw RC, et al. Clinical response to antibiotic impregnated polymethyl methacrylate bead implantation of dogs with severe infections after limb sparing and allograft replacement—18 cases (1994-1996). Vet Comp Orthop Traumatol. 1989;11:94-99.
22. Gogia JS, Meehan JP, Di Cesare PE, et al. Local antibiotic therapy in osteomyelitis. Semin Plast Surg. 2009;23:100-107.
23. Miliani K, L'Heriteau F, Astagneau P. Non-compliance with recommendations for the practice of antibiotic prophylaxis and risk of surgical site infection: results of a multilevel analysis from the INCISO Surveillance Network. J Antimicrob Chemother. 2009;64:1307-1315.
24. Serhan H, Slivka M, Albert T, et al. Is galvanic corrosion between titanium alloy and stainless steel spinal implants a clinical concern? Spine J. 2004;4:379-387.
25. Soares Magalhaes RJ, Loeffler A, Lindsay J, et al. Risk factors for methicillin-resistant *Staphylococcus aureus* (MRSA) infection in dogs and cats: a case-control study. Vet Res. 2010;41:55.
26. Schultz RM, Johnson EG, Wisner ER, et al. Clinicopathologic and diagnostic imaging characteristics of systemic aspergillosis in 30 dogs. J Vet Intern Med. 2008;22:851-859.
27. Packer RA, Coates JR, Cook CR, et al. Sublumbar abscess and discospondylitis in a cat. Vet Radiol Ultrasound. 2005;46:396-399.
28. Norsworthy GD. Discospondylitis as a cause of posterior paresis. Feline Pract. 1979;9:39-40.
29. Aroch I, Shamir M, Harmelin A. Lumbar discospondylitis and meningomyelitis caused by *Escherichia coli* in a cat. Feline Pract. 1999;27:20-22.
30. Watson E, Roberts RE. Discospondylitis in a cat. Vet Radiol. 1993;34:397-398.
31. Malik RM, Latler M, Love DN. Bacterial discospondylitis in a cat. J Small Anim Pract. 1990;31:404-406.
32. Harris JM, Chen AV, Tucker RL, et al. Clinical features and magnetic resonance imaging characteristics of diskospondylitis in dogs: 23 cases (1997-2010). J Am Vet Med Assoc. 2013;242:359-365.
33. Kerwin SC, Lewis DD, Hribernik TN, et al. Discospondylitis associated with *Brucella canis* infection in dogs: 14 cases (1980-1991). J Am Vet Med Assoc. 1992;201:1253-1257.
34. Davis MJ, Dewey CW, Walker MA, et al. Contrast radiographic findings in canine bacterial discospondylitis: a multicenter, retrospective study of 27 cases. J Am Anim Hosp Assoc. 2000;36:81-85.
35. Carrera I, Sullivan M, McConnell F, et al. Magnetic resonance imaging features of discospondylitis in dogs. Vet Radiol Ultrasound. 2011;52:125-131.
36. Garcia RS, Wheat LJ, Cook A, et al. Sensitivity and specificity of a blood and urine galactomannan antigen assay for diagnosis of systemic aspergillosis in dogs. J Vet Intern Med. 2012:Epub.
37. Gendron K, Doherr MG, Gavin P, et al. Magnetic resonance imaging characterization of vertebral endplate changes in the dog. Vet Radiol Ultrasound. 2012;53:50-56.
38. Fischer A, Mahaffey MB, Oliver JE. Fluoroscopically guided percutaneous disk aspiration in 10 dogs with discospondylitis. J Vet Intern Med. 1997;11:284-287.
39. Marchevsky AM, Read RA. Bacterial septic arthritis in 19 dogs. Aust Vet J. 1999;77:233-237.
40. Clements DN, Owen MR, Mosley JR, et al. Retrospective study of bacterial infective arthritis in 31 dogs. J Small Anim Pract. 2005;46:171-176.

CHAPTER 86

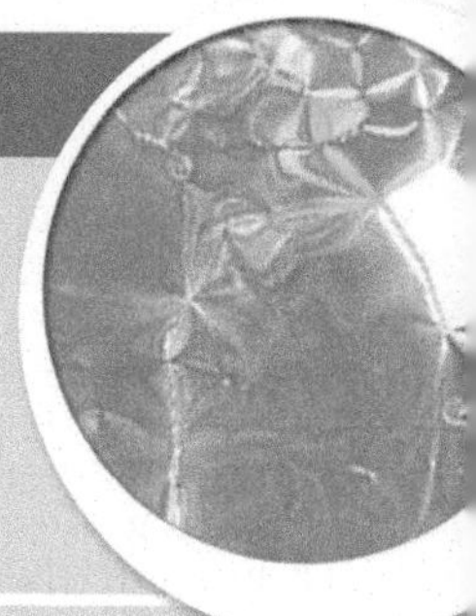

Infections of the Cardiovascular System

Jane E. Sykes and Steven Epstein

> **Overview of Cardiovascular System Infections**
>
> Causes: Most often staphylococci, streptococci, and *Escherichia coli* are involved. Gram-negative bacterial etiologies predominate in cats. Culture-negative infections of the bloodstream may be caused by *Bartonella* spp. or other fastidious bacteria. Anaerobes and mycobacteria are less commonly involved. *Rickettsia rickettsii* can cause vasculitis and myocarditis. Viruses (e.g., parvoviruses), fungi, and protozoal organisms can also infect the bloodstream and myocardium.
>
> Geographic Distribution: Worldwide
>
> Major Clinical Signs: Highly variable. Fever, inappetence, lethargy, and tachycardia are common. Vomiting and/or diarrhea can also occur. Additional findings in infective endocarditis include cardiac murmurs, arrhythmias, lameness, and neurologic signs due to thromboembolic disease. Spinal pain, paresis, or paralysis may occur when discospondylitis complicates bacteremia or fungemia.
>
> Differential Diagnoses: Noninfectious conditions that can mimic sepsis include pancreatitis, trauma, hypoadrenocorticism, heat stroke, anaphylaxis, pulmonary thromboembolism, hemorrhage, cardiac tamponade, and some toxicities. Dogs with primary immune-mediated disorders may show clinical signs that resemble those of chronic bacteremia and infective endocarditis. For suspected infectious pericarditis, the major differential diagnoses are idiopathic or benign pericardial effusion and neoplastic disorders.
>
> Human Health Significance: Dogs and cats with cardiovascular infections may be infected with pathogens that have the potential to cause disease in humans, such as *Salmonella*, *Bartonella*, and *Brucella* spp.

Etiologic Agents, Epidemiology, and Clinical Features

Bacterial infections of the cardiovascular system include bacteremia, infective endocarditis, myocarditis, and infectious pericarditis. These infections are frequently associated with *sepsis*, or the host systemic inflammatory response to infection. When sepsis is associated with hypotension and distant organ dysfunction, the terms *septic shock* and *severe sepsis* are used, respectively. These terms have been clearly defined in human medicine[1] and adapted for use in small animals (Table 86-1). *Septicemia* is a term that has been used interchangeably with bacteremia by veterinary medical and medical professionals, but it is incompletely defined, and as a result, the use of this term is no longer recommended.

Bacteremia

Bacteremia can be divided into *uncomplicated* and *complicated bacteremia* (see Table 86-1). Transient, low-level (≤10 CFU/mL) subclinical bacteremia follows a variety of procedures such as dental prophylaxis, endoscopy, gastrointestinal surgery, and catheter placement. This is typically cleared rapidly (within 15 to 30 minutes) by a functional mononuclear phagocyte system. However, persistent release of large numbers of bacteria into the bloodstream can overwhelm the host immune response and culminate in clinically significant bacteremia. Overwhelming bacteremia can occur with disorders such as pyelonephritis, pyothorax, severe pyoderma, bacterial peritonitis, pyometra, pneumonia, pancreatitis, a variety of gastrointestinal disorders, bite wounds, orthopedic infections, or catheter-related infections. Underlying immune system dysfunction (such as occurs with diabetes mellitus, malignancy, and neutropenia) also predisposes to clinically significant bacteremia, because bacteria multiply unhindered in the bloodstream.

The most common organisms isolated from the blood of sick, bacteremic dogs are *Staphylococcus* spp., *Streptococcus* spp. (especially *Streptococcus canis*), and *Escherichia coli* (Table 86-2).[2] Less than 10% of bacteremic dogs in the author's hospital are infected with anaerobes, but in a study of critically ill dogs and cats from Colorado, anaerobes were isolated from 31% of 39 dogs and 40% of 10 cats.[3] With the exception of *Bartonella* and hemoplasmas, bacteremia is less commonly recognized in cats than in dogs and usually results from infection with gram-negative bacterial pathogens.[2] Polymicrobial infections of the blood are common and typically occur in 10% to 20% of dogs and cats with positive blood culture results. Mixed infections with two or more different strains of a single bacterial species can also occur. Polymicrobial infections often occur when anaerobes are involved or when bacteremia develops secondary to compromise of the gastrointestinal tract.

In addition to sepsis and septic shock, bacteremia may be followed by the development of infective endocarditis (IE), discospondylitis, and metastatic abscess formation in a variety of tissues. Chronic bacteremia may trigger secondary immune-mediated disorders, especially immune-mediated polyarthritis or glomerulonephritis, and rarely immune-mediated hemolytic anemia. This can result in erroneous diagnosis of a primary immune-mediated disorder and inappropriate treatment with immunosuppressive drugs, sometimes with a fatal outcome.

TABLE 86-1
Definitions That Apply to Cardiovascular Infections in Dogs and Cats

Term	Definition
Bacteremia	The presence of viable or cultivable bacteria in the bloodstream
Uncomplicated bacteremia	Positive blood culture results and exclusion of endocarditis; no implants; negative follow-up cultures 2-4 days after the initial set; defervescence within 72 hours of initiation of effective treatment; and no evidence of metastatic sites of infection
Complicated bacteremia	Animals with positive blood culture results that do not meet the criteria for uncomplicated bacteremia
Fungemia	The presence of viable fungi in the bloodstream
Systemic inflammatory response syndrome (SIRS)	The clinical manifestation of systemic inflammation due to both noninfectious and infectious etiologies. Criteria for dogs and cats have been adapted from those in human medicine, but these have varied slightly in the cutoff values used. A single definition for dogs or cats has not been widely accepted. SIRS criteria are nonspecific and must be interpreted in light of an underlying disease. Dogs: 2 of 4 of temperature <100°F or >103.0°F (hypothermia or fever), HR > 140 beats/min, nonpanting RR > 30 breaths/min or PCO_2 < 32 mm Hg (venous or arterial), WBC <6000 or > 16,000 cells/μL, or >3% band neutrophils Cats: 3 of 4 of temperature <100°F or >103.5°F, HR < 140 or >225 bpm, RR > 40 breaths/min, WBC > 19,500 or <5000 cells/μL, or >5% band neutrophils
Sepsis	SIRS due to a proven or clinically suspected infection
Severe sepsis	Sepsis that is accompanied by dysfunction of organs remote from the site of infection, or sepsis-induced tissue hypoperfusion
Sepsis-induced tissue hypoperfusion	Sepsis that is accompanied with hypotension, an elevated lactate concentration, or oliguria either before or after adequate fluid loading
Septic shock	Sepsis that is accompanied by hypotension (systolic blood pressure < 90 mm Hg or mean arterial pressure < 70 mm Hg) that does not resolve with fluid resuscitation alone (i.e., vasopressor therapy is required)
Multiple organ dysfunction syndrome (MODS)	Dysfunction of two or more organ systems (distant to site of infection) in an animal with SIRS/sepsis
Infective endocarditis	Infection of one or more endocardial surfaces of the heart; almost always involves a cardiac valve

Sepsis

Bacteremia does not need to be present for sepsis to occur, but the clinical signs of bacteremia reflect the presence of sepsis (i.e., the host inflammatory response to infection). An understanding of the pathogenesis of sepsis has been critical for the development of drugs to improve survival, but it is complex and not fully understood. In summary, sepsis occurs when components of microbes (known as *pathogen-associated molecular pattern molecules*, or PAMPs) activate a host inflammatory response when they bind to pattern-recognition receptors (PRRs) such as Toll-like receptors (TLRs) and nucleotide-binding domain, leucine-rich repeat containing proteins (NLRs).[3a] The lipid A portion of bacterial lipopolysaccharide (LPS) is especially well known for its ability to stimulate this response (see Chapter 36), but other molecules, such as peptidoglycan, flagellin, DNA, and viral double-stranded RNA, may also be involved. Superantigens of gram-positive bacteria induce a cytokine cascade through simultaneous activation of large numbers of T cells (see Chapter 34). Bacterial LPS binds to an acute phase reactant protein called *LPS binding protein*, which transfers the LPS to CD14, a receptor on the surface of phagocytes.[4] CD14 then transfers the LPS to TLR4, which transmits the signal to the cell interior. This leads to activation of NF-κB and the secretion of cytokines such as TNF-α and Il-1β. The released cytokines induce fever (which may serve to limit bacterial growth), and cause further lymphocyte activation and release of proinflammatory cytokines. Damaged host cells also release molecules (*damage-associated molecular pattern molecules*, or DAMPs) that bind to TLRs and stimulate cytokine release. Important DAMPs recognized in humans include a chromatin-associated protein known as *high mobility group box-1* (HMGB1) and cellular DNA. The cascade of cytokines that is produced in response to DAMPs and PAMPs in turn induces the release and activation of a huge variety of mediators, such as complement, colony stimulating factors, prostacyclin, thromboxane, platelet-activating factor, coagulation factors, histamine, serotonin, nitric oxide, angiotensin II, and endothelin-1. Many of these mediators serve to recruit large numbers of immune cells and trigger fibrin deposition in order to localize, control, and ultimately eliminate the infection. Other molecules, such as cortisol and epinephrine, act to control the inflammatory response. Endothelial cell damage results in increased exposure of tissue factor (which activates the extrinsic coagulation pathway) as well as von Willebrand's factor. Endothelial cell damage also results in decreased expression of thrombomodulin, an important anticoagulant that normally binds thrombin and prevents it from cleaving fibrinogen.

TABLE 86-2

Organisms That May Be Cultured Using Routine Blood Culture Methods from the Bloodstream of Dogs and Cats with Bacteremia*

	Dogs	Cats
Common (>10% of isolates)	• *Staphylococcus* spp., including *S. pseudintermedius*, *S. aureus*, and coagulase-negative staphylococci • *Streptococcus* spp., especially *S. canis*, but also *S. bovis* complex organisms and rarely other streptococci • *Escherichia coli*	• *Escherichia coli* • Other Enterobacteriaceae (*Klebsiella pneumoniae*, *Citrobacter freundii*, *Enterobacter cloacae*) • Anaerobes
Uncommon (1% to 10% of isolates)	• *Enterococcus* spp. • *Klebsiella pneumoniae*, *Serratia* spp., *Enterobacter cloacae* • *Pasteurella canis* and *Pasteurella dagmatis* • *Pseudomonas aeruginosa* • Anaerobes (*Clostridium perfringens*, *Prevotella* spp., *Bacteroides* spp., *Fusobacterium* spp., *Actinomyces* spp., *Peptostreptococcus* spp.)	• *Salmonella* spp. • Non-Enterobacteriaceae gram-negative bacteria (*Pasteurella multocida*, *Pseudomonas aeruginosa*, *Acinetobacter baumannii*) • Staphylococci • Streptococci
Rare (≤1% of isolates)	• *Erysipelothrix* spp. • *Brucella* spp. • *Citrobacter freundii* • *Acinetobacter* spp. • *Salmonella* spp. • *Mycobacterium* spp. • *Campylobacter* spp. • Other nosocomial pathogens, e.g., *Ralstonia pickettii*, *Burkholderia cepacia*	• *Enterococcus* spp.

*Not including fastidious organisms such as *Bartonella* spp.

The thrombomodulin-thrombin complex also activates protein C, which binds to protein S; the activated protein C–protein S complex degrades activated coagulation factors Va and VIIIa and prevents coagulation. Recombinant activated protein C has been the subject of much attention and controversy as a specific treatment for sepsis in human patients (see Treatment).

When the inflammatory response to infection is not effectively controlled or localized, the end result is systemic hypotension, tachycardia, increased vascular permeability, leukocytosis, activation of the coagulation cascade, and disordered tissue perfusion as a result of microcirculatory disturbances, volume depletion, and depressed myocardial function. This leads to further damage to host cells, lactic acidosis, and multiple organ dysfunction. Impaired perfusion, tissue hypoxia, and endothelial cell damage may have a wide range of effects on organ function (Table 86-3). Cats may be particularly susceptible to acute lung injury in sepsis, whereas gastrointestinal and/or hepatic dysfunction is often observed in dogs. Clinical signs of severe sepsis in dogs often include fever, obtundation, tachycardia, bounding or weak pulses, bright red mucous membranes, shortened capillary refill time, icterus, and tachypnea. However, many dogs with sepsis are evaluated when in the hypodynamic phase, with tachycardia, poor pulse quality, prolonged capillary refill time, and cold extremities. Cats may show obtundation, pale mucous membranes or icterus, abdominal pain, poor pulse quality, bradycardia, and/or tachypnea and may either be febrile or hypothermic.[5]

Infective Endocarditis

The reported incidence of canine IE has ranged from fewer than 0.1% of cases seen at veterinary teaching hospitals to approximately 1% of cases presenting to veterinary cardiologists.[6-9] IE is uncommonly diagnosed in cats. Dogs with IE are typically middle aged to older, large-breed dogs such as German shepherds, golden and Labrador retrievers, Weimaraners, mastiffs, and Rottweilers. For unclear reasons, male dogs are affected approximately twice as often as females. Factors that predispose to IE are similar to those that predispose to continuous bacteremia. However, virulence factors possessed by bacteria subsequently affect whether IE develops, which explains why some bacterial species (especially gram-positive bacteria) are more likely to produce IE than others (gram-negative bacteria). Although valvular heart defects, especially congenital defects such as subaortic stenosis, may predispose young dogs to development of IE, the vast majority of dogs with subaortic stenosis never develop IE, and more than 80% of dogs with IE have no identifiable underlying cardiac abnormality.[8,10] Furthermore, IE is rarely diagnosed in small-breed dogs, which are predisposed to myxomatous mitral valve degeneration. One study also found no association between periodontal disease and IE in dogs.[10]

The most commonly reported etiologic agents in canine IE are streptococci, staphylococci, and, to a lesser extent, gram-negative rods, enterococci, and *Bartonella* spp. (Table 86-4).[7,10-13] Organisms that are less commonly incriminated include fungi, gram-positive rods, mycobacteria, and anaerobes. In dogs, the mitral and/or the aortic valves are most commonly affected (Figure 86-1). The larger, septal leaflet of the mitral valve is more commonly affected than the mural leaflet.[8] The tricuspid valve and ventricular wall are rarely involved. This distribution correlates with the degree of pressure that rests on each closed valve. Classically, vegetative lesions develop along the line of valve closure.

TABLE 86-3

Potential Effects of Sepsis on Organ Function

Organ	Clinical Abnormalities
Neurologic system	Obtundation, rarely focal signs and seizures; autonomic dysfunction
Heart	Heart rate variability, arrhythmias (ventricular or supraventricular), decreased contractility
Vasculature	Hypotension despite adequate fluid loading
Lungs	Acute lung injury or acute respiratory distress syndrome
Kidneys	Azotemia, oliguria, anuria
Gastrointestinal tract	Impaired barrier function and bacterial translocation, gastrointestinal ulceration, diarrhea, vomiting
Pancreas	Pancreatitis
Endocrine system	Adrenal insufficiency, hypoglycemia
Liver	Cholestatic jaundice
Immune system	Immunosuppression
Coagulation	Disseminated intravascular coagulation with or without hemorrhage

TABLE 86-4

Causes of Infective Endocarditis in Dogs

Microorganism	Prevalence[11]
Streptococci (primarily *S. canis* but also *S. bovis* group organisms)	29%
Bartonella spp.	20%
Staphylococci (*S. pseudintermedius*, *S. aureus*, and coagulase-negative staphylococci)	15%
Gram-negative rods (most commonly *E. coli*, but also *Pseudomonas aeruginosa*, *Salmonella* spp., *Citrobacter freundii*, *Klebsiella pneumoniae*, *Proteus* spp., *Pasteurella* spp., *Brucella* spp.)	15% (7% *E. coli*; <5% other species)
Other gram-positive bacteria (*Erysipelothrix* spp., *Granulicatella adiacens*, *Actinomyces* spp., *Corynebacterium* spp., *Mycobacterium* spp.)	7% (<5% each species)
Enterococcus spp.	5%
Fungi (e.g., *Aspergillus* spp.)	<5%

The development of IE begins with colonization of a heart valve by bacteria and deposition of fibrin, platelets, leukocytes, and erythrocytes. Colonization may be facilitated by changes in the valve surface as a result of turbulent blood flow, which results in the deposition of platelets, fibrin, and fibronectin; the end result is a sterile vegetation, or *nonbacterial thrombotic endocarditis*. Bacteria then adhere to this matrix, induce inflammatory cytokine and tissue factor release, and become covered with additional layers of platelets and fibrin, which promote bacterial growth to extremely high densities in an environment that is protected from the immune system. Properties of bacteria known to promote valve colonization include adhesins such as *fimA* in streptococci and clumping factor and fibronectin-binding proteins in staphylococci,[14,15] as well as factors that cause platelet aggregation. Portions of the vegetation can then dislodge and embolize in a variety of different tissues, especially the kidneys, spleen, brain, joints, and muscles, with an enormous spectrum of associated clinical manifestations. Thromboembolic complications are more likely to occur in dogs with mitral valve involvement than in those with aortic valve IE.[8] Regardless of the valve affected, valvular dysfunction can lead to impaired cardiac output and congestive heart failure (CHF).

As in humans, IE in dogs may be best classified on the basis of the etiologic agent involved, because the etiologic agent often determines the clinical course of disease, disease manifestations, prognosis, and the most appropriate antimicrobial drugs for treatment. For example, *Bartonella* IE is more likely to involve the aortic valve than the mitral valve, often occurs in the absence of fever, has a high prevalence of CHF when

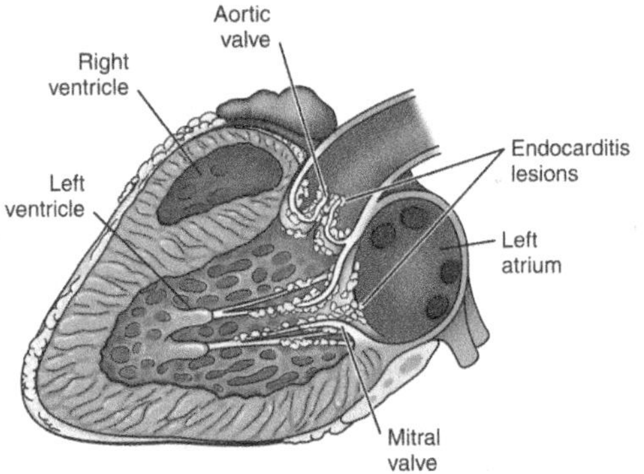

FIGURE 86-1 Infective endocarditis. Vegetations are attached to the mitral and aortic valves and may be mobile or sessile.

compared with IE caused by other bacterial pathogens, and is negatively correlated with survival (see Figure 52-3). In contrast, *Streptococcus canis* IE usually involves the mitral valve and is often associated with secondary polyarthritis. Dogs with gram-negative IE may be less likely to develop CHF than those with IE caused by other pathogens.[11]

The clinical signs and physical examination abnormalities that occur with IE are extremely variable and depend not only on the causative organism, but also on the valve affected, the presence or absence of thromboembolic complications, and the sites and extent of thromboembolism. Common historical findings include lethargy; inappetence; locomotory problems such as lameness, shifting lameness, joint pain, stiffness, reluctance to move, and inability to walk; and vomiting, weight loss, respiratory difficulty, and/or cough. Locomotory abnormalities can result from peripheral arterial thromboembolism, embolic or immune-mediated polyarthritis, neurologic abnormalities, and rarely, hypertrophic osteopathy.

TABLE 86-5

Physical Examination Findings in 70 Dogs with Infective Endocarditis Seen at the University of California, Davis, Veterinary Medical Teaching Hospital

Physical Examination Finding	Number Affected (%)
Cardiac murmur	41 (59)
Tachycardia	34 (50)
Fever	26 (38)
Tachypnea	24 (35)
Abnormal lung sounds	24 (34)
Recumbency	21 (30)
Mental dullness	19 (27)
Neurologic signs (ataxia, delayed or absent placing reactions, strabismus, nystagmus, head tilt, obtundation)	16 (23)
Swollen joints	15 (21)
Stiffness or lameness	13 (19)
Arrhythmias	14 (19)
Dehydration	11 (16)
Bounding pulses	10 (14)
Muscle atrophy	10 (14)
Thin body condition	9 (13)
Weak pulses	8 (11)
Reluctance to stand	8 (11)
Peripheral edema	7 (10)
Spinal pain	7 (10)
Abdominal pain, mucosal pallor, red mucous membranes, muscle pain, weakness, cyanosis, cool or cold limbs, oral ulceration, abdominal enlargement, hepatomegaly, icterus, uveitis, petechial or ecchymotic hemorrhages, cutaneous ulceration	6 or fewer (<10)

Modified from Sykes JE, Kittleson MD, Chomel BB, et al. Clinicopathologic findings and outcome in dogs with infective endocarditis: 71 cases (1992-2005). J Am Vet Med Assoc. 2006;228:1735-1747.

The most common initial physical examination findings are fever, tachycardia, and a cardiac murmur (Table 86-5).[8] In one study of dogs with IE, fever was present in the history or serial physical examinations of only 41 (60%) of 68 dogs with IE, and a cardiac murmur in only 53 (76%) of 70 dogs with IE, so an absence of fever or cardiac murmur does not rule out IE.[8] Although diastolic murmurs are suggestive of IE, more than 90% of dogs with murmurs due to IE have systolic murmurs.

Infectious Myocarditis

Infectious myocarditis in dogs and cats usually results from hematogenous spread of microorganisms to the myocardium or extension of endocarditis lesions to the myocardium. Viruses, bacteria, protozoa, or fungi may be involved. Some organisms have a particular tropism for the myocardium (Table 86-6). Infectious myocarditis is rare in cats.

TABLE 86-6

Infectious Causes of Myocarditis in Dogs and Cats

Pathogen Type	Examples	Affected Host Species
Viruses	West Nile virus	D
	Canine parvovirus 2 variants	D
	Feline panleukopenia virus	C
	Pseudorabies virus	D
Bacteria	Gram-negative and gram-positive bacteria (e.g., extension of endocarditis)	D, C
	Bartonella spp.	D, C
	Borrelia burgdorferi	D
	Rickettsia rickettsii	D
Fungi	*Blastomyces dermatitidis*	D
	Candida albicans	D
	Cryptococcus neoformans	D
	Aspergillus spp.	D
	Paecilomyces variotii	D
Algae	*Prototheca* spp.	D
Protozoa	*Trypanosoma cruzi*	D
	Sarcocystis felis	C
	Leishmania	D
	Neospora caninum	D
	Hepatozoon americanum	D
	Toxoplasma gondii	D, C

C, Cat; D, dog.

Myocarditis may be subclinical or result in arrhythmias, CHF, or sudden death. Simultaneous infection of a variety of other organs is frequent for most pathogens that cause myocarditis, so clinical signs of systemic infection (fever, lethargy) and other organ dysfunction are often present.

Infectious Pericarditis

Infectious pericarditis may result from direct inoculation of organisms into the pericardium (such as occurs with penetrating wounds), extension of infection from adjacent organs such as the pleural space or lungs, or hematogenous dissemination of viral, bacterial, or fungal pathogens to the pericardium. Bite wounds or grass awn migration usually result in mixed aerobic-anaerobic infections that involve organisms such as *Actinomyces* spp. (see Chapter 42). Infectious pericarditis as a result of hematogenous spread of pathogens is rare; idiopathic pericardial effusion and heart-base neoplasia are the most common causes of inflammatory or hemorrhagic pericardial effusion in dogs. Pathogens with particular tropism for the pericardial sac include feline infectious peritonitis virus and *Coccidioides* spp. (see Chapters 20 and 63). Pericarditis results in diastolic cardiac dysfunction with subsequent development of right-sided heart failure, which is manifested as weak pulses, tachycardia, jugular venous distention, ascites, and pleural effusion. Muffled heart sounds may be detected on cardiac auscultation as a result of pericardial and/or pleural effusion.

BOX 86-1

Reasons to Consider Blood Culture in Dogs and Cats

Fever (especially when viral infection is not likely or underlying immunosuppression or barrier disruption is present)
Unexplained peripheral edema in dogs
Evidence of thromboembolism in dogs (e.g., organ infarction, cold limbs)
Neutrophilic polyarthritis in dogs
Discospondylitis in dogs
Echocardiographic evidence of infective endocarditis or new heart murmur
Neutrophilic lymphadenitis
Severe pneumonia or pyothorax
Peritonitis
Development of leukopenia, bandemia, or leukocytosis in association with immunosuppression, catheters, or other devices
Thrombophlebitis in association with an indwelling catheter
Sepsis in a patient in which a culture cannot be obtained from the suspected source (e.g., pneumonia in a severely hypoxemic patient, gastrointestinal bacterial translocation)
Immune-mediated hemolytic anemia or thrombocytopenia

TABLE 86-7

Modified Duke Criteria Used for Diagnosis of Infective Endocarditis in Dogs and Cats[8,20]

Major Criteria	Minor Criteria
Identification of a typical organism using blood culture • *Streptococcus* spp. • *Staphylococcus* spp. • *Escherichia coli*	Predisposing heart condition (congenital valvular malformation)
All 3, or most of 4, separate blood cultures positive, with first and last specimens drawn at least 1 hour apart	New or worsening heart murmur
Two positive blood cultures for any microorganism, when blood cultures are drawn more than 12 hours apart	Fever (≥103°F [39.4°C])
Findings on echocardiogram positive for infective endocarditis	Presence of vascular/embolic phenomena
	Immunologic phenomena: nondegenerate neutrophilic polyarthritis, glomerulonephritis, immune-mediated hemolytic anemia
	Microbiologic phenomena: positive blood culture not meeting major criteria, *or* serologic evidence of infection with a typical organism, *or* detection of a typical organism using PCR technology

Definite endocarditis: 2 major criteria, or histopathologic confirmation of endocarditis.
Possible endocarditis: Positive echocardiographic findings and 1 minor criterion, or 1 major and 3 minor criteria, or 5 minor criteria. In recent human guidelines, 1 major and 3 minor criteria, or 5 minor criteria, are considered sufficient evidence for diagnosis of definitive endocarditis.[19]

Diagnosis

Antemortem diagnosis of bacteremia is based on culture of bacteria from the bloodstream. Reasons to consider blood culture are shown in Box 86-1. The diagnosis of sepsis is based on the presence of the systemic inflammatory response syndrome (SIRS) together with suspected or proven infection (see Table 86-1). A number of biomarkers have been investigated for discrimination of sepsis from SIRS in dogs,[16-18] but as yet, highly sensitive and specific biomarkers for sepsis have not been identified. The diagnosis of IE is based on a set of criteria modified from the Duke criteria used for diagnosis of IE in human patients, which consider the results of blood culture and echocardiography as major criteria, and other clinical manifestations of IE as minor criteria (Table 86-7).[8,19,20] Diagnosis of infective pericarditis relies on echocardiography and the results of cytologic examination and culture of pericardial fluid, or alternatively, histopathologic examination and culture of pericardial biopsies obtained during thoracotomy or thoracoscopy. In dogs and cats, infectious myocarditis is usually a necropsy diagnosis because myocardial biopsy is rarely performed. However, bacterial myocarditis may be suspected based on echocardiographic abnormalities, the presence of arrhythmias, and positive blood cultures.

Laboratory Abnormalities

Complete Blood Count

Common CBC findings in dogs and cats with bloodstream infections are mild nonregenerative anemia, neutrophilia with a left shift and neutrophil toxicity, lymphopenia, and/or monocytosis. Degenerative left shifts may be present, and dogs and cats with disseminated intravascular coagulation (DIC) may be thrombocytopenic or have evidence of schistocytosis. Rarely, bacteria are seen within circulating leukocytes on blood smear examination.

Serum Biochemical Tests

The serum chemistry profile in dogs and cats with bloodstream infection may show evidence of organ dysfunction as a result of severe sepsis or bacterial embolization and infarction. Abnormalities include azotemia, increased activities of liver enzymes, mild to moderate hyperbilirubinemia (usually <5 mg/dL), and electrolyte and acid-base abnormalities (such as a high anion gap metabolic acidosis due to azotemia or lactic acidosis). Hyperglycemia may be present early in septic shock. Hypoglycemia can also be present as a result of decreased hepatic gluconeogenesis or upregulation of non–insulin dependent glucose transporters. Hypoalbuminemia occurs in most dogs with IE, ranges from mild to severe, and may result from decreased hepatic production, from increased vascular permeability, or as part of the inflammatory response (albumin is a negative acute-phase reactant protein). Dogs with thromboemboli to skeletal muscle may have markedly increased activity of serum creatine kinase.

Urinalysis

Urinalysis findings in dogs and cats with bacteremia or IE include proteinuria, pyuria, cylindruria, microscopic hematuria, and/or bacteriuria. Severe proteinuria (urine protein:creatinine

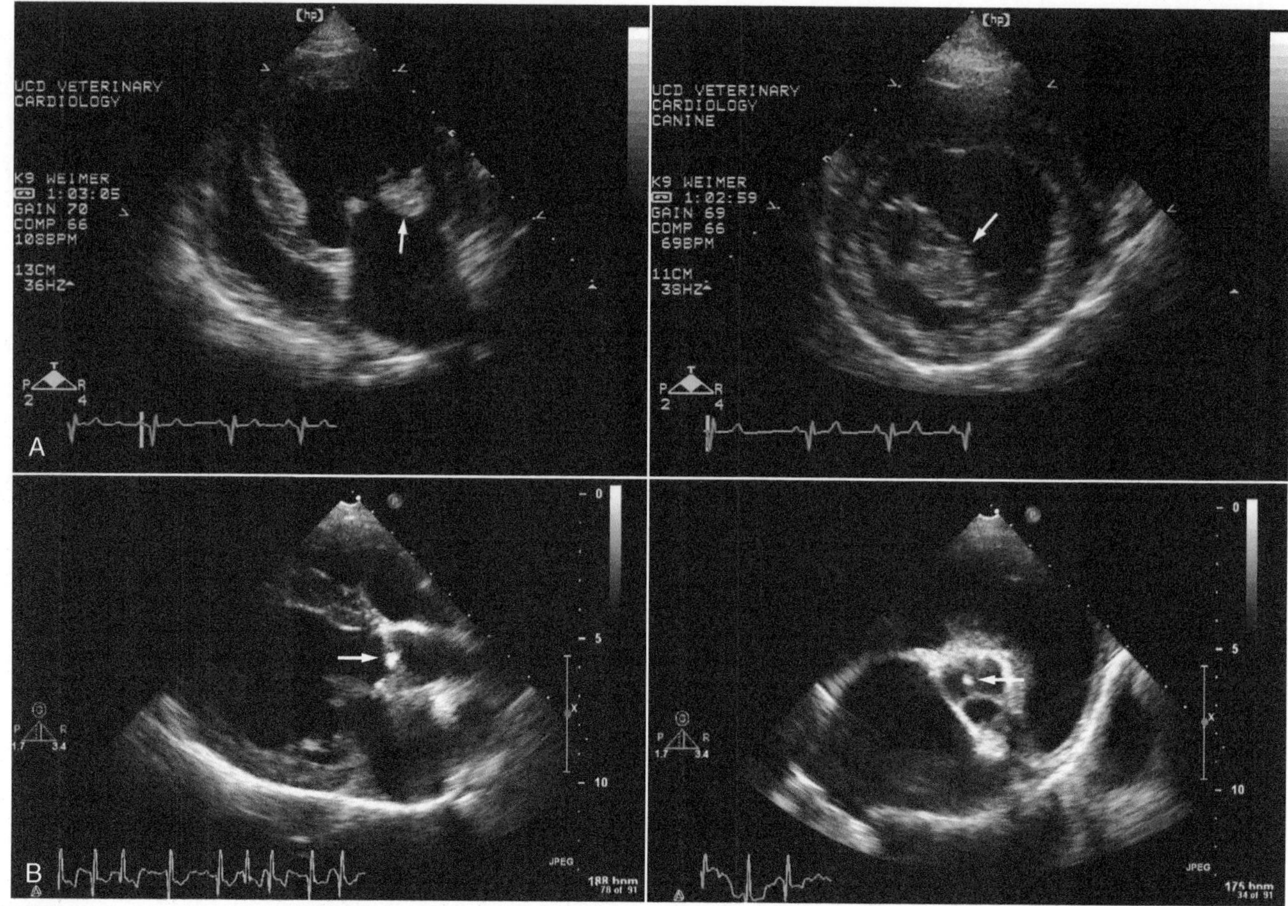

FIGURE 86-2 **A,** Parasternal *(left)* and short-axis *(right)* views of the mitral valve of a 7-year-old male neutered Weimaraner with *Enterococcus faecium* endocarditis that was diagnosed after a perineal urethrostomy procedure. There is a large vegetative lesion attached to the mitral valve *(arrow)*. A smaller lesion is attached to the septal leaflet of the valve. **B,** Parasternal *(left)* and short-axis *(right)* views of the aortic valve of a 4-year-old intact male Doberman with culture-negative endocarditis. The aortic valve cusps are thickened and a hyperechoic nodule is evident *(arrow)*. (Images courtesy University of California, Davis Veterinary Cardiology Service.)

ratio >5) may occur as a result of glomerular damage in dogs with IE.

Coagulation Profile

Dogs and cats with sepsis and DIC may have prolonged APTT and PT, increased concentrations of fibrin degradation products or D-dimers, and/or decreased concentrations of plasma fibrinogen and antithrombin. If thromboelastography is used, either hyper- or hypocoagulability may be documented in dogs.[21] In dogs with IE, PT is often shortened, and fibrinogen concentration is often increased.[8]

Diagnostic Imaging

Plain Radiography

Thoracic radiographs in dogs with IE often show no detectable abnormalities. When present, abnormal findings include pulmonary infiltrates as a result of pneumonia, acute respiratory distress syndrome (ARDS), or CHF; generalized cardiomegaly; left atrial enlargement; pulmonary venous distention; mild pleural effusion; and, occasionally, even microcardia or vascular attenuation (see Figure 52-4). Infectious pericarditis may be associated with radiographic evidence of pleural effusion or cardiomegaly. Changes to the intervertebral disc spaces that suggest discospondylitis may also be detected in dogs with bacteremia or IE (see Chapter 85).

Echocardiography

Echocardiography is indicated when infective endocarditis, myocarditis, or pericarditis is suspected based on the history and physical examination findings (such as fever, arrhythmias, a new murmur, or signs of left- or right-sided CHF). It is also indicated for all dogs and cats with bacteremia, even in the absence of a cardiac murmur or arrhythmia; for dogs with neutrophilic polyarthritis; and for dogs and cats with evidence of systemic thromboembolic disease. Echocardiographic findings in IE can include valvular hyperechogenicity, thickening and irregularity of the valves, and valvular vegetations, which may be nodular, discrete, or have a shaggy or moth-eaten appearance (Figure 86-2 and see Figure 52-5). Large vegetations can oscillate or vibrate, and follow-up echocardiography sometimes reveals sudden disappearance of a vegetative lesion in association with thromboembolism. Mild or severe valvular regurgitation or insufficiency may be present in association with the lesions. Other echocardiographic findings include left ventricular eccentric hypertrophy, chamber dilation, mural hyperechogenicity, ruptured chordae tendineae, acquired defects in the valves or myocardium, and mild pericardial effusion. Echocardiography is a sensitive tool for diagnosis of IE (in one study, its sensitivity was 88% when necropsy was used as the gold standard),[8] but negative results do not completely rule out the

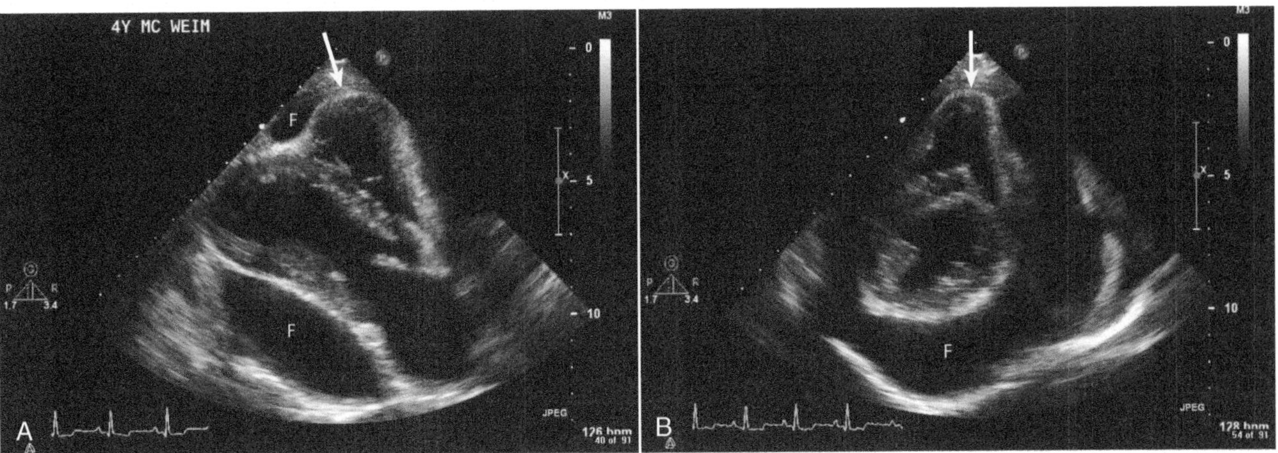

FIGURE 86-3 Long-axis **(A)** and short-axis **(B)** echocardiographic images that show pericarditis in a 4-year-old male neutered Weimaraner with disseminated coccidioidomycosis. The epicardium is adhered to the pericardium *(arrow)*, and a moderate quantity of anechoic pericardial fluid *(F)* can be appreciated. The cardiac chambers are distorted. (Images courtesy University of California, Davis Veterinary Cardiology Service.)

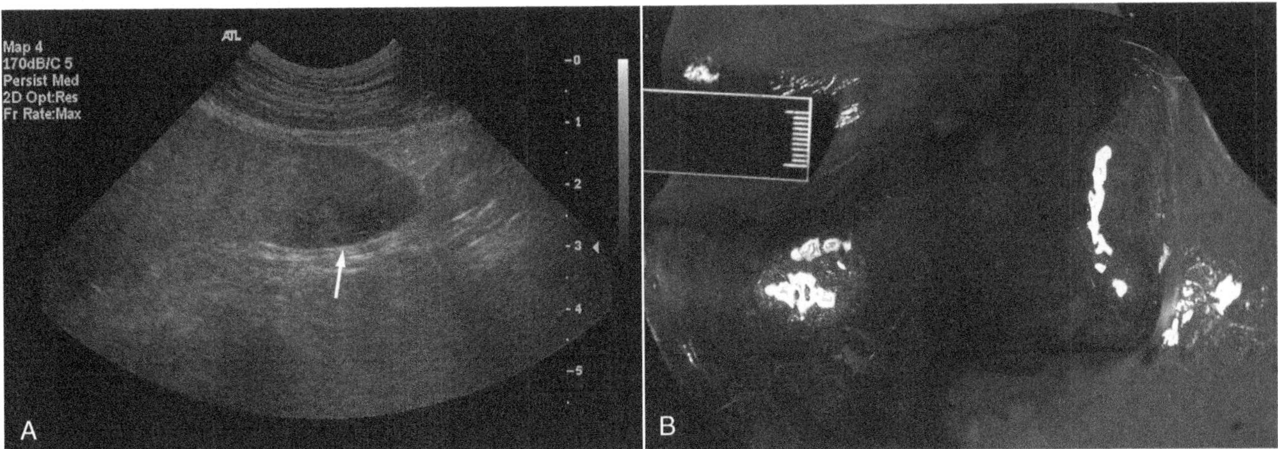

FIGURE 86-4 **A,** Abdominal ultrasound image that shows a splenic infarct *(arrow)* in a 6-year-old female spayed bouvier des Flandres with *Staphylococcus aureus* infective endocarditis. **B,** Splenic infarct at necropsy. (Image courtesy University of California, Davis Veterinary Anatomic Pathology Service.)

possibility of IE. Echocardiography is also useful for monitoring treatment of IE.

Echocardiographic findings in infectious pericarditis include pericardial effusion, adhesions of the pericardium to the epicardium, and sometimes focal or diffuse pericardial thickening and hyperechogenicity (Figure 86-3). Restrictive disease is characterized by impairment of diastole, with decreased left ventricular internal dimensions during diastole, and variation of blood flow velocity across the mitral valve with the respiratory cycle (increased with expiration and decreased with inspiration). In addition, deviation of the interventricular septum into the left ventricle can occur during inspiration and into the right ventricle during expiration.

Abdominal Sonographic Findings

Sonographic abnormalities can be present in a variety of organs in dogs with IE and may reflect underlying disease processes (such as neoplasia or bacterial peritonitis) or septic thromboembolism. Infarction and hemorrhage secondary to thromboembolism can result in focal cavitary or hypoechoic lesions in the spleen (Figure 86-4) or focal hyperechoic or hypoechoic lesions in the kidney. Thrombi may be found in the iliac arteries or aorta.

Microbiologic Tests

Culture

Routine blood cultures assist in identification of infecting pathogens and permit susceptibility testing. Ideally, at least three blood cultures should be obtained from separate sites within a 24-hour period. A suggested protocol for blood cultures is outlined in Chapter 3 (see Box 3-2). The use of separate venipuncture sites has been suggested but is not considered essential for diagnosis of human IE, although collection of specimens from indwelling catheters should be avoided.[19] If a catheter-related bloodstream infection is suspected, collection of paired specimens has been recommended in humans, with one specimen collected from the catheter before removal and the other collected from a peripheral site.[22] The skin should be prepared in the same manner used for surgery, and utmost care should be taken to avoid contamination with commensal bacteria. Because IE is generally associated with continuous bacteremia, positive results in only one of multiple bottles should be interpreted with caution. Positive results for *Bacillus* spp. or coagulase-negative staphylococci in a single bottle generally reflect contamination.

The decision to perform anaerobic blood culture should be considered in light of the animal's underlying disease process and client financial constraints. For example, anaerobic culture may not be cost effective in dogs with IE, given the rare involvement of anaerobes in this condition. Anaerobes are more likely to be present in dogs with histories that suggest involvement of plant awn foreign bodies, bite wounds, or gastrointestinal compromise.

False-negative blood cultures may occur as a result of low-level bacteremia or fungemia, the presence of fastidious or unculturable organisms such as *Bartonella* or anaerobes, insufficient specimen size, suboptimal specimen transport conditions, or recent antimicrobial treatment. Nevertheless, blood culture is still indicated in animals with a history of antimicrobial treatment, especially if antimicrobials have only been administered for 2 to 3 days. If an animal with IE is in stable condition, discontinuation of existing antibiotic treatment for several days (ideally 7 to 10 days) could be considered before blood cultures are obtained. Specific culture and serology for *Bartonella* is also indicated in dogs and cats with IE or suspected myocarditis (see Chapter 52). This should be considered even if routine blood cultures are positive, because polymicrobial infections that include *Bartonella* spp. and other bacteria can occur.[11] Special media used to isolate *Bartonella* spp. (*Bartonella* α-Proteobacteria growth medium [BAPGM]) may also yield other fastidious bacteria such as *Sphingomonas* spp., the clinical significance of which requires further study.[23] Serologic testing for *Aspergillus* antigen and *Brucella* antibody could also be considered for dogs with culture-negative IE (see Chapters 53 and 65).

Attempts should also be made to isolate causative organism(s) from other sites that are suspected to be a source of infection based on the history and clinical findings. Appropriate specimens could include transtracheal or bronchoalveolar lavage specimens, urine, ascites fluid, wounds, or pleural effusion. Urinary tract infections may reflect ascending pyelonephritis or spread of bacteria from the blood into the urine. However, bacteria cultured from the urine do not always reflect those present in the bloodstream,[11] so blood cultures should always be performed even when urine cultures are positive. Isolation of the same organism from the blood as well as an additional site facilitates interpretation of the significance of a single positive blood culture and aids decisions regarding appropriate antimicrobial drug treatment.

Molecular Diagnosis Using the Polymerase Chain Reaction

PCR assays have been used to rapidly detect bacterial DNA within whole blood and especially valvular tissue (obtained at necropsy) of animals with IE and are especially useful for detection of fastidious bacteria such as *Bartonella* spp. within heart valves (see Chapter 52). These assays use broad-range primers that target bacterial 16S ribosomal subunit DNA, and the identity of the organism is determined by sequence analysis of resulting PCR products.

In one prospective study that examined the performance of a conventional broad-range bacterial PCR assay on whole blood for diagnosis of the etiology of IE in 18 dogs, there was no difference in the overall sensitivity of the PCR assay and culture, but the combined use of the PCR assay and blood culture was more sensitive than the use of either assay alone.[20] This was because the PCR assay detected several fastidious organisms, which included *Bartonella vinsonii, Brucella,* and *Granulicatella adiacens*, but appeared less sensitive than culture for detection of less fastidious organisms such as streptococci. Studies that include larger numbers of dogs and cats and that examine the performance of other PCR assays such as real-time PCR assays are required before broad-range bacterial PCR can be recommended for routine diagnosis of bacteremia and IE in dogs and cats, but PCR assays show promise when used in conjunction with blood cultures. Of major concern is the possibility of false positives with highly sensitive PCR assays due to detection of contaminating bacteria. Even in human medicine, evidence is considered insufficient to recommend the routine use of whole blood or serum real-time PCR assays for the diagnosis of culture-negative IE.[19]

Pathologic Findings

There are no specific pathologic findings in sepsis or bacteremia, but underlying causes such as pneumonia, pyometra, or peritonitis may be apparent. Microabscesses may be present in multiple tissues. Isolation of the same bacterial species from multiple different tissues supports a diagnosis of bacteremia. Pathologic findings in IE include valvular vegetations; avulsion or perforation of valvular structures; and gross and histopathologic evidence of infarction, widespread thrombosis, and CHF (Figure 86-5). The inflammatory process may be chronic, with lymphoplasmacytic and histiocytic cell infiltrates and fibrosis; or acute, suppurative, and fibrinous, with or without microscopically visible intralesional bacteria (see Figure 34-6). *Bartonella* IE is characterized by chronic inflammation and may be associated with valvular mineralization (Figure 52-6), whereas IE due to other microorganisms may be acute or chronic and is rarely associated with mineralization.[11] Use of tissue gram stains and silver stains can reveal organisms within valvular vegetations. Necrotizing vasculitis may also be present in the lungs, myocardium, kidney, spleen, liver, and/or brain. Erythrophagocytosis has been described in reticuloendothelial tissues of dogs with IE due to gram-positive cocci. Membranoproliferative, membranous, or necrosuppurative glomerulonephritis may also be identified.[8]

Gross examination of the heart in animals with myocarditis may reveal focal or multifocal areas of myocardial pallor and/or friability. The pericardium of dogs and cats with pericarditis may be thickened and discolored, and pericardial effusion may be present. Histopathology reveals acute or chronic inflammatory infiltrates, depending on the underlying cause, sometimes with intralesional bacteria, protozoa, or fungi.

Treatment and Prognosis

The mainstay of treatment of bacteremia, IE, sepsis, and bacterial myocarditis or pericarditis is early antimicrobial drug treatment. The initial choice of antimicrobial drugs should be based on knowledge of the prevalent bacterial species and their antimicrobial drug susceptibilities for each hospital and/or geographic region, as well as the likely source of infection (which can provide information about the likely bacterial species involved) (Tables 86-8 and 86-9). The presence or absence of IE and/or severe sepsis also affects treatment recommendations.

In addition to antimicrobial drug therapy, the underlying cause of infection or chronic bacteremia should be identified and removed if possible. All catheters or devices should be removed and replaced at new sites if they are still needed. An attempt should be made to locate foreign bodies such as grass awns with imaging techniques and surgically remove them. Surgery may be required to resolve gastrointestinal compromise, such as occurs with foreign bodies, intestinal neoplasia, or torsion. Underlying immunosuppressive disease such as neoplasia or diabetes mellitus should be identified and treated if possible.

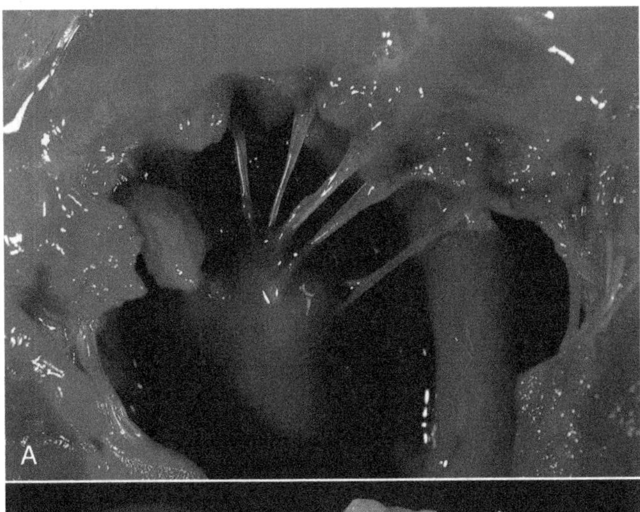
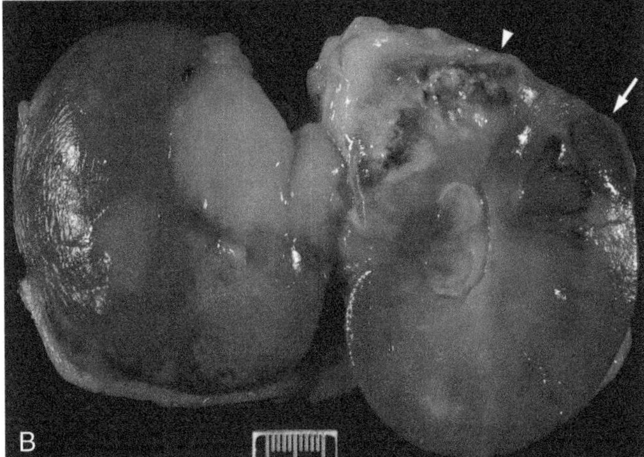
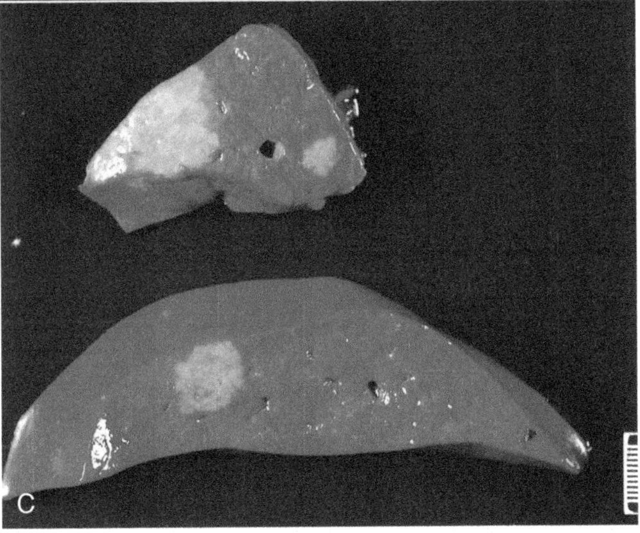

FIGURE 86-5 Gross pathology findings in a 12-year-old male neutered Irish water spaniel with *Enterococcus durans* infective endocarditis and widespread thromboembolic disease. **A,** Mitral valve. The leaflets are thickened and nodular. **B,** Left kidney. Multiple, variably sized, well-demarcated red foci with dark red rims and numerous well-demarcated tan slightly depressed foci are present. On cut surface, these foci extend to and beyond the corticomedullary junction as wedge-shaped lesions *(white arrow)*. On one pole there is a 2.0 cm × 1.5 cm × 1.4 cm tan to brown-green abscess *(white arrowhead)*. **C,** Spleen. Several well-demarcated lesions that measured 0.3 to 0.5 cm in diameter are present. (Courtesy the University of California, Davis, Veterinary Anatomic Pathology Service.)

Maintenance of optimal oxygen delivery to tissues and adequate tissue perfusion is essential for effective treatment of severe sepsis and septic shock. The use of goal-directed therapy for the management of severe sepsis/septic shock in the emergency room during the first 6 hours of hospitalization reduces mortality in humans.[24] The first priority is to rapidly correct blood volume deficits. Liberal administration of IV crystalloids is a critical treatment for dogs and cats with sepsis. Colloids could also be used, but studies of human patients with septic shock have shown either no additional benefit of synthetic colloids such as hetastarch and the possibility of increased mortality[25] or increased risk of development of acute kidney injury.[26] Because hypoalbuminemia is common and affected animals often have increased vascular endothelial permeability, fresh frozen plasma may be needed to maintain appropriate intravascular volume. Excessive fluid administration may be associated with increased mortality, so careful monitoring of central venous pressure (CVP) is optimal. The endpoints of fluid resuscitation should be mean arterial pressure (MAP) of at least 65 mm Hg, adequate perfusion on physical examination, and a lactate clearance of at least 10% or a plasma lactate concentration less than 2 mmol/L.[27] Fluid support is provided until a maximal target CVP of 8 to 12 mm Hg is reached or the listed goals are met.

Tight glycemic control (targeting a blood glucose of <150 mg/dL) has been shown to increase the risk of serious adverse effects in humans and is not recommended at this time.[26] However, blood glucose concentrations must be monitored and hypoglycemia avoided by the addition of supplemental dextrose to IV fluids. Bicarbonate therapy is not recommended to treat metabolic acidosis associated with tissue hypoperfusion because acidosis may be protective. Animals that develop acute lung injury (ALI) or ARDS (bilateral pulmonary interstitial to alveolar infiltrates that are not due to left-sided congestive heart failure with a P_aO_2/F_iO_2 ratio less than 300 [ALI] or less than 200 [ARDS]) may benefit from mechanical ventilation. For less severely affected animals, supplemental oxygen to maintain a SpO_2 of at least 95% or P_aO_2 of at least 80 mm Hg is indicated.

Arterial blood pressure must be monitored either by direct (arterial catheter) or indirect (oscillometric) means and maintained through treatment at or above 65 mm Hg. If hypotension persists despite adequate fluid loading as described previously, a diagnosis of septic shock is made and treatment with vasopressors such as dopamine, norepinephrine, or vasopressin may be indicated. The decision to use inotropes (such as dobutamine) first is based on echocardiographic evidence of impaired myocardial contractility (decreased fractional shortening on echocardiogram, or direct measurement of cardiac output via pulmonary artery catheter or other techniques). If inotropes are not indicated, then vasopressors should be prescribed to achieve an adequate blood pressure. Often treatment with dopamine (5-15 µg/kg/min) is attempted first. If an adequate MAP cannot be obtained, then norepinephrine (0.1-1 µg/kg/min), or vasopressin (0.5-4 mU/kg/min) can be added; additional vasopressors are always added and not substituted. If MAP cannot be maintained with norepinephrine, then vasopressin is added (or vice versa).

Treatment of severe sepsis and septic shock with hydrocortisone has been controversial in human medicine. High doses of hydrocortisone increase mortality and should not be used.[28,29] Relative adrenal insufficiency has been identified in dogs and cats[30] with an apparent reversal of signs of shock

TABLE 86-8

Suggested Empiric Antimicrobial Drug Choices for IV Use in Dogs and Cats with Severe Sepsis or Septic Shock Pending the Results of Blood Culture and Susceptibility*

Antimicrobial Drug	Spectrum	Suspected Source of Infection	Comments
Ampicillin or clindamycin *and* an aminoglycoside†	Activity against most gram-negative bacteria, methicillin-resistant staphylococci, streptococci, enterococci, and most anaerobes	Urinary tract, abdomen	Good first choice for most infections, except when the respiratory tract is involved. Consider use of ampicillin-sulbactam instead of ampicillin or addition of metronidazole if infection with penicillinase-producing anaerobes is possible (e.g., gastrointestinal compromise or plant foreign body, IE absent).
Ampicillin or clindamycin *and* a fluoroquinolone	Active against most anaerobes, streptococci, susceptible staphylococci, and aerobic gram-negative rods. Not active against some methicillin-resistant staphylococci, enterococci, and MDR gram-negative bacteria.	Lung, urinary tract, abdomen, pyothorax	Consider when MDR gram-negative bacteria, enterococci, or methicillin-resistant staphylococci are *unlikely* based on local resistance patterns and aminoglycosides are contraindicated because of toxicity or concerns related to drug penetration. Consider use of ampicillin-sulbactam instead of ampicillin or addition of metronidazole if infection with penicillinase-producing anaerobes is likely.
A carbapenem *or* piperacillin-tazobactam *or* ticarcillin-clavulanate	Active against aerobic gram-negative rods including *Pseudomonas*, anaerobes, streptococci. Not active against methicillin-resistant staphylococci and some enterococci.	Abdomen, aspiration pneumonia	Use when infection with MDR gram-negative bacteria and anaerobes is likely but *aminoglycosides are contraindicated because of toxicity or concerns related to drug penetration* (e.g., airway involvement). Consultation with a veterinary clinical specialist with a focused interest in infectious disease or antimicrobial pharmacology recommended before use.
Vancomycin *and* a carbapenem	Active against methicillin-resistant staphylococci, streptococci, MDR aerobic gram-negative bacilli, and anaerobes.	Skin/soft tissue, urinary tract, abdomen	Last line for treatment of life-threatening mixed infection with MDR gram-negative bacteria, MDR enterococci, anaerobes, and methicillin-resistant staphylococci *when aminoglycosides are contraindicated because of toxicity or concerns related to inadequate drug penetration.* Consultation with a veterinary clinical specialist with a focused interest in infectious disease or antimicrobial pharmacology recommended before use.

Dosages for IV administration (normal renal function). See Chapter 8 for precautions.
Amikacin, 15 mg/kg q24h (dogs), 10 mg/kg q24h (cats)
Ampicillin sodium, 20 mg/kg q6h
Ampicillin-sulbactam, 20 mg/kg q6-8h (dose based on ampicillin component)
Clindamycin phosphate, 10 mg/kg q12h (dilute 1:10 in sterile saline and give slowly over 30 min)
Gentamicin sulfate, 14 mg/kg q24h (dogs), 8 mg/kg q24h (cats)
Ciprofloxacin hydrochloride, 10 mg/kg q24h
Enrofloxacin, 5-20 mg/kg q24h (dogs); avoid in cats and never exceed 5 mg/kg, see important cautionary notes in Chapter 8
Imipenem-cilastatin, 5 mg/kg q6h (dilute in 100 mL sterile saline and give slowly over 30 min)
Meropenem, 25 mg/kg q8h
Piperacillin-tazobactam, 40 mg/kg q6h
Ticarcillin-clavulanate, 50 mg/kg q6h
Vancomycin, 15 mg/kg q8h (dilute in sterile saline and give slowly over 30 min)
MDR, Multidrug-resistant.
*Spectrum should be reduced once culture and susceptibility results become available.
†In human patients, amikacin is less nephrotoxic than gentamicin and may be preferable for treatment of dogs and cats with severe sepsis or septic shock.

TABLE 86-9

Suggested Empiric Antimicrobial Drug Treatment for IV Use in Dogs and Cats with Infective Endocarditis Pending the Results of Blood Culture and Susceptibility*

Antimicrobial Drug	Spectrum	Comments
Ampicillin *and* gentamicin	Streptococci, *Bartonella*, methicillin-resistant staphylococci, enterococci, aerobic gram-negative rods	Covers all major causes of IE including most MDR gram-negative rods. Consider substitution of gentamicin with a fluoroquinolone if impairment of renal function is present.
Vancomycin *and* a carbapenem	Methicillin-resistant staphylococci, enterococci, gram-negative aerobes	Use only when infection with methicillin-resistant staphylococci is likely, local susceptibility patterns preclude use of other antimicrobials, *and aminoglycosides are contraindicated because of toxicity* (e.g., refractory pyoderma; history of orthopedic surgery, antimicrobial treatment, or hospitalization in the last year; or contact with other animals or humans known to have methicillin-resistant staphylococcal infections). Consultation with a veterinary clinical specialist with a focused interest in infectious disease or antimicrobial pharmacology recommended before use.

For drug doses, see bottom of Table 86-8.
*Spectrum should be reduced once culture and susceptibility results become available.

with the treatment of hydrocortisone in one reported case.[31] Current recommendations for human patients are to consider hydrocortisone therapy when hypotension responds poorly to adequate fluid resuscitation and vasopressors. Hydrocortisone is preferred to dexamethasone and dosed at 1 mg/kg IV q6h.

Other supportive treatments could include the H2 blocker famotidine or proton pump inhibitors to manage gastrointestinal ulceration. The use of red blood cell transfusions to maintain a hemoglobin concentration above 7.0 g/dL may be beneficial. Recombinant activated protein C (drotrecogin alfa) was the only approved drug specifically indicated to treat severe sepsis in human patients, but was withdrawn from the market after a worldwide trial showed that it failed to improve outcome for severe sepsis and septic shock.[32] An anti-TLR4 receptor compound, eritoran tetrasodium, also failed to improve outcome. Human intravenous immunoglobulin has been used to treat humans with sepsis, with improved survival. Whether this also translates to dogs and cats is not known.[33,34]

Bacteremia and Septic Shock

It is well established in human patients that the earlier appropriate antimicrobial drug treatment is initiated in sepsis, the lower the mortality. With every hour that antimicrobial drug therapy is delayed after documented hypotension, mortality in affected people increases by 8%.[35] Because of the urgent need to initiate antimicrobial drug treatment, initial treatment should be intravenous, bacteriocidal and broad spectrum, and should occur within an hour of diagnosis of severe sepsis and septic shock, pending the results of culture and susceptibility. Reasonable initial choices for septic shock in dogs and cats are outlined in Table 86-8. *In order to avoid overuse of antimicrobial drugs reserved for treatment of resistant bacterial infections, the drug spectrum should be reduced according to the results of culture and susceptibility as soon as those results are available.* Treatment should be continued for at least 2 weeks, although the optimum duration of treatment may vary depending on the underlying cause. Repeat blood cultures could be considered if fever or clinical abnormalities that suggest ongoing infection persist after 7 days of treatment, but the need for and timing of follow-up blood cultures in animals that are responding adequately to treatment requires further study.

Infective Endocarditis

Guidelines for the treatment of IE in humans have been published and updated.[19,36] However, many factors considered for treatment of human patients do not apply to dogs and cats, including the availability of valve replacement; penicillin allergy in some patients; the higher incidence of infections with methicillin-resistant staphylococci and vancomycin-resistant enterococci; evidence that supports use of specific antimicrobial drugs or drug combinations; and the possibility of long hospitalization times for parenteral antimicrobial drug therapy. Indications for cardiac surgery in humans include severe acute regurgitation or valve obstruction with refractory pulmonary edema; uncontrolled infection with enlarging vegetations; persistent fever and positive blood culture for at least 10 days after appropriate antimicrobial drug treatment is commenced; infection caused by fungi or multidrug-resistant bacteria; large vegetations (>10 mm) in association with embolic episodes or other complications; and isolated large vegetations (>15 mm).[19]

For dogs and cats, valve replacement is not generally possible, so treatment must rely on antimicrobial drugs and resolution of any predisposing factors. Where the local prevalence of multiresistant gram-negative bacteria and methicillin-resistant staphylococci is low, a combination of ampicillin and an aminoglycoside is a good choice for empiric treatment of IE pending the results of culture and susceptibility. Where bloodstream infections with multiresistant gram-negative bacteria and methicillin-resistant staphylococci are locally prevalent, empiric recommendations made for human patients could be considered for dogs and cats pending the results of culture and susceptibility, provided there is a chance of treatment success in the absence of valve replacement. When severe sepsis is absent and IE follows an indolent

TABLE 86-10

Suggested Antimicrobial Drugs for Treatment of Major Causes of Infective Endocarditis in Dogs and Cats Once Cause is Known*

Cause	Preferred Treatment	Oral Equivalent
Methicillin-susceptible *Staphylococcus* spp.	Ampicillin IV Flucloxacillin IV (β-lactamase producer) Ampicillin-sulbactam IV (β-lactamase producer)	Amoxicillin PO Flucloxacillin PO Clavulanic acid–amoxicillin PO
Methicillin-resistant but rifampin-susceptible *Staphylococcus* spp.	Gentamicin IV and rifampin PO *or* Vancomycin IV* and rifampin; IV trimethoprim-sulfas, chloramphenicol or doxycycline with or without rifampin could also be considered if tolerated and the organism is susceptible.	None
Streptococcus spp.	Benzylpenicillin IV Ampicillin IV	Amoxicillin PO
Penicillin-susceptible enterococci	Ampicillin IV	Amoxicillin PO
Penicillin-resistant enterococci	Vancomycin IV* and gentamicin IV. If possible, consider other options based on culture and susceptibility.	None. Linezolid could be considered as an oral alternative.*
Aerobic gram-negative rods	Ampicillin IV and gentamicin IV Ampicillin IV and fluoroquinolone IV Imipenem-cilastatin or meropenem IV* Or base on susceptibility (other options, such as injectable cephalosporines, piperacillin-tazobactam, or ticarcillin-clavulanate may be effective)	Base on susceptibility
Bartonella spp.	Ampicillin IV and gentamicin IV Doxycycline IV and rifampin PO	Doxycycline PO and rifampin PO
Aspergillus spp.	Voriconazole or posaconazole	Voriconazole or posaconazole

*In part based on recommendations for treatment of human IE. The reader is referred to the text for precautionary statements on the use of vancomycin, linezolid, and carbapenems such as meropenem in animals.

course, it is recommended in human patients that antimicrobial treatment be withheld pending the results of culture and susceptibility, or a combination of penicillin with or without low-dose gentamicin (1 mg/kg IV q12h) be administered until results are available. Aminoglycosides are used at this low dose, twice daily for their synergistic activity with penicillin against enterococci and viridans streptococci, which are uncommon causes of IE in dogs. Empiric treatment protocols that have activity against drug-resistant bacteria are used in human patients pending results of culture and susceptibility when severe sepsis is present, such as vancomycin and low-dose gentamicin (no risk factors present for gram-negative bacterial infection), or vancomycin and meropenem (risk factors present for multiresistant Enterobacteriaceae and *Pseudomonas* infection). However, the use of vancomycin and meropenem in dogs and cats has been controversial and may not be permitted or feasible in some geographic locations.

Recommendations for treatment of IE in dogs once the microbial etiology is known are shown in Table 86-10. Intravenous antimicrobial drugs should be continued in the hospital for as long as possible (ideally at least 7 to 10 days). A switch to oral medications is not recommended for human IE patients because of poor activity when compared with intravenous medications.[19] However, oral antibiotic treatment has been used with success to treat some dogs with IE and may be the only viable option. At-home treatment with intravenous drugs through peripheral indwelling catheters, vascular access ports, or subcutaneous injections may be possible for some dogs, but dog, owner, and drug factors should be considered very carefully and proper client education is critical. If oral antimicrobial drugs are used, bacteriocidal drugs with good and reliable oral bioavailability are preferable.

Medical treatment should be continued for at least 4 to 6 weeks, until the underlying disease process has resolved and valvular lesions have also resolved based on echocardiographic examinations. Echocardiography should be repeated after 4 weeks, or earlier if there is evidence of complications (CHF, embolic disease) or inadequate treatment response. Successful resolution of IE is associated with reduction in size and consolidation of valvular vegetations and increase in valvular echogenicity. With unsuccessful treatment, lesions enlarge or remain unchanged, and/or new lesions may appear on other valves.[8]

Infective Pericarditis

In addition to specific antimicrobial drug treatment, surgery may be required in dogs with infective pericarditis in order to debride the pericardium and restore cardiac diastolic function. This carries a significant risk of mortality; if feasible, referral to an experienced cardiac surgeon is recommended.

Prognosis

The prognosis for dogs and cats that develop septic shock, severe sepsis, IE, myocarditis, or pericarditis is guarded, and depends on underlying disease processes, the severity of organ damage, and the etiologic agent or agents. In a study of 114 dogs seen at a veterinary teaching hospital with sepsis secondary to gastrointestinal tract leakage, overall mortality rate was 47.4%.[37] The mortality rate was 40/57 (70%) for dogs with MODS and 14/57 (25%) for dogs without MODS; 50% of the dogs in the study had MODS. In another study, mortality rate in dogs due to IE was at least 40/71 (56%), and median survival time was only 54 days.[8] Factors strongly associated with negative outcome in dogs with IE were thrombocytopenia, increased serum creatinine concentration, renal complications, thromboembolic complications, and *Bartonella* infection.

Prevention

Methods to prevent bloodstream infections and sepsis include limiting the use of invasive devices and catheters unless absolutely necessary and attention to routine hygiene in the hospital to minimize nosocomial infections. Other measures include management of immunosuppressive disorders such as diabetes mellitus, minimizing use of immunosuppressive drugs such as glucocorticoids, and prompt attention to wounds or other underlying infections that have the potential to spread to the bloodstream.

The role of prophylactic antimicrobial drugs to prevent bacteremia and sepsis has been controversial. Beneficial outcomes have been reported when antimicrobials are used to prevent infection after chemotherapy. In one study, the use of a 14-day course of trimethoprim-sulfadiazine reduced morbidity in dogs with osteosarcoma or lymphoma during the first 14 days after treatment with doxorubicin.[38] In human patients a 7-day course of a fluoroquinolone during the expected neutropenic period after chemotherapy for solid tumors and lymphomas reduced the incidence of fever, probable infection, and hospitalization.[39] Prophylactic treatment with antimicrobial drugs could be considered for animals with severe neutropenia (<500 cells/μL), although more studies are required that examine the prevalence of bacteremia in neutropenic animals and the benefits of prophylactic antimicrobial drug treatment. Finally, prophylactic antimicrobial drug treatment has been suggested for dogs and cats with congenital heart defects that undergo dental procedures, but evidence to support the need for this practice is lacking.

Public Health Aspects

Dogs with bloodstream infections may harbor bacteria such as methicillin-resistant *Staphylococcus aureus* that have the potential to colonize humans; these bacteria may not only be present in the bloodstream, but also at other anatomic sites of colonization such as the gastrointestinal tract or nasal cavity. Therefore, routine precautions should be taken when these dogs are handled, with special attention to hand hygiene and fomite disinfection. Dogs and cats with signs of cardiovascular infection may also be infected with important human pathogens such as *Salmonella* spp., *Bartonella* spp., *Brucella* spp., and *Rickettsia rickettsii*, so caution should be taken when handling blood from animals with cardiovascular infections, and needle-stick injuries should be avoided.

CASE EXAMPLE

Signalment: "Betsy," a 6-year-old female spayed bouvier des Flandres from Fallon, NV

History: Betsy was seen at the UC, Davis, VMTH emergency service for treatment of possible sepsis. One week before she was evaluated she had been lethargic and reluctant to stand while on a camping trip. Over the next 2 days she lost interest in food and water and seemed disoriented and unable to see, then developed dark, liquid diarrhea. She was taken to the local veterinary clinic 3 days later where her temperature was 106.3°F (41.3°C), she was unable to stand, and blood work showed moderate thrombocytopenia and hypoglycemia. An injection of ceftiofur (unknown dose), cephalexin (15.4 mg/kg PO q8h), and cimetidine (4.5 mg/kg PO q12h) were prescribed and she was referred for further evaluation. Betsy was up to date on vaccinations for distemper, canine adenovirus, parvovirus, and rabies.

Physical Examination:

Body Weight: 64 kg.

General: Obtunded, laterally recumbent, T = 106.2°F (41.2°C), HR = 170 beats/min, RR = 50 breaths/min, mucous membranes dark red, CRT <1 s.

Eyes, Ears, Nose, and Throat: Hypopyon and conjunctivitis were present in both eyes, and there was marked mucopurulent ocular discharge bilaterally. Serous nasal discharge was present bilaterally. There was moderate dental calculus and gingivitis. Several small gingival ulcerations were present.

Integument: Generalized cutaneous petechiation was noted.

Musculoskeletal: The dog was nonambulatory and unable to stand. Body condition score was 7/9.

Cardiovascular: No arrhythmias or murmurs were auscultated. Very strong, synchronous femoral pulses were palpated bilaterally.

Respiratory: Increased bronchovesicular sounds were present in all fields.

Abdominal Palpation: Moderate abdominal distention was noted. Palpation was difficult because of recumbency and the large size of the patient.

All Other Systems: No abnormalities detected.

Laboratory Findings:

Venous Blood Gas: pH 7.351, pCO_2 31 mm Hg, pO_2 41.4 mm Hg, base deficit 7.8 mmol/L, ionized calcium 1.14 mmol/L, bicarbonate 16.3 mmol/L, lactate 4.2 mmol/L, glucose 59 mg/dL.

CBC:

HCT 47.8% (40%-55%)
MCV 68.5 fL (65-75 fL)
MCHC 36.2 g/dL (33-36 g/dL)
WBC 25,250 cells/μL (6000-13,000 cells/μL)
Neutrophils 17,675 cells/μL (3000-10,500 cells/μL)
Band neutrophils 3030 cells/μL
Lymphocytes 505 cells/μL (1000-4000 cells/μL)

Monocytes 3788 cells/μL (150-1200 cells/μL)
Platelets 23,000 platelets/μL (150,000-400,000 platelets/μL)
Marked neutrophil toxicity was evident.

Serum Chemistry Profile:
Anion gap 25 mmol/L (10-24 mmol/L)
Sodium 146 mmol/L (145-154 mmol/L)
Potassium 3.8 mmol/L (3.6-5.3 mmol/L)
Chloride 113 mmol/L (108-118 mmol/L)
Bicarbonate 12 mmol/L (16-26 mmol/L)
Phosphorus 2.9 mg/dL (3.0-6.2 mg/dL)
Calcium 10.3 mg/dL (9.7-11.5 mg/dL)
BUN 34 mg/dL (5-21 mg/dL)
Creatinine 1.6 mg/dL (0.3-1.2 mg/dL)
Glucose 59 mg/dL (64-123 mg/dL)
Total protein 5.9 g/dL (5.4-7.6 g/dL)
Albumin 3.0 g/dL (3.0-4.4 g/dL)
Globulin 2.9 g/dL (1.8-3.9 g/dL)
ALT 58 U/L (19-67 U/L)
AST 130 U/L (19-42 U/L)
ALP 356 U/L (21-170 U/L)
Cholesterol 377 mg/dL (135-361 mg/dL)
Total bilirubin 0.7 mg/dL (0-0.2 mg/dL)

Urinalysis: SGr 1.028; pH 8.0, 3+ protein (SSA), 1+ bilirubin, 2+ hemoprotein, no glucose or ketones, 1-3 WBC/HPF, 4-10 RBC/HPF, 0-2 granular casts, few triple phosphate crystals, no bacteria seen.

Coagulation Panel: PT 8.3 s (7.5-10.5 s), PTT 19.3 s (9.0-12.0 s), fibrinogen 506 mg/dL (90-255 mg/dL), D-dimer >2.0 μg/mL (0-0.25 μg/mL).

Arterial Blood Gas (Post–Fluid Bolus)(FiO_2 65%): pH 7.278, pCO_2 40 mm Hg, pO_2 62.7 mm Hg, oxygen saturation 82.3%, ionized calcium 1.36 mmol/L, bicarbonate 17.6 mmol/L, base deficit 7.5 mmol/L, lactate 2.8 mmol/L.

Imaging Findings:

Abdominal Ultrasound: The liver was hypoechoic and enlarged. The gallbladder wall was edematous. Bright mesentery surrounded the left limb of the pancreas. There was a dilated, fluid-filled duodenum. Multiple splenic infarcts were identified, some of which were anechoic, consistent with the presence of fluid (see Figure 86-4). The spleen was enlarged, and a splenic venous thrombus was present.

Echocardiography: The left ventricle and atrium were normal in size. There was laminar flow through the pulmonary artery and aorta. The right heart chambers were subjectively normal in size. There was no tricuspid regurgitation. There was a hyperechoic, oscillating vegetative lesion associated with the anterior mitral valve leaflet and possibly with the aortic valve. A small jet of mitral regurgitation was observed. No aortic insufficiency was observed.

Microbiologic Testing: Aerobic urine culture (cystocentesis specimen): No growth.

Aerobic and anaerobic blood culture (3 specimens): Large numbers of *Staphylococcus aureus* from the first 2 of 3 bottles. The isolate was susceptible to all antimicrobials tested.

Treatment and Outcome: Before the results of diagnostic tests were available, treatment was initiated with shock doses of IV fluids (6 liters of lactated Ringer's solution IV as a bolus over 1 hour). Ticarcillin-clavulanate (50 mg/kg IV q6h), enrofloxacin (10 mg/kg IV q24h), famotidine (0.5 mg/kg IV q12h), prednisolone acetate ophthalmic suspension (1 drop in each eye [OU] q6h), and atropine ophthalmic solution (1 drop OU q12h) were administered. Temperature, respiratory rate, and perfusion parameters were monitored by physical examination after each liter of fluid was administered. Systolic blood pressure was 180 mm Hg throughout the resuscitation period. Lactated Ringer's solution with 30 mEq KCl/L and 2.5% dextrose was then continued at 4.7 mL/kg/hr, with monitoring of arterial blood pressure and urine output. Three units of fresh frozen plasma were administered because total plasma protein dropped to 4.2 g/dL, colloid osmotic pressure was 11.6 mm Hg, and further volume resuscitation was indicated. When severe hypoxemia in the face of maximal supplemental oxygen administration (P_aO_2/FiO_2 ratio = 65) was identified on arterial blood gas analysis, the dog was anesthetized and mechanical ventilation commenced. Mean arterial pressure (measured via an arterial catheter) dropped to 45 mm Hg, so a dopamine constant rate infusion was administered to maintain arterial blood pressure >65 mm Hg; a diagnosis of septic shock was made. Subsequently, diagnoses of DIC, hypoglycemia, ARDS, and MODS became apparent. The dog developed melena, and hemorrhagic fluid with a PCV of 15% appeared in the endotracheal tube. Despite additional colloid support with fresh frozen plasma and hetastarch, colloid osmotic pressure remained low and pitting edema of the distal limbs developed. Creatinine increased to 2.6 mg/dL, albumin dropped to 1.4 mg/dL, globulin to 1.3 g/dL, PCV to 22%, and liver enzyme activities increased (ALT 299 U/L, AST 408 U/L, ALP 617 U/L, total bilirubin 5.4 mg/dL). Ultimately, the dog became oliguric (urine output 0.35 mL/kg/hr). Furosemide and mannitol constant rate infusions had no effect to increase urine output. Because of the poor prognosis, euthanasia was elected.

Necropsy Findings: Gross necropsy findings included mucosal petechiations throughout the oral cavity, hemorrhagic nasal discharge, generalized icterus, subcutaneous edema, and 2 liters of cloudy, dark red fluid with floating fibrin strands within the abdomen. The spleen was enlarged and contained a large infarct (see Figure 86-4). A large infarct was also identified in one kidney, and there were multiple foci up to 5 mm in diameter throughout both kidneys. Multiple, slightly depressed, and nodular foci up to 1 cm in diameter were present on the surface of the liver and extended into the parenchyma. The mitral valve leaflets were thickened and rough, with thick fibrin clots adhering to their surfaces. Ecchymoses were present on the left ventricular wall. The lungs were diffusely wet, firm, and red and failed to collapse when the thorax was opened. They also contained multiple 2- to 4-mm tan foci. Histopathology revealed moderate chronic, active neutrophilic mitral valve endocarditis with a few gram-positive intralesional cocci; acute multifocal neutrophilic and necrotizing myocarditis; acute multifocal neutrophilic and necrotizing pneumonia with hemorrhage; acute diffuse alveolar septal necrosis with hemorrhage, fibrin, and hyaline membrane formation (ARDS); multifocal acute necrotizing and neutrophilic hepatitis, tubulointerstitial nephritis, and splenitis with thrombi and infarcts; hepatic congestion and bile stasis; and severe neutrophilic endophthalmitis with hypopyon. *Enterococcus* spp. and

Continued

Acinetobacter spp. were cultured in enrichment broth from the heart valve.

Diagnosis: *Staphylococcus aureus* IE with septic shock.

Comments: This dog had mitral valve IE and widespread thromboembolic complications as a result of overwhelming *S. aureus* infection. Notably, a heart murmur was absent; echocardiography was performed when infarction was recognized on abdominal sonography. MODS with septic shock was present based on the diagnosis of sepsis (endocarditis with positive blood cultures and 4 of 4 SIRS criteria met) and dysfunction of the coagulation, hepatic, cardiovascular, and pulmonary systems. Aggressive treatment with broad-spectrum antimicrobial drugs, fluids, colloids, pressors, and mechanical ventilation was not successful despite the in vitro susceptibility of the *S. aureus* isolated. The significance of the *Enterococcus* spp. and *Acinetobacter* spp. isolated from the valve at necropsy is unclear; they may have represented contaminants or may have been present as part of a polymicrobial infection. The source of bacteremia and endocarditis was not apparent. The blood culture results became available the day the dog was euthanized.

SUGGESTED READINGS

Greiner M, Wolf G, Hartmann K. A retrospective study of the clinical presentation of 140 dogs and 39 cats with bacteraemia. J Small Anim Pract. 2008;49:378-383.

Lewis DH, Chan DL, Pinheiro D, et al. The immunopathology of sepsis: pathogen recognition, systemic inflammation, the compensatory anti-inflammatory response, and regulatory T cells. J Vet Intern Med. 2012;234:457-482.

Sykes JE, Kittleson MD, Chomel BB, et al. Clinicopathologic findings and outcome in dogs with infective endocarditis: 71 cases (1992-2005). J Am Vet Med Assoc. 2006;228:1735-1747.

Sykes JE, Kittleson MD, Pesavento PA, et al. Evaluation of the relationship between causative organisms and clinical characteristics of infective endocarditis in dogs: 71 cases (1992-2005). J Am Vet Med Assoc. 2006;228:1723-1734.

REFERENCES

1. American College of Chest Physicians/Society of Critical Care Medicine Consensus Conference: definitions for sepsis and organ failure and guidelines for the use of innovative therapies in sepsis. Crit Care Med. 1992;20:864-874.
2. Greiner M, Wolf G, Hartmann K. A retrospective study of the clinical presentation of 140 dogs and 39 cats with bacteraemia. J Small Anim Pract. 2008;49:378-383.
3. Dow SW, Curtis CR, Jones RL, et al. Bacterial culture of blood from critically ill dogs and cats: 100 cases (1985-1987). J Am Vet Med Assoc. 1989;195:113-117.

3a. Lewis DH, Chan DL, Pinheiro D, et al. The immunopathology of sepsis: pathogen recognition, systemic inflammation, the compensatory anti-inflammatory response, and regulatory T cells. J Vet Intern Med. 2012;234:457-482.

4. Schumann RR. Old and new findings on lipopolysaccharide-binding protein: a soluble pattern-recognition molecule. Biochem Soc Trans. 2011;39:989-993.
5. Brady CA, Otto CM, Van Winkle TJ, et al. Severe sepsis in cats: 29 cases (1986-1998). J Am Vet Med Assoc. 2000;217:531-535.
6. Lombard CW, Buergelt CD. Vegetative bacterial endocarditis in dogs; echocardiographic diagnosis and clinical signs. J Small Anim Pract. 1983;24:325-339.
7. MacDonald KA, Chomel BB, Kittleson MD, et al. A prospective study of canine infective endocarditis in northern California (1999-2001): emergence of *Bartonella* as a prevalent etiologic agent. J Vet Intern Med. 2004;18:56-64.
8. Sykes JE, Kittleson MD, Chomel BB, et al. Clinicopathologic findings and outcome in dogs with infective endocarditis: 71 cases (1992-2005). J Am Vet Med Assoc. 2006;228:1735-1747.
9. Taboada J, Palmer GH. Renal failure associated with bacterial endocarditis in the dog. J Am Anim Hosp Assoc. 1989;25:243-251.
10. Peddle GD, Drobatz KJ, Harvey CE, et al. Association of periodontal disease, oral procedures, and other clinical findings with bacterial endocarditis in dogs. J Am Vet Med Assoc. 2009;234:100-107.
11. Sykes JE, Kittleson MD, Pesavento PA, et al. Evaluation of the relationship between causative organisms and clinical characteristics of infective endocarditis in dogs: 71 cases (1992-2005). J Am Vet Med Assoc. 2006;228:1723-1734.
12. Calvert CA. Valvular bacterial endocarditis in the dog. J Am Vet Med Assoc. 1982;180:1080-1084.
13. Sisson D, Thomas WP. Endocarditis of the aortic valve in the dog. J Am Vet Med Assoc. 1984;184:570-577.
14. Que YA, Haefliger JA, Piroth L, et al. Fibrinogen and fibronectin binding cooperate for valve infection and invasion in *Staphylococcus aureus* experimental endocarditis. J Exp Med. 2005;201:1627-1635.
15. Piroth L, Que YA, Widmer E, et al. The fibrinogen- and fibronectin-binding domains of *Staphylococcus aureus* fibronectin-binding protein A synergistically promote endothelial invasion and experimental endocarditis. Infect Immun. 2008;76:3824-3831.
16. Declue AE, Sharp CR, Harmon M. Plasma inflammatory mediator concentrations at ICU admission in dogs with naturally developing sepsis. J Vet Intern Med. 2012;26:624-630.
17. Osterbur K, Whitehead Z, Sharp CR, et al. Plasma nitrate/nitrite concentrations in dogs with naturally developing sepsis and non-infectious forms of the systemic inflammatory response syndrome. Vet Rec. 2011;169:554.
18. DeClue AE, Osterbur K, Bigio A, et al. Evaluation of serum NT-pCNP as a diagnostic and prognostic biomarker for sepsis in dogs. J Vet Intern Med. 2011;25:453-459.
19. Gould FK, Denning DW, Elliott TS, et al. Guidelines for the diagnosis and antibiotic treatment of endocarditis in adults: a report of the Working Party of the British Society for Antimicrobial Chemotherapy. J Antimicrob Chemother. 2012;67:269-289.
20. Meurs KM, Heaney AM, Atkins CE, et al. Comparison of polymerase chain reaction with bacterial 16S primers to blood culture to identify bacteremia in dogs with suspected bacterial endocarditis. J Vet Intern Med. 2011;25:959-962.
21. Wiinberg B, Jensen AL, Johansson PI, et al. Thromboelastographic evaluation of hemostatic function in dogs with disseminated intravascular coagulation. J Vet Intern Med. 2008;22:357-365.
22. Mermel LA, Allon M, Bouza E, et al. Clinical practice guidelines for the diagnosis and management of intravascular catheter-related infection: 2009 update by the Infectious Diseases Society of America. Clin Infect Dis. 2009;49:1-45.
23. Davenport AC, Mascarelli PE, Maggi RG, et al. Phylogenetic diversity of bacteria isolated from sick dogs using the BAPGM enrichment culture platform [Abstract]. J Vet Intern Med. 2012;26:786-787.

24. Rivers E, Nguyen B, Havstad S, et al. Early goal-directed therapy in the treatment of severe sepsis and septic shock. N Engl J Med. 2001;345:1368-1377.
25. Reinhart K, Perner A, Sprung CL, et al. Consensus statement of the ESICM task force on colloid volume therapy in critically ill patients. Intensive Care Med. 2012;38:368-383.
26. Brunkhorst FM, Engel C, Bloos F, et al. Intensive insulin therapy and pentastarch resuscitation in severe sepsis. N Engl J Med. 2008;358:125-139.
27. Jones AE, Shapiro NI, Trzeciak S, et al. Lactate clearance vs central venous oxygen saturation as goals of early sepsis therapy: a randomized clinical trial. JAMA. 2010;303:739-746.
28. Annane D, Bellissant E, Bollaert PE, et al. Corticosteroids in the treatment of severe sepsis and septic shock in adults: a systematic review. JAMA. 2009;301:2362-2375.
29. Moran JL, Graham PL, Rockliff S, et al. Updating the evidence for the role of corticosteroids in severe sepsis and septic shock: a Bayesian meta-analytic perspective. Crit Care. 2010;14:R134.
30. Burkitt JM, Haskins SC, Nelson RW, et al. Relative adrenal insufficiency in dogs with sepsis. J Vet Intern Med. 2007;21:226-231.
31. Peyton JL, Burkitt JM. Critical illness-related corticosteroid insufficiency in a dog with septic shock. J Vet Emerg Crit Care. 2009;19:262-268.
32. Xigris [drotrecogin alfa (activated)]: Market Withdrawal—Failure to Show Survival Benefit. 2011. http://www.fda.gov/Safety/MedWatch/SafetyInformation/SafetyAlertsforHumanMedicalProducts/ucm277143.htm, Last accessed January 23, 2013.
33. Turgeon AF, Hutton B, Fergusson DA, et al. Meta-analysis: intravenous immunoglobulin in critically ill adult patients with sepsis. Ann Intern Med. 2007;146:193-203.
34. Kreymann KG, de Heer G, Nierhaus A, et al. Use of polyclonal immunoglobulins as adjunctive therapy for sepsis or septic shock. Crit Care Med. 2007;35(12):2677-2685.
35. Kumar A, Roberts D, Wood KE, et al. Duration of hypotension before initiation of effective antimicrobial therapy is the critical determinant of survival in human septic shock. Crit Care Med. 2006;34:1589-1596.
36. Habib G, Hoen B, Tornos P, et al. Guidelines on the prevention, diagnosis, and treatment of infective endocarditis (new version 2009): the Task Force on the Prevention, Diagnosis, and Treatment of Infective Endocarditis of the European Society of Cardiology (ESC). Endorsed by the European Society of Clinical Microbiology and Infectious Diseases (ESCMID) and the International Society of Chemotherapy (ISC) for Infection and Cancer. Eur Heart J. 2009;30:2369-2413.
37. Kenney EM, Rozanski EA, Rush JE, et al. Association between outcome and organ system dysfunction in dogs with sepsis: 114 cases (2003-2007). J Am Vet Med Assoc. 2010;236:83-87.
38. Chretin JD, Rassnick KM, Shaw NA, et al. Prophylactic trimethoprim-sulfadiazine during chemotherapy in dogs with lymphoma and osteosarcoma: a double-blind, placebo-controlled study. J Vet Intern Med. 2007;21:141-148.
39. Cullen M, Steven N, Billingham L, et al. Antibacterial prophylaxis after chemotherapy for solid tumors and lymphomas. N Engl J Med. 2005;353:988-998.

CHAPTER 87

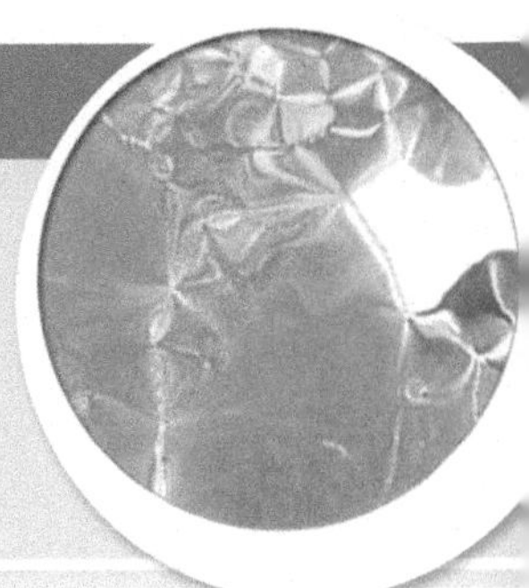

Bacterial Bronchopneumonia and Pyothorax

Jane E. Sykes

> **Overview of Bacterial Tracheobronchitis and Bronchopneumonia Secondary to Invasion by Resident Bacteria**
>
> Causes: Frequently isolated secondary bacterial invaders in respiratory tract infections are *Escherichia coli, Pasteurella* spp., *Mycoplasma* spp., and anaerobes. *Pseudomonas* spp., *Staphylococcus* spp., and *Streptococcus* spp. may also be isolated.
>
> Geographic Distribution: Worldwide
>
> Mode of Transmission: Aspiration of gastrointestinal or oropharyngeal bacteria, opportunistic invasion of commensals as a result of impaired bronchopulmonary immune defenses
>
> Major Clinical Signs: Lethargy, fever, cough, nasal discharge, tachypnea, respiratory distress, cyanosis, increased lung sounds (pneumonia)
>
> Differential Diagnoses: Viral, protozoal, fungal, algal, or parasitic pneumonia; pneumonia caused by primary bacterial pathogens such as *Bordetella, Mycobacterium, Leptospira, Nocardia,* or *Yersinia;* aspiration pneumonitis (chemical injury); toxicity (e.g., paraquat); inflammatory lung diseases (e.g., eosinophilic bronchopneumopathy); pulmonary hemorrhage or edema; foreign body pneumonia; neoplasia
>
> Human Health Significance: Multidrug-resistant bacteria that infect the lungs of dogs and cats may have the potential to colonize human patients, but this requires further study. Some primary bacterial causes of pneumonia in dogs and cats are directly zoonotic.

BACTERIAL TRACHEOBRONCHITIS AND BRONCHOPNEUMONIA

Etiology, Epidemiology, and Pathogenesis

Bacterial tracheobronchitis or bronchopneumonia may be acute or chronic and varies considerably in severity from subclinical through to fulminant and immediately life threatening. Infection of the airways and pulmonary parenchyma can occur secondary to (1) aspiration of gastrointestinal or oropharyngeal bacteria; (2) opportunistic invasion of commensal bacteria as a result of impaired bronchopulmonary immune defenses; (3) hematogenous spread of bacteria to the bronchopulmonary tree from extrapulmonary sites; or (4) aerosol or oronasal transmission of primary respiratory pathogens. Bronchitis and bronchopneumonia that result from invasion by commensal bacteria are the focus of this section. Organisms maintained in the environment (and/or in reservoir hosts) such as *Nocardia, Mycobacterium, Leptospira, Rickettsia rickettsii,* and *Yersinia* can also cause pneumonia in dogs or cats. The reader is referred to Chapters 30, 43, 44, 50 and 55 in Section 2 for more information on these infections. Information on *Bordetella, Mycoplasma,* and *Streptococcus* infections (as part of Canine Infectious Respiratory Disease Complex) is provided in Chapters 34, 38 and 40 in Section 2. *Bordetella, Mycoplasma* and some *Streptococcus* strains have the potential to be contagious pathogens that most often cause disease in young (or young adult) dogs and cats and those housed in overcrowded environments.

Many aerobic and anaerobic commensal bacterial species have been isolated from dogs and cats with opportunistic tracheobronchitis and bronchopneumonia (Figure 87-1 and Box 87-1).[1-13] The relative prevalence of each bacterial species may be affected by the underlying condition(s) that predisposes to bacterial invasion, the population of animals studied (see Figure 87-1), and the methods used to collect and culture specimens from the respiratory tract.

Aspiration Pneumonia

Secondary bacterial infection after aspiration of gastrointestinal or oropharyngeal contents is a common underlying reason for bacterial bronchopneumonia in adult dogs, but is rare in cats. Chemical damage to the lungs results from inhalation of acidic gastric fluid and particulate matter ("aspiration pneumonitis"). In some cases this is followed by development of bacterial bronchopneumonia. Conditions that predispose dogs to aspiration pneumonitis include brachycephalic obstructive syndrome; laryngeal paralysis, laryngeal surgery, or laryngeal foreign bodies; esophageal disorders such as megaesophagus, decreased esophageal motility, or esophageal foreign bodies; hiatal hernia; decreased mentation, seizures, or recumbency secondary to neurologic disease, sedation, or anesthesia; tracheostomy tube placement; vomiting; and swallowing disorders such as cricopharyngeal achalasia.[11,13-15] More than 30% of dogs in one study had more than one abnormality that predisposed to aspiration; the combination of esophageal and neurologic disease was most common.[11] In cats, most bacterial pneumonia follows viral infections or hematogenous spread of bacteria to the respiratory tract; aspiration pneumonia is rarely reported.[4,6,12] Aspiration pneumonia has been described rarely in association with dysautonomia[16] and arytenoid lateralization for treatment of laryngeal paralysis.[17] Systemic immune compromise can predispose to life-threatening bacterial infection after aspiration in both dogs and cats.

In a study of 47 dogs with aspiration that had airway lavage specimens cultured (primarily by transtracheal wash), 77% of specimens yielded bacterial organisms.[13] The most prevalent species was *Escherichia coli.* Other frequently isolated

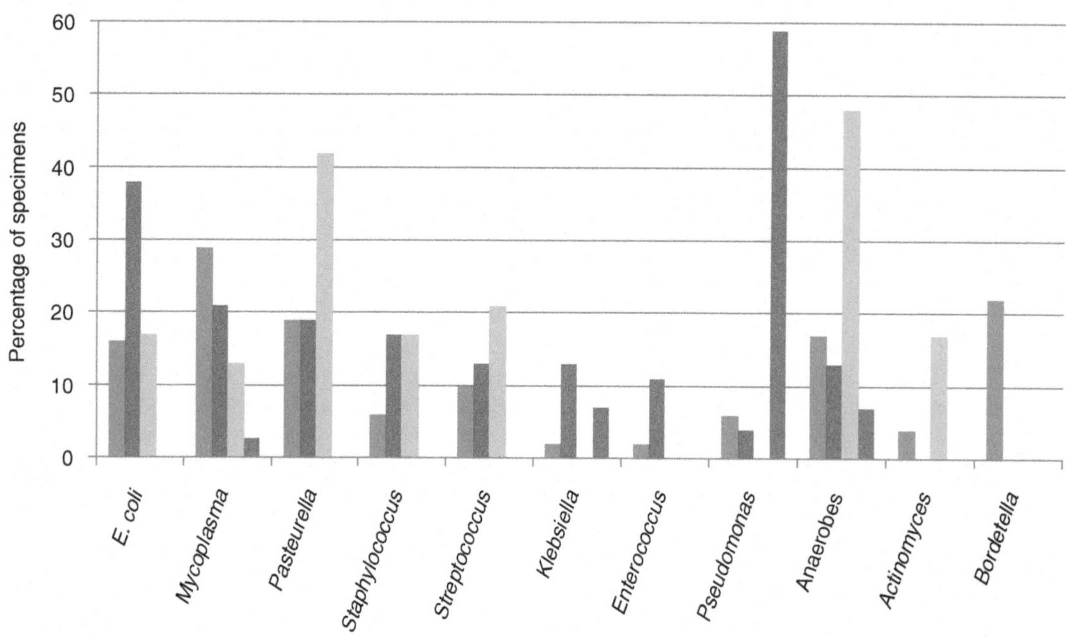

FIGURE 87-1 Prevalence of bacterial species isolated from respiratory lavage specimens from dogs with lower respiratory infection (BAL, blue), aspiration (transtracheal lavage or BAL, red), foreign body pneumonia (BAL, green), and dogs with bronchoscopically diagnosed tracheal collapse (BAL, purple). (Compiled from references 7, 9, 10, and 13.)

BOX 87-1

Bacteria That May Be Isolated from Cats with Lower Respiratory Tract Infection[1,3,4,12,37]

Mycoplasma spp.
Pasteurella spp.
Escherichia coli
Streptococcus spp. (especially *S. canis*)
Enterobacter spp.
Anaerobes (e.g., *Fusobacterium, Peptostreptococcus, Porphyromonas*)
Other gram-positive bacteria (e.g., *Staphylococcus* spp., *Enterococcus, Corynebacterium*)
Other gram-negative bacteria (e.g., *Pseudomonas, Acinetobacter, Klebsiella, Proteus, Bordetella bronchiseptica, Moraxella, Alcaligenes, Neisseria* spp.)

organisms from dogs with aspiration pneumonia were *Mycoplasma* spp., *Pasteurella* spp., *Staphylococcus* spp., *Klebsiella* spp., and *Enterococcus* spp.[13] Overall, gram-negative aerobes are more likely to be present than gram-positive aerobes in dogs with aspiration pneumonia. Anaerobes are also frequently isolated, and many dogs have mixed bacterial infections. Infections with *Pseudomonas aeruginosa*, *Acinetobacter baumannii*, and *Corynebacterium* species such as *Corynebacterium ulcerans* have also been described.[13,18] Some of these infections may be acquired from the hospital environment.

Tracheobronchitis and Bronchopneumonia Secondary to Impaired Local Airway Defenses

Conditions that impair local airway defenses predispose to opportunistic invasion of the tracheobronchial tree and pulmonary parenchyma by commensal bacteria. These conditions include ciliary dyskinesia, viral infections (especially persistent viral infections such as canine distemper virus or feline calicivirus infection), tracheobronchial collapse, tracheal stent placement, eosinophilic bronchopneumopathy, airway foreign bodies or neoplasia, chronic bronchitis, and bronchiectasis.[5,7,9,12,18-21] Chronic bronchitis and bronchiectasis either may be sterile inflammatory processes that predispose to opportunistic bacterial invasion, or alternatively they occur secondary to chronic bacterial infections of the airways (e.g., as a result of chronic low-grade aspiration secondary to laryngeal paralysis). However, in many dogs with disorders such as tracheobronchial collapse, eosinophilic bronchopneumopathy, or chronic bronchitis, concurrent bacterial infection is not present.

In one study of dogs with tracheal collapse that underwent bronchoscopy and bronchoalveolar lavage (BAL), *Pseudomonas* was the most prevalent opportunistic bacterial species isolated (see Figure 87-1).[9] In contrast, *Pseudomonas* is an uncommon isolate from dogs with opportunistic lower respiratory infection.[10] In dogs with airway foreign bodies (usually grass awns), anaerobes, *Pasteurella*, gram-positive cocci, and *Actinomyces* predominate.[7]

Clinical Features

Signs and Physical Examination Findings

Dogs with bacterial bronchitis may have no clinical signs, or cough may be present. Other systemic signs such as fever, lethargy, or inappetence are usually absent. Involvement of the pulmonary parenchyma may be associated with more severe signs such as fever (as high as 107°F [41.6°C]), anorexia, lethargy, dehydration, weakness, weight loss, a moist and/or productive cough, serous to mucopurulent nasal discharge, tachypnea, tachycardia, respiratory distress, increased or harsh lung sounds on thoracic auscultation, crackles, wheezes, reduced lung sounds (due to lung consolidation), and/or cyanosis.[13,22] Some animals with pneumonia show no signs or only a few of these signs. Uncommonly, hemoptysis is reported.[23] Clinical signs of the underlying illness (such as vomiting, regurgitation, neurologic signs, or septic shock) may also be identified.[13]

Cats with bacterial bronchopneumonia may show only fever, lethargy, and/or inappetence. Respiratory signs, and especially cough, are often absent.[12]

Diagnosis

Bacterial bronchitis or bronchopneumonia is usually suspected based on a history of underlying predisposing conditions, clinical signs, and radiographic findings. Antemortem diagnosis of *infection* is most often based on cytologic examination in conjunction with culture and susceptibility of airway lavage specimens. Procedures for collection of airway lavage specimens include transtracheal wash, endotracheal wash, or BAL. Fine-needle aspiration of consolidated lung tissue may also be useful to rule out other disorders such as neoplasia or fungal pneumonia but carries some risk of iatrogenic pneumothorax.[4,24,25] The risk of pneumothorax may be reduced if ultrasound guidance is used. Assessment of laryngeal function (with doxapram stimulation) should be considered in any dog anesthetized for bronchoscopy and airway lavage. In some instances, the diagnosis of bacterial bronchopneumonia is made by histopathology and culture of a lung biopsy specimen collected during surgery or tissue specimens collected at necropsy.

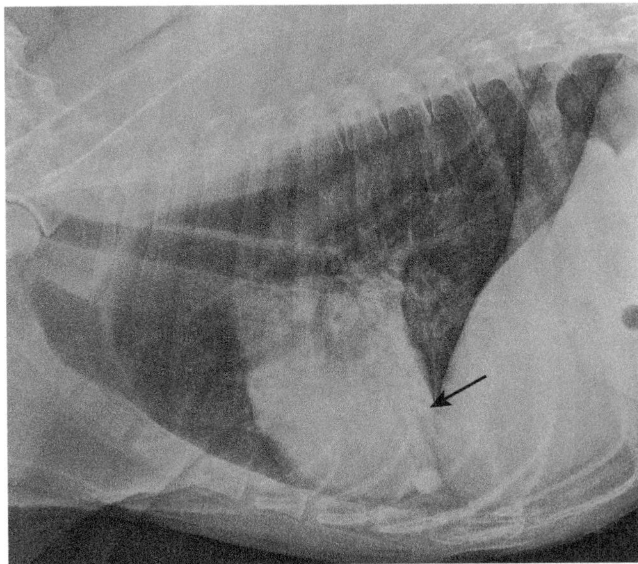

FIGURE 87-2 Left lateral thoracic radiograph from a 12-year-old male neutered German shepherd dog with a history of regurgitation, cough, and pyrexia. Air bronchograms (*arrow*) can be seen overlying the cardiac silhouette, which were less apparent on the right lateral view. The presence of an alveolar pattern in the ventral portions of the left and right cranial lung lobes in this dog was consistent with a diagnosis of aspiration pneumonia. Air is also visible in the esophagus.

Laboratory Abnormalities

Complete Blood Count, Serum Biochemistry Profile, and Urinalysis

Most dogs and cats with bacterial bronchopneumonia have leukocytosis due to a neutrophilia, often with bandemia and toxic neutrophil changes.[4,5,12,13,22] Leukopenia may also occur, but some animals have a normal leukogram. Anemia of inflammatory disease may also be present. The serum biochemistry profile and urinalysis can be unremarkable or may have changes that reflect the presence of concurrent systemic disease.

Arterial Blood Gas Analysis

Arterial blood gas analysis provides the most accurate assessment of oxygenation status in animals with bronchopneumonia. Hypoxemia ($PaO_2 \leq 80$ mm Hg at sea level) can be detected in around 75% of dogs with aspiration pneumonia,[13,22] with a mean PaO_2 of 69 to 77 mm Hg.[5,13,22] Hypocapnia may also be present. The alveolar-arterial (A-a) oxygen gradient may be increased (up to 83 mm Hg with a median around 41 mm Hg; for room air, values >15 mm Hg indicate lung dysfunction).[13,22]

Diagnostic Imaging

Plain Radiography

Thoracic radiographs in dogs with bacterial bronchitis may reveal a diffuse bronchial pattern and there may be evidence of underlying airway disease, such as tracheobronchial collapse or bronchiectasis. Plain thoracic radiographs are insensitive for diagnosis of bacterial bronchitis, and dogs with severe bronchitis can have normal findings.

Dogs with aspiration bronchopneumonia may have bronchointerstitial to alveolar changes in one or more lung lobes. Most often an alveolar pattern is present (Figure 87-2).[13,22] The most commonly affected lung lobe is the right middle lung lobe, and so a left lateral projection as well as right lateral and ventrodorsal projections in full inspiration are important to identify changes in this lobe. The left and right cranial lung lobes are also frequently affected.[13,22] Radiographic changes can lag behind the aspiration event for up to 24 hours. Clues to underlying causes of bronchopneumonia, such as megaesophagus or situs inversus (ciliary dyskinesia), may also be evident.

Dogs and cats with plant awn pneumonia may have a focal interstitial to alveolar pattern that tends to involve the caudal and accessory lung lobes, and to a lesser extent the right middle and left and right cranial lung lobes.[26] Less often, pneumothorax, consolidation of affected lung lobes, and/or pleural effusion (see Pyothorax) are identified.

Advanced Imaging

Because of increased sensitivity over plain radiography, computed tomography (CT) may be useful to evaluate the airways and pulmonary parenchyma when thoracic radiographs are unremarkable or underlying plant awn pneumonia is suspected. Airway thickening and bronchiectasis may be evident in dogs with bronchitis. Focal interstitial to alveolar pulmonary opacities and pleural thickening are the most common finding in animals with migrating plant foreign bodies; other findings include pneumothorax and/or pneumomediastinum, mild enlargement and contrast enhancement of thoracic lymph nodes, lung lobe opacification, mediastinal or thoracic wall masses, and/or pleural effusion (Figure 87-3).[26] CT may be useful to guide subsequent bronchoscopy and BAL fluid collection for animals with focal bronchopneumonia.

Bronchoscopy

On bronchoscopic examination, dogs and cats with bacterial bronchitis or bronchopneumonia may have edematous and hyperemic airways, accumulation of mucus or mucopurulent secretions, and/or mucosal irregularity.[5,6] Other findings include airway collapse, airway stenosis, and bronchiectasis. Foreign bodies such as plant awns may be identified and removed (see Figure 87-3, *B*);[7] if not, identification and localization of a focal accumulation of pus in an airway may direct subsequent surgical removal of a lobe affected by a migrating plant awn.

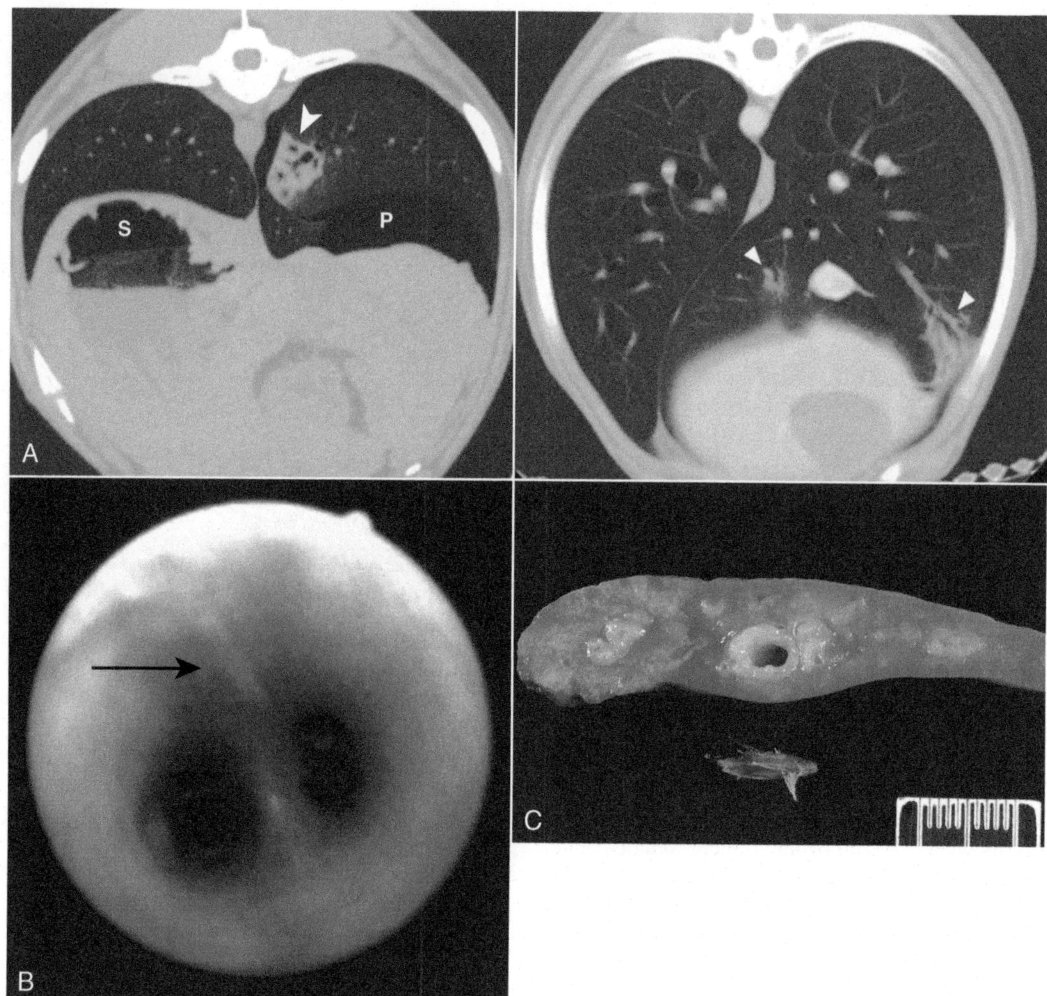

FIGURE 87-3 Migrating plant awn foreign bodies. **A,** CT scan images from a 1-year-old female spayed German shorthaired pointer dog. Pneumothorax (*left, P*) and multifocal pulmonary opacities (*white arrowheads*) are present (*S* = stomach). **B,** Bronchoscopic image showing a plant awn in a bronchus of a 2-year-old male neutered Belgian Malinois. **C,** Portion of the right middle lung lobe of a 2-year-old female spayed Labrador retriever, which was removed during thoracotomy. A 1-cm plant awn was removed from a pocket of mucoid material within a bronchus. (**C,** Image courtesy University of California, Davis, Veterinary Anatomic Pathology Service.)

Microbiologic Tests

Cytologic Examination

Cytologic examination of airway lavage specimens or fine-needle aspirates of the lung in dogs and cats with bacterial bronchopneumonia usually reveals a mixed inflammatory response with a predominance of neutrophils. The presence of degenerate neutrophils should increase suspicion for bacterial infection. In some animals, one or more bacterial populations may be seen intracellularly and extracellularly, but culture is considerably more sensitive than cytologic examination for detection of bacteria in airway lavage specimens.

Culture

Ideally, airway lavage specimens should be collected and submitted for aerobic, anaerobic, and *Mycoplasma* cultures before treatment with antimicrobial drugs is commenced, although this may not be feasible if severe respiratory compromise is present. The need for anaerobic cultures is controversial because anaerobes are difficult to isolate and tend to have predictable susceptibilities. Anaerobes are most likely to be present in dogs with aspiration pneumonia or grass awn foreign bodies. *Mycoplasma* species may also be difficult to isolate (see Chapter 40). False-negative culture results can also occur if low numbers of bacteria are present, if the specimen is small, fastidious organisms are present, or if antimicrobial drugs have recently been administered.

Because a variety of gram-positive and gram-negative bacteria as well as *Mycoplasma* spp. can be found in low numbers in the lower respiratory tracts of healthy dogs and cats,[3,27-29] a positive culture on a respiratory lavage specimen alone is not diagnostic for bacterial bronchitis or bronchopneumonia. However, a positive culture in conjunction with cytologic evidence of leukocytosis with intracellular bacteria supports the presence of infection. When quantitative bacterial cultures on BAL fluid can be performed, it has been suggested that growth greater than 1.7×10^3 CFU/mL is likely to be clinically significant.[5] BAL is more likely to identify clinically significant bacteria, but collection of specimens by transtracheal wash is sufficient if diffuse disease is present and bronchoscopy is not available or not affordable.[30] Care should be taken not to overinterpret the significance of few organisms, or minimally pathogenic organisms (e.g., *Bacillus* spp. or coagulase-negative staphylococci) that may represent airway contaminants.

Some animals with bacterial pneumonia may have positive blood cultures. If airway lavage is not possible because of severe respiratory compromise, blood cultures should be considered in order to obtain information about the identity and susceptibility of bacteria involved. Further study is required to determine the sensitivity and specificity of blood culture for diagnosis of bacterial pneumonia in dogs or cats.

Pathologic Findings

The lung lobes of animals with bacterial bronchopneumonia may be diffusely mottled red or dark pink, firm, and ooze fluid on cut section. The airway mucosa also may be diffusely reddened, with evidence of mucus accumulation. Intraluminal food accumulation may be present in animals with acute aspiration pneumonia. Evidence of predisposing causes such as neoplasia, plant material, or bronchiectasis may be present. Histopathology most often reveals focal, multifocal, or diffuse suppurative and necrotizing inflammation, sometimes with intralesional bacteria. In chronic infections, histiocytic infiltrates may be present.

Treatment and Prognosis

Antimicrobial Drugs

Selection of antimicrobial drugs for treatment of secondary bacterial tracheobronchitis and bronchopneumonia in dogs and cats should ideally be based on the results of culture and susceptibility testing. For dogs with secondary bacterial tracheobronchitis, treatment should be withheld until the results are available, or empiric treatment with doxycycline (first choice) or amoxicillin–clavulanic acid (second choice) is suggested (Table 87-1). Amoxicillin–clavulanic acid is not active against *Mycoplasma,* so if *Mycoplasma* infection is suspected, doxycycline is a more appropriate choice. The optimal duration of treatment is unknown, but if a clinical response to treatment occurs in the first 7 to 10 days, treatment could be continued for a week beyond resolution of clinical signs.[30]

Animals with severe bronchopneumonia may require hospitalization and parenteral treatment with broad-spectrum antimicrobial drugs such as a combination of a fluoroquinolone and a β-lactam (ampicillin, ampicillin-sulbactam) or clindamycin (Table 87-2). Clindamycin may be a good choice if lung consolidation is present and/or anaerobes are suspected, because of its good tissue penetration, although some anaerobes and *Pasteurella* are resistant to clindamycin. If fluoroquinolone resistance is likely based on the regional prevalence of bacterial resistance, drugs other than a fluoroquinolone with activity against gram-negative bacteria may be indicated based on culture and susceptibility test results or the regional prevalence of bacterial resistance. Examples include aminoglycosides, third-generation cephalosporines, carbapenems such as meropenem, or ticarcillin–clavulanic acid. The spectrum of antimicrobial activity should be narrowed once the results of culture and susceptibility are available.

The optimum duration of treatment requires further study. Traditionally, at least 4 weeks of treatment have been recommended for lower respiratory infections, or for at least 1 week after radiographic resolution of pulmonary lesions. Shorter periods of treatment are used in human patients and may also be effective in dogs and cats.

Surgery

In some cases, surgery is required to remove abscessed lung lobes that fail to improve with medical therapy, or plant awn foreign bodies that cannot be retrieved using bronchoscopy.[7] The development of pneumothorax in association with migrating foreign bodies may also be an indication for surgical intervention.

TABLE 87-1

Antimicrobial Drugs That May Be Useful to Treat Secondary Bacterial Tracheobronchitis in Dogs

Drug	Dose (mg/kg)	Route	Interval (hours)	Duration (days)
Doxycycline	5	PO	12	1 week beyond resolution of signs
Amoxicillin-clavulanic acid	22	PO	12	1 week beyond resolution of signs

TABLE 87-2

Suggested Empiric Antimicrobial Drug Choices for IV Use in Dogs or Cats with Bacterial Bronchopneumonia Pending the Results of Culture and Susceptibility*

Drug	Dose (mg/kg)	Route	Interval (hours)
Ampicillin *or*	20	IV	6
Ampicillin-sulbactam† *or*	20	IV	8
Clindamycin phosphate *and*	10	IV	12*
Enrofloxacin‡	5-10 (dogs)	IV	24

*Spectrum should be reduced once the results of culture and susceptibility are available.

†Dose based on ampicillin component.

‡Other fluoroquinolones such as pradofloxacin (which also has activity against anaerobes) should be considered for treatment of cats because of the risk for retinal toxicity in this species, although parenteral formulations are not available. Other drugs with activity against gram-negative bacteria (e.g., meropenem, third-generation cephalosporines, aminoglycosides) could also be considered for parenteral treatment of cats or if the regional prevalence of fluoroquinolone resistance is high. See also Chapter 86.

Supportive Care

Other supportive treatments that may be needed for dogs and cats with severe bronchopneumonia include supplemental humidified oxygen, intravenous fluid therapy, nebulization, and coupage to aid in the mobilization of secretions. Animals that are hypoventilating or that fail to respond to supplemental oxygen therapy may require mechanical ventilation.

Prognosis

The survival rate to discharge for aspiration pneumonia in one study was 77%,[11] with a mean duration of hospitalization of 5 days (range, 1 to 23 days). In one study of dogs with aspiration pneumonia, dogs with two or more affected lung lobes had a worse outcome than dogs with single lung lobe involvement.[13] However, in another study, there was no correlation between radiographic findings and survival.[11] No correlation has been found between survival and the identity of bacterial species present, the number of bacterial species present, the underlying cause of aspiration, or the presence of multiple underlying causes of aspiration.[11,13] Identification and management of the underlying cause, when possible, is critical to prevent recurrence.

Prevention

Prevention of bacterial bronchitis and bronchopneumonia relies on identification and management of underlying causes. Aspiration pneumonia can be prevented by fasting before sedation or anesthesia and proper use of cuffed endotracheal tubes for anesthesia. Upright feeding may be used in an attempt to prevent recurrent aspiration for dogs with laryngeal and esophageal disorders, but the extent to which upright feeding prevents aspiration in these conditions is not known. Antiemetics should be administered to control vomiting in patients that are vomiting secondary to underlying disorders such as pancreatitis or uremia. If a feeding tube is in place, care should be taken to minimize the chance of vomiting and aspiration by slow, frequent feeding of small amounts of food that do not overwhelm gastric capacity. Prophylactic antimicrobial drugs are not recommended because they may predispose dogs to infection by drug-resistant bacteria.

Public Health Aspects

Multidrug-resistant bacteria can be isolated from the airways of some dogs with opportunistic bronchitis and bronchopneumonia.[18] Whether these organisms can colonize humans has not been clearly established. Some causes of pneumonia in dogs or cats, such as *Pasteurella* species, *B. bronchiseptica, Streptococcus equi* subsp. *zooepidemicus, Mycobacterium tuberculosis,* and *Capnocytophaga* and *Yersinia* species are potentially zoonotic pathogens, and immunocompromised humans may be at higher risk for development of infection or serious illness. As for every patient, routine precautions such as hand washing should be used before and after handling dogs and cats with suspected bacterial bronchopneumonia. Dogs with bronchopneumonia should not be allowed to lick in-contact humans.

PYOTHORAX

Etiology, Epidemiology, and Pathogenesis

Pyothorax is defined as the presence of pus within the pleural space. Multiple underlying conditions lead to pyothorax in dogs and cats. These include penetrating injuries to the thoracic wall (such as bite wounds or migrating plant awns), esophageal perforation, or spread of infection from the lungs to the pleural space secondary to rupture of lung abscesses or necrotic pulmonary neoplasia. Rarely, pyothorax occurs secondary to aspiration pneumonia.[31,32] Pathogens may also spread hematogenously to the pleural space as part of a disseminated infection. In many animals with pyothorax, the underlying cause or route of bacterial entry is not clear.

Overview of Bacterial Pyothorax

Causes: Primarily anaerobic bacteria and *Pasteurella* species in cats; anaerobes, aerobic gram-negative enteric bacteria, and *Pasteurella* in dogs. Other bacterial species are involved less commonly.

Geographic Distribution: Worldwide

Mode of Transmission: Traumatic inoculation of bacteria into the pleural space (e.g., bite wounds, foreign bodies), spread from sites of pneumonia (e.g., rupture of lung abscesses), hematogenous spread

Major Clinical Signs: Lethargy, fever, inappetence, tachypnea, rapid and shallow respiratory pattern, decreased lung and heart sounds. Hypothermia, bradycardia, and hypersalivation may be identified in cats.

Differential Diagnoses: Chylothorax, hemothorax, neoplasia, fungal pyothorax (e.g., *Aspergillus, Candida, Cryptococcus*), feline infectious peritonitis (cats), congestive heart failure

Human Health Significance: Bacteria that cause pyothorax are typically commensal organisms found in the oral cavities of healthy cats and dogs.

Pyothorax in Cats

Pyothorax is a common cause of pleural effusion in cats.[33] Cats with pyothorax are usually FeLV and FIV negative and tend to be young to middle-aged adults with outdoor exposure, although cats of any age may be affected.[31,33-35] There is no sex or breed predisposition,[31,35] but residence in a multicat household may increase the risk for pyothorax.[35] In some cats, pyothorax develops after puncture or bite wounds to the thorax or when plant foreign bodies are inhaled or penetrate the thorax.[31,35] However, other cats that develop pyothorax are housed indoors and have no history of exposure to other cats. Ruptured lung abscesses have been identified in some cats.[33,35,36] Occasionally, migrating parasites (*Cuterebra, Aelurostrongylus, Toxocara*) are detected in the lungs of affected cats.[31,35] Other cats have a history of upper respiratory tract infection.[1,3,4,12,37] It has been suggested that pyothorax in these cats occurs secondary to bronchopneumonia.[31]

Oropharyngeal bacterial species, primarily a mixture of anaerobic bacterial species and/or *Pasteurella,* are most often isolated from pleural fluid (Table 87-3).[33-35,38,39] A mixture of anaerobic and facultative bacteria is isolated from over 40% of affected cats.[38]

Pyothorax in Dogs

In dogs, bacterial pyothorax develops secondary to penetrating thoracic wall trauma, migrating grass awn foreign bodies, esophageal perforation, or bite wounds. Young adult, medium to large-breed dogs (especially spaniels, pointers, retrievers, and Border collies) with outdoor exposure are most often affected, but the disease can occur in dogs of any age or breed.[32,34,38,40,41] In some studies, male dogs slightly outnumber female dogs. Obligate anaerobes and gram-negative enterics such as *E. coli* and *Klebsiella pneumoniae* are often isolated, with mixed anaerobic-aerobic infections in at least one third of affected dogs.[32,38,41] Other frequently isolated bacteria include *Actinomyces, Streptococcus canis, Pasteurella,* and *Nocardia.*[32,34,38,37] Less often, other bacterial species are isolated (see Table 87-3).[32,34,38,41,42] Obligate

TABLE 87-3
Bacterial Causes of Pyothorax in Dogs and Cats

Prevalence*	Cats	Dogs
Common (>75% of cases)	*Pasteurella multocida* Obligate anaerobes (*Peptostreptococcus, Bacteroides, Fusobacterium, Porphyromonas, Prevotella, Filifactor villosus*, and *Clostridium*)	Obligate anaerobes Enterobacteriaceae (especially *E. coli, Klebsiella pneumoniae*)
Occasional (25%-75% of cases)	*Actinomyces* spp. *Streptococcus* spp. *Mycoplasma* spp.	*Pasteurella* spp. *Actinomyces* spp. *Streptococcus canis* *Nocardia* spp.
Uncommon to rare (<25% of cases)	*Staphylococcus* spp. Gram-negative bacteria other than *Pasteurella* *Nocardia* spp. *Rhodococcus equi*	*Mycoplasma* spp. *Staphylococcus* spp. *Enterococcus* spp. *Corynebacterium* spp. *Bacillus* spp. *Enterobacter* spp. *Arcanobacterium pyogenes* *Acinetobacter* spp. *Capnocytophaga* spp. *Kluyvera* spp. *Stenotrophomonas maltophilia* *Aeromonas hydrophila* *Achromobacter xylosoxidans* *Serratia marcescens* *Pseudomonas* spp. *Listeria monocytogenes*

*Percentages are approximate, because prevalences of bacteria listed in the occasional and uncommon groups vary between studies.

anaerobes, *Actinomyces* spp., and *Streptococcus canis* infections may be more prevalent where grass awn exposure is common.

Clinical Features

The severity and duration of clinical signs in cats and dogs with pyothorax are extremely variable. Illness durations of months to up to a year can occur, with a median duration of 14 days.[34] Cats can be found dead within 24 hours of having a normal appetite and activity level.[43] Systemic signs of illness are common and include fever, lethargy, weakness, inappetence, weight loss, and/or dehydration.[31,32,34,35,41,42] Clinical signs referable to the respiratory tract include tachypnea with a rapid and shallow respiratory pattern and orthopnea. Physical examination may also reveal decreased lung sounds on auscultation of the ventral thorax, and muffled heart sounds.[31,34,42] Less often, cough or hemoptysis occurs.[33,34] Vomiting and diarrhea occur in a minority of affected dogs,[41] and vomiting, hypersalivation, halitosis, and/or oculonasal discharge may be present in cats.[31,35,39] Cats with severe sepsis may have mucosal pallor and be obtunded, bradycardic, and hypothermic with poor pulse quality.[35,36]

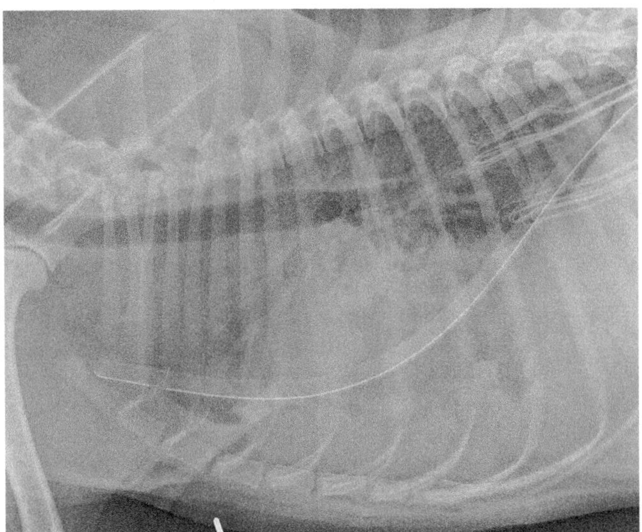

FIGURE 87-4 Lateral thoracic radiograph from a 3-year-old female spayed Labrador retriever mix with pyothorax. A right-sided thoracostomy tube had been placed on an emergency basis. The cardiac silhouette is obscured by the presence of exudate. Cytology of the fluid revealed a mixed bacterial population.

Diagnosis

Diagnosis of pyothorax is based on radiographic findings and gross and cytologic examination of pleural fluid. Imaging may be useful to identify underlying causes such as lung abscessation or esophageal perforation. Culture and susceptibility of the pleural fluid permits identification of the bacteria involved and can guide antimicrobial drug treatment.

Laboratory Abnormalities

Complete Blood Count, Serum Biochemical Tests, Urinalysis

Most dogs and cats with pyothorax have mild to marked leukocytosis with increased numbers of toxic band neutrophils and sometimes a degenerative left shift or metamyelocytes on the CBC.[31,34,35,37,42] The CBC may also be unremarkable. Nonregenerative anemia may be present,[31,34] and animals with severe sepsis and disseminated intravascular coagulation may be thrombocytopenic. The serum biochemistry panel may reveal electrolyte abnormalities such as hyponatremia or hypochloremia, as well as hypoalbuminemia and/or hyperglobulinemia. Mild hyperbilirubinemia can be present in cats.[35] Serum creatine kinase activity may be increased if pyothorax is secondary to trauma to the thoracic wall.

Diagnostic Imaging

Plain Radiography

Findings on plain thoracic radiography in dogs and cats with pyothorax include mild to severe pleural effusion and mass lesions in the pleural space or pulmonary parenchyma (Figure 87-4). Most (>75%) of affected cats and dogs have bilateral effusion, but unilateral effusions also occur.[31,32,34,35,41] Sternal or tracheobronchial lymphadenomegaly may also be evident. In dogs, tracheobronchial lymphadenomegaly may be severe when *Actinomyces*, *Nocardia*, or filamentous fungi such as *Aspergillus* spp. are present.

Sonographic Findings

Thoracic ultrasound of dogs and cats with pyothorax can reveal the presence of echogenic pleural fluid, fibrinous tags adhered to pleural surfaces, pericardial thickening and effusion, consolidated lung lobes, and lung lobe abscessation.[35,41] Occasionally, plant awn foreign bodies are identified in the thoracic wall.[26,44]

Advanced Imaging

CT may be more sensitive than plain radiography for identification of pulmonary mass lesions and esophageal disease and can raise suspicion for the presence of plant awn foreign bodies,[26] and so can assist in surgical decision making. Findings in dogs and cats with pyothorax include unilateral or bilateral pleural effusion, gas within the pleural space secondary to thoracocentesis or foreign body migration, pleural thickening, and focal, single, or multiple soft tissue opacities within the pulmonary parenchyma.[40,43] Mediastinal lymphadenomegaly may also be identified (Figure 87-5). The presence of foreign material may be suspected based on the results of CT, although CT is insensitive for detection of plant foreign bodies. Findings on CT in dogs with pyothorax correlate well with surgical findings, although CT is probably more sensitive for detection of abnormalities within the lung parenchyma.[40]

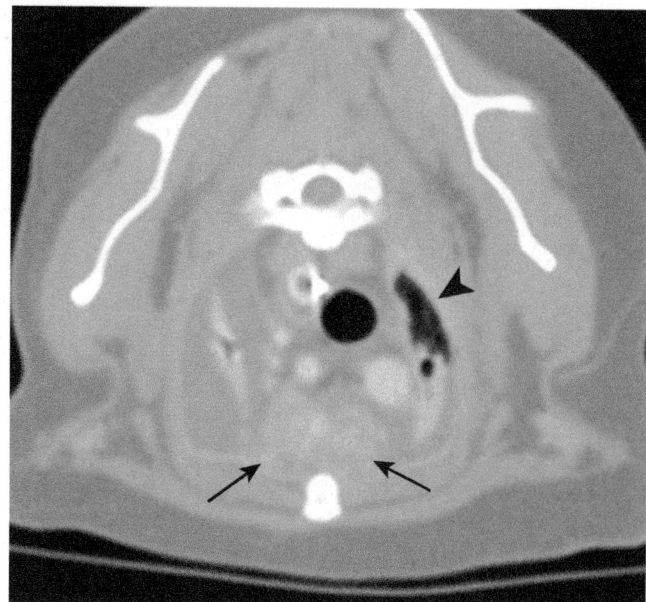

FIGURE 87-5 Thoracic post contrast CT scan image from a 5-year-old male neutered, indoor-outdoor domestic shorthair cat that was evaluated for pyothorax. The cat was hypoventilating after placement of a thoracostomy tube, and mechanical ventilation was required. Culture revealed clindamycin-resistant *Pasteurella multocida*, small numbers of coagulase-negative staphylococci, an *Actinomyces*-like organism, and abundant mixed anaerobic growth that included *Fusobacterium* and β-lactamase–producing *Bacteroides/Prevotella*. Serial thoracic radiographs showed progressive lung lobe consolidation and persistent pleural effusion. The CT scan showed persistent pleural effusion and collapse of the cranial and caudal portion of the left cranial lung lobe, right middle lung lobe, and accessory lung lobe. Three large nodules were present in the ventrocranial thorax that enhanced heterogeneously with contrast; these were interpreted to be enlarged lymph nodes. Two of the nodules are shown (*arrows*), and a small portion of the right cranial lung lobe is aerated (*arrowhead*). Two long plant awns were removed from the mediastinum during exploratory thoracotomy. The thorax was debrided and lavaged and the severely consolidated caudal portion of the left lung lobe was resected. The cat recovered fully.

Microbiologic Tests

Cytologic Examination

Thoracocentesis typically yields fluid that is purulent, flocculent, and/or hemorrhagic; it may also have a fetid odor due to the presence of anaerobes. Sulfur granules may be grossly visible within the fluid if *Actinomyces* or *Nocardia* are present. Cytologic examination of the fluid shows large numbers of leukocytes, most often with a predominance of degenerate neutrophils.[34] Erythrocytes and histiocytes may also be present. Bacteria are visualized in approximately 80% of pleural fluid specimens, either as a mixture of rods, cocci, and filamentous organisms or as a monomorphic bacterial population (Figure 87-6; see also Figure 37-6).[31,34]

Culture

Pleural fluid should be submitted for Gram staining and aerobic and anaerobic bacterial culture and susceptibility. Because *Mycoplasma* spp. can be isolated from dogs and cats with pyothorax, specific culture for *Mycoplasma* spp. could also be considered. Although the sensitivity of effusion culture in dogs and cats with pyothorax is generally high (>69%),[32,34,35] false negatives can occur as a result of recent antibiotic treatment or the presence of fastidious bacteria such as anaerobes and *Mycoplasma*. Because isolation of *Nocardia* and *Actinomyces* can require prolonged incubation and specialized growth conditions, the laboratory should be alerted that these organisms may be present.

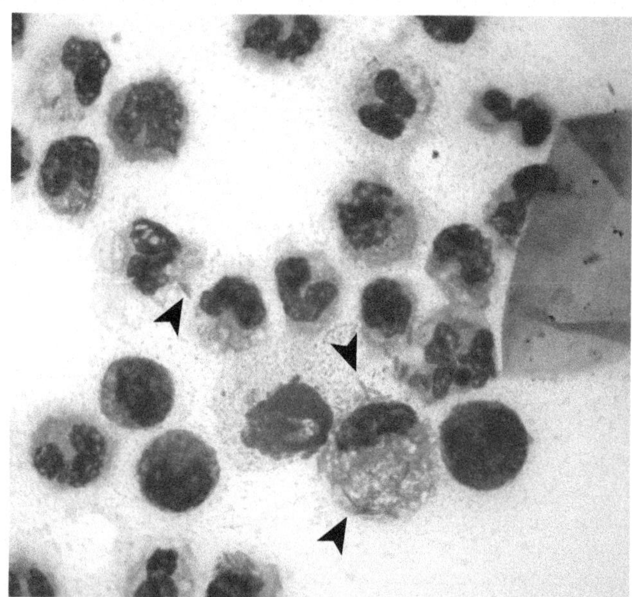

FIGURE 87-6 Cytology of pleural effusion from a 3-year-old male neutered domestic shorthair with pyothorax. There are many variably karyolytic neutrophils. Many contain bacterial rods, which can also be seen extracellularly (*arrowheads*). Anaerobic bacterial culture yielded *Fusobacterium russii*. Aerobic culture was negative.

Pathologic Findings

Gross findings in dogs and cats with pyothorax consist of variable quantities of hemorrhagic to purulent fluid within the thoracic cavity, enlarged thoracic lymph nodes, pleural thickening and irregularity, and mottled and consolidated lung lobes. Plant foreign bodies or lung abscesses may be found. The pleural fluid may contain sulfur granules or fibrinous material (Figure 87-7). Histopathology reveals a fibrinonecrotic to pyogranulomatous inflammatory response in the pleura and sometimes also the mediastinum, pericardium, and/or lungs. Intralesional bacteria may be seen.

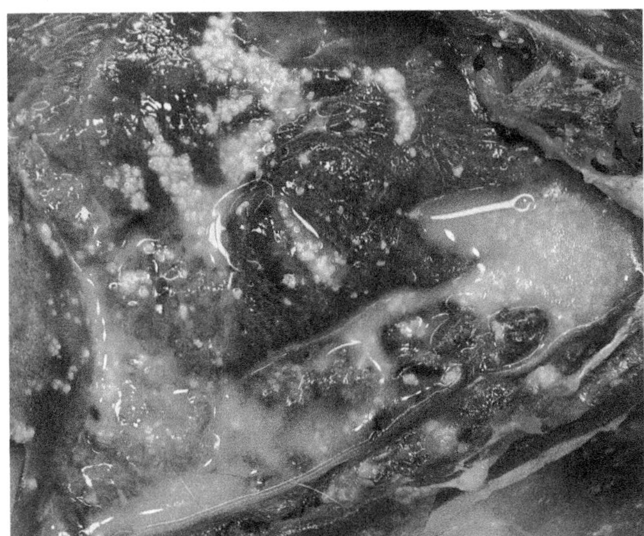

FIGURE 87-7 Thoracic contents of a 5-year-old male neutered domestic shorthair with pyothorax at necropsy. The cat had a 5-day history of progressive inappetence, weakness, and vomiting and on physical examination was stuporous, hypothermic, and in respiratory distress. Creamy white to yellow fluid was present in the thoracic cavity that contains gritty white flecks of material (sulfur granules). The fluid was malodorous. Culture of the fluid yielded *Bacteroides fragilis*, an anaerobic gram-positive rod, and an *Actinomyces* species. (Image courtesy University of California, Davis, Veterinary Anatomic Pathology Service.)

Treatment and Prognosis

Treatment of pyothorax involves a combination of drainage of pus from the thoracic cavity (with or without lavage), combined with targeted antimicrobial drug therapy and supportive care.

Drainage and Lavage

Treatment of pyothorax with antimicrobial drugs alone is generally ineffective, and drainage is required to facilitate drug penetration. This is most often accomplished by unilateral or bilateral placement of indwelling thoracostomy tubes followed by continuous or intermittent suction. Suction is generally continued until cytologic and microbiologic evidence of infection resolves in the pleural fluid. This may take from days to up to 3 weeks, with a median duration of approximately 5 to 7 days.[31,32,34,35] While the thoracostomy tubes are in place, lavage may be performed through the tubes with warm isotonic saline (e.g., 10 to 20 mL/kg administered over 5 to 10 min). The frequency of intrapleural lavage has ranged from q5h to q24h.[31,32,34] Currently, there is no clear evidence that lavage influences outcome in animals with pyothorax, or that instillation of heparin or antimicrobial drugs into the pleural space influences outcome. Ultrasound-guided drainage via a single, unilateral thoracocentesis without lavage has been successful when the pleural effusion is not excessively thick or granular.[37] Exploratory thoracotomy and resection of affected tissues may be required after initial stabilization if there is extensive fibrous tissue formation, pulmonary parenchymal abscessation, known or suspected presence of a foreign body, esophageal perforation, large accumulations of inspissated purulent material that obstructs drainage, or failure to respond to medical therapy.[34,41] Surgical treatment in both dogs and cats has been associated with improved outcomes when compared with medical treatment alone.[35,41] However, thoracotomy is associated with increased cost and length of hospital stay, pain, and anesthetic risk, so it is generally reserved for those animals in which medical management with thoracostomy tube drainage is failing or likely to fail.

Antimicrobial Drug Therapy

Parenteral administration of antimicrobial drugs with activity against *Pasteurella*, *Actinomyces*, and anaerobes is indicated. Ampicillin-sulbactam may be sufficient in most cats. Addition of a fluoroquinolone could be considered in dogs (where gram-negative enteric species such as *E. coli* are more likely to be present), or when the possibility of *Mycoplasma* spp. infection exists. Ampicillin alone or clindamycin may be effective, but some anaerobes are resistant to ampicillin and clindamycin and some *Pasteurella* isolates are clindamycin resistant. Antibiotic choice should then be tailored to the organism(s) present based on culture and susceptibility. If combination therapy was initiated and the bacterial isolates are susceptible to both drugs, the fluoroquinolone should be discontinued. If organisms are grown that are resistant to one of the drugs, that antimicrobial should be discontinued. Drugs that are inactivated by purulent material, such as trimethoprim-sulfamethoxazole, should be avoided. Oral antimicrobial therapy is continued after the animal leaves the hospital.

The optimal duration of treatment for pyothorax is not known and may depend on the severity and chronicity of the disease. Most animals are treated for a minimum of 3 weeks. Serial thoracic radiographs may be useful to determine whether antimicrobial drug treatment should be continued, but whether persistent radiographic abnormalities correlate with the need for additional antimicrobial drug treatment requires further study. If the pyothorax persists or reoccurs after cessation of antibiotic treatment, pleural fluid should again be submitted for culture and susceptibility testing, because the organism(s) involved may change.

Supportive Care

Intravenous fluid therapy and oxygen supplementation is frequently required in the initial stages of management of pyothorax. Early placement of a feeding tube should also be considered if inappetence is present. Rarely, mechanical ventilation is required.

Prognosis

The first 48 hours of hospitalization is the most critical period for dogs and cats with pyothorax.[34,35] Thereafter, prognosis improves considerably.

In general, the prognosis for recovery in dogs with pyothorax is fair to good. Short-term (survival to discharge) and long-term survival rates of 74% and 63% have been reported.[32] Death usually results from complications related to respiratory function or septic shock. The bacterial species present and volume of pleural effusion do not seem to affect survival.[32] In a minority of dogs (≤20%), recurrence of pyothorax occurs for up to 5 years, but most often, months after discharge from the hospital.

The survival rate for cats with pyothorax in one study was 48%; 18% of cats died and 34% were euthanized.[35] The presence of hypersalivation or bradycardia were negative prognostic signs.[35] Serum cholesterol concentration and total white cell counts were significantly lower in cats that died. In another study, 78% of cats were treated successfully, although long-term follow-up was not available.[31]

Prevention

Housing cats indoors and restricting access of dogs and cats to areas where plant awns are abundant may help to prevent pyothorax.

CASE EXAMPLE

Signalment: "Frank", a 3-year-old male neutered domestic shorthair cat from Woodland, CA, was presented for acute onset of respiratory distress of approximately 30 minutes duration. Frank was a barn cat and was outdoors with more than 20 other barn cats. Also on the property were five dogs, horses, and cattle. Other cats in the barn had previously been attacked by "wild animals" and had been diagnosed with a variety of injuries that included abscesses and septic peritonitis. There was no previous medical history and Frank was up to date on routine feline vaccinations (feline herpesvirus-1, calicivirus, panleukopenia virus, rabies and FeLV).

Physical Examination:

Body Weight: 5.6 kg.

General: Obtunded, but ambulatory, dehydrated. T = 103.7°F (39.8°C), HR = 140 beats/min, panting. Mucous membranes were pale pink, CRT = 2 s.

Integument: Some flea excrement was present.

Eyes, Ears, Nose, and Throat: Mild gingivitis was present with halitosis and hypersalivation. No other clinically significant abnormalities were detected.

Musculoskeletal: Body condition score was 4/9.

Cardiovascular: No murmurs or arrhythmias were detected, and pulses were strong and synchronous.

Respiratory: Respiratory difficulty with open mouth breathing was noted. Lung sounds were dull ventrally on auscultation of both sides of the thorax.

All Other Systems: No clinically significant abnormalities.

Laboratory Findings:

Venous Blood Gas: pH 7.273, pCO_2 37.9 mm Hg, pO_2 40.9 mm Hg, base deficit/base excess −8.6 mmol/L, bicarbonate 16.8 mm Hg, ionized calcium 1.3 mmol/L, lactate 4.4 mmol/L, PCV 26%, total plasma protein 6.7 g/dL.

CBC:

HCT 29.8% (30%-50%)
MCV 43.4 fL (42-53 fL)
MCHC 32.2 g/dL (30-33.5 g/dL)
Reticulocytes 15,200 cells/μL
WBC 16,650 cells/μL (4500-14,000 cells/μL)
Neutrophils 4995 cells/μL (2000-9000 cells/μL)
Band neutrophils 7992 cells/μL
Lymphocytes 3497 cells/μL (1000-7000 cells/μL)
Monocytes 167 cells/μL (50-600 cells/μL)
Eosinophils 0 cells/μL (150-1100 cells/μL)
Platelets 345,000/μL (180,000-500,000 platelets/μL)

Serum Chemistry Profile:

Sodium 153 mmol/L (151-158 mmol/L)
Potassium 4.4 mmol/L (3.6-4.9 mmol/L)
Chloride 123 mmol/L (117-126 mmol/L)
Bicarbonate 18 mmol/L (15-21 mmol/L)
Phosphorus 5.7 mg/dL (3.2-6.3 mg/dL)
Calcium 8.3 mg/dL (9.0-10.9 mg/dL)
BUN 18 mg/dL (18-33 mg/dL)
Creatinine 0.8 mg/dL (1.1-2.2 mg/dL)
Glucose 81 mg/dL (63-118 mg/dL)
Total protein 4.9 g/dL (6.6-8.4 g/dL)
Albumin 1.9 g/dL (2.2-4.6 g/dL)
Globulin 3.0 g/dL (2.8-5.4 g/dL)
ALT 29 U/L (27-101 U/L)
AST 86 U/L (17-58 U/L)
ALP 3 U/L (14-71 U/L)
GGT < 3 U/L (0-4 U/L)
Cholesterol 99 mg/dL (89-258 mg/dL)
Total bilirubin 1.9 mg/dL (0-0.2 mg/dL)
Creatine kinase 1532 U/L (73-260 U/L)

In-Clinic FeLV Antigen and FIV Antibody Serology: Negative.

Initial Treatment: Supplemental oxygen was administered. A brief thoracic ultrasound examination confirmed the presence of large amounts of pleural effusion. Thoracocentesis yielded 170 mL of opaque red fluid. Cytologic examination of the fluid in the emergency room revealed numerous degenerate neutrophils and macrophages with filamentous bacterial rods. The fluid was submitted for further analysis and culture. Treatment with intravenous fluids (150 mL bolus of lactated Ringer's solution, then 50 mL/hr of lactated Ringer's solution with 20 mEq/L KCl), enrofloxacin (5 mg/kg IV q24h), and ampicillin (22 mg/kg IV q8h) was initiated. Packed red blood cells were administered because the PCV dropped to 21%. Frank was anesthetized and a 12F chest tube placed on the left side of the thorax.

Thoracic Radiography: Moderate bilateral pleural effusion and irregular scalloping of the ventral lung margins were present. On the lateral projection, several rounded gas lucencies were superimposed over the ventral thorax and apex of the heart. On the ventrodorsal (VD) projection, there was increased opacity to the left of the cardiac silhouette superimposed over the pulmonary parenchyma. A chest tube was present extending into the left cranial hemithorax. Impressions: Moderate bilateral pleural effusion with irregular lung margination, findings consistent with the clinical diagnosis of pyothorax. The increased opacity superimposed over the left lung on the VD projection was thought to represent focal pulmonary infiltrates or pocketing effusion. Slight pneumothorax, likely iatrogenic.

Microbiologic Testing:

Cytologic Examination (Pleural Fluid): Total protein 3.5 g/dL; RBC 240,000 cells/μL; total nucleated cells 206,160 cells/μL with 66% neutrophils, 11% small mononuclear cells, and 23% large mononuclear cells. The neutrophils were variably karyolytic, and many contained intracellular bacteria. The bacterial population was a monomorphic population of long, thin, and linear rods (see Figure 87-6). These bacteria were noted extracellularly and intracellularly.

Aerobic and Anaerobic Bacterial Culture (Pleural Fluid): Small numbers of *Fusobacterium russii* (identified by DNA sequencing), negative for β-lactamase production.

Mycoplasma Culture (Pleural Fluid): Negative.

Diagnosis: Anaerobic bacterial pyothorax.

Outcome: Over the course of day 1, 70 mL/kg of fluid was removed from the thoracostomy tube. Treatment with antimicrobial drugs, intravenous fluids, mechanical intermittent (q4h) suction through the thoracostomy tube, and opioid analgesia was continued. On day 2, fluid production from the tube dropped to 1 mL/kg/hr, yet thoracic radiographs showed persistent pleural effusion. Intrapleural lavage with 60 mL of warm saline was performed.

On day 3, Frank became progressively more obtunded with increased respiratory rate (60 breaths/min) and effort. Cytologic examination of the pleural fluid showed persistent bacterial infection. An exploratory thoracotomy by median sternotomy was performed. Entry into the mediastinum was followed by escape of a large amount of mucopurulent material that contained caseous material and fibrin clots. The mediastinal, pericardial, and sterno-pericardial fat were necrotic and were easily stripped from the pericardium and other mediastinal structures. There was no evidence of communication with the trachea or esophagus and no evidence of plant awn foreign bodies. The right middle and accessory lung lobes were atelectatic. Fibrinous material coated the pleural surfaces. Additional mucopurulent material was present in both pleural cavities. Following mediastinectomy, the pus was suctioned from the thoracic cavity and vigorous lavage and suction applied. Mechanical debridement was performed using moist gauze sponges. Gentle decortication of the right middle lung lobe was performed, resulting in partial re-inflation, and 16F thoracic drains were placed bilaterally.

The following day Frank was more alert and began to eat. Intermittent suction (q6h) and thoracic lavage were performed through the thoracostomy tubes (30 mL warm saline each side q12h). A CBC revealed 79,520 WBC/μL, 16,699 band neutrophils/μL, and 54,074 neutrophils/μL, with moderate neutrophil toxicity. The antibiotic treatment was changed to amoxicillin-clavulanic acid (20 mg/kg PO q8h). After an additional 48h, the thoracostomy tubes yielded only small amounts of mildly hemorrhagic fluid, and so they were removed. Frank was discharged on day 7 of hospitalization, when he was alert and eating well. Antibiotic treatment was continued for 6 weeks. He continued to improve at home and was followed for an additional 2 years with no evidence of recurrence.

Comments: This cat had severe pyothorax likely secondary to thoracic wall trauma (e.g., a bite wound) that was fortunately discovered and treated rapidly. The cat was bradycardic and had ptyalism and low-normal serum cholesterol concentration, all negative prognostic indicators in one study.[35] A thoracotomy was needed because of inspissated pus within the thorax that failed to drain effectively with medical management. The spectrum of antimicrobials used may have been excessive based on the results of culture and susceptibility testing (amoxicillin alone should have been active), but it is possible that other anaerobes may also have been present that failed to grow. Note that the use of parenteral enrofloxacin is off-label for cats and has the potential to cause blindness.

SUGGESTED READINGS

Barrs VR, Beatty JA. Feline pyothorax–new insights into an old problem. Vet J. 2009;179(2):163-178.

Demetriou JL, Foale RD, Ladlow J, et al. Canine and feline pyothorax: a retrospective study of 50 cases in the UK and Ireland. J Small Anim Pract. 2002;43:388-394.

Tart KM, Babski DM, Lee JA. Potential risks, prognostic indicators, and diagnostic and treatment modalities affecting survival in dogs with presumptive aspiration pneumonia: 125 cases (2005-2008). J Vet Emerg Crit Care (San Antonio). 2010;20:319-329.

Waddell LS, Brady CA, Drobatz KJ. Risk factors, prognostic indicators, and outcome of pyothorax in cats: 80 cases (1986-1999). J Am Vet Med Assoc. 2002;221:819-824.

REFERENCES

1. Schulz BS, Wolf G, Hartmann K. Bacteriological and antibiotic sensitivity test results in 271 cats with respiratory tract infections. Vet Rec. 2006;158:269-270.
2. Jameson PH, King LA, Lappin MR, et al. Comparison of clinical signs, diagnostic findings, organisms isolated, and clinical outcome in dogs with bacterial pneumonia: 93 cases (1986-1991). J Am Vet Med Assoc. 1995;206:206-209.
3. Dye JA, McKiernan BC, Rozanski EA, et al. Bronchopulmonary disease in the cat: historical, physical, radiographic, clinicopathologic, and pulmonary functional evaluation of 24 affected and 15 healthy cats. J Vet Intern Med. 1996;10:385-400.
4. Sauve V, Drobatz KJ, Shokek AB, et al. Clinical course, diagnostic findings and necropsy diagnosis in dyspneic cats with primary pulmonary parenchymal disease: 15 cats (1996-2002). J Vet Emerg Crit Care. 2005;15:38-47.
5. Peeters DE, McKiernan BC, Weisiger RM, et al. Quantitative bacterial cultures and cytological examination of bronchoalveolar lavage specimens in dogs. J Vet Intern Med. 2000;14:534-541.
6. Johnson LR, Vernau W. Bronchoscopic findings in 48 cats with spontaneous lower respiratory tract disease (2002-2009). J Vet Intern Med. 2011;25:236-243.
7. Tenwolde AC, Johnson LR, Hunt GB, et al. The role of bronchoscopy in foreign body removal in dogs and cats: 37 cases (2000-2008). J Vet Intern Med. 2010;24:1063-1068.
8. Epstein SE, Mellema MS, Hopper K. Airway microbial culture and susceptibility patterns in dogs and cats with respiratory disease of varying severity. J Vet Emerg Crit Care (San Antonio). 2010;20:587-594.
9. Johnson LR, Fales WH. Clinical and microbiologic findings in dogs with bronchoscopically diagnosed tracheal collapse: 37 cases (1990-1995). J Am Vet Med Assoc. 2001;219:1247-1250.
10. Johnson LR, Queen EV, Vernau W, et al. Microbiologic and cytologic assessment of bronchoalveolar lavage fluid from dogs with lower respiratory tract infection: 105 cases (2001-2011). J Vet Intern Med. 2013;27:259-267.
11. Kogan DA, Johnson LR, Sturges BK, et al. Etiology and clinical outcome in dogs with aspiration pneumonia: 88 cases (2004-2006). J Am Vet Med Assoc. 2008;233:1748-1755.
12. Macdonald ES, Norris CR, Berghaus RB, et al. Clinicopathologic and radiographic features and etiologic agents in cats with histologically confirmed infectious pneumonia: 39 cases (1991-2000). J Am Vet Med Assoc. 2003;223:1142-1150.
13. Tart KM, Babski DM, Lee JA. Potential risks, prognostic indicators, and diagnostic and treatment modalities affecting survival in dogs with presumptive aspiration pneumonia: 125 cases (2005-2008). J Vet Emerg Crit Care (San Antonio). 2010;20:319-329.
14. Java MA, Drobatz KJ, Gilley RS, et al. Incidence of and risk factors for postoperative pneumonia in dogs anesthetized for diagnosis or treatment of intervertebral disk disease. J Am Vet Med Assoc. 2009;235:281-287.
15. Nicholson I, Baines S. Complications associated with temporary tracheostomy tubes in 42 dogs (1998 to 2007). J Small Anim Pract. 2012;53:108-114.

16. Novellas R, Simpson KE, Gunn-Moore DA, et al. Imaging findings in 11 cats with feline dysautonomia. J Feline Med Surg. 2010;12:584-591.
17. Hardie RJ, Gunby J, Bjorling DE. Arytenoid lateralization for treatment of laryngeal paralysis in 10 cats. Vet Surg. 2009;38:445-451.
18. Sykes JE, Mapes S, Lindsay LL, et al. *Corynebacterium ulcerans* bronchopneumonia in a dog. J Vet Intern Med. 2010;24:973-976.
19. Cavrenne R, De Busscher V, Bolen G, et al. Primary ciliary dyskinesia and situs inversus in a young dog. Vet Rec. 2008;163:54-55.
20. Clercx C, Peeters D, Snaps F, et al. Eosinophilic bronchopneumopathy in dogs. J Vet Intern Med. 2000;14:282-291.
21. Sura PA, Krahwinkel DJ. Self-expanding Nitinol stents for the treatment of tracheal collapse in dogs: 12 cases (2001-2004). J Am Vet Med Assoc. 2008;232:228-236.
22. Kogan DA, Johnson LR, Jandrey KE, et al. Clinical, clinicopathologic, and radiographic findings in dogs with aspiration pneumonia: 88 cases (2004-2006). J Am Vet Med Assoc. 2008;233:1742-1747.
23. Bailiff NL, Norris CR. Clinical signs, clinicopathological findings, etiology, and outcome associated with hemoptysis in dogs: 36 cases (1990-1999). J Am Anim Hosp Assoc. 2002;38:125-133.
24. Teske E, Stokhof AA, van den Ingh T, et al. Transthoracic needle aspiration biopsy of the lung in dogs with pulmonary diseases. J Am Anim Hosp Assoc. 1991;27:289-294.
25. Wood EF, O'Brien RT, Young KM. Ultrasound-guided fine-needle aspiration of focal parenchymal lesions of the lung in dogs and cats. J Vet Intern Med. 1998;12:338-342.
26. Schultz RM, Zwingenberger AL. Radiographic, computed tomographic, and ultrasonographic findings with migrating intrathoracic grass awns in dogs and cats. Vet Radiol Ultrasound. 2008;49:249-255.
27. Lindsey JO, Pierce AK. An examination of the microbiologic flora of normal lung of the dog. Am Rev Respir Dis. 1978;117:501-505.
28. McKiernan BC, Smith AR, Kissil M. Bacterial isolates from the lower trachea of clinically healthy dogs. J Am Anim Hosp Assoc. 1984;20:139-142.
29. Padrid PA, Feldman BF, Funk K, et al. Cytologic, microbiologic, and biochemical analysis of bronchoalveolar lavage fluid obtained from 24 healthy cats. Am J Vet Res. 1991;52:1300-1307.
30. Antimicrobial Guidelines Working Group of the International Society for Companion Animal Infectious Diseases (ISCAID). Antimicrobial use guidelines for treatment of respiratory tract disease in dogs and cats. In preparation.
31. Barrs VR, Allan GS, Martin P, et al. Feline pyothorax: a retrospective study of 27 cases in Australia. J Feline Med Surg. 2005;7:211-222.
32. Boothe HW, Howe LM, Boothe DM, et al. Evaluation of outcomes in dogs treated for pyothorax: 46 cases (1983-2001). J Am Vet Med Assoc. 2010;236:657-663.
33. Davies C, Forrester SD. Pleural effusion in cats: 82 cases (1987 to 1995). J Small Anim Pract. 1996;37:217-224.
34. Demetriou JL, Foale RD, Ladlow J, et al. Canine and feline pyothorax: a retrospective study of 50 cases in the UK and Ireland. J Small Anim Pract. 2002;43:388-394.
35. Waddell LS, Brady CA, Drobatz KJ. Risk factors, prognostic indicators, and outcome of pyothorax in cats: 80 cases (1986-1999). J Am Vet Med Assoc. 2002;221:819-824.
36. Brady CA, Otto CM, Van Winkle TJ, et al. Severe sepsis in cats: 29 cases (1986-1998). J Am Vet Med Assoc. 2000;217:531-535.
37. Johnson MS, Martin MW. Successful medical treatment of 15 dogs with pyothorax. J Small Anim Pract. 2007;48:12-16.
38. Walker AL, Jang SS, Hirsh DC. Bacteria associated with pyothorax of dogs and cats: 98 cases (1989-1998). J Am Vet Med Assoc. 2000;216:359-363.
39. Love DN, Jones RF, Bailey M, et al. Isolation and characterisation of bacteria from pyothorax (empyaemia) in cats. Vet Microbiol. 1982;7:455-461.
40. Swinbourne F, Baines EA, Baines SJ, et al. Computed tomographic findings in canine pyothorax and correlation with findings at exploratory thoracotomy. J Small Anim Pract. 2011;52:203-208.
41. Rooney MB, Monnet E. Medical and surgical treatment of pyothorax in dogs: 26 cases (1991-2001). J Am Vet Med Assoc. 2002;221:86-92.
42. Robertson SA, Stoddart ME, Evans RJ, et al. Thoracic empyema in the dog; a report of twenty-two cases. J Small Anim Pract. 1983;24:103-119.
43. Sykes JE. Unpublished observations, 2012.
44. Gnudi G, Volta A, Bonazzi M, et al. Ultrasonographic features of grass awn migration in the dog. Vet Radiol Ultrasound. 2005;46:423-426.

CHAPTER 88

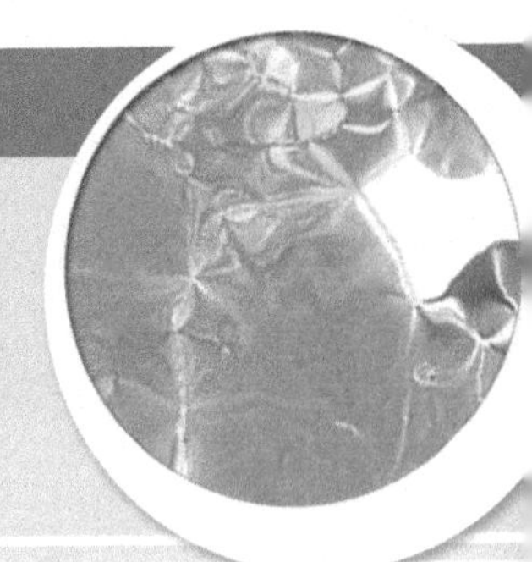

Intra-abdominal Infections

Jane E. Sykes

> **Overview of Bacterial Intra-abdominal and Hepatobiliary Infections**
>
> Causes: Most commonly *Escherichia coli*, *Enterococcus* spp., and anaerobes; less often other gram-negative aerobes, *Streptococcus*, and *Staphylococcus* spp.
>
> Mode of Transmission: Opportunistic invasion by commensal bacteria of the gastrointestinal and urogenital tracts
>
> Major Clinical Signs: Inappetence, fever, vomiting, diarrhea, abdominal pain
>
> Differential Diagnoses: Nonbacterial causes of pancreatitis, peritoneal effusion, hepatitis, or extrahepatic biliary tract obstruction (especially neoplasia and inflammatory disorders but also viral, protozoal, or fungal infections)
>
> Human Health Significance: Enteric bacteria involved may be multidrug-resistant organisms that have the potential to colonize humans.

INFECTIOUS GASTROENTERITIS

Gastroenteritis in dogs and cats may be caused by an enormous array of microorganisms that include viral, bacterial, fungal, and protozoal pathogens (Table 88-1[1-5]). Other parasites (such as nematodes) should also be considered on the differential diagnosis list. Enteropathogenic bacteria cause diarrhea by adhesion to or destruction of enterocytes, secretion of a variety of potent enterotoxins, and stimulation of the host inflammatory response. Many of these microbes can be detected in the feces of apparently healthy animals as well as the feces of those with clinical signs of diarrhea. Therefore, it may be difficult to ascertain the role that these organisms play in disease in a single patient. Clinical signs of diarrhea may be more likely to occur when multiple organisms are present simultaneously ("polyparasitism"). In addition, other host factors (such as nutritional status or age) and bacterial virulence factors influence whether clinical signs develop. When outbreaks occur in dog and cat populations, collection of specimens from multiple affected and in-contact animals may be useful to determine the significance of one or more organisms involved. Use of antibiotics to treat bacterial diarrhea should be reserved for animals with systemic signs of illness such as fever, lethargy, and leukocytosis on the CBC.[6] Other infections are self-limiting, and the mainstay of treatment is proper fluid therapy and supportive care.

The reader is referred to other chapters in this book for detailed information on pathogenesis, clinical signs, diagnosis, and treatment for the organisms that are most commonly involved. References are also provided in Table 88-1 for information on pathogens that are uncommon or rarely identified or that have uncertain pathogenicity.

BACTERIAL PERITONITIS

Etiology and Epidemiology

Peritonitis may be focal or diffuse and can also be classified as *primary* or *secondary peritonitis*. Primary peritonitis is peritonitis that has no identifiable underlying cause. In secondary peritonitis, a reason for bacterial leakage into the abdomen can be identified.

In humans, primary peritonitis has also been referred to as *spontaneous bacterial peritonitis* and most often complicates development of ascites (e.g., secondary to cirrhosis, hepatitis, or congestive heart failure).[7,8] In contrast, conditions that predispose to ascites are rarely present in the history of dogs and cats with primary peritonitis. Some primary peritonitis in dogs or cats may result from hematogenous spread of bacteria to the peritoneum or bacterial translocation from the gastrointestinal tract.[7]

Secondary peritonitis is the most common form of peritonitis in dogs and cats and occurs when bacteria are introduced into the peritoneal space as a result of gastrointestinal perforation, penetration of the abdominal wall, rupture of the genitourinary tract, rupture of intra-abdominal abscesses, gallbladder rupture, or ascending infection of the umbilicus in neonates (Table 88-2).[7,9-15] In dogs, low preoperative total protein or serum albumin concentrations are risk factors for development of bacterial peritonitis after gastrointestinal surgery.[16]

The bacterial species involved in peritonitis reflect the normal flora of the gastrointestinal tract. Mixed aerobic-anaerobic infections, with up to four different bacterial species, occur in more than 50% of affected dogs and cats.[7,10] *Escherichia coli* is the most common isolate from both dogs and cats, followed by *Enterococcus* and *Clostridium* spp.[7,10,11,14,15,17,18] Other isolates include staphylococci, streptococci, *Pseudomonas aeruginosa* or *Acinetobacter* spp., a variety of anaerobes, gram-negative Enterobacteriaceae (*Proteus, Citrobacter, Serratia, Klebsiella,* or *Enterobacter*), *Actinomyces,* or in cats, *Pasteurella multocida*. In one study, a greater proportion of dogs with primary peritonitis had gram-positive bacterial infections than dogs with secondary peritonitis.[7] Uncommonly, *Candida albicans* can be involved, especially if there is a history of antibiotic treatment (see Chapter 67).

The mean age of dogs with peritonitis is around 5 to 7 years, and the mean age of cats is 7 to 10 years, although dogs and cats of any age can be affected.[9,12,19] Age was not found

TABLE 88-1

Examples of Potential Infectious Causes of Enterocolitis in Dogs and Cats

Organism Type	Dogs	Cats
Viruses	Canine parvovirus Canine enteric coronavirus Canine distemper virus Rotaviruses Astroviruses Adenoviruses Caliciviruses	Feline panleukopenia virus Feline coronavirus Feline calicivirus FeLV FIV Rotaviruses Astroviruses Torovirus-like agent Reoviruses
Bacteria	*Salmonella* spp. *Clostridium perfringens* *Clostridium difficile* *Campylobacter* spp. *Helicobacter* spp. *Escherichia coli* *Klebsiella pneumoniae*[1] *Enterococcus* spp.[2] *Yersinia enterocolitica* *Brachyspira pilosicoli*[3] *Mycobacterium* spp. (e.g., *M. avium*) *Leptospira* spp. *Neorickettsia helminthoeca*	*Salmonella* spp. *C. perfringens* *C. difficile* *Campylobacter* spp. *Helicobacter* spp. *Escherichia coli* *Enterococcus* spp.[4] *Y. enterocolitica* *Anaerobiospirillum*[5] *Mycobacterium* spp. (e.g., *M. bovis*)
Protozoa	*Giardia* spp. *Entamoeba histolytica* *Balantidium coli* *Isospora* spp. *Hammondia heydorni* *Cryptosporidium* spp. *Leishmania* spp. *Tritrichomonas foetus*	*Giardia* spp. *E. histolytica* *Isospora* spp. *Cryptosporidium* spp. *Tritrichomonas foetus*
Fungi	*Histoplasma capsulatum* *Cryptococcus neoformans* *Blastomyces dermatitis* *Candida albicans* *Aspergillus* spp. Zygomycetes *Pythium insidiosum* *Prototheca* spp.	*Histoplasma capsulatum* *Candida albicans*
Other parasites	*Toxocara canis* and *Toxascaris leonina* (roundworms) *Ancylostoma* and *Uncinaria* spp. (hookworms) *Trichuris vulpis* (whipworms) Tapeworms (diphyllobothriidean)	*Toxocara cati* and *Toxascaris leonina* (roundworms) *Ancylostoma* and *Uncinaria* spp. (hookworms) Tapeworms (diphyllobothriidean)

TABLE 88-2

Underlying Causes of Secondary Peritonitis in Dogs

Organ System Affected	Disease Process
Gastrointestinal system	Gastrointestinal surgical site dehiscence (e.g., resection and anastomosis) Penetrating abdominal trauma Nonsteroidal or steroidal anti-inflammatory drug toxicity Foreign bodies Gastrointestinal neoplasia Eosinophilic gastroenteritis Torsion Intussusception
Genitourinary tract	Ruptured pyometra Surgical site dehiscence (e.g., ovariohysterectomy) Ruptured prostatic abscess Necrotizing bacterial cystitis
Hepatobiliary system	Gallbladder rupture (especially animals with necrotizing bacterial cholecystitis) Hepatic abscess rupture
Other abdominal organs	Abscess rupture
Umbilicus	Ascending infection in neonates

to relate to development of primary versus secondary peritonitis in dogs or cats.[7] There is no known breed or sex predisposition. In one study, three quarters of affected cats were indoor-only.[10]

Clinical Features

The most common historical signs in dogs and cats with bacterial peritonitis are lethargy, anorexia, vomiting, and diarrhea.[7,10,15] Weakness and collapse can also occur.[14] Diarrhea and vomiting may result from intestinal hypermotility or ileus or may be secondary to underlying intestinal disease.

Physical examination findings include dull mentation, fever (up to 108°F or 42°C), dehydration, mucosal pallor, abdominal pain, thin body condition, and/or abdominal enlargement and a palpable fluid wave due to ascites.[7,10,14] Tachypnea or tachycardia may be present as a result of abdominal pain. However, some affected animals, and especially cats, show none of these signs. More than one third of cats lack any evidence of abdominal pain.[10,15] Signs of septic shock may be present, such as tachycardia, tachypnea, weak pulses, and injected mucous membranes in dogs, or hypothermia and bradycardia in cats (see Chapter 86).[10,15]

Diagnosis

Diagnosis of bacterial peritonitis is based on abdominal imaging findings, cytologic examination of peritoneal fluid, and aerobic and anaerobic bacterial culture of the fluid.

Laboratory Abnormalities

Complete Blood Count and Serum Biochemical Tests

Frequent findings on the CBC in dogs and cats with bacterial peritonitis are leukocytosis due to neutrophilia, a mild to severe bandemia, and monocytosis.[7,10,12] Neutrophil toxicity is often present. Some animals are leukopenic (as low as 270 cells/μL in cats and 1000 cells/μL in dogs).[7,10,15] Anemia of inflammatory disease may be identified. Thrombocytopenia may be present in animals with septic shock and DIC. The serum biochemistry panel often shows electrolyte and acid-base abnormalities and/or hypoalbuminemia due to inflammation or third-space losses. Mild to moderate increases in liver enzyme activities, hypoglycemia, or hyperglycemia may be detected; hyperbilirubinemia can be present in cats.[7,10] Assessment of acid-base status in both dogs and cats most often reveals acidemia; hyperlactatemia is present in at least 50% of affected animals.[7,10,15]

Coagulation Profile

Dogs and cats that develop DIC may have prolongations of PT or APTT, increased plasma D-dimer or fibrin degradation product concentrations, and/or decreased plasma antithrombin concentration.

Diagnostic Imaging

Plain Radiography

Abdominal radiographs in dogs and cats with peritonitis may show a focal or diffuse loss of abdominal detail due to variable amounts of peritoneal effusion. In some animals, pneumoperitoneum is identified secondary to rupture of an abdominal viscus or penetrating abdominal trauma. Evidence of gastrointestinal obstruction or intestinal mass lesions may also be present.[10,14] In tachypneic animals, thoracic radiographs should be considered to determine whether a pulmonary problem (such as acute respiratory distress syndrome or pulmonary thromboembolism) is contributing to respiratory distress.

Sonographic Findings

Findings on abdominal ultrasound examination include focal or diffuse hyperechogenicity of the mesentery and the presence of ascites fluid (Figure 88-1). The latter may have an echogenic appearance if it is an exudate. Evidence of underlying disease may be present, such as intestinal mass lesions or foreign bodies. The presence of pneumoperitoneum; dilated, air-filled bowel loops; or severe abdominal pain may interfere with complete ultrasound examination of some patients. CT examination is preferred to ultrasound for evaluation of human patients with bacterial peritonitis,[7,8] but its usefulness for diagnosis and treatment of peritonitis in dogs and cats requires further investigation.

Microbiologic Tests

Cytologic Examination

Specimens for cytologic examination from animals with peritonitis may be collected by blind or ultrasound-guided abdominocentesis or diagnostic peritoneal lavage (DPL). With the increased availability and sensitivity of ultrasound to detect and guide collection of small quantities of undiluted intra-abdominal fluid, DPL is now uncommonly performed in the author's practice. Peritoneal fluid from dogs and cats with bacterial peritonitis is typically a modified transudate or exudate, although fluid from dogs with primary peritonitis may be more likely to be a modified transudate or transudate.[7] Fluid analysis from most animals with peritonitis reveals a high protein concentration and an increased erythrocyte and total nucleated cell count (usually >500 cells/μL and up to 160,000 cells/μL). There is typically a predominance of neutrophils that may have a degenerate appearance, and foreign material and/or intracellular and extracellular bacteria may be seen. The presence of intracellular bacteria is generally considered diagnostic for bacterial peritonitis. Because an absence of bacteria does not rule out bacterial peritonitis, submission of fluid for culture is essential.[10,14] A blood-to-fluid glucose difference greater than 20 mg/dL was 100% sensitive and 100% specific for a diagnosis of bacterial peritonitis in one study of dogs and cats.[18]

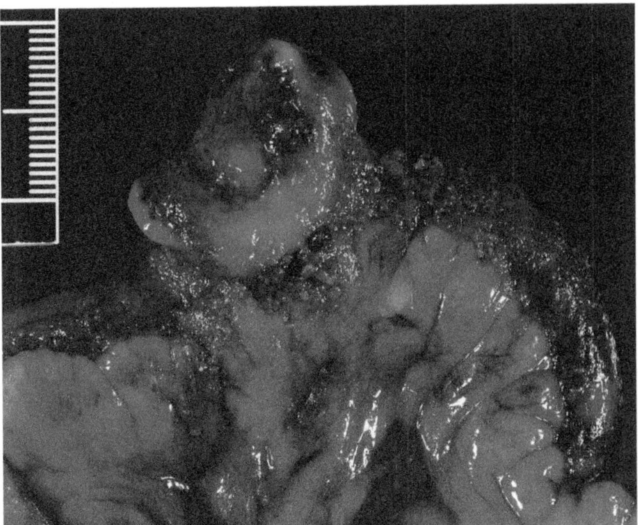

FIGURE 88-1 Necropsy image from a 7-year-old terrier mix with severe bacterial peritonitis secondary to perforated intestinal lymphoma. The dog had acute onset of diarrhea and collapse before being brought to the veterinary clinic in cardiorespiratory arrest. On ultrasound examination there was a large volume of echogenic peritoneal effusion and the mesentery was severely hyperechoic. The stomach, small intestine, and colon were fluid distended, hypomotile, and had thickened, corrugated walls with diminished blood flow. At necropsy, the omentum was discolored dark red to purple, and a segment of jejunum had an intramural mass with a central depression that communicated with the intestinal lumen. (Courtesy University of California, Davis, Veterinary Anatomic Pathology Service.)

Culture

If bacterial peritonitis is suspected, abdominal fluid specimens should be submitted for aerobic and anaerobic bacterial culture and susceptibility testing. Inoculation of blood culture bottles with ascites fluid could be considered if there is to be any delay in transport of the specimen to the laboratory.

Treatment and Prognosis

Treatment of peritonitis involves a combination of antibiotic treatment, supportive care, and surgery. The goal of surgery is to identify and correct the source of leakage and to lavage and drain the abdomen. The latter is critical for effective antibiotic penetration. Cytologic evidence of inflammation with intracellular bacteria in peritoneal fluid specimens and/or the identification of free air within the abdomen (in the absence of a history of surgery or abdominocentesis) are indications for surgical exploration.

TABLE 88-3

Suggested Empiric Antimicrobial Drug Choices for IV Use in Dogs and Cats with Bacterial Peritonitis Pending the Results of Culture and Susceptibility*

Antimicrobial Drug	Spectrum	Comments
Ampicillin-sulbactam *and* a fluoroquinolone (e.g., enrofloxacin, marbofloxacin)	Activity against gram-negative bacteria, some methicillin-resistant staphylococci, streptococci, enterococci, and most anaerobes	Replace the fluoroquinolone with an aminoglycoside (amikacin or gentamicin) if the regional prevalence of fluoroquinolone resistance is high.
Metronidazole *and* a fluoroquinolone	Activity against susceptible gram-negative and gram-positive bacteria and anaerobes	Replace the fluoroquinolone with an aminoglycoside (amikacin or gentamicin) or a third-generation cephalosporine if the regional prevalence of fluoroquinolone resistance is high.
Ticarcillin–clavulanic acid	Activity against susceptible gram-positive and gram-negative aerobes (including *Pseudomonas aeruginosa*) and some anaerobes	Not active against methicillin-resistant staphylococci
Carbapenem (meropenem or imipenem-cilastatin)	Activity against susceptible gram-positive and gram-negative aerobes and anaerobes	Not active against methicillin-resistant staphylococci. Reserve use for when multidrug-resistant gram-negative bacterial infection is suspected.
Piperacillin-tazobactam	Activity against susceptible gram-positive and gram-negative aerobes, including *Pseudomonas aeruginosa,* and some anaerobes	Not active against methicillin-resistant staphylococci. Reserve use for when multidrug-resistant gram-negative bacterial infection is suspected.

*If appropriate, reduce spectrum once the results of culture and susceptibility are available.

Dosages for IV administration (normal renal function). See Chapter 8 for precautions.

Amikacin 15-30 mg/kg q24h (dogs), 10-14 mg/kg q24h (cats)
Ampicillin-sulbactam, 20 mg/kg q6-8h (dose based on ampicillin component)
Gentamicin sulfate, 14 mg/kg q24h (dogs), 8 mg/kg q24h (cats)
Ciprofloxacin hydrochloride, 10 mg/kg q24h
Enrofloxacin, 5-20 mg/kg q24h (dogs); avoid in cats and never exceed 5 mg/kg, see important cautionary notes in Chapter 8
Imipenem-cilastatin, 5 mg/kg q6h (dilute in 100 mL sterile saline and give slowly over 30 min)
Meropenem, 25 mg/kg q8h
Piperacillin-tazobactam, 40 mg/kg q6h
Ticarcillin-clavulanate 50 mg/kg q6h

Antimicrobial Treatment

Parenteral antimicrobial drug treatment should be initiated as soon as possible after diagnosis of peritonitis, because delayed antimicrobial drug treatment in severe sepsis and septic shock may increase mortality (see Chapter 86). The initial choice of antimicrobial drugs in dogs and cats with bacterial peritonitis should include a broad-spectrum combination of antimicrobials with activity against both obligate anaerobes and facultative anaerobes (especially *E. coli* and *Enterococcus*) (Table 88-3). Subsequently, treatment should be adjusted on the basis of cytology and culture and susceptibility results. Because obligate anaerobes may not grow reliably in the laboratory and are commonly involved, continued use of an antibiotic that provides activity against anaerobes is recommended even when anaerobic cultures are negative.

Surgical Treatment

Careful surgical exploration for a site of bacterial leakage is indicated after initial stabilization with fluids, vasopressors, and antimicrobial drug treatment. The underlying cause must be surgically corrected (e.g., intestinal resection and anastomosis), and the peritoneum should be debrided and lavaged thoroughly with warm isotonic saline. The need for subsequent drainage is controversial. Drainage is generally selected when debridement and lavage cannot adequately reduce contamination. Methods of drainage include primary closure with closed suction drains, open peritoneal drainage, and, most recently, vacuum-assisted peritoneal drainage.[10,12,17,20-22] In retrospective studies, no significant differences in survival have been identified among methods, but prospective studies are required. Complications of drainage are ascending nosocomial infection, obstruction of closed suction drains by omentum, and hypoproteinemia. Evisceration and bowel desiccation have the potential to occur with open peritoneal drainage, and fluid production cannot be quantified. Dogs and cats that undergo open drainage are also more likely to require plasma or blood transfusions and may have longer hospitalization times.[17] Frequent sedation or anesthesia for bandage changes is also required.

Supportive Care

Supportive care for cats and dogs with bacterial peritonitis generally includes intensive crystalloid and colloid fluid therapy, administration of vasopressors, and enteral or parenteral nutritional support. Blood transfusions may also be required. Dogs that received early nutritional support had significantly shorter hospitalization times than those for which nutritional support was delayed.[13]

Prognosis

Survival rates of 32% to 67% have been reported in dogs with secondary peritonitis.[7,9,11,12,16,21,22] Survival rates of 44% to

70% after surgery have been reported for cats.[7,10,15] Typically hospitalization is required for 3 to 16 days (median around 5 to 6 days). When death occurs, it usually results from septic shock, DIC, or multiple organ dysfunction. Negative prognostic indicators identified in dogs with bacterial peritonitis include a diagnosis of primary as opposed to secondary peritonitis[7]; preoperative anemia, leukocytosis, or hypoproteinemia[16]; and postoperative administration of glucocorticoids.[16] Low preoperative systolic blood pressure was a negative prognostic factor in a study that included both dogs and cats.[14] Low preoperative median serum ALT activity (56 U/L for surviving cats compared with 179 U/L for non-survivors) was the only positive prognostic indicator in one study of cats with peritonitis.[10] Age, preoperative heart rate, rectal temperature, the results of other laboratory parameters, or the presence of polymicrobial infection did not affect survival. In another study, a high plasma lactate concentration was a negative prognostic indicator in cats with bacterial peritonitis.[15]

HEPATOBILIARY INFECTIONS

Etiology and Epidemiology

Hepatobiliary infections include hepatic abscesses; a variety of viral, bacterial, protozoal, or fungal infections that have spread hematogenously to the liver as part of a systemic infection; ascending infections of the biliary tree; and possibly bacterial translocation from the portal circulation. The focus of this section is bacterial infections of the biliary tree; hepatic abscesses are considered in a separate section that follows.

Bacterial infections of the hepatobiliary system occur occasionally in cats and are rare in dogs. The main mechanism thought to be involved is ascending infections of the biliary tree, although hematogenous spread and bacterial translocation from the portal system are other proposed mechanisms.[23] They have been associated with suppurative cholangitis/cholangiohepatitis, cholecystitis, choledochitis, and cholelithiasis.[24-31] *Cholangitis* is inflammation of intrahepatic bile ducts, whereas *cholangiohepatitis* is inflammation of the bile ducts that has spread to the adjacent liver parenchyma. The use of the term "cholangitis" (rather than "cholangiohepatitis") has been recommended by the WSAVA Liver Diseases and Pathology Standardization Group, because of the variable existence of hepatic involvement, so this term will be used from this point onward. In cats, cholangitis has been classified histologically as *neutrophilic cholangitis, lymphocytic cholangitis,* or *chronic cholangitis associated with liver fluke infestation.* Neutrophilic cholangitis can be further subclassified as acute or chronic depending on the presence of fibrosis, fibroplasia, or bile duct proliferation.[32] Neutrophilic cholangitis is thought to develop as a result of ascending bacterial infection from the gastrointestinal tract, which may occur secondary to inflammatory bowel disease (IBD) and/or pancreatitis (Figure 88-2). It is hypothesized that the common entry of the pancreatic and common bile ducts into the intestine in cats may predispose them to concurrent intestinal, pancreatic, and biliary disease due to pancreatic and hepatobiliary reflux in the face of IBD ("triaditis"). However, not all cats with cholangitis have histologic evidence of associated pancreatitis or IBD. Cats with acute neutrophilic cholangitis tend to be younger than those with chronic neutrophilic cholangitis.[32,33] Retrovirus infection does not appear to be a predisposing factor. The cause of lymphocytic cholangitis is unclear; currently it is thought to be an immune-mediated condition.[34] Chronic cholangitis associated with liver fluke infestation is rare and is primarily reported from regions with subtropical climates such as the southeastern United States and Hawaii, but disease can occur in non-endemic areas in traveled cats. Several different fluke species may be involved, but the most prevalent appears to be *Platynosomum concinnum.*[35]

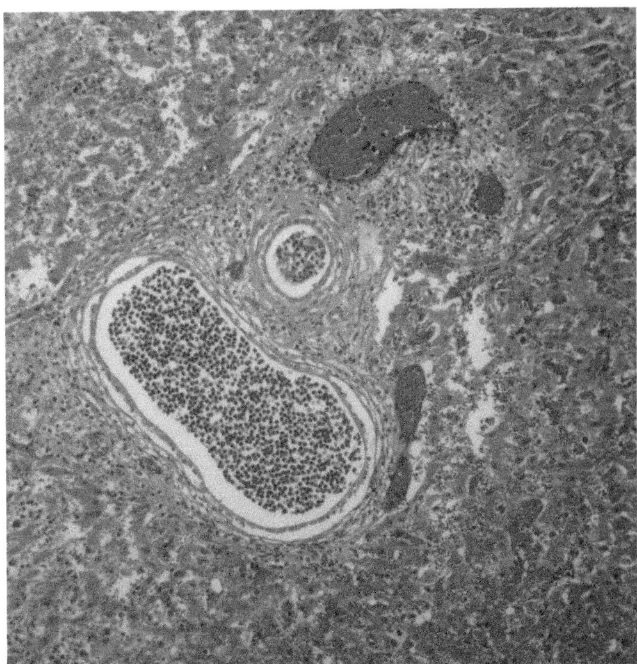

FIGURE 88-2 Histopathology showing severe, acute neutrophilic cholangitis in a 20-year-old female spayed domestic shorthair. Bile ducts are expanded by neutrophils. *Escherichia coli* was isolated from the liver in large numbers at necropsy. Concurrent diseases found at necropsy were pulmonary adenocarcinoma and moderate multifocal glomerulonephritis.

Choledochitis is inflammation of the common bile duct. *Cholecystitis* is inflammation of the gallbladder and may or may not be associated with cholangitis or choledochitis. In some instances, necrotizing and/or emphysematous cholecystitis can develop, which may lead to perforation of the gallbladder wall and septic bile peritonitis. *Cholelithiasis* is stone formation within the biliary tree. In some instances, cholelithiasis or neoplasia of the biliary tree may predispose to cholangitis and necrotizing cholecystitis.[28,29] Alternatively, it has been suggested that bacterial cholecystitis predisposes to stone formation through bacterial deconjugation of soluble bilirubin glucuronide to insoluble unconjugated bilirubin and glucuronic acid.[27] Smaller breed (dachshunds, poodles, miniature schnauzers) female dogs were predisposed to cholelithiasis in one study.[27]

Biliary cultures are more likely to be positive than hepatic cultures in both dogs and cats with hepatobiliary disease. In one large study, approximately 30% of biliary cultures were positive in dogs and cats, whereas hepatic cultures were positive in 14% of cats and 5% of dogs.[31] In cats, more than 80% of biliary cultures yielded a single bacterial species, whereas multiple bacterial species were isolated from approximately 50% of dogs. Bacterial species isolated from cats include obligate anaerobes, a variety of Enterobacteriaceae, *Enterococcus, Streptococcus,* or *Staphylococcus* species.[24,31,32] Dogs are most commonly infected with mixtures of *E. coli, Enterococcus* spp., and anaerobes, primarily *Bacteroides* and *Clostridium* species.[25-29,31]

Staphylococcus spp., other gram-negative aerobes (*Klebsiella, Enterobacter, Citrobacter,* and *Pseudomonas aeruginosa*), and *Streptococcus* spp. may also be isolated from dogs. *Salmonella* in cats and *Campylobacter* in dogs have also been associated with cholecystitis. Although rare, emphysematous cholecystitis in dogs and cats is usually associated with *Clostridium* spp. and/or *E. coli* infection.[36]

Clinical Features

Clinical Signs and Physical Examination Abnormalities

The most common clinical signs of hepatobiliary infection in both dogs and cats are lethargy, inappetence, vomiting, weight loss, and diarrhea.[24,25,30,32,33] These signs may be chronic, acute, and rarely peracute.[25,37] Peracute disease can occur with necrotizing cholecystitis and rupture of the gallbladder wall and may be associated with clinical signs of septic shock. Hypersalivation may be evident in cats with neutrophilic cholangitis.[24] Physical examination may reveal fever, lethargy, dehydration, icterus, thin body condition, and/or pain on palpation of the abdomen. Hepatomegaly may also be identified.[32] Some animals are tachycardic or tachypneic.

Diagnosis

Laboratory Abnormalities

Complete Blood Count

The CBC in dogs and cats with hepatobiliary infections may show leukocytosis due to a neutrophilia, bandemia, and sometimes monocytosis.[24-26,30,32,33,37] Some cats with cholangitis are leukopenic.[24,32] Lymphopenia and/or anemia may also be present.

Serum Biochemical Tests

Dogs with cholangitis or cholecystitis typically have increased activities of serum ALT, ALP, and GGT and hyperbilirubinemia. At least 50% of cats with cholangitis have mild to moderate increases in the activity of ALT and/or ALP (usually <1000 U/L). Increased activity of GGT may also be present. However, some cats with cholangitis have normal serum ALT, ALP, and GGT activities.[32] Hyperbilirubinemia is present in approximately two thirds of cats. Electrolyte abnormalities may be present secondary to gastrointestinal losses in animals with vomiting or diarrhea.[24,33] Hypocholesterolemia, hyperglobulinemia, and hypoalbuminemia are uncommonly identified. Hypercholesterolemia may be present in dogs with cholestasis or bile duct obstruction but is uncommonly present in cats.[26,28,30]

Urinalysis

Urinalysis in animals with hepatobiliary infections may be unremarkable or show evidence of bilirubinuria.[24,26,38]

Coagulation Profile

Coagulation abnormalities such as prolongations of PT and PTT may be present in dogs and cats with hepatobiliary infections, either secondary to impaired absorption of vitamin K secondary to biliary obstruction, or potentially as a result of liver dysfunction.[25,33]

Diagnostic Imaging

Plain Radiography

The most common finding on abdominal radiography in dogs and cats with cholecystitis and cholangitis is hepatomegaly,

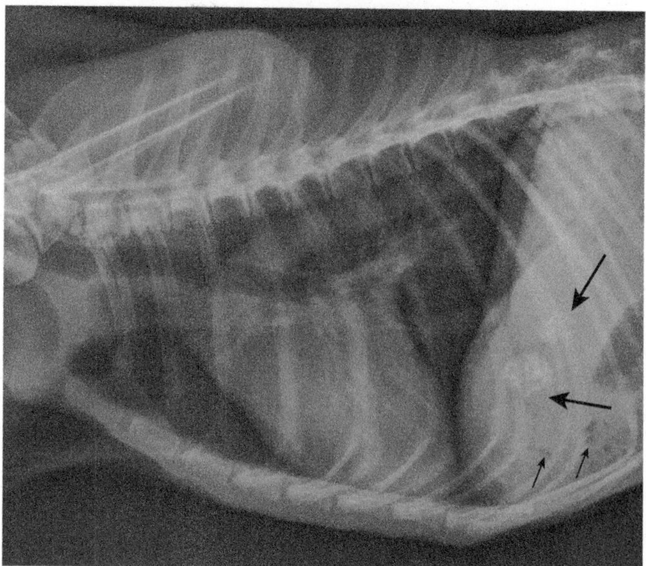

FIGURE 88-3 Lateral thoracic radiograph from a 4-year-old male neutered Chihuahua with a 3-month history of vomiting, lethargy, weight loss, and progressive icterus. Within the viewable abdomen, multiple irregular mineral opacities are present in the region of the gallbladder (*large arrows*). In this region, there are also multiple small irregular gas opacities (*small arrows*). A diagnosis of necrotizing cholecystitis and secondary bile peritonitis was made based on ultrasound and abdominal fluid analysis. Exploratory laparotomy revealed multiple choleliths, and a cholecystectomy was performed. Histopathology revealed severe, subacute to chronic, transmural suppurative and necrotizing cholecystitis.

which is variable.[30,33] Uncommonly, single or multiple radiopaque choleliths are visible (Figure 88-3), although choleliths may also be radiolucent.[26-28] In some animals, no abnormalities are detected. Emphysematous cholecystitis is characterized by the presence of gas in the liver in the region of the gallbladder. Loss of abdominal detail may be present if gallbladder rupture and septic bile peritonitis have occurred.[25]

Sonographic Findings

Abdominal ultrasound findings in dogs and cats with cholangitis are similar and include hepatomegaly, normal or abnormal hepatic echotexture with a homogenous or heterogenous increase in echogenicity, prominent portal vasculature, a thickened and hyperechogenic gallbladder wall, and sediment within the gallbladder.[24-26,30,32,39,40] The gallbladder wall may also appear irregular and contain polypoid mass lesions. Abdominal pain in the right cranial quadrant may be evident during the procedure. Choleliths are occasionally identified within the biliary tract as hyperechoic masses that shadow. Distention of the biliary tract may be evident, sometimes with tortuosity of the cystic and common bile ducts.[24,25,39] Evidence of concurrent pancreatic and/or intestinal wall disease may be present in cats.[32] Gas may be identified in the gallbladder wall of animals with emphysematous cholecystitis (Figure 88-4).

Microbiologic Tests

Cytologic Examination

Cytologic examination of bile collected by percutaneous ultrasound-guided cholecystocentesis (or intraoperative cholecystocentesis) in animals with hepatobiliary infection may reveal increased numbers of degenerate neutrophils, small and/or large mononuclear cells, and in some cases, a mixed or monomorphic bacterial population.[24] Cholecystocentesis carries some risk of

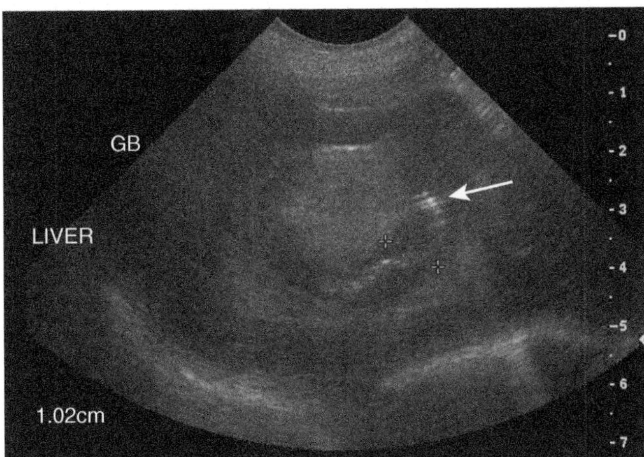

FIGURE 88-4 Abdominal ultrasound image of the gallbladder of a 6-year-old female spayed American Eskimo dog with emphysematous cholecystitis. The gallbladder wall is markedly thickened (1 cm), is diffusely hypoechoic, and the gallbladder contains homogenous sludge. Multiple hyperechoic foci were identified tracking throughout the wall *(arrow)*. The hepatic parenchyma immediately adjacent to the gallbladder was poorly characterized because of a large amount of markedly hyperechoic inflamed mesentery within the cranial abdominal region.

gallbladder leakage or rupture and should be avoided if there is evidence of gas in the gallbladder wall. As much bile should be removed as possible to minimize the chance of leakage. It is possible that percutaneous drainage of infected bile may have a therapeutic benefit, although this requires further study.

Culture

Aerobic and anaerobic bacterial culture can be performed on bile collected by ultrasound-guided or intraoperative cholecystocentesis or liver biopsies. Culture of bile is more likely to yield positive results than culture of liver biopsies. Although it is generally accepted that bile is sterile in healthy dogs and cats,[23,41] transient cytologic and microbiologic evidence of bactibilia has been identified in healthy dogs.[42] Liver tissue from healthy dogs can also harbor a variety of enteric bacterial species.[43] Thus, the results of bile culture must be interpreted in light of clinical and cytologic findings. Antimicrobial drug resistance among bacteria isolated from the bile of dogs and cats with cholecystitis and cholangitis has been described in several studies, and so culture and susceptibility testing should be performed whenever possible. When cholecystocentesis is undesirable because of concerns for gallbladder rupture (see Cytologic Examination), blood cultures may be useful, although the utility of blood culture in dogs and cats with cholecystitis has not been studied. In human patients, bile cultures are positive in 50% to 95% of patients with acute cholecystitis, and blood cultures are positive in 30% to 40% of patients.[44]

Pathologic Findings

On histopathology, neutrophilic cholangitis in cats varies in severity, chronicity, and the extent of associated hepatic parenchymal involvement.[32,38] Concurrent hepatic lipidosis may also be present. In a small percentage of affected cats, complete or partial biliary obstruction is identified as a result of inflammation, neoplasia, or cholelithiasis. Other findings in affected cats include acute or chronic pancreatitis (65% of cats in one study), inflammatory bowel disease and/or intestinal lymphoma (46% of cats). Histopathology of the gallbladder wall in both dogs and cats with cholecystitis may reveal mucosal and glandular hyperplasia and thickening and neutrophilic or lymphoplasmacytic inflammation of the gallbladder wall.[26,30,32]

Choleliths in cats are most often composed of calcium carbonate, although they also may be a mixture of cholesterol, calcium bilirubinate, and calcium carbonate.[26,28] In dogs they are often composed of calcium bilirubinate, bilirubin, or a mixture of bilirubin and cholesterol.

Treatment and Prognosis

Treatment of cholangitis and cholecystitis is usually with supportive care and antimicrobial drug administration. Dogs and cats with necrotizing or emphysematous cholecystitis require cholecystectomy. Cholecystectomy could also be considered to prevent recurrence of cholelithiasis in animals with chronic cholecystitis. Cholecystectomy, biliary stenting procedures, and/or biliary diversion surgery may be required for animals with obstructive processes such as cholelithiasis, biliary neoplasia, or obstructive cholangitis.[27,28] Because cholecystotomy or biliary diversion surgery often results in dehiscence and septic bile peritonitis if bacterial cholecystitis or choledochitis is present, cholecystectomy has been recommended for dogs with cholelithiasis as opposed to cholecystotomy.[27] When compared with other surgical biliary procedures, cholecystectomy has been associated with good clinical outcomes in dogs and cats, but any condition that requires biliary surgery carries a guarded prognosis.

Antimicrobial Drug Treatment and Supportive Care

Empirically used antibiotics should target gram-negative enteric bacterial species and anaerobes and be concentrated in bile. Suitable antibiotics include ampicillin-sulbactam or amoxicillin-clavulanic acid, or a fluoroquinolone with metronidazole, although resistance to amoxicillin-clavulanic acid or enrofloxacin has been documented among biliary isolates from dogs and cats.[30] Pradofloxacin also has a favorable spectrum of activity, because of its activity against anaerobes (see Chapter 8). In human patients, specific treatment of *Enterococcus* biliary infections when they are combined with other bacterial infections may not be necessary, since they tend to resolve when the other infections are treated.[44] Supportive treatments that could be considered include intravenous crystalloid fluids with or without colloids, nutritional support by parenteral or enteral means (with a restricted fat diet), ursodiol, *S*-adenylmethionine, antiemetics, antacids, and parenteral vitamin K supplementation.

Prognosis

The prognosis for cats with neutrophilic cholangitis is fair to good, with mean survival times longer than 1 year.[24,33] Poor outcomes may be related to the presence of underlying disease that contributes to mortality such as neoplasia.[28,33] The presence of septic bile peritonitis was associated with mortality in one study of dogs that underwent extrahepatic biliary surgery; more than half of dogs with septic bile peritonitis died.[29] In another study, 9 of 23 dogs with necrotizing cholecystitis died.[25]

HEPATIC ABSCESSES

Hepatic abscesses are uncommon in dogs and very rare in cats.[45,46] They may be associated with ascending bacterial infection of the biliary tree, translocation of portal bacteria, or hematogenous spread of bacteria to the liver, although the source of bacteremia in some animals is unclear. Because bacteria can be found in the liver of healthy dogs, abscessation may also develop when these bacteria proliferate secondary to compromise of normal defenses (such as hepatic necrosis).[43] Affected animals are typically middle aged to older;[45,46] the mean age of affected dogs or cats is 10 years. The abscesses may be acute or chronic, single or multiple, and macroabscesses or microabscesses may form. Pancreatitis, diabetes mellitus, other hepatobiliary disease, neoplasia, colonic surgery, cholelithiasis, or chronic phenobarbital or glucocorticoid administration have been in the histories of affected dogs.[46-48] Migrating plant awn foreign bodies may also be an underlying cause.[48] Concurrent conditions in affected cats have included IBD, pancreatitis, hepatobiliary neoplasia, chronic cholecystitis, colonic surgery, or congestive heart failure.[45] Many cats have concurrent bacterial urinary tract infections.

The most common bacterial species isolated from hepatic abscesses in both dogs and cats is *E. coli.* In dogs, other species have included *K. pneumoniae, Staphylococcus,* and *Clostridium* spp. In cats, *Bacteroides, Enterococcus,* and *Streptococcus* spp. have been isolated, often in mixed infections with *E. coli.* Blood cultures are also often positive.[45,46] Clinical signs and laboratory abnormalities are similar to those for other hepatobiliary infections, except that severe illness and signs of septic shock are often present. Evidence of bleeding diatheses may be present. Marked neutrophilia or neutropenia, bandemia, toxic neutrophils, anemia, lymphopenia, and thrombocytopenia may be present on the CBC. Hypoalbuminemia and coagulation abnormalities are common.[45,46] Abdominal radiographs may be unremarkable, or they may show hepatomegaly or a hepatic mass effect, poor abdominal detail, and/or pneumoperitoneum if abscess rupture has occurred (Figure 88-5). Thoracic radiography often reveals interstitial, bronchiolar, or alveolar lung infiltrates,[44,46] which may result from associated embolic or aspiration pneumonia. Ultrasonographic examination of the abdomen reveals one or more hypoechoic, anechoic, or heteroechoic hepatic masses, with or without peritoneal effusion. In some cases, gas is evident within the masses.

Antemortem diagnosis of hepatic abscesses usually relies on cytologic examination of ultrasound-guided fine-needle aspirates of the masses, which reveals large numbers of degenerate neutrophils. Abscesses may also be discovered during exploratory laparotomy (e.g., in dogs and cats with bacterial peritonitis). Culture and susceptibility of aspirates of the liver abscesses, free peritoneal fluid, and/or blood should be performed. Effective treatment of solitary abscesses relies on appropriate antimicrobial drug treatment together with complete or partial liver lobectomy, or abscess drainage and omentalization. With the exception of microabscesses, antimicrobial drug therapy alone is often ineffective. Aggressive supportive care in an intensive care unit may be required. Initial antimicrobial drug treatment should be broad

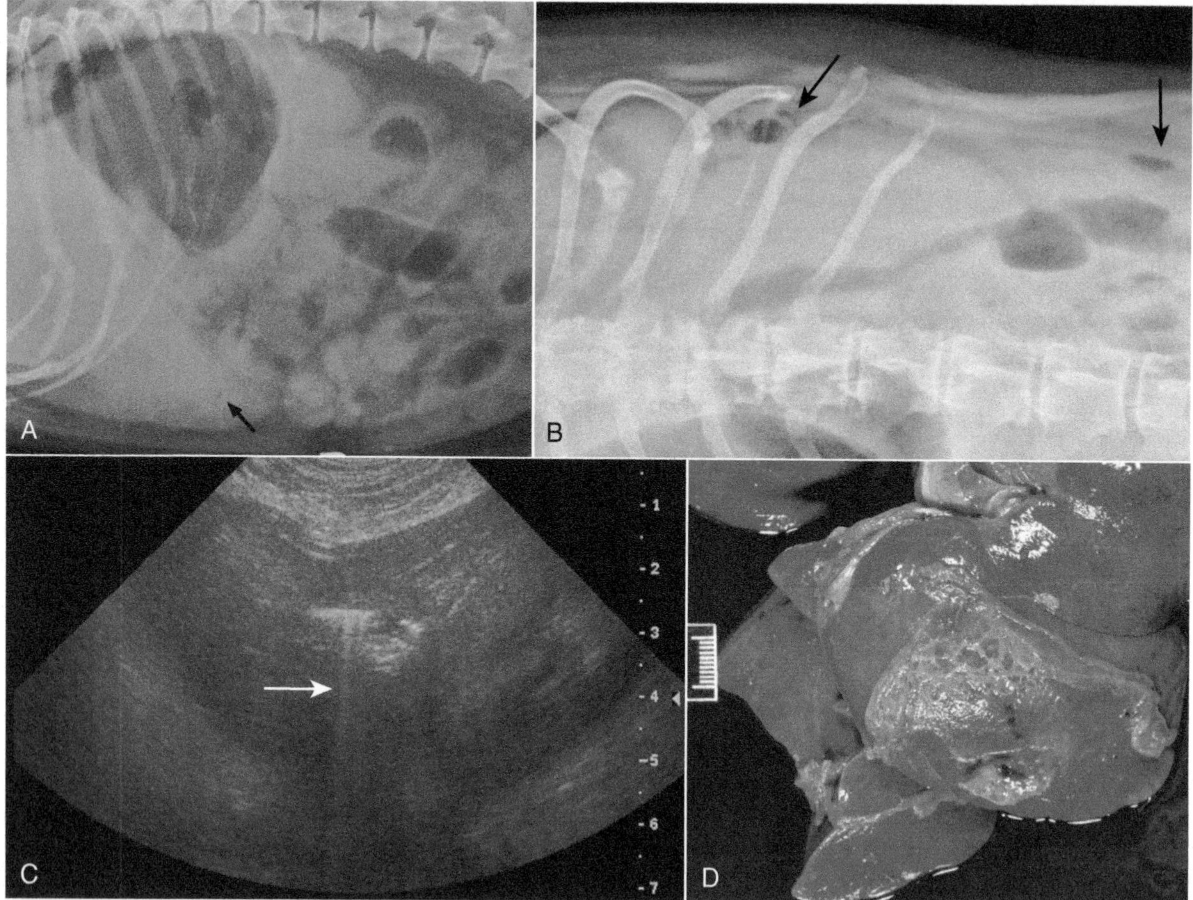

FIGURE 88-5 Ruptured hepatic abscess. **A,** Right lateral abdominal radiograph from a 15-year-old male neutered dachshund with acute onset of vomiting and diarrhea secondary to a ruptured hepatic abscess. There is a diffuse loss of serosal detail as well free peritoneal gas present throughout the abdomen. The liver is enlarged. There are multiple small rounded gas opacities present over the ventral and right aspects of the liver *(arrow).* Multiple small intestinal loops contain gas and fluid, some of which measure at the upper limits or over the upper limit of normal. **B,** Free peritoneal air can be seen clearly *(arrows)* using a horizontal beam view. **C,** Comet-tail artifact *(arrow)* due to the presence of gas within the liver on ultrasound examination. **D,** Hepatic abscess from the same dog at necropsy.

spectrum, after which it should be adjusted based on the results of culture and susceptibility. Mortality rates of 50% and 79% have been reported for dogs and cats, respectively.[45] The prognosis is especially poor when multiple abscesses are present.[45,46]

Pancreatitis and Pancreatic Abscesses

In dogs and cats, pancreatitis and pancreatic abscess formation most often appears to be a sterile process that results from tissue destruction and necrosis by pancreatic enzymes. Experimentally, necrotizing pancreatitis can be complicated by secondary bacterial invasion due to ascending infection from the duodenum or bacterial translocation,[49,50] although the extent to which this occurs in dogs and cats with naturally-occurring pancreatitis remains unclear. Occasionally, pancreatitis results from hematogenous spread of bacteria to the pancreas, usually in addition to other organs (see Table 86-2). Other microorganisms known to cause pancreatitis as a result of systemic infection include *Leptospira* species, *Toxoplasma gondii,* and fungi such as *Cryptococcus neoformans.* In cats, pancreatitis can also result from invasion by flukes *(Eurytrema procyonis)*.[51] When a primary infectious cause of pancreatitis cannot clearly be identified, the use of antimicrobial drugs to treat pancreatitis in dogs and cats is controversial. If used, the primary goal of antimicrobial treatment is to prevent or treat secondary ascending bacterial infection or bacterial translocation; treatment should target enteric bacteria. However, no evidence currently exists that use of antimicrobials alters outcome in dogs and cats with naturally occurring pancreatitis, and it has the potential to select for infection by multidrug-resistant enteric pathogens. In addition, many widely used antimicrobial drugs in veterinary medicine (such as β-lactams and aminoglycosides) penetrate inflamed pancreatic tissue poorly. Suitable choices include fluoroquinolones (for gram-negative aerobes), third-generation cephalosporines, and metronidazole (for anaerobes).

CASE EXAMPLE

Signalment: "George," a 16-year-old male neutered domestic shorthair from northern California

History: George was evaluated for a 2-day history of vomiting and progressive lethargy and inappetence. The owners reported that the vomiting occurred six times at the onset of illness and was associated with apparent abdominal pain but had since ceased. The day he became ill, he was seen at an emergency clinic where a CBC showed only a mild left shift (479 band neutrophils), a chemistry panel showed mild hypokalemia (3.1 mmol/L, reference range 3.6-4.9 mmol/L), and a total serum T4 concentration was increased (10.2 μg/dL, reference range, 1.1-3.3 μg/dL). Pancreatitis was suspected and George was initially treated with subcutaneous lactated Ringer's solution (200 mL SC q24h), mucosal buprenorphine (0.02 mg/kg PO q8h to q12h), and ondansetron (0.2 mg/kg PO q12h) pending the results of laboratory testing. However, because George became inappetent and lethargic, he was returned for reevaluation the following day.

Other medical history: George had been diagnosed with pancreatitis 8 months previously. He was also diagnosed with a biliary cystadenoma at that time. He had been hospitalized for 9 days and treated with jejunostomy tube feeding. Since then, he had been well until this recent onset of illness.

Physical Examination:

Body Weight: 6.1 kg.

General: Quiet, alert, hydrated. T = 103.8°F (39.9°C), HR = 240 beats/min, RR = 32, mucous membranes pink and moist, CRT = 1 s.

Eyes, Ears, Nose, and Throat: Palpable thyroid nodule.

Musculoskeletal: Body condition score was 5/9. The cat was ambulatory with normal gait.

Cardiovascular: A gallop rhythm was present. No murmurs or arrhythmias were auscultated. Femoral pulses were strong and synchronous.

Genitourinary/Gastrointestinal: Soft, mildly painful abdomen. The urinary bladder was small.

Other Systems, Including Peripheral Lymph Nodes: No clinically significant findings.

Imaging Findings:

Abdominal Ultrasound: The margins of the kidneys were irregular, and there was decreased corticomedullary distinction. In the region of the left limb of the pancreas, the mesentery was markedly hyperechoic and hyperattenuating. There was diffuse thickening of the muscularis of the small bowel. There was no evidence of mesenteric lymphadenomegaly. There was a small amount of free anechoic peritoneal fluid.

Thoracic Radiographs: The cardiac silhouette appeared mildly enlarged. There was a mild bronchointerstitial pattern throughout the thorax. There was poor serosal detail within the viewable cranial abdomen.

Outcome: George was treated supportively for pancreatitis with intravenous fluids (lactated Ringer's solution with 20 mEq/L KCl at 15 mL/hr), buprenorphine (0.01 mg/kg IV q6h), famotidine (0.5 mg/kg IV q12h), and ondansetron (0.5 mg/kg IV q12h). His temperature normalized, but he showed no interest in food or his surroundings. Cytologic examination of an ultrasound-guided liver aspirate on day 2 of hospitalization showed moderate hepatic lipidosis and mild mixed inflammation. Laboratory testing was reevaluated and an echocardiogram was performed on the third day of hospitalization in preparation for anesthesia and placement of an esophageal feeding tube. The echocardiogram was unremarkable; the gallop rhythm was suspected to result from a systolic click. New findings on the CBC were mild, nonregenerative anemia (HCT 29.9%, RR 30%-50%), with a WBC of 11,580 cells/μL (4500-14,000 cells/μL), 4053 neutrophils/μL (2000-9000 cells/μL), bandemia (3242 cells/μL), and circulating metamyelocytes (232 cells/μL). Findings on the serum biochemistry panel included a bicarbonate of 24 mmol/L (15-21 mmol/L), calcium of 8.3 mg/dL (9.0-10.9 mg/dL), BUN of 20 mg/dL (18-33 mg/dL), creatinine of 0.8 mg/dL (1.1-2.2 mg/dL), glucose of 114 mg/dL (63-118 mg/dL), total protein of 5.3 g/dL (6.6-8.4 g/dL), albumin of 2.0 g/dL (2.2-4.6 g/dL), globulin of 3.3 g/dL (2.8-5.4 g/dL), ALT of 57 U/L (27-101 U/L), AST of 46 U/L (17-58 U/L), ALP of 26 U/L (14-71 U/L), GGT of <3 U/L (0-4 U/L), cholesterol of 109 mg/dL (89-258 mg/dL), and total bilirubin of 0.4 mg/dL (0-0.2 mg/dL). Urinalysis showed a specific gravity of 1.015; pH 7.0, protein 25 mg/dL, no bilirubin, 25 erythrocytes/µL hemoprotein, 1-3 WBC/HPF, 1-6 RBC/HPF, and many lipid droplets. Serum vitamin B_{12} and folate concentrations were 383 ng/L (279-1254 ng/L) and 7.5 ng/mL (10.4-20.7 ng/mL), respectively.

Because of the severely left-shifted neutrophil count and mild hyperbilirubinemia, bacterial cholecystitis was suspected. Findings on abdominal ultrasonography were unchanged from the previous examination. Ultrasound-guided cholecystocentesis was performed while George was under anesthesia for esophagostomy tube placement, and a small volume of the scant peritoneal fluid present was also collected.

Microbiologic Testing:

Cytologic Examination (Bile): Smears had light blue backgrounds and contained a moderate amount of unidentified material. Nucleated cells were not found, but many short, plump coccobacilli were seen. Most of the bacteria were in large clusters, but a few groups were in chains.

Peritoneal Fluid Analysis: Grossly the fluid was pink and cloudy, and it had a yellow, clear supernatant. The total protein concentration was 2.8 g/dL and there were 100,000 RBC/µL. There were 5380 nucleated cells/µL, with 70% nondegenerate neutrophils, 6% small and well-differentiated lymphocytes, 7% foamy macrophages, and 17% eosinophils. No infectious agents were identified.

Aerobic and Anaerobic Bacterial Culture (Bile): Large numbers of *Enterococcus faecium*. No anaerobes were cultured. The isolate was susceptible to amoxicillin-clavulanic acid (≤4 µg/mL), ampicillin (≤0.25 µg/mL), penicillin (0.12 µg/mL), chloramphenicol (≤4 µg/mL), doxycycline (≤2 µg/mL), imipenem (≤1 µg/mL); had intermediate susceptibility to erythromycin (1 µg/mL); and was resistant to rifampin (>2 µg/mL).

Aerobic and Anaerobic Bacterial Culture (Peritoneal Fluid): Very small numbers of *Enterococcus faecium*. The antibiogram was identical to the isolate from the bile.

Diagnosis: Peritonitis and suspected bacterial cholecystitis caused by *E. faecium*; pancreatitis and secondary hepatic lipidosis.

Treatment: Medical treatment with ampicillin-sulbactam (20 mg/kg [ampicillin component] IV q8h) and enrofloxacin (5 mg/kg slow IV q24h) was commenced on day 3 of hospitalization, before the results of culture and susceptibility were available. Treatment was also continued with intravenous fluids, buprenorphine, famotidine, ondansetron, and nutrition through the esophageal feeding tube with a slurry of a commercially available gastroenteric diet (Purina EN Feline Formula, q4h). Surgery was considered, but because George was stable and the amount of free peritoneal fluid was scant, a decision was made to continue medical treatment with close observation and serial CBC and abdominal ultrasound examinations. Within 12 hours of antibiotic treatment, George was brighter. A repeat abdominal ultrasound showed no changes except that mildly enlarged and hypoechoic mesenteric lymph nodes were identified. The CBC showed persistent nonregenerative anemia (HCT of 26.4%), 10,181 neutrophils/µL, 5553 bands/µL, 185 metamyelocytes/µL, and a normal platelet count (305,000/µL) with moderately toxic neutrophils. On day 5 of hospitalization, ultrasonography showed a decrease in the amount of peritoneal fluid. The enrofloxacin was discontinued when the results of culture and susceptibility became available. On day 6, the CBC showed a stable HCT, 9366 neutrophils/µL, 2810 bands/µL, moderately toxic neutrophils, and no metamyelocytes. A serum chemistry panel was unremarkable, and the total bilirubin was 0.1 mg/dL. On day 8, George began eating a small amount of food on his own, and the CBC showed further improvement with 6048 neutrophils/µL, 336 bands/µL, mild monocytosis (896 cells/µL), and no toxic neutrophils. He was discharged from the hospital the following day with instructions to continue tube feeding, ondansetron (0.3 mg/kg PO q24h), famotidine (0.5 mg/kg PO q12h), and amoxicillin–clavulanic acid (15 mg/kg PO q12h). At a recheck 1 week later, the owner reported that George had been doing well at home, although he had vomited three times over the course of the week. Physical examination was unremarkable, apart from the thyroid nodule and mild weight loss (body weight, 5.6 kg compared with 5.9 kg at discharge). A CBC showed a HCT of 30%, 10,592 neutrophils/µL, and 132 bands/µL. A serum chemistry panel was within normal limits, and the total T4 concentration was 8.2 µg/dL. Treatment with methimazole (1.25 mg q12h) was initiated for the hyperthyroidism, but because of continued vomiting, this was discontinued after three doses. George continued to improve. A week later he was eating canned and dry food on his own with no vomiting, a CBC showed no abnormalities, and the antibiotics were discontinued. The esophageal tube was removed 3 weeks later, and methimazole was reinstituted, after which his T4 normalized. Six months later George was still doing well.

Comments: In this cat, bacterial peritonitis and suspected cholecystitis were diagnosed based on cytologic and microbiologic analysis of bile and peritoneal fluid. However, there were no ultrasonographic abnormalities within the biliary tract, and cytologic evidence of inflammation in the bile was absent. Pancreatitis may have predisposed the cat to ascending infection of the biliary tract, and/or infection may have resulted from bacterial translocation. The lack of an inflammatory reaction in the bile was unusual, but it may have resulted from marked neutrophil degeneration in a toxic environment. Isolation of the same organism from both the bile and the peritoneal fluid and the rapid clinical response to antibiotic treatment suggested that *Enterococcus* played a role in disease in this cat, although some of the clinical signs and hematologic abnormalities may also have resulted from severe pancreatitis and hepatic lipidosis. Surgery was postponed with careful monitoring because the peritonitis appeared to be very low grade and there was concern it might exacerbate pancreatitis. Fortunately, the cat made a complete recovery. See Chapter 8 for precautions regarding administration of enrofloxacin to cats.

SUGGESTED READINGS

Callahan Clark JE, Haddad JL, Brown DC, et al. Feline cholangitis: a necropsy study of 44 cats (1986-2008). J Feline Med Surg. 2011;13:570-576.

Costello MF, Drobatz KJ, Aronson LR, et al. Underlying cause, pathophysiologic abnormalities, and response to treatment in cats with septic peritonitis: 51 cases (1990-2001). J Am Vet Med Assoc. 2004;225:897-902.

Culp WT, Zeldis TE, Reese MS, et al. Primary bacterial peritonitis in dogs and cats: 24 cases (1990-2006). J Am Vet Med Assoc. 2009;234:906-913.

Wagner KA, Hartmann FA, Trepanier LA. Bacterial culture results from liver, gallbladder, or bile in 248 dogs and cats evaluated for hepatobiliary disease: 1998-2003. J Vet Intern Med. 2007;21:417-424.

REFERENCES

1. Roberts DE, McClain HM, Hansen DS, et al. An outbreak of *Klebsiella pneumoniae* infection in dogs with severe enteritis and septicemia. J Vet Diagn Invest. 2000;12:168-173.
2. Collins JE, Bergeland ME, Lindeman CJ, et al. *Enterococcus (Streptococcus) durans* adherence in the small intestine of a diarrheic pup. Vet Pathol. 1988;25:396-398.
3. Hidalgo A, Rubio P, Osorio J, et al. Prevalence of *Brachyspira pilosicoli* and "Brachyspira canis" in dogs and their association with diarrhoea. Vet Microbiol. 2010;146:356-360.
4. Lapointe JM, Higgins R, Barrette N, et al. *Enterococcus hirae* enteropathy with ascending cholangitis and pancreatitis in a kitten. Vet Pathol. 2000;37:282-284.
5. De Cock HE, Marks SL, Stacy BA, et al. Ileocolitis associated with *Anaerobiospirillum* in cats. J Clin Microbiol. 2004;42:2752-2758.
6. Marks SL, Rankin SC, Byrne BA, et al. Enteropathogenic bacteria in dogs and cats: diagnosis, epidemiology, treatment, and control. J Vet Intern Med. 2011;25:1195-1208.
7. Culp WT, Zeldis TE, Reese MS, et al. Primary bacterial peritonitis in dogs and cats: 24 cases (1990-2006). J Am Vet Med Assoc. 2009;234:906-913.
8. Levison ME, Bush LM. Peritonitis and intra-peritoneal infections. In: Mandell GL, Bennett JE, Dolin R, eds. Principles and Practice of Infectious Diseases. 7th ed. Philadelphia, PA: Elsevier; 2010:1011-1034.
9. Hosgood G, Salisbury SK. Generalized peritonitis in dogs: 50 cases (1975-1986). J Am Vet Med Assoc. 1988;193:1448-1450.
10. Costello MF, Drobatz KJ, Aronson LR, et al. Underlying cause, pathophysiologic abnormalities, and response to treatment in cats with septic peritonitis: 51 cases (1990-2001). J Am Vet Med Assoc. 2004;225:897-902.
11. Greenfield CL, Walshaw R. Open peritoneal drainage for treatment of contaminated peritoneal cavity and septic peritonitis in dogs and cats: 24 cases (1980-1986). J Am Vet Med Assoc. 1987;191:100-105.
12. Lanz OI, Ellison GW, Bellah JR, et al. Surgical treatment of septic peritonitis without abdominal drainage in 28 dogs. J Am Anim Hosp Assoc. 2001;37:87-92.
13. Liu DT, Brown DC, Silverstein DC. Early nutritional support is associated with decreased length of hospitalization in dogs with septic peritonitis: a retrospective study of 45 cases (2000-2009). J Vet Emerg Crit Care (San Antonio). 2012;22:453-459.
14. Mueller MG, Ludwig LL, Barton LJ. Use of closed-suction drains to treat generalized peritonitis in dogs and cats: 40 cases (1997-1999). J Am Vet Med Assoc. 2001;219:789-794.
15. Parsons KJ, Owen LJ, Lee K, et al. A retrospective study of surgically treated cases of septic peritonitis in the cat (2000-2007). J Small Anim Pract. 2009;50:518-524.
16. Grimes JA, Schmiedt CW, Cornell KK, et al. Identification of risk factors for septic peritonitis and failure to survive following gastrointestinal surgery in dogs. J Am Vet Med Assoc. 2011;238:486-494.
17. Staatz AJ, Monnet E, Seim 3rd HB. Open peritoneal drainage versus primary closure for the treatment of septic peritonitis in dogs and cats: 42 cases (1993-1999). Vet Surg. 2002;31:174-180.
18. Ludwig LL, McLoughlin MA, Graves TK, et al. Surgical treatment of bile peritonitis in 24 dogs and 2 cats: a retrospective study (1987-1994). Vet Surg. 1997;26:90-98.
19. Culp W, Holt D. Septic peritonitis. Compend Contin Educ Vet. 2010;32:E1-E15.
20. Cioffi KM, Schmiedt CW, Cornell KK, et al. Retrospective evaluation of vacuum-assisted peritoneal drainage for the treatment of septic peritonitis in dogs and cats: 8 cases (2003-2010). J Vet Emerg Crit Care. (San Antonio) 2012;22:601-609.
21. Buote NJ, Havig ME. The use of vacuum-assisted closure in the management of septic peritonitis in six dogs. J Am Anim Hosp Assoc. 2012;48:164-171.
22. Woolfson JM, Dulish ML. Open abdominal drainage in the treatment of generalized peritonitis in 25 dogs and cats. Vet Surg. 1986;15:27-32.
23. O'Neill EJ. Bacterial cholangitis in the dog. In: Proceedings of the 21st ECVIM-CA Congress. Sevilla, Spain, 2011.
24. Brain PH, Barrs VR, Martin P, et al. Feline cholecystitis and acute neutrophilic cholangitis: clinical findings, bacterial isolates and response to treatment in six cases. J Feline Med Surg. 2006;8:91-103.
25. Church EM, Matthiesen DT. Surgical treatment of 23 dogs with necrotizing cholecystitis. J Am Anim Hosp Assoc. 1998;24:305-310.
26. Eich CS, Ludwig LL. The surgical treatment of cholelithiasis in cats: a study of nine cases. J Am Anim Hosp Assoc. 2002;38:290-296.
27. Kirpensteijn J, Fingland RB, Ulrich T, et al. Cholelithiasis in dogs: 29 cases (1980-1990). J Am Vet Med Assoc. 1993;202:1137-1142.
28. Mayhew PD, Holt DE, McLear RC, et al. Pathogenesis and outcome of extrahepatic biliary obstruction in cats. J Small Anim Pract. 2002;43:247-253.
29. Mehler SJ, Mayhew PD, Drobatz KJ, et al. Variables associated with outcome in dogs undergoing extrahepatic biliary surgery: 60 cases (1988-2002). Vet Surg. 2004;33:644-649.
30. O'Neill EJ, Day MJ, Hall EJ, et al. Bacterial cholangitis/cholangiohepatitis with or without concurrent cholecystitis in four dogs. J Small Anim Pract. 2006;47:325-335.
31. Wagner KA, Hartmann FA, Trepanier LA. Bacterial culture results from liver, gallbladder, or bile in 248 dogs and cats evaluated for hepatobiliary disease: 1998-2003. J Vet Intern Med. 2007;21:417-424.
32. Callahan Clark JE, Haddad JL, Brown DC, et al. Feline cholangitis: a necropsy study of 44 cats (1986-2008). J Feline Med Surg. 2011;13:570-576.
33. Gagne JM, Armstrong PJ, Weiss DJ, et al. Clinical features of inflammatory liver disease in cats: 41 cases (1983-1993). J Am Vet Med Assoc. 1999;214:513-516.
34. Warren A, Center S, McDonough S, et al. Histopathologic features, immunophenotyping, clonality, and eubacterial fluorescence in situ hybridization in cats with lymphocytic cholangitis/cholangiohepatitis. Vet Pathol. 2011;48:627-641.
35. Haney DR, Christiansen JS, Toll J. Severe cholestatic liver disease secondary to liver fluke (*Platynosomum concinnum*) infection in three cats. J Am Anim Hosp Assoc. 2006;42:234-237.
36. Armstrong JA, Taylor SM, Tryon KA, et al. Emphysematous cholecystitis in a Siberian husky. Can Vet J. 2000;41:60-62.
37. Neer TM. A review of disorders of the gallbladder and extrahepatic biliary tract in the dog and cat. J Vet Intern Med. 1992;6:186-192.
38. Hirsch VM, Doige CE. Suppurative cholangitis in cats. J Am Vet Med Assoc. 1983;182:1223-1226.
39. Hittmair KM, Vielgrader HD, Loupal G. Ultrasonographic evaluation of gallbladder wall thickness in cats. Vet Radiol Ultrasound. 2001;42:149-155.
40. Newell SM, Selcer BA, Girard E, et al. Correlations between ultrasonographic findings and specific hepatic diseases in cats: 72 cases (1985-1997). J Am Vet Med Assoc. 1998;213:94-98.

41. Savary-Bataille KC, Bunch SE, Spaulding KA, et al. Percutaneous ultrasound-guided cholecystocentesis in healthy cats. J Vet Intern Med. 2003;17:298-303.
42. Kook PH, Schellenberg S, Grest P, et al. Microbiologic evaluation of gallbladder bile of healthy dogs and dogs with iatrogenic hypercortisolism: a pilot study. J Vet Intern Med. 2010;24:224-228.
43. Niza MM, Ferreira AJ, Peleteiro MC, et al. Bacteriological study of the liver in dogs. J Small Anim Pract. 2004;45:401-404.
44. Sifri CD, Madoff LC. Infections of the liver and biliary system. In: Mandell GL, Bennett JE, Dolin R, eds. Principles and Practice of Infectious Diseases. 7th ed. Philadelphia, PA: Elsevier; 2010:1035-1044.
45. Sergeeff JS, Armstrong PJ, Bunch SE. Hepatic abscesses in cats: 14 cases (1985-2002). J Vet Intern Med. 2004;18:295-300.
46. Farrar ET, Washabau RJ, Saunders HM. Hepatic abscesses in dogs: 14 cases (1982-1994). J Am Vet Med Assoc. 1996;208:243-247.
47. Grooters AM, Sherding RG, Biller DS, et al. Hepatic abscesses associated with diabetes mellitus in two dogs. J Vet Intern Med. 1994;8:203-206.
48. Sykes JE. Unpublished observations, 2012.
49. Widdison AL, Alvarez C, Chang YB, et al. Sources of pancreatic pathogens in acute pancreatitis in cats. Pancreas. 1994;9:536-541.
50. Kazantsev GB, Hecht DW, Rao R, et al. Plasmid labeling confirms bacterial translocation in pancreatitis. Am J Surg. 1994;167: 201-206: discussion 206-207.
51. Vyhnal KK, Barr SC, Hornbuckle WE, et al. *Eurytrema procyonis* and pancreatitis in a cat. J Feline Med Surg. 2008;10:384-387.

CHAPTER 89

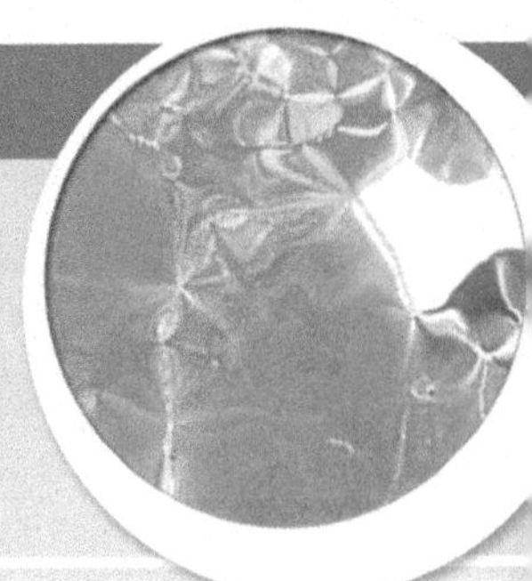

Bacterial Infections of the Genitourinary Tract

Jane E. Sykes and Jodi L. Westropp

> **Overview of Bacterial Infections of the Genitourinary Tract**
>
> Causes: The most common cause of genitourinary tract infections is *Escherichia coli*, but other gram-negative bacteria, staphylococci, and streptococci may also be involved. Anaerobic bacterial infections are rare causes of genitourinary tract infections but may be involved in pyometra.
>
> Geographic Distribution: Worldwide
>
> Major Clinical Signs: Dysuria, hematuria, or pollakiuria may occur with lower urinary tract infection, although some infections are subclinical. Acute pyelonephritis, prostatitis, and pyometra may be accompanied by fever or abdominal pain. Lethargy, inappetence, vomiting, or diarrhea may occur if sepsis develops. Pyometra may be accompanied by abdominal distention and/or a vaginal discharge. Prostatitis may be accompanied by dysuria, dyschezia, and a purulent or hemorrhagic urethral discharge.
>
> Differential Diagnoses: Differential diagnoses for suspected bacterial cystitis include idiopathic/interstitial cystitis (cats), bladder neoplasia, or cystolithiasis. Differentials for bacterial pyelonephritis include nephrotoxin exposure, leptospirosis, fungal pyelonephritis, or protozoal nephritis. Pregnancy, mucometra, or hydrometra are differentials for pyometra, and benign prostatic hyperplasia, paraprostatic cysts, and prostatic neoplasia are differentials for prostatitis.
>
> Human Health Significance: Multidrug-resistant uropathogens from dogs and cats may have the potential to colonize human patients, but this requires further study.

Bacterial infections of the genitourinary tract include uncomplicated and complicated lower urinary tract infections (UTIs); prostatitis; pyelonephritis; renal abscesses; epididymitis and orchitis; and vaginitis, metritis, and pyometra. Infections of the genitourinary tract usually follow impairment of normal host defenses and invasion by bacteria that are part of the normal flora. Less commonly, infection results from hematogenous spread of bacteria to urogenital organs. Specific pathogens such as *Leptospira* spp. that injure the kidneys secondary to systemic infection are described elsewhere in this book.

In healthy dogs and cats, bacteria are not found in the upper urinary tract, urinary bladder, proximal urethra, and prostate gland. Factors that prevent bacterial colonization of the bladder include the glycosaminoglycan layer that covers bladder transitional epithelium, frequent voiding, the normal urethral microflora, antimicrobial properties of urine, an appropriate host immune response, and a functional urethral sphincter. Commensal bacteria that reside in the distal urethra, prepuce, and vagina invade opportunistically when these mechanisms are disturbed. The most common pathogen involved in all genitourinary tract infections is *Escherichia coli*, which has a particular propensity to adhere to epithelial cells of the genitourinary tract. Others include coagulase-positive and coagulase-negative staphylococci; *Enterococcus* spp.; other aerobic gram-negative bacilli such as *Klebsiella, Proteus, Enterobacter,* and *Pseudomonas aeruginosa; Corynebacterium* spp.; streptococci; and mycoplasmas. Anaerobic bacteria can also be found in the genital tracts of female dogs and can contribute to pyometra and metritis when host defenses are impaired. In addition to impaired host defenses, a variety of bacterial virulence factors influence the ability of certain bacteria to ultimately invade tissues and cause disease. Virulence factors of uropathogenic *E. coli* are described in more detail in Chapter 36.

LOWER AND UPPER URINARY TRACT INFECTIONS

Etiology and Epidemiology

Bacterial UTIs are commonly diagnosed in dogs. Although mixed bacterial infections can occur, the vast majority of UTIs involve a single bacterial species.[1] The most common uropathogen isolated is *E. coli*, which accounts for approximately 50% of all isolates, followed by *Staphylococcus, Proteus, Klebsiella, Enterococcus,* and *Streptococcus* species. Mycoplasmas have also been isolated from dogs with UTIs, although their clinical significance can be unclear because they are usually isolated from dogs that have other disorders of the lower urinary tract, such as underlying neoplasia or cystolithiasis. Spayed females and older dogs are at increased risk for bacterial UTIs; the mean age at diagnosis is 7 to 8 years of age.[1,2] As a result of breakdown in host defense mechanisms, systemic disorders such as acute or chronic kidney disease, hyperadrenocorticism, diabetes mellitus, and systemic neoplasia also predispose dogs to UTIs (Table 89-1).

In cats, bacterial UTIs are less common than in dogs. The prevalence of bacterial UTI in cats with lower urinary tract signs (i.e., stranguria, hematuria, pollakiuria, or dysuria; hereafter referred to as LUTS) evaluated by referral institutions has ranged from just 1% to 3%,[3-5] although the prevalence was higher (23% of cystocentesis-collected specimens) in a study from Norway.[6] Most young cats with LUTS have disorders such as feline interstitial cystitis, which are not associated with bacterial infection. When UTIs do occur in *young* adult cats, they are generally secondary to catheterization, perineal urethrostomy, or rarely, congenital anatomical defects. In older cats,

TABLE 89-1

Factors That May Predispose (or Contribute) to Development of Urinary Tract Infections in Dogs and Cats

Dogs	Cats
Recessed vulva or excess vulvar folds	Perineal urethrostomy
Diabetes mellitus	Hyperthyroidism
Hyperadrenocorticism	Diabetes mellitus
Renal failure	Renal disease
Urinary catheterization	Micturition abnormalities (urinary incontinence or urinary retention)
Ectopic ureters	Urinary catheterization
Micturition abnormalities (urinary incontinence or urinary retention)	Urolithiasis
Tube cystostomy	Urinary neoplasia (rare)
Glucocorticoid treatment and possibly treatment with other immunosuppressive drugs	Immunosuppressive drug treatment?
Urethrostomy	
Urolithiasis	
Urinary neoplasia	
Proliferative urethritis	
Polypoid cystitis	

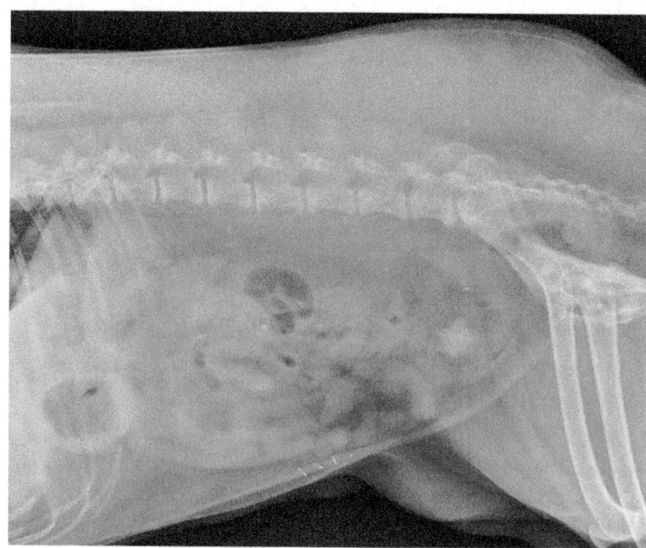

FIGURE 89-1 Lateral abdominal radiograph from a 10-year-old female spayed miniature schnauzer with emphysematous cystitis and a large, irregular cystic calculus. Irregular gas densities can see throughout the urinary bladder wall. *Escherichia coli* was cultured from a urine specimen that was obtained by cystocentesis.

UTIs often accompany diabetes mellitus, hyperthyroidism, and/or chronic kidney disease (CKD). The prevalence of UTIs in cats with diabetes mellitus is 11% to 13%.[7,8] At two referral institutions, positive aerobic bacterial urine cultures were found in 17% and 22% of cats with CKD and 22% and 12% of cats with hyperthyroidism.[7,9] Other factors that may predispose cats to UTI are breed (Persians or Abyssinians), female sex, older age, and lower body weight,[5,8,9] although some of these risk factors may also be associated with the comorbidities mentioned earlier. As in dogs, *E. coli* is the most common infecting species in cats. Other potential uropathogens in cats include *Streptococcus* spp., *Staphylococcus* spp., *Enterococcus* spp., *Klebsiella* spp., *Pasteurella* spp., and *Enterobacter* spp.[1,8,9] Mycoplasmas are very rarely isolated from the urine of cats.[9]

Uncommon forms of bacterial UTI in dogs and cats are *encrusting cystitis* and *emphysematous cystitis*. Encrusting cystitis is caused by the gram-positive bacterium *Corynebacterium urealyticum*. Urease production by this organism leads to precipitation of large amounts of struvite and calcium phosphate within the bladder and along the bladder and urethral mucosa, and in some cases within the ureters and renal pelvis as well.[10-12] Most animals with *C. urealyticum* infections have severe LUTS. Emphysematous cystitis is characterized by the production of gas by bacteria within the urinary bladder wall (Figure 89-1). The most common cause is *E. coli*, but *Clostridium* spp. may also be involved.[13,14] Most dogs and cats that develop *E. coli* emphysematous cystitis have glucosuria (usually secondary to diabetes mellitus), and gas production may result from fermentation of glucose to gas products by *E. coli*. In the absence of glucose, proteins such as albumin may be fermented to gas. Emphysematous cystitis caused by *Clostridium perfringens* occurs in the absence of diabetes mellitus.[13,14]

Definitions applied to infections of the urinary and genital tract are shown in Table 89-2. *Simple uncomplicated UTI* is a

TABLE 89-2

Definitions Applied to Urinary Tract Infections

Term	Definition
Simple uncomplicated UTI	Sporadic bacterial infection of the urinary bladder in an otherwise apparently healthy individual with normal urinary tract anatomy and function
Complicated UTI	UTI that occurs in the presence of an anatomic or functional abnormality or comorbidity that predisposes to persistent UTI, recurrent infection, or treatment failure
Recurrent UTI	Three or more episodes of UTI during a 12-month period
Refractory UTI	Isolation of the same microorganism more than once in the face of treatment, despite in vitro susceptibility to the antimicrobial drug used
Relapsing UTI	Isolation of the same microorganism within 6 months of apparent clearance of the infection with treatment in between positive cultures
Re-infection	Isolation of a different microorganism within 6 months of apparent resolution of a previous infection
Subclinical bacteriuria	Presence of bacteria in the urine as determined by a positive bacterial culture, in the absence of LUTS; differentiation from subclinical UTI may be difficult

sporadic bacterial infection of the bladder in an otherwise apparently healthy individual with normal urinary tract anatomy and function.[15] It has been estimated that uncomplicated UTI occurs in 14% of dogs that visit a veterinarian during their lifetime.[16] However, the actual prevalence of simple uncomplicated UTI may actually be lower, because abnormalities in host defenses probably go unrecognized in many dogs. As noted earlier, uncomplicated UTI is rare in cats. *Complicated UTIs* are associated with concurrent disorders that predispose to recurrent or persistent UTI (see Table 89-1).

Recurrence of UTI may reflect refractory (or persistent) infection, relapsing infection, or re-infection (see Table 89-2). Without the use of molecular techniques (e.g., pulsed field gel electrophoresis), it is not possible to definitively distinguish between relapse of infection and re-infection if the same bacterial species is isolated repeatedly, because different strains may be present. *Enterococcus* spp. and *Pseudomonas* spp. are isolated more commonly from dogs with persistent or recurrent UTIs than from dogs with simple uncomplicated UTIs.[2] *E. coli* can invade and form microcolonies within uroepithelial cells,[17] which may contribute to persistent infection in the face of antimicrobial treatment. Bacteria may also be able to form biofilms in association with the bladder wall ("deep seated" infections), but studies that document this in the dog are lacking.

Subclinical (or asymptomatic) bacteriuria is a term used in human medicine to describe the presence of bacteria in the urine as determined by a positive bacterial culture, in the absence of LUTS. This has generally been referred to as *subclinical UTI* in the veterinary literature. The use of the term *subclinical bacteriuria* in animals and its distinction from *infection* (which implies invasion of host tissues by bacteria and the associated inflammatory response) has been controversial, because subtle signs of infection (such as bladder pain, pollakiuria, or intermittent hematuria) may not always be detected. The term *subclinical UTI* could perhaps be applied to dogs and cats if cytologic evidence of infection (e.g., pyuria or hematuria) is present,[15] but in human patients, the term subclinical bacteriuria is used even when pyuria is present. Subclinical bacteriuria or subclinical UTIs are commonly detected in dogs and cats, especially those with underlying endocrinopathies, renal failure, or neurologic disease, as well as dogs treated with glucocorticoids or cyclosporine.[7,8,18-20] In a study of dogs treated with glucocorticoids for dermatologic disorders, 18% of 127 dogs had bacteriuria in the absence of clinical signs, whereas none of 94 dogs that had not received glucocorticoids had bacteriuria.

Pyelonephritis most often occurs when bacteria ascend into the renal pelvis and parenchyma from the lower urinary tract. Less commonly, hematogenous spread to the kidney occurs. A single bacterial species (most often *E. coli*) is isolated from the urine of approximately three quarters of dogs with pyelonephritis; two species are isolated in fewer than 10% of dogs and three species from fewer than 5% of dogs. Pyelonephritis may be acute or chronic. Strains of *E. coli* that cause pyelonephritis have greater ability to adhere to cells than strains that cause cystitis. Adhesins located on the tip of *E. coli* fimbriae (P fimbriae) adhere to glycolipid residues on tubular, collecting duct, and bladder epithelial cells. In human pyelonephritis, both P and type I fimbriae are important in colonization of the renal pelvis.[21,22] Other *E. coli* virulence factors associated with pyelonephritis include hemolysin, cytotoxic necrotizing factor, the iron scavenger aerobactin, and a serum protease known as Sat. Fimbriae are also important in the pathogenesis of *Proteus* pyelonephritis.[23] The renal medulla is more sensitive to colonization than the cortex, possibly owing to impaired host defenses in a high osmolality, low pH, and low blood flow milieu. Organisms adhere to pelvic, distal, and proximal tubular epithelium and have been observed intracellularly. Considerable renal injury results from the inflammatory response to infection. Aggregation of neutrophils within capillaries and induction of vascular spasm by bacterial toxins and/or cytokines can contribute to renal ischemia.

Clinical Features

Clinical Signs

Clinical signs of lower UTI may be absent, or include signs such as dysuria, hematuria, stranguria, and pollakiuria. Cats may urinate outside the litter box (periuria or inappropriate urination). Rarely, animals with lower UTIs may be lethargic, but fever and inappetence are not present. Acute or acute-on-chronic pyelonephritis may result in inappetence, lethargy, variable fever, hematuria, and clinical signs of uremia, such as vomiting and diarrhea. Polyuria and polydipsia may also be present, or dogs with severe disease may be anuric. Dogs and cats with chronic pyelonephritis may show no signs, or only polyuria and polydipsia.

Physical Examination Findings

Physical examination findings in dogs or cats with lower UTIs may be unremarkable, or urine or urine scalding may be identified around the perineum. A strong ammonia-like odor may be present. Sometimes, pain can be detected on palpation of the urinary bladder of dogs or cats with bacterial cystitis, and abdominal or flank pain may be noted in animals with acute pyelonephritis. The urinary bladder is often small as a result of pollakiuria. A thickened bladder wall may also be palpated. If a large, turgid bladder is present in dogs or cats with a UTI, urethral obstruction due to neoplasia, calculi, proliferative urethritis, or encrusting cystitis should be suspected. Underlying disorders that predispose to lower UTIs may also be apparent (such as vulvar fold dermatitis).

Dogs and cats with severe pyelonephritis may show signs of lethargy, dehydration, variable fever, and evidence of severe sepsis or septic shock (e.g., tachycardia or bradycardia, tachypnea, or prolonged capillary refill time).

Diagnosis

Diagnosis of UTIs is based on the clinical signs present, laboratory abnormalities, imaging findings, and culture of urine. The presence of fever or leukocytosis in addition to a positive bacterial urine culture should increase suspicion for concurrent bacterial pyelonephritis, prostatitis, or pyometra (see relevant sections later in this chapter). Ultrasound examination findings also can support the diagnosis and assist in the identification of underlying disorders such as neoplasia, anatomic abnormalities, or the presence of calculi or foreign material. At a minimum, collection of urine by cystocentesis followed by complete urinalysis (with sediment examination) and quantitative aerobic bacterial urine culture are recommended to properly confirm the presence of bacterial UTI for dogs or cats with signs of lower urinary tract disease.[15] Additional diagnostics are indicated for animals that have recurrent LUTS or those with systemic signs such as fever, weight loss, or inappetence. The owners of animals diagnosed with what appears to be uncomplicated UTI should be advised that other underlying disease may be present.

Laboratory Abnormalities

Complete Blood Count and Serum Biochemical Tests

Animals with infections confined to the lower urinary tract typically have no hematologic or serum biochemistry abnormalities. Animals with pyelonephritis may have mild anemia, leukocytosis due to a neutrophilia, bandemia, and monocytosis. A degenerative left shift, toxic neutrophils, and thrombocytopenia may also be present. The serum biochemistry panel may show azotemia and sometimes hypoalbuminemia and/or electrolyte abnormalities.

Urinalysis

Findings on the urinalysis in dogs and cats with UTIs include isosthenuria, pyuria, hematuria, proteinuria, and/or bacteriuria. Animals with pyelonephritis may have cylindruria, and small amounts of glucose may be present as a result of altered proximal tubular function. However, the urinalysis can also be normal, even in dogs and cats with pyelonephritis. Infections with urease-producing bacteria such as staphylococci, *Proteus* spp., and *C. urealyticum* can be associated with a high urine pH and struvite crystalluria.

Coagulation Profile

Evidence of coagulation abnormalities may be present in animals with severe pyelonephritis that develop severe sepsis or septic shock (see Chapter 86).

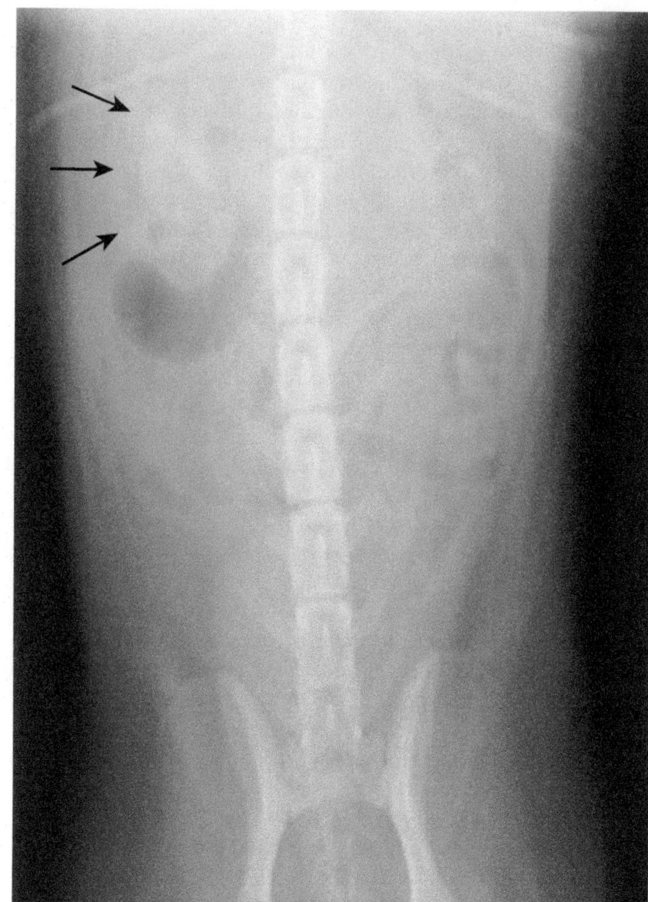

FIGURE 89-2 Dorsoventral radiograph of a 6-year-old female spayed shih tzu mix with a urinary tract infection caused by *Proteus mirabilis* and *Enterococcus faecalis* and nephrolithiasis. An opacity ("staghorn" calculus) occupies the right renal pelvis (*arrows*).

Diagnostic Imaging

Plain Radiography

Dogs or cats with bacterial cystitis generally have no radiographic abnormalities. The urinary bladder may be small if pollakiuria is present. Emphysematous cystitis is characterized by the presence of radiolucencies within the bladder lumen and/or in association with the bladder wall (see Figure 89-1). Radiopaque cystic or renal ("staghorn") calculi may be visible in dogs with struvite calculi secondary to *Staphylococcus* spp. or *Proteus* spp. infections (Figure 89-2).

Renomegaly may be present with acute pyelonephritis, which is typically mild. The kidneys may be small and irregular in dogs or cats with chronic pyelonephritis.

Contrast Radiography

Contrast cystourethrography can be useful for diagnosis of conditions that predispose to recurrent or persistent UTIs, such as anatomic abnormalities, diverticuli, bladder or urethral neoplasia, proliferative urethritis, polypoid cystitis, or nonradiopaque calculi. Intravenous contrast urography has been used to identify pyelectasia and assist in the diagnosis of pyelonephritis, but has largely been replaced by abdominal ultrasound for this purpose, which is less invasive.

Sonographic Findings

Ultrasound examination of the urogenital tract provides information about the extent and severity of disease and underlying causes such as neoplasia, calculi, or foreign bodies. *It does not permit visualization of the entire urethra*, and so urethral abnormalities may be overlooked in some animals if only ultrasound is used to image the lower urinary tract. Ultrasound examination of the urinary bladder may be unremarkable or show a mild to moderately thickened bladder wall in dogs or cats with bacterial cystitis. Echogenicity of the urine may be present. Rarely, the bladder wall is severely thickened (Figure 89-3). Animals with emphysematous cystitis may have a hyperechoic urinary bladder wall with acoustic shadow artifacts. Shadow artifacts also occur when cystic calculi are present.

Dogs or cats with pyelonephritis may have a normal abdominal ultrasound examination; or blunting of the renal papilla, pyelectasia, irregularity of the renal contour, and/or hydronephrosis may be seen (Figure 89-4). However, pyelectasia can occur in animals with normal renal function, diuresis, and outflow tract obstruction, and there is considerable overlap in the extent of dilatation between groups.[24] The renal pelvis of dogs and cats with severe pyelonephritis may contain hyperechoic debris.[25] Sometimes the surrounding mesentery is hyperechoic, and perinephric anechoic fluid is present as a result of localized peritonitis. Other nonspecific findings in pyelonephritis include increased renal cortical echogenicity and decreased corticomedullary definition.

Cystoscopy

Cystoscopy can be a useful diagnostic procedure to identify underlying causes of recurrent UTIs in dogs and cats, after

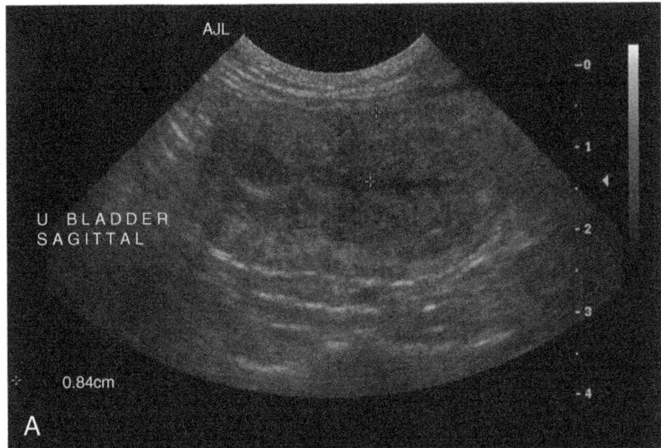

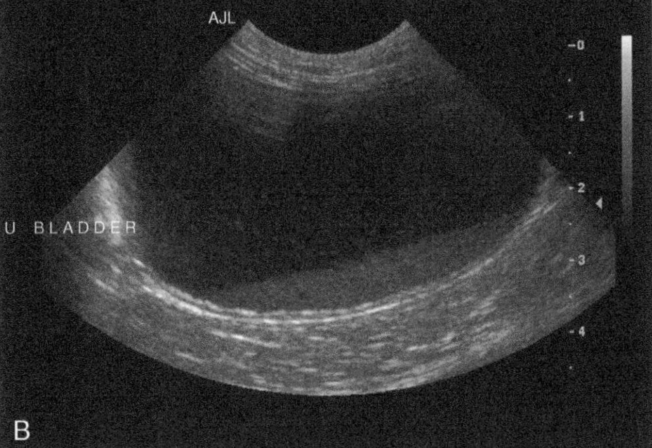

FIGURE 89-3 Ultrasound images of the bladder of an 18-year-old female spayed domestic shorthair cat with diabetes mellitus, generalized osteoarthritis, a cervical myelopathy, and L4-L6 disc space compression and recurrent urinary tract infections. The cat had severe lower urinary tract signs (hematuria, pollakiuria, and stranguria), and a hemolytic *Escherichia coli* was isolated from the urine. **A,** The wall of the urinary bladder is markedly thickened. **B,** Resolution of bladder wall thickening after treatment with marbofloxacin for 3 weeks, which also resolved the clinical signs.

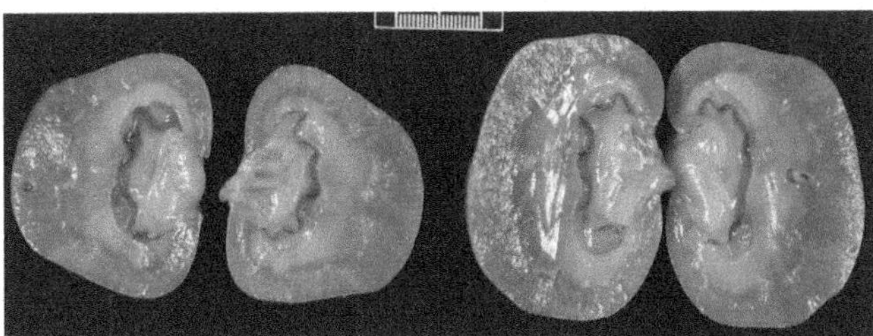

FIGURE 89-4 Kidneys of a 2-year-old male neutered German shepherd with diabetes mellitus and chronic pyelonephritis secondary to *Klebsiella pneumoniae* infection. The kidneys are bilaterally asymmetrical; the right kidney is larger than the left. There are several small, cortical subcapsular cysts, and the kidneys have an irregular conformation with markedly shrunken poles and are fibrotic. The renal parenchyma at the poles is markedly collapsed from the capsule to the pelvis, and the pelvis is uniformly dilated. (Image courtesy University of California, Davis, Veterinary Anatomic Pathology Service.)

evaluation has been performed first to evaluate for metabolic abnormalities such as renal failure, hyperadrenocorticism, or diabetes mellitus. Cystoscopy or contrast computed tomography are the most sensitive diagnostic tests for identification of ectopic ureters. Cystoscopy can also be used to obtain mucosal uroepithelial biopsies for histopathology and culture.

Microbiologic Tests

Isolation and Identification

Quantitative aerobic bacterial culture and susceptibility is always indicated for dogs or cats with UTIs before starting antimicrobial drugs, because of the possibility of antimicrobial drug resistance, which is well recognized among *E. coli* strains isolated from dogs and cats with UTIs.[26,27] Guidelines for diagnosis of bacterial UTIs in dogs and cats have been published.[15] Ideally, urine should be collected by cystocentesis; if this is not possible, urethral catheterization can be used. Although any pathogens isolated from specimens collected by cystocentesis are likely significant, bacterial contamination from the skin is possible; therefore, the presence of more than 10^3 CFU/mL of bacteria is considered clinically significant. If specimens are collected via catheterization, colony counts that exceed 10^4 CFU/mL for male dogs and 10^5 CFU/mL for female dogs are considered clinically significant.[15] Free-catch (midstream voiding) specimen collection should not be used for dogs or cats because it is highly susceptible to contamination. A positive aerobic bacterial culture of a cystocentesis-collected urine specimen confirms the presence of bacterial infection in animals that have LUTS. Culture can also help to differentiate re-infection from relapse should a UTI return; if the second isolate is a different bacterial species or has a different antibiotic susceptibility pattern (also known as an *antibiogram*), reinfection is likely.[15] Specimens for culture should be refrigerated immediately and submitted to the laboratory as soon as possible. For specimens that reach the laboratory more than 24 hours after collection, culture results should be interpreted with caution, because false-negative and false-positive test results can occur. For dogs and cats with recurrent UTIs that undergo surgery, culture of a bladder wall biopsy or of cystoliths should be considered.

Inexpensive urine "paddles" are available for in-house veterinary diagnosis of UTIs. One type consists of two different types of agar on either side of a plastic paddle (see also Chapter 3, Figure 3-6). The media are inoculated with urine collected by cystocentesis, and the paddles are then incubated and examined daily for growth. These paddles can be useful screening tools when client finances do not permit submission of specimens to a microbiology laboratory for culture, and they allow identification of significant bacterial growth by comparison of colony numbers to a chart provided by the manufacturer. They also reduce the effect of delays in submission of specimens to a laboratory. However, they may be inaccurate for identification of bacterial species involved, especially when mixed infections are present.[28] Paddles may not yield reliable results if submitted to a laboratory for confirmation and minimum inhibitory concentration (MIC) testing. If used, and growth is detected on the paddle within 24 hours, saved (refrigerated) urine or a freshly collected urine specimen should be submitted to a microbiology laboratory for culture and susceptibility testing. Another type of in-house culture system provides limited information on bacterial antibiotic susceptibility (Flexicut Vet, Atlantic Diagnostics), but requires further study. In-house bacterial cultures should only be performed in clinics with appropriate laboratory facilities, proper biosafety level containment and waste management, and adequately trained personnel.[15] Accurate susceptibility testing is difficult to perform and interpret, and whenever possible, submission to a veterinary diagnostic laboratory that adheres to Clinical and Laboratory Standards Institute (CLSI) guidelines is recommended.

For animals with indwelling urinary catheters, some bacteriuria is expected due to compromise of host immune defenses. Culture is indicated if clinical signs of infection are present (e.g., gross hematuria, pyuria, or suspected bacteremia).[15] Optimally, the catheter should be removed and cystocentesis performed after the bladder is allowed to fill with urine. Alternatively, the catheter could be removed, replaced with a new catheter, and a urine specimen collected through the catheter after several milliliters of urine are removed to clear the catheter. Urine culture should never be submitted from specimens collected from the urine bag, and there is no indication to culture the catheter tip.

When pyelonephritis is present, bacteria cultured from the urine are usually those present in the upper tract. A negative urine culture does not rule out bacterial pyelonephritis. In some cases, cytology and culture of ultrasound-guided aspirates of the renal pelvis (pyelocentesis) may assist in the diagnosis of pyelonephritis. Blood cultures could also be considered in animals with acute pyelonephritis, especially when signs of sepsis are present.

Laboratories that perform and report susceptibility testing for uropathogens should adhere to local regulatory guidelines (such as the CLSI). Breakpoints for systemic infections also apply to UTIs (see Chapter 3 for a discussion of breakpoints). However, many antimicrobials achieve much higher concentrations in the urine than they do in the serum. Therefore, if routine serum susceptibility testing is performed for a dog or cat with a lower UTI and normal renal function, some antimicrobials may eradicate the UTI, despite in vitro resistance. This is especially true for treatment of staphylococcal UTIs with penicillins and cephalosporines. Urinary breakpoints are available for ampicillin or amoxicillin in dogs (≤8 µg/mL), amoxicillin-clavulanate in dogs and cats (<8/4 µg/mL), and nitrofurantoin. Urinary breakpoints (reported as urine MICs by the laboratory) should be used only when infection is confined to the lower urinary tract.

Pathologic Findings

Pathologic findings in dogs with bacterial cystitis and pyelonephritis depend on the chronicity of the infection, the underlying cause, and the uropathogens present. Acute infections are associated with a dense neutrophilic infiltrate in tissues on histopathology and intralesional bacteria may be identified. Chronic infections may be associated with histiocytic or lymphoplasmacytic infiltrates.

Treatment and Prognosis

Treatment of UTIs consists of removal or management of the underlying cause(s) of infection, followed by antimicrobial drug treatment. Antimicrobial drug treatment alone without attention to an underlying cause frequently leads to recurrent infection and selection for resistant bacteria. Because of the increasing prevalence of multidrug-resistant (MDR) *E. coli* and staphylococci in dogs and cats with UTIs, consideration should be given to delaying antimicrobial drug treatment until the results of culture and susceptibility are available, provided the patient is stable and sepsis is absent. This is especially true for dogs and cats with recurrent UTIs that have a history of antimicrobial drug treatment. Empiric treatment while awaiting the results of culture and susceptibility could be considered to relieve discomfort, if present; however, some dogs respond well to analgesic therapy (e.g., tramadol) pending susceptibility test results. When sepsis is present, initial treatment should be broad-spectrum and cover MDR gram-negative bacteria (see Chapter 86).

Uncomplicated UTIs

In most situations, rational choices for initial treatment of uncomplicated UTIs include amoxicillin or trimethoprim-sulfonamide (TMS) (Table 89-3), although TMS has the potential to cause significant adverse effects in dogs. Amoxicillin–clavulanic acid could be considered if practice/regional susceptibility trends suggest a high (>10%) prevalence of β-lactamase production by uropathogens isolated (i.e., >10% of bacteria isolated in a practice show susceptibility to amoxicillin–clavulanic acid but not amoxicillin).[15] However, amoxicillin–clavulanic acid may need to be given q8h to ensure significant concentrations of clavulanic acid in the urine. Once culture and susceptibility results are available, the chosen antimicrobial drug should either be continued (if a clinical response has occurred) or switched to an alternative drug with activity against the pathogen that enters urine in high concentrations. A treatment duration of 7 days has been suggested.[15] One study showed that treatment of dogs that had uncomplicated UTIs with high-dose enrofloxacin (20 mg/kg) for 3 days was not inferior to treatment with amoxicillin–clavulanic acid for 14 days.[29] Additional studies of dogs with naturally occurring UTI that evaluate short durations of treatment with other antimicrobial drugs such as amoxicillin or TMS are needed. Studies are also needed to evaluate the need for posttreatment cultures to determine whether resolution of infection has occurred.[15]

Complicated UTIs

Investigation to identify an underlying cause is strongly recommended for animals with complicated UTIs. Referral should be considered for advanced imaging and diagnostic tests to evaluate the patient for predisposing factors. The choice of antimicrobial drug should be based on culture and susceptibility test

TABLE 89-3

Suggested Initial Treatment for Stable Dogs or Cats with Genitourinary Tract Infections Pending Culture and Susceptibility Results

Disease	Drug	Dose (mg/kg)	Route	Interval (hours)
Bacterial cystitis or pyometra	Amoxicillin *or*	11-15	PO	8
	Trimethoprim-sulfadiazine *or*	15*	PO	12
	Amoxicillin–clavulanic acid	12.5-25	PO	8
Pyelonephritis, prostatitis	Enrofloxacin *or*	10-20 (dogs)	PO	24
	Marbofloxacin *or*	2.7-5.5	PO	24
	Orbifloxacin	7.5	PO	24

See Table 86-8 for options for severe sepsis.
*Based on trimethoprim plus sulfadiazine concentration.

results, and preference should be given to drugs that are excreted in the urine in active form. If excreted in the urine, drugs with intermediate susceptibility could be used to treat UTIs that are resistant to other appropriate drug choices; however, a higher dose (for concentration-dependent antimicrobials) or dosing frequency (for time-dependent antimicrobials) should be considered in these circumstances. Use of nitrofurantoin could be considered for lower UTIs that are resistant to other oral antimicrobial drugs that are excreted in the urine. When mixed infections are present, ideally antimicrobial drug treatment should be directed at all organisms present. In mixed infections that involve *Enterococcus* spp., anecdotal evidence suggests that the *Enterococcus* spp. infection will resolve when the other organisms are successfully treated.[15] Typically, 4 weeks of treatment is recommended for complicated UTIs, but shorter courses may be effective. Urine culture could be considered 5 to 7 days after initiating treatment to ensure the infection is not persistent and is recommended 7 days after treatment has been discontinued. If follow-up cultures are positive, further investigation to identify an underlying cause may be required. If no clinical signs are present, management should be as for subclinical bacteriuria (see later discussion).

There is no evidence that direct instillation of antimicrobials, antiseptics, glycosaminoglycans, or dimethyl sulfoxide (DMSO) directly into the bladder via a urinary catheter is effective for treatment of recurrent UTIs in dogs. These compounds are rapidly eliminated from the bladder when the animal urinates and may be locally irritating, which may predispose further to infection with drug-resistant bacteria. Approaches used in an attempt to prevent recurrence are detailed in the Prevention section.

Subclinical Bacteriuria

Treatment may not be required for dogs or cats that lack LUTS, but could be considered for dogs or cats that have underlying immunosuppressive disorders or are receiving glucocorticoids or chemotherapeutics (which may predispose them to ascending or systemic infection). However, some animals with disorders that predispose to bacterial colonization of the bladder are continuously bacteriuric, and treatment with antimicrobial drugs only selects for colonization by resistant organisms. More evidence that supports the need for diagnosis and treatment of subclinical bacteriuria when accompanied by specific disorders such as hyperadrenocorticism, diabetes mellitus, or chronic glucocorticoid treatment is required. Bacterial virulence factors may determine whether systemic invasion occurs.[30] MDR organisms are often of low virulence and may be replaced by susceptible bacteria when antimicrobial drug pressure is removed. After that, treatment may be possible if clinical signs develop or if there is concern for ascending infection. In human patients, treatment of asymptomatic bacteriuria associated with *Enterococcus* spp. infection is not recommended.[31] Whether this is also an appropriate recommendation in dogs and cats is unclear.

Pyelonephritis

Treatment of dogs with acute pyelonephritis should be initiated immediately, without waiting for culture and susceptibility test results. Cytologic examination of stained urine sediment may assist in initial selection of an antimicrobial drug (i.e., based on the presence of rods versus cocci). The use of a fluoroquinolone that is excreted in the urine in active form (i.e., not difloxacin) is recommended for gram-negative bacterial pyelonephritis, provided regional susceptibility data do not show widespread resistance to fluoroquinolones.[15] The dosage used may need to be reduced if severe renal impairment is present. If combination treatment is initiated and antimicrobial susceptibility test results show susceptibility to only one drug, the other drug should be discontinued. Treatment for 4 to 6 weeks is recommended, although shorter periods of treatment may be effective and require further study. Dogs with acute pyelonephritis may need hospitalization and treatment with intravenous fluids and other medications for acute renal failure or sepsis. Urinalysis and culture should ideally be performed after 7 days of treatment and again 7 days after treatment has been discontinued, to ensure that infection has been eliminated. If the same organism is isolated again, then an additional antimicrobial drug with in vitro activity against the organism could be added. Struvite nephrolithiasis (such as "staghorn" calculi) or struvite cystoliths may dissolve with antimicrobial treatment, although dietary intervention may also be needed in some cases. When stones are present, antimicrobial treatment should be continued until there is no radiographic or ultrasonographic evidence of calculi and the urine is sterile. Other calculi such as calcium oxalate, urate and cystine can predispose animals to recurrent bacterial infections and, if possible, should be removed. While dissolution protocols are described for urate and cystine, they often are not as rewarding as struvite. Calcium oxalate stones are not amenable to dissolution with dietary or antimicrobial therapy.

Prevention

Prevention of lower UTIs involves identification and reversal of underlying causes of infection, such as vulvar fold dermatitis or congenital abnormalities such as ectopic ureter. Urinary catheterization should be used only when necessary and should be performed in a manner that maintains sterility as much as possible. Intermittent catheterization is preferred to placement of an indwelling catheter. If indwelling catheterization is required, a closed sterile collection system should always be used, and the catheter should be removed as soon as it is no longer required, because the risk of ascending infection increases with every day the catheter is left in place. Treatment of catheterized animals with antimicrobial drugs may increase the risk for infection[32] and so should be done only when necessary; antimicrobial drugs should not be used in an attempt to prevent urinary catheter infection. Routine antimicrobial treatment after catheter removal is not indicated unless clinical signs of UTI develop, because colonization that follows catheterization is cleared once the catheter is removed and host defenses are restored.

Many treatments for prevention of UTIs in dogs and cats with a history of recurrent disease have been considered. Currently there is no evidence that urinary antiseptics (such as methenamine) or nutritional supplements (such as cranberry juice extract) are effective in dogs or cats. Some studies of the use of cranberry extract in human patients have shown no effect.[33,34] Evidence that intermittent (pulse) therapy or chronic, low-dose antimicrobial treatment prevent recurrent UTIs is anecdotal; because it may select for resistant organisms, it is not generally recommended.

Public Health Aspects

Dogs and cats with UTIs have a potential to act as a source of MDR bacteria for humans. Similarities between uropathogenic *E. coli* isolates from dogs and those from humans have been identified,[35,36] but differences also exist.[37] Owners of pets with MDR UTIs should always wash their hands after handling their pets and wear gloves when medications are administered, and pets should be taken to urinate away from other people and animals.

ORCHITIS, EPIDIDYMITIS, AND PROSTATITIS

Etiology and Epidemiology

Orchitis and epididymitis may occur in association with bacterial UTIs or penetrating foreign bodies (e.g., plant awns) in intact male dogs, but this is rare. Infection with *Brucella canis* should always be suspected in dogs with epididymitis (see Chapter 53).

E. coli accounts for most cases of bacterial prostatitis in dogs. Occasionally other gram-negative or gram-positive bacteria, including atypical organisms such as *Mycoplasma* spp. and *Brucella* spp., cause prostatitis. Bacterial prostatitis is extremely rare in cats.[38]

Clinical Features

Signs and Their Pathogenesis

Bacterial prostatitis in dogs may be acute or chronic. It can occur secondary to benign prostatic hyperplasia or prostatic neoplasia, most likely as a result of ascending infection secondary to altered urinary defense mechanisms. Bacterial prostatitis should be suspected in any intact male dog that develops a UTI. Dogs with bacterial prostatitis may show infertility, fever, lethargy, inappetence, weight loss, LUTS, purulent or hemorrhagic urethral discharge, abdominal pain, and sometimes a stiff gait. Tenesmus, vomiting, and diarrhea also occur in some dogs. Acute bacterial prostatitis can be accompanied by severe sepsis or septic shock (see Chapter 86). Formation of prostatic abscesses may be followed by abscess rupture and peritonitis. Dogs with chronic prostatitis may be lethargic or have no clinical signs of illness.

Physical Examination Findings

Dogs with acute bacterial prostatitis may exhibit pain on palpation of the prostate during physical examination. The prostate may be normal in size and shape, or enlarged or irregularly shaped. Fluctuant regions may be palpated if abscesses are present. Palpation should always be performed cautiously when acute bacterial prostatitis is suspected to avoid rupture of prostatic abscesses. Hemorrhagic or purulent discharge may be seen at the urethral orifice. Dogs with severe acute prostatitis may be dehydrated, febrile, obtunded, and show other signs of severe sepsis or septic shock (e.g., tachycardia or bradycardia, tachypnea, prolonged capillary refill time). Intact male dogs with bacterial orchitis or epididymitis may have testicular enlargement, hyperemia, and pain on palpation of the testicles. These findings may be present in association with prostatitis.

Diagnosis

Diagnosis of bacterial prostatitis is based on clinical signs, laboratory abnormalities, imaging findings, and culture of urine or prostatic secretions.

Laboratory Abnormalities

Dogs with acute prostatitis may have mild anemia and leukocytosis due to a neutrophilia, bandemia, and monocytosis. A degenerative left shift, toxic neutrophils, and thrombocytopenia may be present in severely affected dogs. Hypoalbuminemia and electrolyte abnormalities may be present, or there be evidence of organ dysfunction in dogs with septic shock. Hyperglobulinemia can be present in dogs with chronic prostatitis. The urinalysis may reveal abnormalities consistent with UTI.

Diagnostic Imaging

Plain and Contrast Radiography

Plain radiography is of limited value for diagnosis of bacterial prostatitis. Dogs with prostatic abscesses may have prostatomegaly (a prostate diameter >70% of the distance between the pubis and the sacral promontory), with ventral and cranial displacement of the urinary bladder.[39] Prostatic mineralization rarely accompanies chronic bacterial prostatitis in intact dogs, but when present in a neutered dog, mineralization strongly supports the presence of prostatic neoplasia.[40] Extravasation of contrast material into the prostate during retrograde contrast cystourethrography supports a diagnosis of prostatitis or prostatic neoplasia.

Sonographic Findings

Sonographic abnormalities in dogs with prostatitis include prostatic irregularity, mixed echogenicity, and focal accumulations of anechoic or hypoechoic fluid, with distance enhancement (prostatic cysts or abscessation) (Figure 89-5).[41]

Microbiologic Tests

Isolation and Identification

Many dogs with prostatitis shed bacteria into the urine, and therefore bacteria cultured from the urine are usually those involved in prostatitis. However, a negative urine culture does not rule out bacterial prostatitis, and occasionally the organisms isolated from the urine differ from those isolated from the prostate.

Collection of prostatic fluid via ejaculation, prostatic wash, or aspiration of the prostate or prostatic cysts may also be helpful

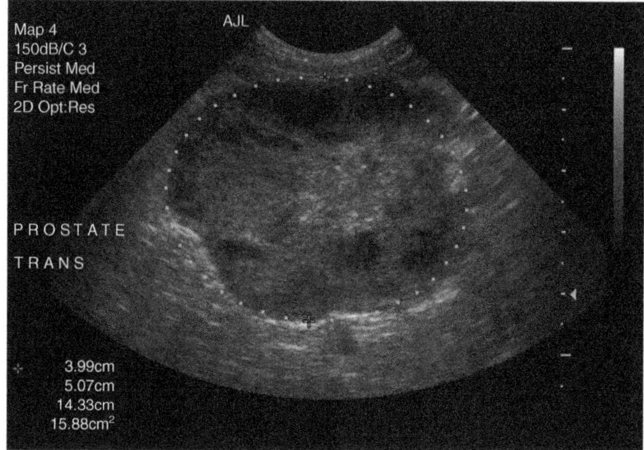

FIGURE 89-5 Ultrasound image of the prostate of a 12-year-old intact male beagle dog that had acute prostatitis due to *Escherichia coli* and associated bacterial peritonitis. The dog was seen for acute onset of anorexia and vomiting. Bloodwork revealed 2254 neutrophils/μL, 1160 band neutrophils/μL, mild hypoalbuminemia (2.4 g/dL; reference range, 2.9-4.2 g/dL), increased serum ALP activity (1338 U/L; reference range, 15-127 U/L) and increased serum total bilirubin concentration (0.5 mg/dL, reference range, 0-0.4 mg/dL). The prostate was significantly increased in size on sonographic examination and contained multiple hypoechoic nodules. There was a small quantity of ascites, which were localized in the caudal abdomen in the region of the prostate. Hemolytic *E. coli* was isolated from urine and from a prostatic aspirate. The owners elected euthanasia. Acute prostatitis and peritonitis were confirmed at necropsy.

for the diagnosis of bacterial prostatitis. Aspirates of the prostate for culture and cytology (if clinically indicated) can be done in dogs with acute and chronic prostatitis; however, dogs with acute prostatitis may require sedation for patient comfort. The presence of large numbers of bacteria (>10^5 CFU/mL) together with an inflammatory response suggests infection. Cytologic examination and culture of ultrasound-guided aspirates of prostatic abscesses has been used to assist diagnosis, but there is a risk of localized peritonitis when abscessed tissues are aspirated.

Pathologic Findings

Dogs with acute prostatitis may have infiltrates of neutrophils with or without intralesional bacteria in the prostate on histopathology. Chronic infections may be associated with histiocytic or lymphoplasmacytic infiltrates. In some cases, prostatic hyperplasia or abscess formation are identified.

Treatment and Prognosis

Acute prostatitis should be treated with an appropriate antimicrobial drug for 4 weeks. If the dog is septic, parenteral antimicrobial administration may initially be required. If inflammation is severe, any drug appropriate for treatment of UTIs may still penetrate the prostate in the acute phase.

Drug penetration is impaired in dogs with chronic prostatitis because of the blood–prostatic fluid barrier. Drugs that effectively cross the prostatic barrier of dogs include enrofloxacin, ofloxacin, marbofloxacin, trimethoprim, and chloramphenicol. Because trimethoprim-sulfamethoxazole and chloramphenicol are more likely to be associated with adverse effects when administered for prolonged periods, a fluoroquinolone such as enrofloxacin is the drug of choice for initial treatment of gram-negative bacterial prostatitis. If the MIC of the organism is between 0.5 and 1.0 µg/mL, the highest dose of enrofloxacin is recommended (20 mg/kg q24h). Clindamycin may be a reasonable choice for dogs with gram-positive bacterial prostatitis, although this is uncommon. Treatment of dogs with chronic prostatitis should continue for at least 6 weeks. Organisms may persist within the prostate of dogs with chronic prostatitis despite appropriate antimicrobial drug treatment. Cure may not be possible without castration.

Surgical castration is recommended for dogs with prostatitis and should be performed as soon as the dog is stable to undergo anesthesia and surgery. The efficacy of drugs that cause prostatic involution, such as finasteride, is not clear, but finasteride enhanced resolution of infection in a rat model of chronic prostatitis when administered with a fluoroquinolone.[42] Prostatic abscesses also must be treated surgically, although ultrasound-guided drainage together with antimicrobial drug treatment can be effective for small (e.g., <2.5 cm) abscesses. Castration and antimicrobial drug treatment alone do not effectively resolve prostatic abscesses; surgical drainage is required. Long-term, once-daily treatment with antimicrobial drugs that enter the prostate has been suggested for dogs that fail to respond to medical and surgical treatment of chronic prostatitis, as used to treat humans.[43]

Follow-up should consist of a recheck 7 to 10 days after initiating treatment. Aerobic bacterial urine culture should be considered at this time if a positive urine culture was initially present. A recheck should also be performed 1 week after discontinuation of treatment, at which time physical examination, urinalysis, urine culture, and prostatic fluid cytology and culture should be performed. Where available, prostatic ultrasound may also provide useful information at these follow-up times and, if possible, should be performed 1 week after discontinuation of antimicrobial drugs.

Prevention

Routine castration reduces the risk of prostatitis, but prostatitis can still occur in neutered animals.

VAGINITIS, METRITIS, AND PYOMETRA

Etiology and Epidemiology

Bacterial vaginitis in adult bitches is usually secondary to an underlying disorder such as neoplasia, foreign bodies (e.g., grass awn), UTI, or anatomic abnormalities such as strictures. Puppy vaginitis is thought to be a consequence of immaturity rather than bacterial infection.

Metritis results from ascending infection of the uterus. It usually occurs shortly after parturition (e.g., within a week) or after obstetrical procedures. It may be associated with clinical signs of lethargy, fever, decreased appetite, and purulent vaginal discharge.

Pyometra is an accumulation of pus within the uterus (Figure 89-6). The pathogenesis of pyometra is incompletely understood. However, in contrast to metritis, pyometra most often seems to occur as a result of increased serum progesterone concentrations, which cause cystic endometrial hyperplasia (CEH), impaired immune function, and decreased uterine contractility. The end result for some dogs and cats is opportunistic bacterial invasion, most often by *E. coli* strains that have virulence factors typical of uropathogenic isolates.[35,44] Other bacterial species that cause pyometra are similar to those that cause UTIs, with the exception that anaerobes are more often involved in pyometra, usually in mixed infections with other bacteria. CEH is not an absolute requirement for development of pyometra, and some animals with CEH never develop pyometra. Exogenous administration of estrogen (used to treat mismating) or progesterone has also been associated with pyometra.[45] Rarely, pyometra occurs in conjunction with uterine

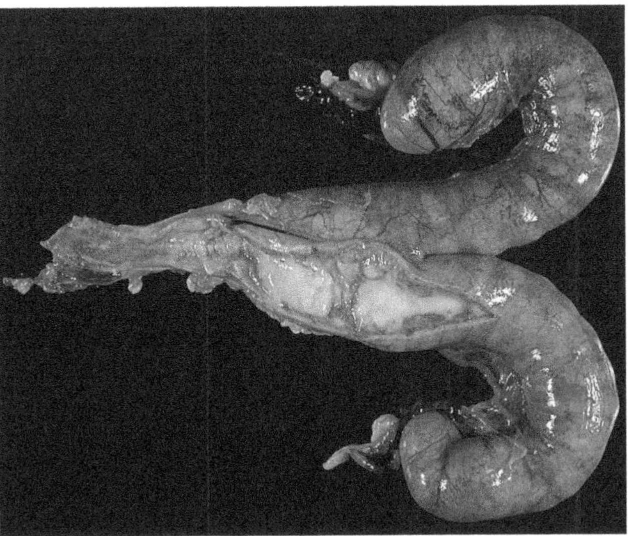

FIGURE 89-6 Uterus of an 11-year-old female spayed Pomeranian with pyometra after ovariohysterectomy. The uterine horns were severely dilated and fluid-filled. (Image courtesy University of California, Davis, Veterinary Anatomic Pathology Service.)

neoplasia.[46] Emphysematous pyometra has been reported in dogs but is uncommon.[47-49] Etiologic agents in emphysematous pyometra include *C. perfringens, Citrobacter diversus,* and *P. aeruginosa.*

In dogs, pyometra usually occurs in diestrus, but it can occur in anestrus. Middle-aged to older (mean age around 9 years), intact female dogs are most often affected, but pyometra has been reported in dogs as young as 8 months of age. Older dogs develop pyometra as a result of chronic, repeated exposure to progesterone with cycling over many years. In contrast, younger dogs tend to develop pyometra as a result of treatment of mismatings with estrogens. Pyometra is prevalent wherever routine ovariohysterectomy of dogs is not widely performed. In a study from Scandinavia, breeds of dogs with increased risk included collies, Rottweilers, Bernese mountain dogs, Cavalier King Charles spaniels, English cocker spaniels, and golden retrievers.[50,51] Nulliparous bitches are at increased risk for development of pyometra when compared with those that have had litters, but false pregnancy does not influence the risk for pyometra in dogs.

In cats, CEH also seems to underlie pyometra. Although cats with pyometra are generally more than 3 years of age (mean, 5 years), pyometra can occur in cats of any age.

Clinical Features

Clinical Signs

Clinical signs of pyometra in dogs usually occur 2 to 10 weeks after estrus or breeding, but occasionally occur as long as 15 weeks after estrus (mean, 7 weeks). In both dogs and cats, clinical signs may be acute or chronic and include lethargy, polyuria and polydipsia, vomiting, weight loss, inappetence, diarrhea, fever, and/or abdominal pain. Some dogs or cats show no signs of illness. Animals with *open-cervix pyometra,* the most common form of pyometra (>60% of dogs), usually have purulent vaginal discharge. The discharge may have a fetid odor and it may be mucopurulent, purulent, or contain blood. Dogs or cats with *closed-cervix pyometra* do not have vaginal discharge, but abdominal distention may be present. Animals with closed pyometra are more likely to have severe signs of systemic illness than those with open pyometra. Concurrent glomerular and tubulointerstitial disease and/or the effects of *E. coli* endotoxin may also contribute to signs of polyuria and polydipsia.[52,53] In some dogs or cats, pyometra is accompanied by severe sepsis or septic shock. When disease is severe the uterus can rupture, which leads to peritonitis.

Stump pyometra is an uncommon form of pyometra. It sometimes occurs after remnants of the ovaries are inadvertently left in place after ovariohysterectomy, but this is not always the case. Stump pyometra occurs most commonly in dogs, but has been reported in the cat.[54] Clinical signs are similar to animals with pyometra. Stump pyometras can also contribute to recurrent lower UTIs.

Physical Examination Findings

Purulent vaginal discharge, sometimes with a putrid odor, may be present in animals with bacterial vaginitis or open pyometra. Fever is most likely to be identified in animals with closed-cervix pyometra. Abdominal pain may be present on palpation of the abdomen. Abdominal palpation should always be performed cautiously when pyometra is suspected so that uterine rupture does not occur. Dogs and cats with severe pyometra may be lethargic, dehydrated, and show signs of severe sepsis or septic shock.

Diagnosis

Diagnosis of vaginitis, metritis, and pyometra is based on signalment, history, clinical signs, laboratory abnormalities, imaging findings, and, in some cases, bacterial culture of the urine or uterine contents obtained during surgery. Blind cystocentesis should never be performed if pyometra is suspected because of the risk of inadvertent puncture and rupture of the uterus. This also has the potential to occur with ultrasound-guided cystocentesis, but the risk is lower.

Laboratory Abnormalities

Acute metritis or pyometra (especially closed-cervix pyometra) may be associated with anemia, leukocytosis due to a neutrophilia, bandemia, a degenerate left shift, toxic neutrophils, and monocytosis. Thrombocytopenia and signs of organ dysfunction (such as azotemia, increased serum ALP activity, and coagulation abnormalities) may be detected in dogs with severe sepsis or septic shock. Azotemia may result from severe dehydration or concurrent pyelonephritis. Hypoalbuminemia and electrolyte abnormalities such as low serum sodium-to-potassium ratios may be present.[55,56] Dogs and cats with chronic pyometra can have few laboratory abnormalities; some animals are hyperglobulinemic. On urinalysis, abnormalities consistent with UTI may be present. Urine protein-to-creatinine ratios may be increased as a result of renal tubular or glomerular injury.[53]

Diagnostic Imaging

Plain Radiography

Abdominal radiographs in dogs with pyometra may reveal the presence of a large coiled or tubular mass in the caudal and mid-abdomen that displaces the small intestine cranially and dorsally. The uterus may not be visible in dogs with open pyometra. Differentiation of pyometra from pregnancy may require ultrasound examination. Localized or generalized loss of abdominal detail may be present in dogs with peritonitis secondary to uterine rupture.

Sonographic Findings

Ultrasound is the imaging technique of choice for diagnosis of pyometra and differentiation of pyometra from pregnancy. However, it may not effectively distinguish pyometra from mucometra or hydrometra. Dogs with pyometra have an enlarged uterus, which is immediately dorsal to the bladder. The uterus may be thin-walled and distended with echogenic intraluminal fluid, or have a thickened wall with anechoic areas due to glandular proliferation and enlargement.[57] Stump pyometra may be recognized as a hypoechoic structure that is located dorsal and caudal to the urinary bladder (Figure 89-7).

Microbiologic Tests

Isolation and Identification

Fine-needle aspiration of the uterus is contraindicated in animals with suspected pyometra because of the risk of uterine rupture. Instead, the bacteria involved in pyometra are initially identified through bacterial culture of the urine, which frequently contains the same bacteria as those involved in the pyometra. However, a negative urine culture does not rule out pyometra, and

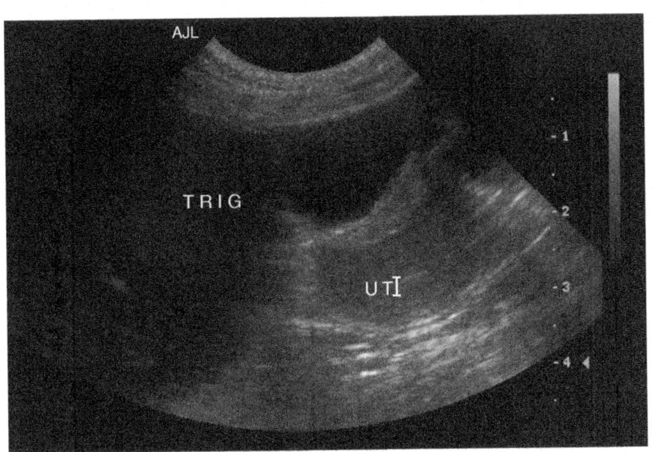

FIGURE 89-7 Ultrasound image of the urinary bladder and uterine stump in a 3-year-old female spayed mixed-breed dog that had vaginal discharge with a putrid odor due to a stump pyometra. An oval structure (*UT*) that contained flocculent material is present within the pelvic inlet caudal to and dorsal to the anechoic urinary bladder (*TRIG*, trigone). A cystic structure was seen in the region of the left ovary that represented a left ovarian remnant (not shown).

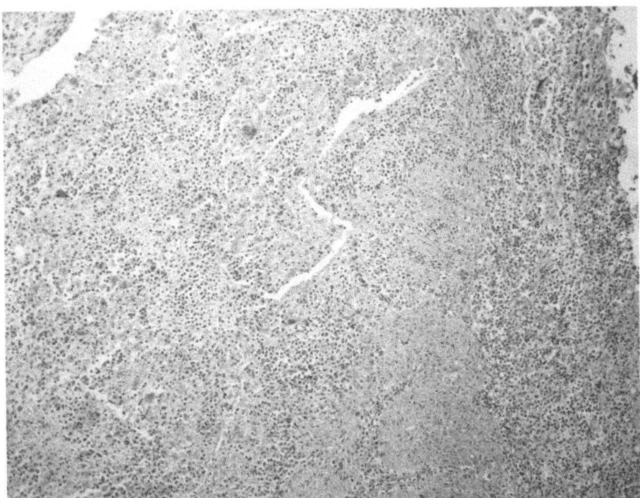

FIGURE 89-8 Histopathology of the uterus from a 7-year-old female poodle with pyometra. The dog was seen for vomiting, inappetence, obtundation, nystagmus, collapse, and abdominal distention. The owner elected euthanasia. Severe, chronic, suppurative metritis with uterine perforation and septic peritonitis was found at necropsy. The myometrium (pink) is almost completely replaced by large numbers of inflammatory cells. Aerobic and anaerobic bacterial culture of the abdominal fluid yielded mixed growth that consisted of *Escherichia coli* and a non-enteric gram-negative aerobic bacterial species, a *Bacteroides levii*–like anaerobe, *Bacteroides fragilis*, *Prevotella heparinolyticus*, *Fusobacterium nucleatum*, and *Peptostreptococcus anaerobius*. H&E stain.

occasionally the organisms isolated from the urine differ from those causing the pyometra. For animals with open pyometra, culture of a swab specimen collected from the cranial vaginal vault could be considered, but the bacteria cultured may or may not be the same as those present within the uterus. Tissues removed surgically can be submitted for culture and susceptibility testing. This should be performed despite administration of broad-spectrum antimicrobial drugs before surgery, because these drugs are unlikely to penetrate pus within the uterus. If possible, both anaerobic and aerobic bacterial cultures should be submitted. Blood cultures could be considered when signs of severe sepsis are present.

Pathologic Findings

As for other urogenital infections, acute pyometra is associated with a dense neutrophilic infiltrate on histopathology (Figure 89-8), and intralesional bacteria may be identified; chronic infections may be associated with histiocytic or lymphoplasmacytic infiltrates. CEH (expansion of the endometrium with hyperplastic and dilated or cystic glands) and corpora lutea may be identified.

Treatment and Prognosis

Sick dogs or cats with metritis or pyometra should be treated aggressively with intravenous fluids and broad-spectrum parenteral antimicrobial drugs that have activity against gram-negative bacteria and anaerobes, such as a combination of clindamycin or metronidazole and a fluoroquinolone. Ovariohysterectomy is strongly recommended for animals with pyometra and may need to be performed on an emergency basis to resolve sepsis or septic shock. Caution is required to avoid rupture of a distended or friable uterus during surgery, because this has been associated with an increase in mortality (from <10% to approximately 50%). Reevaluation should be performed 1 week after discharge from hospital and should include physical examination, a CBC, biochemistry panel, and urinalysis. Usually there is a rapid response to treatment and hematologic and biochemical abnormalities resolve within this time period. The white cell count can increase dramatically after surgery before it returns to normal, because of sudden removal of the leukocyte "sink". Antimicrobial drug treatment should be continued for 7 to 10 days after ovariohysterectomy.

In conjunction with antimicrobial drug treatment, medical treatment with natural or synthetic prostaglandin $F_2\alpha$ ($PGF_2\alpha$) is an alternative option to surgery, especially for dogs with open pyometra that are young (<6 years of age) and otherwise in good health (Table 89-4[58-60]). This treatment causes lysis of the corpora lutea with expulsion of uterine contents. Medical treatment for pyometra without surgery is not recommended for dogs that are systemically unwell, and the possibility of pregnancy must first be ruled out with ultrasound. Medical treatment is less attractive for dogs with closed pyometra because (1) it risks uterine rupture; (2) it is less effective than in dogs with open pyometra; and (3) dogs are often systemically unwell. Nevertheless, it has been used with success in some dogs with closed pyometra. Medical treatment is most

TABLE 89-4

Published Treatment Protocols for Medical Therapy of Pyometra in Dogs and Cats[58-60]

Drug	Dose
Natural $PGF_{2\alpha}$ (Lutalyse)	0.1 mg/kg SC once (day 1), 0.2 mg/kg SC once (day 2), 0.25 mg/kg SC q24h days 3 to 7
Aglepristone	10 mg/kg SC once on days 1, 2, and 7
Aglepristone and cloprostenol	Aglepristone: 10 mg/kg SC once on days 1, 2, and 8 Cloprostenol: 1 μg/kg SC for 5 days on days 3 through 7

likely to be successful in dogs in late diestrus (>5 weeks after the end of estrus). Improvement is generally not evident for at least 48 hours, and adverse reactions to $PGF_2\alpha$ are common and include restlessness, hypersalivation, panting, vocalization, vomiting, diarrhea, mydriasis, fever, and rarely, signs of shock. As a result, treatment should be given in the morning on an empty stomach, hospitalization and observation are recommended for at least 4 hours after the injection (or throughout the treatment period in dogs with closed pyometra), and the dose should be carefully calculated and appropriate for the product used. Walking dogs for 20 to 40 minutes after drug administration (while adverse effects occur) may lessen the adverse effects and promotes close observation.[58] The severity of signs tends to decrease with each injection administered. For dogs with closed pyometra, serial abdominal ultrasound examinations are recommended every 2 days during treatment to evaluate for evidence of peritonitis. $PGF_2\alpha$ can also be used to treat postpartum metritis.

Aglepristone, a progesterone receptor antagonist that is available in Europe, appears to be a safe and effective alternative to $PGF_2\alpha$ for treatment of pyometra in both dogs and cats.[59] Addition of low-dose cloprostenol (a synthetic $PGF_2\alpha$ derivative) to aglepristone in one study increased success rate in dogs with open pyometra from 60% to 84%.[60]

All dogs treated medically should be reevaluated 2 weeks after treatment. If signs of pyometra persist, culture of a swab specimen from the cranial vaginal vault could be performed to determine if resistance to antimicrobials is present, and treatment should be repeated a second time or surgery performed. The measurement of serum progesterone to monitor effective treatment is not necessary, because it does not change treatment recommendations. After successful treatment, the dog or cat should be bred at each subsequent cycle until pregnancy occurs. The chance that subsequent pregnancy will occur is over 80%, and the vast majority of dogs that respond go on to have more than one litter. Once the dog or cat is no longer required as a breeding animal, it should be neutered.

Prevention

Routine ovariohysterectomy reduces the risk of pyometra. Although stump pyometra can still occur in neutered animals, it is relatively rare. There is no known treatment for CEH. Use of estrogens to treat mismatings is not recommended.

CASE EXAMPLE

Signalment: "Molly", a 6-year-old female spayed shih tzu mix from Sacramento, CA

History: Molly was brought to the UC Davis VMTH for evaluation of recently diagnosed nephrolithiasis and hematuria. Three weeks previously, the owners had observed blood in Molly's urine. There had been no stranguria, polyuria, polydipsia, or change in the frequency of urination. They took her to their local veterinary clinic, where blood work was performed; her hematocrit was 56.5% and thrombocytopenia (86,000 platelets/μL) was present. A urine dipstick analysis revealed 2+ protein, a pH of 8, hematuria, and pyuria. Urine specific gravity was 1.014. Abdominal radiographs revealed a 3-cm opacity in the right renal pelvis that was consistent with a nephrolith (see Figure 89-2). The kidneys had a mildly irregular shape but were normal in size. Treatment with amoxicillin was initiated (23 mg/kg PO q12h for 10 days). Twelve days later, the dog was returned for dental prophylaxis. A CBC showed a hematocrit of 50% and persistent thrombocytopenia (51,000 platelets/μL). An abdominal ultrasound showed a 2.9-cm right renal pelvic nephrolith and a 7-mm left renal pelvic nephrolith. The kidneys were normal in size but had a mildly irregular shape. There was moderate thickening of the apical wall of the urinary bladder, with a small (4-mm) apical polyp. Moderate flocculent suspended debris was present within the urine and multiple sand-like calculi were present. All other organs evaluated were within normal limits. The dental procedure was canceled and Molly was referred for further evaluation.

Other Medical History: Molly had traveled frequently to Oregon and Nevada. She was fed a stone dissolution diet (Royal Canin Urinary SO), which had been prescribed 4 years ago when crystals were seen in her urine on urinalysis, as part of a wellness examination. She was also occasionally fed dog treats. She had been vaccinated using a 3-yearly protocol for canine distemper virus, canine adenovirus, canine parvovirus, and rabies; and yearly for *Bordetella bronchiseptica*, canine coronavirus, leptospirosis, and Lyme disease. Her last vaccination was more than 8 months previously. She was treated with imidacloprid and ivermectin for flea and heartworm prophylaxis, respectively, each month.

Physical Examination:

Body Weight: 10.8 kg.

General: Bright and alert, hydrated. T = 101.6°F (38.7°C), HR = 128 beats/min, RR = 32, mucous membranes pink and moist, CRT < 1 s.

Eyes, Ears, Nose, and Throat: Mild epiphora was present bilaterally and there was mild dental calculus and gingivitis. No other clinically significant abnormalities were detected.

Integument: The abdomen was clipped from the previous ultrasound examination with healing clipper wounds. There was a 1-cm ecchymosis on the ventral abdomen.

Musculoskeletal: Body condition score was 7/9. The dog was ambulatory with normal gait.

Genitourinary/Gastrointestinal: The dog had a soft and mildly painful abdomen on palpation. The urinary bladder was moderately sized. Rectal examination was unremarkable. There was no vulvar discharge and no evidence of perivulvar dermatitis. A slightly recessed vulva was present.

All Other Systems: No clinically significant findings.

Laboratory Findings:

CBC:

HCT 49.1% (40%-55%)
MCV 70.3 fL (65-75 fL)
MCHC 35.0 g/dL (33-36 g/dL)
nRBC 1/100 WBC

WBC 10,200 cells/µL (6000-13,000 cells/µL)
Neutrophils 7140 cells/µL (3000-10,500 cells/µL)
Band neutrophils 102 cells/µL
Lymphocytes 1632 cells/µL (1000-4000 cells/µL)
Monocytes 816 cells/µL (150-1200 cells/µL)
Platelets 12,000 platelets/µL (150,000-400,000 platelets/µL)
MPV 21.6 fL (7-13 fL)
Many macroplatelets were reported on smear evaluation.

Serum Chemistry Profile:
Sodium 148 mmol/L (145-154 mmol/L)
Potassium 4.0 mmol/L (3.6-5.3 mmol/L)
Chloride 111 mmol/L (108-118 mmol/L)
Bicarbonate 23 mmol/L (16-26 mmol/L)
Phosphorus 3.6 mg/dL (3.0-6.2 mg/dL)
Calcium 10.1 mg/dL (9.7-11.5 mg/dL)
BUN 12 mg/dL (5-21 mg/dL)
Creatinine 0.9 mg/dL (0.3-1.2 mg/dL)
Glucose 92 mg/dL (64-123 mg/dL)
Total protein 6.1 g/dL (5.4-7.6 g/dL)
Albumin 3.4 g/dL (3.0-4.4 g/dL)
Globulin 2.7 g/dL (1.8-3.9 g/dL)
ALT 42 U/L (19-67 U/L)
AST 16 U/L (19-42 U/L)
ALP 85 U/L (21-170 U/L)
Cholesterol 257 mg/dL (135-361 mg/dL)
Total bilirubin 0.1 mg/dL (0-0.2 mg/dL)

Urinalysis: SGr 1.013; pH 8.0, 2+ protein (SSA), 1+ bilirubin, 4+ hemoprotein, no glucose, no ketones, >100 WBC/HPF, 30-50 RBC/HPF, no crystals or casts, many rods, rafts of atypical transitional cells, many degenerated cells.

Coagulation Panel: PT 9.9 s (7.5-10.5 s), PTT 8.4 s (9.0-12.0 s), fibrinogen 395 mg/dL (90-255 mg/dL).

Microbiologic Testing: Direct smear of urine: Moderate numbers of gram-negative rods and gram-positive cocci were visualized.

Aerobic bacterial urine culture and susceptibility (cystocentesis specimen): 10^5 CFU/mL *Proteus mirabilis*, *Proteus mirabilis* (nonswarming strain), and *Enterococcus faecalis*. Both *Proteus* spp. were resistant to ampicillin (≥256 µg/mL) but susceptible to amoxicillin–clavulanic acid (4 µg/mL), cephalexin (8 µg/mL), chloramphenicol (≤16 µg/mL), enrofloxacin (≤1 µg/mL), tetracycline (64 µg/mL), and trimethoprim-sulfamethoxazole (≤4 µg/mL). The *E. faecalis* was susceptible to ampicillin, amoxicillin–clavulanic acid (≤2 µg/mL), chloramphenicol (≤16 µg/mL), enrofloxacin (≤1 µg/mL), and tetracycline (16 µg/mL).

Diagnosis: *Proteus mirabilis* and *Enterococcus faecalis* cystitis and suspected pyelonephritis with nephrolithiasis, with possible secondary immune-mediated thrombocytopenia.

Treatment: Molly was treated with enrofloxacin (7 mg/kg PO q24h). The following day her platelet count increased to 31,000 platelets/µL, and by day 3 of treatment it was 64,000 platelets/µL. After 7 days of treatment, a CBC showed a neutrophil count of 5700/µL and no band neutrophils, and the platelet count was 79,000 platelets/µL. A urine culture obtained by cystocentesis at this time showed 10^4 CFU/mL of *E. coli* and *E. faecalis*. The *E. coli* was resistant to ampicillin, cephalexin, enrofloxacin, tetracycline, and trimethoprim-sulfamethoxazole, but susceptible to amoxicillin–clavulanic acid (64 µg/mL). The susceptibility of the *E. faecalis* had not changed, with the exception that the MIC for tetracycline was 32 µg/mL. Treatment was changed to amoxicillin–clavulanic acid (23 mg/kg PO q12h). When reevaluated 3 weeks later, Molly had no clinical signs of illness. A CBC showed only mild thrombocytopenia (146,000 platelets/µL, with an MPV of 12.6 fL). However, bacteria and large numbers of white blood cells were still present in the urine sediment, the urine pH was 8.0, and *E. coli* with the same susceptibility pattern was again isolated from the urine. An extended panel showed susceptibility to amikacin (≤4 µg/mL) and imipenem-cilastatin (≤1 µg/mL), but resistance to cefazolin, cefoxitin, cefpodoxime, cephalothin, gentamicin, marbofloxacin, orbifloxacin, and ticarcillin–clavulanic acid. The dosage of clavulanic amoxicillin–clavulanic acid was increased to 23 mg/kg PO q8h. The diet was changed to a commercial urolith dissolution diet (Hill's s/d Canine Dissolution diet). After an additional month, urinalysis findings were unchanged and the same *E. coli* was again isolated from the urine. The platelet count was 244,000 platelets/µL and a biochemistry panel was unremarkable. Abdominal radiographs and ultrasound showed no evidence of nephrolithiasis, but multiple small, rounded mineral opacities were present in the region of the right ureter.

Antimicrobial drug treatment was ultimately changed to amikacin (15 mg/kg SC q24h) 2 weeks later because an *E. coli* was isolated that was resistant to clavulanic acid–amoxicillin. Kidney values were monitored every 2 weeks during amikacin treatment to evaluate for nephrotoxicity. The urine then became sterile, and ultrasound examination showed disappearance of all urinary calculi over a 2-month period, after which antimicrobial drug treatment was discontinued and the diet was changed to a maintenance diet. Because of the recessed vulva and the dog's excess body condition, a weight loss program was discussed with the owner. Molly was diagnosed with a subclinical *Enterobacter aerogenes* UTI 2 months later, which was broadly susceptible to antimicrobial drugs and treated with enrofloxacin. The platelet count was within the reference range. Further evaluation for underlying conditions predisposing to recurrent UTIs (contrast cystourethrography and cystoscopy), followed by vulvoplasty if no other abnormalities were detected, were offered to the owners but they declined further treatment and evaluation. The dog remained alive, untreated, and without clinical signs 4 years later, at which time CBC and biochemistry panel results were unremarkable but MDR *E. coli* was repeatedly isolated from the urine.

Comments: This is an interesting case of bacterial cystitis and pyelonephritis associated with struvite nephrolithiasis, and probable secondary immune-mediated thrombocytopenia. The struvite urolithiasis was likely secondary to the *P. mirabilis* infection, because *P. mirabilis* produces urease. Months of antimicrobial treatment were necessary because of bacterial sequestration within urinary calculi. This may have explained continued isolation of bacteria from the urine in the face of antimicrobial drug treatment, although ultimately resolution of the *E. coli* infection quickly followed the change in antimicrobial drug choice. Meropenem would have been another appropriate choice based on the susceptibility of the organism isolated, but its use in animals is controversial because it is an important

Continued

option for treatment of serious resistant bacterial infections in humans. Fortunately, dissolution of the nephroliths occurred in this case with antimicrobial and dietary therapy, and surgery to remove infected uroliths was not required. Continued UTIs were a likely sequela in this dog in the absence of successful identification and treatment of an underlying cause. Although treatment of the UTI was necessary during nephrolith dissolution, treatment of the subclinical *E. aerogenes* infection may not have been necessary.

SUGGESTED READINGS

Ling GV, Norris CR, Franti CE, et al. Interrelations of organism prevalence, specimen collection method, and host age, sex, and breed among 8,354 canine urinary tract infections (1969-1995). J Vet Intern Med. 2001;15:341-347.

Weese JS, Blondeau JM, Boothe D, et al. Antimicrobial use guidelines for treatment of urinary tract disease in dogs and cats: Antimicrobial Guidelines Working Group of the International Society for Companion Animal Infectious Diseases. Vet Med Int. 2011;2011:263768.

REFERENCES

1. Ling GV, Norris CR, Franti CE, et al. Interrelations of organism prevalence, specimen collection method, and host age, sex, and breed among 8,354 canine urinary tract infections (1969-1995). J Vet Intern Med. 2001;15:341-347.
2. Seguin MA, Vaden SL, Altier C, et al. Persistent urinary tract infections and reinfections in 100 dogs (1989-1999). J Vet Intern Med. 2003;17:622-631.
3. Buffington CA, Chew DJ, Kendall MS, et al. Clinical evaluation of cats with nonobstructive urinary tract diseases. J Am Vet Med Assoc. 1997;210:46-50.
4. Kruger JM, Osborne CA, Goyal SM, et al. Clinical evaluation of cats with lower urinary tract disease. J Am Vet Med Assoc. 1991;199:211-216.
5. Lekcharoensuk C, Osborne CA, Lulich JP. Epidemiologic study of risk factors for lower urinary tract diseases in cats. J Am Vet Med Assoc. 2001;218:1429-1435.
6. Eggertsdottir AV, Lund HS, Krontveit R, et al. Bacteriuria in cats with feline lower urinary tract disease: a clinical study of 134 cases in Norway. J Feline Med Surg. 2007;9:458-465.
7. Mayer-Roenne B, Goldstein RE, Erb HN. Urinary tract infections in cats with hyperthyroidism, diabetes mellitus and chronic kidney disease. J Feline Med Surg. 2007;9:124-132.
8. Bailiff NL, Nelson RW, Feldman EC, et al. Frequency and risk factors for urinary tract infection in cats with diabetes mellitus. J Vet Intern Med. 2006;20:850-855.
9. Bailiff NL, Westropp JL, Nelson RW, et al. Evaluation of urine specific gravity and urine sediment as risk factors for urinary tract infections in cats. Vet Clin Pathol. 2008;37:317-322.
10. Bailiff NL, Westropp JL, Jang SS, et al. *Corynebacterium urealyticum* urinary tract infection in dogs and cats: 7 cases (1996-2003). J Am Vet Med Assoc. 2005;226:1676-1680.
11. Gomez A, Nombela C, Zapardiel J, et al. An encrusted cystitis caused by *Corynebacterium urealyticum* in a dog. Aust Vet J. 1995;72:72-73.
12. Cavana P, Zanatta R, Nebbia P, et al. *Corynebacterium urealyticum* urinary tract infection in a cat with urethral obstruction. J Feline Med Surg. 2008;10:269-273.
13. Middleton DJ, Lomas GR. Emphysematous cystitis due to *Clostridium perfringens* in a non-diabetic dog. J Small Anim Pract. 1979;20:433-438.
14. Sherding RG, Chew DJ. Nondiabetic emphysematous cystitis in two dogs. J Am Vet Med Assoc. 1979;174:1105-1109.
15. Weese JS, Blondeau JM, Boothe D, et al. Antimicrobial use guidelines for treatment of urinary tract disease in dogs and cats: Antimicrobial Guidelines Working Group of the International Society for Companion Animal Infectious Diseases. Vet Med Int. 2011;2011:263768.
16. Ling GV. Therapeutic strategies involving antimicrobial treatment of the canine urinary tract. J Am Vet Med Assoc. 1984;185: 1162-1164.
17. Dhakal BK, Kulesus RR, Mulvey MA. Mechanisms and consequences of bladder cell invasion by uropathogenic *Escherichia coli*. Eur J Clin Invest. 2008;38(suppl 2):2-11.
18. McGuire NC, Schulman R, Ridgway MD, et al. Detection of occult urinary tract infections in dogs with diabetes mellitus. J Am Anim Hosp Assoc. 2002;38:541-544.
19. Peterson AL, Torres SM, Rendahl A, et al. Frequency of urinary tract infection in dogs with inflammatory skin disorders treated with ciclosporin alone or in combination with glucocorticoid therapy: a retrospective study. Vet Dermatol. 2012;23:201–e43.
20. Torres SM, Diaz SF, Nogueira SA, et al. Frequency of urinary tract infection among dogs with pruritic disorders receiving long-term glucocorticoid treatment. J Am Vet Med Assoc. 2005;227:239-243.
21. Melican K, Sandoval RM, Kader A, et al. Uropathogenic *Escherichia coli* P and Type 1 fimbriae act in synergy in a living host to facilitate renal colonization leading to nephron obstruction. PLoS Pathog. 2011;7:e1001298.
22. Lane MC, Mobley HL. Role of P-fimbrial-mediated adherence in pyelonephritis and persistence of uropathogenic *Escherichia coli* (UPEC) in the mammalian kidney. Kidney Int. 2007;72:19-25.
23. Rocha SP, Pelayo JS, Elias WP. Fimbriae of uropathogenic *Proteus mirabilis*. FEMS Immunol Med Microbiol. 2007;51:1-7.
24. D'Anjou MA, Bedard A, Dunn ME. Clinical significance of renal pelvic dilatation on ultrasound in dogs and cats. Vet Radiol Ultrasound. 2011;52:88-94.
25. Choi J, Jang J, Choi H, et al. Ultrasonographic features of pyonephrosis in dogs. Vet Radiol Ultrasound. 2010;51:548-553.
26. Cohn LA, Gary AT, Fales WH, et al. Trends in fluoroquinolone resistance of bacteria isolated from canine urinary tracts. J Vet Diagn Invest. 2003;15:338-343.
27. Ball KR, Rubin JE, Chirino-Trejo M, et al. Antimicrobial resistance and prevalence of canine uropathogens at the Western College of Veterinary Medicine Veterinary Teaching Hospital, 2002-2007. Can Vet J. 2008;49:985-990.
28. Ybarra WL, Sykes JE, Zingale YW, et al. Accuracy of Uricult Vet paddles for the diagnosis and identification of bacterial cystitis in dogs and cats [Abstract]. J Vet Intern Med. 2012;26:799.
29. Westropp JL, Sykes JE, Irom S, et al. Evaluation of the efficacy and safety of a high dose short duration enrofloxacin treatment regimen for uncomplicated urinary tract infections in dogs. J Vet Intern Med. 2012;26:506-512.
30. Marschall J, Zhang L, Foxman B, et al. Both host and pathogen factors predispose to *Escherichia coli* urinary-source bacteremia in hospitalized patients. Clin Infect Dis. 2012;54:1692-1698.
31. Lin E, Bhusal Y, Horwitz D, et al. Overtreatment of enterococcal bacteriuria. Arch Intern Med. 2012;172:33-38.
32. Bubenik LJ, Hosgood GL, Waldron DR, et al. Frequency of urinary tract infection in catheterized dogs and comparison of bacterial culture and susceptibility testing results for catheterized and noncatheterized dogs with urinary tract infections. J Am Vet Med Assoc. 2007;231:893-899.
33. Barbosa-Cesnik C, Brown MB, Buxton M, et al. Cranberry juice fails to prevent recurrent urinary tract infection: results from a randomized placebo-controlled trial. Clin Infect Dis. 2011;52:23-30.

34. Opperman EA. Cranberry is not effective for the prevention or treatment of urinary tract infections in individuals with spinal cord injury. Spinal Cord. 2010;48:451-456.
35. Chen YM, Wright PJ, Lee CS, et al. Uropathogenic virulence factors in isolates of *Escherichia coli* from clinical cases of canine pyometra and feces of healthy bitches. Vet Microbiol. 2003;94:57-69.
36. Kurazono H, Nakano M, Yamamoto S, et al. Distribution of the usp gene in uropathogenic *Escherichia coli* isolated from companion animals and correlation with serotypes and size-variations of the pathogenicity island. Microbiol Immunol. 2003;47:797-802.
37. Wilson RA, Keefe TJ, Davis MA, et al. Strains of *Escherichia coli* associated with urogenital disease in dogs and cats. Am J Vet Res. 1988;49:743-746.
38. Roura X, Camps-Palau MA, Lloret A, et al. Bacterial prostatitis in a cat. J Vet Intern Med. 2002;16:593-597.
39. Feeney DA, Johnston GR, Klausner JS, et al. Canine prostatic disease—comparison of radiographic appearance with morphologic and microbiologic findings: 30 cases (1981-1985). J Am Vet Med Assoc. 1987;190:1018-1026.
40. Bradbury CA, Westropp JL, Pollard RE. Relationship between prostatomegaly, prostatic mineralization, and cytologic diagnosis. Vet Radiol Ultrasound. 2009;50:167-171.
41. Feeney DA, Johnston GR, Klausner JS, et al. Canine prostatic disease–comparison of ultrasonographic appearance with morphologic and microbiologic findings: 30 cases (1981-1985). J Am Vet Med Assoc. 1987;190:1027-1034.
42. Lee CB, Ha US, Yim SH, et al. Does finasteride have a preventive effect on chronic bacterial prostatitis? Pilot study using an animal model. Urol Int. 2011;86:204-209.
43. Barsanti JA. Genitourinary infections. In: Greene CE, ed. Infectious Diseases of the Dog and Cat. 4th ed. St. Louis, MO: Elsevier Saunders; 2012:1013-1044.
44. Siqueira AK, Ribeiro MG, Leite Dda S, et al. Virulence factors in *Escherichia coli* strains isolated from urinary tract infection and pyometra cases and from feces of healthy dogs. Res Vet Sci. 2009;86:206-210.
45. Whitehead ML. Risk of pyometra in bitches treated for mismating with low doses of oestradiol benzoate. Vet Rec. 2008;162:746-749.
46. Tsioli VG, Gouletsou PG, Loukopoulos P, et al. Uterine leiomyosarcoma and pyometra in a dog. J Small Anim Pract. 2011;52:121-124.
47. Hernandez JL, Besso JG, Rault DN, et al. Emphysematous pyometra in a dog. Vet Radiol Ultrasound. 2003;44:196-198.
48. Thilagar S, Vinita WP, Heng HG, et al. What is your diagnosis? Small intestinal and colonic obstruction; emphysematous pyometra. J Small Anim Pract. 2006;47:687-688.
49. Chang J, Jung J, Jeong Y, et al. What is your diagnosis? Emphysematous pyometra with a large amount of gas. J Small Anim Pract. 2007;48:717-719.
50. Egenvall A, Hagman R, Bonnett BN, et al. Breed risk of pyometra in insured dogs in Sweden. J Vet Intern Med. 2001;15:530-538.
51. Niskanen M, Thrusfield MV. Associations between age, parity, hormonal therapy and breed, and pyometra in Finnish dogs. Vet Rec. 1998;143:493-498.
52. Whitney JC. Polydipsia in the dog—symposium. 2. Polydipsia and its relationship to pyometra. J Small Anim Pract. 1969;10:485-489.
53. Maddens B, Heiene R, Smets P, et al. Evaluation of kidney injury in dogs with pyometra based on proteinuria, renal histomorphology, and urinary biomarkers. J Vet Intern Med. 2011;25:1075-1083.
54. Rota A, Pregel P, Cannizzo FT, et al. Unusual case of uterine stump pyometra in a cat. J Feline Med Surg. 2011;13:448-450.
55. Roth L, Tyler RD. Evaluation of low sodium:potassium ratios in dogs. J Vet Diagn Invest. 1999;11:60-64.
56. Pak SI. The clinical implication of sodium-potassium ratios in dogs. J Vet Sci. 2000;1:61-65.
57. Bigliardi E, Parmigiani E, Cavirani S, et al. Ultrasonography and cystic hyperplasia-pyometra complex in the bitch. Reprod Domest Anim. 2004;39:136-140.
58. Feldman EC, Nelson RW. Cystic endometrial hyperplasia/pyometra complex. Canine and Feline Endocrinology and Reproduction. 3rd ed. St. Louis, MO: Saunders; 2004:852-867.
59. Nak D, Nak Y, Tuna B. Follow-up examinations after medical treatment of pyometra in cats with the progesterone-antagonist aglepristone. J Feline Med Surg. 2009;11:499-502.
60. Fieni F. Clinical evaluation of the use of aglepristone, with or without cloprostenol, to treat cystic endometrial hyperplasia-pyometra complex in bitches. Theriogenology. 2006;66:1550-1556.

CHAPTER 90

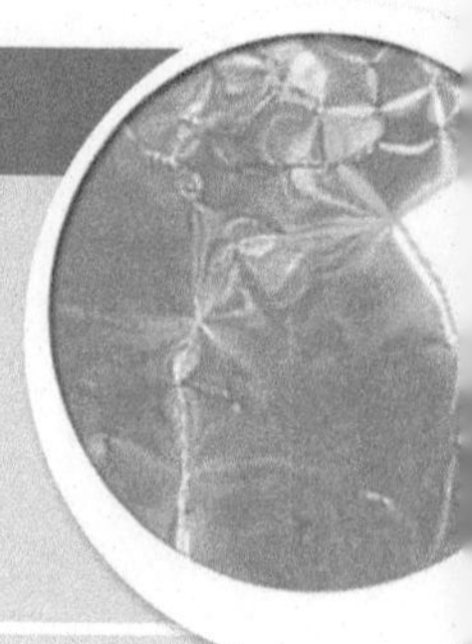

Bacterial Meningitis

Craig E. Greene

Overview of Canine and Feline Bacterial Meningitis

Cause: Bacterial meningitis is caused by a variety of pyogenic bacteria that enter the subdural space. Organisms are usually microfloral species or from environmental contamination of penetrating objects.

Affected Hosts: Dogs and cats of all ages are affected.

Geographic Distribution: Worldwide

Mode of Transmission: Bacteria can spread to the meninges from (1) sites of infection in the nasal sinuses, retrobulbar tissues, or middle or inner ear when host immune defenses are compromised; (2) sites of traumatic focal penetration; (3) sites of infection in adjacent venous sinuses or bony structures; or (4) via hematogenous arterial dissemination.

Major Clinical Signs: Fever, reluctance to move, stiff gait, and muscle spasms are the most common clinical signs. Paraspinal hyperesthesia and progressive neurologic dysfunction are progressive features.

Differential Diagnoses: Meningeal inflammation caused by nonbacterial microorganisms and immune-mediated causes should be considered. Myeloid or lymphoid neoplasias that affect the meninges may cause similar diffuse signs of inflammation.

Human Health Significance: None. The organisms that cause bacterial meningitis are indigenous microflora or environmental contaminants. Precautions should always be taken in collecting or handling cerebrospinal fluid potentially laden with microorganisms during diagnostic medical procedures.

Etiology and Epidemiology

Bacterial meningitis involves inflammation of the subdural covering of the brain and spinal cord, including the arachnoid membrane, subarachnoid space, pia mater, and cerebrospinal fluid (CSF), in response to a bacterial infection. The subarachnoid space projects into the nervous tissue alongside penetrating blood vessels. Bacterial infections can spread into the meningeal spaces from natural orifices such as the nasal sinuses, retrobulbar tissues,[1-3] and middle or inner ear.[4] Bacteria that proliferate in middle or inner ear infections can enter the cranial vault and produce cranial meningitis or subdural abscess formation (empyema) and, frequently, central vestibular dysfunction.[5-8] Bacteria can also enter the meningeal spaces through traumatic focal penetration (foreign bodies or bite wounds),[9,10] spread from sites of infection in adjacent venous sinuses or bony structures, or spread via hematogenous arterial dissemination.[11,12] Vascular spread can result in lodgment of bacteria in the endothelial cells of capillaries or the choroid plexus, which results in bacterial invasion of the parenchyma of the central nervous system (CNS) or colonization of the CSF, respectively. In the CSF, bacteria have adequate nutrients and a paucity of phagocytes and immunoglobulin, and they can proliferate, which produces a progressive inflammatory process that can readily spread along CSF pathways.

Bacteria that cause meningitis in dogs or cats are varied and can include aerobic, microaerophilic, and anaerobic species. Staphylococci, streptococci, *Pasteurella* spp., *Actinomyces* spp., *Nocardia* spp., and a variety of anaerobic bacteria have been isolated.[5,13-15]

Clinical Features

Signs and Their Pathogenesis

On entry into the CSF, bacteria can replicate to a moderate degree before they trigger a host protective response, because the immune response in this area is slow. The immune response of the host, rather than virulence of the pathogen, is usually responsible for most of the subsequent pathologic events. Toll-like receptors (TLRs), which are present on astrocytes, neurons, microglia, and oligodendrocytes, initiate innate recognition of the microorganisms. TLR signals initiate the release of a wide variety of proinflammatory mediators including reactive intermediates, cytokines, and chemokines within the CNS tissues and CSF spaces.[16] Within the nervous tissue, inflammatory processes lead to increased expression of TNF-α; thus, higher CSF concentrations of TNF-α have been used to distinguish bacterial from aseptic meningitis in humans.[17,18] Immunologic damage to bacteria leads to the release of breakdown products into the CSF and local CNS tissue. This further stimulates release of cytokines and prostaglandins, which are chemotactic for leukocytes and contribute to meningeal and ependymal inflammation. Subsequent inflammation leads to vascular injury and vascular thrombosis; tissue inflammation, edema, and necrosis; and increased CNS pressure within the confines of the dura mater and bony spaces. Inflammatory processes may also lead to adhesions and obstruction to CSF flow, resulting in obstructive internal or external hydrocephalus.[19]

Hyperesthesia from nerve root irritation is an important clinical sign of meningitis from any cause. Any stretching of extremities or palpation of muscles, especially of the paraspinal region, can lead to hyperesthesia and muscle spasm. The gait of animals with meningitis is often choppy and stiff. With progression, the inflammatory process may penetrate the spinal cord and brain parenchyma, which results in additional neurologic deficits. Manifestations of intracranial deficits include seizures,

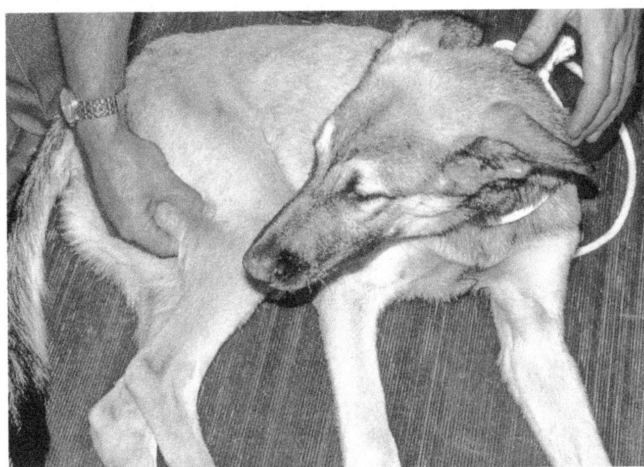

FIGURE 90-1 Dog with meningitis that had hyperesthesia on palpation of its spine and extremities. (Courtesy Craig Greene, Copyright 2012, University of Georgia Research Foundation Inc.)

behavioral abnormalities, and progressive decline in mental status until coma occurs.

Physical Examination Findings

Elevated rectal temperature may be found on examination because of fever, as well as excessive muscular exertional activity. Animals walk with a short stiff stride. Often the back of affected dogs is arched and the neck is outstretched with the head pointing in a downward direction. Paraspinal and extremity hyperesthesia is present with limb and spinal manipulation (Figure 90-1). When inflammation is confined to the meninges, postural reactions that involve motor responses are often stilted. As the inflammation progresses into the CNS parenchyma, deficits in sensory and motor responses are observed. Delayed placing reactions, paresis, and ataxia can be observed if cerebrospinal pathways are affected. Cranial nerve deficits are often observed on neurologic examination. Further signs of cerebral dysfunction include signs such as altered mentation (depression, aggression) or seizures. Myotatic and flexor reflexes may be difficult to elicit because of increased muscle tone from the animal's extreme tenderness and unwillingness to relax. Loss of reflex function occurs if spinal nerves become damaged in the inflammatory process.

Diagnosis

Inflammation or compression of muscle, bone, and joints can be initially confused with that of nerve root or peripheral nerve inflammation. The differential diagnosis for bacterial meningitis includes other infectious causes of meningeal irritation including that caused by viral, rickettsial, fungal, protozoal, and algal organisms (Table 90-1).[20] Feline infectious peritonitis is probably the most common cause of meningomyelitis in cats.[21,22] When parenchymal neurologic dysfunction is apparent, such as evidenced by delayed placing reactions, then protozoal meningoencephalomyelitis should also be considered. Frequently, more localized hyperesthesia associated with upper or lower motor neuron deficits can be observed with epidural empyema, discospondylitis, or paraspinal osteomyelitis. Steroid-responsive meningitis-arteritis in dogs can mimic all the signs of bacterial meningitis.[23] Diseases associated with myositis (such as American canine hepatozoonosis and leptospirosis) can also produce clinical signs that resemble those of meningitis.

TABLE 90-1

Examples of Infectious Agents That Can Cause Meningitis in Dogs and Cats*

	Dogs	Cats
Viruses	Canine distemper virus Arboviruses Suid herpesvirus 1 (pseudorabies)	Feline infectious peritonitis virus Borna disease virus Suid herpesvirus 1 (pseudorabies)
Bacteria	*Staphylococcus* spp. *Streptococcus* spp. *Pasteurella multocida* Enterobacteriaceae (including *Salmonella* spp.) *Actinomyces* spp. *Nocardia* spp. *Mycoplasma* spp. Anaerobes *Brucella canis* *Bartonella* spp.? *Borrelia burgdorferi*? *Leptospira* spp.? *Anaplasma phagocytophilum*? *Rickettsia rickettsii* *Neorickettsia helminthoeca* *Ehrlichia canis*	*Streptococcus* spp. *Pasteurella multocida* *Nocardia* spp. *Mycoplasma* spp. Anaerobes
Fungi	*Blastomyces dermatitidis*† *Coccidioides* spp. *Cryptococcus* spp.† *Aspergillus* spp.† *Candida* spp. *Histoplasma* spp. Phaeohyphomycoses Hyalohyphomycoses (e.g., *Paecilomyces* spp.)	*Cryptococcus* spp.†
Protozoa	*Toxoplasma gondii* *Neospora caninum* *Leishmania* spp. *Balamuthia mandrillaris* *Acanthamoeba* spp.	*Toxoplasma gondii*
Algae	*Prototheca* spp.	

*Many of the listed agents also cause encephalitis or encephalomyelitis in association with meningitis.

†Via dissemination or cribriform plate destruction as a result of extension of nasal cavity disease.

Laboratory Abnormalities

Although there are no hematologic or biochemical abnormalities that are specific for bacterial meningitis, the CBC may reveal leukocytosis, often with a left shift, especially if the process that leads to the meningitis resulted from hematogenous spread; however, an absence of neutrophilic leukocytosis is common in dogs or cats with meningitis.[15] Serum chemistry abnormalities are variable and nonspecific and can include increased ALT and ALP activities, hyperglycemia, and variable changes in serum electrolytes.

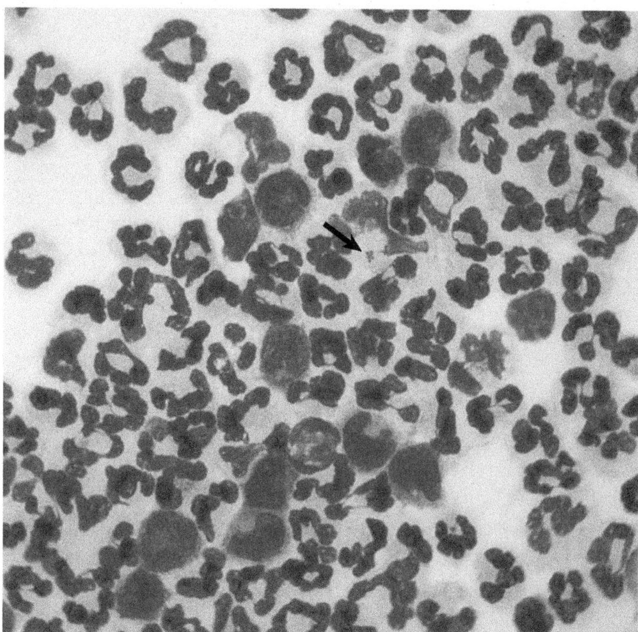

FIGURE 90-2 Cytologic appearance of CSF (cytospin preparation) in a 3-year-old male neutered Labrador retriever with bacterial meningitis. There is a large population of nondegenerate to moderately degenerate neutrophils. Many of the neutrophils contained intracellular cocci to pleomorphic short rod-shaped bacteria found in pairs and small aggregates *(arrow)*. Moderate numbers of foamy macrophages and reactive lymphocytes are also present. CSF analysis revealed a total protein of 402 mg/dL (reference range, <25 mg/dL), 100 red blood cells/μL, and 5200 white cells/μL, 92% of which were neutrophils.

Definitive diagnosis of bacterial meningitis requires evaluation of the CSF. Precautions should be taken not to remove too much fluid if CSF pressures could be increased. If imaging capabilities are available, they should be performed and evaluated before CSF removal, since they may reveal evidence of increased intracranial pressure. However, findings on medical imaging should not be used to eliminate CNS inflammatory disease, because CSF findings have the highest sensitivity for its detection.[24] Abnormalities found on CSF analysis in animals with bacterial meningitis usually consist of marked neutrophilic pleocytosis (Figure 90-2), and CSF protein concentration is increased. CSF protein concentration (often >100 mg/dL) and leukocyte numbers (usually >100 cells/μL) tend to be greatest in suppurative meningitis (especially of infectious origin) as compared to other CNS diseases; however, the electrophoretic patterns of the proteins are not specific for a diagnosis.[25] Neutrophils generally predominate; however, especially in chronicity or with concurrent antimicrobial use, monocytes, lymphocytes, or eosinophils may be observed. In human bacterial meningitis, glucose levels in the CSF are reduced because of inflammatory cell utilization, and lactic acid levels may be increased. Further studies are needed to determine if these can be used in dogs and cats to differentiate bacterial from other causes of meningeal inflammation. Finding organisms in the CSF on cytologic examination is exceedingly rare, and isolation of organisms in culture is also uncommon despite their visible presence on histopathologic examination.

Diagnostic Imaging

Plain Radiography

Plain radiographic findings are unremarkable in dogs or cats with bacterial meningitis unless a bacterial osteomyelitis of paraspinal or cranial bones is a source of infection. Bulla radiography is a valuable procedure for animals with suspected otogenic sources for their CNS infection; however, advanced imaging procedures are preferred when available.

Computed Tomography

Computed tomography of the brain or spinal cord in dogs or cats with bacterial meningitis may reveal contrast-enhancing lesions on the meningeal or ependymal surfaces. Focal areas of enhancement in areas of abscess formation or edema may also be present.

Magnetic Resonance Imaging

Purulent exudates that cover the CNS tissue may be visualized by MRI in animals with meningitis using T2-weighted sequences while suppressing the signal from CSF (high fluid attenuation inversion recovery [FLAIR]) (Figure 90-3, *A*). This method results in enhancement of signal intensity found in the meninges.[26] In more advanced cases, using T2-weighted or post-contrast T1-weighted images, meningeal enhancement (signal hyperintensity) indicates thickening of the meninges and edema of adjacent CNS tissue.[27] Occasionally, plaque-like densities are found that compress nervous tissue, which represent abscesses.

Microbiologic Tests

The main microbiologic assays used for diagnosis of bacterial meningitis in dogs and cats are aerobic bacterial culture and PCR assay of cerebrospinal fluid. False-negative results occur because organism numbers in CSF of dogs and cats are often low. Depending on the sensitivity of the PCR assay used and the viability of the bacteria in the specimen, culture may be positive when PCR results are negative, and vice versa.

Bacterial Culture

Bacteria may be isolated using routine aerobic and anaerobic bacterial culture media and conditions. At least 0.5 mL of CSF should be submitted for aerobic and anaerobic bacterial culture if possible. Organisms are uncommonly cultured from CSF because of their low number and the small amounts of fluid that are typically available; however, when successful, subsequent susceptibility testing assists in appropriate antimicrobial drug selection. Because of the infrequency of positive culture results despite the histopathologic presence of organisms at necropsy,[15] empiric antibacterial therapy should be employed based on a suspected site of origin of infection (see Antimicrobial Treatment, later).

Molecular Diagnosis Using the Polymerase Chain Reaction

Sensitive and specific real-time PCR assays for detection of bacteria in the CSF have been described.[28] However, as with culture methods, their sensitivity is low. The use of PCR to document bacterial infection of the CSF has been implemented in human medicine.[29,30] Although it has been used on a clinical basis on CSF of dogs and cats,[31] further studies are needed to document the sensitivity and specificity of various PCR assays for detection of microorganisms in CSF.

Pathologic Findings

Gross Pathologic Findings

At necropsy, sites of infection in animals with bacterial meningitis may be found in organs outside the CNS, such as the skin or mucous membranes, respiratory tract, internal organs,

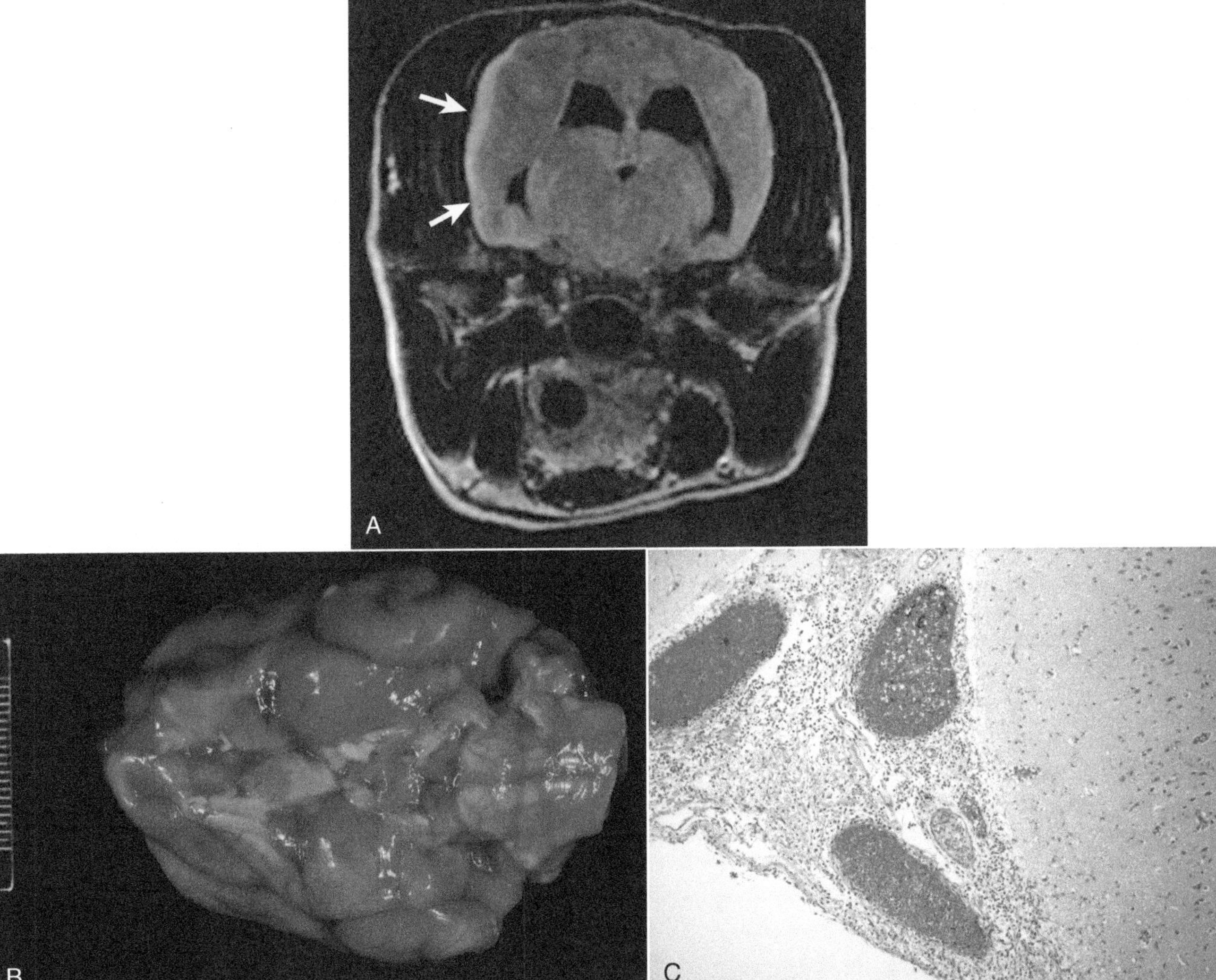

FIGURE 90-3 Clinical images from a 4-year-old female spayed Yorkshire terrier with bacterial meningitis. The dog had a 12-hour history of hypersalivation, generalized seizures, and vomiting. Small numbers of *Corynebacterium* spp. were isolated in culture from the meninges. **A,** MRI (FLAIR image). There is marked hyperintensity of the meninges on the left side *(white arrows)*. **B,** Gross pathologic findings. Ventral aspect of the brain. Purulent material covered the cerebellum and left cerebral cortex and pooled on the floor of the calvarium. The right cerebral vasculature was markedly engorged (shown). Cerebellar herniation was also found (not shown). **C,** Histopathologic appearance of meningitis. The meninges and Virchow-Robin spaces are expanded with inflammatory cells. The diagnosis was chronic, suppurative meningitis. H&E stain, 100× magnification. (Courtesy University of California, Davis, Veterinary Anatomic Pathology Service.)

external or middle ear, or ocular tissues. Gross pathologic findings in the CNS are generally minimal in dogs or cats with early inflammatory changes. As the infection progresses in the parenchyma, the meninges may appear congested and nervous tissue parenchyma in the regions adjacent to CSF surfaces may be discolored or opaque (Figure 90-3, *B*). Focal accumulations of pus may occasionally be observed in the meningeal spaces or adjacent nervous tissue. In late stages, ischemic infarction of CNS tissue may occur as a result of severe vascular inflammation and necrosis. Occasionally, obstructive hydrocephalus occurs if the inflammatory process occludes the mesencephalic aqueduct.

Histopathologic Findings

Microscopic findings in bacterial meningitis consist of a suppurative inflammatory response that is prominent in the meningeal spaces and the penetrating sulci that contain blood vessels (Virchow-Robin spaces) (Figure 90-3, *C*). With tissue gram stains, bacteria may be observed within inflammatory cells, blood vessels, or neural tissues, in association with inflammation of the meninges and adjacent neural parenchyma.

Treatment and Prognosis

Antimicrobial Treatment

Because of the low sensitivity of culture and/or PCR assays in bacterial meningitis and the turnaround time involved, treatment must be instituted following the neurologic examination and availability of the results of CSF analysis (Table 90-2). The earlier the drug is administered, the better the chance that parenchymal damage will be minimized. Anti-inflammatory agents have been recommended, with some caution and on a temporary basis, to reduce intracranial pressure. Almost all drugs, either ionic or lipid-soluble, penetrate acutely inflamed meninges. However, as the inflammation subsides, only lipid-soluble drugs are effective. Where parenchymal abscesses are present, antibacterial drugs may not effectively penetrate affected tissue.

TABLE 90-2

Antibacterial Drugs that Penetrate Central Nervous System Tissues and Fluids*

High	Intermediate	Low
Trimethoprim-sulfonamide, chloramphenicol, doxycycline, metronidazole	Third-generation penicillins, third-generation cephalosporines, fluoroquinolones	Penicillin, first-generation cephalosporines, aminoglycosides, clindamycin

*During acute inflammation, penetration is adequate for most drugs; however, as treatment progresses and inflammation subsides, the penetration becomes limited.

In these cases, neurosurgical drainage is required in addition to systemic antibacterial therapy.

Antiinflammatory Therapy

In addition to antimicrobial therapy, control of the immune response and resultant inflammation in CNS tissues is critical when intracranial or intraspinal pressures are elevated. Control of CNS edema is usually achieved with targeted dosages of glucocorticoids; however, therapy must be judicious, since these medications are immunosuppressive and nonspecific in their effect on the host.[32]

Supportive Care and Prognosis

The prognosis for dogs with early acute bacterial meningitis is good, provided that minimal CNS parenchymal tissue is damaged. Dogs with severe hyperesthesia should be treated with muscle relaxants to help reduce the increase in body temperature. Anticonvulsant medications may be needed for animals with signs of cerebrocortical irritation.

Prevention

Bacterial meningitis is a result of exogenous or endogenous factors that allow bacterial organisms to gain access to the subdural spaces. Although these insults cannot be completely prevented, injuries or lesions that occur close to the cranial or paraspinal spaces potentially predispose to CNS infection. Animals with wounds or infections in these areas or with systemic bacteremia should be treated appropriately then monitored closely for CNS signs and placed on judicious antimicrobial therapy if meningitis is highly suspected or documented. Although the signs of bacterial meningitis are confused with those of immune-mediated meningitis, continued use of immunosuppressive drugs may lead to detrimental progression of a bacterial disease process.

Public Health Aspects

There are minimal, if any, public health risks associated with bacterial meningitis in dogs or cats—that is, unless veterinary staff inadvertently inoculate themselves with organisms being collected for culture or PCR assays. *Haemophilus influenzae*, *Streptococcus pneumoniae*, and *Neisseria meningitidis*, which cause contagious respiratory disease and subsequent complicating hematogenous-origin meningitis in humans, do not readily infect dogs or cats.

CASE EXAMPLE

Signalment: "Jake," a 10-month-old male Weimaraner from North Georgia, USA

History: Jake was evaluated for a 2-week history of reluctance to move, in association with anorexia and fever. He had been treated with oral enrofloxacin and clindamycin for 2 days; however, the signs of discomfort returned 2 days after medication was discontinued. Jake also had a history of external ear inflammation and pruritic skin disease for the previous month. The dog was up to date on routine vaccinations, lived indoors and outdoors, and traveled outdoors locally with the owner.

Physical Examination: The dog was alert, but held his head down with his neck extended. He was reluctant to stand or walk, and appeared painful when his head was elevated or lifted; however, no further discomfort could be elicited by more caudal paraspinal palpation. T = 103.5°F (39.7°C), HR = 110 beats/min, RR = 30 breaths/min, with shallow breathing. Body condition score was 3/9 and body weight was 31 kg. Mild erythema of the external ear canals was present and small amount of yellow-colored exudate was noted in the ear canals bilaterally. With the exception of the neurologic examination, no other abnormalities were detected.

Neurologic Examination: The dog held its neck extended and head down and walked with a short, stiff gait. Placing reactions were present in all limbs, but initiation and follow-through were stilted. In lateral recumbency, the dog did not relax, and myotatic reflexes were difficult to elicit because of excessive muscle tone. Discomfort was elicited by paraspinal palpation and application of traction on the extremities or with deep muscle palpation. No deficits in cranial nerve responses or reflexes were observed.

Imaging Findings: Cervical spinal radiographs without anesthesia showed no detectable abnormalities.

Laboratory Findings: Hematologic and biochemical findings: The only abnormality of the CBC was a low MCV (65.5 fL; reference range 66-77 fL) and mild leukocytosis (13,200 cells/µL; reference range 5100-13,000 cells/µL). Serum alkaline phosphatase activity was increased (267 IU/L; reference range 13-122 IU/L). No abnormalities were found on urinalysis.

Arthrocentesis: Synovial fluid was pink and hazy. Nucleated cell count was slightly increased (3.2×10^3 cells/µL in the stifle joint). Nondegenerate neutrophils predominated; no intracellular inclusions or LE cells observed. Impressions: Mild purulent inflammation.

CSF analysis findings (specimen collected from cisterna magna): Clear, RBC = 26 cells/µL, WBC = 462 cells/µL (reference range, <5 cells/µL), total protein 72.6 mg/dL (reference range, 15-35 mg/dL). Differential cell count: Lymphocytes 4%, macrophages 18%, neutrophils 78%, occasional RBC, no bacteria observed in this specimen. Impressions: Marked purulent inflammation.

Microbiologic Testing: Aerobic bacterial culture (CSF): Negative. Anaerobic culture was not done.

Outcome: The dog was treated with chloramphenicol (35 mg/kg IV q8h) for 5 days and was then discharged on oral therapy for 3 weeks. The dog made a complete recovery from the signs when monitored for over 1 year.

Diagnosis: Meningitis (antibacterial-responsive) caused by suspected unidentified bacterial organisms.

Comments: Bacterial meningitis was suspected in this dog based on the history, clinical signs, laboratory findings, and response to chloramphenicol. Systemic spread of infection from a hematogenous route was suspected based on some of the inflammatory indicators in the hematologic and biochemical profile and evidence of mild suppurative polyarthritis that was found. The original treatment with enrofloxacin and clindamycin may have been subtherapeutic since it was short-lived and may not have penetrated the CNS tissues and fluids as well as chloramphenicol. Furthermore, IV dosing with chloramphenicol for the first days of therapy allowed for very high levels of drug in the CNS. Although an organism was not observed or isolated, bacterial infection was suspected based on the dramatic response to antibacterial therapy alone. In bacterial meningitis of dogs and cats, organisms are not often identified by cytologic or cultural examination of CSF. Response to antibacterial therapy should be considered presumptive evidence of bacterial infection.

SUGGESTED READINGS

Griffin JF, Levine JM, Levine GJ, et al. Meningomyelitis in dogs: a retrospective review of 28 cases (1999-2007). J Small Anim Pract. 2008(49):509-517.

Radaelli ST, Platt SR. Bacterial meningoencephalomyelitis in dogs: a retrospective study of 23 cases (1990-1999). J Vet Intern Med. 2002(16):159-163.

Tipold A, Stein VM. Inflammatory diseases of the spine in small animals. Vet Clin North Am Small Anim Pract. 2010;40:871-879.

REFERENCES

1. Oliver JAC, Llabrés-Diaz FJ, Gould DJ, et al. Central nervous system infection with *Staphylococcus intermedius* secondary to retrobulbar abscessation in a dog. Vet Ophthalmol. 2009;12:333-337.
2. Fletcher DJ, Snyder JM, Messinger JS, et al. Ventricular pneumocephalus and septic meningoencephalitis secondary to dorsal rhinotomy and nasal polypectomy in a dog. J Am Vet Med Assoc. 2006;229:240-245.
3. Britton AP, Davies JL. Rhinitis and meningitis in two shelter cats caused by *Streptococcus equi* subspecies *zooepidemicus*. J Comp Pathol. 2010;143:70-74.
4. Cook LB, Bergman RL, Bahr A, et al. Inflammatory polyp in the middle ear with secondary suppurative meningoencephalitis in a cat. Vet Radiol Ultrasound. 2003;44:648-651.
5. Sturges BK, Dickinson PJ, Kortz GD, et al. Clinical signs, magnetic resonance imaging features, and outcome after surgical and medical treatment of otogenic intracranial infection in 11 cats and 4 dogs. J Vet Intern Med. 2006;20:648-656.
6. Spangler EA, Dewey CW. Meningoencephalitis secondary to bacterial otitis media/interna in a dog. J Am Anim Hosp Assoc. 2000;36:239-243.
7. Klopp LS, Hathcock JT, Sorjonen DC. Magnetic resonance imaging features of brain stem abscessation in two cats. Vet Radiol Ultrasound. 2000;41:300-307.
8. Barrs VR, Nicoll RG, Chrucher RK, et al. Intracranial empyema: literature review and two novel cases in cats. J Small Anim Pract. 2007;48:449-454.
9. Dennis MM, Pearce LK, Norrdin RW, et al. Bacterial meningoencephalitis and ventriculitis due to migrating plant foreign bodies in three dogs. Vet Pathol. 2005;42:840-844.
10. Mateo I, Lorenzo V, Muñoz A, et al. Brainstem abscess due to plant foreign body in a dog. J Vet Intern Med. 2007;21:535-538.
11. Bach JF, Mahony OM, Tidwell AS, et al. Brain abscess and bacterial endocarditis in a Kerry Blue terrier with a history of immune-mediated thrombocytopenia. J Vet Emerg Crit Care. 2007;17:409-415.
12. Bilderback AL, Faissler D. Surgical management of a canine intracranial abscess due to a bite wound. J Vet Emerg Crit Care (San Antonio). 2009;19:507-512.
13. Dow SW, Lecouteur RA, Henik RA, et al. Central nervous-system infection associated with anaerobic bacteria in 2 dogs and 2 cats. J Vet Intern Med. 1988;2:171-176.
14. Messer JS, Kegge SJ, Cooper ES, et al. Meningoencephalomyelitis caused by *Pasteurella multocida* in a cat. J Vet Intern Med. 2006;20:1033-1036.
15. Radaelli ST, Platt SR. Bacterial meningoencephalomyelitis in dogs: a retrospective study of 23 cases (1990-1999). J Vet Intern Med. 2002;16:159-163.
16. Hanke ML, Kielian T. Toll-like receptors in health and disease in the brain: mechanisms and therapeutic potential. Clin Sci. 2011;121:367-387.
17. Glimaker M, Kragsbjerg P, Forsgren M, et al. Tumor necrosis factor-α (TNF-α) in cerebrospinal fluid from patients with meningitis of different etiologies: high levels of TNF-α indicate bacterial meningitis. J Infect Dis. 1993;167:882-889.
18. Nelson RP. Bacterial meningitis and inflammation. Curr Opin Neurol. 2006;19:369-373.
19. Dewey CW. External hydrocephalus in a dog with suspected bacterial meningoencephalitis. J Am Anim Hosp Assoc. 2002;38:563-567.
20. Griffin JF, Levine JM, Levine G, et al. Meningomyelitis in dogs: a retrospective review of 28 cases (1999-2007). J Small Anim Pract. 2008;49:509-517.
21. Rand JS, Parent J, Percy D, et al. Clinical, cerebrospinal fluid, and histological data from twenty-seven cats with primary inflammatory disease of the central nervous system. Can Vet J. 1994;35:103-110.
22. Bradshaw JM, Pearson GR, Gruffydd-Jones TJ. A retrospective study of 286 cases of neurological disorders of the cat. J Comp Path. 2004;131:112-120.
23. Irving G, Chrisman CL. Long-term outcome of five cases of corticosteroid-responsive meningomyelitis. J Am Anim Hosp Assoc. 1990;26:324-328.
24. Bohn AA, Wills TB, West CL, et al. Cerebrospinal fluid analysis and magnetic resonance imaging in the diagnosis of neurologic disease in dogs: a retrospective study. Vet Clin Pathol. 2006;35:315-320.
25. Behr S, Trumel C, Cauzinille L, et al. High resolution protein electrophoresis of 100 paired canine cerebrospinal fluid and serum. J Vet Intern Med. 2006;20:657-662.
26. Negrin A, Lamb CR, Cappello R, et al. Results of magnetic resonance imaging in 14 cats with meningoencephalitis. J Feline Med Surg. 2007;9:109-116.

27. Mellema LM, Samii VF, Vernau KM, et al. Meningeal enhancement on magnetic resonance imaging in 15 dogs and 3 cats. Vet Radiol Ultrasound. 2002;43:10-15.
28. Messer JS, Wagner SO, Baumwart RD, et al. A case of canine streptococcal meningoencephalitis diagnosed using universal bacterial polymerase chain reaction assay. J Am Anim Hosp Assoc. 2008;44:205-209.
29. Poppert S, Essig A, Stoehr B, et al. Rapid diagnosis of bacterial meningitis by real-time PCR and fluorescence in situ hybridization. J Clin Microbiol. 2005;43:3390-3397.
30. Schuurman T, de Boer RF, Kooistra-Smid AM, et al. Prospective study of use of PCR amplification and sequencing of 16S ribosomal DNA from cerebrospinal fluid for diagnosis of bacterial meningitis in a clinical setting. J Clin Microbiol. 2004;42:734-740.
31. Barber RM, Li Q, Diniz PPVP, et al. Evaluation of brain tissue or cerebral spinal fluid with broadly reactive polymerase chain reaction for *Ehrlichia, Anaplasma*, spotted fever-group *Rickettsia, Bartonella*, and *Borrelia* species in canine neurological diseases (109 cases). J Vet Intern Med. 2010;24:372-378.
32. de Gans J, van de Beek BD. Dexamethasone in adults with bacterial meningitis. N Engl J Med. 2002;347:1549-1556.

APPENDIX

Vaccination Schedules for Dogs and Cats

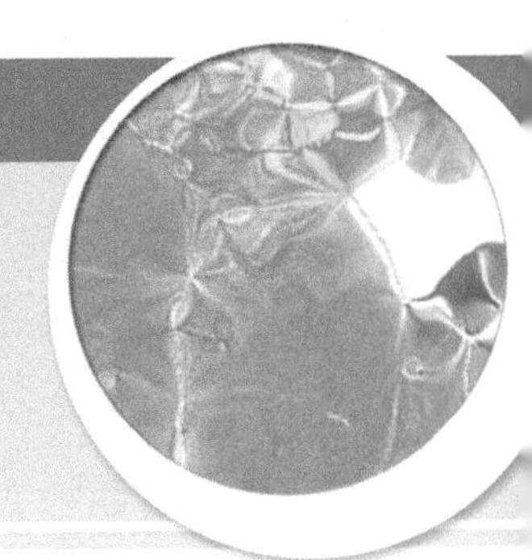

The schedules provided in this appendix are guidelines for immunization of dogs and cats against major viral and bacterial agents. These assume the availability of (1) client resources and (2) suitable products for immunization. The schedules are based on guidelines written by the WSAVA, AAHA, AAFP, and ABCD[1-11] and on information available at the time of writing. These are *general guidelines*, because the vaccine types recommended and the frequency of immunization vary depending on the lifestyle of the pet being immunized—that is, indoor versus outdoor pets, shelter animals, travel plans, kennel/boarding plans, and underlying disease conditions such as immune-mediated diseases or preexisting infections such as FIV infection. Because these factors may change over time, the vaccination plan for individual pet animals should be decided by the owner at routine annual examinations, after a discussion between the veterinarian and the client regarding the animal's lifestyle in the year ahead and the advantages and disadvantages of vaccination. This discussion should be documented in the medical record. A previous history of vaccine reactions in an individual pet will also affect recommendations for immunization. Considerable research is still required to generate optimal recommendations for vaccination of dogs and cats.

Guidelines for Vaccination of Individual Pet Dogs and Cats

Guidelines for vaccination of individual pet dogs and cats are summarized in Tables A-1 and A-2, respectively.

TABLE A-1

Guidelines for Vaccination of Individual Pet Dogs

	Initial Vaccination			
Vaccine	**Age ≤ 16 Weeks**	**Age > 16 Weeks**	**Booster Schedule**	**Comments**
CPV-2 (A, SC)	6-8 weeks of age, then every 3-4 weeks until no sooner than 14-16 weeks (16-20 weeks in breeding kennels)	Two doses 3-4 weeks apart recommended, but one dose is considered protective	1 year, then every 3 years thereafter	***Core.*** Protection after the 12-month booster may be lifelong. Administer with vaccines for CDV and CAV-2.
CPV-2 (I, SC)				Not recommended when attenuated vaccines are available and indicated
CDV (A, SC)	6-8 weeks of age, then every 3-4 weeks until no sooner than 14-16 weeks (16-20 weeks in breeding kennels)	Two doses 3-4 weeks apart recommended, but one dose is considered protective	1 year, then every 3 years thereafter	***Core.*** Protection after the 12-month booster may be lifelong. Administer with CPV and CAV-2 vaccines.
CDV (Recombinant, SC)	6-8 weeks of age, then every 3-4 weeks until no sooner than 14-16 weeks (16-20 weeks in breeding kennels)	Two doses 3-4 weeks apart recommended, but one dose is considered protective	1 year, then every 3 years thereafter	***Core.*** Can be interchanged with the attenuated live vaccine. May immunize in the face of maternal antibody. Administer with CAV2 and CPV vaccines.
CAV-2 (A, SC)	6-8 weeks of age, then every 3-4 weeks until no sooner than 14-16 weeks	Two doses 3-4 weeks apart recommended, but one dose is considered protective	1 year, then every 3 years thereafter	***Core.*** Administer with CDV and CPV vaccines.

Continued

TABLE A-1

Guidelines for Vaccination of Individual Pet Dogs—cont'd

Vaccine	Initial Vaccination: Age ≤ 16 Weeks	Initial Vaccination: Age > 16 Weeks	Booster Schedule	Comments
CAV-2 (A, IN)	One dose as early as 3 weeks of age	Single dose	Annual	Parenteral CAV-2 vaccines preferred for protection against CAV-1. Administered with IN CPiV and *B. bronchiseptica* vaccines
CAV-1 (A and I, SC)				Not recommended when CAV2 available because of adverse effects
Rabies (I, SC)	One dose as early as 3 months of age depending on local regulations	Single dose	1 year, then every 3 years thereafter with an approved product for 3-yearly immunization. Local regulations may dictate alternate protocols.	**Core.** In endemic areas or where required by local regulations
CPiV (A, SC)	6-8 weeks of age, then every 3-4 weeks until no sooner than 14-16 weeks	Single dose	Annual or within 6 months of boarding, and at least 1 week before boarding	**Noncore.** Use as a monovalent product or in combination with other noncore vaccines for annual boosters
CPiV (A, IN)	One dose as early as 3 weeks of age; consider second dose 2-4 weeks later if initial immunization occurs at < 6 weeks of age	One dose	Annual or within 6 months of boarding, and at least 1 week before boarding	**Noncore.** Potential to provide improved local mucosal immunity over SC products. Available in combination with IN *B. bronchiseptica*.
Bordetella bronchiseptica (I, SC)	Two doses 3-4 weeks apart as early as 6 weeks of age	Two doses, 3-4 weeks apart	Annual or within 6 months of boarding, and at least 1 week before boarding	**Noncore**
B. bronchiseptica (cell wall antigen extract, SC)	Two doses 3-4 weeks apart starting at 8 weeks of age	Two doses, 4 weeks apart	Annual or within 6 months of boarding, and at least 1 week before boarding	**Noncore**
B. bronchiseptica (Avirulent live, IN)	One dose as early as 3 weeks of age	One dose	Annual or within 6 months of boarding, and at least 1 week before boarding	**Noncore.** Potential to provide improved local mucosal immunity over SC products. Never administer SC, as may cause fatal hepatic necrosis.
Borrelia burgdorferi (I, SC or recombinant OspA, SC)	Two doses 3-4 weeks apart starting at 12 weeks of age	Two doses, 3-4 weeks apart	Annual. Revaccinate 1 month before the onset of the local *Ixodes* tick season	**Noncore**
Canine influenza (I, SC)	Two doses 3-4 weeks apart starting at 6 weeks of age	Two doses, 3-4 weeks apart	Annual	**Noncore.** For dogs at risk of exposure such as co-housed dogs, or before import to certain countries as dictated by regulations.

TABLE A-1

Guidelines for Vaccination of Individual Pet Dogs—cont'd

Vaccine	Initial Vaccination: Age ≤ 16 Weeks	Initial Vaccination: Age > 16 Weeks	Booster Schedule	Comments
Leptospira (I, SC)	Two doses 3-4 weeks apart starting at 12 weeks of age	Two doses, 3-4 weeks apart	Annual. Revaccinate 1 month before the onset of the season if disease occurs seasonally.	***Noncore.*** For dogs at risk of exposure. If available, a 4-serovar vaccine is preferred because protection is serovar-specific
Canine coronavirus (I and A, SC)				Not recommended because disease is mild and immunization of unproven benefit

A, Attenuated live; I, inactivated whole organism; IN, intranasal; SC, subcutaneous.

TABLE A-2

Guidelines for Vaccination of Individual Pet Cats

Vaccine	Initial Vaccination: Age ≤ 16 Weeks	Initial Vaccination: Age > 16 Weeks	Booster Schedule	Comments
FPV (A, SC; I, SC; A, IN)	6-8 weeks of age, then every 3-4 weeks until no sooner than 16 weeks (16-20 weeks in breeding catteries)[4]	Two doses, 3-4 weeks apart	1 year, then every 3 years thereafter	***Core.*** Protection after the 12-month booster is strong and may be lifelong. Provides cross-protection to CPV2.[12] Do not give attenuated live vaccines to pregnant cats. Inactivated vaccines are for pregnant cats (if absolutely necessary) and cats with retrovirus infection. Inactivated and intranasal FPV vaccines should be avoided for routine vaccination in heavily contaminated environments such as shelters.
FHV-1 (A, SC; I, SC; A, IN)	6-8 weeks of age, then every 3-4 weeks until no sooner than 14-16 weeks	Two doses, 3-4 weeks apart	1 year, then every 3 years thereafter. Annual revaccination may be indicated in heavily contaminated environments.	***Core.*** Does not provide complete protection. Attenuated live vaccines preferred if available and indicated. Inactivated vaccines are for pregnant queens (if absolutely necessary) and in retrovirus-infected cats. Intranasal vaccines may be associated with transient upper respiratory signs. One dose of IN vaccine may be sufficient to reduce clinical signs due to FHV-1 infection.
FCV (A, SC; I, SC; A, IN)	6-8 weeks of age, then every 3-4 weeks until no sooner than 14-16 weeks	Two doses, 3-4 weeks apart	1 year, then every 3 years thereafter. Annual revaccination may be indicated in heavily contaminated environments.	***Core.*** Does not provide complete protection. Attenuated live vaccines preferred if available and indicated. Inactivated vaccines are for pregnant queens (if absolutely necessary) and in retrovirus-infected cats. Intranasal vaccines may be associated with transient upper respiratory signs. One dose of IN vaccine may be sufficient to reduce clinical signs due to FCV.

Continued

TABLE A-2

Guidelines for Vaccination of Individual Pet Cats—cont'd

Vaccine	Initial Vaccination: Age ≤ 16 Weeks	Initial Vaccination: Age > 16 Weeks	Booster Schedule	Comments
Hypervirulent FCV (I, SC)	Two doses, 3-4 weeks apart starting at 8 weeks of age	Two doses, 3-4 weeks apart	Annual	Not generally recommended. Hypervirulent strains have differed for every outbreak, and outbreaks are effectively halted after institution of disinfection and quarantine programs.
Rabies (I, SC)	One dose as early as 3 months of age depending on local regulations	Single dose	1 year, then every 3 years thereafter with an approved product for 3-yearly immunization. Local regulations may dictate alternate protocols.	Core in endemic areas or where required by local regulations. Provides strong protection. Vaccine-associated sarcoma task force recommended immunization as distal as possible in the right pelvic limb.
Rabies (recombinant canarypox, SC)	Single dose as early as 8 weeks of age depending on local regulations	Single dose	Annual	Core in endemic areas or where required by local regulations. Provides strong protection. Vaccine-associated sarcoma task force recommended administration as distal as possible in the right pelvic limb
FeLV (I, SC)	Two doses 3-4 weeks apart starting at 8 weeks of age	Two doses, 3-4 weeks apart	1 year, then every 3 years thereafter when risk is ongoing. Beyond 1 year of age, age-related resistance may provide protection.	***Noncore.*** *Only for FeLV-negative cats. FeLV testing before administration mandatory before first administering the vaccine to kittens and if exposure was likely before, booster immunization is required. Can provide strong protection.[13] Vaccine-associated sarcoma task force recommended administration as distal as possible in the left pelvic limb
FeLV (recombinant canarypox, SC)	Two doses 3-4 weeks apart starting at 8 weeks of age	Two doses, 3-4 weeks apart	Annual when risk is ongoing.† Beyond 1 year of age, age-related resistance may provide protection.	***Noncore.*** *Only for FeLV-negative cats (see FeLV (I, SC)). More data are required on relative efficacy and whether these are associated with a reduced risk of injection-site sarcomas. Vaccine-associated sarcoma task force recommended administration as distal as possible in the left pelvic limb.
FeLV (subunit, SC)	Two doses, 3 weeks apart, starting at 8 weeks of age	Two doses, 3 weeks apart	Annual when risk is ongoing.† Beyond 1 year of age, age-related resistance may provide additional protection.	Inactivated whole virus vaccines may provide superior protection.[13] See above.
FIV (I, SC)	Three doses, 3 weeks apart, starting at 8 weeks of age	Three doses, 3 weeks apart	Annual	Not generally recommended. Immunization does not provide complete protection and interferes with interpretation of antibody test results, and PCR is insufficiently sensitive for accurate diagnosis. The first dose should only be given to FIV-negative cats. Antibodies may also be passed to kittens in colostrum and interfere with testing up to 12 weeks of age.

TABLE A-2

Guidelines for Vaccination of Individual Pet Cats—cont'd

Vaccine	Initial Vaccination: Age ≤ 16 Weeks	Initial Vaccination: Age > 16 Weeks	Booster Schedule	Comments
FIP (A, IN)	Two doses, 3-4 weeks apart, starting at 16 weeks of age	Two doses, 3-4 weeks apart	Annual	Not generally recommended. Only sero-negative cats have the potential to be protected. Benefit and risks currently unclear
Chlamydia felis (I and A, SC)	Two doses, 3-4 weeks apart, starting at 9 weeks of age	Two doses, 3-4 weeks apart	Annual	*Noncore.* Provides incomplete protection. Could be used as part of a control program in multiple cat households where infection is confirmed using appropriate diagnostic tests as endemic. Vaccination may be associated with adverse effects.
B. bronchiseptica (A, IN)	One dose as early as 8 weeks of age	One dose	Annual, but young cats are most at risk	*Noncore.* Provides incomplete protection. Use as part of a control program in multiple-cat households where infection is confirmed using appropriate diagnostic tests as endemic. Never administer parenterally.

A, attenuated live; I, inactivated whole organism; IN, intranasal; SC, subcutaneous.
*The AAFP highly recommends immunization of all kittens for FeLV.[2]
†Annual vaccination of adult cats for FeLV is controversial. The ABCD and WSAVA suggest boosters every 2 to 3 years in view of the significant lower susceptibility of older cats, even with recombinant and subunit vaccines.

Guidelines for Immunization of Dogs and Cats in Shelter Environments

For shelter animals, attenuated live core vaccines apart from rabies should be given before or immediately on entry to the shelter. Optimally, immunization for CPV and CDV should occur at least 3 days before entry to a shelter environment, but immunization even hours before entry has the potential to make a difference. When outbreaks of known parvovirus disease or canine distemper are present, vaccines can be administered as early as 4 to 5 weeks of age, but they should not be administered earlier than this because of the possibility of vaccine-induced disease and immunosuppression. In the absence of an outbreak situation, immunization for these pathogens should be performed no earlier than 6 weeks of age. In a shelter situation, the benefits and risks of vaccination of individual pregnant animals with attenuated live vaccines must be carefully assessed. Immunization with an inactivated vaccine is probably better than no vaccine for pregnant animals that enter a shelter, but inactivated vaccines should not be administered to other animals in the shelter environment, because the onset of immunity is slower than with attenuated live vaccines. Attenuated live vaccines should be administered if ovariohysterectomy is to be performed during pregnancy. If pregnant animals are not immunized, they should be strictly isolated from the rest of the shelter animal population. The use of rapid in-house serologic tests that determine the immune status of pregnant animals may be helpful in this situation (see Chapter 12).

Revaccination should be performed no more frequently than at intervals of 2 to 3 weeks, because vaccine administration that occurs within 3 to 14 days of another immunization attempt with attenuated live vaccines can interfere with development of immune responses. Further study is required to determine optimum revaccination intervals in shelter environments. Revaccination is most important for pups and kittens younger than 16 weeks of age and is performed to maximize the chance of immunization as soon as possible after the disappearance of maternal antibody interference. Puppies and kittens should also be physically separated from the rest of the shelter animal population and handled with strict attention to quarantine protocols.

Intranasal vaccines are preferred for management of upper respiratory tract disease in shelter environments because of the potential for improved local immunity, the possibility of administration to very young animals, more rapid onset of protection, and improved protection in the face of maternal antibody. However, they also have been associated with vaccine-induced upper respiratory disease, which may be more severe in debilitated animals and can be difficult to distinguish from natural infection. In addition, field studies have yet not shown benefit of intranasal over parenteral vaccines for prevention of respiratory disease.[14] Intranasal *Bordetella bronchiseptica* vaccines should never be given parenterally. This is an emergency situation that requires immediate treatment. See Chapter 12 for specific instructions for how to manage accidental parenteral administration of these vaccines.

In endemic areas, if possible, a rabies vaccine could be administered at the time of discharge from the facility.[1] Administration of a 3-year product is preferred, but regardless of the product used, booster immunization must be performed no later than 1 year after the initial immunization. Rabies immunization must be properly documented, and a veterinarian must usually be present at the time of immunization. Otherwise, the number of vaccines should be limited to those that can assist control of disease that is confirmed to exist within the shelter. This will avoid excessive immune suppression that may worsen the severity of illness due to other pathogens in the shelter for which vaccines are nonexistent.

TABLE A-3

Guidelines for Vaccination of Dogs in Shelter Environments

Vaccine	Initial Vaccination		Recommendations for Booster at Exit	Comments
	Age ≤ 16 Weeks	Age > 16 Weeks		
CPV-2 (A, SC)	On entry no earlier than 6 weeks of age,* then every 2-3 weeks until no sooner than 16 weeks (and up to 20 weeks if outbreaks occur)	Two doses 2-3 weeks apart recommended, but one dose is considered protective	1 year, then every 3 years thereafter.	***Core.*** Potential to provide strong protection. Do not use in pregnancy. Administer with vaccines for CDV and CAV-2.
CDV (A, SC)	On entry no earlier than 6 weeks of age,* then every 2-3 weeks until no sooner than 16 weeks (up to 20 weeks when outbreaks occur)	Two doses 2-3 weeks apart recommended, but one dose is considered protective	1 year, then every 3 years thereafter	***Core.*** Potential to provide strong protection. Do not use in pregnancy. Administer with CPV and CAV-2 vaccines.
CDV (recombinant, SC)	On entry no earlier than 6 weeks of age,* then every 2-3 weeks until no sooner than 16 weeks (up to 20 weeks when outbreaks occur)	Two doses 2-3 weeks apart recommended, but one dose is considered protective	1 year, then every 3 years thereafter	***Core.*** Administer with CPV and CAV-2. Potential to provide strong protection and immunize pups in the face of maternal antibody. More studies needed that compare the relative efficacy of recombinant and live attenuated CDV vaccines in dogs of all ages in shelter environments.
CAV-2 (A, SC)	On entry no earlier than 6 weeks of age,* then every 2-3 weeks until no sooner than 16 weeks	Two doses 2-3 weeks apart recommended, but one dose is considered protective	1 year, then every 3 years thereafter.	***Core.*** Administer with CDV and CPV vaccines. Do not use in pregnancy.
Rabies (I, SC)	If at all, one dose on exit from the shelter as early as 3 months depending on local regulations	If at all, one dose on exit from the shelter	1 year, then every 3 years thereafter with an approved product for 3-yearly immunization. Local regulations may dictate alternate protocols.	Use in endemic areas. Local regulations can dictate the need for rabies immunization.
CPiV (A, SC)	On entry no earlier than 6 weeks of age,* then every 2-3 weeks until no sooner than 16 weeks	Two doses 2-3 weeks apart recommended, but one dose is considered protective	Annual or within 6 months of boarding, and at least 1 week before boarding with monovalent SC or IN respiratory disease vaccines	If the SC vaccine is used, it can be administered in shelters in combination with CDV, CPV, and CAV-2. Administer with a vaccine for *B. bronchiseptica.*

TABLE A-3

Guidelines for Vaccination of Dogs in Shelter Environments—cont'd

Vaccine	Initial Vaccination: Age ≤ 16 Weeks	Initial Vaccination: Age > 16 Weeks	Recommendations for Booster at Exit	Comments
CPiV (A, IN)	Two doses 2-3 weeks apart starting as early as 3 weeks, although one dose may be sufficient	Two doses 2-3 weeks apart, although one dose may be sufficient	Annual or within 6 months of boarding, and at least 1 week before boarding	Potential to provide improved local mucosal immunity over SC products, but further study required. Available in combination with IN *B. bronchiseptica*
B. bronchiseptica (A, IN)	Two doses 2-3 weeks apart starting as early as 3 weeks, although one dose may be sufficient	Two doses 2-3 weeks apart, although one dose may be sufficient	Annual or within 6 months of boarding, and at least 1 week before boarding	Potential to provide improved local mucosal immunity over SC products, but further study required. Provides more rapid immunization than SC products and improved likelihood of immunization in the face of maternal antibody compared with SC products available at the time of writing. Never administer SC. Available in combination with CPiV
Canine influenza (I, SC)	On entry, two doses 3 weeks apart starting at 6 weeks of age	Two doses, 3 weeks apart	Annual if risk is ongoing	For dogs at risk of exposure in shelters in endemic regions of the United States. Maximal protection does not occur until approximately one week after the second vaccine.

A, attenuated live; I, inactivated whole organism; IN, intranasal; SC, subcutaneous.
*Immunization can be performed as early as 4-5 weeks in the face of an outbreak.

TABLE A-4

Guidelines for Vaccination of Cats in Shelter Environments

Vaccine	Initial Vaccination: Age ≤ 16 Weeks	Initial Vaccination: Age > 16 Weeks	Recommendations for Booster at Exit	Comments
FPV (A, SC)	On entry and no earlier than 4-6 weeks of age, then every 2-3 weeks until no sooner than 16 weeks (up to 20 weeks when outbreaks occur)[4]	Two doses 3 weeks apart recommended, but one dose is considered protective	1 year, then every 3 years thereafter.	Potential to provide strong protection against FPV and CPV-2.[12] Administer alone or with SC vaccines for FHV-1 and FCV. Do not use in pregnant queens. The use of IN FPV vaccines is not recommended in shelters.
FHV-1 (A, SC; A, IN)	On entry and no earlier than 4-6 weeks of age, then every 2-3 weeks until no sooner than 14-16 weeks	Two doses 3 weeks apart recommended, but one dose is considered protective	1 year, then every 3 years thereafter. Annual revaccination may be indicated in contaminated environments.	Does not provide complete protection. Avoid use in pregnancy. Intranasal vaccines may be associated with transient upper respiratory signs. Administer with FCV. One dose of the IN vaccine may be sufficient.

Continued

TABLE A-4

Guidelines for Vaccination of Cats in Shelter Environments—cont'd

Vaccine	Initial Vaccination: Age ≤ 16 Weeks	Initial Vaccination: Age > 16 Weeks	Recommendations for Booster at Exit	Comments
FCV (A, SC; A, IN)	On entry and no earlier than 4-6 weeks of age, then every 2-3 weeks until no sooner than 14-16 weeks	Two doses 2-3 weeks apart recommended, but one dose is considered protective	1 year, then every 3 years thereafter. Annual revaccination may be indicated in contaminated environments.	Does not provide complete protection. Avoid use in pregnancy. Intranasal vaccines may be associated with transient upper respiratory signs. Administer with FHV-1. One dose of the IN vaccine may be sufficient.
Rabies (I, SC)	If at all, one dose on exit from the shelter as early as 3 months depending on local regulations	If at all, one dose on exit from the shelter	1 year, then every 3 years thereafter with an approved product for 3-yearly immunization. Local regulations may dictate alternate protocols.	For use in endemic areas. Local regulations may dictate the need for rabies immunization.

A, attenuated live; I, inactivated whole organism; IN, intranasal; SC, subcutaneous.

REFERENCES

1. Day MJ, Horzinek MC, Schultz RD. WSAVA guidelines for the vaccination of dogs and cats. J Small Anim Pract. 2010;51(6):1-32.
2. Richards JR, Elston TH, Ford RB, et al. The 2006 American Association of Feline Practitioners Feline Vaccine Advisory Panel Report. J Am Vet Med Assoc. 2006;229(9):1405-1441 (also http://www.aafponline.org/resources/practice_guidelines.htm).
3. American Animal Hospital Association (AAHA) Canine Vaccine Taskforce. 2006 AAHA canine vaccine guidelines. J Am Anim Hosp Assoc. 2006;42(2):80-89.
4. Truyen U, Addie D, Belák S, et al. Feline panleukopenia. ABCD guidelines on prevention and management. J Feline Med Surg. 2009;11(7):538-546.
5. Thiry E, Addie D, Belák S, et al. Feline herpesvirus infection. ABCD guidelines on prevention and management. J Feline Med Surg. 2009;11(7):547-555.
6. Radford AD, Addie D, Belák S, et al. Feline calicivirus infection. ABCD guidelines on prevention and management. J Feline Med Surg. 2009;11(7):556-564.
7. Lutz H, Addie D, Belák S, et al. Feline leukemia. ABCD guidelines on prevention and management. J Feline Med Surg. 2009;11(7):565-574.
8. Frymus T, Addie D, Belák S, et al. Feline rabies. ABCD guidelines on prevention and management. J Feline Med Surg. 2009;11(7):585-593.
9. Addie D, Belák S, Boucraut-Baralon C, et al. Feline infectious peritonitis. ABCD guidelines on prevention and management. J Feline Med Surg. 2009;11(7):594-604.
10. Gruffydd-Jones T, Addie D, Belák S, et al. *Chlamydophila felis* infection. ABCD guidelines on prevention and management. J Feline Med Surg. 2009;11(7):605-609.
11. Egberink H, Addie D, Belák S, et al. *Bordetella bronchiseptica* infection in cats. ABCD guidelines on prevention and management. J Feline Med Surg. 2009;11(7):610-614.
12. Chalmers WS, Truyen U, Greenwood NM, et al. Efficacy of feline panleucopenia vaccine to prevent infection with an isolate of CPV2b obtained from a cat. Vet Microbiol. 1999;69(1-2):41-45.
13. Torres AN, O'Halloran KP, Larson LJ, et al. 2009. Feline leukemia virus immunity induced by whole inactivated vaccination. Vet Immunol Immunopathol. 2010;134(1-2):122-131.
14. Larson LJ, Newbury S, Schultz RD. Canine and feline vaccinations and immunology. In: Miller L, Hurley K, eds. Infectious Disease Management in Animal Shelters. Ames, IA: Wiley-Blackwell; 2009:61-82.

Index

Page numbers followed by *f* indicate figures, *t* tables, and *b* boxes.

N

O